The American Psychiatric Press
Textbook of Psychopharmacology

Second Edition

The American Psychiatric Press

Textbook of Psychopharmacology

Second Edition

Edited by

Alan F. Schatzberg, M.D., and
Charles B. Nemeroff, M.D., Ph.D.

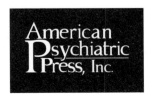

Washington, DC
London, England

Note: The authors have worked to ensure that all information in this book concerning drug dosages, schedules, and routes of administration is accurate as of the time of publication and consistent with standards set by the U.S. Food and Drug Administration and the general medical community. As medical research and practice advance, however, therapeutic standards may change. For this reason and because human and mechanical errors sometimes occur, we recommend that readers follow the advice of a physician who is directly involved in their care or the care of a member of their family.

After this textbook went to press, fenfluramine and dexfenfluramine were withdrawn from the U.S. market because of concerns regarding cardiac toxicity. The textbook still contains references to fenfluramine and dexfenfluramine.

In addition, the manufacturer of the atypical antipsychotic sertindole has recently decided not to release the drug in the United States. The textbook still includes material about this drug; the Appendix on new agents ("New Psychotropic Drugs for Axis I Disorders: Recently Arrived, in Development, and Never Arrived") correctly describes its status.

Readers should check the manufacturer's package insert for the most reliable information about the currently recommended dosing strategies, side-effect warnings, contraindications, etc. Also, this book is intended to provide background information only, and dosages should be rechecked for accuracy with the manufacturer's package insert.

Books published by the American Psychiatric Press, Inc., represent the views and opinions of the individual authors and do not necessarily represent the policies and opinions of the Press or the American Psychiatric Association.

Diagnostic criteria included in this book are reprinted, with permission, from the *Diagnostic and Statistical Manual of Mental Disorders*, 4th Edition. Copyright 1994, American Psychiatric Association.

Copyright © 1998 American Psychiatric Press, Inc.
ALL RIGHTS RESERVED
Manufactured in the United States of America on acid-free paper
01 00 99 98   4 3 2 1
Second Edition
American Psychiatric Press, Inc.
1400 K Street, N.W., Washington, DC   20005
www.appi.org

Library of Congress Cataloging-in-Publication Data
The American Psychiatric Press textbook of psychopharmacology / edited
   by Alan F. Schatzberg and Charles B. Nemeroff. — 2nd ed.
       p.   cm.
   Includes bibliographical references and index.
   ISBN 0-88048-817-4
   1. Mental illness—Chemotherapy.   2. Psychotropic drugs.
3. Psychopharmacology.   I. Schatzberg, Alan F.   II. Nemeroff,
Charles B.
   [DNLM: 1. Psychotropic Drugs—pharmacology.   2. Psychotropic
Drugs—therapeutic use.   3. Mental Disorders—drug therapy.   QV
77.2 A512 1998]
RC483.A515   1998
615'.78—dc21
DNLM/DLC
for Library of Congress   98-10616
                                                                                              CIP

British Library Cataloguing in Publication Data
A CIP record is available from the British Library.

Cover designed by David Ryner, Echo Communications, Bethesda, Maryland

Contents

SECTION I

Principles of Psychopharmacology
Joseph T. Coyle, M.D., Section Editor

ONE

TWO

THREE

FOUR

FIVE

SIX

SECTION II

Classes of Psychiatric Treatments: Animal and Human Pharmacology
Dennis S. Charney, M.D., and
Herbert Y. Meltzer, M.D., Section Editors

Antidepressants and Anxiolytics

Drugs for Treatment of Bipolar Disorder

TWENTY

TWENTY-ONE

TWENTY-TWO

Other Agents

TWENTY-THREE

TWENTY-FOUR

TWENTY-FIVE

FORTY-EIGHT

APPENDIX

Contributors

W. Stewart Agras, M.D.
Professor of Psychiatry, Department of Psychiatry and Behavioral Sciences, Stanford University School of Medicine, Stanford, California

James C. Ballenger, M.D.
Professor and Chair, Department of Psychiatry and Behavioral Sciences; and Director, Institute of Psychiatry, Medical University of South Carolina, Charleston

Joseph M. Bebchuk, M.D., F.R.C.P.C.
Assistant Professor of Psychiatry, Wayne State University School of Medicine, Detroit, Michigan

Joseph K. Belanoff, M.D.
Acting Assistant Professor of Psychiatry and Behavioral Sciences, Department of Psychiatry and Behavioral Sciences, Stanford University School of Medicine, Stanford, California

S. Paul Berger, M.D.
Associate Professor of Psychiatry, University of Cincinnati, Cincinnati, Ohio

Robert M. Berman, M.D.
Assistant Professor of Psychiatry, Yale University School of Medicine, New Haven, Connecticut

David R. Borchelt, Ph.D.
Department of Pathology, Division of Neuropathology, The Johns Hopkins University School of Medicine, Baltimore, Maryland

Charles L. Bowden, M.D.
Nancy U. Karren Professor and Chairman, Department of Psychiatry; and Professor, Department of Pharmacology, The University of Texas Health Science Center at San Antonio

Joel Bregman, M.D.
Associate Clinical Professor of Psychiatry, University of Connecticut; and Assistant Professor of Child Psychiatry, Yale University, New Haven, Connecticut

Karen Britton, M.D., Ph.D.
Professor, Department of Psychiatry, San Diego VA Medical Center, University of California, San Diego, School of Medicine

Benjamin S. Bunney, M.D.
Charles B.G. Murphy Professor and Chairman, Department of Psychiatry; and Professor of Pharmacology, Yale University School of Medicine, New Haven, Connecticut

Adam B. Burrows, M.D.
Assistant Professor of Medicine, Boston University School of Medicine; and Medical Director, Elder Service Plan, Upham's Corner Health Center, Boston, Massachusetts

Katie A. Busch, M.D.
Assistant Professor of Psychiatry, Rush-Presbyterian-St. Luke's Medical Center, Chicago, Illinois

Regina C. Casper, M.D.
Professor of Psychiatry, Department of Psychiatry and Behavioral Sciences, Stanford University School of Medicine, Stanford, California

Dennis S. Charney, M.D.
Professor of Psychiatry, Yale University School of Medicine, New Haven, Connecticut

Jonathan O. Cole, M.D.
Professor of Psychiatry, Harvard Medical School, Boston, Massachusetts; and Senior Staff Consultant, McLean Hospital, Affective Disorders Program, Belmont, Massachusetts

Barbara Cordell, Ph.D.
Vice President, Research, Scios, Inc., Mountain View, California

James W. Cornish, M.D.
Assistant Professor of Psychiatry and Director of Pharmacotherapy, Treatment Research Center, University of Pennsylvania and Department of Veterans Affairs Medical Center, Philadelphia, Pennsylvania

Joseph T. Coyle, M.D.
Chairman, Department of Psychiatry, Eben S. Draper Professor of Psychiatry and Neuroscience, Harvard Medical School, Boston and Belmont, Massachusetts

Kenneth L. Davis, M.D.
Professor and Chairman, Department of Psychiatry, Mt. Sinai School of Medicine, New York City

Karon Dawkins, M.D.
Assistant Professor, Department of Psychiatry, University of North Carolina, Chapel Hill

Charles DeBattista, D.M.H., M.D.
Assistant Professor, Department of Psychiatry and Behavioral Sciences, Stanford University School of Medicine, Stanford, California

William C. Dement, M.D., Ph.D.
Lowell W. and Josephine Q. Berry Professor, Department of Psychiatry and Behavioral Sciences, Stanford University School of Medicine, Stanford, California; and Director, Stanford Sleep Disorders Center, Palo Alto, California

C. Lindsay DeVane, Pharm.D.
Professor of Psychiatry and Behavioral Sciences and Professor of Pharmaceutical Sciences, Medical University of South Carolina, Charleston

Marie deVegvar, M.D.
Fellow, Department of Psychiatry, Mt. Sinai School of Medicine, New York City

Steven L. Dubovsky, M.D.
Professor of Psychiatry and Medicine and Vice Chairman, Department of Psychiatry, University of Colorado Health Sciences Center, Denver

Mina K. Dulcan, M.D.
Margaret C. Osterman Professor of Child Psychiatry, Children's Memorial Hospital, Northwestern University Medical School, Chicago, Illinois

Dwight L. Evans, M.D.
Professor and Chairman, Department of Psychiatry, University of Pennsylvania School of Medicine, Philadelphia

S. Hossein Fatemi, M.D., Ph.D.
Associate Professor, Departments of Psychiatry, Cell Biology, and Neuroanatomy, Division of Neuroscience Research, University of Minnesota Medical School, Minneapolis

Jan Fawcett, M.D.
Professor and Chairman, Department of Psychiatry, Rush-Presbyterian-St. Luke's Medical Center; and Grainger Director, Rush Institute for Mental Well-Being, Chicago, Illinois

Gary S. Figiel, M.D.
Director, The Mood Disorders Center, Eastside Heritage Center, Atlanta, Georgia

Ira D. Glick, M.D.
Professor of Psychiatry and Behavioral Sciences, Department of Psychiatry and Behavioral Sciences, Stanford University School of Medicine, Stanford, California

Robert N. Golden, M.D.
Professor and Chair, Department of Psychiatry, University of North Carolina, Chapel Hill

Rueben A. Gonzales, Ph.D.
Associate Professor, Department of Pharmacology, College of Pharmacy, University of Texas, Austin

Jack M. Gorman, M.D.
Professor of Psychiatry, Department of Psychiatry, Columbia University; and Deputy Director, New York State Psychiatric Institute, New York City

Anthony A. Grace, Ph.D.
Professor of Neuroscience and Psychiatry, Department of Neuroscience, University of Pittsburgh, Pittsburgh, Pennsylvania

Robert E. Hales, M.D., M.B.A.
Professor and Vice Chair, Department of Psychiatry, University of California, Davis, School of Medicine; and Medical Director, Sacramento County Mental Health Services

Sherri M. Hansen-Grant, M.D.
Assistant Professor, Director, Adult Consultation/Liaison Psychiatry, University of Wisconsin Medical School, Madison

Stephan Heckers, M.D.
Instructor, Department of Psychiatry, Massachusetts General Hospital and Harvard Medical School, Boston, Massachusetts

Stephen C. Heinrichs, Ph.D.
Staff Scientist, Neurocrine Biosciences, Inc., San Diego, California

Ned H. Kalin, M.D.
Hedberg Professor and Chair, Department of Psychiatry; and Director, Health Emotions Research Institute, University of Wisconsin Medical School, Madison

Claudia H. Kawas, M.D.
Departments of Pathology, Neurology, The Johns Hopkins University School of Medicine, Baltimore, Maryland

Paul E. Keck, Jr., M.D.
Associate Professor of Psychiatry and Pharmacology, and Vice Chairman for Research, Department of Psychiatry, University of Cincinnati College of Medicine, Cincinnati, Ohio

Justine M. Kent, M.D.
Fellow, Affective and Anxiety Disorders Research Program, New York State Psychiatric Institute; and Department of Psychiatry, Columbia University, New York City

Clinton D. Kilts, Ph.D.
Associate Professor, Department of Psychiatry and Behavioral Sciences, Emory University School of Medicine, Atlanta, Georgia

Richelle Kirrane, M.D.
Fellow, Mood and Personality Disorder Research Program, Mt. Sinai Medical Center, Mt. Sinai Hospital School of Medicine, New York City

Donald F. Klein, M.D.
Director, Psychiatric Research, Office of Mental Health, New York State Psychiatric Institute, New York City

Joel E. Kleinman, M.D., Ph.D.
Deputy Chief, Clinical Brain Disorders Branch; and Chief, Section on Neuropathology, National Institute of Mental Health, Division of Intramural Research Programs, Washington, D.C.

Michael B. Knable, D.O.
Senior Staff Fellow, National Institute of Mental Health, Division of Intramural Research Programs, Clinical Brain Disorders Branch, Washington, D.C.

Christine Konradi, Ph.D.
Assistant Professor, Department of Psychiatry, Harvard Medical School, Boston, Massachusetts

George F. Koob, Ph.D.
Professor, Department of Neuropharmacology, The Scripps Research Institute, La Jolla, California

K. Ranga Rama Krishnan, M.D.
Professor of Psychiatry; Head, Division of Biological Psychiatry; and Director, Affective Disorders Program, Duke University Medical Center, Durham, North Carolina

David J. Kupfer, M.D.
Thomas Detre Professor and Chair, Department of Psychiatry; and Director of Research, Western Psychiatric Institute and Clinic, University of Pittsburgh Medical Center, Pittsburgh, Pennsylvania

Michael K. Lee, Ph.D.
Department of Pathology, Division of Neuropathology, The Johns Hopkins University School of Medicine, Baltimore, Maryland

Robert H. Lenox, M.D.
Professor of Psychiatry, Pharmacology and Neuroscience; and Director of Molecular Neuropsychopharmacology Program, University of Florida College of Medicine and Brain Institute, Gainesville

Juan F. López, M.D.
Assistant Professor, Department of Psychiatry; and Research Investigator, Mental Health Research Institute, University of Michigan, Ann Arbor

Husseini K. Manji, M.D., F.R.C.P.C.
Director, Molecular Pathophysiology Program, and Schizophrenia and Mood Disorders Clinical Research Division, Departments of Psychiatry and Behavioral Neurosciences, and Pharmacology, Wayne State University School of Medicine, Detroit, Michigan

Alfred Mansour, Ph.D.
Research Investigator, Mental Health Research Institute, University of Michigan, Ann Arbor

Stephen R. Marder, M.D.
Professor and Vice Chair, Department of Psychiatry and Biobehavioral Sciences, UCLA School of Medicine; and Chief, Psychiatry Department, West Los Angeles Veterans Affairs Medical Center, Los Angeles, California

Deborah B. Marin, M.D.
Assistant Professor, Department of Psychiatry, Mt. Sinai School of Medicine, New York City

W. Vaughn McCall, M.D.
Associate Professor, Bowman-Gray School of Medicine, Winston-Salem, North Carolina

William M. McDonald, M.D.
Assistant Professor, Department of Psychiatry, Emory University School of Medicine, Atlanta, Georgia

Susan L. McElroy, M.D.
Associate Professor of Psychiatry, and Director, Biological Psychiatry Program, Department of Psychiatry, University of Cincinnati College of Medicine, Cincinnati, Ohio

Laura F. McNicholas, M.D., Ph.D.
Assistant Professor of Psychiatry, University of Pennsylvania; and Director, Department of Veterans Affairs Center of Excellence in Substance Abuse Treatment, Philadelphia, Pennsylvania

James H. Meador-Woodruff, M.D.
Associate Professor of Psychiatry and Senior Associate Research Scientist, Mental Health Research Institute, University of Michigan, Ann Arbor

Herbert Y. Meltzer, M.D.
Professor of Psychiatry and Pharmacology and Director of Psychopharmacology Division, Department of Psychiatry, Vanderbilt University School of Medicine, Nashville, Tennessee

Roger E. Meyer, M.D.
Clinical Professor of Psychiatry, Georgetown University, Washington, D.C.; and Senior Consultant on Clinical Research, Association of American Medical Colleges

Emmanuel Mignot, M.D., Ph.D.
Associate Professor of Psychiatry and Behavioral Sciences, Stanford University School of Medicine, Stanford, California; and Director, Center for Narcolepsy, Stanford Sleep Research Center, Palo Alto, California

Andrew H. Miller, M.D.
Associate Professor, Department of Psychiatry and Behavioral Sciences, Emory University School of Medicine, Atlanta, Georgia

Helen L. Miller, M.D.
Department of Psychiatry, Veterans Administration Connecticut Healthcare System, West Haven Campus, West Haven, Connecticut

Joseph D. Miller, Ph.D.
Associate Professor, Department of Pharmacology, Texas Tech University Health Sciences Center, Lubbock, Texas

Michael G. Moran, M.D.
Associate Professor, University of Colorado; and National Jewish Medical and Research Center, Denver, Colorado

Greer M. Murphy, Jr., M.D., Ph.D.
Assistant Professor, Department of Psychiatry and Behavioral Sciences, Stanford University School of Medicine, Stanford, California

Dominique L. Musselman, M.D.
Assistant Professor, Department of Psychiatry and Behavioral Sciences, Emory University School of Medicine, Atlanta, Georgia

Kalpana I. Nathan, M.D.
Director of Outpatient Substance Abuse Service, San Francisco General Hospital, Department of Psychiatry, San Francisco, California

Charles B. Nemeroff, M.D., Ph.D.
Reunette W. Harris Professor and Chairman, Department of Psychiatry and Behavioral Sciences, Emory University School of Medicine, Atlanta, Georgia

Linda Nicholas, M.D.
Assistant Professor, Department of Psychiatry, University of North Carolina, Chapel Hill

Philip T. Ninan, M.D.
Associate Professor, Department of Psychiatry and Behavioral Sciences; and Director, Mood and Anxiety Disorders Program, Emory University School of Medicine, Atlanta, Georgia

Seiji Nishino, M.D., Ph.D.
Senior Research Scientist of Psychiatry and Behavioral Sciences, Stanford University School of Medicine, Stanford, California; and Associate Director, Center for Narcolepsy, Stanford Sleep Research Center, Palo Alto, California

Charles P. O'Brien, M.D., Ph.D.
Professor and Vice Chairman, Department of Psychiatry, University of Pennsylvania; ACOS, Behavioral Health Services, Department of Veterans Affairs Medical Center, Philadelphia, Pennsylvania

Michael J. Owens, Ph.D.
Associate Professor, Department of Psychiatry and Behavioral Sciences, Laboratory of Neuropsychopharmacology, Emory University School of Medicine, Atlanta, Georgia

Carmine M. Pariante, M.D.
Maudsley Hospital, Denmark Hill, London, England

Elaine R. Peskind, M.D.
Associate Professor, Department of Psychiatry and Behavioral Sciences, University of Washington School of Medicine, and Veterans Affairs Puget Sound Health Care System, Seattle, Washington

William Z. Potter, M.D., Ph.D.
Lilly Research Fellow, Lilly Research Laboratories, Eli Lilly and Company, Indianapolis, Indiana

Donald L. Price, M.D.
Departments of Pathology, Neurology, and Neuroscience, Division of Neuropathology, The Johns Hopkins University School of Medicine, Baltimore, Maryland

Murray A. Raskind, M.D.
Professor and Vice Chair, Department of Psychiatry and Behavioral Sciences, University of Washington School of Medicine, and Veterans Affairs Puget Sound Health Care System, Seattle, Washington

Martin Reite, M.D.
Professor of Psychiatry, University of Colorado Health Sciences Center, Denver

S. Craig Risch, M.D.
Professor of Psychiatry and Behavioral Sciences, Department of Psychiatry and Behavioral Sciences, Clinical Neuropharmacology Program, Medical University of South Carolina, Charleston

Jerrold F. Rosenbaum, M.D.
Director of Outpatient Psychiatry, and Chief, Clinical Psychopharmacology Unit, Massachusetts General Hospital, Boston

Matthew V. Rudorfer, M.D.
Assistant Chief, Adult and Geriatric Treatment and Preventive Interventions Research Branch, National Institute of Mental Health, Rockville, Maryland

Carl Salzman, M.D.
Professor of Psychiatry, Harvard Medical School; and Director of Education and Director of Psychopharmacology, Massachusetts Mental Health Center, Boston

Andrew Satlin, M.D.
Associate Director, Nervous System Clinical Research, Novartis Pharmaceuticals Corporation, East Hanover, New Jersey

Alan F. Schatzberg, M.D.
Kenneth T. Norris, Jr., Professor in Psychiatry and Behavioral Sciences; and Chairman, Department of Psychiatry and Behavioral Sciences, Stanford University School of Medicine, Stanford, California

Larry J. Siever, M.D.
Professor of Psychiatry and Director, Out-Patient Psychiatry Division, Mt. Sinai School of Medicine, Bronx VA Medical Center, New York City

Jonathan M. Silver, M.D.
Chief, Ambulatory Services, Department of Psychiatry, Lenox Hill Hospital; and Clinical Professor of Psychiatry, New York University School of Medicine, New York City

George M. Simpson, M.D.
Professor of Psychiatry, Director of Research Psychiatry, and Interim Chair, Department of Psychiatry, University of Southern California School of Medicine, Los Angeles

Sangram S. Sisodia, Ph.D.
Departments of Pathology, Neuroscience, Division of Neuropathology, The Johns Hopkins University School of Medicine, Baltimore, Maryland

Joseph K. Stanilla, M.D.
Department of Psychiatry, MCP-Hahnemann School of Medicine at Eastern Pennsylvania Psychiatric Institute, and Allegheny University–Norristown State Hospital, Clinical Research Unit at Norristown State Hospital, Norristown, Pennsylvania

Murray B. Stein, M.D., F.R.C.P.C.
Associate Professor of Psychiatry In-Residence, Department of Psychiatry, University of California, San Diego, La Jolla, California

Alan Stoudemire, M.D.
Department of Psychiatry, Emory University School of Medicine, Atlanta, Georgia

Zachary N. Stowe, M.D.
Department of Psychiatry and Behavioral Sciences, Department of Gynecology and Obstetrics, Emory University School of Medicine, Atlanta, Georgia

James R. Strader, Jr., B.S.
Department of Psychiatry and Behavioral Sciences, Emory University School of Medicine, Atlanta, Georgia

C. Barr Taylor, M.D.
Professor of Psychiatry, Department of Psychiatry and Behavioral Sciences, Stanford University School of Medicine, Stanford, California

Gopal Thinakaran, Ph.D.
Department of Pathology, Division of Neuropathology, The Johns Hopkins University School of Medicine, Baltimore, Maryland

Gary D. Tollefson, M.D., Ph.D.
Vice President, Lilly Research Laboratories, Eli Lilly and Company, Indianapolis, Indiana

Robert L. Trestman, Ph.D., M.D.
Associate Professor, Department of Psychiatry, Mt. Sinai School of Medicine, New York City

Juan C. Troncoso, M.D.
Departments of Pathology, Neurology, Division of Neuropathology, The Johns Hopkins University School of Medicine, Baltimore, Maryland

Michael J. Tueth, M.D.
Associate Professor of Psychiatry, University of Florida College of Medicine, Gainesville

Thomas W. Uhde, M.D.
Professor and Chair, Department of Psychiatry and Behavioral Neurosciences, Wayne State University School of Medicine, Detroit, Michigan

Stanley J. Watson, Jr., Ph.D., M.D.
Co-Director, Mental Health Research Institute, University of Michigan, Ann Arbor

Daniel R. Weinberger, M.D.
Chief, Clinical Brain Disorders Branch, National Institute of Mental Health, Division of Intramural Research Programs, Washington, D.C.

Jay M. Weiss, Ph.D.
Jenny C. Adams Professor, Department of Psychiatry and Behavioral Sciences, Emory University School of Medicine; and Director of Research, Georgia Mental Health Institute, Atlanta

Elizabeth B. Weller, M.D.
Professor of Psychiatry, University of Pennsylvania, Philadelphia

Ronald Weller, M.D.
Professor of Psychiatry, University of Pennsylvania, Philadelphia

Richard E. Wilcox, Ph.D.
Professor and Doluisio Fellow of Pharmacology, College of Pharmacy and Institute for Neuroscience, University of Texas, Austin

Philip C. Wong, Ph.D.
Department of Pathology, Division of Neuropathology, The Johns Hopkins University School of Medicine, Baltimore, Maryland

Ann Marie Woo-Ming, M.D.
Fellow, Department of Psychiatry, Mt. Sinai School of Medicine, New York City

Kimberly A. Yonkers, M.D.
Assistant Professor, Departments of Psychiatry and Obstetrics and Gynecology, University of Texas Southwestern Medical Center, Dallas

Stuart C. Yudofsky, M.D.
D.C. and Irene Ellwood Professor and Chairman, Department of Psychiatry and Behavioral Sciences, Baylor College of Medicine; and Chief, Psychiatry Service, The Methodist Hospital, Houston, Texas

Charles Zorumpski, M.D.
Professor and Chairman, Department of Psychiatry, Washington University School of Medicine, St. Louis, Missouri

Introduction

Psychopharmacology has developed as a medical discipline over approximately the past four decades. The discoveries of the earlier effective antidepressants, antipsychotics, and mood stabilizers were frequently based on serendipitous observations. The repeated demonstration of efficacy of these agents then served as an impetus for considerable research into the neurobiological bases of their therapeutic effects and of emotion and cognition themselves, as well as the biological basis of the major psychiatric disorders. Moreover, the emergence of an entire new multidisciplinary field, neuropsychopharmacology, which has led to newer specific agents to alter maladaptive central nervous system processes or activity, was another byproduct of these early endeavors. The remarkable proliferation of information in this area—coupled with the absence of any comparable, currently available text—led us to edit the first edition of *The American Psychiatric Press Textbook of Psychopharmacology*. The response to that edition was overwhelmingly positive. However, psychopharmacology is still a burgeoning field; in this second edition, we expand considerably on the first edition, covering a number of areas in much greater detail, adding several new chapters, and updating all of the previous material.

In order for the reader to appreciate and integrate the rich amount of information about pharmacological agents, we attempted in the first edition to provide sufficient background material to understand more easily how drugs work and why, when, and in whom they should be used. We maintain this overall structure in the second edition. The textbook consists of four major sections. The first section, "Principles of Psychopharmacology," provides a theoretical background for the ensuing sections and still includes chapters on neurotransmitters, molecular neurobiology, neuroanatomy, electrophysiology, animal models of depression and schizophrenia, and pharmacokinetics. All these chapters have been extensively revised or rewritten by new authors. Also, we have added to this section chapters on animal models of anxiety disorders and Alzheimer's disease and a chapter on psychoneuroendocrinology/psychoneuroimmunology.

The second section, "Classes of Psychiatric Treatments: Animal and Human Pharmacology," presents information by classes of drugs. For each drug within a class, data are reviewed on preclinical and clinical pharmacology, pharmacokinetics, indications, dosages, and the like. This section is pharmacopoeia-like. We include data on currently available drugs in the United States and medications that will almost certainly become available in the near future. We have added new chapters or subsections on electroconvulsive therapy, new antipsychotics, new antidepressants (e.g., dual reuptake inhibitors), and nonbenzodiazepine anxiolytics.

The third section, "Clinical Psychobiology and Psychiatric Syndromes," reviews data on the biological underpinnings of specific disorders—for example, major depression, bipolar disorder, and panic disorder. The authors in this section comprehensively review the biological alterations described for each of the major psychiatric disorders, allowing the reader to better understand current psychopharmacological approaches as well as to anticipate future developments. These chapters have been updated in great detail, and the chapters on Alzheimer's disease and personality disorders are entirely new.

The fourth section, "Psychopharmacological Treatment," reviews state-of-the-art therapeutic approaches to patients with major psychiatric disorders as well as to those in specific age groups or circumstances: childhood disorders, emergency psychiatry, pregnancy and postpartum, medically ill patients, and so forth. This section provides the reader with specific information about drug selection and their prescription. We have added a new chapter on insomnia. In addition, an Appendix on promising new psychotropic drugs for Axis I disorders is once again included.

This textbook would not have been possible without the superb editorial work of the section editors—Joseph T. Coyle, M.D., Dennis S. Charney, M.D., Herbert Y. Meltzer, M.D., David J. Kupfer, M.D., and Donald F. Klein, M.D.—as well as, of course, the authors of the chapters who so generously gave of their time. In addition, we wish to thank Claire Reinburg of the American Psychiatric Press and her staff for their editorial efforts. In particular, we appreciate the major efforts of Stacy Jobb, Acquisitions Assistant, and our Project Editor, Alisa Guerzon. Finally, we extend our thanks to Gertrud Cory at Stanford University and Anne Griswell at Emory University for their invaluable assistance.

Alan F. Schatzberg, M.D.

Charles B. Nemeroff, M.D., Ph.D.

SECTION I

Principles of Psychopharmacology

Joseph T. Coyle, M.D., Section Editor

ONE

Introduction to Neurotransmitters, Receptors, Signal Transduction, and Second Messengers

Richard E. Wilcox, Ph.D.,
Rueben A. Gonzales, Ph.D., and Joseph D. Miller, Ph.D.

In this chapter, we consider prototypes of each class of signaling molecule and then discuss other key members of the class comparatively—the horizontal approach shown in Figure 1–1. This discussion should provide the reader with a solid core of information with which to approach the more detailed discussions in later chapters of this book that focus on the vertical approach of transmitter systems. To achieve the status accorded a signaling molecule within its class, a potential signal substance must meet certain criteria. To highlight this concept, the sections on neurotransmitters and second messengers begin with a brief overview of the criteria that potential signal molecules have met for inclusion within these classes. The discussion within each section focuses on a few fundamental principles by which the reader can compare signaling molecules within and between functional classes.

NEUROTRANSMITTERS

Core Transmitters and the Prototype for Discussion

We consider acetylcholine, dopamine, norepinephrine, serotonin, glutamate, and γ-aminobutyric acid (GABA) as key transmitters implicated in psychiatric disease and its

pharmacological therapy. Dopamine, which plays a major role in schizophrenia and its pharmacotherapy (Seeman 1995), is considered as the prototype, and other core transmitters are compared with it.

Criteria for a Neurotransmitter

Following the format of McGeer et al. (1987) is useful in stating the criteria for a transmitter within anatomical, chemical, physiological, and pharmacological domains. Dopamine fulfills the *anatomical criterion* by being unevenly distributed within the brain, where it is especially enriched in nerve terminals and differentially distributed across brain regions. Indeed, it was the difference in the brain distributions of dopamine and norepinephrine that first suggested an independent transmitter role for dopamine. The *chemical criteria* for dopamine are also fulfilled by the presence of the enzymes necessary for dopamine synthesis (tyrosine hydroxylase and aromatic amino acid decarboxylase; Nagatsu 1991) in terminals of dopamine neurons and by the calcium-dependent and potassium-stimulated release of endogenous dopamine from pinched-off nerve endings (synaptosomes) from the corpus striatum of the basal ganglia (Leslie et al. 1985).

Local microinjections of dopamine by needle-guide cannula (chemitrode), iontophoresis, pressure pulse, and microdialysis tube infusion mimic the actions produced by

Information flow

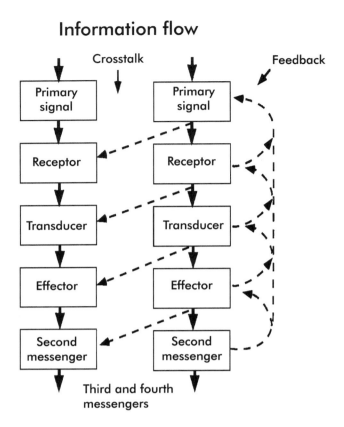

Figure 1–1.   Schematic representation of the elements that mediate information processing in the central nervous system. Boldface arrows indicate "vertical" or direct transfer of information across classes of signaling molecules. Dashed arrows indicate examples of some of the potential points of integration that involve interactions between and within classes of signaling molecules. For simplicity, only a few of the many possible types of integration are shown in the figure. These processes involve regulation, modulation, or fine-tuning of direct signals. Emphasized in the figure are feedback processes, in which information can flow from distal to proximal portions of a biochemical information pathway (i.e., from effector to receptor), and "crosstalk," in which information can be transferred between parallel biochemical pathways through common linkages

stimulation of the nigrostriatal dopamine tract and other dopamine-containing pathways, such as the ventral tegmental dopaminergic projection to mesolimbic and mesocortical brain regions. This fulfills the basic *physiological criterion* for transmitter status. Finally, the effects of drugs on the several possible sites of action within the dopaminergic synapse (discussed in the next section) should alter behavior in ways predictable from stimulating or lesioning tracts containing dopamine in the brain. This is indeed the case and fulfills the *pharmacological criterion* for dopamine's transmitter status.

Major Sites of Drug Action— Steps in Chemical Transmission

Tyrosine from dietary sources is taken up into dopaminergic nerve terminals through a process of facilitated diffusion. Subsequently, it is acted on by the cytoplasmic enzyme tyrosine hydroxylase to yield L-dopa and then dopamine. This occurs through the action of an L-aromatic amino acid decarboxylase enzyme (also termed *dopa-decarboxylase*) (Figure 1–2).

From there, the dopamine is taken into presynaptic vesicles. The *neurotransmitter presynaptic vesicle transport proteins* are neurotransmitter–H$^+$ antiporters in which transmitter movement into the presynaptic vesicle is linked to an outward movement of a hydrogen ion (proton). These proteins have 12 membrane-spanning regions, and the aminoterminal (N-terminal) and carboxyterminal (C-terminal) of the transporter are located outside the vesicle proper (Usdin et al. 1995). The vesicular transport protein found within dopamine nerve terminals recovers dopamine that has been removed from the synapse by the neuronal transporter (see below). It is important to distinguish such vesicular transporters from the plasma membrane transporter (see below).

The dopamine is protected from degradation within the presynaptic terminal by storage in membranous vesicles. The dopamine remains within the vesicles until an action potential arrives at the terminal and induces a voltage-dependent calcium ion entry that induces transmitter release (stimulus-secretion coupling). As a result of calcium entry, the vesicular contents (including dopamine and several proteins) are extruded into the immediately adjacent synaptic cleft. Within the cleft, dopamine diffuses to stimulate dopamine receptors. These receptors may be on the nerve terminal (axon terminal autoreceptors, named so because they respond to the neuron's own transmitter) or on the nondopaminergic target cell (postsynaptic heteroceptors, named so because these neurons do not secrete dopamine; Wolf and Roth 1987). Similarly, dopamine release from the dendrites or cell body can stimulate another class of impulse-flow-regulating receptors (dendritic or somal autoreceptors, respectively; Roth 1984).

Clearly, dopamine cannot be released unless it is synthesized and stored properly; thus, complete inhibition of either of the above enzymatic reactions (tyrosine hydroxylation or dopa-decarboxylation) can prevent dopamine production. Such inhibition will reduce dopamine release into the synaptic cleft. This process illustrates the principle of *synaptic effect:* effects of a drug or a disease on dopamine synthesis become relevant to behavior only if such

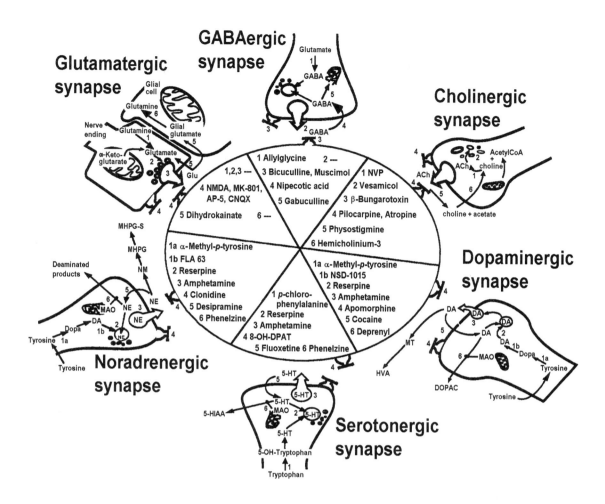

Figure 1–2. Sites of drug action for several neurotransmitter systems. The six panels of the rosette show synapses for γ-aminobutyric acid (GABA), acetylcholine (ACh), dopamine (DA), serotonin (5-HT), norepinephrine (NE), and glutamate (Glu). In general, each of the steps in synaptic transmission offers a potential target for therapeutic intervention by a drug. These steps (sites) include synthesis, vesicular uptake, transmitter release, receptor binding, cellular uptake, and transmitter metabolism. For each synapse, drugs are shown that act at the sites indicated by the numbers on the scheme. AP-5 = 2-amino-5-phosphonopentanoic acid; CNQX = 6-cyano-7-nitroquinoxaline-2,3-dione; NMDA = *N*-methyl-D-aspartate; MAO = monoamine oxidase; NM = normetanephrine; MHPG = 3-methoxy-4-hydroxyphenylglycol; MHPG-S = MHPG sulfate; 5-HIAA = 5-hydroxyindoleacetic acid; MT = 3-methoxytyramine; HVA = homovanillic acid; DOPAC = 3,4-dihydroxyphenylacetic acid; 8-OH-DPAT = 8-hydroxydipropylaminotetralin; MK-801, FLA-63, and NSD-1015 are chemical code names designated by pharmaceutical companies.

changes also somehow alter the amount of dopamine that is released into the synaptic cleft and available to stimulate its receptors. Dopamine is both a transmitter and a precursor for the synthesis of two other transmitters—norepinephrine and epinephrine. Thus, inhibition of dopamine synthesis also inhibits norepinephrine and epinephrine synthesis.

The hydroxylation of tyrosine is the rate-limiting step in dopamine synthesis; its inhibition by α-methylparatyrosine (AMPT) reduces the active pool of dopamine, the disappearance of which can serve as an index of the rate at which dopamine is "turned over" (utilized) within a particular brain region. Also, AMPT administration appears capable of inducing a behavioral quieting consistent with reduced dopamine synthesis. Activity of this enzyme, thus, sets the pace of dopamine synthesis (Cooper et al. 1996).

A marked behavioral activation is induced by enhancing synaptic dopamine levels through the actions of cocaine or dextroamphetamine (see discussion later in this section). Interestingly, some of the symptoms of schizophrenia appear linked to reduced dopamine activity within cortical portions of the limbic system of the forebrain. Methylphenidate, an agent with a mechanism of action like that of cocaine (which inhibits the uptake of dopamine into the nerve terminal; see below), has been used to treat these "negative" symptoms. (This topic is discussed in Marder, Chapter 17, in this volume.) Amphetamine-like agents also have other uses in psychiatry, including management of attention-deficit/hyperactivity disorder (ADHD) (see Fawcett and Busch, Chapter 25, in this volume).

In animals, dopamine synthesis can be reasonably estimated either from the decline in dopamine levels after tyrosine hydroxylase inhibition or from the increase in L-dopa accumulation after inhibition of dopa-decarboxylase (by agents such as NSD1015; Vaughn et al. 1990). Clinically, the normally high levels of brain tyrosine preclude attempts to enhance dopamine synthesis by making more of this precursor amino acid available because the enzyme is already fully saturated. In humans, dopamine synthesis and the functional integrity of the nigrostriatal dopamine nerve terminals may be estimated with positron-emission tomography (PET) (Hall et al. 1992; Laihinen et al. 1992) from changes in the specific radioactivity of ^{18}F-fluorodopa after administration of an intravenous tracer dose.

People with Parkinson's disease have insufficient dopamine in the nigrostriatal pathway of the brain. However, replacement therapy with dopamine itself is ineffective because dopamine does not cross the blood-brain barrier. The dopamine precursor L-dopa, however, is transported across the blood-brain barrier, where it may be converted to dopamine. In people with Parkinson's disease, inhibition of the other enzyme involved in dopamine synthesis, dopa-decarboxylase, may be achieved by an agent such as carbidopa. Carbidopa is an effective enzyme inhibitor; however, carbidopa does not cross the blood-brain barrier. Therefore, carbidopa cannot prevent the conversion of L-dopa to dopamine in brain but can do so only in the peripheral nervous system. This action causes most of a dose of L-dopa to reach the brain.

Newly synthesized dopamine is stored in a functional "pool," which is preferentially released on nerve stimulation by a calcium-dependent process and which can be modified by agonists and antagonists acting at axon terminal autoreceptors. This pool is especially sensitive to inhibition by the actions of AMPT. Other (earlier synthesized) dopamine, which composes the great majority of the transmitter content of a dopamine nerve terminal, is stored in a less labile pool that is sensitive to the drug reserpine. Those synaptic vesicles closest to the neuronal (plasma) membrane are those which are the most likely sites of transmitter release. Thus, proximity to the plasma membrane within the terminal may help to define the releasable and storage pools anatomically. A third pool of dopamine consists of the cytoplasmic transmitter not yet taken up into the presynaptic vesicles (McMillen 1983).

Physiological dopamine release depends on the concentration of external calcium ion, because it is calcium influx down its steep concentration gradient into the nerve terminal that couples the voltage changes associated with axon potentials to the secretion of transmitter. It is convenient to study release processes in vitro by using either pinched-off nerve endings (synaptosomes) or tissue slices. Biophysical properties of the preparations dictate that synaptosomes are typically depolarized by potassium stimulation, whereas slices are depolarized by either potassium or electrical stimulation. In either instance, increasing the amount of depolarization increases the net calcium influx and dopamine release from the nerve terminal (Leslie et al. 1985). In contrast to the physiological release process, certain psychostimulants, such as dextroamphetamine and methamphetamine, can enhance the release of dopamine and some other transmitters through a calcium-independent release mechanism (Robinson and Becker 1986). Such non-calcium-dependent release is thought to occur via a process called *exchange diffusion* (McMillen 1983). According to this hypothesis, the amphetamine molecules are transported into the nerve terminal by the dopamine uptake carrier and exchange places with endogenous dopamine within one of the storage pools of the transmitter; the amphetamine then diffuses through the membrane out of the terminal into the synaptic cleft, producing an increased dopamine release.

Released dopamine can stimulate autoreceptors, which appear to be of the D_2 subfamily, located on dopamine nerve terminals. Such stimulation initiates a negative feedback effect on dopamine synthesis to reduce further release of dopamine. The consequences of dopamine stimulation are thought to involve a change in the kinetics of tyrosine hydroxylase (Saller and Salama 1986). This regulatory process illustrates the principle of *autoregulation* (synaptic homeostasis), whereby release of dopamine, elevating synaptic levels above baseline, initiates a set of events that tends to restore dopamine levels to their basal values. Some dopamine agonists, such as the prototype agent apomorphine or its congener N-n-propylnorapomorphine (NPA), can stimulate autoreceptors somewhat selectively in low doses. Autoreceptor stimulation turns off dopamine synthesis by inhibiting tyrosine hydroxylase activity, thereby reducing synaptic dopamine levels without stimulating postsynaptic dopamine receptors. NPA has been used in open studies to reduce the enhanced levels of limbic system dopamine thought to be associated with the delusions and hallucinations of psychosis. Released dopamine from dendritic or somal sites can similarly exert a negative feedback action to inhibit firing of dopaminergic neurons (Chiodo 1992; Grace and Onn 1989).

In the nigrostriatal dopamine system of the brain, increases in impulse flow produce complex actions on dopamine synthesis, turnover, and metabolite levels. For example, antipsychotic drugs increase neuronal firing rate of dopamine neurons early in their administration, whereas they induce increases in dopamine metabolite levels later in treatment. Adaptations to antipsychotic administration within striatum include a depolarization inactivation, which may actually lead to reductions in metabolite levels (see Chapter 17). However, in contrast to most other systems, decreases in impulse flow in this dopamine pathway, which lead to increases in dopamine content within the terminal, also lead to dramatic increases in dopamine synthesis (Bannon and Roth 1983; Deutch and Roth 1990). Although this at first seems paradoxical, there is a potential explanation. Decreased neural firing reduces dopamine in the synaptic cleft, which reduces stimulation of the autoreceptors on the axon terminal. Less autoreceptor stimulation activates tyrosine hydroxylase by altering its kinetics for its pteridine cofactor. As a result, newly synthesized dopamine is increased.

Released dopamine can also stimulate postsynaptic receptors in target neurons to cause a variety of changes, depending on the type of dopamine receptor that is activated. Drugs that mimic dopamine by stimulating its receptors—*direct agonists* (such as some of the agents used to treat parkinsonism)—can reduce dopamine synthesis and release in the corpus striatum through negative feedback (Severson et al. 1990; Wilcox et al. 1990). However, striatal dopamine synthesis is also reduced after antiparkinsonian drug administration through stimulation of axon terminal autoreceptors. Antipsychotic drugs that block dopamine receptors—acting as *antagonists*—prevent the actions of dopamine at these receptor sites. As described in detail in Chapter 10 in this volume (Potter et al.), this general action appears to be responsible for the major use of these drugs in psychiatry—that is, treatment of symptoms of psychosis. In Chapter 17, the author discusses the problems associated with long-term administration of antipsychotic agents, including induction of an iatrogenic (drug-induced) disorder termed *tardive dyskinesia*. Acute administration of antipsychotics typically halts the negative feedback action of dopamine on its synthesis and release, leading to marked increases in both actions in corpus striatum (Bartholini et al. 1989). Very low doses of antipsychotic agents appear able to block autore-

ceptors selectively, leading to elevated synaptic dopamine concentrations in the absence of significant postsynaptic blockade (Bannon et al. 1986). As such, these very low antipsychotic drug doses would not be expected to reduce psychotic symptoms such as delusions and hallucinations and could actually worsen these symptoms.

Stimulation of postsynaptic receptors by dopamine is a key event in the synaptic transmission process. Dopamine can activate at least five major subtypes of dopamine receptors (some of which have splice- or allelic-variants), which is discussed in detail below in the section, "Receptors" (Bunzow et al. 1988; Civelli et al. 1991; Dearry et al. 1990; Seeman 1995; Sibley and Monsma 1992; Sunahara et al. 1991). Note that the amount of dopamine bound to the receptor is directly proportional to the concentration of dopamine. In marked contrast, the cellular actions of dopamine (i.e., cellular response) increase to their maximum as a nonlinear, monotonic function of increasing amounts of the dopamine-receptor complex (i.e., cellular stimulus) (Mak et al. 1996; Randall 1988). In other words, a single drug–receptor complex may activate multiple transduction proteins, each of which activates many effector enzymes (see "Adenylate Cyclase" in the section, "Signal Transduction," later in this chapter), constituting a considerable amplification of the signal. The system behaves as if "spare" receptors actually exist, although current knowledge suggests that all of the receptors of a given class are functionally equivalent (i.e., that any receptor is as likely to be occupied by dopamine as any other) and that only a small fraction of them need to be activated to produce a maximal cellular response. This illustrates the dose dependence of biological responses. Also, because dopamine's stimulation of its receptors produces a specific sequence of cellular events, it is important to realize that the peak time for the biological effects of a transmitter (or drug) depends on the agent's ability to get to its sites of action.

Of great relevance to the clinician is the adaptation of receptor systems to previous exposure to drugs. For example, chronic blockade of D_2 dopamine receptors leads to an approximate 30% increase in receptor density and to changes in postreceptor events. These changes increase the system's sensitivity to endogenous dopamine and to the actions of dopamine agonists (*sensitization*) but decrease the sensitivity to some of the biological consequences of receptor blockade. Repeated stimulation of dopamine receptors by dopamine or dopamine agonists leads to the converse situation—that is, a reduction in dopamine receptor numbers (*downregulation*) or an uncoupling of the receptors from their signal-transducing proteins (*desensitization*) and an enhanced effect of receptor blockers

(Riffee et al. 1982; Severson et al. 1990; Vaughn et al. 1990). It is important to understand that sensitization and desensitization need not only follow chronic exposure to exogenous agents. Both can occur with a single brief exposure to a drug or hormone (Mak et al. 1996; Severson et al. 1990) and, indeed, probably play a significant role in allowing motor, emotional, and cognitive systems to adapt to changing stimuli, as has been shown for sensory systems. Furthermore, circadian rhythms (~24 hours) in endogenous transmitter synthesis and release dynamically modulate receptor function over time.

Understanding the therapeutic actions of psychoactive agents requires knowledge of how the nervous system adapts to repeated exposure to the drug. The operational phenomenon of *tolerance*, whereby exposure to an agonist induces a smaller response to subsequent agonist doses (partially via the process of desensitization), reflects the longitudinal response of the nervous system to changes in receptor stimulation, signal transduction, and gene expression (Sibley and Lefkowitz 1985).

These adaptive changes to drug exposure illustrate the principle of *synaptic resilience*, which is a form of homeostasis. In this process, the nervous system attempts to maintain a balanced level of receptor activation and cellular responsiveness despite marked changes in formation of drug-receptor complexes. This is accomplished by altering receptor densities (through changes in gene expression), coupling of receptor to signal transduction pathways (often through phosphorylation; see section, "Gene Regulation and Fourth-Messenger Systems—Phospho-CREB" later in this chapter), and releasing transmitters. Faulty feedback among components of a biochemical pathway extending from a cell-surface receptor through second messengers and associated genes may contribute to disease symptoms (Montmayeur and Borrelli 1991). Similarly, altered balances between presynaptic and postsynaptic elements of a synapse may also contribute to manifestations of psychiatric disorders (Cole et al. 1992). In both instances, the mechanism is a disruption of synaptic resilience.

The idea that two properties of primary importance to the potential therapeutic use of a given drug are its affinity for a given receptor and its ability to induce an activated receptor state (the drug's efficacy) has been introduced. However, the therapeutic benefits (or lack thereof) arising from administration of a given compound also depend on the drug's selectivity of binding to various receptors. Clozapine is more effective in reducing the negative symptoms of schizophrenia than are other available antipsychotics. Clozapine binds with high affinity to no fewer than six receptors of potential importance to schizophre-

nia, and it may be this very lack of specificity that provides its unique therapeutic profile. The indications for use of this agent and the unusually broad spectrum of receptor blockade by this compound are considered in Chapter 17.

Dopamine binds to and dissociates from its receptors more rapidly than do dopamine antagonists, such as spiperone, which has a dissociation rate constant of -0.078 min^{-1} at the D_2 receptor (R. E. Wilcox, unpublished data, October 1978). Subsequently, the synaptic dopamine concentration declines because of an active reuptake process mediated by a sodium-dependent plasma membrane transporter protein, which recently has been cloned and sequenced (Eshleman et al. 1994; Kilty et al. 1991). The disappearance of synaptic dopamine via active reuptake by a plasma membrane transporter is one of two mechanisms for transmitter inactivation, the other being metabolic degradation.

Many plasma membrane transporters contain 12 membrane-spanning regions. The plasma membrane transporters for dopamine, norepinephrine, and serotonin also have both the C- and the N-terminals in the cytoplasm. These transport proteins have a large extracellular loop between regions M3 and M4, which appears to represent the binding site for pharmacological agents and may be involved in selecting the appropriate transmitter to transport. For example, this region of the dopamine transporter contains the binding site for cocaine and for the neurotoxin MPP^+ (1-methyl-4-phenylpyridinium ion), which can cause a Parkinson's disease–like syndrome by inducing destruction of the nigrostriatal pathway in healthy young adults who have ingested MPTP (1-methyl-4-phenyl-1,2,5,6-tetrahydropyridine) (Amara and Kuhar 1993). Uptake into the nerve terminal is the major means by which the released dopamine is removed from the synapse.

Drugs that inhibit the plasma membrane uptake carrier include the widely abused stimulant cocaine and the therapeutically used stimulant methylphenidate (Nestler 1992; Self et al. 1996). Note that although both cocaine and dextroamphetamine have similar abilities to enhance the synaptic content of dopamine, which leads to increased dopamine receptor stimulation, they do so by different molecular mechanisms (primarily plasma membrane uptake inhibition and increased release, respectively).

Once inside the nerve terminal, cytoplasmic dopamine is subject to metabolism by monoamine oxidase (MAO), located in the outer mitochondrial membrane. Thus, dopamine levels available for further release would tend to decline, because of catabolism by MAO, were no other processes operative. However, a second uptake carrier located in synaptic vesicle membranes (representing a gene product that appears to be distinct from that in the neuronal membrane; see above) removes the dopamine from the cytoplasm to the protected vesicular environment. Reserpine is an inhibitor of the vesicular uptake of dopamine and certain other transmitters. Administration of this drug causes the dopamine removed from the synapse to be subject to degradation by MAO. This leads to a profound reduction in stores of the transmitter. Although cocaine and reserpine have somewhat similar mechanisms (uptake inhibition), they actually have opposite effects on synaptic dopamine levels: cocaine increases these levels, whereas reserpine decreases them. This is because the two uptake carrier proteins are distinct in not only amino acid sequence but also location and, hence, function. Thus, although inhibition of transport occurs with both cocaine and reserpine, cocaine's inhibition increases synaptic dopamine, whereas reserpine's inhibition increases cytoplasmic dopamine, thereby exposing it to degradation by MAO.

Inhibition of the B form of MAO by deprenyl (selegiline) potentiates the actions of dopamine. In contrast, inhibition of the A form of MAO, which preferentially acts on serotonin-like substrates, provides an important action in the treatment of depression refractory to standard agents (Racagni et al. 1992). In particular, serotonin (5-hydroxytryptamine, 5-HT) systems of the limbic forebrain appear to undergo substantial changes in people with depression. (These changes are discussed in Musselman et al., Chapter 27, in this volume.)

O-Methylation by the enzyme catechol-O-methyltransferase (COMT) appears to play a minor role in the metabolism of catecholamines (including dopamine), because drugs that block the actions of COMT, such as tropolone or pyrogallol, have relatively little effect on levels of transmitters or metabolites. Also, inhibitors of COMT do not alter basal dopamine levels extracellularly in brain microdialysates. However, some of the newer inhibitors of COMT do appear able to potentiate the behavioral actions of systemically administered L-dopa. Thus, a complete evaluation of the therapeutic importance of COMT inhibition awaits the results of further research.

Agents that depend on an intact neuron for their action are defined as *indirect acting*. In contrast, drugs that bypass the neuron and directly activate or block receptors are defined as *direct acting*. These two types of agents respond in dramatically different ways to alterations in neuronal function or integrity. For example, loss of the nigrostriatal dopamine tract projecting to the basal ganglia, as occurs in parkinsonism, leads to a loss of effectiveness of indirect-acting agonists, such as dextroamphetamine, co-

caine, and methylphenidate. In contrast, the actions of direct-acting agonists may actually be enhanced because of sensitization of receptor and postreceptor elements, as discussed earlier in this chapter (synaptic resilience).

Comparison of Dopamine and Serotonin Systems in the Brain

Clinicians should be aware of similarities and differences among the key transmitters most relevant to biological psychiatry. In this section, we briefly review the serotonin system. The actions of serotonin are quite broad, including roles in affective disorders, suicide, impulsive behavior, and aggression, which has led to myriad uses of agents that alter serotonin function in psychiatry. (For example, Tollefson and Rosenbaum, Chapter 11, and Krishnan, Chapter 12, in this volume, discuss the uses of compounds that inhibit neuronal uptake of serotonin and serotonin breakdown by MAO, respectively.)

Serotonin synthesis depends on facilitated transport of tryptophan, which competes with other large neutral amino acids for entry into the brain. Serotonin synthesis also depends on a rate-limiting synthetic step: hydroxylation of tryptophan by tryptophan hydroxylase. This enzyme has a K_m (a kinetic measure of the affinity of the enzyme for its substrate) for tryptophan that is greater than the normal biological concentrations of the amino acid. Under these conditions, the availability of the substrate (tryptophan) becomes rate limiting. These conditions allow changes in dietary tryptophan composition to alter the synthesis of brain serotonin by altering precursor availability. (This is in contrast to the situation in the dopamine system, in which tyrosine availability is not rate limiting.)

Serotonin is produced from 5-hydroxytryptophan (5-HTP) through the action of 5-HTP-decarboxylase. This enzyme is part of a family of closely related L-aromatic amino acid decarboxylases (with a broad substrate profile) that includes dopa-decarboxylase. In contrast to what is observed within the dopamine system, 5-HTP administration does not inhibit tryptophan hydroxylase activity, indicating that end product (serotonin) inhibition of serotonin synthesis is not normally an important controlling factor in regulation of this transmitter. However, impulse flow in serotonergic neurons may initiate changes in the affinity of tryptophan hydroxylase for its pteridine cofactor, as we saw for the dopamine system and tyrosine hydroxylase kinetics.

There appears to be some subtype specificity in serotonergic axon terminal autoreceptors, such that they are composed of primarily the 5-HT$_{1B/1D}$ receptor subtype, whereas somatodendritic autoreceptors appear to be predominantly 5-HT$_{1A}$. This finding contrasts with that of the dopamine autoreceptor system, in which both axon terminal and somatodendritic autoreceptors appear to be of the same subtype (D$_2$, possibly D$_3$). Thus, serotonergic neurons can self-regulate synaptic transmitter concentrations and receptor stimulation through negative feedback. Termination of serotonergic receptor stimulation is achieved by neuronal uptake. For example, inhibition of serotonin uptake into the nerve terminal by fluoxetine increases synaptic transmitter levels to exert a clinically significant antidepressant action (Siever et al. 1991). (Chapter 10 provides a discussion of the affinities of various antidepressant drugs for neuronal transport proteins and amine receptors, and Chapter 11 compares the various selective serotonin reuptake inhibitors for their selectivity on the neuronal transporters.)

Recent immunocytochemical studies with antibodies against serotonin suggest that two anatomically distinguishable varieties of serotonin terminals may be present in brain: fine axons with small varicosities arising from the dorsal raphe nuclei and beaded axons with large spherical varicosities originating from the median raphe (Cooper et al. 1996). This is of some importance clinically because of the greater sensitivity of the fine axons to the neurotoxic effects of 3,4-methylenedioxyamphetamine (MDMA, "ecstasy"; Mamounas et al. 1992). Similarly, serotonin degradation by MAO-A can be prevented by enzyme inhibitors such as iproniazid, which also exerts an important antidepressant action in treatment of patients refractory to other types of agents.

Sites of Clinically Important Actions of Other Major Transmitters in Brain

More detailed discussions of the therapeutically significant actions of the major transmitters are provided in subsequent chapters. Here, it is important to highlight some of the more significant differences between those transmitters not yet discussed and dopamine and serotonin. Dopamine's status as the immediate precursor of norepinephrine suggests that most aspects of noradrenergic neuronal regulation should be similar to those observed for dopamine systems, which is the case. However, all known noradrenergic systems and some brain dopamine systems (such as the mesoprefrontal tract) lack autoreceptors modulating transmitter synthesis. This lack differentiates these pathways from the nigrostriatal dopamine pathway, which has synthesis-modulating autoreceptors. Thus, the former (autoreceptor-deficient) systems do not increase transmitter synthesis when impulse flow is interrupted, whereas the latter (autoreceptor-containing) system does (Bannon and Roth 1983).

Acetylcholine synthesis, like that of serotonin, is regulated primarily by availability of the precursor, choline, and the activity of the sodium-dependent, high-affinity choline uptake carrier. A second salient characteristic of cholinergic neurons is the extremely rapid termination of acetylcholine action, which occurs by enzymatic degradation. This degradation occurs through the activity of the acetylcholinesterase enzyme. Thus, inhibition of acetylcholine metabolism—in contrast to that of dopamine, serotonin, and norepinephrine—is clinically significant and has been used in attempts to treat symptoms of Alzheimer's disease and in standard therapy of myasthenia gravis (Summers et al. 1986; P. Taylor 1990). (Marin and Davis, Chapter 23, in this volume, provide an interesting discussion of various types of drugs, including acetylcholinesterase inhibitors, as cognition enhancers for treating dementias, especially Alzheimer's disease.)

The major amino acid transmitters include glutamate, the prototype excitatory substance, and GABA, the prototype inhibitory mediator. These signaling molecules offer several major contrasts to other key transmitters considered in this chapter. First, the number of synapses using these transmitters is much greater than those using all other types of monoamines and peptide transmitters combined. Second, both glutamate- and GABA-containing neurons are very widely distributed within brain, in contrast to the more restricted distribution of dopaminergic, serotonergic, and noradrenergic neurons. Third, glutamate (but not GABA) has other biochemical and metabolic actions in the body in addition to its transmitter functions. These actions include its highly important roles in intermediary metabolism in neurons and glial cells. Thus, glutamate serves as a precursor to both GABA and α-ketoglutarate in the production of ammonium ion (which is subsequently converted into urea). These characteristics of brain glutamate and/or GABA systems have major implications for biological psychiatry. The first implication is that the ubiquity of these transmitters makes it likely that some of their pathways will be dysfunctional in most diseases affecting behavior. The second implication is that this same feature renders difficult the standard pharmacotherapeutic approaches that increase or decrease synaptic levels of either transmitter. The third implication is that successful pharmacotherapy to alter either glutamate or GABA functions in brain must take advantage of advances in receptor pharmacology derived from the cloning of the genes for glutamate and GABA receptors and, perhaps, transporters (Cotman et al. 1995; Paul 1995). In this instance, new drugs that can selectively stimulate or block subtypes of these amino acid transmitter receptors at restricted sites could thereby yield a therapeutically useful balance between symptomatic relief and side effects.

RECEPTORS

A *receptor* is one of the key elements in normal synaptic transmission and in the action of psychopharmacological agents. In fact, this site is the most likely target for most clinically available psychoactive agents, because the receptor proteins appear to show the most selectivity in their interactions with small molecules. By interacting with receptors, drugs can alter cellular function and may thus bring a dysfunctional system back toward normal. The existence of a number of receptors was originally predicted from examination of pharmacological data. However, with the advent of modern biochemical techniques, including molecular cloning, receptors are now known to exist in a bewildering diversity.

Definition of a Receptor

A receptor is a protein that binds a signaling molecule (hormone or transmitter), becomes activated, and activates a signal transduction pathway. Thus, the basic function of any receptor is molecular recognition of a signaling molecule, resulting in signal transduction. In contrast, a *binding site* potentially interacts with endogenous signaling molecules or drugs with high affinity but is not directly linked to signal transduction. The statement of the operational basis of a receptor explicitly distinguishes a receptor from a binding site. The study of binding sites associated with a receptor may provide important information about the pharmacological characteristics or location of the receptor. However, it is important to keep in mind that the existence of a binding site does not necessitate the existence of a receptor. Recognition of the appropriate signal by the receptor causes its activation, which begins the process of signal transduction. The transduction process (discussed in more detail in the section, "Signal Transduction," below) either involves another set of proteins or may be intrinsic to the receptor's structure. On a molecular level, receptor activation is accomplished by a change in the three-dimensional structure of the receptor protein.

The first basic characteristic of a receptor that we discuss is the ability of the receptor to recognize specific molecules. Numerous signaling molecules exist in the brain. Each signaling molecule, or primary messenger, has evolved as a member of a complex of transmitter, receptor, signal transducer, and effector to carry a specific type of information, which is then used in the process of integration to produce a response such as behavior. Receptors have evolved to recognize specific signals to begin the integration process for neuronal information. The initial event in this process is molecular recognition, which occurs through the chemical interactions between the primary messenger and the receptor protein. During synaptic transmission, the molecular recognition at many types of receptors occurs within the transmembrane region of the receptor but still within the extracellular space. However, other receptors, such as hormone receptors, may exist within the cell.

For all receptors, the recognition site is intrinsic to the three-dimensional structure of the receptor protein. Therefore, the primary amino acid sequence of the protein determines the nature of the recognition site, the type of receptor, and the receptor activation mechanism(s). Receptor polypeptides are generally transmembrane molecules with the amino acid chain looping through the membrane several times, offering a good membrane anchor. Although the primary amino acid sequence of many receptors is known, we are only beginning to understand how various amino acids participate in the binding of the primary messenger molecule and, hence, the molecular recognition process in receptors such as the dopaminergic, β_2-adrenergic, and nicotinic cholinergic receptor proteins (Bunzow et al. 1988; Changeux et al. 1992; Hollenberg 1991; van Rhee and Jacobson 1996). For example, the agonist-binding site in the prototype of the G-protein-linked receptor, the β_2-adrenergic receptor, is composed of several amino acids that reside on several interacting transmembrane domains located on a single polypeptide chain. In contrast, the agonist-binding site in the prototype of the ligand-gated ion channel receptor, the nicotinic receptor, is localized primarily to amino acid residues near the N-terminal extracellular portion of a single subunit in a heteromeric complex. Models of receptors for classic neurotransmitters that are being proposed share this feature: the amino acids that form the binding site are located at or near the extracellular face of the protein. This location is consistent with the function of the receptors in synaptic transmission—that is, to receive hormones or transmitters.

Classification of Receptors

Receptors can be classified based on their primary amino acid sequence or through differences in pharmacology (i.e., their ability to interact with specific drugs). Before the initial determination of the amino acid sequence of a receptor, the nicotinic cholinergic receptor (Noda et al. 1983), the only classification scheme available was pharmacological. With the knowledge of the primary amino acid sequences of many neurotransmitter receptors, it has become clear that some receptors are more closely related than previously indicated by the pharmacological classification schemes (Andersen et al. 1990; Civelli et al. 1991; Sibley and Monsma 1992). In addition, in most cases more receptor subtypes are known from differences in primary amino acid structure than can be determined from pharmacological studies alone. For example, some drugs can readily distinguish between two types of dopamine receptors previously known as D_1 and D_2 (Andersen et al. 1990). However, to date there are five separate primary dopamine receptor subtypes with distinct primary amino acid sequences that form two receptor subfamilies: D_1-like and D_2-like.

Discordance between the number of receptor subtypes from molecular biological analysis and pharmacological studies has been found for most neurotransmitter receptors covered in this textbook. This lack of correspondence between molecular biology and pharmacology with regard to receptor classification indicates the need for newer and more selective pharmacological agents. As these newer agents are developed, the hope is that the additional selectivity achieved will translate into better therapeutic agents with fewer side effects. Until we reach this point, however, we must rely on classic pharmacological methods for receptor classification in whole animal and clinical experiments, with the knowledge that a number of receptor subtypes may contribute to the overall clinical response (Albert et al. 1990; Neve et al. 1989). To this end, we discuss some general aspects of receptor pharmacology for purposes of receptor classification. Various well-documented changes in brain dopamine receptor densities occur during normal aging and in several disorders. (For example, changes in dopamine receptors in schizophrenia are described in Knable et al., Chapter 28, in this volume.)

Drug Affinity and Efficacy

The binding of a neurotransmitter or drug (generally referred to as a ligand) to a receptor involves the interaction between the electronic forces associated with the ligand molecule and those associated with some of the projecting amino acid residues of the receptor protein. Figure 1–3 shows the electrostatic potential surface of an agonist drug, dihydrexidine, as it binds to the active site on the D_{1A} dopamine receptor. The *affinity* of a ligand for a particular receptor refers to the steady-state concentration between the ligand and the receptor. In turn, this depends on the ratio of the ligand's dissociation (off) rate to its association (on) rate for the receptor. Thus, the affinity of a ligand-receptor interaction depends only on the chemical characteristics of the drug and the receptor and may be derived solely through information obtained from binding experiments. A common measure of the affinity of a ligand for a receptor is the concentration of the ligand that is necessary to occupy one-half of the total number of receptors available (K_d, similar to the K_m from enzyme kinetics, is the reciprocal of the affinity). This parameter can be determined experimentally from radioligand binding experiments conducted on tissue homogenates or whole cells (Limbird 1986; Vaughn et al. 1990; Wilcox et al. 1990).

Different drugs have different affinities for particular receptors because of the varied strengths of interactions of their respective electronic fields. These differences are reflected in the electrostatic (charge) and steric (bulk) features presented to the receptor when aligned in a common binding conformation (Brusniak et al. 1996). Figure 1–4A shows a series of compounds aligned in their probable binding conformations at the recombinant D_{1A} dopamine receptor. Figure 1–4B shows a fairly rigid partial D_{1A} agonist drug in its probable binding conformation in relation to the electrostatic fields of the receptor that favor or disfavor positive charge on the drug. When the affinities of a series of drugs for different receptors are compared, the affinities of the drugs can be ranked from highest to lowest. The drugs with highest affinity will bind to the receptor at lower concentrations (i.e., a lower concentration of the drug is needed to occupy half of the receptor sites). Each receptor is pharmacologically characterized by a series of drugs with a range of affinities from high to low. Appropriate computational models of the drug-receptor interaction can predict drug affinity quite efficiently, as is shown in the scatter plot of Figure 1–5 (Brusniak et al. 1996). This information can be used to define and identify particular receptors. The ability of a receptor to distinguish different drugs by their affinities is the basis of molecular recognition (P. Taylor and Insel 1990). Hormones and transmitters tend to have lower overall affinity for their receptors than do many drugs, because they bind to a "resting" conformation of the receptor, in which the receptor's ability to initiate signal transduction is reduced compared with the agonist-induced "active" state. This overall mechanism of rapid transmitter dissociation from the receptor appears to allow the transmitter-receptor complex to dissociate ("reset" to its resting state) rapidly and, thus, adapt quickly to a changing environment. For those receptors that couple to independent membrane proteins called guanine nucleotide binding proteins (G proteins), neurotransmitter binding to the receptor induces the receptor to change its conformation, which allows the agonist-

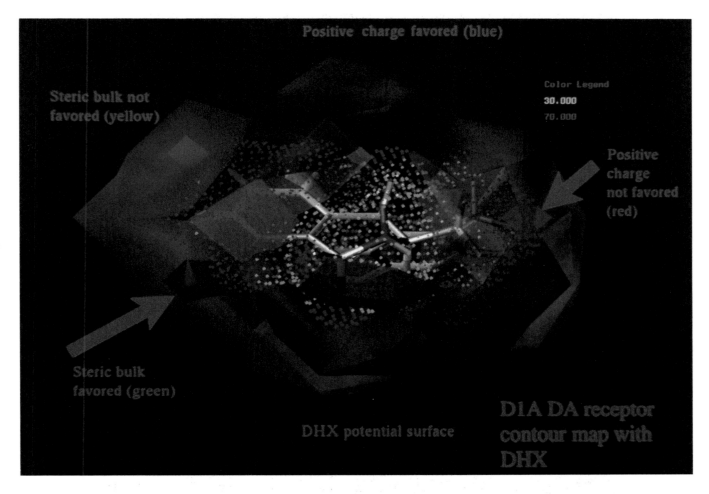

Figure 1–3.   Electrostatic potential surface of dihydrexidine (DHX). The positive charge surface, which the dopamine (DA) agonist DHX presents when binding to the recombinant D_{1A} dopamine receptor, is shown. Also shown are the regions in space where positive charge or steric bulk would tend to favor high affinity or make high-affinity binding less likely.
Source.   R. E. Wilcox, unpublished observations, September 1996.

receptor complex to bind to a third component, the G protein. The receptor can then bind to the agonist with high affinity.

Drug affinity depends only on the chemical interaction between the drug and the receptor. Therefore, knowing the affinity of a drug does not divulge its *activity* (i.e., what the drug does to the cell, tissue, organ, or behavior of the organism). The activity of a drug is determined by completing an experiment in which a response, such as biochemical (cellular) or behavioral, is measured. The ability of a drug to elicit a response per unit of receptors occupied is referred to as the drug's *intrinsic efficacy* (McGonigle and Molinoff 1989; Ruffalo 1982). Because the efficacy of a given drug is usually measured against that of a reference compound (such as the transmitter itself), with a correction for binding affinity, biological activity is measured as *relative intrinsic efficacy* (Mak et al. 1996).

Strong full agonists produce the maximum response of which the tissue is capable when occupying a small fraction of the total receptors. In contrast, weaker full agonists may need to occupy a substantial fraction of the total receptors to produce the maximum tissue response. Strong partial agonists may also produce the maximum tissue response but only when occupying a greater proportion of the receptors than do full agonists. Weak partial agonists may not be able to produce a maximum tissue response, even when occupying all receptors (Mak et al. 1996). Competitive antagonists have zero efficacy and, thereby, prevent or reverse the effects of agonists without themselves inducing the response. Like competitive antagonists, partial agonists can prevent or reverse the effects of high transmitter concentrations. In fact, partial agonists may substitute for a deficient transmitter in one part of the brain (e.g., frontal and prefrontal cortex) because they

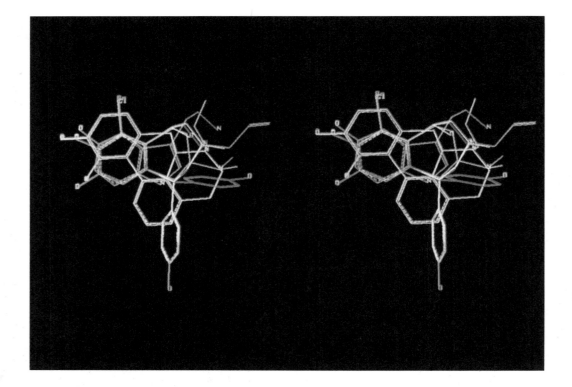

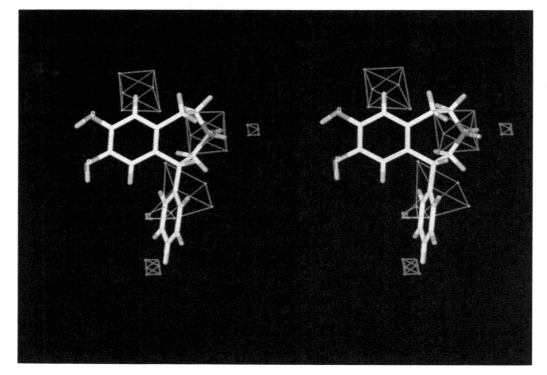

Figure 1–4.   Structure-activity relations for agonist affinity at recombinant D_{1A} dopamine receptors. (Additional details are provided in the original paper.)

A: Structures of drugs aligned in their probable binding conformations.

B: Contour map of electrostatic fields for binding.

Source.   Reprinted from Brusniak M-Y, Pearlman R, Neve KA, et al: "Comparative Molecular Field Analysis (CoMFA) and Agonist Affinity at Recombinant D1A vs. D2A Dopamine Receptors." *Journal of Medicinal Chemistry* 39:850–859, 1996. Copyright 1996, American Chemical Society. Used with permission.

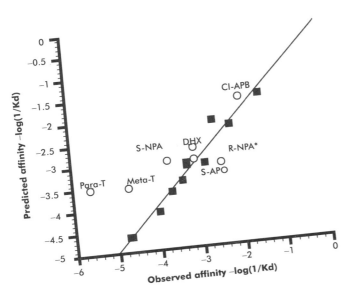

Figure 1–5. Scatterplot relating observed affinity for agonists at recombinant D_{1A} dopamine receptors to affinity predicted by Comparative Molecular Field Analysis (CoMFA). *Affinity measured in rat C6 glioma cells. NPA = N-n-propylnorapomorphine; DHX = dihydrexidine; APO = apomorphine; Cl-APB = SKF-82958. (Additional details are provided in original paper.)
Source. Redrawn from Brusniak M-Y, Pearlman R, Neve KA, et al: "Comparative Molecular Field Analysis (CoMFA) and Agonist Affinity at Recombinant D1A vs. D2A Dopamine Receptors." *Journal of Medicinal Chemistry* 39:850–859, 1996. Copyright 1996, American Chemical Society. Used with permission.

have efficacy at the receptor. In contrast, they can reduce net activity at the receptor when endogenous transmitter activity is high in another part of the brain (e.g., cingulate gyrus) by displacing the transmitter.

Such "biological buffering" has been shown at the level of second-messenger functions of recombinant receptors in intact cells (Avalos et al. 1997). It provides a possible mechanistic explanation for the potential of partial D_2 dopamine agonists to treat symptoms caused by both a dopamine excess and a dopamine deficiency in schizophrenic patients. These individuals are thought to express "positive" symptoms of delusions and hallucinations because of an excess of dopamine activity within subcortical portions of the limbic system and "negative" symptoms of flattened affect and social withdrawal because of deficient dopamine activity within cortical portions of the limbic system (Coward et al. 1989). Another interesting potential use of partial agonists is in the treatment of the "craving" for ethanol and psychostimulants (e.g., amphetamine and cocaine) in addicted persons (Wilcox and McMillen 1996).

The loss of control over drug-seeking behavior may reflect a sensitization process within the limbic system caused by chronically elevated release of dopamine within the medial forebrain bundle pathway. Full agonists may worsen the dependence, whereas partial agonists can mask the dependence, whereas partial agonists can mask the tonically elevated dopamine levels while maintaining enough residual "dopaminergic tone" (through partially mimicking the cellular response) to allow function within the pleasure pathway. One way to screen for possible anticraving effects of novel agents with animal models involves a conditioned place preference test (described in Meyer and Berger, Chapter 31, in this volume).

The pharmacological definition of efficacy differs from the clinical use of the term, which refers to the ability of a drug to elicit a therapeutic response. In this latter instance, both agonists and antagonists may have clinical efficacy, as in the use of dopamine agonists to treat Parkinson's disease symptoms and the use of dopamine antagonists to treat schizophrenia symptoms. The pharmacological efficacy of a drug also may be used to a limited degree for receptor classification, but drug affinity is a more reliable measure for this purpose. The clinical efficacy of a drug depends on both pharmacological efficacy and affinity. Because drug efficacy depends on the ability of a drug to induce a conformational change in the receptor that it activates, leading to a cellular response, efficacy may depend on proteins other than the receptor (e.g., G proteins). Note that at least some of the potential therapeutic benefits of partial agonists may be associated with differential actions at pre- and postsynaptic receptors (see above).

Molecular Structure of Receptors

As indicated in the above section, "Classification of Receptors," until the mid-1980s, the only means to classify and identify receptors was pharmacological. In 1983, Noda and colleagues reported the initial determination of the primary amino acid sequence of a receptor subunit of the multiple subunit nicotinic acetylcholine receptor. Since then, the other subunits of this receptor have been identified, and their primary amino acid sequences have been reported (Changeux et al. 1992; Figure 1–6). Numerous other receptor proteins have been isolated and purified, and their DNA has been sequenced and their amino acid sequences deduced. This new information from biochemical and molecular biological analyses of receptor structure has led to new ways of thinking about receptor structure and classification. Several general patterns are now apparent from this type of analysis, which will influence the future pharmacological analysis of receptors. For example, in virtually every case in which subtypes of re-

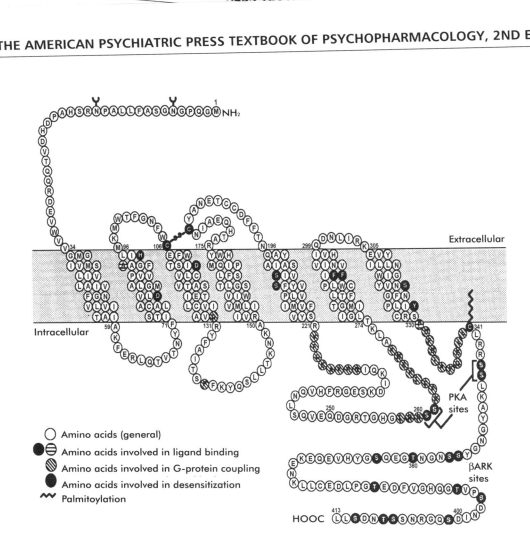

○ Amino acids (general)

●⊜ Amino acids involved in ligand binding

▨ Amino acids involved in G-protein coupling

● Amino acids involved in desensitization

〰 Palmitoylation

Figure 1–7. Amino acid sequence of the β_2-adrenergic receptor.

A: The deduced amino acid sequence of the human β_2-adrenergic receptor. Also shown are amino acid residues thought to be involved in binding of adrenergic ligands to the active site, in coupling with the stimulatory G protein, G_s, in desensitization after exposure to an agonist, and in anchoring the receptor to the membrane via palmitoylation. Regulatory regions of the receptor are also highlighted in the figure as consensus sequences that are phosphorylated by the enzymes protein kinase A (PKA) and β-adrenergic receptor kinase (βARK) during cyclic adenosine monophosphate (cAMP)–dependent and –independent desensitization, respectively.

Source. Reprinted from Schwinn DA, Caron MG, Lefkowitz RJ: "The Beta-Adrenergic Receptor as a Model for Molecular Structure-Function Relationships in G-Protein-Coupled Receptors," in *The Heart and Cardiovascular System,* 2nd Edition. Edited by Fozzard HA, et al. New York, Raven, 1992, pp. 1657–1684. Copyright 1992, Lippincott-Raven Publishers. Used with permission.

B: A model of the possible alignment of the seven transmembrane regions of the β_2-adrenergic receptor. This model is based on a similarity to bacteriorhodopsin in the purple membrane of *Holobacterium halobium,* measured by X-ray crystallography. Animation of Figure 1–7B may be viewed at the following URL: http://www.utexas.edu/pharmacy/divisions/pharmtox./faculty/wilcox.html.

Source. Adapted from Henderson R, Unwin PN: "Three Dimensional Model of Purple Membrane Obtained by Electron Microscopy." *Nature* 257:28–32, 1975.

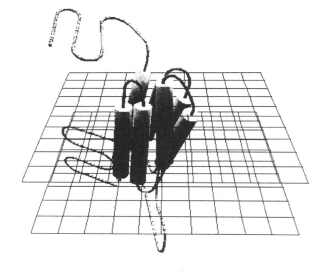

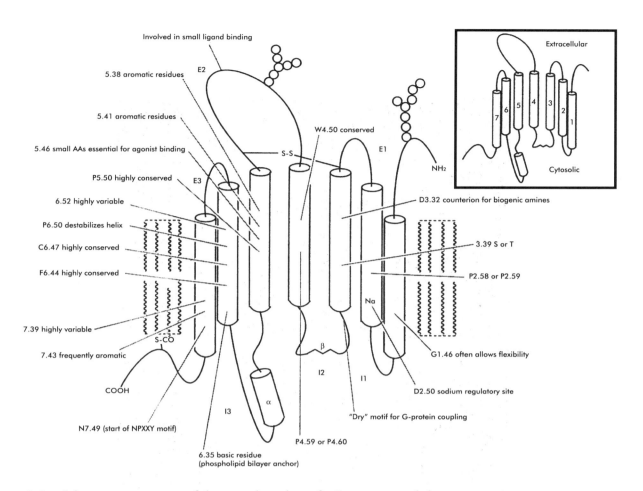

Figure 1–8. Schematic presentation of the general topology of a G-protein-coupled receptor.
Inset: Numbers of the seven transmembrane (TM) regions. AAs = amino acids; NT = N-terminal region (glycosylation has been shown to occur at the NT and/or E2); CT = C-terminal region; Ix = intracellular loop X; Ex = extracellular loop X; α = a proposed α-helical fragment of I3; β = a proposed β-pleated sheet substructure in I2; S-S = a possible cystine bond between TM3 and TM5; stacked circles = possible ribosylation sites; S-CO = a proposed acylation site in the CT. (Additional details are provided in the original paper.)
Source.   Reprinted from van Rhee AM, Jacobson KA: "Molecular Architecture of G Protein-Coupled Receptors." *Drug Development Research* 37:1–38, 1996. Copyright 1996, Wiley-Liss, Inc., a subsidiary of John Wiley & Sons, Inc. Used with permission.

proof that G-protein-linked receptors conform to this model awaits the crystallization of the receptor proteins and analysis by X-ray crystallography. However, this evidence has been obtained for a closely related protein, bacteriorhodopsin, from the purple membrane of *Holobacterium halobium*, where it acts as a proton pump (Figure 1–7; Probst et al. 1992; Smith 1989). This model G-protein-linked receptor is a single polypeptide containing seven transmembrane domains that consist of stretches of hydrophobic amino acids arranged in α-helical structures. The α helices are arranged with the N-terminal extending into the extracellular fluid and the C-terminal extending into the cytoplasm of the neuron. Knowledge of the amino acid sequences of many G-protein-linked receptors has al-

lowed the methods of site-directed mutagenesis and construction of chimeric proteins to be applied to their study (see Konradi et al., Chapter 2, in this volume). This study has led to a further increase in the understanding of the functions of specific portions of these proteins.

The *site-directed mutagenesis* method allows the deletion, insertion, or alteration of one or more amino acids within particular domains of the protein (Cox et al. 1992; Mansour et al. 1992; Neve et al. 1991). The *chimeric receptor* method involves combining large portions of one receptor with a hypothesized function (e.g., ligand binding) and a portion of another receptor potentially associated with another function (e.g., G-protein coupling; Kozell et al. 1992). Expression of the mutated receptors, measurement of their ligand-binding characteristics, and coupling to signal transduction molecules and effectors have helped to identify sites on the proteins that play important functional roles. This knowledge, coupled with the information on the structure of bacteriorhodopsin, has led to the development of several elegant models for such receptors (Teeter et al. 1994). As indicated in Figure 1–9, the ligand-binding site is thought to lie within a pocket formed by the

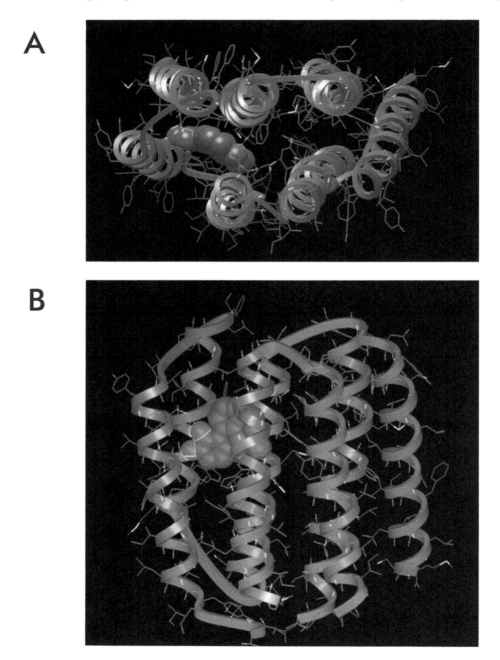

Figure 1–9. Docking of the dopamine agonist apomorphine to the D_{2A} dopamine receptor. In both panels, the transmembrane regions of the receptor are shown by solid ribbons, and the drug is shown in a space-filling representation. (Additional details are provided in the original paper.)

A: View looking down the transmembrane regions from the extracellular space.

B: Side view in the plane of the transmembrane regions from within the membrane.

Source.   Reprinted from Teeter MM, Froimowitz M, Stec B, et al: "Homology Modeling of the Dopamine D_2 Receptor and Its Testing by Docking of Agonists and Tricyclic Antagonists." *Journal of Medicinal Chemistry* 37:2874–2888, 1994. Copyright 1994, American Chemical Society. Used with permission.

seven transmembrane domains (Probst et al. 1992; Teeter et al. 1994; van Rhee and Jacobson 1996). Interaction of the receptor with the G protein depends, in part, on a chain of amino acids that compose part of the third cytoplasmic loop between the fifth and sixth transmembrane domain and, in some instances, several amino acids in the C-terminal region (Probst et al. 1992). Many of these details are summarized in Figure 1–7A; further discussion of these details may be found in the figure caption.

Changes in receptor activation, caused by blockade by competitive antagonists, may also induce changes in gene expression. For example, Chapter 2 provides a discussion of the effects on gene expression of blockade of brain dopamine receptors by antipsychotic drugs.

Differences in the structural features among receptor subtypes discussed earlier in this chapter may be important functionally and behaviorally. The long and short forms of the D_{2A} dopamine receptor differ by only 29 amino acids within the third cytoplasmic loop as a result of alternative messenger RNA (mRNA) splicing (Chio et al. 1990). As a result, the long D_{2A} receptor produces almost double the inhibition of cyclic adenosine monophosphate (cAMP) production stimulated by calcitonin gene–related peptide than that observed with the short D_{2A} receptor (Hayes et al. 1992). Furthermore, Van Tol et al. (1992) reported that a 48-base pair sequence in the third loop of the D_4 dopamine receptor exists in at least three polymorphic variants: two repeats, four repeats, or seven repeats are the most common. The receptor forms with these various repeats differ from one another with respect to their ability to bind classical (spiperone) and atypical (clozapine) antipsychotic drugs (Seeman 1995).

Other superfamilies.   We briefly described some of the structural and functional characteristics of the two major superfamilies of receptors that are targets for traditional psychotherapeutic agents. However, other receptor superfamilies may become important targets as new knowledge of their roles in neuronal function is forthcoming. For example, hormones that act as general homeostatic and metabolic regulators throughout the body may have unique roles to play in control of neuronal excitability. Hormone receptors tend to be intracellular (although the melatonin-1A receptor is extracellular) but generally act through molecular recognition and separate signal transduction mechanisms that involve changes in gene expression (McEwen et al. 1986). In addition, growth factors not only may be important in development of the brain but also may play a role in the maintenance of synaptic connections throughout adult life. Receptors for several growth factors have been cloned. Their sequence analysis has revealed structural similarities, such as the presence of a tyrosine kinase motif (i.e., these receptors have the ability to phosphorylate other proteins, including themselves) (Aaronson 1991).

To date, 7 distinct classes of serotonin receptors have been cloned, consisting of at least 13 distinct subtypes. The 5-HT_3 receptor is a ligand-gated ion channel, whereas all the others are G-protein-linked receptors. Initially, investigators thought that the major G-protein-linked signal transduction mechanisms for 5-HT involved either stimulation of phospholipase C activity (5-HT_2 subfamily) or inhibition of adenylate cyclase (5-HT_1 subfamily). However, many of the most recently discovered receptors (5-HT_4, 5-HT_6, and 5-HT_7) are positively coupled to adenylate cyclase (Watson and Girdlestone 1995). (The effector actions associated with serotonin receptor stimulation are discussed in Weiss and Kilts, Chapter 5, in this volume.)

As additional sequences for receptors become available, it seems clear that new classes of receptors will be recognized. For example, receptors for immunomodulators such as interleukins have been cloned and found to have unique structural motifs that can be combined in various ways. Many of these mediators and their receptors are also found in the brain and are potential targets for therapeutic intervention. In some cases, the receptor molecule has been identified and sequenced, but sequences that code for sites that couple to known signal transduction mechanisms have not been identified. This suggests that additional transduction mechanisms are yet to be detected.

SIGNAL TRANSDUCTION

Cellular information processing begins at the most basic level with a signal transduction mechanism. Signals are constantly being initiated, transduced, and integrated throughout every cell in the body. In the central nervous system, information processing and integration are clearly major functions. Therefore, understanding how signals are carried through a cell membrane is of fundamental importance. In the neuron, signals consist of changes in voltage across a membrane or changes in concentration of specific molecules or ions. We focus on biochemical signal transduction systems that convert an extracellular primary signal into an intracellular second messenger. (In Chapter 4 in this volume, Grace and Bunney consider more fully the electrophysiology of neurons.)

Ion-Based Signaling

The excitable nature of neurons is a result of the formation of ionic gradients from outside compared with inside the cell (Kandel et al. 1991; Kuffler et al. 1984). These gradients are initiated and maintained by the energy-dependent ion pumps located in the plasma membrane (e.g., sodium concentration is higher outside the cell, whereas potassium concentration is higher inside the cell). Once the ionic gradient forms, the difference in ion concentration across the membrane, in conjunction with the selective permeability of the membrane to certain ions, maintains the resting membrane potential of the neuron. Under resting conditions, these properties of the neuron create a measurable voltage across the membrane, and the neuron is polarized. A polarized neuron can be excited by an appropriate stimulus. Excitation is often the result of the change in permeability of the plasma membrane toward ions such as sodium, potassium, chloride, and calcium. These permeability changes are often sudden and result from the opening of ion channels embedded in the neuron's plasma membrane.

A sudden change in the concentration of an ion across the membrane alters the membrane potential, and the neuron may become depolarized or hyperpolarized. Ligand-gated ion channels are a common signal transduction mechanism for altering neuronal excitability as a part of normal synaptic transmission. In this case, the primary signal is the concentration of neurotransmitter stimulating the receptor on the cell surface. The transduction mechanism involves a single molecule—the ligand-gated ion channel. The second messenger for a ligand-gated ion channel is the ion that passes into the cell. The nicotinic cholinergic receptor discussed earlier in this chapter is an example of this type of transduction mechanism. Ultimately, the increase in sodium and calcium within the neuron causes depolarization of the neuron, which may cause the cell to fire an action potential.

G-Protein-Linked Signaling

In contrast to the change in intracellular ion concentration mediated by ligand-gated ion channels, specific molecules play a second-messenger role inside cells. These molecules are generally formed through the action of an effector enzyme controlled by receptor activation. In contrast to standard enzyme catalytic mechanisms, one advantage of the G-protein-linked pathways is the potential for amplification of the transmitter signal at several steps. In addition, this pathway is a point at which neurotransmitter signals can be integrated because different transmitters can activate or inhibit the same enzyme. The best-known

second-messenger molecules are probably cAMP, inositol triphosphate (IP_3), and diacylglycerol (DAG), although many others have been proposed, such as metabolites of arachidonic acid and, more recently, nitric oxide. Nitric oxide, synthesized by nitric oxide synthase, is an unusual neuromodulator in many ways. It is not stored inside presynaptic vesicles prior to release. Nitric oxide has no conventional receptors and no neuronal uptake system. Additionally, nitric oxide is lipid soluble and therefore diffuses freely to an effective distance of approximately 1 mm from its release sites to affect distant neurons. Nitric oxide's major actions include modulation of guanylate cyclase activity and alteration of calcium flux through N-methyl-D-aspartate (NMDA) channels (Marletta 1994; Nathan and Xie 1994; Schmidt and Walter 1994; Schuman and Madison 1994).

We discuss the actions of second messengers in more detail in the next section. In this chapter, the phrase *second messenger* is used loosely to refer to a signaling molecule or system that is downstream from the receptor. We discuss not only classic second messengers, including cAMP and other small intracellular signaling molecules, but also third and fourth messengers. It is now clear that, among the many diverse receptors that use second messengers as part of the signal transduction mechanism, the actual transduction process involves a set of transducing proteins called G proteins (Lamb and Pugh 1992; Spiegel 1992). Most of the known transmitters and known receptors appear to produce their effects inside the cell through the mediation of G proteins. Within this type of transduction system, the G protein itself is a molecular switch-timer, which when turned on alters cellular functions in a specific way until its timer runs out and it turns itself off. The various G proteins show preferential interactions with certain receptors, maintaining the specificity of the signal (Senogles et al. 1990). Molecular biological analysis of these and related proteins indicates that the family of G proteins involved in signal transduction is part of a larger superfamily of enzymes that contain guanosine triphosphate (GTP)ase activity (the ability to hydrolyze GTP; Figure 1–10; Bourne et al. 1991; Gilman 1987). Figure 1–10 highlights some of the features of a model GTPase (the proto-oncogene *Ras;* see Chapter 2 for a discussion of oncogenes), which are involved in its functions, including the extent to which the conformation of the protein can be altered during the exchange of GTP for guanosine diphosphate (GDP) on its binding site. From detailed studies of the coupling of receptors to effectors such as adenylate cyclase and phospholipase C, a general mechanism has emerged and may be applicable to the formation of other second-messenger molecules. Recently, X-ray crystallographic analyses have

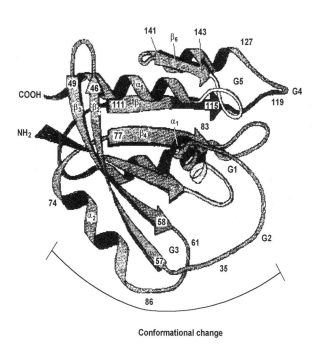

Conformational change

Figure 1–10.   Model of a guanine nucleotide-binding signal-transducing protein (G protein). Shown is a schematic version of the initial 166 amino acid residues of the proto-oncogene (p21^{ras}), a paradigm of the guanosine triphosphate (GTP)ase family of enzymes of which G proteins are a part. Overall, the core of the protein consists of six β sheets, which are connected to one another by α helices and hydrophilic loops. Five regions of the protein, encoded G1–G5, are critical in the reactions of this protein. The nucleotide exchange reaction, in which guanosine diphosphate (GDP) is exchanged for GTP as a result of transmitter binding to a receptor on the cell surface, the conformational resulting change in the G protein, and the hydrolysis of GTP that inactivates the G protein are all associated with various combinations of the G1–G5 regions. Also shown in the figure is the approximate magnitude of the conformational change in the protein that occurs with nucleotide exchange.
Source.   Reprinted from Bourne HR, Sanders DA, McCormick F: "The GTPase Superfamily: Conserved Structure and Molecular Mechanism." *Nature* 349:117–127, 1991. Copyright 1991, Macmillan Magazines Limited. Used with permission.

been done for two important G proteins—transducin (G$_t$), the G protein that mediates the signal due to photons interacting with rhodopsin in retinal rod photoreceptors, and guanine nucleotide inhibitory binding protein (G$_i$), which plays an important role in mediating the functions of dopamine receptors, implicated in psychiatric conditions (Manji 1992). Furthermore, the psychiatric implications of altered G-protein regulation are now becoming evident

(Manji 1992; Okada et al. 1991). In particular, how the G protein is activated by guanine nucleotides has now been resolved with clear evidence for the changes that occur in various portions of the molecule. Figure 1–11 shows a ribbon and coil scheme diagram of the α subunit of the inhibitory G protein, G$_{i1}$, and highlights the helical domain that is not present in the Ras protein.

Adenylate Cyclase

Hormone-sensitive adenylate cyclase activity has been shown to require just three proteins: the receptor, the heterotrimeric (three-part) G protein, and the catalytic unit of the adenylate cyclase enzyme itself. Thus, these three proteins constitute a basic pathway for transmitter stimulation of cAMP synthesis (Figure 1–12; Bates et al. 1991; Strulovici et al. 1984). Activation or inhibition of the adenylate cyclase enzyme (effector) by an agonist depends on the formation of a three-component intermediate complex of agonist, receptor, and G protein. The hypothesis of a ternary complex of agonist, receptor, and G protein as a regulator of second-messenger function and high-affinity agonist binding to the receptor was first suggested for the hepatic glucagon receptor and, subsequently, for the β-adrenergic receptors. More generally, all hormones and neurotransmitters that act at the cell surface to stimulate or inhibit adenylate cyclase appear to function via this ternary complex (Iyengar and Birnbaumer 1987). A similar approach to the pituitary D$_2$ receptor and the striatal D$_1$ and D$_2$ receptors supports the ternary complex hypothesis for these systems. Furthermore, it is now well established that in striatum, activation of D$_1$ receptors stimulates the cyclase, whereas D$_2$ receptor activation inhibits it (Hess and Creese 1987). From this viewpoint, the major role of a receptor is to modulate G-protein activation through agonist binding.

At the molecular level, the best characterized of all ternary complex systems is the β$_2$-adrenergic receptor associated with adenylate cyclase via a stimulatory G protein (G$_s$) (Collins et al. 1991; Schwinn et al. 1992). Reconstitution studies of the β$_2$ receptor and G$_s$ have confirmed that agonist binding to the receptor is sensitive to guanine nucleotides. The low-affinity agonist-binding conformation of the receptor reflects the receptor dissociated from G$_s$ (resting state), whereas the high-affinity conformation reflects the receptor-G$_s$ complex (activated state; Coleman et al. 1994; Gilman 1987). The agonist-receptor-G$_s$ complex is considered to be a relatively stable intermediate. However, its half-life is short in the presence of physiological concentrations of GTP. In the β$_2$-adrenergic receptor system, agonist binding stimulates dissociation of GDP

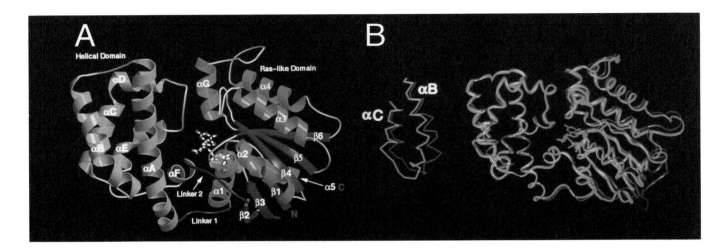

Figure 1–11. X-ray crystal structure of a G-protein subunit ($G_{i1-\alpha}$). (Additional details are provided in the original paper.)
A: Ribbon and coil schematic view of the $G_{i1-\alpha}$. α-Helices are shown as coiled ribbons, and β-pleated sheets are shown as arrows. The Ras-like domain is shown in the right-hand portion of *Panel A* and corresponds to the Ras protein shown in Figure 1–10. The Ras protein does not have a helical domain, whereas the $G_{i1-\alpha}$ helical domain is shown in the left-hand portion of *Panel A.*
B: Comparison of the structures of $G_{i1-\alpha}$ and $G_{t-\alpha}$ (α-transducin).
Source. Reprinted from Coleman DE, Berghuis AM, Lee E, et al: "Structures of Active Conformations of $G_{i\alpha1}$ and the Mechanism of GTP Hydrolysis." *Science* 265:1405-1412, 1994. Copyright 1994, American Association for the Advancement of Science. Used with permission.

from the G_s protein and stimulates the binding of GTP to G_s. A guanine nucleotide binding site has been described to function as if "closed" in the absence of agonist-receptor complex and "open" (allowing nucleotide exchange) in its presence (Gilman 1987), and this has now been directly confirmed with X-ray crystallographic methods (Coleman et al. 1994; see Figure 1–11). Thus, high-affinity agonist binding is GTP sensitive in this system. Binding of GTP causes dissociation of the ternary complex and of G_s into its α and βγ subunits, and the molecular switch is turned to the "on" position, which starts the molecular timer. Concomitantly, GTP binding also shifts the receptor from a high- to low-affinity agonist-binding conformation, thus resetting the system, to allow further agonist binding.

Once the α subunit of G_s is activated, it can then move laterally in the plane of the membrane until it interacts with adenylate cyclase. Adenylate cyclase is an integral membrane-bound protein with a channel- or transporter-like structure. The adenylate cyclase catalytic unit is activated by $G_{s\alpha}$–GTP (Krupinski 1992; Krupinski et al. 1989). The substrate for this reaction is adenosine triphosphate (ATP; in the presence of magnesium), which is normally present in sufficient concentrations through energy-producing reactions in the cell. Thus, the major process for production of cAMP is through the pathway of agonist-activated receptor through a G protein activated by the agonist-receptor complex to activated effector (adenylate cyclase).

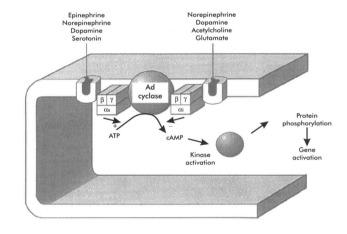

Figure 1–12. Adenylate (Ad)-cyclase-linked signal transduction. Agonists can stimulate or inhibit adenylate cyclase activity through separate receptors and G proteins. Activation of a receptor linked to a stimulatory G protein, G_s, increases the intracellular concentration of cyclic adenosine monophosphate (cAMP). Conversely, activation of a receptor linked to an inhibitory G protein, G_i, lowers the intracellular concentration of cAMP. ATP = adenosine triphosphate.

A receptor-activated inhibitory pathway also exists for control of cAMP levels. This pathway requires activation of a receptor by agonist binding, ternary complex formation, and involvement of a different G protein called G_i, which must be activated by nucleotide exchange by the agonist-bound receptor. The α_2-adrenergic, D_2 dopamine, and 5-HT$_{1A}$ serotonin receptors mediate this action. One aspect of the transduction mechanism may be more complex in this inhibitory pathway relative to that described above for stimulation of adenylate cyclase. As above, dissociation of G_i into $G_{i\alpha}$ and $G_{i\beta\gamma}$ subunits causes the accumulation of $G_{\beta\gamma}$ subunits. However, both G_ia and $G_{i\beta\gamma}$ subunits may play roles in the transduction process as follows. The $G_{i\alpha}$ plays its normal role to interact with the catalytic subunit of adenylate cyclase; however, binding of $G_{i\alpha}$ to the enzyme inactivates it, thereby inhibiting its ability to produce cAMP. In addition, the $\beta\gamma$ subunits also induce reassociation of the G_s (stimulatory) heterotrimer (α-β-γ), thereby preventing G_s from activating the adenylate cyclase. This is because $\beta\gamma$ subunits from one G protein appear able to substitute to some extent for $\beta\gamma$ subunits from another G protein (Spiegel et al. 1992). An important feature common to both stimulatory and inhibitory G-protein signaling is that after a time determined by the structure of the α subunit of the G protein, the molecular switch is turned off by hydrolysis of the bound GTP to GDP, which causes the G protein α subunits to reassociate with the $\beta\gamma$ subunits, thereby reversing the G-protein activation.

A general principle of signal transduction through "second messenger" (the quotation marks are meant to remind the reader that we are using the term loosely to refer to the portion of the signal transduction pathway downstream from the receptor and G protein) formation is the concept of *amplification* of the primary signal. Thus, the signal is not merely passed from the cell surface to the cell interior by the transduction process but also may grow in magnitude. Specifically, formation of one agonist-receptor complex may be sufficient to activate several G-protein molecules before the agonist dissociates from the receptor. Additionally, a single activated molecule of G protein may be sufficient to activate adenylate cyclase to produce many molecules of cAMP from ATP before the G protein is inactivated. Thus, a dramatic (pmoles of cAMP produced) change occurs in cellular function ultimately resulting from a modest (fmoles of agonist-receptor complex) binding of agonist to a small percentage (perhaps <5%) of the cell's receptors. In G-protein-linked signaling, amplification may occur at several levels (Alousi et al. 1991). Molecular recognition may be one source of amplification whereby the transmitter may activate several receptors before it diffuses away to its sites for uptake or catabolism. The activation of G protein via formation of the GTP-bound $G_{s\alpha}$ is another point at which amplification may occur. Also, a single $G_{s\alpha}$ may stimulate many effector

enzyme molecules before GTP hydrolysis renders the G-protein α subunit unable to do so. Finally, the activated adenylate cyclase may produce many molecules of cAMP before it returns to its resting state. In pharmacological terms, signal transduction activated by the drug-receptor interaction determines the ability of the drug to produce a response for a given receptor occupancy (the drug's efficacy).

To date, evidence suggests that dopaminergic, muscarinic, and some serotonergic receptor–G-protein–adenylate cyclase systems in brain behave similarly to the adenylate cyclase systems coupled to the β-adrenergic receptor (Savarese and Fraser 1992). Because many neurotransmitter-receptor systems use common signal transduction mechanisms, the transduction mechanism may not be a good target for therapeutic intervention in a dysfunctional brain. However, a newly recognized diversity in these signal transduction pathways appears to be the result of differences in the subtypes of G proteins that are required for stimulation by specific receptors and differential activation of second-messenger pathways by separate G proteins. Furthermore, it is now known that there is a complex regulation of receptors and effectors by a variety of molecules (including the $\beta\gamma$ subunits of G proteins) plus a localization of regulator and regulated proteins to the same part of the cell. Together, this suggests that there may be greater specificity to transduction than was first assumed. Additionally, the α subunit of the G protein is itself regulated, in part by the binding of receptor, $\beta\gamma$ subunits, magnesium ion, guanine nucleotide, and certain toxins to specific sites on its surface. These findings suggest that selectivity of psychotherapeutic drugs targeted toward signal transduction may be achieved some day. Evidence suggests that some psychiatric drugs such as lithium may target the transduction systems associated with G proteins (Atack et al. 1995; Avissar and Schreiber 1989). This finding is consonant with the potential changes in G proteins that may be associated with psychiatric disorders such as schizophrenia (Manji 1992; Okada et al. 1991).

Phospholipase C

Another major G-protein-linked signal transduction mechanism is the phosphoinositide (PI) hydrolysis pathway (Figure 1–13; Berridge 1989). Emerging evidence suggests that the general steps described above for the adenylate cyclase system also operate for the PI pathway. In other words, the transduction process is initiated when an agonist binds to and activates a receptor on the cell surface. The activated agonist-receptor complex forms a ternary complex with a G protein, which turns on the G-

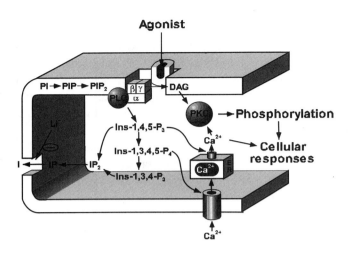

Figure 1–13. Phosphoinositide (PI)-linked signal transduction. An agonist binds to its receptor and initiates the G-protein-linked signal pathway. The effector enzyme is a PI-specific phospholipase C (PLC), which hydrolyzes membrane phosphatidylinositol-4,5-bisphosphate (PIP_2) into inositol-1,4,5-triphosphate ($Ins-1,4,5-P_3$) and diacylglycerol (DAG). $Ins-1,4,5-P_3$ then acts to release calcium (Ca^{2+}) from an endoplasmic reticulum–like store, and calcium can then activate a variety of calcium-dependent enzymes. DAG, which stays associated with the membrane, activates protein kinase C (PKC), which causes phosphorylation of specific proteins leading to cellular responses. $Ins-1,4,5-P_3$ can be phosphorylated to $Ins-1,3,4,5-P_4$, which has been proposed to control influx of extracellular calcium. A series of dephosphorylation reactions control the levels of inositol phosphates. The inositol monophosphatase is inhibited by therapeutic concentrations of lithium (Li^+) and can disrupt the normal function of the PI cycle.
Source. Redrawn from Berridge 1989.

protein switch through nucleotide exchange and initiates the intrinsic timer mechanism of the G protein. Hence, we describe only the major differences between this pathway and the adenylate cyclase system. Within the PI hydrolysis pathway, the receptor, G protein, and effector are required and may be sufficient for the process to operate. The effector enzyme is a PI-specific phospholipase C (Berridge 1989; Fisher et al. 1992).

It is now clear that several classes of G proteins serve as transducers for the PI system, and these are distinct from those that couple receptors to adenylate cyclase. For example, G proteins called G_q and G_{11} are active in coupling receptors to phospholipase C. The phospholipase C involved in the receptor-activated transduction pathway exists in several different isoforms that may play unique roles in specific pathways (Rhee 1991). This enzyme uses phosphatidylinositol-4,5-bisphosphate (PIP_2) as sub-

strate. PIP_2 is a phospholipid that makes up a small portion of the plasma membrane where it is produced from other phospholipids. Phospholipase C breaks down PIP_2 into two second messengers: DAG and IP_3. In this way, the PI pathway results in a bifurcating signaling system inside the cell (Fowler and Tiger 1991). As with the adenylate cyclase transduction pathway, the phospholipase C–mediated production of DAG and IP_3 is halted when the G-protein timer goes off, allowing GTP hydrolysis and a return of the system to its resting state. According to our loose use of the term second messengers, DAG and IP_3 qualify as second messengers because they are diffusible cytosolic substances that can ultimately modulate the activity of protein kinases (PKs).

Other Effectors

It is now clear that additional signal transduction systems are operative in the central nervous system and that the molecular diversity that occurs within a single pathway may soon be matched by various pathways. In most cases, the exact receptor-coupling mechanisms or roles that these novel pathways play in the control of neuronal function and ultimate behaviors are not known. For example, guanylate cyclase is an enzyme found in the brain in several different forms, some of which may be membrane bound and some of which appear to be cytoplasmic (Schulz et al. 1991). Stimulation of this enzyme, which results in the formation of cyclic guanosine monophosphate (GMP), may occur through direct activation of a receptor (membrane-bound form) or through intervening steps that may involve additional signaling molecules. Phospholipase A_2 is a well-established enzyme involved in signal transduction in lymphocytes, but it may also play a role in neuronal function. Receptor-activated phospholipase A_2 produces arachidonic acid, which can be metabolized to several potential intracellular-messenger molecules (Shimizu and Wolfe 1990; see section, "Arachidonic Acid Intracellular-Messenger Pathway," later in this chapter). (Arachidonic acid is included within the second-messenger category because of size and ability to activate PKs indirectly.)

Several growth factors that stimulate neuron growth and maintenance transduce their signals via tyrosine phosphorylation, which then participates in the activation of an isozyme (γ form) of PI-specific phospholipase C (Rhee 1991). The mitogen-activated protein kinase (MAPK) also may be activated by growth factors (see section, "General Aspects of Third Messengers," later in this chapter).

A recent addition to the growing list of signal transduction systems is the pathway leading to the novel signaling molecule nitric oxide. Studies have shown that pathways that lead to an increase in intracellular calcium cause activation of nitric oxide synthase, which leads to nitric oxide production. Nitric oxide then stimulates guanylate cyclase activity, ultimately leading to increased levels of cyclic GMP. This pathway may play a role in strengthening certain synapses in an activity-dependent manner, as in learning (Snyder 1992). Nitric oxide would then qualify as a second messenger that indirectly leads to PK activation through cyclic GMP.

INTRACELLULAR MESSENGERS

In this section, we focus on two types of intracellular messengers—the prototype cAMP and three "second messengers" derived from membrane phospholipids: IP_3, DAG, and arachidonic acid metabolites. First, we discuss criteria for considering a substance a second messenger and then discuss the prototype. We describe each second-messenger system from the perspective of a few basic organizing principles to allow comparison among them and other such systems that will be encountered by the reader. We also discuss briefly the third- and fourth-messenger systems whose actions are modulated by the second messengers.

Criteria for Establishing Intracellular-Messenger Function

1. *Specific enzymes for the production of the substance* (Northup 1989): for example, cytosolic adenylate cyclase converts ATP to cAMP in the presence of a magnesium ion.
2. *A specific removal pathway:* cAMP breakdown is catalyzed by a specific cyclic nucleotide phosphodiesterase with high activity in the nervous system (Conti et al. 1992).

   Together, these two criteria allow a cellular substance to be present in controlled amounts in response to specific signals. This provides an optimum set of conditions for the intracellular messenger to regulate cellular enzymatic functions and for altering gene expression (by acting on a cAMP response element within the DNA of certain genes).
3. *Transmitter responsiveness:* for instance, stimulation of a receptor (such as D_1 dopamine) by the transmitter should yield a predictable change in cellular content of the substance (in this example, cAMP).
4. *Mimicry-potentiation:* basically, application of analogues of the substance (e.g., cAMP analogues that are resistant to hydrolysis, such as dibutyryl-cAMP or 8-bromo-cAMP) should yield cellular actions that mimic those of the transmitter (stimulation of cAMP-dependent PK activity; see next section). Similarly, inhibitors of breakdown of the substance (by using phosphodiesterase inhibitors such as theophylline or caffeine) should potentiate the cellular actions of the transmitter.
5. *Existence of a specific output,* such as cAMP-dependent PK (an important enzyme that is activated by binding of cAMP, thereby allowing it to add phosphate groups to cellular proteins): in this context, it is interesting that blockade of dopamine receptors with antipsychotic drugs also changes cAMP levels (Kaneko et al. 1992).

Adenylate Cyclase and Protein Kinase Systems

The cAMP pathway is the prototype of an intracellular signaling system. A soluble substance (cAMP) exerts its primary actions within the cytosol on a tetrameric PK enzyme, cAMP-dependent PK (Gao and Gilman 1991). Although cAMP may be considered a second messenger, the PK system acts as a third-messenger system in the cytosol. After cAMP is produced by adenylate cyclase, four cAMP molecules bind to the two regulatory subunits of the cAMP-dependent PK to initiate one of the major actions of the second messenger. The cAMP binding causes the two catalytic subunits of the protein kinase A (PKA) holoenzyme to be freed to phosphorylate various target proteins. Among the target proteins for PKA action is the cell surface receptor itself (Hausdorff et al. 1990; Sibley and Lefkowitz 1988). Stimulation of a β-adrenergic receptor by an agonist activates both a productive pathway (which causes cAMP to be formed) and a regulatory pathway (which changes the ease with which the receptor can be activated by subsequent agonist binding) inside the cell. The productive pathway activates adenylate cyclase, which stimulates cAMP production. The regulatory pathway (or pathways) includes the feedback influences that activation of the cAMP-dependent PK can have on the β-adrenergic receptor by virtue of phosphorylating it and, thus, changing its ability to be activated by the agonist. As with the phospholipase C pathway (see section, "Inositol Lipid-Based Second and Third Messengers," later in this chapter), multiple isoforms (at least eight) of adenylate cyclase exist, leading to myriad possible distributions of receptor, G protein, and enzyme. Clear differences in regulation of several recombinant receptors have been linked to differences in the expression of various adenylate cyclase isoforms. Together, this view of the β-adrenergic receptor–G protein–adenylate cyclase–PKA system provides a further example of the homeostatic consequences of activation of an intracellular-messenger pathway.

Several isoforms of the regulatory PKA subunits have in common three functional domains: two cAMP binding sites per subunit near the C-terminal region, one portion of the N-terminal region to which the other regulatory subunit binds, and another portion of the N-terminal region that normally inhibits the attached catalytic subunit (S. Taylor et al. 1990). Each of the catalytic subunits contains an ATP binding site and a substrate (target) protein-binding site. The cellular target of cAMP is PKA. The activity of cellular protein targets of PKA is altered (either enhanced or reduced) by PKA-mediated phosphorylation. This arrangement potentially allows the catalytic subunit of PKA to interact with specific amino acid sequences in several proteins. Just as the receptor can amplify the agonist signal by interacting with several of the more numerous G-protein molecules within the membrane, further signal amplification occurs inside the cell as each catalytic subunit of the PKA transfers the γ-phosphoryl group of ATP to the hydroxyl groups of specific serine and threonine residues of many target protein molecules.

cAMP levels are regulated through the action of two basic kinds of enzymes. Several phosphodiesterases convert active cAMP to the inactive AMP to terminate the second-messenger action. Various protein phosphatases remove phosphate groups from the target proteins (dephosphorylate) to terminate the cellular responses that are mediated by proteins in their phosphorylated states. Thus, kinases and phosphatases act in concert to dynamically regulate the phosphorylation state of cellular proteins. Phosphorylation may cause some proteins to be activated but others (such as β_2-adrenergic receptors) to be less active. Also, an autophosphorylation reaction, found with many PKs, causes at least some isoforms of the regulatory domain of the PKA molecule to be phosphorylated by its own catalytic subunits. This autophosphorylation causes a slower rate of interaction between regulatory and catalytic subunits than would otherwise occur (Walaas and Greengard 1991).

It is significant that multiple transmitters produce at least some of their cellular actions through increasing or decreasing cAMP levels inside the cell. This action illustrates the principle of *convergent processing* of information in the nervous system (refer back to Figure 1–1). Furthermore, as discussed earlier in this chapter, multiple steps are involved in the cAMP-PKA intracellular-messenger

pathway, including formation of a bimolecular complex of agonist and receptor, formation of a ternary complex, activation of a G protein, dissociation of the ternary complex and G-protein heterotrimer, activation of the catalytic unit of the cyclase enzyme, and activation of PKA. Because of the several chemical reactions involved in cAMP production and its subsequent effects on PKA, a significantly greater time is required for changes in cAMP levels than for changes in conductances of an ion channel intrinsic to the nicotinic cholinergic receptor. However, the cellular consequences of adenylate cyclase activation or inhibition often outlast those associated with altered ion fluxes through membrane channels. Together, these observations illustrate the principle of *latency/duration of action* (i.e., whereby second-messenger activity determines the temporal nature of the target cellular response).

cAMP formation is not an end point for the cell but an intermediate reaction. The cellular response to a change in second-messenger level is a change in activity of other cellular proteins (often through changes in their phosphorylation state mediated by PK "third" messengers; Garattini 1992). As discussed earlier in this section, increases in cAMP accumulation inside the cell activate the cAMP-dependent PK by releasing its regulatory subunits from the catalytic subunits. In fact, most of the known actions of cAMP result from activation of PKs, illustrating the principle of *PK output*.

Also, *regulatory pathway participation* is a principle that refers to the observation that second-messenger pathways consist of two kinds of loops: a productive pathway and one or more regulatory pathways. As described above for cAMP, activation of the productive loop in the β-adrenergic receptor system increases cAMP levels inside the cell. However, the increases in cAMP activate PKA, which phosphorylates the receptor and, thereby, limits its ability to respond to further agonist stimulation. Stimulation of PKA by cAMP causes phosphorylation of residues within the cytoplasmic portion of the β-adrenergic receptor and makes it less able to couple to the G_s transducer. The receptor becomes less able to respond to agonist binding (desensitization). Another consequence of agonist stimulation of the β_2 receptor that is not cAMP dependent but dependent on previous agonist occupancy is activation of the β-adrenergic receptor kinase. This novel type of enzyme phosphorylates residues on the receptor different from those phosphorylated by PKA and induces modulation of the receptor by another protein, β-arrestin (Arriza et al. 1992; Attramadal et al. 1992; Benovic et al. 1986; Lohse et al. 1990). Binding of β-arrestin to the receptor contributes to its desensitization. This example demonstrates one means by which activation of a signal transduction pathway not only produces a cellular response (increased cAMP) but also reduces the response to further activation (desensitization; Sibley and Lefkowitz 1985, 1988).

Inositol Lipid-Based Second and Third Messengers

As discussed in the earlier section, "Phospholipase C," the hydrolysis of PIP_2 forms both a membrane-associated DAG and an IP_3 second messenger (Berridge 1989). DAG is the primary lipid regulator of a phospholipid-dependent enzyme, protein kinase C (PKC), which it activates. As we observed above with the cAMP-PKA system, the DAG-PKC system involves activation of a third-messenger system (i.e., PKC) by a second messenger (i.e., DAG). PKC actually is an enzyme family that phosphorylates serine and threonine residues in a variety of target protein substrates, both membranous and cytosolic (Kikkawa et al. 1989). Thus, like all PK enzymes, PKC adds phosphate groups to target proteins at specific sites. Of the 10 known isozymes of PKC, the 4 major forms contain lipid- and calcium-binding sites within the N-terminal region, whereas the catalytic domain of the molecule resides in the C-terminal region. The 4 so-called minor forms of the enzyme are structurally similar but lack the calcium-binding site. In the presence of ATP, the activated PKC phosphorylates substrate proteins, producing phosphoproteins with altered activity compared with that of the unphosphorylated state. To be activated by DAG, PKC must shift from a cytosolic location to a membrane position because phospholipid is required for the activation process. This shift of PKC from the cytosol to the membrane is one of many examples of intracellular protein trafficking, which appears to play a major role in the activation and deactivation of protein functions.

IP_3 is a soluble product of PIP_2 cleavage and is a messenger with a short half-life (<10 seconds; however, its duration of action is longer than that of many ion channels). IP_3 acts by binding to a specific IP_3 receptor within membrane organelles such as endoplasmic or sarcoplasmic reticulum. The IP_3 receptor protein contains both an IP_3 binding site and a calcium channel. These receptors are 260 kDa proteins consisting of four similar subunits (a homotetramer), each with six transmembrane regions. The N- and C-terminals are both located within the cytoplasm. IP_3 binds to a region near the N-terminal (Mikoshiba 1993). Increased IP_3 levels release calcium from intracellular stores. The released calcium subsequently interacts with various cellular components such as calmodulin. This calcium-binding protein then can acti-

vate calcium- and calmodulin-dependent PKs to phosphorylate target proteins (Miller 1991). Calcium may also facilitate its own release from ryanodine receptor-gated calcium pools.

Central to the regulatory roles of IP_3 and DAG is their recycling, which is controlled by specific enzymes (Berridge 1989). DAG may be phosphorylated to phosphatidic acid, which combines with cytidine triphosphate to form cytidine diphosphate–DAG. The cytidine diphosphate–DAG then reacts with inositol to regenerate PIs. The phosphatidylinositol can then be phosphorylated to PIP_2. An alternative degradative pathway for DAG involves its hydrolysis to glycerol and constituent fatty acids. One of these is often arachidonic acid, which is itself a precursor to another important lipid-derived second messenger (see next section). IP_3 breakdown is catalyzed by the sequential action of phosphatases (enzymes that remove phosphate groups). The last of the dephosphorylations, catalyzed by an inositol monophosphatase, is inhibited by millimolar lithium concentrations (Berridge 1989). This action of lithium disrupts the entire cascade of reactions because the production of DAG and IP_3 is dependent on the regeneration of PIP_2. Because inositol cannot cross the blood-brain barrier, only locally available inositol can be used for PIP_2 production. Investigators have speculated that at least a part of the antimanic action of lithium ion may be mediated by its effects on the regeneration of inositol phospholipids (Atack et al. 1995; Berridge 1989). In Chapter 20 in this volume, Lenox and Manji provide a thorough discussion of the many actions of lithium cation on neurotransmission.

The principle of convergent processing is shown for DAG and IP_3 because many transmitters act through the phospholipase C pathway. The latency and duration of action of DAG and IP_3 are also greater than those typically observed for ionic conductance changes. PK output is obvious for DAG because of its direct action on PKC; that for IP_3 is less direct, but also significant, because of the activation of calcium-calmodulin-dependent PKs, ultimately by IP_3. Finally, regulatory pathway participation is shown for both of the lipid-derived second messengers. These products of phospholipid hydrolysis can feed back to regulate both their own production and that of other cytosolic messengers, including cAMP. For example, haloperidol, a prototypic antipsychotic drug, appears to alter both cAMP and IP_3 accumulation (Kaneko et al. 1992). This suggests interactions between adenylate cyclase and phospholipase C pathways in brain (Figure 1–1). Convergent processing is discussed further later in this chapter (see section, "Gene Regulation and Fourth-Messenger Systems—Phospho-CREB").

Arachidonic Acid Intracellular-Messenger Pathway

Arachidonic acid is a fatty acid that is typically found in the ester form at position 2 in brain phospholipid molecules. Thus, stimulation of receptors that activate the enzyme phospholipase A_2 releases arachidonic acid from the membrane, where it is quickly converted to several active eicosanoid metabolites. The term *eicosanoid* refers to one of a class of compounds, including the prostaglandins, thromboxanes, and leukotrienes, all of which are derived from arachidonic acid (also called eicosatetraenoic acid; Figure 1–14). Cyclooxygenase metabolism of arachidonic acid produces the prostaglandins and thromboxanes, whereas the actions of several lipoxygenases on arachidonic acid yield the leukotrienes and several other metabolites (Shimizu and Wolfe 1990). Thus, their relative place in signal transduction suggests that these arachidonic acid derivatives function in a manner similar to that of cAMP, DAG, and IP_3 as second messengers. A further significant aspect of arachidonic acid pathway function is that each of the active metabolic products must be created on demand to function both inside and outside the target cells, because these substances are not stored. It is interesting that levels of prostaglandins and thromboxanes are increased during electroconvulsive shock, acute cerebral ischemia, and trauma, whereas levels of a lipoxygenase product (hydroperoxyeicosatrienoic acid; HPETE) are elevated after depolarization of brain slices with potassium, glutamate, or NMDA (Schwartz and Kandel 1991). Because drugs acting on the arachidonic acid metabolite systems of brain are not currently used in psychiatry, they are not discussed in detail. However, arachidonic acid metabolites do appear to fulfill the criteria required for second messengers, and their actions also appear consonant with the principles of convergent processing, latency/duration of action, and regulatory pathway participation.

General Aspects of Third Messengers

One of the themes of modern molecular neuroscience is that the functional activity of many cellular proteins depends on their state of phosphorylation. As noted earlier in this chapter, kinases phosphorylate substrate proteins, often with a considerable degree of selectivity, whereas phosphatases dephosphorylate such proteins. Thus, the activity of the protein reflects some weighted sum of the kinases and phosphatases that act on it. Three important observations are as follows:

1. Phosphorylation can either increase or decrease substrate protein functional activity.

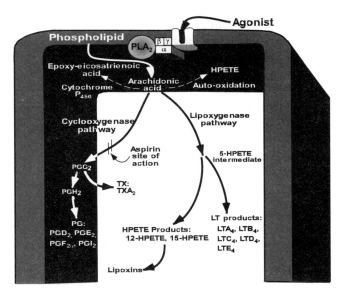

Figure 1-14.   Signal transduction linked to arachidonic acid (AA). An agonist binds to a cell-surface receptor and activates a G protein, in a manner similar to that shown for the adenylate cyclase and phosphoinositide systems in other figures. The effector enzyme is phospholipase A_2, which converts membrane phospholipids to AA. The AA is then rapidly converted to several active metabolites, including prostaglandins (PG), thromboxanes (TX), leukotrienes (LT), hydroperoxy acid products (e.g., hydroperoxyeicosatrienoic acid, HPETE), and lipoxins. Two major pathways are shown, reflecting the actions of cyclooxygenase and lipoxygenase. Information in the figure is not intended to be complete but to illustrate some of the major known active products resulting from the actions of cyclooxygenase and lipoxygenase on AA to produce second messengers on demand. Note the important roles of PGG_2 and PGH_2 as intermediates in the cyclooxygenase pathway and of 5-HPETE in the lipoxygenase pathway. Note also that aspirin acts to inhibit the cyclooxygenase pathway. PLA_2 = phospholipase A_2.

2. Many, if not most, kinases and phosphatases are cytoplasmic.
3. The activity of most isoforms of these enzymes depends on second messengers such as cAMP and calcium.

Together, these results imply that it would be reasonable to call kinases and phosphatases *third messengers*. Usually, however, the term refers to the kinase systems.

Kinases may be divided into three main classes, depending on which amino acid residues they can phosphorylate on substrate proteins: 1) serine/threonine kinases, 2) tyrosine kinases, and 3) "dual-specificity" kinases, which phosphorylate serine, threonine, or tyrosine residues. Serine/threonine kinases include cAMP-activated PKA, cyclic GMP–activated protein kinase G (PKG), calcium-calmodulin-dependent kinase, and DAG-activated PKC. Tyrosine kinases may be part of growth factor receptors (receptor tyrosine kinases) or cytosolic. A well-known example of a dual-specificity kinase is MAPK. Multiple isoforms of most of these kinases have been characterized.

The PKA serine/threonine kinases were discussed earlier in this chapter (see section, "Adenylate Cyclase and Protein Kinase Systems") as examples of the general class of kinase enzymes. Here, we point out that growth factors such as insulin (Lazar et al. 1995) can activate tyrosine kinases, which can activate elements of an MAPK cascade in which MAPK kinase kinase (also known as Raf) can phosphorylate MAPK kinase (also known as MEK), which can phosphorylate MAPK. The final targets of MAPK include transcription factors (fourth messengers; see next section) and phospholipase A_2. It is already apparent that tyrosine kinases have a role in long time course or persistent central nervous system–mediated phenomena such as long-term potentiation (O'Dell et al. 1991) and circadian rhythmicity (Roberts et al. 1992).

Gene Regulation and Fourth-Messenger Systems—Phospho-CREB

Transmitters are the cell's first messengers; small intracellular molecules, including cAMP and DAG, are among the cell's second messengers; and various PKs form a third-messenger system. So-called fourth messengers constitute the next level of signal transduction in the cell (Curran et al. 1988). These fourth messengers are transcription factors that can be translocated into the nucleus, where they bind to DNA at sites that can cause downstream transcription of target genes.

The fourth messenger is often sensitive to modulation by second and third messengers. For example, the calcium/cAMP response element binding (CREB) protein is sensitive to elevations in either intracellular calcium (Bading et al. 1993) or cAMP. An increase in calcium levels activates the calcium-calmodulin-dependent PK, or perhaps PKC, which can phosphorylate CREB (Sheng et al. 1990). Similarly, an increase in cAMP will activate PKA, which can phosphorylate CREB. Phospho-CREB is translocated into the nucleus, where it binds to the calcium/cAMP response element (Ca/CRE). The Ca/CRE lies in the promoter region for downstream transcriptional control of genes such as *c-fos* and *jun B* (Sheng and Greenberg 1990). Because these genes tend to be expressed rapidly, they are often called *immediate early genes*. The protein products of *c-fos* (FOS) and *jun B* (JUN) can dimerize to form complexes called *activator proteins*. These proteins can then bind to yet other genomic sites (AP-1 sites), which can

regulate expression of target genes such as peptide neurotransmitters (e.g., vasoactive intestinal polypeptide) (Fink et al. 1991). Such a transcriptional/translational cascade may not be complete for hours or even days. Physiological processes that appear to require some form of long-lasting biochemical "memory" (long-term potentiation, circadian rhythmicity) do indeed seem to use such fourth-messenger cascades (Kornhauser et al. 1996).

SUMMARY

General Summary

In this chapter, we focus on the use of model systems to provide the reader with an approach to understanding transmitters, receptors, signal-transducing proteins, intracellular messengers, and their target proteins.

Neurotransmitters—First Messengers

In this brief review of brain signaling, we have seen that certain key principles may be applied to each of the four fundamental steps in the chemical signaling process—neurotransmission, receptor binding, signal transduction, and second-messenger activation. Thus, we examined several principles of neurotransmission in brain.

The first principle of neurotransmission was that of *synaptic effect*, such that each of the steps in synaptic transmission is relevant to psychopharmacology only to the extent that it alters the synaptic transmitter content (and, hence, the amount of transmitter available to bind to receptors). Any effect of disease or drug that does not change the synaptic content of a transmitter does not alter behavior.

The second principle of neurotransmission was that of *self-regulation* (synaptic homeostasis), in which each pulse of released transmitter tends to reduce its subsequent release by initiating feedback processes within its neuron.

The third principle of neurotransmission was that of *dose dependence*, whereby the stimulation of receptors by hormones, neurotransmitters, and drugs is proportional to the concentration.

The fourth principle of neurotransmission was that the biological effects of any chemical mediator have a characteristic *latency* and *duration of action*.

The fifth principle of neurotransmission was that of *synaptic resilience*, in which partial damage to one portion of a nerve terminal or to one aspect of a neuron's functions tends to be associated with compensatory changes in neuronal activity.

These principles were considered briefly in relation to

the several sites of drug action—synthesis, storage, release, binding, reuptake, and metabolism. Just as each of these sites of drug action applies in principle to any transmitter or modulator system, so do the five fundamental principles of neurotransmission. The psychopharmacologist must determine how best to utilize these principles with respect to the sites of drug action in dealing with symptoms of the diseases discussed in subsequent chapters.

Receptors

Receptor proteins are the initial component of a signal-transduction system for transferring the message of the neurotransmitter across the neuronal membrane into the cell. Molecular recognition of receptors for drugs or neurotransmitters is the basis of pharmacological selectivity. Receptors can be classified based on pharmacological, structural, and functional criteria. Elucidation of the primary amino acid sequences for a growing number of receptors has revealed that a few general features are used by most of these proteins and that they can be separated into superfamilies on this basis. The G-protein-linked superfamily contains seven transmembrane domains in a single polypeptide. The nicotinic receptor type of the ligand-gated ion channel superfamily exists as a complex of five subunits, each of which contains four transmembrane domains.

Signal Transduction

Activation of the receptor by an agonist initiates the process of signal transduction. G-protein-linked receptors use a G protein to couple to the effector enzyme. The transduction process involves exchange of GDP for GTP (nucleotide exchange) and dissociation of the heterotrimeric G protein into α and $\beta\gamma$ subunits. The activated, GTP-bound α subunit may stimulate the activity of enzymes such as adenylate cyclase or PI-specific phospholipase C to produce second messengers (cAMP or IP_3 and DAG) inside the cell. Signal transduction through ligand-gated ion channels involves the movement of ions into or out of the cell, which alters the membrane potential and, thus, the excitability of the neuron.

Intracellular Second, Third, and Fourth Messengers

The first fundamental principle of intracellular messengers discussed was that of *convergent processing*, in which information conveyed by many neurotransmitters is funneled and integrated into the action of a few intracellular messengers. *Latency/duration of action* distinguishes the rapid mediation of biological activity by ligand-gated ion channels from the slower, but more lasting, actions of cellular second messengers such as cAMP. *PK output* is an action shared by cellular second messengers, which leads, through phosphorylation of target proteins to phosphoproteins (a third-messenger action), to a variety of direct and indirect actions on the target proteins inside the cell. These actions may include effects at some distance from the site of second-messenger production, especially those that involve changes in gene transcription mediated by the fourth-messenger systems of the cell. Finally, *regulatory pathway participation* is the principle whereby second messengers play a significant role in altering the ability of hormones, neurotransmitters, and drugs to change cellular second-messenger levels (i.e., change their own levels). This is accomplished by feedback actions to desensitize the receptor–signal-transducer system and by feedforward actions to alter gene expression. Third and fourth messengers provide a further downstream level of signal transduction and information integration to modulate extracellular signals beyond the actions mediated by second messengers.

REFERENCES

Aaronson SA: Growth factors and cancer. Science 254: 1146–1153, 1991

Albert PR, Neve KA, Bunzow JR, et al: Coupling of a cloned rat dopamine-D2 receptor to inhibition of adenylyl cyclase and prolactin secretion. J Biol Chem 265: 2098–2104, 1990

Alousi AA, Jasper JR, Insel PA, et al: Stoichiometry of receptor-G_s-adenylate cyclase interactions. FASEB J 5:2300–2303, 1991

Amara SG, Kuhar M: Neurotransmitter transporters. Annu Rev Neurosci 16:73–93, 1993

Andersen PH, Gingrich JA, Bates MD, et al: Dopamine receptor subtypes: beyond the D1/D2 classification. Trends Pharmacol Sci 11:231–236, 1990

Arriza JL, Dawson TM, Simerly RB, et al: The G-protein-coupled receptor kinases βARK1 and βARK2 are widely distributed at synapses in rat brain. J Neurosci 12: 4045–4055, 1992

Atack JR, Broughton HB, Pollack SJ: Inositol monophosphatase—a putative target for Li^+ in the treatment of bipolar disorder. Trends Neurosci 18:343–349, 1995

Attramadal H, Arriza JL, Aoki C, et al: β-Arrestin2, a novel member of the arrestin/β-arrestin gene family. J Biol Chem 267:17882–17890, 1992

Avalos M, Mak C, Randall P, et al: Prototype and novel antipsychotic drug interactions with dopamine in C6 glioma cells selectively and stably expressing D2S dopamine receptors. Society for Neuroscience Abstracts 23:1778, 1997

Avissar S, Schreiber G: Muscarinic receptor subclassification and G-proteins: significance for lithium action in affective disorders and for the treatment of the extrapyramidal side effects of neuroleptics. Biol Psychiatry 26:113–130, 1989

Bading H, Ginty DD, Greenberg ME: Regulation of gene expression in hippocampal neurons by distinct calcium signaling pathways. Science 260:181–186, 1993

Bannon MJ, Roth R: Pharmacology of mesocortical dopamine neurons. Pharmacol Rev 35:53–68, 1983

Bannon MJ, Freeman AS, Chiodo LA, et al: The pharmacology and electrophysiology of mesolimbic dopamine neurons, in Handbook of Psychopharmacology, Vol 19. Edited by Iversen LL, Iversen SD, Snyder SH. New York, Plenum, 1986, pp 329–374

Bartholini G, Zivkovic B, Scatton B: Dopaminergic neurons: basic aspects, in Handbook of Experimental Pharmacology, Vol 90/11. Edited by Trendelenburg U, Weiner N. Berlin, Springer-Verlag, 1989, pp 277–317

Bates MD, Senogles SE, Bunzow JR, et al: Regulation of responsiveness at D2 dopamine receptors by receptor desensitization and adenylyl cyclase sensitization. Mol Pharmacol 35:55–63, 1991

Benovic JL, Strasser RH, Caron MG, et al: β-Adrenergic receptor kinase: identification of a novel protein kinase that phosphorylates the agonist-occupied form of the receptor. Proc Natl Acad Sci U S A 83:2797–2801, 1986

Berridge MJ: Inositol triphosphate and diacylglycerol: two interacting second messengers. Annu Rev Biochem 56:159–193, 1989

Bourne HR, Sanders DA, McCormick F: The GTPase superfamily: conserved structure and molecular mechanism. Nature 349:117–127, 1991

Brusniak M-Y, Pearlman R, Neve KA, et al: Comparative Molecular Field Analysis (CoMFA) and agonist affinity at recombinant D1A vs. D2A dopamine receptors. J Med Chem 39:850–859, 1996

Bunzow JR, Van Tol HHM, Grandy DK, et al: Cloning and expression of a rat D2 dopamine receptor cDNA. Nature 336:783–787, 1988

Burt DR, Kamatchi GL: GABA$_A$ receptor subtypes: from pharmacology to molecular biology. FASEB J 5:2916–2923, 1991

Changeux J-P, Devillers-Thiery A, Galzi J-L, et al: New mutants to explore nicotinic receptor functions. Trends Pharmacol Sci 13:299–301, 1992

Chio CL, Hess GF, Graham RS, et al: A second molecular form of D2 dopamine receptor in rat and bovine caudate nucleus. Nature 343:266–269, 1990

Chiodo LA: Dopamine autoreceptor signal transduction in the DA cell body: a "current view." Neurochem Int 20:815–845, 1992

Civelli O, Bunzow JR, Grandy DK, et al: Molecular biology of the dopamine receptors. Eur J Pharmacol 207:277–286, 1991

Cole AJ, Bhat RV, Patt C, et al: D1 dopamine receptor activation of multiple transcription factor genes in rat striatum. J Neurochem 58:1420–1426, 1992

Coleman DE, Berghuis AM, Lee E, et al: Structures of active conformations of $G_{i\alpha1}$ and the mechanism of GTP hydrolysis. Science 265:1405–1412, 1994

Collins S, Caron MG, Lefkowitz RJ: Regulation of adrenergic receptor responsiveness through modulation of receptor gene expression. Annu Rev Physiol 53:497–508, 1991

Conti M, Swinnen JV, Tsikalas KE, et al: Structure and regulation of the rat high-affinity cyclic AMP phosphodiesterases: a family of closely related enzymes. Adv Second Messenger Phosphoprotein Res 25:87–99, 1992

Cooper JR, Bloom FE, Roth RH: The Biochemical Basis of Neuropharmacology, 7th Edition. New York, Oxford University Press, 1996

Cotman CW, Kahle JS, Miller SE, et al: Excitatory amino acid neurotransmission, in Psychopharmacology: The Fourth Generation of Progress. Edited by Bloom FE, Kupfer DJ. New York, Raven, 1995, pp 75–85

Coward DM, Dixon K, Enz A, et al: Partial brain dopamine D2 receptor agonists in the treatment of schizophrenia. Psychopharmacol Bull 25:393–397, 1989

Cox BA, Henningsen RA, Spanoyannis A, et al: Contributions of conserved serine residues to the interactions of ligands with dopamine D2 receptors. J Neurochem 59:627–635, 1992

Curran T, Rauscher FJ, Cohen DR, et al: Beyond the second messenger: oncogenes and transcription factors. Cold Spring Harb Symp Quant Biol 53:769–777, 1988

Dearry A, Gingrich JA, Falardeau P, et al: Molecular cloning and expression of the gene for a human D1 dopamine receptor. Nature 347:72–76, 1990

Deutch AY, Roth RH: The determinants of stress-induced activation of the prefrontal cortical dopamine system. Prog Brain Res 85:367–403, 1990

Dixon RAF, Kobilka BK, Strader DJ, et al: Cloning of the gene and cDNA for mammalian β-adrenergic receptor and homology and rhodopsin. Nature 321:75–79, 1986

Eshleman AJ, Henningsen RA, Neve KA, et al: Release of dopamine via the human transported. Mol Pharmacol 45:312–316, 1994

Fink JS, Verhave M, Walton K, et al: Cyclic AMP- and phorbol ester-induced transcriptional activation are mediated by the same enhancer element in the human vasoactive intestinal peptide gene. J Biol Chem 266:3882–3887, 1991

Fisher SK, Heacock AM, Agranoff BW: Inositol lipids and signal transduction in the nervous system: an update. J Neurochem 58:18–38, 1992

Fowler CJ, Tiger G: Modulation of receptor-mediated inositol phospholipid breakdown in the brain. Neurochem Int 19:171–206, 1991

Gao B, Gilman AG: Cloning and expression of a widely distributed (type IV) adenylyl cyclase. Proc Natl Acad Sci U S A 88:10178–10182, 1991

Garattini S: Pharmacology of second messengers: a critical appraisal. Drug Metab Rev 24:125–194, 1992

Gasic GP, Hollmann M: Molecular neurobiology of glutamate receptors. Annu Rev Physiol 54:507–536, 1992

Gilman AG: G proteins: transducers of receptor-generated signals. Annu Rev Biochem 56:615–649, 1987

Grace AA, Onn S-P: Morphology and electrophysiological properties of immunocytochemically identified rat dopamine neurons recorded *in vitro*. J Neurosci 9:3463–3481, 1989

Hall H, Farde L, Halldin C, et al: Imaging of dopamine receptors using PET and SPECT. Neurochem Int 20:329S–333S, 1992

Hausdorff WP, Caron MG, Lefkowitz RJ: Turning off the signal: desensitization of β-adrenergic receptor function. FASEB J 4:2881–2889, 1990

Hayes G, Bident TJ, Selbie LA, et al: Structural subtypes of the dopamine D2 receptor are functionally distinct: expression of the cloned D_{2A} and D_{2B} subtypes in a heterologous cell line. Mol Endocrinol 6:920–926, 1992

Hess EJ, Creese I: Biochemical characterization of dopamine receptors, in Dopamine Receptors. Edited by Creese I, Graser CM. New York, Alan R Liss, 1987, pp 1–28

Hollenberg MD: Structure-activity relationships for transmembrane signaling: the receptor's turn. FASEB J 5:178–186, 1991

Iyengar R, Birnbaumer L: Signal transduction by G-proteins. ISI Atlas of Science: Pharmacology 1: 213–221, 1987

Kandel ER, Schwartz JH, Jessell TM (eds): Principles of Neural Science, 3rd Edition. New York, Elsevier, 1991

Kaneko M, Sato K, Horikoshi R, et al: Effect of haloperidol on cyclic AMP and inositol triphosphate in rat striatum *in vivo*. Prostaglandins Leukot Essent Fatty Acids 46:53–57, 1992

Kikkawa U, Kishimoto A, Nishizuka Y: The protein kinase C family: heterogeneity and its implications. Annu Rev Biochem 58:31–44, 1989

Kilty JE, Lorang D, Amara SG: Cloning and expression of a cocaine-sensitive rat dopamine transporter. Science 254:578–579, 1991

Kornhauser JM, Ginty DD, Greenberg ME, et al: Light entrainment and activation of signal transduction pathways in the SCN. Prog Brain Res 3:133–146, 1996

Kozell L, Starr S, Machida C, et al: Agonist induced changes in density of D1, D2, and chimeric D1/D2 receptors. Society for Neuroscience Abstracts 18:276, 1992

Krupinski J: The adenylyl cyclase family. Mol Cell Biochem 104:73–79, 1992

Krupinski J, Coussen F, Bakalyar HA, et al: Adenylyl cyclase amino acid sequence: possible channel- or transporter-like structure. Science 244:1558–1564, 1989

Kuffler SW, Nicholls JG, Martin AR: From Neuron to Brain: A Cellular Approach to the Function of the Nervous System, 2nd Edition. Sunderland, MA, Sinauer Associates, 1984

Laihinen A, Rinne JO, Rinne UK, et al: (^{18}F)-6-Fluorodopa PET scanning in Parkinson's disease after selective COMT inhibition with nitecapone (OR-462). Neurology 42:199–203, 1992

Lamb TD, Pugh EN Jr: G-protein cascades: gain and kinetics. Trends Neurosci 15:291–298, 1992

Lazar DF, Wiese RJ, Brady MJ, et al: Mitogen-activated protein kinase inhibition does not block the stimulation of glucose utilization by insulin. J Biol Chem 270:20801–20807, 1995

Leslie S, Woodward J, Wilcox R: Correlation of rates of calcium entry and endogenous dopamine release in mouse striatal synaptosomes. Brain Res 325:99–105, 1985

Limbird LE: Cell Surface Receptors: A Short Course on the Theory and Methods. Boston, MA, Martinus Nijhoff Publishing, 1986

Lohse MJ, Benovic JL, Codina J, et al: β-Arrestin: a protein that regulates β-adrenergic receptor function. Science 248: 1547–1550, 1990

Maelicke A, Albuquerque EX: New approach to drug therapy in Alzheimer's dementia. Drug Discovery Today 1:53–59, 1996

Mak C, Avalos M, Randall P, et al: Improved models for pharmacological null experiments: calculation of drug efficacy at recombinant D1A dopamine stably expressed in clonal cell lines. Neuropharmacology 5:549–570, 1996

Mamounas LA, Mullen CA, O'Hearn E, et al: Dual serotonergic project to forebrain in the rat: morphologically distinct 5HT axon terminals exhibit differential vulnerability to neurotoxic amphetamine derivatives. J Comp Neurol 314:558–586, 1992

Manji HK: G proteins: implications for psychiatry. Am J Psychiatry 149:746–760, 1992

Mansour A, Meng F, Meador-Woodruff JH, et al: Site-directed mutagenesis of the human dopamine D2 receptor. Eur J Pharmacol 227:205–214, 1992

Marletta MA: Nitric oxide synthase: aspects concerning structure and catalysis. Cell 78:927–930, 1994

McEwen BS, DeKloet ER, Rostene W: Adrenal steroid receptors and actions in the nervous system. Physiol Rev 66:1121–1188, 1986

McGeer PL, Eccles JC, McGeer EG: Molecular Neurobiology of the Mammalian Brain, 2nd Edition. New York, Plenum, 1987

McGonigle P, Molinoff P: Quantitative aspects of drug–receptor interactions, in Basic Neurochemistry, 4th Edition. Edited by Siegel G, Agranoff B, Albers RW, et al. New York, Raven, 1989, pp 183–202

McMillen BA: CNS stimulants: two distinct mechanisms of action for amphetamine-like drugs. Trends Pharmacol Sci 4:429–432, 1983

Mikoshiba K: Inositol 1,4,5-triphosphate receptor. Trends Pharmacol Sci 14:86–89, 1993

Miller RJ: The control of neuronal Ca^{2+} homeostasis. Prog Neurobiol 37:225–285, 1991

Montmayeur J-P, Borrelli E: Transcription mediated by a cAMP-responsive promoter element is reduced upon activation of dopamine D_2 receptors. Proc Natl Acad Sci U S A 88:3135–3139, 1991

Nagatsu T: Genes for human catecholamine-synthesizing enzymes. Neurosci Res 12:315–345, 1991

Nathan C, Xie Q-W: Nitric oxide synthases: rules, tolls and controls. Cell 78:915–918, 1994

Nestler EJ: Molecular mechanisms of drug addiction. J Neurosci 12:2439–2450, 1992

Neve KA, Henningsen RA, Bunzow JR, et al: Functional characterization of a rat dopamine D-2 receptor cDNA expressed in a mammalian cell line. Mol Pharmacol 36:446–451, 1989

Neve KA, Cox BA, Henningsen RA, et al: Pivotal role of aspartate-80 in the regulation of dopamine D2 receptor affinity for drugs and inhibition of adenylyl cyclase. Mol Pharmacol 39:733–739, 1991

Noda M, Takahashi H, Tanabe T, et al: Structural homology of *Torpedo californica* acetylcholine receptor subunits. Nature 302:528–532, 1983

Northup JK: Regulation of cyclic nucleotides in the nervous system, in Basic Neurochemistry, 4th Edition. Edited by Siegel G, Agranoff B, Albers RW, et al. New York, Raven, 1989, pp 349–364

O'Dell TJ, Kandel ER, Grant SGN: Long-term potentiation in the hippocampus is blocked by tyrosine kinase inhibitors. Nature 353:558–560, 1991

Okada F, Crow RJ, Roberts GW: G proteins (Gi, Go) in the medial temporal lobe in schizophrenia: preliminary report of a neurochemical correlate of structural change. J Neural Transm Gen Sect 84:147–153, 1991

Paul SM: GABA and glycine, in Psychopharmacology: The Fourth Generation of Progress. Edited by Bloom FE, Kupfer DJ. New York, Raven, 1995, pp 87–94

Probst WC, Snyder LA, Schuster DI, et al: Sequence alignment of the G-protein coupled receptor superfamily. DNA Cell Biol 11:1–20, 1992

Racagni G, Brunello N, Tinelli D, et al: New biochemical hypotheses on the mechanism of action of antidepressant drugs: cAMP-dependent phosphorylation system. Pharmacopsychiatry 25:51–55, 1992

Randall PK: Quantitative analysis of behavioral pharmacological data. Ann N Y Acad Sci 515:124–139, 1988

Rhee SG: Inositol phospholipid-specific phospholipase C: interaction of the $_\gamma 1$ isoform with tyrosine kinase. Trends Biochem Sci 16:297–301, 1991

Riffee WH, Wilcox RE, Vaughn DM, et al: Dopamine receptor sensitivity after chronic dopamine agonists: striatal (3H)-spiroperidol binding in mice after chronic administration of high doses of apomorphine, N-n-propyl-norapomorphine, and dextroamphetamine. Psychopharmacology 77:146–149, 1982

Roberts MH, Towles JA, Leader NK: Tyrosine kinase regulation of a molluscan circadian clock. Brain Res 592:170–174, 1992

Robinson TE, Becker JB: Enduring changes in brain and behavior produced by chronic amphetamine administration: a review and evaluation of animal models of amphetamine psychosis. Brain Res Rev 11:157–198, 1986

Roth R: CNS dopamine autoreceptors: distribution, pharmacology, and function. Ann N Y Acad Sci 430:27–55, 1984

Ruffalo RR Jr: Important concepts of receptor theory. J Auton Pharmacol 2:277–295, 1982

Sakmann B: Elementary steps in synaptic transmission revealed by currents through single ion channels. Science 256:503–512, 1992

Saller CF, Salama AI: Apomorphine enantiomers' effects on dopamine metabolism: receptor and non-receptor related actions. Eur J Pharmacol 121:181–188, 1986

Savarese TM, Fraser CM: *In vitro* mutagenesis and the search for structure-function relationships among G protein-coupled receptors. Biochem J 283:1–19, 1992

Schmidt HHHW, Walter U: NO at work. Cell 78:919–925, 1994

Schulz S, Yuen PST, Garbers DL: The expanding family of guanylyl cyclases. Trends Pharmacol Sci 12:116–120, 1991

Schuman EM, Madison DV: Nitric oxide and synaptic function. Annu Rev Neurosci 17:153–183, 1994

Schwartz JH, Kandel ER: Synaptic transmission mediated by second messengers, in Principles of Neural Science, 3rd Edition. Edited by Kandel ER, Schwartz JA, Jessell TM. New York, Elsevier, 1991, pp 173–193

Schwinn DA, Caron MG, Lefkowitz RJ: The beta-adrenergic receptor as a model for molecular structure-function relationships in G-protein-coupled receptors, in The Heart and Cardiovascular System, 2nd Edition. Edited by Fozzard HA, et al. New York, Raven, 1992, pp 1657–1684

Seeman P: Dopamine receptors and psychosis. Sci Am Sept/Oct:2–11, 1995

Self DW, Barnhart WJ, Lehman DA, et al: Opposite modulation of cocaine seeking behavior by D1- and D2-like dopamine receptor agonists. Science 271:1586–1589, 1996

Senogles SE, Spiegel AM, Padrell E, et al: Specificity of receptor-G protein interactions. J Biol Chem 265:4507–4514, 1990

Severson J, Randall P, Wilcox RE: Single apomorphine pretreatment results in a rapid decline in high-affinity dopamine binding to the striatal D2 receptor. Eur J Pharmacol 188:283–286, 1990

Sheng M, Greenberg ME: The regulation and function of c-*fos* and other immediate early genes in the nervous system. Neuron 4:477–485, 1990

Sheng M, McFadden G, Greenberg ME: Membrane depolarization and calcium induce c-*fos* transcription via phosphorylation of transcription factor CREB. Neuron 4:571–582, 1990

Shimizu T, Wolfe LS: Arachidonic acid cascade and signal transduction. J Neurochem 55:1–15, 1990

Sibley DR, Lefkowitz RJ: Molecular mechanisms of receptor desensitization using the β-adrenergic receptor-coupled adenylate cyclase system as a model. Nature 317:124–129, 1985

Sibley DR, Lefkowitz RJ: Biochemical mechanisms of β-adrenergic receptor regulation. ISI Atlas of Science: Pharmacology 2:66–70, 1988

Sibley DR, Monsma FJ Jr: Molecular biology of dopamine receptors. Trends Pharmacol Sci 13:61–69, 1992

Siever LJ, Kahn RS, Lawlor BA, et al: Critical issues in defining the role of serotonin in psychiatric disorders. Pharmacol Rev 43:509–525, 1991

Smith CUM: Elements of Molecular Neurobiology. New York, Wiley, 1989

Snyder SH: Nitric oxide: first in a new class of neurotransmitters? Science 257:494–496, 1992

Spiegel AM: Heterotrimeric GTP-binding proteins: an expanding family of signal transducers. Med Res Rev 12:55–71, 1992

Spiegel A, Shenker A, Weinstein L: Receptor–effector coupling by G proteins: implications for normal and abnormal signal transduction. Endocr Rev 13:536–565, 1992

Strulovici B, Cerione RA, Kilpatrick BF, et al: Direct demonstration of impaired functionality of a purified desensitized β-adrenergic receptor in a reconstituted system. Science 225:837–840, 1984

Summers WK, Majovski V, Marsh GM, et al: Oral tetrahydroaminoacridine in long-term treatment of senile dementia, Alzheimer type. N Engl J Med 315:1241–1245, 1986

Sunahara R, Guan H-C, O'Dowd BF, et al: Cloning of the gene for a human dopamine D5 receptor with higher affinity for dopamine than D1. Nature 350:614–619, 1991

Taylor P: Anticholinesterase agents, in Goodman and Gilman's The Pharmacological Basis of Therapeutics, 8th Edition. Edited by Gilman AG, Rall TW, Nies AS, et al. New York, Pergamon, 1990, pp 131–150

Taylor P, Insel PA: Molecular basis of pharmacologic selectivity, in Principles of Drug Action, 3rd Edition. Edited by Pratt WB, Taylor P. New York, Churchill Livingstone, 1990, pp 1–102

Taylor S, Buechler J, Yonemoto W: cAMP-dependent protein kinase: framework for a diverse family of regulatory enzymes. Annu Rev Biochem 59:971–1005, 1990

Teeter MM, Froimowitz M, Stec B, et al: Homology modeling of the dopamine D2 receptor and its testing by docking of agonists and tricyclic antagonists. J Med Chem 37:2874–2888, 1994

Usdin TB, Eiden LE, Bonner TI, et al: Molecular biology of the vesicular ACh transporter. Trends Neurosci 18:218–224, 1995

van Rhee AM, Jacobson KA: Molecular architecture of G protein-coupled receptors. Drug Discovery Research 37:1–38, 1996

Van Tol HHM, Wu CM, Guan H-C, et al: Multiple dopamine D4 receptor variants in the human population. Nature 358:149–152, 1992

Vaughn D, Severson J, Woodward J, et al: Behavioral sensitization following subchronic apomorphine treatment—possible neurochemical basis. Brain Res 526:37–44, 1990

Walaas SI, Greengard P: Protein phosphorylation and neuronal function. Pharmacol Rev 43:299–350, 1991

Watson S, Girdlestone D: Tips on nomenclature. Trends Pharmacol Sci 16:15–16, 1995

Wilcox RE, McMillen BA: The rationale development of drugs as adjuncts to the treatment of the alcoholisms: a commentary. Alcohol (in press)

Wilcox RE, Severson J, Woodward J, et al: Behavioral sensitization following a single apomorphine treatment—selective effects on the dopamine release process. Brain Res 528:109–113, 1990

Wolf ME, Roth RH: Dopamine autoreceptors, in Dopamine Receptors. Edited by Creese I, Fraser DM. New York, Alan R Liss, 1987, pp 45–96

TWO

Molecular Biology

Christine Konradi, Ph.D., Stephan Heckers, M.D., and
Joseph T. Coyle, M.D.

Molecular biology is transforming all areas of biomedical research and has assumed the dominant role as the paradigm for understanding disease processes and their treatment. Thus, it is quite appropriate that a review of the advances in psychopharmacology should include a discussion of the application of molecular biology in this discipline. Molecular biology is closely allied with molecular genetics, and it offers powerful tools for dissecting the function of specific proteins in the nervous system. It has facilitated the identification of families of receptors, such as the five dopamine receptors, three more than standard pharmacological techniques had suggested. Through the exploration of recombinant DNA technology, molecular biology can now manipulate the mouse genome so that specific genes can be inactivated or inserted to characterize their function (Paigen 1995; Rossant and Nagy 1995; Shuldiner 1996). Recently, methods have been developed so that these inserted genes can be turned on or off at will in regionally specific areas of the brain (Morris and Morris 1997; Rossant and Nagy 1995; Tsien et al. 1996a, 1996b).

At the same time, as the Human Genome Project advances (Watson 1990), the ability to map loci of heritable vulnerability to disorders improves steadily as increasing numbers of genetic markers are identified on human chromosomes at progressively shorter intervals (Schuler et al. 1996). This improvement has a considerable effect on the search for heritable risk factors for psychiatric disorders and complex behavioral traits. Thus, clinical genetic studies are providing evidence that heritable factors contribute to risk for an expanding number of Axis I disorders (see Table 2–1) and for personality characteristics and temperament.

Molecular neurobiology and molecular genetics advance hand in hand as genetic loci of risk are identified at the same time that genes encoding proteins of interest are mapped on human and mouse genomes. The knowledge acquired discloses final common pathways from genotype to phenotype and provides specific targets for pharmacological intervention. Thus, molecular models will replace serendipity as the method of neuropsychotropic drug discovery.

In this chapter, we take two approaches to explicate the use of molecular biology in psychopharmacology. First, we review the basic principles for moving from gene to protein and the methods for understanding and manipulating these processes. Second, we consider several examples of brain disorders in which molecular strategies have been used to understand pathophysiology and to develop pharmacological interventions.

BASIC PRINCIPLES OF MOLECULAR BIOLOGY

The Molecular Substrate of Inherited Traits: From DNA to RNA to Proteins

Inherited traits are defined by their ability to be passed on from one generation to the next. They include biological properties responsible for visible likeness of offspring to parents (e.g., hair and eye color, facial shape) and psychological properties such as personality traits. Inherited traits are not restricted to features promoting optimal adaptation to the environment, which is important for the survival of the species, but may include attributes that are counterproductive to this objective (e.g., inherited diseases).

The sum of all inherited traits constitutes the genetic composition—the *genotype* of an organism. However, not all of these traits are necessarily apparent. Thus, the genotype of the organism is distinguished from the *phenotype*, which reflects the apparent characteristics of an individual and which results from the interaction of the genotype with the environment.

DNA. The blueprint for all inherited traits can be found in every cell of the body in a structure called *DNA* (deoxyribonucleic acid), which specifies the primary characteristics of all proteins that constitute the organism. DNA in humans contains 46 double strands of polynucleotide chains linked by phosphodiester bonds. Each nucleotide consists of a base—either the purines adenine (A) and guanine (G) or the pyrimidines cytosine (C) and thymine (T)—linked to a sugar (deoxyribose) and a phosphate group (Figure 2–1). Each base is linked to a complementary counterbase by an opposing polynucleotide strand (Figure 2–2). Purines always face pyrimidines in A-T or G-C base pairs (bp), which are connected by hydrogen bonds (Figure 2–2). The two strands form a helical structure—*double helix* (Watson and Crick 1953) (Figure 2–2)—which is coiled around protein complexes (*histones*), forming *nucleosomes* (Wolffe 1994). Nucleosomes

are further condensed into 300Å filaments.

During cell division, each of the 46 double helices is replicated (Figure 2–2) and folded into chromosomes. The 46 human chromosomes comprise 22 pairs of autosomes and 2 sex chromosomes, either XX for females or XY for males. During *genetic recombination*, a process taking place during meiosis in the gonads, the chromosome pairs *cross over* and reciprocally exchange pieces of DNA. Ge-

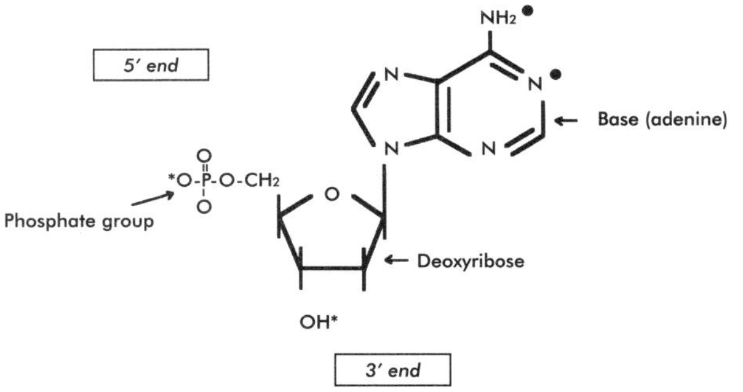

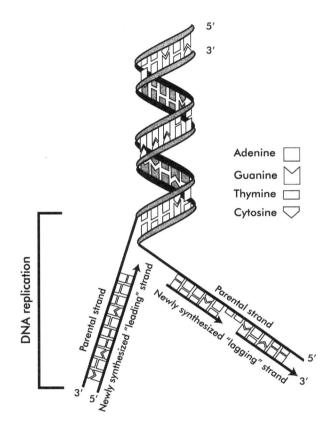

Figure 2–2. Double-helical structure of DNA. The most common structure of DNA is the double helix, composed of two polymeric nucleotide chains of complementary sequence—adenine (A) facing thymine (T) and guanine (G) facing cytosine (C). The complementary polynucleotide chains are linked by hydrogen bonds, with two hydrogen bonds linking A to T (see Figure 2–1) or three hydrogen bonds linking G to C. A full helical turn consists of approximately 10 nucleotide pairs. The two polynucleotide chains run in opposite directions, with one strand running 5′ to 3′ and the other strand running 3′ to 5′. During replication of DNA, each of the two original (parental) strands serves as a template for a newly synthesized, complementary strand (semiconservative replication). Because DNA is synthesized in a unidirectional manner (3′ to 5′ phosphodiesterase linkage), one new strand (the "lagging" strand) can be synthesized only in fragments, which are later connected by DNA polymerase I and DNA ligase.

Figure 2–1. Structure of the nucleotide deoxyadenosine monophosphate. The molecular components of DNA, the *nucleotides*, are composed of deoxyribose linked to a phosphate group and one of four bases (adenine, guanine, cytosine, and thymine). During DNA synthesis, nucleotides are added by their 5′ phosphate group at the 3′ end of the nucleotide chain (3′ to 5′ phosphodiester linkage).
* = atoms involved in phosphodiester bonds, which link the polynucleotide chain together; ● = atoms involved in hydrogen bonds between the complementary DNA strands (see Figure 2–2).

netic mapping, a powerful tool in *linkage analysis* (see sub-section, "Reverse Genetics and Positional Cloning," later in this chapter) is based on the statistical likelihood of crossover events.

Transcription: from DNA to mRNA.   DNA is not directly translated into proteins but rather is transcribed by specific enzymes into a complementary strand of RNA (ribonucleic acid). RNA is synthesized in a 5′ to 3′ fashion (similar to that shown in Figure 2–2). Three RNA species are found in eukaryotic cells:

1. *Ribosomal RNA (rRNA)*, the building blocks of ribosomes
2. *Messenger RNA (mRNA)*, the templates for proteins
3. *Transfer RNA (tRNA)*, the form used to assist in the translation from mRNA to proteins

Like DNA, RNA consists of four nucleotides, adenine (A), guanine (G), cytosine (C), and uracil (U), which are linked to the sugar ribose and a phosphate group. Uracil substitutes for thymine and is the complementary base to adenine. RNA predominantly forms a single-stranded chain by phosphodiester bonds.

mRNA is transcribed from DNA by the enzyme RNA polymerase II, with an intermediate product termed *heterogeneous nuclear RNA* (hnRNA) (Figure 2–3). RNA polymerase II binds to a generic promoter, the TATA box (a region rich in the nucleotides thymidine and adenosine), with the help of accessory transcription factors (McKnight and Yamamoto 1992). The TATA box is a common motif approximately 25 bp upstream of the transcription start site (Figures 2–3 and 2–4) (Grosschedl et al. 1981; Mathis and Chambon 1981). In addition, a multitude of *enhancer elements* in various DNA locations can bind transcription factors, which can help to recruit RNA polymerase II to the TATA box (Figure 2–4) (Tjian and Maniatis 1994). Enhancer elements confer cell-specific and stimulus-dependent expression of hnRNA. The newly synthesized hnRNA is chemically modified by capping at the 5′ end and addition of a poly (A) sequence at the 3′ end (Figure 2–3), before it is transported out of the nucleus into the cytoplasm. During the process of transport out of the nucleus, hnRNA is converted into mRNA (Figure 2–3). hnRNA is usually larger in size than cytoplasmic mRNA because of the presence of stretches of RNA (*introns*), which are excised by a process called *splicing* (Figure 2–3) (Aloni et al. 1978; Cech 1983; Crick 1979; P. A. Sharp 1994). The linked *exons* constitute mRNA.

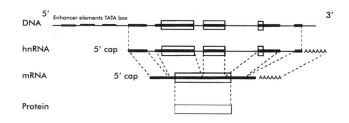

Figure 2–3.   From DNA to RNA to protein. RNA polymerase II is recruited to the TATA box located 5′ of the transcription initiation site. Enhancer elements (see Figure 2–4) can aid in the recruitment of RNA polymerase II. RNA polymerase II transcribes DNA into heterogeneous nuclear RNA (hnRNA), which is methylated at the 5′ end (cap) and polyadenylated at the 3′ end. During the process of splicing, introns are removed, leaving the messenger RNA (mRNA) product. The coding sequence of mRNA (open box) is then translated into protein with the help of transfer RNA (tRNA) (Figure 2–5) and ribosomes.

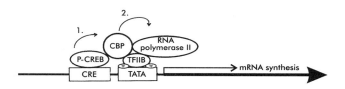

Figure 2–4.   Enhancer elements in various DNA locations can bind transcription factors (TFs), which can help recruit RNA polymerase II to the TATA box. The CRE enhancer element is bound by the transcription factor cyclic adenosine monophosphate (cAMP) response element binding (CREB). 1. Phosphorylation of CREB leads to the binding of the CREB binding protein (CBP), a transcriptional coactivator of CREB (Arias et al. 1994; Chrivia et al. 1993; Kwok et al. 1994). 2. CBP binds RNA polymerase II (Kee et al. 1996), which leads to increased messenger RNA (mRNA) synthesis in the presence of transcription factors of the TFII protein family. Thus, it may be important that CBP can also interact with the basal transcription factor TFIIB (Kwok et al. 1994).
TF = TFII members of the transcription initiation complex.
P-CREB = phosphorylated CREB.

Translation: from mRNA to proteins.   In the cytoplasm, mRNA is translated into proteins with the assistance of ribosomes and tRNA. tRNA has a cloverleaf structure (Figure 2–5), with three nucleotides on the top leaf forming a complementary codon (*anticodon*) to each of three adjoining, nonoverlapping mRNA nucleotides (*triplet*). Each tRNA binds a specific amino acid (amino acids are the modules for proteins) opposite the antico-

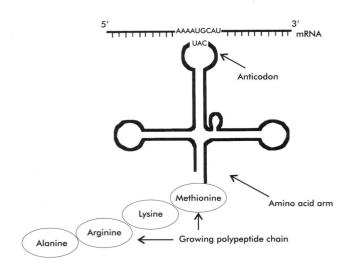

Figure 2–5.   Structure of transfer RNA (tRNA). tRNA has a cloverleaf structure, with the anticodon triplet on one side and the amino acid arm with the respective amino acid (determined by the anticodon) on the opposite side. The amino acid is added to the growing polypeptide chain within the ribosomes by peptide bond formation. Methionine-aminoacyl-tRNA is shown as example. mRNA = messenger RNA; A = adenine; U = uracil; G = guanine, C = cytosine.

don, thus allowing each mRNA nucleotide triplet (*codon*) to code for a specific amino acid. tRNA carrying an amino acid is termed *aminoacyl-tRNA* (Figure 2–5).

The vast majority of proteins found in living organisms are composed of 20 different amino acids assembled in a specific order depending on the individual protein. If a triplet of 3 nucleotides codes for 1 amino acid, 4^3 (64) different options are available. Thus, most amino acids are coded by more than 1 nucleotide triplet, with the defining emphasis on the first 2 nucleotides. Only 61 triplets code for amino acids, whereas 3 triplets signal termination of translation (*stop codons*). Translation is always initiated at the sequence AUG (in RNA, or ATG in DNA; see above) which codes for methionine, both at the start of translation and during protein elongation. Surprisingly, only 1 nucleotide triplet (AUG) codes for methionine. However, methionine-aminoacyl-tRNA involved in initiating protein synthesis is distinct from methionine-aminoacyl-tRNA (Figure 2–5) involved in protein elongation.

Anticodons of aminoacyl-tRNAs are paired with mRNA codons in *ribosomes*. Ribosomes are a combination of rRNA and enzymes needed for translation. They can be dissociated into two subunits of unequal size. Before the smaller subunit is joined by the larger subunit, it binds to the initiator methionine-aminoacyl-tRNA and to mRNA in the presence of initiation factors. Assembled ribosomes travel along mRNA templates and provide all functions required for protein synthesis. The presentation of a stop codon ends the synthesis of a particular protein with the help of release factors.

Regulatory Mechanisms: Regulation of Gene Expression and Posttranslational Modification

Regulatory mechanisms are best known for their role in development. However, because all cells within an organism have identical blueprints for proteins, regulatory mechanisms are needed to ensure continuous tissue- and cell-specific expression (Tjian and Maniatis 1994). Moreover, regulation of protein synthesis and modification of protein function provide important mechanisms to secure the proper operation of the cell. However, the numerous regulatory mechanisms also provide potential for malfunction and add to the number of parameters that must be considered when investigating the cause of brain disorders. Although the expression of proteins in a cell is regulated at DNA and RNA levels, the function of specific proteins may depend further on posttranslational modification.

Regulation of gene expression.   Gene expression is tightly controlled in many ways from transcription to translation. Common control mechanisms include the following:

To make DNA accessible to enzymes involved in transcription, adjustments in the chromatin structure are necessary. Decondensation of chromatin and adjustments in the DNA-histone complex render DNA accessible to RNA polymerase II and transcription factors (Wolffe 1994).

Methylation of cytosines at 5′ CG 3′ positions represses transcription (Bestor and Tycko 1996). DNA locations with high transcriptional activity are generally less methylated. Genetic *imprinting*, a process by which particular paternal or maternal genes are inactivated throughout a species, is at least partly controlled by DNA methylation (Barlow 1995). One of the abnormalities of the gene causing fragile X syndrome (*FMR-1*), a common cause of mental retardation in males, is the excessive methylation and transcriptional inhibition of the mutated version of the *FMR-1* gene (Bell et al. 1991; McConkie-Rosell et al. 1993; Steyaert et al. 1996).

The DNA promoter is particularly regulated and controls cell type and stimulus-specific expression of genes (Tjian and Maniatis 1994). The activity of the DNA promoter can be influenced by specified sequences known as enhancer elements, which bind transcription factors and can increase the efficiency of RNA polymerase II (Figure 2–4) (McKnight and Yamamoto 1992; Tjian and Maniatis 1994). Some DNA binding proteins may also inhibit promoter activity. The activity of most transcription factors is regulated through second-messenger pathways. A common gene-regulating pathway involves cyclic adenosine monophosphate (cAMP), a second messenger activated by agonists of several neurotransmitter receptors, such as the β-adrenergic receptor and the dopamine D_1 receptor, or by inhibitors of the dopamine D_2 receptor (Figure 2–6) (Cote et al. 1982; Levitzki 1988; Monsma et al. 1990). Various genes are regulated by cAMP pathways, many of which are relevant for brain function (e.g., *proenkephalin, somatosta-tin, prodynorphin, tyrosine hydroxylase*) (Comb et al. 1986; Douglass et al. 1994; Montminy and Bilezikjian 1987; Montminy et al. 1990). Intracellular increases in cAMP levels (e.g., via stimulation of G_s protein–coupled receptors) lead to the activation of protein kinase A (PKA) (Figure 2–6) (Levitzki 1988). PKA can phosphorylate the transcription factor cAMP response element binding (CREB) protein, which is constitutively bound at specific DNA enhancer elements (Figures 2–4 and 2–6) (Montminy and Bilezikjian 1987). With the aid of other transcription factors, phosphorylated CREB can recruit RNA polymerase II with high efficiency to the promoter (Figure 2–4) (Arias et al. 1994; Chrivia et al. 1993; Kwok et al. 1994).

Protein expression can be regulated at the RNA level. Some hnRNAs may code for more than one protein, and alternative splicing determines which protein is synthesized (Bingham et al. 1988). Defective processing of hnRNA can lead to neurological disorders, as is implicated in Friedreich's ataxia (Campuzano et al. 1996).

The half-life and stability of hnRNA and mRNA can be regulated and will determine how much protein is synthesized.

Posttranslational modification. Posttranslational modifications determine proper function of proteins and thus present another level of regulation. Common posttranslational modifications include the following mechanisms:

- Enzymatic conversion of preproteins to the final product allows preproteins to be processed in a tissue-specific manner. For example, *pro-opio-melanocortin* is enzymatically cleaved into various biologically active peptides, including β-endorphin, adrenocorticotropic hormone, β- and γ-lipotropic hormones, and α-, β-, and γ-melanocyte-stimulating hormones (Dores 1990). This type of posttranslational processing reflects the differential activity of cell-specific proteases.

- Organization into the three-dimensional structure of the protein is important for proper protein function.

- Allosteric regulation through interaction with cofactors (e.g., nicotinamide adenine dinucleotide [NADH], cAMP) determines enzymatic function.

- Interactions with ions (e.g., Ca^{2+}, Cu, Zn) may be needed for protein and enzymatic function (e.g., superoxide dismutase).

- Assembly with other proteins may be necessary to form functional complexes. Ion channels and receptors are often assembled from different proteins. In

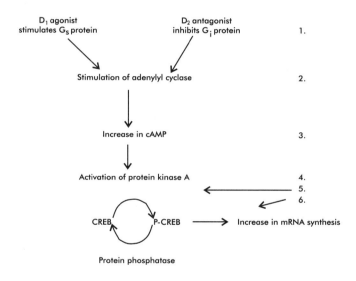

Figure 2–6. Drugs interacting with neurotransmitter receptors can induce long-term effects by altering neuronal gene expression. 1. Dopamine D_1 receptor agonists (e.g., indirect dopamine agonists amphetamine and cocaine) stimulate cyclic adenosine monophosphate (cAMP) production through D_1 receptor–linked G proteins, which (2.) activate adenylyl cyclase (G_s proteins). Dopamine D_2 receptor antagonists (e.g., haloperidol) stimulate cAMP production through an opposite mechanism: D_2 receptors are coupled to G_i proteins, which inhibit adenylyl cyclase activity. Inhibition of the inhibitory receptors leads to an activation of adenylyl cyclase (2.). 3. cAMP activates (4.) protein kinase A, which is translocated to the nucleus and phosphorylates the transcription factor cAMP response element binding (CREB) protein at [133]Ser (Gonzalez and Montminy 1989) (5.). As shown in Figure 2–4, CREB recruits other transcription factors, which enable RNA transcription (6.). A variety of genes are susceptible to changes in cAMP levels and are regulated by CREB.

fact, redundancies of receptor protein subtypes are common. Depending on the cell type, the protein subtypes can vary and thus contribute to cell type specificity.

- Chemical modifications control the function of specific proteins. Glycosylation (addition of sugar groups), phosphorylation (addition of phosphate groups), and acetylation (addition of acyl groups) are some of the modifications that may influence the ability of proteins to control, gain, or retain their function. Protein phosphorylation, for instance, can be regulated by the activation of protein kinases through second-messenger pathways (see the example of the transcription factor CREB above and Figures 2–4 and 2–6). The properties of both ion channels and receptors are dramatically changed through phosphorylation. Thus, phosphorylation provides a mechanism to convert short-term neurotransmitter-receptor interactions into long-lasting cellular changes and is an important factor in memory formation (Schacher et al. 1990).

Tools to Investigate the Genome

Certain genetic alterations affect brain function and cause neuropsychiatric disorders. Scientists have attempted to develop methods to help unravel disease mechanisms by comparing the genome of healthy individuals with that of patients with neuropsychiatric disorders. Some disorders may involve a single mutation in one gene, which leads to a change in the function of a single protein (e.g., Huntington's disease—see subsection, "Huntington's Disease," later in this chapter; Alzheimer's disease and β-amyloid protein—see subsection, "Alzheimer's Disease," later in this chapter). "Change in function" does not necessarily imply a loss or decrease of function but also could involve the gain of a new, undesired function. In fact, dominantly inherited disorders often reflect the acquisition of an altered, unwanted role of the mutated protein, providing it with powerful new properties to disrupt normal cell function (e.g., in Huntington's disease, amyotropic lateral sclerosis). Inherited brain disorders are not necessarily caused by mutations in protein coding genes but could be caused by mutations in noncoding areas, which may affect regulation, processing, or stability of proteins (Friedreich's ataxia—see subsection, "Reverse Genetics and Positional Cloning," later in this chapter and Campuzano et al. 1996).

The most challenging molecular analysis involves complex traits (see subsections, "Complex Traits" and "Schizophrenia and Bipolar Disorder," later in this chap-

ter). Most traits of psychiatric relevance do not follow a simple *monogenic* pattern of inheritance (one gene—one trait). Thus, detecting a single mutation that is present in all affected individuals is impossible. There may be one or more predisposing genes that—only in combination and possibly only in the presence of certain environmental factors—lead to the clinical presentation of the disorder. Nevertheless, new and powerful methods are being developed to clarify the molecular genetics of complex traits; thus, psychiatry will finally be able to move to the heart of molecular biology.

Cloning of DNA.   The original term *cloning* referred to the production of genetically identical organisms. Derived from that meaning, *cloning of DNA* connotes the ability to replicate and amplify individual pieces of DNA. Cloning can be done with *genomic* DNA (nuclear DNA) or *complementary* DNA (cDNA). cDNA is synthesized from mRNA with the aid of the viral enzyme *reverse transcriptase*. Thus, genomic DNA may contain any stretch of DNA, either expressed as protein or not (e.g., introns, exons, regulatory sequences), whereas cDNA consists of exons only. For cloning, pieces of DNA (subsequently referred to as DNA *insert*) are fused with the DNA of genetically engineered *vectors* or *plasmids* and introduced into various *hosts*. A *DNA library* consists of cloned random pieces of genomic DNA (genomic library) or cDNA. Good cDNA libraries contain all mRNA molecules expressed in a certain tissue (e.g., brain cDNA libraries).

Genetically engineered vectors possess all functions needed for the host to accept and replicate vector DNA and DNA insert and additional functions that help in the cloning process (e.g., *polylinkers* that provide various options for insertion of DNA or markers that differentiate between empty vectors and vectors containing DNA inserts). Because many control sequences are species specific, vectors are tailored for their hosts. Common hosts are bacteria, bacteriophages or other viruses, yeast, mammalian cell lines, and transgenic animals. Vectors for all these hosts are commercially available. However, in choosing a perfect vector, scientists consider various facts, including

- *Simplicity to raise and maintain the host:* The easiest hosts to maintain are bacteria and bacteriophages.
- *Length of the insert:* Bacteria are limited in the amount of plasmid DNA that they can accept. Most cDNAs fit within bacteria. For large pieces of DNA, especially genomic DNA, bacteriophages, bacterial artificial chromosome (BAC) vectors, or yeast artificial chromosomes (YACs) are commonly used (For-

get 1993; Monaco and Larin 1994; Schlessinger 1990).

■ *Need for posttranscriptional or posttranslational modification:* If the studies with the cloned DNA require correct posttranscriptional (e.g., splicing) or posttranslational modifications, eukaryotic hosts (e.g., mammalian cell lines) will be necessary. RNA splicing is a process that was acquired by eukaryotic cells during evolution (Aloni et al. 1978).

Forward genetics. The most straightforward approach to the cloning of disease genes involves the cloning of DNA of known disease-causing proteins in a process called *forward genetics*. Proteins can be extracted, purified, and partially sequenced, and the nucleic acid sequence can be deduced from the amino acid sequence (see subsection, "Transcription: From DNA to mRNA," earlier in this chapter). The deduced DNA sequence is synthesized, and cDNA libraries (see subsection, "Cloning of DNA," above) are screened for a complete clone. Alternatively, antibodies raised against the purified protein can be used to screen a cDNA library transfected into bacteriophages. Bacteria that are transfected with the bacteriophages and the cDNA they carry will translate the cDNA into protein (Figure 2–7). Antibodies can be used to screen for the protein of interest, the bacteriophages containing the respective cDNA can be retrieved, and the sequence of the cDNA can be analyzed (Figure 2–7).

Reverse genetics and positional cloning. For the vast majority of inherited diseases, no underlying defective protein has been identified by biochemical analysis. In these cases, recombinant DNA techniques must be applied to identify the defective gene. *Reverse genetics* refers to the search for genes that cause inherited diseases and does not require any knowledge about their biological function (Gusella 1986, 1989). Disease genes are isolated based on their physical location on the chromosomes, a process referred to as *positional cloning*. In the simpler cases, the chromosomal location already may be known (e.g., affected individuals have obvious chromosomal dislocations or deletions), or the disease is X-linked and affects predominantly males, as in fragile X syndrome (Bell et al. 1991; McConkie-Rosell et al. 1993; Steyaert et al. 1996).

Positional cloning is made possible through a genetic map of unique DNA segments or genes (*genetic markers*), with known chromosomal locations, that exist in several alternative forms (*alleles*). Allelic variations are referred to as *polymorphisms*. Initially, the approximate distance of the genetic markers from one another is determined in the

general population by *linkage analysis*. Linkage analysis is based on the assumption that the likelihood that two genes will be passed on together in progeny decreases with increasing physical distance between them as a result of crossover events (recombination). It is not surprising that statistics is at the heart of linkage analysis. In reverse genetics, linkage analysis is used to examine the inheritance pattern of a particular trait or disease within large families by studying its relationship to the inheritance pattern of the mapped genetic markers. The closer a marker is to the gene of interest, the smaller is the likelihood for crossover events between them. In other words, a marker in the vicinity of the disease-causing gene does not distribute randomly with the risk for disorder, which is contrary to markers located on other chromosomes or markers located on the same chromosome but distant from the disease-causing gene. Thus, nearby markers will *cosegregate* with the gene, and the same marker allele will be shared by the affected individuals within a family. The disease gene and markers in the vicinity are in *linkage disequilibrium*. The closer a marker is to the disease locus, the larger is the linkage disequilibrium. If a genetic disorder originated from a mutation in a single founder (e.g., Huntington's dis-

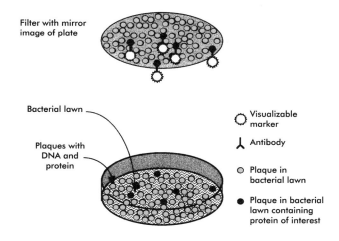

Figure 2–7. Screening complementary DNA (cDNA) libraries with antibodies. A lawn of bacteria transfected with bacteriophages that carry cDNA is grown on a petri dish. Bacteriophages will lyse the bacteria and transfect surrounding bacteria. Because of spreading bacterial lysis, small indentations (plaques) appear in the bacterial lawn at bacteriophage locations. When a filter is gently laid on the plate and removed, a replica of the plaques and the proteins they contain is created. The antibody (linked to a visualizable marker) is used to find plaques containing the protein the antibody was raised against. The original plaque on the plate contains the bacteriophages, which can be used to amplify and sequence the DNA of the protein of interest.

ease—see subsection, "Huntington's Disease," later in this chapter), linkage disequilibrium can be used to pinpoint the gene in seemingly unrelated families, an important statistical opportunity to increase the sample size.

Originally, restriction fragment length polymorphism (RFLP) was the method to determine allelic variations (Gusella 1986). RFLPs are based on the activity of *restriction endonucleases*, enzymes that cut double-stranded DNA at specific sequences. A single base change eliminates cleavage at that site. Thus, RFLPs differentiate two allele states: 1) restriction site present and 2) restriction site absent. More recently, highly polymorphic genetic markers were discovered. These markers are repeated sequences (e.g., $(CpG)_n$) embedded in unique sequences (Jeffreys et al. 1993; Sutherland and Richards 1995). The number of repeats is highly variable but follows Mendelian rules. Repeat sequences enable researchers to establish an abundant number of alleles, making the statistical power superior to that of RFLPs.

The more markers that are available, the more polymorphic they are, and the closer they are together, the easier it is to narrow down the location of the gene of interest. The goal of the *Human Genome Project* (Watson 1990) was to define enough markers on enough chromosomes to facilitate the search for disease-causing genes. Obviously, as increasing numbers of genes and genomic markers are identified on various chromosomes (Schuler et al. 1996), the ease of identifying new genes increases progressively.

Once the chromosomal location of the defect has been ascertained, the area can be cloned (e.g., into YACs) (Forget 1993; Monaco and Larin 1994; Schlessinger 1990) and further analyzed with various techniques. Because less than 1% of human DNA actually encodes proteins, techniques that specifically amplify gene-coding areas (e.g., *exon trapping, exon amplification*) (Datson et al. 1996; Duyk et al. 1990) are particularly useful. However, inherited diseases are not necessarily caused by mutations in coding areas of the gene, as is the case in Friedreich's ataxia, in which the mutation occurs in the first intron (Campuzano et al. 1996).

The identification of trinucleotide tandem repeat disorders is an important accomplishment of reverse genetics. In many disorders, a triplet sequence of bases such as $(CAG)_n$ may be excessively repeated, causing an abnormal expansion of a gene (Rosenberg 1996; Ross 1995; Sutherland and Richards 1995). A repeat located within the noncoding region (e.g., intron) could disrupt the expression of the gene, whereas a repeat in the coding region results in an expansion in a series of amino acids such as glutamine (polyglutamine repeat) (Ross 1995). The latter is the case for Huntington's disease, in which the mutation causes an increase in the length of a polyglutamine sequence from 36 to several hundred glutamines (The Huntington's Disease Collaborative Research Group 1993). Interestingly, trinucleotide repeat disorders do not follow the rules of Mendelian inheritance because the size of the repeat can vary (usually increase) from one generation to the next. The increase in severity and/or earlier age at onset of the disorder in successive generations is known as *anticipation* (Sutherland and Richards 1995). Trinucleotide repeat disorders have a proclivity for affecting the brain and include Huntington's disease (see subsection, "Huntington's Disease," later in this chapter), myotonic dystrophy (Brook et al. 1992; Mahadevan et al. 1992), fragile X syndrome (Bell et al. 1991; McConkie-Rosell et al. 1993; Steyaert et al. 1996), and Friedreich's ataxia (Campuzano et al. 1996). A common mechanism by which trinucleotide repeats cause neurodegeneration has not yet been detected, but these types of disorders have gained a lot of deserved attention. Anticipation has been described in affective disorders and schizophrenia (Bassett and Honer 1994; Gorwood et al. 1996; Thibaut et al. 1995); thus, interest in searching for expanded trinucleotide repeats in these psychiatric disorders is justified.

Transgenic and knockout mice. One of the most powerful experimental systems for mammalian research is provided by transgenic mice (Paigen 1995). With the advent of reverse genetics, the defective genes of an increasing number of neuropsychiatric disorders have been identified, yet their function may remain a mystery. Because the complexity of the human genome cannot be recreated in simple nonmammalian systems, manipulation of genes of interest in mice can serve as a model for characterizing their function. Thus, if a known gene defect in humans can be imitated in the mouse, a powerful system is available to study the effects of this gene defect and to learn about the parameters involved in the disease process. Eventually, this process can lead to the identification of molecular targets for therapeutic interventions and even to gene therapy (Suhr and Gage 1993).

The mouse genome can be manipulated in various ways: mouse genes can be deleted (*knockout*), mouse genes can be replaced by mutated genes, or genes can be added and overexpressed. Moreover, cell-specific gene regulation can be studied by linking regulatory elements (e.g., enhancer elements—see subsection, "Transcription: From DNA to mRNA," earlier in this chapter) of known genes to *reporter genes*, genes of which the expression can easily be visualized on a cellular level in the nervous system (e.g., Robertson et al. 1995).

In recent years, elegant methods used to generate *ge-*

netically engineered mice have been established. Genes within the mouse genome specifically can be targeted by *homologous recombination* and either rendered nonfunctional (in knockout mice) or replaced by a mutated version of the gene. Vectors containing the gene of interest are introduced into *embryonic stem cells*. Embryonic stem cells are undifferentiated cells derived from the mouse embryo that can be maintained indefinitely in culture. The vectors are engineered to allow for easy selection of mutated cells (e.g., only mutated cells will survive the culture conditions). Mutated cells are introduced into early mouse embryos, leading to *chimeric* mice, with patches of tissue, including germ cells, derived from the mutated embryonic stem cell. Chimeras with the mutated gene in their germ cells can be bred to attain homozygosity of the mutation in subsequent generations.

MOLECULAR NEUROBIOLOGY

Molecular biology has revolutionized the approach toward disorders of the brain. The ultimate goal of the molecular approach to neuropsychiatric disorders is to identify genes and proteins that determine normal and abnormal brain function and from this knowledge to develop pharmacological treatments that specifically correct the pathological consequences of mutant genes or alleles. In this section, we highlight three areas of recent research that exemplify the power of molecular techniques in the study of the brain.

First, we describe the success of positional cloning in the understanding of two diseases: Huntington's disease and Alzheimer's disease. This process has led to the discovery of disease genes and new proteins that have an unknown role in the etiology of the diseases. Second, we examine the genetics of some complex traits such as memory, nurturing behavior, novelty seeking, and anxiety. This area is potentially of great interest for understanding more complex brain function in humans. Finally, we review the current status of the genetics of two major psychiatric disorders: schizophrenia and bipolar disorder.

Huntington's Disease

Huntington's disease is characterized by a selective degeneration of neurons, particularly in the striatum, resulting in abnormal involuntary movements and personality changes. The typical symptoms (i.e., progressive cognitive decline, dysarthria, choreoathetosis, dystonia, and rigidity) have a mean age at onset of about 40 years, but symptoms may occur as early as age 2 years and as late as age 80 or 90 years (Young 1995). Huntington's disease is caused by a highly penetrant autosomal dominant gene. In the United States, 25,000 persons are affected by Huntington's disease, and approximately 150,000 persons are at a 50% risk for the disease. Because Huntington's disease is a *completely dominant* disorder (i.e., Huntington's disease homozygotes do not differ clinically from Huntington's disease heterozygotes), it became the first disorder from which to isolate a disease gene with positional cloning (Gusella et al. 1993).

In 1983, Gusella and his colleagues described a linkage between a polymorphic DNA marker, D4S10, on the short arm of chromosome 4 and the disease locus for Huntington's disease. The Huntington's disease gene was mapped to location 4p16.3. An unprecedented collaborative effort of 10 years was required to isolate the Huntington's disease gene. Genetic and physical maps of the candidate region were created on chromosome 4, and variable nucleotide tandem repeats were analyzed to identify more informative polymorphisms.

In 1993, the Huntington's Disease Collaborative Research Group found that Huntington's disease chromosomes contain an expanded and unstable trinucleotide $(CAG)_n$ repeat within the gene, termed *IT15* or *huntingtin*. The same repeat is present in normal chromosomes but is shorter, ranging from 11 to 34 copies of the repeat, and stably transmitted. In patients with Huntington's disease, the range of the repeat lengths extends from 37 to more than 100 repeats, with the number of repeats changing in meiotic transmissions. This increase in $(CAG)_n$ repeats is more marked during transmission from father to child (Gusella et al. 1993). The group also showed that increased length of the Huntington's disease trinucleotide repeat is associated with a younger age at onset of the disorder. Thus, juvenile-onset Huntington's disease has the longest trinucleotide repeats.

The gene affected in Huntington's disease, *IT15* or *huntingtin*, is expressed in several brain regions, with high levels of expression in the cerebellum and hippocampus and moderate levels in the striatum (Young 1995). All neuronal cells of the striatum, the proposed site of major pathology in Huntington's disease, express the *huntingtin* mRNA. Huntington's disease cases express a 350 kDA huntingtin protein, which contains the polyglutamine sequence translated from the $(CAG)_n$ repeat (A. H. Sharp et al. 1995). However, the Huntington's disease gene is not overexpressed in Huntington's disease. Furthermore, transgenic mice in which the *huntingtin* gene has been "knocked out" do not have the neuropathology of Huntington's disease (Ross 1995). These findings indicate that the expanded polyglutamine sequence in *huntingtin* confers a gain of function to the mutant gene product.

In parallel with the search for the gene responsible for Huntington's disease, neuroscientists were characterizing mechanisms responsible for neurodegeneration. Activation of glutamate ionotropic receptors on neurons caused a delayed, selective degeneration of neurons (Coyle and Schwarcz 1976). Intrastriatal injection of N-methyl-D-aspartate (NMDA) receptor agonists in experimental animals faithfully reproduced the pattern of neuronal degeneration that occurs in Huntington's disease (Beal et al. 1986). Furthermore, systemic treatment with agents that disrupt the mitochondrial electron transport chain and thereby impair oxidative metabolism caused striatal neuronal degeneration mediated by NMDA receptors (Coyle and Puttfarcken 1993).

These findings provide a neurobiological context for understanding how the mutant *huntingtin* might selectively sensitize striatal neurons for neuronal degeneration. Investigators recently showed that both the normal and the abnormal huntingtin proteins bind to another protein, huntingtin-associated protein (HAP), which is enriched in brain (Li et al. 1995; Trottier et al. 1995). Interestingly, the binding of HAP to huntingtin is increased by an expanded polyglutamine repeat in huntingtin. Furthermore, the polyglutamine repeat region in huntingtin also binds to glyceraldehyde phosphate dehydrogenase (Barinaga 1996; Burke et al. 1996; Gusella et al. 1993). Such an interaction might disrupt the energy state of striatal neurons analogous to that of mitochondrial toxins. Regardless of the precise mechanism whereby mutant huntingtin kills striatal neurons, these studies will inevitably provide clear targets for the development of pharmacological agents to arrest and even prevent this process.

Alzheimer's Disease

Alzheimer's disease is a neurodegenerative disorder characterized initially by a decline in memory that typically progresses to profound deterioration in cognitive and language functions and the appearance of apraxias. Currently, Alzheimer's disease affects more than 4 million people in the United States. The pathological hallmarks of Alzheimer's disease are amyloid deposits around blood vessels and in many brain areas, intraneuronal neurofibrillary tangles, neuronal cell loss, and brain atrophy. The cause and the time sequence for the development of these pathological markers are unknown, but most evidence supports the hypothesis that pathological deposition of amyloid is the initiating event in Alzheimer's disease. Recently, four genes have been linked to Alzheimer's disease: most cases of early-onset familial Alzheimer's disease are caused by mutations in genes on chromosomes 1, 14, and 21. Late-onset Alzheimer's disease, both sporadic and familial, has been linked to a gene on chromosome 19 (Table 2–1) (Hisama and Schellenberg 1996).

Advances in the molecular biology of Alzheimer's disease reflect the application of both forward and reverse genetics. On the one hand, the observation of Alzheimer's disease neuropathology in patients older than 30 with Down's syndrome led researchers to test for linkage between Alzheimer's disease and markers on chromosome 21. In 1987, St. George-Hyslop et al. reported such linkage for chromosome 21 in four large pedigrees affected by early-onset Alzheimer's disease. On the other hand, the amyloid protein was purified from the brains of patients with Alzheimer's disease and Down's syndrome and characterized as a polypeptide of 40–42 amino acids. Screening of a human cDNA library with the predicted sequence for amyloid yielded a gene coding for a much larger protein, the amyloid precursor protein (APP), which contained within it the amyloid motif. The APP gene was mapped to chromosome 21 (Kang et al. 1987; Tanzi et al. 1987). Subsequently, several mutations of the APP gene were identified in pedigrees with several cases of Alzheimer's disease or a related condition, hereditary cerebral hemorrhage with amyloidosis—Dutch type (Hisama and Schellenberg 1996). The different mutations of the APP gene (involving codons 670–671, 692, 693, 717, and 770) cluster around the A β segment (codon 672–714). Although it was exciting to link a mutation in one gene to the occurrence of Alzheimer's disease, mutations of the APP gene occur

Table 2–1.   Genes linked to Alzheimer's disease

Gene	Gene type	Chromosome	Chromosome location	Protein	Age at onset	% of familial cases	% of all cases
β*APP*	AD	21	q21	APP	Early	2–3	<1
PS1	AD	14	q24	S182 (=PS1)	Early	50	5–10
PS2	AD	1	q31–42	STM2 (=PS2)	Early		?
APOE	Risk factor	19	q13	APOE-ε4	Late	?	40–50

Note.   APP = amyloid precursor protein; PS1 = Presenilin 1; PS2 = Presenilin 2; APOE = apolipoprotein E.

in fewer than 5% of all familial Alzheimer's disease cases.

A substantial portion (i.e., about 70%) of familial cases of Alzheimer's disease showed an association with a second locus, found by linkage on chromosome 14 (Schellenberg et al. 1992). In 1995, Sherrington et al. found that a novel gene—initially termed *S182* and now called *Presenilin 1 (PS1)*—caused this linkage. Shortly after the *PS1* gene was described, a third locus for familial Alzheimer's disease was found on chromosome 1 in families descended from the Volga Germans (Levy-Lahad et al. 1995a, 1995b; Rogaev et al. 1995). This gene, *Presenilin 2 (PS2)*, has 67% homology with *PS1* at the amino acid level. More than 30 point mutations have been found in *PS1* and several in *PS2* that cosegregate with early-onset familial Alzheimer's disease, which strongly indicates a causative role for both genes.

The presenilins code for a seven transmembrane protein, similar to G-protein coupled receptors, but the biological functions are as yet unknown. They resemble two proteins found in the small nematode *Caenorhabditis elegans*, *sel-12* and *spe-4*, which are involved in cell fate decisions and intracellular protein trafficking. Researchers are now studying whether *PS1* and *PS2* play a role in programmed cell death or the processing of β-amyloid protein. For example, overexpression of *PS2* in nerve growth factor–differentiated PC12 cells increases apoptosis induced by trophic factor withdrawal or β-amyloid (Wolozin et al. 1996). Cells transfected with *PS1* double their secretion of amyloid, especially the Aβ1-42 form that appears to be particularly toxic.

Mutations in *APP, PS1,* and *PS2* appear to account for most early-onset, hereditary Alzheimer's disease; however, most Alzheimer's disease has a late onset and weak familial patterns. Strittmatter et al. (1993) reported a highly significant association of the apolipoprotein E type ε4 (APOE-ε4) allele on the long arm of chromosome 19 and late-onset familial Alzheimer's disease. Several series of sporadic Alzheimer's disease cases showed a similar association (Saunders et al. 1993). APOE, cholesterol-binding protein, exists in three major isoforms: the two uncommon forms, ε2 and ε4, and the predominant form, ε3. In patients with Alzheimer's disease, the frequency of the ε4 isoform was significantly higher than that in control subjects. The APOE-ε4 allele is neither necessary nor adequate to develop Alzheimer's disease: many individuals with Alzheimer's disease do not have the APOE-ε4 allele, and many individuals who carry the allele do not develop Alzheimer's disease. However, the APOE-ε4 allele confers a greater risk to develop Alzheimer's disease. For example, the risk for Alzheimer's disease increased from 20% to 90% and mean age at onset decreased from 84 to 68 years with increasing number of APOE-ε4 alleles in 42 families with late-onset Alzheimer's disease (Corder et al. 1993). APOE is localized in senile plaques and binds avidly to β-amyloid protein; thus, APOE probably is involved in the processing of APP and the generation of amyloid plaques (Strittmatter et al. 1993).

Since several genes responsible for Alzheimer's disease have been identified, researchers are focusing on potential interactions of these genes' normal and mutant proteins in brain and in cell culture systems. Evidence is mounting that these mutations or allelic variations favor a catabolic pathway for APP that generates amyloid and not one that prevents the secretion of amyloid (Yankner 1996). Furthermore, with the creation of transgenic mice that overexpress human mutant APP, the sequence of events from amyloid deposition through neuronal degeneration can be characterized. These studies are yielding molecular targets for drug development—for example, by inhibiting the pathogenic protease involved in the secretion of amyloid, by interfering with APOE-ε4's role in the aggregation of amyloid, or by protecting against the cytotoxic consequences of amyloid (Selkoe 1997).

Complex Traits

Studying the genetic basis of complex behaviors (e.g., memory, affect, or interpersonal interaction) is obviously much more demanding than analyzing a disease with dominant inheritance such as Huntington's disease. However, recent studies, one using experiments in transgenic mice and another investigating the effects of genes on quantifiable traits of human behavior, have reported that complex behavior can be dissected at the genetic level. Generally, this research is a variant of forward genetics, which takes advantage of rapid advances in developmental and cellular neurobiology. As specific proteins are identified, their genes are cloned, offering two possible strategies: 1) transgenic methods produce mice that differ from wild types (i.e., normal mice) only in the expression of the target gene and often show no discernible anatomical or gross behavioral differences, and 2) investigators search for allelic variants that may correlate with behavioral phenotypes consistent with the identified function of the protein.

Transgenic methods were used to produce mice that did not express the enzyme α-calcium-calmodulin-dependent kinase II (CaMKII). These mice were unable to produce long-term potentiation (LTP) in the hippocampus (Silva et al. 1992b) and thus were unable to learn new spatial memory when tested in a Morris water maze (Silva et al. 1992a). Although this behavioral deficit was consistent with the hypothesized role of CaMKII in modulating glutamatergic neurotransmission, alternative explanations could not be ruled out. For example, CaMKII may be essential for normal brain development so that memory impairment in the transgenic mice simply resulted from disrupted neuronal circuitry. Or, because CaMKII is broadly expressed in the brain, the behavioral impairment might have resulted from a global disruption of neuronal function unrelated to CaMKII's function in the hippocampus.

Recently, researchers used refined transgenic methods to produce animals with spatially and temporally restricted expression of target genes (Mayford et al. 1996; Tsien et al. 1996a). First, expression of a mutant version of CaMKII, resulting in constant autophosphorylation and activation of this kinase only in the hippocampus and only for a limited time during adulthood, resulted in a specific and reversible loss of LTP and spatial memory deficit (Mayford et al. 1996). Second, deletion of the NMDA receptor 1 gene (*NMDAR1*), which encodes the essential subunit of the NMDA receptor, in the hippocampal CA1 sector after the hippocampus had been developed abolished NMDA-receptor-mediated synaptic currents and LTP, which resulted in impaired spatial memory (Tsien et al. 1996b). These results indicate that functional CaMKII and NMDA receptor in specific subsectors of the hippocampus are prerequisites for the formation of spatial memory.

Another interesting, almost serendipitous finding was reported for mice that lack the *fosB* gene, an immediate early gene that codes for a transcription factor involved in the regulation of gene expression. Surprisingly, these mice appeared to have normal brains at microscopic inspection and a normal repertoire of behaviors, including the ability to mate. However, female mice that lacked the *fosB* gene completely disregarded their pups, which led to starvation and early death of the offspring (Brown et al. 1996). Exposure of the normal female mice to their pups resulted in the induction of fosB protein expression in the preoptic area of the hypothalamus, an area that was known to be involved in nurturing behavior from previous lesion experiments (Numan et al. 1988). Thus, activation of *fosB* in a specific neuronal circuit seems to be involved in the mediation of nurturing behavior, and the loss of the gene disrupts nurturing behavior in a specific manner. Although complex behavior cannot be reduced to the expression of just one gene, the *CaMKII* and *fosB* knockout experiments point to at least a genetic component in complex behavior.

Gene deletion and the study of its effects are not possible in humans. Therefore, researchers use a different strategy to study the genetic basis of complex traits in humans. Large sets of genetic data, typically the individual pattern of polymorphic markers, are correlated with behavioral data sets (e.g., scores from rating scales of normal or abnormal behavioral traits). Such a strategy successfully showed an association between a dopamine D_4 receptor gene polymorphism on the short arm of chromosome 11 and novelty-seeking scores (Benjamin et al. 1996; Ebstein et al. 1996). Total heritability of novelty seeking is about 40%, and the D_4 receptor polymorphism appears to account for about 10% of the genetic variation in the trait of novelty seeking. The link of novelty seeking to the D_4 receptor is intriguing because previous studies had shown increased blood flow and uptake of 18-fluoro-dopa in the striatum and high prolactin levels, indicating enhanced dopaminergic tone in such individuals (Cloninger et al. 1996).

Another recent study proposed an association between anxiety-related traits and a polymorphism in the serotonin transporter gene regulatory region (Lesch et al. 1996). The polymorphism gives rise to two alleles: the short (s) and long (l) allele. The l allele leads to a higher expression of the transporter protein. Interestingly, the subjects with the l allele scored significantly higher on the subscale for neuroticism. The polymorphism accounts for 3%–4% of total variation and 7%–9% of inherited variance in anxiety-related personality traits. Again, the linkage is intriguing because it associates a well-studied personality trait with a neurotransmitter system (i.e., the serotonergic system) that has been implicated in the origin and pharmacological manipulation of anxiety. It seems reasonable to anticipate that such research designs, linking quantifiable behavioral traits to genetic factors, should also contribute to the understanding of schizophrenia and bipolar disorder (Lander and Schork 1994; Plomin et al. 1994; Risch and Merikangas 1996).

Schizophrenia and Bipolar Disorder

Schizophrenia is a psychotic disorder of complex inheritance that is characterized by varying degrees of delusions, hallucinations, cognitive deficits, and flattening of affect. The risk of developing schizophrenia is 1% in the general population but approximately 50% for the monozygotic twin of an affected proband, about 10% for a sibling or a parent, and about 3% for a niece or nephew. Schizophrenia does not fit the pattern seen for a single (dominant, additive, or recessive) disease gene in which the risk to develop the disease would decrease by one-half as one progresses to the next more distant family member. However, it seems to fit the pattern of oligogenic inheritance (i.e., there is an interaction between a few genes) (Risch and Merikangas 1996).

In 1988, Sherrington et al. reported the first evidence for linkage between a schizophrenia locus and two markers on the long arm of chromosome 5. Unfortunately, subsequent studies basically ruled out a linkage in several other pedigrees (Detera-Wadleigh et al. 1989; Kennedy et al. 1988; McGuffin et al. 1990; St Clair et al. 1989). Other investigators reported conflicting results for linkage between a schizophrenia locus and markers on chromosomes 5, 8, 11, and 22 (Karayiorgou and Gogos 1997). The most robust finding so far in the search for a schizophrenia disease gene was reported for the short arm of chromosome 6, involving several markers in the region 6p21–24 (Antonarakis et al. 1995; Diehl et al. 1994; Moises et al. 1995; Schwab et al. 1995; Straub et al. 1995; Wang et al. 1995). However, other reports did not confirm a linkage (Gurling et al. 1995; Mowry et al. 1995).

Bipolar disorder is a mood disorder characterized by manic episodes and in most cases intermittent depressive episodes. Family studies have reported a 7% risk for first-degree relatives of bipolar probands compared with a 1% lifetime prevalence rate in the general population. The concordance is 65% for monozygotic twins and 15% for dizygotic twins.

In 1987, Egeland et al. reported linkage between a bipolar disorder locus and a marker on chromosome 11 in an Old Order Amish pedigree, but subsequent studies excluded a linkage (Kelsoe et al. 1989; McInnis 1997). Several other chromosomes have been implicated to carry a disease locus for bipolar disorder (McInnis 1997). Reports of a susceptibility locus near the pericentromeric region of chromosome 18 are particularly encouraging (Berrettini et al. 1994; McInnis 1997).

In contrast to the success story of molecular biology in the study of Huntington's disease and Alzheimer's disease, the search for a genetic basis of schizophrenia or bipolar disorder has not yet yielded a single disease locus or gene, and researchers have not identified any protein that could be implicated in the pathophysiology of the diseases. The failure to replicate linkage of potential disease loci with schizophrenia and bipolar disorder among different pedigrees is not surprising given the experience with Alzheimer's disease, in which several genes are implicated. Psychiatric disorders more typically may reflect complex disease traits, in which several genes interact and contribute to the risk of the disorder. However, the elucidation of such vulnerability genes will set the stage for clarifying their role in neuronal function, the mechanisms of interactions, and the final common pathway to the behavioral phenotype, as has been done with Alzheimer's disease research.

RELEVANCE OF MOLECULAR BIOLOGY TO NEUROPSYCHOPHARMACOLOGY

The search for the location of disease-causing genes and the subsequent analysis of the function of these disease-causing genes apparently have important implications for the establishment of therapeutic interventions for neuropsychiatric disorders (Roses 1996). Gene therapy, for example, is a potentially potent newer method of treating several brain disorders (Suhr and Gage 1993).

Molecular biology can provide the means to elucidate unique neuronal pathways of drug response, is centrally involved in the function of drugs, and can be used in the search for new drug strategies. In schizophrenia research, for example, the two major hypotheses that have emerged implicate either the dopaminergic system or the glutamatergic system in the primary pathophysiology. With the help of molecular biology, common denominators can be identified to link both hypotheses. Data recently established in our laboratories suggest a strong intraneuronal cooperation of second-messenger pathways activated by glutamate and dopamine receptors (Konradi et al. 1996). Thus, pharmacological intervention (e.g., at the dopamine receptor) will affect the neuronal response to glutamate.

Another example of the role of molecular biology in pharmacology concerns drugs of abuse. Most psychotropic drugs have an immediate action (e.g., a receptor ligand inhibits or activates the receptor) and a delayed action. The delayed action may not be apparent immediately, can last for a period exceeding hours or even months, and may persevere long after withdrawal of the drug. For instance, drugs of abuse (e.g., amphetamine or cocaine) have long-lasting effects such as drug dependence and drug tolerance. Based on the prolonged time course of drug dependence and drug tolerance, these processes almost certainly involve drug-induced alterations in gene expression. Not surprisingly, amphetamine (and cocaine) regulates the expression of several genes, including *prodynorphin* (Cole et al. 1995) and *c-fos* (Graybiel et al. 1990). Moreover, amphetamine induces phosphorylation of transcription factor CREB in rat in vivo (Konradi et al. 1994). Because CREB has been implicated in the activation of several immediate early genes and several neuropeptide genes (see also Figures 2–4 and 2–6), CREB phosphorylation is an important nuclear event capable of mediating long-term consequences of amphetamine or cocaine abuse (Konradi et al. 1994).

Likewise, neuroleptics and antidepressants have delayed therapeutic effects, which constitute a major part of their therapeutic properties (Manji et al. 1995). These delayed drug actions can only be explained by structural or functional changes in the neurons responsive to these drugs. The events that enable neurons to adapt to altered stimulation and to manifest long-lasting changes are the core of molecular biology. How neurons memorize a previous drug action and how the response adapts to temporal and quantitative exposure can only be explained by mechanisms inherent to molecular biology.

CONCLUSION

In summary, molecular biology is transforming the approach to drug discovery in clinical psychopharmacology. As the characterization of the chromosomal location and function of a rapidly increasing number of brain proteins (i.e., forward genetics) advances in tandem with the localization of heritable risk factors for psychopathology (i.e., reverse genetics), the ability to understand molecular mechanisms will progressively accelerate. This knowledge will reveal complex gene-environment interactions that lead to the behavioral phenotypes that are operationally categorized in DSM-IV (American Psychiatric Association 1994). Understanding the converging pathways in neuronal function that result in the behavioral phenotype will disclose molecular targets that should permit the development of more effective and specific drugs. Finally, drug selection will likely depend on molecular diagnosis in conjunction with clinical assessment.

REFERENCES

Aloni Y, Bratosin S, Dhar R, et al: Splicing of SV40 mRNAs: a novel mechanism for the regulation of gene expression in animal cells. Cold Spring Harb Symp Quant Biol 42 (pt 1):559–570, 1978

American Psychiatric Association: Diagnostic and Statistical Manual of Mental Disorders, 4th Edition. Washington, DC, American Psychiatric Association, 1994

Antonarakis SE, Blouin J-L, Pulver AE, et al: Schizophrenia susceptibility and chromosome 6p24-22. Nat Genet 11:235–236, 1995

Arias J, Alberts AS, Brindle P, et al: Activation of cAMP and mitogen responsive genes relies on a common nuclear factor. Nature 370:226–229, 1994

Barinaga M: An intriguing new lead on Huntington's disease [news]. Science 271:1233–1234, 1996

Barlow DP: Gametic imprinting in mammals. Science 270:1610–1613, 1995

Bassett AS, Honer WG: Evidence for anticipation in schizophrenia. Am J Hum Genet 54:864–870, 1994

Beal MF, Kowall NW, Ellison DW, et al: Replication of the neurochemical characteristics of Huntington's disease by quinolinic acid. Nature 321:168–172, 1986

Bell MV, Hirst MC, Nakahori Y, et al: Physical mapping across the fragile X: hypermethylation and clinical expression of the fragile X syndrome. Cell 64:861–866, 1991

Benjamin J, Li L, Patterson C, et al: Population and familial association between the D4 dopamine receptor gene and measures of novelty seeking. Nat Genet 12:81–84, 1996

Berrettini WH, Ferraro TN, Goldin LR, et al: Chromosome 18 DNA markers and manic-depressive illness: evidence for a susceptibility gene. Proc Natl Acad Sci U S A 91: 5918–5921, 1994

Bestor TH, Tycko B: Creation of genomic methylation patterns. Nat Genet 12:363–367, 1996

Bingham PM, Chou TB, Mims I, et al: On/off regulation of gene expression at the level of splicing. Trends Genet 4:134–138, 1988

Brook JD, McCurrach ME, Harley HG, et al: Molecular basis of myotonic dystrophy: expansion of a trinucleotide (CTG) repeat at the 3′ end of a transcript encoding a protein kinase family member. Cell 68:799–808, 1992

Brown JR, Ye H, Bronson RT, et al: A defect in nurturing in mice lacking the immediate early gene *fosB*. Cell 86:297–309, 1996

Burke JR, Enghild JJ, Martin ME, et al: Huntingtin and DRPLA proteins selectively interact with the enzyme GAPDH. Nature Medicine 2:347–350, 1996

Campuzano V, Montermini L, Molto MD, et al: Friedreich's ataxia: autosomal recessive disease caused by an intronic GAA triplet repeat expansion [see comments]. Science 271:1423–1427, 1996

Cech TR: RNA splicing: three themes with variations. Cell 34:713–716, 1983

Chrivia JC, Kwok RP, Lamb N, et al: Phosphorylated CREB binds specifically to the nuclear protein CBP. Nature 365:855–859, 1993

Cloninger CR, Adolfsson R, Svrakic NM: Mapping genes for human personality. Nat Genet 12:3–4, 1996

Cole RL, Konradi C, Douglass J, et al: Neuronal adaptation to amphetamine and dopamine: molecular mechanisms of prodynorphin gene regulation in rat striatum. Neuron 14:813–823, 1995

Comb M, Birnberg NC, Seasholtz A, et al: A cyclic AMP- and phorbol ester-inducible DNA element. Nature 323:353–356, 1986

Corder EH, Saunders AM, Strittmatter WJ, et al: Gene dose of apolipoprotein E type 4 allele and the risk of Alzheimer's disease in late onset families. Science 261:921–923, 1993

Cote TE, Eskay RL, Frey EA, et al: Biochemical and physiological studies of the beta-adrenoceptor and the D-2 dopamine receptor in the intermediate lobe of the rat pituitary gland: a review. Neuroendocrinology 35:217–224, 1982

Coyle JT, Puttfarcken P: Oxidative stress, glutamate, and neurodegenerative disorders. Science 262:689–695, 1993

Coyle JT, Schwarcz R: Lesions of striatal neurones with kainic acid provides a model for Huntington's chorea. Nature 263:244–246, 1976

Crick F: Split genes and RNA splicing. Science 204:264–271, 1979

Datson NA, van de Vosse E, Dauwerse HG, et al: Scanning for genes in large genomic regions: cosmid-based exon trapping of multiple exons in a single product. Nucleic Acids Res 24:1105–1111, 1996

Detera-Wadleigh SD, Goldin LR, Sherrington R, et al: Exclusion of linkage to 5q11-13 in families with schizophrenia and other psychiatric disorders. Nature 340:391–393, 1989

Diehl SR, Wang S, Detera-Wadleigh S, et al: Evidence suggesting possible SCA1 gene involvement in schizophrenia (abstract). Am J Hum Genet 55 (suppl):867, 1994

Dores RM: The proopiomelanocortin family. Prog Clin Biol Res 342:22–27, 1990

Douglass J, McKinzie AA, Pollock KM: Identification of multiple DNA elements regulating basal and protein kinase A-induced transcriptional expression of the rat prodynorphin gene. Mol Endocrinol 8:333–344, 1994

Duyk GM, Kim SW, Myers RM, et al: Exon trapping: a genetic screen to identify candidate transcribed sequences in cloned mammalian genomic DNA. Proc Natl Acad Sci U S A 87:8995–8999, 1990

Ebstein RP, Novick O, Umansky R, et al: Dopamine D4 receptor (D4DR) exon III polymorphism associated with the human personality trait of novelty seeking. Nat Genet 12:78–80, 1996

Egeland JA, Gerhard DS, Pauls DL, et al: Bipolar affective disorders linked to DNA markers on chromosome 11. Nature 325:783–787, 1987

Forget BG: YAC transgenes: bigger is probably better. Proc Natl Acad Sci U S A 90:7909–7911, 1993

Gonzalez GA, Montminy MR: Cyclic AMP stimulates somatostatin gene transcription by phosphorylation of CREB at serine 133. Cell 59:675–680, 1989

Gorwood P, Leboyer M, Falissard B, et al: Anticipation in schizophrenia: new light on a controversial problem. Am J Psychiatry 153:1173–1177, 1996

Graybiel AM, Moratalla R, Robertson HA: Amphetamine and cocaine induce drug-specific activation of the c-fos gene in striosome-matrix compartments and limbic subdivisions of the striatum. Proc Natl Acad Sci U S A 87:6912–6916, 1990

Grosschedl R, Wasylyk B, Chambon P, et al: Point mutation in the TATA box curtails expression of sea urchin H2A histone gene in vivo. Nature 294:178–180, 1981

Gurling H, Kalsi G, Hui-Sui Chen A, et al: Schizophrenia susceptibility and chromosome 6p24-22. Nat Genet 11:234–235, 1995

Gusella JF: DNA polymorphism and human disease. Annu Rev Biochem 55:831–854, 1986

Gusella JF: Location cloning strategy for characterizing genetic defects in Huntington's disease and Alzheimer's disease. FASEB J 3:2036–2041, 1989

Gusella JF, MacDonald ME, Ambrose CM, et al: Molecular genetics of Huntington's disease. Arch Neurol 50:1157–1163, 1993

Hisama FM, Schellenberg GD: Progress in molecular genetics of Alzheimer's disease. The Neuroscientist 2:3–6, 1996

The Huntington's Disease Collaborative Research Group: A novel gene containing a trinucleotide repeat that is expanded and unstable on Huntington's disease chromosomes. Cell 72:971–983, 1993

Jeffreys AJ, Monckton DG, Tamaki K, et al: Minisatellite variant repeat mapping: application to DNA typing and mutation analysis. EXS 67:125–139, 1993

Kang J, Lemaire H-G, Unterbeck A, et al: The precursor of Alzheimer's disease amyloid A4-protein resembles a cell-surface receptor. Nature 325:733–736, 1987

Karayiorgou M, Gogos JA: A turning point in schizophrenia genetics. Neuron 19:967–979, 1997

Kee BL, Arias J, Montminy MR, et al: Adaptor-mediated recruitment of RNA polymerase II to a signal-dependent activator. J Biol Chem 271:2373–2375, 1996

Kelsoe JR, Ginns EI, Egeland JA, et al: Re-evaluation of the linkage relationship between chromosome 11p loci and the gene for bipolar affective disorder in the Old Order Amish. Nature 342:238–243, 1989

Kennedy JL, Giuffra LA, Moises HW, et al: Evidence against linkage of schizophrenia to markers on chromosome 5 in a northern Swedish pedigree. Nature 336:167–170, 1988

Konradi C, Cole RL, Heckers S, et al: Amphetamine regulates gene expression in rat striatum via transcription factor CREB. J Neurosci 14:5623–5634, 1994

Konradi C, Leveque JC, Hyman SE: Amphetamine and dopamine-induced immediate early gene expression in striatal neurons depends upon postsynaptic NMDA receptors and calcium. J Neurosci 16:4231–4239, 1996

Kwok RP, Lundblad JR, Chrivia JC, et al: Nuclear protein CBP is a coactivator for the transcription factor CREB [see comments]. Nature 370:223–226, 1994

Lander ES, Schork NJ: Genetic dissection of complex traits. Science 265:2037–2048, 1994

Lesch K-P, Bengel D, Heils A, et al: Association of anxiety-related traits with a polymorphism in the serotonin transporter gene regulatory region. Science 274:1527–1531, 1996

Levitzki A: From epinephrine to cyclic AMP. Science 241:800–806, 1988

Levy-Lahad E, Wasco W, Poorkaj P, et al: Candidate gene for the chromosome 1 familial Alzheimer's disease locus. Science 269:973–977, 1995a

Levy-Lahad E, Wijsman EM, Nemens E, et al: A familial Alzheimer's disease locus on chromosome 1. Science 269:970–973, 1995b

Li X-J, Li S-H, Sharp AH, et al: A Huntington-associated protein enriched in brain with implications for pathology. Nature 378:398–402, 1995

Mahadevan M, Tsilfidis C, Sabourin L, et al: Myotonic dystrophy mutation: an unstable CTG repeat in the 3′ untranslated region of the gene. Science 255:1253–1255, 1992

Manji HK, Potter WZ, Lenox RH: Signal transduction pathways: molecular targets for lithium's actions. Arch Gen Psychiatry 52:531–543, 1995

Mathis DJ, Chambon P: The SV40 early region TATA box is required for accurate in vitro initiation of transcription. Nature 290:310–315, 1981

Mayford M, Bach ME, Huang Y-Y, et al: Control of memory formation through regulated expression of a CaMKII transgene. Science 274:1678–1683, 1996

McConkie-Rosell A, Lachiewicz AM, Spiridigliozzi GA, et al: Evidence that methylation of the FMR-I locus is responsible for variable phenotypic expression of the fragile X syndrome. Am J Hum Genet 53:800–809, 1993

McGuffin P, Sargeant M, Hett G, et al: Exclusion of a schizophrenia susceptibility gene from the chromosome 5q11-q13 region: new data and a re-analysis of previous reports. Am J Hum Genet 47:524–535, 1990

McInnis MG: Recent advances in the genetics of bipolar disorder. Psychiatric Annals 27:482–488, 1997

McKnight S, Yamamoto Y: Transcriptional Regulation. Cold Spring Harbor, NY, Cold Spring Harbor Laboratory Press, 1992

Moises HW, Yang L, Kristbjarnarson H, et al: An international two-stage genome-wide search for schizophrenia susceptibility genes. Nat Genet 11:321–324, 1995

Monaco AP, Larin Z: YACs, BACs, PACs and MACs: artificial chromosomes as research tools. Trends in Biotechnology 12:280–286, 1994

Monsma FJ Jr, Mahan LC, McVittie LD, et al: Molecular cloning and expression of a D1 dopamine receptor linked to adenylyl cyclase activation. Proc Natl Acad Sci U S A 87:6723–6727, 1990

Montminy MR, Bilezikjian LM: Binding of a nuclear protein to the cyclic-AMP response element of the somatostatin gene. Nature 328:175–178, 1987

Montminy MR, Gonzalez GA, Yamamoto KK: Regulation of cAMP-inducible genes by CREB. Trends Neurosci 13:184–188, 1990

Morris RGM, Morris RJ: Memory floxed. Nature 385:680–681, 1997

Mowry BJ, Nancarrow DJ, Lennon DP, et al: Schizophrenia susceptibility and chromosome 6p24-22. Nat Genet 11:233–234, 1995

Numan M: A neural circuitry analysis of maternal behavior in the rat. Acta Paediatr Suppl 397:19–28, 1988

Paigen K: A miracle enough: the power of mice. Nature Medicine 1:215–220, 1995

Plomin R, Owen MJ, McGuffin P: The genetic basis of complex human behaviors. Science 264:1733–1739, 1994

Risch N, Merikangas K: The future of genetic studies of complex human diseases. Science 273:1516–1517, 1996

Robertson LM, Kerppola TK, Vendrell M, et al: Regulation of c-fos expression in transgenic mice requires multiple interdependent transcription control elements. Neuron 14:241–252, 1995

Rogaev EI, Sherrington R, Rogaeva EA, et al: Familial Alzheimer's disease in kindreds with missense mutations in a gene on chromosome 1 related to the Alzheimer's disease type 3 gene. Nature 376:775–778, 1995

Rosenberg RN: DNA-triplet repeats and neurologic disease. N Engl J Med 335:1222–1224, 1996

Roses AD: From genes to mechanisms to therapies: lessons to be learned from neurological disorders [see comments]. Nature Medicine 2:267–269, 1996

Ross CA: When more is less: pathogenesis of glutamine repeat neurodegenerative diseases. Neuron 15:493–496, 1995

Rossant J, Nagy A: Genome engineering: the new mouse genetics. Nature Medicine 1:592–594, 1995

Saunders AM, Strittmatter WJ, Schmechel D, et al: Association of apolipoprotein E allele ε4 with late-onset familial and sporadic Alzheimer's disease. Neurology 43:1467–1472, 1993

Schacher S, Glanzman D, Barzilai A, et al: Long-term facilitation in Aplysia: persistent phosphorylation and structural changes. Cold Spring Harb Symp Quant Biol 55:187–202, 1990

Schellenberg GD, Bird TD, Wijsman EM, et al: Genetic linkage evidence for a familial Alzheimer's disease locus on chromosome 14. Science 258:668–671, 1992

Schlessinger D: Yeast artificial chromosomes: tools for mapping and analysis of complex genomes. Trends Genet 6:248, 255–258, 1990

Schuler GD, Boguski MS, Hudson TJ, et al: Genome maps 7: the human transcript map (wall chart). Science 274:547–562, 1996

Schwab SG, Albus M, Hallmayer J, et al: Evaluation of a susceptibility gene for schizophrenia on chromosome 6p by multipoint affected sib-pair linkage analysis. Nat Genet 11:325–327, 1995

Selkoe DJ: Alzheimer's disease: genotypes, phenotypes, and treatments. Science 275:630–631, 1997

Sharp AH, Loev SJ, Schilling G, et al: Widespread expression of Huntington's disease gene (IT15) protein product. Neuron 14:1065–1074, 1995

Sharp PA: Split genes and RNA splicing. Cell 77:805–815, 1994

Sherrington R, Brynjolfsson J, Petursson H, et al: Localization of a susceptibility locus for schizophrenia on chromosome 5. Nature 336:164–167, 1988

Sherrington R, Rogaev EI, Liang Y, et al: Cloning of a gene bearing missense mutations in early onset familial Alzheimer's disease. Nature 375:754–760, 1995

Shuldiner MD: Molecular medicine: transgenic animal. N Engl J Med 334:653–655, 1996

Silva AJ, Paylor R, Wehner JM, et al: Impaired spatial learning in α-calcium-calmodulin kinase II mutant mice. Science 257:206–211, 1992a

Silva AJ, Stevens CF, Tonegawa S, et al: Deficient hippocampal long-term potentiation in α-calcium-calmodulin kinase II mutant mice. Science 257:201–206, 1992b

St Clair D, Blackwood D, Muir W, et al: No linkage of chromosome 5q11-13 markers to schizophrenia in Scottish families. Nature 339:305–307, 1989

Steyaert J, Borghgraef M, Legius E, et al: Molecular-intelligence correlations in young fragile X males with a mild CGG repeat expansion in the FMR1 gene. Am J Med Genet 64:274–277, 1996

St. George-Hyslop P, Tanzi RE, Polinsky RJ, et al: The genetic defect causing familial Alzheimer disease maps on chromosome 21. Science 235:885–889, 1987

Straub RE, MacLean CJ, O'Neill FA, et al: A potential vulnerability locus for schizophrenia on chromosome 6p24-22: evidence for genetic heterogeneity. Nat Genet 11:287–293, 1995

Strittmatter WJ, Saunders AM, Schmechel D, et al: Apolipoprotein E: high-avidity binding to β-amyloid and increased frequency of type 4 allele in late-onset familial Alzheimer's disease. Proc Natl Acad Sci U S A 90:1977–1981, 1993

Suhr ST, Gage FH: Gene therapy for neurologic disease. Arch Neurol 50:1252–1268, 1993

Sutherland GR, Richards RI: Simple tandem DNA repeats and human genetic disease. Proc Natl Acad Sci U S A 92:3636–3641, 1995

Tanzi RE, Gusella JF, Watkins PC, et al: Amyloid b-protein gene: cDNA, mRNA distributions and genetic linkage near the Alzheimer locus. Science 235:880–884, 1987

Thibaut F, Martinez M, Petit M, et al: Further evidence for anticipation in schizophrenia. Psychiatry Res 59:25–33, 1995

Tjian R, Maniatis T: Transcriptional activation: a complex puzzle with few easy pieces. Cell 77:5–8, 1994

Trottier Y, Lutz Y, Stevanin G, et al: Polyglutamine expansion as a pathological epitope in Huntington's disease and four dominant cerebellar ataxias. Nature 378:403–406, 1995

Tsien JZ, Chen DF, Gerber D, et al: Subregion- and cell type-restricted gene knockout in mouse brain. Cell 87:1317–1326, 1996a

Tsien JZ, Huerta PT, Tonegawa S: The essential role of hippocampal CA1 NMDA receptor-dependent synaptic plasticity in spatial memory. Cell 87:1327–1338, 1996b

Wang S, Sun CE, Walczak CA, et al: Evidence for a susceptibility locus for schizophrenia on chromosome 6pter-p22. Nat Genet 10:41–46, 1995

Watson JD: The Human Genome Project: past, present, and future. Science 248:44–49, 1990

Watson JD, Crick FHC: A structure for deoxyribonucleic acid. Nature 171:737–738, 1953

Wolffe AP: Transcription: in tune with the histones. Cell 77:13–16, 1994

Wolozin B, Iwasaki K, Vito P, et al: Participation of presenilin 2 in apoptosis: enhanced basal activity conferred by an Alzheimer mutation. Science 274:1710–1713, 1996

Yankner BA: Mechanisms of neuronal degeneration in Alzheimer's disease. Neuron 16:921–932, 1996

Young AB: Huntington's disease: lessons from and for molecular neuroscience. The Neuroscientist 1:51–58, 1995

THREE

Biochemical Anatomy: Insights Into the Cell Biology and Pharmacology of the Dopamine and Serotonin Systems in the Brain

Alfred Mansour, Ph.D., James H. Meador-Woodruff, M.D., Juan F. López, M.D., and Stanley J. Watson, Jr., Ph.D., M.D.

This volume contains numerous chapters focused on a range of clinical conditions that involve many regions of the central nervous system (CNS) and require a wide variety of drugs and approaches. This single chapter, therefore, cannot possibly describe the relevant cellular biology and anatomy for all these conditions and the therapeutic compounds discussed. Ideally, one could provide an overview of the 30–50 most relevant neurotransmitter systems and their associated cell biology and anatomy in order to fill these needs. Such an undertaking would require several volumes in its own right and is obviously impractical here. Rather, we have opted to focus this chapter on two major neurotransmitter systems—dopamine and serotonin—each of which is thought to be central to the current theories of certain psychiatric illnesses and the drugs used to treat them.

The primary aim of this chapter, then, is to provide the conceptual links between the neurotransmitter systems in the brain and the modes of action of psychotherapeutic drugs by using the dopamine and serotonin systems as prototypical examples. These links occur at several different levels of neuronal organization and require a knowledge of gross neuroanatomy, neuronal circuitry, synaptic regulation, and cellular biology. We discuss each of these levels in this chapter, with a particular emphasis on neuronal circuits, because they are fundamental to understanding the biological basis of drug action.

Early anatomists recognized that the brain is a complex organ. Gross anatomical criteria suggested that it could be divided into several regions, including the brain stem, cerebellum, midbrain, hypothalamus, thalamus, and cerebral cortex. In addition to gross anatomical divisions, differences were noted in cell morphology. For example, pyramidal neurons in the cerebral cortex were observed to be structurally different from the small, round neurons in the suprachiasmatic nucleus of the hypothalamus and the large pigmented neurons of the substantia nigra. More recently, neuroscientists reported that neurons can be classified by biochemical and structural criteria, which revolutionized anatomy and heralded the era of biochemical neuroanatomy. Investigators can now clearly demonstrate that neurons in the CNS have specific complements of neurotransmitters, transporters, receptors, guanine nucleotide binding proteins (G proteins), and other signal transduction molecules. Identifying neurons in the CNS in terms of their biochemical constituents and examining how they may form functional networks or circuits are, in fact, major functions of present-day neuroanatomists and are a focus of this chapter.

DOPAMINE-SYNTHESIZING CELL GROUPS

Brain dopamine projections are organized into four major circuits—the nigrostriatal, mesolimbic, tuberoinfundibular, and incertohypothalamic systems. Each system has specific anatomical and biochemical characteristics, and their activity regulates specific components of brain function.

The nigrostriatal circuit is one of the most extensive dopamine systems in the brain (Figure 3–1). Its importance in brain functioning is evidenced by the dramatic deficits in motor function observed in individuals with Parkinson's disease, a disorder that results in the destruction of most of the dopaminergic neurons in this circuit. Two groups of dopaminergic neurons, A8 and A9, form the presynaptic components of this circuit. A8 cells are located in the mesencephalic reticular formation and are closely associated with the A9 dopaminergic neurons. A9 dopaminergic neurons are located in the pars compacta region of the substantia nigra. The A8 and A9 neurons give rise to axons that travel to the forebrain through the medial forebrain bundle. These axons terminate mainly in the caudate nucleus and putamen, with a small group of axons also providing dopamine to the central amygdaloid nucleus (Anden et al. 1964; Ungerstedt 1971).

Neurons in the A10 cell group are the point of origin for the mesolimbic system. A10 dopaminergic neurons are located in the midbrain, medial to the A9 cells in the ventral tegmental area. This system runs parallel to the nigrostriatal system, with its axons ascending through the lateral hypothalamus in the medial forebrain bundle (Figure 3–1). Unlike the nigrostriatal system, the mesolimbic dopaminergic projection has a more diverse group of targets, including the nucleus accumbens, olfactory tubercle, bed nucleus of the stria terminalis, lateral septum, hippocampus, and the frontal, cingulate, and entorhinal regions of the cerebral cortex (Lindvall 1975; Lindvall et al. 1974; Moore 1978; Nauta et al. 1978; Ungerstedt 1971).

The tuberoinfundibular system consists of the dopaminergic cells in the arcuate nucleus of the hypothalamus and their projections. These A12 neurons send axons from their ventromedial location in the caudal hypothalamus to the external layer of the median eminence, where they terminate in the region of the hypothalamo-hypophyseal portal vessels (Hökfelt 1967; Hökfelt et al. 1976). This dopaminergic cell group is in a strategic position to influence the output of endocrine cells in the pituitary gland, especially prolactin-secreting cells.

Cells in the A11, A13, A14, and A15 groups make up the incertohypothalamic dopaminergic system of the diencephalon. A11 cells are located in the caudal periventricular hypothalamus dorsal to the A12 cells, which are found in the infundibular region of the hypothalamus. The zona incerta, a region of the dorsolateral caudal hypothalamus, contains the A13 dopaminergic cells. The A14 cells are located in the periventricular hypothalamus rostral to the A11 periventricular dopaminergic cells. Finally, the A15 dopaminergic neurons of the hypothalamus are found rostral, dorsal, and lateral to the A14 cells in the region of the paraventricular and supraoptic hypothalamic nuclei (Pearson et al. 1990). This diffuse dopamine system modulates many aspects of hypothalamic function.

In rats, the olfactory bulbs contain the only group of dopaminergic cells in the telencephalon. This group of cells is referred to as A16. Unlike other dopaminergic cells that in some cases have quite extensive projections, A16 cells are interneurons and participate only in local olfactory bulb circuitry. A vestige of this olfactory dopamine system, however, is observed in humans. These A16 cells are located in the substantia innominata region of the rostral forebrain (Pearson et al. 1990).

DOPAMINE RECEPTOR TYPES AND THEIR NEUROANATOMICAL DISTRIBUTIONS

Most of what we know about the distribution of dopamine in the CNS was well established in the 1970s with what are now conventional histochemical techniques. With development of selective ligands and binding conditions for the dopamine systems, we have been able to examine the

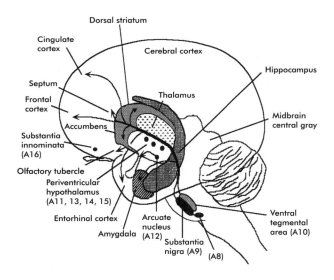

Figure 3–1. Dopaminergic cell groups and their projections. Presynaptic receptors are found on dopamine-producing cells, and postsynaptic receptors are found in their projection fields. See the text and Table 3–2 for details on dopamine binding and mRNA distributions.

other side of the synapse and selectively label the receptors to which dopamine can bind. It was not until the application of molecular biological techniques to the CNS in the 1980s, however, that we had a real appreciation of the complexity and diversity of the dopamine and serotonin receptors in the brain and the way drugs may interact to produce their physiological and behavioral effects. This technology has allowed the identification of many families and types of receptors, including the dopamine and serotonin receptors, as well as neurotransmitter transporters and G proteins that were previously unappreciated with conventional techniques.

Numerous behavioral and pharmacological studies initially identified two types of dopamine receptors: D_1 and D_2. Each receptor type has a distinct anatomical distribution (Bouthenet et al. 1987; Boyson et al. 1986; Charuchinda et al. 1987; Dawson et al. 1988; Mansour et al. 1990; Wamsley et al. 1989) and pharmacology and has been associated with different behavioral effects (Clark and White 1987; Stoof and Kebabian 1984). With the advent of molecular biological approaches, the number of proteins that can bind dopamine has increased to five and is likely to expand further. The five dopamine receptor types (D_1–D_5) can be divided into D_1 and D_2 receptor families and appear to be part of the superfamily of seven-transmembrane, G-protein-coupled receptors. The D_1 family consists of D_1 and D_5 receptors (Dearry et al. 1990; Monsma et al. 1990; Sunahara et al. 1990, 1991; Zhou et al. 1990), whereas the D_2 family consists of D_2, D_3, and D_4 receptors (Bunzow et al. 1988; Sokoloff et al. 1991; Van Tol et al. 1991).

The D_1 family can be differentiated from the D_2 family in its affinity for experimental drugs SCH23390 (antagonist) and SKF39383 (agonist) that do not bind to the D_2 family of receptors. The D_1 and D_5 subtypes can be differentiated from each other in terms of their anatomical distribution (Fremeau et al. 1991; Mansour et al. 1991; Meador-Woodruff et al. 1991, 1992; Mengod et al. 1991) and their affinity for dopamine; the D_5 receptor has a higher affinity for the endogenous ligand (Sunahara et al. 1991). Although the D_2 receptor family may be more important to psychiatry because of the large number of therapeutic compounds that bind to these sites, the D_1 receptor family should not be ignored. A great deal of pharmacological and electrophysiological evidence suggests an interaction between D_1-like and D_2-like receptors, with D_1 sites having enabling or modulating effects on D_2-mediated activities (Clark and White 1987).

The D_2 receptor family has a high affinity for antipsychotic drugs, such as haloperidol, chlorpromazine, and clozapine, and has been shown to be negatively coupled (D_2,

D_3, D_4) to the second messenger adenylate cyclase. Within the D_2 family, each receptor has its own pharmacologically distinct profile (Table 3–1). For example, D_3 receptors have a relatively higher affinity for dopamine and quinpirole as compared with D_2, and D_4 receptors have a 10-fold higher affinity for clozapine as compared with D_2 and D_3. Similarly, raclopride has a far greater affinity for D_2 and D_3 than for D_4. Many of the clinically used antipsychotic drugs (particularly at higher doses) clearly affect all three of these dopamine receptors, and further research is necessary to develop truly selective dopamine antagonists for therapeutic use. Interestingly, the atypical antipsychotics (especially clozapine), although potentially active at a number of receptors, show the highest affinity for the D_4 receptor of all of the dopamine receptors. As we discuss below, this receptor is primarily localized in limbic brain structures but has no appreciable expression in extrapyramidal motor structures, which may explain why the atypical antipsychotics have a low incidence of extrapyramidal side effects. On the other hand, most typical neuroleptics have high affinities for the D_2 receptor in addition to the D_3 and D_4 sites. The high level of D_2 receptor expression in the extrapyramidal system (discussed below) might explain why typical antipsychotic agents are often associated with extrapyramidal side effects.

The D_1 and D_2 families of receptors can be further differentiated with respect to their gene structures. Members of the D_2 receptor family have multiple introns in the coding regions of their genes that lead to the production of multiple messenger RNA (mRNA) variants by alternative

Table 3–1. Drug dissociation constants (K_i values [nM])

Agonists	D_2	D_3	D_4
Bromocriptine	5.3	7.4	340.0
Apomorphine	24.0	20.0	4.1
Dopamine	474.0	25.0	28.0
Quinpirole	576.0	5.1	46.0
Antagonists			
Haloperidol	0.45	9.8	5.1
Spiperone	0.07	0.6	0.05
(-) Sulpiride	9.2	25.0	52.0
Raclopride	1.8	3.5	237.0
Clozapine	56.0	180.0	9.0
Chlorpromazine	2.8	6.1	37.0
Pimozide	2.4	3.7	43.0

Note. The K_i values were derived from Bunzow et al. 1988 and Van Tol et al. 1991. The lower the numerical value, the higher the affinity a drug has for a receptor subtype. Relative selectivities may be estimated from ratios of K_i values across receptor subtype.

DNA splicing. Two functional forms of the D_2 receptor that differ by 29 amino acids have been identified (Dal Toso et al. 1989; Giros et al. 1989; Monsma et al. 1989), and two additional variants of the D_3 receptor have been described (Giros et al. 1991). Multiple nucleic acid repeats also have been reported for the D_4 receptor within the putative third intracelluar loop (Van Tol et al. 1992). This region of the receptor is critical for G-protein coupling, and receptor-binding studies suggest that the receptors with the highest number of repeats have the lowest affinity for dopaminergic drugs. The D_1 and D_5 receptor genes, on the other hand, have no introns in their coding regions, which results in single D_1 and D_5 receptor proteins. Pseudogenes of the D_5 receptor that encode truncated forms of the D_5 receptor have been described in humans (Weinshank et al. 1991), but these pseudogenes do not appear to be functional.

Anatomically, the dopamine receptor subtypes have five distinct distributions (Bouthenet et al. 1991; Mansour et al. 1990, 1991; Meador-Woodruff et al. 1989, 1991, 1992; Mengod et al. 1991; O'Malley et al. 1992; Weiner et al. 1991), supporting the notion that they may play functionally different roles in the CNS. However, before we review their anatomy, a brief discussion of the methods used to identify these receptors is necessary to put these data into perspective. Brain receptors can be anatomically characterized in one of three ways: 1) with in situ hybridization techniques to localize their mRNA, 2) with receptor autoradiographic techniques to localize the binding sites, and 3) with immunohistochemical techniques to localize the receptor proteins themselves.

In situ hybridization allows the selective identification of the mRNAs of each receptor and, thus, the cell bodies that synthesize these receptors. Receptor autoradiographic techniques, on the other hand, rely on the pharmacological identification of binding sites that may be present on both cell bodies and fibers in the CNS. Immunohistochemical techniques directly label the receptor protein, which may be localized in cell bodies and fibers, but use antibodies generated to selective amino acid stretches of the receptors. In situ hybridization provides excellent cellular resolution and mRNA quantitation but little information about cellular projections when used alone. Receptor autoradiography provides a measure of receptor quantitation and allows the mapping of possible brain projections when used in combination with in situ hybridization and immunohistochemical methods. This technique is dependent, however, on the development of selective ligands that currently do not exist for the D_4 and D_5 receptors. Immunohistochemical identification of receptors provides excellent cellular resolution of the receptor protein and can be applied to any known amino acid sequence, but it is not quantitative, and certain antibodies are often difficult to develop. It is clear that each method has limitations and advantages, and the integration of information from mRNA, binding site, and protein studies is needed for an accurate understanding of the anatomy of these receptors.

Note that the same amount of information is not available for each of the dopamine receptors and that much of the distribution information that is available is derived from studies with rats as animal models. This situation is changing rapidly, however, with major discoveries in the localization of the human dopamine receptors. The distributions of D_1 and D_2 have been studied most extensively, partially because of their relatively high levels of mRNA and protein expression in brain. The D_3, D_4, and D_5 receptors are less abundant, and we are likely detecting signals only in those regions of highest mRNA expression. Further research is necessary to develop more selective and sensitive means of measuring these receptors.

Despite these limitations, a great deal of evidence indicates that the five dopamine receptors have different and often complementary distributions in the CNS (Table 3–2). We describe thoroughly the dopamine receptor mRNA distributions in the rat brain and then present some of the most recent salient findings in humans. Because the D_2 receptor was cloned first, we have the best appreciation of its distribution in the brain. High levels of D_2 mRNA, binding, and immunohistochemical staining can be observed in many dopaminergic projection fields, including the caudate-putamen, nucleus accumbens, olfactory tubercle, and lateral septum, in addition to being localized in the dopamine-producing cells of the substantia nigra, ventral tegmental area, olfactory bulb, and zona incerta (Mansour et al. 1990; Meador-Woodruff and Mansour 1991; Meador-Woodruff et al. 1989, 1991; Mengod et al. 1992; Najlerahim et al. 1989; Weiner et al. 1991). Such a distribution would suggest both a postsynaptic and an autoreceptor function of the D_2 receptor (Nagy et al. 1978). Receptors located on dopamine-producing cells are referred to as *autoreceptors* because they are thought to regulate dopamine release. Autoreceptors have also been described for the serotonergic system and are discussed later in this chapter.

The distribution of these receptors often is not homogeneous throughout an anatomical region. For example, in the caudate-putamen, mediolateral, rostral-caudal, and dorsoventral regions, gradients have been observed. D_2 receptor binding and mRNA are most concentrated dorsolaterally and in the more rostral portion of the caudate-putamen. These differences, as well as a wealth of other anatomical data, suggest that the striatum may be subdi-

Table 3–2. Dopamine receptor messenger RNA (mRNA) distribution

	D_1	D_5	D_2	D_3	D_4
Anatomical distribution	Highest mRNA levels in caudate-putamen, olfactory tubercle, nucleus accumbens, amygdala, and cortex; no detectable mRNA in substantia nigra and pituitary	mRNA localized in the parafascicular nucleus of the thalamus, hippocampus, and dentate gyrus; in human brain, mRNA also localized in many cortical fields	Highest mRNA levels in basal ganglia, including caudate-putamen, olfactory tubercle, nucleus accumbens, and substantia nigra; D_2 mRNA levels also high in pituitary	D_3 mRNA has a more "limbic" distribution, with high levels in olfactory tubercle and nucleus accumbens; only low levels in caudate-putamen, and no D_3 detected in pituitary	mRNA levels difficult to detect in the rat; in human brain, however, mRNA is enriched in cortical fields, including prefrontal and temporal cortex, and hippocampus and dentate gyrus
Pre- or postsynaptic	Postsynaptic	Postsynaptic	Pre- and postsynaptic	Pre- and postsynaptic	Postsynaptic

vided further into anatomically and biochemically defined compartments that may be functionally distinct. The core of the nucleus accumbens and the dorsal caudate-putamen have been implicated, for example, in motor control and integration, whereas the shell of the nucleus accumbens and the ventral caudate-putamen are associated with limbic functions (Heimer et al. 1991). Other regions in which D_2 receptor binding and mRNA have been reported include the hippocampus, lateral preoptic area, anterior and lateral hypothalamus, lateral mammillary nuclei, and periaqueductal gray matter.

Despite the related pharmacology of the D_3 receptor, its distribution varies markedly from that of D_2 and D_4. Like the D_2 receptor, D_3 receptor mRNA and binding have been localized to both dopaminoceptive (or postsynaptic) and dopamine-containing cells. The two distributions differ in that the D_3 dopamine receptors appear to be more concentrated in dopaminoceptive fields associated with limbic function, such as the islands of Calleja, stria terminalis, ventral caudate-putamen, and nucleus accumbens. These regions receive dopaminergic projections from the ventral tegmental area and are part of the mesolimbic dopamine system. These regions also receive nondopaminergic projections from other limbic structures, including the prefrontal cortex and amygdala. Some investigators report a localization of D_3 mRNA in the ventral tegmental area and substantia nigra (lateral division), which suggests that, like the D_2 receptor, the D_3 receptor may serve an autoreceptor function in addition to its role as a postsynaptic dopamine receptor. Given its more "limbic" distribution, drugs selective for D_3 may be less apt to produce the extrapyramidal side effects often seen with D_2 antagonists. Other areas with D_3 receptors include the medial septum, hippocampus, medial mammillary nuclei of the hypothalamus, and lobules 9 and 10 of the cerebellum (Bouthenet et al. 1991; Landwehrmeyer et al. 1993; Mengod et al. 1992; Sokoloff et al. 1991). The D_3 receptor clearly should be considered as a possible site of action when evaluating the effects of antipsychotic drugs previously thought to function by antagonizing D_2 receptors.

D_4 receptor pharmacology is similar to that of D_2 and D_3 receptors; it differs in affinities for only a few compounds such as clozapine (Van Tol et al. 1991). Of the D_2-like family, D_4 has been the most difficult to characterize because of its relatively low levels in the rat CNS, but it may be the most interesting receptor from a psychiatric point of view. Several polymorphic variants of the D_4 receptor have been described in humans (Van Tol et al. 1992). Each consists of 16 amino acid repeats in the putative third cytosolic loop of the D_4 receptor. One-, four-, and sevenfold repeats that have been described appear to differ in their affinity for clozapine and spiperone as well as in their ability to couple to G proteins. Perhaps with the development of selective D_4 antibodies for immunohistochemistry and ligands for receptor binding, the distribution and function of this receptor will be better understood. The D_4 receptors are more abundant in the human brain than in the rodent brain (O'Malley et al. 1992) and, as discussed later in this chapter, may play a comparatively larger role in dopaminoceptive transmission.

The D_1 receptor distribution overlaps partially with that of the D_2-like family of receptors, especially in the basal forebrain, but represents a fourth dopaminergic receptor distribution. One distinguishing feature of the D_1 receptor is that it is not an autoreceptor (Table 3–2) and therefore is not localized in dopamine-producing cells of the substantia nigra, ventral tegmental area, hypothalamus, and olfactory bulb. D_1 receptor mRNA and binding are more widespread in the CNS as compared with the D_2-like family of receptors, with detectable levels of mRNA in the caudate-putamen, nucleus accumbens, olfactory tubercle, neo- and allocortex, dentate gyrus, amygdala (basolateral, central, medial, and cortical nuclei), suprachiasmatic nucleus of the hypothalamus, and cerebellum. Marked discrepancies between high levels of D_1 receptor binding and no receptor mRNA are found in several structures, including the globus pallidus, entopeduncular and subthalamic nuclei, and substantia nigra (pars reticulata), which likely reflect receptor transport from its cell of origin in the striatum to their terminals. Other regions containing D_1 receptor binding and no mRNA include the medial septum, stratum moleculare of the hippocampus, superior and inferior colliculi, and periaqueductal gray matter.

As is the case with the D_2 receptor family, D_1 receptor mRNA and binding are differentially distributed within specific brain nuclei (Fremeau et al. 1991; Mansour et al. 1991; Meador-Woodruff et al. 1991; Mengod et al. 1991; Weiner et al. 1991). For example, higher levels of D_1 mRNA are found in the dorsomedial and ventrolateral caudate-putamen and in the deeper layers (V, VI) of neocortex. Similarly, differences in D_1 mRNA levels can be detected between the core and shell of the nucleus accumbens, which have been associated with limbic and motor functions, respectively. As with D_2, a rostral-caudal gradient occurs in D_1 mRNA and binding in the nucleus accumbens, with the highest levels observed rostrally.

In contrast to the D_1 receptor, the distribution of the D_5 receptor is far more restricted. In situ hybridization studies suggest that the D_5 receptor is restricted in rats to the hippocampus and parafascicular nucleus of the thalamus (Meador-Woodruff et al. 1992; Tiberi et al. 1991).

Despite the 10-fold greater sensitivity of the D_5 receptor for dopamine compared with D_1, it does not appear to be localized in traditional dopaminergic projection regions. Rather, the D_5 receptor localization in the parafascicular nucleus suggests an integrative role because this thalamic nucleus receives afferent projections from the substantia nigra and has efferent projections to the striatum.

Dopamine Receptor Expression in the Human Brain

The most exciting findings in dopamine receptor anatomy in the last few years have been generated from studies of the human brain (Meador-Woodruff et al. 1994a, 1994b, 1996). As seen in the rat, all five dopamine receptor mRNAs have distinct anatomical distributions, which are likely associated with specific functional roles. Of the receptor mRNAs, D_1 and D_2 are the most widely distributed in the CNS, with D_3, D_4, and D_5 expressing cells localized in more limited cortical or limbically related regions.

As seen in the rat, the dopamine receptors are localized in both dopamine-synthesizing and dopaminoceptive cells. Their localization varies with receptor subtype and anatomical region. In the substantia nigra, for example, D_2 and D_3 receptor transcripts are the most prominent; thus, these receptors may serve an autoreceptor function. As observed in the rat, D_1, D_4, and D_5 mRNAs cannot be detected in the midbrain dopamine neurons and are unlikely to mediate an autoreceptor function.

Postsynaptically, D_1, D_2, and D_3 are the primary mRNA transcripts seen in the human striatum, as has been the case in the rat. D_1 and D_2 mRNAs are distributed more homogeneously in the striatum, whereas D_3 mRNA is expressed in the ventral striatum, which suggests that it has a role in mediating limbic functions. D_4 mRNA, if present, is found at extremely low levels and localized to the medial aspects of the nucleus accumbens. In the prefrontal cortex, D_1 and D_4 receptor mRNAs are the most abundant, although the other three transcripts are seen at lower levels. D_1 and D_4 mRNAs are enriched in the deep layers of the prefrontal cortex, with lower levels seen in superficial lamina. Also of psychiatric relevance, the same pattern of dopamine receptor mRNA expression is seen in the temporal cortex, where D_1 and D_4 receptor mRNAs predominate, with lower levels of D_2, D_3, and D_5 detected. In the hippocampal formation, D_2, D_3, D_4, and D_5 mRNAs are localized in the dentate gyrus and the CA1–4 pyramidal fields of Cajal, but D_1 expression is limited to the CA1 field, with only faint labeling in CA2–4.

Despite some similarities to the rodent, important species differences in the human brain must be considered in understanding the pharmacological complexity of this neurotransmitter system. In the cortex, for example, although the D_2 receptor distribution in the rat and human is similar, the expression of D_3, D_4, and D_5 receptors is notably different. In contrast to the rat, in the human cortex, D_4 receptor mRNA is enriched and, in some cases, may be the predominant form of D_2-like receptor. Furthermore, the D_5 receptor mRNA distribution in the human cortex parallels that of D_2; this result is completely unexpected based on data from the rat. Unlike the rat, D_2 receptor mRNA in the human midbrain is localized exclusively in the substantia nigra (A9) and does not extend to the dopaminergic cells of the ventral tegmental area and retrorubral field (A8, A10). This finding suggests that in the human, only the nigrostriatal projections may have autoreceptors (Meador-Woodruff et al. 1994a). D_3 receptor mRNA, which is less abundant than D_2 in the midbrain, is similarly localized only in the A9 cells of the substantia nigra and is not seen in the ventral tegmental and retrorubral areas. The relative lack of dopamine autoreceptors in the limbic, but not motor, systems of humans has important implications in terms of understanding the pathophysiology of psychiatric disorders and in developing rational pharmacological approaches to treat these diseases. Cumulative anatomical and pharmacological evidence suggests that in schizophrenia, in which dopaminergic transmission is dysfunctional, the D_3 receptors in the mesolimbic system and the D_2 and D_4 receptors in the mediotemporal and limbic cortical areas may be primarily involved.

Dopamine Receptor Colocalization

Although each dopamine receptor has a distinct distribution, regions of overlap exist, particularly in forebrain and midbrain structures such as the caudate-putamen, nucleus accumbens, olfactory tubercle, hippocampus, and substantia nigra. Thus, there may be a colocalization of multiple dopamine receptors within the same cells. This issue has been controversial, and the true extent of colocalization is unclear. Behavioral, electrophysiological, and pharmacological evidence suggest extensive colocalization of D_1, D_2 (for review, see Clark and White 1987), and possibly D_3 receptors within the caudate-putamen and nucleus accumbens. Unfortunately, the anatomical data are divided from extreme viewpoints of little or no colocalization of D_1 and D_2 in the striatum (Gerfen et al. 1991) to complete colocalization of D_1, D_2, D_3, and D_4 in nigrostriatal projecting neurons (Surmeier et al. 1992). Studies in our laboratory indicated that depending on the anatomical methods used, colocalization of D_1 and D_2 in the dorsal striatum can vary from 30% (Meador-Woodruff et

al. 1991) to as little as 10% (Curran and Watson 1995). More research is necessary to determine how regional differences may contribute to the extent of colocalization and the relative colocalization with D_3 and D_4 receptors. Investigators recently used dual mRNA labeling techniques to report a high level of D_1 and D_3 receptor colocalization within subregions of the ventral striatum (Curran and Watson 1995). This is of critical functional significance in understanding the role of the dopamine receptors in the nigrostriatal and mesolimbic systems and in the cellular regulation of the striatum by psychotropic drugs.

SEROTONIN-SYNTHESIZING CELL GROUPS

The serotonin-synthesizing neurons consist of a heterogeneous population of cells in the brain stem (Figure 3–2). Based on the original description by Dahlstrom and Fuxe (1964) in rat brain stem, serotonergic cell groups were coded B_1–B_9 with respect to their rostral-caudal location (B_9 is the most rostral supralemniscal region). These serotonergic nuclei can be further divided into rostral and caudal subdivisions with respect to target projection areas. The rostral division, localized in the midbrain and pons, provides ascending projections to the forebrain, whereas the caudal division, located in the medulla oblongata, sends descending projections to the spinal cord. In this

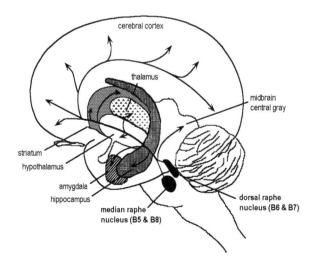

Figure 3–2. Serotonergic cell groups and their projections. Presynaptic receptors are found on serotonin-producing cells, and postsynaptic receptors are found in their projection fields. See the text and Table 3–4 for details on serotonin receptor binding and mRNA distributions.

chapter, we focus on the ascending serotonergic system.

Most ascending serotonergic projections originate in the dorsal (B_6 and B_7) and median (B_5 and B_8) raphe nuclei of the brain stem. However, both the caudal linear nucleus (B_8) of the midbrain and the more ventral supralemniscal (B_9) cell group contribute to rostral serotonergic afferents (for review, see Tork 1985). The dorsal raphe nucleus, located in the ventral portion of the periaqueductal gray matter, contains the largest number of serotonin neurons in the brain (estimated at 165,000 in humans). Based on cell densities and morphology, several subregions are identifiable within this nucleus: interfascicular, ventral, ventrolateral, dorsal (lateral and medial), and caudal (Steinbusch and Nieuwenhuys 1983; Tork 1985). The dorsal subnucleus, which extends into the periaqueductal gray matter, contains the largest number of serotonergic neurons in this region. The median raphe nucleus is located in the central portion of the pons, ventral to the dorsal raphe nucleus. The morphology of cells in this nucleus is similar to that found in the dorsal raphe nucleus. Here, however, serotonin cells are found along the midline and are only one-third of those found in the dorsal raphe (Tork 1990).

Unlike the distinct subsystems involved in dopaminergic circuitry, virtually every area of the brain receives projections from the raphe nuclei described above (Figure 3–2). Therefore, serotonin is involved in a diverse array of cognitive and behavioral functions. Ascending projections travel initially in the medial forebrain bundle before branching to innervate specific target regions, including the hippocampus, hypothalamus, cerebral cortex, septal nuclei, caudate-putamen, and thalamus. The ascending serotonergic system can be thought of as a dual projection system, with projection areas receiving input that originates in both dorsal and median raphe nuclei. However, the proportion of projection fibers arising from each nucleus varies considerably in different brain structures. For example, the vast majority of fibers innervating the dentate gyrus originate within the median raphe nucleus with very little apparent input from the dorsal raphe cells. On the other hand, striatal innervation arises predominantly from dorsal raphe cells with minimal input from median raphe cells (Tork 1990). Thus, the median raphe–hippocampal system may be considered important in relation to serotonergic influence of limbic hippocampal function, whereas dorsal raphe–striatal projections relate to basal ganglia function.

In each projection area, serotonergic input has a distinct innervation pattern. Thus, within the hippocampal formation, serotonin fibers are particularly concentrated within stratum laconosum moleculare and stratum oriens of CA subfields but sparse across the pyramidal cell layer of the CA subfields and the granule cell layer of dentate gyrus (Tork 1985). In a similar fashion, raphe input to the cerebral cortex in rats is concentrated in superficial lamina, and fewer axons are found in deeper layers (Lidov et al. 1980). Comparison of serotonin fiber distributions with specific serotonin receptor localization in anatomical subregions (see following section) provides valuable insight into the role of serotonin receptor subtypes within specific serotonin circuits. This information is useful in considering the action of serotonergic drugs in the brain.

SEROTONIN RECEPTOR TYPES AND THEIR DISTRIBUTIONS

Like dopamine, the actions of serotonin are mediated by multiple receptors. Serotonin receptors were originally divided into two subtypes—$5\text{-}HT_1$ and $5\text{-}HT_2$—on the basis of pharmacological profile (Peroutka and Snyder 1979). However, more recent pharmacological and biochemical data indicate the presence of at least seven major serotonin receptor families or classes: $5\text{-}HT_1$, $5\text{-}HT_2$, $5\text{-}HT_3$, $5\text{-}HT_4$, $5\text{-}HT_5$, $5\text{-}HT_6$, and $5\text{-}HT_7$, and some families have multiple subtypes (Hoyer and Martin 1996; Humphrey et al. 1993). This complex pharmacology has been confirmed and extended with molecular cloning techniques (Albert et al. 1990; Hamblin and Metcalf 1991; Julius et al. 1988; McAllister et al. 1992; Voigt et al. 1991). Indeed, the speed at which nucleic acid sequences for serotonin-like receptors have become available has far outpaced the availability of specific serotonergic pharmacological tools; this situation is similar to that of the dopamine receptors.

Serotonin receptors are currently classified according to their structural and functional characteristics and their linkage to second messenger systems. Thus, the $5\text{-}HT_1$ receptor family, defined as having high affinity for serotonin, was originally subdivided into six receptor subtypes: $5\text{-}HT_{1A-1F}$. However, the $5\text{-}HT_{1C}$ receptor was reclassified as $5\text{-}HT_{2C}$ because, like other members of the $5\text{-}HT_2$ family, it activates the phospholipase C pathway. The other members of the $5\text{-}HT_1$ family are preferentially coupled to inhibition of adenylate cyclase. Members of the $5\text{-}HT_1$ family have not only a common transduction mechanism but also intronless genes (Humphrey et al. 1993).

Based on sequence information and pharmacological profiles, at least 14 serotonin receptors have been identified in the brain to date (Table 3–3). In a similar fashion to dopamine receptors, most cloned serotonin receptors belong to the superfamily of G-protein-coupled receptors, which appear to span the plasma membrane seven times.

A notable exception is the 5-HT$_3$ receptor, which belongs to the ligand-gated ion channel family. The physiological role of the most recently cloned receptors (e.g., 5-HT$_5$, 5-HT$_6$, and 5-HT$_7$) is still under investigation. Of interest is that some of these newly discovered receptors (5-HT$_6$ and 5-HT$_7$) have a very high affinity for clozapine, which suggests a role for serotonin systems in antipsychotic activity (Roth et al. 1994; Tricklebank 1996). The Serotonin Receptor Nomenclature Committee (Hoyer and Martin 1996) recommends that new recombinant receptors be described in lowercase letters (i.e., 5-ht$_n$) until a physiological role for the receptor is confirmed. At the time this chapter was written, only 5-ht$_{1E}$, 5-ht$_{1F}$, 5-ht$_{5A}$, and 5-ht$_{5B}$ are described this way.

A detailed description of the anatomical distribution of all known serotonin receptors is beyond the scope of this chapter; therefore, only their cellular mRNA distribution is included in Table 3–4. A brief discussion of the distribution of the 5-HT$_1$, 5-HT$_2$, 5-HT$_3$, and 5-HT$_4$ receptors follows because they are particularly relevant in understanding the actions of psychotherapeutic drugs with serotonergic properties. For purposes of clarity, the serotonin receptors have been divided into their pre- and postsynaptic localization. Although most available distribution data are derived from rat brain studies, human mapping studies indicate that serotonin receptor binding sites have a similar distribution in both species.

Serotonin receptors (5-HT$_{1B}$ and 5-HT$_{1D}$) located presynaptically are responsible for negative feedback control of serotonin release from serotonergic terminals. Consistent with this finding, 5-HT$_{1B}$ and 5-HT$_{1D}$ receptor mRNAs have been detected within both dorsal and median raphe nuclei of mouse and rat brain, whereas 5-HT$_{1B}$ binding sites are found predominantly in raphe projection areas such as the neocortex (Maroteaux et al. 1992; Voigt et al. 1991). The 5-HT$_{1D}$ receptor was thought to represent a variant of the 5-HT$_{1B}$ receptor that was present in human brain but not in mouse or rat brain. However, it is now clear that this proposed species dichotomy is inaccurate because a 5-HT$_{1B}$ receptor has been cloned from human brain (Jin et al. 1992), and a gene encoding a 5-HT$_{1D}$-like receptor has been found in rat brain (Hamblin et al. 1992). Thus, *both* of these receptors may act to control serotonin release within serotonin circuits.

Presynaptic serotonergic activity is also controlled by serotonin autoreceptors located on the soma and/or dendrites of serotonin cells. Electrophysiological data indicate that activation of 5-HT$_{1A}$ receptors on raphe neurons results in decreased firing of serotonin cells (Sprouse and Aghajanian 1987). In keeping with these findings, 5-HT$_{1A}$ receptor mRNA and 5-HT$_{1A}$ receptors are both found in raphe neurons (Chalmers and Watson 1991), which suggests a local synthesis of these sites. These receptors represent important sites for presynaptic regulation of serotonergic circuitry because they may act to modulate serotonergic "tone" within brain systems. Consequently, these somatodendritic 5-HT$_{1A}$ receptors may be important sites for serotonergic drug action (see section, "Synap-

Table 3–3. Pharmacological characteristics of serotonin (5-HT) receptors

	5-HT$_{1A}$	5-HT$_{1B}$	5-HT$_{1D}$	5-ht$_{1E}$	5-ht$_{1F}$
Selective pharmacological agents	Azaperones (8-OH-DPAT, ipsapirone)	CP-93,129	GR 127935	None	None
Radioligands	[^{3}H]8-OH-DPAT	[^{125}I]GTI	[^{125}I]GTI	[^{3}H]5-HT	[^{125}I]LSD
	5-HT$_{2A}$	**5-HT$_{2B}$**	**5-HT$_{2C}$**	**5-HT$_3$**	**5-HT$_4$**
Selective pharmacological agents	DOB, DOI, ketanserin, ritanserin	5-MeOT, LY 53857	5-MeOT, mesulergine, LY 53857	m-Chlorophenil-biguanide, ondansetron	5-MeOT, renzapride
Radioligands	[^{3}H]Ketanserin	[^{3}H]5-HT	[^{3}H]Mesulergine	[^{3}H]Zacopride	[^{3}H]GR 113808
	5-ht$_{5A}$	**5-ht$_{5B}$**	**5-HT$_6$**	**5-HT$_7$**	
Selective pharmacological agents	None	None	None	None	
Radioligands	[^{125}I]LSD	[^{125}I]LSD	[^{125}I]LSD [^{3}H]5-CT	[^{125}I]LSD [^{3}H]5-CT	

Note. 8-OH-DPAT = 8-hydroxy-N, N-dipropyl, 2-aminotetraline; GTI = serotonin-O-carboxymethylglycyl-iodotyrosinamide; 5-CT = 5-carboxyamidotryptamine; DOB = 4-bromo-2,5-dimethoxyamphetamine; DOI = 4-iodo-2,5-dimethoxyamphetamine; 5-MeOT = 5-methoxytryptamine; LSD = lysergic diethylamide.

Table 3–4. Serotonin receptor messenger RNA (mRNA) distribution

	5-HT$_{1A}$	5-HT$_{1B}$	5-HT$_{1D}$	5-ht$_{1E}$	5-ht$_{1F}$
Anatomical distribution	mRNA localized in hippocampus, septum, amygdala, and raphe nuclei	mRNA expression in raphe neurons, hippocampus (CA1), striatum, and cortex	mRNA present in hippocampus, striatum, and amygdala	mRNA present in amygdala, caudate-putamen, and cortex	High mRNA levels in hippocampal formation, claustrum, and cortical areas
Pre- or postsynaptic	Pre- and postsynaptic	Pre- and postsynaptic	Pre- and postsynaptic	Postsynaptic	Postsynaptic
	5-HT$_{2A}$	5-HT$_{2B}$	5-HT$_{2C}$	5-HT$_3$	5-HT$_4$
Anatomical distribution	mRNA localized in neocortex (1V), claustrum, pontine nuclei, and hippocampus	Very low mRNA levels in human cortex, cerebellum, amygdala, caudate, thalamus, and hypothalamus	High mRNA levels in choroid plexus; also expressed in subiculum, dorsal raphe, and hypothalamus	mRNA expression in cortex, hippocampus (CA1), amygdala, and dorsal raphe	High mRNA expression in striatum, hippocampus, thalamus septal region, and midbrain
Pre- or postsynaptic	Postsynaptic	Postsynaptic?	Postsynaptic/ presynaptic?	Pre-and postsynaptic	Postsynaptic
	5-ht$_{5A}$	5-ht$_{5B}$	5-HT$_6$	5-HT$_7$	
Anatomical distribution	mRNA expression in piriform cortex, septum, amygdala, hypothalamus, and hippocampus	Abundant mRNA levels in hippocampus (CA1), habenula, and raphe nuclei	mRNA present in hippocampus, nucleus accumbens, striatum, and olfactory tubercle	mRNA expression in thalamus, hippocampus (CA3), septum, amygdala, and periaqueductal gray	
Pre- or postsynaptic	Postsynaptic	Postsynaptic/ presynaptic?	Postsynaptic	Postsynaptic	

tic Regulation," below). In addition to 5-HT$_{1A}$ receptors, both 5-HT$_{1B}$ and 5-HT$_{2C}$ receptors may be present on serotonergic cells in raphe nuclei (Hoffman and Mezey 1989; Voigt et al. 1991). However, the functional role of these sites in this region remains to be clarified.

In situ hybridization histochemistry indicates that 5-HT$_{1A}$ receptor mRNA is abundant in the hippocampus, septal nuclei, amygdaloid nuclei, and entorhinal cortex (Chalmers and Watson 1991), which are key anatomical structures related to limbic function. The presence of 5-HT$_{1A}$ receptors in these anatomical regions confirms a local postsynaptic localization for these sites. Therefore, any drugs acting at 5-HT$_{1A}$ sites may alter function within multiple anatomical components of circuitry associated with emotional control. In addition to the 5-HT$_{1A}$ receptor, the 5-HT$_{2C}$ receptor is expressed within limbic areas, particularly the ventral hippocampus, septum, amygdala, and cingulate cortex (Hoffman and Mezey 1989). Again, such an anatomical distribution suggests that this receptor may play a role in serotonergic regulation of affect. However, the extremely high level (10 times greater than in limbic structures) of 5-HT$_{2C}$ mRNA expression in epithe-

lial cells of the choroid plexus indicates that the primary role of this receptor may relate to cerebrospinal fluid production.

Early receptor binding experiments with [^{3}H]spiperone indicated a high level of 5-HT$_2$ receptors in the neocortex. Autoradiographic studies with the selective 5-HT$_{2A}$ antagonist ketanserin found high levels of receptor binding within laminae I and V of the neocortex and within the claustrum and other parts of the basal ganglia. More recent in situ hybridization studies have confirmed the synthesis of 5-HT$_{2A}$ receptors within neocortical cells (Mengod et al. 1990), which indicates that these sites are indeed present on intrinsic cortical cells. The morphology of 5-HT$_{2A}$-immunoreactive cells in this region (Morilak et al. 1992) indicates that 5-HT$_{2A}$ receptors are most likely localized on γ-aminobutyric acid (GABA)ergic interneurons or cholinergic cells within the neocortex.

In addition to their role as autoreceptors, 5-HT$_{1B}$ and 5-HT$_{1D}$ receptors likely act as postsynaptic serotonin receptors in some brain regions. 5-HT$_{1B}$ receptor transcripts are found in cells within CA1 and subicular subfields of the hippocampus and layer IV of the neocortex and entorhinal cortex (Voigt et al. 1991). Thus, these sites not only may regulate presynaptic serotonergic input to limbic areas but also may participate in mediating postsynaptic serotonergic effects. In fact, studies have implicated postsynaptic 5-HT$_{1B}$ receptors in modulating impulsive and aggressive behavior (Ramboz et al. 1996; Sijbesma et al. 1991).

The relatively high abundance of 5-HT$_3$ and 5-HT$_4$ receptors in the mesolimbic system points to a role of these receptors in modulating dopamine function and perhaps antipsychotic activity (Kilpatrick et al. 1996). High levels of 5-HT$_3$ binding are found in limbic and cortical areas—in particular, in the terminal regions of the mesolimbic system. The mesolimbic and nigrostriatal pathways also have high levels of 5-HT$_4$ receptors (Kilpatrick et al. 1996). In fact, functional studies strongly suggested that these two receptors can modulate dopamine function, either directly or through GABA neurons.

SYNAPTIC REGULATION

The number of dopamine and serotonin receptor subtypes and the lack of selective ligands have made it difficult to determine exactly which receptors and circuits may be activated after pharmacological treatments. As is shown in Table 3–1, many drugs previously thought to bind to the D$_2$ receptor actually bind to D$_2$, D$_3$, and D$_4$ sites at different levels of occupancy depending on the drug concentration. Similarly, all drugs examined thus far that bind D$_1$ with high affinity also bind D$_5$ receptors (Sunahara et al. 1991; Weinshank et al. 1991). Receptor-specific compounds are also absent within the serotonergic system, in which, to date, most serotonin receptor subtypes are characterized in terms of agonist profiles, and very few receptor-specific ligands are available (Table 3–3).

Despite these kinds of limitations, the issues of synaptic regulation can be examined on a more conceptual level. When a clinician administers a drug, he or she should view it not only as interacting with a specific receptor or family of receptors but also as activating or inhibiting specific cell groups or circuits. The smallest functional units of such circuits are synapses, and one mode of drug action is the modulation of neurotransmission across synapses. The dopamine and serotonin receptor distributions described here may be thought of as potential sites of synaptic transmission that should be kept in mind in understanding psychotropic drug action. When selective D$_3$ or D$_4$ antagonists become clinically available, they will activate entirely different sets of synapses than do D$_2$ antagonists, given the differences in their distributions. Similarly, D$_5$ antagonists will likely have markedly different sites of action as compared with D$_1$ drugs because the receptors are differentially distributed.

Presynaptic Mechanisms

Presynaptic mechanisms control the level of neurotransmitter released into the synapse and can be modulated by drugs that affect neurotransmitter synthesis, breakdown, release, and reuptake. Figures 3–3 and 3–4 illustrate pre- and postsynaptic mechanisms of regulation.

Neurotransmitter Synthesis

In the case of dopaminergic neurons, the conversion of tyrosine to dihydroxyphenylalanine (DOPA) by tyrosine hydroxylase is the rate-limiting step in dopamine production. Therefore, the amount of dopamine in the synapse is affected by drugs such as α-methyl-*p*-tyrosine, an effective tyrosine hydroxylase inhibitor used to reduce catecholamine levels. In an analogous fashion, inhibition of tryptophan hydroxylase by *para*-chlorophenylalanine blocks the conversion of tryptophan to 5-hydroxytryptophan, the rate-limiting step in serotonin synthesis. These drugs are not given clinically but have been used in animal research paradigms.

Neurotransmitter Breakdown

Drugs that inhibit the oxidative breakdown of catecholamines and indoleamines, such as monoamine oxidase inhibitors (MAOIs), can be used clinically to elevate monoamine levels, as in the drug treatment of depression. The antidepressants pargyline, phenelzine, and tranylcypromine act to inhibit the action of monoamine oxidase, thereby blocking the catabolism of dopamine and serotonin. This process increases monoamine content within the brain, which presumably leads to augmentation of monoaminergic tone.

Neurotransmitter Release

Release of neurotransmitters is controlled by several factors. The more proximal determinant of release is intracellular calcium (Ca^{2+}) levels. As Ca^{2+} levels increase, the levels of neurotransmitter release increase. In the long term, however, release of neurotransmitters depends on the presence of autoreceptors. Autoreceptors are specific receptors found on neurotransmitter-producing cell bodies or presynaptic terminals that, when stimulated, inhibit transmitter release. Members of the D$_2$ and 5-HT$_1$ families of receptors are examples of autoreceptors.

A feature of dopamine neurons is that they can release dopamine not only from presynaptic terminals but also

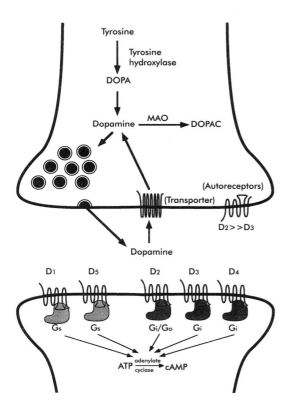

Figure 3–3. Schematic representation of a dopaminergic synapse. Dopaminergic cells synthesize dopamine from dihydroxyphenylalanine (DOPA), which is synthesized from tyrosine. The conversion of tyrosine to DOPA by tyrosine hydroxylase is the rate-limiting step in the synthesis of dopamine. Once dopamine is synthesized, it is packaged into secretory granules until it is released into the synapse. Once released, dopamine can interact with postsynaptic receptors (D_1-D_5) or presynaptically located autoreceptors (predominantly D_2, some D_3). These receptors are members of the seven-transmembrane domain, G-protein-coupled superfamily. The D_1 and D_5 receptors are coupled to adenylate cyclase via G_s. D_2 can be coupled to adenylate cyclase through either G_i or G_o, whereas D_3 and D_4 appear to be coupled via G_i. Dopamine can also undergo reuptake into the synthesizing cell for repackaging into granules via a transporter molecule that is located in the presynaptic cell membrane. Dopamine catabolism can occur intracellularly: monoamine oxidase (MAO) metabolizes dopamine to dihydroxyphenylacetic acid (DOPAC). ATP = adenosine triphosphate; cAMP = cyclic adenosine monophosphate.

from their cell bodies and dendrites (Geffen et al. 1976). Consistent with this characteristic, D_2 and D_3 receptors have been identified in several dopaminergic cell groups. D_2 receptors are perhaps the best documented in this regard and have been identified in the midbrain dopamine cells of the substantia nigra, zona incerta, and olfactory bulb. Whether specific members of the D_2 family may pre-

dominate in particular dopamine-producing cell groups is unclear. For example, D_2 may be the dominant dopamine receptor subtype in the zona incerta, whereas D_2 and D_3 may act as autoreceptors in the substantia nigra.

The actions of the dopamine autoreceptors have been best explored in the substantia nigra; here, dopamine agonists have been shown to inhibit dopamine release and cell firing (Aghajanian and Bunney 1977; Skirboll et al. 1979; White and Wang 1984). Many antipsychotics have, in fact, been specifically designed to activate the autoreceptors selectively, thereby reducing dopamine activity without producing extrapyramidal side effects. To some extent, these drugs have been successful, but whether they are superior to conventional pharmacological therapies is unknown because clinical data are inadequate. It was hoped with the original cloning of the D_2 receptor and the subsequent identification of a longer isoform that one form of D_2 would be the postsynaptic D_2 receptor, and the other form would be the D_2 autoreceptor. However, the multiple forms of the D_2 receptor appear to have identical anatomical distributions in the brain (Meador-Woodruff and Mansour 1991; Snyder et al. 1991).

5-HT_{1A}, 5-HT_{1B}, 5-HT_{1D}, and 5-HT_{2C} receptors are localized on the serotonin-containing cells of the brain stem. As indicated earlier in this chapter, these sites most likely act to regulate presynaptic serotonergic activity. A recently purified peptide, 5-HT-moduline, has been shown to interact with presynaptic 5-HT_{1B} receptors and may modulate serotonin release in the synapse (Fillion et al. 1996). The role of this peptide in modulating in vivo serotonin activity has not yet been determined.

Neurotransmitter Reuptake

Specific proteins have been identified that selectively remove neurotransmitters from the synapse back into the cell cytosol and subsequently to storage granules. To date, specific transporter molecules have been described for dopamine, serotonin, norepinephrine, GABA, glycine, and glutamate (see Amara 1992). Two types of dopamine transporters have been identified. One is localized in storage vesicles and is important in the relatively nonspecific reuptake into monoamine storage granules. A second is localized in the presynaptic membrane and is responsible for the selective reuptake of neurotransmitter released into the synaptic cleft. For the dopamine and serotonin transporters, neurotransmitter influx is linked to cotransport of sodium and chloride ions across the cell plasma membrane.

A number of drugs can affect levels of transmitter by binding to the uptake sites and effectively controlling syn-

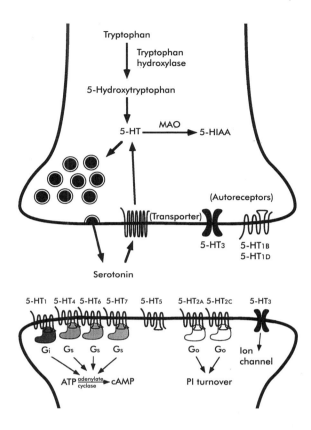

Figure 3–4. Schematic representation of a serotonergic synapse. Serotonin- (5-HT) and dopamine-synthesizing cells have many similarities: serotonin is synthesized from 5-hydroxytryptophan, which is synthesized from tryptophan. The conversion of tryptophan to 5-hydroxytryptophan by tryptophan hydroxylase is the rate-limiting step in serotonin synthesis. Like dopamine, serotonin is packaged into secretory granules after synthesis. Once released, serotonin can interact with a complement of postsynaptic receptors and autoreceptors or undergo reuptake by a transporter similar to the dopamine transporter. Most of the serotonin receptors are also members of the seven-transmembrane domain, G-protein-coupled superfamily. All of the 5-HT$_1$ receptors (i.e., 5-HT$_{1A}$, 5-HT$_{1B}$, 5-HT$_{1D}$, 5-ht$_{1E}$, and 5-ht$_{1F}$) are coupled to adenylate cyclase through G$_i$. The 5-HT$_4$, 5-HT$_6$, and 5-HT$_7$ receptors are also coupled to adenylate cyclase but via G$_s$. Rather than being coupled to adenylate cyclase, the 5-HT$_{2A}$ and 5-HT$_{2C}$ receptors are linked to phosphoinositide (PI) turnover via G$_o$. The structurally unique 5-HT$_3$ receptor appears to be a ligand-gated ion channel. The 5-HT$_5$ receptor appears to be a seven-transmembrane domain receptor molecule, but its coupling to a transduction system has not yet been determined. The 5-HT$_{1B}$, 5-HT$_{1D}$, and 5-HT$_3$ receptors have also been shown to serve as autoreceptors. 5-HT$_{1A}$ may also serve as an autoreceptor in somatodendritic synapses. Serotonin can serve as a substrate for monoamine oxidase (MAO), resulting in the formation of the metabolite 5-hydroxyindoleacetic acid (5-HIAA). ATP = adenosine triphosphate; cAMP = cyclic adenosine monophosphate.

aptic levels of neurotransmitter. Cocaine, for example, binds to the dopamine, serotonin, and norepinephrine transporters in the presynaptic membrane; inhibits reuptake; and thereby increases the levels of monoamines in the synaptic cleft. Some evidence suggests that this may, in fact, represent the underlying mechanism related to cocaine-reinforced behavior (Ritz et al. 1987). Similarly, the tricyclic antidepressants, such as imipramine and amitriptyline, and the newer selective serotonin reuptake inhibitors, such as fluoxetine, sertraline, and paroxetine, can act to block the action of the serotonin transporter, preventing the reuptake of serotonin from the synapse and prolonging the action of serotonin at synaptic receptors.

Postsynaptic Mechanisms

Unlike presynaptic forms of regulation, in which the emphasis is on the amount of neurotransmitter released into the synapse, postsynaptic mechanisms of regulation involve the ability of a neurotransmitter to produce biophysical changes in the postsynaptic membrane. As is the case for the presynaptic cell, transduction of information in the postsynaptic cells can be modulated at various levels.

Dopamine antagonists have been used to treat psychotic disorders for nearly 40 years. Many antipsychotics used today are believed to derive their therapeutic efficacy, at least in part, from their ability to block dopaminergic transmission by acting as antagonists at postsynaptic dopamine receptor sites. Typical antipsychotics are likely to have their effects at predominantly D$_2$ and D$_3$ and, to a lesser extent, D$_4$ receptors. Patients resistant to typical antipsychotics are often given atypical antipsychotics, such as clozapine, which may act predominantly at the D$_4$ receptor (Seeman 1992). Antipsychotic drugs clearly also have potent effects on other nondopaminergic receptors, such as muscarinic, adrenergic, and serotonergic receptors, which should not be ignored in understanding their mechanism of action. For example, although clozapine has a high affinity for D$_4$, it also has a good affinity for D$_2$ and a number of nondopamine receptors, including serotonergic and muscarinic receptors (Fitton and Heel 1990).

REGULATION

Acute administration of a dopamine receptor agonist or antagonist has little or no effect on receptor number. With repeated administration, however, dopamine antagonists, such as haloperidol, produce long-lasting increases in D$_2$ receptor number in rats (Boyson et al. 1988; Hess et al. 1988) that may be associated with the extrapyramidal side effects occasionally seen in humans. It is unclear whether this represents a change at the gene transcription level, however, because changes in mRNA after chronic haloperidol treatment are inconsistent. Some investigators suggest that after chronic antagonist treatment, the D_2 receptor protein may become more stabilized rather than undergo increased biosynthesis (Srivastava et al. 1990; Van Tol et al. 1990). Of the studies reporting an increase in D_2 mRNA after chronic haloperidol treatment (Buckland et al. 1992; Kopp et al. 1992), one study suggested that the shorter isoform of D_2 mRNA is particularly increased (Arnauld et al. 1991). D_1 receptor binding has also been reported to increase with chronic D_1 antagonist treatment (Creese and Chen 1985), but whether this represents a transcriptional change is unclear. Only one study (Buckland et al. 1992) of D_3 is available that shows an increase in D_3 mRNA levels after chronic antagonist treatment; no reports on the regulation of D_4 or D_5 receptors by dopamine agonists or antagonists are available. The tools to measure these receptors, however, have only recently become available.

With regard to the serotonin system, although the acute effects of both MAOIs and reuptake blockers are to increase the concentration of serotonin within the brain, the therapeutic effects of these drugs occur only after subchronic treatment (at least 2–3 weeks). The mechanism responsible for this delayed response is unclear. However, some evidence supports the long-standing theory that drug action is related to slowly developing adaptive changes in postsynaptic serotonergic elements in response to alterations in presynaptic input. For example, cortical 5-HT_{2A} receptors are downregulated after chronic antidepressant treatment (Goodwin et al. 1984). The number of hippocampal 5-HT_{1A} receptors has been reported to be increased after chronic treatment with a tricyclic antidepressant (Welner et al. 1989), although this finding has not been replicated after administration of other antidepressants (Hensler et al. 1991). Interestingly, the reported increase in hippocampal 5-HT_{1A} receptors after tricyclic treatment appears to have a functional correlate, because tricyclics also enhance the suppressant effect of 5-HT_{1A} activation on hippocampal pyramidal cells (deMontigny and Aghajanian 1978). Bearing in mind the importance of the hippocampus in limbic circuitry, alterations in 5-HT_{1A} receptors in this anatomical region may contribute to the beneficial effects of selective antidepressants (i.e., enhancing serotonergic input to hippocampal cells).

Somatodendritic 5-HT_{1A} receptors located presynaptically on serotonergic cell bodies also appear to be sensitive to regulation by specific antidepressants. Both MAOIs and selective serotonin reuptake inhibitors desensitize 5-HT_{1A} autoreceptors in raphe nuclei after chronic treatment (Blier and deMontigny 1983, 1985). Such a receptor response may act to disinhibit serotonergic cells and consequently enhance serotonergic input to projection areas. Desensitization of somatodendritic 5-HT_{1A} receptors may also be the mode of action by which 5-HT_{1A} agonists such as buspirone and gepirone produce anxiolytic and antidepressant effects (Welner et al. 1989). However, these drugs may produce their effects by regulating postsynaptic 5-HT_{1A} receptors in regions expressing high levels of these sites (i.e., hippocampus and other limbic structures).

The high levels of 5-HT_{2A} receptors within neocortical regions, particularly the claustrum, may underlie the hallucinogenic effects of 5-HT_{2A} agonists. Some 5-HT_{2A} antagonists, such as ritanserin, have been shown to have therapeutic effects in generalized anxiety and to reduce negative symptoms in schizophrenia (Leysen and Pauwels 1990). The mechanism of action for these effects is unclear but may be related to transsynaptic effects of the drugs or serotonergic/dopaminergic interactions in selective circuits. 5-HT_3 receptor antagonists have potent antiemetic properties, which relate to the high concentration of these receptors in both the nucleus tractus solitarius and the area postrema (Tyers 1990). Some evidence suggests that certain 5-HT_3 antagonists may be anxiolytic (Briley and Chopin 1991).

RECEPTOR COUPLING

Regulation of receptor number is not the only means by which a cell can control the level of signal transmission. Many dopamine and serotonin receptors, as we indicated earlier in this chapter, are coupled to G proteins. When agonists bind to these receptors, they are thought to undergo a conformational change that allows G proteins to bind tightly to the receptor, which initiates a cascade of events including the activation of a host of second messengers (e.g., adenylate cyclase) (Vallar and Meldolesi 1989). Effectiveness of signal transduction depends on not only the number of receptors and their affinity for the ligand but also the efficiency of coupling to G proteins and the ability to activate second messenger systems. For example, with lesions of dopamine cells in the substantia nigra, as occurs in Parkinson's disease, D_1 receptor number or affinity does not change, but the receptor uncouples from adenylate cyclase in striatal cells (Ariano 1989). It is also apparent that various antidepressants regulate the expression of G proteins in several brain regions after chronic administration (Lesch and Manji 1992).

The best information available to date is that D_2, D_3, and D_4 are coupled to a subset of inhibitory G proteins referred to as G_i and G_o, whereas D_1 and D_5 are coupled to a stimulatory set referred to as G_s (Figure 3–3). In studies with stably transfected cell lines, D_2 receptors were coupled to $G_{\alpha i2}$ and $G_{\alpha i3}$ but not to $G_{\alpha i1}$ (O'Hara et al. 1996). Even though it is clear that D_4 receptors are coupled to one or more inhibitory G proteins, the precise subtype has been elusive. The best evidence we have thus far suggests that they are not the same G-protein subtypes to which the D_2 receptors are coupled (O'Hara et al. 1996). However, as the family of G proteins grows, this description is too simplistic, and receptor G-protein coupling will likely depend on the cell type in which these receptors are found. In the future, drugs may be targeted to specific receptor subtypes as well as to particular G proteins to which they are coupled.

It should be kept in mind that adenylate cyclase is not the only second messenger in the brain. Dopamine D_2 receptor activation has also been linked to decreases in phospholipase C, changes in potassium (K^+) and Ca^{2+} currents, and increases in arachidonic acid (Freedman et al. 1988; Lledo et al. 1992; Pionelli et al. 1991). Similarly, in addition to adenylate cyclase inhibition, 5-HT_{1A} receptors are also linked to K^+ and Ca^{2+} channels, likely via a G protein. As stated above, the rest of the 5-HT_1 receptor family is also linked to inhibition of adenylate cyclase, whereas 5-HT_{2A}, 5-HT_{2B}, and 5-HT_{2C} receptors are coupled to inositol phosphate production (Figure 3–4). 5-HT_4, 5-HT_6, and 5-HT_7 are linked to adenylate cyclase activation via G_s. The second messenger effector pathway for the 5-ht_{5A} and 5-ht_{5B} receptors has not yet been determined (Hoyer and Martin 1996).

CONCLUSION

In emphasizing receptor selectivities and pre- and postsynaptic mechanisms, it is often easy to forget that these receptors and cells are part of complicated circuits. Despite their importance, we know only a small fraction of the potential circuits in the CNS. Neuronal circuits can be identified with traditional anterograde and retrograde anatomical tracing techniques. A newer way to measure functional circuits is the visualization and quantification of what are known as *immediate early genes* (e.g., *c-fos* and *c-jun*). Under basal conditions, the mRNA and protein levels of these molecules are very low and difficult, if not impossible, to detect. Within minutes after cellular activation or inhibition that would result from drug administration or behavioral treatment, the expression levels of these immediate early genes increase dramatically. Maps

of the cells and circuits that are transcriptionally active can be generated by examining the cellular expression of these genes before and after experimental treatments. For example, investigators have used these techniques to examine the effects of amphetamine and have demonstrated the activation of a specific subpopulation of cells in various brain areas, including the caudate-putamen, nucleus accumbens, and specific cortical areas (Graybiel et al. 1990). By colocalizing these immediate early gene products and specific receptor subtypes, one can begin to develop an appreciation of which circuits are activated during pharmacological treatment.

Perhaps the most important lesson to be learned from the preceding analysis of the dopamine and serotonin systems is the prevalence of, if not the requirement for, diversity in the CNS. This diversity is manifest in the number of receptor families, receptor subtypes, coupling mechanisms, and possible second messenger systems that can be stimulated under normal physiological conditions or with the administration of drugs. This diversity is further amplified when complex anatomical and biochemical circuitry and the colocalization of multiple receptors and neurotransmitters occur within the same cells. The obvious question is, "Why have mammals evolved such a complicated means of neuronal communication?" It may well be an adaptive mechanism to maximize the processing and integration of information. This is the primary function of the CNS and what differentiates humans from invertebrates.

This analysis has been restricted to the dopamine and serotonin systems, but it could easily have focused on a number of other neurotransmitter or neuropeptide systems. The concepts would have been the same. An emphasis on neuronal circuitry, synaptic regulation, and cellular and molecular biology would also apply to many other neurotransmitter systems. Research on the organization of the dopamine and serotonin receptor systems has made great strides in the last 5 years and promises to further the understanding of the CNS and the physiological basis of mental disorders.

REFERENCES

Aghajanian GK, Bunney BS: Dopamine autoreceptors: pharmacological characterization by microintophoretic single cell recording studies. Naunyn Schmiedebergs Arch Pharmacol 297:1–7, 1977

Albert PR, Zhou QY, Van Tol HHM, et al: Cloning, functional expression and mRNA tissue distribution of the rat 5-hydroxytryptamine$_{1A}$ receptor gene. J Biol Chem 265:5825–5832, 1990

Amara SG: A tale of two families. Nature 360:420–421, 1992

Anden NE, Dahlstrom A, Fuxe K, et al: Demonstration and mapping out of nigroneostriatal dopamine neurons. Life Sci 3:523–530, 1964

Ariano MA: Long term changes in striatal D_1 dopamine receptor distribution after dopaminergic deafferentation. J Neurosci 32:203–212, 1989

Arnauld E, Arsaut J, Demotes-Mainard J: Differential plasticity of the dopaminergic D_2 receptor mRNA isoforms under haloperidol treatment, as evidenced by in situ hybridization in rat anterior pituitary. Neurosci Lett 130:12–16, 1991

Blier P, deMontigny C: Electrophysiological investigations on the effect of repeated zimelidine administration on serotonergic transmission in the rat. J Neurosci 3:1270–1278, 1983

Blier P, deMontigny C: Serotonergic but not noradrenergic neurons in rat CNS adapt to long term treatment with monoamine oxidase inhibitors. Neuroscience 16:949–955, 1985

Bouthenet M-L, Martres MP, Sales N, et al: A detailed mapping of dopamine D_2 receptors in rat CNS by autoradiography with [^{125}I] Iodosulpride. Neuroscience 20:117–155, 1987

Bouthenet M-L, Souil E, Matres M-P, et al: Localization of dopamine D_3 receptor mRNA in the rat brain using in situ hybridization histochemistry: comparison with D_2 receptor mRNA. Brain Res 564:203–219, 1991

Boyson SJ, McGonigle P, Molinoff PB: Quantitative autoradiographic localization of the D_1 and D_2 subtypes of dopamine receptors in rat brain. J Neurosci 6:3177–3188, 1986

Boyson SJ, McGonigle P, Luthin GR, et al: Effects of chronic administration of neuroleptic and anticholinergic agents on the densities of D_2 dopamine and muscarinic cholinergic receptors in rat striatum. J Pharmacol Exp Ther 244:987–993, 1988

Briley M, Chopin P: Serotonin in anxiety: evidence from animal models, in 5-Hydroxytryptamine in Psychiatry: A Spectrum of Ideas. Edited by Sandler M, Coppen A, Harnett S. Oxford, NY, Oxford Medical Publications, 1991, pp 177–197

Buckland PR, O'Donovan MC, McGuffin P: Changes in D_1, D_2, and D_3 receptor mRNA levels in rat brain following antipsychotic treatment. Psychopharmacology 106:479–483, 1992

Bunzow JR, Van Tol HHM, Grandy DK, et al: Cloning and expression of a rat D_2 dopamine receptor cDNA. Nature 336:783–787, 1988

Chalmers DT, Watson SJ: Comparative anatomical distribution of 5-HT_{1A} receptor mRNA and 5-HT_{1A} binding in rat brain—a combined in situ hybridization/in vitro receptor autoradiographic study. Brain Res 561:51–60, 1991

Charuchinda C, Supavilai P, Karobath M, et al: Dopamine D_2 receptors in the rat brain: autoradiographic visualization using a high affinity selective agonist ligand. J Neurosci 7:1352–1360, 1987

Clark D, White FJ: Review: D_1 dopamine receptor—the search for a function; a critical evaluation of the D_1/D_2 dopamine classification and its functional implications. Synapse 1:345–388, 1987

Creese I, Chen A: Selective D_1 dopamine receptor increase following chronic treatment with SCH23390. Eur J Pharmacol 109:127–128, 1985

Curran EJ, Watson SJ Jr: Dopamine receptor mRNA expression patterns by opioid peptide cells in the nucleus accumbens of the rat: a double in situ hybridization study. J Comp Neurol 361:57–76, 1995

Dahlstrom A, Fuxe K: Evidence for the existence of monoamine-containing neurons in the CNS, I: demonstration of monoamines in cell bodies of brain stem neurons. Acta Physiol Scand Suppl 232:1–55, 1964

Dal Toso R, Sommer B, Ewert M, et al: The dopamine D_2 receptor: two molecular forms generated by alternative splicing. EMBO J 8:4025–4034, 1989

Dawson TM, Barone P, Sidhu A, et al: The D_1 dopamine receptor in the rat brain: quantitative autoradiographic localization using an iodinated ligand. Neuroscience 26:83–100, 1988

Dearry A, Gingrich JA, Falardeau P, et al: Molecular cloning and expression of the gene for a human D_1 dopamine receptor. Nature 347:72–76, 1990

deMontigny C, Aghajanian GK: Tricyclic antidepressants: long term treatment increases responsivity of rat forebrain neurons to serotonin. Science 202:1303–1306, 1978

Fillion G, Rousselle J-C, Massot O, et al: A new peptide, 5-HT-moduline, isolated and purified from mammalian brain specifically interacts with 5-$HT_{1B/1D}$ receptors. Behav Brain Res 73:313–317, 1996

Fitton A, Heel RC: Clozapine—a review of pharmacological properties, and therapeutic use in schizophrenia. Drug 40:722–747, 1990

Freedman JE, Weight FF: Simple K$^+$ channels activated by D_2 dopamine receptors in acutely dissociated neurons from rat corpus striatum. Proc Natl Acad Sci U S A 85:3618–3622, 1988

Fremeau RT, Duncan GE, Fornaretto M-G, et al: Localization of D_1 dopamine receptor mRNA in brain supports a role in cognitive, affective, and neuroendocrine aspects of dopaminergic neurotransmission. Proc Natl Acad Sci U S A 88:3772–3776, 1991

Geffen LB, Jessell TM, Cuello AC, et al: Release of dopamine from dendrites in rat substantia nigra. Nature 260:258–261, 1976

Gerfen CR, McGinty JF, Young WS: Dopamine differentially regulates dynorphin, substance P, and enkephalin expression in striatal neurons: in situ hybridization histochemical analysis. J Neurosci 11:1016–1031, 1991

Giros B, Sokoloff P, Martes M-P, et al: Alternative splicing directs the expression of two D_2 dopamine receptor isoforms. Nature 342:923–926, 1989

Giros B, Martes M-P, Pilon C, et al: Shorter variants of the D$_3$ dopamine receptor produced through various patterns of alternative splicing. Biochem Biophys Res Commun 176:1584–1592, 1991

Goodwin GM, Green AR, Johnson P: 5-HT$_2$ receptor characteristics in frontal cortex and 5-HT$_2$ receptor-mediated head twitch behaviour following antidepressant treatment to mice. Br J Pharmacol 83:235–242, 1984

Graybiel AM, Moratalla R, Robertson HA: Amphetamine and cocaine induce drug specific activation of the c-fos gene in striosome-matrix compartments and limbic subdivisions of the striatum. Proc Natl Acad Sci U S A 87:6912–6919, 1990

Hamblin MW, Metcalf MA: Primary structure and functional characterization of a human 5-HT$_{1D}$ serotonin receptor. Mol Pharmacol 40:143–148, 1991

Hamblin MW, McGuffin RW, Metcalf MA, et al: Distinct 5-HT$_{1B}$ and 5-HT$_{1D}$ serotonin receptors in rat: structural and pharmacological comparison of the two cloned receptors. Mol Cell Neurosci 3:578–587, 1992

Heimer L, Zahm DS, Churchill L, et al: Specificity in the projection patterns of accumbal core and shell in the rat. Neuroscience 41:89–125, 1991

Hensler JG, Kovachich GB, Frazer A: A quantitative autoradiographic study of serotonin1A receptor regulation: effect of 5,7-dihydroxytryptamine and antidepressant treatments. Neuropsychopharmacology 4:131–144, 1991

Hess EJ, Norman AB, Cresse I: Chronic treatment with dopamine receptor antagonists: behavioral and pharmacologic effects of D$_1$ and D$_2$ dopamine receptors. J Neurosci 8:2361–2370, 1988

Hoffman BJ, Mezey E: Distribution of serotonin 5-HT$_{1C}$ receptor mRNA in adult rat brain. FEBS Lett 247:453–462, 1989

Hökfelt T: The possible ultrastructural identification of tubero-infundibular dopamine containing nerve endings in the median eminence of the rat. Brain Res 5:121–123, 1967

Hökfelt T, Johansson O, Fuxe K, et al: Immunohistochemical studies on the localization and distribution of monoamine neuron systems in the rat brain, I: tyrosine hydroxylase in the mes and diencephalon. Med Biol Eng Comput 54:427–453, 1976

Hoyer D, Martin GR: Classification and nomenclature of 5-HT receptors: a comment on current issues. Behav Brain Res 73:263–268, 1996

Humphrey PPA, Hartig P, Hoyer D: A proposed new nomenclature for 5-HT receptors. Trends Pharmacol Sci 14:233–236, 1993

Jin H, Oksenberg D, Ashkenazi A, et al: Characterization of the human 5-hydroxytryptamine$_{1B}$ receptor. J Biol Chem 267:5735–5738, 1992

Julius D, McDermott R, Axel R, et al: Molecular characterization of a functional cDNA encoding the serotonin 1c receptor. Science 241:558–564, 1988

Kilpatrick GJ, Hagan RM, Gale JD: 5-HT3 and 5-HT4 receptors in terminal regions of the mesolimbic system. Behav Brain Res 73:11–13, 1996

Kopp J, Lindefors N, Brene S, et al: Effect of raclopride on dopamine D$_2$ receptor mRNA expression in rat brain. Neuroscience 47:771–779, 1992

Landwehrmeyer B, Mengod G, Palacios JM: Differential visualization of dopamine D$_2$ and D$_3$ receptor sites in rat brain: a comparative study using in situ hybridization histochemistry and ligand binding autoradiography. Eur J Neurosci 5:145–153, 1993

Lesch KP, Manji HK: Signal-transducing G proteins and antidepressant drugs: evidence for modulation of alpha subunit gene expression in rat brain. Biol Psychiatry 32:549–579, 1992

Leysen JE, Pauwels PJ: 5-HT$_2$ receptors, roles and regulation, in The Neuropharmacology of Serotonin. Edited by Whitaker-Azmitia PM, Peroutka S. New York, New York Academy of Sciences, 1990, pp 183–193

Lidov HGW, Grzanna R, Molliver ME: The serotonin innervation of the cerebral cortex in the rat—an immunohistochemical analysis. Neuroscience 5:207–227, 1980

Lindvall O: Mesencephalic dopamine afferents to the lateral septal nucleus of the rat. Brain Res 87:89–95, 1975

Lindvall O, Bjorkland A, Moore A, et al: Mesencephalic dopamine neurons projecting to the neocortex. Brain Res 81:325–331, 1974

Lledo PM, Hornburger V, Bockaert J, et al: Differential G-protein-mediated coupling of D$_2$ dopamine receptors to K$^+$ and Ca^{2+} currents in rat anterior pituitary cells. Neuron 8:455–463, 1992

Mansour A, Meador-Woodruff JH, Bunzow JR, et al: Localization of dopamine D$_2$ receptor mRNA and D$_1$ and D$_2$ receptor binding in the rat brain and pituitary: an in situ hybridization-receptor autoradiographic analysis. J Neurosci 10:2587–2600, 1990

Mansour A, Meador-Woodruff JH, Zhou Q-Y, et al: A comparison of D$_1$ receptor binding and mRNA in rat brain using receptor autoradiographic and in situ hybridization techniques. Neuroscience 45:359–371, 1991

Maroteaux L, Saudou F, Amlaiky N, et al: Mouse 5-HT1B serotonin receptor: cloning, functional expression and localization in motor control centers. Proc Natl Acad Sci U S A 89:3020–3024, 1992

McAllister G, Charlesworth A, Snodin C, et al: Molecular cloning of a serotonin receptor from human brain (5-HT$_{1E}$): a fifth 5-HT1-like subtype. Proc Natl Acad Sci U S A 89:5517–5521, 1992

Meador-Woodruff JH, Mansour A: Expression of the dopamine D$_2$ receptor gene in brain. Biol Psychiatry 30:985–1007, 1991

Meador-Woodruff JH, Mansour A, Bunzow JR, et al: Distribution of D$_2$ dopamine receptor mRNA in rat brain. Proc Natl Acad Sci U S A 86:7625–7628, 1989

Meador-Woodruff JH, Mansour A, Healy DJ, et al: Comparison of the distributions of D_1 and D_2 dopamine receptor mRNAs in the rat brain. Neuropsychopharmacology 5:231–242, 1991

Meador-Woodruff JH, Mansour A, Grandy DK, et al: Distribution of D_5 dopamine receptor mRNA in rat brain. Neurosci Lett 145:209–212, 1992

Meador-Woodruff JH, Damask SP, Watson SJ Jr: Differential expression of autoreceptors in the ascending dopamine systems of the human brain. Proc Natl Acad Sci U S A 91:8297–8301, 1994a

Meador-Woodruff JH, Grandy DK, Van Tol HHM, et al: Dopamine receptor gene expression in the human medial temporal lobe. Neuropsychopharmacology 10:239–248, 1994b

Meador-Woodruff JH, Damask SP, Wang J, et al: Dopamine receptor mRNA expression in human striatum and neocortex. Neuropsychopharmacology 15:17–29, 1996

Mengod G, Pompeiano M, Inocencia M, et al: Localization of the mRNA for the 5-HT_2 receptor by in situ hybridization histochemistry: correlation with the distribution of receptor sites. Brain Res 524:139–143, 1990

Mengod G, Vilaró MT, Niznik HB, et al: Visualization of a dopamine D_1 receptor mRNA in human and rat brain. Molecular Brain Research 10:185–191, 1991

Mengod G, Villaró MT, Landwehrmeyer GB, et al: Visualization of dopamine D_1, D_2, and D_3 receptor mRNAs in human and rat brain. Neurochem Int 20 (suppl):33S–43S, 1992

Monsma FJ, McVittie LD, Gerten CR, et al: Multiple D_2 dopamine receptors produced by alternative RNA splicing. Nature 342:926–929, 1989

Monsma FJ, Mahan LC, McVittie LD, et al: Molecular cloning and expression of a D_1 dopamine receptor linked to adenylyl cyclase activation. Proc Natl Acad Sci U S A 87:6723–6727, 1990

Moore RY: Catecholamine innervation of the basal forebrain, I: the septal area. J Comp Neurol 177:665–684, 1978

Morilak DA, Garlow SJ, Ciaranello RD: Localization and description of 5-HT_2 immunoreactive neurons in the rat brain. Society for Neuroscience Abstracts 18:212, 1992

Nagy JI, Lee T, Seeman P, et al: Direct evidence for presynaptic and postsynaptic dopamine receptors in brain. Nature 274:278–281, 1978

Najlerahim A, Barton AJL, Harrison PJ, et al: Messenger RNA encoding the D_2 dopaminergic receptor detected by in situ hybridization histochemistry in rat brain. FEBS Lett 255:335–339, 1989

Nauta WJH, Smith GP, Faull RLM, et al: Efferent connections and nigral afferents of the nucleus accumbens septi in the rat. Neuroscience 3:385–401, 1978

O'Hara CM, Tang L, Taussig R, et al: Dopamine D_{2L} receptor couples to $G_{\alpha i2}$ and $G_{\alpha i3}$ but not $G_{\alpha i1}$, leading to the inhibition of adenylate cyclase in transfected cell lines. J Pharmacol Exp Ther 278:354–360, 1996

O'Malley KL, Harmon S, Tang L, et al: The rat dopamine D_4 receptor: sequence, gene structure, and demonstration of expression in the cardiovascular system. New Biologist 4:137–146, 1992

Pearson J, Halliday G, Sakamoto N, et al: Catecholeminergic neurons, in The Human Nervous System. Edited by Paxinos G. San Diego, CA, Academic Press, 1990, pp 1023–1050

Peroutka SJ, Snyder SH: Multiple serotonin receptors: differential binding of [^{3}H]-5-hydroxytryptamine, [^{3}H]-lysergic acid diethylamide and [^{3}H]-spiperidol. Mol Pharmacol 16:687–699, 1979

Pionelli D, Pilon C, Giros B, et al: Dopamine activation of the arachidonic acid cascade via a modulatory mechanism as a basis of D_1/D_2 receptor synergism. Nature 353:164–167, 1991

Ramboz S, Saudou F, Amara DA, et al: 5-HT1B receptor knock out-behavioral consequences. Behav Brain Res 73:305–312, 1996

Ritz MC, Lamb RJ, Goldberg SR, et al: Cocaine receptors on dopamine transporters are related to self administration of cocaine. Science 237:1219–1223, 1987

Roth BL, Craigo SC, Salman Choudary M, et al: Binding of typical and atypical antipsychotic agents to 5-hydroxytryptamine-6 and 5-hydroxytryptamine-7 receptors. J Pharmacol Exp Ther 268:1404–1410, 1994

Seeman P: Dopamine receptor sequences—theraputic levels of neuroleptics occupy D_2 receptors, clozapine occupies D_4. Neuropsychopharmacology 7:261–284, 1992

Sijbesma H, Schipper J, De Kloet ER, et al: Postsynaptic 5-HT1 receptors and offensive aggression in rats: a combined behavioural and autoradiographic study with eltoprazine. Pharmacol Biochem Behav 38:447–458, 1991

Skirboll LR, Grace AA, Bunney BS: Dopamine auto- and postsynaptic receptors: electrophysiological evidence for differential sensitivity to dopamine agonists. Science 206:80–82, 1979

Snyder LA, Roberts JL, Sealfon SC: Distribution of dopamine D_2 receptor mRNA splice variants in the rat by solution hybridization/protection assay. Neurosci Lett 122:37–40, 1991

Sokoloff P, Giros B, Martes M-P, et al: Molecular cloning and characterization of a novel dopamine receptor (D_3) as a target for neuroleptics. Nature 347:146–151, 1991

Sprouse JS, Aghajanian GK: Electrophysiological responses of serotonergic dorsal raphe neurons to 5-HT_{1A} and 5-HT_{1B} agonists. Synapse 1:3–9, 1987

Srivastava LK, Morency MA, Bajwa SB, et al: Effect of haloperidol on expression of dopamine D_2 receptor mRNAs in rat brain. J Mol Neurosci 2:155–161, 1990

Steinbusch HWM, Nieuwenhuys R: The raphe nuclei of the rat brain stem: a cytoarchitectonic and immunohistochemical study, in Chemical Neuroanatomy. Edited by Emson PC. New York, Raven, 1983, pp 131–207

Stoof JC, Kebabian JW: Two dopamine receptors: biochemistry, physiology and pharmacology. Life Sci 35:2281–2296, 1984

Sunahara RK, Niznik HB, Weiner DM, et al: Human dopamine D_1 receptor encoded by an intronless gene on chromosome 5. Nature 347:80–83, 1990

Sunahara RK, Guan H-C, O'Dowd BF, et al: Cloning of the gene for a human dopamine D_5 receptor with higher affinity for dopamine than D_1. Nature 350:614–619, 1991

Surmeier DJ, Eberwine J, Wilson CJ, et al: Dopamine receptor subtypes co-localize in rat striatonigral neurons. Proc Natl Acad Sci U S A 89:10178–10182, 1992

Tiberi M, Jarvie KR, Silvia C, et al: Cloning, molecular characterization, and chromosomal assignment of a gene encoding a second D_1 dopamine receptor subtype: differential expression pattern in rat brain compared with the D_{1A} receptor. Proc Natl Acad Sci U S A 88:7491–7495, 1991

Tork I: Raphe nuclei and serotonin containing systems, in The Rat Nervous System, Vol 2. Edited by Paxinos G. Sydney, Academic Press, 1985, pp 43–78

Tork I: Anatomy of the serotonergic system, in The Neuropharmacology of Serotonin. Edited by Whitaker-Azmitia P, Peroutka S. New York, New York Academy of Sciences, 1990, pp 9–35

Tricklebank MD: The antipsychotic potential of subtype selective 5-HT receptor ligands based on interactions with mesolimbic dopamine systems. Behav Brain Res 73:15–17, 1996

Tyers MB: 5-HT$_3$ receptors, in The Neuropharmacology of Serotonin. Edited by Whitaker-Azmitia PM, Peroutka S. New York, New York Academy of Sciences, 1990, pp 194–205

Ungerstedt U: Stereotaxic mapping of the monoamine pathways in the rat brain. Acta Physiol Scand Suppl 367:1–49, 1971

Vallar L, Meldolesi J: Mechanisms of signal transduction at the dopamine D_2 receptor. Trends Pharmacol Sci 10:74–77, 1989

Van Tol HHM, Riva M, Civelli O, et al: Lack of effect of chronic dopamine receptor mRNA level. Neurosci Lett 111:303–308, 1990

Van Tol HHM, Bunzow JR, Guan H-C, et al: Cloning of the gene for a human dopamine D_4 receptor with high affinity for the antipsychotic clozapine. Nature 350:610–614, 1991

Van Tol HHM, Wu CM, Guan H-C, et al: Multiple dopamine D_4 receptor variants in the human population. Nature 358:149–152, 1992

Voigt MM, Laurie DJ, Seeburg PH, et al: Molecular cloning and characterization of a rat brain cDNA encoding a 5-hydroxytryptamine$_{1B}$ receptor. EMBO J 10:4017–4023, 1991

Wamsley JK, Gehlert DR, Filloux FM, et al: Comparison of the distribution of D_1 and D_2 dopamine receptors in the rat brain. J Comp Neuroanatomy 2:119–137, 1989

Weiner DM, Levey AI, Sunahara RK, et al: D_1 and D_2 dopamine receptor mRNA in rat brain. Proc Natl Acad Sci U S A 88:1859–1863, 1991

Weinshank RL, Adham N, Macchi M, et al: Molecular cloning and characterization of a high affinity dopamine receptor (D_{1B}) and its pseudogene. J Biol Chem 266:22427–22435, 1991

Welner SA, deMontigny C, Desroches J, et al: Autoradiographic quantification of serotonin$_{1A}$ receptors in rat brain following antidepressant drug treatment. Synapse 4:347–352, 1989

White FJ, Wang RY: Pharmacological characterization of dopamine autoreceptors in the rat ventral tegmental area: microiontophoretic studies. J Pharmacol Exp Ther 231:275–280, 1984

Zhou QY, Grandy DK, Thambi L, et al: Cloning and expression of human and rat D_1 dopamine receptors. Nature 347:76–80, 1990

FOUR

Electrophysiology

Anthony A. Grace, Ph.D., and
Benjamin S. Bunney, M.D.

Several approaches can be used to analyze the structure and function of the nervous system in health and disease. Many of these techniques—for example, the biochemical analysis of neurotransmitter and metabolite levels, anatomical studies of axonal projection sites or neurotransmitter enzymes, and molecular biological studies of messenger levels and turnover—examine the nervous system at the level of groups or populations of neurons. In contrast, by its very nature, electrophysiology is oriented toward the physiological analysis of individual neurons. In this chapter, we describe preparations and techniques that are in a general sense applicable to many systems, with specific examples drawn from the dopaminergic system to draw on our field of expertise.

The use of electrophysiological techniques for the analysis of neuronal physiology depends on the unique properties of the neuronal membrane. Like many other cell types, the neuron possesses an electrochemical gradient across its membrane. The electrochemical gradient itself is a product of two forces: an electrical potential force that is derived from the voltage difference between the inside and the outside of the cell and a chemical potential force that results from the unequal distribution of ions across the membrane. Cells set up and maintain this electrochemical gradient because of the selective permeability of their membranes to particular ionic species. Thus, the membrane has a rather high degree of permeability to ions such as potassium but is relatively impermeable to ions such as sodium and calcium.

In the resting state, cells have a very low internal concentration of sodium and calcium. To achieve this state, the cell must expend energy (in the form of adenosine tri-phosphate [ATP] hydrolysis) to extrude sodium from the intracellular space in exchange for potassium ions. The extrusion of sodium sets up both a chemical gradient (because sodium attempts to exist in equal concentrations across the membrane) and an electrical gradient (because sodium is positively charged and is not freely permeable across the membrane; thus, net positive charges are being removed from inside the cell). To partially counter this electrical gradient, potassium—which is more permeable—flows down the electrical gradient to become concentrated inside the cell. However, during this process, it is also setting up an opposing chemical gradient because it is achieving higher concentrations within the cell when compared with the extracellular environment. When the electrical force drawing potassium into the cell balances the chemical force of the concentration gradient forcing potassium out of the cell, the membrane is at equilibrium—with high extracellular sodium concentrations, relatively high intracellular potassium concentrations, and a transmembrane potential causing the inside of the cell to be negatively charged with respect to its environment.

A typical resting membrane potential for a neuron is rather small, being on the order of -70 mV with respect to the extracellular fluid. In actuality, potassium itself is not freely permeable. A small electrochemical gradient exists in most neurons that attempts to force potassium out of the cell and draw the membrane potential to more negative values. Although the scenario is somewhat more complicated than this (e.g., involving charged proteins and other ionic species with selective permeabilities), this description approximates how a cell gains an electrochemical gradient via the energy-dependent extrusion of sodium.

Note that neurons are not the only cells that have

transmembrane potentials. In fact, all living cells have an electrochemical gradient across their membranes that they use for transporting glucose and other essential materials and accumulating them against a concentration gradient. Such energy-dependent processes are usually coupled to other gradients from which they derive this energy. For example, a compound may be taken up and concentrated by linking its transport to sodium, which itself has a large electrochemical gradient in the opposite direction. What makes the neuron unique is its ability to rapidly change the permeability of its membrane to one or more ion species in a regenerative manner. This process underlies the generation of an action potential, sets up active propagation of an action potential down an axon, and triggers the procedure that ultimately results in neurotransmitter release. It also provides the electrophysiologist with a measure of neuronal activity that can be assayed by recording the electrical activity generated by the neuron.

The *action potential* is an active, regenerative phenomenon, which means that the events that initiate the action potential also serve as the force that drives this event to completion. Normally, a given neuron receives information in the form of synaptic potentials. For example, an axon terminal synapsing on the neuron releases a neurotransmitter, which binds to the neuron and selectively alters the permeability of its membrane by opening ion channels linked to its binding site. An ion channel that opens in response to a neurotransmitter is referred to as a *ligand-gated channel*. If the neurotransmitter activates a channel that increases the permeability of the membrane to a negatively charged ion present in high concentrations in the extracellular fluid (e.g., chloride), the influx of chloride down its electrochemical gradient causes a negative shift in the membrane potential of the cell, thereby increasing the potential difference across the membrane, or a hyperpolarization of the cell. If activation of this channel causes a positively charged ion such as sodium to flow down its electrochemical gradient and into the cell, it will cause a brief decrease in the membrane potential (i.e., a depolarization) of the neuron.

Because a change in the membrane potential alters the electrochemical gradient of potassium across the membrane, potassium ions will flow through their respective channels to restore the membrane to its resting level. Thus, a neurotransmitter that depolarizes the membrane causes an efflux of potassium ions and a return of the membrane potential to resting levels. However, if the depolarization is large enough, another type of channel is activated—the *voltage-gated* or *voltage-dependent sodium channel*. In response to a given level of depolarization, this channel increases its permeability to sodium to allow more of this ion

to enter the cell. The result is a further depolarization of the membrane and consequently increased activation of this voltage-dependent channel. Because of the positive feedback nature of this event, it is referred to as regenerative because the depolarization augments the very factor that causes the cell to be depolarized. The membrane potential at which this regenerative process is initiated is thus the threshold potential for action potential generation, with a hyperpolarization of the cell causing a decrease in its excitability and a depolarization increasing the likelihood that it will generate an action potential.

The regenerative depolarization of the membrane has limits, however. One limit is the equilibrium potential for sodium. The *equilibrium potential* is the membrane potential at which the electrochemical gradient for a particular ion is zero, with no net flux of the ion across a membrane. This would occur when the membrane potential is sufficiently positive to oppose the further influx of the positively charged sodium ion across its concentration gradient. Although this potential is usually about +40 mV in many cells, the action potential does not actually reach this value. Instead, another voltage-activated channel that is selectively permeable to potassium is activated. The resultant massive increase in potassium permeability starts to return the membrane potential to its original state, thereby inactivating the regenerative sodium conductance. The increased potassium permeability is sufficient to drive the membrane potential negative to the resting potential and toward the equilibrium potential for potassium (i.e., approximately −80 to −90 mV) before the subsequent decrease in voltage-dependent potassium conductance returns the membrane to its original resting state.

The equilibrium potential of an ion determines the net effect that opening its associated ion channels will have on the neuron. The equilibrium potential occurs when the membrane is depolarized or hyperpolarized sufficiently to offset exactly the effects of the concentration gradient on the ion; as a result, no net flux of this ion crosses the membrane. For example, because of the very high concentration of sodium outside of the neuron compared with inside the cell, the large concentration gradient for sodium across the membrane attempts to force sodium into the neuron. Therefore, to oppose this concentration gradient, the membrane potential of the neuron would have to be highly positive to provide an electrical gradient of equivalent force. This occurs at approximately +40 mV for sodium. However, potassium's equilibrium potential is about 10–20 mV more negative than its resting potential, which is partly the result of ATP hydrolysis that exchanges extruded sodium for potassium. As a result, increasing potassium permeability causes a hyperpolarization of the neuron because of an efflux of potassium down its concentration gradient.

Chloride is another common ionic species. This ion is negatively charged and therefore has an electrical gradient that would act against it entering the cell. However, the concentration of chloride is so much higher in the extracellular fluid that the chemical gradient predominates. As a result, opening chloride ion channels causes chloride to flow into the cell, hyperpolarizing the membrane (Figure 4–1). In fact, the opening of chloride ion channels is the mechanism through which the primary inhibitory neurotransmitter in the brain (i.e., γ-aminobutyric acid [GABA]) decreases neuronal activity.

Neurons within the vertebrate nervous system have additional conductances that provide them with unique functions. One of these conductances is the voltage-gated calcium conductance. Like sodium, calcium exists in higher concentrations outside of the neuron compared with inside the cell. However, the gradient is even more extreme than it is for sodium. Even though much less calcium than sodium is present in the extracellular fluid, the equilibrium potential for calcium is almost +240 mV because of the extremely low intracellular concentration of this ion. The neuron maintains this low intracellular concentration so as to use this ion for specialized purposes. Thus, calcium influx causes neurotransmitter release, activates calcium-gated ion channels, and triggers second-messenger systems (e.g., calcium-regulated protein kinase). Calcium channels, like their sodium counterparts, are also voltage gated and cause calcium influx into the neuron during the action potential. Furthermore, calcium can influence the excitability of the cell by activating the calcium-activated potassium current, which then causes a large membrane hyperpolarization after the spike, known as an *afterhyperpolarization*, that delays the occurrence of a subsequent spike in that neuron. After entering the neuron, calcium is rapidly sequestered into intracellular organelles to terminate its action and reset the neuron before the next event. Therefore, calcium can alter the physiological activity and the biochemical properties of the neuron it affects (Llinás 1988).

ELECTROPHYSIOLOGICAL TECHNIQUES

By using a broad range of electrophysiological techniques to assess information about a neuron, such as that described earlier in this chapter, experiments can be designed to investigate differences in the physiological properties of neurons of interest, the interaction between neurotransmitter systems that are involved in behavioral or pathological conditions, and the mode of action of pathomimetic or psychotherapeutic agents. In attempting to gain such information, it is important to note that there is no "best" technique. Each approach has its relative strengths and weaknesses, and only through integrating information gained at these various levels will a more complete comprehension of neuronal function be achieved.

Numerous parameters of neuronal activity can be assessed electrophysiologically. These parameters can be selectively assessed depending on the method of recording used. Six recording methods are reviewed here: electroencephalographic (EEG) recordings, field potential recordings, single unit extracellular recordings, intracellular recordings, patch clamp recordings, and whole-cell recordings. Which parameter is measured is essentially a function of the type of electrode used.

Electroencephalographic Recordings

In recording EEGs, the desired signal is very small in amplitude; thus, a large electrode that sums activity over large regions of the brain surface is used. Although this technique is less invasive than others, the information it yields is comparatively narrow, in that a large array of neurons must be simultaneously activated for the potentials to be recorded at the scalp. As a result, stimulus presentation and EEG averaging are typically required to separate the signal desired from the background noise.

Field Potential Recordings

The next level of analysis is the recording of field potentials. This method uses a recording electrode with a smaller tip and a higher resistance than that for EEG electrodes, and the electrophysiological measures are confined to a small population of neurons surrounding the electrode tip. This technique still depends on the simultaneous activation of a number of cells; however, because the electrode is inserted into the brain, the cells do not have to be at the surface of the skull as in the EEG recordings. Furthermore, the activation can consist of stimulation of an afferent pathway. Nonetheless, the array of neurons sampled must have a common orientation for the massed activity to be measurable. Therefore, such measures are typically restricted to cortical structures such as the neocortex and hippocampus. With this method, the current resulting from the parallel activation of excitatory and inhibitory afferents can be measured as well as the electrophysiological response of a population of neurons to such stimulation. However, as with EEG recordings, such an approach is of limited value in psychopharmacological research.

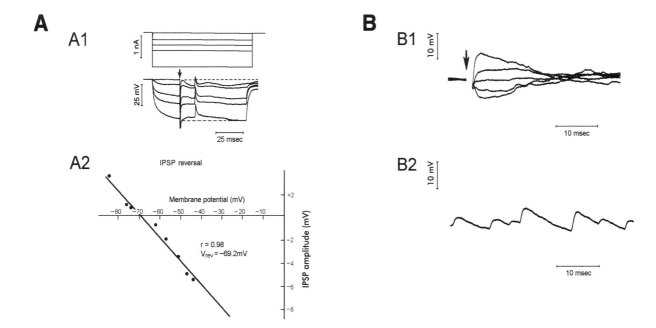

Figure 4–1. At least three techniques can be used to determine the ionic species that mediates a synaptic response: determining the reversal potential of the ion, reversing the membrane potential deflection produced by changing the concentration gradient of the ion across the membrane, and determining the reversal potential (or blocking the synaptic response) after applying a specific ion channel blocker.

In this figure, three techniques are used to illustrate the involvement of a chloride ion conductance increase evoked in dopamine-containing neurons by stimulation of the striatonigral γ-aminobutyric acid (GABA)ergic projection.

A: The reversal potential of a response may be determined by examining the amplitude of the response as the membrane potential of the neuron is varied. In this example, we superimposed several responses of the neuron evoked at increasingly hyperpolarized membrane potentials (top traces), with the membrane potential altered by injecting current through the electrode and into the neuron (bottom traces = current injection). *Panel A1:* A synaptic response in the form of an inhibitory postsynaptic potential (IPSP) is evoked in a dopamine neuron by stimulating the GABAergic striatonigral pathway (arrow). When increasing amplitudes of hyperpolarizing current (lower traces) are injected into the neuron through the electrode, a progressive hyperpolarization of the membrane occurs (top traces). As the membrane is made more negative, the IPSP diminishes in amplitude, eventually being replaced by a depolarizing response. *Panel A2:* Plotting the amplitude of the evoked response (y-axis) against the membrane potential at which it was evoked (x-axis) illustrates how the synaptic response changes with membrane potential. The membrane voltage at which the synaptic response is equal to zero (i.e., −69.2 mV in this case) is the reversal potential of the ion mediating the synaptic response (i.e., the potential at which the electrochemical forces working on the

ion are zero). Therefore, there is no net flux of ions that cross the membrane. At more negative membrane potentials, the flow of the ion is reversed, causing the chloride ion (in this case) to exit the cell and result in a depolarization of the membrane.

B: The flow of an ion across a membrane may also be altered by changing the concentration gradient of the ion across the membrane. Normally, chloride ions flow from the outside of the neuron (where they are present at a higher concentration) to the inside of the neuron (where their concentration is lower), causing the membrane potential to become more negative. In this case, the concentration of chloride ions across the membrane of the dopamine neuron is reversed by using potassium chloride as the electrolyte in the intracellular recording electrode. *Panel B1:* Soon after the neuron is impaled with the potassium chloride-containing electrode, stimulation of the striatonigral pathway (arrow) evokes an IPSP (bottom trace). However, as the recording is maintained, chloride is diffusing from the electrode into the neuron, causing the electrochemical gradient to decrease progressively over time. As a result, each subsequent stimulation pulse evokes a smaller IPSP, eventually causing the IPSP to reverse to a depolarization (top trace). The depolarization is caused by an efflux of chloride ions out of the neuron and down its new electrochemical gradient. This has caused the reversal potential of the chloride-mediated response to change from a potential that was negative to the resting potential to one that is now positive to the resting potential. *Panel B2:* After injecting chloride ions into the neuron, spontaneously occurring IPSPs that were not readily observed in the control case are now readily seen as reversed IPSPs (i.e., depolarizations) occurring in this dopamine neuron recorded in vivo.

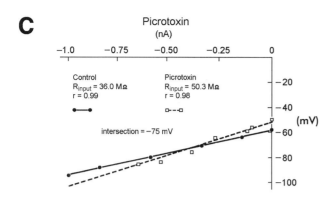

Figure 4–1. *(continued)* **C:** Another means for determining the ionic conductance involved in a response is by using a specific ion channel blocker. This can be done in two ways: by using the drug to block an evoked response or (as shown in this example) by examining the effects of administering the drug on the neuron to determine whether the cell is receiving synaptic events that alter the conductance of the membrane to this ion. To do this, the current/voltage relationship of the cell is first established. This is done by injecting hyperpolarizing current pulses into the neuron (x-axis) and recording the membrane potential that is present during the current injection (y-axis). These values are then plotted on the graph (filled circles), with the resting membrane potential being the membrane potential at which no current is being injected into the neuron (y-intercept). The slope of the resultant regression line (solid line) is equal to the input resistance of the neuron (R_{input} = 36 megohms). After administration of the chloride ion channel blocker picrotoxin (open boxes), a new current/voltage relationship is established in a similar manner. Picrotoxin caused a depolarization of the membrane (y-intercept of dashed line is more positive) and an increase in the neuron input resistance (the slope of the dashed line is larger). The intersection of the membrane current/voltage plots obtained before and after picrotoxin administration is then calculated. By definition, this point of intersection (i.e., –75 mV) is the reversal potential of the response to picrotoxin, because a neuron at this membrane potential would show no net change in membrane potential on drug administration.

Source. Adapted from Grace AA, Bunney BS: "Opposing Effects of Striatonigral Feedback Pathways on Midbrain Dopamine Cell Activity." *Brain Research* 333:271–284, 1985. Used with permission.

Single Unit Extracellular Recordings

The next level of recording involves examining the electrophysiology of individual neurons with extracellular single unit recording techniques. This technique requires that an electrode be placed in close proximity to a single neuron to record its spike discharge. An electrode with a smaller tip and a higher resistance than those used for recording field potentials results in the sampling of a smaller volume of tissue (i.e., the somata of individual neurons). Because the region sampled by the electrode is small, the signal is larger in amplitude and the background noise is less. This allows easy recording of the spontaneous spike discharge of a single neuron within the brain of a living (but typically anesthetized) animal. The cells examined are located by the use of an atlas and a stereotaxic apparatus. The stereotaxic apparatus holds the head of the animal in a precise orientation so that a brain atlas may be used to place the recording electrodes accurately within the region of the brain desired. Furthermore, if a dye is dissolved in the electrolyte within the recording pipette, the dye may be ejected into the recording site for subsequent histological verification of the region recorded.

Because the recording electrode is placed near the outside surface of the neuron, there is less of a concern that the activity recorded is a result of damage to the neuron itself, as may be the case with intracellular recording techniques. Furthermore, many neurons may be sampled in a given animal. However, as a consequence, the amount of information that can be obtained from a neuron is limited. Typically, the research is relegated to recording information related to action potential firing (e.g., the firing rate of the neuron, its pattern of spike discharge, and how these states of activity may be affected by stimulation of an afferent pathway or administration of a drug [Figure 4–2]). Nonetheless, when combined with the appropriate pharmacological techniques, extracellular recording has yielded a substantial amount of valuable information related to drug action or neuronal interconnections of physiologically important neuronal types. For example, by using a series of coordinated pharmacological and physiological techniques, we were able to define a unique extracellular waveform as that associated with the discharge of a dopamine-containing neuron (Bunney et al. 1973; Grace and Bunney 1983). This provided the basis for studies that yielded information defining the mode of action of antipsychotic drugs (Bunney and Grace 1978; Grace 1992).

Extracellular recordings from neurons measure the current flow generated around a neuron as it generates spikes. For this reason, extracellular action potentials generally are composed of two components: a positive-going component followed by a negative-going component. The positive-going component is a reflection of the ion flux across the neuronal membrane surrounding the electrode that occurs during the depolarizing phase of the action potential, with the negative phase reflecting the repolarization. Because the extracellular recording electrode is

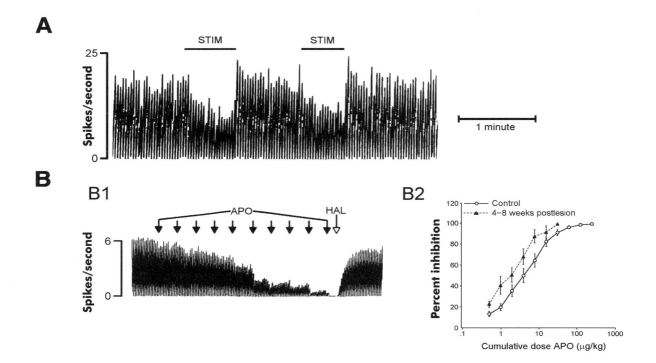

Figure 4–2. Extracellular recording techniques are an effective means of assessing the effects of afferent pathway stimulation or drug administration on neuron activity. On the other hand, the measurements that can be made are typically restricted to changes in firing rates or in the pattern of spike discharge.

A: This firing rate histogram illustrates the response of a substantia nigra–zona reticulata neuron to stimulation of the γ-aminobutyric acid (GABA)ergic striatonigral pathway. A common method for illustrating how a manipulation affects the firing rate of a neuron is by constructing a firing rate histogram. This is typically done by using some type of electronic discriminator and counter to count the number of spikes that a cell fires in a given time. In this example, the counter counts spikes over a 10-second interval and converts this number to a voltage, which is then plotted on a chart recorder. The counter then resets to zero and begins counting spikes over the next 10-second interval. Therefore, in this firing rate histogram, the height of each vertical line is proportional to the number of spikes that the cell fires during each 10-second interval, with the calibration bar on the left showing the equivalent firing frequency in spikes per second. During the period at which the striatonigral pathway is stimulated (horizontal bars above trace marked "STIM"), the cell is inhibited, as reflected by the decrease in the height of the vertical lines. When the stimulation is terminated, a rebound activation of cell firing is observed.

Source. Adapted from Grace AA, Bunney BS: "Opposing Effects of Striatonigral Feedback Pathways on Midbrain Dopamine Cell Activity." *Brain Research* 333:271–284, 1985. Used with permission.

B: In this figure, a similar histogram is used to illustrate the effects of a drug on the firing of a neuron. *Panel B1:* This figure shows the well-known inhibition of dopamine neuron firing rate on administration of the dopamine agonist apomorphine (APO). Each of the filled arrows represents the intravenous administration of a dose of APO. After the cell is completely inhibited, the specificity of the response is tested by examining the ability of the dopamine antagonist haloperidol (HAL [open arrow]) to reverse this response. Typically, drug sensitivity is determined by administering the drug in a dose-response fashion. This is done by giving an initial drug dose that is subthreshold for altering the firing rate of the cell. The first dose is then repeated, with each subsequent dose given being twice that of the previous dose. This is continued until a plateau response is achieved (in this case, a complete inhibition of cell discharge). *Panel B2:* The drug is administered in a dose-response manner to facilitate the plotting of a *cumulative* dose-response curve, with drug doses plotted on a logarithmic scale (i.e., a log dose-response curve). To compare the potency of two drugs or the sensitivity of two cells to the same drug, a point on the curve is chosen during which the fastest rate-of-change of the response is obtained. The point usually chosen is that at which the drug dose administered causes 50% of the maximal change obtained (i.e., the ED_{50}). As is shown in this example, the dopamine neurons recorded after a partial dopamine depletion (dashed line) are substantially more sensitive to inhibition by APO than the dopamine neurons recorded in control (solid line) rats.

Source. Adapted from Pucak ML, Grace AA: "Partial Dopamine Depletions Result in an Enhanced Sensitivity of Residual Dopamine Neurons to Apomorphine." *Synapse* 9:144–155, 1991. Used with permission.

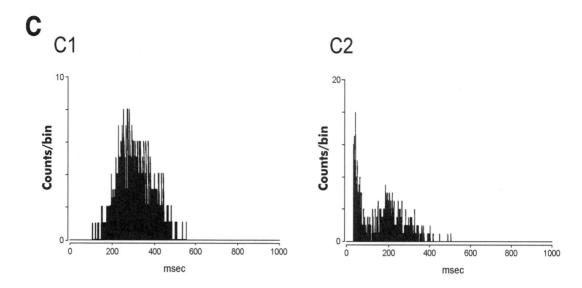

Figure 4–2. *(continued)* **C:** In addition to determining the firing rate of a neuron, extracellular recording techniques may be used to assess the effects of drugs on the pattern of spike discharge. This is typically done by plotting an interspike interval histogram. In this paradigm, a computer is connected to a spike discriminator, and a train of about 500 spikes is analyzed. The computer is used to time the delay between subsequent spikes in the train (i.e., the time interval between spikes) and plots this in the form of a histogram, in which the x-axis represents time between subsequent spikes, and the y-axis shows the number of interspike intervals that had a specific delay (bin = range of time; e.g., for 1-msec bins, all intervals between 200.0 and 200.99 msec).
Panel C1: The cell is firing irregularly (as shown by the primarily normal distribution of intervals around 200 msec),

with some spikes occurring after longer-than-average delays (i.e., bins greater than 400 msec, probably caused by spontaneous inhibitory postsynaptic potentials [IPSPs] delaying spike occurrence). *Panel C2:* In contrast, this cell is firing in bursts, which consists of a series of 3–10 spikes with comparatively short interspike intervals (i.e., approximately 70 msec) separated by long delays between bursts (i.e., events occurring at greater than 150-msec intervals). The computer determined that, in this case, the cell was discharging 79% of its spikes in bursts, compared with 0% in *Panel C1.*

Source. Adapted from Grace AA, Bunney BS: "The Control of Firing Pattern in Nigral Dopamine Neurons: Single Spike Firing." *Journal of Neuroscience* 4:2866–2876, 1984a. Used with permission.

measuring current across the membrane occurring in concert with changes in intracellular membrane potential and because current is defined in terms of the first derivative (i.e., rate of change) of voltage, the extracellularly recorded action potential (or "spike") waveform is typically a first derivative of the action potential voltage with respect to time (Terzuolo and Araki 1961). This phenomenon underlies the biphasic nature of the extracellularly recorded event (Figure 4–3). Furthermore, the recorded spike is largest when the recording electrode is placed near the active site of spike generation because the current density is greatest (and thus the voltage drop induced across the electrode largest) at this site.

Intracellular Recordings

With intracellular recording, an electrode with a much smaller tip and a much higher electrical resistance than

that used with extracellular recording is inserted into the membrane of the neuron. Although the tip of the electrode is smaller, the signal measured is much larger than that with extracellular recording, because it measures the potential difference across the membrane directly rather than relying on transmembrane current density changes outside of the neuron. As a result, electrical activity occurring within the neuron can be measured, which would be nearly impossible to measure extracellularly, such as spontaneously occurring or evoked (via afferent pathway stimulation) electrical potentials generated by neurotransmitter release (or postsynaptic potentials). Furthermore, because the membrane potential of the neuron may be altered by injecting depolarizing or hyperpolarizing current into the cell through the electrode, the equilibrium potential (also known as the reversal potential) of the response may be determined. In addition, the overall conductance of the membrane may be measured by injecting

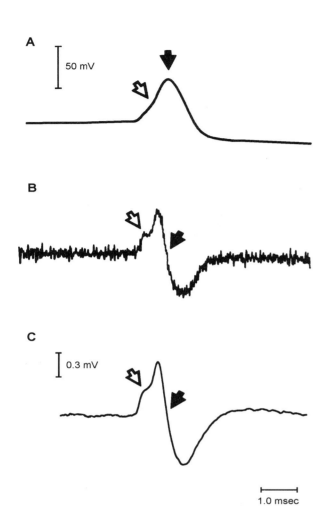

Figure 4–3.   Relationship between action potentials recorded intracellularly and those recorded extracellularly from dopamine-containing neurons.

A: During intracellular recordings, an action potential is initiated from a negative resting membrane potential (e.g., −55 mV), reaches a peak membrane potential (solid arrow), and is followed by a repolarization of the membrane and usually an afterhyperpolarization. An inflection in the rising phase of the spike (open arrow) is often observed. This reflects the delay between the initial segment spike that initiates the action potential (occurring prior to the open arrow) and the somatodendritic action potential that it triggers (occurring after the open arrow).

B: A computer was used to differentiate the membrane voltage deflection occurring in the action potential in *Panel A* with respect to time, resulting in a pattern that shows the rate of change of membrane voltage. Note that the inflection is exaggerated (open arrow), and the peak of the action potential crosses zero (solid arrow), because at the peak of a spike, the rate of change reaches zero before reversing to a negative direction.

C: A trace showing a typical action potential in a dopamine neuron recorded extracellularly. The extracellular action potential resembles the differentiated intracellular action potential in *Panel B*. This is because the extracellular electrode is actually measuring the current crossing the membrane during the action potential and is therefore, by definition, equivalent to the absolute value of the first derivative of the voltage trace in *Panel A*. The amplitude of the extracellular spike is indicated in volts, because the parameter measured is actually the voltage drop produced across the electrode tip by the current flux and is therefore much smaller than the actual membrane voltage change that occurs in *Panel A*.

Source.   Adapted from Grace AA, Bunney BS: "Intracellular and Extracellular Electrophysiology of Nigral Dopaminergic Neurons, I: Identification and Characterization." *Neuroscience* 10:301–315, 1983. Used with permission.

known levels of current and measuring the membrane voltage deflection produced. By applying this information using Ohm's law, the input resistance of the cell can be determined. This could be important in assessing drug effects. A drug could increase the input resistance of the membrane, making it more responsive to current generated by afferent synapses, without changing the membrane potential of the neuron. Indeed, such a condition has been proposed to underlie the mechanism through which norepinephrine exerts a "modulatory" action—that is, increasing the amplitude of the response of a neuron to a stimulus without affecting its basal firing rate (which has also been described as increasing its "signal-to-noise" ratio; Freedman et al. 1977; Woodward et al. 1979).

The intracellular recording electrode can also be used to inject specific substances into the neuron. For example, second messengers or calcium chelators may be introduced into the neuron to examine how they alter neuronal physiology or the neuron's response to drugs. Furthermore, by injecting the neuron with a fluorescent dye or enzymatic marker, the morphology of the specific cell impaled may be recovered and examined (Figure 4–4). This technique can be combined with immunocytochemistry to examine the neurotransmitter synthesized by the cell under study (e.g., Grace and Onn 1989).

Inserting an electrode into the membrane of a cell to measure transmembrane voltage and manipulating its membrane by injecting current are commonly known as *current clamp*, because the amount and direction of ionic

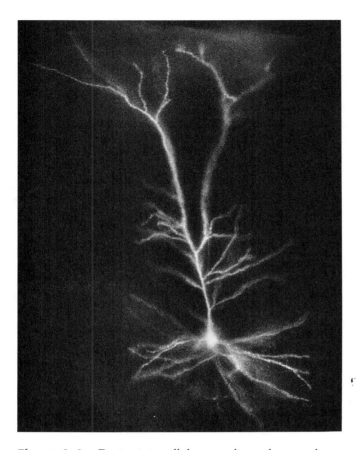

Figure 4–4. During intracellular recordings, the recording pipette is filled with an electrolyte to enable the transmission of membrane voltage deflections to the preamplifier. The electrode may also be filled with substances, such as a morphological stain, for injection into the impaled neuron. In this example, the electrode was filled with the highly fluorescent dye Lucifer yellow. Because this dye has a negative charge at neutral pH, it may be ejected from the electrode by applying a negative current across the electrode, with the result that the Lucifer yellow carries the negative current flow from the electrode and into the neuron. Because this dye diffuses rapidly in water, it quickly fills the entire neuron impaled. The tissue is then fixed in a formaldehyde compound, the lipids clarified by dehydration-defatting or by using dimethylsulfoxide (Grace and Llinás 1985), and the tissue examined under a fluorescence microscope. In this case, a brightly fluorescing pyramidal neuron in layer 3 of the neocortex of a guinea pig is recovered.

current crossing the membrane of the cell can be controlled by the experimenter, such as when determining the reversal potential of a response. Another technique that is effective in neurophysiological research is the use of *voltage clamps*. With voltage clamping, the membrane potential of the neuron is maintained at a set voltage level by injecting current into the cell. This is achieved by rapid feedback electronics that adjusts the current injected to accurately offset any factors that may act to change this

potential. Thus, when the neuron is exposed to a drug that opens ion channels, the effect of the ionic influx is precisely counterbalanced by altering the current injected into the neuron by the voltage clamp device. The amount of additional current that must be injected into the neuron to maintain the membrane potential at its set point is therefore the inverse of the transmembrane current generated in response to the drug. By using specific ion channel blockers or by altering the extracellular ionic environment of the neuron, the precise ionic mechanism and conductance changes induced in a neuron by a drug or neurotransmitter may be determined.

Patch Clamp Recordings

A final level of analysis to be discussed is one directed at assessing the response of individual ionic channels in the membrane of a neuron. Actually, this technique may be described more as a type of high-resolution extracellular recording. In this method, a glass pipette with a comparatively large tip is drawn, and the tip is fire-polished until it is very smooth. The electrode tip is then placed against the membrane surface of a neuron under visual control. Typically, the neuronal membrane is first cleaned of debris with a jet of fluid to permit a tight seal between the electrode and the membrane. A small suction is then applied to the pipette to tighten its seal with the membrane. Because such an attachment provides a high-resistance junction with the membrane, the minute transmembrane currents that are generated as a result of the opening and closing of individual ionic channels may be monitored. The biophysical characteristics (e.g., open time, inactivation rate) of specific ion channels and how they may be modified by drugs applied via the pipette lumen or to other regions of the neuron being studied can be determined.

Whole-Cell Recordings

A recent widely used technique is whole-cell recordings. This technique is a modification of the patch clamp technique. The membrane patch underlying the electrode is ruptured, typically by applying a small suction through the pipette, which results in the interior of the electrode becoming continuous with the intracellular fluid. The combination of a tight, giga-ohm seal around the electrode–cell membrane junction and the very low resistance of the electrode–intracellular patch has two major advantages: the recordings are very low noise, and the transmembrane potential can be more accurately controlled over extended regions of the cell's interior surface.

When combined with infrared video microscopy techniques, which allow both the large electrode tip and the cell to which it is to be attached to be visualized, recordings can be made from specific cell types or from cells that had been labeled by a retrogradely transported fluorescent dye. Although such a preparation has many unique and powerful advantages, this low-resistance junction is also subject to the introduction of artifacts. This is particularly true in cases in which the response to be measured is mediated by diffusable second messengers: the large bore of the attached electrode has been reported to dialyze intracellular constituents from the cell into the electrode. When this process happens, the experimenter often observes a rundown of the response, in which the current gradually decreases with time as a result of loss of the intracellular milieu. To test for this possibility, investigators often rely on a "perforated patch" technique, in which the patch pipette is filled with the ionophore nystatin. When a patch pipette of this type is attached to the cell surface, these channel ionophores are incorporated into the membrane section adjacent to the bore of the electrode. As a result, a low-resistance access to the intracellular space is obtained without the need for rupturing the membrane.

PREPARATIONS USED IN ELECTROPHYSIOLOGICAL RESEARCH

As with the various types of recordings that can be done, several preparations also can be used in this analysis. No single preparation is "best"; instead, each has specific advantages and shortcomings. A more complete picture of the functioning of a system can be gained by taking advantage of the unique perspective provided by each preparation and designing the experiments accordingly. Except for the first category listed below, all preparations pertain to the mammalian vertebrate.

Simpler Nervous Systems—Invertebrates and Lower Vertebrate Preparations

We include a reference to simpler nervous systems for completeness; more comprehensive reviews of the use of nonmammalian model systems can be found elsewhere (Kandel 1978). However, depending on the application, use of these preparations may yield varying degrees of relevance. With respect to the use of phylogenetically lower species as models for psychopharmacological studies in humans, much of the data related to anatomy, cellular physiology, and behavior would be of limited value. The nervous system of these organisms is substantially different from those of vertebrates and humans, even at the sin-

gle neuronal level. As a result, information derived from these systems is likely to be substantially less applicable to behavioral control in the mammalian class. Nonetheless, several unique advantages are associated with the study of the nervous systems of these organisms: the nervous system is more accessible, the small number of neurons allows for simple and replicable identification of specific neurons, the large neuronal size enables more stable impalement and more complex procedures, and so on. Furthermore, information about the study of some second-messenger systems or receptor transduction mechanisms appears to be more directly transferable to the vertebrate. Thus, it appears that nature is more likely to conserve the most basic functional units of neurotransmitter actions throughout phylogeny, with decreasing levels of homology as the functional units are assembled into more complex systems of neurons and networks.

In Vivo Electrophysiological Recordings

Protocols that use the in vivo preparation focus on the living, intact, anesthetized animal as the subject of the study. Recording the activity of neurons in the intact animal has numerous advantages over studies of isolated tissues. For example, the health of the tissue or neuron under study is more easily maintained and monitored. Furthermore, the neuron can be examined in its normal ionic and cellular microenvironment, with its normal complement of afferent connections intact. In addition, neurons recorded in vivo are more likely to be spontaneously active, facilitating the use of extracellular recordings and investigations into the actions of inhibitory neurotransmitters.

With respect to psychopharmacological research, the in vivo preparation provides the most direct link between neurophysiology and behavior. A drug that elicits a characteristic behavioral response can be administered systemically to examine how the drug affects neurons that are likely to participate in the behavioral response. For similar reasons, this preparation is also the most effective for investigating the mode of action of psychotherapeutic drugs on specific neuronal systems. Although the precise locus of action through which the systemically administered drugs act to achieve these effects may be difficult to determine directly, whether a given drug ultimately influences the activity of a neuronal system of interest can be determined.

Experimental parameters present difficulties that, although not insurmountable, add complexity to the experimental paradigm. For example, the researcher cannot visually identify the nucleus or the cell to be recorded and must often rely on indirect techniques for cell identification. However, methods are available to enhance the ability to identify cell types. Thus, unlike the in vitro preparations, cells may be identified with respect to the projection sites of their axons by employing antidromic activation—that is, stimulation of the axon terminal region to evoke an action potential that is conducted back down the axon and subsequently recorded at the soma. Furthermore, by using in vivo intracellular recording, the neuron in question may be stained with dye and its location, morphology, and neurotransmitter content identified post hoc by various histochemical and immunocytochemical techniques (e.g., Grace and Bunney 1983; Onn et al. 1994). In addition, although the precise locus of action of systemically administered drugs cannot be determined, the drug effects obtained can be compared with those produced by directly applying the drug to the neuron through microiontophoresis (Figure 4–5 [Bloom 1974]).

On the other hand, the properties that confer distinct advantages on the in vivo preparation with respect to ex-

amining how drugs act in the intact organism also limit the type of data that may be collected. Regarding drug administration, some drugs do not readily cross the blood-brain barrier or do not exert their actions on neurons via an effect on peripheral organs. Thus, although dopamine cells can be excited by microiontophoretic administration of cholecystokinin (Skirboll et al. 1981), the excitation produced by systemic administration of this peptide is mediated peripherally and affects the brain via the vagus (Hommer et al. 1985). In addition, the inability to control the microenvironment of the neuron restricts the analysis of the ionic mechanisms underlying cell firing or drug action because the researcher cannot administer ion channel blockers to the entire neuron surface or change the ionic composition of the extracellular fluid. Therefore, whereas the in vivo preparation affords many advantages with respect to examining how behaviorally or therapeutically effective drugs may exert their actions through defined neuronal

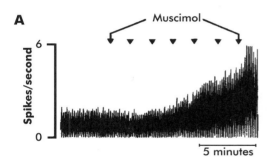

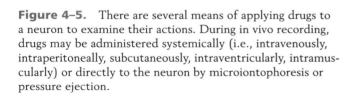

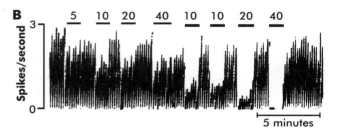

Figure 4–5. There are several means of applying drugs to a neuron to examine their actions. During in vivo recording, drugs may be administered systemically (i.e., intravenously, intraperitoneally, subcutaneously, intraventricularly, intramuscularly) or directly to the neuron by microiontophoresis or pressure ejection.

A: Systemic administration of a drug is useful for determining how a drug affects neurons in the intact organism, regardless of whether the action is direct or indirect. In this case, intravenous administration of the γ-aminobutyric acid (GABA) agonist muscimol (solid arrows) causes a dose-dependent increase in the firing rate of this dopamine-containing neuron.

B: In contrast, direct administration of a drug to a neuron will provide information about the site of action of the drug, at least as it concerns the discharge of the neuron under study. In this case, GABA is administered directly to a dopamine neuron by microiontophoresis. In this technique, several drug-containing pipettes are attached to the recording electrode. The pH of the drug solutions is adjusted to ensure that the drug molecules are in a charged state (e.g., GABA is

used at pH = 4.0 to give it a positive charge), and the drug is ejected from the pipette tip by applying very small currents to the drug-containing pipette. Because the total diameter of the microiontophoretic pipette tip is only about 5 µm, the drugs ejected typically affect only the cell being recorded. In this case, GABA is applied to a dopamine neuron by microiontophoresis; the horizontal bars show the time during which the current is applied to the drug-containing pipette, and the amplitude of the current (indicated in nA) is listed above each bar. Note that, unlike the excitatory effects produced by a systemically administered GABA agonist in *Panel A*, direct application of GABA will *inhibit* dopamine neurons. This has been shown to be caused by inhibition of a much more GABA-sensitive inhibitory interneuron by the systemically administered drug and illustrates the need to compare systemic drug administration with direct drug administration to ascertain the site of action of the drug of interest.

Source. Adapted from Grace AA, Bunney BS: "Opposing Effects of Striatonigral Feedback Pathways on Midbrain Dopamine Cell Activity." *Brain Research* 333:271–284, 1985. Used with permission.

systems, examination of the site of action or the membrane mechanisms underlying these responses is more readily accessible with in vitro systems.

In Vitro Electrophysiological Recordings From Brain Slices

Recordings of neurons maintained in vitro have led to significant advances in understanding the ionic mechanisms underlying neurotransmitter and drug action. This preparation consists of slices 300–400 µm thick cut from the brain of an animal soon after decapitation. If this procedure is done carefully and the brain slices are rapidly placed into oxygenated physiological saline, the neurons within the slices will remain alive and healthy, often for 10 hours or more. Because the neurons are recorded in a chamber with oxygenated media superfused over the slice, several advantages may be realized:

1. Both intracellular and extracellular recordings are more stable because blood and breathing pulsations are absent.
2. Visual control over electrode placement is achieved.
3. The ionic composition of the microenvironment may be controlled precisely.
4. Little interference from the activity of long-loop afferents occurs, and the near-absence of spontaneous spike discharge limits the contribution of local circuit neurons to the responses.

Furthermore, in contrast to microiontophoresis, the concentration of drug in the solution can be controlled precisely. This preparation is also the most complex that can be used for patch clamp recordings because debris may be removed and the patch pipette placed on selected neurons under visual control with a high-resolution optics system (Edwards et al. 1989).

Nonetheless, because of the isolated nature of this system, the results obtained may not precisely reflect the physiology of the intact system. For example, dopamine neurons recorded in vivo have been characterized by their burst-firing discharge pattern (Grace and Bunney 1984b), which appears to be important in regulating neurotransmitter release (Gonon 1988). However, dopamine neurons recorded in vitro do not fire in bursting patterns (Grace and Onn 1989 [Figure 4–6]). On the other hand, this distinction provides what may be an ideal system for examining the factors that cause in vivo burst firing. Therefore, the most complete model of the functioning of a system or of its response to drug application can be derived by comparing the results obtained in vitro with those in the intact organism.

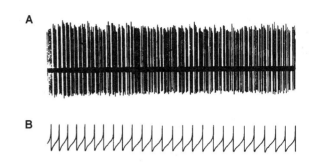

Figure 4–6. Variation (sometimes substantial) in patterns of activity of a neuron type, depending on the preparation in which it is recorded.

A: Extracellular recordings of a dopamine neuron in an intact, anesthetized rat (i.e., in vivo) illustrate the typical irregular firing pattern of the cell, with single spikes occurring intermixed with bursts of action potentials.

B: In contrast, intracellular recordings of a dopamine neuron in an isolated brain slice preparation (i.e., in vitro) illustrate the pacemaker pattern that occurs exclusively in identified dopamine neurons in this preparation. For dopamine neurons, a pacemaker firing pattern is rarely observed in vivo, and burst firing has never been observed in the in vitro preparation. However, although the activity recorded in vitro is obviously an abstraction compared with the firing pattern of this neuron in vivo, a comparative study in each preparation does provide the opportunity to examine factors that may underlie the modulation of firing pattern in this neuronal type.

Source. Adapted from Grace AA: "The Regulation of Dopamine Neuron Activity as Determined by In Vivo and In Vitro Intracellular Recordings, in *The Neurophysiology of Dopamine Systems.* Edited by Chiodo LA, Freeman AS. Detroit, MI, Lake Shore Publications, 1987, pp. 1–67; and Grace AA, Bunney BS: "Intracellular and Extracellular Electrophysiology of Nigral Dopaminergic Neurons, I: Identification and Characterization." *Neuroscience* 10:301–315, 1983. Used with permission.

Recordings From Dissociated Neurons and Neuronal Cell Cultures

Recordings from isolated neurons are actually a subset of in vitro recording methods, with many of the same advantages in terms of accessibility and stability. Furthermore, because the neurons can be completely visualized, advanced techniques such as patch clamping are more easily done. A unique advantage of this system can be obtained by coculturing different neuronal populations. For example, defining the effects of a noradrenergic synapse on a hippocampal pyramidal neuron more precisely may be possible by coculturing these cell types and allowing them to make synapses. In this way, the researcher has visual control over impaling neurons that constitute a presynaptic and postsynaptic pairing. On the other hand, the synapses formed are not necessarily limited to those that occur naturally in the intact organism, in terms of both the location of the synapse on the neuron and the classes of neurons that are interconnected. Furthermore, the altered neuronal morphology present in these preparations may modify the response of the neurons to drugs. Nonetheless, when the analysis is limited to well-defined responses, such as second-messenger actions or ion channel measures, this system affords an unparalleled level of accessibility.

RELATIONSHIP BETWEEN BIOCHEMICAL AND ELECTROPHYSIOLOGICAL MEASURES OF NEURONAL ACTIVITY

The methods outlined here are directed at analyzing the activity of individual neurons as a means of assessing their role in pharmacological responses or behavioral actions. This is based on the premise that the discharge of a neuron in some manner reflects its release of a transmitter onto a postsynaptically located target neuron. As such, biochemical measures of neurotransmitter levels would be predicted to correspond to the activity changes occurring during electrophysiological recordings from neurons (Roth 1987). In several cases, such approaches have helped to define the physiological relevance of recorded neuron activity. One case in which this has proven valuable is in the analysis of firing pattern. For example, dopamine neurons, like many other cell types in the central nervous system, are capable of discharging trains of action potentials in two patterns of activity: single spiking and burst firing. However, their range of firing rates is comparatively restricted, with most cells firing only between 2 and 8 Hz. Nonetheless, information on the temporal relationship between spikes and bursts (Grace and Bunney 1984b) has been used in in vivo voltammetry studies to measure dopamine levels. Dopamine cells firing in bursts will release two to three times more neurotransmitter per spike from their terminals than those discharging at similar frequencies but in a steady firing pattern (Gonon 1988). Therefore, in this case, knowledge of the physiological firing pattern provided information to the electrochemist that resulted in the elucidation of the physiological consequence of burst firing in this system.

However, the extrapolation between biochemical and electrophysiological measures may not always be valid.

Thus, recordings from single neurons may not necessarily reflect the activity across the population of neurons of interest. Therefore, a drug that exerts an action via activation of the nonfiring population of neurons may be overlooked if its actions are assessed on single spontaneously discharging neurons (Bunney and Grace 1978; Grace and Bunney 1984a). Furthermore, the response may be confined to a topographically defined subset of neurons mediating a particular response (e.g., a change in the activity of neurons regulating movement of the leg would not be predicted if the response involves a reaching movement of the arm). With respect to biochemical measurements, actions of transmitters at presynaptic terminals could dramatically alter the amount of neurotransmitter they release independent of neuronal discharge (e.g., Grace 1991). On the other hand, electrophysiological measurements enable researchers to examine responses that occur very rapidly. Indeed, a massive but transient activation of spike discharge in a neuronal system may evoke a substantial behavioral response, whereas biochemical measurements of neurotransmitter release performed over a long time course may dilute the impact of the transient event. Therefore, although the results obtained from each measure may not be directly comparable, the electrophysiological measurements are better optimized for detecting transient events.

SUMMARY

In this chapter, we reviewed several electrophysiological techniques and preparations used in the analysis of nervous system function. Each approach is characterized by a set of unique advantages and potential shortcomings inherent in the method. Nonetheless, it should be apparent that no single technique has an overwhelming advantage in psychopharmacological research. Instead, by matching the preparation to the question at hand, and through the judicious comparison of data obtained from intact versus isolated preparations, the various limitations may be systematically overcome to yield a more broadly applicable model of psychopharmacological action.

REFERENCES

Bloom FE: To spritz or not to spritz: the doubtful value of aimless iontophoresis. Life Sci 14:1819–1834, 1974

Bunney BS, Grace AA: Acute and chronic haloperidol treatment: comparison of effects on nigral dopaminergic cell activity. Life Sci 23:1715–1728, 1978

Bunney BS, Walters JR, Roth RH, et al: Dopaminergic neurons: effect of antipsychotic drugs and amphetamine on single cell activity. J Pharmacol Exp Ther 185:560–571, 1973

Edwards FA, Konnerth A, Sakmann B, et al: A thin slice preparation for patch clamp recordings from neurons of the mammalian central nervous system. Pflugers Arch 414:600–612, 1989

Freedman R, Hoffer BJ, Woodward DJ, et al: Interaction of norepinephrine with cerebellar activity evoked by mossy and climbing fibers. Exp Neurol 55:269–288, 1977

Gonon FG: Nonlinear relationship between impulse flow and dopamine released by rat midbrain dopaminergic neurons as studied by in vivo electrochemistry. Neuroscience 24:19–28, 1988

Grace AA: The regulation of dopamine neuron activity as determined by in vivo and in vitro intracellular recordings, in The Neurophysiology of Dopamine Systems. Edited by Chiodo LA, Freeman AS. Detroit, MI, Lake Shore Publications, 1987, pp 1–67

Grace AA: Phasic versus tonic dopamine release and the modulation of dopamine system responsivity: a hypothesis for the etiology of schizophrenia. Neuroscience 41:1–24, 1991

Grace AA: The depolarization block hypothesis of neuroleptic action: implications for the etiology and treatment of schizophrenia. J Neural Transm 36 (suppl):91–131, 1992

Grace AA, Bunney BS: Intracellular and extracellular electrophysiology of nigral dopaminergic neurons, I: identification and characterization. Neuroscience 10:301–315, 1983

Grace AA, Bunney BS: The control of firing pattern in nigral dopamine neurons: single spike firing. J Neurosci 4:2866–2876, 1984a

Grace AA, Bunney BS: The control of firing pattern in nigral dopamine neurons: burst firing. J Neurosci 4:2877–2890, 1984b

Grace AA, Bunney BS: Opposing effects of striatonigral feedback pathways on midbrain dopamine cell activity. Brain Res 333:271–284, 1985

Grace AA, Llinás R: Dehydration-induced morphological artifacts in intracellularly stained neurons: circumvention using rapid DMSO clearing. Neuroscience 16:461–475, 1985

Grace AA, Onn SP: Morphology and electrophysiological properties of immunocytochemically identified rat dopamine neurons recorded in vitro. J Neurosci 9:3463–3481, 1989

Hommer DW, Palkovits M, Crawley JN, et al: Cholecystokinin-induced excitation in the substantia nigra: evidence for peripheral and central components. J Neurosci 5:1387–1392, 1985

Kandel ER: A Cell-Biological Approach to Learning (Grass Lecture Monograph 1). Bethesda, MD, Society for Neuroscience, 1978, pp 1–90

Llinás RR: The intrinsic electrophysiological properties of mammalian neurons: a new insight into CNS function. Science 242:1654–1664, 1988

Onn SP, Berger TW, Grace AA: Identification and characterization of striatal cell subtypes using in vivo intracellular recording and dye-labelling in rats, III: morphological correlates and compartmental localization. Synapse 16:231–254, 1994

Pucak ML, Grace AA: Partial dopamine depletions result in an enhanced sensitivity of residual dopamine neurons to apomorphine. Synapse 9:144–155, 1991

Roth RH: Biochemical correlates of the electrophysiological activity of dopaminergic neurons: reflections on two decades of collaboration with electrophysiologists, in Neurophysiology of Dopaminergic Systems—Current Status and Clinical Perspectives. Edited by Chiodo LA, Freeman AS. Detroit, MI, Lake Shore Publications, 1987, pp 187–203

Skirboll LR, Grace AA, Hommer DW, et al: Peptide-monoamine coexistence: studies of the actions of a cholecystokinin-like peptide on the electrical activity of midbrain dopamine neurons. Neuroscience 6:2111–2124, 1981

Terzuolo CA, Araki T: An analysis of intra- versus extracellular potential changes associated with activity of single spinal motoneurons. Ann N Y Acad Sci 94:547–558, 1961

Woodward DJ, Moises HC, Waterhouse BD, et al: Modulatory actions of norepinephrine in the central nervous system. Federation Proceedings 38:2109–2116, 1979

FIVE

Animal Models of Depression and Schizophrenia

Jay M. Weiss, Ph.D., and Clinton D. Kilts, Ph.D.

Animal models of both depression and schizophrenia have played a significant role in the development of current treatments for these disorders. Despite this, animal models of these disorders have yet to achieve more than a small percentage of their ultimate promise because existing models remain imperfect approximations of their target pathologies. However, the ability to study physiological and environmental processes under experimental control that is not possible when human patients are the subject population makes animal models of such value for development of effective treatments that efforts to improve animal models are continually ongoing. In this chapter, we summarize the development of such models to date.

TYPES OF ANIMAL MODELS

Animal models can be divided into two categories. The first category can be called *animal assay* models. Models in this category use behavioral and/or physiological responses of animals to assess processes, usually physiological processes, that existing evidence indicates are important in a disorder. For example, evidence from drug and other studies indicates that alteration in the activity of the neurotransmitter dopamine is important in schizophrenia and Parkinson's disease. Rats show turning (rotational) behavior when receptors for dopamine in the brain are stimulated. The sensitivity of receptors and/or activity of the dopaminergic neurons can be assessed in animals by measuring turning behavior; thus, this response of the animal serves as an assay for a physiological process of impor-

tance in behavioral pathology. It can be noted that the responses observed and/or measured in an animal assay model, being essentially a "readout" of some process of interest, may bear no resemblance to what is seen in the disorder that the model is relevant to. The second category can be called *homologous* models. These models endeavor to re-create the human disorder in animals. In these models, treatments are administered to animals in the hope of causing the animals to resemble individuals who are afflicted with the disorder. In contrast to animal assay models, the responses seen in homologous models are usually distinctly similar to what is seen in the relevant human disorder.

Both animal assay and homologous models are very useful. Animal assay models find their major use in drug screening and development of new drugs. By permitting researchers to determine how various compounds affect physiological processes that are important in pathology, animal assay models make it possible to assess rapidly the potential usefulness of drug compounds and, in some cases, to discover new drugs that unexpectedly affect an important physiological process. Of course, a limitation of this type of model is that it assumes a priori that a particular physiological process is important in a disorder, and the usefulness of the model rests on this assumption.

Homologous models are also valuable, perhaps even more so than animal assay models. Once perfected, a homologous model reproduces a human disorder (as closely as can be done) in an animal. Unlike the animal assay type, a homologous model is not designed with the assumption that a particular physiological abnormality underlies a disorder. Consequently, because the perfected homologous model reproduces a disorder, the model can then be studied as a means to identify the underlying cause (i.e., the physiological defect) of the disorder. In addition, such a model can be used to test for *totally novel treatments* of the disorder; that is, because a perfected homologous model reproduces the disorder without making any assumptions about its physiological basis, researchers can test any potential treatment on the animal model to determine whether it can reverse the disorder. Because the physiological basis of a disorder can be discovered if a disorder is produced in animals, and because completely new treatments may be tested as well, major advances in the understanding and treatment of a disorder will rapidly follow the development of an adequate homologous model.

CRITERIA FOR EVALUATING ANIMAL MODELS

Soon after animal models of behavioral disorders, particularly depression, came into use, criteria were proposed by which such models could be evaluated. Although these criteria have been developed primarily for evaluation of homologous models, animal assays also can be evaluated by applying those aspects of the criteria applicable to such models. Interestingly, a considerable degree of consensus has developed with regard to one particular set of criteria, which has been widely accepted in the field despite the occasional recommendations for some modifications.

Criteria Proposed by McKinney and Bunney

The criteria that have been widely accepted are those proposed by McKinney and Bunney (1969). They proposed that the usefulness and/or validity of an animal model of any behavioral disorder could be determined on the basis of the similarity of the animal model to the human disorder with respect to four criteria:

1. Etiology
2. Symptomatology
3. Biochemistry
4. Response to treatment

In other words, the "goodness" or validity of an animal model of any behavioral, psychological, or psychiatric disorder can be determined by the extent to which the animal model 1) is produced by etiological factors similar to those that produce the human disorder, 2) resembles the human disorder in manifestations or symptomatology, 3) has an underlying pathophysiological basis similar to that of the

human disorder, and 4) responds as does the disorder in humans to appropriate therapeutic treatments. Before commenting further on these particular criteria, we examine other suggestions and/or amplifications.

Criteria Proposed by Abramson and Seligman

In a book that reviewed a wide variety of animal models, Abramson and Seligman (1977) proposed a different set of criteria:

1. Is the analysis of the laboratory phenomenon (model) thorough in describing the essential features of its cause, prevention, and cure?
2. Is the similarity of symptoms convincingly demonstrated?
3. To what extent are physiology, cause, cure, and prevention similar to the human disorder?
4. Does the model describe in all instances a naturally occurring psychopathology or only a subgroup?

In actuality, these criteria do not suggest anything markedly different from those proposed by McKinney and Bunney (1969) but appear to address issues such as the quality of the research that is carried out to establish the model (i.e., Is the analysis thorough enough? Are symptoms convincingly demonstrated?). The third criterion seems to repeat those proposed by McKinney and Bunney, with the exception that etiology is omitted from this particular list. Finally, the last criterion simply asks for judgment regarding whether the model reproduces a particular subgroup of a disorder; however, once this issue is settled, the same criteria would be used to evaluate the model, whether it represented some disorder globally or a subgroup of the disorder.

Criteria Proposed by Willner

The most significant attempt to improve the simple schema of McKinney and Bunney (1969) was offered by Willner (1984). This investigator suggested that animal models should be evaluated for different types of validity—predictive validity, face validity, and construct validity. Each of these categories was said to possess five characteristics. Predictive validity is determined by whether a model correctly identifies 1) pharmacological antidepressant treatments of 2) different types 3) without showing false-positive results or 4) false-negative results, and by whether 5) drug dosages that are effective in the model correlate in potency with those found to be effective in the clinic. Face validity is determined by whether 1) antidepressant effects are present only on chronic administration and by whether the symptoms of the model 2) resemble a number of the symptoms of depression that are 3) specific to depression and 4) found in a particular subtype of depression, and 5) the model should not show characteristics that are not seen clinically. Finally, construct validity requires that 1) the behavioral features of the model and 2) the features of depression that the model seeks to reproduce can be unambiguously interpreted, 3) are homologous, and 4) stand in an established empirical and 5) theoretical relationship to depression.

Although these criteria are long and detailed, it is unclear how they add constructively to those proposed by McKinney and Bunney (1969). For example, predictive validity, which Willner (1984) applies only to antidepressant medications, would seem to be subsumed under the McKinney and Bunney criterion of response to treatment. Moreover, the first characteristic listed by Willner under face validity—that antidepressant medication has therapeutic effects only as a result of chronic administration—would seem to be an aspect of this criterion rather than of another. Thus, what Willner describes as predictive validity as well as the chronicity requirement for the effects of drugs could well be seen simply as a more elaborate description of McKinney and Bunney's last general criterion. (Also, note that Willner's schema omits any mention of nonpharmacological treatments, which not only are effective in ameliorating depression but also could conceivably be modeled in an animal.) A similar judgment could be made regarding face validity, which would seem to be subsumed under McKinney and Bunney's requirement of symptom similarity. Moreover, the specific requirements proposed by Willner for this category may be excessively restrictive. In particular, it is unclear why a model that includes all salient clinical features of depression (which presumably are also reversible by antidepressant treatment) would be of lesser value if the model showed additional changes as well; depression in humans is rarely uncontaminated by other changes or disturbances.

Although predictive validity and face validity seem to be variations or elaborations of criteria already present in McKinney and Bunney's schema, a potentially significant contribution is embodied in Willner's (1984) suggestion that construct validity also should be considered. However, not all aspects of this criterion represent additions. For instance, by pointing out the need to define characteristics clearly and unambiguously, Willner draws attention to the fact that attributes of the human disorder are often poorly described, which makes modeling exceedingly difficult. The need for construct validity in this respect could be said to apply to every aspect of both the animal response

being generated (and measured) and the human behavior that researchers attempt to match in an animal model, all of these characteristics falling within the criteria of McKinney and Bunney (1969). In other words, these aspects of construct validity, like many of the Abramson and Seligman (1977) criteria, appear to set requirements for how any criterion, including those proposed by McKinney and Bunney, should be established and/or evaluated, but such requirements do not themselves expand the actual list of criteria proposed by McKinney and Bunney.

There is, however, one important exception to this judgment in regard to Willner's use of construct validity. It is the aspect of construct validity that stipulates that responses seen in the animal model should "stand in theoretical relationship to depression." This stipulation could be regarded as trivial—one that might be fulfilled, for example, by conceptually linking reduced motor activity in rats to psychomotor retardation in humans. However, defining a theoretical basis for a model would ordinarily be understood to require more than this. What would be expected by this requirement is *to establish a link across different levels of analysis*, such as linking a syndrome of different behaviors to an underlying generalized cognitive deficit or physiological defect. Thus, this criterion potentially expands the scope of homologous models by promoting modeling not only of responses and/or syndromes of responses but also of *processes* involved in abnormal behavior. For example, researchers might model deficits in the appreciation of pleasure (for depression) or the inability to properly exclude irrelevant stimuli (for schizophrenia). Moreover, it can be argued that ultimately the most appropriate and satisfactory models for behavioral disorders reflect critical underlying processes.

But despite potential positive attributes of this suggestion, it is also important to consider the appreciable dangers in using the criterion described above. To model a critical process, two major assumptions must be made: 1) that the particular process one attempts to study is affected (disturbed) in the disorder and 2) that the behavioral change measured in the animal validly represents that process rather than the change being caused by some other unrelated influence. In short, adopting this approach means that researchers are no longer strictly bound by symptom similarity of the behavior seen in the model to that seen in the disorder; the link to the disorder is accomplished through a series of theoretical formulations. In considering this course, it should be recalled that the field of abnormal psychology is emerging from a long period during which disorders were defined by hypothetical underlying processes. In the past, these processes were usually psychodynamic in nature. Today, proponents of theoretically based models are likely to have replaced psychodynamic processes with physiological ones as the appropriate basis for abnormal psychology. For example, in the case of depression, "anger turned inward" is likely to be replaced by "deficits in brain dopaminergic transmission mediating pleasure." However, although aspects of the latter formulation may be easier (and more fashionable) to measure than the former, the underlying concerns with respect to modeling are similar. This is because even a physiologically based formulation of an underlying deficit, like the earlier psychodynamic formulations, remains a conjecture at present. It must be emphasized that little is actually known at present about the pathophysiology underlying abnormal psychology. No reliable physiological abnormalities demarcate any diagnostic group. The wealth of information available in the physiological realm relates largely to drug action that describes processes involved in counteracting or ameliorating abnormal responses, which ultimately may relate only indirectly to what physiological processes are disturbed in the affected patient. As a result, although theoretically based models are likely to provide interesting and valuable information about the relation of certain behaviors to physiological changes, they face no fewer fundamental problems in establishing their validity as models of diagnostic categories than did the psychodynamic formulations they have replaced.

The thrust of DSM-III, DSM-III-R, and DSM-IV (American Psychiatric Association 1980, 1987, 1994) has been to move away from diagnosis related to theoretical constructs and toward diagnosis based on directly observable markers. This trend is accentuated in the call for basing the diagnosis of depression on behavioral "signs" rather than even on reported symptoms (Mitchell and Potter 1993; Parker et al. 1990). Consequently, reproducing the symptoms or "signs" of abnormal psychological conditions in animal models, and finding these symptoms to be ameliorated by effective treatments, must continue to be the goal of current models, or researchers risk slipping back to pre-DSM-III diagnosis. *The appropriate goal for models is to achieve empirical validity, regardless of theoretical validity.* For depression, this pursuit is aided by the considerable repertoire of motor and vegetative symptoms found in this disorder. For schizophrenia, on the other hand, symptoms and signs in the human disorder are predominantly evidence of cognitive disturbance, so that reproducing these specific symptoms in an animal model is much more difficult. As is seen in the discussion of models for schizophrenia, attempting to duplicate disturbed processes appears to be the most productive avenue at present, despite the conceptual risks.

In conclusion, the concise, straightforward schema

proposed by McKinney and Bunney (1969) appears to be the most adequate set of criteria yet suggested for evaluating animal models. As Sir Martin Roth (1976) commented in addressing diagnosis of affective disorders, "good classifications are simple and parsimonious" (p. 86).

MODELS OF DEPRESSION

In this section, each model is described. These descriptions begin by focusing on procedural aspects by which the model is produced, and then attributes of the model are summarized, particularly those that permit evaluation according to the criteria of McKinney and Bunney (1969). The allocation of models to either the animal assay category or the homologous model category can occasionally be somewhat arbitrary, but heavy emphasis is placed here on face validity with respect to symptomatology. For example, in accord with the view that a fundamental aspect of depression is a slowing, or retardation, of function (e.g., Cohen et al. 1982; Nelson and Charney 1981; Parker et al. 1990), models are classified here as homologous when reduced motor activity is the primary symptom shown by the animal, although the model may be deficient in other ways. Conversely, models of depression are not classified as homologous when hyperactivity is a significant feature, except in those cases in which the model shows evidence that functioning is otherwise generally retarded and/or that the hyperactivity seen in the model is caused by agitation.

Animal Assay Models

As stated earlier in this chapter, animal assay models are essentially used to screen antidepressant drugs. Consequently, these models are described in terms of their ability to detect pharmacological agents useful in the treatment of depression. This includes not only how models respond to effective antidepressant drugs or treatments but also whether models respond to drugs that are not antidepressant in nature and/or do not respond to known antidepressant treatments. Whether a model responds to acute or long-term drug administration is also noted.

Muricide. Some rats will spontaneously kill mice when the mice are presented to them. Horovitz and colleagues (1965) noted that administration of imipramine and iproniazid (a monoamine oxidase inhibitor [MAOI]) blocked the tendency of such rats to kill mice and that this effect could not be attributed to drug-induced debilitation or sedation. However, these investigators observed that dextroamphetamine, which is not considered to be an effective antidepressant drug, had a similar effect. Subsequent studies confirmed that tricyclic antidepressants (TCAs; i.e., desipramine [DMI], imipramine) and MAOIs have this effect, as do amphetamines and antihistamines (Sofia 1969a, 1969b). It should be noted that antidepressants produced this effect when administered acutely.

Yohimbine lethality. The drug yohimbine can be administered to mice in dosages that are lethal; administration of sublethal doses was found to be lethal when accompanied by the administration of TCAs and MAOIs (Quinton 1963). Malick (1981) reported that atypical antidepressants (i.e., bupropion, nomifensine, mianserin, iprindole) also produced this effect, whereas antipsychotics and most tranquilizers did not. An important exception is that electroconvulsive therapy (ECT) does not potentiate lethality, but anticholinergics and antihistaminics do. The drugs produce these effects when administered acutely.

Amphetamine potentiation. Amphetamine produces a number of effects in rats, including hyperthermia, increased locomotor activity, and improved shuttle box avoidance performance. Antidepressants, both TCAs and MAOIs, have been found to potentiate these responses (Carlton 1961; Halliwell et al. 1964; Morpurgo and Theobald 1965). As with the models previously described, these effects are observed after acute administration of drug. The various effects measured in conjunction with this test derive from the catecholamimetic action of amphetamine; consequently, the ability of a drug or treatment to potentiate these effects of amphetamine primarily detects ability to potentiate catecholaminergic neurotransmission.

Kindling. Electrical stimulation of certain brain regions (e.g., amygdala, cortex) apparently sensitizes the brain region to initiate seizure activity, so that following such stimulation, considerably less electrical stimulation delivered to the brain region is required to initiate seizure activity than is the case when that brain region has not received electrical stimulation. Babington and Wedeking (1973) reported that TCAs reduced the likelihood of development of seizures in "kindled" animals. Other drugs such as tranquilizers and sedatives also blocked kindled seizures. However, only the antidepressants tested (i.e., amitriptyline, nortriptyline, imipramine) blocked seizures initiated in the amygdala at considerably lower doses than were needed to block seizures kindled in the neocortex; all other drugs tested were equipotent against seizures initiated at both sites. Subsequently, ECT was

found to produce the same effect (Babington 1975), but MAOIs did not. Drugs are effective in this model when given acutely.

Circadian rhythm readjustment. Rats are normally active during the dark period of the day and are quiet (less active) during the light period. If the light-dark periods are switched, the animals must readjust their activity to this shift in the light-dark cycle. The rapidity with which animals will shift their activity to the new dark period and decrease their activity in the new light period is facilitated by administration of the TCA imipramine or the MAOI pargyline (Baltzer and Weiskrantz 1975). A stimulant (amphetamine) and a tranquilizing agent (chlordiazepoxide) were not effective. In treatments reported to be effective, drugs were administered repeatedly (i.e., for 10 days before the light-dark shift and for approximately 2 weeks thereafter).

Lesioning of the olfactory bulbs. Bilateral lesions of the olfactory bulbs produce a number of behavioral effects. This procedure generally results in hyperactivity in novel situations such as the open field (Janscar and Leonard 1980) and exaggerated responses to excitatory stimuli (Cairncross et al. 1977). Effects that may be related to the hyperactivity in animals with olfactory bulb lesions include deficits in passive avoidance performance (Archer et al. 1984; Rigter et al. 1977) as well as superior performance in the two-way shuttle avoidance task (Archer et al. 1984) that is highly dependent on high levels of motor activity for good acquisition (e.g., Weiss et al. 1968). However, olfactory bulb lesions also produce poor performance in one-way avoidance (King and Cairncross 1974), suggesting that decreased fearfulness may contribute to both poor passive avoidance and enhanced shuttle avoidance (i.e., shuttle avoidance is performed better in animals whose fear level is low). Activity in the Porsolt swim test has been reported to be unaffected by bulbectomy (Gorka et al. 1985), but bulbectomy increased activity in a swim task that emphasized escape attempts (Stockert et al. 1988). Lesioning of the olfactory bulbs was initially reported to produce a sustained elevation of circulating corticosterone in the rat, thus mimicking the hypocortisolemia seen in severe depression, but this response may have been generated as an acute reaction to the measurement procedures (see discussion in van Riezen and Leonard 1991).

Regarding pharmacological tests, deficits in avoidance behavior, particularly passive avoidance, produced by bulbectomy were found to be reversed by TCAs (i.e., amitriptyline, imipramine, clomipramine), atypical antidepressants (i.e., mianserin, viloxazine), and a serotonin uptake inhibitor, whereas these deficits were exaggerated by tranquilizers and neuroleptics (Cairncross et al. 1975a, 1977; Rigter et al. 1977; van Riezen et al. 1977). Drugs were effective in such tests when administered chronically. Increased open-field activity of bulbectomized animals was diminished by selective serotonin reuptake inhibitors (SSRIs), which were effective when given acutely as well as chronically (Earley and Leonard 1985).

Differential operant responding for low reinforcement (DRL). Seiden, O'Donnell, and colleagues screened a wide variety of drugs for their effects on rats whose low rate of response is reinforced. In this task, an animal is taught to press a lever to receive a food reward. After the response is learned, the animal is placed on a "differential reinforcement of low rate 72 second" (or DRL72) schedule, which requires the animal to wait 72 seconds after making a response before making another response to obtain the food reward; making a second response in less than 72 seconds after the first produces no reinforcement and simply resets the timing sequence so that the animal must wait an additional 72 seconds before responding to receive a reward.

In several studies, McGuire and Seiden (1980a, 1980b) and O'Donnell and Seiden (1982, 1983, 1985) found that ECT and various antidepressant drugs, including TCAs (i.e., DMI, imipramine, nortriptyline, clomipramine), MAOIs (i.e., tranylcypromine, iproniazid, phenelzine), atypical antidepressants (i.e., iprindole, mianserin, trazodone), and SSRIs (i.e., zimeldine, fluoxetine), all improved the ability of animals to inhibit responding and obtain rewards. Danysz and colleagues (1988) found similar detection of antidepressants. This effect was usually seen with acute administration of drug, but further improvements in performance were seen when the drug was administered repeatedly. Antipsychotic, psychomotor stimulant, narcotic analgesic, anxiolytic, antihistaminic, and anticholinergic agents did not improve performance.

Seiden and O'Donnell (1985) described findings indicating that the improved ability to obtain rewards on a DRL schedule could not be explained simply by the possibility that antidepressant treatment decreased response rate. These data showed that anxiolytics and phenothiazines also decreased response rate but did so to such an extent that the number of reinforcements decreased dramatically. However, Pollard and Howard (1986) found in two studies that nonantidepressant drugs (i.e., chlorpromazine, haloperidol, buspirone) could reduce response rate moderately to produce an increase in reinforcements

similar to what is seen with antidepressants, and they argued that this test is not specific for antidepressant drugs. (Note that the absolute magnitude of an effect seen in this test situation is often small—for example, reinforcements may increase from an average of 15 under "no-drug" conditions to 20–25 under "drug" conditions—so that the results are quite sensitive to small changes in response rate. On the other hand, the lever-press response that is used permits investigators to test the same animals repeatedly and under all conditions, so that small effects can be discerned and become statistically significant.)

Seiden and colleagues (1985) have tested animals to determine whether a specific monoamine neurotransmitter might be responsible for the increase in reinforced responding on a DRL72 schedule that occurs when antidepressants are given. Lesions of the dorsal bundle noradrenergic system that innervates the forebrain (i.e., lesioning the axons originating from the locus coeruleus [LC]) did not block the ability of DMI to increase the number of rewards obtained, but partial lesioning of brain dopamine did reduce this effect somewhat. Such results point to dopamine as the important catecholamine neurotransmitter (O'Donnell and Seiden 1984); however, 1) partial lesions of brain dopamine are of uncertain functional effect and can even result in enhancement of dopaminergic neurotransmission, and 2) bupropion, which preferentially potentiates dopamine by blocking its reuptake, was ineffective in increasing reinforced responding in the test (Seiden et al. 1985). Consequently, the neurotransmitter basis of the phenomenon has not yet been clarified.

Isolation-induced hyperactivity. When rats were housed individually as soon as they were weaned, as adults they were found to be hyperactive when tested in a novel environment. Garzon and Del Rio (1981; Garzon et al. 1979) found that this hyperactivity (i.e., increased activity of isolated rats relative to nonisolated rats) was attenuated or abolished by TCAs (i.e., amitriptyline, clomipramine, DMI), MAOIs (i.e., phenelzine, clorgiline), and atypical antidepressants (i.e., iprindole, mianserin, trazodone). The hyperactivity of isolated rats was not affected by antipsychotic medication (i.e., chlorpromazine, haloperidol), anxiolytics (i.e., chlordiazepoxide, diazepam), and amphetamine.

These investigators tested several drugs in an attempt to elucidate the neurotransmitter mechanism underlying the hyperactivity. The activity difference between isolated and nonisolated rats was abolished by the postsynaptic dopamine receptor agonist apomorphine and also by higher doses of nomifensine, which blocks dopamine and norepinephrine reuptake. Interestingly, the lowest dose of nomifensine used (5 mg/kg intraperitoneally) markedly increased the difference between isolated and nonisolated animals. Hyperactivity of isolated animals was also blocked by cyproheptadine, a serotonin receptor antagonist, and by salbutamol, a β-adrenergic receptor stimulant. Based on this array of pharmacological results, the nature of isolation-induced hyperactivity does not appear easily explained in relation to any one particular monoamine. All of the drug effects described here were seen with acute administration. One potential concern in the use of this testing procedure, which was emphasized by the investigators and considered throughout their studies, is that many of the drugs used will affect motor activity of normal (i.e., nonisolated) animals, so that drugs can eliminate differences between isolated and nonisolated animals by either markedly increasing or decreasing activity in general. Therefore, care must be taken to use drug doses that do not considerably change normal motor patterns when this model is used.

Summary Observations Regarding Animal Assay Models

Animal assays are, almost by definition, useful (or not useful) depending on their ability to screen for drugs or other potential treatments for depression. As can be noted from the preceding descriptions, many of these models detect antidepressant medication when the drug is administered acutely. The first observation is that, although this might at first appear to be a deficiency because antidepressant medication is effective in patients only after repeated administration, this is not a defect for an animal assay model. A drug screen can be viewed as most useful if it specifically detects effective antidepressant medication when the drug is given only once and is therefore highly efficient in detecting antidepressant compounds. In evaluating animal assays, it should be kept in mind that such assays use responses of animals, whether behavioral or physiological, in a manner similar to that of an in vitro assay; that is, the response of the animal, even if it is a behavioral one, is no more than a "readout" of drug action. As researchers increasingly require that the drug mimic the effects observed in human patients (i.e., drug effectiveness only when administered chronically), they are moving toward criteria that are applicable to homologous models and requiring that the behavioral response of the animal resembles the behavioral response of the depressed patient. Consequently, an animal assay that responds to acute administration of a treatment is as useful as, and perhaps more useful than, one that requires chronic administration of the treatment.

Lesioning of the olfactory bulbs produces one of the more interesting models described under the category of animal assays. This model has one of the best profiles for detection of known antidepressants, responding to TCAs and atypical antidepressants as well as to serotonin uptake inhibitors, whereas stimulants (amphetamine) and the anticholinergic atropine were ineffective; however, the single MAOI that was tested, tranylcypromine, was ineffective. The ability of olfactory bulbectomy to act as a screen for antidepressant medication may appear anomalous at first given the nature of the manipulation, but studies have determined that neurotransmitter changes resulting from lesions of the olfactory bulbs may account for the ability of this seemingly unusual procedure to generate a model relevant to depression. For instance, all effective TCAs potentiate the effects of released norepinephrine by blocking reuptake (e.g., Richelson and Pfenning 1984), which was a key observation that led to the catecholamine hypothesis of depression (Bunney and Davis 1965; Schildkraut and Kety 1967). This hypothesis originally proposed that a deficit in brain norepinephrine, which noradrenergic reuptake blockers and MAOIs corrected, was responsible for depression. Lesioning of the olfactory bulbs produces a marked depletion of norepinephrine in the forebrain, possibly by interruption of noradrenergic axons as they course by the olfactory bulbs in projecting to the neocortex (Cairncross et al. 1973, 1975b). Moreover, Shipley and colleagues (1985) reported that 40% of neurons of the LC, the major noradrenergic cell-body group in the brain, project to the rat olfactory bulb, which is 10 times as many LC cells as project to any other part of the cerebral cortex; consequently, altered activity of a significant number of the noradrenergic cells that innervate the forebrain is likely to follow a lesion of the olfactory bulbs.

However, as could be expected, the consequences of bulbectomy are not simple. Lesions of the olfactory bulbs affect not only norepinephrine but also serotonergic, cholinergic, and γ-aminobutyric acid (GABA)ergic systems (see review by Leonard and Tuite 1981). Moreover, the behavioral effects of bulbectomy cannot be reproduced simply by reducing forebrain norepinephrine levels. This last point was made in a particularly illuminating series of experiments by Archer and colleagues (1984), who used the drug DSP-4 to destroy forebrain noradrenergic terminals on axons of LC cells and found that this procedure did not mimic effects seen after olfactory bulbectomy. In contrast to manipulating noradrenergic systems, Cairncross and colleagues administered neurotoxins that destroy serotonergic neurons (i.e., 5,6- and 5,7-dihydroxytryptamine) and produced behavioral effects similar to those seen with bulbectomy (reviewed in Cairncross et al. 1979), which suggests that the deficit induced by bulbectomy might be serotonergic in nature. However, Leonard and Tuite (1981) argued that the effects of these neurotoxins are notably smaller in magnitude than those produced by bulbectomy. In addition, taking into account that these effects of serotonergic neurotoxins can be reversed by treatment with mianserin (Wren 1976, reported in Leonard and Tuite 1981), a drug that blocks α_2-adrenergic receptors (Robson et al. 1978), it appears that, at the least, both norepinephrine and serotonin need to be considered in the eventual resolution of how the bulbectomy model is generated.

Homologous Models

As was stated earlier in this chapter, the models discussed in this section represent those in which the animal shows responses similar to those seen in clinical depression. Inclusion of the model in this section does not require the symptom profile to be extensive—the animal may manifest only one particular response that appears similar to that seen in clinical depression—although animal models included here may also reproduce a number of changes, behavioral or physiological, that can be related to depressive responses.

Reserpine-induced reduction of motor activity.
Reserpine and reserpine-like compounds, such as tetrabenazine, inactivate the ability of synaptic vesicles to retain monoamines; as a consequence of this action, release of monoamines follows administration of these drugs, and then a long-term reduction in monoamine stores occurs, resulting in depletion of dopamine, norepinephrine, epinephrine, and serotonin in the brain and periphery. The depletion of amines produces a variety of physiological and behavioral effects, and antidepressants have been shown to counteract some of these. Domenjoz and Theobald (1959) first reported that imipramine could block the ability of reserpine to potentiate hypnotic effects. Costa and colleagues (1960) then reported that imipramine blocked reserpine-induced decreases in rectal temperature and heart rate and increases in diarrhea and ptosis. These effects would ordinarily cause this model to be classified as an animal assay, but reserpine also decreases motor activity, and antidepressants counteract this effect as well. Vernier and colleagues (1962) reported that imipramine would antagonize reserpine-induced sedation, which was quantified largely by decreased motor activity. In addition to imipramine, other TCAs also antagonize reserpine-induced (or tetrabenazine-induced) reduction of motor activity. MAOIs have a similar effect (Howard et al. 1981). The "reserpinized rodent" consti-

tutes one of the earliest animal models of depression. The observation that reserpine suppresses motor activity was apparently a key factor in suggesting the catecholamine hypothesis of depression.

Given the ability of TCAs and MAOIs to potentiate the action of monoamines, in retrospect it is not surprising that these substances antagonize the effects of reserpine on a variety of responses, including reserpine's ability to depress motor activity. On the other hand, a variety of compounds that do not appear to be effective antidepressant medications, such as amphetamine and cocaine, also yield positive results in antagonizing reserpine-induced reduction of motor activity. Thus, this test apparently detects the ability of a treatment or drug to potentiate central aminergic transmission rather than to have specific antidepressant action. The effects described here are also seen with acute administration of drug rather than requiring chronic administration. Finally, the test is not known to detect non-TCAs such as iprindole.

Depression of active responding induced by 5-hydroxtryptophan.
Based on early studies suggesting that lysergic acid diethylamide (LSD) produced psychoactive effects by interacting with serotonergic receptors, Aprison hypothesized that serotonin might be importantly involved in behavioral states. Consequently, Aprison and colleagues injected the serotonin precursor 5-hydroxtryptophan (5-HTP) into pigeons, and subsequently rats, and observed that the treatment produced marked suppression of active responding for food reinforcement (summarized in Aprison et al. 1978). This reduction in active behavior seen following increased serotonin release due to administration of 5-HTP was blocked by TCAs (i.e., amitriptyline, imipramine) as well as by non-TCAs (i.e., mianserin, iprindole) (Nagayama et al. 1981). Two features of the model do not reproduce what is seen in depression: 1) acute administration of the antidepressants was effective in blocking the behavioral depression, and 2) drugs that block serotonin reuptake (e.g., fluoxetine) increased 5-HTP-induced behavioral depression markedly (Nagayama et al. 1980), so that this class of antidepressants exacerbates rather than prevents depression in this model.

Swim-test immobility.
A test proposed by Porsolt and colleagues involves placing a rodent (a rat or mouse) into a beaker of water and determining the amount of time that the animal remains immobile. The typical procedure that has been used is to place the animal in the tank for 15 minutes on day 1; as a result of this exposure, active coping attempts are extinguished so that the animal ceases

movement by the end of the session. The following day, the animal is returned to the water tank for 5 minutes, and immobility is timed. Between the first and second exposure to the swim tank, the drug (or other treatment) is given, often a single drug administration shortly before the immobility test or two or three drug administrations during the 24 hours between the first and second exposures to the swim tank. Effective antidepressants cause animals to show less immobility on the second (test) exposure than is shown by vehicle-treated or untreated animals. The test situation with an animal showing the immobile response is illustrated in Figure 5–1.

This test detects a wide range of potential antidepressant treatments, including all TCAs tested (i.e., imipramine, DMI, amitriptyline, nortriptyline), MAOIs (i.e., nialamide, iproniazid), atypical antidepressants

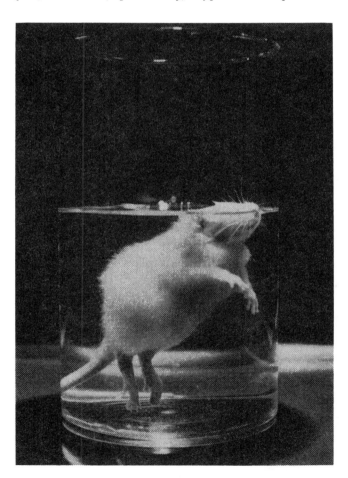

Figure 5–1. Rat showing characteristic posture of immobility.
Source. Reprinted from Porsolt RD: "Behavioral Despair," in *Antidepressants: Neurochemical, Behavioral, and Clinical Perspectives.* Edited by Enna SJ, Malick JB, Richardson E. New York, Raven, 1981, pp. 121–139. Copyright 1981, Raven Press. Used with permission.

(i.e., iprindole, mianserin, nomifensine), and ECT (Porsolt et al. 1978; see also review by Borsini and Meli 1988). This test also detects deprivation of rapid eye movement (REM) sleep, which is therapeutic in depression (Hawkins et al. 1980). The test does not detect anxiolytics or phenothiazines (these drugs increase, not decrease, immobility). However, it will show false-positive results to various substances (for a complete list, see De Pablo et al. 1989), particularly stimulants (i.e., amphetamine and caffeine). Also, a significant weakness of this test, given the current preference for antidepressant medication, is its poor detection of SSRIs, which was noted early on by Porsolt and colleagues (1979; Satoh et al. 1984).

Perhaps because of its ease of use and ability to detect drugs of antidepressant potential, the Porsolt swim test is currently the most widely used pharmacological test for antidepressants. Several interesting and significant characteristics of this model have been discovered. First, drugs work when given acutely, which does not reproduce the clinical response to antidepressant drugs that requires repeated administration. However, larger effects are often seen when drugs have been given repeatedly before testing. Second, although the test was initially described as "behavioral despair," little evidence indicates that exposure of animals to this test situation produces a significant degree of anything that might be called despair. Rather, immobility in the standard test situation appears to be explained, at least in part, by the animal's learning to adopt an immobile posture with the rear feet or tail balanced on the bottom of the swim tank, thereby supporting the head above the top of the water (see Figure 5–1; see also De Pablo et al. 1989; Hawkins et al. 1978). Thus, effective drugs appear to cause the animal on the test day to attempt active behavior instead of continuing to practice a previously learned immobile posture. Modifications of the original test situation using deeper water to prevent the animal from standing on the bottom of the tank have been used in several situations (e.g., Abel 1991; De Pablo et al. 1989; Weiss et al. 1981); under these conditions, the immobility that is measured represents more unambiguously a loss of motivation to engage in active coping attempts than is the case when the animal can partially resolve its dilemma by standing on the floor of the tank. Third, although "despair" has not been shown to characterize the model, stress may well be involved in the model's ability to detect antidepressant effects. Borsini and colleagues (1989) showed that the initial exposure of the rat to the swim tank, although typically done to extinguish active behavior, produces consequences similar to those produced by known stressors (i.e., cold, restraint, footshock) and that exposing the rat to the swim tank on the day before the test considerably enhances the capacity of the test to detect antidepressant effects. Thus, the swim test, as usually conducted, appears to determine how treatments counteract "stress-induced" immobility. Supporting the idea that the initial exposure to the swim tank functions as a stressor, Jordan et al. (1994) found that release of monoamines in the brain (measured by microdialysis) is considerably higher during and after exposure to the swim tank on the second day (i.e., the test day) than it is during and after the initial exposure on the previous day. Fourth, antidepressant medication particularly increases "escapelike" motor activity that occurs early in the swim test, which can be discriminated from general increases in motor activity that can be detected late in swim tests of long duration (Armario et al. 1988; Kitada et al. 1981). Thus, looking at different types of motor responses may be a way to discriminate between antidepressant action and nonspecific stimulation of motor activity in the swim test.

Various investigators have examined the neurochemical basis of swim-test immobility by studying antidepressant-treated animals to try to obtain possible clues to neurophysiological pathology underlying depression. Depression-like behavior (i.e., swim-test immobility) was increased by potentiating cholinergic transmission (Hasey and Hanin 1991) and by blocking catecholamine synthesis with α-methyl-p-tyrosine (Gil et al. 1992). To decrease swim-test immobility, several investigators have focused, not surprisingly, on brain dopamine, which is prominently related to motor activity. Activity in the swim test has been increased by 1) blocking dopamine reuptake and stimulating dopamine D_2 receptors (Borsini et al. 1988), 2) stimulating the ventral tegmental cell bodies projecting to forebrain dopaminergic regions (Plaznik et al. 1985a), and 3) infusing into the nucleus accumbens norepinephrine, phenylephrine (α_1 receptor stimulant), isoproterenol (β-adrenergic receptor stimulant), and apomorphine (dopamine receptor stimulant) (Plaznik et al. 1985b). Plaznik and colleagues (1985a) argued that only the noradrenergic manipulations specifically affect activity in the swim test that represents escapelike responses, whereas stimulation of dopamine directly decreases swim-test immobility by increasing motor activity in general. Finally, Murua and Molina (1990) suggested that opiate mechanisms may be involved in producing immobility because they found that naloxone reduced immobility in stressed rats.

The swim test also has been used to attempt to determine the mechanism of action of antidepressant drugs; these studies have focused on analyzing DMI's mode of action. The therapeutic (anti-immobility) effect of DMI in the swim test can be blocked by the dopamine receptor (D_2) antagonist sulpiride (Cervo and Samanin 1987) and lesions of the LC (by the neurotoxin 6-hydroxydopamine) (Plaznik et al. 1985a). The latter finding indicates that norepinephrine is essential for the therapeutic effect of DMI; this is perhaps not surprising given the extreme potency with which DMI blocks norepinephrine reuptake (Richelson and Pfenning 1984). Kitada and colleagues (1986) showed that pharmacological stimulation of adrenergic β receptors attenuated the anti-immobility effects of DMI; this suggests that an important function of norepinephrine in DMI's therapeutic effect is to downregulate β receptors, a long-held theory of why certain antidepressants are effective (Sulser 1979; Vetulani et al. 1976).

Clonidine withdrawal. Acute administration of the drug clonidine causes rats to be inactive for a brief period in the swim test. However, long-lasting inactivity can be produced in this test in drug-free animals by clonidine administration as well. Hoffman and Weiss (1986) reported a procedure to accomplish this. When clonidine was administered to rats for 2 weeks and then was withdrawn abruptly, the animals, which were now drug-free, showed a depression of activity in the swim test that lasted for several weeks. The long-lasting nature of this reduction in motor activity permits examination of the effects of long-term treatment regimens. Only DMI has been tested to date. When given daily for 2 weeks, DMI reversed the depression of swim-test activity seen in this model; when chronic DMI administration was halted, activity in the swim test again became depressed. Also, DMI did not increase swim-test activity after being given for only 1 day. Further studies of this model have not been conducted.

Tail suspension test. When a mouse is suspended in the air by its tail, it will struggle to free itself. Steru and colleagues (1985) reported that antidepressant drugs increase the amount of time spent in such struggling. Struggling is increased by TCAs, MAOIs, and atypical antidepressants but is not increased by neuroleptics, anxiolytics, or anticholinergics. However, struggling time is also increased by psychostimulants (dextroamphetamine). Drugs work in this test when given acutely; therefore, this model has been proposed to be, and has been used exclusively as, a screening technique for pharmacological treatments. However, because effective treatments counteract a form of immobility (i.e., cessation of struggling), the test is thought to be related to the Porsolt swim test and is therefore listed here as a homologous model.

Neonatal clomipramine. In the neonatal clomipramine model, rat pups are injected with clomipramine (15 mg/kg) twice daily on postnatal days 8 through 21.

When tested at age 90+ days, these animals have decreased sexual activity, intracranial self-stimulation, aggressive behavior, and motor hyperactivity in a novel situation (Hartley et al. 1990; Neill et al. 1990; Vogel et al. 1990a). Relative to control animals that had been injected neonatally with saline, clomipramine-injected rats also showed changes in sleep behavior that have been associated with depression, including reduced latency to enter REM sleep following sleep onset and frequent onset of REM periods (Vogel et al. 1988, 1990c). Based on these behavioral effects, the investigators who developed the procedure proposed it as a means to model endogenous, as opposed to reactive, depression (Vogel et al. 1990b). One drawback to this model appears to be the hyperactivity evidenced by the animals in that patients manifesting "endogenous" depression are likely to be the most seriously depressed and will show psychomotor retardation rather than hyperactivity. Testing of treatment efficacy on this model has been very limited; preliminary data (Vogel et al. 1990b) indicated that imipramine treatment for 4 days reduced locomotor hyperactivity of the animals treated neonatally with clomipramine. Although this treatment uses an inducing stimulus that seems to have little relation to normal physiological conditions that may give rise to susceptibility to depression, the hypothesis offered by the investigators is that a physiological defect is present in endogenous depression, and neonatal administration of clomipramine somehow reproduces this defect.

Lesioning of the dorsomedial amygdala in dogs.

When the dorsomedial amygdala is lesioned electrolytically in dogs, one of the most dramatic syndromes resembling severe depression is produced. Fonberg (1969a, 1969b; summarized in Fonberg 1972) reported that these animals display lethargy, negativism, reluctance to eat, and, to the extent that this can be judged in a dog, saddened facial expression. In terms of symptom profile, the appearance of these animals ranks with the "monkey separation" model (see next section) as producing the most similarity to what is observed in severe retarded depression (see Figure 5–2). The effect of antidepressant medication on this syndrome has not yet been reported. Despite its dramatic appearance, the model has been little studied and perhaps is likely to remain so given the problems of using dogs as subjects. Also, some questions can be raised as to its relevance. Fonberg reported that lesioning of the lateral hypothalamus, which is now well known to disturb dopaminergic axons ascending to the striatum and frontal brain, produces in the dog a similar phenomenon, which raises the question of whether the dorsolateral amygdala lesions simply produce a variant of the lateral

hypothalamic syndrome that is produced by lesioning of dopamine inputs of the basal ganglia. If this is the case, it would mean that either the model is unrelated to clinical depression or the resemblance of these dogs' symptoms to those seen in very severe retarded depression indicates that clinical depression involves disturbance of these dopaminergic systems, which is simply seen in extreme form when the brain lesions are made in the dogs.

Isolation- and separation-induced depression in monkeys.

Behavioral responses that appear similar to those seen in severe depression have been elicited by separating young monkeys from their mothers and normal social setting or from their juvenile peers. Following separation, animals initially display high activity accompanied by much vocalization; this is labeled as the stage of *agitation* or *protest* and usually lasts 24–36 hours. Following this stage, the behavioral pattern changes markedly—the ani-

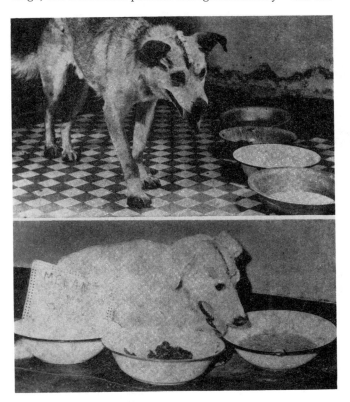

Figure 5–2. Two dogs (upper and lower) after bilateral dorsomedial amygdala damage. Note the animals' lack of interest in the various kinds of food presented and their sad appearance.
Source. Reprinted from Fonberg E: "Control of Emotional Behaviour Through the Hypothalamus and Amygdaloid Complex," in *Physiology, Emotion and Psychosomatic Illness (Ciba Foundation Symposium 8)*. Edited by Porter R, Knight J. Amsterdam, Elsevier, 1972, pp 131–161. Copyright 1972, the Ciba Foundation. Used with permission.

mal shows decreased activity, huddling and self-clasping, dejected and saddened facial expression, and generally decreased exploration (e.g., Kaufman and Rosenblum 1967; McKinney et al. 1971) (see Figures 5–3 through 5–7). This constellation of depressive-type behaviors can persist for 5 or 6 days before gradually remitting; however, in some cases, it lasts even longer. Depression-related behaviors are diminished by long-term administration of imipramine, and symptoms reappear if the drug is withheld (Suomi et al. 1978). Also, the drug appears not to work soon after it is administered but requires long-term administration, thus paralleling what is seen with antidepressant administration in humans.

Studies exploring underlying biochemical changes in this model are of interest. Kraemer (1986) and colleagues found that animals that are isolated for long periods have norepinephrine levels in the cerebrospinal fluid (CSF) that are approximately half the levels seen in nonisolated animals. These investigators also reported that animals with low CSF levels of norepinephrine were more susceptible to depressive-like symptoms when separated than were animals with higher levels of norepinephrine. Porsolt and colleagues (1984) reported that acute administration of imipramine, which blocks norepinephrine reuptake, increased both motor activity and vocalizations during the protest stage, making responses during this initial stage more extreme. These data suggest that norepinephrine and adrenergic receptors in the brain are importantly involved in this type of depression, suggesting such hypotheses as 1) decreased CSF norepinephrine in susceptible animals is indicative of low norepinephrine release and, consequently, supersensitive adrenergic receptors in these animals, and 2) animals prone to depression, with low CSF norepinephrine, are vulnerable to norepinephrine depletion in the brain when subjected to stress, which results in depression.

Separation of Siberian hamsters. Siberian dwarf hamsters (*Phodopus sungorus pallas*) form stable male-female mating pairs that ordinarily remain together even after pups are born, with the male participating in rearing activities. Crawley (1984) developed a model in which Siberian hamster pairs, maintained in the laboratory, were separated 3–4 weeks after they had formed mating pairs, and thereafter the animals were housed in individual cages. During the period after separation (3–4 weeks was generally monitored), the male hamsters showed decreased daily running-wheel activity, decreased activity when tested in an open field, increased body weight, and decreased social interaction when an unfamiliar animal of the opposite sex was introduced into the cage. Separated

females showed a smaller decrease in running-wheel activity compared with males but no change in the other measures. All of these changes could be reversed by reuniting the separated pair. The changes in behavior described here could not be attributed to the isolation (i.e., single housing) of animals after separation because similar changes were not seen in animals that had been maintained in single-sex groups and were then individually housed. Effects of one antidepressant, imipramine, were tested in this model. Administration of imipramine (10 mg/kg/day) for 2 weeks after separation eliminated some activity-related changes shown by male hamsters in the open field (but not the decrease in total distance traversed in the open field). Imipramine administration also did not eliminate the increase in body weight or the decrease in social interaction with an unfamiliar animal of the opposite sex. Regarding neurochemical differences, males showed evidence of decreased serotonin turnover (possibly decreased release), as indicated by lower 5-hydroxyindoleacetic acid (5-HIAA)-to-serotonin ratios in cortex, diencephalon, and mesencephalon (Crawley 1983). Further studies of this model have not been reported.

Exhaustion stress. Hatotani and colleagues (1982) exposed female rats to forced running in an activity wheel until the animals were exhausted, as indicated by rectal temperature reaching 33°C or lower (37.5°C is normal). After exposure to three sessions of forced running, each separated by a 24-hour rest period, spontaneous motor activity in the rats was markedly depressed for several weeks. This depression of motor activity was marked by complete suppression of the diurnal peaks in spontaneous motor activity seen in nonstressed animals. Motor activity returned to normal after daily injections of imipramine; a therapeutic response was seen only after the drug was administered for longer than 10 days. The other characteristic described for this model is that a marked increase in intensity of histochemical fluorescence of noradrenergic cell bodies in the brain accompanies the exhaustion-induced decrease in motor activity, thereby indicating that activation of noradrenergic neurons in the brain appears to be increased by the exhaustion-stress procedure. Conversely, fluorescence of dopamine neurons of the tuberoinfundibular system in the hypothalamus was much weaker in stressed animals, which was thought to indicate decreased activity in these dopaminergic neurons.

Chronic mild stress model. First introduced by Katz, Roth, and Carroll, the chronic mild stress model is generated by exposing rats to a succession of different stressful con-

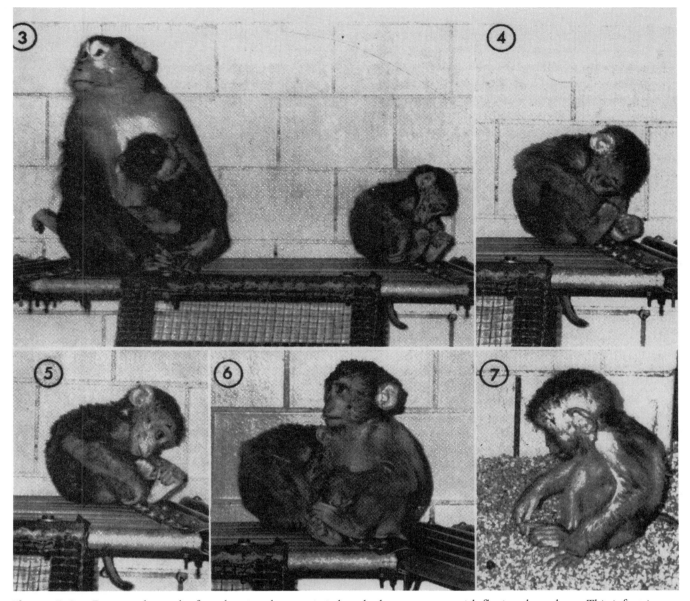

Figure 5–3. Depressed pigtail infant showing characteristic hunched-over posture with flexion throughout. This infant is completely disengaged from the mother and infant nearby who are in ventral-ventral contact.

Figure 5–4. Depressed pigtail infant showing characteristic posture including head between legs. Note slightly opened eyes as he sucks his penis.

Figure 5–5. Depressed pigtail infant showing characteristic posture and dejected expression on face.

Figure 5–6. Two depressed pigtail infants. The one in rear shows characteristic hunched-over posture. The one in front has lifted his head to look across pen. Despite their passive contact, they are not engaged with each other.

Figure 5–7. Depressed pigtail infant showing aimless, tentative exploration of bedding during early stages of recovery.

Source.   Reprinted from Kaufman IC, Rosenblum LA: "The Reaction to Separation in Infant Monkeys: Anaclitic Depression and Conservation-Withdrawal." *Psychosomatic Medicine* 29:648–675, 1967. Copyright 1967, Williams & Wilkins. Used with permission.

ditions (i.e., mild uncontrollable footshock, cold swim, change in housing conditions, reversal of light and dark periods, and food and water deprivation) over a period of either 2 weeks (Roth and Katz 1981) or 3 weeks (Katz et al.

1981a). The sequence of stressors concludes with exposure to noise at 95 decibels and bright light for 1 hour, followed by testing of spontaneous motor activity in an open field; the effect measured in these studies is a decrease in open-field activity seen in chronically stressed animals relative to animals that have not been exposed to the chronic stress regimen. Although changes were sometimes of small magnitude (20%–30% relative to nonstressed animals), a reduction in open-field activity nevertheless reliably characterized chronically stressed animals in a number of studies. Katz and colleagues principally analyzed effects of treatment (Katz 1981; Katz and Baldrighi 1982; Katz and Hersh 1981; Katz and Sibel 1982a, 1982b; Katz et al. 1981b). They showed that the decrease in activity in the open field could be reduced by TCAs (i.e., imipramine, amitriptyline), an MAOI (i.e., tranylcypromine), atypical antidepressants (i.e., mianserin, bupropion, iprindole), and ECT, and was not consistently reversed by an anticholinergic, antihistaminic, anxiolytic, or neuroleptic drug. This profile indicated that the decreased activity in the open field produced by chronic stress is selectively responsive to antidepressant medications. Katz and colleagues also reported that stress-induced elevations in corticosteroids were antagonized by antidepressant medication.

An interesting effect reported in one paper of the series has been followed up by a considerable amount of research because of its hypothesized relevance to depression. Katz (1982) reported that the chronic stress regimen decreased the hedonic value of a stimulus and that this change could be reversed by treatment with imipramine. It was found in this study that normal rats would ingest increasingly larger amounts of fluid that contained progressively larger concentrations of sucrose or saccharin but that consumption of more palatable solutions was not greater when consumption was measured within 24–48 hours after conclusion of the 3-week chronic stress regimen. When chronically stressed rats were treated with imipramine during the 3-week stress procedure, the amount of sucrose solution they ingested was equivalent to that ingested by unstressed animals, although the interpretation of this therapeutic effect is complicated by the fact that the imipramine treatment decreased saccharin consumption in the control animals that were exposed to no stress at all. Nevertheless, these results indicate that the tendency of rats to take in larger than normal amounts of a palatable solution was reduced by the chronic stress regimen.

Subsequent studies have followed up on this result on the assumption that it may model what Klein (1975) termed the principal characteristic of depression: the inability to experience pleasurable events. Reward and hedonic effects have been related to the dopaminergic system of the brain (e.g., Wise and Rompre 1989). Tekes et al. (1986) showed that the chronic stress regimen decreased indicants of dopamine turnover in the brain, and that these changes in dopamine turnover were antagonized by chronic treatment with a TCA (amitriptyline) and an MAOI (deprenyl). Moreau and colleagues (1992) found that a similar stress regimen increased the threshold for electrical self-stimulation through electrodes in the ventral tegmental area of the brain (dopamine cell body region), and that this reduction in self-stimulation was countered by DMI. Willner and colleagues (Muscat et al. 1988, 1990, 1992; Sampson et al. 1991; Willner et al. 1992) have published a number of articles showing that chronic mild stress decreases intake of palatable solutions, that these effects can be counteracted by treatment with antidepressants, and that chronic stress alters dopamine turnover and dopamine receptors in the brain. Although these studies make clear that the chronic stress regimen does alter various aspects of dopaminergic systems in the brain, the interpretation of changes in intake that were observed is more ambiguous. For example, studies do not appear to confirm that animals exposed to the chronic stress regimen ever lose their preference for palatable substances (e.g., sucrose, saccharin) in comparison with tap water; rather, only the degree to which they will overconsume these palatable substances in comparison with tap water decreases in animals exposed to chronic stress. Thus, the chronic stress regimen may have simply decreased total consumption rather than affected preference. It is well known that stressful conditions will decrease consumption of both food and liquid (e.g., Pare 1965; Weiss 1968). From the clinical perspective, the emphasis of these studies on the dopaminergic system raises the question of why antidepressants that preferentially potentiate dopaminergic transmission (e.g., bupropion) appear to be no faster acting or better (and perhaps less so) than the classic TCAs that block norepinephrine uptake or the SSRIs.

Uncontrollable shock (or the "learned helplessness") model. In the late 1960s, several studies showed that exposing animals, both rats and dogs, to electric shocks that they could not control resulted in quite different responses from those seen in animals that received the same shocks but that they could control. Overmier and Seligman (1967), Seligman and Maier (1967), and Seligman et al. (1971) found that exposing dogs to uncontrollable shock made the animals unable to acquire an active (shuttle) avoidance-escape response. At the same time, Weiss (1968) observed that exposure of rats to uncontrollable shock decreased subsequent food and water intake in the home cage and caused body weight loss; these changes were virtually absent in animals that received the same shocks while exerting control over them. In these studies, the rats also became more fearful after receiving uncontrollable shock than they did after receiving controllable shock. In the mid-1970s, both Seligman and Maier found that the avoidance-escape deficit resulting from uncontrollable shock could be produced in rats (Maier et al. 1973; Seligman and Beagley 1975). In 1974, Seligman hypothesized that exposure to uncontrollable events produces a depression-like response and that exposure of animals to uncontrollable shock therefore constituted a model for the study of depression. Subsequently, Weiss and colleagues (1981) showed that uncontrollable shock, but not controllable shock, decreased active behavior and increased immobility in a swim test. Figure 5–8

shows an experimental setting that generates this model.

Perhaps because it has been studied more widely than any other model, the uncontrollable shock model has reproduced the largest list of symptoms found in human depression. In 1982, Weiss and colleagues listed the various effects of uncontrollable shock and showed that these symptoms correspond closely with those listed in DSM-III (which was then the standard for diagnosis of mental disorders) for diagnosis of depression in humans. The symptoms produced by uncontrollable shock now include 1) decreases in food and water consumption, 2) loss of body weight, 3) loss of ability to initiate normal active behavior,

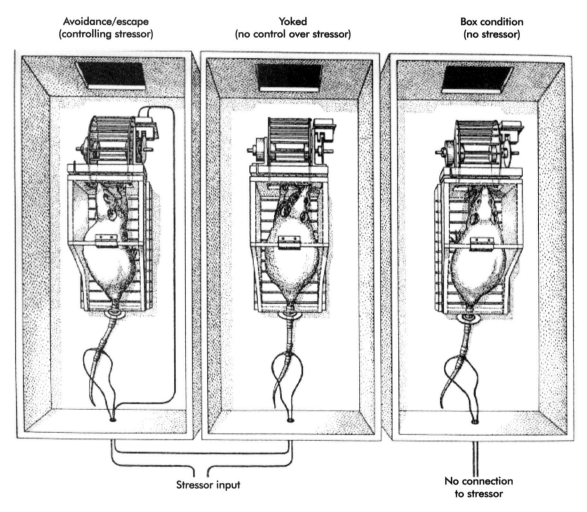

Figure 5–8. Conditions used to generate the uncontrollable shock model. At left, the animal can terminate (avoid and/or escape) the stressor (electric shock to the tail) by turning the wheel at the front of its box enclosure. At center, the "yoked" animal receives exactly the same shocks (through fixed tail electrodes wired in series with the avoidance-escape animal), but its wheel-turn responses have no effect on shock. At right, the "no-stressor" animal simply remains in the box apparatus with no tail-shock stressor being received throughout the procedure. After this procedure, the yoked animal at center shows depression-related behavioral changes, whereas the avoidance-escape and box-condition animals do not show these behavioral changes. *Source.* Reprinted from Weiss JM, Goodman PA, Losito BG, et al: "Behavioral Depression Produced by an Uncontrollable Stressor: Relationship to Norepinephrine, Dopamine, and Serotonin Levels in Various Regions of the Rat Brain." *Brain Research: Brain Research Reviews* 3:167–205, 1981. Copyright 1981, Elsevier Science Publishers B.V. Used with permission.

4) loss of normal grooming activity, 5) loss of normal competitiveness and playlike activities, 6) alteration of sleep patterns, particularly marked by early-morning awakening, 7) loss of responding for rewarding brain stimulation, and 8) increase in errors in discrimination tasks (for references, see Weiss 1991).

Responsivity to antidepressant treatment of animals exposed to uncontrollable shock has been examined by various investigators. All studies concerned with this issue have measured the ability of antidepressant treatment to reverse the deficit in avoidance-escape performance produced by uncontrollable shock. Poor performance of active avoidance-escape responses following uncontrollable shock was first reported to be reversed by DMI (Leshner et al. 1979) and then by nortriptyline (Telner and Singhal 1981). Sherman and colleagues (1982) then conducted a large study in which the avoidance-escape deficit was reversed by a wide variety of antidepressant medications—including TCAs, atypical antidepressants, and MAOIs—and ECT, but it was not corrected by stimulants or antipsychotic medications. P. Martin et al. (1990) also found that deficits were reversed by SSRIs as well as by TCAs and MAOIs (P. Martin et al. 1987). In these studies, drugs were generally given for only 1–3 days between the uncontrollable shock and the testing, although Leshner and colleagues (1979) tested effects after 7 days of drug administration. Although these findings might suggest beneficial effects of acute drug administration, Telner and Singhal (1981) reported no effects early in drug administration but positive effects later. A difficulty with establishing efficacy after long-term (i.e., 2 weeks) drug administration is that the symptoms in this model tend to dissipate (see last paragraph in this section).

Regarding the pathophysiology that underlies the behavioral symptoms produced by uncontrollable shock, investigations have again focused on reduced motor activity produced by uncontrollable shock. Studies of the physiological mechanism underlying this deficit have been extensive, with disturbance of central noradrenergic, serotonergic, cholinergic, GABAergic systems, and endorphins and enkephalins hypothesized by different investigators to be responsible for the deficit. Of these various formulations, the most well-developed hypotheses are those emphasizing disturbance of norepinephrine and serotonin; these hypotheses not only are based on data showing that pharmacological manipulation of these systems can produce and/or reverse the behavioral deficit but, most important, also include studies showing that uncontrollable shock alters the implicated neurotransmitter system to produce changes potentially able to mediate the behavioral deficit observed after shock.

The hypothesis relating effects of uncontrollable shock to noradrenergic changes is the most detailed and specific one offered at present. It states that strong uncontrollable shock depletes norepinephrine in terminals of the LC region, which causes increased burst firing of LC cells by reducing transmitter available to stimulate inhibitory somatodendritic α_2 receptors on LC cell bodies (summarized in Weiss 1991). Thus, this formulation attributes depression produced by uncontrollable shock to disinhibition of LC neurons. If LC neurons are disinhibited (and therefore hyperactive), then depressive symptomatology in the uncontrollable shock model may result from an excess of norepinephrine released in the terminal regions to which the LC neurons project (e.g., hippocampus, cortex, forebrain). It can also be noted that this formulation appears to complement the findings of Henn and colleagues, who reported that β-adrenergic receptors are upregulated in animals that are susceptible to the behavior-depressing effects of uncontrollable shock (Henn et al. 1985; J. V. Martin et al. 1990). Both higher-than-normal release of norepinephrine from LC terminals and upregulated β receptors would potentiate postsynaptic noradrenergic activity.

The data relating serotonin to deficits produced by uncontrollable shock are currently less clear than those supporting the noradrenergic hypothesis. Although serotonergic receptors are altered by uncontrollable shock (J. V. Martin et al. 1990), the investigators who have studied these changes point out this change does not appear well correlated with the behavioral deficit. Also, the data are contradictory regarding whether serotonin release in the brain is increased (Edwards et al. 1992; Petty et al. 1990) or decreased (Petty and Sherman 1983) as a consequence of uncontrollable shock. Thus, serotonin seems affected, but the nature of the change is unclear.

Finally, it should be mentioned that deficits in responding for electrical (rewarding) brain stimulation that occur after uncontrollable shock seem related to changes in dopaminergic mesocorticolimbic regions (e.g., Zacharko and Anisman 1991).

A significant drawback to the uncontrollable shock model is that most of the depression-like symptoms produced in the model (described previously in this section) do not last beyond 48–72 hours after exposure to uncontrollable shock; in some instances, the loss of symptoms at about this time is rather abrupt (e.g., Desan et al. 1988; Overmier and Seligman 1967; Weiss et al. 1981; Zacharko et al. 1983). Although the lack of persistence of the symptoms appears to be a deficiency in this model, it may be a clue to the model's underlying pathophysiology. Weiss et al. (1981) noted that the disappearance of behavioral depression at 2–3 days postshock corresponds to the time at which the enzyme tyrosine hydroxylase, whose activity is the primary determinant of norepinephrine synthesis, shows a marked increase specifically in the LC. Thus, salient behavioral symptoms disappear at the same time as a rise in norepinephrine synthesis capacity occurs in the LC, based on a well-known biochemical correlate of the habituation (i.e., induction of tyrosine hydroxylase) in that brain region. Although induction of tyrosine hydroxylase in the LC is surely only one of many neurophysiological changes occurring at the time when behavior normalizes in animals subjected to uncontrollable shock, the correspondence of these events points to the possibility that specific compensatory changes in noradrenergic systems participate in the cessation of depressive symptomatology. With respect to habituation, the chronic stress model described previously may be an extension of the uncontrollable shock model that avoids habituation and its therapeutic consequences by continually exposing animals to mild and varied stressors. In this event, the two models would be based on the same fundamental mechanisms.

A final point relevant to this model concerns the controversial issue of interpretation. The model produced by exposure of animals to uncontrollable shock is often called the *learned helplessness* model, a term derived from the original interpretation offered by Seligman and Maier (1967) and Seligman and colleagues (1971). These investigators hypothesized that the poor avoidance responding following exposure to uncontrollable shock occurred because the animals learned that they were helpless during exposure to the shock—that "nothing I do matters." This cognition was said to cause the various consequences that followed uncontrollable shock; in fact, Seligman's (1974) original hypothesis linking the consequences of uncontrollable shock to depression argued that, consistent with the "learned helplessness" explanation, depressed persons made many comments indicative of their feelings of helplessness. In contrast, Weiss (1980; Weiss et al. 1970) and others (e.g., Anisman and Bignami 1978; Anisman et al. 1991) argued that the inference of the "I am helpless" cognition to nonhuman animals was extremely difficult, if not impossible, to test, and that a simpler explanation was available—that exposure to uncontrollable shock (as opposed to shock that can be controlled) is extremely stressful, and the depression-like symptoms observed are produced by this high degree of stress. According to this view, the depression-like symptoms resulting from uncontrollable shock are stress induced.

Investigators have sought to test these alternatives. A potentially important development occurred when the last symptom listed in the second paragraph of this subsection—that uncontrollable shock causes increased errors in discrimination tasks—was reported to occur in rats. When first described, this finding was thought to demonstrate that exposure to uncontrollable shock diminished an animal's ability to make associations as would be predicted if uncontrollable shock indeed led to a "learned helplessness" cognition (Jackson et al. 1978). However, Minor and colleagues (1984, 1988) carefully analyzed the phenomenon in further studies and found that the deficits in learning ability seen in these experiments could be accounted for by increased emotionality and/or fearfulness produced by uncontrollable shock. These studies linked the effects to changes in the concentration of norepinephrine in the forebrain, thus suggesting that deficits in discrimination learning were produced by a stress-induced change (Minor et al. 1984, 1988). Despite the durability of the "learned helplessness" label for the model discussed here, there is as yet no substantial evidence that the consequences of uncontrollable shock in animals involve a "learned helplessness" cognition.

Models Using Selective Breeding (Genetic Selection)

Despite the ability of homologous models to approximate symptoms seen in depression and to respond to treatments effective in combating human clinical depression, each of the various models described here nevertheless lacks elements found in the human disorder. For example, the uncontrollable shock model, which appears to reproduce the most complete symptom profile of any animal model of depression, does not generate symptoms that last long enough to reproduce the longevity of human clinical depression; that is, certain significant depression-like features in this animal model disappear within 48–72 hours (see previous section). Attempts to correct this and other shortcomings of existing animal models have given rise to a salient development in this area—the use of selective-breeding procedures to attempt to produce populations of animals that either 1) have a higher likelihood of showing the appropriate characteristics than is the case in a normal population of animals or 2) show characteristics of the disorder to a more pronounced extent than is seen in normal populations. Thus, investigators are now attempting to incorporate into their models the clinical observation that not all individuals appear to be equally likely to become depressed in that there is often a genetic component to the expression of behavioral disorders.

It should be noted that the models described in this section often use standard procedures described earlier in this chapter for various models (e.g., uncontrollable shock, swim test); therefore, the models included here could have been described under previously defined models. However, because genetic selection procedures constitute recent, and perhaps the most promising, developments now being conducted in the generation of animal models of depression, these models are addressed here in a separate section.

Models using animals selected for response to stress. The first model considered is one in which animals were selectively bred for susceptibility and resistance to a behavioral deficit produced by uncontrollable shock (Henn et al. 1985). Henn and colleagues exposed animals to uncontrollable grid shock and then tested animals for their ability to depress a lever to escape from grid shock. In a normal population of Sprague-Dawley rats used by these investigators, only 5%–20% of the animals showed impaired escape behavior (i.e., long latencies of more than 20 seconds to escape) after receiving uncontrollable shock. Long latencies, which the investigators termed *failure to escape*, can be attributed to decreased motor activity and, hence, constitute a depression-like symptom generated in the uncontrollable shock model. These investigators repeatedly tested for, and then bred, animals that showed failure to escape after uncontrollable shock, and they also bred animals that performed the escape response quite well (i.e., showed short escape latencies). After four generations of selective breeding, the proportion of animals showing failure to escape had increased to 45% among offspring bred for this characteristic, whereas 0% of animals bred for rapid escape showed poor escape performance. The authors also reported that, among animals bred for susceptibility to poor escape performance, uncontrollable shock also reduced appetite and caused weight loss.

Effects of antidepressant treatment have been evaluated in animals selectively bred for poor escape performance. Henn et al. (1985) reported that when such animals were given placebo (or vehicle), they showed normal escape performance after 3–5 weeks of repeated escape training. In contrast, antidepressant treatment was reported to produce normal escape performance after 5 days. Effective antidepressants were reported to include TCAs, MAOIs, and atypical antidepressants, although details were not given.

These investigators have also sought to uncover brain mechanisms that might underlie the poor escape performance of animals selectively bred for this characteristic. They reported that poor performance after uncontrollable shock was accompanied by upregulation of β-adrenergic receptors in the hippocampal region and by exaggerated cyclic adenosine monophosphate (cAMP) responses to norepinephrine. This physiological characteristic of animals selectively bred for depression-related symptomatology appears consistent with a well-known action of antidepressants, which is to downregulate β receptors. However, a significant question remains concerning all of these studies (as well as a number of others by this group) in which physiological differences have been examined in animals that show escape deficits after uncontrollable shock in contrast with those that do not show such deficits (Edwards et al. 1991a, 1991b, 1992; Lachman et al. 1993; J. V. Martin et al. 1990; Papolos et al. 1993). When animals fail to escape in the lever-press test, these particular animals always receive considerably more grid shock than do animals that do not fail to escape, so that a difference observed in any physiological parameter might have resulted from these animals receiving a large amount of grid shock during the test rather than the difference having predisposed these animals to perform poorly. This issue needs to be clarified in order to determine whether the various differences reported in these studies are produced by differential amounts of shock received during testing or whether they are inherent in the animals before the shock experience and are somehow involved in mediating the poor performance.

Another model that has utilized breeding of animals that differ in their response to stress was described by Scott et al. (1996). These investigators selectively bred animals that showed large reductions in motor activity in a swim test after they were exposed to uncontrollable electric shock (called swim-test-susceptible rats) and also bred animals that were very resistant to showing any decrease in motor activity in a swim test after they were exposed to the shock (swim-test-resistant rats). Interestingly, subsequent studies found that while the swim-test-susceptible rats showed large reductions in swim-test activity after stress, the swim-test-resistant rats showed very large reductions in spontaneous ambulation in the home cage as well as reductions of food intake after uncontrollable shock, and these reductions were accompanied by the sequence of changes that Weiss and colleagues identified as the basis of stress-induced behavioral depression: depletion of norepinephrine in the LC region and LC neuronal hyperactivity. This experiment indicates that different subpopulations of rats, which can be isolated by selective breeding, will manifest depression-like symptomatology to a greater or lesser extent depending on the nature of the testing situation used.

Taking advantage of the vulnerability of swim-test-susceptible rats to showing decreased activity in the swim test, these investigators have used this line of rats in a screening technique for antidepressant treatments; these findings illustrate the promise of using selectively bred animals. Additional selective breeding of the animals described in the Scott et al. (1996) article produced swim-test-susceptible rats with heightened vulnerability such that, by the tenth generation, susceptible rats showed reduced struggling in the swim test when exposed to a much milder stressor than uncontrollable shock—they showed reduced struggling after a 30-minute exposure to a novel environment in which there was white noise of moderate intensity (95 decibels).

To assess the effects of antidepressants, these rats were exposed to the "novel environment plus noise" stressor and tested after receiving drugs or vehicle for 14 days via subcutaneous Alzet minipumps. The results, reported by West and Weiss (1995), are shown in Figure 5–9. In vehicle-treated (i.e., normal) susceptible rats, exposure to the stressor decreased struggling activity in the swim test

as expected. This stress-induced decrease in struggling activity was not seen in the animals that were given any of the antidepressant drugs. Electroconvulsive shock (administered twice, 1 week apart, with testing 1 week after the last shock) also blocked the decrease in struggling. Regarding other drugs, as pointed out earlier in this chapter, a significant limitation of the swim test as an accurate screening technique for antidepressant drugs is that a variety of nonantidepressant drugs, particularly stimulants, antihistamines, and anticholinergics, produce positive responses (i.e., false-positive results) in the swim test (see Porsolt et al. 1978, 1991). When drugs that commonly produce these false-positive results in the swim test, including the stimulant amphetamine, the antihistamine chlorpheniramine, the anticholinergic scopolamine, and the anxiolytic chlordiazepoxide, were tested in the above-described paradigm, all of these drugs failed to eliminate the stress-induced decrease in struggling behavior, and thus none

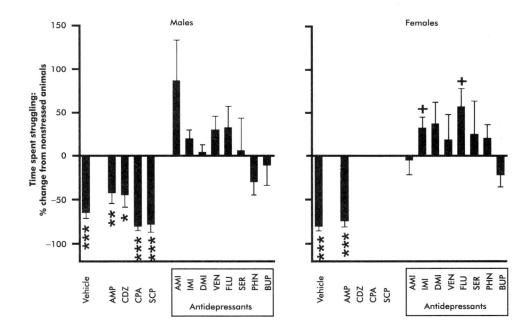

Figure 5–9. Effect of exposure to 30-minute "novel environment plus noise" stressor on the struggling behavior in a swim test of "swim-test susceptible" male and female rats after the animals have been treated chronically (for 14 days) with various drugs (via subcutaneous minipump). Groups of animals received a vehicle or one of the following antidepressant drugs: amitriptyline (AMI; 10 mg/kg/day), imipramine (IMI; 10 mg/kg/day), desipramine (DMI; 10 mg/kg/day), venlafaxine (VEN; 20 mg/kg/day), fluoxetine (FLU; 16 mg/kg/day), sertraline (SER; 25 mg/kg/day), phenelzine (PHN; 5 mg/kg/day), and bupropion (BUP; 20 mg/kg/day); or nonantidepressant drugs: amphetamine [stimulant] (AMP; 2 mg/kg/day), chlordiazepoxide [anxiolytic] (CDZ; 2 mg/kg/day), chlorpheniramine [antihistamine] (CPA; 10 mg/kg/day), and scopolamine [anticholinergic] (SCP; 2 mg/kg/day). For each drug, the struggling time of stressed rats that received that drug is shown, which is expressed as a percent of the mean struggling time of rats that received the same drug but were not exposed to the stressor condition. Percent change values show the effectiveness of antidepressant drugs to block stress-induced decreases in struggling behavior. Significant differences between struggling time of stressed animals and that of nonstressed animals are indicated as follows: for decreases, by *P < .05, **P < .01, ***P < .001; for increases, by +P < .05.

showed a positive response. Also, when three antidepressants that were effective after chronic treatment (imipramine, fluoxetine, and phenelzine) were administered acutely (i.e., for 1 day prior to the test), they were likewise ineffective. Finally, chronic treatment with antidepressant drugs had no effects on behavior of the swim-test-resistant rats, showing that detection of effective treatments requires the susceptible strain.

As an additional comment, Figure 5–9 shows that this model has been tested in both male and female rats; thus, this is the first model validated on female rats as well as male rats, which seems highly desirable in view of the high prevalence of depression in females. In summary, based on the initial data, the model described here appears to represent a selective and specific screen for potential antidepressant medications; in fact, at the present stage of testing, it is the most specific screen available for these treatments.

Models using animals selected for response to drugs.

Another model derives from rats initially selected for being highly responsive to cholinergic agonists (reviewed in Overstreet 1993). In this model, animals originally were differentiated by the extent to which various responses (i.e., decreased body temperature, body weight, drinking behavior) were affected by potentiation of acetylcholine (by use of the anticholinesterase drug diisopropylfluorophosphate). Selective breeding was then undertaken for animals that were sensitive or resistant to pharmacological manipulation of cholinergic activity.

Two lines have been developed—the Flinders sensitive line (FSL) and the Flinders resistant line (FRL). Based on the hypothesis that depressed individuals are hypersensitive to cholinergic agonists, it was suspected that the FSL rats would have an increased propensity for depressive symptomatology. Consistent with this hypothesis, the FSL rats showed reduced motor activity (measured in the open field and the swim test) relative to FRL rats, and this difference was exaggerated by exposure to uncontrollable footshock (Overstreet 1986). FSL rats also show increased REM sleep (Shiromani et al. 1988), which may relate to differences in REM shown by depressed patients.

This model also has been reported to respond to several different antidepressant drugs, including SSRIs (Overstreet 1993). Of considerable interest regarding underlying pathophysiology, studies indicate that despite the initial selection of these animals because of sensitivity to cholinergic agonists, affecting cholinergic receptors pharmacologically does not alter the reduced motor activity shown in the model, whereas intervening with drugs that affect norepinephrine (imipramine, DMI) does counter-

act this symptom (Schiller et al. 1992). Thus, the hypoactivity in the model appears related to classic catecholaminergic systems that previously had been linked to depression.

Models using other inbred lines of animals.

Overstreet and colleagues (1992) have also explored the possibility that the fawn-hooded rat might be used as a model of depression and have compared fawn-hooded animals with rats of the Flinders lines described above. The fawn-hooded rat has reduced sensitivity to serotonergic drugs and consequently has been characterized as showing deficient serotonergic neurotransmission (Aulakh et al. 1988; Wang et al. 1988). In view of the antidepressant effects of SSRIs, it has been suggested that the fawn-hooded animal may constitute a depression-susceptible rat.

Overstreet et al. (1992) found that the fawn-hooded rat showed decreased motor activity after exposure to uncontrollable shock, although the extent of this deficiency was not as great as that found in the FSL. The researchers observed that the fawn-hooded rat, as opposed to its normal progenitor (the Wistar rat), had a marked preference for alcohol. Consequently, the investigators argued that the fawn-hooded rat may also be used as an animal model for alcoholism. Antidepressant drugs have not yet been tested in this model.

Finally, in a series of brief reports, Golda and Petr proposed that the spontaneous hypertensive rat (derived from the Wistar line) could be used as an animal model of depression. They reported that exposure of the hypertensive rats to grid shock resulted in a decrease in motor activity that could be seen up to 9 weeks after exposure to the shock (Golda and Petr 1986). The stress-induced suppression of motor activity has been dissociated from changes in spontaneous exploratory activity (Golda and Petr 1987a) and threshold for reaction to shock (Golda and Petr 1987c). Golda and Petr (1987a, 1987b) reported the effects of various drugs in reversing this shock-induced decrease in motor activity; however, only one drug related to classic antidepressants (an MAOI) was tested (and showed positive results). A significant question that remains regarding this model is whether the reduction in motor activity described in these studies represents a response other than that produced by conditioned fear (i.e., freezing behavior by the rats). The brief reports that present the findings do not make clear whether motor activity was tested in a location different from the one in which the animals initially received inescapable grid shock. If the location was the same, the phenomenon being investigated (i.e., long-term suppression of motor activity) could simply reflect the expected durability of conditioned fear and consequently could be unrelated to reduced motor activity that is analogous to a depression-like symptom.

Summary Observations Regarding Homologous Models of Depression

Neither an overall summary of depression models nor an evaluation of the strengths and weaknesses of such models is undertaken here; this endeavor should be the prerogative of the reader based on the preceding material. As an aid to this process, the attributes of the various homologous models are summarized in Table 5–1, with the characteristics of each described according to the criteria of McKinney and Bunney (1969).

One additional point, an observation that arises from surveying the various animal models of depression, is offered here. One of the most useful functions of animal models is to explore potential pathophysiology underlying depression as well as neurochemical mechanisms underlying antidepressant drug action. In addressing these issues, investigators have almost always focused on single neurotransmitter systems to explain changes seen in any model. This is good science in the reductionist tradition because such theories have led to clear, specific hypotheses that could then be tested. This having been said, the message that now can be gleaned from the considerable number of relevant studies using animal models is that explaining depression-related behavior as well as the action of drugs appears to require reference to multiple transmitter systems interacting with one another.

As a specific example of how interacting neurochemical systems must be considered, one can examine what research indicates about the mechanism by which DMI exerts antidepressant action as revealed in the swim test. Studies show that DMI potently reduces immobility in the swim test through noradrenergic mechanisms. Although this conclusion might be conjectured from the dominant norepinephrine reuptake blocking action of the drug, it is further indicated by the ability of neurotoxic lesions of the LC to block completely the therapeutic (i.e., antiimmobility) effect of DMI (Plaznik et al. 1985a) as well as by the attenuation of this effect by stimulation of β-adrenergic receptors (Kitada et al. 1986) that norepinephrine presumably downregulates. In addition, Platt and Stone (1982) showed that repeated exposure to a stressor produces the therapeutic (anti-immobility) effect in the swim test, which further implicates norepinephrine because this amine system shows by far the most distinct habituational changes of the various monoamines in the brain. But despite compelling evidence that changes in norepinephrine and adrenergic receptors are involved in how DMI decreases immobility in the swim test, it is not evident how norepinephrine acting independently anywhere in the brain could accomplish this effect because this transmitter has little claim to direct action on motor systems (see discussion in Weiss et al. 1980). When we add to this the several studies showing that stimulation of dopamine and dopaminergic receptors, particularly in the nucleus accumbens, can initiate motor activity (Plaznik et al. 1985b) and, most important, that blockade of D_2 receptors will block the effects of DMI (Cervo and Samanin 1987), one is led to conclude that limbic dopamine is needed to produce DMI's therapeutic effects. On the other hand, increasing dopamine release did not counteract immobility in the swim test (Borsini et al. 1988), so that simply potentiating dopaminergic transmission in any manner is not sufficient for a therapeutic effect; in contrast, infusing norepinephrine and adrenergic receptor agonists into the nucleus accumbens did accomplish this effect (Plaznik et al. 1985b). All of this leads to the conclusion that neither norepinephrine nor dopamine alone can currently explain the action of DMI; rather, the therapeutic effect of DMI requires norepinephrine to influence limbic dopamine. Both elements appear necessary to orchestrate the antidepressant response that animals show to DMI. In conclusion, also note that when other models responsive to diverse pharmacological agents that affect different neurochemical systems are examined, there is no instance in which a manipulation restricted to only one neurotransmitter system is able to reproduce pathophysiology or therapeutic drug action (e.g., Danysz et al. 1988; Plaznik et al. 1988).

To summarize, the value of animal models is to permit, relative to examining the human patient, rapid and detailed physiological studies. A considerable body of work of this nature has been done, and these studies suggest that we will not solve the problem of treating depression without paying attention to the interaction of neurotransmitter systems. The metaphor of Parkinson's disease, with its specific pathophysiological defect related to dopamine in the basal ganglia, appears inadequate for addressing the problem of depression.

MODELS OF SCHIZOPHRENIA

The disruption of normal cognitive operations is the hallmark of schizophrenia. As such, it can be argued that schizophrenia is a uniquely human disorder that cannot be modeled in animals. At the very least, it can be asserted that the inability of animal models to incorporate elements of language that are invaluable to the expression

Table 5–1. Homologous animal models of depression

	Etiology	Symptomatology	Responsiveness to treatment	Biochemistry
Reserpine-induced depression	?	Decreased motor activity	*Responds to TCAs and MAOIs **Responds to acute drug administration; also responds to stimulants, α-adrenergic agonists, β-blockers, and antihistamines	Disruption of monoaminergic neurotransmission
5-HTP-induced depression	?	Decreased active responding (for food reward)	*Responds to various antidepressants (amitriptyline, imipramine, iprindole, mianserin, trazodone) **Responds to acute drug pretreatment; also responds to methysergide; responds negatively to fluoxetine	Augmentation of serotonergic neurotransmission
Swim-test immobility	"Behavioral despair," but more evidence points to learned inactivity and/or stress-induced inactivity	Decreased motor activity	*Responds to TCAs, MAOIs, atypical antidepressants, ECT, and REM sleep deprivation; has weak response to 5-HT reuptake inhibitors; responds to chronic drug administration **Responds to acute drug administration; also responds to stimulants, anticholinergics, and antihistamines	Decreased motor activity produced by potentiating cholinergic transmission or blocking catecholamines; decreased activity counteracted by increased catecholaminergic transmission and (in stressed animals) blocking opiate receptors
Clonidine withdrawal	?	Decreased motor activity	*Responds to chronic but not acute DMI administration	(?) Subsensitivity of α₂ receptors
Tail suspension	?	Decreased escape-related motor activity	*Responds to TCAs, MAOIs, and atypical antidepressants **Responds to acute drug administration; also responds to stimulants (D-amphetamine)	
Neonatal clomipramine	?	Decreased sexual activity, aggression, responding for brain stimulation, and REM latency; motor hyperactivity	**Responds to imipramine (decreases motor hyperactivity)	
Dorsomedial amygdala lesion in dogs	?	Decreased appetite (feeding and drinking) and grooming; lethargy and "negativism"		(?) Decreased DA in forebrain

Separation-induced depression in primates	Separation	Agitation, sleeplessness, "protest" followed by decreased activity, social activity, appetite, and play; self-clasping, hunched posture, and "sad" facial expression	*Chronic imipramine decreases some symptoms (self-clasping, vocalizations); acute imipramine has opposite effect (i.e., exacerbates "protest" reactions)	Decreased NE in CSF; i.e., (?) decreased noradrenergic activity in brain
Separation of Siberian hamsters	Separation	Decreased social interaction and exploratory activity; increase in body weight in males	*Responds (some symptoms) to repeated imipramine administration	Decreased 5-HT turnover in males
Exhaustion stress	Exposure to a highly stressful, uncontrollable situation (i.e., forced exercise)	Decreased spontaneous motor activity; loss of body weight; hypothermia; loss of normal estrous cycling	*Responds (i.e., more rapid recovery of motor activity) to imipramine	Elevation of NE in brain stem noradrenergic cell body regions in animals with reduced spontaneous activity; also decreased hypothalamic DA
Chronic, mild stress	Exposure to series of stressful, uncontrollable conditions during a 2- to 3-week period	Decreased active behavior (in open field); failure to respond to pleasurable stimuli (but possibly decreased consumption?); elevated steroids	*Responds to TCAs, MAOIs, atypical antidepressants, and ECT; does not respond to stimulants, antihistamines, or anxiolytics	Decreased mesocorticolimbic dopaminergic activity linked to deficit in responding for brain stimulation and (?) nonresponse to pleasurable stimuli
Uncontrollable shock–induced depression	Exposure to a highly stressful, uncontrollable situation	Decreased appetite (feeding and drinking); loss of body weight; decreased motor activity in a variety of tests; decreased grooming, play, competitiveness; decreased sleep marked by early-morning awakening; decreased responding for electrical brain stimulation	*Responds (deficit in active responding) to TCAs, MAOIs, atypical antidepressants, and ECT but not to antipsychotics, stimulants (amphetamine and caffeine), or antihistamines; does not respond to anxiolytics except when given during exposure to uncontrollable shock	Deficit in active behavior linked to 1) decreased NE release in the region of the LC leading to (?) increased NE release in projection regions of the LC; 2) increased concentration of β-adrenergic receptors in the hippocampal region; and 3) altered serotonergic release in forebrain (cortex and septum). Decreased responding for brain stimulation linked to deficit in mesocorticolimbic dopaminergic activity

Note. ? = relationship to depression is unclear, uncertain, or conjectural. (?) = statement that follows is an extrapolation or derivation from other results, has not been directly observed or measured, or is a theoretical hypothesis. Under "Responsiveness to treatment," effects listed after * are consistent with changes seen in human clinical depression; effects listed after ** are not consistent.

CSF = cerebrospinal fluid; DA = dopamine; DMI = desipramine; ECT = electroconvulsive therapy; 5-HT = serotonin; 5-HTP = 5-hydroxytryptophan; LC = locus coeruleus; MAOI = monoamine oxidase inhibitor; NE = norepinephrine; REM = rapid eye movement; TCA = tricyclic antidepressant.

and examination of schizophrenia creates an enormous barrier to model development. Nevertheless, the potential benefits for understanding the neurobiology and improving treatment that would accrue from the study of valid models of a disorder as prevalent and debilitating as schizophrenia have resulted in the proposal of a variety of related animal models (for reviews, see Dunn et al. 1990; Lyon 1990). Animal assay models exist for screening of antipsychotic drugs, although the newer generation of antipsychotic medications has necessitated the redevelopment of assay models. In addition, various animal models of schizophrenia that can be classified as homologous have been generated based on hypotheses that describe underlying deficits in schizophrenia in both physiological and psychological terms.

Animal Assay Models

Animal behavioral models stressing their predictive pharmacology represent by far the greatest effort expended in the development and use of animal models of schizophrenia. The confirmed efficacy of neuroleptics, both phenothiazine and nonphenothiazine drugs, in the treatment of psychosis (e.g., Cott and Kurtz 1987; Kane 1987) established the basis for describing the effects of these drugs on responses of animals and then for screening of potentially new antipsychotic medications by assessing their ability to produce similar effects. As with animal assays for depression, such models reflect pharmacological similarity of the responses that are measured to the pharmacology of schizophrenia; these responses observed in the animal may bear little or no relevance to the symptoms of schizophrenia.

Conditioned avoidance responding. Perhaps the most studied pharmacological model has been the inhibitory effects of neuroleptic antipsychotics on conditioned avoidance responding (CAR) to aversive stimuli (Cook and Catania 1964; Worms et al. 1983). In this test, animals (usually rodents) are conditioned to make an active response (e.g., locomotion in a shuttle box, pole climbing) to avoid or escape footshock. Neuroleptic administration results in a deficit in avoidance responding, with escape behavior impaired only by greater drug doses. The differential effect of neuroleptics on avoidance and escape behavior distinguishes neuroleptics from other avoidance-disrupting drugs such as barbiturates, MAOIs, and benzodiazepines that have overlapping dose-effect relations for avoidance and escape behavior (Arnt 1982). In addition to drug specificity, CAR paradigms show significant positive correlations between the potency of neuroleptic antipsy-

chotics to inhibit avoidance responding (ED_{50} values) and their clinical potency as reflected in their average administered daily dose (Kuribara and Tadokoro 1981).

However, this model has several features that limit its relationship to the pharmacology of schizophrenia. First, neuroleptic antipsychotic use to inhibit avoidance responding leads to tolerance with repeated drug administration (Fregnan and Chieli 1980; Moller Nielsen et al. 1974; Sanger 1985). Second, the atypical antipsychotic drug clozapine is not effective in the CAR test (Sanger 1985). CAR paradigms have use as a screening technique for neuroleptic antipsychotics, but they appear to be of limited value in identifying mechanistically novel antipsychotics.

Catalepsy test. The induction of catalepsy (the inability to correct an externally imposed body posture) (Sanberg et al. 1988) represents an additional animal behavioral screen for neuroleptic antipsychotics (Worms et al. 1983). However, drug-induced catalepsy is neither specific nor sensitive for antipsychotic drugs, shows tolerance with repeated neuroleptic administration, and has a poor correlation with the therapeutic potency of antipsychotics (Dunn et al. 1990). Despite having virtually no strength as an animal behavioral model of antipsychotics, catalepsy tests do have value in the study of the neuropharmacology of extrapyramidal function (Sanberg et al. 1988) and as a rapid behavioral screen for predicting the motor side effects of potential antipsychotic drugs.

Paw test. The paw test (Ellenbroek et al. 1987), a pharmacological behavioral model related to schizophrenia, reflects the effect of drug administration to rats on the spontaneous retraction of their extended forelimbs and hindlimbs (Ellenbroek and Cools 1988). Neuroleptic antipsychotics increase the time to retraction of the hindlimb and forelimb, with equipotent effects for both limbs, whereas atypical antipsychotics increase hindlimb retraction time (HRT) at lower doses than those required to increase forelimb retraction time (FRT). From these observations, it was proposed that drug effects on HRT and FRT are separate measures of the antipsychotic potential and liability for extrapyramidal side effects (EPS), respectively, of tested drugs. The paw test appears superior to previously developed screening techniques in that it distinguishes neuroleptics from atypical antipsychotics; members of the latter class show positive rather than false-negative effects in the test.

As a pharmacological model of schizophrenia, the paw test shows specificity of antipsychotic drugs and lack of anticholinergic drug effects on the HRT. Another positive aspect of the model is that drug-induced increases in the HRT do not develop tolerance with repeated administration of antipsychotic drugs (Ellenbroek and Cools 1988). Although additional tests of antipsychotic drug sensitivity and specificity are needed to establish the predictive strength of this model, the paw test appears to represent a unique behavioral screen for the distinct clinical pharmacology of neuroleptic and atypical antipsychotics (Kane et al. 1988).

Self-stimulation paradigms. Neuroleptic administration produces an inhibition of operantly conditioned lever pressing for intracranial electrical stimulation (Worms et al. 1983) and increased lever pressing for intravenous doses of cocaine (Roberts and Vickers 1984). Both paradigms appear to be models of the dopaminergic pharmacology of brain reward mechanisms, and drug effects are typically interpreted as an induction of an anhedonic state (Ettenberg et al. 1981). Intracranial electrical self-stimulation (ICSS) paradigms may also (or alternatively) model the effects of neuroleptics on motor function, as the inhibitory effects of flupenthixol on ICSS obtained when ICSS is delivered after lever pressing are not observed in rats that obtain ICSS by nose poking, a motorically simple task (Ettenberg et al. 1981). Many neuroleptic and atypical antipsychotics cause an inhibition of ICSS and an increase in cocaine self-administration (Roberts and Vickers 1984; Worms et al. 1983). A notable exception is clozapine, which actually decreases cocaine self-administration (Roberts and Vickers 1984). These authors also reported an excellent correlation (for a limited number of antipsychotics other than clozapine) between potency for increasing cocaine intake by self-administration and daily clinical dose for antipsychotic effects. Antipsychotic drug specificity and tolerance development represent unresolved issues for both self-stimulation paradigms. Collectively, these self-stimulation paradigms would seem better able to predict the negative effect of a drug on dopamine-mediated reward mechanisms than its antipsychotic potential.

Homologous Models

Homologous models aspire to a direct relevance between the behavior shown in the animal model and behavioral responses seen in schizophrenia and/or underlying processes that are thought to define schizophrenia. Homologous animal models of schizophrenia can be subdivided into three types. The first type reflects the previously made point that the signs and symptoms of schizophrenia express disturbances in cognitive operations, and these can only be represented in nonhuman animals by theoretically based constructs. Modeling of psychophysiological processes that are believed to be disturbed in schizophrenia has largely focused on deficits in information processing and stimulus filtering (Braff and Geyer 1990; Freedman et al. 1991; Nuechterlein and Dawson 1984). As might be expected, such animal models do not necessarily reproduce observable consequences (i.e., symptoms) seen in the disorder. Moreover, it has been shown that deficits in these processes and the diagnostic symptoms of schizophrenia in patients may not covary over time (Penn et al. 1993). The second type of homologous model reproduces a salient symptom seen in schizophrenia—the disturbance of social behavior. Finally, the third type of model reproduces physiological disturbances linked theoretically to the etiology of schizophrenia.

With respect to these latter models, it should be noted that progression from knowledge of etiology to development of models represents the most rational approach to establishing models but that pharmacological models of schizophrenia are an excellent example of the reverse progression (Iversen 1987). A defect of brain dopamine function (i.e., overactivity), which neuroleptic medication presumably counteracts, has been taken as an etiological fact of schizophrenia, and models then reproduce the "hyperdopaminergic" state in animals to study the consequences of this state.

Latent inhibition paradigms. The latent inhibition of conditioned responses by preexposure to a to-be-conditioned stimulus is a well-studied model of selective attention (Lubow et al. 1982). Operationally, it is proposed that the neutral presentation of a stimulus retards the subsequent learning of conditioned associations to the stimulus (Lubow 1973). Conceptually, latent inhibition paradigms are models of the ability to categorize a stimulus accurately based on its changing salience. The phenomenon of latent inhibition attempts to reproduce attentional deficits in schizophrenia that are expressed as the use of inefficient and inflexible processing strategies to filter stimuli. Latent inhibition also contains parallels with nonattentional constructs of schizophrenia such as deficits in the control of behavior by context (Lubow 1989) and the influence of experience on the perception of current events (Hemsley 1987).

The empirical strength of latent inhibition paradigms as models of brain functions affected by schizophrenia is derived from animal behavioral pharmacology and human behavioral studies. Initial interest in latent inhibition paradigms stemmed from their being affected by amphetamine (Solomon et al. 1981; Weiner et al. 1984), a drug thought to induce psychosis (see subsection, "Chronic Amphetamine Intoxication," later in this chapter). More recent studies of latent inhibition have emphasized the response of these paradigms to antipsychotic drugs (Christison et al. 1988; Dunn et al. 1993; Feldon and Weiner 1991; Weiner and Feldon 1987). For example, administering haloperidol to rats facilitates the latent inhibition of conditioned response suppression by stimulus preexposure (Christison et al. 1988; Weiner and Feldon 1987). The facilitation of latent inhibition by haloperidol has a potency similar to the clinical potency of haloperidol, is self-limiting at higher doses, and does not lead to tolerance with repeated drug administration (Dunn et al. 1993). Haloperidol administration also enhances latent inhibition in nonschizophrenic human subjects (Williams et al. 1996). Also, latent inhibition is enhanced by structurally diverse neuroleptic antipsychotics (see Figure 5–10). Of interest is the observation that latent inhibition appears to be markedly less sensitive to the administration of atypical antipsychotic drugs. Our group has consistently noted a lack of effect or even decreased latent inhibition following the administration of clozapine or olanzapine to inbred rat strains. The collective effects of clozapine (Moran et al. 1996; Weiner et al. 1996, 1997), sertindole (Weiner et al. 1994), and remoxipride (Trimble et al. 1997) indicate an enhancement of only small latent inhibition effects (resulting from small numbers of stimulus preexposures or increased numbers of conditioned stimulus–unconditioned stimulus associations) and poor dose-response relationships for drug-induced facilitation of latent inhibition (Gosselin et al. 1996). Drug effects on latent inhibition were, however, consistently enhanced when defined against an amphetamine-disrupted latent inhibition baseline. Whether this enhancement reflects simply a lesson in dopamine receptor pharmacology or an interesting dependence of drug effects on deficit states of latent inhibition remains to be seen.

Significantly, the effects of neuroleptic and atypical antipsychotics on latent inhibition, although distinct, are confined to stimulus preexposure effects on conditioned suppression. Conditioned responses in the absence of stimulus preexposures were unaffected by drug administration (Dunn et al. 1993). This pattern of effect is not mimicked by anxiolytics, sedative-hypnotics, antidepressants, a nonantipsychotic phenothiazine, or morphine (Dunn et al. 1993). A challenge for this model will be to define conditions (e.g., a deficit in latent inhibition) that produce a convergence for all efficacious antipsychotic drugs on a common behavioral effect or an appreciation of the mechanisms (e.g., serotonin-dopamine actions) underlying the distinct effects on latent inhibition of neuro-

leptic compared with atypical antipsychotics as a key to understanding their distinct clinical pharmacology (Kane et al. 1988).

Human behavioral studies lend further support to latent inhibition phenomena as animal models of symptoms or psychopathological constructs of schizophrenia. Baruch and colleagues (1988a) used a variation of latent inhibition paradigms used in animals to show that latent inhibition of a learned stimulus association by stimulus preexposure was absent in patients with acute schizophrenia; control subjects without schizophrenia and a group of subjects with chronic schizophrenia had clear latent inhibition. These results led to the proposal that latent inhibition paradigms represent a model of the positive symptoms and causal mechanisms (i.e., hyperdopaminergic states) of acute but not chronic schizophrenia (Baruch et al. 1988a). Note that all three groups readily learned the stimulus association in the absence of stimulus preexposure. The further evidence that acutely ill schizophrenic patients (N. S. Gray et al. 1995; Guterman et al. 1996; but see Swerdlow et al. 1996) and schizotypal individuals (De la Casa and Ruiz 1993) have significantly impaired performance compared with healthy subjects in a latent inhibition paradigm indicates that latent inhibition tasks also fulfill elements of construct validity as an animal behavioral model of specific attentional processes impaired in schizophrenia. A plausible assumption based on the animal pharmacology of latent inhibition is that differences in latent inhibition between acute and chronically ill patients are attributable to a stabilizing effect of antipsychotic medication. However, the observation of comparable latent inhibition in neuroleptic-naive patients with schizophrenia and healthy volunteers (N. S. Gray et al. 1995) suggests that latent inhibition returns over time because of the progression of the illness rather than medication effects.

Dopamine receptors negatively modulate latent inhibition in both animal and human paradigms. The administration of apomorphine, amphetamine, and D_1 or D_2/D_3 dopamine receptor agonists inhibits latent inhibition in rats in a dose-dependent manner (Dunn et al. 1991), and amphetamine administration inhibits latent inhibition in nonschizophrenic human subjects (N. S. Gray et al. 1992; Thornton et al. 1996). Latent inhibition paradigms appear to be promising models of brain functions sensitive to schizophrenia, antipsychotic drugs, and dopamine receptor activation.

Blocking paradigms.   Blocking paradigms, like latent inhibition tasks, represent models of selective attention and the influence of context and experience on current perception and learning (J. A. Gray et al. 1991). Blocking

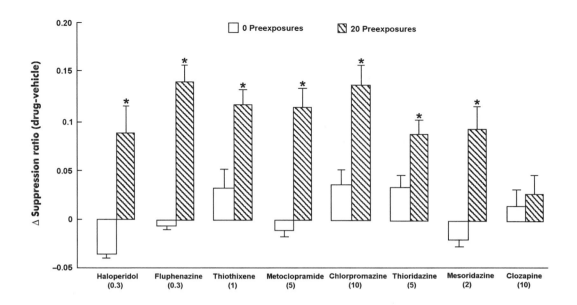

Figure 5–10. Effect of structurally diverse neuroleptic antipsychotics and clozapine on the latent inhibition (LI) of conditioned response suppression by 20 stimulus preexposures. (See Dunn et al. 1993 for details of the LI paradigm.) Preexposure to the to-be-conditioned stimulus (house light) weakens its ability to serve as a conditioned stimulus (CS) in classical conditioning with the unconditioned stimulus (footshock), so that stimulus-preexposed animals have a decreased conditioned response (suppression of spout licking) to the CS relative to nonpreexposed subjects. The amount of suppression that occurs is expressed as a ratio that is calculated by A/A + B, where A represents the time to complete licks 81–90 prior to the onset of the CS and B represents the time to complete licks 91–100 after the onset of the CS. Results represent the difference (delta, Δ) in ratio that was measured in drug-treated groups relative to control animals that were given vehicle (i.e., vehicle-treated ratio subtracted from drug-treated ratio). All neuroleptic antipsychotics tested enhanced the LI effect, as reflected in a significantly greater delta suppression ratio. Numbers in parentheses are the mg/kg dose administered daily for 7 consecutive days before stimulus preexposures. An asterisk (*) denotes statistical significance ($P < .05$) compared with delta suppression ratios calculated in the absence of stimulus preexposure.

tasks also involve a stimulus preexposure, conditioning, and behavioral testing component (Kamin 1969). Stimulus preexposure, unlike that in latent inhibition paradigms, involves the conditioned association of the stimulus (CS-A) with an unconditioned stimulus. In conditioning, a compound stimulus (CS-A plus CS-B) is presented, followed by the same unconditioned stimulus. In testing, the conditioned response to CS-B is measured; preexposure (prior association of CS-A and the unconditioned stimulus) weakens (or blocks) the response to CS-B. As models of the differential processing of stimuli of different relevance, blocking and latent inhibition tasks differ in the simultaneous presentation of different stimuli (blocking) compared with sequential processing of the same stimulus (latent inhibition).

Blocking tasks were used initially as models of amphetamine-induced or -exacerbated psychosis (Crider et al. 1982). The negative effect of amphetamine on the blocking effect was antagonized by haloperidol adminis-

tration (Crider et al. 1982). However, the ability of blocking tasks to detect a range of antipsychotic drugs has not yet been tested. Testing of humans indicates the presence of a deficit in the stimulus blocking effect in schizophrenia (Jones et al. 1992). Blocking of conditioned associations to CS-B by CS-A does not occur in acutely ill schizophrenic patients; a clear blocking effect is seen in nonschizophrenic control subjects and patients with anxiety disorder or chronic schizophrenia. The validation of blocking behavior as an animal model (distinct from latent inhibition) of brain functions relevant to schizophrenia must await the study of the sensitivity, specificity, and potency of the effects of antipsychotic drugs and the assessment of tolerance development with repeated drug administration.

Prepulse inhibition of the startle reflex. An additional animal model of the information processing/stimulus filtering deficits of schizophrenia is represented by the inhibition of the startle reaction to an acoustic or tactile stimulus when the startling stimulus is preceded by a weak prestimulus (hence, prepulse inhibition, or PPI) (Braff et al. 1978). The PPI effect is often proposed to represent an animal behavior model of sensorimotor gating functions. Induced deficits in PPI (see below) are proposed to model a psychopathological construct of schizophrenia—impaired sensorimotor gating. Based on this contention, PPI has been used to probe the neural and pharmacological substrates of schizophrenia (Braff and Geyer 1990; Swerdlow et al. 1986, 1990, 1994). Parallels between rats and humans in the graded response and threshold for PPI defined by a range of prepulse intensities and in the startle stimuli (Swerdlow et al. 1994) support the contention that similar operations underlie PPI in both species. Unlike latent inhibition and blocking paradigms, PPI does not involve associative learning tasks. Like latent inhibition and blocking paradigms, PPI (of an eye blink reflex) is absent or dramatically reduced in patients with schizophrenia compared with nonschizophrenic control subjects (Braff and Geyer 1990; Braff et al. 1978, 1992). Like latent inhibition (Baruch et al. 1988b; De la Casa and Ruiz 1993), PPI is diminished in psychosis-prone individuals (Simmons 1990). However, deficits in PPI are not unique to schizophrenia but are also observed in patients with Huntington's disease or obsessive-compulsive disorder (Swerdlow et al. 1993, 1994).

As behavioral models of stimulus filtering functions that are disrupted by schizophrenia, PPI paradigms differ from latent inhibition paradigms with respect to modulation by dopamine receptors and effects of antipsychotic drugs, neural substrates, and early life stressors. PPI is inhibited by the administration of D_2 but not D_1 receptor agonists, although D_1 receptor agonists potentiate the disruptive effects of D_2 receptor activation on PPI (Peng et al. 1990). In contrast, the latent inhibition of conditioned response suppression by stimulus preexposure is inhibited by the activation of either D_1 or D_2/D_3 dopamine receptors in the absence of apparent interactive effects between receptor subtypes (C. D. Kilts, L. Dunn, R. J. Scibilia, unpublished data, 1996). The specific dopamine projections involved in modulating PPI and latent inhibition also appear to differ. The selective activation of dopamine receptors in the nucleus accumbens (Swerdlow et al. 1990, 1991) or their antagonism in the medial prefrontal cortex (Ellenbroek et al. 1996) inhibits PPI of the startle reflex but does not affect latent inhibition (Ellenbroek et al. 1996; Killcross and Robbins 1993). Finally, early social isolation in rats inhibited PPI without disrupting latent inhibition (Wilkinson et al. 1994). These differences suggest that latent inhibition and PPI of the startle reflex represent distinct aspects of stimulus filtering with different neural

mechanisms. These paradigms would therefore have distinct strengths and applications as models of the psychobiological "symptom" of information processing deficits in schizophrenia.

Differences between latent inhibition and PPI are also seen in response to antipsychotic drugs. Latent inhibition in normally functioning animals is significantly affected by antipsychotic drug administration; neuroleptic antipsychotics enhance the negative effect of stimulus preexposure on associative learning. In contrast, sensorimotor gating measured by PPI is not consistently affected by the administration of antipsychotic drugs to normally functioning animals (Johansson et al. 1995; Swerdlow et al. 1994). Antipsychotic drugs do antagonize decreases in PPI of the startle reflex produced by apomorphine (Swerdlow and Geyer 1993; Swerdlow et al. 1991, 1994) or isolation rearing (Geyer et al. 1993). That a deficit in PPI is needed to identify an effect of antipsychotic drugs may represent a source of strength for the PPI model because the substrates of drug action in schizophrenia are those brain functions that are degraded by the genetic and psychosocial factors unique to this disorder. In other words, a "defect state" may be a requirement of valid animal models of antipsychotic drug effects in schizophrenia. Interestingly, the disruptive effects of phencyclidine are opposed by the administration of atypical (Bakshi and Geyer 1995; Swerdlow et al. 1996) but not typical (Swerdlow et al. 1996) antipsychotic drugs. These observations extend the use of deficits in PPI to explore the distinct processes underlying the differences between typical and atypical antipsychotics in the treatment of schizophrenia.

The contention that antipsychotic drug effects on induced deficits in PPI in animals represent a model of the pharmacology of sensorimotor gating abnormalities in schizophrenia (Swerdlow et al. 1991, 1994) is weakened by the apparently negligible effect of antipsychotic medication on PPI deficits in schizophrenic patients (Braff and Geyer 1990). This inconsistency highlights a means for validating animal models—the testing of predictions from the model in human behavioral studies. Are the modeled behaviors (e.g., PPI, latent inhibition) affected differently in distinct symptom subtypes of schizophrenia, by different classes of antipsychotic drugs in a within-subject crossover design, or by the patients' sex? The attempt to correlate results of clinical behavioral research with animal behavioral models represents both the best effort in model testing and the ultimate goal of animal modeling—to learn about the clinical condition. The study of PPI phenomena in humans may reveal highly useful information about the neurobiology of stimulus-processing deficits in schizophrenia but not about the mode of action of antipsychotic drugs. Perhaps Carlton's (1978) assessment of the restricted relevance of animal behavioral models is partly correct in that a *complete* relation between an animal model and schizophrenia is not required and places too much strain on the model.

Rodent interaction. The degradation of social skills in schizophrenia is a hallmark of this disorder (Mueser et al. 1991) and the distinguishing feature of subgroups of schizophrenia (Carpenter et al. 1988; Kibel et al. 1993). Deterioration of social skills is associated with the chronic phase of schizophrenia and its deficit form (Carpenter et al. 1988) or negative syndrome (Kibel et al. 1993). A modification of the rat social interaction paradigm, developed and tested as an animal behavioral model of anxiolytic drug activity (Gardner and Guy 1984), has been proposed as an animal model of the effects of antipsychotic drugs on social behaviors affected by schizophrenia (Corbett et al. 1993).

Active, nonaggressive behavioral interactions between pairs of familiar or unfamiliar rats were timed following the acute administration of antipsychotic or nonantipsychotic drugs. Antipsychotic drug administration significantly altered social interaction behaviors between unfamiliar, but not familiar, pairs compared with vehicle-injected control pairs; neuroleptic antipsychotics decreased social interaction, whereas atypical antipsychotics increased social interaction. As a comparison, diazepam administration enhanced social interaction in both familiar and unfamiliar pairs of rats. Social interaction paradigms thus have possible use as behavioral screens for drugs of potential value in the treatment of the deficits in social skills observed in schizophrenia. Several considerations, however, support a cautious use of these models. The effectiveness of clozapine in this test may be explained in part by the anxiolytic properties of this drug (Spealman et al. 1982). Also, the negative influence of neuroleptic antipsychotics on social interaction is difficult to reconcile with their beneficial (i.e., ameliorative) effects on negative symptoms (Labarca et al. 1993; Meltzer et al. 1986).

A critical test of the model strength of social interaction to the field of schizophrenia research will be the determination of antipsychotic drug effects after chronic drug administration and on disrupted social interaction behavior. The putative psychotomimetics phencyclidine and amphetamine decrease social interactions in humans and animals. In rats, drug effects reflect a voluntary avoidance of social interactions (Kuppinger et al. 1996). The phencyclidine-induced stereotyped behaviors and social isolation have been proposed as behavioral models of the positive and negative symptoms, respectively, of schizo-

phrenia (Sams-Dodd 1996). The repeated daily administration (21 days) of clozapine (Sams-Dodd 1996) or of related atypical antipsychotic drugs (Sams-Dodd 1997) to rats inhibited phencyclidine-induced social isolation and stereotyped behaviors. Further assessment of the specificity of antipsychotic drug effects on phencyclidine-induced behaviors is needed to establish this paradigm as a valid model of the clinical pharmacology of schizophrenia.

Social behavior in monkeys. An obvious limitation of the use of social interaction models is the conceptual distance between interactive behavior in rodent pairs and deficits in social skills and social withdrawal in schizophrenic patients in complex human social contexts. These deficiencies have been addressed by an ethological analysis of monkeys in the context of their complex, well-organized social structure (Ellenbroek 1991). Observed social interactions are compiled into a behavioral ethogram. Monkeys show a wide and rich repertoire of social behaviors; as a result, they approximate the social setting of humans better than do rodents. For instance, drug effects on the interactive behavior of the alpha and beta males and the females of a social group can be described and changes analyzed in terms of group social structure or individual social bonds (Ellenbroek et al. 1989). Monkey social behavior in models of schizophrenia has largely been studied in conjunction with amphetamine-induced social isolation (Arnett et al. 1989; Ellenbroek et al. 1989; Miczek and Yoshimura 1982), which is thought to be analogous to social withdrawal symptoms seen in the negative (or deficit) forms of schizophrenia.

Amphetamine administration to monkeys markedly reduces the duration and number of both active and passive social behaviors, with a resulting increase in spatial distance between socially living monkeys (Arnett et al. 1989; Ellenbroek 1991; Ellenbroek et al. 1989). Amphetamine-induced social isolation is observed following either chronic or acute drug administration, and different social behaviors are differentially affected. For instance, acute amphetamine administration 1) decreased behavioral items of the ethogram, such as grooming and huddling; 2) had no significant effect on looking at other animals; and 3) increased submissive behaviors (Ellenbroek et al. 1989; Miczek and Yoshimura 1982). The social withdrawal observed in monkeys following amphetamine administration and the complex pattern (compared with that of rodents) of drug-induced stereotyped behaviors have been proposed as models of both negative and positive symptoms, respectively, of schizophrenia in a single paradigm (Ellenbroek 1991). The amphetamine-induced social isolation in monkeys has characteristics of a deficient ability to interpret communicative signals and/or a hyperdopaminergic state.

The validity of this model has not been established beyond a shared lack of effect of noradrenergic and opiate receptor antagonists, benzodiazepines, and neuroleptic antipsychotics on deficits in social function in schizophrenia and this animal behavioral model (Ellenbroek 1991). However, the assertion that neuroleptics lack effect is dubious for both the clinical symptoms and the animal behaviors. The needed test of efficacy for the atypical antipsychotics on amphetamine-induced social isolation in monkeys apparently has not been conducted. The fact that this model is produced by a dopaminomimetic drug limits its application as a screen for novel antipsychotics and as a tool for studying the mechanism of schizophrenia. However, this animal model is unique in reproducing the degraded complex social behaviors of the negative, or deficit, form of schizophrenia. A more systematic analysis of the monkey behaviors associated with social withdrawal induced by other nonpharmacological means, and a more thorough analysis of the behavioral pharmacology of antipsychotic drugs, would seem worthwhile in the development and testing of such a model.

Chronic amphetamine intoxication.   Animal behavioral models based on an induced hyperdopaminergic state derive from the long-held belief in the involvement of the neurotransmitter dopamine in the neurochemical pathology of schizophrenia (Carlson 1988; Davis et al. 1991). Indirect evidence for a hyperactivity of dopamine neurons innervating the subcortical limbic system in schizophrenia is inferred from the behavioral symptoms of patients, exacerbation of symptoms by dopaminomimetics (Angrist et al. 1985; Davidson et al. 1987), and therapeutic response of symptoms to antidopaminergic treatment (Creese et al. 1976). More recent reformulations of the dopamine hypothesis of schizophrenia include postulating a hypoactivity of dopamine neurons innervating the prefrontal cortex as the neural basis of the negative/deficit symptom complex in schizophrenia (Davis et al. 1991). The behavioral effects of the drug-induced activation of brain dopamine receptors have long been proposed as an animal model of psychotic symptoms (Ellinwood and Kilbey 1977; Ellinwood et al. 1972; Ellison et al. 1978).

Chronic amphetamine intoxication models in cats and monkeys have focused on elicited behaviors that are interpreted as parallels of motor and cognitive symptoms of schizophrenia (Ellinwood and Kilbey 1977; Nielsen et al. 1983). Motor disturbances observed in the end stage of chronic amphetamine administration in animals include

restless shifting and awkward postures; behavioral effects include fragmented, perseverative, or abortive behaviors with situationally irrelevant responses and reduced or inappropriate social behaviors. Nielsen and associates (1983) also described apparent amphetamine-induced hallucinatory behavior consisting of behavioral sequences oriented toward nonexistent stimuli in monkeys. Not surprisingly, treatment with neuroleptic antipsychotics resulted in a rapid cessation of these effects of chronic amphetamine administration. Chronic amphetamine intoxication models thus produce animal behavioral analogues of even the most human of the positive and negative symptoms of schizophrenia. Historically, these models have added considerable momentum to the purported role of dopamine in the neurochemical pathology of schizophrenia. However, a caution in interpreting these models is worth noting because effects of amphetamine and other dopaminomimetics may reflect actions on neural mechanisms related to treatment but not to etiology. The use of in vivo functional brain imaging techniques (e.g., positron-emission tomography) may demonstrate parallels between the functional neuroanatomy of schizophrenia (Liddle et al. 1992; Tamminga et al. 1992) and that of chronic amphetamine intoxication and thus may strengthen the model beyond its behavioral parallels.

Hippocampal damage.   Animal models of schizophrenia involving experimentally induced damage of the hippocampus have gained added significance with the confirmation that changes in the volume of the hippocampus (and amygdala) currently represent the most consistently observed component of the neuropathology of schizophrenia (Bogerts et al. 1993; Shenton et al. 1992). Bilateral lesions of the hippocampus in animals affect specific behaviors (e.g., attention, arousal, habituation), cognitive operations (e.g., learning, memory), and physiological reactions (e.g., skin conductance) that parallel a constellation of deficits associated with schizophrenia (Schmajuk 1987). Behavioral deficits following hippocampal lesioning can be reversed by administration of clinically efficacious antipsychotics (Schmajuk 1987).

More recent formulations of the hippocampal lesion model have shown that it reproduces diverse phenomenological aspects of schizophrenia. Bilateral lesions of the ventral hippocampus of young adult (42-day-old) rats produced by intracerebral microinjection of the excitatory amino acid neurotoxin ibotenic acid resulted in changes in postoperative behavior as well as in pharmacological and biochemical estimates of brain dopamine systems (Lipska et al. 1992). Specifically, hippocampal damage increased spontaneous exploratory behavior and amphetamine-induced locomotion and induced an increase in the estimated activity of dopamine neurons innervating the limbic (ventral) striatum and a decrease in the activity of dopamine neurons of the medial prefrontal cortex. Hippocampal damage in these studies was not associated with an altered behavioral responsivity to environmental stimuli (i.e., stressors).

The hippocampal damage paradigm has also been strengthened by the documentation of developmentally delayed consequences. Schizophrenia is a disorder with a defined developmental latency. The index episode typically occurs at postpubertal ages in late adolescence or early adulthood (Kendler et al. 1987). Moreover, the neuroanatomical alterations associated with schizophrenia (e.g., decreased volume of the amygdaloid-hippocampal complexes of the temporal lobes) are thought to represent early developmental pathology that remains functionally quiescent until adolescence or adulthood (Crow 1990; Weinberger 1987). In the animal model described here, ibotenic acid–induced hippocampal damage of rats at postnatal day 7 resulted in a delayed emergence of an enhanced (relative to sham-operated controls) locomotor response to a novel environment, an intraperitoneal injection of saline or amphetamine, or a swim stressor (Lipska et al. 1993). Behavioral effects of lesions were noted at postpubertal postnatal day 56, but not prepubertal day 35, following lesioning on postnatal day 7. Behavioral effects were interpreted as being suggestive of an enhanced response of mesolimbic dopamine neurons to stressful environmental and pharmacological stimuli. The neonatal hippocampal damage model thus possesses analogues of the postpubertal onset and stress vulnerability of schizophrenia and of the neurochemical construct of limbic dopamine dysregulation (Lipska et al. 1993). Neonatal hippocampal damage is also associated with postpubertal deficits in sensorimotor gating. An increased sensitivity to the disruptive effects of apomorphine on PPI (Swerdlow et al. 1995) and reduced basal PPI (Lipska et al. 1995) were observed in adults after neonatal ventral hippocampal lesions.

Note that, despite the similarities described here, the observed changes in hippocampal volume (Bogerts et al. 1993; Shenton et al. 1992) or cytoarchitecture (Conrad et al. 1991) in adult schizophrenic patients represent subtle, asymmetric changes, in contrast to the robust loss of neuropil, gliosis, and cavitation observed in the hippocampus of lesioned animals. Also, changes in neuroanatomy associated with schizophrenia are not confined to the hippocampal formation. Regardless, the neonatal hippocampal damage model of the brain structural and functional deficits associated with schizophrenia increasingly gains support

through its behavioral, neurochemical, and developmental parallels to schizophrenia.

High ambient pressure.   The psychotogenic effects of exposure to high ambient pressure (Stoudemire et al. 1984) have led to the conclusion that high-pressure-induced changes in neurotransmission and behavior represent a method by which schizophreniform psychosis can be produced (Abraini et al. 1993). Deep-sea divers experiencing very high pressure show not only neurological and other psychiatric symptoms but also neuroleptic-reversible delusions, hallucinations, paranoid thoughts, and agitation (Stoudemire et al. 1984). Rats exposed to environments of high ambient pressure manifest neuroleptic-reversible increases in spontaneous locomotor activity and correlated increases in the dopamine content of the nucleus accumbens and caudate putamen (Abraini et al. 1993). The high-pressure-induced model has its strength in parallels with a long-standing behavioral/neurochemical construct of schizophrenia—the hypothetical overactivity of mesolimbic dopamine neurons. An additional strength of the model is that the inducing condition (i.e., high pressure) does not involve a presumption of underlying causes of schizophrenia and thus enables studies of the mechanistic bases and pharmacology of schizophrenia's consequences in an attempt to understand these aspects of psychotic disorders. An obvious weakness of the model is its lack of relevance to inducing conditions of schizophrenia.

Genetic Models

Genetic animal models of human disorders represent powerful approaches to the study of their determinants. The study of the genotypic and phenotypic correlates of experimentally induced alterations in gene expression provides valuable clues as to the biological bases of specific behavior and of behavioral disorders. Such alterations are most frequently induced by selective breeding for a behavioral phenotype. This approach is essentially the same as that used to breed animals for desirable agricultural or esthetic characteristics. Typically, lines of mice or rats are generated by systematically mating pairs of animals with an extreme of the selection phenotype. The genetic consequence of artificial selection is an increase in the gene frequencies of alleles that affect the behavioral trait in either a positive way or a negative way when lines are also bred for the absence of the trait. If successful, the relevant alleles will become homozygously fixed in each selected line, and the frequency of alleles at all trait-irrelevant genes will theoretically be unaffected by selective breeding. The subsequent understanding of the gene products (e.g., behavior, neurotransmitters, receptors) of the affected alleles furnishes novel clues as to the biological determinants of the selected behavior. Interested readers are referred to excellent reviews from Crabbe et al. (1990) and Crabbe and Li (1995) of the methods of selective breeding in deriving animal behavioral models.

An additional valid approach in genetic animal models research is the study of existing inbred strains of animals. After many generations of brother-sister matings, all members of the resulting inbred strain are genetically identical. More than 100 inbred rat and mouse strains are currently available. The comparison of the varying expression of a behavioral trait in different inbred strains helps to define its genetic determinant and, by defining strain differences in neurotransmission, its biological determinants. The study of the consequences of the overexpression or deletion of specific gene sequences in transgenic mice and the study of the results of movement of genes responsible for a trait to a strain that does not express the trait in generating (by backcrossing) a congenic line are increasingly used approaches to the identification of the neurobiology of behavior.

Even those animal models of schizophrenia that are arguably best able to reproduce symptoms or psychophysiological constructs of schizophrenia (e.g., latent inhibition, blocking, PPI) have significant shortcomings. An example is the apomorphine-induced deficit in PPI of the startle reflex, in which an induced behavioral deficit is a prerequisite for demonstrating antipsychotic drug effects (Swerdlow et al. 1994). This manipulation produces a short-lived behavioral deficit that differs from the enduring deficiencies that characterize schizophrenia. As with animal models of depression, behavioral genetic techniques offer a promising approach by which models may be improved. However, the technique has not yet been used extensively.

That behavioral paradigms, such as PPI, have genotypic determinants is suggested by a comparison of inbred strains. Inbred rat strains differed in acoustic startle response amplitude (Acri et al. 1995), sensitivity of PPI to the prepulse stimulus (Varty and Higgins 1994), and response of startle amplitude and PPI to apomorphine and phencyclidine, respectively (Varty and Higgins 1994). These strain differences support the use of selective breeding techniques to evolve genetic animal models of enduring deficits in PPI and of the pharmacology and neurobiology of PPI disruptions associated with schizophrenia. Such selection studies have not yet been initiated for the PPI phenotype. Comparative studies of inbred rat strains also support a critical role for genetic factors in defining the phenotypic response in the previously discussed neonatal

hippocampal damage model of schizophrenia. The spontaneous and amphetamine-induced locomotor response to early induced hippocampal damage was dramatically dependent on the specific rat strain examined (Lipska and Weinberger 1995). A significant interaction between strain and extent of hippocampal damage was shown: Lewis rats had no significant locomotor effect of hippocampal damage, and Fischer 344 rats had hyperlocomotion in response to small ventral hippocampal lesions; large, but not small, hippocampal lesions affected locomotor responses in Sprague-Dawley rats.

One area of schizophrenia research in which genetic selection techniques have been applied is drug response. As explained earlier in this chapter, drug-produced interference with CAR has been used as a screening technique for antipsychotic medication. Genetically distinct inbred strains of mice differ greatly in the effect of neuroleptic antipsychotics on CAR (Fuller 1970) and induction of catalepsy (Fink et al. 1982), and these observations constituted the impetus for developing pharmacogenetic models of response to neuroleptic antipsychotics. A significant proportion (7%–30%) of newly admitted patients with schizophrenia have little or no therapeutic response to neuroleptic therapy (Kane et al. 1988; Kolakowska et al. 1985), whereas a smaller subgroup of patients have a rapid and robust response to neuroleptic antipsychotics (Garver et al. 1984). Selective breeding programs have been used to develop genetic animal models of neuroleptic response and nonresponse in gerbils (Upchurch and Schallert 1983) and in mice (Hitzemann et al. 1991). Use of the cataleptic response to haloperidol administration as the selected behavior produces a significant bidirectional response to selection in mice. By the seventh generation, the haloperidol-nonresponsive line had negligible catalepsy after haloperidol (2 mg/kg) administration, whereas the haloperidol-responsive line had a robust cataleptic response of long duration to 1 mg/kg of haloperidol (Hitzemann et al. 1991). Behavioral differences between lines in drug response to haloperidol were not attributable to differences in the pharmacokinetics of haloperidol. The response to selection generalized to D_2 dopamine receptor antagonists other than haloperidol, suggesting that alterations in brain D_2 receptor density or function may underlie the difference in response. Further study of these selected lines and of inbred mouse strains showed the power of genetic models to explore the mechanisms of neuroleptic drug response and nonresponse. An analysis of genetic and phenotypic correlations for pairs of traits found modest and complex associations between haloperidol response and the number of striatal cholinergic neurons (Dains et al. 1996).

In addition, note that selective breeding techniques for good and poor CAR learning have long been known to result in the generation of distinct lines of rats (Bignami 1965; Brush 1991; Brush et al. 1979). The three major strains of rats resulting from successful bidirectional selection for CAR acquisition are the Roman, Syracuse, and Australian High and Low Avoidance strains (Brush 1991). Although these breeding programs have convincingly demonstrated the hereditary influences on CAR, the effect of genetic selection on the response of CAR to antipsychotic drug administration has not been systematically examined. Finally, the use of selective breeding to induce genetic selection pressure on the latent inhibition phenotype in N/Nih rats has provided initial support for the heritability of stimulus-filtering ability and for the differential effects of antipsychotic drugs on disrupted versus intact stimulus filtering ability (C. D. Kilts, unpublished data, November 1997).

Summary Observations Regarding Models of Schizophrenia

The signs and symptoms of schizophrenia reflect cognitive disturbances that have no prima facie duplication in animal behavior. As such, animal behavioral models of schizophrenia have sought validation in pharmacological parallels as well as in parallels with psychophysiological and neurochemical constructs of schizophrenia. The utility of such models in elucidating the neurobiology of schizophrenia and as targets for the development of mechanistically novel antipsychotics with improved efficacy and decreased side effects is dependent on an increased number of facts of schizophrenia that may be modeled. Noninvasive in vivo imaging techniques will play a major role in the discovery of the neurobiological facts of schizophrenia. The application of improved techniques of magnetic resonance imaging has identified a neuropathology of schizophrenia (Breier et al. 1992; Shenton et al. 1992) that suggests a disturbance in neocortical-limbic communication. Similarly, the application of functional brain imaging techniques to schizophrenia has found that schizophrenia has a functional neuroanatomy represented by alterations in functional neural circuits (Liddle et al. 1992; Tamminga et al. 1992). Recent positron-emission tomography evidence of selective decreases in D_1 dopamine receptors in the frontal cortex of patients with schizophrenia (Okubo et al. 1997) highlights the evolving picture of the in vivo neurochemistry of schizophrenia. In solving the mysteries of schizophrenia, these findings provide important clues as to the "what," "where," and "how" of the effects of schizophrenia on the brain and offer leads in defining why such effects occur and how they affect cognitive processes. These findings also furnish needed facts about the neurobiology of schizophrenia for use as targets for animal modeling and model validation.

Finally, future animal behavioral models related to schizophrenia should manifest "appropriate" deficits in psychophysiology before these models are used to probe the neurochemistry, neuroanatomy, and pharmacology of schizophrenia. The reverse order has typically been pursued. In particular, researchers should recognize that the psychopharmacology of schizophrenia is often unique, because drugs interact with the abnormalities in neurochemistry and neuroanatomy that underlie the disorder. The dependency of pharmacology on a "defect state" for accurate assessment suggests that the search for novel treatments of schizophrenia by using animal models needs to proceed from the development of valid symptom models.

REFERENCES

Abel EL: Alarm substance emitted by rats in the forced-swim test is a low volatile pheromone. Physiol Behav 50:723–727, 1991

Abraini JH, Ansseau M, Fechati T: Pressure-induced disorders in neurotransmission and spontaneous behavior in rats: an animal model of psychosis. Biol Psychiatry 34:622–629, 1993

Abramson LY, Seligman MEP: Modeling psychopathology in the laboratory: history and rationale, in Psychopathology: Experimental Models. Edited by Maser JD, Seligman MEP. San Francisco, CA, WH Freeman, 1977, pp 1–26

Acri JB, Brown KJ, Saah MI, et al: Strain and age differences in acoustic startle responses and effects of nicotine in rats. Pharmacol Biochem Behav 50:191–198, 1995

American Psychiatric Association: Diagnostic and Statistical Manual of Mental Disorders, 3rd Edition. Washington, DC, American Psychiatric Association, 1980

American Psychiatric Association: Diagnostic and Statistical Manual of Mental Disorders, 3rd Edition, Revised. Washington, DC, American Psychiatric Association, 1987

American Psychiatric Association: Diagnostic and Statistical Manual of Mental Disorders, 4th Edition. Washington, DC, American Psychiatric Association, 1994

Angrist B, Pedselow E, Rubinstein M, et al: Amphetamine response and relapse risk after depot neuroleptic discontinuation. Psychopharmacology (Berl) 85:277–301, 1985

Anisman H, Bignami G: A comparative neurochemical, pharmacological, and functional analysis of aversively motivated behaviors: caveats and general consideration, in Psychopharmacology of Aversively Motivated Behavior. Edited by Anisman H, Bignami G. New York, Plenum, 1978, pp 487–512

Anisman H, Shanks N, Zakman S, et al: Multisystem regulation of performance deficits induced by stressors: an animal model of depression, in Animal Models in Psychiatry, Vol 2. Edited by Iverson MTM. Clifton, NJ, Humana Press, 1991, pp 1–55

Aprison MH, Takahashi R, Tachiki K: Hypersensitive serotonergic receptors involved in clinical depression—a theory, in Neuropharmacology and Behavior. Edited by Haber B, Aprison MH. New York, Plenum, 1978, pp 23–53

Archer T, Soderberg U, Ross SB, et al: Role of olfactory bulbectomy and DSP4 treatment in avoidance learning in the rat. Behav Neurosci 98:496–505, 1984

Armario A, Gavalda A, Marti O: Forced swimming test in rats: effect of desipramine administration and the period of exposure to the test on struggling behavior, swimming, immobility and defecation rate. Eur J Pharmacol 158:207–212, 1988

Arnett L, Ridley R, Gamble S, et al: Social withdrawal following amphetamine administration to marmosets. Psychopharmacology (Berl) 99:222–229, 1989

Arnt J: Pharmacology specificity of conditioned avoidance response inhibition in rats: inhibition by neuroleptics and correlation to dopamine receptor blockade. Acta Pharmacologica et Toxicologica 51:321–329, 1982

Aulakh CS, Wozniak KM, Hill JL, et al: Differential neuroendocrine responses to the 5-HT agonist m-chlorophenylpiperazine in fawn-hooded rats relative to Wistar and Sprague-Dawley rats. Neuroendocrinology 48:401–406, 1988

Babington RG: Antidepressives and the kindling effect, in Antidepressants. Edited by Fielding S, Lal H. Mount Kisco, NY, Futura Publishing, 1975, pp 113–124

Babington RG, Wedeking PW: The pharmacology of seizures induced by sensitization with low intensity brain stimulation. Pharmacol Biochem Behav 1:461–467, 1973

Bakshi VP, Geyer MA: Antagonism of phencyclidine-induced deficits in prepulse inhibition by the putative atypical olanzapine. Psychopharmacology 122:198–201, 1995

Baltzer V, Weiskrantz L: Antidepressant agents and reversal of diurnal activity cycles in the rat. Biol Psychiatry 10:199–209, 1975

Baruch I, Hemsley DR, Gray JA: Differential performance of acute and chronic schizophrenics in a latent inhibition task. J Nerv Ment Dis 176:598–606, 1988a

Baruch I, Hemsley DR, Gray JA: Latent inhibition and "psychotic proneness" in normal subjects. Personality and Individual Differences 9:777–783, 1988b

Bignami G: Selection for high rates and low rates of avoidance conditioning in rat. Animal Behavior 13:221–227, 1965

Bogerts B, Lieberman JA, Ashtari M, et al: Hippocampus-amygdala volumes and psychopathology in chronic schizophrenia. Biol Psychiatry 33:236–246, 1993

Borsini F, Meli A: Is the forced swimming test a suitable model for revealing antidepressant activity? Psychopharmacology (Berl) 94:147–160, 1988

Borsini F, Lecci A, Mancinelli A, et al: Stimulation of dopamine D_2 but not D_1 receptors reduces immobility time of rats in the forced swimming test: implication for antidepressant activity. Eur J Pharmacol 148:301–307, 1988

Borsini F, Lecci A, Sessarego A, et al: Discovery of antidepressant activity by forced swimming test may depend on pre-exposure of rats to a stressful situation. Psychopharmacology (Berl) 97:183–188, 1989

Braff DL, Geyer MA: Sensorimotor gating and schizophrenia: human and animal model studies. Arch Gen Psychiatry 47:181–188, 1990

Braff D, Stone C, Callaway E, et al: Prestimulus effects on human startle reflex in normals and schizophrenics. Psychophysiology 15:339–343, 1978

Braff DL, Grisson C, Geyer MA: Gating and habituation of the startle reflex in schizophrenic patients. Arch Gen Psychiatry 49:206–215, 1992

Breier A, Buchanan RW, Elkashef A, et al: Brain morphology and schizophrenia. Arch Gen Psychiatry 49:921–926, 1992

Brush FR: Genetic determination of individual differences in avoidance learning: behavioral and endocrine characteristics (review). Experientia 47:1039–1050, 1991

Brush FR, Froehlich JC, Sakellaris PC: Genetic selection for avoidance behavior in the rat. Behav Genet 9:309–316, 1979

Bunney WE Jr, Davis JM: Norepinephrine in depressive reactions: a review. Arch Gen Psychiatry 13:483–494, 1965

Cairncross KD, Schofield S, King HG: The implication of noradrenaline in avoidance learning in the rat. Prog Brain Res 39:481–485, 1973

Cairncross KD, King MG, Schofield SPM: Effect of amitriptyline on avoidance learning in rats following olfactory bulb ablation. Pharmacol Biochem Behav 3:1063–1067, 1975a

Cairncross KD, Schofield SPM, Bassett JR: Endogenous brain norepinephrine levels following bilateral olfactory bulb ablation. Pharmacol Biochem Behav 3:425–427, 1975b

Cairncross KD, Cox B, Forster C, et al: The olfactory bulbectomized rat: a simple model for detecting drugs with antidepressant potential (proceedings). Br J Pharmacol 61:497P, 1977

Cairncross KD, Cox B, Forster C, et al: Olfactory projection systems, drugs and behaviour: a review. Psychoneuroendocrinology 4:253–272, 1979

Carlson A: The current status of the dopamine hypothesis of schizophrenia. Neuropsychopharmacology 1:179–186, 1988

Carlton PL: Potentiation of the behavioral effects of amphetamine by imipramine. Psychopharmacologia 2:364–376, 1961

Carlton PL: Theories and models in psychopharmacology, in Psychopharmacology: A Generation of Progress. Edited by Lipton MA, DiMascio A, Killam KF. New York, Raven, 1978, pp 553–561

Carpenter WT, Heinrichs DW, Wagman AMI: Deficit and non-deficit forms of schizophrenia: the concept. Am J Psychiatry 145:578–601, 1988

Cervo L, Samanin R: Evidence that dopamine mechanisms in the nucleus accumbens are selectively involved in the effect of desipramine in the forced swimming test. Neuropharmacology 26:1469–1472, 1987

Christison GW, Atwater GE, Dunn LA, et al: Haloperidol enhancement of latent inhibition: relation to therapeutic action? Biol Psychiatry 23:746–749, 1988

Cohen RM, Weingartner H, Smallberg SA, et al: Effort and cognition in depression. Arch Gen Psychiatry 39:593–597, 1982

Conrad AJ, Abebe T, Austin R, et al: Hippocampal pyramidal cell disarray in schizophrenia as a bilateral phenomenon. Arch Gen Psychiatry 48:413–417, 1991

Cook L, Catania AC: Effects of drugs on avoidance and escape behavior. Federation Proceedings 23:818–835, 1964

Corbett R, Hartman H, Kerman LL, et al: Effects of atypical antipsychotic agents on social behavior in rodents. Pharmacol Biochem Behav 45:9–17, 1993

Costa E, Garattini S, Valzelli L: Interactions between reserpine, chlorpromazine, and imipramine. Experientia 16:461–463, 1960

Cott JM, Kurtz NM: New pharmacological treatments for schizophrenia, in Handbook of Schizophrenia, Vol 2: Neurochemistry and Neuropharmacology of Schizophrenia. Edited by Henn FA, DeLisi LE. New York, Elsevier, 1987, pp 203–207

Crabbe JC, Li T-K: Genetic strategies in preclinical substance abuse research, in Psychopharmacology: The Fourth Generation of Progress. Edited by Bloom FE, Kupfer DJ. New York, Raven, 1995, pp 799–811

Crabbe JC, Phillips TJ, Kosobud A, et al: Estimation of genetic correlation: interpretation of experiments using selectively bred and inbred animals. Alcohol Clin Exp Res 14:141–151, 1990

Crawley JN: Preliminary report of a new rodent separation model of depression. Psychopharmacol Bull 19:537–541, 1983

Crawley JN: Evaluation of a proposed hamster separation model of depression. Psychiatry Res 11:35–47, 1984

Creese I, Burt DR, Snyder SH: Dopamine receptor binding predicts clinical and pharmacological potencies of antipsychophrenic drugs. Science 192:481–483, 1976

Crider A, Solomon PR, McMahon MA: Disruption of selective attention in the rat following chronic *d*-amphetamine administration: relationship to schizophrenic attention disorder. Biol Psychiatry 17:351–360, 1982

Crow TJ: Temporal lobe asymmetries as the key to the etiology of schizophrenia. Schizophr Bull 16:433–443, 1990

Dains K, Hitzemann B, Hitzemann R: Genetics, neuroleptic response and the organization of cholinergic neurons in the mouse striatum. J Pharmacol Exp Ther 279:1430–1438, 1996

Danysz W, Plaznik A, Kostowski W, et al: Comparison of desipramine, amitriptyline, zimeldine and alaproclate in six animal models used to investigate antidepressant drugs. Pharmacol Toxicol 62:42–50, 1988

Davidson MK, Lindsey JR, Davis JK: Requirements and selection of an animal model. Isr J Med Sci 23:551–555, 1987

Davis KL, Kahn RS, Ko G, et al: Dopamine in schizophrenia: a review and reconceptualization. Am J Psychiatry 148:1474–1486, 1991

De la Casa LG, Ruiz G: Latent inhibition and recall/recognition of irrelevant stimuli as a function of pre-exposure duration in high and low psychotic-prone normal subjects. Br J Psychol 84:119–132, 1993

De Pablo JM, Parra A, Segovia S, et al: Learned immobility explains the behavior of rats in the forced swimming test. Physiol Behav 46:229–237, 1989

Desan PH, Silbert LH, Maier SF: Long-term effects of inescapable stress on daily running activity and antagonism by desipramine. Pharmacol Biochem Behav 30:21–29, 1988

Domenjoz R, Theobald W: Zur pharmakologie des Tofranil (*N*-(3-dimethylaminopropyl)-iminodibenzylhydrochlorid). Arch Int Pharmacodyn Ther 120:450–489, 1959

Dunn LA, Kilts CD, Nemeroff CB: Animal behavioral models for drug development in psychopharmacology, in Modern Drug Discovery Technology. Edited by Moos WH, Clark JS. Chichester, England, VCH and Ellis Horwood, 1990, pp 259–280

Dunn LA, Scibilia RJ, Franks JA, et al: Comparison of the effect on latent inhibition of dopamine agonists and atypical antipsychotics in rats. Society for Neuroscience Abstracts 17:99, 1991

Dunn LA, Atwater GE, Kilts CD: Effects of antipsychotic drugs on latent inhibition: sensitivity and specificity of an animal behavioral model of clinical drug action. Psychopharmacology (Berl) 112:315–323, 1993

Earley B, Leonard BE: Effect of two specific-serotonin reuptake inhibitors on the behaviour of the olfactory bulbectomized rat in the "open field" apparatus, in Clinical and Pharmacological Studies in Psychiatric Disorders. Edited by Burrows GD, Norman TR, Dennerstein L. London, John Libby, 1985, pp 234–240

Edwards E, Harkins K, Wright G, et al: Modulation of [^{3}H]paroxetine binding to the 5-hydroxytryptamine uptake site in an animal model of depression. J Neurochem 56:1581–1586, 1991a

Edwards E, Harkins K, Wright G, et al: 5-HT$_{1b}$ receptors in an animal model of depression. Neuropharmacology 30:101–105, 1991b

Edwards E, Kornrich W, Van Houtten P, et al: In vitro neurotransmitter release in an animal model of depression. Neurochem Int 21:29–35, 1992

Ellenbroek BA: The ethological analysis of monkeys in a social setting as an animal model for schizophrenia, in Animal Models in Psychopharmacology (Advances in Pharmacological Sciences Series). Edited by Olivier B, Mos J, Slangen JL. Basel, Switzerland, Birkhäuser Verlag, 1991, pp 265–284

Ellenbroek B, Cools AR: The paw test: an animal model for neuroleptic drugs which fulfills the criteria for pharmacological isomorphism. Life Sci 42:1205–1213, 1988

Ellenbroek BA, Peeters BW, Honig WM, et al: The paw test: a behavioural paradigm for differentiating between classical and atypical neuroleptic drugs. Psychopharmacology (Berl) 93:343–348, 1987

Ellenbroek BA, Willemen APM, Cools AR: Are antagonists of dopamine D_1 receptors drugs that attenuate both positive and negative symptoms of schizophrenia? Neuropsychopharmacology 2:191–199, 1989

Ellenbroek BA, Budde S, Cools AR: Prepulse inhibition and latent inhibition: the role of dopamine in the medial prefrontal cortex. Neuroscience 75:535–542, 1996

Ellinwood EH Jr, Kilbey MM: Chronic stimulant intoxication models of psychosis, in Animal Models in Psychiatry and Neurology, Vol I. Edited by Hanin I, Usdin E. Oxford, England, Pergamon, 1977, pp 61–74

Ellinwood EH Jr, Sudilovsky A, Nelson LM: Behavioral analysis of chronic amphetamine intoxication. Biol Psychiatry 4:215–225, 1972

Ellison G, Eison MS, Huberman HS: Stages of constant amphetamine intoxication: delayed appearance of paranoid-like behaviors in rat colonies. Psychopharmacology (Berl) 56:293–299, 1978

Ettenberg A, Koob ZGF, Bloom FE: Response artifact in the measurement of neuroleptic induced anhedonia. Science 213:357–359, 1981

Feldon J, Weiner I: The latent inhibition model of schizophrenic attention disorder: haloperidol and sulpiride enhance rats' ability to ignore irrelevant stimuli. Biol Psychiatry 29:635–646, 1991

Fink JS, Swerdloff A, Reis DJ: Genetic control of dopamine receptors in mouse caudate nucleus: relationship of cataleptic response to neuroleptic drugs. Neurosci Lett 32:301–306, 1982

Fonberg E: Effects of small dorsomedial amygdala lesions on food intake and acquisition of instrumental alimentary reactions in dogs. Physiol Behav 4:739–743, 1969a

Fonberg E: The role of the hypothalamus and amygdala in food intake, alimentary motivation and emotional reaction. Acta Biologiae Experimentalis 29:335–358, 1969b

Fonberg E: Control of emotional behaviour through the hypothalamus and amygdaloid complex. Ciba Found Symp 8:131–161, 1972

Freedman R, Waldo MR, Bickford-Wimer P, et al: Elementary neuronal dysfunctions in schizophrenia. Schizophr Res 4:233–243, 1991

Fregnan GB, Chieli T: Classical neuroleptics and deconditioning activity after single or repeated treatments. Arzneimittelforschung 30:1865–1870, 1980

Fuller JL: Strain differences in the effects of chlorpromazine and chlordiazepoxide upon active and passive avoidance in mice. Psychopharmacologia 16:261–271, 1970

Gardner C, Guy A: A social interaction model of anxiety sensitive to acutely administered benzodiazepines. Drug Development Research 4:207–216, 1984

Garver DL, Zemlan F, Hirschowitz J, et al: Dopamine and nondopamine psychoses. Psychopharmacology (Berl) 84:138–145, 1984

Garzon J, Del Rio J: Hyperactivity induced in rats by long-term isolation: further studies on a new model for the detection of antidepressants. Eur J Pharmacol 74:287–294, 1981

Garzon J, Fuentes JA, Del Rio J: Antidepressants selectively antagonize the hyperactivity induced in rats by long-term isolation. Eur J Pharmacol 59:293–296, 1979

Geyer MA, Wilkinson LS, Humby T, et al: Isolation rearing of rats produces a deficit in prepulse inhibition of acoustic startle similar to that in schizophrenia. Biol Psychiatry 34:361–372, 1993

Gil M, Marti J, Armario A: Inhibition of catecholamine synthesis depresses behavior of rats in the holeboard and forced swim tests: influence of previous chronic stress. Pharmacol Biochem Behav 43:597–601, 1992

Golda V, Petr R: Behaviour of genetically hypertensive rats in an animal model of depression and in an animal model of anxiety. Activitas Nervosa Superior 28:274–275, 1986

Golda V, Petr R: Animal model of depression: drug induced changes independent of changes in exploratory activity. Activitas Nervosa Superior 29:114–115, 1987a

Golda V, Petr R: Animal model of depression: effect of nicotergoline and metergoline. Activitas Nervosa Superior 29:115–117, 1987b

Golda V, Petr R: Animal model of depression: retention of motor depression not predictable from the threshold of reaction to the inescapable shock. Activitas Nervosa Superior 29:113–114, 1987c

Gorka Z, Earley B, Leonard BE: Effect of bilateral olfactory bulbectomy in the rat, alone or in combination with antidepressants, on the learned immobility model of depression. Neuropsychobiology 13:26–30, 1985

Gosselin G, Oberling P, Di Scala G: Antagonism of amphetamine-induced disruption of latent inhibition by the atypical antipsychotic olanzapine in rats. Behavioural Pharmacology 7:820–826, 1996

Gray JA, Feldon J, Rawlins JNP, et al: The neuropsychology of schizophrenia. Behavior and Brain Sciences 14:1–35, 1991

Gray NS, Pickering AD, Hemsley DR, et al: Abolition of latent inhibition by a single 5 mg dose of d-amphetamine in man. Psychopharmacology (Berl) 307:425–430, 1992

Gray NS, Pilowsky LS, Gray JA, et al: Latent inhibition in drug naive schizophrenics: relationship to duration of illness and dopamine D2 binding using SPET. Schizophr Res 17:95–107, 1995

Guterman Y, Josiassen RC, Bashore TE, et al: Latent inhibition effects reflected in event-related brain potentials in healthy controls and schizophrenics. Schizophr Res 20:315–326, 1996

Halliwell G, Quinton RM, Williams FE: A comparison of imipramine, chlorpromazine and related drugs in various tests involving autonomic functions and antagonism of reserpine. Br J Pharmacol 23:330–350, 1964

Hartley P, Neill D, Hagler M, et al: Procedure- and age-dependent hyperactivity in a new animal model of endogenous depression. Neurosci Biobehav Rev 14:69–72, 1990

Hasey G, Hanin I: The cholinergic-adrenergic hypothesis of depression reexamined using clonidine, metoprolol, and physostigmine in an animal model. Biol Psychiatry 29:127–138, 1991

Hatotani N, Nomura J, Kitayama I: Changes in brain monoamines in the animal model for depression, in New Vistas in Depression, Advances in the Biosciences, Vol 40. Edited by Langer SZ, Takahashi R, Segawa T, et al. Oxford, England, Pergamon, 1982, pp 65–72

Hawkins J, Hicks RA, Phillips N, et al: Swimming rats and human depression (letter). Nature 274:512, 1978

Hawkins J, Phillips N, Moore JD, et al: Emotionality and REMD: a rat swimming model. Physiol Behav 25:167–171, 1980

Hemsley DR: An experimental psychological model for schizophrenia, in Search for the Causes of Schizophrenia. Edited by Hafner H, Gattaz WF, Janzarik W. Berlin, Springer-Verlag, 1987, pp 179–188

Henn FA, Johnson J, Edwards E, et al: Melancholia in rodents: neurobiology and pharmacology. Psychopharmacol Bull 21:443–446, 1985

Hitzemann R, Daines K, Bier-Langing CM, et al: On the selection of mice for haloperidol response and non-response. Psychopharmacology (Berl) 103:244–250, 1991

Hoffman LJ, Weiss JM: Behavioral depression following clonidine withdrawal: a new animal model of long-lasting depression? Psychopharmacol Bull 22:943–949, 1986

Horovitz ZP, Ragozzino PW, Leaf RC: Selective block of rat mouse-killing by antidepressants. Life Sci 4:1909–1912, 1965

Howard JL, Soroko FE, Cooper BR: Empirical behavioral models of depression, with emphasis on tetrabenazine antagonism, in Antidepressants: Neurochemical, Behavioral, and Clinical Perspectives. Edited by Enna SJ, Malick JB, Richardson E. New York, Raven, 1981, pp 107–120

Iversen SD: Is it possible to model psychotic state in animals? Journal of Psychopharmacology 1:154–156, 1987

Jackson RL, Maier SF, Rapaport PM: Exposure to inescapable shock produces both activity and associative deficits in the rat. Learning and Motivation 9:69–98, 1978

Janscar S, Leonard BE: The effects of olfactory bulbectomy on the behaviour of rats in the open field. Isr J Med Sci 149:80–81, 1980

Johansson C, Jackson DM, Zhang J, et al: Prepulse inhibition of acoustic startle, a measure of sensorimotor gating: effects of antipsychotics and other agents in rats. Pharmacol Biochem Behav 52:649–654, 1995

Jones SH, Gray JA, Hemsley DR: Loss of the Kamin blocking effect in acute but not chronic schizophrenics. Biol Psychiatry 32:739–755, 1992

Jordan S, Kramer GL, Zukas PK, et al: Previous stress increases in vivo biogenic amine response to swim stress. Neurochem Res 19:1521–1525, 1994

Kamin LJ: Predictability, surprise, attention and conditioning, in Punishment and Aversive Behaviour. Edited by Campbell BA, Church RM. New York, Appleton-Century-Crofts, 1969, pp 279–296

Kane JM: Neuroleptic treatment of schizophrenia, in Handbook of Schizophrenia, Vol 2: Neurochemistry and Neuropharmacology of Schizophrenia. Edited by Henn FA, DeLisi LE. New York, Elsevier, 1987, pp 179–226

Kane J, Honigfeld G, Singer J, et al: Clozapine for the treatment resistant schizophrenic. Arch Gen Psychiatry 45:789–796, 1988

Katz RJ: Animal model of depression: effects of electroconvulsive shock therapy. Neurosci Biobehav Rev 5:273–277, 1981

Katz RJ: Animal model of depression: pharmacological sensitivity of a hedonic deficit. Pharmacol Biochem Behav 16:965–968, 1982

Katz RJ, Baldrighi G: A further parametric study of imipramine in an animal model of depression. Pharmacol Biochem Behav 16:969–972, 1982

Katz RJ, Hersh S: Amitriptyline and scopolamine in an animal model of depression. Neurosci Biobehav Rev 5:265–271, 1981

Katz RJ, Sibel M: Animal model of depression: tests of three structurally and pharmacologically novel antidepressant compounds. Pharmacol Biochem Behav 16:973–977, 1982a

Katz RJ, Sibel M: Further analysis of the specificity of a novel animal model of depression—effects of an antihistaminic, antipsychotic and anxiolytic compound. Pharmacol Biochem Behav 16:979–982, 1982b

Katz RJ, Roth KA, Carroll BJ: Acute and chronic stress effects on open field activity in the rat: implications for a model of depression. Neurosci Biobehav Rev 5:247–251, 1981a

Katz RJ, Roth KA, Schmaltz K: Amphetamine and tranylcypromine in an animal model of depression: pharmacological specificity of the reversal effect. Neurosci Biobehav Rev 5:259–264, 1981b

Kaufman IC, Rosenblum LA: The reaction to separation in infant monkeys: anaclitic depression and conservation-withdrawal. Psychosom Med 29:648–675, 1967

Kendler KS, Tsuang MT, Hays P: Age at onset in schizophrenia. Arch Gen Psychiatry 44:881–890, 1987

Kibel DA, Lafont I, Liddle PF: The composition of the negative syndrome of chronic schizophrenia. Br J Psychiatry 162:744–750, 1993

Killcross AS, Robbins TW: Differential effects of intra-accumbens and systemic amphetamine on latent inhibition using an on-baseline, within-subject conditioned suppression paradigm. Psychopharmacology (Berl) 110:479–489, 1993

King MG, Cairncross KD: Effects of olfactory bulb section on brain noradrenaline, corticosterone and conditioning in the rat. Pharmacol Biochem Behav 2:347–353, 1974

Kitada Y, Miyauchi T, Satoh A, et al: Effects of antidepressants in the rat forced swimming test. Eur J Pharmacol 72:145–152, 1981

Kitada Y, Miyauchi T, Kosasa T, et al: The significance of β-adrenoceptor down regulation in the desipramine action in the forced swimming test. Naunyn Schmiedebergs Arch Pharmacol 333:31–35, 1986

Klein DF: Differential diagnosis and treatment of the dysphorias, in Depression: Behavioral, Biochemical, Clinical and Treatment Concepts. Edited by Simpson GM, Gallant DM. New York, Spectrum, 1975, pp 127–154

Kolakowska T, Williams AO, Arden M, et al: Schizophrenia with good and poor outcome, I: early clinical features, response to neuroleptics and signs of organic dysfunction. Br J Psychiatry 146:229–239, 1985

Kraemer GW: Causes of changes in brain noradrenaline systems and later effects on responses to social stressors in rhesus monkeys: the cascade hypothesis. Ciba Found Symp 123:216–233, 1986

Kuppinger HE, Harrington A, Kaczmerek MJ, et al: The effects of phencyclidine and amphetamine on social behavior in tether-restrained and freely moving rats. Experimental and Clinical Psychopharmacology 4:77–81, 1996

Kuribara H, Tadokoro S: Correlation between antiavoidance activities of antipsychotic drugs in rats and daily clinical doses. Pharmacol Biochem Behav 14:181–192, 1981

Labarca R, Silva H, Jerez S, et al: Differential effects of haloperidol on negative symptoms in drug-naive schizophrenic patients: effects on plasma homovanillic acid. Schizophr Res 9:29–34, 1993

Lachman HM, Papolos DF, Boyle A, et al: Alterations in glucocorticoid inducible RNAs in the limbic system of learned helpless rats. Brain Res 609:110–116, 1993

Leonard BE, Tuite M: Anatomical, physiological, and behavioral aspects of olfactory bulbectomy in the rat. Int Rev Neurobiol 22:251–286, 1981

Leshner AI, Remler H, Biegon A, et al: Desmethylimipramine (DMI) counteracts learned helplessness in rats. Psychopharmacology (Berl) 66:207–208, 1979

Liddle PF, Firston KJ, Frith CD, et al: Patterns of cerebral blood flow in schizophrenia. Br J Psychiatry 160:179–186, 1992

Lipska BK, Weinberger DR: Genetic variation in vulnerability to the behavioral effects of neonatal hippocampal damage in rats. Proc Natl Acad Sci U S A 92:8906–8910, 1995

Lipska BK, Jaskiw GE, Chrapusta S, et al: Ibotenic acid lesion of the ventral hippocampus differentially affects dopamine and its metabolites in the nucleus accumbens and prefrontal cortex in the rat. Brain Res 585:1–6, 1992

Lipska BK, Jaskiw GE, Weinberger DR: Postpubertal emergence of hyperresponsiveness to stress and amphetamine after neonatal excitotoxic hippocampal damage: a potential animal model of schizophrenia. Neuropsychopharmacology 9:67–75, 1993

Lipska BK, Swerdlow NR, Geyer MA, et al: Neonatal excitotoxic hippocampal damage in rats causes post-pubertal changes in prepulse inhibition of startle and its disruption by apomorphine. Psychopharmacology (Berl) 122:35–43, 1995

Lubow RE: Latent inhibition. Psychol Bull 79:398–407, 1973

Lubow RE: Latent Inhibition and Conditioned Attention Theory. New York, Cambridge University Press, 1989

Lubow RE, Weiner I, Feldon J: An animal model of attention, in Behavioral Models and the Analysis of Drug Action. Edited by Spiegelstein MY, Levy A. Amsterdam, Elsevier, 1982, pp 89–107

Lyon M: Animal models of mania and schizophrenia, in Behavioral Models in Psychopharmacology: Theoretical, Industrial and Clinical Perspectives. Edited by Wilner P. Cambridge, England, Cambridge University Press, 1990, pp 253–310

Maier SF, Albin RW, Testa TJ: Failure to learn to escape in rats previously exposed to inescapable shock depends on nature of escape response. Journal of Comparative and Physiological Psychology 85:581–592, 1973

Malick JB: Yohimbine potentiation as a predictor of antidepressant action, in Antidepressants: Neurochemical, Behavioral, and Clinical Perspectives. Edited by Enna SJ, Malick JB, Richardson E. New York, Raven, 1981, pp 141–155

Martin JV, Edwards E, Johnson JO, et al: Monoamine receptors in an animal model of affective disorder. J Neurochem 55:1142–1148, 1990

Martin P, Soubrie P, Simon P: The effect of monoamine oxidase inhibitors compared with classical tricyclic antidepressants on learned helplessness paradigm. Prog Neuropsychopharmacol Biol Psychiatry 11:1–7, 1987

Martin P, Soubrie P, Puech AJ: Reversal of helpless behavior by serotonin uptake blockers in rats. Psychopharmacology (Berl) 101:403–407, 1990

McGuire PS, Seiden LS: Differential effects of imipramine in rats as a function of DRL schedule value. Pharmacol Biochem Behav 13:691–694, 1980a

McGuire PS, Seiden LS: The effects of tricyclic antidepressants on performance under a differential-reinforcement-of-low-rates schedule in rats. J Pharmacol Exp Ther 214:635–641, 1980b

McKinney WT, Bunney WE: Animal model of depression. Arch Gen Psychiatry 21:240–248, 1969

McKinney WT, Suomi SJ, Harlow HF: Depression in primates. Am J Psychiatry 127:49–56, 1971

Meltzer HY, Sommers AA, Luchins DJ: The effect of neuroleptics and other psychotropic drugs on negative symptoms in schizophrenia. J Clin Psychopharmacol 6:329–338, 1986

Miczek KA, Yoshimura H: Disruption of primate social behavior by *d*-amphetamine and cocaine: differential antagonism by antipsychotics. Psychopharmacology (Berl) 76: 163–171, 1982

Minor TR, Jackson RL, Maier SF: Effects of task-irrelevant cues and reinforcement delay on choice-escape learning following inescapable shock: evidence for a deficit in selective attention. J Exp Psychol Anim Behav Process 10:543–556, 1984

Minor TR, Pelleymounter MA, Maier SF: Uncontrollable shock, forebrain norepinephrine, and stimulus selection during choice-escape learning. Psychobiology 16:135–145, 1988

Mitchell PB, Potter WZ: Major depression: the validity of a diagnosis (letter). Depression 1:180, 1993

Moller Nielsen I, Fjalland B, Pedersen V, et al: Pharmacology of neuroleptics upon repeated administration. Psychopharmacology (Berl) 34:95–104, 1974

Moran PM, Fischer TR, Hitchcock JM, et al: Effects of clozapine on latent inhibition in the rat. Behavioural Pharmacology 7:42–48, 1996

Moreau JL, Jenck F, Martin JR, et al: Antidepressant treatment prevents chronic unpredictable mild stress-induced anhedonia as assessed by ventral tegmentum self-stimulation behavior in rats. Eur J Pharmacol 2:43–49, 1992

Morpurgo C, Theobald W: Influence of imipramine-like compounds and chlorpromazine on the reserpine-hypothermia in mice and the amphetamine-hyperthermia in rats. Medicina et Pharmacologia Experimentalis 12:226–232, 1965

Mueser KT, Bellack AS, Douglas MS, et al: Prevalence and stability of social skill deficits in schizophrenia. Schizophr Res 5:167–176, 1991

Murua VS, Molina VA: An opiate mechanism involved in conditioned analgesia influences forced swim-induced immobility. Physiol Behav 48:641–645, 1990

Muscat R, Towell A, Willner P: Changes in dopamine autoreceptor sensitivity in an animal model of depression. Psychopharmacology (Berl) 94:545–550, 1988

Muscat R, Sampson D, Willner P: Dopaminergic mechanism of imipramine action in an animal model of depression. Biol Psychiatry 28:223–230, 1990

Muscat R, Papp M, Willner P: Antidepressant-like effects of dopamine agonists in an animal model of depression. Biol Psychiatry 31:937–946, 1992

Nagayama H, Hingtgen JN, Aprison MH: Pre- and postsynaptic serotonergic manipulations in an animal model of depression. Pharmacol Biochem Behav 13:575–579, 1980

Nagayama H, Hingtgen JN, Aprison MH: Postsynaptic action by four antidepressive drugs in an animal model of depression. Pharmacol Biochem Behav 15:125–130, 1981

Neill D, Vogel G, Hagler M, et al: Diminished sexual activity in a new animal model of endogenous depression. Neurosci Biobehav Rev 14:73–76, 1990

Nelson JC, Charney DS: The symptoms of major depressive illness. Am J Psychiatry 138:1–13, 1981

Nielsen EB, Lyon M, Ellison G: Apparent hallucinations in monkeys during around-the-clock amphetamine for seven to fourteen days: possible relevance to amphetamine psychosis. J Nerv Ment Dis 171:222–233, 1983

Nuechterlein KH, Dawson ME: Information processing and attentional functioning in the developmental course of schizophrenic disorders. Schizophr Bull 10:160–203, 1984

O'Donnell JM, Seiden LS: Effects of monoamine oxidase inhibitors on performance during differential reinforcement of low response rate. Psychopharmacology (Berl) 78:214–218, 1982

O'Donnell JM, Seiden LS: Differential-reinforcement-of-low-rate 72-second schedule: selective effects of antidepressant drugs. J Pharmacol Exp Ther 224:80–88, 1983

O'Donnell JM, Seiden LS: Altered effects of desipramine on operant performance after 6-hydroxydopamine-induced depletion of brain dopamine or norepinephrine. J Pharmacol Exp Ther 229:629–635, 1984

O'Donnell JM, Seiden LS: Effect of the experimental antidepressant AHR-9377 on performance during differential reinforcement of low response rate. Psychopharmacology (Berl) 87:283–285, 1985

Okubo Y, Suhara T, Suzuki K, et al: Decreased prefrontal dopamine D1 receptors in schizophrenia revealed by PET. Nature 385:634–636, 1997

Overmier JB, Seligman MEP: Effects of inescapable shock upon subsequent escape and avoidance learning. Journal of Comparative and Physiological Psychology 63:28–33, 1967

Overstreet DH: Selective breeding for increased cholinergic function: development of a new animal model of depression. Biol Psychiatry 21:49–58, 1986

Overstreet DH: The Flinders sensitive line rats: a genetic animal model of depression. Neurosci Biobehav Rev 17:51–68, 1993

Overstreet DH, Rezvani AH, Janowsky DS: Genetic animal models of depression and ethanol preference provide support for cholinergic and serotonergic involvement in depression and alcoholism. Biol Psychiatry 31:919–936, 1992

Papolos DF, Edwards E, Marmur R, et al: Effects of the antiglucocorticoid RU 38486 on the induction of learned helpless behavior in Sprague-Dawley rats. Brain Res 615:304–309, 1993

Pare WP: Stress and consummatory behavior in the albino rat. Psychol Rep 16:399–405, 1965

Parker G, Hadzi-Pavlovic D, Boyce P, et al: Classifying depression by mental state signs. Br J Psychiatry 157:55–65, 1990

Peng RY, Mansbach RS, Braff DL, et al: A D_2 dopamine receptor agonist disrupts sensorimotor gating in rats: implications for dopaminergic abnormalities in schizophrenia. Neuropsychopharmacology 3:211–217, 1990

Penn DL, Van Der Dose AJW, Spaulding WD, et al: Information processing and social cognitive problem solving in schizophrenia. J Nerv Ment Dis 181:13–20, 1993

Petty F, Sherman AD: Learned helplessness induction decreases in vivo cortical serotonin release. Pharmacol Biochem Behav 18:649–650, 1983

Petty F, Kramer GL, Phillips TR, et al: Learned helplessness and serotonin: in vivo microdialysis. Society for Neuroscience Abstracts 16:752, 1990

Platt JE, Stone EA: Chronic restraint stress elicits a positive antidepressant response on the forced swim test. Eur J Pharmacol 82:179–181, 1982

Plaznik A, Danysz W, Kostowski W: Mesolimbic noradrenaline but not dopamine is responsible for organization of rat behavior in the forced swim test and an anti-immobilizing effect of desipramine. Pol J Pharmacol Pharm 37:347–357, 1985a

Plaznik A, Danysz W, Kostowski W: A stimulatory effect of intraaccumbens injections of noradrenaline on the behavior of rats in the forced swim test. Psychopharmacology (Berl) 87:119–123, 1985b

Plaznik A, Tamborska E, Hauptmann M, et al: Brain neurotransmitter systems mediating behavioral deficits produced by inescapable shock treatment in rats. Brain Res 447:122–132, 1988

Pollard GT, Howard JL: Similar effects of antidepressant and non-antidepressant drugs on behavior under an interresponse-time >72-s schedule. Psychopharmacology (Berl) 89:253–258, 1986

Porsolt RD: Behavioral despair, in Antidepressants: Neurochemical, Behavioral, and Clinical Perspectives. Edited by Enna SJ, Malick JB, Richardson E. New York, Raven, 1981, pp 121–139

Porsolt RD, Anton G, Blavet N, et al: Behavioural despair in rats: a new model sensitive to antidepressant treatments. Eur J Pharmacol 47:379–391, 1978

Porsolt RD, Bertin A, Blavet N, et al: Immobility induced by forced swimming in rats: effects of agents which modify central catecholamine and serotonin activity. Eur J Pharmacol 57:201–210, 1979

Porsolt RD, Roux S, Jalfre M: Effects of imipramine on separation-induced vocalizations in young rhesus monkeys. Pharmacol Biochem Behav 20:979–981, 1984

Porsolt RD, Lenègre, McArthur RA: Pharmacological models of depression, in Animal Models in Psychopharmacology. Edited by Olivier B, Mos J, Slangen JL. Basel, Switzerland, Birkhäuser Verlag, 1991, pp 137–159

Quinton RM: The increase in the toxicity of yohimbine induced by imipramine and other drugs in mice. Br J Pharmacol 21:51–66, 1963

Richelson E, Pfenning M: Blockade by antidepressants and related compounds of biogenic amine uptake into rat brain synaptosomes: most antidepressants selectively block norepinephrine uptake. Eur J Pharmacol 104:277–286, 1984

Rigter H, van Riezen H, Wren A: Pharmacological validation of a new test for the detection of antidepressant activity of drugs. Br J Pharmacol 59:451–452, 1977

Roberts DCS, Vickers G: Atypical neuroleptics increase self-administration of cocaine: an evaluation of a behavioural screen for antipsychotic activity. Psychopharmacology (Berl) 82:135–139, 1984

Robson RD, Antonaccio MJ, Saelens JK, et al: Antagonism by mianserin and classical α-adrenoceptor blocking drugs of some cardiovascular and behavioral effects of clonidine. Eur J Pharmacol 47:431–442, 1978

Roth KA, Katz RJ: Further studies on a novel animal model of depression: therapeutic effects of a tricyclic antidepressant. Neurosci Biobehav Rev 5:253–258, 1981

Roth M: A classification of affective disorders based on a synthesis of new and old concepts, in Research in the Psychobiology of Human Behavior. Edited by Meyer E, Brady JV. Baltimore, MD, Johns Hopkins University Press, 1976, pp 75–114

Sampson D, Willner P, Muscat R: Reversal of antidepressant action by dopamine antagonists in an animal model of depression. Psychopharmacology (Berl) 104:491–495, 1991

Sams-Dodd F: Phencyclidine-induced stereotyped behaviour and social isolation in rats: a possible animal model of schizophrenia. Behavioural Pharmacology 7:3–23, 1996

Sams-Dodd F: Effect of novel antipsychotic drugs on phencyclidine-induced stereotyped behaviour and social isolation in the rat social interaction test. Behavioural Pharmacology 8:196–215, 1997

Sanberg PR, Bunsey MD, Giordano M, et al: The catalepsy test: its ups and down. Behav Neurosci 102:748–759, 1988

Sanger DJ: The effect of clozapine on shuttle box avoidance responding in rats: comparison with haloperidol and chlordiazepoxide. Pharmacol Biochem Behav 23:231–236, 1985

Satoh H, Mori J, Shimomura K, et al: Effect of zimelidine, a new antidepressant, on the forced swimming test in rats. Jpn J Pharmacol 35:471–473, 1984

Schildkraut JJ, Kety SS: Biogenic amines and emotion. Science 156:23–33, 1967

Schiller GD, Pucilowski O, Wienicke C, et al: Immobility-reducing effects of antidepressants in a genetic animal model of depression. Brain Res Bull 28:821–823, 1992

Schmajuk NA: Animal models of schizophrenia: the hippocampally lesioned animal. Schizophr Bull 13:317–327, 1987

Scott PA, Cierpial MA, Kilts CD, et al: Susceptibility and resistance of rats to stress-induced decreases in swim test activity: a selective breeding study. Brain Res 725:217–230, 1996

Seiden LS, O'Donnell JM: Effects of antidepressant drugs on DRL behaviour, in Behavioural Pharmacology: The Current Status. Edited by Seiden LS, Balster RL. New York, Alan R Liss, 1985, pp 323–338

Seiden LS, Dahms JL, Shaughnessy RA: Behavioral screen for antidepressants: the effects of drugs and electroconvulsive shock on performance under a differential-reinforcement-of-low-rate schedule. Psychopharmacology (Berl) 86:55–60, 1985

Seligman MEP: Depression and learned helplessness, in The Psychology of Depression: Contemporary Theory and Research. Edited by Friedman RJ, Katz MM. Washington, DC, VH Winston, 1974, pp 83–125

Seligman MEP, Beagley G: Learned helplessness in the rat. Journal of Comparative and Physiological Psychology 88:534–541, 1975

Seligman MEP, Maier SF: Failure to escape traumatic shock. J Exp Psychol 74:1–9, 1967

Seligman MEP, Maier SF, Solomon RL: Unpredictable and uncontrollable aversive events, in Aversive Conditioning and Learning. Edited by Brush FR. New York, Academic Press, 1971, pp 347–400

Shenton ME, Kikinis R, Jolesz FA, et al: Abnormalities of the left temporal lobe and thought disorder in schizophrenia. N Engl J Med 327:604–612, 1992

Sherman AD, Sacquitne JL, Petty F: Specificity of the learned helplessness model of depression. Pharmacol Biochem Behav 16:449–454, 1982

Shipley MT, Halloran FJ, De La Torre J: Surprisingly rich projection from locus coeruleus to the olfactory bulb in the rat. Brain Res 329:294–299, 1985

Shiromani PJ, Overstreet D, Levy D, et al: Increased REM sleep in rats selectively bred for cholinergic hyperactivity. Neuropsychopharmacology 1:127–133, 1988

Simmons RF: Schizotypy and startle prepulse inhibition (abstract). Psychophysiology 27 (suppl):S6, 1990

Sofia RD: Effects of centrally active drugs on four models of experimentally induced aggression in rodents. Life Sci 8:705–716, 1969a

Sofia RD: Structural relationship and potency of agents which selectively block mouse killing (muricide) behavior in rats. Life Sci 8:1201–1210, 1969b

Solomon CR, Crider A, Winkleman JW, et al: Disrupted latent inhibition in the rat with chronic amphetamine or haloperidol-induced supersensitivity: relationship to schizophrenic attention disorder. Biol Psychiatry 16:519–537, 1981

Spealman RD, Kelleher RT, Goldberg SR, et al: Behavioral effects of clozapine: comparison with thioridazine, chlorpromazine, haloperidol and chlordiazepoxide in squirrel monkeys. J Pharmacol Exp Ther 224:127–134, 1982

Steru L, Chermat R, Thierry B, et al: The tail suspension test: a new method for screening antidepressants in mice. Psychopharmacology (Berl) 85:367–370, 1985

Stockert M, Serra J, DeRobertis E: Effect of olfactory bulbectomy and chronic amitriptyline treatment in rats: ^{3}H-imipramine binding and behavioral analysis by swimming and open field tests. Pharmacol Biochem Behav 29:681–686, 1988

Stoudemire A, Miller J, Schmitt F, et al: Development of an organic affective syndrome during a hyperbaric diving experiment. Am J Psychiatry 141:1251–1254, 1984

Sulser F: New perspectives on the mode of action of antidepressant drugs. Trends Pharmacol Sci 1:92–94, 1979

Suomi SJ, Seaman SF, Lewis JK, et al: Effects of imipramine treatment of separation-induced social disorders in rhesus monkeys. Arch Gen Psychiatry 35:321–325, 1978

Swerdlow NR, Geyer MA: Clozapine and haloperidol in an animal model of sensorimotor gating deficits in schizophrenia. Pharmacol Biochem Behav 44:741–744, 1993

Swerdlow NR, Geyer M, Braff D, et al: Central dopamine hyperactivity in rats mimics abnormal acoustic startle in schizophrenics. Biol Psychiatry 21:23–33, 1986

Swerdlow NR, Braff DL, Masten VL, et al: Schizophrenic-like sensorimotor gating abnormalities in rats following dopamine infusion into the nucleus accumbens. Psychopharmacology (Berl) 101:414–420, 1990

Swerdlow NR, Keith VA, Braff DL, et al: The effects of spiperone, raclopride, SCH 23390 and clozapine on apomorphine-inhibition of sensorimotor gating of the startle response in the rat. J Pharmacol Exp Ther 256:530–536, 1991

Swerdlow NR, Benbow CH, Zisook S, et al: A preliminary assessment of sensorimotor gating in patients with obsessive compulsive disorder. Biol Psychiatry 33:298–301, 1993

Swerdlow NR, Braff DL, Taaid N, et al: Assessing the validity of an animal model of deficient sensorimotor gating in schizophrenic patients. Arch Gen Psychiatry 51:139–154, 1994

Swerdlow NR, Lipska BK, Weinberger DR, et al: Increased sensitivity to the sensorimotor gating-disruptive effects of apomorphine after lesions of medial prefrontal cortex or ventral hippocampus in adult rats. Psychopharmacology 122:27–34, 1995

Swerdlow NR, Bakshi V, Geyer MA: Seroquel restores sensorimotor gating in phencyclidine-treated rats. J Pharmacol Exp Ther 279:1290–1299, 1996

Tamminga CA, Thaker GK, Buchanan R, et al: Limbic system abnormalities identified in schizophrenia using position emission tomography with fluorodeoxyglucose and neocortical alteration with deficit syndrome. Arch Gen Psychiatry 49:522–530, 1992

Tekes K, Tothfalusi T, Magyar K: Irregular chronic stress related selective presynaptic adaptation of dopaminergic system in rat striatum: effects of (−) deprenyl and amitriptyline. Acta Physiol Pharmacol Bulg 12:21–28, 1986

Telner JI, Singhal RL: Effects of nortriptyline treatment on learned helplessness in the rat. Pharmacol Biochem Behav 14:823–826, 1981

Thornton JC, Dawe S, Lee C, et al: Effects of nicotine and amphetamine on latent inhibition in human subjects. Psychopharmacology 127:164–173, 1996

Trimble KM, Bell R, King DJ: Enhancement of latent inhibition in the rat by the atypical antipsychotic agent remoxipride. Pharmacol Biochem Behav 56:809–816, 1997

Upchurch M, Schallert T: A behavioral analysis of the offspring of "haloperidol-sensitive" and "haloperidol-resistant" gerbils. Behavioral and Neural Biology 39:221–228, 1983

van Riezen H, Leonard BE: Effects of psychotropic drugs on the behavior and neurochemistry of olfactory bulbectomized rats, in Psychopharmacology of Anxiolytics and Antidepressants. Edited by File SE. New York, Pergamon, 1991, pp 231–250

van Riezen H, Schnieden H, Wren AF: Olfactory bulb ablation in the rat: behavioural changes and their reversal by antidepressant drugs. Br J Pharmacol 60:521–528, 1977

Varty GB, Higgins GA: Differences between three rat strains in sensitivity to prepulse inhibition of an acoustic startle response: influence of apomorphine and phencyclidine pretreatment. Journal of Psychopharmacology 8:148–156, 1994

Vernier VG, Hanson HM, Stone CA: The pharmacodynamics of amitriptyline, in Psychosomatic Medicine: The First Hahnemann Symposium. Edited by Nodine JH, Moyer JH. Philadelphia, PA, Lea & Febiger, 1962, pp 683–690

Vetulani J, Stawarz RJ, Dingell JV, et al: A possible mechanism of action of antidepressant treatments. Naunyn Schmiedebergs Arch Pharmacol 293:109–114, 1976

Vogel G, Hartley P, Neill D, et al: Animal depression model by neonatal clomipramine: reduction of shock induced aggression. Pharmacol Biochem Behav 31:103–106, 1988

Vogel G, Neill D, Hagler M, et al: Decreased intracranial self-stimulation in a new animal model of endogenous depression. Neurosci Biobehav Rev 14:65–68, 1990a

Vogel G, Neill D, Hagler M, et al: A new animal model of endogenous depression: a summary of present findings. Neurosci Biobehav Rev 14:85–91, 1990b

Vogel G, Neill D, Kors D, et al: REM sleep abnormalities in a new animal model of endogenous depression. Neurosci Biobehav Rev 14:77–83, 1990c

Wang P, Aulakh CS, Hill JL, et al: Fawn-hooded rats are subsensitive to the food intake suppressant effects of 5-HT agonists. Psychopharmacology (Berl) 94:558–562, 1988

Weinberger DR: Implications of normal brain development for the pathogenesis of schizophrenia. Arch Gen Psychiatry 44:660–669, 1987

Weiner I, Feldon J: Facilitation of latent inhibition by haloperidol in rats. Psychopharmacology (Berl) 91:248–253, 1987

Weiner I, Lubow RE, Feldon J: Abolition of expression but not acquisition of latent inhibition by chronic amphetamine in rats. Psychopharmacology (Berl) 83:194–199, 1984

Weiner I, Kidron R, Tarrasch R, et al: The effects of the new antipsychotic sertindole on latent inhibition in rats. Behavioural Pharmacology 5:119–124, 1994

Weiner I, Shadach E, Tarrasch R, et al: The latent inhibition model of schizophrenia: further validation using the atypical neuroleptic, clozapine. Biol Psychiatry 40:834–843, 1996

Weiner I, Shadach E, Barkai R, et al: Haloperidol- and clozapine-induced enhancement of latent inhibition with extended conditioning: implications for the mechanism of action of neuroleptic drugs. Neuropsychopharmacology 16:42–50, 1997

Weiss JM: Effects of coping responses on stress. Journal of Comparative and Physiological Psychology 65:251–260, 1968

Weiss JM: Coping behavior: explaining behavioral depression following uncontrollable stressful events. Behav Res Ther 18:485–504, 1980

Weiss JM: Stress-induced depression: critical neurochemical and electrophysiological changes, in Neurobiology of Learning, Emotion and Affect. Edited by Madden J IV. New York, Raven, 1991, pp 123–154

Weiss JM, Krieckhaus EE, Conte R: Effects of fear conditioning on subsequent avoidance and movement. Journal of Comparative and Physiological Psychology 65:413–421, 1968

Weiss JM, Stone EA, Harrell N: Coping behavior and brain norepinephrine level in rats. Journal of Comparative and Physiological Psychology 72:153–160, 1970

Weiss JM, Bailey WH, Pohorecky LA, et al: Stress-induced depression of motor activity correlates with regional changes in brain norepinephrine but not in dopamine. Neurochem Res 5:9–22, 1980

Weiss JM, Goodman PA, Losito BG, et al: Behavioral depression produced by an uncontrollable stressor: relationship to norepinephrine, dopamine, and serotonin levels in various regions of the rat brain. Brain Res Brain Res Rev 3:167–205, 1981

Weiss JM, Bailey WH, Goodman PA, et al: A model for neurochemical study of depression, in Behavioral Models and the Analysis of Drug Action. Edited by Spiegelstein MY, Levy A. Amsterdam, Elsevier, 1982, pp 195–223

West CHK, Weiss JM: A new, sensitive and potentially selective test for antidepressant therapeutic agents (abstract). American College of Neuropsychopharmacology 34:247, 1995

Wilkinson LS, Killcross SS, Humby T, et al: Social isolation in the rat produces developmentally specific deficits in prepulse inhibition of the acoustic startle response with disrupting latent inhibition. Neuropsychopharmacology 10:61–72, 1994

Williams JH, Wellman NA, Geaney DP, et al: Antipsychotic drugs effects in a model of schizophrenic attentional disorder: a randomized controlled trial of the effects of haloperidol on latent inhibition in healthy people. Biol Psychiatry 40:1135–1143, 1996

Willner P: The validity of animal models of depression. Psychopharmacology (Berl) 83:1–16, 1984

Willner P, Muscat R, Papp M: Chronic mild stress-induced anhedonia: a realistic animal model of depression. Neurosci Biobehav Rev 16:525–534, 1992

Wise RA, Rompre PP: Brain dopamine and reward. Annu Rev Psychol 40:191–225, 1989

Worms P, Broekkamp CLE, Lloyd KG: Behavioral effects of neuroleptics, in Neuroleptics: Neurochemical, Behavioral, and Clinical Perspectives. Edited by Coyle JT, Enna SJ. New York, Raven, 1983, pp 93–117

Wren AF: Master's thesis, Manchester University, United Kingdom, 1976 (reported in Leonard and Tuite 1981)

Zacharko RM, Anisman H: Stressor-induced anhedonia in the mesocorticolimbic system. Neurosci Biobehav Rev 15:391–405, 1991

Zacharko RM, Bowers WJ, Kokkinidis L, et al: Region-specific reductions of intracranial self-stimulation after uncontrollable stress: possible effects of reward processes. Behav Brain Res 9:129–141, 1983

SIX

Animal Models of Anxiety Disorders

George F. Koob, Ph.D.,
Stephen C. Heinrichs, Ph.D., and
Karen Britton, M.D., Ph.D.

Anxiety is a common emotion and an integral response to the vicissitudes of life. Anxiety is adaptive when mild but may be incapacitating and terrifying when extreme. To the clinician, anxiety appears in several clinically recognizable forms. Patients who experience persistent, diffuse psychological feelings of dread, unremitting nervousness, tension, and worry, accompanied by motor tension, vigilance, and autonomic hyperactivity in the absence of obvious external stressors, are differentiated from patients who are relatively symptom free until paroxysmal acute anxiety or panic attack occurs. Panic attacks are accompanied by subjective feelings of terror, apprehension, and fear of dying. Somatic symptoms occur in multiple physiological systems and include dyspnea, sweating, faintness, and trembling. The signs and symptoms of panic disorder are similar to those occurring during a life-threatening situation or during intense physical exercise. Further diagnostic distinctions are made among patients with anxiety due to posttraumatic stress disorder

(PTSD), obsessive-compulsive disorder, and phobic disorders, as reflected in DSM-IV (American Psychiatric Association 1994). Anxiety is also a prominent component of other psychiatric disorders, including schizophrenia, affective illness, and substance abuse and withdrawal.

ANIMAL MODELS OF ANXIETY

Animal models of anxiety are preparations that attempt to mimic some aspect of the anxious state. The most ambitious type of model attempts to mimic most or all of the signs and symptoms of the psychiatric syndrome (homologous model—face validity). This approach is difficult and misleading because many of the parameters that define anxiety (e.g., worry, apprehension, dread) are subjective. Another approach is to develop a model that mimics only specific aspects of the disorder rather than the entire syndrome. The particular aspect being studied may

The authors thank Mike Arends for his valuable assistance with manuscript preparation.

not even be symptomatic for anxiety, but it must be operationally defined. Another more limited approach is to develop an animal model of anxiety that is intended to reflect the efficacy of known antianxiety therapeutic agents and that leads to the discovery of new pharmaceutical therapies (pharmacological isomorphism). This approach may or may not model the actual psychiatric disorder.

Regardless of the type of model, predictive validity and reliability are essential (Geyer and Markou 1995). *Predictive validity* is the ability to make consistent predictions about anxiety based on an animal's performance in the model. Many animal models of anxiety have been used in a narrow sense, in which predictive validity refers to the model's ability to identify compounds with potential therapeutic usefulness. However, these same animal models have also led to the identification of variables that have enhanced the understanding of the neurobiology of anxiety and specific anxiety disease states. Other types of validity that are important to consider are

- ▪ *Face validity:* the apparent similarity between the behavior observed in the model and the specific symptoms of the anxiety disorder
- ▪ *Convergent validity:* the degree to which the model correlates with other models of anxiety
- ▪ *Etiological validity:* the same etiologies are found for the anxiety disorder in the animal model and in the human condition
- ▪ *Construct validity:* the accuracy with which the model measures what it is intended to measure

The state of clinical anxiety research has evolved rapidly over the past decade with the identification of several subtypes of clinically specific anxiety states. Whether these subtypes and their distinctive signs and symptoms reflect a single phenomenon or are independent syndromes with separate neurobiological substrates is unknown. Unfortunately, few, if any, animal models have been sufficiently validated to discriminate among the various subtypes of anxiety disorders. A future challenge will be to develop animal models that reflect some aspect of these clinical anxiety syndromes.

SELECTED ANIMAL MODELS OF GENERALIZED ANXIETY

Operant Conflict Test

One of the most widely used animal models of anxiety is the operant conflict test. This model is based on pairings of positive reinforcement (e.g., food or water) and punishment (e.g., shock). The test has proven uniquely useful in identifying drugs that have antianxiety effects in humans.

Historically, the conflict paradigm was based on the approach-avoidance tests developed by Masserman and Yum (1946), but the first operant configuration was introduced by Geller and Seifter (1960). Animals are first trained to press a lever for food reinforcement. At discrete time intervals, a tone signals the onset of a "conflict" period, during which lever presses are simultaneously reinforced with food and punished with electric shock. Rats pretreated with antianxiety agents, such as diazepam and chlordiazepoxide, elect to accept significantly more electric shocks during the conflict period than do control rats (Figure 6–1).

Studies using a variety of drugs have reported that behavior on the conflict test is highly selective for and sensitive to anxiolytic agents with a rank order of potency similar to that observed clinically (Cook and Sepinwall 1975). Neuroleptic phenothiazines and butyrophenones do not produce a release of punished behavior (Cook and Sepinwall 1975). Stimulants, such as amphetamine, also decrease the frequency of punished behavior (Geller and Seifter 1960). Analgesics, such as morphine, do not disinhibit punished behavior in this test (Kelleher and Morse 1964). Antidepressants and antipanic drugs, such as imipramine and amitriptyline, are similarly ineffective (Rastogi and McMillan 1985). The serotonin-1A (5-HT$_{1A}$) agonists produce inconsistent results (Martin et al. 1993; Yamashita et al. 1995) (Table 6–1).

Thus, in general, the Geller-Seifter conflict test is pharmacologically similar to the human state of generalized anxiety and has good predictive validity and reliability in identifying potentially useful pharmacotherapies for anxiety.

It has been argued that approach-avoidance models such as the conflict test have some face validity as models of human anxiety (Blackwell and Whitehead 1975; Brady 1968; Howard and Pollard 1977). This theory is based on the fact that approach-avoidance situations produce fear in the animal, and the aversive stimulation or anticipation of it is viewed as a basic cause of anxiety. However, little evidence supports this contention, and, in general, little effort has been made to explore this assertion or to draw other parallels between human anxiety and animal behavior in the conflict test.

Another version of the operant conflict model of anxiety is the Vogel conflict test (Vogel et al. 1971). In this model, water licking in fluid-restricted animals is paired with an electric shock. The two conflict models show fairly good convergent validity, but the Vogel procedure lacks a component that measures potential nonspecific effects (e.g., sedation, ataxia, general malaise) that can confound interpretation of results and produce false-negative results. However, the models appear to assess processes mediated by the same neurobiological substrates (Howard and Pollard 1991).

The use of operant conflict models has some disadvantages. An inherent limitation of all such drug-correlational models is that they may only identify compounds that act at the γ-aminobutyric acid (GABA)-benzodiazepine receptor complex. Second, the training procedures are often time-consuming. Third, the conflict models rely on an animal's motivation to consume food or water. Critics have argued that a drug-induced increase in appetite (or thirst)

might be sufficient to account for an antipunishment effect and thus confounds interpretation of the results. However, an examination of the literature shows that all the classic antianxiety compounds, including benzodiazepines and barbiturates (Cooper 1989), 3-α-hydroxylated pregnane steroids (Chen et al. 1996), and (acutely) ethanol (Beazell and Ivy 1949), produce some degree of hyperphagia. In a direct test of the hypothesis that the conflict test measures food motivation rather than anxiety, Pollard and Howard (1994) tested food-deprived rats over several days in the conflict model and compared their responses with those of rats receiving chlordiazepoxide. Hunger produced a significant rise in nonpunished responding but only a slight increase in conflict responding.

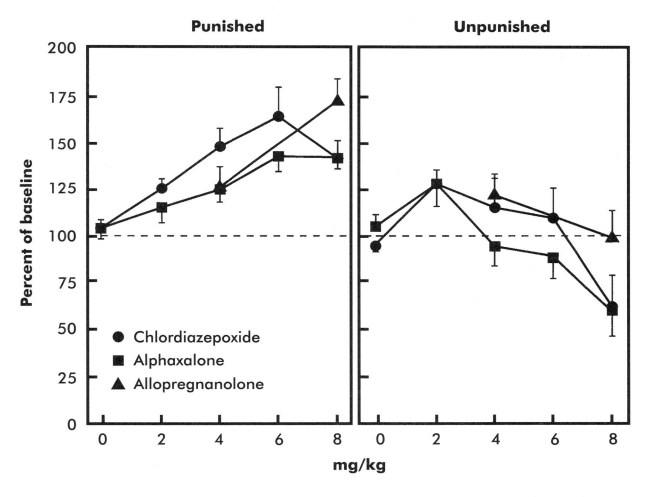

Figure 6–1. Effects of the benzodiazepine, chlordiazepoxide; the synthetic steroid, alphaxalone; and the natural steroid, allopregnanolone, on punished (conflict) and unpunished (random interval) responding in an operant conflict test. Results are expressed as the percentage of baseline response from the previous 2 days (mean ± SEM; n = 5–10 for each group).
Source. Reprinted from Britton KT, Page M, Baldwin H, et al: "Anxiolytic Activity of the Steroid Anesthetic Alphaxalone." *Journal of Pharmacology and Experimental Therapeutics* 258:124–129, 1991 and Brot MD, Akwa Y, Purdy RH, et al: "The Anxiolytic-Like Effects of the Neurosteroid Allopregnanolone: Interactions With GABA_A Receptors." *European Journal of Pharmacology* 325:1–7, 1997. Used with permission.

Table 6–1. Anxiolytic and anxiogenic treatment effects in conflict animal model of anxiety

Treatment	Conflict	References
Benzodiazepines	+	Cook and Sepinwall 1975; Howard and Pollard 1991
Benzodiazepine inverse agonists	–	Petersen et al. 1982; Prado de Carvalho et al. 1983
Corticotropin-releasing factor	–	Thatcher-Britton and Koob 1986
Progesterone abstinence	ND	
Serotonin autoreceptor agonists	±	Martin et al. 1993; Yamashita et al. 1995
Septal lesions	–	Yadin et al. 1993
Cocaine or amphetamine	–	Geller and Seifter 1960

Note. ND = not determined; + = anxiolytic efficacy; – = anxiogenic efficacy.

These results suggest that enhanced food motivation alone is not sufficient to account for the release of punished responding produced by anxiolytic compounds. In addition, the conflict test has good convergent validity with other models of anxiety that do not use either food reinforcement or shock. Why most anxiolytic compounds also produce hyperphagia remains to be elucidated.

The operant conflict test also is sensitive to anxiogenic pharmacological treatments, but these treatments often, if not always, generalize to a decrease in unpunished responding when measured (Koob et al. 1986). A proconflict effect has been observed with the benzodiazepine inverse agonists in a rat conflict test (De Boer et al. 1992; Prado de Carvalho et al. 1983), in the water-lick conflict test (Corda and Biggio 1986), and in a mouse conflict test (Petersen et al. 1982). Proconflict effects in the conflict test also have been observed with administration of other drugs that modulate the GABA receptor complex to decrease function (Koob et al. 1988), with administration of corticotropin-releasing factor (CRF) into the central nervous system (Thatcher-Britton and Koob 1986), and with administration of various stimulant drugs (Geller and Seifter 1960).

Elevated Plus-Maze Test

The elevated plus-maze test, an ethologically based exploratory model of anxiety, measures how animals, typically rats and mice, respond to a novel approach-avoidance situation—that is, relative exploration of two distinct en-

vironments: a lit and exposed runway compared with a dark and walled runway. Both runways are elevated and intersect in the form of a plus sign. No motivational constraints are necessary, and the animal is free to remain in the darkened arm or venture out onto the open arms. This type of approach-avoidance situation is a classic animal model of "emotionality" (Archer 1973) and is very sensitive to treatments that produce disinhibition (e.g., sedative-hypnotic drugs) and stress (Dawson and Tricklebank 1995) (Figure 6–2; Table 6–2). Moreover, the simplicity of the plus-maze test is very useful for measuring emotional reactivity to experimental treatments. Accordingly, the plus-maze test has been the subject of several hundred studies of rodent emotionality since the description and validation of the modern testing protocol in 1984–1985 (Handley and Mithani 1984; Pellow et al. 1985).

Early papers (Handley and Mithani 1984; Pellow et al. 1985) emphasized the significance of innate fearlike processes that motivated subjects consistently to prefer the enclosed maze arms at the expense of open-arm exploration. This contention of built-in aversive properties of the plus-maze test was supported by evidence of stresslike pituitary-adrenal activation (Pellow et al. 1985), nonopioid antinociception (Lee and Rodgers 1990), and broad central nervous system activation (Silveira et al. 1993) in subjects not given drugs and examined after exposure to the apparatus. Experimental treatments (Table 6–2) such as GABA inverse agonists, which reduce open-arm visitation, are identified as anxiogenic-like in the plus-maze test, whereas drugs such as GABA agonists, which increase open-arm exploration, are judged to be anxiolytic (Pellow and File 1986).

More recently, several dedicated reviews (Handley and McBlane 1993; Reibaud and Böhme 1993) offered critical examination of the validity of the plus-maze model of anxiety. For instance, the plus-maze test is sensitive, as expected, to serotonergic ligands (Treit et al. 1993a); however, the effects of 5-HT$_{1A}$ receptor agonists are equivocal (File et al. 1996; Handley et al. 1993), perhaps because of motor effects of this drug class that confound the measurement of emotionality (Dawson and Tricklebank 1995). Accordingly, caution should be exercised in modeling clinical anxiety disorders with the plus-maze test. Some benzodiazepine-sensitive anxiety states, such as ethanol withdrawal, are modeled quite well by the plus-maze test (Baldwin et al. 1991; File et al. 1991); however, the plus-maze test is apparently not sensitive to agents that induce panic in the clinical setting (Rodgers and Cole 1993). Agoraphobia, the fear of being in places or situations from which escape might be difficult (American Psychiatric Association 1994), is one anxiety disorder that may have

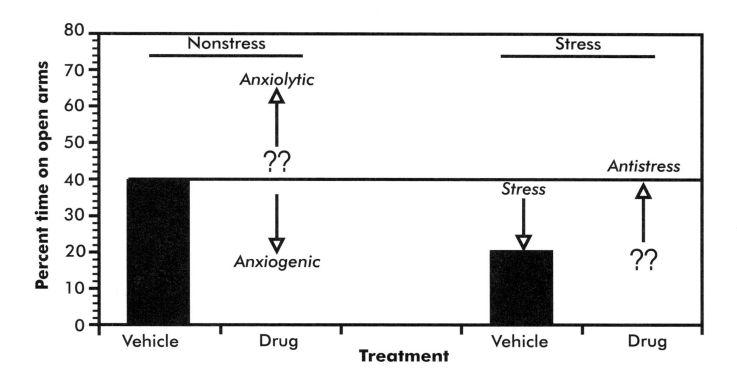

Figure 6–2. Plus-maze model of anxiety: effects of a stressor and test drug. Hypothetical data using a validated measure of emotionality, percent time spent exploring the open arms of the elevated plus-maze, which reflects the baseline 40% time exploration of well-handled, nondrugged control rats and the suppression of open-arm visitation by exposure to an experimental stressor. Drug and treatment effects can then be evaluated either on or off baseline to answer a specific experimental hypothesis. *Source.* Adapted from Brot MD, Akwa Y, Purdy RH, et al: "The Anxiolytic-Like Effects of the Neurosteroid Allopregnanolone: Interactions With GABA_A Receptors." *European Journal of Pharmacology* 325:1–7, 1997. Copyright 1997, Elsevier Science-NL.

Table 6–2. Anxiolytic and anxiogenic treatment effects in three unconditioned escape/withdrawal animal models of anxiety

Treatment	Plus-maze	Defensive withdrawal	Defensive burying	References
Benzodiazepines	+	+	+	Pellow and File 1986; Tsuda et al. 1988; Yang et al. 1992
Benzodiazepine inverse agonists	−	ND	ND	Grahn et al. 1995
Corticotropin-releasing factor	−	−	−	Diamant et al. 1992; Korte et al. 1994
Progesterone abstinence	ND	−	−	Gallo and Smith 1993
Serotonin autoreceptor agonists	±	ND	+	Handley et al. 1993; Korte et al. 1992
Septal lesions	+	ND	+	Pesold and Treit 1992
Cocaine or amphetamine	−	−	±	Parker 1988; Rogerio and Takahashi 1992; Yang et al. 1992

Note. ND = not determined; + = anxiolytic efficacy; − = anxiogenic efficacy.

face validity for the plus-maze test given the fear of open spaces inherent in this test (Treit et al. 1993b), but see section, "Animal Tests and State, Trait, and Different Kinds of Anxiety," later in this chapter.

The documented sensitivity of the plus-maze test to anxiogenic- and anxiolytic-like drug effects also confers the ability to detect environmental threats, including exposure to experimental stressors (Figure 6–2). For instance, pretest exposure to various stressors, including prolonged social isolation, electric footshock, forced swimming, surgery, novelty, and social defeat, significantly increases behavioral indexes of anxiety in the plus-maze test (Dawson and Tricklebank 1995; Rodgers and Cole 1993). Moreover, plus-maze performance appears to be exquisitely sensitive to seasonal variability (Reibaud and Böhme 1993), differences in apparatus construction or testing protocol (Handley and McBlane 1993), pretest handling of experimental subjects, and the novelty of the maze (Pellow et al. 1985). Thus, many environmental conditions, which may or may not be under experimental control, likely contribute to the experimental results. An excellent resource for the design and execution of the plus-maze test for rats and mice is available (Handley et al. 1993).

Defensive Withdrawal Test

The defensive withdrawal test consists of an illuminated open field with a small enclosed and darkened chamber situated near one corner of the field (Gorman and Dunn 1993). The extent to which subjects, typically rats and mice, remain in the enclosure without venturing to explore the open-field environment is taken as a measure of fearlike behavior. The defensive withdrawal test evolved from so-called timidity tests (Archer 1973), in which latency to emerge from a sheltered environment is recorded. The particular species-typical behavior modeled in emergence tests is the tendency for rodents in a diverse environment to seek physical protection from real or potentially threatening stimuli (Takahashi et al. 1989). Benzodiazepines decrease the latency to emerge and decrease the amount of defensive withdrawal, whereas anxiogenic treatments have opposite effects. For example, the adrenergic agonist isoproterenol significantly increased defensive withdrawal, whereas the β-adrenergic antagonist propranolol prevented the isoproterenol-induced defensive withdrawal, suggesting that the effect of isoproterenol resulted from stimulation of the β-adrenergic receptors (Gorman and Dunn 1993). Anxiety disorders that may have face validity with the emergence tests include agoraphobia, because defensive withdrawal constitutes a pas-

sive immobility response to environmental novelty, but see see section, "Animal Tests and State, Trait, and Different Kinds of Anxiety," later in this chapter.

The defensive withdrawal test also detects antistress properties of CRF antagonists. When injected centrally, both CRF agonists and competitive CRF receptor antagonists modify behavior in the defensive withdrawal paradigm (Takahashi et al. 1989) (Table 6–2). In particular, intracerebrovascular administration of CRF in animals familiarized with the apparatus increases both the latency to emerge from the small chamber and the mean time spent in the chamber during the 15-minute session. Infusion of CRF into the locus coeruleus produces similar changes in defensive withdrawal behavior; therefore, the interaction of CRF with noradrenergic neurons seems to be involved in defensive withdrawal behavior in rats (Butler et al. 1990). Conversely, intracerebrovascular administration of competitive CRF receptor antagonists reverses the CRF-like effect of restraint or swim stressors in a familiar environment (Rodríguez de Fonseca et al. 1996) and significantly decreases both the latency to emerge and the mean time spent in the chamber in animals unfamiliar with the apparatus (Yang et al. 1990). Details related to design and execution of the defensive withdrawal test are available (Gorman and Dunn 1993; Takahashi et al. 1989).

Defensive Burying Test

Rodents have a natural defense reaction to unfamiliar and potentially dangerous objects; they spray bedding material to cover the object. The best-known procedure uses a metal prod protruding into the cage and on which, at first contact, a mild electric shock is delivered (Andrews and Broekkamp 1993). Total time spent burying the prod, total number of burying acts, and height of bedding material deposited over the prod all serve as validated measures of emotionality in this test (Bowers et al. 1992; Korte et al. 1994). In an environment without bedding material, where the active burying option is not possible, subjects adopt a passive strategy by remaining immobile in locations away from the prod (Korte and Bohus 1990).

One variant of this procedure is to test subjects 24 hours after shock so that the conditioned rather than direct effects of shock can be studied. For example, the defensive burying test has been used to profile serotonergic anxiolytic drugs. The 5-HT$_{1A}$ receptor agonist ipsapirone dose-dependently decreases the duration of burying behavior both immediately and 24 hours after shock, thereby suggesting serotonergic involvement in unconditioned and conditioned anxiety situations that elicit an active coping behavior (Korte et al. 1992). The anxiety disorder most effectively modeled in terms of face validity by the defensive burying task may be specific phobia (formerly simple phobia), the essential feature of which is a marked and persistent fear of clearly discernible, circumscribed objects or situations (American Psychiatric Association 1994).

Alternative models of defensive burying use nonelectrified objects that provoke burying spontaneously (Njung'e and Handley 1991) (Table 6–2). For instance, rats will bury noxious materials such as food pellets that are coated with bitter-tasting quinine, drinking spouts that dispense hot pepper sauce, or flashcubes that discharge nearby. Mice do the same (for instance, burying harmless objects such as glass marbles), and the behavior is particularly vigorous in new cages with clean bedding material. Anxiolytic drugs, such as diazepam, inhibit this behavior by decreasing the duration and extent of marble burying (Njung'e and Handley 1991). The lack of extinction of burying behaviors with repeated exposure to the inducing stimuli has invited comparison (Broekkamp and Jenck 1989) of this animal model of anxiety with obsessive-compulsive disorders, the symptomatology for which includes repetitive acts aimed at preventing or reducing distress (American Psychiatric Association 1994). A specific protocol for performing the shock-prod and glass marble variants of the defensive burying test in rats and mice is available (Andrews and Broekkamp 1993).

Social Interaction Test

The social interaction test in rats measures the time spent in social investigation by pairs of male rats (File and Hyde 1978). The pairs of male rats are placed in an experimental arena, and the time that they spend in active social interaction (e.g., sniffing, grooming) is measured. The addition of infrared beams in the testing arena allows automated measures of locomotor activity and rearing and provides a measure of specificity. When rats are unfamiliar with these test environments, or when the test environment is highly illuminated, the overall level of social interaction is suppressed.

Anxiolytic compounds dose-dependently increase the social interaction in the unfamiliar, bright environment (Table 6–3) (File 1980; File and Hyde 1978). The social interaction test is sensitive to the anxiolytic properties of GABAergic agonists, such as benzodiazepines, ethanol, and barbiturates. Other anxiolytic compounds (e.g., steroids, opioids, and serotonergic drugs) can produce anxiolytic-like effects in the social interaction test, but the effects differ as conditions such as the lighting or the novelty of the testing situation change (for a review, see File 1993).

Chronic administration of antidepressants is ineffec-

tive (Johnston and File 1988). The social interaction test is also sensitive to anxiogenic-like treatments. Administration of CRF produces an anxiogenic-like action in the social interaction test (Dunn and File 1987).

The social interaction test has been validated behaviorally, physiologically, and pharmacologically for male rats (File 1980, 1988; File and Hyde 1978). However, attempts to develop a similar test for mice have largely failed because mice have a tendency to produce aggression, and mice do not respond to the familiarity of the test arena (De Angelis and File 1979). Similarly, the test has not been successful for female rats because of a decreased response to the familiarity of the test arena (Johnson and File 1991).

Pentylenetetrazol (PTZ) Cue Discrimination Test

The PTZ cue discrimination test is an operant test that uses drug discrimination to reflect a given emotional state. Animals are trained to discriminate between the presence and absence of a psychoactive drug, usually a drug with an anxiogenic-like profile, and use it as a cue for differential responding in an operant task (Lal and Sherman 1980). Rats are trained to press one lever after PTZ and another lever after saline. The stability of the PTZ discrimination is then assessed after different psychoactive drugs are administered. Anxiolytic compounds reliably suppress PTZ discrimination in a dose-dependent manner (Lal and Sherman 1980).

Table 6–3. Anxiolytic and anxiogenic treatment effects in the social interaction animal model of anxiety

Treatment	Social interaction	References
Benzodiazepines	+	File and Hyde 1978
Benzodiazepine inverse agonists	−	File et al. 1985
Corticotropin-releasing factor	−	Dunn and File 1987
Progesterone abstinence	ND	
Serotonin autoreceptor agonists	±	File and Andrews 1994; File et al. 1996
Septal lesions	+	Clarke and File 1982
Cocaine or amphetamine	−	File and Hyde 1979

Note. ND = not determined; + = anxiolytic efficacy; − = anxiogenic efficacy.

ANIMAL TESTS AND STATE, TRAIT, AND DIFFERENT KINDS OF ANXIETY

One major difference between animal models of anxiety and clinical disorders is that most patients requiring drug treatment for anxiety present with high trait anxiety, whereas all animal tests are based on conditions that presumably reflect transient changes in state. The tests described above measure adaptive responses to a test situation, not a pathological state. However, as long as these tests are predictive for various aspects of the pathological state, then they have validity as animal models (Geyer and Markou 1995). Clearly, the use of specific genetic strains and molecular genetic manipulations, as is currently under way with mouse models, will allow exploration of state versus trait similarities or differences.

An equally challenging question is whether different clinical syndromes, such as generalized anxiety disorder and panic disorder, can be discriminated by current animal models and whether such discrimination can be validated. Animal models are, of course, limited by the soundness of the relevant clinical literature (Segal and Geyer 1985), and whether panic disorder reflects the same underlying pathology as that of generalized anxiety disorder, only differing in intensity and severity, or is truly a nosological entity remains to be determined (File 1991).

Another approach to the question of what is being measured in animal models of anxiety has been the use of statistical procedures, such as factor analysis, to extract factor loadings from measures taken in various tests. In one such analysis, a modified hole-board apparatus was used to measure motor activity and head-dipping to measure exploration (File and Wardill 1975). Comparing the hole-board measures to the plus-maze and the social interaction test with factor analysis revealed three factors: 1) an index of anxiety, 2) an index of exploration, and 3) an index of motor activity (File 1991). Others who used comparable analyses reached similar conclusions (Belzung and Le Pape 1994; Hilakivi and Lister 1990; Lister 1987; Ramos et al. 1997; Trullas and Skolnick 1993).

Incorporating the Vogel punished drinking test extracted additional independent unspecified factors (File 1991). Although the activity factors appeared to differ significantly among tests, within each test, measures of anxiety and motor activity were separated adequately. Most interesting was that no common factor of anxiety-like state emerged—each test produced an independent anxiety-like factor (File 1991). Similar factor loadings were extracted after treatment with the benzodiazepine chlordiazepoxide (File 1991). Thus, these three animal tests—plus-maze, social interaction, and conflict—appear to be measuring different types of anxiety-like states.

Similar conclusions were made in comparing the light-dark box, plus-maze, hole-board, exploration with an object, and exploration without an object tests (Blackwell and Whitehead 1975), although the authors argued for extraction of state (exploration) and trait (novelty reaction) factors.

ANIMAL MODELS OF PANIC DISORDER, OBSESSIVE-COMPULSIVE DISORDER, AND POSTTRAUMATIC STRESS DISORDER

Little evidence exists to show that particular animal tests are analogues of particular clinical types of anxiety. However, the fact that different tests appear to measure different anxiety-like states in rodents, the explosion of basic research of the neurobiological basis of these anxiety-like measures, and the effects of clinically relevant drugs on these measures will ultimately provide the database with which to validate such hypotheses.

Despite the availability of specific treatments for panic disorder (tricyclic antidepressants, serotonin reuptake inhibitors), no generally accepted animal models of panic disorder exist. Recently, Cuccheddu et al. (1995) reported that a brief inhalation of carbon dioxide produces an anxiogenic-like effect in the Vogel conflict test. Because carbon dioxide inhalation produces subjective feelings of anxiety in some humans (e.g., Papp et al. 1993), this report may have some face validity. However, further work is needed to validate the procedure as a model of panic disorder. In addition, chronic treatment with several types of antidepressants, including tricyclics and monoamine oxidase inhibitors (MAOIs), has reversed conditioned suppression of drinking in rats, suggesting a potential predictive model for the use of antidepressants in panic disorder and generalized anxiety disorder (Fontana and Commissaris 1988; Fontana et al. 1989).

A model that has been proposed for obsessive-compulsive disorder is schedule-induced polydipsia (SIP). Food-deprived rats drink excessively when exposed to a schedule in which small amounts of food are delivered intermittently. Falk (1977) hypothesized that SIP develops as a displacement behavior to stress, similar to other displacement behaviors described by the ethologist Tinbergen (1952). Both displacement behaviors and SIP may serve a stress-reduction function. Selective serotonin reuptake inhibitors, such as fluoxetine and clomipramine, decrease SIP after 14–21 days of treatment, suggesting that SIP may be pharmacologically similar to the human condition (Roehr et al. 1995; Woods-Kettelberger et al. 1996). Although this possibility is intriguing and appears to have some face validity, other data are inconsistent with this hypothesis. For example, low doses of benzodiazepines increase SIP (Sanger and Corfield-Sumner 1979), and the anxiogenic-like compound CRF has been reported to attenuate SIP (Cole and Koob 1994), the opposite of what might be expected.

Several animal models of PTSD have been proposed, including sensitization models, fear-potentiated startle paradigms, and learned helplessness (for review, see Rasmusson and Charney 1997). PTSD involves a broad range of behaviors occurring together, and no specific pharmacological treatment for the syndrome is available. The challenge may be to isolate particular aspects of the syndrome in order to understand them more completely and to investigate them in terms of their origin, their context, and their responsiveness to selective interventions. Alternatively, recent studies on rodent defensive reactions (rat and mouse defensive test batteries) and more detailed analysis of defensive strategies in established procedures have provided a separation of reactions to proximal threat (e.g., freezing, burying) from reactions to distal threat (e.g., avoidance, flight) (Blanchard et al. 1993; Rodgers 1997). Drugs effective in generalized anxiety disorder may show greater effects on proximal threat behaviors, and drugs effective in panic disorder may show greater effects on distal threat behavior (Rodgers 1997).

CONCLUSION

Most animal models of anxiety have been developed to identify anxiolytic drugs and to reject nonanxiolytic drugs. Most of the standard models reviewed seem to have good predictive validity for drugs that are effective in the treatment of generalized anxiety disorder. Each model has its strengths and weaknesses that must be recognized, and use of multiple models provides convergent validation of the findings.

Clearly, more work is needed to develop and validate animal models of panic disorder, obsessive-compulsive disorder, simple phobias, and PTSD. Potential pharmacological treatments that reverse some of the disorders (panic, obsessive-compulsive) have not been adequately tested. Animal models for PTSD and simple phobias are fraught with difficulty because no specific treatments are available. Models for these disorders may need to be nonpharmacologically based and focus on theory-driven and mechanistic approaches.

REFERENCES

American Psychiatric Association: Diagnostic and Statistical Manual of Mental Disorders, 4th Edition. Washington, DC, American Psychiatric Association, 1994

Andrews JS, Broekkamp CLE: Procedures to Identify Anxiolytic or Anxiogenic Agents. Oxford, United Kingdom, IRL Press, 1993, pp 37–54

Archer J: Tests for emotionality in rats and mice: a review. Animal Learning and Behavior 21:205–235, 1973

Baldwin HA, Rassnick S, Rivier J, et al: CRF antagonist reverses the "anxiogenic" response to ethanol withdrawal in the rat. Psychopharmacology 103:227–232, 1991

Beazell JM, Ivy AC: The influence of alcohol in the digestive tract. Quarterly Journal of Studies on Alcohol 1:45, 1949

Belzung C, Le Pape G: Comparison of different behavioral test situations used in psychopharmacology for measurement of anxiety. Physiol Behav 56:623–628, 1994

Blackwell B, Whitehead W: Behavioral evaluation of antianxiety drugs, in Predictability in Psychopharmacology: Preclinical and Clinical Correlations. Edited by Sudilovsky A, Gershon S, Beer B. New York, Raven, 1975, pp 121–138

Blanchard RJ, Yudko EB, Rodgers RJ, et al: Defense system psychopharmacology: an ethological approach to the pharmacology of fear and anxiety. Behav Brain Res 58:155–165, 1993

Bowers RL, Herzog CD, Stone EH, et al: Defensive burying following injections of cholecystokinin, bombesin and LiCl in rats. Physiol Behav 51:969–972, 1992

Brady JP: Drugs in behavior therapy, in Psychopharmacology: A Review of Progress. Edited by Efron DH. Washington, DC, U.S. Government Printing Office, 1968, pp 271–280

Britton KT, Page M, Baldwin H, et al: Anxiolytic activity of the steroid anesthetic alphaxalone. J Pharmacol Exp Ther 258:124–129, 1991

Broekkamp CL, Jenck F: The relationship between various animal models of anxiety, fear-related psychiatric symptoms and response to serotonergic drugs, in Behavioral Pharmacology of 5-HT. Edited by Bevan P, Cools R, Archer T. Hillsdale, NJ, Lawrence Erlbaum, 1989, pp 321–325

Brot MD, Akwa Y, Purdy RH, et al: The anxiolytic-like effects of the neurosteroid allopregnanolone: interactions with $GABA_A$ receptors. Eur J Pharmacol 325:1–7, 1997

Butler PD, Weiss JM, Stout JC, et al: Corticotropin-releasing factor produces fear-enhancing and behavioral activating effects following infusion into the locus coeruleus. J Neurosci 10:176–183, 1990

Chen S-W, Rodriguez L, Davies MF, et al: The hyperphagic effect of 3-alpha-hydroxylated pregnane steroids in male rats. Pharmacol Biochem Behav 53:777–782, 1996

Clarke A, File SE: Selective neurotoxin lesions of the lateral septum: changes in social and aggressive behaviours. Pharmacol Biochem Behav 17:623–628, 1982

Cole BJ, Koob GF: Corticotropin-releasing factor and schedule-induced polydipsia. Pharmacol Biochem Behav 47:393–398, 1994

Cook L, Sepinwall J: Behavioral analysis of the effects and mechanism of action of benzodiazepines, in Mechanisms of Action of Benzodiazepines. Edited by Costa E, Greengard P. New York, Raven, 1975, pp 1–28

Cooper S: Benzodiazepine receptor-mediated enhancement and inhibition of taste reactivity, food choice, and intake. Ann N Y Acad Sci 575:321–336, 1989

Corda MG, Biggio G: Proconflict effect of GABA receptor complex antagonists: reversal by diazepam. Neuropharmacology 25:541–544, 1986

Cuccheddu T, Floris S, Serra M, et al: Proconflict effect of carbon dioxide inhalation of rats. Life Sci 56:PL321–PL324, 1995

Dawson GR, Tricklebank MD: Use of the elevated plus maze in the search for novel anxiolytic agents. Trends Pharmacol Sci 16:33–36, 1995

De Angelis L, File SE: Acute and chronic effects of three benzodiazepines in the social interaction anxiety test in mice. Psychopharmacology 64:127–129, 1979

De Boer SF, Katz JL, Valentino RJ: Common mechanisms underlying the proconflict effects of corticotropin-releasing factor, a benzodiazepine inverse agonist and electric footshock. J Pharmacol Exp Ther 262:335–342, 1992

Diamant M, Croiset G, De Wied D: The effect of corticotropin-releasing factor (CRF) on autonomic and behavioral responses during shock-prod burying test in rats. Peptides 13:1149–1158, 1992

Dunn AJ, File SE: Corticotropin-releasing factor has an anxiogenic action in the social interaction test. Horm Behav 21:193–202, 1987

Falk JL: The origin and functions of adjunctive behavior. Animal Learning and Behavior 5:325–335, 1977

File SE: The use of social interaction as a method for detecting anxiolytic activity of chlordiazepoxide-like drugs. J Neurosci Methods 2:219–238, 1980

File SE: The contribution of behavioural studies to the neuropharmacology of anxiety. Neuropharmacology 26:877–886, 1987

File SE: How good is social interaction as a test of anxiety?, in Selected Models of Anxiety, Depression and Psychosis. Edited by Simon P, Soubrie P, Wildlocher D. Basel, Switzerland, Karger, 1988, pp 151–166

File SE: Interactions of anxiolytic and antidepressant drugs with hormones of the hypothalamic-pituitary-adrenal axis, in Psychopharmacology of Anxiolytics and Antidepressants. Edited by File SE. New York, Pergamon, 1991, pp 39–55

File SE: The social interaction test of anxiety, in Neuroscience Protocols (Protocol Number 93-010-01-010-07). Edited by Wouterlood FG. Amsterdam, Elsevier, 1993, pp 1–7

File SE, Andrews N: Anxiolytic-like effects of 5-HT$_{1A}$ agonists in drug-naive and in benzodiazepine-experienced rats. Behavioural Pharmacology 5:99–102, 1994

File SE, Hyde JR: Can social interaction be used to measure anxiety? Br J Pharmacol 62:19–24, 1978

File SE, Hyde JRG: A test of anxiety that distinguishes between the actions of benzodiazepines and those of other minor tranquillisers and of stimulants. Pharmacol Biochem Behav 11:65–69, 1979

File SE, Wardill AG: Validity of head-dipping as a measure of exploration in a modified hole-board. Psychopharmacologia 44:53–59, 1975

File SE, Pellow S, Braestrup C: Effects of the β-carboline, FG7142, in the social interaction test of anxiety and the holeboard: correlations between behaviour and plasma concentrations. Pharmacol Biochem Behav 22:941–944, 1985

File SE, Zharkovsky A, Gulati K: Effects of baclofen and nitrendipine on ethanol withdrawal responses in the rat. Neuropharmacology 30:183–190, 1991

File SE, Andrews N, Hogg S: New developments in animal tests of anxiety, in Advances in the Neurobiology of Anxiety. Edited by Westenberg HGM, Den Boer JA, Murphy DL. Chichester, England, Wiley, 1996, pp 61–79

Fontana DJ, Commissaris RL: Effects of acute and chronic imipramine administration on conflict behavior in the rat: a potential "animal model" for the study of panic disorder. Psychopharmacology 95:147–150, 1988

Fontana DJ, Carbary TJ, Commissaris RL: Effects of acute and chronic anti-panic drug administration on conflict behavior in the rat. Psychopharmacology 98:157–162, 1989

Gallo MA, Smith SS: Progesterone withdrawal decreases latency to and increases duration of electrified prod burial: a possible rat model of PMS anxiety. Pharmacol Biochem Behav 46:897–904, 1993

Geller I, Seifter J: The effect of meprobamate, barbiturates, d-amphetamine and promazine on experimentally induced conflict in the rat. Psychopharmacologia 1:482–491, 1960

Geyer MA, Markou A: Animal models of psychiatric disorders, in Psychopharmacology: The Fourth Generation of Progress. Edited by Bloom FE, Kupfer DJ. New York, Raven, 1995, pp 787–798

Gorman AL, Dunn AJ: Beta-adrenergic receptors are involved in stress-related behavioral changes. Pharmacol Biochem Behav 45:1–7, 1993

Grahn RE, Kalman BA, Brennan FX, et al: The elevated plus-maze is not sensitive to the effect of stressor controllability in rats. Pharmacol Biochem Behav 52:565–570, 1995

Handley SL, McBlane JW: An assessment of the elevated x-maze for studying anxiety and anxiety-modulating drugs. J Pharmacol Toxicol Methods 29:129–138, 1993

Handley SL, Mithani S: Effects of alpha-adrenoceptor agonists and antagonists in a maze-exploration model of "fear"-motivated behavior. Naunyn Schmiedebergs Arch Pharmacol 327:1–5, 1984

Handley SL, McBlane JW, Critchley MAE, et al: Multiple serotonin mechanisms in animal models of anxiety: environmental, emotional and cognitive factors. Behav Brain Res 58:203–210, 1993

Hilakivi LA, Lister RG: Correlations between behavior of mice in Porsolt's swim test and in tests of anxiety, locomotion, and exploration. Behavioral and Neural Biology 53:153–159, 1990

Howard JL, Pollard GT: The Geller conflict test: a model of anxiety and a screening procedure for anxiolytics, in Animal Models in Psychiatry and Neurology. Edited by Hanin I, Usdin E. Oxford, England, Pergamon, 1977, pp 269–278

Howard JL, Pollard GT: Effects of drugs on punished behavior: preclinical test for anxiolytics, in Psychopharmacology of Anxiolytics and Antidepressants. Edited by File SE. New York, Pergamon, 1991, pp 131–153

Johnson AL, File SE: Sex differences in animal tests of anxiety. Physiol Behav 49:245–250, 1991

Johnston AL, File SE: Profiles of the antipanic compounds, triazolobenzodiazepines and phenelzine, in two animal tests of anxiety. Psychiatry Res 25:81–90, 1988

Kelleher RT, Morse WH: Escape behavior and punished behavior. Federation Proceedings 23:808–817, 1964

Koob GF, Braestrup C, Britton KT: The effects of FG 7142 and RO 15-1788 on the release of punished responding produced by chlordiazepoxide and ethanol in the rat. Psychopharmacology 90:173–178, 1986

Koob GF, Mendelson WB, Schafer J, et al: Picrotoxinin receptor ligand blocks anti-punishment effects of alcohol. Alcohol 5:437–443, 1988

Korte SM, Bohus B: The effect of ipsapirone on the behavioural and cardiac responses in the shock-probe/defensive burying test in male rats. Eur J Pharmacol 181:307–310, 1990

Korte SM, Bouws GAH, Koolhaas JM, et al: Neuroendocrine and behavioral responses during conditioned active and passive behavior in the defensive burying-probe avoidance paradigm: effects of ipsapirone. Physiol Behav 52:355–361, 1992

Korte SM, Korte-Bouws GAH, Bohus B, et al: Effect of corticotropin-releasing factor antagonist on behavioral and neuroendocrine responses during exposure to defensive burying paradigm in rats. Physiol Behav 56:115–120, 1994

Lal H, Sherman GT: Interoceptive discriminative stimuli in the development of CNS drugs and a case of an animal model of anxiety. Annual Reports in Medicinal Chemistry 15:51–58, 1980

Lee C, Rodgers RJ: Antinociceptive effects of elevated plus-maze exposure: influence of opiate receptor manipulations. Psychopharmacology 102:507–513, 1990

Lister RG: The use of a plus-maze to measure anxiety in the mouse. Psychopharmacology 92:180–185, 1987

Martin JR, Moreau JL, Jenck F, et al: Acute and chronic administration of buspirone fails to yield anxiolytic-like effects in a mouse operant punishment paradigm. Pharmacol Biochem Behav 46:905–910, 1993

Masserman JH, Yum KS: An analysis of the influence of alcoholism experimental neuroses in cats. Psychosom Med 8:36–52, 1946

Njung'e K, Handley SL: Evaluation of marble-burying behavior as a model of anxiety. Pharmacol Biochem Behav 38:63–67, 1991

Papp LA, Klein DF, Martinez J, et al: Diagnostic and substance specificity of carbon dioxide-induced panic. Am J Psychiatry 150:250–257, 1993

Parker LA: Defensive burying of flavors paired with lithium but not amphetamine. Psychopharmacology 96:250–252, 1988

Pellow S, File SE: Anxiolytic and anxiogenic drug effects on exploratory activity in an elevated plus-maze: a novel test of anxiety in the rat. Pharmacol Biochem Behav 24:525–529, 1986

Pellow S, Chopin P, File SE, et al: Validation of open:closed arm entries in an elevated plus-maze as a measure of anxiety in the rat. J Neurosci Methods 14:149–167, 1985

Pesold C, Treit D: Excitotoxic lesions of the septum produce anxiolytic effects in the elevated plus-maze and the shock-prod burying tests. Physiol Behav 52:37–47, 1992

Petersen EN, Paschelke G, Kehr W, et al: Does the reversal of the anticonflict effect of phenobarbital by β-CCE and FG 7142 indicate benzodiazepine receptor-mediated anxiogenic properties? Eur J Pharmacol 82:217–221, 1982

Pollard GT, Howard JC: Comparison of chlordiazepoxide and food deprivation on punished and unpunished responding maintained by food. Experimental and Clinical Psychopharmacology 2:37–42, 1994

Prado de Carvalho L, Grecksch G, Chapouthier G, et al: Anxiogenic and non-anxiogenic benzodiazepine antagonists. Nature 301:64–66, 1983

Ramos A, Berton O, Mormede P, et al: A multiple-test study of anxiety-related behaviours in six inbred rat strains. Behav Brain Res 85:57–69, 1997

Rasmusson AM, Charney DS: Animal models of relevance to PTSD. Ann N Y Acad Sci 821:332–351, 1997

Rastogi SK, McMillan DE: Effects of some typical and atypical antidepressants on schedule-controlled responding in rats. Drug Development Research 5:243–250, 1985

Reibaud M, Böhme A: Evolution of putative anxiolytics in the elevated plus-max, in Methods in Neurosciences, Vol 14: Paradigms for the Study of Behavior. Edited by Conn M. San Diego, CA, Academic Press, 1993, pp 230–239

Rodgers RJ: Animal models of "anxiety": where next? Behavioural Pharmacology 8:477–496, 1997

Rodgers RJ, Cole JC: Anxiety enhancement in the murine elevated plus maze by immediate prior exposure to social stressors. Physiol Behav 53:383–388, 1993

Rodríguez de Fonseca F, Rubio P, Menzaghi F, et al: Corticotropin-releasing factor (CRF) antagonist [D-phe[12], Nl[21,38], C[α]MeLeu[37]] CRF attenuates the acute actions of the highly potent cannabinoid receptor agonist Hu-210 on defensive-withdrawal behavior in rats. J Pharmacol Exp Ther 276:56–64, 1996

Roehr J, Woods A, Corbett R, et al: Changes in paroxetine binding in the cerebral cortex of polydipsic rats. Eur J Pharmacol 278:75–78, 1995

Rogerio R, Takahashi RN: Anxiogenic properties of cocaine in the rat evaluated with the elevated plus-maze. Pharmacol Biochem Behav 43:631–633, 1992

Sanger DJ, Corfield-Sumner PK: Schedule-induced drinking and thirst: a pharmacological analysis. Pharmacol Biochem Behav 10:471–474, 1979

Segal DS, Geyer MA: Animal models of psychopathology, in Psychobiological Foundations of Clinical Psychiatry. Edited by Judd LL, Groves PM. Philadelphia, PA, JB Lippincott, 1985, pp 1–21

Silveira MCL, Sandner G, Graeff FG: Induction of Fos immunoreactivity in the brain by exposure to the elevated plus-maze. Behav Brain Res 56:115–118, 1993

Takahashi LK, Kalin NH, Vandenburgt JA, et al: Corticotropin-releasing factor modulates defensive-withdrawal and exploratory behavior in rats. Behav Neurosci 103:648–654, 1989

Thatcher-Britton KT, Koob GF: Alcohol reverses the proconflict effect of corticotropin-releasing factor. Regul Pept 16:315–320, 1986

Tinbergen N: "Derived" activities: their causation, biological significance and emancipation during evolution. Q Rev Biol 27:1–32, 1952

Treit D, Menard J, Royan C: Anxiogenic stimuli in the elevated plus-maze. Pharmacol Biochem Behav 44:463–469, 1993a

Treit D, Robinson A, Rotzinger S, et al: Anxiolytic effects of serotonergic interventions in the shock-probe burying test and the elevated plus-maze test. Behav Brain Res 54:23–34, 1993b

Trullas R, Skolnick P: Differences in fear motivated behaviors among inbred mouse strains. Psychopharmacology 111:323–331, 1993

Tsuda A, Ida Y, Tanaka M: The contrasting effects of diazepam and yohimbine on conditioned defensive burying in rats. Psychobiology 16:213–217, 1988

Vogel JR, Beer B, Clody DE: A simple and reliable conflict procedure for testing anti-anxiety agents. Psychopharmacologia 21:1–7, 1971

Woods-Kettelberger AT, Smith CP, Corbett R, et al: Besipiridone (HP 749) reduces schedule-induced polydipsia in rats. Brain Res Bull 41:125–130, 1996

Yadin E, Thomas E, Grishkat HL, et al: The role of the lateral septum in anxiolysis. Physiol Behav 53:1077–1083, 1993

Yamashita S, Oishi R, Gomita Y: Anti-conflict effects of acute and chronic treatments with buspirone and gepirone in rats. Pharmacol Biochem Behav 50:477–479, 1995

Yang XM, Gorman AL, Dunn AJ: The involvement of central nonadrenergic systems and corticotropin-releasing factor in defensive-withdrawal behavior in rats. J Pharmacol Exp Ther 255:1064–1070, 1990

Yang XM, Gorman AL, Dunn AJ, et al: Anxiogenic effects of acute and chronic cocaine administration: neurochemical and behavioral studies. Pharmacol Biochem Behav 41:643–650, 1992

SEVEN

Animal Models of Alzheimer's Disease

Donald L. Price, M.D., Sangram S. Sisodia, Ph.D.,
Claudia H. Kawas, M.D., David R. Borchelt, Ph.D.,
Philip C. Wong, Ph.D., Michael K. Lee, Ph.D.,
Gopal Thinakaran, Ph.D., and Juan C. Troncoso, M.D.

As more people reach old age (Olshansky et al. 1993), the prevalence of disorders that affect the elderly has increased significantly; the most common major disability in this age group is impairments in cognitive and memory processes. The most frequent cause of this problem is Alzheimer's disease (AD) (Evans et al. 1989; Katzman 1997; Khachaturian 1985; McKhann et al. 1984). The prevalence of AD—approximately 10% in persons older than 65 years (i.e., 4 million individuals in the United States) (Bachman et al. 1993; Evans et al. 1989; Pfeffer et al. 1987)—is increasing because of significant shifts in life expectancy and demographic parameters. In 1900, 1% of the world's population was older than 65 years; in 1992, that figure was 6.2%; in 2050, it is estimated that 25% of the population will be older than 65 years (Olshansky et al. 1993). Because of the increasing prevalence and the magnitude of the morbidity and mortality of AD, it is imperative to understand the etiologies and pathogeneses of this disease and to develop effective treatments to ameliorate or prevent this illness.

In this chapter, we discuss some of the recent advances that have been made in studies of animal models relevant to aging and AD (Price and Sisodia, in press; Price et al. 1996). Animal models for AD are important for several reasons. First, they provide an in vivo system for preclinical testing of new potential agents for the treatment of AD. Second, transgenic or gene-targeted animals allow researchers to examine the effects of modified expression of individual genes relevant to AD pathophysiology. Third, animal models help investigators examine the relationship between neurochemical or neuropathological changes in the brain and behavioral changes. Despite the advances that have been made in animal models for AD, it should be emphasized that neither the neuropathological features nor the clinical changes that occur in humans with AD have been reproduced in their entirety in animals.

GENETICALLY MODIFIED ANIMAL MODELS FOR ALZHEIMER'S DISEASE

Familial AD with an autosomal dominant inheritance accounts for approximately 10% of all AD cases. Subsets of

The authors gratefully acknowledge discussions with Drs. Linda C. Cork, Mortimer Mishkin, Cheryl A. Kitt, Lary C. Walker, Peter R. Mouton, John D. Gearhart, Bruce T. Lamb, Chun-I Sze, and Mary Lou Voytko.
This work was supported by grants from the U.S. Public Health Service (AG 05146, NS 20471, AG 08325, AG 14248) as well as the Adler Foundation, the Alzheimer's Association, the Develbiss fund, the American Health Assistance Foundation, and Merck, Sharp and Dohme. Drs. Price and Borchelt are the recipients of a Leadership and Excellence in Alzheimer's Disease (LEAD) award (AG 07914); Dr. Price is the recipient of a Javits Neuroscience Investigator Award (NS 10580).

early-onset familial AD cases are linked to mutations of specific genes, including the amyloid precursor protein (APP) and presenilin 1 and 2 (PS1, PS2) genes (Bird 1994; Haass 1997; Hardy 1997; Schellenberg 1995). A subset of late-onset familial cases as well as some sporadic (nonfamilial) AD cases are associated with the presence of the apolipoprotein E (ApoE, the protein; *APOE*, the gene) ε4 allele (Roses 1995). (These genetic associations are covered in detail in Murphy and Cordell, Chapter 30, in this volume.) Here, we discuss transgenic and gene-targeted ("knockout") animals designed to model altered expression of wild-type or mutant APP and/or presenilin proteins. These models have led to important insights into the roles of APP and presenilins in AD.

Transgenic Mice

APP transgenic mice.   A histological hallmark of AD is the presence in amygdala, hippocampus, and neocortex of senile plaques (Khachaturian 1985; McKhann et al. 1984; Probst et al. 1987, 1991) composed of dystrophic neurites in proximity to thioflavin S/Congo red–positive deposits of amyloid consisting of principally the amyloid β protein (Aβ; also called β amyloid). This approximately 4-kD peptide is derived from APP, a type I single transmembrane glycoprotein expressed in many cells, including neurons, and encoded by a gene on chromosome 21 (Glenner and Wong 1984; Goldgaber et al. 1987; Kang et al. 1987; Kitaguchi et al. 1988; Masters et al. 1985; Ponte et al. 1988; Robakis et al. 1987; Tanzi et al. 1988). Aβ species are deposited in the neural parenchyma (as diffuse or compact amyloid in plaques) and around blood vessels (congophilic angiopathy) (Glenner and Wong 1984; Iwatsubo et al. 1994; Lemere et al. 1996; Roher et al. 1986). Aβ-containing peptide species include Aβ40 and Aβ42(43), with the longer forms of Aβ42 deposited early. Aβ42 is the principal component in diffuse or compact amyloid plaques (Iwatsubo et al. 1994). These Aβ fibrillar aggregates act as a nidus for subsequent deposits of additional proteins, including α_1-antichymotrypsin, components of the complement cascade, ApoE and J, and cholinesterases (Abraham et al. 1988, 1989; Johnson et al. 1992; Mesulam and Geula 1994; Mesulam et al. 1992; Rogers et al. 1988; Schmechel et al. 1993; Snow et al. 1988; Strittmatter et al. 1993; Wisniewski and Frangione 1992). Aβ amyloidogenesis in AD is discussed further in Chapter 30.

To generate animal models of Aβ amyloidogenesis and the associated histopathology of AD, many groups have created transgenic mice that express wild-type APP, familial AD–linked APP variants, carboxyterminal (C-terminal) fragments of APP, and Aβ itself (Borchelt et al.

1997; Buxbaum et al. 1993; Games et al. 1995; Higgins et al. 1994; Hsiao et al. 1995, 1996; Irizarry et al. 1997; Kammesheidt et al. 1992; LaFerla et al. 1995; Lamb et al. 1993, 1997; Masliah et al. 1996; Moran et al. 1995; Nalbantoglu et al. 1997; Neve et al. 1992). These efforts have produced multiple lines of transgenic mice, and to illustrate the approach, we reviewed several models that recapitulate some of the neuropathological features of human AD (Games et al. 1995; Hsiao et al. 1996). Studies of these lines of transgenic mice as well as lines produced in future experiments will be valuable for investigating mechanisms for testing therapies. To illustrate the approach and outcomes, we have selected several studies for discussion.

In one line of mice, the platelet-derived growth factor β-promoter was used to drive the expression of a human APP minigene that encodes the familial AD–linked APP (717V→F) mutation in an outbred strain; the construct contained portions of APP introns 6–8 that allow alternative splicing of exons 7 and 8. Levels of human APP messenger RNA (mRNA) and protein significantly exceeded levels of endogenous murine APP. The transcripts encoded the three major splicing variants, particularly the Kunitz protease inhibitor coding APP isoform (KPI; see Chapter 30), and levels of the transgene (Tg) product were four to five times higher than levels of endogenous APP (Games et al. 1995). The brain showed diffuse Aβ deposits, and plaques with dystrophic neurites were found around Aβ cores (Masliah et al. 1996).

In a second line of transgenic mice, the hamster prion protein (PrP) promoter overexpressed human APP 695.swe (the "Swedish" familial AD APP mutation; Hsiao et al. 1996; see Chapter 30). These mice were given two memory tests (spatial reference and alternation tasks); at age 9–10 months, animals were impaired on these tasks. The interpretation of these observations has been challenged (Routtenberg 1997) and defended (Hsiao et al. 1997). In brain, levels of Aβ40 and Aβ42 were increased 5-fold and 14-fold, respectively; dystrophic neurites and Aβ deposits were conspicuous in amygdala, hippocampus, and cortex. Although abnormalities were detected in the neuropil of the hippocampus, neuronal loss in CA1 was not evident (Irizarry et al. 1997). Similar strategies using a mouse PrP promoter have recently produced two additional lines of human APPswe transgenic mice that develop Aβ deposits at age 17–20 months (Borchelt et al. 1997).

In transgenic mice containing yeast artificial chromosomes (YACs) within which resides the entire 400 kD human APP gene with the "Swedish" mutation, Lamb and colleagues (1997) showed that the levels of Aβ peptides were increased in the brain and that the levels of α-secretase-generated soluble APP derivatives (nonpathogenic products of APP metabolism; see Chapter 30) were diminished. In contrast, levels of the longer, pathogenic Aβ peptides (i.e., Aβ42, 43) were elevated in the YAC transgenic mice expressing the APPV717I mutation. Thus, in vivo, both familial AD mutations influence APP processing to increase levels of the amyloidogenic Aβ42, 43 fragments, with the APPswe transgenic mice showing increased levels of all Aβ peptides, and the APPV717I transgenic mice showing selective elevations in levels of Aβ42 (Lamb et al. 1997).

In all lines of APP transgenic animals with increased levels of Aβ, the mutant APP transgene was expressed at high levels in nervous tissue, and the mice lived well into adult life. Findings in the APP transgenic mice are consistent with studies of other successful Tg models that have reproduced familial amyotrophic lateral sclerosis, prion diseases, and SCA-1 by overexpressing mutant superoxide dismutase 1 (SOD1), PrP, and ataxin-1, respectively (Burright et al. 1995; Hsiao et al. 1990; Wong et al. 1995).

PS1 and APP transgenic mice. PS1 and PS2, encoded by genes on chromosomes 14 and 1, respectively, are highly homologous proteins (Sherrington et al. 1995) predicted to contain eight transmembrane helices (Doan et al. 1996a). Mutations in the PS1 gene appear to be the cause of up to 50% of cases of early-onset familial AD (Alzheimer's Disease Collaborative Group 1995; Sherrington et al. 1995; St George-Hyslop et al. 1992). Approximately 50% of PS1 mutations occur within or immediately adjacent to the predicted loop domain (Alzheimer's Disease Collaborative Group 1995; Doan et al. 1996b; Sherrington et al. 1995). Patients with the Glu 280 Ala mutation show massive deposits of Aβ42 in many brain regions (Lemere et al. 1996). The PS2 gene shows substantial homology to PS1, and PS2 mutations have been reported to cause autosomal dominant AD in Volga German kindreds and in an Italian pedigree (Levy-Lahad et al. 1995a, 1995b; Li et al. 1995; Rogaev et al. 1995).

The mechanisms by which mutations in PS1 and PS2 predispose individuals to familial AD are not clear, but recent studies indicate that the mutation in PS1 influences levels of Aβ42: plasma and conditioned media from fibroblasts obtained from carriers of PS1 and PS2 mutations have elevated levels of Aβ42 species as compared with samples from unaffected family members (Scheuner et al. 1996); in vitro studies of transfected cell lines expressing PS1 mutations (A246E, M146L, or ΔE9) have increased Aβ42-to-Aβ40 ratios as compared with ratios in media of cells expressing wild-type PS1 (Borchelt et al. 1996).

Thus, one mechanism by which these mutant PS1 could cause AD is to influence APP processing to increase the extracellular concentration of Aβ42 peptides prone to deposition/aggregation and thought to be toxic Aβ species.

Studies using transgenic PS1 mice support this hypothesis. In the brains of young (2–3 month) transgenic mice that express human PS1 harboring familial AD–linked mutations, the Aβ42:40 ratio is increased (Borchelt et al. 1996; Citron et al. 1997; Duff et al. 1996; Thinakaran et al. 1996). In our studies, we coexpressed A246E human PS1 and a chimeric mouse/human APP695 harboring a human Aβ domain as well as mutations (K595N, M596L) linked to APPswe familial AD pedigrees (Borchelt et al. 1996). At age 12 months, transgenic animals that coexpress A246E human PS1 and APPswe contained numerous amyloid deposits (Borchelt et al. 1997), many of which were associated with dystrophic neurites and reactive astrocytes. Parallel analyses of brains from age-matched animals that express APP695.swe alone or mice that express A246E human PS1 alone were free of amyloid deposits (Borchelt et al. 1997). These observations indicate that A246E human PS1 acts synergistically with APPswe to accelerate the rate of amyloid deposition. Our findings suggest that the principal mechanism by which mutations in PS1 cause disease is through elevating extracellular concentrations of Aβ1–42 and, thereby, accelerating the deposition of amyloid.

Gene-Targeted Mice

APP knockout mice. When compared with hemizygous APP or wild-type littermates, homozygous APP knockout mice were fertile and viable but had subtle decreases in locomotor activity and forelimb grip strength as well as reactive astrogliosis (Zheng et al. 1995). The absence of substantial phenotypes in APP knockout mice may be related to functional redundancy provided by homologous amyloid precursor-like proteins (APLP1 and APLP2), molecules expressed at high levels with developmental and cellular distributions similar to those of APP (Slunt et al. 1994; Wasco et al. 1992, 1993).

PS1 knockout mice. Homozygous mutant mice failed to survive beyond the early postnatal period (Shen et al. 1997; Wong et al. 1997). The most striking phenotype observed in PS1$^{-/-}$ embryos was a severe perturbation in the development of the axial skeleton and ribs. The failed development of the axial skeleton in PS1$^{-/-}$ animals was traced to defects in somitogenesis; in E8.5 and E9.5 embryos, somites were irregularly shaped and misaligned along the entire length of the neural tube and largely absent at the caudalmost regions. The abnormal somite patterns in PS1[-/-] embryos are highly reminiscent of somite segmentation defects described in mice with functionally inactivated Notch1 and Dll1 (encoding a Notch ligand) alleles (Conlon et al. 1995; Hrabe de Angelis et al. 1997). Remarkably, the expression of mRNA that encodes Notch1 and Dll1 is reduced considerably in the presomitic mesoderm of PS1[-/-] mice (Wong et al. 1997). In addition, all PS1[-/-] embryos had intraparenchymal hemorrhages after day 11 of gestation. It has also been reported that, in the brains of PS1[-/-] mice, the ventricular zone is thinner by day 14.5, and the massive neuronal loss in specific subregions is apparent after day 16.5. Shen and colleagues (1997) interpreted these observations to indicate that PS1 is required for normal neurogenesis and neuronal survival, but, in the face of confounding cerebral hemorrhage, this interpretation may not be correct. A more satisfying model, in which the PS1 gene is ablated in a conditional manner, is required to clarify this issue.

AGED NONHUMAN PRIMATES

Although transgenic and knockout rodent models for AD have been extremely informative, aged wild-type mice and rats do not develop behavioral or neuropathological changes analogous to those seen in human aging and AD. In contrast, behavioral and neuropathological changes that occur in aged nonhuman primates closely resemble those occurring in aged humans and in patients with AD (Presty et al. 1987; Rapp and Amaral 1992; Walker et al. 1988a). Our laboratory has behaviorally characterized a colony of rhesus monkeys ages 3–34 years (Bachevalier et al. 1991; Presty et al. 1987) by using behavioral tasks chosen on the basis of previous research showing that the successful performance of each task requires the integrity of relatively specific regions of brain. The delayed nonmatching-to-sample task assesses visual object recognition memory. Performance deteriorates when memory is challenged by increasing delay and list length, and impairments in this task are most significant in the oldest group of monkeys. Because successful performance of the delayed nonmatching-to-sample task depends on the integrity of the parahippocampal gyrus, hippocampus, inferior temporal cortex, ventromedial prefrontal cortex, medial thalamus, and basal forebrain cholinergic system, aged monkeys showing deficits in recognition memory are thought to have lesions in one or more of these brain regions. This theory is significant in that many of these brain regions show extensive neurodegeneration in humans with AD as well (Braak and Braak 1991, 1994; Braak et al.

1996a, 1996b; D'Amato et al. 1987; De Souza et al. 1986; Hyman et al. 1984, 1986, 1990; Kemper 1984; Vogels et al. 1990; Whitehouse et al. 1982; Zweig et al. 1988).

This cohort of monkeys was also tested on several other tasks, including delayed response (spatial learning), 24-hour concurrent discrimination learning (habit formation), route following (visuospatial orientation), and simple visual discrimination. Declines in short-term memory on the delayed-response task appear when monkeys are in their late teens and early 20s (Bachevalier et al. 1991; Rapp and Amaral 1992). These spatial deficits suggest that abnormalities may exist in the dorsolateral prefrontal cortex and/or dorsal part of the caudate nucleus. Aged rhesus monkeys are also impaired on a concurrent object discrimination task, which is a measure of habit formation (Bachevalier et al. 1991). This problem has been attributable to abnormalities of the inferior temporal cortex and, possibly, the caudoventral portion of the neostriatum. Aged monkeys are also less adept than younger monkeys at performing a route-following test of visuospatial orientation (Bachevalier et al. 1991). In contrast, tests for simple visual discrimination detect no significant differences between young and old animals. These behavioral investigations indicate that cognitive and memory deficits in rhesus monkeys appear in the late teens and become more evident in the mid- to late 20s (Bachevalier et al. 1991; Walker et al. 1988b). Impairments in performance of certain spatial abilities occur in some animals in their late teens; however, in other test categories, behavior is not altered until the 20s.

Aged monkeys have neuropathological changes similar to those occurring in older humans and in individuals with AD, including senile plaques, abnormal neurites, diffuse Aβ deposits, congophilic angiopathy/tau-immunoreactive neurofibrillary tangles (see Chapter 30), reduced numbers of subsets of neurons, and a decrease in several markers of transmitter systems (Abraham et al. 1989; Brizzee et al. 1980; Cork et al. 1990; Selkoe et al. 1987; Struble et al. 1982, 1985; Walker et al. 1987, 1988b, 1990; Wisniewski and Terry 1973b). The senile plaques, composed of neurites and deposits of Aβ40 and 42, in aged monkeys are virtually identical to those in aged humans and in individuals with AD (Abraham et al. 1989; Selkoe et al. 1987; Struble et al. 1985; Walker et al. 1987; Wisniewski and Terry 1973a, 1973b). Enlarged neurites (i.e., distal axons, nerve terminals, and dendrites) and preamyloid deposits in the parenchyma of cortex appear early in the third decade of life (Cork et al. 1990; Selkoe et al. 1987; Struble et al. 1982, 1985; Walker et al. 1988b; Wisniewski and Terry 1973b). These neurites are derived from cholinergic, monoaminergic, serotonergic, γ-aminobutyric acid

(GABA)ergic, and peptidergic populations of neurons (Kitt et al. 1984, 1985, 1989; Walker et al. 1985, 1987, 1988b). In individual plaques, neurites may be derived from more than one transmitter-specific system (Walker et al. 1988b). Neurites accumulate a variety of constituents, including membranous elements, mitochondria (some degenerating), lysosomes, APP, phosphorylated neurofilaments, acetylcholinesterase, transmitter markers, and synaptophysin (Martin et al. 1991). In individual plaques, APP- and synaptophysin-immunoreactive structures are often surrounded by a halo of distorted neuropil that, in adjacent sections, contains Aβ immunoreactivity. The presence of APP-like immunoreactivity in neuronal perikarya, axons, and some neurites within Aβ-containing plaques suggests that neurons (i.e., neurites, dendrites, and degenerating cell bodies) serve as one source for some of the Aβ deposited in the brains of these aged animals. The proximity of Aβ to reactive cells (including astrocytes and microglia) and to vascular elements suggests that several nonneuronal populations of cells participate in the formation of Aβ (Frackowiak et al. 1992; Martin et al. 1991; Masters et al. 1985; Wisniewski et al. 1992).

In older rhesus monkeys, cholinergic and monoaminergic markers are reduced in some regions of cortex (Beal et al. 1991; Goldman-Rakic and Brown 1981; Wagster et al. 1990; Wenk et al. 1989). Cholineacetyltransferase activity is decreased in some regions in the oldest animals, and concentrations of both muscarinic and nicotinic receptor binding sites decline with increasing age (Beal et al. 1991; Wagster et al. 1990; Walker et al. 1988a). In the brains of some older monkeys, concentrations of dopamine and norepinephrine are decreased in certain regions of cortex (Beal et al. 1991; Goldman-Rakic and Brown 1981; Wenk et al. 1989). These studies suggest that alterations in certain neurotransmitter systems are partly responsible for cognitive impairments in some aged animals. The distributions and severities of lesions vary among different animals of the same age, and performances on specific behavioral tasks are probably related to patterns of brain abnormalities in individual animals. These findings are significant in that patients with AD show pathological changes in cholinergic brain function (Arendt et al. 1983; Armstrong et al. 1986; DeKosky et al. 1992; Francis et al. 1985; Pearson et al. 1983; E. K. Perry 1986; R. H. Perry et al. 1982; Vogels et al. 1990; Whitehouse et al. 1982, 1986) and in monoaminergic brain systems (Bondareff et al. 1982; Curcio and Kemper 1984; D'Amato et al. 1987; Tomlinson et al. 1981).

In summary, some behavioral, neuropathological, and neurochemical changes characteristic of AD are also present in aged nonhuman primates. However, the low reproductive rate, long generation time, and high care costs of nonhuman primates preclude large-scale use of these animals in screening new compounds for the treatment of AD.

CONCLUSION

Over the past decade, significant progress has been made in establishing diagnostic criteria for AD; in understanding the character, evolution, and mechanisms of the cellular pathology; and in defining genes implicated in familial AD. The discovery that mutations in genes encoding APP, PS1, and PS2 are linked to familial AD has ushered in a new and exciting era of research aimed at clarifying the relationships of genetic abnormalities to the pathogenesis of AD. Other mutant genes await discovery. In this chapter, we discussed information gained from the analyses of models of AD, including transgenic and knockout mice and nonhuman primates. We are particularly enthusiastic about the availability of transgenic animal models that will allow investigators to define the relationships between alterations in behavioral performance and neuropathological or biochemical abnormalities in brain, to test pathogenic hypotheses more rapidly, and to develop and test treatment strategies to prevent or retard specific pathological processes (e.g., Aβ42 deposition, neuronal degeneration).

REFERENCES

Abraham CR, Selkoe DJ, Potter H: Immunocytochemical identification of the serine protease inhibitor α₁-antichymotrypsin, in the brain amyloid deposits of Alzheimer's disease. Cell 52:487–501, 1988

Abraham CR, Selkoe DJ, Potter H, et al: α₁-antichymotrypsin is present together with the β-protein in monkey brain amyloid deposits. Neuroscience 32:715–720, 1989

Alzheimer's Disease Collaborative Group: The structure of the presenilin 1 (*S182*) gene and identification of six novel mutations in early onset AD families. Nat Genet 11:219–222, 1995

Arendt T, Bigl V, Arendt A, et al: Loss of neurons in the nucleus basalis of Meynert in Alzheimer's disease, paralysis agitans, and Korsakoff's disease. Acta Neuropathol (Berl) 61:101–108, 1983

Armstrong DM, Bruce G, Hersh LB, et al: Choline acetyltransferase immunoreactivity in neuritic plaques of Alzheimer brain. Neurosci Lett 71:229–234, 1986

Bachevalier J, Landis LS, Walker LC, et al: Aged monkeys exhibit behavioral deficits indicative of widespread cerebral dysfunction. Neurobiol Aging 12:99–111, 1991

Bachman DL, Wolf PA, Linn RT, et al: Incidence of dementia and probable Alzheimer's disease in a general population: the Framingham study. Neurology 43:515–519, 1993

Beal MF, Walker LC, Storey E, et al: Neurotransmitters in neocortex of aged rhesus monkeys. Neurobiol Aging 12:407–412, 1991

Bird TD: Clinical genetics of familial Alzheimer disease, in Alzheimer Disease. Edited by Terry RD, Katzman R, Bick KL. New York, Raven, 1994, pp 65–74

Bondareff W, Mountjoy CQ, Roth M: Loss of neurons of origin of the adrenergic projection to cerebral cortex (nucleus locus ceruleus) in senile dementia. Neurology 32:164–168, 1982

Borchelt DR, Thinakaran G, Eckman CB, et al: Familial Alzheimer's disease-linked presenilin 1 variants elevate Aβ1-42/1-40 ratio in vitro and in vivo. Neuron 17:1005–1013, 1996

Borchelt DR, Ratovitski T, Van Lare J, et al: Accelerated amyloid deposition in the brains of transgenic mice co-expressing mutant presenilin 1 and amyloid precursor proteins. Neuron 19:939–945, 1997

Braak H, Braak E: Alzheimer's disease affects limbic nuclei of the thalamus. Acta Neuropathol 81:261–268, 1991

Braak H, Braak E: Pathology of Alzheimer's disease, in Neurodegenerative Diseases. Edited by Calne DB. Philadelphia, PA, WB Saunders, 1994, pp 585–613

Braak H, Braak E, Bohl J, et al: Age, neurofibrillary changes, Aβ-amyloid and the onset of Alzheimer's disease. Neurosci Lett 210:87–90, 1996a

Braak H, Braak E, Yilmazer D, et al: Pattern of brain destruction in Parkinson's and Alzheimer's diseases. J Neural Transm 103:455–490, 1996b

Brizzee KR, Ordy JM, Bartus RT: Localization of cellular changes within multimodal sensory regions in aged monkey brain: possible implications for age-related cognitive loss. Neurobiol Aging 1:45–52, 1980

Burright EN, Clark HB, Servadio A, et al: SCA1 transgenic mice: a model for neurodegeneration caused by an expanded CAG trinucleotide repeat. Cell 82:937–948, 1995

Buxbaum JD, Christensen JL, Ruefli AA, et al: Expression of APP in brains of transgenic mice containing the entire human APP gene. Biochem Biophys Res Commun 197:639–645, 1993

Citron M, Westaway D, Xia W, et al: Mutant presenilins of Alzheimer's disease increase production of 42-residue amyloid β-protein in both transfected cells and transgenic mice. Nature Medicine 3:67–72, 1997

Conlon RA, Reaume AG, Rossant J: Notch 1 is required for the coordinate segmentation of somites. Development 121:1533–1545, 1995

Cork LC, Masters C, Beyreuther K, et al: Development of senile plaques: relationships of neuronal abnormalities and amyloid deposits. Am J Pathol 137:1383–1392, 1990

Curcio CA, Kemper T: Nucleus raphe dorsalis in dementia of the Alzheimer type: neurofibrillary changes and neuronal packing density. J Neuropathol Exp Neurol 43:359–368, 1984

D'Amato RJ, Zweig RM, Whitehouse PJ, et al: Aminergic systems in Alzheimer's disease and Parkinson's disease. Ann Neurol 22:229–236, 1987

DeKosky ST, Harbaugh RE, Schmitt FA, et al: Cortical biopsy in Alzheimer's disease: diagnostic accuracy and neurochemical, neuropathological, and cognitive correlations. Ann Neurol 32:625–632, 1992

De Souza EB, Whitehouse PJ, Kuhar MJ, et al: Reciprocal changes in corticotrophin-releasing factor (CRF)-like immunoreactivity and CRF receptors in cerebral cortex of Alzheimer's disease. Nature 319:593–595, 1986

Doan A, Thinakaran G, Borchelt DR, et al: Protein topology of presenilin 1. Neuron 17:1023–1030, 1996a

Doan A, Thinakaran G, Lanahan A, et al: Identification and characterization of a presenilin 1 interacting protein (abstract). Society for Neuroscience Abstracts 22:728, 1996b

Duff K, Eckman C, Zehr C, et al: Increased amyloid-β42(43) in brains of mice expressing mutant presenilin 1. Nature 383:710–713, 1996

Evans DA, Funkenstein HH, Albert MS, et al: Prevalence of Alzheimer's disease in a community population of older persons: higher than previously reported. JAMA 262:2551–2556, 1989

Frackowiak J, Wisniewski HM, Wegiel J, et al: Ultrastructure of the microglia that phagocytose amyloid and the microglia that produce β-amyloid fibrils. Acta Neuropathol 84:225–233, 1992

Francis PT, Palmer AM, Sims NR, et al: Neurochemical studies of early onset Alzheimer's disease: possible influence on treatment. N Engl J Med 313:7–11, 1985

Games D, Adams D, Alessandrini R, et al: Alzheimer-type neuropathology in transgenic mice overexpressing V717F β-amyloid precursor protein. Nature 373:523–527, 1995

Glenner GG, Wong CW: Alzheimer's disease: initial report of the purification and characterization of a novel cerebrovascular amyloid protein. Biochem Biophys Res Commun 120:885–890, 1984

Goldgaber D, Lerman MI, McBride OW, et al: Characterization and chromosomal localization of a cDNA encoding brain amyloid of Alzheimer's disease. Science 235:877–880, 1987

Goldman-Rakic PS, Brown RM: Regional changes of monoamines in cerebral cortex and subcortical structures of aging rhesus monkeys. Neuroscience 6:177–187, 1981

Haass C: Presenilins: genes for life and death. Neuron 18:687–690, 1997

Hardy J: Amyloid, the presenilins and Alzheimer's disease. Trends Neurosci 20:154–159, 1997

Higgins LS, Holtzman DM, Rabin J, et al: Transgenic mouse brain histopathology resembles early Alzheimer's disease. Ann Neurol 35:598–607, 1994

Hrabe de Angelis M, McIntyre J, Gossler A: Maintenance of somite borders in mice requires the *Delta* homologue *Dll1*. Nature 386:717–721, 1997

Hsiao KK, Scott M, Foster D, et al: Spontaneous neurodegeneration in transgenic mice with mutant prion protein. Science 250:1587–1590, 1990

Hsiao KK, Borchelt DR, Olson K, et al: Age-related CNS disorder and early death in transgenic FVB/N mice overexpressing Alzheimer amyloid precursor proteins. Neuron 15:1203–1218, 1995

Hsiao K, Chapman P, Nilsen S, et al: Correlative memory deficits, Aβ elevation and amyloid plaques in transgenic mice. Science 274:99–102, 1996

Hsiao K, Chapman P, Nilsen S, et al: Measuring memory in a mouse model of Alzheimer's disease. Science 277:840–841, 1997

Hyman BT, Van Hoesen GW, Damasio AR, et al: Alzheimer's disease: cell-specific pathology isolates the hippocampal formation. Science 225:1168–1170, 1984

Hyman BT, Van Hoesen GW, Kromer LJ, et al: Perforant pathway changes and the memory impairment of Alzheimer's disease. Ann Neurol 20:472–481, 1986

Hyman BT, Van Hoesen GW, Damasio AR: Memory-related neural systems in Alzheimer's disease: an anatomic study. Neurology 40:1721–1730, 1990

Irizarry MC, McNamara M, Fedorchak K, et al: App$_{Sw}$ transgenic mice develop age-related Aβ deposits and neuropil abnormalities, but no neuronal loss in CA1. J Neuropathol Exp Neurol 56:965–973, 1997

Iwatsubo T, Odaka A, Suzuki N, et al: Visualization of Aβ42(43)-positive and Aβ40-positive senile plaques with end-specific Aβ-monoclonal antibodies: evidence that an initially deposited Aβ species is Aβ1-42(43). Neuron 13:45–53, 1994

Johnson SA, Lampert-Etchells M, Pasinetti GM, et al: Complement mRNA in the mammalian brain: responses to Alzheimer's disease and experimental brain lesioning. Neurobiol Aging 13:641–648, 1992

Kammesheidt A, Boyce FM, Spanoyannis AF, et al: Deposition of β/A4 immunoreactivity and neuronal pathology in transgenic mice expressing the carboxyterminal fragment of the Alzheimer amyloid precursor in the brain. Proc Natl Acad Sci U S A 89:10857–10861, 1992

Kang J, Lemaire H-G, Unterbeck A, et al: The precursor of Alzheimer's disease amyloid A4 protein resembles a cell-surface receptor. Nature 325:733–736, 1987

Katzman R: The aging brain: limitations in our knowledge and future approaches. Arch Neurol 54:1201–1205, 1997

Kemper T: Neuroanatomical and neuropathological changes in normal aging and in dementia, in Clinical Neurology of Aging. Edited by Albert ML. New York, Oxford University Press, 1984, pp 9–52

Khachaturian Z: Diagnosis of Alzheimer's disease. Arch Neurol 42:1097–1105, 1985

Kitaguchi N, Takahashi Y, Tokushima Y, et al: Novel precursor of Alzheimer's disease amyloid protein shows protease inhibitory activity. Nature 331:530–532, 1988

Kitt CA, Price DL, Struble RG, et al: Evidence for cholinergic neurites in senile plaques. Science 226:1443–1445, 1984

Kitt CA, Struble RG, Cork LC, et al: Catecholaminergic neurites in senile plaques in prefrontal cortex of aged nonhuman primates. Neuroscience 16:691–699, 1985

Kitt CA, Walker LC, Molliver ME, et al: Serotoninergic neurites in senile plaques in cingulate cortex of aged nonhuman primate. Synapse 3:12–18, 1989

LaFerla FM, Tinkle BT, Bieberich CJ, et al: The Alzheimer's Aβ peptide induces neurodegeneration and apoptotic cell death in transgenic mice. Nat Genet 9:21–30, 1995

Lamb BT, Sisodia SS, Lawler AM, et al: Introduction and expression of the 400 kilobase *precursor amyloid protein* gene in transgenic mice. Nat Genet 5:22–30, 1993

Lamb BT, Call LM, Slunt HH, et al: Altered metabolism of familial Alzheimer's disease-linked amyloid precursor protein variants in yeast artificial chromosome transgenic mice. Hum Mol Genet 6:1535–1541, 1997

Lemere CA, Lopera F, Kosik KS, et al: The E280A presenilin 1 Alzheimer mutation produces increased Aβ42 deposition and severe cerebellar pathology. Nature Medicine 2:1146–1150, 1996

Levy-Lahad E, Wasco W, Poorkaj P, et al: Candidate gene for the chromosome 1 familial Alzheimer's disease locus. Science 269: 973–977, 1995a

Levy-Lahad E, Wijsman EM, Nemens E, et al: A familial Alzheimer's disease locus on chromosome 1. Science 269:970–973, 1995b

Li J, Ma J, Potter H: Identification and expression analysis of a potential familial Alzheimer disease gene on chromosome 1 related to *AD3*. Proc Natl Acad Sci U S A 92: 12180–12184, 1995

Martin LJ, Sisodia SS, Koo EH, et al: Amyloid precursor protein in aged nonhuman primates. Proc Natl Acad Sci U S A 88:1461–1465, 1991

Masliah E, Sisk A, Mallory M, et al: Comparison of neurodegenerative pathology in transgenic mice overexpressing V717F β-amyloid precursor protein and Alzheimer's disease. J Neurosci 16:5795–5811, 1996

Masters CL, Multhaup G, Simms G, et al: Neuronal origin of a cerebral amyloid: neurofibrillary tangles of Alzheimer's disease contain the same protein as the amyloid of plaque cores and blood vessels. EMBO J 4:2757–2763, 1985

McKhann G, Drachman D, Folstein M, et al: Clinical diagnosis of Alzheimer's disease: report of the NINCDS-ADRDA Work Group under the auspices of the Department of Health and Human Services Task Force on Alzheimer's Disease. Neurology 34:939–944, 1984

Mesulam M-M, Geula C: Butyrylcholinesterase reactivity differentiates the amyloid plaques of aging from those of dementia. Ann Neurol 36:722–727, 1994

Mesulam M, Carson K, Price B, et al: Cholinesterases in the amyloid angiopathy of Alzheimer's disease. Ann Neurol 31:565–569, 1992

Moran PM, Higgins LS, Cordell B, et al: Age-related learning deficits in transgenic mice expressing the 751-amino acid isoform of human β-amyloid precursor protein. Proc Natl Acad Sci U S A 92:5341–5345, 1995

Nalbantoglu J, Tirado-Santiago G, Lahsaïni A, et al: Impaired learning and LTP in mice expressing the carboxy terminus of the Alzheimer amyloid precursor protein. Nature 387:500–505, 1997

Neve RL, Kammesheidt A, Hohmann CF: Brain transplants of cells expressing the carboxyl-terminal fragment of the Alzheimer amyloid protein precursor cause specific neuropathology in vivo. Proc Natl Acad Sci U S A 89:3448–3452, 1992

Olshansky SJ, Carnes BA, Cassel CK: The aging of the human species. Sci Am 268:46–52, 1993

Pearson RCA, Sofroniew MV, Cuello AC, et al: Persistence of cholinergic neurons in the basal nucleus in a brain with senile dementia of the Alzheimer's type demonstrated by immunohistochemical staining for choline acetyltransferase. Brain Res 289:375–379, 1983

Perry EK: The cholinergic hypothesis—ten years on. Br Med Bull 42:63–69, 1986

Perry RH, Candy JM, Perry EK, et al: Extensive loss of choline acetyltransferase activity is not reflected by neuronal loss in the nucleus of Meynert in Alzheimer's disease. Neurosci Lett 33:311–315, 1982

Pfeffer RI, Afifi AA, Chance JM: Prevalence of Alzheimer's disease in a retirement community. Am J Epidemiol 125:420–436, 1987

Ponte P, Gonzalez-DeWhitt P, Schilling J, et al: A new A4 amyloid mRNA contains a domain homologous to serine proteinase inhibitors. Nature 331:525–532, 1988

Presty SK, Bachevalier J, Walker LC, et al: Age differences in recognition memory of the rhesus monkey (Macaca mulatta). Neurobiol Aging 8:435–440, 1987

Price DL, Sisodia SS: Mutant genes in familial Alzheimer's disease and transgenic models. Annu Rev Neurosci (in press)

Price DL, Kawas CH, Sisodia SS: Aging of the brain and dementia of the Alzheimer's type, in Principles of Neural Science. Edited by Kandel ER, Schwartz JH, Jessell TM. New York, Elsevier, 1996

Probst A, Brunnschweiler H, Lautenschlager C, et al: A special type of senile plaque, possibly an initial stage. Acta Neuropathol 74:133–141, 1987

Probst A, Langui D, Ipsen S, et al: Deposition of β/A4 protein along neuronal plasma membranes in diffuse senile plaques. Acta Neuropathol 83:21–29, 1991

Rapp PR, Amaral DG: Individual differences in the cognitive and neurobiological consequences of normal aging. Trends Neurosci 15:340–345, 1992

Robakis NK, Ramakrishna N, Wolfe G, et al: Molecular cloning and characterization of a cDNA encoding the cerebrovascular and the neuritic plaque amyloid peptides. Proc Natl Acad Sci U S A 84:4190–4194, 1987

Rogaev EI, Sherrington R, Rogaeva EA, et al: Familial Alzheimer's disease in kindreds with missense mutations in a gene on chromosome 1 related to the Alzheimer's disease type 3 gene. Nature 376:775–778, 1995

Rogers J, Luber-Narod J, Styren SC, et al: Expression of immune system-associated antigens by cells of the human central nervous system: relationship to the pathology of Alzheimer's disease. Neurobiol Aging 9:339–349, 1988

Roher A, Wolfe D, Palutke M, et al: Purification, ultrastructure, and chemical analysis of Alzheimer disease amyloid plaque core protein. Proc Natl Acad Sci U S A 83:2662–2666, 1986

Roses AD: Apolipoprotein E genotyping in the differential diagnosis, not prediction, of Alzheimer's disease. Ann Neurol 38:6–14, 1995

Routtenberg A: Measuring memory in a mouse model of Alzheimer's disease. Science 277:839–840, 1997

Schellenberg GD: Progress in Alzheimer's disease genetics. Curr Opin Neurol 8:262–267, 1995

Scheuner D, Eckman C, Jensen M, et al: Secreted amyloid β-protein similar to that in the senile plaques of Alzheimer's disease is increased *in vivo* by the presenilin 1 and 2 and *APP* mutations linked to familial Alzheimer's disease. Nature Medicine 2:864–870, 1996

Schmechel DE, Saunders AM, Strittmatter WJ, et al: Increased amyloid β-peptide deposition in cerebral cortex as a consequence of apolipoprotein E genotype in late-onset Alzheimer's disease. Proc Natl Acad Sci U S A 90:9649–9653, 1993

Selkoe DJ, Bell DS, Podlisny MB, et al: Conservation of brain amyloid proteins in aged mammals and humans with Alzheimer's disease. Science 235:873–877, 1987

Shen J, Bronson RT, Chen DF, et al: Skeletal and CNS defects in *presenilin-1*-deficient mice. Cell 89:629–639, 1997

Sherrington R, Rogaev EI, Liang Y, et al: Cloning of a gene bearing missense mutations in early onset familial Alzheimer's disease. Nature 375:754–760, 1995

Slunt HH, Thinakaran G, von Koch C, et al: Expression of a ubiquitous, cross-reactive homologue of the mouse β-amyloid precursor protein (APP). J Biol Chem 269:2637–2644, 1994

Snow AD, Mar H, Nochlin D, et al: The presence of heparan sulfate proteoglycans in the neuritic plaques and congophilic angiopathy in Alzheimer's disease. Am J Pathol 133:456–463, 1988

St George-Hyslop PH, Haines P, Rogaev E, et al: Genetic evidence for a novel familial Alzheimer's disease locus on chromosome 14. Nat Genet 2:330–334, 1992

Strittmatter WJ, Saunders AM, Schmechel D, et al: Apolipoprotein E: high-avidity binding to β-amyloid and increased frequency of type 4 allele in late-onset familial Alzheimer disease. Proc Natl Acad Sci U S A 90:1977–1981, 1993

Struble RG, Cork LC, Whitehouse PJ, et al: Cholinergic innervation in neuritic plaques. Science 216:413–415, 1982

Struble RG, Price DL Jr, Cork LC, et al: Senile plaques in cortex of aged normal monkeys. Brain Res 361:267–275, 1985

Tanzi RE, McClatchey AI, Lampert ED, et al: Protease inhibitor domain encoded by an amyloid protein precursor mRNA associated with Alzheimer's disease. Nature 331:528–530, 1988

Thinakaran G, Borchelt DR, Lee MK, et al: Endoproteolysis of presenilin 1 and accumulation of processed derivatives *in vivo*. Neuron 17:181–190, 1996

Tomlinson BE, Irving D, Blessed G: Cell loss in locus coeruleus in senile dementia of Alzheimer type. J Neurol Sci 49:419–428, 1981

Vogels OJM, Broere CAJ, Ter Laak HJ, et al: Cell loss and shrinkage in the nucleus basalis Meynert complex in Alzheimer's disease. Neurobiol Aging 11:3–13, 1990

Wagster MV, Whitehouse PJ, Walker LC, et al: Laminar organization and age-related loss of cholinergic receptors in temporal neocortex of rhesus monkey. J Neurosci 10:2879–2885, 1990

Walker LC, Kitt CA, Struble RG, et al: Glutamic acid decarboxylase-like immunoreactive neurites in senile plaques. Neurosci Lett 59:165–169, 1985

Walker LC, Kitt CA, Schwam E, et al: Senile plaques in aged squirrel monkeys. Neurobiol Aging 8:291–296, 1987

Walker LC, Kitt CA, Cork LC, et al: Multiple transmitter systems contribute neurites to individual senile plaques. J Neuropathol Exp Neurol 47:138–144, 1988a

Walker LC, Kitt CA, Struble RG, et al: The neural basis of memory decline in aged monkeys. Neurobiol Aging 9:657–666, 1988b

Walker LC, Masters C, Beyreuther K, et al: Amyloid in the brains of aged squirrel monkeys. Acta Neuropathol 80:381–387, 1990

Wasco W, Bupp K, Magendantz M, et al: Identification of a mouse brain cDNA that encodes a protein related to the Alzheimer disease–associated amyloid-beta-protein precursor. Proc Natl Acad Sci U S A 89:10758–10762, 1992

Wasco W, Gurubhagavatula S, Paradis MD, et al: Isolation and characterization of *APLP2* encoding a homologue of the Alzheimer's associated amyloid β protein precursor. Nat Genet 5:95–99, 1993

Wenk GL, Pierce DJ, Struble RG, et al: Age-related changes in multiple neurotransmitter systems in the monkey brain. Neurobiol Aging 10:11–19, 1989

Whitehouse PJ, Price DL, Struble RG, et al: Alzheimer's disease and senile dementia: loss of neurons in the basal forebrain. Science 215:1237–1239, 1982

Whitehouse PJ, Martino AM, Antuono PG, et al: Nicotinic acetylcholine binding sites in Alzheimer's disease. Brain Res 371:146–151, 1986

Wisniewski T, Frangione B: Apolipoprotein E: a pathological chaperone protein in patients with cerebral and systemic amyloid. Neurosci Lett 135:235–238, 1992

Wisniewski HM, Terry RD: Morphology of the aging brain, human and animal. Prog Brain Res 40:167–186, 1973a

Wisniewski HM, Terry RD: Reexamination of the pathogenesis of the senile plaque, in Progress in Neuropathology. Edited by Zimmerman HM. New York, Grune & Stratton, 1973b, pp 1–26

Wisniewski HM, Wegiel J, Wang KC, et al: Ultrastructural studies of the cells forming amyloid in the cortical vessel wall in Alzheimer's disease. Acta Neuropathol 84:117–127, 1992

Wong PC, Pardo CA, Borchelt DR, et al: An adverse property of a familial ALS-linked SOD1 mutation causes motor neuron disease characterized by vacuolar degeneration of mitochondria. Neuron 14:1105–1116, 1995

Wong PC, Zheng H, Chen H, et al: Presenilin 1 is required for *Notch1* and *Dll1* expression in the paraxial mesoderm. Nature 387:288–292, 1997

Zheng H, Jiang M-H, Trumbauer ME, et al: β-Amyloid precursor protein-deficient mice show reactive gliosis and decreased locomotor activity. Cell 81:525–531, 1995

Zweig RM, Ross CA, Hedreen JC, et al: The neuropathology of aminergic nuclei in Alzheimer's disease. Ann Neurol 24:233–242, 1988

EIGHT

Principles of Pharmacokinetics and Pharmacodynamics

C. Lindsay DeVane, Pharm.D.

The dose and the frequency of dosing necessary to produce the desired pharmacological response from psychoactive drugs differ widely among patients. This variability in the drug dose-effect relationship is not surprising given the large differences in patients' physiology, ages, range of severity of illness, and other variables. Thus, a rational approach toward drug dosage regimen design based on scientific principles is needed to reach therapeutic objectives without either underdosing and obtaining an unsatisfactory response or overdosing and risking toxicity (DeVane and Jusko 1982).

Pharmacokinetics is defined as the study of the time course of drugs and their metabolites through the body. This discipline is closely linked with *pharmacodynamics*, which is defined as the study of the time course and intensity of pharmacological effects of drugs. Pharmacokinetic and pharmacodynamic variability is a major determinant of the dose-effect relationship in patients (see Figure 8–1). Knowledge of these areas is essential in the drug development process and can be instrumental in individualizing dosage regimens for specific patients.

The interface between pharmacokinetics and pharmacodynamics, where drugs interact with receptors at an effect site (Figure 8–1), is increasingly becoming the focus of research. In psychiatry, measurements of plasma drug concentration are far more accurate than measurements of pharmacological effects. Sensitive analytical methods including gas and liquid chromatography and mass spectroscopy are routinely applied in animal and human studies to quantify drug disposition. Computer methods for applying observed data to mathematical models are helpful in

relating theoretical effect site concentrations to pharmacological effects (Holford and Sheiner 1982). Simple correlational methods suffice when pharmacological effects are direct and reversible, but many data sets in psychopharmacology require nonlinear models, which use more sophisticated analyses. These kinetic-dynamic models can help explain indirect pharmacological effects, delayed effects in time, and nonlinear effects that occur from graded drug exposure (Dingemanse et al. 1988; Stanski 1992).

The purpose of this chapter is to explain the basic principles of pharmacokinetics and pharmacodynamics that can aid in developing drug dosage regimens and to provide insight into observed dose-effect relationships. The presence of pharmacologically active metabolites, the pharmacogenetic differences between patients, and the interactions of concurrently administered drugs contribute to the variability in the dose-effect relationship. I review these areas of active research.

PHARMACOKINETICS

A human pharmacokinetic study typically results in a mathematical description of drug concentration changes in plasma over time. The value of these data and of their use varies according to patient circumstances. During drug development, this knowledge is essential to develop guidelines for ensuring safe and effective dosage regimens in clinical trials. In clinical practice, plasma concentration measurements are useful to guide dosage adjustments to reach targeted steady-state concentrations of lithium, the anticonvulsant mood stabilizers, and some tricyclic anti-

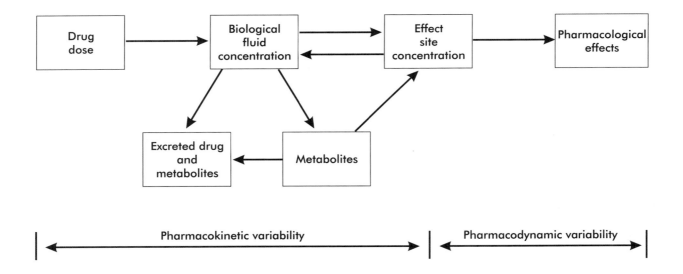

Figure 8–1. Pharmacokinetic and pharmacodynamic variability as determinants of the dose-effect relationship.

depressants and antipsychotics. Population estimates of drug and metabolite half-life can predict washout from the body when switching among antidepressants. This information is useful when prescribing fluoxetine, for example, which produces an active metabolite, norfluoxetine, with an elimination half-life estimated between 4 and 16 days. Thus, an interval as long as a month may be necessary after discontinuing fluoxetine before initiating treatment with a monoamine oxidase inhibitor to minimize the possibility of developing a serotonin syndrome. The fundamental description of drug disposition begins with studies of single drug doses.

Single-Dose Drug Disposition

Absorption. The route of administration is a major determinant of the onset and duration of a drug's pharmacological effects. Intravenous injection ensures that all of the administered drug is available to the circulation. The rate of drug injection or infusion can be used to control completely the rate of drug availability. However, few psychopharmacological drugs are administered intravenously. Rapid tranquilization with intravenous haloperidol or other neuroleptics generally has been replaced by intramuscular lorazepam (see Tueth et al., Chapter 44, in this volume; Salzman et al. 1991). Intramuscular administration is commonly thought to produce a rapid onset of effects, but exceptions are recognized. Drug absorption by this route can be slow and erratic with chlordiazepoxide (Greenblatt et al. 1974). Most psychoactive drugs are

highly lipophilic compounds, which are well absorbed when taken orally.

Drug absorption is usually a passive process occurring in the small intestine. The efficiency of oral absorption is influenced by the physiological state of the patient, by formulation factors, and by the timing of administration around meals. Most drugs are best absorbed on an empty stomach. The presence of food or antacids in the stomach usually decreases the rate of drug absorption. The physical characteristics of drug molecules may delay their entry into solution, which is a necessary step before absorption across gastrointestinal membranes. Under these conditions, the peak drug concentration achieved in blood or plasma is reduced and the time is prolonged following an oral dose to reach the maximum plasma concentration. The absolute amount of drug absorbed may or may not be affected.

The rate of drug absorption is important when a rapid onset of effect is needed. Antianxiety and sedative-hypnotic effects are examples. The effects of several benzodiazepines depend on the rate of absorption (Greenblatt et al. 1978). Acute drug effects are facilitated by administration apart from meals, but the anxiolytic effects of chronic benzodiazepine therapy should not change when the completeness of absorption is unaltered.

Formulation factors are especially meaningful when a drug effect is associated with achieving a minimal effective concentration (MEC) in plasma. Figure 8–2 shows the predicted plasma concentration curves of a drug following a rapid intravenous injection (I), an oral formulation that is completely absorbed with no presystemic elimination (II), an incompletely absorbed oral formulation (III), and a formulation that results in slow release and absorption of drug (IV). A formulation with poor bioavailability (III) may not result in a plasma concentration above the MEC, whereas a drug whose absorption is delayed (IV) may retard the onset of effect but maintain an effective concentration for a period similar to the more rapidly available formulations (I, II). A general rank order of dosage formulations providing the most rapid to the slowest rate of drug release for oral absorption is solutions, suspensions, tablets, enteric- or film-coated tablets, and capsules. Regardless of the dosage formulation selected, the last several hours of declining drug concentration in plasma occur in parallel, because drug elimination rate is unaffected by its rate or extent of absorption (Figure 8–2).

Drugs with short elimination half-lives, which must be given multiple times per day to maintain an effective concentration, may be formulated into sustained- or slow-release tablets or capsules for once- or twice-daily administration. Examples include venlafaxine and bupropion. For sustained-release formulations, the apparent elimination rate may actually reflect the absorption rate.

Many drugs undergo extensive metabolism as they move from the gastrointestinal tract to the systemic circulation (i.e., as they pass through the gastrointestinal membranes and hepatic circulation during absorption). This process is known as the *first-pass effect* or *presystemic*

elimination. A first-pass effect is usually indicated by either a decreased amount of parent drug reaching the systemic circulation or an increased quantity of metabolites after oral administration compared with parenteral dosing. This process is important in the formation of active metabolites for psychoactive drugs and is a major source of pharmacokinetic variability (George et al. 1982).

Gut wall metabolism of drugs is extensively accomplished by cytochrome P450 (CYP) enzymes in the luminal epithelium of the small intestine (Kolars et al. 1992). CYP3A4 represents approximately 70% of total cytochrome P450 in human intestine. Several useful psychopharmacological drugs are CYP3A4 substrates. These drugs are listed in Table 8–1 along with substrates, inhibitors, and inducers of the major human cytochrome P450 isoenzymes. The liver contains about two- to fivefold greater amounts of CYP3A protein (nmol/mg protein) compared with the intestine (de Waziers et al. 1990). Nevertheless, intestinal CYP3A4 has a profound effect on presystemic drug metabolism. Up to 43% of orally administered midazolam, for example, is metabolized as it passes through the intestinal mucosa (Paine et al. 1996). The exposure of drugs to gut CYP3A4 is not limited by binding to plasma proteins as can occur with hepatic metabolism. Differences in blood flow may also contribute to intestinal metabolism, thereby compensating for the lower quantity of CYP3A4 in gut compared with liver. CYP3A metabolism in the gut may be inhibited by grapefruit juice, which contains naringin and other flavonoids (Fuhr and Kummert 1995). One goal of current research is to reduce the intersubject variability of pharmacological effects by decreasing the variability in presystemic drug elimination through coadministration of nonabsorbable CYP3A4 inhibitors.

In summary, an important pharmacokinetic principle is that the choice of drug formulation and the route of administration can determine the rate at which the drug appears in the systemic circulation. This rate may be manipulated to retard the magnitude of the peak plasma drug concentration when it appears to be related to the occurrence of adverse effects. For example, a slow-release lithium formulation reduces gastrointestinal side effects. Alternatively, rapid absorption may be desirable to achieve immediate pharmacological effects.

Distribution.   Drug distribution to tissues begins almost simultaneously with absorption into the systemic circulation. The rate at which distribution occurs will partially influence the onset of pharmacological response. Access to effect sites depends on membrane permeability, the patient's state of hydration, regional blood flow, and other physiological variables. Physicochemical properties

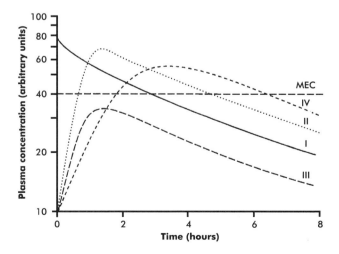

Figure 8–2.   Predicted plasma concentration curves following single doses of a drug by rapid intravenous injection (I), a dosage form with complete bioavailability (II), a dosage form with reduced bioavailability (III), and a dosage form that reduces the rate but not the completeness of absorption (IV). MEC = minimal effective concentration.

Table 8–1.   Substrates, inhibitors, and inducers of the major human liver cytochrome P450 (CYP) enzymes involved in drug metabolism

P450 enzyme	Substrates	Inhibitors[a]	Inducers
CYP1A2	Caffeine,[b] clozapine, haloperidol,[b] imipramine,[b] phenacetin, tacrine, theophylline,[b] verapamil,[b] warfarin[b]	Ciprofloxacin, fluvoxamine	Charcoal-broiled beef, cigarette smoke, cruciferous vegetables, marijuana smoke, omeprazole
CYP2A6	Coumarin, nicotine		Barbiturates
CYP2C9	Amitriptyline,[b] metoclopramide, phenytoin, propranolol,[b] tetrahydrocannabinol, [b] tolbutamide, warfarin[b]	Sulfaphenazole	Rifampin
CYP2C19	Amitriptyline,[b] clomipramine,[b] desmethyldiazepam,[b] diazepam,[b] diclofenac, ibuprofen, imipramine,[b] mephenytoin, moclobemide, naproxen, omeprazole,[b] piroxicam, tenoxicam	Omeprazole	Rifampin
CYP2D6	Amitriptyline,[b] codeine,[b] debrisoquin, desipramine, dextromethorphan, haloperidol,[b] imipramine,[b] metoclopramide, metoprolol, mexiletine, nortriptyline, ondansetron,[b] orphenadrine, paroxetine, pindolol, propafenone, propranolol,[b] risperidone, sparteine, thioridazine, timolol, venlafaxine[b]	Fluoxetine, paroxetine, quinidine, sertraline	
CYP2E1	Caffeine,[b] dapsone,[b] ethanol	Disulfiram	Ethanol
CYP3A4	Alprazolam, amiodarone, amitriptyline,[b] astemizole, bupropion, caffeine,[b] carbamazepine, cisapride, clarithromycin, clonazepam, codeine,[b] cortisol, cyclosporin, dapsone,[b] desmethyldiazepam,[b] diazepam,[b] diltiazem, erythromycin, estradiol, ethinylestradiol, fluoxetine, haloperidol,[b] imipramine,[b] lidocaine, loratadine, lovastatin, midazolam, nefazodone, nicardipine, nifedipine, omeprazole,[b] ondansetron, orphenadrine, progesterone, quinidine, rifampin, sertraline, tamoxifen, terfenadine, testosterone, trazodone, triazolam, venlafaxine,[b] verapamil,[b] zolpidem	Fluoxetine, fluvoxamine, ketoconazole, naringenin, nefazodone, sertraline	

[a]Inhibitory potency varies greatly (see text).
[b]More than one P450 enzyme is known to be involved in the metabolism of these drugs.
Source.   Ketter et al. 1995; Nemeroff et al. 1996; Schmider et al. 1996.

influencing the rate of drug distribution to effect sites include lipid solubility, ionizability, and affinity for plasma proteins and tissue components. Diazepam is highly lipophilic, and its onset of effect is rapid as a result of its entry into the brain within minutes after oral administration (Greenblatt et al. 1980).

The concentration of diazepam at its effect site may fall so precipitously as a result of redistribution that its duration of action after an initial dose is shorter than would be expected based on its elimination half-life. Frequently, the intensity and duration of the pharmacological effect of a second drug dose, taken immediately after cessation of the effect of the first dose, is greater and longer, respectively, than the intensity and duration of the effect of the first dose. This effect occurs with diazepam because of a sustained concentration at its effect site.

The predicted time course of drug concentration in plasma and in tissue following a single intravenous drug injection is shown in Figure 8–3. Drug concentration in plasma rapidly declines consistent with extensive distribution out of the systemic circulation. Drug concentration in tissue rapidly increases during this time. Pharmacological effects may not occur immediately but may be delayed until the tissue concentration at the effect site rises above an MEC. An equilibrium eventually occurs between drug in plasma and in tissue. Concentrations from this time forth

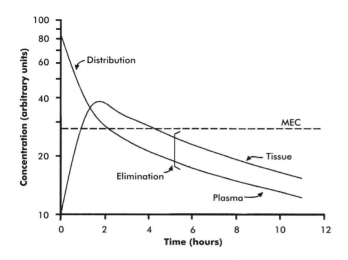

Figure 8–3. Predicted concentration of a drug in plasma and tissue following a rapid intravenous injection. MEC = minimal effective concentration.

decline in parallel during a terminal elimination phase.

The observed time course of drug concentration changes in plasma has frequently been considered in the pharmacokinetic literature to confer the characteristics on the body of a two-compartment mathematical model (Gibaldi and Perrier 1975). Many drugs appear to be absorbed into a central compartment composed of the circulation and rapidly equilibrating tissues and then distributed to less accessible tissues, which collectively form a peripheral compartment. This compartmentalization of drug concentration greatly aids mathematical analysis of pharmacokinetic data but is clearly an oversimplification because drug concentrations determined in animal studies can vary over orders of magnitude among different tissues (DeVane and Simpkins 1985).

Even though the drug concentration can vary widely among tissues, equilibrium eventually occurs between drug concentration in plasma and in tissue (Figure 8–3). For this reason, an MEC determined from plasma data may reflect an MEC at the effect site. The distribution of a drug in the body largely depends on the drug's relative binding affinity to plasma proteins and tissue components and the capacity of tissues for drug binding. This pharmacokinetic principle is illustrated in Figure 8–4. Only unbound drug is capable of distributing between plasma and tissues. Different degrees of plasma protein binding among antidepressants, for example, cannot be used to draw valid conclusions about the availability of drug to exert pharmacological effects at the site of action (DeVane 1994). The nonspecific binding of drugs to tissue components compli-

cates the interpretation of the significance of plasma protein binding differences among drugs. Drug binding in tissues cannot be measured directly in vivo and must be inferred using mathematical models and/or in vitro methods (Pacifici and Viani 1994).

Displacement of drug from plasma protein-binding sites may result from drug-drug interactions. This situation should lead to more unbound drug being available for distribution to peripheral tissues (Figure 8–4). As a result, potentially greater pharmacological effects may be expected. When plasma protein binding is restrictive regarding the drug's hepatic and/or renal elimination, then the increased free drug concentration in plasma will be a transient effect as more free (non protein bound) drug becomes available for elimination. Total (bound plus free) drug concentration in plasma will eventually return to a predisplacement value. Plasma protein-binding displacement interactions are rarely a major source of variability in psychopharmacology (Sellers 1979). Several reviews thoroughly examine this issue (MacKichan 1984; Wilkinson 1983). Drug interactions involving inhibition of drug metabolism are more common and are discussed below.

Elimination. Drugs are eliminated or cleared from the body primarily through renal excretion in an unchanged form, by biotransformation in the liver to polar metabolites, or both (Figure 8–1). *Clearance* is defined as the volume of blood or other fluid from which drug is irreversibly removed per unit of time. Thus, clearance units are volume per time. Drug clearance is analogous to creatinine clearance by the kidney. From the blood that delivers drug to the liver, or any other eliminating organ, an extraction occurs as blood travels through the organ. Drug extraction by the liver and other organs is rarely 100%, so the portion that escapes presystemic elimination reaches the systemic

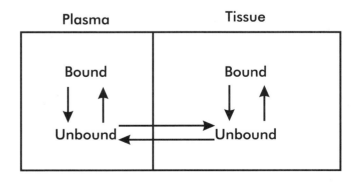

Figure 8–4. The effect of protein binding on distribution of drug between plasma and tissue.

circulation intact. Plasma protein binding, as mentioned above, can restrict the organ extraction process depending on the specific drug. If a drug were to be completely extracted, then clearance would equal the blood flow to the organ. An average hepatic blood flow is 1,500 mL/minute. When drug is eliminated by additional organs, the total clearance is an additive function of all the individual organ clearances. Clearance values reported in excess of 1,500 mL/minute for many psychopharmacological drugs are reflective of presystemic elimination (DeVane 1994). When the drug dose and bioavailability are constant, then clearance is the pharmacokinetic parameter that determines the extent of drug accumulation in the body. In contrast, elimination half-life reflects the rate of drug accumulation.

Elimination half-life is defined as the time required for the amount of drug in the body, or drug concentration, to decline by 50% and is commonly determined after a single-dose pharmacokinetic study or after drug discontinuation in a multiple-dose study. In either situation, drug concentration decline in plasma can be followed by multiple blood sampling. Half-life is easily determined by graphical means or by inspection, as long as data are used from the terminal, log-linear portion of the elimination curve (Figures 8–2 and 8–3). Knowledge of a drug's elimination half-life is useful for designing multiple-dosing regimens (DeVane and Jusko 1982).

Multiple Dosing to Steady State

Multiple drug doses usually are required in the pharmacotherapy of mental illness. During a multiple-dosing regimen, second and subsequent drug doses are usually administered before sufficient time has elapsed for the initial dose to be completely eliminated from the body. This process results in drug accumulation as illustrated in Figure 8–5. When drug elimination follows a linear or first-order process, then the amount of drug eliminated over time is proportional to the amount of drug available for elimination (Gibaldi and Perrier 1975). Accumulation does not occur indefinitely; rather, it reaches a steady state. A *steady state* exists when the amount of drug entering the body is equal to the amount leaving the body. From a practical standpoint, this definition means that after a period of continuous dosing, the body retains a pool of drug molecules from several doses, and the drug eliminated each day is replaced by an equivalent amount of newly administered drug. The time required from the first administered dose until an approximate steady state occurs is equivalent to the total of four to five elimination half-lives. The same amount of time is required to achieve

a new steady state after an increase or decrease in the daily dosing rate or for a drug to wash out of the body after dosing is discontinued (Figure 8–5).

The term steady state is a misnomer in that a true drug steady state occurs only with a constant-rate intravenous infusion. Because of the concurrent processes of drug absorption, distribution, and elimination, drug concentration is constantly changing in plasma during an oral dosing regimen. A peak and trough concentration occurs within each dosage interval. The average steady-state concentration occurs somewhere between these extremes and is determined by the daily dose and the drug's total body clearance for that individual.

On reaching a steady-state concentration, the average concentration and the magnitude of the peaks and troughs may be manipulated according to established pharmacokinetic principles. Figure 8–6 shows the predicted plasma concentration changes based on drug doses given every 24 hours. The selected dose does not produce a high enough average steady-state concentration to reach the desired concentration range between an MEC and a concentration threshold associated with an increased risk of toxicity. By doubling the dose and keeping the dosage interval constant, the average steady-state concentration increases, but the magnitude of the peak and trough concentration difference also increases. These changes are consistent with the pharmacokinetic principles of super-

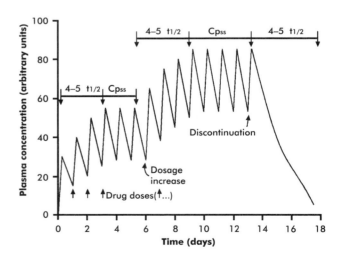

Figure 8–5. Accumulation of drug during multiple dosing. It takes four to five half-lives (4–5 $t_{1/2}$) to achieve initial steady state (Cp_{ss}) on a constant dosage regimen, to achieve a new steady state after an increase in dosage, or to wash out drug from the body after discontinuation. The average steady-state concentration lies somewhere between the peaks and troughs of drug concentration during a dosage interval.

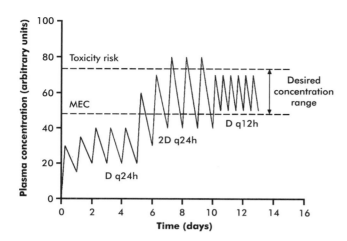

Figure 8–6. Predicted plasma concentration changes from administering either a selected dose (D) every 24 hours (D q24h), twice the dose every 24 hours (2D q24h), or the original dose every 12 hours (D q12h). MEC = minimal effective concentration.

position and linearity (Gibaldi and Perrier 1975).

Linearity refers to maintaining a stable clearance across the usual dosage range. Within the linear dose range, the magnitude of a dosage increase results in a proportional change in steady-state concentration (Figure 8–6). The size of the dose change theoretically superimposes on the new peak and trough concentration. In Figure 8–6, doubling the daily dose results in an adequate average steady-state concentration, but the new peak and trough concentration values cause both an increased risk of toxicity and an inadequate concentration declining below the MEC for a portion of each dosage interval. An alternative is to increase the total daily dose and divide it into more frequent administrations. This is accomplished by administering the original dose every 12 hours instead of every 24 hours. The new average steady-state concentration remains within the desired range, and the differences between the peak and trough concentrations are reduced to an acceptable fluctuation.

Selection of a proper drug dosage regimen must consider both the amount of drug administered and the frequency. Some drugs with half-lives long enough to be administered once daily may not be suitable for administration every 24 hours because toxicity may be precipitated by an excessive peak concentration in a single dose. Examples include lithium, bupropion, and clozapine. Once-daily dosing with lithium may produce gastrointestinal intolerance, and bupropion and clozapine are dosed multiple times each day to avoid peak concentrations that might predispose to seizure activity.

PHARMACODYNAMICS

Pharmacodynamic variability may exceed pharmacokinetic variability (Figure 8–1). The drug dose or concentration that produces a pharmacological effect differs widely among patients. Similarly, pharmacological effects can vary widely among patients with a comparable plasma concentration of drug.

The principles of dosage regimen design discussed above rely heavily on the existence of a functional relationship between concentration at an effect site and the intensity of the response produced. Many observed processes in nature behave according to the sigmoid relationship shown in Figure 8–7. At a low dose or concentration, only a marginal effect is produced. As drug dose or concentration increases, the intensity of effect (E) increases until a maximum effect (E_{max}) is achieved. This response is observed as a plateau in the sigmoid dose-effect curve (Figure 8–7). Further dose increases do not produce a greater effect.

The sigmoid dose-effect relationship in Figure 8–7 has practical applications to psychopharmacology. The increase in drug response that results from an increase in dosage depends on the shape and steepness of the theoretical dose-response curve for each patient and the starting point on the curve when a dosage is changed. At low doses or concentrations, a substantial dose increase may be necessary to achieve an effect. In a linear part of the relationship, dosage increases should result in proportional increases in effect. In the higher dose or concentration range, a further increase will not produce a significant increase in effect because of diminishing returns. This phenomenon is likely caused by the saturation of enzyme-binding sites or receptors by drug molecules above a critical concentration.

The general equation shown in Figure 8–7 describes the sigmoid relationship between concentration and response or intensity of effect. The response is usually measured as a percent change or the difference from the baseline effect. C is the drug concentration, and EC_{50} is the effective concentration that produces half of the E_{max}. Theoretically, n is an integer reflecting the number of molecules that bind to a specific drug receptor. Practically, it is a parameter that determines the sigmoid shape of the concentration-effect relationship. Pharmacokinetic-pharmacodynamic models have found wide application in psychopharmacology; for example, relating concentration to electroencephalogram parameters, psychomotor reaction times, and subjective effects from drugs of abuse (Dingemanse et al. 1988).

Drugs rarely have a single pharmacological effect or interact with only a single receptor population. Drugs often

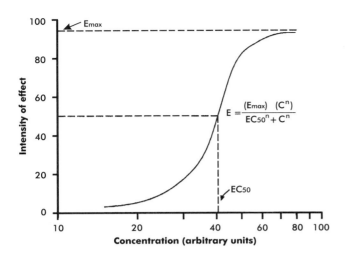

Figure 8–7. The sigmoid maximum effect (E_{max}) pharmacodynamic model relates concentration (C) to intensity of effect (E). EC_{50} is the concentration that produces half of the E_{max}, and n is an exponent that relates to the shape of the curve.

have affinity for multiple receptors; therefore, several theoretical concentration-effect relationships can exist for a given drug. Dose-response curves are shown in Figure 8–8 for a drug that produces a therapeutic effect and mild and severe toxicity. The greater the separation between the curves for therapeutic and toxic effects, the safer the drug can be administered in increasing doses to achieve therapeutic goals. Estimates of these interrelationships are made in preclinical animal studies and Phase 1 human studies for drugs in development. In clinical practice, the degree of separation between these curves and their steepness will show both inter- and intraindividual variability. Concurrent medical illness may predispose to side effects by effectively causing a shift to the left in one or both of the concentration-toxicity curves. This narrows the range over which doses can be safely administered without incurring adverse effects. The EC_{50} in Figure 8–8 produces negligible toxicity. Increasing the concentration with a dosage increase to gain an increased response can only be accomplished at the expense of mild toxicity. As the dosage and concentration increase, therapeutic effects approach a plateau, and small increments in concentration result in a disproportionate change in toxicity.

The pharmacodynamic relationships considered above are most reproducible when pharmacological effects are direct and closely related to plasma concentration. In Figure 8–9, the concentration-effect relationship is shown as a function of drug concentration changes over time. In Figure 8–9A, the changes in effect are almost superimposible with the increase and decrease in concentra-

tion. This type of relationship often reflects a direct action of the drug with a single receptor. This straightforward relationship is generally not observed in psychopharmacology.

In Figure 8–9B, the response has begun to diminish with time before concentration begins to decline. This type of plot is known as a *clockwise hysteresis curve*. The observed effect may be explained by the development of tolerance. The time course of tolerance to psychoactive drug effects varies from minutes to weeks. Acute tolerance to some euphoric effects of cocaine can occur following a single dose (Foltin and Fischman 1991). Tolerance to the sedative-hypnotic effects of barbiturates may take weeks. The mechanisms operative in the development of tolerance include acute depletion of a neurotransmitter or cofactor and homeostatic changes such as β-receptor downregulation in cerebral cortex as occurs following chronic antidepressant therapy.

A time delay in response occurs when effects are increasing and are maintained despite decreasing plasma drug concentration (Figure 8–9C). This results in a *counterclockwise hysteresis curve*. A pharmacokinetic explanation of this lag in response may involve a delay in reaching the critical drug MEC at the effect site until the plasma concentration has already begun to decline. Alternatively, response may depend on multiple "downstream" receptor effects. This theory likely accounts for the counterclockwise hysteresis curve observed between plasma drug concentration and growth hormone response in plasma after an intravenous alprazolam challenge (Osmon et al. 1991).

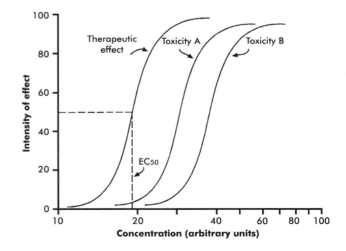

Figure 8–8. Concentration-effect curves for a drug that produces a therapeutic effect and mild (A) and severe (B) toxicity. The concentration is shown for a therapeutic effect that produces 50% of the maximum effect (EC_{50}).

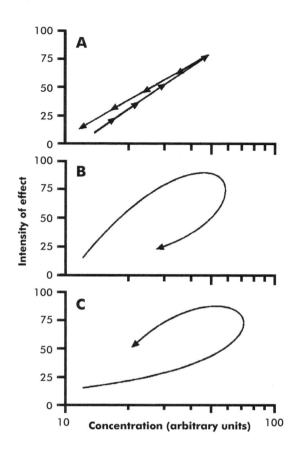

Figure 8–9. Theoretical relationships of drug concentration versus intensity of effect. Drug concentration changes occur in the direction of the arrow. Effects superimposible on concentration changes (A) suggest a direct and reversible interaction between drug and receptor, a clockwise hysteresis curve (B) suggests the development of tolerance, and a counterclockwise curve (C) suggests an indirect effect or the presence of an active metabolite.

Response may increase despite a decreasing drug concentration when a metabolite contributes to the observed effects. To overcome these complications, kinetic dynamic models can incorporate an "effect" compartment (Figure 8–1; Holford and Sheiner 1982). The effect site equilibrates with plasma after a finite time, which can be assigned a half-life. Models can also incorporate the presence of metabolites (Dingemanse et al. 1988).

VARIABILITY IN THE DOSE-EFFECT RELATIONSHIP

A major challenge of treating mental illness with drugs is that both pharmacokinetic and pharmacodynamic variability complicate the dose-effect relationship. The presence of active metabolites, the influence of pharmacogenetics, and the effects of combining two or more drugs contribute to variability. Noncompliance with the prescribed treatment plan on the part of the patient can seriously undermine reliability in the expected effects from pharmacotherapy. Physiological differences between patients are another source of variability. The effects of age, weight, and hepatic and other disease states are major factors in pharmacokinetics and pharmacodynamics that indicate the need for individualization of therapy. Several reviews (Blouin et al. 1994; McLean and Morgan 1991; Woodhouse 1994) summarize the influence of these variables.

Active Metabolites

With the exception of lithium, which is renally excreted, drugs used in clinical psychopharmacology are cleared partially or completely by metabolism, primarily in the liver. Many psychoactive drugs produce pharmacologically active metabolites that distribute to the effect sites (Figure 8–1) to produce pharmacological effects. Like their precursors, metabolites may have multiple pharmacological effects that may be similar to or different from those of the parent drug. The secondary amine tricyclic antidepressants (nortriptyline and desipramine) have anticholinergic effects similar to those of their parent drugs (amitriptyline and imipramine, respectively) but are more noradrenergic and less serotonergic in their ability to inhibit the uptake of monoamines presynaptically. Sertraline's metabolite, desmethylsertraline, has about 10% of the activity of sertraline in inhibiting serotonin (5-HT) reuptake, but the metabolite is equipotent with sertraline in its affinity for the hepatic isoenzyme CYP2D6 (Fuller et al. 1995).

When switching therapy from one drug or drug class to another, the presence of any active metabolites should be considered (Garattini 1985). Norfluoxetine, for example, has an average half-life of 8–9 days, much longer than the average of 2–3 days for fluoxetine, its parent drug (DeVane 1994), and is an equipotent serotonin reuptake inhibitor. It may take several weeks for this metabolite to clear the body after discontinuation of fluoxetine (Pato et al. 1991).

Metabolites will accumulate to a steady state in the body in relation to their elimination half-lives and not those of their parent drugs. Desmethyldiazepam, for example, will reach a steady-state concentration long after that of diazepam (Greenblatt et al. 1980). Thus, for some drugs, direct pharmacological effects may not be expected until the drug and any important active metabolites have all accumulated to their steady state. For drugs producing indirect effects when the response depends on second messengers or a cascade of receptor actions, the waiting period for fully expressed effects may be even longer.

Pharmacogenetics

Inheritance accounts for a large part of the variations observed in the ability to eliminate drugs (Figure 8–1) among individuals. This forms the basis of *pharmacogenetics*, which is defined as the study of the genetic contribution to the variability in drug response (Kalow et al. 1986; Price Evans 1993). The genetic differences in pharmacokinetics that have been detected apply almost totally to drug metabolism. The renal clearance of drugs appears to be similar in age- and weight-matched healthy subjects with no defined genetic polymorphisms. Genetic polymorphism has been identified and defined for several hepatic enzymes important in metabolism of many drugs used in psychopharmacology. These genetic polymorphisms are summarized in Table 8–2.

Genetic polymorphism in a drug-metabolizing enzyme results in a subpopulation of people who are poor metabolizers for substrates of the affected enzyme. Poor metabolizers constitute at least 1% of the population, but the majority of subjects are normal or rapid metabolizers. The genetic polymorphisms in Table 8–2 were identified mostly as a result of adverse drug reactions.

For example, a severe attack of hypotension following ingestion of debrisoquin led Smith (1986) in 1975 to observe that most individuals who did not have a similar reaction had a substantially greater amount of 4-hydroxydebrisoquine relative to unchanged debrisoquin in their urine. This observation led to a systematic investigation to uncover the cause. Subsequent studies have used debriso-

quin, sparteine, and dextromethorphan to calculate a metabolic ratio (MR) as an index of the relative ability of an individual to metabolize CYP2D6 substrates. The MR is equal to the concentration of parent drug divided by the concentration of the major metabolite determined in the urine excreted during a timed interval following an oral dose. Similar methodology has been applied to study the metabolism of prototype substrates for a variety of hepatic enzymes (Price Evans 1993).

The results of many pharmacogenetic studies appear similar to the frequency distribution histograms in Figure 8–10. The frequency in Figure 8–10A is expected when enzyme activity is distributed normally within a population without genetic polymorphisms. The range of values for the MR may be broad, which reflects a large variability in oxidation reaction capacity in the study population. Thus, vastly different dosages are required for many patients. The bimodal distribution in Figure 8–10B is a typical finding for an enzyme that has a genetic polymorphism. Values above the antimode for the reference, or "probe," drug define poor metabolizers, which are clearly differentiated from normal or extensive metabolizers. The probe drug need not be metabolized by only one enzyme, which characterizes the use of caffeine for phenotyping the enzyme activity of *N*-acetyltransferase, but the overlap of other enzymes should be minimal to produce the specific metabolite of interest (Denaro et al. 1996). Comparison of MRs between many patients of different ethnic origins has yielded measures of variability in enzyme activity in the population (Lin et al. 1996).

The potential clinical consequences of being a poor metabolizer will vary according to the activity of the administered drug and any active metabolites. When the drug is active and a pathway is affected, which usually pro-

Table 8–2. Some genetically determined variations in drug-metabolizing enzymes

Enzyme	Frequency of poor metabolizers	Clinical consequences	Example substrates
CYP2D6	5%–10% Caucasians 3% Blacks 1% Asians 1% Arabs	High drug concentrations; possible toxicity	Desipramine, nortriptyline, codeine, dextromethorphan
CYP2C19	3%–5% Caucasians 15%–20% Asians	High drug concentrations; increased sedation and possible toxicity	Diazepam
NAT-2	40%–60% Caucasians 10%–20% Asians and Eskimos	Greater toxicity; peripheral neuritis; skin eruptions	Procainamide, hydralazine
Plasma	<1% ; many atypical cholinesterase forms	Prolonged apnea	Succinylcholine

Note. CYP = cytochrome P450; NAT-2 = *N*-acetyltransferase.
Source. Kalow and Genest 1957; Lockridge 1990; Meyer et al. 1990; Price Evans 1993; Relling et al. 1991.

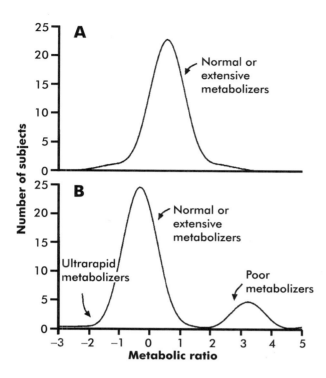

Figure 8–10. Theoretical frequency histograms of the distribution of the metabolic ratio of a model substrate showing a unimodal distribution among a population of normal or extensive metabolizers (A) and a bimodal distribution among a population including poor metabolizers and ultrarapid metabolizers (B).

duces an inactive metabolite, higher drug concentrations can be expected. This result can lead to an exaggerated response and potential toxicity. The most serious consequences would be expected from drugs with a narrow therapeutic window (Table 8–1). For example, when perphenazine (a drug with a narrow therapeutic window) was given to elderly patients who were CYP2D6 poor metabolizers, extrapyramidal side effects were exaggerated (Pollock et al. 1995). If the therapeutic effects depend on an active metabolite, then diminished response can be expected from a lower concentration of metabolite in poor metabolizers. For example, normal doses of codeine, which is partially metabolized to the more potent morphine, may provide an inadequate analgesic effect.

For CYP2D6, the poor metabolizer status is inherited as an autosomal recessive trait. CYP2D6 is not expressed in poor metabolizers, and most are homozygous or heterozygous for the CYP2D6-A, CYP2D6-B, or CYP2D6-D allele (Kagimoto et al. 1990). As many as 28 different alleles have been defined for the *CYP2D6* gene (Gonzalez and Idle 1994). Methods such as polymerase chain reaction (PCR) have a high sensitivity for detecting the mutant

alleles and can unequivocally establish one's CYP2D6 genotype. This procedure can be beneficial in drug development to test compounds that are CYP2D6 substrates and in some forensic circumstances to help establish the cause of excessive drug concentrations. Genetic phenotyping is potentially more clinically useful than genotyping and can be done when patients are drug free to characterize their relative ability to metabolize CYP2D6 substrates. The outcome of phenotyping should aid in the initial selection of drugs and drug doses to achieve a plasma concentration that is both safe and effective (Pollock et al. 1995).

About 1% of Caucasians are ultrarapid metabolizers because of an amplification of the functional *CYP2D6* gene (Johansson et al. 1993). These patients have the lowest MR when phenotyped with a CYP2D6 substrate with a high urinary concentration of metabolite and a low parent drug concentration (Figure 8–10B). The implication is that these individuals will often require very high drug doses. This is an active area of pharmacogenetic investigation, and limited data are available.

Of the human cytochrome P450 enzymes, three families (CYP1, CYP2, and CYP3) are involved in drug metabolism (Guengerich 1992; Wrighton and Stevens 1992). The enzymes most relevant to psychopharmacology are listed in Table 8–1. Interindividual differences in the expression and catalytic activities of cytochrome P450 result in a large variation in the in vivo metabolism of drugs. The average immunoquantified levels of the various specific P450s in 60 human liver microsomal samples were reported by Shimada et al. (1994). Benet et al. (1996) and Wrighton and Stevens (1992) estimated the participation of the liver cytochrome P450s in drug metabolism based on known substrates and pathways (Table 8–1). These values are compared in Table 8–3. CYP3A has the highest level of P450 in the liver and participates in the metabolism of the largest number of drugs. Together, CYP3A and CYP2D6 participate in the metabolism of an estimated 80% of currently used drugs.

In summary, recent pharmacogenetic investigations have yielded fruitful data relating to the causes of pharmacokinetic variability in the dose-effect relationship. In comparison, much less is known of the pharmacogenetics of drug receptors in the brain as a source of pharmacodynamic variability. Pharmacogenetic studies have extensively used metabolic phenotyping with model substrates for specific enzymes to characterize several genetic polymorphisms (Table 8–2). The practical implications of metabolic phenotyping are most meaningful when the metabolic pathways of therapeutically administered drugs are known and when drug concentration has been correlated to either therapeutic or toxic effects (Gonzalez and

Table 8–3. Comparison of average immunoquantified levels of the various P450s in liver microsomes with the estimated participation in drug metabolism

Cytochrome P450	Average immunoquantified level of P450 in human liver microsomal samples (%)[a]	Estimated participation in drug metabolism (%)[b]
1A2	13	<10
2A6	4	<10
2B6	0.2	(Marginal)
2E1	7	<10
2C	18	10
2D6	1.5	30
3A	29	50
Unidentified	27.3	
Total	**100**	

[a]Shimada et al. 1994.
[b]Benet et al. 1996; Wrighton and Stevens 1992.

Idle 1994). In this situation, knowledge of enzyme activity will serve as a guide to initial dosing and also allow a prediction of the significance of potential drug-drug interactions.

Drug Interactions

Drugs are frequently coadministered to achieve therapeutic effects from the combined actions at effect sites or to treat the adverse effects caused by one drug with another. Drug combinations include sedatives and antidepressants, anticholinergic-antiparkinsonian drugs and high-potency antipsychotics, and benzodiazepines and selective serotonin reuptake inhibitors (SSRIs). When more than one drug is administered concurrently to a patient, they may interact in a negative or undesired way because of either pharmacokinetic or pharmacodynamic mechanisms.

Pharmacodynamic interactions are likely to occur when the combination of a monoamine oxidase inhibitor and an SSRI produces a serotonin syndrome and when the combination of ethanol and a benzodiazepine leads to psychomotor impairment. Two drugs may have affinity for the same receptor sites in the brain and produce additive, or synergistic, effects, or their actions may oppose each other through antagonistic interactions at receptor sites. Most often, pharmacodynamic mechanisms are not such obvious causes of drug interactions and are usually less easily determined and investigated than pharmacokinetic interactions.

The kinetics of drug interactions has been extensively described and is the focus of much research (Brosen 1996;

Rowland and Matin 1973). Two major mechanisms of drug interactions involve an alteration of metabolism through either induction or inhibition of hepatic cytochrome P450 enzymes. Major differences exist in the pharmacokinetic consequences of these interactions. The expected changes are illustrated in Figures 8–11 and 8–12. In Figure 8–11, the steady-state plasma concentration of drug A following continuous intermittent dosing is altered by the addition of an enzyme inducer. When the inducer is started, the effects on the steady-state concentration of drug A do not occur for several days while additional enzyme that metabolizes drug A is synthesized. Ultimately, an increase in the metabolic clearance of drug A accompanied by a decrease in its steady-state plasma concentration occurs. The degree to which clearance is increased will depend on the relative importance of the particular induced enzymes in the overall elimination of drug A and the dose and potency of the inducer. Examples of this type of interaction include the loss of oral contraceptive effect by carbamazepine induction of CYP3A4 and the loss of antipsychotic effect from induction of antipsychotic metabolism. The time for a new steady state of drug A to occur following enzyme induction and the extent to which plasma concentrations decrease will depend on how marked a change in clearance occurs and the resulting change in drug half-life.

In contrast to the delayed effects of an inducer on drug A, the addition of an inhibitor causes an immediate increase in the plasma concentration of drug A (Figure 8–12). This increase occurs as a result of a competitive inhibition of the relevant hepatic enzyme. Drug A's plasma

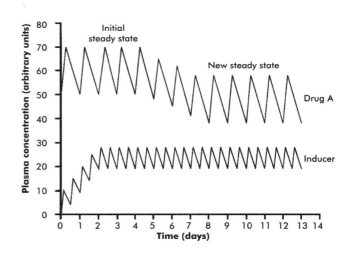

Figure 8–11. Predicted plasma concentration changes from the coadministration of an inducer of the metabolism of drug A.

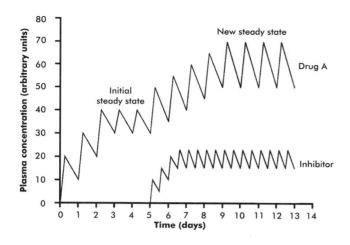

Figure 8–12. Predicted plasma concentration changes from the coadministration of an inhibitor of the metabolism of drug *A*.

concentration rises to a new steady state consistent with a change in its clearance. The time to achieve the new steady state is greater than the time to achieve the initial steady state, because the half-life is now prolonged from its original value. The full effect of an inhibitory interaction may not be realized until the inhibitor also reaches a steady state, because the degree of inhibition will also depend on the concentration of the inhibitor (Houston 1994; von Moltke et al. 1994, 1995).

Drug interactions are graded phenomena. The degree of interaction depends on the concentration of interacting drugs and, therefore, on the dose and timing of administration. Drug interactions are most likely to be detected when therapy with an interacting drug is initiated or discontinued. The clinical significance will depend on the particular drugs involved, the physiological state of the patient, the presence of concurrent illness, and other factors. Drugs with a narrow concentration range over which therapeutic effects are present without incurring toxicity are more likely to be involved in clinically significant drug interactions. These drugs include theophylline, some anticonvulsants, and antiarrhythmics (Table 8–1).

When selecting a specific drug from a class of drugs to treat mental illness, efficacy, safety, cost, and a history of response are pertinent considerations. The introduction of the SSRIs has emphasized the critical importance of also considering potential drug interactions (Brosen 1996). These antidepressants have been shown in vitro and in vivo to be potent inhibitors of some cytochrome P450 isoenzymes (Crewe et al. 1992; Nemeroff et al. 1996; von Moltke et al. 1994, 1995). The most thoroughly studied

reaction is the competitive inhibition of CYP2D6. Pharmacokinetic studies in healthy volunteers have provided a rank order of the potency for increasing the plasma concentration of model substrates. Case reports in patients have confirmed the existence of some interactions, and many others remain theoretical possibilities. Table 8–4 provides an overall ranking of the cytochrome P450 inhibitory potential of the newer antidepressants based on both in vitro and in vivo data. The rational selection of an antidepressant should include consideration of its potential enzyme inhibition when therapy is to be combined with substrates listed in Table 8–1, which may be inhibited by the specific antidepressant. Reviews (Harvey and Preskorn 1996; Nemeroff et al. 1996) describe the specific in vivo reports in more detail.

The selection of a drug based on its cytochrome P450 inhibitory potential should not be limited to the newer antidepressants (Table 8–4). Combining any two drugs that are substrates for the same enzyme increases the likelihood of competitive enzyme inhibition. All of the substrates listed in Table 8–1 are potential inhibitors. For example, nortriptyline, desipramine, and thioridazine are potent inhibitors of CYP2D6. In vitro methods using microsomal incubations to predict in vivo interactions have appeared and are based on accepted pharmacokinetic principles (Gillette 1971; Houston 1994; von Moltke et al. 1994, 1995). These screening techniques are now used extensively in the pharmaceutical industry in drug development. The knowledge of isoenzyme-specific metabo-

Table 8–4. Newer antidepressants and P450 enzyme inhibitory potential

Drug	CYP1A2	CYP2C	CYP2D6	CYP3A4
Fluvoxamine	++++	++	0	+++
Fluoxetine	0	++	++++	++
(metabolite)			(++++)	(+++)
Sertraline	0	++	+	++
(metabolite)		(++)	(++)	(++)
Paroxetine	0	0	++++	0
Citalopram	0	0	0	0
Nefazodone	0	0	0	++++
Venlafaxine	0	0	0	0
(metabolite)			(+)	
Bupropion	0	0	0	0
Mirtazapine	0	0	0	0

Note. 0 = unknown or insignificant; + = mild and usually insignificant; ++ = moderate and possibly significant; +++ = moderate and usually significant; ++++ = potent.
Source. In vivo and in vitro results: Crewe et al. 1992; Nemeroff et al. 1996; von Moltke et al. 1994, 1995.

lism of new and established drugs is expanding rapidly and holds promise for further enabling the selection of combined pharmacotherapy based on pharmacokinetic principles.

CONCLUSION

The use of drugs in psychopharmacology can be problematic as a result of pharmacokinetic and pharmacodynamic variability in the dose-effect relationship. Some sources of variability can be controlled through application of pharmacokinetic principles in dosage regimen design and therapeutic drug monitoring. Understanding of pharmacodynamic principles contributes to individualization of dosage regimens. The database is rapidly expanding on the genetic contribution to drug response and the interactions between drugs. Future application of this knowledge will further enhance pharmacotherapy for mentally ill patients.

REFERENCES

Benet LZ, Kroetz DL, Sheiner LB: Pharmacokinetics: the dynamics of drug absorption, distribution, and elimination, in Goodman and Gilman's Pharmacologic Basis of Therapeutics. Edited by Hardman JG, Limbird LE. New York, McGraw-Hill, 1996, pp 3–27

Blouin RA, Kolpek JH, Mann HJ: Influence of obesity on drug disposition. Clinical Pharmacy 6:706–714, 1994

Brosen K: Are pharmacokinetic drug interactions with the SSRIs an issue? Int Clin Psychopharmacol 11 (suppl 1):23–27, 1996

Crewe HK, Lennard MS, Tucker GT, et al: The effect of selective serotonin re-uptake inhibitors on cytochrome P4502D6 (CYP2D6) activity in human liver microsomes. Br J Clin Pharmacol 34:262–265, 1992

Denaro CP, Wilson M, Jacob III P, et al: Validation of urine caffeine metabolite ratios with use of stable isotope-labeled caffeine clearance. Clin Pharmacol Ther 59:284–296, 1996

DeVane CL: Pharmacokinetics of the newer antidepressants: clinical relevance. Am J Med 97 (suppl 6A):13–23, 1994

DeVane CL, Jusko WJ: Dosage regimen design. Pharmacol Ther 17:143–164, 1982

DeVane CL, Simpkins JM: Pharmacokinetics of imipramine and its major metabolites in pregnant rats and their fetuses treated with a single dose. Drug Metab Dispos 13:438–442, 1985

de Waziers I, Cugnenc PH, Yang CS, et al: Cytochrome P450 isoenzymes, epoxide hydrolase and glutathione transferases in rat and human hepatic and extrahepatic tissues. J Pharmacol Exp Ther 253:287–294, 1990

Dingemanse J, Danhof M, Briemer DD: Pharmacokinetic-pharmacodynamic modeling of CNS drug effects: an overview. Pharmacol Ther 38:1–52, 1988

Foltin RW, Fischman MW: Smoked and intravenous cocaine in humans: acute tolerance, cardiovascular and subjective effects. J Pharmacol Exp Ther 257:247–261, 1991

Fuhr U, Kummert AL: The fate of naringin in humans: a key to grapefruit juice-drug interactions? Clin Pharmacol Ther 58:365–373, 1995

Fuller RW, Hemrick-Luecke SK, Litterfield ES, et al: Comparison of desmethylsertraline with sertraline as a monoamine uptake inhibitor in vivo. Life Sci 19:135–149, 1995

Garattini S: Active drug metabolites: an overview of their relevance in clinical pharmacokinetics. Clin Pharmacokinet 19:216–227, 1985

George CF, Shand DG, Renwick AG (eds): Presystemic Drug Elimination. London, Butterworth Scientific, 1982

Gibaldi M, Perrier D: Pharmacokinetics. New York, Marcel Dekker, 1975

Gillette JR: Techniques for studying drug metabolism in vitro, in Fundamentals of Drug Metabolism. Edited by La Du BN, Mandel HG, Way EL. Baltimore, MD, Williams & Wilkins, 1971, pp 400–418

Gonzalez FJ, Idle JR: Pharmacogenetic phenotyping and genotyping: present status and future potential. Clin Pharmacokinet 26:59–70, 1994

Greenblatt DJ, Shader RI, Koch-Wiser J, et al: Slow absorption of intramuscular chlordiazepoxide. N Engl J Med 291:1116–1118, 1974

Greenblatt DJ, Allen MD, MacLaughlin DS, et al: Diazepam absorption: effect of antacids and food. Clin Pharmacol Ther 24:600–609, 1978

Greenblatt DJ, Allen MD, Harmatz JS, et al: Diazepam disposition determinants. Clin Pharmacol Ther 27:301–312, 1980

Guengerich FP: Human cytochrome P-450 enzymes. Life Sci 50:1471–1478, 1992

Harvey AT, Preskorn SH: Cytochrome P450 enzymes: interpretation of their interactions with selective serotonin reuptake inhibitors, part I. J Clin Psychopharmacol 16:273–285, 1996

Holford NHG, Sheiner LB: Kinetics of pharmacologic response. Pharmacol Ther 16:143–166, 1982

Houston JB: Utility of in vitro drug metabolism data in predicting in vivo metabolic clearance. Biochem Pharmacol 47:1469–1479, 1994

Johansson I, Lundqvist E, Bertilsson L, et al: Inherited amplification of an active gene in the cytochrome P450 CYP2D locus as a cause of ultrarapid metabolism of debrisoquin. Proc Natl Acad Sci U S A 90:11825–11829, 1993

Kagimoto M, Heim M, Kagimoto K, et al: Multiple mutations of the human cytochrome P450IID6 gene (CYP2D6) in poor metabolizers of debrisoquine. J Biol Chem 265:17209–17214, 1990

Kalow W, Genest K: A method for the detection of atypical forms of human serum cholinesterase. Canadian Journal of Biochemistry and Physiology 35:339–346, 1957

Kalow W, Goedde WH, Agarwal DP: Ethnic Differences in Reactions to Drugs and Xenobiotics. New York, Alan R Liss, 1986

Ketter TA, Flockhart DA, Post RM, et al: The emerging role of cytochrome P450 3A in psychopharmacology. J Clin Psychopharmacol 15:387–398, 1995

Kolars JC, Schmiedlin-Ren P, Schuetz JD, et al: Identification of rifampin-inducible P450IIIA4 (CYP3A4) in human small bowel enterocytes. J Clin Invest 90:1871–1878, 1992

Lin K-M, Poland RE, Wan Y-JY, et al: The evolving science of pharmacogenetics: clinical ethnic perspectives. Psychopharmacol Bull 32:205–217, 1996

Lockridge O: Genetic variants of human serum cholinesterase influence metabolism of the muscle relaxant succinylcholine. Pharmacol Ther 47:35–60, 1990

MacKichan JJ: Pharmacokinetic consequences of drug displacement from blood and tissue proteins. Clin Pharmacokinet 9 (suppl 1):32–41, 1984

McLean AJ, Morgan DJ: Clinical pharmacokinetics in patients with liver disease. Clin Pharmacokinet 21:42–69, 1991

Meyer UA, Zanger UM, Grant D, et al: Genetic polymorphisms of drug metabolism. Advances in Drug Research 19:197–241, 1990

Nemeroff CB, DeVane CL, Pollock BG: Newer antidepressants and the cytochrome P450 system. Am J Psychiatry 153:311–320, 1996

Osmon OT, DeVane CL, Greenblatt DJ, et al: Pharmacokinetic and dynamic correlates of intravenous alprazolam challenge. Clin Pharmacol Ther 50:656–662, 1991

Pacifici GM, Viani A: Methods of determining plasma and tissue binding of drugs: pharmacokinetic consequences. Clin Pharmacokinet 29:449–468, 1994

Paine MF, Shen DD, Kunze KL, et al: First-pass metabolism of midazolam by the human intestine. Clin Pharmacol Ther 60:14–24, 1996

Pato M, Murphy DL, DeVane CL: Sustained plasma concentrations of fluoxetine and/or norfluoxetine four and eight weeks after fluoxetine discontinuation. J Clin Psychopharmacol 11:224–225, 1991

Pollock BG, Mulsant BH, Sweet RA, et al: Prospective cytochrome P450 phenotyping for neuroleptic treatment in dementia. Psychopharmacol Bull 31:327–331, 1995

Price Evans DA: Genetic Factors in Drug Therapy. Cambridge, MA, Cambridge University Press, 1993

Relling MV, Cherrie J, Schell MJ, et al: Lower prevalence of the debrisoquin oxidative poor metabolizer phenotype in American black versus white subjects. Clin Pharmacol Ther 50:308–313, 1991

Rowland M, Matin SB: Kinetics of drug-drug interactions. J Pharmacokinet Biopharm 1:553–567, 1973

Salzman C, Solomon D, Miyawaki E, et al: Parenteral lorazepam versus parenteral haloperidol for the control of psychotic disruptive behavior. J Clin Psychiatry 52:177–180, 1991

Schmider J, Greenblatt DJ, von Moltke LL, et al: Relationship of in vitro data on drug metabolism to in vivo pharmacokinetics and drug interactions: implications for diazepam disposition in humans. J Clin Psychopharmacol 16:267–272, 1996

Sellers EM: Plasma protein displacement interactions are rarely of clinical significance. Pharmacology 18:225–227, 1979

Shimada T, Yamazaki H, Mimura M, et al: Interindividual variations in human liver cytochrome P-450 enzymes involved in the oxidation of drugs, carcinogens and toxic chemicals: studies with liver microsomes of 30 Japanese and 30 Caucasians. J Pharmacol Exp Ther 270:414–423, 1994

Smith RL: Human genetic variations in oxidative drug metabolism. Xenobiotica 16:361–365, 1986

Stanski DR: Pharmacodynamic modeling of anesthetic EEG drug effects. Annu Rev Pharmacol Toxicol 32:423–447, 1992

von Moltke LL, Greenblatt DJ, Cotreau-Bibbo MM, et al: Inhibition of desipramine hydroxylation in vitro by serotonin-reuptake-inhibitor antidepressants, and by quinidine and ketoconazole: a model system to predict drug interactions in vivo. J Pharmacol Exp Ther 268:1278–1283, 1994

von Moltke LL, Greenblatt DJ, Court MH, et al: Inhibition of alprazolam and desipramine hydroxylation in vitro by paroxetine and fluvoxamine: comparison with other selective serotonin reuptake inhibitor antidepressants. J Clin Psychopharmacol 15:125–131, 1995

Wilkinson GR: Plasma and tissue binding considerations in drug disposition. Drug Metab Rev 14:427–465, 1983

Woodhouse K: Drug and the liver, part III: ageing of the liver and the metabolism of drugs. Biopharm Drug Dispos 13:311–320, 1994

Wrighton SA, Stevens JC: The human hepatic cytochromes P450 involved in drug metabolism. Crit Rev Toxicol 22:1–21, 1992

NINE

Neuroendocrine and Immune System Pathology in Psychiatric Disease

Sherri M. Hansen-Grant, M.D., Carmine M. Pariante, M.D., Ned H. Kalin, M.D., and Andrew H. Miller, M.D.

The neuroendocrine and immune systems play critical roles in the maintenance of homeostasis and in the integration of responses of the body to the external environment. The immune system also provides defense against invading pathogens and neoplastically transformed cells. As the knowledge of the basic physiology and molecular biology of these two systems has evolved, recognition of the potential role of hormones and immune processes in the development, course, and outcome of psychiatric disorders has increased. Greater understanding of the specific contributions that hormones and the immune system make to psychiatric disease will lead to pharmacological treatment strategies targeted at specific regulatory peptides and cytokines. This chapter is designed to provide a foundation for integrating the neuroendocrine and immune systems into the formulation of the causes and consequences of psychiatric diseases and evaluating the potential clinical relevance of this area of research.

NEUROENDOCRINE MANIFESTATIONS OF PSYCHIATRIC DISEASE

Research over the last 50 years has established an association between neuropsychiatric illnesses and alterations in endocrine systems. Harvey Cushing made one of the earliest links between endocrine alterations and psychiatric symptoms in his demonstration of psychiatric symptoms in patients who secreted excessive amounts of cortisol (Cushing 1981). Later, in the 1940s, Hans Selye de-

scribed the relationship among stress, adaptation, and activation of the adrenal cortex (Selye 1973). Since then, numerous investigators have pursued this relationship as well as other neuroendocrine alterations that may be associated with stress-related and neuropsychiatric disorders. Studies have focused on not only the hypothalamic-pituitary-adrenal (HPA) system but also thyroid hormones, growth hormone (GH), sex hormones, and prolactin.

Understanding the link between neuroendocrine alterations and neuropsychiatric illnesses is important not only because endocrine alterations may provide markers for specific psychiatric illnesses but also because these endocrine changes may play a role in the pathophysiology of these illnesses. Because neuroendocrine systems are regulated by brain neurotransmitters, neuroendocrine alterations can provide insight into changes in neurotransmitter systems underlying neuropsychiatric illnesses. In this section, we provide an overview of the physiology of neuroendocrine function, review findings linking neuropsychiatric illnesses with neuroendocrine abnormalities, and discuss the clinical implications of these findings.

Basic Neuroendocrine Principles

In the late 1940s, Guillemin and Schally separately proposed that substances existed in the hypothalamus that served to control the pituitary's release of trophic factors (Mornex 1978). Ultimately, these hypothesized releasing factors were discovered, and subsequent work identified a series of peptides, including thyrotropin-releasing hor-

Alterations in peripheral corticosteroid receptors have also been found in depressed patients. Corticosteroids have two intracellular receptors. The Type I receptor, or the mineralocorticoid receptor, has a high affinity for circulating cortisol and is believed to be involved in maintaining the circadian rhythm (Reul and de Kloet 1985). The Type II receptor, or the glucocorticoid receptor, has a lower affinity for cortisol and, therefore, is believed to play a role in mediating the feedback effects of high (stress-induced) levels of cortisol as well as the effects of dexamethasone. Functionally, alterations in corticosteroid receptors may occur during episodes of depression, either as a result of hyperactivity of the HPA axis or as a primary defect. The latter hypothesis assumes that depression is associated with an alteration in corticosteroid receptors leading to "glucocorticoid resistance," in which cells are less sensitive to the effects of adrenocortical hormones. In this model, glucocorticoid hormones would be unable to exert their feedback action efficiently at one or more of the various levels of the HPA axis, including the synthesis and release of CRH or ACTH, thus resulting in persistent HPA axis activation. Glucocorticoid resistance in patients with depression may also provide an explanation for the lack of the typical physical stigmata such as moon faces, truncal obesity, and abdominal striae observed in other patients with elevated cortisol levels, such as those with Cushing's disease.

Several studies have directly examined glucocorticoid receptor number and function in depression. Although some studies have found decreased glucocorticoid receptor number in depressed patients (Gormley et al. 1985; Sallee et al. 1995; Whalley et al. 1986; Yehuda et al. 1993), most have not (for review, see Pariante et al. 1995). Nevertheless, studies investigating glucocorticoid receptor function have consistently found that cells from depressed patients—especially nonsuppressors on the dexamethasone suppression test—are significantly less sensitive to the inhibitory effects of glucocorticoids on functional endpoints than are cells from healthy control subjects. For example, immune cells from depressed patients, compared with control subjects, exhibit a reduced inhibition of mitogen-induced lymphocyte proliferation or natural killer (NK) cell activity after either oral dexamethasone or in vitro incubation with dexamethasone or cortisol. This in vitro glucocorticoid resistance, which seems to normalize in recovered patients, is consistent with the in vivo data showing nonsuppression of HPA axis function after dexamethasone administration. In further support of the hypothesis that abnormalities in the glucocorticoid receptor contribute to the pathophysiology of major depression, recent studies have suggested that a possible mechanism by which

antidepressants exert their effect is through direct modulation of the glucocorticoid receptor. In fact, a number of animal studies have reported that long-term in vivo treatment with a range of tricyclic and nontricyclic antidepressants or electroconvulsive therapy can enhance glucocorticoid feedback inhibition (as evidenced by decreased basal and/or stress-induced glucocorticoid secretion) and/or increase glucocorticoid receptor binding and mRNA in key brain regions including the hippocampus (Holsboer and Barden 1996). Of note is that the modification in glucocorticoid receptors following antidepressant administration seems to occur after approximately 2–3 weeks of treatment, the same amount of time that antidepressants usually take to produce their clinical benefits in depressed patients.

An in vitro study using a fibroblast cell line showed that acute treatment with the tricyclic antidepressant desipramine was capable of inducing upregulation of glucocorticoid receptor protein after 72 hours of treatment (Pepin et al. 1992); more recently, 24-hour in vitro desipramine treatment of a different fibroblast cell line led to enhancement of glucocorticoid receptor function (glucocorticoid receptor translocation from the cytoplasm to the nucleus) (Pariante et al. 1997c). These findings suggest that one important aspect of the effects of antidepressants in vivo may be to facilitate glucocorticoid receptor–mediated feedback inhibition on the HPA axis—by increasing glucocorticoid receptor number and/or function—and thereby reverse glucocorticoid hypersecretion in depression. Therefore, the return to normal HPA functioning, which typically has been related to recovery from the illness, may be the result of a direct effect of antidepressant therapy on the glucocorticoid receptor.

Extrahypothalamic CRH systems function and are regulated differently from hypothalamic CRH systems. Measurements of cerebrospinal fluid (CSF) CRH concentrations likely reflect the activity of the extrahypothalamic CRH system (Kalin et al. 1987), and CSF CRH concentrations are elevated in some depressed patients (Kling et al. 1991). Postmortem studies of depressed suicide victims show a reduction in frontal cortical CRH receptors (Nemeroff 1988). Taken together, these findings suggest that outside of the hypothalamus, depression is associated with an increased presynaptic release of CRH followed by a downregulation of postsynaptic CRH receptors.

Numerous animal studies confirm that intraventricular and/or site-specific CRH administration results in anxiety and depressive-like behaviors (Glowa and Gold 1991). In addition, the administration of CRH antagonists blocks fear-related and anxiety-like behavioral responses. Finally, work with neonatal animals has shown that early developmental experiences play a critical role in dictating CRH responsiveness in adulthood, thereby potentially sensitizing animals to stress-related disorders later in life (Ladd et al. 1996; Plotsky and Meaney 1993). Together, these studies form the basis for the idea that increased brain CRH may underlie depressive and anxiety symptoms as well as disorders.

Hypothalamic-Pituitary-Adrenal Axis and Other Psychiatric Disorders

Other Disorders

Overactivity of the HPA system has also been identified in a significant number of patients with anorexia nervosa (Licinio et al. 1996), anxiety disorders (Schreiber et al. 1996), and Alzheimer's disease (Nasman et al. 1996). However, the extent to which these findings are due to the presence of comorbid depression or other nonspecific factors affecting the HPA system is unclear. In addition, anorexia nervosa and Alzheimer's disease are frequently associated with malnourishment, which can account for HPA alterations and other disturbances in endocrine function. Patients with Alzheimer's disease generally have a high rate of dexamethasone nonsuppression (Hatzinger et al. 1995; Miller et al. 1994a). In contrast to depressed patients, Alzheimer's patients are not reported to have elevated CSF CRH levels (Heilig et al. 1995). In addition, postmortem studies in patients with Alzheimer's disease revealed decreased concentrations of CRH in cortical regions, whereas CRH receptors remained unchanged (Ferrier and Leake 1990).

Patients with posttraumatic stress disorder (PTSD) are thought to have HPA alterations that are opposite to those of patients with depression. Patients with PTSD have lower levels of cortisol and also seem to be hyperresponsive to dexamethasone administration, suggesting enhanced negative feedback (Yehuda et al. 1993). In addition, these patients have increased lymphocyte glucocorticoid receptors (Yehuda et al. 1995). Some reports indicate that patients with PTSD have a blunted ACTH response to CRH administration (Smith et al. 1989), and increased CSF CRH levels have recently been detected in patients with PTSD (Bremnar et al. 1997). Metyrapone given to patients with PTSD also causes a significantly greater increase in ACTH compared with that in subjects without PTSD (Yehuda et al. 1996). Imaging techniques have identified a reduced hippocampal volume in patients with PTSD and depression (Bremnar et al. 1995; Grillon et al. 1996). Because research in animals has demonstrated neurotoxic effects of increased glucocorticoids, it is of interest to speculate about the effects of prolonged cortisol elevations or increased sensitivity to cortisol in mediating these hippocampal changes.

Hypothalamic-Pituitary-Thyroid Axis and Psychiatric Disease

Organization of the hypothalamic-pituitary-thyroid (HPT) axis is similar to that of the HPA axis (Table 9–1). TRH, a 3-amino-acid peptide, is released from hypothalamic neurons into the pituitary-portal vasculature and stimulates thyroid-stimulating hormone (TSH)-containing cells in the anterior pituitary to release TSH. In the peripheral circulation, TSH induces the release of thyroxine (T_4) and 3,5,3-triiodothyronine (T_3) from the thyroid gland. Outside the thyroid gland, T_4 can be converted to T_3. Biologically active levels of thyroid hormone, which constitute the non-protein-bound fraction, are in part regulated by thyroid-binding globulin. Thyroid hormones have a major role in regulating metabolism, and circulating levels of T_3 and T_4 regulate TSH and TRH release via inhibitory negative feedback mechanisms.

Diseases of the thyroid gland are often associated with a variety of neuropsychiatric symptoms. Signs and symptoms of anxiety, fatigue, depression, and emotional lability most commonly occur during hyperthyroidism. In primary hypothyroidism, the clinical picture overlaps significantly with that of major depression, with symptoms of psychomotor slowing, fatigue, decreased libido, depressed mood, and suicidality. The frequent occurrence of increased sleep and weight gain in patients with hypothyroidism may lead to a misdiagnosis of atypical depression (Pariante et al. 1997b).

In patients with hypothyroidism, depressive symptoms do not respond to antidepressants unless the hormone deficiency has been resolved. Moreover, combined therapy with a tricyclic antidepressant and T_3 has been shown repeatedly to be efficacious in refractory depressed patients (Pariante et al. 1997b). Relatively high doses of T_4 have been reported to be effective in treating both the depression and the mania associated with rapid-cycling bipolar disease (Pariante et al. 1997b). Studies have also indicated that antithyroid antibodies are increased in patients with bipolar disorder (Oomen et al. 1996).

In depressed patients, the circadian pattern of thyroid hormone secretion may be blunted or absent (Garbutt et al. 1994; Kjellman et al 1985; Weeke and Weeke 1978). Some studies have found a decrease in mean nocturnal serum TSH and mean serum T_3 concentrations (Rubin et al. 1987). However, decreased TSH can also occur secondary to sleep deprivation, which is a common symptom in patients with major depression (Parker et al. 1987). A blunted TSH response to TRH has been reported in depressed patients, manic patients, and alcoholic patients (Loosen 1985; Loosen and Prange 1982; Nemeroff 1989). However, alcohol use and starvation may also increase TRH (Brown 1989).

TSH blunting may be secondary to chronic hypersecretion of hypothalamic TRH such that thyrotropic cells may become hyporesponsive to TRH possibly via downregulation of TRH receptors (Loosen 1987). Consistent with this notion, some depressed patients have elevated CSF TRH concentrations (Banki et al. 1988). A recent preliminary report indicates that TRH administered directly into the CSF may have acute antidepressant effects (Marangell et al. 1997). This finding suggests that the elevated CSF TRH levels in depressed patients may reflect a compensatory hypersecretion of TRH in response to the depressed state.

In patients with anorexia nervosa, studies of thyroid abnormalities have reported inconsistent results (Pariante et al. 1997b). For example, the TSH response to TRH has been observed to be normal, delayed, and blunted in patients who were underweight and in patients who gained weight (Pariante et al. 1997b). As in depression, a blunted TSH response could be associated with TRH hypersecretion and a consequent downregulation of the receptors. However, CSF TRH concentrations have been reported to be persistently reduced in anorexic patients, both when they were underweight and when they attained goal weight. The persistence of this finding suggests that this abnormality could be a trait marker for the illness.

Growth Hormone and Psychiatric Disease

The regulation of the hypothalamic-pituitary-GH system follows that of the HPA and HPT axes (Table 9–1). Neurons in the hypothalamus manufacture two peptides that play a pivotal role in stimulating the release and inhibition of GH. GHRH, when released from the hypothalamus into the portal vasculature, stimulates secretion of GH from the basophilic cells of the anterior pituitary. Somatostatin, also released from the hypothalamus, acts on the basophilic cells to inhibit GH secretion. In the periphery, GH produces some actions, such as antagonism of insulin directly, whereas other actions, such as somatic growth, are produced through hepatic manufacture of insulin-like growth factor 1 (IGF-1; also known as somatomedin-C). GH and IGF-1 provide negative feedback to the pituitary and hypothalamus. GH secretion is greater in women than in men and declines in both sexes with advanced age. GH secretion follows a circadian pattern and is most active at

night, especially during Stage 4 sleep. It is responsive to stress, exercise, hypoglycemia, and gonadal hormones, which cause an increase in GH secretion. Many other hormones and neurotransmitters stimulate the release of GH, including dopamine, norepinephrine, and acetylcholine.

Basal studies of GH in depression have found a blunting of the slow-wave sleep-related nocturnal secretion of GH (Jarrett et al. 1994; Mendlewicz et al. 1985). This alteration in GH release may be caused by the fragmented sleep architecture that often accompanies major depression (Schildkraut et al. 1975). Pharmacological challenge studies have identified a blunted GH response to clonidine (an α_2 agonist) and apomorphine (a dopamine D_2 agonist) in some patients with depression (Brown et al. 1983; Corn et al. 1984; Grof et al. 1982). However, these findings can vary depending on age, sex, stress, and the female menstrual cycle (Brown et al. 1983). Depressed patients also have blunted GH responses to other provocative stimuli, including insulin-induced hypoglycemia, L-dopa, 5-hydroxytryptamine (5-HTP), amphetamine, and desipramine (Charney et al. 1982; Thakore and Dinan 1994). Somatotropin release-inhibiting factor has been noted to be increased in depression (Rubinow et al. 1987).

In other psychiatric illnesses, studies have found paradoxical GH responses to GHRH in some male adolescent schizophrenic patients. However, these studies have been inconsistent and difficult to interpret. Somatostatin has been found in the CSF of patients with Alzheimer's disease (Molchan et al. 1993; Nemeroff et al. 1989). The GHRH stimulation test has also been tried in a variety of psychiatric diseases but has not yielded consistent results (Skare et al. 1994).

Prolactin and Psychiatric Disease

Prolactin is secreted by the anterior pituitary and is under the inhibitory control of dopamine released from the tuberoinfundibular neurons originating in the arcuate nucleus (Bevan et al. 1992) (Table 9–1). TRH is thought to play a major role in stimulating the release of prolactin (Kjellman et al. 1985). Prolactin stimulates lactation, and prolactin secretion may be induced by suckling, nipple stimulation, sexual intercourse, exercise, and stress. In contrast, hyperglycemia inhibits prolactin secretion. Prolactin secretion follows a circadian rhythm pattern and is elevated during sleep and reduced during wakefulness.

Changes in the amount of prolactin secreted and alterations in the circadian pattern of its secretion have also been identified in major depression (Mendlewicz et al. 1980; Rubin 1989). In depressed patients, a decreased prolactin response to hypoglycemia (Grof et al. 1982) and opioid agonists (Judd et al. 1982; Zis et al. 1985), as well as to the serotonergic agents tryptophan and fenfluramine, has been noted (Rubin 1989). Theoretically, this decreased response may be the result of alterations in brain serotonin and/or opioids. Other studies have reported no difference between depressed patients and control subjects in the amount of prolactin secreted, the circadian pattern of prolactin secretion, or the prolactin responses to TRH and other challenges (Rubin et al. 1987).

Hypothalamic-Pituitary-Gonadotropin Axis and Psychiatric Disease

GnRH is secreted by the hypothalamus and is responsible for the pulsatile secretion of LH and FSH (Table 9–1). Increased nocturnal secretion of GnRH is one of the first critical hormonal changes that result in puberty. The release of LH and FSH from the anterior pituitary is critical for sexual development and maintenance of sexual functioning in both males and females. In nonpregnant females, secretion of LH and FSH varies with the phase of the menstrual cycle, with a surge of both just before ovulation. LH and FSH function to induce the release of the sex steroids, such as estrogen, progesterone, and testosterone. In women, estrogen is sexually and mentally activating, and in recent reports, estrogen replacement therapy in postmenopausal women has been associated with improved outcome following medication therapy for depression and a decreased risk for the development of Alzheimer's disease (Paganini-Hill and Henderson 1996; Schneider et al. 1997). In men, the role of estrogen is unclear, except for a feminizing influence on secondary sex characteristics. Progesterone is an inhibitory hormone that can reduce sensation and sexual desire in both men and women. Testosterone promotes sex drive, assertiveness, and aggression in both sexes and sexual responsiveness in men.

The regulation of LH and FSH is subject to feedback regulation by ovarian and testicular hormones. Ovarian and testicular failure lead to an increase in LH and FSH. Increased sex hormones impose negative feedback on both the hypothalamus and the pituitary gland except during the follicular phase of the menstrual cycle when there is positive feedback. Stress, possibly via an inhibitory effect of cortisol, can decrease LH secretion.

Studies in patients with premenstrual dysphoric disorder characterized by symptoms of depressed mood, anxiety, and decreased energy have not found differences in hormonal levels in affected women compared with nonaffected control subjects (Giannini et al. 1990). It was once believed that this disorder was caused by a relative deficiency of progesterone, but progesterone suppositories have not been found to be effective in its treatment (Magos 1990; Schmidt et al. 1991).

Following childbirth, estrogen and progesterone levels decline precipitously. Fifty percent to 80% of women experience "baby blues," which is characterized by emotional lability, dysphoria, anxiety, insomnia, and irritability. These symptoms generally resolve within 2 weeks after delivery (Robinson and Stewart 1993). However, 10% of women have a more severe nonpsychotic postpartum depression, and 0.1% of women develop florid psychotic symptoms (Robinson and Stewart 1993). Studying the endocrine alterations, such as hypercortisolism and dexamethasone nonsuppression, is difficult after childbirth because these alterations are common postpartum (Pariante et al. 1997b).

Oxytocin and Vasopressin and Psychiatric Disease

Oxytocin and vasopressin are both secreted from the posterior pituitary into the systemic circulation. Oxytocin stimulates uterine contractions during parturition and milk letdown during lactation. Vasopressin regulates salt and water balance in the body. In the CSF of schizophrenic patients, oxytocin levels have been found to be increased and decreased (Beckmann et al. 1985; Glovinsky et al. 1994) and have been associated with chronic neuroleptic treatment. In bipolar disorder, oxytocin levels were decreased, and vasopressin levels were significantly higher in patients with mania (Legros and Ansseau 1989). No difference in these hormones was found between unipolar depressed patients and control subjects. CSF oxytocin levels were significantly lower in anorexic patients than in control subjects (Demitrack 1990). Plasma vasopressin levels have been increased and CSF vasopressin levels have been decreased in anorexic patients (Gold et al. 1983). Studies have also shown that oxytocin, but not vasopressin, is increased in the CSF of patients with obsessive-compulsive disorder without tics (Leckman et al. 1994a, 1994b). Theories have been posited that oxytocin may play a role in some forms of obsessive-compulsive disorder.

Summary

A wide variety of neuroendocrine hormones act directly on the central nervous system (CNS) to influence and modify human behavior. Moreover, a rich database has shown that the various neuroendocrine axes are altered in psychiatric disorders. Major depression has been the most extensively studied regarding neuroendocrine function, and the HPA axis has been the most extensively studied neuroendocrine system. Many of the alterations in the HPA axis, such as CRH hypersecretion and dexamethasone nonsuppression, are considered integral components of the pathophysiological process of the illness. The interactions between antidepressants, glucocorticoid receptors, and CRH will likely provide novel information on the mechanism of action of antidepressants. Alterations in the HPT axis and in GH secretion have also been found in depressed patients and are believed to play an important role in the pathophysiology and treatment of this disorder.

Evidence that neuroendocrine alterations play a preeminent role in the pathogenesis of other psychiatric disorders discussed is lacking. For anorexia nervosa, the main difficulty is determining whether the endocrine changes are primary and related to the disease or are a result of weight loss and malnutrition. For other neuroendocrine systems, whether alterations are responsible for the behavioral signs and symptoms of these diseases is unclear, and continued research in these areas is needed to understand their implications.

THE IMMUNE SYSTEM AND PSYCHIATRIC DISEASE

Over the past few decades, numerous studies have documented that the immune system and the CNS represent a bidirectional communication network with a host of shared transmitters, hormones, and peptides. Given the extensive intercommunication between these two systems, attention has been focused on the relevance of nervous system–immune system interactions to psychiatry.

At least two major factors must be considered when examining the potential role of the immune system in psychiatric diseases. First, the potential effects that psychiatric disorders (e.g., major depression) and psychological events (e.g., severe life stress) have on immune function must be considered. Because the neuroendocrine system appears to be involved in immune regulation, it is logical to consider that psychological/psychiatric states that alter hormonal systems (as described above) may contribute to the development, course, and outcome of diseases involving the immune system, including infectious diseases and cancer. Second, in the context of bidirectional communication between the nervous and immune systems, immune system mediators (e.g., cytokines) and immune processes (e.g., infectious, paraneoplastic, and autoimmune processes) may affect the nervous and endocrine systems and thereby play a role in the pathophysiology of psychiatric

disorders. In the following sections, we review the data documenting the relevance of the immune system to psychiatry. This information is designed to provide a foundation for further understanding the role of the immune system in psychiatric diseases.

Evidence of Interactions Between the CNS and the Immune System

To establish that meaningful interactions occur between the brain and the immune system, investigators have proceeded along several lines of investigation that have provided the foundation for the work described below (Table 9–3). Extensive data have clearly demonstrated that the necessary "hardware" is in place for brain–immune system communication. Immune cells express receptors for a host of transmitters, hormones, and peptides typically associated with the nervous system, including the monoamines, glucocorticoids, sex steroids, thyroid hormones, prolactin, GH, CRH, ACTH, and opioids (Ader et al. 1991; Miller and Spencer 1995). As described in more detail below, the immune system also has a rich innervation by autonomic nervous system (ANS) fibers; those emanating from the sympathetic branch have been best characterized. Studies that used a range of CNS manipulations, including selective brain lesions, have also established that discreet brain regions are involved in immune regulation (Ader et al. 1991; Miller and Spencer 1995). Robert Ader (who coined the term *psychoneuroimmunology* for the study of brain–immune system interactions) has demonstrated the capacity of the immune system to be conditioned in both positive and negative directions (N. Cohen et al. 1994). Finally, many studies have documented the bidirectional nature of brain–immune system interactions through the characterization of the profound effect of cytokines on the neuroendocrine system and a variety of behaviors (Besedovsky and del Rey 1996).

Table 9–3. Evidence of central nervous system (CNS) and immune system interactions

---

Immune cells express receptors for neuropeptides, neurotransmitters, and hormones.

Immune tissues are innervated by nerve fibers from the autonomic nervous system.

CNS lesions, stress, and psychiatric disorders are associated with altered immune function.

The immune system can be conditioned in a classical conditioning paradigm.

Soluble immune factors (cytokines) influence neuroendocrine function, neurotransmission, and behavior.

Effect of Stress and Depression on the Immune System

Probably the most well-established phenomenon in the context of CNS effects on the immune system is the capacity of stress to modulate a wide range of immune responses as well as the expression of diseases involving the immune system. Although much of the interest has been on the negative effect of stress on immune function, studies have shown that stressors can both enhance and inhibit immune responses, and many of these qualitative issues appear to be related to whether the stress is acute or chronic and which immune response in what immune compartment (e.g., blood, spleen, lymph nodes, gut, skin, lung) is being examined. In addition, stressors may have differential effects depending on the particular type of immune response that is being elicited by the pathogen (e.g., humoral versus cellular response).

Psychological Stress and the Immune System

One of the first studies to link stressful life events and the immune system in humans was conducted by Bartrop and colleagues (1977), who found that bereaved individuals had lower mitogen-stimulated lymphocyte proliferation compared with control subjects. Schleifer and co-workers (1983) confirmed these findings in a later prospective study of men whose wives were dying from advanced breast carcinoma. In this study, lymphocyte proliferative responses to the mitogens, phytohemagglutinin (PHA), concanavalin A, and pokeweed mitogen, were significantly lower during the first 2 months postbereavement compared with prebereavement responses. No differences in lymphocyte subpopulations were found. The impaired proliferative responses were still present, in some of the men, up to 1 year after their spouses had died.

Kiecolt-Glaser and Glaser (1991) also investigated the association of a range of stressful life events with the immune response in humans. Studies initially focused on academic stress among medical students as a common stressful situation. NK cell activity was decreased during the final examination period as compared with preexamination baseline responses. Examination stress was also associated with decreased number of T cells, decreased mitogen responses, decreased interferon production, increased antibody titers to latent herpesviruses (a putative marker of decreased cellular immune function), and reduced antibody responses to recombinant hepatitis B vaccine (Glaser et al. 1992). The effects of chronic life stressors, such as caregiving for patients with Alzheimer's disease, also were evaluated; lymphocyte subpopulations were altered, and titers for herpes simplex virus were increased (Kiecolt-Glaser et al. 1987). In a prospective study, caregivers of patients with Alzheimer's disease also had decreased proliferative responses to mitogens and more days of illness from infectious disease compared with matched control subjects (Kiecolt-Glaser et al. 1991). Finally, and most noteworthy from a clinical point of view, subjects with high levels of stress had impaired antibody responses to influenza vaccine (Kiecolt-Glaser et al. 1996) and prolonged latency of wound healing (Kiecolt-Glaser et al. 1995).

Depression and the Immune System

In studies examining bereavement stress, the level of depression has been found to be an important predictor of altered immune parameters (Irwin et al. 1987; Zisook et al. 1994). Therefore, considerable interest has evolved concerning the effect of depression (as a clinical syndrome) on the immune system.

In the early 1980s, two reports that appeared in the literature indicated that patients with major depression had decreased cellular immune responses (decreased proliferative response to mitogens) compared with healthy control subjects (Kronfol et al. 1983; Schleifer et al. 1984). Since then, numerous studies have examined immune parameters in depression; however, the relationship between depression and the immune system has turned out to be much more complicated than initially anticipated (Miller et al. 1993; Stein et al. 1991). For example, although a number of investigators have reported depression-related alterations in peripheral blood immune cell numbers and decreases in peripheral blood mitogen responses, these findings have not been reliably replicated. Alterations in the immune system do not appear to be a specific biological correlate of depression but appear to occur in subgroups of depressed patients who are older, more severely depressed, and male. For example, in a large study of 91 depressed patients and 91 control subjects, Schleifer et al. (1989) found no mean differences in immune measures between the groups. However, in that study, both advancing age and severity of depression were associated with decreases in CD4+ cell numbers and mitogen responsiveness of peripheral blood lymphocytes in depressed patients compared with control subjects.

Two studies reported sex differences in immune function of depressed patients. For example, one study, which reported decreased NK cell activity in males, found no changes in females (Evans et al. 1992), whereas two other studies found no changes in depressed men but increased NK cell activity in depressed women compared with their respective female control subjects (Miller et al. 1991; Pariante and Miller 1995). Some immune parameters, especially NK cell activity, appear to be more reliably altered than others (e.g., mitogen responses).

Because cortisol secretion is frequently altered in depressed patients, several studies have examined the relation between measures of cortisol secretion and the immune response in depressed patients. No clear association between these variables has emerged (Miller et al. 1993), although, as previously discussed, many depressed patients may show resistance to the inhibitory effects of glucocorticoids on immune function.

The Role of Age in Stress- and Depression-Mediated Changes in Immune Parameters

The interactions among stress, depression, and age are particularly important because older people show age-related alterations in immune function (immunosenescence), which may leave them more vulnerable to stress-induced immune alterations and the development of immune-related diseases. Moreover, advancing age has been shown to increase responsivity to the physiological effects of stress and depression on the neuroendocrine and immune systems. Data from experimental studies with laboratory animals suggest that older animals have a greater sensitivity to stress-induced immune alterations (Lorens et al. 1990), as well as an impaired capacity to terminate the HPA axis (Sapolsky et al. 1986) and sympathetic nervous system (Lorens et al. 1990; Milakofsky et al. 1993) response to stress. In humans, age also has been shown to interact with chronic stress and social support in determining the cardiovascular reactivity to stress (Uchino et al. 1992). Noteworthy in this regard are the findings reported by Pariante et al. (1997a), who examined female caregivers of persons with disabilities. Caregivers had a significantly lower percentage of T cells, a significantly higher percentage of T-suppressor/cytotoxic cells, and a significantly lower ratio of T-helper (Th) to T-suppressor cells. Interestingly, older caregivers (>45 years, median age) had not only lower numbers of T cells and Th cells but also higher antibody titers for cytomegalovirus. Finally, as mentioned earlier in this chapter, the largest study to date investigating immune abnormalities in major depression (Schleifer et al. 1989) failed to find between-group differences but revealed significant age-related differences.

Mechanisms of the Effects of Stress and Depression on the Immune System

Primary biological components of the response to stress are the HPA axis and the ANS. Both of these systems have been shown to have profound immunoregulatory effects and, therefore, are likely to be operative in determining stress-induced alterations in immune parameters.

HPA axis. Corticosteroids, the final product of HPA axis activation, have potent effects on the immune system and can both decrease immune cell function and induce lymphocyte subset redistribution between blood and other bodily compartments. As noted earlier in this chapter, immune cells and tissues have corticosteroid receptors, but the high degree of heterogeneity among immune cells and tissues in receptor expression allows for cell- and tissue-specific responses to stress. For example, consistent with the exquisite sensitivity of the thymus to involution following exogenous or endogenous glucocorticoid exposure, the thymus expresses one of the highest concentrations of glucocorticoid receptors in the body (~1,000 fmol/mg protein), followed by the spleen (~500 fmol/mg protein) and peripheral blood mononuclear cells (~250 fmol/mg protein) (Miller et al. 1990; Spencer et al. 1991). In addition, whereas only the glucocorticoid receptor is expressed in the thymus, both glucocorticoid receptors and mineralocorticoid receptors are expressed in the spleen (Miller et al. 1990; Spencer et al. 1991). Clinically, pharmacological doses of corticosteroids (including their synthetic analogues) are used because of their well-known "immunosuppressive" and antiinflammatory effects, mainly secondary to the inhibition of the synthesis of cytokines and mediators of inflammation (Schleimer et al. 1989). However, under physiological conditions, corticosteroids have important modulatory effects on immunity (McEwen et al. 1997). For example, by regulating the production of specific interleukins, it has been hypothesized that glucocorticoids shift the balance of an ongoing immune reaction from a Th1-directed (cell-mediated) response toward a Th2-directed (antibody-mediated) response (Mason 1991; Mosmann and Coffman 1989).

One of the best characterized effects of corticosteroids on the immune system is their ability to influence blood leukocyte distribution. Dhabhar et al. (1994, 1995, 1996) recently studied the effects of diurnal cycle, acute stress, and corticosteroid secretion on immune cell distribution. A mild, acute stressor (1 hour of restraint) caused significant and selective changes in peripheral blood cell distribution, including decreased numbers of white blood cells and decreased numbers and percentages of monocytes and lymphocytes—namely, B cells, NK cells, and, to a lesser degree, T cells—and slightly increased numbers and percentages of neutrophils. The changes were associated with a concomitant increase in plasma corticosterone and were almost completely abolished by adrenalectomy or administration of a glucocorticoid synthesis inhibitor. Administration of corticosterone (both mineralocorticoid receptor and glucocorticoid receptor agonist) or of the selective glucocorticoid receptor agonist RU28362 to adrenalectomized animals resulted in close replication of the stress-induced changes observed in intact animals, thus suggesting that the glucocorticoid receptor plays the major role in stress-induced leukocyte redistribution (Miller et al. 1994b). Finally, stress-induced changes in leukocyte subpopulations were remarkably similar to those obtained in nonstressed animals at the beginning of their active period, when corticosteroids reach their highest peak during the diurnal cycle (Dhabhar et al. 1994).

Note that stress-induced changes in immune cell numbers and distribution between the blood and various immune compartments may have profound effects on the effectiveness and functioning of the immune system. For example, it has been suggested that circadian variation in lymphocyte responsiveness to mitogens (Tavadia et al. 1975) is related to diurnal changes in peripheral blood leukocyte subsets (Dhabhar et al. 1994) and that stress-induced suppression of splenic and peripheral blood NK cell activity is related to stress-induced migration of NK cells out of these compartments (Ghoneum et al. 1987). Lymphocyte redistribution implies that cells are directed toward various immune compartments (i.e., lymph nodes, spleen, mucosa, skin) where they may be more likely to encounter antigens (Dhabhar and McEwen 1996; Dhabhar et al. 1994).

Autonomic nervous system. A second fundamental outflow pathway of the stress response, the ANS, also plays a relevant role in the immune response to stress. Historically, the identification of nerve fibers derived from the ANS in immune tissues was one of the first indications that communication between the CNS and immune system was possible.

Parasympathetic and sympathetic nerve fibers have been identified in organs that are responsible for the development, education, and function of lymphocytes, including the bone marrow, thymus, spleen, and lymph nodes (Bellinger et al. 1997; Felten et al. 1987). As mentioned earlier in this chapter, sympathetic nerve fibers have been the most extensively characterized and typically enter lymphoid tissues in association with the vascular supply. Inside the organs, the nerves are associated with smooth muscle cells of the blood vessels, where they play a role in vascular tone, and in the parenchyma, where they are associated with lymphocytes and other immune cells. Therefore, within the various immune compartments, ANS nerve fibers can influence the immune system either by changing the vascular tone and blood flow or by directly effecting the local release of neurotransmitters (norepinephrine, acetylcholine, neuropeptide Y, substance P, vasoactive intestinal peptide, calcitonin gene-related peptide) that interact with specific receptors on nearby immune cells (Bellinger et al. 1992, 1997).

Indeed, animal studies have shown that surgical or chemical sympathectomy alters immune responses in rodents as well as abrogates stress-induced immune changes, especially in the spleen (Hori et al. 1995).

In humans, the sympathetic nervous system appears to play a role in immune changes induced by brief experimental stressors, as suggested by the rapid onset of these changes and the greater immune changes in those subjects with increased cardiovascular responses (mediated by catecholamines) (Herbert et al. 1994). Elevated sympathetic activity also has been evident in subjects experiencing chronic stress (Uchino et al. 1992); therefore, the sympathetic nervous system may play a role in some of the immune changes occurring in association with naturalistic (life) stressors as well.

CRH. As noted earlier in this chapter, CRH is a pivotal neuropeptide in the regulation of the HPA axis and the sympathetic nervous system. Therefore, a series of studies has examined the effect of CRH on the immune system. Intracerebroventricular administration of CRH was first shown to have a powerful immunosuppressive effect on NK cell activity in the rat spleen (Irwin et al. 1988, 1990). Follow-up studies found that CRH can also inhibit in vivo and in vitro antibody formation, including the generation of an immunoglobulin G (IgG) response to immunization with keyhole limpet hemocyanin (Irwin 1993; Leu and Singh 1993). The influence of CRH on antibody responses is also apparent in CRH-overproducing mice whose immune deficits are characterized by a profound decrease in the number of B cells and severely diminished primary and memory antibody responses (Stenzel-Poore et al. 1996). Chronic intracerebroventricular administration of CRH and acute infusion of CRH into the locus coeruleus suppress lymphocyte proliferative responses to nonspecific mitogens and T-cell receptor antibody (anti-CD3) (Caroleo et al. 1993; Labeur et al. 1995; Rassnick et al. 1994). Interestingly, CRH has also been found to stimulate the release of proinflammatory cytokines in both laboratory animals and humans. For example, chronic intracerebroventricular administration of CRH to rats led to induction of interleukin-1 (IL-1β) mRNA in splenocytes, and intravenous infusion of CRH in humans led to an almost fourfold induction of IL-1α (Labeur et al. 1995, Schulte et al. 1994). Both treatments also led to significant increases in the immunoregulatory cytokine IL-2 (Labeur et al. 1995; Schulte et al. 1994). The proinflammatory effects of CRH are also manifest in the direct autocrine or paracrine inflammatory actions of this peptide at peripheral sites of inflammation, such as in an inflamed arthritic joint (Karalis et al. 1997). Taken together, these results indicate that CRH has well-documented immunosuppressive effects on in vivo cellular and humoral responses and a stimulatory effect on cytokine production and local inflammation.

The mechanism by which centrally administered CRH influences the immune response has been an active area of investigation. As noted, in the hypothalamus, CRH stimulates two major outflow pathways: the sympathetic nervous system, which releases catecholamines, and the HPA axis, which ultimately releases glucocorticoids. As indicated above, both catecholamines and glucocorticoids are well known to influence multiple aspects of the cellular and humoral immune response as well as the production and release of cytokines (McEwen et al. 1997).

Activation of the sympathetic nervous system by intracerebroventricular CRH has been found to be a major regulator of the effects of CRH on splenic NK activity, particularly through the use of the sympathetic ganglionic blocker chlorisondamine, which reversed the inhibitory effect of intracerebroventricular CRH on NK activity in the spleen (Irwin et al. 1988).

The HPA axis is also involved in CRH immune effects. Labeur and co-workers (1995) showed that the effects of chronic intracerebroventricular CRH on splenocyte proliferative responses were eliminated by adrenalectomy. In addition, the B-cell decreases found in CRH-overproducing mice are very consistent with the marked reduction of rodent B cells found after chronic exposure to glucocorticoids (Miller et al. 1994b).

Although both outflow pathways are clearly involved in CRH effects on the immune system, the relative contributions of the sympathetic nervous system and the HPA axis to immune changes in specific immune compartments as a function of length of exposure (acute versus chronic) have not been well characterized.

Studies of the effects of stress on the immune response indicate that various neuroendocrine mechanisms can be operative in different immune compartments, such that immune responses in the peripheral blood seem to be more influenced by glucocorticoids, whereas immune responses in the spleen (and possibly the immune tissues in general) seem to be more sensitive to locally released catecholamines. This differential sensitivity of these two immune compartments has been well demonstrated in studies by Rabin et al. (1990) and Cunnick et al. (1990). These

investigators found that the inhibitory immunological effects of acute stress on lymphocyte proliferative responses in the blood were reversed by adrenalectomy, whereas stress-induced inhibition of proliferative responses in the spleen was blocked by the administration of a β-adrenergic receptor antagonist.

Other factors.   HPA axis hormones and catecholamines (as regulated by CRH) are not the only factors involved in the modulation of the immune response following stress. In fact, studies conducted on hypophysectomized rats (Keller et al. 1988) showed that the stress-induced suppression of peripheral blood lymphocyte proliferative response to the mitogen PHA is significantly more pronounced in stressed hypophysectomized animals than in stressed intact animals. These findings suggest that pituitary hormones may be involved in counteracting stress-induced immunosuppressive mechanisms. The specific pituitary-dependent mitigating or compensating hormones are unknown but probably involve multiple hormones with immunoenhancing properties, such as GH and prolactin (Bernton et al. 1991; Kelley 1991). These findings also suggest that a regulatory network of hormonal and nonhormonal systems is involved in the maintenance of immunological capacity following exposure to stressors.

Nitric oxide.   Regarding the biochemical mechanisms of the immunological effects of stress, nitric oxide recently has been shown to be involved in the physiological and pathological responses to stress in various tissues, including immune tissues. Nitric oxide is a ubiquitous molecule that is involved in very different phenomena such as blood vessel tone, gastric mucosa protection, neurotoxicity, and macrophage function. Acute stress has influenced nitric oxide production in the immune system in rats (Persoons et al. 1995). Moreover, stress-induced changes in nitric oxide production by macrophages are indeed relevant to stress-induced decreases in lymphocyte proliferative responses, because both the depletion of macrophages and the addition of a nitric oxide synthesis inhibitor attenuated stress-induced immune suppression (Coussons-Read et al. 1994).

Consequences of Stress and Depression on Medical Illnesses

Because stress and depression have been associated with alterations in the immune response, there has been considerable interest in the possibility that stress and depression in humans may contribute to the development, course, and outcome of immune-based diseases. However, studies in humans confirming that stress and depression are associated with increased morbidity or mortality through direct effects on the immune system are lacking. For example, convincing evidence indicates that psychological stress is associated with an increased number and severity of infectious episodes in otherwise healthy individuals (S. Cohen et al. 1991; Graham et al. 1986; Kiecolt-Glaser et al. 1991). However, the role of stress-induced changes in the immune system in determining these findings is still unknown. Nevertheless, whether stressful events or depression are relevant to the progression or outcome of severe medical illness involving the immune system, especially cancer and acquired immunodeficiency syndrome (AIDS), remains a matter of great interest.

Depression and Cancer

To date, epidemiological studies have not supported the idea that depressive symptoms or mood disorders are associated with an increased risk of cancer morbidity and mortality. Although a prospective study of 2,018 male employees of the Western Electric Company has often been cited to support a relation between depressive symptoms and cancer (Persky et al. 1987), at least four subsequent reports with larger samples of subjects have not found such a relation (Hahn and Petitti 1988; Kaplan and Reynolds 1988; Linkins and Comstock 1990; Zonderman et al. 1989). Moreover, results from several studies that have examined mortality in large numbers of patients with psychiatric disorders suggest that psychiatric disorders are significantly associated not with death from natural causes but, rather, with unnatural mortality, such as suicide and accidental death.

Clearly, depression does not cause cancer; however, in individuals with cancer, depression not only is a common comorbid condition, occurring in 25%–50% of patients depending on the site, but also is associated with reduced quality of life. Moreover, psychiatric treatment of cancer patients has revealed some intriguing data on the effect of depression and psychosocial factors on disease outcome, including long-term survival.

The possibility that psychosocial interventions (e.g., group therapy) could improve survival in patients with cancer was elegantly demonstrated by two independent series of studies conducted by Spiegel et al. (1981, 1989) and Fawzy et al. (1990a, 1990b, 1993). Both series used a randomized study design to describe the influence of psychosocial interventions on the well-being and course of illness in patients with different kinds of cancer. Spiegel et al. (1989) used weekly group therapy to treat women with metastatic breast cancer. The intervention focused on encouraging the discussion of how to cope with cancer and the expression of feelings about the illness and its physical consequences and increasing social supports by developing relationships with other group members. Self-hypnosis was used for pain control, but the patients did not use imagery of the immune system fighting the tumor, and they were never told that the group therapy might affect the course of their illness. Following the first report in which Spiegel et al. (1981) described the usefulness of this approach in improving the quality of life of the patients, a randomized study compared 1 year of the psychosocial treatment with that in a control group (both undergoing routine oncological care). After a 10-year follow-up, the survival time of patients in the intervention group was almost double that of control subjects (36.6 months vs. 18.9 months, starting from the onset of the intervention). The divergence in survival was not evident during the treatment but appeared 20 months after study entry, almost 8 months after the end of the treatment.

Fawzy et al. (1990a, 1990b, 1993) also used a group therapy approach in the treatment of patients with malignant melanoma, but the intervention consisted of a short-term (6 weeks) structured approach focused on health education, enhancement of problem-solving skills, stress management with relaxation techniques, and psychological support. The authors reported at 6-month follow-up that this intervention (compared with a control group obtained by randomized assignment) was not only effective in reducing psychological distress of patients, including depressive symptoms, but also capable of inducing changes in immune parameters, including an increase in NK cell percentage and NK cytotoxic activity (two assays that could be relevant in the reaction of the immune system against cancer cells) and a small decrease in CD4+ (T-helper) cells (Fawzy et al. 1990a, 1990b). In addition, after 5–6 years of follow-up (Fawzy et al. 1993), patients who underwent the psychosocial intervention had a lower rate of death and cancer recurrence than did control subjects. However, the relation between immune parameters and outcome was not conspicuous (i.e., the baseline NK activity was predictive of only recurrence, not of survival), and the changes of the immune parameters over time had no evident effect on the course of the illness.

Although these studies testify to the positive effect of psychosocial interventions on the course of illness (and quality of life) of cancer patients, the role of putative changes in the immune system in determining this influence has not yet been established.

Psychological Variables and Viral Infections

As for the effects of stress on viral infections, data have confirmed that individuals who have high levels of perceived life stress are significantly more likely to be infected and develop a "cold" following intranasal inoculation of standardized doses of a series of respiratory viruses than are low-stressed individuals (S. Cohen et al. 1991).

Recently, great efforts have been devoted to determining the influence of stressful life events on the immune system and disease progression in subjects infected with human immunodeficiency virus (HIV), especially asymptomatic HIV-positive subjects. This issue is not trivial, because the hypothesis that psychological factors might influence the progression from the seropositive asymptomatic state to the AIDS state has led to the development of strategies for avoiding exposure to stressful events or for controlling the psychological reaction to these events (Kessler et al. 1991). However, the scientific evidence of an association between psychosocial factors and disease progression remains controversial, and contrasting findings have been reported on the effects of stress on immune parameters in this population. For example, three studies have not found an influence of psychosocial factors—distress levels and/or depression—on CD4+ cells alone (Kessler et al. 1991; Rabkin et al. 1991), CD4+ and CD8+ cells (Perry et al. 1992), and markers of disease progression, including the onset of fever and thrush (Kessler et al. 1991). Therefore, evidence suggesting that depression increases the progression of HIV disease appears to be lacking (Perry and Fishman 1993).

However, two recent studies found that HIV-positive subjects who experienced severe stress had relevant changes in immune parameters. In one study (Evans et al. 1995) of HIV-positive asymptomatic homosexual men, the presence of severe stress in the previous 6 months was associated with lower CD8+ and lower NK cell count, whereas no such association was evident in a control group of HIV-negative subjects. In another study (Kemeny et al. 1995), HIV-positive and HIV-negative homosexual men were followed up prospectively to evaluate the effect of the death of their intimate partners on immune parameters. Those who experienced bereavement during the follow-up had a significant increase in the level of serum neopterin (a marker of immune activation) and a significant decrease in the proliferative response to PHA compared with their prebereavement evaluation. These changes did not occur in the control groups composed of HIV-positive and HIV-negative nonbereaved men. Interestingly, the latter study did not show any effect of stress on lymphocyte subsets, including CD4+, CD8+, and NK cells.

Several methodological issues may account for the discrepancies in the literature, such as differences in the stage of illness, behavioral influences on the immune system, and above all, differences in the immune measures evaluated (Goodkin et al. 1994). In fact, negative studies by Rabkin et al. (1991) and Perry et al. (1992) evaluated mainly CD4+ cells, a lymphocyte subset that is heavily damaged by HIV infection. Indeed, the studies by Evans et al. (1995) and Kemeny et al. (1995) also failed to find any influence of stress on this immune parameter. These negative findings regarding the CD4+ subset count are intriguing, given the importance of this cell subset as a marker of progression of the illness. However, this immune measure may simply not be appropriate or meaningful in this context, because the relevant role of HIV virulence in determining the CD4+ level might confound the influence of psychosocial factors (Stein et al. 1991). On the other hand, the studies by Evans et al. (1995) and Kemeny et al. (1995) in HIV-positive subjects showed that stress influences CD8+ cells, NK cells, serum neopterin, and proliferative responses to PHA. Each of these parameters could be relevant to disease progression: the CD8+, cytotoxic T lymphocyte, and NK cells are important in the immune responses against viral infections and thus may have a role in controlling HIV infection, whereas both increased neopterin levels and decreased PHA proliferation in HIV-positive subjects have predicted the development of AIDS. In fact, recent work by Evans et al. (1997) supports the notion that severe life stress through effects on the immune system predicts early disease progression in HIV-infected individuals.

Contribution of the Immune System to the Pathogenesis of Psychiatric Diseases

Aside from the effect of stress and psychiatric illnesses on the immune system, interest has been increasing in the possibility that immune mediators and immune effectors may contribute to the pathophysiology of several neuropsychiatric diseases, including depression, schizophrenia, and Alzheimer's disease.

The Immune System in the CNS

The idea that infectious agents can lead to psychiatric disorders has been well established (Mohammed et al. 1993). Obvious examples include the mental retardation that occurs after congenital infection with rubella or cytomegalovirus; the delirium that accompanies acute meningoencephalitis after CNS infection by herpes simplex virus type I; the dementia that is caused by prion-related disease, such as kuru and Creutzfeldt-Jakob disease; and the neuropsychiatric manifestations that occur during neurosyphilis. Altered CNS function usually results from a combination of the direct effects of an injurious event or an infectious agent on various cell types and the effects of the immune/inflammatory response elicited by the injury or pathogen (cytokines and other inflammatory mediators). Thus, the brain has developed a specialized immune system to maintain the tenuous balance between protecting neurons from invading pathogens on the one hand and preventing damage mediated by the immune response on the other. In fact, the brain has historically been considered "immune privileged" because it lacks conventional lymphatics, has extremely low levels of major histocompatibility complex (MHC) expression, and is resistant to the transmigration of immune cells. Nevertheless, invading pathogens or other forms of injury can elicit a pronounced inflammatory response (Fabry et al. 1994). During an infection, extracellular antigens can drain to cervical lymphatics, glia are induced to express MHC class I and II, and activated T cells enter the CNS. Local induction of cytokines helps orchestrate the immune response, and adhesion molecules are upregulated on endothelium and perivascular glia to facilitate the entry of macrophages and other leukocytes. In addition to being a major source of proinflammatory cytokines, astrocytes and microglia become activated during inflammation and can produce other diffusible mediators such as nitric oxide, prostaglandins, and excitatory amino acids. Such inflammatory reactions can occur even in the absence of an infectious agent, as exemplified in postischemic brain injury in which a rapid induction of cytokines, extravasation of leukocytes, and gliosis occur. It remains to be determined which aspects of this immune reaction are deleterious rather than the immunological accoutrements of repair.

Cytokines and CNS Function

Beginning with the early work of Besedovsky and colleagues (1983), there has been increasing appreciation for the capacity of immune responses (which are not necessarily directed against brain pathogens or brain antigens) to affect CNS function. Early studies characterized alterations in the release of glucocorticoids and norepinephrine turnover in the hypothalamus during an immune response to sheep red blood cells, and more recent studies have extensively characterized the ability of cytokines to activate the HPA axis at virtually every level, most notably, through the effects of cytokines (IL-1β being the most potent) on CRH (Besedovsky and del Rey 1996). Cytokines also mediate a host of neurotransmitter changes in the brain and can modulate a series of behaviors including

feeding, activity levels, sleep, and social interactions (Besedovsky and del Rey 1996; Kent et al. 1992). Because data indicate that cytokine effects on behavior are mediated within the CNS and cytokines do not readily cross the blood-brain barrier in the absence of CNS infection, the mechanisms by which peripherally released cytokines communicate with the brain have received considerable attention. Four major pathways have been described: 1) active transport of cytokines across the blood-brain barrier (Banks et al. 1995); 2) access of cytokines to brain areas where the blood-brain barrier does not exist or is "leaky," such as the organum vasculosum of the lamina terminalis (Schobitz et al. 1994); 3) conversion of cytokine signals into prostaglandin or nitric oxide signals by endothelial cells lining the blood vessels in the brain (Rivier 1995); and 4) transmission of cytokine signals (through cytokine receptor binding) along sensory afferents to the nucleus of the solitary tract and then to relevant brain regions including the PVN in the hypothalamus (Cunningham et al. 1990; Ericsson et al. 1994; Watkins and Maier 1995). Note that cytokines and their receptors are constitutively expressed in neurons throughout the CNS, and whether cytokines play a role as neurotransmitters is an area of active investigation (Besedovsky and del Rey 1996; Schobitz et al. 1994).

Although definitive data regarding the participation of immune processes in the development of psychiatric disorders is only beginning to be collected, considerable attention has been focused on the role of immune factors in the expression of psychiatric diseases.

Depression

One of the first lines of evidence suggesting a role of the immune system (proinflammatory cytokines and immune activation, in particular) in the pathogenesis of depression was derived from clinical observations that administration of various cytokines in clinical trials for immune-based diseases was associated with the development of numerous behavioral symptoms, including depressed mood. Specifically, these symptoms have been described as part of a behavioral syndrome referred to as *sickness behavior* (Kent et al. 1992). This syndrome is induced by increased levels of proinflammatory cytokines, including IL-1, IL-6, and tumor necrosis factor, as well as IL-2 and interferon-α/β. Symptoms include weakness, malaise, listlessness, anhedonia, hypersomnia, anorexia, social isolation, hyperalgesia, and poor concentration. This syndrome typically occurs during infections but may occur in a wide variety of clinical settings, including any medical condition that leads to significant inflammation and the release of proinflammatory cytokines, as well as when cytokines are administered exogenously for therapy in neoplastic or viral diseases.

Along these lines, data indicate that stress can induce the release of proinflammatory cytokines in the absence of a more formal immune challenge (i.e., a pathogen). For example, different mild stressors such as open-field exposure, electric footshock, and restraint induce an elevation in plasma levels of IL-6 (LeMay et al. 1990; Zhou et al. 1993) that appears to be secondary to the release of catecholamines. IL-6 is an important proinflammatory mediator of the acute phase response and the inflammatory response and presumably may play a role in the various stress-related changes in immune function. However, like the other proinflammatory cytokines, IL-6 has profound neuroendocrine effects, including stimulation of the release of HPA axis hormones CRH and ACTH (Besedovsky and del Rey 1996). In this regard, stress-induced IL-6 production may participate in the neuroendocrine response to stress. Moreover, induction of proinflammatory cytokines by stress may contribute to some of the behavioral consequences of stress that also have features similar to depression.

Support for the notion that the immune system may contribute to the biochemical and molecular biological changes that characterize depression comes from studies reporting elevated serum concentrations of the proinflammatory cytokine IL-6 and increased acute phase proteins, including haptoglobin, C-reactive protein, and α_1-acid glycoprotein, in patients with major depression (Maes 1993; Maes et al. 1993; Sluzewska et al. 1996). The acute phase response may contribute to decreased availability of L-tryptophan (Hasselgren et al. 1988), which leads to reduced serotonin in the brain. In addition, in vivo and in vitro studies suggest that proinflammatory cytokines, especially IL-1, may induce resistance of tissues to circulating glucocorticoid hormones through direct inhibitory effects on glucocorticoid receptor expression and/or function (Hill et al. 1986, 1988; Pariante et al. 1996). Therefore, increased levels of proinflammatory cytokines may induce glucocorticoid resistance in depressed patients and, therefore, contribute to HPA axis hyperactivity caused by impaired feedback inhibition.

Schizophrenia

A number of investigators have considered the role of the immune system in schizophrenia, including evaluation of both an infectious and an autoimmune etiology.

Several lines of evidence suggest that viral infection during neural development may be involved in the pathogenesis of some cases of schizophrenia. The data include

- An excess number of patient births in the late winter and early spring, suggesting possible exposure to viral infection in utero during the fall and winter peak of viral illnesses
- An association between exposure to viral epidemics while in utero and the later development of schizophrenia
- An increased likelihood for schizophrenic patients to have had older siblings in the household (a potential source of viral infections) compared with control subjects
- The presence of gliosis, a process known to accompany infection and inflammation, in some brain areas of schizophrenic patients (Kirch 1993; Wright and Murray 1995)

Unfortunately, attempts to isolate infectious agents, especially viruses and viral DNA, from schizophrenic patients have been unsuccessful. However, because the initial neuronal abnormalities in schizophrenia have been proposed to arise during neurodevelopment, a perinatal viral infection could insidiously disrupt development and then be cleared by the immune system before clinical diagnosis. In such a scenario, host factors such as cytokines could be responsible for causing the developmental abnormality by interacting with growth factors or adhesion molecules. For example, IL-1 and glucocorticoids can regulate the production of brain-derived neurotropic factor (Smith 1996). Because certain inhibitory neurons are dependent on this factor for their normal differentiation, this mechanism could explain the decrease in subpopulations of inhibitory interneurons reported in schizophrenia. Alternatively, antibodies produced by a pregnant woman who has a viral infection may cross the placenta and cross-react with antigen localized in the brain. Because these antibodies would exert their damage early in intrautero life, it would not be surprising to find no trace of virus and/or antibody in the adult patient.

Interestingly, investigators have reported various alterations in immune markers, including increased interferon levels, decreased IL-2 production, and increased IL-2 receptors, in schizophrenic patients (Ganguli et al. 1993). CSF immunoglobulins have also been increased in some studies. Although those immune findings in schizophrenic patients may indicate evidence of immune system activation secondary to infection, they also may indicate that an autoimmune process is involved in the disorder. However, studies trying to isolate autoantibodies to CNS tissue constituents in schizophrenic patients have yielded inconsistent results. Moreover, because schizophrenia may involve various forms of CNS tissue damage, with the resultant release of brain antigens, autoantibodies to CNS tissues in those instances may be the result of CNS pathology rather than the cause.

Nevertheless, several autoimmune disorders, including thyroid disorders and collagen vascular diseases such as systemic lupus erythematosus, can indirectly or nonspecifically alter CNS function; however, only a few autoimmune conditions directly involve brain antigens. Neural cells are the target for autoantibodies in the paraneoplastic syndromes. For example, autoantibodies to cytoplasmic proteins of Purkinje cells are associated with subacute cortical cerebellar degeneration, which is a rare complication of breast or ovarian cancers (Posner and Furneaux 1990). Autoantibodies to γ-aminobutyric acid (GABA)ergic neurons in the serum and CSF appear to be the mechanism behind at least some cases of the stiff-man syndrome, a rare disorder characterized by progressive rigidity, accompanied by recurrent painful muscle spasms (Lernmark 1996). Antineuronal antibodies can also arise following group A β-hemolytic streptococcal infections, as exemplified by Sydenham's chorea (Swedo et al. 1997). Considering that children with Sydenham's chorea frequently have obsessive-compulsive symptoms, emotional lability, and hyperactivity, a spectrum of pediatric autoimmune neuropsychiatric disorders may be associated with streptococcal infections (Swedo et al. 1997). The basal ganglia have been suggested as a possible target of the autoimmune response in pediatric autoimmune neuropsychiatric disorders associated with streptococcal infections.

Alzheimer's Disease

Although Alzheimer's disease is not considered to be primarily an inflammatory disease, emerging evidence indicates that the immune system may contribute to its pathogenesis. The discovery that amyloid plaques are associated with acute phase proteins, such as complement proteins, α_1-antichymotrypsin, and C-reactive protein, suggests the possibility of an ongoing immune response (Aisen and Davis 1994). Furthermore, gliosis and increased levels of proinflammatory cytokines are also found in and around plaques. Interestingly, the induction of IL-6 has been proposed to precede neuritic degeneration in nascent (diffuse) plaques, and IL-1β can increase mRNA for amyloid precursor protein (Goldgaber et al. 1989; Hull et al. 1996). Thus, immune mediators have been theorized to have an early role in plaque formation. Moreover, microglial cells that produce IL-1 and other proinflammatory cytokines have also been described to synthesize amyloid precursor protein (LeBlanc et al. 1997). Finally, the idea that inflammatory processes are involved in Alzheimer's

disease has been bolstered by recent studies showing that the long-term use of nonsteroidal antiinflammatory drugs is negatively correlated with the development of Alzheimer's disease (Breitner 1996).

Summary

Clearly, the nervous, endocrine, and immune systems interact in a meaningful way that may be involved in the pathophysiology of both nervous system and immune system diseases. Further understanding of the basic physiology of brain–endocrine–immune system interactions in conjunction with further characterization of these interactions in psychiatric diseases will provide the foundation for the development of new treatment strategies that will address the participation of hormones and cytokines in the expression of behavioral disorders.

REFERENCES

Abelson JL, Curtis GC, Cameron OG: Hypothalamic-pituitary-adrenal axis activity in panic disorder: effects of alprazolam on 24 hr secretion of adrenocorticotrophin and cortisol. J Psychiatr Res 30:79–83, 1996

Ader R, Cohen N, Felten D (eds): Psychoneuroimmunology II. New York, Academic Press, 1991

Aisen PS, Davis KL: Inflammatory mechanisms in Alzheimer's disease: implications for therapy. Am J Psychiatry 151:1105–1113, 1994

Axelson DA, Doraiswamy PM, Boyko O, et al: In vivo assessment of pituitary volume with magnetic resonance imaging and systematic stereology: relationship to dexamethasone suppression test results in patients. Psychiatry Res 44:63–70, 1992

Banki CM, Bissette G, Arato M, et al: Elevation of immunoreactive CSF-TRH in depressed patients. Am J Psychiatry 145:1526–1531, 1988

Banks WA, Kastin AJ, Broadwell RD: Passage of cytokines across the blood-brain barrier. Neuroimmunomodulation 2:241–248, 1995

Bartrop RW, Lazarus L, Luckherst E, et al: Depressed lymphocyte function after bereavement. Lancet 1:834–836, 1977

Baxter JD, Tyrrell JB: The adrenal cortex, in Endocrinology and Metabolism. Edited by Felig P, Baxter JD, Broadus AE, et al. New York, McGraw-Hill, 1987, pp 511–650

Beck-Friis J, Ljunggren JG, Thoren M, et al: Melatonin, cortisol, and ACTH in patients with major depressive disorder and healthy human with special reference to the outcome of the dexamethasone suppression test. Psychoneuroendocrinology 10:173–186, 1985

Beckmann H, Lang RF, Gattaz WF: Vasopressin-oxytocin in cerebrospinal fluid of schizophrenic patients and normal controls. Psychoneuroendocrinology 10:187–191, 1985

Bellinger DL, Felten SY, Felten DL: Neural-immune interactions, in American Psychiatric Association Annual Review, Vol 11. Edited by Tasman A. Washington, DC, American Psychiatric Press, 1992, pp 127–144

Bellinger DL, Felten SY, Lorton D, et al: Innervation of lymphoid organs and neurotransmitter-lymphocyte interactions, in Immunology of the Nervous System. Edited by Keane RW, Hickey W. New York, Oxford University Press, 1997, pp 226–329

Bernton EW, Bryant HU, Holaday JW: Prolactin and immune function, in Psychoneuroimmunology, 2nd Edition. Edited by Ader R, Felten DL, Cohen N. New York, Academic Press, 1991, pp 403–428

Besedovsky HO, del Rey A: Immune-neuro-endocrine interaction: facts and hypotheses. Endocr Rev 17:64–102, 1996

Besedovsky H, del Rey A, Sorkin E, et al: The immune response evokes changes in brain noradrenergic neurons. Science 221:564–566, 1983

Bevan JS, Webster J, Burke CW, et al: Dopamine agonists and pituitary tumor shrinkage. Endocr Rev 13:220–240, 1992

Breitner JCS: Inflammatory processes and antiinflamatory drugs in Alzheimer's disease: a current appraisal. Neurobiol Aging 17:789–794, 1996

Bremnar JD, Randall P, Scott TM, et al: MRI-based measurement of hippocampal volume in patients with combat-related post-traumatic stress disorder. Am J Psychiatry 152:973–981, 1995

Bremnar JD, Licinio J, Darnell A, et al: Elevated CSF corticotropin-releasing factor concentration in PTSD. Am J Psychiatry 154:624–629, 1997

Brown GM: Psychoneuroendocrinology of depression. Psychiatric Journal of the University of Ottawa 14:344–348, 1989

Brown GM, Clayhorn JM, Boyne TS: Psychoneuroendocrinology of growth hormone: an update, in The Anterior Pituitary Gland. Edited by Bhatnager AS. New York, Raven, 1983, pp 393–403

Caroleo MC, Pulvirenti L, Arbitrio M, et al: Evidence that CRH microinfused into the locus coeruleus decreases cell-mediated immune response in rats. Funct Neurol 8:271–277, 1993

Carroll BJ, Feinburg M, Greden JF, et al: Diagnosis of endogenous depression: comparison of clinical, research, and neuroendocrine criteria. J Affect Disord 2:177–194, 1980

Charney DS, Henniger GR, Steinberg DE, et al: Adrenergic receptor sensitivity in depression: effects of clonidine in depressed patients and healthy subjects. Arch Gen Psychiatry 39:290–294, 1982

Cohen N, Moynihan JA, Ader R: Pavlovian conditioning of the immune system. Int Arch Allergy Immunol 105:101–106, 1994

Cohen S, Tyrrell DA, Smith AP: Psychological stress and susceptibility to the common cold. N Engl J Med 325:606–612, 1991

Corn TH, Hale AS, Thompson C, et al: A comparison of the growth hormone responses to clonidine and apomorphine in the same patients with endogenous depression. Br J Psychiatry 144:636–639, 1984

Coussons-Read ME, Maslonek KA, Fecho K, et al: Evidence for the involvement of macrophage-derived nitric oxide in the modulation of immune status by a conditioned aversive stimulus. J Neuroimmunol 50:51–58, 1994

Cunnick JE, Lysle DT, Kucinski BJ, et al: Evidence that shock induced immune suppression is mediated by adrenal hormones and peripheral beta-adrenergic receptors. Pharmacol Biochem Behav 36:645–651, 1990

Cunningham ET, Bohn MC, Sawchenko PE: Organization of adrenergic inputs to the paraventricular and supraoptic nuclei of the hypothalamus in the rat. J Comp Neurol 292:651–667, 1990

Curtis GC, Abelson JL, Gold PW: Adrenocorticotropic hormone and cortisol responses to CRH: changes in panic disorder and effects of alprazolam treatment. Biol Psychiatry 41:76–85, 1997

Cushing H: Medical classic: the functions of the pituitary body: Harvey Cushing. Am J Med Sci 281:70–78, 1981

Demitrack MA: CSF oxytocin in anorexia nervosa and bulimia nervosa: clinical and pathophysiological considerations. Am J Psychiatry 147:882–886, 1990

Dhabhar FS, McEwen BS: Stress-induced enhancement of antigen-specific cell-mediated immunity. J Immunol 156:2608–2615, 1996

Dhabhar FS, Miller AH, Stein M, et al: Diurnal and acute stress-induced changes in distribution of peripheral blood leukocyte subpopulations. Brain Behav Immun 8:66–79, 1994

Dhabhar FS, Miller AH, McEwen BS, et al: Effects of stress on immune cell distribution: dynamics and hormonal mechanisms. J Immunol 154:5511–5527, 1995

Dhabhar FS, Miller AH, McEwen BS, et al: Stress-induced changes in blood leukocyte distribution: role of adrenal steroid hormones. J Immunol 157:1638–1644, 1996

Ericsson A, Kovacs J, Sawchenko PE: A functional anatomical analysis of central pathways subserving the effects of interleukin-1 on stress-related neuroendocrine neurons. J Neurosci 14:897–913, 1994

Evans DL, Folds JD, Petitto JM, et al: Circulating natural killer cells phenotypes in men and women with major depression: relation to cytotoxic activity and severity of depression. Arch Gen Psychiatry 49:388–395, 1992

Evans DL, Leserman J, Perkins DO, et al: Stress-associated reductions of cytotoxic T lymphocytes and natural killer cells in asymptomatic HIV infection. Am J Psychiatry 152:543–550, 1995

Evans DL, Leserman J, Perkins DO, et al: Severe life stress as a predictor of early disease progression in HIV infection. Am J Psychiatry 154:630–634, 1997

Fabry Z, Raine CS, Hart MN: Nervous tissue as an immune compartment: the dialect of the immune response in the CNS. Immunol Today 15:218–224, 1994

Fawzy FI, Cousins N, Fawzy NW, et al: A structured psychiatric intervention for cancer patients, I: changes over time in methods of coping and affective disturbance. Arch Gen Psychiatry 47:720–725, 1990a

Fawzy FI, Kemeny ME, Fawzy NW, et al: A structured psychiatric intervention for cancer patients, II: changes over time in immunological measures. Arch Gen Psychiatry 47:729–735, 1990b

Fawzy FI, Fawzy NW, Hyun CS, et al: Malignant melanoma: effects of an early structured psychiatric intervention, coping, and affective state on recurrence and survival 6 years later. Arch Gen Psychiatry 50:681–689, 1993

Felten DL, Felten SY, Bellinger DL, et al: Noradrenergic sympathetic neural interactions with the immune system: structure and function. Immunol Rev 100:225–260, 1987

Ferrier IN, Leake A: Peptides in the neocortex in Alzheimer's disease and ageing. Psychoneuroimmunology 15:89–95, 1990

Ganguli R, Brar JS, Chengappa KR, et al: Autoimmunity in schizophrenia: a review of recent findings (Special Section: Psychoneuroimmunology). Ann Med 25:489–496, 1993

Garbutt JC, Mayo JP, Little KY, et al: Dose-response studies with protirelin. Arch Gen Psychiatry 51:875–883, 1994

Ghoneum M, Gill G, Assanah P, et al: Susceptibility of natural killer cell activity of old rats to stress. Immunology 60:461–465, 1987

Giannini AJ, Martin DM, Turner CE: Beta-endorphin decline in late luteal phase dysphoric disorder. Int J Psychiatry Med 97:279–284, 1990

Glaser R, Kiecolt-Glaser JK, Bonneau RH, et al: Stress-induced modulation of the immune response to recombinant hepatitis B vaccine. Psychosom Med 54:22–29, 1992

Glovinsky D, Kalogeras KT, Kirch DG, et al: Cerebrospinal fluid oxytocin concentration in schizophrenic patients does not differ from control subjects and is not changed by neuroleptic medication. Schizophr Res 11:273–276, 1994

Glowa JR, Gold PW: Corticotropin releasing hormone produces profound anorexigenic effects in the rhesus monkey. Neuropeptides 18:55–61, 1991

Gold PW, Kaye W, Robertson GL, et al: Abnormalities in plasma and cerebrospinal-fluid arginine vasopressin in patients with anorexia nervosa. N Engl J Med 308:1117–1123, 1983

Gold PW, Lichinio J, Wong M, et al: Corticotropin releasing hormone in the pathophysiology of melancholic and atypical depression in the mechanism of action of antidepressant drugs. Ann N Y Acad Sci 771:716–729, 1995

Goldgaber D, Herbert WH, Hla T, et al: Interleukin 1 regulates synthesis of amyloid β-protein precursor mRNA in human endothelial cells. Proc Natl Acad Sci U S A 86:7606–7610, 1989

Goodkin K, Mulder CL, Blaney NT, et al: Psychoneuroimmunology and human immunodeficiency virus type 1 infection revisited. Arch Gen Psychiatry 51:246–247, 1994

Gormley GJ, Lowy MT, Reder AT, et al: Glucocorticoid receptors in depression: relationship to the dexamethasone suppression test. Am J Psychiatry 142:1278–1284, 1985

Graham NMH, Douglas RM, Ryan P: Stress and acute respiratory infection. Am J Epidemiol 124:389–401, 1986

Grillon C, Southwick SM, Charney DS: The psychobiological basis of post-traumatic stress disorder. Molecular Psychiatry 4:278–297, 1996

Grof E, Brown GM, Arato M, et al: Investigations of melatonin secretion in man. Prog Neuropsychopharmacol Biol Psychiatry 6:487–490, 1982

Hahn RC, Petitti DB: Minnesota Multiphasic Personality Inventory–rated depression and the incidence of breast cancer. Cancer 61:845–848, 1988

Hasselgren PO, Pederssen P, Sax HC, et al: Current concepts of protein turnover and amino acid transport in liver and skeletal muscle during sepsis. Arch Surg 123:992–999, 1988

Hatzinger M, Z'brun A, Hemmeter U, et al: Hypothalamic-pituitary-adrenal system function in patients with Alzheimer's disease. Neurobiol Aging 16:205–209, 1995

Heilig M, Sjogren M, Blennow K, et al: Cerebrospinal fluid neuropeptides in Alzheimer's disease and vascular dementia. Biol Psychiatry 38:210–216, 1995

Herbert TB, Cohen S, Marsland AL, et al: Cardiovascular reactivity and the course of immune response to an acute psychological stressor. Psychosom Med 56:337–344, 1994

Heuser I, Yassouridis A, Hosboer F: The combined dexamethasone/CRH test: a refined laboratory test for psychiatric disorders. J Psychiatr Res 28:341–356, 1994

Hill MR, Stith RD, McCallum RE: Interleukin 1: a regulatory role in glucocorticoid-regulated hepatic metabolism. J Immunol 137:858–862, 1986

Hill MR, Stith RD, McCallum RE: Human recombinant IL-1 alters glucocorticoid receptor function in Reuber hepatoma cells. J Immunol 141:1522–1528, 1988

Holsboer F, Barden N: Antidepressants and hypothalamic-pituitary-adrenocortical regulation. Endocr Rev 17:187–205, 1996

Hori T, Katafuchi T, Take Shimizu, et al: The autonomic nervous system as a communication channel between the brain and the immune system. Neuroimmunomodulation 2:203–215, 1995

Hull M, Strauss S, Berger M: Inflammatory mechanisms in Alzheimer's disease. Eur Arch Psychiatry Clin Neurosci 246:124–128, 1996

Irwin M: Brain corticotropin-releasing-hormone- and interleukin-1β-induced suppression of specific antibody production. Endocrinology 133:1352–1360, 1993

Irwin M, Daniels M, Bloom ET, et al: Life events, depressive symptoms, and immune function. Am J Psychiatry 144:437–441, 1987

Pariante CM, Miller AH: Natural killer cell activity in major depression: a prospective study of the in vivo effects of desmethylimipramine treatment. Eur Neuropsychopharmacol 1 (suppl):83–88, 1995

Pariante CM, Nemeroff CB, Miller AH: Glucocorticoid receptors in depression. Isr J Med Sci 31:705–712, 1995

Pariante CM, Pearce BD, Pisell TL, et al: Interleukin-1 a inhibits nucleocytoplasmic traffic of the glucocorticoid receptor. Third International Congress of the International Society of Neuroimmunomodulation, Bethesda, MD, November 1996

Pariante CM, Carpiniello B, Orru' MG, et al: Chronic caregiving stress alters peripheral blood immune parameters: the role of age and severity of stress. Psychother Psychosom 66:199–207, 1997a

Pariante CM, Nemeroff CB, Miller AH: Hormonal regulation of behavior, in Current Psychiatric Therapy II. Edited by Dunner DL. Philadelphia, PA, WB Saunders, 1997b, pp 44–51

Pariante CM, Pearce BD, Pisell TL, et al: Steroid-independent translocation of the glucocorticoid receptor by the antidepressant desipramine. Mol Pharmacol 52:571–581, 1997c

Parker DC, Rossman LG, Pekary AE, et al: Effect of 64-hour sleep deprivation on the circadian wave form of thyrotropin (TSH): further evidence of sleep-related inhibition of TSH release. J Clin Endocrinol Metab 64:157–161, 1987

Pepin M-C, Govindan MV, Barden N: Increased glucocorticoid receptor gene promoter activity after antidepressant treatment. Mol Pharmacol 41:1016–1022, 1992

Perry S, Fishman B: Depression and HIV: how does one affect the other? JAMA 270:2609–2610, 1993

Perry S, Fishman B, Jacobsberg L, et al: Relationships over 1 year between lymphocyte subsets and psychosocial variables among adults with infection by human immunodeficiency virus. Arch Gen Psychiatry 49:396–401, 1992

Persky VW, Kempthorne-Rawson J, Shekelle RB: Personality and risk of cancer: 20-year follow-up of the Western Electric Study. Psychosom Med 49:435–449, 1987

Persoons JHA, Schornagel K, Breve J, et al: Acute stress affects cytokines and nitric oxide production by alveolar macrophages differently. Am J Respir Crit Care Med 152:619–624, 1995

Pfohl B, Sherman B, Schlechte J, et al: Pituitary-adrenal axis rhythm disturbances in psychiatric depression. Arch Gen Psychiatry 42:897–903, 1985

Plotsky PM, Meaney MJ: Early, postnatal experience alters hypothalamic corticotropin-releasing factor (CRF) mRNA, median eminence CRF content and stress-induced release in adult rats. Molecular Brain Research 18:195–200, 1993

Posner JB, Furneaux HM: Paraneoplastic syndromes, in Immunologic Mechanisms in Neurologic and Psychiatric Disease. Edited by Waksman BH. New York, Raven, 1990, pp 187–219

Raadsheer FC, Hoogendijk WJ, Stam FC, et al: Increased numbers of CRH expressing neurons in the hypothalamic paraventricular nucleus of depressed patients. Neuroendocrinology 60:436–444, 1994

Raadsheer FC, Van Heerikhuize JJ, Lucassen PJ, et al: Corticotropin-releasing hormone mRNA levels in the paraventricular nucleus of patients with Alzheimer's disease and depression. Am J Psychiatry 152:1372–1376, 1995

Rabin BS, Cunnick JE, Lysle DT: Stress-induced alteration of immune function. Progress in NeuroEndocrinImmunology 2:116–124, 1990

Rabkin JG, Williams JBW, Remien RH, et al: Depression, distress, lymphocyte subsets, and human immunodeficiency virus symptoms on two occasions in HIV-positive homosexual men. Arch Gen Psychiatry 48:111–119, 1991

Rassnick S, Sved AF, Rabin BS: Locus coeruleus stimulation by corticotropin-releasing hormone suppresses in vitro cellular immune responses. J Neurosci 14:6033–6040, 1994

Reul JM, de Kloet ER: Two receptor systems for corticosterone in rat brain: microdistribution and differential occupation. Endocrinology 117:2505–2511, 1985

Rivier C: Influence of immune signals on the hypothalamic-pituitary axis of the rodent. Front Neuroendocrinol 16:151–182, 1995

Robinson GA, Stewart DE: Postpartum disorders, in Psychological Aspects of Women's Health Care: The Interface Between Psychiatry and Obstetrics and Gynecology. Edited by Stewart DG, Stotland NL. Washington, DC, American Psychiatric Press, 1993

Rubin RT: Pharmacoendocrinology of major depression. Eur Arch Psychiatry Neurol Sci 238:259–267, 1989

Rubin RT, Poland RE, Lesser IM, et al: Neuroendocrine aspects of primary endogenous depression, IV: pituitary-thyroid axis activity in patients and matched control subjects. Psychoneuroendocrinology 12:333–347, 1987

Rubin RT, Phillips JS, McCracken JT, et al: Adrenal gland volume in major depression: relationship to basal and stimulated pituitary-adrenal cortical axis function. Biol Psychiatry 40:89–97, 1996

Rubinow DR, Post RD, Davis CL, et al: Somatostain and GHRH: mood and behavioral regulation. Adv Biochem Psychopharmacol 43:137–152, 1987

Sallee FR, Nesbitt L, Dougherty D, et al: Lymphocyte glucocorticoid receptor: predictor of sertraline response in adolescent major depressive disorder (MDD). Psychopharmacol Bull 31:339–345, 1995

Sapolsky RM, Krey LC, McEwen BS: The neuroendocrinology of stress and aging: the glucocorticoid cascade hypothesis. Endocr Rev 7:284–301, 1986

Schildkraut R, Chandra O, Osswald M, et al: Growth hormone release during sleep and with thermal stimulation in depressed patients. Neuropsychobiology 1:70–79, 1975

Schleifer SJ, Keller SE, Camerino M, et al: Suppression of lymphocyte stimulation following bereavement. JAMA 250:374–377, 1983

Schleifer SJ, Keller SE, Meyerson AT, et al: Lymphocyte function in major depressive disorder. Arch Gen Psychiatry 41:484–486, 1984

Schleifer SJ, Keller SE, Bond RN, et al: Major depressive disorder and immunity: role of age, sex, severity and hospitalization. Arch Gen Psychiatry 46:81–87, 1989

Schleimer RP, Claman HN, Oronsky A (eds): Anti-Inflammatory Steroid Action, Basic and Clinical Aspects. San Diego, CA, Academic Press, 1989

Schmidt P, Nieman R, Grover G, et al: Lack of effect of induced menses on symptoms in women with premenstrual syndrome. N Engl J Med 324:1174–1179, 1991

Schneider LS, Small GW, Hamilton SH, et al: Estrogen replacement and response to fluoxetine in a multicenter geriatric depression trial. American Journal of Geriatric Psychiatry 5:97–106, 1997

Schobitz B, De Kloet ER, Holsboer F: Gene expression and function of interleukin-1, interleukin 6 and tumor necrosis factor in the brain. Prog Neurobiol 44:397–432, 1994

Schreiber W, Lauer CJ, Krumrey K, et al: Dysregulation of the hypothalamic-pituitary-adrenocortical system in panic disorder. Neuropsychopharmacology 15:7–15, 1996

Schulte HM, Bamberger CM, Elsen H, et al: Systemic interleukin-1 alpha and interleukin-2 secretion in response to acute stress and to corticotropin-releasing hormone in humans. Eur J Clin Invest 24:773–777, 1994

Selye H: The evolution of the stress concept. American Scientist 61:692–699, 1973

Skare SS, Dysken MW, Billington CJ: A review of the GHRH stimulation test in psychiatry. Biol Psychiatry 36:249–265, 1994

Sluzewska A, Rybakowsky J, Bosmans E, et al: Indicators of immune activation in major depression. Psychiatry Res 64:161–167, 1996

Smith MA: Hippocampal vulnerability to stress and aging: possible role of neurotrophic factors. Behav Brain Res 78:25–36, 1996

Smith MA, Davidson J, Ritchie JC, et al: The corticotropin releasing hormone test in patients with post-traumatic stress disorder. Biol Psychiatry 26:349–355, 1989

Spencer RL, Miller AH, Stein M, et al: Corticosterone regulation of type I and type II adrenal steroid receptors in brain, pituitary and immune tissue. Brain Res 549:236–246, 1991

Spiegel D, Bloom JR, Yalom ID: Group support for patients with metastatic cancer: a randomized outcome study. Arch Gen Psychiatry 38:527–533, 1981

Spiegel D, Bloom JR, Kraemer HC, et al: Effects of psychosocial treatment on survival of patients with metastatic breast cancer. Lancet 2:888–891, 1989

Stein M, Miller AH, Trestman RL: Depression, the immune system, and health and illness. Arch Gen Psychiatry 48:171–177, 1991

Stenzel-Poore M, Duncan JE, Rittenberg MB, et al: CRH overproduction in transgenic mice: behavioral and immune system modulation. Ann N Y Acad Sci 780:36–48, 1996

Stokes PE: The potential role of excessive cortisol induced by HPA hypersecretion in the pathogenesis of depression. Eur Neuropsychopharmacol 5 (suppl):77–82, 1995

Stokes PE, Sikes CR: The hypothalamic-pituitary-adrenocortical axis in major depression. Endocrinol Metab Clin North Am 17:1–19, 1988

Swedo SE, Leonard HL, Mittleman BB, et al: Identification of children with pediatric autoimmune neuropsychiatric disorders associated with streptococcal infections by a marker associated with rheumatic fever. Am J Psychiatry 154:110–112, 1997

Tavadia HB, Fleming KA, Hume PD, et al: Circadian rhythmicity of human plasma cortisol and PHA-induced lymphocyte transformation. Clin Exp Immunol 22:190–193, 1975

Thakore JH, Dinan TG: Subnormal growth hormone responses to acutely administered dexamethasone in depression. Clin Endocrinol (Oxf) 40:623–627, 1994

Uchino BN, Kiecolt-Glaser JK, Cacioppo JT: Age-related changes in cardiovascular response as a function of a chronic stressor and social support. J Pers Soc Psychol 63:839–846, 1992

Vale W, Spiess J, Rivier C, et al: Characterization of a 41-residue ovine hypothalamic peptide that stimulates secretion of corticotropin and beta-endorphin. Science 213:1394–1397, 1981

Watkins LR, Maier SF: Cytokine-to-brain communication: a review and analysis of alternative mechanisms. Life Sci 57:1011–1026, 1995

Weeke A, Weeke J: Disturbed circadian variation of serum thyrotropin in patients with endogenous depression. Acta Psychiatr Scand 57:281–289, 1978

Whalley LJ, Borthwick N, Copolov D, et al: Glucocorticoid receptors and depression. BMJ 292:859–861, 1986

Wright P, Murray RM: Prenatal influenza, immunogenesis and schizophrenia: a hypothesis and some recent findings, in The Neurodevelopmental Basis of Schizophrenia. Edited by Waddington JL, Buckley PF. New York, RG Landes, 1995, pp 43–60

Yehuda R, Boisoneau D, Mason JW, et al: Glucocorticoid receptor number and cortisol excretion in mood, anxiety and psychotic disorders. Biol Psychiatry 34:18–25, 1993

Yehuda R, Boisoneau D, Lowy MT, et al: Dose-response changes in plasma cortisol and lymphocyte glucocorticoid receptors following dexamethasone administration in combat veterans with and without post-traumatic stress disorder. Arch Gen Psychiatry 52:583–593, 1995

Yehuda R, Levengood RA, Schmeidler J, et al: Increased pituitary activation following metyrapone administration in post-traumatic stress disorder. Psychoneuroendocrinology 21:1–16, 1996

Young EA, Lopez JF, Murphy-Weinburg V, et al: Normal pituitary response to metyrapone in the morning in depressed patients: implications for circadian regulation of corticotropin-releasing hormone secretion. Biol Psychiatry 41:1149–1155, 1997

Zhou D, Kusnecov AW, Shurin MR, et al: Exposure to physical and psychological stressors elevates plasma interleukin 6: relationship to the activation of the hypothalamic-pituitary-adrenal axis. Endocrinology 133:2523–2530, 1993

Zis AP, Haskett RF, Albala AA, et al: Prolactin response to morphine in depression. Biol Psychiatry 20:287–292, 1985

Zisook S, Shuchter SR, Irwin M, et al: Bereavement, depression, and immune function. Psychiatry Res 52:1–10, 1994

Zonderman AB, Costa PT Jr, McCrae RR: Depression as a risk for cancer morbidity and mortality in a nationally representative sample. JAMA 262:1191–1195, 1989

SECTION II

Classes of Psychiatric Treatments: Animal and Human Pharmacology

Dennis S. Charney, M.D., and
Herbert Y. Meltzer, M.D., Section Editors

TEN

Tricyclics and Tetracyclics

William Z. Potter, M.D., Ph.D.,
Husseini K. Manji, M.D., F.R.C.P.C., and
Matthew V. Rudorfer, M.D.

From the 1960s until the late 1980s, tricyclic antidepressants (TCAs) represented the major pharmacological treatment for depression in the United States. They still provide the surest antidepressant response for moderately to severely nondelusionally depressed patients, especially those with a primary depression of the endogenous or melancholic type who may be candidates for hospitalization (Potter et al. 1991). Furthermore, the original tertiary amine tricyclics—first imipramine, then amitriptyline and clomipramine (in Europe)—all included in their biochemical spectrum of effects at least a moderate degree of serotonin reuptake inhibition at therapeutic doses. It was the recognition of this fact that led to the development of the selective serotonin reuptake inhibitors (SSRIs). Thus, the clinical pharmacology of the tricyclics forms the basis of the current understanding of how to best use most antidepressants and of theories on mechanisms of action.

In this chapter, we selectively review what has been learned about tricyclics and the subsequently introduced heterocyclics in both clinical and preclinical studies over the past three decades. We focus on their comparative pharmacology and on those findings most relevant to deciding when to treat a patient's condition with any of these compounds.

HISTORY AND DISCOVERY

The synthesis of iminodibenzyl, the "tricyclic" core of imipramine, and the description of its chemical characteristics date to 1889 (Baldessarini 1985). As Baldessarini noted, it was only after 1948, when Hafliger and Schindler synthesized a series of more than 40 derivatives of iminodibenzyl to be screened as possible antihistamines, sedatives, analgesics, and antiparkinsonian drugs, that the pharmacological properties were investigated. Out of this effort emerged imipramine, a dibenzazepine compound, which was distinguished from the phenothiazines only by replacement of the sulfur with an ethylene linkage. Interestingly, the best-known phenothiazine, chlorpromazine, was not synthesized until 1952, although attempts to use promethazine (which had been available for some time) to reduce motor agitation had been carried out for more than a decade (Laborit et al. 1952). Following their screening in animals, a few iminodibenzyl derivatives, including imipramine, were selected on the basis of their sedative or hypnotic properties for therapeutic trials as agents to calm agitated and/or psychotic patients.

In the meantime, and starting with reports in 1952 and 1953, a wide variety of clinical effects of chlorpromazine were described, including an ameliorative effect on psychosis. Thus, with a view toward imipramine as a pheno-

The authors thank Melanie Wadman for her editorial assistance in preparing this chapter revision.

thiazine analogue, Kuhn (1958) later assessed its ability to quiet agitated psychotic patients but found it relatively ineffective. On the other hand, he noticed that imipramine seemed to produce remarkable improvement in a subset of patients who were identified as depressed. Kuhn followed up on this chance observation with subsequent administration of imipramine to patients with various depressive syndromes. He suggested that imipramine was most useful in "endogenous" depressions characterized by regression and inactivity, an impression not that different from what is held by most clinicians today after more than three decades of controlled trials (see next section).

STRUCTURE-ACTIVITY RELATIONS

As shown in Figure 10–1, nine drugs are marketed in the United States as antidepressants that may be classified as tricyclic, and one drug (maprotiline) is classified as tetracyclic. (In the case of the tricyclic clomipramine, it has been approved only for treatment of obsessive-

compulsive disorder.) This simplistic and loose classification is a product of convention and implies somewhat greater similarity of structure and function than actually exists. In most instances, the nature of the side chain rather than the cyclic structure is most easily related to function.

To clarify this point, the first two compounds in Figure 10–1, imipramine and desipramine, are distinguished only by a methyl group on the propylamine side chain. As we discuss in detail in both the "Pharmacological Profile" and the "Side Effects and Toxicology" sections later in this chapter, this simple alteration from a tertiary amine ($3°$; e.g., imipramine) to a secondary amine ($2°$; e.g., desipramine) side chain has widespread effects. This is the case in terms of both monoamine uptake inhibition— $3°$ amines are more potent as inhibitors of serotonin, and $2°$ amines are more potent as inhibitors of norepinephrine uptake—and interaction with α_1-adrenergic, histaminergic, and muscarinic receptors—$3°$ amines are more than an order of magnitude more potent. Interestingly, the core dibenzapine (tricyclic) structure—the same iminodibenzyl synthesized a century ago, which is common to both imipramine and desipramine—has no significant pharmacological activity in concentrations similar to those required for imipramine to produce effects in preclinical "antidepressant" models (Bickel and Brodie 1964).

Consideration of the next two compounds in Figure 10–1, amitriptyline and nortriptyline, makes these concepts about the structure-activity relation even clearer. The core tricyclic structure is a dibenzocycloheptadiene that must be presumed to occupy more or less the same molecular space as iminodibenzyl. Given the same propylamine side chains, the profile of pharmacological effects is qualitatively the same for the respective $3°$ and $2°$ amine forms, amitriptyline and nortriptyline, as for imipramine and desipramine. However, absolute potencies in terms of monoamine reuptake and receptor inhibitions are affected by modification of the tricyclic structure. For instance, amitriptyline is more potent than imipramine in terms of cholinergic, α_1-adrenergic, and histaminergic receptor blockade, as well as serotonin uptake inhibition (but less potent in terms of norepinephrine uptake inhibition).

The fifth compound, clomipramine, differs from imipramine only in the addition of a chloride atom to one of the tricyclic benzene rings. This confers an increase in potency as an inhibitor of serotonin reuptake as well as an inhibitor of histaminergic receptors and some loss of potency as an inhibitor of norepinephrine uptake (Hall and Ogren 1981). Clomipramine's demethylated $2°$ amine metabolite, however, is a potent norepinephrine uptake

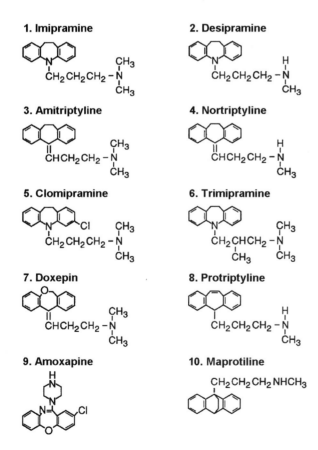

Figure 10–1. Drugs marketed in the United States as tricyclics (1–9) and tetracyclic (10).

inhibitor and is formed extensively in humans (see section, "Pharmacokinetics," later in this chapter).

Trimipramine, the sixth compound in Figure 10–1, is also closely related to imipramine with the addition of a methyl group to the second carbon of the propylamine side chain. Precise comparisons of the pharmacodynamics of trimipramine with that of other tricyclics are limited, but available data show that in its parent form trimipramine is somewhat less potent than imipramine as a norepinephrine uptake inhibitor (Randrup and Braestrup 1977) but more potent as an antihistamine (Psychoyos 1981). In some preparations it has been claimed to have significant potency as a dopamine uptake inhibitor, although this property is not established in humans (Randrup and Braestrup 1977).

Doxepin, the seventh compound, is most closely related to amitriptyline; the only difference is an oxygen in place of a carbon, such that the central cycloheptadiene ring is converted to an oxepinylidene. Consistent with the principles previously described, this modification affects only the potency of the 3° amine's actions. Serotonin uptake inhibition is decreased in comparison to that produced by amitriptyline, and norepinephrine uptake inhibition is somewhat increased (Pinder et al. 1977). In other words, doxepin's biochemical profile most closely resembles that of imipramine, consistent with the retention of the 3° amine side chain.

The eighth compound in Figure 10–1, protriptyline, is closely related to nortriptyline, from which it is distinguished by desaturation of two saturated central ring carbons. This change further enhances this 2° amine's potency as a norepinephrine uptake inhibitor. Through some unknown mechanism, it also greatly reduces the metabolism, such that protriptyline has a three- to fourfold longer half-life than nortriptyline (Moody et al. 1977; Ziegler et al. 1978) and achieves steady-state concentrations similar to those achieved with nortriptyline at one-third of the dose.

The last tricyclic in the figure, amoxapine, deviates the most because it is derived more directly from an active neuroleptic, loxapine, which has a very different middle ring. Although amoxapine has two benzene rings (one with a chlorine as for clomipramine), the central ring and side chain have little similarity to the other tricyclic structures. Nonetheless, amoxapine does share the property of potent norepinephrine uptake inhibition (Richelson and Pfenning 1984), which could not be predicted from its structure. What could be expected more, given its close relationship to loxapine, is that amoxapine and its metabolite, 7-hydroxyamoxapine, produce dopamine receptor blockade at therapeutic doses (Coupet et al. 1979).

The last compound shown in Figure 10–1, maprotiline, has been called a heterocyclic, although this appellation is ultimately misleading, given the abundance of "hetero"-cyclic drugs not included. Even the term *tetracyclic* is confusing and is used only to relate maprotiline to the "classic" tricyclics (compounds 1–8 in Figure 10–1). Maprotiline has an ethylene-type bridge between the two central carbons of a six-member middle ring that produces a more rigid core structure but a compound similar in biochemical properties to desipramine, nortriptyline, and protriptyline, given the presence of the identical 2° amine side chain (Wells and Gelenberg 1981). Maprotiline appears to achieve somewhat greater *selectivity* (but not potency) as a norepinephrine uptake inhibitor, according to a report that it has negligible effects as a serotonin uptake inhibitor following its chronic administration in humans (Turner and Ehsanullah 1977).

PHARMACOLOGICAL PROFILE

Primary Biochemical Effects

As we have defined them, the classic TCAs are imipramine, amitriptyline, and their close structural analogues. Observations of their ability to block the reuptake of the neurotransmitters serotonin and norepinephrine into their respective nerve terminals formed the basis of the monoamine hypothesis of depression (Bunney and Davis 1965; Prange 1965; Schildkraut 1965). These biochemical activities are still considered the pharmacological essence of their therapeutic effect. Amitriptyline and imipramine are metabolized to the 2° amines (on the side chain) nortriptyline and desipramine, which are themselves marketed as antidepressants (Figure 10–1).

Of these four compounds, desipramine is the most biochemically selective with respect to both neurotransmitter uptake inhibition and relative lack of interaction with other systems for a given plasma concentration. In actual clinical use, nortriptyline is almost as specific. It is effective at substantially lower plasma concentrations (see below); also, as we noted in the earlier discussion of structure-activity relations, the so-called heterocyclic maprotiline is relatively specific for norepinephrine uptake inhibition. Compared with most other tricyclic compounds, desipramine and maprotiline block the reuptake of norepinephrine at low concentrations unlikely to affect the uptake of serotonin. Moreover, desipramine has little affinity for muscarinic-cholinergic, histaminergic, and α-adrenergic receptors (Table 10–1), although its potency in these cases is still considerably higher than that seen with the SSRIs, bupropion, venlafaxine, and nefazodone.

The availability of TCAs that showed relative specificity and/or potency with regard to inhibition of norepinephrine or serotonin uptake, together with the clinical impression that different compounds were effective in different patients, led to the theory that there were noradrenergic and serotonergic forms of depression (Beckmann and Goodwin 1975; Maas et al. 1972). Convincing evidence to support this hypothesis has not been forthcoming. Treatment responses to desipramine (the most selective norepinephrine reuptake inhibitor) compared with those of an early SSRI, zimeldine, and later with those of fluoxetine and other SSRIs have not been consistently different (Potter 1984). Another study in which patients who did not respond to desipramine were to be crossed over to clomipramine (the most potent tricyclic serotonin uptake inhibitor) could not be completed because the failure rate of endogenomorphically depressed patients to desipramine was extremely low (Stewart et al. 1980). Thus, specific pharmacology has not translated into specific antidepressant effects.

The rationale for selecting a tricyclic on the basis of its specific biochemical pharmacology is weakened further by findings that even drugs with *acute* biochemical specificity have common effects on multiple biochemical systems with *chronic* administration in humans. For example, both norepinephrine and serotonin uptake inhibitors reduce the production of the neurotransmitters' respective metabolites, 3-methoxy-4-hydroxyphenylglycol (MHPG) and 5-hydroxyindoleacetic acid (5-HIAA), in cerebrospinal fluid (Aberg-Wistedt et al. 1982; Potter et al. 1985). Moreover,

other antidepressants, such as monoamine oxidase inhibitors (MAOIs) and bupropion (which has no clearly defined mechanism of action), can at least reduce output of norepinephrine (Golden et al. 1988). Finally, recent experiments in animals have shown that antidepressant drugs and electroconvulsive shock alter the density and function of receptors for both norepinephrine and serotonin in the brain after 1–2 weeks of administration (see section, "Mechanism of Action," later in this chapter). Therefore, the administration of any currently available drug as a test for biochemical specificity of effect in depression is not warranted.

This brings us to a consideration of the diverse biochemical effects associated with the use of tricyclic compounds, most of which have at least some physiological relevance if no direct relation to antidepressant outcome. These medications are considered pharmacologically "dirty drugs." That is, in addition to exertion of their presumed desired mode of action (i.e., inhibition of monoamine neurotransmitter uptake), they interact with a host of receptors in the brain and periphery (Table 10–1), with consequent unwanted actions. The relationships of these diverse biochemical actions to side effects and toxicity are discussed in the next section.

PHARMACOKINETICS

From a clinical point of view, the most important advances from studying the pharmacology of TCAs have emerged from studies of their pharmacokinetics (Amsterdam et al.

Table 10–1.   In vitro acute biochemical activity of tricyclic antidepressants[a]

	Reuptake inhibition			Receptor affinity				
	NE	**5-HT**	**DA**	α_1	α_2	**H$_1$**	**MUSC**	**D$_2$**
Imipramine	+	+	0	++	0	+	++	0
Desipramine	+++	0	0	+	0	0	+	0
Amitriptyline	±	++	0	+++	±	++++	++++	0
Nortriptyline	++	±	0	+	0	+	++	0
Clomipramine	+	+++	0	++	0	+	++	0
Trimipramine	+	0	0	++	±	+++	++	+
Doxepin	++	+	0	++	0	+++	++	0
Protriptyline	++	0	0	+	0	+	++	0
Amoxapine	++	0	0	++	±	±	0	++
Maprotiline	++	0	0	+	0	++	+	0

Note.   NE = norepinephrine; 5-HT = serotonin; DA = dopamine; α_1 = α_1-adrenergic receptor; α_2 = α_2-adrenergic receptor; H$_1$ = histamine-1 receptor; MUSC = muscarinic cholinergic receptor; D$_2$ = dopamine-2 receptor.
+ to ++++ = active to strongly active; ± = weakly active; 0 = lacking.
[a]Relative potencies from earlier reviews (i.e., Potter 1984; Potter et al. 1991; Richelson and Nelson 1984; Richelson and Pfenning 1984).

1981; Rudorfer and Potter 1987). TCAs are well absorbed following oral administration, although peak plasma levels occur over the relatively wide range of 2–6 hours. Most TCAs have a half-life of approximately 24 hours, which allows for once-a-day dosing (Table 10–2).

Less than 5% of a dose is excreted unchanged; metabolism occurs primarily in the liver through the mixed function oxidases. The tricyclics undergo demethylation, aromatic hydroxylation, and glucuronide conjugation of the hydroxy metabolite (Figure 10–2). The demethylated metabolites of 3° amines are pharmacologically active, as are the hydroxy metabolites of both 3° and 2° amines (Bertilsson et al. 1979; Potter et al. 1979). Conjugation contributes the most to rendering the lipophilic tricyclics water soluble and easier to excrete by the kidneys. The glucuronide metabolites are considered inactive, both because they have no identified effects on biological systems in the concentrations achieved and because they do not cross the blood-brain barrier (reviewed in detail in Potter et al. 1980).

The metabolism rates of TCAs are determined by individual genetics and vary 30- to 40-fold; 7%–9% of a Caucasian population may be classified as "slow hydroxylators" (Brosen et al. 1985; Evans et al. 1980). Great progress has been made recently in understanding the exact source of slow hydroxylation. Individuals can be so classified on the basis of the urinary ratio of debrisoquin to

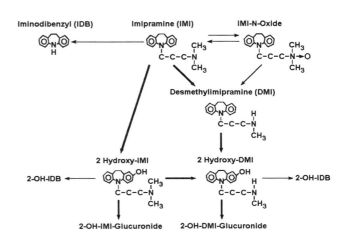

Figure 10–2. Known metabolic pathways for the major tricyclic antidepressant (TCA) imipramine in humans. Similar pathways apply to other TCAs.

4-hydroxydebrisoquin in an 8-hour collection following an oral 10-mg dose of debrisoquin (an antihypertensive). A high ratio means that a person is a "slow hydroxylator."

It was recognized that metabolism of another test compound, sparteine, correlated with that of debrisoquin, and what was known as *sparteine-debrisoquin oxidation polymorphism* is now determined by cytochrome P450-2D6 (CYP2D6), a specific isozyme of the P450 microsomal enzymes. Furthermore, CYP2D6 has been explicitly shown to be responsible for the 2-hydroxylation of imipramine and desipramine, and mutations of the *CYP2D6* gene are responsible for slow metabolism through these pathways (Brosen et al. 1991; Daly et al. 1996). The P450 isozymes involved in TCA demethylation reactions may include CYP1A2, CYP2C19, and CYP3A4 based on in vitro data; the most direct evidence indicates that CYP2C19 is involved in vivo (Madsen et al. 1997; Shen 1997). However, most TCAs appear to depend on the CYP2D6 enzyme for major hydroxylation reactions, which are a necessary prelude to glucuronidation. Of interest, most SSRIs are potent inhibitors of one or another P450 isozymes (Nemeroff et al. 1996). For instance, fluoxetine and norfluoxetine inhibit the CYP2D6 isozyme at therapeutic doses such that parent TCA concentrations can be more than doubled during concurrent use (Brosen and Skjelbo 1991). Paroxetine is also a potent inhibitor of CYP2D6, fluvoxamine is an inhibitor of CYP3A4, and chronic treatment with sertraline (150 mg/day) clearly inhibits CYP2D6 (Kurtz et al. 1997; Shen 1997) (see also section, "Drug-Drug Interactions," later in this chapter).

Some of the demethylated metabolites of TCAs that

Table 10–2. Elimination half-life of tricyclic antidepressants

	Half-life (hours)	
	Mean	**Range**
Imipramine	12	7–22
	28	18–34
Desipramine	18	10–31
Amitriptyline	24	20–30
	36	31–46
Nortriptyline	28	22–39
	33	18–58
Clomipramine	24	20–39
Trimipramine	24	16–38
Doxepin	16	8–24
	17	10–47
Protriptyline	74	54–92
Amoxapine	10	8–18
Maprotiline	43	27–58

Source. Adapted from Rudorfer and Potter 1987 with values from one or more studies using more sensitive high-performance liquid chromatography and/or gas chromatography/mass spectrometry assays, with added information on trimipramine and amoxapine from Abernethy et al. 1984 and Calvo et al. 1985, respectively.

show differential pharmacodynamics as discussed here actually exceed concentrations of the parent compound. For example, the 3° amine and potent serotonin uptake inhibitor clomipramine is metabolized to desmethylclomipramine concentrations that exceed those of the parent compound at steady state (Traskman et al. 1979). Because desmethylclomipramine (as would be expected for a 2° amine) is a potent norepinephrine uptake inhibitor, the in vitro selectivity of clomipramine as a serotonin uptake inhibitor is lost on administration to patients.

Other metabolic pathways may also be relevant to clinical effects (Rudorfer and Potter 1997). Results of both animal and clinical studies suggested that hydroxy-TCA metabolites, which are rarely assayed, may be more cardiotoxic than their parent precursors (Jandhyala et al. 1977; Young et al. 1984); however, the most recent evidence shows that no such generalization is possible. For instance, the clinically predominant E enantiomer of 10-hydroxynortriptyline is considerably *less* toxic than nortriptyline itself, whereas the minor Z-10-OH enantiomer has cardiotoxicity similar to that of the parent 3° amine (Pollock et al. 1992a). A very different type of effect that may be produced by metabolites is indicated in the report that elevated plasma concentrations of E-10-hydroxynortriptyline were associated with poorer antidepressant response (Young et al. 1988).

Although TCA pharmacokinetics also may be influenced by age, changes in pharmacodynamic responses as a function of aging are more important. Elderly patients are more sensitive to at least the anticholinergic and α_1-antagonistic effects of tricyclics, as reflected in drug-induced delirium (Sunderland et al. 1987) and orthostatic hypotension (Glassman et al. 1979, 1987), respectively, independent of any processes that might elevate plasma concentrations. Increased concentrations must, of course, be considered, because secondary decreases in P450 activity and hepatic blood flow are more likely to occur in elderly patients from either concomitant medical illness or medication. Thus, in earlier more naturalistic studies, elevated concentrations of TCAs were sometimes reported as a function of age (Linnoila et al. 1981; Nies et al. 1977; Ziegler and Biggs 1977). However, in more controlled prospective studies, concentrations of parent TCAs or rates of hydroxylation activity do not differ between otherwise healthy old and young subjects (Asberg et al. 1971; Cutler et al. 1981; Pollock et al. 1992b; Young et al. 1984).

With regard to active metabolites, however, the known decline of renal clearance with age predictably reduces the urinary excretion of unconjugated hydroxy metabolites, resulting in substantially increased steady-state concentrations in elderly patients (Kitanaka et al. 1982;

Pollock and Perel 1989; Young et al. 1984). These concentrations, especially in the case of nortriptyline, are elevated to a toxic or countertherapeutic range of hydroxynortriptyline (Young et al. 1988; see previous discussion). At the other end of the spectrum, in many studies of prepubescent children, TCA clearance is higher than that in adults; a lower plasma concentration is often achieved at the same mg/kg dose (Geller 1991; Rapoport and Potter 1981).

Controlling for plasma concentration is, of course, essential to any evaluation of pharmacodynamics. This is particularly important in longer-term studies of clinical response in which problems with compliance are likely. To show compliance, concentrations must be stable over time. This information is also necessary for establishing nonresponse to a TCA, defined as lack of clinical improvement when therapeutic concentrations are present for 4–6 weeks. However, what is considered "therapeutic" is uncertain.

Despite a current appreciation for the great variability in metabolism of tricyclic drugs and a consequent need to individualize treatment, definitive therapeutic concentrations are not well established for all TCAs. Most critical analyses agree that therapeutic levels have been defined for only nortriptyline, imipramine, and desipramine (American Psychiatric Association Task Force 1985; Perry et al. 1987; Rudorfer and Potter 1987). Nonetheless, attempts have been made to provide estimates of reasonable therapeutic ranges for all marketed TCAs based on cumulative experience with therapeutic monitoring rather than on prospective controlled studies (Orsulak 1989). Lack of response, toxicity, minimizing adverse effects by using the minimal effective dose, and suspected pharmacokinetic interactions (e.g., with neuroleptics or SSRIs) are indications for measurement of plasma drug levels. Even without such measurements, daily doses of tricyclic drugs other than nortriptyline or protriptyline can be increased to 300–350 mg of imipramine or the equivalent if side effects allow. Dose increases of nortriptyline require monitoring, because plasma levels greater than 150 ng/mL are as ineffective as those yielding a subtherapeutic (<50 ng/mL) level.

TCAs also have a narrow therapeutic index with considerable risk of significant toxicity when blood concentrations are two to six times therapeutic levels; thus, a 1-week supply may be fatal if taken all at once (Gram 1990; Rudorfer and Robins 1982). In general, concentrations greater than 1,000 ng/mL are associated with prolongation of the QRS interval, an effect that may be seen even at 500 ng/mL (Preskorn and Irwin 1982; Rudorfer and Young 1980b; Spiker et al. 1975). This relatively narrow therapeutic index is of special concern for depressed patients with suicide potential who may intentionally take an overdose. Specific pharmacodynamic properties that might contribute to fatal arrhythmia, for example, are not clearly established in humans with regard to a concentration-response relationship. Nonetheless, TCA blood concentrations may remain elevated for several days after overdose, presenting a cardiac risk even after apparent clinical improvement (Jarvis 1991). Furthermore, central nervous system toxicity in terms of coma, shock, respiratory depression, delirium, seizures, and hyperpyrexia may well contribute as much to fatalities as the quinidine-like effects on cardiac conduction of the TCAs.

MECHANISM OF ACTION

Our discussion of pharmacology so far has been primarily in terms of clomipramine and the four most closely related TCAs marketed in the United States. Despite the 10 examples of this class in Figure 10–1 (if the tetracyclic maprotiline is included) that acutely affect norepinephrine and serotonin uptake to varying extents, the bulk of data on biochemical effects in humans is provided by studies with imipramine, desipramine, nortriptyline, and clomipramine. Because (as we have noted) all of these drugs reduce indices of norepinephrine and serotonin turnover (i.e., total synthesis and metabolism in humans), all other TCAs are assumed to do the same. Given what has been learned from preclinical studies about chronic "adaptive" changes following TCA administration (which we describe below), the commonality of biochemical findings is not so surprising.

Several major flaws in the original hypothesis about the mechanism of action of TCAs as simply enhancing intrasynaptic norepinephrine and/or serotonin began to appear in the mid-1970s and are briefly outlined here. First, compounds with antidepressant activity such as iprindole (never marketed) and bupropion are weak inhibitors of monoamine uptake at best (Ferris et al. 1981; Zis and Goodwin 1979). The recently introduced antidepressants nefazodone and mirtazapine also lack significant activity to inhibit monoamine uptake. Second, several potent reuptake inhibitors, most notably cocaine and amphetamine, do not produce convincing evidence of antidepressant effects in controlled trials. Finally, the most compelling objection—and the one raised most frequently—is the large temporal discrepancy between the rapid drug-induced biochemical effects on monoamine uptake, which occur within hours, and the antidepressant response, which generally occurs after at least 7–14 days.

At this point, we should note that our knowledge

about the complex cascade of events that translate *any* biochemical event into long-term changes in mood and affect is limited. Thus, the temporal discordance discussed here need not represent prima facie evidence against the "classic monoamine hypothesis" of antidepressant drug action. Nevertheless, this has led to extensive research and the formulation of the "receptor sensitivity hypothesis of antidepressant drug action." This postulates that alterations in the sensitivity of various receptors observed only after chronic drug administration are directly related to the mechanism of antidepressant drug action. It is beyond the scope of this chapter to review the extensive literature regarding alterations in various receptor systems, and we highlight only a few major ones here. Several excellent reviews are available (Charney et al. 1991; Heninger and Charney 1987; Sugrue 1983; Sulser 1984). Most recently, alterations of receptor systems have been studied in the context of antidepressant effects on specific messenger RNAs (mRNAs), thereby extending theories of action to long-term molecular changes at the level of the cell nucleus (Duman et al. 1997).

Vetulani and Sulser (1975) were the first to report that chronic (but not acute) administration of various antidepressants to rats reduces the activity of the norepinephrine-stimulated adenylate cyclase in the limbic forebrain. Activation of adenylate cyclase results in an increase in intracellular cyclic adenosine monophosphate (cAMP). cAMP is an important "second messenger" that mediates the physiological effects of various hormones and neurotransmitters. The stimulation of brain adenylate cyclase by norepinephrine is at least partially mediated by β-adrenoceptors (Sulser et al. 1978). Several researchers have since showed that the actual number of forebrain β-adrenoceptors is also reduced following chronic administration of many (but not all) TCAs. Moreover, a reduction in β-adrenoceptors was observed not only with imipramine and desipramine but also with MAOIs and the atypical antidepressants iprindole and mianserin (Sulser et al. 1978).

Chronic administration of all chemically diverse and unrelated antidepressants can decrease the density of β-adrenoceptors and/or the responsiveness of the β-adrenoceptor-coupled adenylate cyclase system. In contrast, other drugs that share common pharmacological properties with the TCAs, such as various anticholinergic and antihistaminergic agents, do not produce similar changes in β-adrenoceptor function. Finally, other neurotransmitter receptors including muscarinic-cholinergic, histaminergic, and dopaminergic receptors are not consistently altered during chronic administration of antidepressants to animals (Hauger and Paul 1983).

The time course of the antidepressant-induced decrease in β-adrenoceptors in animals is in keeping with the delayed therapeutic effects of these drugs in humans. Interestingly, both electroconvulsive therapy (ECT) and rapid eye movement (REM) sleep deprivation (which are both clinically effective antidepressants) decrease cerebral β-adrenoceptors in animals somewhat faster than the chemical antidepressants do (Mogilnicka et al. 1980; Sulser et al. 1978), a finding that may be related to their relatively rapid antidepressant effects in patients. The most intuitively obvious explanation for the decrease in brain β-adrenoceptors following chronic antidepressant administration is that all of these drugs somehow increase the intrasynaptic concentration of norepinephrine.

In addition to reducing the number of central β-adrenoceptors, TCAs (as well as SSRIs and MAOIs) appear to alter the number and/or function of serotonin receptors in various forebrain regions (Charney et al. 1991; Heninger and Charney 1987). Single-unit electrophysiological investigations have consistently shown enhanced serotonergic transmission in various postsynaptic brain regions following chronic antidepressant administration. In particular, evidence indicates that there is increased throughput at the serotonin-1A (5-HT_{1A}) receptor in the hippocampus in the absence of consistent alterations in the density of the receptors themselves, suggesting an enhancement of the coupling to second-messenger-generating systems.

Because many receptor systems homeostatically downregulate and desensitize in response to increased transmitter availability, the antidepressant-induced downregulation of β-receptors has generally been regarded as an "adaptive phenomenon." However, this seemingly parsimonious explanation has several problems, including the lack of β-receptor downregulation in several areas of the brain receiving dense noradrenergic innervation. The ascending serotonergic projections from the midbrain therefore represent another monoaminergic neurotransmitter system that is affected by antidepressants.

Serotonin receptors have multiple subtypes, among them the broadly inclusive 5-HT_2 class as well as the 5-HT_{1A} class referred to previously. Chronic administration of antidepressants to rats decreases the number of 5-HT_2 receptors in the brain, and with some drugs, this reduction is quite dramatic (Peroutka and Snyder 1980). Because acute administration of antidepressants fails to alter 5-HT_2 receptors (Lerer 1987; Vetulani et al. 1981), it is unlikely that this decrease is the result of residual drug present in the membrane preparation. Indeed, many antidepressants are far more potent in reducing 5-HT_2 receptors than β-adrenoceptors (with the possible exception of desipramine, which is more effective in reducing β-

adrenoceptors). However, because the most effective treatment, electroconvulsive shock (ECS), increases the density of rat cortical 5-HT_2 receptors, direct antidepressant properties clearly cannot be ascribed to a reduction in 5-HT_2 receptor numbers.

Evidence also suggests that a functional linkage exists between the noradrenergic and serotonergic neurotransmitter systems, although how this relates to receptor regulation remains to be defined. For instance, destruction of the noradrenergic system (with 6-hydroxydopamine) markedly reduces the ability of several antidepressants (including ECS) to enhance serotonin-mediated behaviors in rats (Green and Deakin 1980). Monoamine neurotransmitter system interactions may provide a basis for unifying several major hypotheses of depression and the mechanism of action of antidepressants (Hsiao et al. 1987; Potter et al. 1985). These interactions also highlight the difficulty in isolating a drug effect to a specific neurotransmitter system; with chronic administration, subtle and permissive interactions between systems are to be expected.

The potential clinical relevance of these studies designed to explore the mechanisms of action of TCAs in comparison with those of other antidepressants lies in their highlighting two phenomena. First, whatever the balance of acute biochemical effects, all TCAs produce qualitatively similar chronic changes and hence would not be expected to show major differences in degree or type of antidepressant efficacy. Second, biochemical changes occur over a period of 1–2 weeks and may take even longer to stabilize with extended escalation of dose—a phenomenon that argues against any therapeutic advantage of one compound over another in speed of response.

The preceding notwithstanding, the possibility remains that norepinephrine (and serotonin) uptake inhibition may not be necessary or a sufficient condition to initiate and sustain the chain of biochemical events leading to therapeutic response. Although the most obvious explanation for the decrease in brain β-adrenoceptors following chronic administration is that antidepressants somehow increase the intrasynaptic concentration of norepinephrine and/or serotonin, we return our discussion to the ability of other atypical antidepressants, such as iprindole, to downregulate β-adrenoceptors, which requires that other mechanism(s) be evoked (Manier et al. 1989). Indeed, several investigators (including us) have shown that chronic in vitro treatment in systems lacking presynaptic input (e.g., human fibroblasts or cultured C6 glioma cells) results in a similar downregulation and desensitization of the β-adrenergic receptor (Manji et al. 1991a). Other complementary in vitro and/or in vivo preclinical studies provide evidence for effects of tricyclics and other antidepressants distal to the receptor whereby coupling of β-adrenoceptors to guanine nucleotide binding proteins (G proteins) (Lesch and Manji 1992; Manji and Potter 1995), coupling of the G protein to the enzyme adenylate cyclase (Chen and Rasenick 1995; Rasenick et al. 1996), and the activity of membrane phospholipases (Manji et al. 1991b; Nakamura 1994; Pandey et al. 1991) and protein kinase C (Li and Hrdina 1997; Morishita and Watanabe 1997; Nalepa and Vetulani 1996) are altered. More recently, novel targets of antidepressant drug action have been explored (discussed in Owens 1996), including glucocorticoid receptors (Barden 1996) and neurotrophic factors (Duman et al. 1997; Smith et al. 1995). In addition, one of the most exciting areas of research pertaining to the mechanisms of action of agents used in the treatment of mood disorders has been the study of these agents at the genomic level. Thus, it has become increasingly appreciated in recent years that any relevant biochemical models proposed for the actions of antidepressants and mood stabilizers must attempt to account for their special temporal clinical profile—in particular, that the therapeutic effects require a lag period for onset of action and are generally not immediately reversed on discontinuation (Duman et al. 1997; Hyman and Nestler 1996; Manji and Lenox 1994; Manji et al. 1995). Patterns of effects requiring such prolonged administration of the drug suggest alterations at the genomic level (Duman et al. 1997; Hyman and Nestler 1996; Manji and Lenox 1994; Manji et al. 1995). In this context, it is noteworthy that the chronic administration of TCAs has been demonstrated to modulate glucocorticoid receptor gene expression (Barden 1996), G protein gene expression (Lesch and Manji 1992), and cAMP response element binding (CREB) protein/cAMP response element directed gene transcription both in vitro and ex vivo (Nibuya et al. 1996; Schwaninger et al. 1995). These changes in gene expression are likely mediated by the downstream effects of converging signal transduction pathways. The rapid technological advances in both biochemistry and molecular biology have greatly enhanced our understanding of the complexities of the regulation of neuronal function; these advances hold much promise for novel improved therapeutics for the treatment of depressive disorder.

Another point to emphasize is that in terms of presumed core biochemical effects, TCAs are best distinguished from SSRIs by their universal ability to potently inhibit norepinephrine uptake and to more variably inhibit serotonin uptake. Thus, a third phenomenon can be highlighted: TCAs are more "broad spectrum" in their effects on neurotransmitter systems than are SSRIs and hence may ultimately prove to have a different spectrum of clinical effects.

In keeping with this suggestion, researchers in a series of Danish studies concluded that SSRIs may not be as effective in treatment of severely depressed inpatients as is clomipramine, although the latter clearly has more severe side effects (Bech 1988; Danish University Antidepressant Group 1990). Indeed, there is a paucity of studies of SSRIs in inpatients; even in outpatients, it is often difficult to distinguish effects of SSRIs from those of placebo. It is appropriate to wonder whether the "classic" patients who participated in studies of TCAs in the 1960s and early 1970s differ substantially from the outpatient groups studied today. If so, generalizations about response to all treatments of depression from studies done 20 years apart are not valid. However, several clinical predictors do help to identify the most appropriate patients to receive TCAs, and some of these are highlighted here.

INDICATIONS

Major Depression and Melancholia

It is now generally accepted that patients with major depressive disorder, with melancholic features, require pharmacotherapy or ECT (Potter et al. 1991). Earlier studies suggested that major depressive disorder, with melancholic features, responded better to TCAs than did depression not meeting the DSM-IV (American Psychiatric Association 1994) criteria for major depressive disorder, with melancholic features (Paykel 1972; Raskin and Crook 1976). However, most recent data do not support such selectivity of response, perhaps reflecting the changing population available for studies (Paykel 1989). After a review, investigators concluded that, allowing for the limitations of the research base, a good premorbid personality (i.e., absence of significant personality pathology), psychomotor retardation, and moderate severity with melancholia predict good response to tricyclic drug therapy (Joyce and Paykel 1989). Severity has long been identified as a predictor of response to TCAs (Stewart et al. 1989), whereas good premorbid personality is consistent with observations that primary depression (i.e., depression not preceded by other psychiatric diagnoses or medical illness) responds best to drugs (Coryell and Turner 1985; Fairchild et al. 1986). Identification of symptoms that most consistently change after treatment with desipramine has been used to develop a scale for measuring response to TCAs that may prove useful in future studies (Nelson and Mazure 1990).

Overall, TCAs produce an antidepressant response rate of 80% in nonpsychotic patients who have major depressive disorder, with melancholic features; have an illness duration of less than 1 year; and are maintained at plasma levels in selected ranges for 4–6 weeks. Estimates of lower response rates in these patients most likely result from inadequate dosage over too short a time. The critical importance of adjusting for wide interindividual differences in the pharmacokinetics of the TCAs has already been described.

Atypical Depression

Atypical forms of depression have been formally considered only in the recent DSM-IV. The term *atypical* previously referred simply to the absence of melancholic features. However, according to DSM-IV, major depressive disorder, with atypical features, is characterized by a combination of mood reactivity (i.e., inability to experience a positive response to favorable events), overeating, oversleeping, and chronic oversensitivity to rejection (Liebowitz et al. 1988). Patients with atypical depression have a lower response rate to TCAs than to MAOIs (Paykel et al. 1982; Quitkin et al. 1991; Ravaris et al. 1980). However, the concept of atypical depression is imprecise, and at least one report suggested that SSRIs may be as effective as MAOIs in its treatment (Pande et al. 1996). Given the probability of shifts in patient populations under study, it seems premature to conclude that TCAs should be systematically avoided in treating atypical features of depression. For instance, desipramine tended to be more effective than phenelzine in a group of outpatients with recurrent depression who had experienced recent moderate to severe stress; this population is not typically included in most research studies of efficacy (Swann et al. 1997).

Delusional (With Psychotic Features) Depression

Patients who have symptoms that meet the criteria for major depression and have delusions (DSM-IV major depressive disorder, severe with psychotic features) show a very poor response rate to monotherapy with traditional TCAs (Glassman et al. 1977; Perry et al. 1982). Successful pharmacotherapy for such delusional or psychotic depressions requires a combination of a neuroleptic and a TCA (Spiker et al. 1985). Because amoxapine, the tricyclic metabolite of loxapine, has dopamine-blocking as well as monoamine-uptake-inhibitory properties, it may be effective alone in treating delusional depression (Anton et al. 1985; Coupet et al. 1979). However, the opportunity to adjust the neuroleptic and antidepressant components independently is lost. A potentially important detail re-

garding combination therapy concerns the ability of some neuroleptic drugs to block the metabolism of TCAs, which necessitates special attention to doses and possibly to blood-level monitoring (Gram et al. 1974). Alternatively, the response rates to ECT among patients with delusional depression are excellent (86% in the aggregate from a dozen studies; Kroessler 1985).

Obsessive-Compulsive Disorder

Only one TCA, clomipramine, has been shown to produce significant therapeutic benefit in patients with obsessive-compulsive disorder, despite attempts to treat this disorder with other members of the drug class such as desipramine for adults and children (Ananth et al. 1981; Insel et al. 1985; Leonard et al. 1989; Thoren et al. 1980). This effect is believed to be a function of the potent serotonin-reuptake-inhibiting properties of clomipramine because most SSRIs tested to date also produce benefit in obsessive-compulsive disorder. It is significant that the specified upper dose limit of clomipramine in United States product labeling is 250 mg because the incidence of seizures is increased at higher doses. Unfortunately, studies reporting seizures did not include data on blood levels, and it is almost certain that those patients who are rapid metabolizers of clomipramine will require higher doses. These higher doses may well be safe in such rapid metabolizers. The experience of European research teams with clomipramine treatment indicates that many patients tolerate doses up to 450 mg/day and experience only those side effects that would be expected from a 3° amine TCA at therapeutic doses (Collins 1973).

Enuresis

Nocturnal enuresis in children can clearly benefit from TCAs. Imipramine is the one member of the class that has received United States product labeling for this indication. Recommended doses are low (i.e., 25–50 mg at bedtime in children younger than 12 years and up to 75 mg in those age 12 years or older). No other TCAs are specifically approved for treatment of enuresis, although others with a 3° amine profile of action may be assumed to share similar effects (see section, "Structure-Activity Relations," earlier in this chapter). The mechanism of action is not known. The beneficial effect may be related to the anticholinergic effect or to modifications of sleep processes. Controlled trials with plasma blood-level monitoring provide strong evidence of an antienuretic effect of imipramine (Rapoport et al. 1980). Earlier studies support the use of amitriptyline and nortriptyline for the treatment of nocturnal enuresis in children (Forsythe and Merrett

1969; Lake 1968). Suggested amitriptyline doses are 10–20 mg at bedtime for children ages 6–10 years and 25–50 mg at bedtime for children age 11 years or older.

Panic Disorder

Although we have referred to tricyclic *antidepressants* in this chapter, at least some members of this class clearly are effective treatments for panic disorder, even in the absence of depression. Note that use of TCAs in the treatment of panic disorder is not included in United States product labeling. Nonetheless, such use has played a considerable role in the treatment of panic disorder (including that with agoraphobia); controlled studies support the use of both the 3° amine imipramine and the 2° amine nortriptyline (Jobson et al. 1978; Munjack et al. 1988; Uhde and Nemiah 1989; Zitrin et al. 1980). Ultimate doses and presumably plasma levels are the same as those used in the treatment of depression.

One special consideration in the treatment of panic disorder with TCAs is that, particularly with the 2° amines, too rapid escalation of dose may increase anxiety and even precipitate a panic attack. Therefore, treatment should begin with low doses (e.g., 10–20 mg) and then build up to typical therapeutic doses (100–250 mg) over weeks rather than days.

Attention-Deficit/Hyperactivity Disorder

As reviewed by Spencer and colleagues (1996), as of 1995, 29 studies of pharmacotherapy for attention-deficit/hyperactivity disorder (ADHD) in children and adolescents ($N = 1,016$) had been done. Most reported modest to robust response rates, at least over a few-week to few-month period. Some controlled studies of imipramine in the treatment of ADHD in children date back more than two decades and reported relatively modest degrees of response (Rapoport et al. 1974), as did a study of desipramine (Donnelly et al. 1986) a decade later.

Subsequent studies in children relied on longer durations of treatment (at least 3–4 weeks) and higher doses (>4 mg/kg in preadolescent children). With this approach, more than two-thirds of children with ADHD treated with desipramine were very much or much improved in contrast to only 10% given placebo (Biederman et al. 1989). A recent comparison of desipramine (200 mg/day or as tolerated) and placebo in adults with ADHD produced very similar results to those observed in children with regard to overall response (Wilens et al.

1996). In light of the short half-life and abuse potential of methylphenidate and dextroamphetamine, TCAs, especially the 2° amine desipramine, are argued to be of use for both children and adults with ADHD (Spencer et al. 1996).

Other Indications

A surprisingly diverse number of uses for TCAs is recorded not only in the clinical literature but also in a current authoritative American reference such as the *United States Pharmacopeia Dispensing Information* (USPDI 1997) and an international pharmacopoeia, *Therapeutic Drugs* (Dollery 1991, 1992). In Table 10–3, those uses of the TCAs referred to in one or the other source are listed in alphabetical order. This list is important for two reasons: 1) in terms of appreciating that many prescriptions of TCAs have nothing to do with the presence of depression or other psychiatric disorders, and 2) in understanding how TCAs are useful in any single condition, which may clarify why it is useful for others and ultimately contribute to knowledge on their pathophysiologies.

Use in Pregnancy

All medications are best avoided during pregnancy and breast-feeding, but when antidepressant treatment is re-

Table 10–3. Uses of one or more tricyclic antidepressants (TCAs) not included in product labeling

Use	Specified TCAs[a]
Anxiety/panic	Clomipramine, desipramine, doxepin, imipramine
Bulimia	Amitriptyline, desipramine, imipramine
Cataplexy/narcolepsy	Clomipramine, desipramine, imipramine, protriptyline
Enuresis	Amitriptyline, clomipramine, nortriptyline
Migraine (prophylaxis)	Amitriptyline
Nausea with chemotherapy	Nortriptyline
Neuralgia (chronic pain)	Amitriptyline, desipramine, doxepin, imipramine, nortriptyline
Peptic ulcer	Amitriptyline, doxepin, imipramine
Urticaria/pruritus	Doxepin, nortriptyline

[a]At least one mention in USPDI (1997) or *Therapeutic Drugs* (Dollery 1991, 1992).

quired at such times, tricyclics have been used safely. Physiological changes during pregnancy lead to a gradual decline in steady-state plasma tricyclic concentrations, requiring upward titration in dosage by mid-pregnancy (Altshuler and Hendrick 1996). Following delivery, TCAs have been used with care in nursing mothers, whose breast milk contains negligible amounts of these drugs and their active hydroxy metabolites (Rudorfer and Potter 1997; Wisner et al. 1997).

SIDE EFFECTS AND TOXICOLOGY

As indicated in Table 10–4, there are distinctions among properties of specific TCAs in the expected frequency and severity of adverse effects. Thus, as predicted from the variety of greater receptor affinities of the 3° amine tricyclics for a variety of receptors (Table 10–1), in general, they produce more pronounced anticholinergic, antihistaminic (H_1 and H_2), sedative, and hypotensive actions than their 2° amine counterparts. We recently reviewed the possible relationships between the various side effects observed in human subjects and the specific biochemical actions of the full range of antidepressants (Rudorfer et al. 1994). We present the salient details regarding TCAs below.

Table 10–4. Possible clinical side effects of blocking various receptors

Property	Possible clinical consequences
Blockade of muscarinic receptors	Blurred vision Dry mouth Sinus tachycardia Constipation Urinary retention Cognitive dysfunction
Blockade of α_1-adrenergic receptors	Potentiation of the anti-hypertensive effect of prazosin and terazosin Postural hypotension, dizziness, drowsiness Reflex tachycardia
Blockade of α_2-adrenergic receptors	Blockade of the antihypertensive effects of clonidine and α-methyldopa
Blockade of dopamine D_2 receptors	Extrapyramidal movement disorders
Blockade of histamine (H_1) receptors	Sedation Weight gain

Cardiovascular Effects

TCAs commonly produce a benign rise in heart rate, often on the order of 15–20 beats per minute. Although this increased heart rate is sometimes ascribed to vagal inhibition, it occurs most consistently after use of 2° amine tricyclics, such as desipramine, for which norepinephrine reuptake blockade clearly plays a role (Ross et al. 1983). α_1-Adrenergic antagonism is more marked after administration of 3° amine TCAs and is now believed to be the most likely basis for any orthostatic hypotension observed with use of those drugs. Such orthostatic hypotension usually produces only transient benign dizziness upon standing in young physically healthy patients but can lead to falls and injury in older individuals (Ray 1992). Some experts prefer nortriptyline among the TCAs to minimize orthostatic hypotension in elderly patients because it has relatively less potency at α_1 receptors and achieves therapeutic effects at low blood levels.

The most potentially dangerous TCA cardiac effect (i.e., of a quinidine-like membrane stabilization resulting in slowed impulse conduction) was discussed in the earlier section, "Pharmacokinetics." Although such slowed impulse conduction produces only an innocuous prolongation of electrocardiogram (ECG) parameters during routine TCA dosing in physically healthy individuals (Laird et al. 1993; Rudorfer and Young 1980b)—and can suppress preexisting premature atrial or ventricular contractions—it may precipitate frank bundle branch or complete heart block in cardiac patients (Glassman et al. 1987), with consequent morbidity or mortality. This property may relate to cases of sudden death in patients taking therapeutic doses of TCAs, such as those reported in several children taking desipramine (Riddle et al. 1993). However, despite comprehensive 24-hour monitoring, no evidence of desipramine-associated cardiac abnormalities was found in a subsequent intensive study of 71 pediatric patients, and cardiac parameters failed to correlate with desipramine dose or plasma level; desipramine metabolites were not assayed (Biederman et al. 1993). In a related study of developmental factors in desipramine pharmacokinetics (Wilens et al. 1992), excessive accumulation of the potentially cardiotoxic desipramine hydroxy metabolite (Rudorfer and Potter 1997) was not found in children or adolescents during routine dosing. Analysis of standard ECGs in that patient sample (Wilens et al. 1993) revealed little relation between ECG parameters and desipramine or OH-desipramine plasma levels in children and adolescents.

Widening of the QRS complex on the ECG, which has been correlated with red blood cell concentrations of tricyclic desmethyl metabolites (Amitai et al. 1993), has become a standard index of serious TCA poisoning, especially in overdose situations (Jarvis 1991). Preskorn and Fast (1991) speculated that the association of serious cardiac conduction slowing with supratherapeutic TCA plasma concentrations may explain some cases of sudden death during tricyclic therapy in presumed slow metabolizers of these drugs. Recent data have raised concern that the risk of sudden death during TCA treatment among patients with ventricular arrhythmias or ischemic heart disease may be greater than previously appreciated (Glassman et al. 1993). And, as we have noted, disturbing reports of sudden death in children treated with TCAs persist (Riddle et al. 1993).

The possibility of TCA-induced impaired left ventricular function may have been overestimated in the past (Glassman et al. 1987) but is reported occasionally in patients with severe underlying heart disease (Dalack et al. 1991). An earlier suggestion of greater cardiac safety of doxepin was refuted by Roose and associates (1991), who showed the usual TCA adverse effects (and consequent poor tolerability) of doxepin in cardiac patients with depression.

Anticholinergic Effects

Especially with 3° amine TCAs, antimuscarinic actions of TCAs are universal, presenting minor annoyances to most young healthy patients but posing major hazards to physically compromised individuals. Even the commonly experienced side effect of dry mouth has been associated with serious dental pathology. Reduced tear flow and impaired visual accommodation, with resultant blurred vision, may impair daily function and pose a hazard to contact lens wearers (reviewed by Nierenberg and Cole 1991). Constipation may be a minor discomfort that responds to increased fluids and bulk laxatives, or it could progress to life-threatening paralytic ileus in medically vulnerable patients. A similar spectrum exists for urinary retention, a major risk of TCA use in older men with prostatic hypertrophy. Narrow-angle glaucoma may constitute a contraindication to the use of medications with any anticholinergic effects.

3° Amine TCAs are particularly prone to produce cognitive toxicity, ranging from confusion and memory impairment to frank delirium in elderly patients who have increased sensitivity to anticholinergics (Sunderland et al. 1987). Although some cases of TCA-related sexual dysfunction have been ascribed to anticholinergic effects, such a correlation was not observed in a recent survey (Balon et al. 1993). Indeed, sexual dysfunction has emerged as a more prominent adverse effect associated with the use of SSRIs. Thus, the potent serotonin-uptake-inhibiting property of clomipramine, rather than its strong anticholinergic effects, may explain the high incidence of sexual dysfunction caused by this TCA (Aizenberg et al. 1991).

Although correlations between TCA plasma levels and anticholinergic effects have been identified (Rudorfer and Young 1980a), these side effects are maximal at subtherapeutic plasma concentrations of 3° amine forms (Preskorn and Fast 1991), rendering dosage adjustment inefficient in combating them. Although counteracting cholinergic agents, such as bethanechol, are sometimes used in the treatment of peripheral antimuscarinic actions of TCAs (Rosen et al. 1993), and symptomatic relief can be obtained with the use of artificial saliva or tears, most clinically significant problems require change of medication. Thus, the 3° amine TCAs should be avoided in standard antidepressant doses, or used judiciously (Rahman et al. 1991), in geriatric patients. Note that even desipramine, which has the lowest anticholinergic activity among the classic tricyclics, still produces appreciable muscarinic blockade at therapeutic blood levels (Ross et al. 1983; Rudorfer and Young 1980a).

Sedation

The sedative action of the tricyclics, reflecting antihistaminic and α-blocking as well as anticholinergic activity—particularly the 3° amines (Table 10–2)—is one of the few side effects that can be used therapeutically in drug selection. Thus, the 3° amine TCAs are commonly used in a once-daily nighttime dose to address symptomatic sleep disturbance in depressed patients with insomnia (Potter et al. 1991). An incidental benefit of antihistaminic potency of the TCAs has been the antiallergic and antiulcer activities noted in Table 10–3, especially for amitriptyline, doxepin, and trimipramine.

Weight Gain

Use of TCAs is often associated with a degree of weight gain, which more than compensates for any prior weight loss associated with depression-related anorexia. This effect is believed to result from the antihistaminic and possibly α-receptor blocking actions of the TCAs, as well as a TCA-induced carbohydrate craving and slowing of metabolism that is still not well understood. In one survey of clinical practice (Berken et al. 1984), outpatients treated with amitriptyline—possibly the worst offender among the TCAs—gained an average of more than 7 kg (with craving for sweets) during 6 months of treatment. Weight gain was related to dose, and subsequent loss of weight occurred after drug discontinuation. This side effect does appear to vary among the TCAs (Fernstrom et al. 1986) and is minimal or absent with the most stimulatory members of the class (e.g., protriptyline and desipramine).

DRUG-DRUG INTERACTIONS

TCAs interact, pharmacodynamically and pharmacokinetically, with a variety of other compounds. The well-established adverse cognitive and psychomotor consequences of combining 3° amine TCAs with alcohol (Shoaf and Linnoila 1991) are primarily of a pharmacodynamic nature, although pharmacokinetics may be relevant. As reviewed by Shoaf and Linnoila (1991), tricyclic clearance is generally decreased by acute dosing with ethanol but increased by chronic alcohol use (in the absence of cirrhotic liver damage). Most adverse TCA pharmacodynamic interactions with other medications involve additive sedative or anticholinergic effects (e.g., with hypnotics or neuroleptics).

The dependence of tricyclics on hepatic metabolism is the basis of pharmacokinetic interactions with drugs that induce or impair the liver cytochrome P450 microsomal enzyme system (Rudorfer and Potter 1987).

Barbiturates and carbamazepine, for example, induce hepatic enzymes, accelerating tricyclic metabolism and reducing steady-state blood levels. On the other hand, valproate, an anticonvulsant increasingly prescribed in bipolar disorder, is associated with reduced TCA clearance in healthy volunteers (Wong et al. 1996). Most recent interest in TCA kinetic interactions with other medications has centered on drugs that interfere with the CYP2D6-mediated hydroxylation and related P450 isoenzyme functions (Rudorfer et al. 1994). For instance, concomitant neuroleptics are associated with elevated TCA levels, apparently by interfering with the hydroxylation pathway of tricyclic metabolism.

Of particular current clinical significance is the competitive inhibition of CYP2D6 by all of the currently marketed SSRIs except fluvoxamine (Bergstrom et al. 1992; Kurtz et al. 1997; Nemeroff et al. 1996; Preskorn et al. 1994). These TCA-SSRI interactions are associated with often-dramatic elevations of steady-state TCA plasma concentrations and with reduced clearance via hydroxylation, but demethylation is unaffected. Nonetheless, such combinations may be safe and effective, provided that tricyclic dosages are adjusted downward (Bergstrom et al. 1992; Nelson et al. 1991; Rudorfer et al. 1994). As newer psychotropic medications are developed and frequently combined with standard treatments such as tricyclics, the range of clinically significant drug-drug inter-

actions will continue to be defined (Rudorfer and Potter, in press).

Potentially Hazardous Interactions

The following listing is a distillation of warnings provided in the USPDI (1997) and/or *Therapeutic Drugs* (Dollery 1991, 1992).

MAOIs. As discussed in most sources, giving TCAs to individuals taking MAOIs may produce stroke, hyperpyrexia, convulsions, and death through a variety of mechanisms. Nonetheless, safely combining most TCAs with MAOIs is possible, especially if treatment begins with a 3° amine compound. The one exception is clomipramine, which (because of its potent serotonin-uptake-inhibiting action) can produce a potentially fatal "serotonin syndrome" when combined with MAOIs.

Norepinephrine and epinephrine. Following administration of the biogenic amines norepinephrine and epinephrine for other medical conditions, unexpectedly large increases in blood pressure and a greater incidence of arrhythmias may occur in individuals taking TCAs.

Phenothiazines. Additive anticholinergic effects may occur with phenothiazines, which may be manifested apace of psychosis and/or agitation, especially in elderly subjects. Nonetheless, combinations of phenothiazines with TCAs are appropriate and necessary for the treatment of delusional depression, as we noted earlier in this chapter (Spiker et al. 1985).

Other Significant Reactions

Barbiturates. Barbiturates can increase the metabolism of TCAs, requiring higher than usual doses of the antidepressant to achieve a therapeutic effect.

Cimetidine. The use of cimetidine can block the metabolism of both 3° and 2° amine TCAs. Lower doses may therefore be appropriate in patients taking this H_2-receptor antagonist. Other H_2-receptor antagonists are not reported to decrease the metabolism of TCAs.

Clonidine. The effects of clonidine are reduced or blocked by desipramine, presumably secondary to its ability to increase norepinephrine in the synapse. Other TCAs can be expected to have a similar effect.

Guanethidine. All TCAs can be expected to block the antihypertensive effects of guanethidine by inhibiting its uptake into nerve endings, although this effect should be most marked with the most potent norepinephrine uptake inhibitors.

Haloperidol. Haloperidol can block the metabolism of TCAs, depending on the dose and sequence of administration, thereby potentially raising their plasma concentrations to a toxic or nontherapeutic range.

Methylphenidate. The use of methylphenidate has been reported to block the metabolism of TCAs but not to the same extent as do antipsychotic drugs.

Phenothiazines. The phenothiazines—in particular, chlorpromazine—can block the metabolism of TCAs, depending on the dose and sequence of administration.

Phenytoin. The concentrations of phenytoin may be elevated to a toxic range by administration of TCAs.

Warfarin. The activity of the anticoagulant warfarin may be increased by administration of TCAs, which are competitive inhibitors of warfarin metabolism.

CONCLUSION

After several decades as the standard medication for treatment of major depression, the TCAs today occupy a narrower role in the psychopharmacological armamentarium. They remain a first-line and, more commonly, second-line intervention for moderate to severe depression, particularly in the presence of melancholic symptoms. In psychotic depression, TCAs are commonly combined with antipsychotic medications. Additionally, one or more tricyclics are used as an effective treatment for a variety of nonaffective disorders, including obsessive-compulsive disorder, enuresis, panic disorder, ADHD, and chronic pain syndromes. These venerable antidepressants also have a current role in combination with SSRIs and other newer antidepressant compounds in treatment-refractory depression. Pharmacokinetic interactions resulting from such combinations have furthered understanding of the metabolism of TCAs and the inducing and inhibiting effects of newer antidepressants on isoenzymes of the hepatic cytochrome P450 system. Finally, continued progress in tracing the multiple postsynaptic steps in the production of the therapeutic activity of TCAs has informed further understanding of possible universal mechanisms of antidepressant action, helping the ongoing search for and development of the next generation of antidepressant treatments.

REFERENCES

Aberg-Wistedt A, Ross SB, Jostell KG, et al: A double-blind study of zimelidine, a serotonin uptake inhibitor, and desipramine, a noradrenaline uptake inhibitor, in endogenous depression, II: biochemical findings. Acta Psychiatr Scand 66:66–82, 1982

Abernethy DR, Greenblatt DJ, Shader RI: Trimipramine kinetics and absolute bioavailability: use of gas-liquid chromatography with nitrogen-phosphorus detection. Clin Pharmacol Ther 35:348–353, 1984

Aizenberg D, Zemishlany Z, Hermesh H, et al: Painful ejaculation associated with antidepressants in four patients. J Clin Psychiatry 52:461–463, 1991

Altshuler LL, Hendrick VC: Pregnancy and psychotropic medication: changes in blood levels. J Clin Psychopharmacol 16:78–80, 1996

American Psychiatric Association: Diagnostic and Statistical Manual of Mental Disorders, 4th Edition. Washington, DC, American Psychiatric Association, 1994

American Psychiatric Association Task Force: Task Force on the Use of Laboratory Tests in Psychiatry: tricyclic antidepressants—blood level measurements and clinical outcome. Am J Psychiatry 142:155–162, 1985

Amitai Y, Erikson T, Kennedy EJ, et al: Tricyclic antidepressants in red cells and plasma: correlation with impaired intraventricular conduction in acute overdose. Clin Pharmacol Ther 54:219–227, 1993

Amsterdam J, Brunswick D, Mendels J: The clinical application of tricyclic antidepressant pharmacokinetics and plasma levels. Am J Psychiatry 137:653–662, 1981

Ananth J, Pecknold JC, Van der Steen N: Double blind comparable study of clomipramine and amitriptyline in obsessive neurosis. Prog Neuropsychopharmacol Biol Psychiatry 5:257–262, 1981

Anton RF, Ressner EL, Hitri A, et al: Efficacy of amoxapine in psychotic depression: relationship to serum prolactin and neuroleptic activity (monograph). J Clin Psychiatry 3:8–13, 1985

Asberg M, Cronholm B, Sjoqvist F, et al: Relationship between plasma levels and therapeutic effect of nortriptyline. BMJ 3:331–334, 1971

Baldessarini RJ: Drugs and the treatment of psychiatric disorders, in The Pharmacological Basis of Therapeutics, 4th Edition. Edited by Gilman AG, Goodman IS, Rall TW, et al. New York, Macmillan, 1985, pp 387–445

Balon R, Yeragani VK, Pohl R, et al: Sexual dysfunction during antidepressant treatment. J Clin Psychiatry 54:209–212, 1993

Barden N: Modulation of glucocorticoid receptor gene expression by antidepressant drugs. Pharmacopsychiatry 29: 12–22, 1996

Bech P: A review of the antidepressant properties of serotonin reuptake inhibitors. Adv Biol Psychiatry 17:58–69, 1988

Beckmann H, Goodwin FK: Antidepressant response to tricyclics and urinary MHPG in unipolar patients. Arch Gen Psychiatry 32:17–22, 1975

Bergstrom RF, Peyton AL, Lemberger L: Quantification and mechanism of the fluoxetine and tricyclic antidepressant interaction. Clin Pharmacol Ther 51:239–248, 1992

Berken GN, Weinstein DO, Stern WC: Weight gain: a side effect of tricyclic antidepressants. J Affect Disord 7:133–138, 1984

Bertilsson L, Mellstrom B, Sjoqvist F: Pronounced inhibition of noradrenaline uptake by 10-hydroxy-metabolites of nortriptyline. Life Sci 25:1285–1291, 1979

Bickel MN, Brodie BB: Structure and antidepressant activity of imipramine analogues. International Journal of Neuropharmacology 3:611–621, 1964

Biederman J, Baldessarini RJ, Wright V, et al: A double-blind placebo controlled study of desipramine in the treatment of ADD, I: efficacy. J Am Acad Child Adolesc Psychiatry 28:777–784, 1989

Biederman J, Baldessarini RJ, Goldblatt A, et al: A naturalistic study of 24-hour electrocardiographic recording and echocardiographic findings in children and adolescents treated with desipramine. J Am Acad Child Adolesc Psychiatry 32:805–813, 1993

Brosen K, Skjelbo E: Fluoxetine and norfluoxetine are potent inhibitors of P_{450}IID6—the source of the sparteine/debrisoquine oxidation polymorphism. Br J Clin Pharmacol 31:136–137, 1991

Brosen K, Otton SV, Gram LF: Sparteine oxidation polymorphism in Denmark. Acta Pharmacol Toxicol 57:357–360, 1985

Brosen K, Zeugin T, Myer UA: Role of P_{450}IID6, the target of the sparteine/debrisoquin oxidation polymorphism, in the metabolism of imipramine. Clin Pharmacol Ther 49:609–617, 1991

Bunney WE, Davis JM: Norepinephrine in depressive reactions: a review. Arch Gen Psychiatry 13:483–494, 1965

Calvo B, Garcia MJ, Pedraz JL, et al: Pharmacokinetics of amoxapine and its active metabolites. Int J Clin Pharmacol Ther Toxicol 23:180–185, 1985

Charney DS, Delgado PL, Southwick SM, et al: Current hypotheses of the mechanism of antidepressant treatments: implications for the treatment of refractory depression, in Advances in Neuropsychiatry and Psychopharmacology, Vol 2. Edited by Amsterdam JD. New York, Raven, 1991, pp 23–41

Chen J, Rasenick MM: Chronic treatment of C6 glioma cells with antidepressant increases functional coupling between a G protein (Gs) and adenylyl cyclase. J Neurochem 64:724–732, 1995

Collins GH: The use of parenteral and oral clomipramine (Anafranil) in the treatment of depressive states. Br J Psychiatry 122:189–190, 1973

Coryell W, Turner R: Outcome with desipramine therapy in subtypes of nonpsychotic major depression. J Affect Disord 9:149–154, 1985

Coupet I, Rauh CE, Szucs-Myers VA, et al: 2-chloro-11(piperazinyl)[b,f][1,4]oxazepine (amoxepine), an antidepressant with antipsychotic properties—a possible role for 7-hydroxyamoxapine. Biochem Pharmacol 28:2514–2515, 1979

Cutler NR, Zavadil AP III, Eisdorfer C, et al: Concentration of desipramine in elderly women. Am J Psychiatry 138:1235–1237, 1981

Dalack GW, Roose SP, Glassman AH: Tricyclics and heart failure (letter). Am J Psychiatry 148:1601, 1991

Daly AK, Brockmoller J, Broly F, et al: Nomenclature for human CYP2D6 alleles. Pharmacogenetics 6:193–201, 1996

Danish University Antidepressant Group: Paroxetine: a selective serotonin reuptake inhibitor showing better tolerance, but weaker antidepressant effect than clomipramine in a controlled multicenter study. J Affect Disord 18:289–299, 1990

Dollery C (ed): Therapeutic Drugs. Edinburgh, Churchill Livingstone, 1991, 1992

Donnelly M, Zametkin AJ, Rapoport JL, et al: Treatment of childhood hyperactivity with desipramine: plasma drug concentration, cardiovascular effects, plasma and urinary catecholamine levels, and clinical response. Clin Pharmacol Ther 39:72–81, 1986

Duman RS, Heninger GR, Nestler EJ: A molecular and cellular theory of depression. Arch Gen Psychiatry 54:597–606, 1997

Evans DAP, Mahgoub A, Sloan TP, et al: A family and population study of the genetic polymorphism of debrisoquine oxidation in a white British population. J Med Genet 17:102–105, 1980

Fairchild CJ, Rush AJ, Vasavada N, et al: Which depressions respond to placebo? Psychiatry Res 18:217–226, 1986

Fernstrom MD, Krowinski RL, Kupfer DJ: Chronic imipramine treatment and weight gain. Psychiatry Res 17:269–273, 1986

Ferris RM, White HL, Cooper BR, et al: Some neurochemical properties of a new antidepressant, bupropion hydrochloride (Wellbutrin). Drug Development Research 1:21–35, 1981

Forsythe WI, Merrett JD: A controlled trial of imipramine and nortriptyline in the treatment of enuresis. Br J Clin Pract 23:210–215, 1969

Geller B: Psychopharmacology of children and adolescents: pharmacokinetics and relationships of plasma/serum levels to response. Psychopharmacol Bull 27:401–409, 1991

Glassman A, Perel J, Shostak M, et al: Clinical implication of imipramine plasma levels for depressive illness. Arch Gen Psychiatry 34:197–204, 1977

Glassman AH, Bigger JT Jr, Giardina EV, et al: Clinical characteristics of imipramine induced orthostatic hypotension. Lancet 1:468–472, 1979

Glassman AH, Roose SP, Giardina EGV, et al: Cardiovascular effects of tricyclic antidepressants, in Psychopharmacology: The Third Generation of Progress. Edited by Meltzer HY. New York, Raven, 1987, pp 1437–1442

Glassman AH, Roose SP, Bigger JT Jr: The safety of tricyclic antidepressants in cardiac patients: risk-benefit reconsidered. JAMA 269:2673–2675, 1993

Golden RN, Markey SP, Risby ED, et al: Antidepressants reduce whole-body norepinephrine turnover while maintaining 6-hydroxymelatonin output. Arch Gen Psychiatry 45:144–149, 1988

Gram LF: Inadequate dosing and pharmacokinetic variability as confounding factors in assessment of efficacy of antidepressants. Clin Neuropharmacol 13 (suppl 1):S35–S44, 1990

Gram LF, Overo KF, Kirk L: Influence of neuroleptics and benzodiazepines on metabolism of tricyclic antidepressants in man. Am J Psychiatry 131:863–866, 1974

Green AR, Deakin JFW: Brain noradrenaline depletion prevents ECS-induced enhancement of serotonin and dopamine-mediated behavior. Nature 285:232–233, 1980

Hall H, Ogren SO: Effects of antidepressant drugs on different receptors in the brain. Eur J Pharmacol 70:393–407, 1981

Hauger RL, Paul SM: Neurotransmitter receptor plasticity: alterations by antidepressants and antipsychotics. Psychiatric Annals 13:399–407, 1983

Heninger GR, Charney DS: Mechanism of action of antidepressant treatments: implications for the etiology and treatment of depressive disorders, in Psychopharmacology: The Third Generation of Progress. Edited by Meltzer HY. New York, Raven, 1987, pp 535–545

Hsiao JK, Agren H, Rudorfer MV, et al: Monoamine neurotransmitter interactions and the prediction of antidepressant response. Arch Gen Psychiatry 44:1078–1083, 1987

Hyman SE, Nestler EJ: Initiation and adaptation: a paradigm for understanding psychotropic drug action. Am J Psychiatry 153:151–162, 1996

Insel TR, Mueller EA, Alterman I, et al: Obsessive-compulsive disorder and serotonin: is there a connection? Biol Psychiatry 20:1174–1188, 1985

Jandhyala B, Steenberg M, Perel JM, et al: Effects of several tricyclic antidepressants on the hemodynamics and myocardial contractility of anesthetized dogs. Eur J Pharmacol 42:403–410, 1977

Jarvis MR: Clinical pharmacokinetics of tricyclic antidepressant overdose. Psychopharmacol Bull 27:541–550, 1991

Jobson K, Linnoila M, Gillam J, et al: Successful treatment of severe anxiety attacks with tricyclic antidepressants: a possible mechanism of action. Am J Psychiatry 135:863–864, 1978

Joyce PR, Paykel ES: Predictors of drug response in depression. Arch Gen Psychiatry 46:89–99, 1989

Kitanaka I, Ross RI, Cutler NR, et al: Altered hydroxydesipramine concentrations in elderly depressed patients. Clin Pharmacol Ther 31:51–55, 1982

Kroessler D: Relative efficacy rates for therapies of delusional depression. Convuls Ther 1:173–182, 1985

Kuhn R: The treatment of depressive states with G22355 (imipramine hydrochloride). Am J Psychiatry 115:459–464, 1958

Kurtz DL, Bergstrom RF, Goldberg MJ, et al: The effect of sertraline on the pharmacokinetics of desipramine and imipramine. Clin Pharmacol Ther 62:145–156, 1997

Laborit H, Huguenard P, Alluaume R: Un nouveau stabilisateur végétatif: le 4560 RP [A new vegetative stabilizer: 4560 RP]. Presse Med 60:206–208, 1952

Laird LK, Lydiard RB, Morton WA, et al: Cardiovascular effects of imipramine, fluvoxamine and placebo in depressed outpatients. J Clin Psychiatry 54:224–228, 1993

Lake B: Controlled trial of nortriptyline in childhood enuresis. Med J Aust 5 (suppl 14):582–585, 1968

Leonard HL, Swedo S, Rapoport JL, et al: Treatment of obsessive compulsive disorder in children and adolescents with clomipramine and desipramine: a double-blind crossover comparison. Arch Gen Psychiatry 46:1088–1092, 1989

Lerer B: Neurochemical and other neurobiological consequences of ECT: implications for the pathogenesis and treatment of affective disorders, in Psychopharmacology: The Third Generation of Progress. Edited by Meltzer HY. New York, Raven, 1987, pp 577–588

Lesch KP, Manji HK: Signal-transducing G proteins and antidepressant drugs: evidence for modulation of alpha subunit gene expression in rat brain. Biol Psychiatry 32:549–579, 1992

Li Q, Hrdina PD: GAP-43 phosphorylation by PKC in rat cerebrocortical synaptosomes: effect of antidepressants. Res Commun Mol Pathol Pharmacol 96:3–13, 1997

Liebowitz MR, Quitkin FM, Stewart JW, et al: Antidepressant specificity in atypical depression. Arch Gen Psychiatry 45:129–137, 1988

Linnoila M, George L, Guthrie S, et al: Effect of alcohol consumption and cigarette smoking on antidepressant levels of depressed patients. Am J Psychiatry 138:841–842, 1981

Maas JW, Fawcett JA, Dekirmenjian H: Catecholamine metabolism, depressive illness, and drug response. Arch Gen Psychiatry 26:353–363, 1972

Madsen H, Rasmussen BB, Brosen K, et al: Imipramine demethylation in vivo: impact of CYP1A2, CYP2C19, and CYP3A4. Clin Pharmacol Ther 61:319–324, 1997

Manier DH, Gillespie DD, Sulser F: Dual aminergic regulation of central beta adrenoreceptors: effect of "atypical" antidepressants and 5-hydroxytryptophan. Neuropsychopharmacology 2:89–95, 1989

Manji HK, Lenox RH: Long-term action of lithium: a role for transcriptional and posttranscriptional factors regulated by protein kinase C. Synapse 16:11–28, 1994

Manji HK, Potter WZ: Emerging strategies in affective disorders, in Emerging Strategies in Neurotherapeutics. Edited by Pullan L, Patel J. Totowa, NJ, Humana Press, 1995, pp 35–83

Manji HK, Chen G, Bitran JA, et al: Chronic exposure of C6 glioma cells to desipramine desensitizes β-adrenoceptors, but increases K_L/K_H ratio. Eur J Pharmacol 206:159–162, 1991a

Manji HK, Chen G, Bitran JA, et al: Down-regulation of beta receptors by desipramine in vitro involves PKC/phospholipase A_2. Psychopharmacol Bull 27:247–253, 1991b

Manji HK, Potter WZ, Lenox RH: Signal transduction pathways: molecular targets for lithium's actions. Arch Gen Psychiatry 52:531–543, 1995

Mogilnicka E, Arbilla S, Depoortere H, et al: Rapid-eye-movement sleep deprivation decreases the density of ³H-dihydroalprenolol and ³H-imipramine binding sites in the rat cerebral cortex. Eur J Pharmacol 65:289–292, 1980

Moody JP, Whyte SF, MacDonald AJ, et al: Pharmacokinetic aspects of protriptyline plasma levels. Eur J Clin Pharmacol 11:51–56, 1977

Morishita S, Watanabe S: Effect of the tricyclic antidepressant desipramine on protein kinase C in rat brain and rabbit platelets in vitro. Psychiatry and Clinical Neuroscience 51:249–252, 1997

Munjack DJ, Usigli R, Zulueta A, et al: Nortriptyline in the treatment of panic disorder and agoraphobia with panic attacks. J Clin Psychopharmacol 8:204–207, 1988

Nakamura S: Effects of phospholipase A2 inhibitors on the antidepressant-induced axonal regeneration of noradrenergic locus coeruleus neurons. Microsc Res Tech 29:204–210, 1994

Nalepa I, Vetulani J: Modulation of electroconvulsive treatment induced beta-adrenergic down-regulation by previous chronic imipramine administration: the involvement of protein kinase C. Pol J Pharmacol 48:489–494, 1996

Nelson JC, Mazure CM: A scale for rating tricyclic response in major depression: the TRIM. J Clin Psychopharmacol 10:252–260, 1990

Nelson JC, Mazure CM, Bowers MB Jr, et al: A preliminary open study of the combination of fluoxetine and desipramine for rapid treatment of major depression. Arch Gen Psychiatry 48:303–307, 1991

Nemeroff CB, DeVane CL, Pollock BG: Newer antidepressants and the cytochrome P450 system. Am J Psychiatry 153:311–320, 1996

Nibuya M, Nestler EJ, Duman RS: Chronic antidepressant administration increases the expression of cAMP response element-binding protein (CREB) in rat hippocampus. J Neurosci 16:2365–2372, 1996

Nierenberg AA, Cole JO: Antidepressant adverse drug reactions. J Clin Psychiatry 52 (suppl):40–47, 1991

Nies A, Robinson DS, Friedman DS, et al: Relationship between age and tricyclic antidepressant plasma levels. Am J Psychiatry 134:790–793, 1977

Orsulak PJ: Therapeutic monitoring of antidepressant drugs: guidelines updated. Ther Drug Monit 11:497–507, 1989

Owens MJ: Molecular and cellular mechanisms of antidepressant drugs. Depression and Anxiety 4:153–159, 1996

Pande AC, Birkett M, Fechner-Bates S, et al: Fluoxetine versus phenelzine in atypical depression. Biol Psychiatry 40:1017–1020, 1996

Pandey SC, Davis JM, Schwertz DW, et al: Effect of antidepressants and neuroleptics on phosphoinositide metabolism in human platelets. J Pharmacol Exp Ther 256:1010–1018, 1991

Paykel ES: Depressive typologies and response to amitriptyline. Br J Psychiatry 120:147–156, 1972

Paykel ES: Treatment of depression: the relevance of research for clinical practice. Br J Psychiatry 155:754–763, 1989

Paykel ES, Rowan PR, Parker RR, et al: Response to phenelzine and amitriptyline in subtypes of outpatient depression. Arch Gen Psychiatry 39:1041–1049, 1982

Peroutka SJ, Snyder SH: Long term antidepressant treatment decreases spiroperidol-labeled serotonin receptor binding. Science 210:88–90, 1980

Perry PJ, Morgan DE, Smith RE, et al: Treatment of unipolar depression accompanied by delusions. J Affect Disord 4:195–200, 1982

Perry PJ, Pfohl BM, Holstad SG: The relationship between antidepressant response and tricyclic antidepressant plasma concentrations. Clin Pharmacokinet 13:381–392, 1987

Pinder RM, Brogden RN, Speight TM, et al: Doxepin up-to-date: a review of its pharmacological properties and therapeutic efficacy with particular reference to depression. Drugs 13:161–218, 1977

Pollock BG, Perel JM: Tricyclic antidepressants: contemporary issues for therapeutic practice. Can J Psychiatry 34:609–617, 1989

Pollock BG, Everett G, Perel JM: Comparative cardiotoxicity of nortriptyline and its isomeric 10-hydroxymetabolites. Neuropsychopharmacology 6:1–10, 1992a

Pollock BG, Perel JM, Altieri LP, et al: Debrisoquine hydroxylation phenotyping in geriatric psychopharmacology. Psychopharmacol Bull 28:163–168, 1992b

Potter WZ: Psychotherapeutic drugs and biogenic amines: current concepts and therapeutic implications. Drugs 28:127–143, 1984

Potter WZ, Calil NM, Manian AA, et al: Hydroxylated metabolites of tricyclic antidepressants: preclinical assessment of activity. Biol Psychiatry 14:601–613, 1979

Potter WZ, Bertilsson L, Sjoqvist F: Clinical pharmacokinetics of psychotropic drugs: fundamental and practical aspects, in The Handbook of Biological Psychiatry. Edited by Van Praag NM, Rafaelson O, Lader O, et al. New York, Marcel Dekker, 1980, pp 71–134

Potter WZ, Scheinin M, Golden RN, et al: Selective antidepressants and cerebrospinal fluid: lack of specificity on norepinephrine and serotonin metabolites. Arch Gen Psychiatry 42:1171–1177, 1985

Potter WZ, Rudorfer MV, Manji HK: The pharmacologic treatment of depression: an update. N Engl J Med 523:633–642, 1991

Prange AI: The pharmacology and biochemistry of depression. Diseases of the Nervous System 25:217–221, 1965

Preskorn SH, Fast GA: Therapeutic drug monitoring for antidepressants: efficacy, safety, and cost effectiveness. J Clin Psychiatry 52 (6, suppl):23–33, 1991

Preskorn SH, Irwin HA: Toxicity of tricyclic antidepressants: kinetics, mechanism, intervention: a review. J Clin Psychiatry 43:151–156, 1982

Preskorn SH, Alderman J, Chung M, et al: Pharmacokinetics of desipramine coadministered with sertraline or fluoxetine. J Clin Psychopharmacol 14:90–98, 1994

Psychoyos S: Antidepressant inhibition of H_1-H_2-histamine-receptor-mediated adenylate cyclase in [2-^{3}H]adenine-prelabeled vesicular preparations from guinea pig brain. Biochem Pharmacol 30:2182–2185, 1981

Quitkin FM, Harrison W, Stewart JW, et al: Response to phenelzine and imipramine in placebo nonresponders with atypical depression. Arch Gen Psychiatry 48:319–323, 1991

Rahman MK, Akhtar MJ, Savla NC, et al: A double-blind randomized comparison of fluvoxamine with dothiepin in the treatment of depression in elderly patients. Br J Clin Pract 45:255–258, 1991

Randrup A, Braestrup C: Uptake inhibition of biogenic amines by newer antidepressant drugs: relevance to the dopamine hypothesis of depression. Psychopharmacology (Berl) 53:309–314, 1977

Rapoport J, Potter WZ: Tricyclic antidepressants: use in pediatric psychopharmacology, in Pharmacokinetics: Youth and Age. Edited by Raskin A, Robinson D. Amsterdam, Elsevier, 1981, pp 105–123

Rapoport JL, Quinn PO, Bradbard G, et al: A double-blind comparison of imipramine and methylphenidate treatments of hyperactive boys. Arch Gen Psychiatry 30:789–793, 1974

Rapoport JL, Mikkelson EJ, Zavadil AP, et al: Childhood enuresis II: psychopathology, tricyclic concentration in plasma and anti-enuretic effect. Arch Gen Psychiatry 37:1146–1152, 1980

Rasenick MM, Chaney KA, Chen J: G protein-mediated signal transduction as a target of antidepressant and antibipolar drug action: evidence from model systems. J Clin Psychiatry 57 (suppl 13):49–55, 1996

Raskin A, Crook TA: The endogenous-neurotic distinction as a predictor of response to antidepressant drugs. Psychol Med 6:59–70, 1976

Ravaris CL, Robinson DS, Ives JO, et al: Phenelzine and amitriptyline in the treatment of depression: a comparison of present and past studies. Arch Gen Psychiatry 37:1075–1080, 1980

Ray WA: Psychotropic drugs and injuries among the elderly: a review. J Clin Psychopharmacol 12:386–396, 1992

Richelson E, Nelson A: Antagonism by antidepressants of neurotransmitter receptors of normal human brain in vitro. J Pharmacol Exp Ther 230:94–102, 1984

Richelson E, Pfenning M: Blockade by antidepressants and related compounds of biogenic amine uptake into rat brain synaptosomes: most antidepressants selectively block norepinephrine uptake. Eur J Pharmacol 130:277–286, 1984

Riddle MA, Geller B, Ryan N: Another sudden death in a child treated with desipramine. J Am Acad Child Adolesc Psychiatry 32:792–797, 1993

Roose SP, Dalack GW, Glassman AH, et al: Is doxepin a safer tricyclic for the heart? J Clin Psychiatry 52:338–341, 1991

Rosen J, Pollock BG, Altieri LP, et al: Treatment of nortriptyline's side effects in elderly patients: a double-blind study of bethanechol. Am J Psychiatry 150:1249–1251, 1993

Ross RI, Zavadil AP, Calil NM, et al: The effects of desmethylimipramine on plasma norepinephrine, pulse and blood pressure in volunteers. Clin Pharmacol Ther 33:429–437, 1983

Rudorfer MV, Potter WZ: Pharmacokinetics of antidepressants, in Psychopharmacology: The Third Generation of Progress. Edited by Meltzer HY. New York, Raven, 1987, pp 1353–1364

Rudorfer MV, Potter WZ: The role of metabolites of antidepressants in the treatment of depression. CNS Drugs 7:273–312, 1997

Rudorfer MV, Potter WZ: Metabolism of tricyclic antidepressants, in Drug Metabolism and Psychiatry: A Special Issue of Cellular and Molecular Neurobiology. Edited by Baker GB. (in press)

Rudorfer MV, Robins E: Amitriptyline overdose: clinical effects of tricyclic antidepressant plasma levels. J Clin Psychiatry 43:457–460, 1982

Rudorfer MV, Young RC: Anticholinergic effects and plasma desipramine levels. Clin Pharmacol Ther 28:703–706, 1980a

Rudorfer MV, Young RC: Desipramine: cardiovascular effects and plasma levels. Am J Psychiatry 137:984–986, 1980b

Rudorfer MV, Manji HK, Potter WZ: Comparative tolerability profiles of the newer versus older antidepressants. Drug Saf 10:18–46, 1994

Schildkraut JJ: The catecholamine hypothesis of affective disorders: a review of supporting evidence. Am J Psychiatry 122:509–522, 1965

Schwaninger M, Schofl C, Blume R, et al: Inhibition by antidepressant drugs of cyclic AMP response element-binding protein/cyclic AMP response element-directed gene transcription. Mol Pharmacol 47:1112–1118, 1995

Shen WW: The metabolism of psychoactive drugs: a review of enzymatic biotransformation and inhibition. Biol Psychiatry 41:814–826, 1997

Shoaf SE, Linnoila M: Interaction of ethanol and smoking on the pharmacokinetics and pharmacodynamics of psychotropic medications. Psychopharmacol Bull 27:577–594, 1991

Smith MA, Makino S, Altemus M, et al: Stress and antidepressants differentially regulate neurotrophin 3 mRNA expression in the locus coeruleus. Proc Natl Acad Sci U S A 92:8788–8792, 1995

Spencer T, Biederman J, Wilens T, et al: Pharmacotherapy of attention-deficit hyperactivity disorder across the life cycle. J Am Acad Child Adolesc Psychiatry 35:409–432, 1996

Spiker D, Weiss A, Chang S, et al: Tricyclic antidepressant overdose: clinical presentation and plasma levels. Clin Pharmacol Ther 18:539–546, 1975

Spiker DG, Weiss JC, Dealy RS, et al: The pharmacologic treatment of delusional depression. Am J Psychiatry 142:430–436, 1985

Stewart JW, Quitkin F, Fyer A, et al: Efficacy of desmethylimipramine in endogenomorphically depressed patients. Psychopharmacol Bull 16:52–54, 1980

Stewart JW, Quitkin FM, Liebowitz MR, et al: Efficacy of desipramine in depressed outpatients: response according to Research Diagnostic Criteria and severity of illness. Arch Gen Psychiatry 40:202–207, 1989

Sugrue MF: Chronic antidepressant therapy and associated changes in central monoaminergic function. Pharmacol Ther 21:1–37, 1983

Sulser F: Antidepressant treatments and regulation of norepinephrine-receptor-coupled adenylate cyclase systems in brain. Adv Biochem Psychopharmacol 39:249–261, 1984

Sulser F, Vetulani J, Mobley PL: Mode of action of antidepressant drugs. Biochem Pharmacol 27:257–261, 1978

Sunderland T, Tariot PN, Cohen RM, et al: Anticholinergic sensitivity in patients with dementia of the Alzheimer type and age-matched controls: a dose-response study. Arch Gen Psychiatry 44:418–426, 1987

Swann AC, Bowden CL, Rush AJ, et al: Desipramine versus phenelzine in recurrent unipolar depression: clinical characteristics and treatment response. J Clin Psychopharmacol 17:78–83, 1997

Thoren P, Asberg M, Cronholm B, et al: Clomipramine treatment of obsessive compulsive disorder: a controlled clinical trial. Arch Gen Psychiatry 37:1281–1289, 1980

Traskman L, Asberg M, Bertilsson L, et al: Plasma levels of clomipramine and its dimethyl metabolite during treatment of depression. Clin Pharmacol Ther 26:600–610, 1979

Turner P, Ehsanullah RSB: Clomipramine and maprotiline on human platelet uptake of 5-hydroxytryptamine and dopamine in vitro: relevance to their antidepressive and other central actions? Postgrad Med J 53 (suppl 4):14–18, 1977

Uhde TW, Nemiah JC: Panic and generalized anxiety disorders, in Comprehensive Textbook of Psychiatry, 5th Edition. Edited by Sadock BJ. Baltimore, MD, Williams & Wilkins, 1989, pp 952–972

United States Pharmacopeia Dispensing Information: Drug Information for the Health Care Professional, 17th Edition. Rockville, MD, United States Pharmacopeial Convention, 1997

Vetulani J, Sulser F: Action of various antidepressant treatments reduces reactivity of noradrenergic cyclic AMP generating systems in limbic forebrain. Nature 257:395–496, 1975

Vetulani J, Lebrecht U, Pilc A: Enhancement of responsiveness of the central system and serotonin-2-receptor density in rat frontal cortex by electroconvulsive treatments. Eur J Pharmacol 76:81–85, 1981

Wells BG, Gelenberg AJ: Chemistry, pharmacology, pharmacokinetics, adverse effects and efficacy of the antidepressant maprotiline hydrochloride. Pharmacotherapy 1:121–139, 1981

Wilens TE, Biederman J, Baldessarini RJ, et al: Developmental changes in serum concentrations of desipramine and 2-hydroxydesipramine during treatment with desipramine. J Am Acad Child Adolesc Psychiatry 31:691–698, 1992

Wilens TE, Biederman J, Baldessarini RJ, et al: Electrocardiographic effects of desipramine and 2-hydroxydesipramine in children, adolescents, and adults treated with desipramine. J Am Acad Child Adolesc Psychiatry 32:798–804, 1993

Wilens TE, Biederman J, Prince J, et al: Six-week, double-blind, placebo-controlled study of desipramine for adult attention deficit hyperactivity disorder. Am J Psychiatry 153:1147–1153, 1996

Wisner KL, Perel JM, Findling RL, et al: Nortriptyline and its hydroxymetabolites in breastfeeding mothers and newborns. Psychopharmacol Bull 33:249–251, 1997

Wong SL, Cavanaugh J, Shi H, et al: Effects of divalproex sodium on amitriptyline and nortriptyline pharmacokinetics. Clin Pharmacol Ther 60:48–53, 1996

Young RC, Alexopoulos GS, Shamoian CA, et al: Plasma 10-hydroxynortriptyline in elderly depressed patients. Clin Pharmacol Ther 35:540–544, 1984

Young RC, Alexopoulous GS, Shindledeker R, et al: Plasma 10-hydroxynortriptyline and therapeutic response in geriatric depression. Neuropsychopharmacology 1:213–215, 1988

Ziegler VE, Biggs JT: Tricyclic plasma levels: effect of age, race, sex, and smoking. JAMA 238:2167–2169, 1977

Ziegler VE, Biggs JT, Wylie LT, et al: Protriptyline kinetics. Clin Pharmacol Ther 23:580–584, 1978

Zis AP, Goodwin FK: Novel antidepressants and the biogenic amine hypothesis of depression: the case of iprindole and mianserin. Arch Gen Psychiatry 36:1097–1107, 1979

Zitrin CM, Klein DF, Woerner MG: Treatment of agoraphobia with group exposure in vivo and imipramine. Arch Gen Psychiatry 37:63–72, 1980

ELEVEN

Selective Serotonin Reuptake Inhibitors

Gary D. Tollefson, M.D., Ph.D., and Jerrold F. Rosenbaum, M.D.

The class of selective serotonin reuptake inhibitors (SSRIs) represents an important advance in pharmacotherapy and has been the catalyst for substantial serotonin-oriented basic and clinical research. Considerable evidence demonstrates that this drug class has a broad spectrum of clinical indications. In general, an advantageous safety profile has propelled these agents to their current level of popularity. Although the members of this category share several common features, we also highlight some of their unique differences.

HISTORY AND DISCOVERY

Serotonin is an indoleamine with wide distribution in plants, animals, and humans. Pioneering histochemistry by Falck and colleagues (1962) found that serotonin was localized within specific neuronal pathways and cell bodies. These originate principally from two discrete nuclei—the medial and dorsal raphe. Across animal species, serotonin innervation is widespread. Although regional variations exist, several limbic structures manifest especially high levels of serotonin (A. H. Amin et al. 1954).

However, serotonin levels in the central nervous system (CNS) represent only a small fraction of that found in the body (Bradley 1989). Because serotonin does not cross the blood-brain barrier, it must be synthesized locally. Serotonin is released into the synapse from the cytoplasmic and vesicular reservoirs (Elks et al. 1979). Following release, serotonin is principally inactivated by reuptake into nerve terminals through a sodium/potassium (Na^+/K^+) adenosine triphosphatase (ATPase)-dependent carrier (Shaskan and Snyder 1970). The transmitter is subse-quently subject to either degradation by monoamine oxidase (MAO) or vesicular restorage. Abnormalities in central serotonin function have been hypothesized to underlie disturbances in mood, anxiety, satiety, cognition, aggression, and sexual drives, to highlight a few. As described by Fuller (1985), there are several loci at which therapeutic drugs might alter serotonin neurotransmission (see Figure 11–1). The recent explosion of knowledge regarding the serotonin system can largely be traced to the development of compounds that block the reuptake of this neurotransmitter.

STRUCTURE-ACTIVITY RELATIONS

Drugs that inhibit serotonin reuptake vary in their selectivity (see Table 11–1). Despite the tendency to lump the contemporary SSRIs into the same class designation, significant structural and activity differences exist. Their structural formulas help illustrate this diversity (see Figure 11–2). Both paroxetine and sertraline exist as single isomers; in contrast, fluoxetine and citalopram are racemic. Fluvoxamine has no optically active forms. Structural differences bestow both pharmacokinetic and pharmacodynamic heterogeneity.

The family of SSRIs manifests diverse structural and activity relations. Such data are in vitro and thus subject to methodological variability (Thomas et al. 1987). Paroxetine appears to be the most potent in vitro SSRI, whereas citalopram may be the most selective. However, note that in vitro potency does not necessarily equate with in vivo dosing experience, clinical efficacy, adverse-event profile, and so on. Of the SSRIs, sertraline is the only class member that is a more potent inhibitor of dopamine than

colleagues (1987) noted that coadministration with mianserin or maprotiline also increased the duration of downregulation. Sertraline induced downregulation of the β receptor and reduced production at the β receptor of the second messenger cAMP (Koe et al. 1987). In contrast, investigations with fluvoxamine, paroxetine, and citalopram have not yielded consistent results. In general, the greater the serotonin selectivity of a compound, the less in vitro evidence for β-norepinephrine downregulation has been seen. Thus, β-norepinephrine downregulation may not be essential for clinical efficacy.

Current data do not support a significant effect on α-norepinephrine receptor affinity or density by the SSRIs. Studies using several different radiolabels to investigate paroxetine (Nelson et al. 1989), fluoxetine (Wong et al. 1985), and citalopram (Nowak 1989) have shown a relative inactivity at this site. Studies with sertraline or fluvoxamine are limited. Fluoxetine has been reported to reduce desipramine-induced release of growth hormone after 4 weeks of treatment (O'Flynn et al. 1991). This effect suggests a possible indirect activity at the $α_2$-norepinephrine receptor.

In summary, most SSRIs do not manifest significant norepinephrine activity. However, relative differences in adrenoceptor affinity exist across the class; the clinical significance of these differences is negligible based on present information.

Dopamine

Animal studies provide evidence that the serotonin system may exert tonic inhibition on the central dopaminergic system. Thus, SSRIs might diminish dopaminergic transmission consistent with anecdotes of extrapyramidal side effects (EPS) during fluoxetine therapy (Bouchard et al. 1989). Serotonin agonists, however, also exert a facilitory influence on dopamine release (Benloucif and Galloway 1991), which can be antagonized by the 5-HT$_1$ blocker pindolol, and evidence suggests that SSRIs may actually sensitize mesolimbic dopamine receptors (Arnt et al. 1984a, 1984b). Many structurally diverse antidepressants are associated with a net enhancement of mesolimbic dopamine (Klimek and Maj 1990). The benefits of antidepressants in an animal model of depression can be antagonized by a dopamine D$_1$ (SCH-23390) or D$_2$ blocker (sulpiride) (Sampson et al. 1991). Repeated administration of several SSRIs increased the hypermotility response to several dopaminergic agents, including amphetamine, methylphenidate (Arnt et al. 1984b), quinpirole (Maj et al. 1984), and apomorphine (Plaznik and Kostowski 1987).

The induction of catalepsy or inhibition of apomorphine-induced catalepsy is not a property of the SSRIs. Within the family of SSRIs, citalopram reportedly downregulated rat striatolimbic D$_1$ receptors (Klimek and Nielsen 1987). Both citalopram and fluoxetine have been inactive in displacing D$_2$ blockers (Peroutka and Snyder 1980). Baldessarini and co-workers (1992) reported that fluoxetine "even at high doses or with repeated treatment" demonstrated "no significant inhibition of the DA [dopamine]-metabolism—increasing actions of haloperidol" (p. 191).

In summary, the SSRIs do not appear to exert a significant effect on the dopamine system. However, in clinical use, a multitude of variables makes simple conclusions regarding dopamine-mediated events unreliable.

Miscellaneous

Neuroendocrine and neurotransmitter dysfunction in major depression has been linked to corticotropin-releasing factor (CRF) in locus coeruleus neurons. Antidepressants have been hypothesized to reverse CRF-related increases in locus coeruleus discharge. Sertraline has been proposed as an acute functional CRF antagonist (Valentino and Curtis 1991). However, net serotonin enhancement by an SSRI would be expected to promote the release of CRF (Fuller 1985). Activity through 5-HT$_{1A}$ receptors has been proposed by Lorens and Van der Kar (1987); the role for SSRIs, however, as CRF antagonists awaits further clarification.

In summary, the SSRIs enhance central serotonin transmission through increased output and/or increased postsynaptic receptor sensitivity (Blier et al. 1987). However, such changes alone do not guarantee a clinically meaningful response (Charney et al. 1984). A change in baseline serotonin function or a "permissive" set of interactions with other colocalized neurotransmitter receptors is likely involved in the highly individualized responses in depressed patients.

PHARMACOKINETICS AND DISPOSITION

Pharmacokinetic variability exists within the SSRI class (Leonard 1992) (Table 11–2). Discussion of drug half-life must also include consideration of the presence or absence of active metabolites. Fluoxetine is principally metabolized to norfluoxetine, which has similar activity to fluoxetine on serotonin reuptake. The elimination half-life of norfluoxetine is longer (4–16 days) than that of fluoxetine (4–6 days). The desmethyl metabolite of sertraline manifests uptake inhibition of serotonin, albeit of a magnitude approximately one-tenth that of the parent

Table 11–2. A comparison of several selective serotonin reuptake inhibitors

	Fluoxetine	Paroxetine	Sertraline	Citalopram	Fluvoxamine
Volume of distribution (L/kg)	3–40	17	20	12–16	>5
Percent protein bound	94	95	99	80	77
Peak plasma level (hours)	6–8	2–8	6–8	1–6	2–8
Parent half-life (hours)	24–72	20	24–26	33	15
Major metabolite half-life	4–16 days	N/A	66 hours	N/A	N/A
Standard dose range (mg)	20–80	10–50	50–200	10–40	50–300
Absorption altered by a fast or fed status	No	No	Yes	No	No
Altered half-life in the geriatric patient	No	Yes	Yes	Yes	No
Reduced clearance in renal patients	±	+	±	±	±

Note. N/A = not applicable.

(Heym and Koe 1988). The elimination half-life of desmethyl sertraline also exceeds that of its parent (66 vs. 24–26 hours) (Doogan and Caillard 1988). The principal desmethyl metabolite of citalopram is approximately 4 times less potent as an SSRI than its parent and 11 times more potent as a norepinephrine uptake inhibitor (Hyttel 1982). However, this metabolite's concentration is typically less than that of citalopram and weakly crosses the blood-brain barrier. Thus, an antidepressant contribution from the metabolite is probably negligible.

In contrast, paroxetine (Haddock et al. 1989) and fluvoxamine (Claassen 1983) have metabolites with minimal or no activity. An SSRI with a relatively long half-life offers greater protection from the discontinuation syndrome associated with abrupt discontinuation or noncompliance related to interruption of treatment. Conversely, those drugs require a more prolonged vigilance for drug-drug interactions following their discontinuation; for example, a 5-week washout from fluoxetine is recommended before initiating an MAOI (Ciraulo and Shader 1990). Variability in drug half-life is associated with a range in time to steady-state plasma concentrations, which does not predict or correlate with onset of antidepressant activity. The time to onset of antidepressant effect is the same for all SSRIs.

MECHANISM OF ACTION

In the absence of pharmacological manipulation, the reuptake of serotonin into the presynaptic nerve terminal typically leads to its inactivation. The SSRIs, through blockade of the reuptake process, acutely enhance serotonergic neurotransmission by permitting serotonin to act for an extended time at synaptic binding sites. A net result is an acute increase in synaptic serotonin. One difference separating the SSRIs from the direct-acting agonists is that the SSRIs are dependent on neuronal release of serotonin for their action. That is, SSRIs can be considered as augmentors of basal physiological signals, but they are not direct stimulators of postsynaptic receptor function and are dependent on presynaptic neuronal integrity; these pharmacodynamic features might explain SSRI nonresponse. If the release of serotonin from presynaptic neuronal storage sites was substantially compromised, and in turn their net synaptic serotonin concentration was negligible, a clinically meaningful response to an SSRI would not be expected.

Serotonin receptors also include a family of presynaptic autoreceptors that suppress the further release of serotonin, thus limiting the degree of postsynaptic receptor stimulation that can be achieved. DeMontigny and colleagues (1989) investigated the mechanism of action of several SSRIs and suggested that the enhanced efficacy of serotonergic synaptic transmission is not the result of increased postsynaptic sensitivity. Rather, longer-term SSRI treatment induced a desensitization of somatodendritic and terminal serotonin autoreceptors. Such a desensitization would permit serotonin neurons to reestablish a normal rate of firing despite sustained reuptake blockade. These neurons could then release a greater amount of serotonin per impulse into the synaptic cleft. This modification reportedly occurs over a time course compatible with the antidepressant response.

INDICATIONS

Depression

A plethora of placebo-controlled, double-blind trials have established the clear superiority of the SSRIs over placebo

(Kasper et al. 1992). Statistically significant reductions from baseline in the Hamilton Rating Scale for Depression (HRSD; Hamilton 1960) score have been seen as early as the second week of treatment; however, the rate and quality of response to an SSRI are highly individualized (range 10–42 days). Overall, the efficacy of the SSRIs compared with that of conventional TCAs has been comparable or slightly better (Feighner et al. 1989; Guelfi et al. 1987; Wernicke et al. 1987) with some exceptions (Peselow et al. 1989; vanPraag et al. 1987). Several trials have also established that the SSRIs may be effective in patients with TCA-resistant depressions (Delgado et al. 1988; Tyrer et al. 1987).

In general, the range for dose titration with most SSRIs is relatively narrow (see Table 11–2), and higher dosages are more often associated with increased adverse events (Altamura et al. 1988; M. Amin et al. 1989). Schweizer and colleagues (1990) reported that in a study of 108 subjects treated with 20 mg of fluoxetine for 3 weeks and then randomized to either 20 mg or 60 mg for another 5 weeks, both groups did equally well after 8 weeks.

However, early implementation of high-dose therapy may be appropriate in some circumstances. Conversion of nonresponders by prescribing at the higher end of the dose range has been described with fluoxetine and paroxetine (Fava et al. 1992; Hebenstreit et al. 1989). However, extreme doses of sertraline (up to 400 mg/day) have been associated with reduced efficacy (W. Guy et al. 1986). Unfortunately, plasma level studies have contributed little toward the understanding of the dose-response relationship. Most studies have failed to confirm any relationship between clinical response and plasma concentration with paroxetine (Tasker et al. 1989), fluoxetine (Kelly et al. 1989), citalopram (Hebenstreit et al. 1989), or fluvoxamine (De-Wilde and Doogan 1982). This suggests that synaptic concentrations and/or pharmacodynamic effects are not accurately reflected by plasma levels. The question of a linear versus curvilinear dose-response pattern with the SSRIs also remains unanswered.

Continued SSRI efficacy during maintenance therapy has been established in several trials (Danion 1989; Dufour 1987; Ferrey et al. 1989; Michelson et al. 1997b; Montgomery et al. 1988). One trial reported a recurrence among 54 of 94 (57%) placebo- versus 23 of 88 (26%) fluoxetine-maintained subjects ($P < .0001$) who had at least 4.5 months of recovery before their randomization (Montgomery et al. 1988). Study participants had been required to have at least two previous episodes. Similar outcomes favoring the SSRI include a blinded trial ($N = 289$) with sertraline (Doogan and Caillard 1988) and open trials

of fluvoxamine (Feldmann and Dunbar 1982) and citalopram (Pedersen et al. 1982).

Although the SSRIs are often thought of as "activating," considerable evidence supports their utility in depression with anxious features. Montgomery (1989a) conducted a meta-analysis of several fluoxetine trials that indicated efficacy in depressions featuring anxiety and psychomotor agitation. Similar findings have been reported by Jouvent et al. (1989) and Beasley et al. (1991). Ravindran and colleagues (1997) reported analogous benefits with paroxetine. Fluvoxamine reduced comorbid anxiety to an extent similar to that of a comparator benzodiazepine in trials conducted by Charbannes and Douge (1989) and Laws and colleagues (1990).

What has emerged from comparative blinded depression trials is that the risk-benefit profile of SSRIs is often superior to that of conventional TCAs (Boyer and Feighner 1991). A favorable comparison to the standard TCAs is particularly noteworthy in light of the HRSD's emphasis on somatic and sleep symptoms, because these items may improve independent of mood status secondary to the characteristic sedative and anticholinergic effects of the TCAs (Montgomery 1989b; Shaw and Crimmins 1989), thus inflating measures of change in depression per se.

From a clinician's perspective, the predominant advantage of the SSRIs is their adverse-event profile. This translates into superior patient acceptance and compliance in most cases. The advantage of at least comparable efficacy and superior tolerability was also evident in the treatment of dysthymia in a placebo-controlled comparison of sertraline and imipramine (Thase et al. 1996). In controlled clinical trials, the rate of early treatment discontinuations with a TCA comparator has been severalfold higher than that with the SSRIs (Jenike et al. 1989a; Shrivastava et al. 1992). Thus, the SSRIs represent a significant addition to the therapeutic armamentarium and have a favorable safety profile and at least similar efficacy compared with the TCAs.

Obsessive-Compulsive Disorder

Clomipramine, a potent inhibitor of both serotonin and norepinephrine reuptake, was observed more than 20 years ago to reduce obsessive-compulsive symptoms (Renynghe de Voxurie 1968). The superior benefit of this potent serotonergic TCA over desipramine represents a cornerstone in the serotonin hypothesis of obsessive-compulsive disorder (Benkelfat et al. 1989). Sertraline (Bick and Hackett 1989), fluvoxamine (Goodman et al. 1989), fluoxetine (Jenike et al. 1989b), and paroxetine (Zohar et al. 1996) have also been shown to be effective in obsessive-compulsive disorder independent of a patient's comorbid mood status. Patients who have obsessive-compulsive disorder may require higher doses of medication and longer treatment periods than do patients with depression to determine response.

A precise explanation of this selective serotonin advantage in obsessive-compulsive disorder is unknown. A heightened level of metabolic activity in the orbital region and caudate dysfunction have been reported by Baxter and colleagues (1992) and may be normalized by either somatic (fluoxetine 60–80 mg) or behavioral interventions. Hypersensitivity of the serotonin system has been theorized. Receptor downregulation, associated with long-term SSRI therapy, has been offered as a potential explanation of clinical response (Zohar et al. 1988). This hypothetical neuroadaptation is supported by a positive correlation between symptomatic improvement from baseline and cerebrospinal fluid (CSF) 5-hydroxyindoleacetic acid (5-HIAA) (Thoren et al. 1980) or platelet serotonin concentration (Flament et al. 1985). Chronic administration of fluoxetine attenuates ipsapirone-induced hypothermia and adrenocorticotropic hormone (ACTH) and cortisol release among patients with primary obsessive-compulsive disorder. Although these data support a model of drug-induced 5-HT_{1A} subsensitivity and/or dampened postreceptor signal, the magnitude of change fails to correlate with the degree of clinical improvement (Lesch et al. 1991). An SSRI-mediated decrease in serotonin responsivity is consistent with the observed latency in symptomatic improvement.

Because obsessive-compulsive disorder is a chronic disorder, prolonged SSRI therapy may be necessary. In patients whose symptoms have been minimally or only moderately reduced with SSRI treatment, numerous augmentation strategies have been proposed, including tryptophan, fenfluramine, lithium, buspirone, trazodone, or a neuroleptic (see Goodman et al. 1992).

Panic Disorder

SSRIs are the drugs of choice in the prevention of panic attacks and the treatment of panic disorder. Positive results from double-blind, placebo-controlled trials in patients with panic disorder are available for paroxetine, fluvoxamine, sertraline, citalopram, and fluoxetine (Lydiard et al. 1997; Sheehan and Harnett-Sheehan 1996). In 1996, paroxetine was the first SSRI approved by the U.S. Food and Drug Administration (FDA) for use in the treatment of panic disorder, followed by sertraline in 1997. In a comparison trial, paroxetine had efficacy similar to that of clomipramine for 12 weeks in 367 patients with panic disorder (Lecrubier et al. 1997a); 176 patients elected to continue their assigned treatment for an additional 36 weeks (Lecrubier et al. 1997b). Paroxetine was significantly better than placebo and again similar to clomipramine. Fewer patients discontinued therapy because of adverse events in the paroxetine-treated than in the clomipramine-treated group.

In general, patients with panic disorder need a low initial dose of an SSRI (fluoxetine 10 mg, paroxetine 10 mg, sertraline 25 mg) but often require a moderate to high dose for optimal response. This initial low dose serves to reduce early somatic symptoms of anxiety and sets the stage for long-term compliance. The recurrent and chronic nature of panic disorder requires individual medication regimens that may include multiple agents as well as variable dosages.

Eating Disorders

Manipulation of central serotonin results in significantly altered feeding behaviors (e.g., an increased satiety response) (Carruba et al. 1986). Blundell (1986) reported that pharmacological enhancement of serotonin reduced meal size, rate of eating, and body weight. The predominant locus of this serotonin effect is likely within the hypothalamus. In general, an antidepressant's ability to diminish appetite and in turn reduce weight is related to its ability to block serotonin uptake (Angel et al. 1988). One exception may be paroxetine, a highly potent serotonin uptake inhibitor that compared with conventional TCAs was associated in clinical trial experience with a similar proportion of subjects reporting weight gain (Dechant and Clissold 1991). Selective 5-HT_{1A} activation in some patients may influence weight gain (Dourish et al. 1986).

Bulimia nervosa. Serotonin involvement in bulimia nervosa has been based on several observations (Jimerson et al. 1989; Kaye et al. 1988). Kaye and colleagues (1988) hypothesized that variations in the ratio of tryptophan to other amino acids consequent to recurrent bingeing and vomiting mediated both satiety and mood. Some patients with bulimia nervosa, independent of mood status, manifest a blunted prolactin response to m-chlorophenylpiperazine (m-CPP). This has been interpreted as evidence of postsynaptic serotonin hypersensitivity within select hypothalamic pathways (Brewerton et al. 1990).

Goldbloom and colleagues (1988) reported that the V_{max} (V_{max} [maximum velocity] is the maximum amount of substrate per unit of time that an enzyme can break down [or synthesize] at saturation [i.e., when all the enzyme's active sites are filled].) of platelet serotonin uptake was increased among nondepressed bulimic patients. Jimerson and colleagues (1989) observed a significant inverse association between CSF 5-HIAA and symptom severity. However, much of the support for a serotonin role in bulimia nervosa comes from pharmacotherapeutic experience. Agents with at least some degree of serotonin uptake inhibition have been useful in bulimia nervosa (see Brewerton et al. 1990). Clinical trials with fluoxetine (Goldstein et al. 1995) have found a positive treatment effect on binge eating and purging behaviors. In a large placebo-controlled trial, Enas and colleagues (1989) studied dosing of 20 mg versus 60 mg of fluoxetine in 382 female outpatients with bulimia. A clinical benefit was observed in binge frequency, purging, mood, and carbohydrate craving. Based on an open trial by Mitchell and co-workers (1989), therapeutic benefits of the SSRIs may also be apparent among patients previously resistant to TCAs.

Anorexia nervosa. A serotonin disturbance in anorexia nervosa was postulated by Fanelli and colleagues (1986). Coppen and colleagues (1976) reported a reduction in plasma L-tryptophan among patients with anorexia. Others have observed that platelet imipramine binding is decreased (Weizman et al. 1986); however, these findings have not been uniformly replicated. Brewerton and colleagues (1990) suggested that hypothalamic serotonin responsivity at or beyond postsynaptic sites is abnormal in subjects with anorexia nervosa.

Pharmacological trials with SSRIs in patients with anorexia nervosa have been relatively sparse. Kaye and colleagues (1991) suggested that fluoxetine may help maintain body weight in patients with anorexia nervosa who have gained weight. This group also completed a similar study with fluoxetine under controlled conditions with positive results (Kaye et al. 1997). Efficacy of the SSRIs has been linked to the food obsessions of many patients with eating disorders.

Schizophrenia

Evidence of a serotonin role in schizophrenia dates to the 1950s (Woolley and Campbell 1962). The chemical similarities between serotonin and several hallucinogenic ergot alkaloids led to the demonstration that lysergic acid diethylamide (LSD) suppressed the firing rate of serotonin neurons in the raphe nucleus (Aghajanian et al. 1970). Several complex interrelationships between the serotonin and dopamine systems have since been described (Korsgaard et al. 1985).

The pharmacotherapy of schizophrenia with selective serotonin agents includes trials with both agonists and an-

tagonists. However, experience with SSRIs has been relatively limited. Stahl and colleagues (1985) reported that the mixed SSRI/releasing agent fenfluramine reduced negative symptoms in 3 of 12 schizophrenic patients. Several preclinical observations call attention to the possible utility of 5-HT$_2$ and 5-HT$_3$ receptor antagonists. Reduction of negative symptoms, independent of mood or extrapyramidal improvements, was observed during a 7-week placebo-controlled trial with fluvoxamine added to a neuroleptic (Silver and Nassar 1992). Similar therapeutic benefits have been reported during open-label experiences with fluoxetine, in which negative symptoms, aggressive behaviors, mood, or psychosis improved (Goff et al. 1990; Goldman and Janecek 1990).

Miscellaneous

A broad variety of other medical disorders may also benefit from SSRIs. However, several of these potential uses are based on anecdotal or open-label experience and thus require confirmation.

Anger. Diminished serotonergic activity has been implicated in the personality features of impulsivity, anger, hostility, and aggression (Coccaro et al. 1989). These clinical attributes best associate with DSM-IV (American Psychiatric Association 1994) Cluster B personality disorders. Fluoxetine reduced impulsivity in small groups of patients with borderline personality disorder (Cornelius et al. 1991; Norden 1989). Similar results were achieved in an open trial with sertraline (Kavoussi et al. 1994). Fluoxetine significantly reduced anger attacks in depressed and nondepressed patients (Fava et al. 1991, 1993, 1996; Rubey et al. 1996; Salzman et al. 1995).

Posttraumatic stress disorder (PTSD). Fluoxetine significantly reduced symptoms of PTSD compared with placebo in 64 patients (veterans and nonveterans) when measured by the Clinician-Administered PTSD Scale (CAPS) (Van der Kolk et al. 1994). Several other smaller open trials with fluvoxamine and sertraline have also shown positive results (Brady et al. 1995; Marmar et al. 1996).

Premenstrual dysphoric disorder (PMDD). Several randomized, blinded, and placebo-controlled trials utilizing various diagnostic criteria and outcome measures have established the efficacy and tolerability of fluoxetine in the treatment of PMDD (Menkes et al. 1993; Pearlstein et al. 1997; Steiner et al. 1995; Su et al. 1993, 1997; Wood et al. 1992). Positive responses have also been reported in controlled and uncontrolled trials with sertraline (Freeman et al. 1996b; Yonkers et al. 1996b), paroxetine (Eriksson et al 1995; Yonkers et al. 1996a), and fluvoxamine (Freeman et al. 1996a).

In the largest study, 313 women with DSM-III-R (American Psychiatric Association 1987)-defined late luteal phase dysphoric disorder received 20 mg of fluoxetine, 60 mg of fluoxetine, or placebo daily for six menstrual cycles after a two-cycle placebo washout period (Steiner et al. 1995). One hundred eighty women completed the study. Both doses of fluoxetine were superior to placebo beginning at the first menstrual cycle and continuing throughout the six cycles. More patients treated with 60 mg of fluoxetine discontinued because of adverse events than patients treated with 20 mg of fluoxetine or placebo. More patients treated with placebo discontinued because of lack of response than patients treated with either fluoxetine dose. In a subsequent study of 34 women, fluoxetine was significantly superior to bupropion and placebo in treating PMDD (Pearlstein et al. 1997).

Premature ejaculation. SSRIs are emerging as an effective treatment of premature ejaculation. Mendels and colleagues (1995) compared sertraline (50–200 mg/day) with placebo for 8 weeks in 52 men. Ejaculation latency time and number of successful attempts at intercourse were significantly improved in patients treated with sertraline. Similar results occurred with fluoxetine and paroxetine in double-blind, controlled trials (Kara et al. 1996; Waldinger et al. 1997). In a 1-year follow-up study, patients treated with fluoxetine (20 mg/day or less) combined with sexual behavior therapy had significantly improved conditions (Graziottin et al. 1996). Clear-cut dosing recommendations have not been clarified, and titration (up or down) may be necessary.

Pain syndromes. Citalopram, fluoxetine, and paroxetine have showed efficacy in reducing pain associated with diabetic neuropathy (Max et al. 1992; Sindrup et al. 1990, 1992a, 1992b). Fluoxetine (20 mg/day) improved scores on the Fibromyalgia Impact Questionnaire (FIQ) over placebo (Goldenberg et al. 1996). The effect of fluoxetine combined with amitriptyline was superior to either agent used alone. In contrast, in patients with fibromyalgia treated with citalopram (20–40 mg/day for 8 weeks), conditions did not improve (Norregaard et al. 1995). Fluoxetine and fluvoxamine reduced the number of attacks in patients with migraine headaches (Bank 1994; Saper et al. 1994).

Alcoholism. A substantial amount of evidence supports a serotonin dysfunction in alcoholism. Animal stud-

ies have shown that increased serotonin levels reduce alcohol consumption (Farren 1995). For example, Murphy and colleagues (1988) reported beneficial effects with fluoxetine and fluvoxamine in reducing alcohol intake in a rat model.

Some clinical trials with SSRIs have reported reduced alcohol consumption in patients with and without depression in contrast to those treated with TCAs, which have less robust efficacy (Cornelius et al. 1997; Lejoyeux 1996). A precise explanation for the role of SSRIs in the treatment of alcohol dependence is not understood. To date, the beneficial effect appears to be independent of antidepressant activity (Naranjo et al. 1986, 1990). More work is needed to determine the specific patient subpopulations that benefit most from the SSRIs (Gorelick 1989).

From a risk-benefit assessment, it is reassuring that SSRIs do not appear to potentiate the effects of ethanol (Lemberger et al. 1985). SSRIs may help selected patients with alcohol dependence in recovery when these drugs are used as part of a multifaceted treatment program.

Obesity. SSRIs have been extensively investigated for an effect on food consumption. This interest stems from evidence that perturbation of serotonin receptors modifies animal feeding behavior (Garattini et al. 1986). This modification appears independent of a local gastrointestinal effect (e.g., the perception of nausea). Serotonin innervation to the hypothalamus influences satiety and may selectively affect carbohydrate consumption (Wurtman et al. 1981). Fluoxetine, fluvoxamine, and sertraline have been evaluated for use in the treatment of obesity (Abell et al. 1986; Darga et al. 1991; Ricca et al. 1996). In the largest trial to date, 458 patients were treated for 52 weeks with fluoxetine (60 mg/day) or placebo (Goldstein et al. 1994). Weight loss was significantly greater in the fluoxetine-treated group at 28 weeks but not at 52 weeks. Long-term benefits may be better sustained when combining fluoxetine with behavior modification (Marcus et al. 1990).

The broad involvement of serotonin systems in modulating behavior and cognition supports the wide potential utility of the SSRIs.

SIDE EFFECTS AND TOXICOLOGY

Safety and a favorable side-effect profile, as well as lack of multiple receptor affinity that mediates adverse events associated with TCAs, distinguish SSRIs from TCAs. SSRIs as a class have a similar side-effect profile.

For most patients, SSRIs are better tolerated, based

on the number of early trial discontinuations attributable to an adverse event, than TCAs (see Boyer and Feighner 1991). In general, for three-arm trials, a 5%–10% incidence of early discontinuations because of an adverse event occurred for the placebo group, 10%–20% for the SSRI group, and 30%–35% for the TCA group. The SSRIs, presumably by enhancement of serotonin within the CNS, may induce agitation, anxiety, sleep disturbance, tremor, sexual dysfunction (primarily anorgasmia), or headache. Baseline clinical features do not appear to predispose to these adverse events (Montgomery 1989b). Although CNS adverse events may occur with the SSRIs, Kerr and colleagues (1991) suggested that these drugs have a more favorable profile of behavioral toxicity overall than do the conventional TCAs.

Because the enteric nervous system is richly innervated by serotonin, adverse events may include altered gastrointestinal motility and nausea. Certain autonomic adverse events, including dry mouth, sweating, and weight change, also occur.

As was discussed earlier in this chapter, SSRIs are unlikely to alter dopamine function. Anecdotal reports of EPS (Meltzer et al. 1979) associated with the SSRIs are not more frequent than has been reported historically with TCAs (Fann et al. 1976; Zubenko et al. 1987), MAOIs (Teusink et al. 1984), or trazodone (Papini et al. 1982). Very rare events, including arthralgia, lymphadenopathy, inappropriate antidiuretic syndrome, agranulocytosis, and hypoglycemia, have been reported during clinical trials or postmarketing surveillance; however, causality typically is uncertain.

One additional rare and life-threatening idiosyncratic event associated with the SSRIs (and, more prominently, their interaction with MAOIs or other serotonin enhancers) is the central serotonin syndrome. This phenomenon appears to represent an overactivation of central serotonin receptors and may manifest with features such as abdominal pain, diarrhea, sweating, fever, tachycardia, elevated blood pressure, altered mental state (e.g., delirium), myoclonus, increased motor activity, irritability, hostility, and mood change. Severe manifestations of this syndrome can induce hyperpyrexia, cardiovascular shock, or death. Realistically, data are inadequate to rate one MAOI or SSRI as more or less likely to be associated with serotonin syndrome. The risk of serotonin syndrome seems to be increased when an SSRI is administered temporally with a second serotonin-enhancing agent (e.g., an MAOI) (Marley and Wozniak 1984a, 1984b). When following an SSRI with an MAOI, drug half-life (and that of any active metabolite, where applicable) should serve as a guide to the length of the washout period. A standard recommendation would be to wait at least five times the half-life of the SSRI or its metabolite, whichever is longer, before administering the next serotonergic agent. (For a review, see Lane and Baldwin 1997.)

Although some variability in adverse event frequency has been reported among the SSRIs, all are characterized by the above-mentioned features. Tolerance to an adverse event may change with dose and/or length of exposure; higher doses are typically associated with higher rates of adverse events (Bressa et al. 1989). Many events such as activation are transient, usually beginning early in the course of therapy and then remitting (Beasley et al. 1991). Comparisons between A.M. and P.M. administration did not identify differences in efficacy (Usher et al. 1991); however, the P.M. dosing was associated with fewer intolerable side effects in a fluvoxamine trial (Siddiqui et al. 1985). Individual patient differences suggest the need for some flexibility in dosing schedules.

TCAs behave like type IA antiarrhythmics and, thus, in a dose-dependent fashion may retard His-Purkinje conduction. SSRIs are essentially devoid of this property. In clinical trials, the incidence of increased heart rate or conduction disturbance has been very uncommon across several of the SSRIs (Edwards et al. 1989; Fisch 1985; S. Guy and Silke 1990). However, very high doses of citalopram reportedly mimicked TCA-like cardiovascular effects only in a specific animal model (Boeck et al. 1984). SSRIs are not associated with α-adrenergic antagonism and thus rarely have been associated with orthostatic hypotension. The above-mentioned properties of the SSRIs translate into a wider safety profile than that of TCAs.

Sleep

Fluoxetine decreases rapid eye movement (REM) and increases nonrapid eye movement (NREM) sleep at dose ranges of 5–40 mg/kg in rodent models (Gao et al. 1992). Citalopram (Hilakivi et al. 1987) and fluvoxamine (Scherschlict et al. 1982) also shorten REM sleep in laboratory animal models. This is a common property of many antidepressant medications. Interestingly, both fluoxetine and sertraline induce higher rates of sedation as dosages are increased. In contrast, paroxetine causes a dose-dependent increase in arousal, wakening, reduced slow-wave sleep, and REM suppression (Kleinlogel and Burki 1987).

Suicidality

Evidence implicating serotonin in suicide or violence is compelling. Reduced CSF 5-HIAA concentrations correlate highly with completed suicides in depressed patients

(Edman et al. 1986; Ninan et al. 1984). In vitro binding assays have shown an increased density (B_{max}) of 5-HT$_2$ receptors in depressed and suicidal individuals (Pandey et al. 1990). Both observations are consistent with a relative state of serotonin depletion among suicidal subjects. The American College of Neuropsychopharmacology (1992) reviewed evidence that antidepressants result in substantial improvement or remission of suicidal ideation and impulses in the vast majority of patients. SSRIs were thought to potentially "carry a lower risk for suicide than older tricyclic antidepressants" (p. 181) when taken in overdose. Furthermore, this task force stated that no evidence indicated that SSRIs triggered emergent suicidal ideation above base rates associated with depression. Also, Warshaw and Keller (1996) determined that fluoxetine use did not increase the rate of suicide in a group of 654 patients with anxiety disorders. In a large retrospective review of patients receiving one or more of 10 antidepressants (including fluoxetine), Jick and colleagues (1995) concluded that the risk for suicide was similar among all agents.

Pregnancy and Lactation

Given the widespread use of SSRIs and the high prevalence of mood disorders during the childbearing years, these agents probably will be used during pregnancy and breast-feeding. Except for fluoxetine, published information about the use and safety of SSRIs in this special population is very limited. Goldstein and colleagues (1997) evaluated the outcomes of 796 prospectively identified pregnancies with confirmed first-trimester exposure to fluoxetine. Historic reports of newborn surveys were used for comparison. Abnormalities were observed in 5% of the fluoxetine-exposed newborns, which was consistent with historic controls.

Pregnancy outcomes and follow-up cognitive and behavioral assessments of 135 children exposed in utero to a TCA or fluoxetine (55 infants) were compared with a control group of infant-mother pairs (Nulman et al. 1997). The incidence of major malformations and perinatal complications was similar among the three groups. No statistically significant differences in mean global intelligence quotient (IQ) scores or language development were found in the children of mothers who received a TCA or fluoxetine or were in the control group. There were also no differences among the groups on several behavioral assessments. The results of children exposed during the first trimester were not different from those of children exposed throughout the pregnancy. Prospectively derived data are not available for paroxetine, sertraline, fluvoxamine, or citalopram.

Fluoxetine is secreted into breast milk. One naturalistic study (Taddio et al. 1996) and two case reports (Burch and Wells 1992; Isenberg 1990) with a total of 13 infants noted no adverse effects in these infants during the short-term study periods. One case report described adverse events in a breast-fed infant whose mother was taking fluoxetine (Lester et al. 1993). In addition, two cases reported no adverse effects and plasma levels that were very low or nondetectable (<2 ng/mL) in 4 breast-fed infants whose mothers were taking sertraline (Altshuler et al. 1995; Mammen et al. 1997).

SSRI Discontinuation Syndrome

Discontinuation symptoms have been described with several antidepressants, including TCAs and MAOIs. SSRI discontinuation symptoms have been reported most frequently with paroxetine (short elimination half-life and no active metabolite) and least frequently with fluoxetine (long elimination half-lives of parent and active metabolite). SSRIs are not drugs of abuse; when these agents are discontinued, patients show neither the characteristic abstinence syndrome of CNS-depressant withdrawal nor drug-seeking behavior. The most common physical symptoms are dizziness, nausea and vomiting, fatigue, lethargy, flulike symptoms (aches and chills), and sensory and sleep disturbances. Psychological symptoms most commonly reported are anxiety, irritability, and crying spells. For most patients, the discontinuation symptoms are different from the adverse effects they may have had while taking an SSRI. Discontinuation symptoms most often emerge within 1–3 days (Schatzberg et al. 1997).

Until recently, most information about the SSRI discontinuation syndrome came from case reports or retrospective analyses. Blomgren and colleagues (1997) compared the effects of a 5- to 8-day abrupt discontinuation period from fluoxetine, paroxetine, or sertraline in three groups of depressed patients receiving maintenance therapy. Patients from the paroxetine and sertraline groups had a significant increase in adverse events, whereas patients in the fluoxetine group had no increase in adverse events.

The effects of a more extended evaluation after abrupt discontinuation of fluoxetine were studied in 195 depressed patients (Michelson et al. 1997a). Patients whose depression remitted on fluoxetine were randomized to continue fluoxetine (20 mg/day) or to discontinue abruptly to placebo and were monitored for 6 weeks. Reports of adverse events were similar for both groups.

SSRIs with short half-lives (paroxetine and fluvoxamine) and related drugs such as venlafaxine should be tapered. Fluoxetine does not require tapering because of its extended half-life.

Drug Overdosage

A major advantage of SSRIs relative to other antidepressants has been their superior therapeutic index (Cooper 1988; Pedersen et al. 1982). The number of deaths per 1 million prescriptions across several SSRIs (0–6) is substantially lower than that of the conventional TCAs (8–53) or the MAOIs (0–61) (Leonard 1992).

Borys and colleagues (1992) reported on 234 cases of fluoxetine overdose (232–1,390 ng/mL) obtained in a prospective multicenter study. Fluoxetine was the sole ingestant in 87 cases and was taken in combination with alcohol and/or other drugs in the remaining 147 cases. Common symptoms included tachycardia, sedation, tremor, nausea, and emesis. These authors concluded that the emergent symptoms were minor and of short duration; thus, aggressive supportive care "is the only intervention necessary" (p. 115).

The SSRIs currently represent an important addition to the therapeutic armamentarium for the depressed patient at risk for a drug overdose.

DRUG-DRUG INTERACTIONS

Although the potential for significant interactions exists, SSRIs are unlikely to be associated with many of the conventional problems seen with the earlier antidepressants. These problems include cumulative CNS-depressant effects with alcohol, anticholinergic agents, or antihistaminic compounds. The structural differences (see Figure 11–2) among the SSRIs offer a basis for some intraclass differences. Paroxetine and fluvoxamine have been associated with increased bleeding time when given with warfarin. Lithium concentrations are generally unaffected.

One potential for clinically relevant antidepressant pharmacokinetic interactions is based on drug effect on the cytochrome P450 (CYP) family of isoenzymes (Brosen and Gram 1989). For example, SSRIs are both substrates and inhibitors for oxidation via CYP2D6. Crewe and colleagues (1992) ranked the potency of CYP2D6 inhibition for serotonin antidepressants from most potent to least: paroxetine, fluoxetine, sertraline, fluvoxamine, citalopram, clomipramine, and amitriptyline.

By inhibition of CYP2D6, the SSRIs may elevate the concentration of concomitantly administered drugs that rely on this isoenzyme for metabolism. This has particular clinical relevance when the second agent has a narrow therapeutic index. Examples of such agents include flecainide, quinidine, carbamazepine, propafenone, TCAs, and several antipsychotics (Rudorfer and Potter 1989). The clinical consequence of such an interaction may either enhance or impair efficacy and/or heighten the adverse-event profile.

SSRIs vary in their effect on the other cytochromes including 1A2, 3A3/4, 2C9, and 2C19. (See DeVane, Chapter 8, in this volume for more details.)

CONCLUSION

The SSRIs have been shown to be a safe and effective drug class. They are frequently better tolerated than conventional TCAs and have a superior safety profile in overdosage for patients with comorbid medical illness. Preliminary evidence suggests a broad utilitarian role for SSRIs across a spectrum of psychopathology. As experience with these compounds broadens, continued advances in scientific knowledge about the serotonin system and its role with human pathophysiology can be expected.

REFERENCES

Abell CA, Farquhar DL, Galloway SM, et al: Placebo-controlled double-blind trial of fluvoxamine maleate in the obese. J Psychosom Res 30:143–146, 1986

Aghajanian JK, Foote WE, Sheard MH: Action of psychotogenic drugs on midbrain raphe neurons. J Pharmacol Exp Ther 171:178–187, 1970

Aghajanian JK, Sprouse JS, Rasmussen K: Electrophysiology of central serotonin receptor subtypes, in The Serotonin Receptors. Edited by Sanders-Bush E. Clifton, NJ, Humana Press, 1988, pp 225–252

Altamura AC, Montgomery SA, Wernicke JF: The evidence for 20 mg a day of fluoxetine as the optimal dose in the treatment of depression. Br J Psychiatry 153:109–112, 1988

Altshuler LL, Burt VK, McMullen M, et al: Breastfeeding and sertraline: a 24-hour analysis. J Clin Psychiatry 56:243–245, 1995

American College of Neuropsychopharmacology: Suicidal behavior and psychotropic medication (consensus statement). Neuropsychopharmacology 8:177–183, 1992

American Psychiatric Association: Diagnostic and Statistical Manual of Mental Disorders, 3rd Edition, Revised. Washington, DC, American Psychiatric Association, 1987

American Psychiatric Association: Diagnostic and Statistical Manual of Mental Disorders, 4th Edition. Washington, DC, American Psychiatric Association, 1994

Amin AH, Crawford TBB, Gaddum JH: The distribution of substance P and 5-hydroxytryptamine in the central nervous system of the dog. J Physiol (Lond) 126:596–618, 1954

Amin M, Lehmann H, Mirmiran J: A double-blind, placebo-controlled, dose-finding study with sertraline. Psychopharmacol Bull 25:164–167, 1989

Angel I, Taranger MA, Claustrey Y, et al: Anorectic activities of serotonin uptake inhibitors: correlation with their potencies at inhibiting serotonin uptake in vivo and with ^{3}H-mazindol binding in vitro. Life Sci 43:651–658, 1988

Arnt J, Hyttel J, Overo FK: Prolonged treatment with the specific 5-HT uptake inhibitor citalopram: effect on dopaminergic and serotonergic functions. Pol J Pharmacol Pharm 36:221–230, 1984a

Arnt J, Overo KF, Hyttel J, et al: Changes in rat dopamine and serotonin function in vivo after prolonged administration of the specific 5-HT uptake inhibitor citalopram. Psychopharmacology (Berl) 84:457–465, 1984b

Asakura M, Tsukamoto T, Kubota H, et al: Role of serotonin in regulation of β-adrenoceptors by antidepressants. Eur J Pharmacol 141:95–100, 1987

Backus LI, Sharp T, Grahame-Smith DJ: Behavioral evidence for a functional interaction between central 5-HT$_2$ and 5-HT$_{1A}$ receptors. Journal of Pharmacology 100:793–799, 1990

Baldessarini RJ, Marsh ER, Kula NS: Interactions of fluoxetine with metabolism of dopamine and serotonin in rat brain regions. Brain Res 579:152–156, 1992

Bank J: A comparative study of amitriptyline and fluvoxamine in migraine prophylaxis. Headache 34:476–478, 1994

Baron BM, Ogden AM, Siegel BW, et al: Rapid down-regulation of β-adrenoceptors by co-administration of desipramine and fluoxetine. Eur J Pharmacol 154:125–134, 1988

Baxter LR, Schwartz JM, Bergman KS, et al: Caudate glucose metabolic rate changes with both drug and behavior therapy for obsessive-compulsive disorder. Arch Gen Psychiatry 49:681–689, 1992

Beasley CM, Sayler ME, Bosomworth JC, et al: High-dose fluoxetine: efficacy and activating-sedating effects in agitated and retarded depression. J Clin Psychopharmacol 11:166–174, 1991

Benkelfat C, Murphy DL, Zohar J, et al: Clomipramine in obsessive-compulsive disorder: further evidence for a serotonergic mechanism of action. Arch Gen Psychiatry 46:23–28, 1989

Benloucif S, Galloway MP: Facilitation of dopamine release in vivo by serotonin agonists: studied with microdialysis. Eur J Pharmacol 200:1–8, 1991

Bergstrom DA, Kellar JK: Adrenergic and serotonergic receptor binding in rat brain after chronic desmethyl imipramine treatment. J Pharmacol Exp Ther 209:256–261, 1979

Bick PA, Hackett E: Sertraline is effective in obsessive-compulsive disorder, in Psychiatry Today: VIII World Congress of Psychiatry Abstracts. Edited by Stefanis CN, Soldatos CR, Rabavilas AD. New York, Elsevier, 1989, p 152

Blier P, deMontigny C, Chaput Y: Modifications of the serotonin system by antidepressant treatments: implications for the therapeutic response in major depression. J Clin Psychopharmacol 7:24S–35S, 1987

Blier P, Chaput Y, deMontigny C: Long-term 5-HT reuptake blockade, but not monoamine oxidase inhibition, decreases the function of terminal 5-HT autoreceptors; an electrophysiological study in the rat brain. Naunyn Schmiedebergs Arch Pharmacol 337:246–254, 1988

Blier P, deMontigny C, Chaput Y: A role for the serotonin system in the mechanism of action of antidepressants. J Clin Psychiatry 51 (suppl 4):14–20, 1990

Blomgren SL, Krebs W, Wilson M, et al: SSRI dose interruption study: interim data. American Psychiatric Association 1997 Annual Meeting New Research Program and Abstracts (NR188). Washington, DC, American Psychiatric Association, 1997, p 118

Blundell JE: Serotonin manipulations and the structure of feeding behaviour. Appetite 7 (suppl):39–56, 1986

Boeck V, Jorgensen A, Overo KF: Comparative animal studies on cardiovascular toxicity of tri- and tetracyclic antidepressants and citalopram; relation to drug plasma levels. Psychopharmacology (Berl) 82:275–281, 1984

Borys DJ, Setzer SC, Ling LJ, et al: Acute fluoxetine overdose: a report of 234 cases. Am J Emerg Med 10:115–120, 1992

Bouchard RH, Pourcher E, Vincent P: Fluoxetine and extrapyramidal side effects. Am J Psychiatry 146:1352–1353, 1989

Boyer WF, Feighner JP: The efficacy of selective serotonin uptake inhibitors in depression, in Selective Serotonin Uptake Inhibitors. Edited by Feighner JP, Boyer WF. Chichester, England, Wiley, 1991, pp 89–108

Bradley PB: Introduction to Neuropharmacology. Boston, MA, Wright, 1989

Brady KT, Sonne SC, Roberts JM: Sertraline treatment of comorbid posttraumatic stress disorder and alcohol dependence. J Clin Psychiatry 56:502–505, 1995

Bressa GM, Brugnoli R, Pancheri P: A double-blind study of fluoxetine and imipramine in major depression. Int Clin Psychopharmacol 4 (suppl 1):69–73, 1989

Brewerton TD, Brandt HA, Lessem MD, et al: Serotonin in eating disorders, in Serotonin in Major Psychiatric Disorders. Edited by Coccaro EF, Murphy DL. Washington, DC, American Psychiatric Press, 1990, pp 153–184

Brosen K, Gram LF: Clinical significance of the sparteine/debrisoquine oxidation polymorphism. Eur J Clin Pharmacol 36:537–547, 1989

Burch KJ, Wells BG: Fluoxetine/norfluoxetine concentrations in human milk. Pediatrics 89:676–677, 1992

Carruba MO, Mantegazza P, Memo M, et al: Peripheral and central mechanisms of action of serotoninergic anorectic drugs. Appetite 7 (suppl):105–113, 1986

Chaput Y, deMontigny C, Blier P: Effects of a selective 5-HT reuptake blocker citalopram on the sensitivity of 5-HT autoreceptors, electrophysiological studies in the rat. Naunyn Schmiedebergs Arch Pharmacol 333:342–348, 1986

Charbannes JP, Douge R: Efficacy on anxiety of fluvoxamine versus prazepam, diazepam with anxiodepressed patients, in Psychiatry Today: VIII World Congress of Psychiatry Abstracts. Edited by Stefanis CN, Soldatos CR, Rabavilas AD. New York, Elsevier, 1989, p 282

Charney DS, Menkes DB, Heninger GR: Receptor sensitivity and the mechanism of action of antidepressant treatment. Arch Gen Psychiatry 38:1160–1180, 1981

Charney DS, Heninger GR, Sternberg DE: Serotonin function and mechanism of action of antidepressant treatment. Arch Gen Psychiatry 41:359–365, 1984

Ciraulo DA, Shader RI: Fluoxetine drug-drug interactions, I: antidepressants and antipsychotics. J Clin Psychopharmacol 10:48–50, 1990

Claassen V: Review of the animal pharmacology and pharmacokinetics of fluvoxamine. Br J Clin Pharmacol 15:349S–355S, 1983

Coccaro EF, Siever LJ, Klar HM, et al: Serotonergic studies in patients with affective and personality disorders: correlated with suicidal and impulsive aggressive behavior. Arch Gen Psychiatry 46:587–599, 1989

Cooper GL: The safety of fluoxetine—an update. Br J Psychiatry 153:77–86, 1988

Coppen AJ, Gupta RK, Eccleston EG, et al: Plasma tryptophan in anorexia nervosa (letter). Lancet 1:961, 1976

Cornelius JR, Soloff PH, Perel JM, et al: A preliminary trial of fluoxetine in refractory borderline patients. J Clin Psychopharmacol 11:116–120, 1991

Cornelius JR, Salloum IM, Ehler JG, et al: Fluoxetine in depressed alcoholics: a double-blind, placebo-controlled trial. Arch Gen Psychiatry 54:700–705, 1997

Cowen PJ: Serotonin receptor subtypes: implications for psychopharmacology. Br J Psychiatry 159 (suppl 12):7–14, 1991

Crewe HK, Lennard MS, Tucker GT, et al: The effect of selective serotonin reuptake inhibitors on the cytochrome P450IID6 activity in human liver microsomes. Br J Clin Pharmacol 34:262–265, 1992

Danion JM: The effectiveness of fluoxetine in acute studies and long-term treatment, in Psychiatry Today: VIII World Congress of Psychiatry Abstracts. Edited by Stefanis CN, Soldatos CR, Rabavilas AD. New York, Elsevier, 1989, p 334

Darga LL, Carroll-Michals L, Botsford SJ, et al: Fluoxetine's effect on weight loss in obese subjects. Am J Clin Nutr 54:321–325, 1991

Dechant KL, Clissold SP: Paroxetine. Drugs 41:225–253, 1991

Delgado PL, Price LH, Charney DS, et al: Efficacy of fluvoxamine in treatment-refractory depression. J Affect Disord 15:55–60, 1988

deMontigny C, Chaput Y, Blier P: Long-term tricyclic and electroconvulsive treatment increases responsiveness of dorsal hippocampus 5-HT$_{1A}$ receptors: an electrophysiological study. Society for Neuroscience Abstracts 15:854, 1989

De-Wilde JE, Doogan DP: Fluvoxamine and clomipramine in endogenous depression. J Affect Disord 4:249–259, 1982

Doogan DP, Caillard V: Sertraline: a new antidepressant. J Clin Psychiatry 49 (suppl):46–51, 1988

Dourish CT, Hutson PH, Kennett GA, et al: 8-OH-DPAT-induced hyperphagia: its neural basis and possible therapeutic relevance. Appetite 7 (suppl):127–140, 1986

Dresse A, Scuvee-Moreau J: The effects of various antidepressants on the spontaneous firing rates of noradrenergic and serotonergic neurons. Clin Neuropharmacol 7 (suppl 1):572–573, 1984

Dufour H: Fluoxetine: long-term treatment and prophylaxis in depression. Paper presented at the International Fluoxetine Symposium, Tyrol, Austria, October 13–17, 1987

Edman G, Asberg M, Levander S, et al: Skin conductance habituation and cerebrospinal fluid 5-hydroxyindoleacetic acid in suicidal patients. Arch Gen Psychiatry 43:586–592, 1986

Edwards JG, Goldie A, Papayanni-Papasthatis S: Effect of paroxetine on the electrocardiogram. Psychopharmacology (Berl) 97:96–98, 1989

Elks ML, Youngblood WW, Kizer JS: Serotonin synthesis and release in brain slices, independence of tryptophan. Brain Res 172:471–486, 1979

Enas GG, Pope HJ, Levine LR: Fluoxetine and bulimia nervosa: double-blind study. American Psychiatric Association 1989 Annual Meeting New Research Program and Abstracts. Washington, DC, American Psychiatric Association, 1989, p 204

Eriksson E, Hedberg MA, Andersch B, et al: The serotonin reuptake inhibitor paroxetine is superior to the noradrenaline reuptake inhibitor maprotiline in the treatment of premenstrual syndrome. Neuropsychopharmacology 12:167–176, 1995

Falck B, Hillarp N-A, Thieme G, et al: Fluorescence of catecholamines and related compounds condensed with formaldehyde. J Histochem Cytochem 10:348–354, 1962

Fanelli FR, Cangiano C, Cecil F, et al: Plasma tryptophan and anorexia in human cancer. Eur J Cancer Clin Oncol 22:89–95, 1986

Fann WE, Sullivan JL, Richman BW: Dyskinesia's associated with tricyclic antidepressants. Br J Psychiatry 128:490–493, 1976

Farren CK: Serotonin and alcoholism: clinical and experimental research. Journal of Serotonin Research 2:9–26, 1995

Fava M, Rosenbaum JF, McCarthy M, et al: Anger attacks in depressed outpatients and their response to fluoxetine. Psychopharmacol Bull 27:275–280, 1991

Fava M, Rosenbaum JF, Cohen L, et al: High dose fluoxetine in the treatment of depressed patients not responsive to a standard dose of fluoxetine. J Affect Disord 25:229–234, 1992

Fava M, Rosenbaum JF, Pava JA, et al: Anger attacks in unipolar depression, part 1: clinical correlates and response to fluoxetine treatment. Am J Psychiatry 150:1158–1163, 1993

Fava M, Alpert J, Nierenberg AA, et al: Fluoxetine treatment of anger attacks: a replication study. Ann Clin Psychiatry 8:7–10, 1996

Feighner JP, Boyer WF, Meredith CH, et al: A placebo-controlled inpatient comparison of fluvoxamine maleate and imipramine in major depression. Int Clin Psychopharmacol 4:239–244, 1989

Feldmann HS, Dunbar HC: Long-term study of fluvoxamine: a new rapid-acting antidepressant. International Pharmacopsychiatry 17:114–122, 1982

Ferrey G, Gailledrau J, Beuzen JN: The interest of fluoxetine in prevention of depressive recurrences, in Psychiatry Today: VIII World Congress of Psychiatry Abstracts. Edited by Stefanis CN, Soldatos CR, Rabavilas AD. New York, Elsevier, 1989, p 99

Fisch C: Effect of fluoxetine on the electrocardiogram. J Clin Psychiatry 46:42–44, 1985

Flament MF, Rapoport JL, Berg CJ, et al: Clomipramine treatment of childhood obsessive-compulsive disorder: a double-blind, controlled study. Arch Gen Psychiatry 42:977–983, 1985

Fraser A, Offord SJ, Lucki I: Regulation of serotonin receptors and responsiveness in the brain, in The Serotonin Receptors. Edited by Sanders-Bush E. Clifton, NJ, Humana Press, 1988, pp 319–362

Freeman EW, Rickels K, Sondheimer SJ: Fluvoxamine for premenstrual dysphoric disorder: a pilot study. J Clin Psychiatry 57 (suppl 8):56–59, 1996a

Freeman EW, Rickels K, Sondheimer SJ, et al: Sertraline versus desipramine in the treatment of premenstrual syndrome: an open-label trial. J Clin Psychiatry 57:7–11, 1996b

Fuller RW: Drugs altering serotonin synthesis and metabolism, in Neuropharmacology of Serotonin. Edited by Green AR. New York, Oxford University Press, 1985, pp 1–20

Fuller RW: Mechanisms and functions of serotonin neuronal systems: opportunities for neuropeptide interactions. Ann N Y Acad Sci 780:176–184, 1996

Gao B, Duncan WC Jr, Wehr ATA: Fluoxetine decreases brain temperature and REM sleep in Syrian hamsters. Psychopharmacology (Berl) 106:321–329, 1992

Garattini S, Mennini T, Bendotti C, et al: Neurochemical mechanism of action of drugs which modify feeding via the serotonergic system. Appetite 7 (suppl):15–38, 1986

Goff DC, Brotman AW, Waites M, et al: Trial of fluoxetine added to neuroleptics for treatment-resistant schizophrenic patients. Am J Psychiatry 147:492–494, 1990

Goldbloom DS, Hicks LK, Garfinkel PE: Platelet serotonin uptake in bulimia nervosa. American Psychiatric Association 1988 Annual Meeting New Research Program and Abstracts. Washington, DC, American Psychiatric Association, 1988, p 137

Goldenberg D, Mayskiy M, Mossey C, et al: A randomized, double-blind crossover trial of fluoxetine and amitriptyline in the treatment of fibromyalgia. Arthritis Rheum 39:1852–1859, 1996

Goldman MB, Janecek HM: Adjunctive fluoxetine improves global function in chronic schizophrenia. J Neuropsychiatry Clin Neurosci 2:429–431, 1990

Goldstein DJ, Rampey AH, Enas GG, et al: Fluoxetine: a randomized clinical trial in the treatment of obesity. Int J Obes 18:129–135, 1994

Goldstein DJ, Wilson MG, Thompson VL, et al: Long-term fluoxetine treatment of bulimia nervosa. Br J Psychiatry 166:660–666, 1995

Goldstein DJ, Corbin LA, Sundell KL: Effects of first-trimester fluoxetine exposure on the newborn. Obstet General 89 (5 pt 1):713–718, 1997

Goodman WK, Price LH, Rasmussen SA, et al: Efficacy of fluvoxamine in obsessive-compulsive disorder: a double-blind comparison with placebo. Arch Gen Psychiatry 46:36–44, 1989

Goodman WK, McDougle CJ, Price LH: Pharmacotherapy of obsessive-compulsive disorder. J Clin Psychiatry 53 (suppl 4):29–37, 1992

Gorelick DA: Serotonin uptake blockers and the treatment of alcoholism. Recent Dev Alcohol 7:267–281, 1989

Graziottin A, Montorsi F, Guazzoni G, et al: Combined fluoxetine and sexual behavioral therapy for premature ejaculation: one-year follow-up analysis of results, complications and success predictors (abstract). J Urol 155 (5 suppl):497A, 1996

Guelfi JD, Dreyfus JF, Pichot P: Fluvoxamine and imipramine: results of a long-term controlled trial. Int Clin Psychopharmacol 2:103–109, 1987

Guy S, Silke B: The electrocardiogram as a tool for therapeutic monitoring: a critical analysis. J Clin Psychiatry 51 (12, suppl B):37–39, 1990

Guy W, Manov G, Wilson WH: Double-blind dose determination study of a new antidepressant—sertraline. Drug Development Research 9:267–272, 1986

Haddock RE, Johnson AM, Langley PE, et al: Metabolic pathway of paroxetine in animals and man and the comparative pharmacological properties of its metabolites. Acta Psychiatr Scand 80 (suppl 350):24–26, 1989

Hall H, Ogren SO: Effects of antidepressant drugs on different receptors in rat brain. Eur J Pharmacol 70:393–407, 1981

Hamilton M: A rating scale for depression. J Neurol Neurosurg Psychiatry 23:56–62, 1960

Hebenstreit GF, Fellerer K, Zoechling R, et al: A pharmacokinetic dose titration study in adult and elderly depressed patients. Acta Psychiatr Scand 80:81–84, 1989

Heym J, Koe BK: Pharmacology of sertraline: a review. J Clin Psychiatry 49 (suppl):40–45, 1988

Hilakivi I, Kovala T, Leppavuori A, et al: Effects of serotonin and noradrenaline uptake blockers on wakefulness and sleep in cats. Pharmacol Toxicol 60:161–166, 1987

Hyttel J: Citalopram—pharmacological profile of a specific serotonin uptake inhibitor with antidepressant activity. Prog Neuropsychopharmacol Biol Psychiatry 6:277–295, 1982

Isenberg KE: Excretion of fluoxetine in human breast milk (letter). J Clin Psychiatry 51:169, 1990

Jenike MA, Baer L, Greist JH: Clomipramine versus fluoxetine in obsessive-compulsive disorder: a retrospective comparison of side effects and efficacy. J Clin Psychopharmacol 10:122–124, 1989a

Jenike MA, Buttolph L, Baer L, et al: Open trial of fluoxetine in obsessive-compulsive disorder. Am J Psychiatry 146:909–911, 1989b

Jick SS, Dean AD, Jick H: Antidepressants and suicide. BMJ 310:215–218, 1995

Jimerson DC, Lesem MD, Kaye WH, et al: Serotonin and symptom severity in eating disorders (abstract). Biol Psychiatry 25 (suppl 7A):141A, 1989

Johnson AM: The comparative pharmacological properties of selective serotonin re-uptake inhibitors in animals, in Selective Serotonin Uptake Inhibitors. Edited by Feighner JP, Boyer WF. Chichester, England, Wiley, 1991, pp 37–70

Jouvent R, Baruch P, Ammar S, et al: Fluoxetine efficacy in depressives with impulsivity vs blunted affect, in Psychiatry Today: VIII World Congress of Psychiatry Abstracts. Edited by Stefanis CN, Soldatos CR, Rabavilas AD. New York, Elsevier, 1989, p 398

Kara H, Aydin S, Agargun MY, et al: The efficacy of fluoxetine in the treatment of premature ejaculation: a double-blind placebo controlled study. J Urol 156:1631–1632, 1996

Kasper S, Fuger J, Moller H-J: Comparative efficacy of antidepressants. Drugs 43 (suppl 2):11–23, 1992

Kavoussi RJ, Liu J, Cocarro EF: An open trial of sertraline in personality disordered patients with impulsive aggression. J Clin Psychiatry 55:137–141, 1994

Kaye WH, Gwirtsman HE, Brewerton TD, et al: Bingeing behavior and plasma amino acids: a possible involvement of brain serotonin in bulimia nervosa. Psychiatry Res 23:31–43, 1988

Kaye WH, Weltzin TE, Hsu LK, et al: An open trial of fluoxetine in patients with anorexia nervosa. J Clin Psychiatry 52:464–471, 1991

Kaye WH, Weltzin TE, Hsu LK, et al: Relapse prevention with fluoxetine in anorexia nervosa: a double-blind placebo-controlled study. American Psychiatric Association 1997 Annual Meeting New Research Program and Abstracts (NR405). Washington, DC, American Psychiatric Association, 1997, p 178

Kelly MW, Perry J, Holstad SG, et al: Serum fluoxetine and norfluoxetine concentrations and antidepressant response. Ther Drug Monit 11:165–170, 1989

Kerr JS, Sherwood N, Hindmarch I: The comparative psychopharmacology of 5-HT reuptake inhibitors. Human Psychopharmacology 6:313–317, 1991

Kleinlogel H, Burki HR: Effects of the selective 5-hydroxytryptamine uptake inhibitors, paroxetine and zimeldine, on EEG sleep and waking changes in the rat. Neuropsychobiology 17:206–212, 1987

Klimek V, Maj J: Repeated administration of antidepressant drugs enhanced agonist affinity for mesolimbic D-2 receptors. J Pharm Pharmacol 41:555–558, 1990

Klimek V, Nielsen M: Chronic treatment with antidepressants decreases the number of [^{3}H]-SCH 23390 binding sites in rat striatum and limbic system. Eur J Pharmacol 139:163–169, 1987

Koe BK, Koch SW, Lebel LA, et al: Sertraline, a selective inhibitor of serotonin uptake, induces subsensitivity of β-adrenoceptor of rat brain. Eur J Pharmacol 141:187–194, 1987

Korsgaard S, Gerlach J, Christensson E: Behavioral aspects of serotonin-dopamine interaction in the monkey. Eur J Pharmacol 118:245–252, 1985

Lane R, Baldwin D: Selective serotonin reuptake inhibitor-induced serotonin syndrome: review. J Clin Psychopharmacol 17:208–221, 1997

Laws D, Ashford JJ, Anstee JA: A multicentre double-blind comparative trial of fluvoxamine versus lorazepam in mixed anxiety and depression treated in general practice. Acta Psychiatr Scand 81:185–189, 1990

Lecrubier Y, Bakker A, Dunbar G, et al: A comparison of paroxetine, clomipramine and placebo in the treatment of panic disorder. Acta Psychiatr Scand 95:145–152, 1997a

Lecrubier Y, Judge R, Collaborative Paroxetine Panic Study Investigators: Long-term evaluation of paroxetine, clomipramine and placebo in panic disorder. Acta Psychiatr Scand 95:153–160, 1997b

Lejoyeux M: Use of serotonin (5-hydroxytryptamine) reuptake inhibitors in the treatment of alcoholism. Alcohol 31 (suppl 1):69–75, 1996

Lemberger L, Rowe H, Bergstrom RF, et al: Effect of fluoxetine on psychomotor performance, physiologic response and kinetics of ethanol. Clin Pharmacol Ther 37:658–664, 1985

Leonard BE: Pharmacological differences of serotonin reuptake inhibitors and possible clinical relevance. Drugs 43 (suppl 2):3–10, 1992

Lesch KP, Hoh A, Schulte HM, et al: Obsessive-compulsive disorder. Psychopharmacology 105:415–420, 1991

Lester BM, Cucca J, Andreozzi BA, et al: Possible association between fluoxetine hydrochloride and colic in an infant. J Am Acad Child Adolesc Psychiatry 32:1253–1255, 1993

Lorens SA, Van der Kar LD: Differential effects of serotonin (5-HT$_{1A}$ and 5-HT$_2$) agonists and antagonists on renin and corticosterone secretion. Neuroendocrinology 45:305–310, 1987

Lydiard RB, Pollack MH, Judge R, et al: Fluoxetine treatment of panic disorder: a randomized, placebo-controlled, multi-center trial (abstract). Presented at the annual meeting of the European College of Neuropsychopharmacology (ECNP), Vienna, Austria, September 1997

Maj J, Rogoz Z, Skuza G, et al: Repeated treatment with antidepressant drugs potentiates the locomotor response to (+)-amphetamine. J Pharm Pharmacol 36:127–130, 1984

Mammen OK, Perel JM, Rudolph G, et al: Sertraline and nor-sertraline levels in three breastfed infants. J Clin Psychiatry 58:100–103, 1997

Marcus MD, Wing RR, Ewing L, et al: Double-blind, placebo-controlled trial of fluoxetine plus behavior modification in the treatment of obese binge eaters and non-binge eaters. Am J Psychiatry 147:876–881, 1990

Marley E, Wozniak KM: Interactions of a non-selective monoamine oxidase inhibitor, phenelzine, with inhibitors of 5-hydroxytryptamine, dopamine or noradrenaline re-uptake. J Psychiatr Res 18:173–189, 1984a

Marley E, Wozniak KM: Interactions of non-selective monoamine oxidase inhibitors, tranylcypromine and niala-mide, with inhibitors of 5-hydroxytryptamine, dopamine or noradrenaline re-uptake. J Psychiatr Res 18:191–203, 1984b

Marmar CR, Schoenfeld F, Weiss DS, et al: Open trial of fluvoxamine treatment for combat-related posttraumatic stress disorder. J Clin Psychiatry 57 (suppl 8):66–72, 1996

Marsden CA: The neuropharmacology of serotonin in the central nervous system, in Selective Serotonin Re-Uptake Inhibitors. Edited by Feighner JP, Boyer WF. Chichester, England, Wiley, 1991, pp 11–35

Marshall EF, Nelson DR, Johnson AM, et al: Desensitisation of central 5-HT$_2$ receptor mechanisms after repeated administration of the antidepressant paroxetine (abstract). Journal of Psychopharmacology (Oxf) 2:194, 1988

Max MB, Lynch SA, Muir J, et al: Effects of desipramine, amitriptyline, and fluoxetine on pain in diabetic neuropathy. N Engl J Med 326:1250–1256, 1992

Meltzer HY, Young M, Metz J, et al: Extrapyramidal side effects and increased serum prolactin following fluoxetine, a new antidepressant. J Neural Transm 45:165–175, 1979

Mendels J, Camera A, Sikes C: Sertraline treatment for premature ejaculation. J Clin Psychopharmacol 15:341–346, 1995

Menkes DB, Taghavi E, Mason PA, et al: Fluoxetine's spectrum of action in premenstrual syndrome. Int Clin Psychopharmacol 8:95–102, 1993

Michelson D, Onawala R, Beasley CM: Abrupt discontinuation of fluoxetine: a randomized, placebo-controlled study. American Psychiatric Association 1997 Annual Meeting New Research Program and Abstracts (NR200). Washington, DC, American Psychiatric Association, 1997a, p 122

Michelson D, Reimherr FW, Beasley CM: Optimal length on continuation therapy: a prospective assessment during fluoxetine long-term treatment of major depressive disorder. American Psychiatric Association 1997 Annual Meeting New Research Program and Abstracts (NR189). Washington, DC, American Psychiatric Association, 1997b

Mitchell JE, Pyle RL, Eckert ED, et al: Response to alternative antidepressants in imipramine nonresponders with bulimia nervosa. J Clin Psychopharmacol 9:291–293, 1989

Montgomery SA: Fluoxetine in the treatment of anxiety, agitation and suicidal thoughts, in Psychiatry Today: VIII World Congress of Psychiatry Abstracts. Edited by Stefanis CN, Soldatos CR, Rabavilas AD. New York, Elsevier, 1989a, p 335

Montgomery SA: New antidepressants and 5-HT uptake inhibitors. Acta Psychiatr Scand 80 (suppl 350):107–116, 1989b

Montgomery SA, Dufour H, Brion S, et al: The prophylactic efficacy of fluoxetine in unipolar depression. Br J Psychiatry 153:69–76, 1988

Murphy JM, Waller MB, Gatto GJ, et al: Effects of fluoxetine on the intragastric self-administration of ethanol in the alcohol preferring P line of rats. Alcohol 5:283–286, 1988

Naranjo CA, Sellers EM, Lawrin MO: Modulation of ethanol intake by serotonin uptake inhibitors. J Clin Psychiatry 47 (suppl 4):16–22, 1986

Naranjo CA, Kadlec KE, Sanhueza P, et al: Fluoxetine differentially alters alcohol intake and other consummatory behaviors in problem drinkers. Clin Pharmacol Ther 47:490–498, 1990

Nelson DR, Thomas DR, Johnson AM: Pharmacological effects of paroxetine after repeated administration to animals. Acta Psychiatr Scand 80 (suppl 350):21–23, 1989

Ninan PT, van-Kammen DP, Scheinin M, et al: CSF 5-hydroxyindoleacetic acid levels in suicidal schizophrenic patients. Am J Psychiatry 141:566–569, 1984

Norden MJ: Fluoxetine in borderline personality disorder. Prog Neuropsychopharmacol Biol Psychiatry 13:885–893, 1989

Norregaard J, Volkmann H, Danneskiold-Samsoe B: A randomized controlled trial of citalopram in the treatment of fibromyalgia. Pain 61:445–449, 1995

Nowak G: Long term effect of antidepressant drugs and electroconvulsive shock (ECS) on cortical α_1-adrenoceptors following destruction of dopaminergic nerve terminals. Pharmacol Toxicol 64:469–470, 1989

Nulman I, Rovet J, Stewart DE, et al: Neurodevelopment of children exposed in utero to antidepressant drugs. N Engl J Med 336:258–262, 1997

O'Flynn K, O'Keane V, Lucey JV, et al: Effect of fluoxetine on noradrenergic mediated growth hormone release: a double-blind, placebo-controlled study. Biol Psychiatry 30:377–382, 1991

Pandey GN, Pandey SC, Janicak PG, et al: Platelet serotonin-2 receptor binding sites in depression and suicide. Biol Psychiatry 28:215–222, 1990

Papini M, Martinetti MJ, Pasquinelli A: Trazodone symptomatic extrapyramidal disorders of infancy and childhood. Ital J Neurol Sci 3:161–162, 1982

Pearlstein TB, Stone AB, Lund SA, et al: Comparison of fluoxetine, bupropion, and placebo in the treatment of premenstrual dysphoric disorder. J Clin Psychopharmacol 17:261–266, 1997

Pedersen OL, Kragh-Sorensen P, Bjerre M, et al: Citalopram, a selective serotonin reuptake inhibitor: clinical antidepressive and long-term effect—a phase II study. Psychopharmacology (Berl) 77:199–204, 1982

Peroutka SJ, Snyder SH: Long-term antidepressant treatment decreases spiroperidol-labelled serotonin receptor binding. Science 210:88–90, 1980

Peselow ED, Filippi AM, Goodnick P, et al: The short- and long-term efficacy of paroxetine HCl, B: data from a double-blind crossover study and from a year-long term trial vs. imipramine and placebo. Psychopharmacol Bull 25:272–276, 1989

Plaznik A, Kostowski W: The effects of antidepressants and electroconvulsive shocks on the functioning of the mesolimbic dopaminergic system: a behavioural study. Eur J Pharmacol 135:389–396, 1987

Ravindran AV, Judge R, Hunter BN, et al: A double-blind, multicenter study in primary care comparing paroxetine and clomipramine in patients with depression and associated anxiety. J Clin Psychiatry 58:112–118, 1997

Renynghe de Voxurie GE: Anafranil (G34586) in obsessive neurosis. Acta Neurol Belg 68:787–792, 1968

Ricca V, Mannucci E, Di Bernardo M, et al: Sertraline enhances the effects of cognitive-behavioral treatment on weight reduction of obese patients. J Endocrinol Invest 19:727–733, 1996

Richelson E: Synaptic effects of antidepressants. J Clin Psychopharmacol 16 (suppl 2):1S–9S, 1996

Rubey RN, Johnson MR, Emmanuel N, et al: Fluoxetine in the treatment of anger: an open clinical trial. J Clin Psychiatry 57:398–401, 1996

Rudorfer MV, Potter WZ: Combined fluoxetine and tricyclic antidepressants. Am J Psychiatry 146:562–564, 1989

Salzman C, Wolfson AN, Schatzberg A, et al: Effect of fluoxetine on anger in symptomatic volunteers with borderline personality disorder. J Clin Psychopharmacol 15:23–29, 1995

Sampson D, Willner P, Muscat R: Reversal of antidepressant action by dopamine antagonists in an animal model of depression. Psychopharmacology (Berl) 104:491–495, 1991

Saper JR, Silberstein SD, Lake AE III, et al: Double-blind trial of fluoxetine: chronic daily headache and migraine. Headache 34:497–502, 1994

Schatzberg AF, Haddad P, Kaplan EM, et al: Serotonin reuptake discontinuation syndrome: a hypothetical definition (discontinuation consensus panel). J Clin Psychiatry 58 (suppl 7):5–10, 1997

Scherschlicht R, Polc P, Schneeberger J, et al: Selective suppression of rapid eye movement sleep in cats by typical and atypical antidepressants. Adv Biochem Psychopharmacol 31:359–364, 1982

Schmidt A, Lebel L, Koe BK, et al: Sertraline patently displaces (+)-[^{3}H]-3-PPP binding to α sites in rat brain. Eur J Pharmacol 165:335–336, 1989

Schweizer E, Rickels K, Amsterdam JD, et al: What constitutes an adequate antidepressant trial for fluoxetine? J Clin Psychiatry 51:8–11, 1990

Shaskan EG, Snyder SH: Kinetics of serotonin accumulation into slices from rat brain: relationship to catecholamine uptake. J Pharmacol Exp Ther 175:404–418, 1970

Shaw DM, Crimmins R: A multicentre trial of citalopram and amitriptyline in major depressive illness, in Citalopram: the New Antidepressant From Lundbeck Research. Edited by Montgomery SA. Amsterdam, Excerpta Medica, 1989, pp 43–49

Sheehan DV, Harnett-Sheehan K: The role of SSRIs in panic disorder. J Clin Psychiatry 57 (suppl 10):51–58, 1996

Shrivastava RK, Shrivastava SHP, Overweg N, et al: Depression. J Clin Psychiatry 53 (suppl 2):48–51, 1992

Siddiqui UA, Chakravarti SK, Jesinger DK: The tolerance and antidepressive activity of fluvoxamine as a single dose compared to a twice-daily dose. Curr Med Res Opin 9: 681–690, 1985

Silver H, Nassar A: Fluvoxamine improves negative symptoms in treated chronic schizophrenia: an add-on double-blind, placebo-controlled study. Biol Psychiatry 31:698–704, 1992

Sindrup SH, Gram LF, Brosen K, et al: The selective serotonin reuptake inhibitor paroxetine is effective in the treatment of diabetic neuropathy symptoms. Pain 42:135–144, 1990

Sindrup SH, Bjerre U, Dejgaard A, et al: The selective serotonin reuptake inhibitor citalopram relieves the symptoms of diabetic neuropathy. Clin Pharmacol Ther 52:547–552, 1992a

Sindrup SH, Brosen K, Gram LF, et al: The relationship between paroxetine and sparteine oxidation polymorphism. J Clin Pharmacol Ther 51:278–287, 1992b

Sleight AJ, Marsden CA, Martin KF, et al: Relationship between extracellular 5-hydroxytryptamine and behaviour following monoamine oxidase inhibition and L-tryptophan. Br J Pharmacol 93:303–310, 1988

Snyder SH, Yamamura HI: Antidepressants and the muscarinic acetylcholine receptor. Arch Gen Psychiatry 34:236–239, 1977

Stahl SM, Uhr SB, Berger PA: Pilot study on the effects of fenfluramine on negative symptoms in twelve inpatients. Biol Psychiatry 20:1098–1102, 1985

Stauderman KA, Gandhi DC, Jones DJ: Fluoxetine-induced inhibition of synaptosomal [^{3}H] 5-HT release: possible calcium-channel inhibition. Life Sci 50:2125–2138, 1992

Steiner M, Steinberg S, Stewart D, et al: Fluoxetine in the treatment of premenstrual dysphoria. N Engl J Med 332:1529–1534, 1995

Stockmeier CA, McLeskey SW, Blendy JA, et al: Electroconvulsive shock but not antidepressant drugs increase α_1-adrenoceptor binding sites in rat brain. Eur J Pharmacol 139:259–266, 1987

Su T-P, Danaceau M, Schmidt PJ, et al: Fluoxetine in the treatment of patients with premenstrual syndrome. Biol Psychiatry 33:159A–160A, 1993

Su T-P, Schmidt PJ, Danaceau MA, et al: Fluoxetine in the treatment of premenstrual dysphoria. Neuropsychopharmacology 16:346–356, 1997

Taddio A, Ito S, Koren G: Excretion of fluoxetine and its metabolite, norfluoxetine, in human breast milk. J Clin Pharmacol 36:42–47, 1996

Tasker TCG, Kaye CM, Zussman BD, et al: Paroxetine plasma levels: lack of correlation with efficacy or adverse events. Acta Psychiatr Scand 80:152–155, 1989

Teusink JP, Alexopoulos GS, Shamoian CA: Parkinsonian side effects induced by a monoamine oxidase inhibitor. Am J Psychiatry 141:118–119, 1984

Thase ME, Fava M, Halbreich U, et al: A placebo-controlled, randomized clinical trial comparing sertraline and imipramine for the treatment of dysthymia. Arch Gen Psychiatry 53:777–784, 1996

Thomas DR, Nelson DR, Johnson AM: Biochemical effects of the antidepressant paroxetine, a specific 5-hydroxytryptamine uptake inhibitor. Psychopharmacology (Berl) 93:193–200, 1987

Thoren P, Asberg M, Bertilsson L, et al: Clomipramine treatment of obsessive-compulsive disorder, II: biochemical aspects. Arch Gen Psychiatry 37:1289–1294, 1980

Tyrer P, Marsden CA, Casey P, et al: Clinical efficacy of paroxetine in resistant depression. J Psychopharmacol 1:251–257, 1987

U'Prichard DC, Greenberg DA, Sheehan PB, et al: Tricyclic antidepressants: therapeutic properties and affinity for α-noradrenergic receptor binding sites in the brain. Science 199:197–198, 1978

Usher RW, Beasley CM, Bosomworth JC: Efficacy and safety of morning versus evening fluoxetine administration. J Clin Psychiatry 52:134–136, 1991

Valentino RJ, Curtis AL: Pharmacology of locus coeruleus spontaneous and sensory evoked activity. Prog Brain Res 88:249–256, 1991

Van der Kolk BA, Dreyfuss D, Michaels M, et al: Fluoxetine in posttraumatic stress disorder. J Clin Psychiatry 55:517–522, 1994

vanPraag HM, Kahn R, Asnis GM, et al: Therapeutic indications for serotonin-potentiating compounds: a hypothesis. Biol Psychiatry 22:205–212, 1987

Waldinger MD, Hengeveld MW, Zwinderman AH: Ejaculation-retarding properties of paroxetine in patients with primary premature ejaculation: a double-blind, randomized, dose-response study. Br J Urol 79:592–595, 1997

Warshaw MG, Keller MB: The relationship between fluoxetine use and suicidal behavior in 654 subjects with anxiety disorders. J Clin Psychiatry 57:158–166, 1996

Weizman R, Carmi M, Tyano S, et al: High affinity [^{3}H] imipramine binding and serotonin uptake to platelets of adolescent females suffering from anorexia nervosa. Life Sci 38:1235–1242, 1986

Wernicke JF, Bremner JD, Bosomworth J, et al: The efficacy and safety of fluoxetine in the long-term treatment of depression. Paper presented at the International Fluoxetine Symposium, Tyrol, Austria, October 13–17, 1987

Wong DT, Reid LR, Bymaster FP, et al: Chronic effects of fluoxetine, a selective inhibitor of serotonin uptake, on neurotransmitter receptors. J Neural Transm 64:251–269, 1985

Wong DT, Threlkeld PG, Robertson DW: Affinities of fluoxetine, its enantiomers, and other inhibitors of serotonin uptake for subtypes of serotonin receptors. Neuropsychopharmacology 5:43–47, 1991

Wood SH, Mortola JF, Chan Y-F, et al: Treatment of premenstrual syndrome with fluoxetine: a double-blind placebo-controlled crossover study. Obstet General 80:339–344, 1992

Woolley DW, Campbell NK: Exploration of the central nervous system serotonin in humans. Ann N Y Acad Sci 90:108–117, 1962

Wurtman JJ, Wurtman RJ, Growdon JH, et al: Carbohydrate craving in obese people: suppression by treatments affecting serotonergic transmission. Int J Eat Disord 1:2–15, 1981

Yonkers KA, Gullion C, Williams A, et al: Paroxetine as a treatment for premenstrual dysphoric disorder. J Clin Psychopharmacol 16:3–8, 1996a

Yonkers KA, Halbreich U, Freeman E, et al: Sertraline in the treatment of premenstrual dysphoric disorder. Psychopharmacol Bull 32:41–46, 1996b

Zohar J, Insel TR, Zohar-Kadouch RC, et al: Serotonergic responsivity in obsessive-compulsive disorder: effects of chronic clomipramine treatment. Arch Gen Psychiatry 45:167–172, 1988

Zohar J, Judge R, OCD Paroxetine Study Investigators: Paroxetine versus clomipramine in the treatment of obsessive-compulsive disorder. Br J Psychiatry 169:468–474, 1996

Zubenko GS, Cohen BM, Lipinski JF: Antidepressant-related akathisia. J Clin Psychopharmacol 7:254–257, 1987

TWELVE

Monoamine Oxidase Inhibitors

K. Ranga Rama Krishnan, M.D.

Monoamine oxidase inhibitors (MAOIs) were first identified as effective antidepressants in the late 1950s. An early report suggested that iproniazid, an antituberculosis agent, had mood-elevating properties in patients who had been treated for tuberculosis (Bloch et al. 1954). Following these observations, two studies confirmed that iproniazid did indeed have antidepressant properties (Crane 1957; Kline 1958). Zeller (1963) reported that iproniazid caused potent inhibition of MAO enzymes both in vivo and in vitro in the brain. He also reported that the medication reversed some of the actions of reserpine. Because reserpine produced significant depression as a side effect, it was suggested that iproniazid might have mood-elevating properties.

The use of iproniazid soon fell into disfavor because of its significant hepatotoxicity. Other MAOIs, both hydrazine derivatives (e.g., isocarboxazid and phenylhydrazine) and nonhydrazine derivatives (e.g., tranylcypromine), were introduced. These MAOIs were not specific for any subtype of MAO enzyme and were irreversible inhibitors of MAO (see next section). Their use has been rather limited, because hypertensive crisis by the MAOIs may occur in some patients from potentiation of the pressor effects of amines (such as tyramine) in food (Blackwell et al. 1967).

In the last few years, there has been a resurgence of interest in the development of new MAOIs—those that are more specific subtypes of MAO enzyme and those that are reversible in nature. Newer MAOIs, such as L-deprenyl (selegiline hydrochloride), an MAO β-inhibitor, have been introduced (Table 12–1).

Reversible MAO α-inhibitors such as moclobemide are currently being evaluated. Moclobemide has been introduced in Europe but is not available in the United States.

MONOAMINE OXIDASE ISOENZYMES

MAO is widely distributed in mammals. Two isoenzymes—monoamine oxidase A (MAO-A) and monoamine oxidase B (MAO-B)—are of special interest to psychiatry (Cesura and Pletscher 1992). Both are present in the central nervous system (CNS) and in some peripheral organs. Both MAO-A and MAO-B are present in discrete cell populations within the CNS. MAO-A is present in both dopamine and norepinephrine neurons, whereas MAO-B is present to a greater extent in serotonin-containing neurons. They are also present in nonaminergic neurons in various subcortical regions of the brain. Glial cells also express MAO-A and MAO-B (Cesura and Pletscher 1992). The physiological function of these two isoenzymes has not been fully elucidated. The main substrates for MAO-A are epinephrine, norepinephrine, and serotonin. The main substrates for MAO-B are phenylethylamine, phenylethanolamine, tyramine, and benzylamine. Dopamine and tryptamine are metabolized by both isoen-

Treatment of Various Psychiatric Disorders

Panic disorder. Both single-blind and double-blind studies have found that phenelzine and iproniazid are effective in treating panic disorder (Lydiard et al. 1989; Quitkin et al. 1990; Tyrer et al. 1973). About 50%–60% of patients with panic disorder respond to MAOIs. In the early stages of treatment, patients may have a worsening of symptoms. This is reduced in clinical practice by combining the MAOI with a benzodiazepine for the initial phase of the study. It has been suggested that phenelzine has an antiphobic action in addition to its antipanic effect (Kelly et al. 1971). The time-course of effect and the dose used are similar to that for major depression.

Social phobia. Liebowitz and colleagues (1992) reported that phenelzine is effective in treating social phobia. In an open-label study, Versiani and colleagues (1988) suggested that tranylcypromine is effective and also demonstrated the efficacy of moclobemide in a double-blind study (Versiani et al. 1992). In clinical experience, about 50% of patients' conditions respond to MAOIs. The onset of response is gradual (usually about 2–3 weeks).

Obsessive-compulsive disorder. Although initial case reports suggested that MAOIs may be effective in the treatment of obsessive-compulsive disorder (Jenike 1981), no double-blind studies indicate efficacy.

Posttraumatic stress disorder. The classic MAOI phenelzine has been proven effective for treatment of posttraumatic stress disorder (PTSD) in both single-blind trials (Davidson et al. 1987b) and a double-blind crossover trial (Kosten et al. 1991).

Generalized anxiety disorder. MAOIs are not usually used to treat generalized anxiety disorder because the risk-benefit ratio favors the use of azaspirones or benzodiazepines. MAOIs are used primarily in treatment-resistant patients with generalized anxiety disorder.

Bulimia nervosa. Both phenelzine and isocarboxazid have been shown to be effective in treating some symptoms of bulimia nervosa (Kennedy et al. 1988; McElroy et al. 1989; Walsh et al. 1985, 1987).

Premenstrual dysphoria. Preliminary studies and clinical experience suggest that MAOIs may be effective in treatment of premenstrual dysphoria (Glick et al. 1991).

Chronic pain. MAOIs are believed to be effective in the treatment of atypical facial pain and other chronic pain syndromes. However, only limited data on these conditions are available.

Neurological diseases. The classic MAOIs have not been found to be effective for treating neurological disorders such as Parkinson's disease and Alzheimer's dementia. However, the MAOI-B selegiline has been shown to be effective in slowing the progression of Parkinson's disease (Cesura and Pletscher 1992), but the mechanism underlying this effect is unknown.

Side Effects of Monoamine Oxidase Inhibitors

Side effects of MAOIs are generally more severe or frequent than for other antidepressants (Zisook 1984). The most frequent side effects include dizziness, headache, dry mouth, insomnia, constipation, blurred vision, nausea, peripheral edema, forgetfulness, fainting spells, trauma, hesitancy of urination, weakness, and myoclonic jerks. Loss of weight and appetite may occur with isocarboxazid use (Davidson and Turnbull 1982). Hepatotoxicity is rarer with the currently available MAOIs compared with iproniazid. However, liver enzymes such as serum glutamic-oxaloacetic transaminase (SGOT) and serum glutamic-pyruvic transaminase (SGPT) are elevated in 3%–5% of patients. Liver function tests must be done only when patients have symptoms such as malaise, jaundice, and excessive fatigue.

Some side effects first emerge during maintenance treatment (Evans et al. 1982). These side effects include weight gain (which occurs in almost half of the patients), edema, muscle cramps, carbohydrate craving, sexual dysfunction (usually anorgasmia), pyridoxine deficiency (Goodheart et al. 1991), hypoglycemia, hypomania, urinary retention, and disorientation. Peripheral neuropathy (Goodheart et al. 1991) and speech blockage (Goldstein and Goldberg 1986) are rare side effects of MAOIs. Weight gain is more of a problem with the hydrazine compounds such as phenelzine than with tranylcypromine. Therefore, weight gain caused by the hydrazine derivatives is an indication to switch to tranylcypromine. Edema is also more common with phenelzine than with tranylcypromine.

The management of some of these side effects can be problematic. Orthostatic hypotension is common with MAOIs. Addition of salt and salt-retaining steroids such as fluorohydrocortisol is sometimes effective in treating orthostatic hypotension. Elastic support stockings are also helpful. Small amounts of coffee or tea taken during the day also keep the blood pressure elevated. The dose of flurohydrocortisol should be adjusted carefully, because in elderly patients, it could provoke cardiac failure resulting from fluid retention.

Sexual dysfunction that occurs with these compounds is also difficult to treat. Common problems include anorgasmia, decreased libido, impotence, and delayed ejaculation (Harrison et al. 1985; Jacobson 1987). Cyproheptadine is sometimes effective in treating sexual dysfunction such as anorgasmia. Bethanechol may also be effective in some patients.

Insomnia occasionally occurs as an intermediate or late side effect of these compounds. Changing the time of administration does not seem to help much, although dosage reduction may be helpful. Adding trazodone at bedtime is effective, but this should be done with caution. Myoclonic jerks, peripheral neuropathy, and paresthesia, when present, are also difficult to treat. When a patient has paresthesia, the clinician should evaluate for peripheral neuropathy and pyridoxine deficiency. In general, patients taking MAOIs should also take concomitant pyridoxine therapy. When myoclonic jerks occur, patients can be treated with cyproheptadine.

MAOIs also have the potential to suppress anginal pain; therefore, coronary artery disease could be overlooked or underestimated. Patients with hyperthyroidism are more sensitive to MAOIs because of their overall sensitivity to pressor amines. MAOIs can also worsen hypoglycemia in patients taking hypoglycemic agents such as insulin.

Dietary Interactions of Monoamine Oxidase Inhibitors

After the MAOIs were introduced, several reports of severe headaches in patients who were taking these compounds were published (Anonymous 1970; Cronin 1965; Hedberg et al. 1966; Simpson and Gratz 1992). These headaches were caused by a drug-food interaction. The risk of such an interaction is highest for tranylcypromine and lower for phenelzine, providing the dose of the latter remains low. The interaction of MAOIs with food has been attributed to increased tyramine levels. Tyramine, which has a pressor action, is present in a number of foodstuffs. It is normally broken down by the MAO enzymes and has both direct and indirect sympathomimetic actions. The classic explanation of this side effect may not be entirely accurate; in fact, it has been suggested that the potentiation of tyramine by an MAOI may be secondary to increased release of noradrenaline rather than MAOIs. Adrenaline would increase the indirect sympathetic activity of tyramine. The spontaneous occurrence of hypertensive crises in a few patients lends support to this hypothesis (O'Brien et al. 1992; Zajecka and Fawcett 1991).

The tyramine effect is potentiated by MAOIs 10- to 20-fold. A mild tyramine interaction occurs with about 6 mg of tyramine; 10 mg can produce a moderate episode, and 25 mg can produce a severe episode, characterized by hypertension, occipital headache, palpitations, nausea, vomiting, apprehension, occasional chills, sweating, and restlessness. On examination, neck stiffness, pallor, mild pyrexia, dilated pupils, and motor agitation may be seen. The reaction usually develops within 20 minutes to 1 hour after ingestion of the food. Occasionally, the reaction can be very severe and may lead to alteration of consciousness, hyperpyrexia, cerebral hemorrhage, and death. Death is exceedingly rare and has been calculated to be about 0.01%–0.02% for tranylcypromine.

The classic treatment of the hypertensive reaction is 5 mg of phentolamine administered intravenously (Youdim et al. 1987; Zisook 1984). More recently, nifedipine, a calcium channel blocker, has been shown to be effective. Nifedipine has an onset of action in about 5 minutes, and it lasts approximately 3–5 hours; in fact, some clinicians have suggested that patients should carry nifedipine with them for immediate use in the event of a hypertensive crisis.

Because of the drug interaction of the classic MAOIs with food, clinicians usually make several dietary recommendations (see Table 12–3). These recommendations are quite varied.

All the MAOI diets recommend restriction of cheese (except for cream cheese and cottage cheese), wine, beer, sherry, liquors, pickled fish, overripe aged fruit, brewer's yeast, fava beans, beef and chicken liver, and fermented products. Other diets also recommend restriction of all alcoholic beverages, coffee, chocolate, colas, tea, yogurt, soy sauce, avocados, and bananas. The more restrictive the diet, the greater the risk of patient noncompliance. Furthermore, many of the compounds (e.g., avocados, bananas) rarely cause hypertensive crisis; for example, an interaction may occur only if overripe fruit is eaten or, in the case of bananas, if the skin is eaten (which is uncommon in the United States). Similarly, unless a person ingests large amounts of caffeine, the interaction is usually not clinically significant.

In evaluating patients who have had a drug-food reaction, it is also important to evaluate the hypertensive reaction and differentiate it from histamine headache, which can occur with an MAOI. Histamine headaches are usually accompanied by hypotension, colic, loose stools, salivation, and lacrimation (Cooper 1967). The clinician should

Table 12–3.   Food restrictions for MAOIs

To be avoided	To be used in moderation
Cheese (except for cream cheese)	Coffee
Overripe aged fruit (banana peel)	Chocolate
	Colas
Fava beans	Tea
Sausage, salami	Soy sauce
Sherry, liquors	Beer, other wines
Sauerkraut	
Monosodium glutamate	
Pickled fish	
Brewer's yeast	
Beef and chicken liver	
Fermented products	
Red wine	

Note.   MAOIs = monoamine oxidase inhibitors.

provide oral instructions as well as printed cards outlining these instructions to patients who are taking classic MAOIs.

In addition to the food interaction, drug interactions are extremely important (see next section). Each patient should be given a card indicating that he or she is taking an MAOI and should be instructed to carry it at all times. A medical bracelet indicating that the wearer takes an MAOI is also a good idea.

Drug Interactions

The extensive inhibition of MAO by MAOI enzymes raises the potential for a number of drug interactions (Table 12–4). These interactions are particularly important because many over-the-counter medications can interact with the MAOIs. These medications include cough syrups containing sympathomimetic agents, which, in the presence of an MAOI, can precipitate a hypertensive crisis.

Another area of caution is the use of MAOIs in patients who need surgery. In this situation, interactions include those with narcotic drugs, especially meperidine. Meperidine administered with MAOIs can produce a syndrome characterized by coma, hyperpyrexia, and hypertension. This syndrome has been reported primarily with phenelzine but also with tranylcypromine (Mendelson 1979; Stack et al. 1988). Stack and colleagues (1988) noted that this syndrome is most likely to occur with meperidine and may be related to its serotonergic properties. Similar reactions have not been reported to any significant extent with other narcotic analgesics such as mor-

phine or codeine. In fact, many patients probably receive these medications without problems. Only a small fraction of patients may have this interaction, and it could reflect an idiosyncratic effect. In general, current opinion favors the use of morphine or fentanyl when intra- or postoperative narcotics are needed in patients taking MAOIs.

The issue of whether directly acting sympathomimetic amines interact with MAOIs is more controversial. Intravenous administration of sympathomimetic amines to patients receiving MAOIs does not provoke hypertension. When a bolus infusion of catecholamines is given to healthy volunteer subjects who have been taking phenelzine or tranylcypromine for a week, a potentiation of the pressor effect of phenylephrine occurs, but no clinically significant potentiation of cardiovascular effects of norepinephrine, epinephrine, or isoproterenol occurs (Wells 1989).

In general, direct sympathomimetic amine–MAOI interactions do not appear to produce significant cardiovascular problems but rather a low incidence of hypertensive episodes in the presence of indirect sympathomimetics. Ideally, these compounds should not be used in patients receiving MAOIs. A direct-acting compound is preferable to an indirect-acting one.

Caution should be exercised when using MAOIs in patients with pheochromocytoma and cardiovascular, cerebrovascular, and hepatic disease. Because phenelzine tablets contain gluten, they should not be given to patients with coeliac disease.

PHENELZINE

Phenelzine, a hydrazine derivative, is a potent MAOI and the best studied among the MAOIs. Phenelzine undergoes acetylation. Thus, the levels are lower in fast acetylators than in slow acetylators. However, because it is an irreversible inhibitor, plasma concentrations are not relevant.

Efficacy

Phenelzine is useful in the treatment of major depression, atypical depression, panic disorder, social phobia, and atypical facial pain. (See general discussion of efficacy in "Monoamine Oxidase Inhibitors" earlier in this chapter.)

Side Effects

The primary side effects of phenelzine are similar to those of other MAOIs. Hepatitis secondary to phenelzine may occur. This effect is quite rare (<1 in 30,000). The most difficult side effect often leading to discontinuation is postural hypotension.

Table 12–4. Drug interactions with MAOIs

Drug	Interaction	Comment
Other MAOIs (e.g., furazolidone, pargyline, and procarbazine)	Potentiation of side effects; convulsions possible	Allow at least 1 week before changing MAOI
Tricyclic antidepressants (TCAs) (e.g., maprotiline, bupropion)	Severe side effects possible, such as hypertension and convulsions	Allow at least 2 weeks before changing MAOI; combinations have been used occasionally for refractory depression
Carbamazepine	Low possibility of interaction; similar to TCAs	Same as for TCAs
Cyclobenzaprine	Low possibility of interaction; similar to TCAs	Same as for TCAs
Selective serotonin reuptake inhibitors	Serotonin syndrome	Avoid combinations; allow at least 2 weeks before changing MAOI and 5 weeks if switching from fluoxetine to MAOI
Stimulants (e.g., methylphenidate, dextroamphetamine)	Potential for increased blood pressure (hypertension)	Avoid combination
Buspirone	Potential for increased blood pressure (hypertension)	Avoid; if used, monitor blood pressure
Meperidine	Severe, potentially fatal interaction possible (see text)	Avoid combination
Dextromethorphan	Reports of brief psychosis	Avoid high doses
Direct sympathomimetics (e.g., L-dopa)	Increased blood pressure	Avoid, if possible; use with caution
Indirect sympathomimetics	Hypertensive crisis possible	Avoid use
Oral hypoglycemics (e.g., insulin)	May worsen hypoglycemia	Monitor blood sugar levels and adjust medications
Fenfluramine	Serotonin syndrome possible	Avoid use
L-Tryptophan	Serotonin syndrome possible	Avoid use

Note. MAOIs = monoamine oxidase inhibitors.

Contraindications

The contraindications to phenelzine include known sensitivity to the drug, pheochromocytoma, congestive heart failure, and history of liver disease (see also sections, "Dietary Interactions of Monoamine Oxidase Inhibitors" and "Drug Interactions," earlier in this chapter).

ISOCARBOXAZID

Isocarboxazid is a hydrazine type of MAOI. Isocarboxazid is rapidly absorbed from the gastrointestinal tract and metabolized in the liver. It is primarily excreted as hippuric acid. Its half-life is of little interest because it is an irreversible MAOI.

Efficacy

Isocarboxazid is the least studied of the MAOIs. Its indications are similar to those of the other MAOIs.

Side Effects

The side effects of isocarboxazid are similar to those of phenelzine. Postural hypotension is the most common problem.

Contraindications

The contraindications to isocarboxazid are similar to those of phenelzine.

TRANYLCYPROMINE

Tranylcypromine, a nonhydrazine reversible MAOI, increases the concentration of norepinephrine, epinephrine, and serotonin in the CNS. When tranylcypromine is discontinued, about 5 days are needed for recovery of MAO function. Tranylcypromine has a mild stimulant effect.

Efficacy

See the general discussion of efficacy in "Monoamine Oxidase Inhibitors" earlier in this chapter.

Side Effects

Tranylcypromine's side effects are similar to those of other MAOIs. In addition, problems with physical dependence on tranylcypromine have been reported. Thus, withdrawal symptoms such as anxiety, restlessness, depression, and headache may occur. Syndrome of inappropriate antidiuretic hormone (SIADH) has been reported with tranylcypromine. Rare cases of toxic hepatitis have been reported. Tranylcypromine can lead to increased agitation, insomnia, and restlessness compared with phenelzine.

Contraindications

The contraindications to tranylcypromine are the same as those for phenelzine. Also, in view of the greater potential for hypertensive episodes, tranylcypromine should be used with particular caution in patients with cerebrovascular or cardiovascular disease.

MOCLOBEMIDE

Moclobemide, a reversible inhibitor of MAO-A enzyme (Amrein et al. 1989), has a higher potency in vivo than in vitro. Therefore, it has been suggested that moclobemide is a prodrug and is metabolized to a form with higher affinity for MAO-A than the parent compound. The recovery of MAO-A activity after single- or repeated-dose moclobemide administration is much shorter than that seen with other MAOIs including clorgiline, an irreversible inhibitor of MAO-A. One of the metabolites of moclobemide does inhibit MAO-B; however, this action is minimally significant in humans. Moclobemide, when administered to rats, increases the concentration of serotonin, norepinephrine, epinephrine, and dopamine in rat brain (see Haefely et al. 1992). These effects are short lasting and parallel the time-course of MAO-A inhibition. In addition, unlike other irreversible inhibitors, repeated administration does not increase the inhibition.

In animals, moclobemide only partially potentiates the blood pressor effect of oral tyramine. The reason for this is that it is a reversible inhibitor with a low affinity for the MAO isoenzymes and is easily displaced by the pressor amines ingested in food. Based on these studies, moclobemide is thought to be safer than other irreversible MAOIs.

Pharmacokinetics

After oral administration of moclobemide, peak plasma concentrations are reached within 1 hour. The drug is about 50% bound to plasma proteins and is extensively metabolized; only 1% of the compound is excreted in the urine, unchanged. The half-life of the compound is approximately 12 hours.

Efficacy

Moclobemide has been studied in all types of depressive disorders (Gabelic and Kuhn 1990; Larsen et al. 1991; Rossel and Moll 1990). Controlled trials have found that it is superior to placebo. In addition, moclobemide has been found to be as effective as imipramine, desipramine, clomipramine, and amitriptyline in the treatment of depression. The dose required is 300–600 mg/day.

Unlike the classic MAOIs, moclobemide has been found to be effective in both endogenous and nonendogenous suppression. In addition, in combination with antipsychotics, the drug appears to be effective in treating psychotic depression (Amrein et al. 1989). Moclobemide has also been effective in treating bipolar endogenous depression.

Versiani and colleagues (1992) compared phenelzine, moclobemide, and placebo and reported that both phenelzine and moclobemide were superior to placebo in treating patients with social phobia. Based on the efficacy of classic MAOIs in the treatment of other psychiatric disorders, such as bulimia, panic disorder, and PTSD, it is likely that these patients would respond to the reversible MAOIs. Additional trials are required to confirm the utility in other psychiatric disorders.

Side Effects

Nausea was the only side effect noted to be greater in patients taking moclobemide compared with those taking placebo. Thus, the profile of the drug appears to be ideal in that it causes few or no major side effects. Case reports have shown no toxicity after overdoses of up to 20 g (Amrein et al. 1989).

Food and Drug Interactions

Intravenous tyramine pressor tests indicate that a single dose of moclobemide increases tyramine sensitivity (Cusson et al. 1991). However, this increase is marginal compared with the increase associated with other MAOIs. Under most conditions, there appears to be limited drug-food interaction. However, to minimize even mild tyramine pressor effects, it would be preferable to administer moclobemide after a meal rather than before it. In a study in which tyramine was administered in dosages up to 100 mg, inpatients pretreated with moclobemide had no significant changes in blood pressure. The drug also has minimal effect on cognitive performance and no effect on body weight or hematological parameters (Wesnes et al. 1989; Youdim et al. 1987).

Drug Interactions

Several studies have examined potential drug interactions with moclobemide, unlike the other MAOIs (Amrein et al. 1992). No drug interaction with lithium or in combination with TCAs has been reported. The drug has also been combined with fluoxetine and other selective serotonin reuptake inhibitors with no significant interaction. No interactions with benzodiazepines or neuroleptics have been reported (Amrein et al. 1992). Parallel data suggest that moclobemide can potentiate the effects of meperidine; therefore, the narcotic-MAOI interaction may occur. Until proven otherwise, it would be prudent to avoid the combination of moclobemide with opiates such as meperidine. A pharmacokinetic interaction has been observed with cimetidine that requires the reduction of the moclobemide dose because cimetidine reduces the clearance of moclobemide.

SELEGILINE HYDROCHLORIDE

Selegiline hydrochloride is an irreversible MAO-B inhibitor (Cesura and Pletscher 1992). Its primary use is in treatment of Parkinson's disease as an adjunct to L-dopa and carbidopa. The average daily dose for Parkinson's disease is 5–10 mg/day. The exact mechanism of action of MAO-B in Parkinson's disease is unknown (Gerlach et al. 1996; Hagan et al. 1997; Lyytinen et al. 1997). Selegiline is metabolized to levoamphetamine, methamphetamine, and *N*-desmethylselegiline.

Efficacy

The efficacy of selegiline in treating depression has not been well studied. The few studies that have examined its utility have been equivocal. The dose required for treating depression may be much higher than that required to treat Parkinson's disease. Clinical experience suggests that doses of 20–40 mg/day are needed. At these doses, dietary interactions could occur. Early studies have reported that selegiline is of modest benefit in patients with Alzheimer's disease (Lawlor et al. 1997).

Side Effects

Selegiline has been found to have no adverse effects when combined with other antidepressants during treatment of depression in patients with Parkinson's disease. The few side effects that have been noted with selegiline include nausea, dizziness, and light-headedness. When the drug is abruptly discontinued, nausea, hallucinations, and confusion have been reported.

Food and Drug Interactions

Because MAO-B is not involved in the intestinal tyramine interaction, at low doses of 5–10 mg/day, dietary interaction with selegiline would probably be minimal; therefore, no drug interactions have been reported. An interaction between selegiline and narcotics has been reported and should be kept in mind.

SUMMARY

Various MAOIs have been shown to be effective in treating a wide variety of psychiatric disorders, including depression, panic disorder, social phobia, and PTSD. The classic MAOIs are currently used only rarely as first-line medication because of potential dietary interaction and other long-term side effects. With the introduction of reversible inhibitors of MAO-A enzyme, such as moclobemide and brofaromine, which have fewer side effects and no dietary restrictions compared with classic MAOIs, first-line use should increase. In fact, the risk-benefit ratio for these compounds is highly favorable compared with other antidepressants. The MAO-B inhibitor selegiline is used to reduce the progression of Parkinson's disease. Its utility in treating other degenerative disorders is currently being assessed. New applications and wider use of these compounds may be found in the near future.

REFERENCES

Amrein R, Allen SR, Guentert TW, et al: Pharmacology of reversible MAOI. Br J Psychiatry 144:66–71, 1989

Amrein R, Guntert TW, Dingemanse J, et al: Interactions of moclobemide with concomitantly administered medication: evidence from pharmacological and clinical studies. Psychopharmacology (Berl) 106:S24–S31, 1992

Anonymous: Cheese and tranylcypromine (letter). BMJ 3(718):354, 1970

Blackwell B, Marley E, Price J, et al: Hypertensive interactions between monoamine oxidase inhibitors and food stuffs. Br J Psychiatry 113:349–365, 1967

Bloch RG, Doonief AS, Buchberg AS, et al: The clinical effect of isoniazid and iproniazid in the treatment of pulmonary tuberculosis. Ann Intern Med 40:881–900, 1954

Cesura AM, Pletscher A: The new generation of monoamine oxidase inhibitors. Prog Drug Res 38:171–297, 1992

Cooper AJ: MAO inhibitors and headache (letter). BMJ 2:420, 1967

Crane GE: Iproniazid (Marsilid) phosphate, a therapeutic agent for mental disorders and debilitating disease. Psychiatry Research Reports 8:142–152, 1957

Cronin D: Monoamine-oxidase inhibitors and cheese (letter). BMJ 5469:1065, 1965

Cusson JR, Goldenberg E, Larochelle P: Effect of a novel monoamine oxidase inhibitor, moclobemide on the sensitivity to intravenous tyramine and norepinephrine in humans. J Clin Pharmacol 31:462–467, 1991

DaPrada M, Kettler R, Burkard WP, et al: Moclobemide, an antidepressant with short-lasting MAO-A inhibition: brain catecholamines and tyramine pressor effects in rats, in Monoamine Oxidase and Disease: Prospects for Therapy With Reversible Inhibitors. Edited by Tipton KF, Dostert P, Strolin Benedetti M. New York, Academic Press, 1984, pp 137–154

DaPrada M, Kettler R, Keller HH, et al: Neurochemical profile of moclobemide, a short-acting and reversible inhibitor of monoamine oxidase type A. J Pharmacol Exp Ther 248:400–414, 1989

Davidson J, Turnbull C: Loss of appetite and weight associated with the monoamine oxidase inhibitor isocarboxazid. J Clin Psychopharmacol 2:263–266, 1982

Davidson J, Raft D, Pelton S: An outpatient evaluation of phenelzine and imipramine. J Clin Psychiatry 48:143–146, 1987a

Davidson J, Walker JI, Kilts C: A pilot study of phenelzine in the treatment of post-traumatic stress disorder. Br J Psychiatry 150:252–255, 1987b

Evans DL, Davidson J, Raft D: Early and late side effects of phenelzine. J Clin Psychopharmacol 2:208–210, 1982

Finberg JPM, Youdim MBH: Reversible monoamine oxidase inhibitors and the cheese effect, in Monoamine Oxidase and Disease: Prospects for Therapy With Reversible Inhibitors. Edited by Tipton KF, Dostert P, Strolin Benedetti M. New York, Academic Press, 1984, pp 479–485

Gabelic I, Kuhn B: Moclobemide (Ro 11–1163) versus tranylcypromine in the treatment of endogenous depression (abstract). Acta Psychiatr Scand Suppl 360:63, 1990

Gerlach M, Youdim MB, Riederer P: Pharmacology of selegiline. Neurology 47 (6 suppl 3):S137–S145, 1996

Glick R, Harrison W, Endicott J, et al: Treatment of premenstrual dysphoric symptoms in depressed women. J Am Med Wom Assoc 46:182–185, 1991

Goldstein DM, Goldberg RL: Monoamine oxidase inhibitor-induced speech blockage (case report). J Clin Psychiatry 47:604, 1986

Goodheart RS, Dunne JW, Edis RH: Phenelzine associated peripheral neuropathy clinical and electrophysiologic findings. Aust N Z J Med 21:339–340, 1991

Haefely W, Burkard WP, Cesura AM, et al: Biochemistry and pharmacology of moclobemide: a prototype RIMA. Psychopharmacology (Berl) 106 (suppl):S6–S15, 1992

Hagan JJ, Middlemiss DN, Sharpe PC, et al: Parkinson's disease: prospects for improved drug therapy. Trends Pharmacol Sci 18:156–163, 1997

Harrison WM, Stewart J, Ehrhardt AA, et al: A controlled study of the effects of antidepressants on sexual function. Psychopharmacol Bull 21:85–88, 1985

Hedberg DL, Gordon MW, Glueck BC Jr: Six cases of hypertensive crisis in patients on tranylcypromine after eating chicken livers. Am J Psychiatry 122:933–937, 1966

Himmelhoch JM, Fuchs CZ, Symons BJ: A double-blind study of tranylcypromine treatment of major anergic depression. J Nerv Ment Dis 170:628–634, 1982

Himmelhoch JM, Thase ME, Mallinger AG, et al: Tranylcypromine versus imipramine in anergic bipolar depression. Am J Psychiatry 148:910–916, 1991

Husain M, Edmondson DE, Singer TP: Kinetic studies on the catalytic mechanism of liver monoamine oxidase. Biochemistry 21:595–600, 1982

Jacobson JN: Anorgasmia caused by an MAOI (letter). Am J Psychiatry 144:527, 1987

Jenike MA: Rapid response of severe obsessive-compulsive disorder to tranylcypromine. Am J Psychiatry 138:1249–1250, 1981

Johnstone EC: Relationship between acetylator status and response to phenelzine. Mod Probl Pharmacopsychiatry 10:30–37, 1975

Johnstone EC, Marsh W: The relationship between response to phenelzine and acetylator status in depressed patients. Proc R Soc Lond B Biol Sci 66:947–949, 1973

Kelly D, Mitchell-Heggs N, Sherman D: Anxiety and the effects of sodium lactate assessed clinically and physiologically. Br J Psychiatry 119:129–141, 1971

Kennedy SH, Warsh JJ, Mainprize E, et al: A trial of isocarboxazid in the treatment of bulimia. J Clin Psychopharmacol 8:391–396, 1988

Kline NS: Clinical experience with iproniazid (Marsilid). Journal of Clinical and Experimental Psychopathology 19 (suppl 1):72–78, 1958

Kosten TR, Frank JB, Dan E, et al: Pharmacotherapy for post-traumatic stress disorder using phenelzine or imipramine. J Nerv Ment Dis 179:366–370, 1991

Larsen JK, Gjerris A, Holm P, et al: Moclobemide in depression: a randomized, multicentre trial against isocarboxazide and clomipramine emphasizing atypical depression. Acta Psychiatr Scand 84:564–570, 1991

Lawlor BA, Aisen PS, Green C, et al: Selegiline in the treatment of behavioural disturbance in Alzheimer's disease. Int J Geriatr Psychiatry 12:319–322, 1997

Liebowitz MR, Schneier F, Campeas R, et al: Phenelzine vs atenolol in social phobia: a placebo-controlled comparison. Arch Gen Psychiatry 49:290–300, 1992

Lydiard RB, Laraia MT, Howell EF, et al: Phenelzine treatment of panic disorder: lack of effect on pyridoxal phosphate levels. J Clin Psychopharmacol 9:428–431, 1989

Lyytinen J, Kaakkola S, Ahtila S, et al: Simultaneous MAO-B and COMT inhibition in L-dopa-treated patients with Parkinson's disease. Mov Disord 12:497–505, 1997

McElroy SL, Keck PE Jr, Pope HG Jr, et al: Pharmacological treatment of kleptomania and bulimia nervosa. J Clin Psychopharmacol 9:358–360, 1989

McGrath PJ, Stewart JW, Harrison W, et al: Phenelzine treatment of melancholia. J Clin Psychiatry 47:420–422, 1986

Mendelson G: Narcotics and monoamine oxidase-inhibitors (letter). Med J Aust 1:400, 1979

Murphy DL, Garrick NA, Aulakh CS, et al: New contribution from basic science of understanding the effects of monoamine oxidase inhibiting antidepressants. J Clin Psychiatry 45:37–43, 1984

Murphy DL, Sunderland T, Garrick NA, et al: Selective amine oxidase inhibitors: basic to clinical studies and back, in Clinical Pharmacology in Psychiatry. Edited by Dahl SG, Gram A, Potter W. Berlin, Springer Verlag, 1987, pp 135–146

O'Brien S, McKeon P, O'Regan M, et al: Blood pressure effects of tranylcypromine when prescribed singly and in combination with amitriptyline. J Clin Psychopharmacol 12:104–109, 1992

Paykel ES, West PS, Rowan PR, et al: Influence of acetylator phenotype on antidepressant effects of phenelzine. Br J Psychiatry 141:243–248, 1982

Pearce LB, Roth JA: Human brain monoamine oxidase type B: mechanism of deamination as probed by steady-state methods. Biochemistry 24:1821–1826, 1985

Quitkin F, Rifkin A, Klein DF: Monoamine oxidase inhibitors: a review of antidepressant effectiveness. Arch Gen Psychiatry 36:749–760, 1979

Quitkin FM, McGrath PJ, Stewart JW, et al: Atypical depression, panic attacks, and response to imipramine and phenelzine: a replication. Arch Gen Psychiatry 47:935–941, 1990

Quitkin FM, Harrison W, Stewart JW, et al: Response to phenelzine and imipramine in placebo nonresponders with atypical depression: a new application of the crossover design. Arch Gen Psychiatry 48:319–323, 1991

Ramsay RR, Singer TP: The kinetic mechanisms of monoamine oxidases A and B. Biochem Soc Trans 19:219–223, 1991

Rossel L, Moll E: Moclobemide versus tranylcypromine in the treatment of depression. Acta Psychiatr Scand Suppl 360:61–62, 1990

Rowan PR, Paykel ES, West PS, et al: Effects of phenelzine and acetylator phenotype. Neuropharmacology 20(12B):1353–1354, 1981

Simpson GM, Gratz SS: Comparison of the pressor effect of tyramine after treatment with phenelzine and moclobemide in healthy male volunteers. J Clin Pharm Ther 52:286–291, 1992

Stack CG, Rogers P, Linter SPK: Monoamine oxidase inhibitors and anaesthesia: a review. Br J Anaesth 60:222–227, 1988

Thase ME, Mallinger AG, McKnight D, et al: Treatment of imipramine-resistant recurrent depression, IV: a double-blind crossover study of tranylcypromine for anergic bipolar depression. Am J Psychiatry 149:195–198, 1992

Tyrer PJ, Candy J, Kelly D: A study of the clinical effects of phenelzine and placebo in the treatment of phobic anxiety. Psychopharmacologia 32:237–254, 1973

Vallejo J, Gasto C, Catalan R, et al: Double-blind study of imipramine versus phenelzine in melancholias and dysthymic disorders. Br J Psychiatry 151:639–642, 1987

Versiani M, Mundim FD, Nardi AE, et al: Tranylcypromine in social phobia. J Clin Psychopharmacol 8:279–283, 1988

Versiani M, Nardi AE, Mundim FD, et al: Pharmacotherapy of social phobia: a controlled study with moclobemide and phenelzine. Br J Psychiatry 161:353–360, 1992

Walsh BT, Stewart JW, Roose SP, et al: A double-blind trial of phenelzine in bulimia. J Psychiatr Res 19(2–3):485–489, 1985

Walsh BT, Gladis M, Roose SP, et al: A controlled trial of phenelzine in bulimia. Psychopharmacol Bull 23:49–51, 1987

Wells DG: MAOI revisited. Can J Anaesth 36:64–74, 1989

Wesnes KA, Simpson PM, Christmas L, et al: Acute cognitive effects of moclobemide and trazodone, alone and in combination with alcohol, in the elderly. Br J Clin Pharmacol 27:647P–648P, 1989

White K, Razani J, Cadow B, et al: Tranylcypromine vs nortriptyline vs placebo in depressed outpatients: a controlled trial. Psychopharmacology (Berl) 82:258–262, 1984

Youdim MBH, DaPrada M, Amrein R (eds): The cheese effect and new reversible MAO-A inhibitors. Proceedings of the Round Table of the International Conference on New Directions in Affective Disorders, Jerusalem, Israel, 5–9 April 1987

Zajecka J, Fawcett J: Susceptibility to spontaneous MAOI hypertensive episodes (letter). J Clin Psychiatry 52:513–514, 1991

Zeller EA: Diamine oxidase, in The Enzymes, Vol 8, 2nd Edition. Edited by Boyer PD, Lardy H, Myrback K. London, Academic Press, 1963, pp 313–335

Zisook S: Side effects of isocarboxazid. J Clin Psychiatry 45(7 part 2):53–58, 1984

Zisook S, Braff DL, Click MA: Monoamine oxidase inhibitors in the treatment of atypical depression. J Clin Psychopharmacol 5:131–137, 1985

decline in trazodone use. The medication is now available in generic formulation.

Structure-Activity Relations

Trazodone is chemically unrelated to other antidepressant drugs, although it does resemble some of the side-chain components of tricyclic antidepressants (TCAs) and the phenothiazines. Its structure (shown in Figure 13–1) includes a triazole moiety that may be critical to its antidepressant activity (Walters 1982).

Pharmacological Profile

Trazodone's effects on serotonergic systems are complex. Trazodone itself is a relatively weak SSRI compared with the more potent SSRIs such as fluoxetine and sertraline (Hyttel 1982). However, it is relatively *specific* for serotonin uptake inhibition, with minimal effects on norepinephrine or dopamine reuptake (Hyttel 1982). In addition, trazodone has some serotonin (5-HT) receptor antagonist activity, particularly at 5-HT_{1A}, 5-HT_{1C}, and 5-HT_2 receptor subtypes (Haria et al. 1994). Furthermore, its active metabolite, m-chlorophenylpiperazine (mCPP), is a potent direct serotonin agonist. Thus, trazodone can be viewed as a mixed serotonergic agonist/antagonist, with the relative amount of mCPP accumulation affecting the relative degree of the predominant agonist activity.

In vivo, trazodone is virtually devoid of anticholinergic activity, and in clinical studies, the incidence of anticholinergic side effects is similar to that seen with placebo (Boschsmans 1987; Schuckit 1987). Trazodone is a relatively weak blocker of presynaptic α_2-adrenergic receptors and a relatively potent antagonist of postsynaptic α_1-adrenergic receptors (Brogden et al. 1981). The latter property probably accounts for trazodone's propensity to cause orthostatic hypotension, as discussed in the section, "Indications," later in this chapter. Trazodone has moderate antihistaminergic (H_1) activity (Marek et al. 1992).

Pharmacokinetics and Disposition

Trazodone is well absorbed after oral administration, with peak blood levels occurring about 1 hour after dosing when the drug is taken on an empty stomach and about

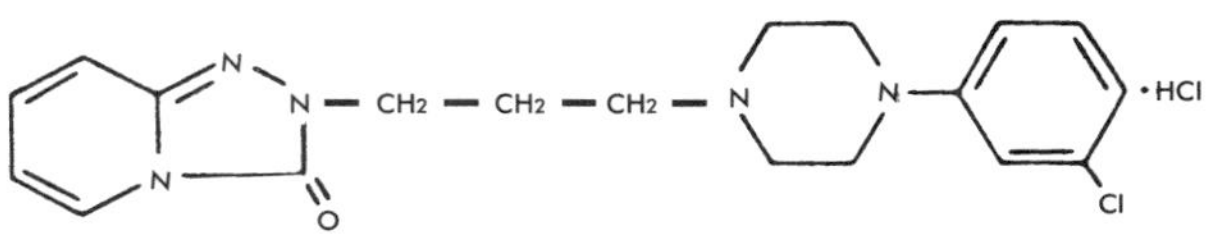

Figure 13–1. Chemical structure for trazodone.

2 hours after dosing when the drug is taken with food. Trazodone is 89%–95% bound to protein in plasma. Elimination appears to be biphasic, consisting of an initial alpha phase followed by a slower beta phase, with half-lives of 3–6 and 5–9 hours, respectively. The area under the plasma concentration-time curve (AUC) following an oral 100-mg dose of trazodone is significantly greater in elderly people compared with young volunteers (Bayer et al. 1983). Other studies, however, suggest that bioavailability is not influenced by age or by food intake, and gender differences appear to be inconsistent (Greenblatt et al. 1987; Nilsen and Dale 1992).

Trazodone undergoes extensive hepatic metabolism, including hydroxylation, splitting at the pyridine ring, oxidation, and N-oxidation (Garattini 1974). Less than 1% of the drug is excreted unchanged in the feces and urine (Caccia et al. 1981). The active metabolite, mCPP (see "Pharmacological Profile" above), is cleared more slowly than the parent compound (4- to 14-hour half-life), and it reaches higher concentrations in the brain than in plasma (Caccia et al. 1981). The cytochrome P450 (CYP) 2D6 isoenzyme appears to be involved in the metabolism of trazodone, suggesting the potential for interaction with other drugs that compete as a substrate for this isoenzyme (Yasui et al. 1995).

The relation between steady-state blood levels and clinical response to trazodone is unclear. In a study of geriatric patients, plasma concentrations of trazodone were lower in responders compared with nonresponders (Spar 1987). However, this study was limited by the lack of a fixed-dose design (increasing the chances that patients who were destined to be nonresponders would have continued dose increases, yielding relatively higher plasma levels) and the small sample size. Another study of geriatric patients found a positive relation between steady-state trazodone plasma concentrations and clinical response in a sample of 11 subjects (Monteleone and Gnocchi 1990). To our knowledge, well-designed studies examining the relation between plasma mCPP concentrations and trazodone levels have not been reported. Such studies could shed light on the question of trazodone's mechanism of action, in which mCPP might play a critical role (see next section).

Mechanism of Action

The ultimate mechanism of action of trazodone remains unclear. The mixed agonist/antagonist profile for its effects on serotonin is interesting. Although the drug is often referred to as a serotonin reuptake inhibitor, such labeling overlooks the complexity of its effects on this neurotransmitter system. For example, binding studies confirm that trazodone has relative selectivity for serotonin reuptake sites (Hyttel 1982); however, in vivo, it blocks the head twitch response induced by classic serotonin agonists in animals (Brogden et al. 1981). In addition, the potent serotonin agonist properties of trazodone's major metabolite, mCPP, probably play a role in the mechanism of action of the parent compound. It is also interesting that trazodone, unlike the vast majority of antidepressants, does not produce downregulation of β-adrenergic receptors in rat cortex (Sulser 1983).

Indications

The primary indication for trazodone is the treatment of major depression. In more than two dozen double-blind, placebo-controlled studies in Europe and the United States, trazodone's efficacy has been consistently superior to that of placebo and equivalent to that of conventional TCAs (Golden et al. 1988a). In a review of the double-blind studies published after trazodone's release in the United States, Schatzberg (1987) found trazodone's therapeutic efficacy to be similar to that of TCAs in patients with either endogenous or nonendogenous depression. Furthermore, the accumulated data suggest that trazodone may have a more pronounced, earlier onset of anxiolytic action compared with conventional antidepressants—perhaps reflecting its potent sedative properties (Schatzberg 1987). Lader's (1987) review of the European literature yielded similar findings: data from open and double-blind trials suggest that trazodone's antidepressant efficacy is comparable to that of amitriptyline, doxepin, and mianserin. Also, trazodone showed anxiolytic properties, low cardiotoxicity, and relatively mild side effects in the European studies (Lader 1987).

Questions have been raised about trazodone's effectiveness in treating severely ill patients, especially those with prominent psychomotor retardation (Klein and Muller 1985). Shopsin et al. (1981) pointed out that in several unpublished, double-blind, controlled studies, independent groups at different institutions found extremely low rates of response to trazodone (i.e., 10%–20%) in depressed patients. Lader (1987) acknowledged that the actual numbers of depressed patients with severe psychomotor retardation that have been reported in individual studies are too small to resolve the continued impression among many clinicians that trazodone's efficacy is limited in this population.

In relatively recent direct comparisons with other second-generation antidepressants, trazodone's performance has been mixed. In a double-blind, placebo-controlled trial, both trazodone and venlafaxine were significantly superior to placebo in terms of mean change from baseline in Hamilton Rating Scale for Depression (Hamilton 1960) scores, yet the final response rates were 55% for placebo, 60% for trazodone, and 72% for venlafaxine. It is not surprising that trazodone was more effective than venlafaxine in ameliorating sleep disturbances and was associated with the most dizziness and somnolence (Cunningham et al. 1994). In a double-blind comparison, trazodone and bupropion response rates were 46% and 58%, respectively. Trazodone was more likely to be associated with somnolence, appetite increase, and edema (Weisler et al. 1994).

Because trazodone has minimal anticholinergic activity, it was especially welcomed as a treatment for depressed geriatric patients when it first became available in 1982. Three double-blind studies reported that trazodone has antidepressant efficacy similar to that of other antidepressants in geriatric patients (Gerner 1987). However, a side effect of trazodone, orthostatic hypotension, which causes dizziness and the risk of falling, can have devastating consequences in elderly patients; thus, this side effect, along with sedation, often makes trazodone less acceptable in this population compared with newer compounds that share its lack of anticholinergic activity but not the rest of its side-effect profile. Still, trazodone is often helpful for depressed geriatric patients with severe agitation and insomnia. In fact, case reports of its use in controlling agitation and hostility associated with dementia in geriatric patients have been published (Greenwald et al. 1986; Simpson and Foster 1986). The use of trazodone to control aggression in nongeriatric patients with organic mental disorders has yielded mixed results in a small number of patients (Gedye 1991; Pinner and Rich 1988).

Trazodone has been reported to have antianxiety properties as well. In a study based in a general practice setting, the anxiolytic efficacy of trazodone was equal to that of chlordiazepoxide (Wheatley 1976). Another study found that trazodone has antianxiety properties in doses as low as 50 mg/day (Schwartz and Blendl 1974). In a randomized, double-blind, placebo-controlled trial, trazodone's anxiolytic efficacy was comparable to that of diazepam in weeks 3 through 8 of treatment for generalized anxiety disorder, although patients treated with diazepam had greater improvement during the first 2 weeks of treatment (Rickels et al. 1993).

Many clinicians use low-dose trazodone as a sleep-promoting agent, especially in patients for whom benzodiazepines may be risky (e.g., patients with sleep apnea or histories of sedative-hypnotic abuse). In a double-blind, placebo-controlled trial of 17 depressed patients with insomnia related to fluoxetine or bupropion pharmacotherapy, trazodone was an effective hypnotic agent at doses of 50–100 mg (Nierenberg et al. 1994). Several case series reported trazodone (25–150 mg) response rates to antidepressant-associated insomnia ranging from 31% to 92% (Jacobsen 1990; Metz and Shader 1990; Nierenberg and Keck 1989).

A limited number of case reports indicate that trazodone is associated with improvement in obsessive-compulsive disorder and associated depression (Baxter 1985; Kim 1987; Lydiard 1986; Prasad 1984), but a double-blind, placebo-controlled study found that trazodone lacked antiobsessional effects (Pigott et al. 1992). A handful of reports describe the use of trazodone in the treatment of bulimia nervosa, including a well-designed, placebo-controlled trial in 42 women that found trazodone to be superior to placebo in reducing the frequency of episodes of binge eating and vomiting (Hudson et al. 1989). Also, alone and in combination with yohimbine, trazodone has been effective in the treatment of erectile dysfunction (Kurt et al. 1994; Lance et al. 1995; Montorsi et al. 1994). Finally, case reports and open trials describe the use of trazodone in a wide variety of neuropsychiatric syndromes, including sleep terror disorder (Balon 1994), disruptive behavior disorders in children (Zubieta and Alessi 1992), trichotillomania (Sunkureddi and Markovitz 1993), posttraumatic stress disorder and dementia-associated disruptive behavior (Hargrave 1993), Alzheimer's disease and other dementias (Lebert et al. 1994; Schneider and Sobin 1992; Tejera and Saravay 1995), and continuous screaming (Pasion and Kirby 1993).

Side Effects and Toxicology

As mentioned earlier in this chapter, trazodone lacks the anticholinergic side effects of TCAs; thus, trazodone is especially useful in those situations in which antimuscarinic effects would be particularly problematic (e.g., patients with prostatic hypertrophy, closed-angle glaucoma, severe constipation). Its propensity to cause sedation is a dual-edged sword. For many patients, the relief from agitation, anxiety, and insomnia can be rapid; for others, including those with considerable psychomotor retardation and feelings of low energy, therapeutic doses of trazodone may not be tolerable because of sedation.

Trazodone elicits orthostatic hypotension in some patients, probably as a consequence of α_1-adrenergic receptor blockade. Trazodone-related syncope in the elderly has been described (Nambudiri et al. 1989). At therapeutic doses, it has no negative inotropic effect on the heart and, therefore, no tendency to cause heart failure. However, case reports have noted cardiac arrhythmias emerging in

apparent relation to trazodone treatment, both in patients with preexisting mitral valve prolapse and in patients with negative personal and family histories of cardiac disease (Janowsky et al. 1983; Lippman et al. 1983).

A relatively rare, but dramatic, side effect associated with trazodone is priapism. More than 200 cases have been reported (Thompson et al. 1990), and the manufacturer estimates the incidence of any abnormal erectile function to be approximately 1 in 6,000 male patients treated with trazodone. The risk for this side effect appears to be greatest during the first month of treatment at low doses (i.e., <150 mg/day). Early recognition of any abnormal erectile function, including prolonged or inappropriate erections, is important and should prompt discontinuation of trazodone treatment. Also, clinical reports have described trazodone-associated psychosexual side effects in women. Three women experienced increased libido above premorbid levels in association with trazodone treatment, and after resolution of their depression, two of them were reluctant to discontinue the medication because of this side effect (Gatrell 1986). There is a single case report of priapism of the clitoris (Pescatori et al. 1993) and of spontaneous orgasms in an elderly postmenopausal woman (Purcell and Ghurye 1995).

Mania has been observed in association with trazodone treatment, as with nearly all antidepressants. The switch to mania has been described in bipolar patients as well as in patients with previous diagnoses of unipolar depression (Arana and Kaplan 1985; Knobler 1986; Lennhoff 1987; Zmitek 1987). In a literature review, Terao (1993) found that the switch process occurs more rapidly in trazodone-treated patients than in fluoxetine-treated patients (average time to onset of mania: 16 days vs. 59 days, respectively).

Other rare side effects that have recently been associated with trazodone treatment include chronic active hepatitis (Beck et al. 1993) and agranulocytosis (Van der Klauw et al. 1993). Considering the worldwide experience with this medication, these toxic syndromes, if not coincidental, are exceedingly rare. Also, serotonin syndrome has been described in patients taking trazodone, usually in combination with other serotomimetic medications (see next section). Clinicians should recognize this potential toxicity when considering the use of trazodone for SSRI-associated insomnia.

Trazodone has an important advantage—a wider therapeutic margin—in comparison with tricyclics, monoamine oxidase inhibitors (MAOIs), and a few other second-generation antidepressants. Trazodone appears to be *relatively* safer than other antidepressants in overdose situations, especially when it is the only agent taken. Fatalities are rare, even with large overdoses; uneventful recoveries have been reported after ingestion of doses as high as 6,000–9,200 mg (Ayd 1984). In one report, 9 of 294 overdose cases were fatal, and all 9 patients had taken other central nervous system (CNS) depressants with trazodone (Gamble and Peterson 1986). When trazodone overdoses occur, clinicians should carefully monitor for hypotension, a potentially serious toxic effect.

Drug-Drug Interactions

Trazodone can potentiate the effects of other CNS depressants. In mice, it increases hexobarbital sleeping time (B. Silvestrini et al. 1968). In a single case report, phenytoin toxicity emerged in association with the addition of trazodone therapy (Dorn 1986). Patients should be warned about increased drowsiness and sedation when trazodone is combined with other CNS depressants, including alcohol.

In theory, the combination of trazodone with other pro-serotonergic agents could result in the development of the *serotonin syndrome* (Sternbach 1991); this toxic syndrome has been reported after the combined use of trazodone and buspirone (Goldberg and Huk 1992), trazodone and an MAOI plus methylphenidate (Bodner et al. 1995), and trazodone and paroxetine (Reeves and Bullen 1995). Lithium potentiation of trazodone treatment has been described, however, without any mention of such toxicity (Birkhimer et al. 1983). The combination of trazodone with an MAOI, as with other antidepressants, should be handled with great caution. However, there are case reports of the successful combination of trazodone with an MAOI in treatment-resistant depressed patients (Zimmer et al. 1984). As Rudorfer and Potter (1989) pointed out, the ability to add trazodone to ongoing MAOI treatment could enable clinicians to use trazodone for MAOI-induced insomnia.

Trazodone inhibits the antihypertensive effects of clonidine (van Zwieten 1977), and for this reason, Georgotas et al. (1982) recommend avoiding the combined use of these two agents. On the other hand, trazodone itself can cause hypotension, especially orthostatic hypotension, and the manufacturer states in the package insert that concomitant administration of Desyrel with antihypertensive therapy may require a reduction in the dose of the antihypertensive agent.

NEFAZODONE

History and Discovery

Nefazodone has selective and unique effects on the serotonin system. Its analogue, trazodone, was found to be an effective second-generation antidepressant. Unfortunately, trazodone is also very sedating and has a propensity to cause postural hypotension (see above subsection, "Side Effects and Toxicology"). A deliberate effort to improve the pharmacological profile of trazodone with receptor-binding techniques led to the discovery of nefazodone (Taylor et al. 1986). It became available for clinical use in the United States in the latter part of 1994.

Structure-Activity Relations

Nefazodone is a phenylpiperazine compound. Its chemical structure, which is similar to that of trazodone, is depicted in Figure 13–2.

Pharmacological Profile

In vitro studies have found that nefazodone is a 5-HT$_2$ receptor antagonist, but it has little affinity for α_2, β-adrenergic, or 5-HT$_{1A}$ receptors (Eison et al. 1990). Nefazodone's inhibition of serotonin reuptake (similar potency to desipramine) and norepinephrine reuptake (similar potency to norfluoxetine) is limited (Bolden-Watson and Richelson 1993). Its affinity for the α_1-adrenergic receptor is less than that of trazodone (Eison et al. 1990). Nefazodone is inactive at most other receptor-binding sites, including muscarinic, H$_1$, dopamine, benzodiazepine, γ-aminobutyric acid, μ-opiate, and calcium channel receptors (Taylor et al. 1986).

Nefazodone has two principal active metabolites—hydroxynefazodone and mCPP. Hydroxynefazodone has similar affinities for 5-HT$_2$ receptors and serotonin reuptake sites compared with nefazodone, whereas mCPP has modest activity at serotonin reuptake sites (Eison et al. 1990) and is a potent direct serotonin agonist. Recently, another human metabolite, triazoledione, has been identified and appears to have pharmacological activity similar to that of nefazodone (Mayol et al. 1994).

Nefazodone's activity in animal models is suggestive of antidepressant activity. For example, it prevents reserpine-induced ptosis in mice and reverses learned

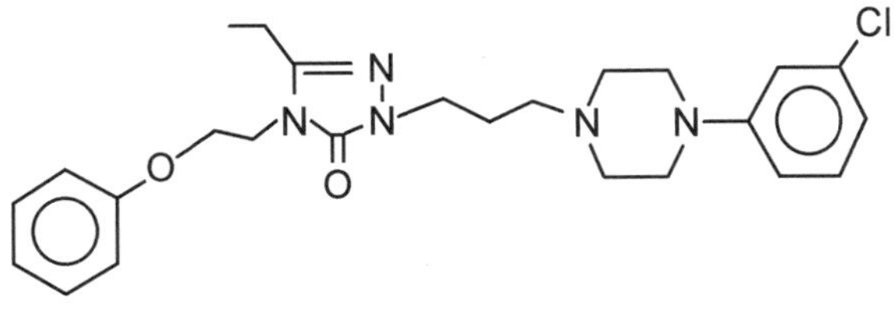

Figure 13–2. Chemical structure for nefazodone.

helplessness in rats (Eison et al. 1990). Nefazodone increases REM sleep in humans, in sharp contrast to most other antidepressants, which typically suppress REM sleep (Sharpley et al. 1992).

Pharmacokinetics and Disposition

Nefazodone is rapidly and completely absorbed from the gastrointestinal tract and has an absolute bioavailability of 15%–23% because of extensive first-pass hepatic metabolism. Peak plasma levels occur between 1 and 3 hours, and steady state is achieved in 3–4 days with a twice-daily dosing regimen. Nefazodone is metabolized primarily by the liver to three metabolites: hydroxynefazodone, desmethyl-hydroxynefazodone (triazoledione), and mCPP (only 3% of the parent compound at peak concentrations). Nefazodone has nonlinear kinetics, which result in greater than proportional mean plasma concentrations with higher doses. Similar kinetics for nefazodone and hydroxynefazodone are seen in poor and extensive metabolizers, whereas mCPP is eliminated more slowly by poor metabolizers. The elimination half-life is 2–4 hours for the parent compound and hydroxynefazodone, 18–33 hours for desmethyl-hydroxynefazodone, and 4–9 hours for mCPP. Nefazodone is extensively (99%) but loosely protein bound. It does not displace chlorpromazine, desipramine, diazepam, diphenylhydantoin, lidocaine, prazosin, propranolol, verapamil, or warfarin (data on file, Bristol-Myers Squibb Pharmaceutical Research Institute, June 1994). In patients with hepatic cirrhosis, single-dose nefazodone and hydroxynefazodone levels are about twice as high as in healthy volunteers, but the difference decreases to approximately 25% at steady state. Exposure to mCPP is about twofold to threefold greater in the cirrhotic patients, and exposure to triazoledione is similar after a single dose and at steady state (Barbhaiya et al. 1995b).

Mechanism of Action

The most likely means by which nefazodone acts as an antidepressant is through its effects on serotonin neurotransmission, but these effects are complex. Nefazodone blocks serotonin reuptake, thereby increasing serotonin availability in the synapse while functioning as a 5-HT$_2$ receptor antagonist. In addition, mCPP, nefazodone's active metabolite, functions as a serotonin agonist. In animal studies, long-term exposure to nefazodone increases the intensity of reciprocal forepaw treading induced by the 5-HT$_{1A}$ agonist 8-hydroxy-2-(di-N-propylamino)-tetralin, suggesting that nefazodone also enhances stimulation of 5-HT$_{1A}$ receptors (Eison et al. 1990). Nefazo-

done's effects on electrophysiological measures of serotonergic systems are similar to those of many other effective antidepressants (Blier et al. 1990).

Indications

Eight double-blind, placebo-controlled trials found that nefazodone is an effective antidepressant. Patients with symptoms meeting DSM-III-R (American Psychiatric Association 1987) criteria for major depression had a 72% response rate when treated with nefazodone in doses of 300–500 mg/day. The response rate dropped to 56% with doses of 200–300 mg/day and to 48% with a dose of 600 mg/day (placebo response rates did not differ significantly from those of the low- or high-dose ranges; Rickels et al. 1995). These findings suggest that nefazodone may have a "therapeutic window" similar to that of nortriptyline.

Nefazodone is effective in both first-episode and recurrent major depression, and several studies have shown that its efficacy is comparable to that of imipramine (Feighner et al. 1989; Fontaine et al. 1994). In one published multicenter comparison, nefazodone and imipramine were significantly superior to placebo in treating major depression. However, the response to the lower dose range of nefazodone (50–250 mg/day) was suboptimal, whereas the higher dose range (100–500 mg/day) produced more robust clinical response. In both nefazodone dose-range groups, fewer side effects were reported than in the imipramine group, and more nefazodone-treated patients completed 6 weeks of therapy than did the imipramine or placebo groups (Fontaine et al. 1994). The lower response rate at lower nefazodone doses has been confirmed by others (Mendels et al. 1995).

In a European study of patients with moderate to severe major depression, the efficacy of amitriptyline (50–200 mg/day) was clearly superior to that of nefazodone (100–400 mg/day) (Ansseau et al. 1994). In another study, both nefazodone and the comparison tricyclic imipramine were superior to placebo during long-term (1 year or longer) continuation therapy (Anton et al. 1994).

At present, published data regarding the use of nefazodone in the treatment of psychiatric disorders other than depression are quite limited. One open-label report described nefazodone's efficacy in the treatment of late luteal phase dysphoric disorder (Freeman et al. 1994). In an open-label study of major depression and comorbid obsessive-compulsive disorder, nefazodone showed only a modest trend toward reducing obsessive-compulsive disorder symptom severity (Nelson 1994). Nefazodone has also been shown to have some analgesic properties and to potentiate morphine analgesia in animal studies, which suggests that it may have a role in pain management (Pick et al. 1992).

Side Effects and Toxicology

Nefazodone has been found to be safe and well tolerated in clinical trials that included approximately 2,250 patients (Fontaine 1993). It has a relatively benign side-effect profile, as expected based on its lack of affinity for muscarinic and histaminic receptors. Its lower affinity, compared with that of trazodone, for α_1-adrenergic receptors suggests that it should have a lower propensity to cause orthostatic hypotension. Side effects that occur more frequently in patients who receive nefazodone, compared with placebo, include dizziness, asthenia, dry mouth, nausea, and constipation (Fontaine 1993). To place these observations into a clinical perspective, many of these side effects (i.e., dry mouth, constipation, sweating, and tremor) occur less often with nefazodone than with imipramine treatment. Also, there was no evidence of cardiac dysfunction or cardiotoxicity in a careful review of more than 2,000 patients. Nefazodone modestly reduced the resting pulse and supine blood pressure, but orthostatic hypotension was rare (Fontaine 1993).

Preskorn (1995) recently compared reported treatment-emergent adverse effects in patients receiving nefazodone and other antidepressants. The total cumulative incidence of treatment-emergent adverse effects for nefazodone was lower than that for imipramine or fluoxetine. The most common placebo-adjusted adverse effects associated with nefazodone were dry mouth (7.5%), somnolence (5.8%), dizziness (5.6%), nausea (5.5%), constipation (3.3%), blurred vision (3.2%), and postural hypotension (2.6%) (Preskorn 1995).

A recent double-blind, placebo-controlled crossover study (van Laar et al. 1995) compared the effects of imipramine with those of nefazodone on highway driving skills, cognitive functions, and daytime sleepiness in 12 adults and 12 elderly healthy subjects. Imipramine had a detrimental effect after a single dose on lateral position control, primarily in the adult group, that diminished after repeated dosing over a 7-day period and also produced continued minor impairment on psychomotor test performance. In contrast, a single dose of nefazodone did not impair highway driving skills and had only minor effects on psychomotor performance. After repeated dosing, however, 200 mg of nefazodone twice a day (but not 100 mg twice a day) produced slight impairment of lateral position control, and dose-related impairment of cognitive and memory functions occurred. Neither drug affected daytime sleepiness, which is surprising in terms of imipra-

mine's usual side-effect profile (van Laar et al. 1995).

In two published case reports of suicide attempts by overdose with nefazodone, involving 3,400 mg and 3,600 mg, life-threatening symptoms did not occur, and both patients recovered without any sequelae (Fontaine 1993). A recently published case report of nefazodone-induced mania suggested that the popular clinical opinion that probably all effective antidepressants can stimulate the switch process may be correct (Jeffries and Al-Jeshi 1995).

Drug-Drug Interactions

Reports on interactions between nefazodone and other drugs are just now emerging. In Phase 2 and 3 trials, the kinetics of alprazolam and triazolam, but not nefazodone, changed when these medications were given together. Recently, the manufacturer of triazolam issued a statement warning that its concurrent use with nefazodone is contraindicated because of nefazodone's significant inhibition of oxidative metabolism mediated by CYP3A. In the Phase 2 and 3 trials, some small increases in the plasma concentration of digoxin occurred with concurrent nefazodone administration. Although the observed increases in plasma digoxin concentrations were modest, the combined administration of the two drugs should be avoided, in light of the narrow therapeutic index for digoxin. No significant pharmacokinetic or pharmacodynamic interactions were noted between nefazodone and cimetidine, propranolol, warfarin, or lorazepam (Barbhaiya et al. 1995a; Salazar et al. 1995). Nefazodone potentiates the analgesic effects of morphine, but not the lethality or gastrointestinal effects, in animal models; thus, a potential use of nefazodone is as an adjunct in the pharmacological management of pain (Pick et al. 1992). Nefazodone does not appear to potentiate the sedative-hypnotic effects of alcohol and causes less disruption of human performance on psychomotor and memory tasks in combination with alcohol when compared with the coadministration of imipramine and alcohol (Frewer and Lader 1993).

BUPROPION

History and Discovery

Nearly three decades ago, a group of pharmacologists decided to search for a new antidepressant compound that was active in conventional antidepressant screening models yet was 1) different chemically, pharmacologically, and biochemically from TCAs; 2) not an inhibitor of monoamine oxidase; 3) not sympathomimetic; 4) not anticholinergic; and 5) not a cardiac depressant. It was believed that the first two characteristics would maximize the chances of developing a unique approach to treating depression, whereas the next three features would provide a compound with a side-effect profile that was far superior to that of existing antidepressant medications (Soroko and Maxwell 1983). The culmination of this intensive research program resulted in the development of bupropion.

Early studies confirmed that bupropion has efficacy comparable to that of conventional antidepressants but a side-effect profile that was generally viewed as milder and safer, with notable lack of substantial anticholinergic toxicity and relatively innocuous effects on cardiovascular function. Then, just as the drug was about to be released in 1986, seizures were reported in a few nondepressed bulimic study patients treated with bupropion. The manufacturer voluntarily withdrew the drug pending further, extensive clinical investigations. Finally, in 1989, bupropion was released for clinical use in the United States.

Structure-Activity Relations

Bupropion's chemical structure is unique among the antidepressants (Figure 13–3). It is a unicyclic aminoketone. The lack of complex heterocyclic fused rings, as well as the more common functional groups (e.g., *N*-methylpiperazine) often found in neuroleptics, is thought to contribute to bupropion's lack of the side effects usually seen in polycyclic antidepressants (Mehta 1983). Bupropion's chemical structure does resemble, in some aspects, that of certain psychostimulants, including amphetamine and the diet pill diethylpropion (Tenuate) (Mehta 1983), which

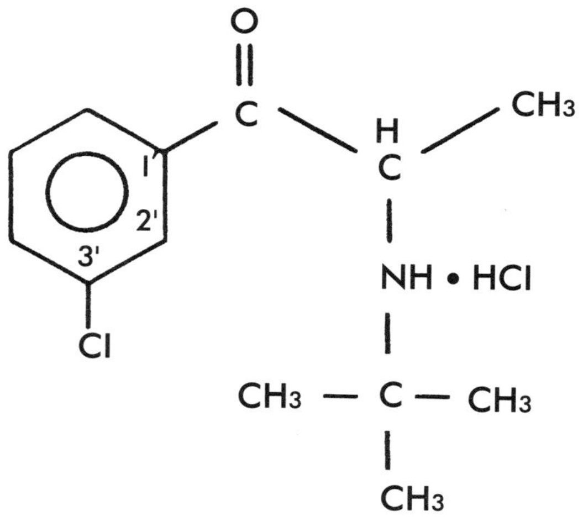

Figure 13–3. Chemical structure for bupropion.

may account for certain shared characteristics (Golden 1988). In fact, in a recent report, bupropion metabolites produced false-positive results on urine amphetamine toxicology screens (Nixon et al. 1995).

Pharmacological Profile

Bupropion is a relatively weak inhibitor of dopamine reuptake, with modest effects on norepinephrine reuptake and no effect on serotonin reuptake (Richelson 1991). It does not appear to be associated with downregulation of postsynaptic β-adrenergic receptors nor does it have significant effects on 5-HT$_2$, α_2-adrenergic, imipramine, or dopaminergic receptors in brain tissue (Ferris and Beaman 1983). It lacks anticholinergic activity and is at least 10-fold weaker than TCAs in terms of cardiac depressant effects (Soroko and Maxwell 1983).

Bupropion is active in the classic animal models for predicting antidepressant activity (Soroko and Maxwell 1983). Furthermore, its active metabolites, especially hydroxybupropion, have been shown to possess antidepressant profiles in mice (Martin et al. 1990). This finding may be relevant to preliminary observations from human studies exploring the roles these metabolites might play in determining clinical outcome (see next section) (Golden 1991).

In humans, bupropion (like nefazodone) does not suppress REM sleep. In fact, it appears to reduce REM latency (which is often abnormally low in depressed patients). In this regard, bupropion is different from most other treatments for depression, including tricyclics, MAOIs, SSRIs, and cognitive-behavior therapy (Nofzinger et al. 1994).

Pharmacokinetics and Disposition

Bupropion is rapidly absorbed after oral administration, with peak blood levels occurring within 2 hours (Lai and Schroeder 1983). Mean protein binding in healthy subjects is 85% (Findlay et al. 1981). The elimination is biphasic, with an initial phase of approximately 1.5 hours and a second phase of about 14 hours.

Bupropion undergoes extensive hepatic metabolism, including a pronounced first-pass effect. Three active metabolites—hydroxybupropion, threo-hydrobupropion, and erythyro-hydrobupropion—predominate over the parent compound in both plasma and cerebrospinal fluid at steady state and may play an important role in determining clinical response (see below) (Golden et al. 1988b).

There does not appear to be a consistent, clear relation between steady-state bupropion plasma concentrations and clinical response (Goodnick 1991). Preskorn (1983) found a curvilinear relationship between antidepressant efficacy and trough bupropion plasma concentrations, with greatest efficacy associated with bupropion plasma concentrations greater than 25 ng/mL but less than 100 ng/mL. On the other hand, Goodnick (1992) reported better response with trough levels of less than 30 ng/mL. In another study, no relation was found between plasma bupropion concentrations and clinical response; however, higher concentrations of each of the three active metabolites, especially hydroxybupropion, were significantly related to poor clinical outcome (Golden et al. 1988b). More clinical studies are required to clarify the potential utility of plasma bupropion metabolite measurements in clinical care. Preskorn (1991) proposed that bupropion should be the next antidepressant to undergo aggressive study for the value of therapeutic drug monitoring.

Mechanism of Action

The mechanism of action for bupropion remains unclear (Ascher et al. 1995). From the start, its effects on dopaminergic function have been a focus of investigation. Some of the behavioral effects of bupropion, including stimulation of locomotor activity and effects on the Porsolt forced swim test, are abolished after dopaminergic neurons are destroyed by 6-hydroxydopamine (Cooper et al. 1980). Bupropion-induced behavioral sensitization in the rat is accompanied by a selective potentiation of the effects of this compound on interstitial dopamine concentrations in the nucleus accumbens (Nomikos et al. 1992). In humans, plasma concentrations of homovanillic acid, a major metabolite of dopamine, increased in patients who did not respond to bupropion treatment but not in clinical responders (Golden et al. 1988d).

Noradrenergic systems may also play a critical role in the mechanism of action of bupropion. In a study investigating the effects of antidepressants on noradrenergic function in hospitalized depressed patients, bupropion, along with the norepinephrine reuptake inhibitor desipramine and MAOIs, increased 24-hour excretion of 6-hydroxymelatonin, a physiological gauge of noradrenergic activity, and simultaneously reduced "whole-body norepinephrine turnover," (i.e., the 24-hour excretion of norepinephrine and its metabolites) (Golden et al. 1988c). Bupropion's active metabolites, especially hydroxybupropion, inhibit the reuptake of norepinephrine into rat cortical tissue (Perumal et al. 1986).

Bupropion's metabolites may be quite important in determining clinical response. In animal models, hydroxybupropion has more potent antidepressant properties than does the parent compound, and threo-hydrobupropion also has some antidepressant activity (Martin et al. 1990). In depressed patients, metabolite concentrations predominate over bupropion concentrations in both plasma and cerebrospinal fluid (Golden et al. 1988b). As mentioned earlier in this section, there is no clear relation between plasma bupropion concentrations and clinical response, but concentrations of its metabolites, especially hydroxybupropion, are significantly greater in nonresponders compared with responders. This observation may reflect untoward effects that are evoked when the hydroxybupropion concentration exceeds a threshold for toxicity. On the other hand, hydroxybupropion may be responsible for bupropion's therapeutic effects, and a curvilinear plasma level–response relationship (similar to that seen with nortriptyline) may exist. However, future investigations of the mechanism of action of bupropion clearly must consider the role played by its active metabolites.

Indications

Bupropion has been shown to be as effective as standard TCAs and SSRIs and superior to placebo in treating hospitalized, as well as ambulatory, depressed patients (Chouinard 1983; Davidson et al. 1983; Feighner et al. 1986, 1991; Mendels et al. 1983; Merideth and Feighner 1983; Pitts et al. 1983). Under double-blind conditions, bupropion was superior to placebo in treating hospitalized patients who were refractory to tricyclics, and in an open-label study, outpatients with a history of either nonresponse or nonresponse plus intolerance to tricyclics had a marked improvement in their conditions after taking bupropion (Stern et al. 1983). In a recent open study of 41 depressed patients who did not respond to well-documented tricyclic treatment, about half responded to bupropion (Ferguson et al. 1994).

One report suggested that bupropion may be particularly promising in treating rapid-cycling bipolar II disorder (Haykal and Akiskal 1990). In that case series, all 6 patients' conditions improved, and 4 had "dramatic" improvement that was sustained after an average of 2 years of treatment. In addition, none of the patients developed hypomania or rapid cycling, in contrast to the experience with conventional antidepressants (Haykal and Akiskal 1990). Although there are case reports of possible bupropion precipitation of mania and a mixed affective state (Masand and Stern 1993; Zubieta and Demitrack 1991), a recent prospective, double-blind trial found that bupropion was less likely to induce hypomania or mania in bipolar depressed patients than was desipramine (Sachs et al. 1994). In contrast, in a series of 11 consecutive bipolar patients, 6 experienced hypomanic or manic symptoms when bupropion was added to their treatment regimen (Fogelson et al. 1992).

In light of bupropion's enhancement of dopaminergic neurotransmission, it is not surprising that it has been applied to conditions in which activation and other psychostimulant-like properties could be useful. Bupropion has been found to be effective in the treatment of attention-deficit/hyperactivity disorder in double-blind studies in children (Barrickman et al. 1995; Casat et al. 1989) and in an open trial in adults (Wender and Reimherr 1990). However, it may exacerbate tics in children with attention-deficit/hyperactivity disorder and comorbid Tourette's disorder (Spencer et al. 1993). Bupropion's activating properties have led to explorations of its potential use in the treatment of chronic fatigue syndrome (Goodnick 1990; Goodnick et al. 1992) and in the treatment of fatigue associated with multiple sclerosis (Duffy and Campbell 1994).

Uncontrolled case reports have described the use of bupropion in treating social phobia (Emmanuel et al. 1991). In a placebo-controlled, double-blind trial in patients with bulimia, bupropion was superior to placebo in reducing episodes of binge eating and purging (Horne et al. 1988). However, because four subjects experienced grand mal seizures during treatment, the use of bupropion in the treatment of bulimia should be avoided (Horne et al. 1988).

Side Effects and Toxicology

Bupropion's side-effect profile is clearly different from that of conventional TCAs. It lacks anticholinergic effects, is clearly not sedating, and suppresses appetite in some patients (Rudorfer and Potter 1989). Unlike several other second-generation antidepressants, bupropion does not cause psychosexual dysfunction (Gardner and Johnston 1985). Patients who experience psychosexual dysfunction in conjunction with fluoxetine treatment report substantially greater satisfaction with their sexual function while taking bupropion (Walker et al. 1993).

Bupropion's cardiovascular profile is especially favorable. It does not cause electrocardiogram changes and does not trigger orthostatic hypotension, even in patients with preexisting heart disease (Roose et al. 1987). Bupropion has been shown to be safer than nortriptyline in regard to cardiovascular side effects (Kiev et al. 1994).

Bupropion appears to be relatively less lethal following overdose than tricyclics and certain other antidepressants (Hayes and Kristoff 1986). In a review of 58 cases of bupropion overdose and 9 cases of combined bupropion/benzodiazepine ingestion, bupropion seemed to lack major cardiovascular toxicity. Neurological toxicity was found, including lethargy, tremors, and seizures (which re-

sponded well to either benzodiazepines or phenytoin) (Spiller et al. 1994). Two fatal overdoses that were reported were associated with peripheral blood levels of 4.0–4.2 mg/L of bupropion and total metabolite levels of 15 and 16.6 mg/L. By history, the estimated lethal doses were less than 10 g (Friel et al. 1993).

Many of bupropion's side effects can be predicted based on its stimulation of dopaminergic systems. Thus, like conventional psychostimulants, bupropion can have activating effects, which are often helpful in patients with psychomotor retardation but can be experienced as agitation or insomnia in others. Appetite suppression is also perceived as an advantage in some patients but a disadvantage in others. Psychotic symptoms, including hallucinations and delusions, can emerge in association with bupropion treatment (Golden et al. 1985). Since the initial description of bupropion-related psychoses, numerous case reports have described similar toxic reactions, including organic mental disorders (Ames et al. 1992), delirium (Dager and Heritch 1990), and catatonia (Jackson et al. 1992). These psychotic reactions may be a consequence of overstimulation of dopaminergic systems, because one series of patients with bupropion-associated psychoses had increased plasma concentrations of homovanillic acid, a major metabolite of dopamine (Golden et al. 1985).

A rare but serious side effect of bupropion is seizure induction. A careful review by Davidson (1989) found the incidence of seizures in patients receiving bupropion at doses of 450 mg/day or less ranged from 0.33% to 0.44%, depending on the method used to make the calculation. The cumulative 2-year risk in patients receiving 450 mg/day or less was 0.48%. To place these observations in the proper context, clinicians should be aware that the estimated frequency of seizures in outpatients with no predisposing factors who are receiving TCAs at modest doses (e.g., 150 mg/day or less) is 0.1% (Jick et al. 1983); at higher doses (e.g., 200 mg/day or greater), it rises to 0.6%–0.9% (Peck et al. 1983). Careful evaluation for risk factors (e.g., history of seizures, recent withdrawal from alcohol or anxiolytic drugs, concomitant therapy with drugs that lower the seizure threshold, history of organic brain disease or abnormal electroencephalogram), conservative dose titration with a maximum dose of 450 mg/day, and use of divided dose schedules (three times a day) should minimize the risk for bupropion-related seizures (Davidson 1989).

Drug-Drug Interactions

Because bupropion undergoes extensive hepatic transformation, other drugs that induce or inhibit hepatic enzyme systems may alter its metabolism. As with most antidepressants, the combined use of bupropion with MAOIs should be approached with caution because of the risk of a hypertensive reaction if bupropion is added to ongoing monoamine oxidase inhibition. Because bupropion provides dopaminergic activation, clinicians treating patients with coexisting Parkinson's disease and depression can often decrease the dose of antiparkinsonian medication when bupropion is added. The combination of bupropion and antiparkinsonian medication should be administered with care. Goetz et al. (1984) reported the emergence of hallucinations, confusion, and dyskinesia following the addition of bupropion to previously therapeutic doses of L-dopa.

The addition of bupropion to fluoxetine treatment has coincided with the onset of delirium (Van Putten and Shaffer 1990) and a grand mal seizure (Ciraulo and Shader 1990). The combination of bupropion and lithium may affect lithium serum levels and has been linked to seizures in three patients (Goodnick 1991), although this combination generally has been safe and well tolerated in a few published studies (Apter and Woolfolk 1990; Goodnick, in press; Haykal and Akiskal 1990). A report of two cases suggests that carbamazepine may decrease bupropion blood levels and increase hydroxybupropion levels, whereas bupropion may increase sodium valproate levels (Popli et al. 1995).

MIRTAZAPINE

History and Discovery

Mirtazapine is the newest antidepressant to become available for clinical use in the United States. It was introduced in the United States in August 1996. Mirtazapine is structurally similar to mianserin, which has been prescribed in several European countries for many years.

Structure-Activity Relations

Mirtazapine is a tetracyclic member of the piperazinoazepine class of compounds. It represents the 6-aza analogue of mianserin. The formulation contains a 50/50 racemic mixture of the R- and S-enantiomers (Davis and Wilde 1996). The chemical structure for mirtazapine is shown in Figure 13–4.

Pharmacological Profile

Mirtazapine has a pharmacological profile that is different from those of the currently available antidepressants. Mirtazapine has a unique pattern of effects on monoamine neurotransmission compared with other available antidepressants. It is a potent antagonist of central α_2-adrenergic auto- and heteroreceptors, is an antagonist of both 5-HT$_2$ and 5-HT$_3$ receptors, and has minimal effects on monoamine reuptake (de Boer 1996).

Mirtazapine enhances noradrenergic transmission but not via reuptake inhibition. Blockade of presynaptic α_2 noradrenergic autoreceptors leads to increased norepinephrine release (de Boer et al. 1988). In addition, it preferentially blocks α_2 heteroreceptors on serotonin neurons, which affects serotonin release (de Boer 1995). Mirtazapine's affinity for central presynaptic noradrenergic α_2 autoreceptors is approximately 10-fold higher than for central postsynaptic and peripheral presynaptic α_2 autoreceptors. In addition, its affinity for central presynaptic α_2 autoreceptors is about 30-fold greater than its affinity for central and peripheral α_1 adrenoceptors (de Boer 1995). Thus, this profile suggests that mirtazapine has selective α_2-adrenergic antagonist properties with a preference for central presynaptic α_2-adrenergic auto- and heteroreceptors.

Blockade of the α_2 heteroreceptors leads to enhanced serotonin release. At the same time, mirtazapine blocks 5-HT$_2$ and 5-HT$_3$ receptors. The net effect is selective enhancement of 5-HT$_1$-mediated neurotransmission (de Boer 1995). This pharmacological profile explains the difference in serotonin-linked side effects of mirtazapine compared with SSRIs, which nonselectively stimulate serotonin receptors (see section, "Side Effects and Toxicology," below). Mirtazapine has low affinity for muscarinic, cholinergic, and dopaminergic receptors. It does have a high affinity for H$_1$ receptors (de Boer 1995). This combination of potent antihistaminic activity and enhanced noradrenergic neurotransmission may explain the clinical

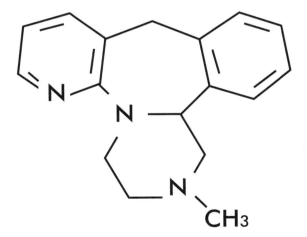

Figure 13–4. Chemical structure for mirtazapine.

observation that mirtazapine is *more* sedating at low doses than at higher doses; antihistaminergic side effects emerge at the lower doses but are somewhat counteracted by activation via noradrenergic stimulation at higher doses.

In preclinical monoamine depletion models of depression, such as the reserpine-induced sedation and hypokinesia, mirtazapine does not show activity. However, it is active in the olfactory bulbectomized rat model (de Boer 1996). Like most antidepressants, mirtazapine suppresses REM sleep (Ruigt et al. 1990).

Pharmacokinetics and Disposition

Bioavailability following single and multiple doses of mirtazapine is approximately 50% (Voortman and Paanakker 1995). Peak plasma concentrations are reached within 2 hours after oral administration (Sitsen and Zikov 1995). The average elimination half-life is 21.5 hours, with a range of 20–40 hours (Sitsen and Zikov 1995). The parent compound is eliminated via hepatic metabolism, with demethylation and oxidation and subsequent conjugation of the metabolites. Demethyl-mirtazapine is approximately three- to fourfold less active than the parent drug. Mirtazapine has linear pharmacokinetics over clinically relevant dose ranges. It is approximately 85% bound to protein in plasma. The relation between plasma concentrations and clinical response has not been determined (Kehoe and Schorr 1996).

Mechanism of Action

The putative mechanism of action of mirtazapine is unique among currently available antidepressant drugs in the United States. Blockade of presynaptic central α_2-adrenergic autoreceptors leads to enhanced noradrenergic neurotransmission via increased noradrenergic cell firing and norepinephrine release. In turn, norepinephrine stimulates α_1 adrenoreceptors on the cell bodies of serotonergic neurons, which leads to increased serotonin cell firing. In addition, mirtazapine blocks α_2-adrenergic heteroreceptors on the synaptic terminals of serotonin neurons, which leads to a further increase in serotonin release (de Boer 1995). Thus, by increasing the serotonergic firing rate and blocking the α_2-adrenergic heteroreceptors on serotonin terminals, mirtazapine increases intracellular serotonin levels. Coupled with its antagonistic properties at 5-HT_{2A}, 5-HT_{2C}, and 5-HT_3 receptors, mirtazapine's stimulation of serotonin release leads to functional enhancement of 5-HT_{1A} neurotransmission (de Boer 1995). The overall effect of these pharmacological actions is increased noradrenergic and 5-HT_{1A} activity.

Indications

Mirtazapine is superior to placebo and comparable to standard antidepressants in the treatment of major depression (Davis and Wilde 1996; Kasper 1995; Zikov et al. 1995). Hamilton Rating Scale for Depression scores begin to improve significantly during the first week of mirtazapine treatment (and during the first week of amitriptyline treatment) compared with placebo (Bremner 1995), probably because of early effects on sleep and anxiety symptoms. When depressed patients are classified on the basis of symptom severity, those with severe depression (i.e., 17-item Hamilton Rating Scale for Depression scores > 24) have the same response to mirtazapine as those with moderate depression, whereas the placebo response rate is lower in the more severely ill patients (Claghorn and Lesem 1995). In a 20-week extension trial, mirtazapine was superior to placebo and amitriptyline in endpoint analyses of symptom severity (Bremner and Smith 1996). In a double-blind, controlled study of elderly depressed patients, mirtazapine and trazodone both had superior efficacy compared with placebo. The trend, which failed to reach statistical significance, was toward greater efficacy in the mirtazapine than in the trazodone treatment group (Halikas 1995).

In a controlled trial, efficacy of mirtazapine was greater than that of placebo in the treatment of patients with ICD-9 primary diagnoses of anxiety states (Sitsen and Moors 1994). In another report, mirtazapine was as effective as diazepam in relieving anxiety and improving the subjective experience of sleep in women who were undergoing gynecological surgery the next day (Sorensen et al. 1985).

Side Effects and Toxicology

A meta-analysis that included all of the patients participating in the mirtazapine clinical trial development program who had received at least one dose of medication compared mirtazapine- and placebo-related side effects. In this sample of 359 mirtazapine- and 328 placebo-treated patients, the following side effects occurred more frequently in association with mirtazapine than with placebo: drowsiness (23% vs. 14%), excessive sedation (19% vs. 5%), dry mouth (25% vs. 16%), increased appetite (11% vs. 2%), and weight gain (10% vs. 2%). Usually, these side effects were mild and transient and often decreased over time despite increases in mirtazapine dosages. No significant increases in cardiovascular side effects (e.g., blood pressure changes, tachycardia) or in psychosexual side effects were associated with mirtazapine compared with placebo (Montgomery 1995). Thus, mirtazapine has antihistaminic side effects, without the cardiovascular side effects or gastrointestinal/psychosexual side effects that are associated with TCAs and SSRIs, respectively.

Geriatric patients are especially vulnerable to side effects of psychoactive medications, in general, and some side effects can lead to devastating sequelae in this group (e.g., hip fractures following a fall related to orthostatic hypotension). In a comparative trial in elderly patients, dry mouth and somnolence occurred more frequently with both mirtazapine and trazodone treatment than with placebo. Compared with placebo, trazodone treatment was linked to a higher incidence of dizziness and amblyopia, whereas mirtazapine was associated with increased appetite and a modest weight gain (Davis and Wilde 1996).

Clinicians may start treatment with many psychoactive medications at rather low doses to allow for accommodation to mild side effects and then gradually increase the dosage as tolerated. Because of the unique pharmacological profile of mirtazapine (see section, "Pharmacological Profile," above), this practice should be avoided. Mirtazapine's affinity for histaminergic receptors is greater than its affinity for α_2-adrenergic receptors. Thus, at doses lower than the recommended 15-mg starting dose, maximum sedation caused by substantial antihistaminergic activity occurs. At 15 mg and higher doses, the enhancement of noradrenergic neurotransmission via α_2-adrenergic receptor blockade leads to activating effects that, at least in part, counteract the antihistaminergic sedation.

A few abnormal laboratory parameters have been rarely associated with mirtazapine treatment. Transient elevations in liver alanine aminotransferase (ALT) levels to greater than three times the upper limit of normal range were reported in about 2% of patients (Davis and Wilde 1996). These enzyme elevations returned to normal after treatment was discontinued. Random plasma total cholesterol levels have been reported to increase by an average of 3%–4% in depressed patients receiving mirtazapine (Davis and Wilde 1996). However, it is very difficult to interpret the meaning of random (i.e., nonfasting) cholesterol levels, which would be expected to increase in relation to improved appetite and increased food intake.

Mirtazapine appears to have a relatively low potential for inducing seizures. Only one patient taking mirtazapine was reported to have a seizure in all of the worldwide clinical trials, and that individual had a history of tricyclic-related seizures (Richou et al. 1995).

To date, the available data suggest that mirtazapine is relatively safe in overdose situations compared with conventional TCAs. In the 10 overdose cases that have been reported, transient excessive somnolence was the only observed symptom. These cases included an 81-year-old patient who ingested a 20-day supply of mirtazapine, along with a 14-day supply of midazolam. No seizures or electrocardiogram changes were observed (Montgomery 1995).

Drug-Drug Interactions

Few drug-drug interactions involving mirtazapine have been described at this point. Mirtazapine can have additive subjective and objective effects on motor and cognitive performance when taken in conjunction with alcohol or diazepam (Kuitunen 1994; Sitsen and Zikov 1995). Mirtazapine is metabolized by several subfamilies of the cytochrome P450 enzyme system, including CYP2DG, CYP1A2, CYP3A4, and CYP2C9. Mirtazapine does not appear to increase plasma concentrations of desipramine (data on file, Organon, July 1996).

SUMMARY

We reviewed the pharmacological properties of four antidepressants that are not readily cataloged within the conventional classifications of antidepressants. One of them, trazodone, was among the first of the second-generation antidepressants, and mirtazapine is the most recent addition to the antidepressant armamentarium. Do any common themes link these medications, other than their relegation to the category of miscellaneous antidepressants?

In a way, trazodone, nefazodone, and bupropion all serve to remind us of the potential importance of metabolites on the clinical profile of pharmacological agents. In the case of trazodone and nefazodone, the active metabolite mCPP may play a role in the mechanism of action, in light of its potent activity as a serotonin agonist. For bupropion, several active metabolites may influence clinical response and/or side effects. Future research should help to clarify the specific roles of these metabolites, including their potential utility in therapeutic blood level monitoring.

Another important theme that has emerged from our review is the important advantage that an understanding of a drug's basic pharmacology provides for clinicians. Many side effects can be understood, or even predicted, based on the pharmacological profiles of the newer agents. Thus, trazodone's propensity to evoke orthostatic hypotension makes sense in light of its effects on α-adrenergic receptors, and many of the side effects associated with bupropion could be anticipated based on its effects on dopaminergic neurotransmission.

Finally, each novel antidepressant adds to our available tools for the treatment of depression. Although we do not have a "perfect" antidepressant therapy that is safe and effective for all patients, all of the compounds, with their various side-effect profiles, provide clinicians with additional options and flexibility in selecting the best available approach for each patient.

REFERENCES

American Psychiatric Association: Diagnostic and Statistical Manual of Mental Disorders, 3rd Edition, Revised. Washington, DC, American Psychiatric Association, 1987

Ames D, Wirshing WC, Szuba MP: Organic mental disorders associated with bupropion in three patients. J Clin Psychiatry 53:53–55, 1992

Ansseau M, Darimont P, Lecoq A, et al: Controlled comparison of nefazodone and amitriptyline in major depressive inpatients. Psychopharmacology (Berl) 115:254–260, 1994

Anton SF, Robinson DS, Roberts DL, et al: Long-term treatment of depression with nefazodone. Psychopharmacol Bull 30:165–169, 1994

Apter JT, Woolfolk RL: Lithium augmentation of bupropion in refractory depression. Ann Clin Psychiatry 2:7–10, 1990

Arana GW, Kaplan GB: Trazodone-induced mania following desipramine-induced mania in major depressive disorders (letter). Am J Psychiatry 142:386, 1985

Ascher JA, Cole JO, Colin JN, et al: Bupropion: a review of its mechanism of antidepressant activity. J Clin Psychiatry 56:395–401, 1995

Ayd FJ Jr: Pharmacology update: which antidepressant to choose, II: the overdose factor. Psychiatric Annals 14:212–214, 1984

Balon R: Sleep terror disorder and insomnia treated with trazodone: a case report. Ann Clin Psychiatry 6:161–163, 1994

Barbhaiya RJ, Sukla UA, Greene DS: Lack of interaction between nefazodone and cimetidine: a steady state pharmacokinetic study in humans. Br J Clin Pharmacol 40:161–165, 1995a

Barbhaiya RJ, Sukla UA, Matarakam CS, et al: Single- and multiple-dose pharmacokinetics of nefazodone in patients with hepatic cirrhosis. Clin Pharmacol Ther 58:390–398, 1995b

Barrickman LL, Perry PJ, Allen AJ, et al: Bupropion versus methylphenidate in the treatment of attention-deficit hyperactivity disorder. J Am Acad Child Adolesc Psychiatry 34:649–657, 1995

Baxter LR Jr: Two cases of obsessive-compulsive disorder with depression responsive to trazodone. J Nerv Ment Dis 173:423–433, 1985

Bayer AJ, Pathy MSJ, Ankier SI: Pharmacokinetic and pharmacodynamic characteristics of trazodone in the elderly. Br J Clin Pharmacol 16:371–376, 1983

Beck PL, Bridges RJ, Demetrick DJ, et al: Chronic active hepatitis associated with trazodone therapy. Ann Intern Med 118:791–792, 1993

Birkhimer LJ, Alderman AA, Schmitt CE, et al: Combined trazodone-lithium therapy for refractory depression (letter). Am J Psychiatry 140:1382–1383, 1983

Blier P, de Montigny C, Chaput Y: A role for the serotonin system in the mechanism of action of antidepressant treatments: preclinical evidence. J Clin Psychiatry 51 (suppl 4):14–20, 1990

Bodner RA, Lynch T, Lewis L, et al: Serotonin syndrome. Neurology 45:219–223, 1995

Bolden-Watson C, Richelson E: Blockade by newly developed antidepressants of biogenic amine uptake into rat brain synaptosomes. Life Sci 52:1023–1029, 1993

Boschmans SA, Perkin MF, Terblanche SE: Antidepressant drugs: imipramine, mianserin and trazodone. Comp Biochem Physiol 86:225–232, 1987

Bremner JD: A double-blind comparison of Org 3770, amitriptyline, and placebo in major depression. J Clin Psychiatry 56:519–525, 1995

Bremner JD, Smith WT: Org 3770 vs amitriptyline in the continuation treatment of depression: a placebo controlled trial. European Journal of Psychiatry 10:5–15, 1996

Brogden RN, Heel RC, Speight TM, et al: Trazodone: a review of its pharmacological properties and therapeutic uses in depression and anxiety. Drugs 21:401–429, 1981

Caccia S, Ballabio M, Fanelli R, et al: Determination of plasma and brain concentrations of trazodone and its metabolite, 1-m-chlorophenylpiperazine, by gas-liquid chromatography. J Chromatogr 210:311–318, 1981

Casat CD, Pleasants DZ, Schroeder DH, et al: Bupropion in children with attention deficit disorder. Psychopharmacol Bull 25:198–201, 1989

Chouinard G: Bupropion and amitriptyline in the treatment of depressed patients. J Clin Psychiatry 44 (sec 2):121–129, 1983

Ciraulo DA, Shader RI: Fluoxetine drug-drug interactions II. J Clin Psychopharmacol 10:213–217, 1990

Claghorn JL, Lesem MD: A double-blind placebo-controlled study of Org 3770 in depressed outpatients. J Affect Disord 34:165–171, 1995

Cohen ML, Fuller RW, Kurz KD: Evidence that blood pressure reduction by serotonin antagonists is related to α receptor blockade in spontaneously hypertensive rats. Hypertension 5:676–681, 1983

Cooper BR, Hester TJ, Maxwell RA: Behavioral and biochemical effects of the antidepressant bupropion (Wellbutrin): evidence for selective blockade of dopamine uptake in vivo. J Pharmacol Exp Ther 215:127–134, 1980

Cunningham LA, Borison RL, Carman JS, et al: A comparison of venlafaxine, trazodone, and placebo in major depression. J Clin Psychopharmacol 14:99–106, 1994

Dager SR, Heritch AJ: A case of bupropion-associated delirium. J Clin Psychiatry 51:307–308, 1990

Davidson J: Seizures and bupropion: a review. J Clin Psychiatry 50:256–261, 1989

Davidson J, Miller R, Fleet JVW, et al: A double-blind comparison of bupropion and amitriptyline in depressed patients. J Clin Psychiatry 44 (sec 2):S115–117, 1983

Davis R, Wilde MI: Mirtazapine: a review of its pharmacology and therapeutic potential in the management of major depression. CNS Drugs 5:389–402, 1996

de Boer T: The effects of mirtazapine on central noradrenergic and serotonergic neurotransmission. Int Clin Psychopharmacol 10 (suppl 4):19–23, 1995

de Boer T: The pharmacological profile of mirtazapine. J Clin Psychiatry 57 (suppl 4):19–25, 1996

de Boer T, Maura G, Raiteri M, et al: Neurochemical and autonomic pharmacological profiles of the 6-aza-analogue of mianserin, mirtazapine and its enantiomers. Neuropharmacology 27:399–408, 1988

Dorn JM: A case of phenytoin toxicity possibly precipitated by trazodone. J Clin Psychiatry 47:89–90, 1986

Duffy JD, Campbell J: Bupropion for the treatment of fatigue associated with multiple sclerosis (letter). Psychosomatics 35:170–171, 1994

Eison AS, Eison MS, Torrente JR, et al: Nefazodone: preclinical pharmacology of a new antidepressant. Psychopharmacol Bull 26:311–315, 1990

Emmanuel NP, Lydiard RB, Ballenger JC: Treatment of social phobia with bupropion (letter). J Clin Psychopharmacol 11:276–277, 1991

Feighner J, Hendrickson G, Miller L, et al: Double-blind comparison of doxepin versus bupropion in outpatients with a major depressive disorder. J Clin Psychopharmacol 6:27–32, 1986

Feighner JP, Pambakian R, Fowler RC, et al: A comparison of nefazodone, imipramine, and placebo in patients with moderate to severe depression. Psychopharmacol Bull 25:219–221, 1989

Feighner JP, Gardner EA, Johnston JA, et al: Double-blind comparison of bupropion and fluoxetine in depressed outpatients. J Clin Psychiatry 52:329–335, 1991

Ferguson J, Cunningham L, Merideth C, et al: Bupropion in tricyclic antidepressant nonresponders with unipolar major depressive disorder. Ann Clin Psychiatry 6:153–160, 1994

Ferris RM, Beaman OJ: Bupropion: a new antidepressant drug, the mechanism of action of which is not associated with down-regulation of postsynaptic β-adrenergic, serotonergic (5-HT$_2$), α$_2$-adrenergic, imipramine and dopaminergic receptors in brain. Neuropharmacology 22:1257–1267, 1983

Findlay JWA, Van Wyck Fleet J, Smith PG, et al: Pharmacokinetics of bupropion, a novel antidepressant agent, following oral administration to healthy subjects. Eur J Clin Pharmacol 21:127–135, 1981

Fogelson DL, Bystritsky A, Pasnau R: Bupropion in the treatment of bipolar disorders: the same old story? J Clin Psychiatry 53:443–446, 1992

Fontaine R: Novel serotonergic mechanisms and clinical experience with nefazodone. Clin Neuropharmacol 16 (suppl 3):S45–S50, 1993

Fontaine R, Ontiveros A, Elie R, et al: A double-blind comparison of nefazodone, imipramine, and placebo in major depression. J Clin Psychiatry 55:234–241, 1994

Freeman EW, Rickels K, Sondheimer SJ, et al: Nefazodone in the treatment of premenstrual syndrome: a preliminary study. J Clin Psychopharmacol 14:180–186, 1994

Frewer LJ, Lader M: The effects of nefazodone, imipramine and placebo, alone and combined with alcohol, in normal subjects. Int Clin Psychopharmacol 8:13–20, 1993

Friel PN, Logan BK, Fligner CL: Three fatal drug overdoses involving bupropion. J Anal Toxicol 17:436–438, 1993

Gamble DE, Peterson LG: Trazodone overdose: four years of experience from voluntary reports. J Clin Psychiatry 47:544–546, 1986

Garattini S: Biochemical studies with trazodone, in Trazodone: Modern Problems of Pharmacopsychiatry, Vol 9. Edited by Ban TA, Silvestrini B. Basel, Karger, 1974, pp 29–46

Gardner EA, Johnston A: Bupropion: an antidepressant without sexual pathophysiological action. J Clin Psychopharmacol 5:24–29, 1985

Gatrell N: Increased libido in women receiving trazodone. Am J Psychiatry 143:781–782, 1986

Gedye A: Serotonergic treatment for aggression in a Down's syndrome adult showing signs of Alzheimer's disease. Journal of Mental Deficiency Research 35:247–258, 1991

Georgotas A, Forsell TL, Mann JJ, et al: Trazodone hydrochloride: a wide spectrum antidepressant with a unique pharmacological profile. Pharmacotherapy 2:255–265, 1982

Gerner RH: Geriatric depression and treatment with trazodone. Psychopathology 20:82–91, 1987

Goetz CG, Tanner CM, Klawans HL: Bupropion in Parkinson's disease. Neurology 34:1092–1094, 1984

Goldberg RJ, Huk M: Serotonin syndrome from trazodone and buspirone (letter). Psychosomatics 33:235–236, 1992

Golden RN: Diethylpropion, bupropion, and psychoses (letter). Br J Psychiatry 153:265–266, 1988

Golden RN: Antidepressant profile of bupropion and three metabolites: clinical and pre-clinical studies (letter). Pharmacopsychiatry 24:68, 1991

Golden RN, James S, Sherer M, et al: Psychoses associated with bupropion treatment. Am J Psychiatry 142:1459–1462, 1985

Golden RN, Brown DO, Miller H, et al: The new antidepressants. N C Med J 49:549–554, 1988a

Golden RN, DeVane L, Laizure SC, et al: Bupropion in depression: the role of metabolites in clinical outcome. Arch Gen Psychiatry 45:145–149, 1988b

Golden RN, Markey SP, Risby ED, et al: Antidepressants reduce whole-body norepinephrine turnover while enhancing 6-hydroxymelatonin output. Arch Gen Psychiatry 45:150–154, 1988c

Golden RN, Rudorfer MV, Sherer M, et al: Bupropion in depression: biochemical effects and clinical response. Arch Gen Psychiatry 45:139–143, 1988d

Goodnick PJ: Bupropion in chronic fatigue syndrome (letter). Am J Psychiatry 147:1091, 1990

Goodnick PJ: Pharmacokinetics of second generation antidepressants: bupropion. Psychopharmacol Bull 27:513–519, 1991

Goodnick PJ: Blood levels and acute response to bupropion. Am J Psychiatry 149:399–400, 1992

Goodnick PJ: Adjunctive lithium treatment with bupropion and fluoxetine: a naturalistic report. Lithium (in press)

Goodnick PJ, Sandoval R, Brickman A, et al: Bupropion treatment of fluoxetine-resistant chronic fatigue syndrome. Biol Psychiatry 32:834–838, 1992

Greenblatt DJ, Friedman H, Burstein ES, et al: Trazodone kinetics: effects of age, gender, and obesity. Clin Pharmacol Ther 42:193–200, 1987

Greenwald BS, Marin DB, Silverman SM: Serotonergic treatment of screaming and banging in dementia. Lancet 2:1464–1465, 1986

Halikas JA: Org 3770 (mirtazapine) versus trazodone: a placebo controlled trial in depressed elderly patients. Human Psychopharmacology 10 (suppl):S125–S133, 1995

Hamilton M: A rating scale for depression. J Neurol Neurosurg Psychiatry 23:56–62, 1960

Hargrave R: Serotonergic agents in the management of dementia and posttraumatic stress disorder. Psychosomatics 34:461–462, 1993

Haria M, Fitton A, McTavish D: Trazodone: a review of its pharmacology, therapeutic use in depression and therapeutic potential in other disorders. Drugs Aging 4:331–335, 1994

Hayes PE, Kristoff CA: Adverse reactions to five new antidepressants. Clinical Pharmacology 5:471–480, 1986

Haykal RF, Akiskal HS: Bupropion as a promising approach to rapid cycling bipolar II patients. J Clin Psychiatry 51:450–455, 1990

Horne RL, Rerguson JM, Pope HG Jr, et al: Treatment of bulimia with bupropion: a multicenter controlled trial. J Clin Psychiatry 49:262–266, 1988

Hudson JI, Pope HG Jr, Keck PE Jr, et al: Treatment of bulimia nervosa with trazodone: short-term response and long-term follow-up. Clin Neuropharmacol 12 (suppl 1):38–46, 1989

Hyttel J: Citalopram-pharmacologic profile of a specific serotonin uptake inhibitor with antidepressant activity. Prog Neuropsychopharmacol Biol Psychiatry 6:277–295, 1982

Jackson CW, Head LA, Kellner CH: Catatonia associated with bupropion treatment (letter). J Clin Psychiatry 53:210, 1992

Jacobsen FM: Low-dose trazodone as a hypnotic in patients treated with MAOIs and other psychotropics: a pilot study. J Clin Psychiatry 51:298–302, 1990

Janowsky D, Curtis G, Zisook S, et al: Ventricular arrhythmias possibly aggravated by trazodone. Am J Psychiatry 140:796–797, 1983

Jeffries JJ, Al-Jeshi A: Nefazodone-induced mania (letter). Can J Psychiatry 40:218, 1995

Jick H, Binan B, Hunter JR, et al: Tricyclic antidepressants and convulsions. J Clin Psychopharmacol 3:128–185, 1983

Kasper S: Clinical efficacy of mirtazapine: a review of meta-analyses of pooled data. Int Clin Psychopharmacol 10 (suppl 4):25–35, 1995

Kehoe WA, Schorr RB: Focus on mirtazapine: a new antidepressant with noradrenergic and specific serotonergic activity. Formulary 31:455–469, 1996

Kiev A, Masco HL, Wenger TL, et al: The cardiovascular effects of bupropion and nortriptyline in depressed outpatients. Ann Clin Psychiatry 6:107–115, 1994

Kim SW: Trazodone in the treatment of obsessive-compulsive disorder: a case report. J Clin Psychopharmacol 7:278–279, 1987

Klein HE, Muller N: Trazodone in endogenous depressed patients: a negative report and a critical evaluation of the pertaining literature. Prog Neuropsychopharmacol Biol Psychiatry 9:173–186, 1985

Knobler H: Trazodone-induced mania. Br J Psychiatry 149:787–789, 1986

Kuitunen T: Drug and ethanol effects on the clinical test for drunkenness: single doses of ethanol, hypnotic drugs and antidepressant drugs. Pharmacol Toxicol 75:91–98, 1994

Kurt U, Ozkardes H, Altug U, et al: The efficacy of anti-serotoninergic agents in the treatment of erectile dysfunction. J Urol 152:407–409, 1994

Lader M: Recent experience with trazodone. Psychopathology 20 (suppl 1):39–47, 1987

Lai AA, Schroeder DH: Clinical pharmacokinetics of bupropion: a review. J Clin Psychiatry 44 (sec 2):82–84, 1983

Lance R, Albo M, Costabile RA, et al: Oral trazodone as empirical therapy for erectile dysfunction: a retrospective review. Urology 46:117–120, 1995

Lebert F, Pasquier F, Petit H: Behavioral effects of trazodone in Alzheimer's disease. J Clin Psychiatry 55:536–538, 1994

Lennhoff M: Trazodone-induced mania. J Clin Psychiatry 48:423–424, 1987

Lippman S, Bedford P, Manshadi M, et al: Trazodone cardiotoxicity (letter). Am J Psychiatry 140:1383, 1983

Lydiard RB: Obsessive-compulsive disorder successfully treated with trazodone. Psychosomatics 27:858–859, 1986

Marek GJ, McDougle CJ, Price LH, et al: A comparison of trazodone and fluoxetine: implications for serotonergic mechanism of antidepressant action. Psychopharmacol 109:2–11, 1992

Martin P, Massol J, Colin JN, et al: Antidepressant profile of bupropion and three metabolites in mice. Pharmacopsychiatry 23:187–194, 1990

Masand P, Stern TA: Bupropion and secondary mania: is there a relationship? Ann Clin Psychiatry 5:271–274, 1993

Mayol RF, Cole CA, Luke GM, et al: Characterization of the metabolites of the antidepressant drug nefazodone in human urine and plasma. Drug Metab Dispos 22:304–311, 1994

Mehta NB: The chemistry of bupropion. J Clin Psychiatry 44 (sec 2):56–59, 1983

Mendels J, Amin MM, Chouinard G, et al: A comparative study of bupropion and amitriptyline in depressed outpatients. J Clin Psychiatry 44 (sec 2):118–120, 1983

Mendels J, Reimherr F, Marcus RN, et al: A double-blind, placebo-controlled trial of two dose ranges of nefazodone in the treatment of depressed outpatients. J Clin Psychiatry 56 (suppl 6):30–36, 1995

Merideth CH, Feighner JP: The use of bupropion in hospitalized depressed patients. J Clin Psychiatry 44 (sec 2):85–87, 1983

Metz A, Shader RI: Adverse interactions encountered when using trazodone to treat insomnia associated with fluoxetine. Int Clin Psychopharmacol 5:191–194, 1990

Monteleone P, Gnocchi G: Evidence for a linear relationship between plasma trazodone levels and clinical response in depression in the elderly. Clin Neuropharmacol 13 (suppl 1):84–89, 1990

Montgomery SA: Safety of mirtazapine: a review. Int Clin Psychopharmacol 10 (suppl 4):37–45, 1995

Montorsi F, Strambi LF, Guazzoni G, et al: Effect of yohimbine-trazodone on psychogenic impotence: a randomized, double-blind, placebo-controlled study. Urology 44:732–736, 1994

Nambudiri DE, Mirchandani IC, Young RC: Two more cases of trazodone-related syncope in the elderly (letter). J Geriatr Psychiatry Neurol 2:225, 1989

Nelson EC: An open-label study of nefazodone in the treatment of depression with and without comorbid obsessive compulsive disorder. Ann Clin Psychiatry 6:249–253, 1994

Nierenberg A, Keck PE: Management of monoamine oxidase inhibitor-associated insomnia with trazodone. J Clin Psychopharmacol 9:42–45, 1989

Nierenberg A, Adler LA, Peselow E, et al: Trazodone for antidepressant-associated insomnia. Am J Psychiatry 151:1069–1072, 1994

Nilsen OG, Dale O: Single dose pharmacokinetics of trazodone in healthy subjects. Pharmacol Toxicol 71:150–153, 1992

Nixon AL, Long WH, Puopolo PR, et al: Bupropion metabolites produce false-positive urine amphetamine results (letter). Am J Psychiatry 152:813, 1995

Nofzinger EA, Reynolds CF III, Thase ME, et al: REM sleep enhancement by bupropion in depressed men. Am J Psychiatry 152:274–276, 1994

Nomikos GG, Damsma G, Wenkstern D, et al: Effects of chronic bupropion on interstitial concentrations of dopamine in rat nucleus accumbens and striatum. Neuropsychopharmacology 7:7–14, 1992

Pasion RC, Kirby SG: Trazodone for screaming (letter). Lancet 341:970, 1993

Peck AW, Stern WC, Watkinson C: Incidence of seizures during treatment with tricyclic antidepressant drugs and bupropion. J Clin Psychiatry 44 (sec 2):197–201, 1983

Perumal AS, Smith TM, Suckow RF, et al: Effect of plasma from patients containing bupropion and its metabolites on the uptake of norepinephrine. Neuropharmacology 25:199–202, 1986

Pescatori ES, Engelman JC, Davis G, et al: Priapism of the clitoris: a case report following trazodone use. J Urol 149:1557–1559, 1993

Pick CG, Paul D, Eison MS, et al: Potentiation of opioid analgesia by the antidepressant nefazodone. Eur J Pharmacol 211:375–381, 1992

Pigott TA, Leheureux F, Rubenstein CS, et al: A double-blind, placebo controlled study of trazodone in patients with obsessive-compulsive disorder. J Clin Psychopharmacol 12:156–162, 1992

Pinner E, Rich CL: Effects of trazodone on aggressive behavior in seven patients with organic mental disorders. Am J Psychiatry 145:1295–1296, 1988

Pitts WM, Fann WE, Halaris AE, et al: Bupropion in depression: a tri-center placebo-controlled study. J Clin Psychiatry 44 (sec 2):95–100, 1983

Popli AP, Tanquary J, Lamparella V, et al: Bupropion and anti-convulsant drug interactions. Ann Clin Psychiatry 7:99–101, 1995

Prasad AJ: Obsessive-compulsive disorder and trazodone. Am J Psychiatry 141:612–613, 1984

Preskorn SH: Antidepressant response and plasma concentrations of bupropion. J Clin Psychiatry 44 (sec 2):137–139, 1983

Preskorn SH: Should bupropion dosage be adjusted based upon therapeutic drug monitoring? Psychopharmacol Bull 27:637–643, 1991

Preskorn SH: Comparison of the tolerability of bupropion, fluoxetine, imipramine, nefazodone, paroxetine, sertraline, and venlafaxine. J Clin Psychiatry 56 (suppl):12–21, 1995

Purcell P, Ghurye R: Trazodone and spontaneous orgasms in an elderly postmenopausal woman: a case report (letter). J Clin Psychopharmacol 15:293–295, 1995

Reeves RR, Bullen JA: Serotonin syndrome produced by paroxetine and low-dose trazodone (letter). Psychosomatics 36:159–160, 1995

Richelson E: Biological basis of depression and therapeutic relevance. J Clin Psychiatry 52 (suppl):4–10, 1991

Richou H, Ruimy P, Charbaut J, et al: A multicentre, double-blind, clomipramine-controlled efficacy and safety study of Org 3770. Human Psychopharmacology 10:263–271, 1995

Rickels K, Downing R, Schweizer E, et al: Antidepressants for the treatment of generalized anxiety disorder: a placebo-controlled comparison of imipramine, trazodone, and diazepam. Arch Gen Psychiatry 50:884–895, 1993

Rickels K, Robinson DS, Schweizer E, et al: Nefazodone: aspects of efficacy. J Clin Psychiatry 56 (suppl 6):43–46, 1995

Roose SP, Glassman AH, Giardina EGV, et al: Cardiovascular effects of imipramine and bupropion in depressed patients with congestive heart failure. J Clin Psychopharmacol 7:247–251, 1987

Rudorfer MV, Potter WZ: Antidepressants: a comparative review of the clinical pharmacology and therapeutic use of the "newer" versus the "older" drugs. Drugs 37:713–738, 1989

Rudorfer MV, Golden RN, Potter WZ: Second generation antidepressants. Psychiatr Clin North Am 7:519–534, 1984

Ruigt GSF, Kemp B, Groenhout CM, et al: Effect of the antidepressant Org 3770 on human sleep. Eur J Clin Pharmacol 38:551–554, 1990

Sachs GS, Lafer B, Stoll AL, et al: A double-blind trial of bupropion versus desipramine for bipolar depression. J Clin Psychiatry 55:391–393, 1994

Salazar DE, Dockens RC, Milbrath RL, et al: Pharmacokinetic and pharmacodynamic evaluation of warfarin and nefazodone coadministration in healthy subjects. J Clin Pharmacol 35:730–738, 1995

Schatzberg AF: Trazodone: a 5-year review of antidepressant efficacy. Psychopathology 20 (suppl 1):48–56, 1987

Schneider LS, Sobin PB: Non-neuroleptic treatment of behavioral symptoms and agitation in Alzheimer's disease and other dementia. Psychopharmacol Bull 28:71–79, 1992

Schuckit MA: United States experience with trazodone: a literature review. Psychopathology 20 (suppl 1):32–38, 1987

Schwartz D, Blendl M: Sedative and anxiety-reducing properties of trazodone, in Trazodone: Modern Problems of Pharmacopsychiatry, Vol 9. Edited by Ban TA, Silvestrini B. Basel, Karger, 1974, pp 29–46

Sharpley AL, Walsh AES, Cowen PJ: Nefazodone—a novel antidepressant—may increase REM sleep. Biol Psychiatry 31:1070–1073, 1992

Shopsin B, Cassano GB, Conti L: An overview of new "second generation" antidepressant compounds: research and treatment implications, in Antidepressants: Neurochemical, Behavioral and Clinical Perspectives. Edited by Enna SJ, Molick J, Richelson E. New York, Raven, 1981, pp 219–251

Silvestrini B: Introductory remarks on trazodone and its position in treatment of psychiatric diseases, in Trazodone: A New Broad-Spectrum Antidepressant (Proceedings of the Symposium of the 11th Congress of the Collegium Internationale Neuro-Psychopharmacologicum, Vienna 1978). Edited by Gershon ES, Rickels K, Silvestrini G. Amsterdam, Excerpta Medica, 1980, pp 34–38

Silvestrini B, Lisciani R: Pharmacology of trazodone, round table discussion—trazodone: a new psychotropic agent. Current Therapeutic Research 15:749–754, 1973

Silvestrini B, Cioli V, Burbert S, et al: Pharmacological properties of AF 1161, a new psychotropic drug. International Journal of Neuropharmacology 7:587–599, 1968

Simpson DM, Foster DL: Improvement in organically disturbed behavior with trazodone treatment. J Clin Psychiatry 47:191–193, 1986

Sitsen JMA, Moors J: Mirtazapine, a novel antidepressant, in the treatment of anxiety symptoms: results from a placebo-controlled trial. Drug Investigations 8:339–344, 1994

Sitsen JMA, Zikov M: Mirtazapine: clinical profile. CNS Drugs 4 (suppl 1):39–48, 1995

Sorensen M, Jorgensen J, Viby-Mogensen J, et al: A double-blind group comparative study using the new antidepressant Org 3770, placebo and diazepam in patients with expected insomnia and anxiety before elective gynaecological surgery. Acta Psychiatr Scand 71:339–346, 1985

Soroko FE, Maxwell RA: The pharmacologic basis for therapeutic interest in bupropion. J Clin Psychiatry 44 (sec 2):67–73, 1983

Spar JE: Plasma trazodone concentrations in elderly depressed inpatients: cardiac effects and short-term efficacy. J Clin Psychopharmacol 7:406–409, 1987

Spencer T, Biederman J, Steingard T, et al: Bupropion exacerbates tics in children with attention-deficit hyperactivity disorder and Tourette's syndrome. J Am Acad Child Adolesc Psychiatry 32:211–214, 1993

Spiller HA, Ramoska EA, Krenzelok EP: Bupropion overdose: a 3-year multi-center retrospective analysis. Am J Emerg Med 12:43–45, 1994

Stern WC, Harto-Truax N, Bauer N: Efficacy of bupropion in tricyclic-resistant or intolerant patients. J Clin Psychiatry 44 (sec 2):148–152, 1983

Sternbach H: The serotonin syndrome. Am J Psychiatry 148:705–713, 1991

Sulser F: Mode of action of antidepressant drugs. J Clin Psychiatry 44 (sec 2):14–20, 1983

Sunkureddi K, Markovitz P: Trazodone treatment of obsessive-compulsive disorder and trichotillomania (letter). Am J Psychiatry 150:523–524, 1993

Taylor DP, Hyslop DK, Riblet A: Trazodone, a new non-tricyclic antidepressant without anticholinergic activity. Biochem Pharmacol 29:2149–2150, 1980

Taylor DP, Smith DW, Hyslop DK, et al: Receptor binding and atypical antidepressant drug discovery, in Receptor Binding in Drug Research. Edited by O'Brien RA. New York, Marcel Dekker, 1986, pp 151–165

Tejera CA, Saravay SM: Treatment of organic personality syndrome with low-dose trazodone. J Clin Psychiatry 56:374–375, 1995

Terao T: Comparison of manic switch onset during fluoxetine and trazodone treatment (letter). Biol Psychiatry 33:477–478, 1993

Thompson JW Jr, Ware MR, Blashfield RK: Psychotropic medication and priapism: a comprehensive review. J Clin Psychiatry 51:430–433, 1990

Van der Klauw MM, Janssen JC, Stricker BH: Agranulocytosis probably induced by trazodone (letter). Am J Psychiatry 150:1563–1564, 1993

van Laar MW, van Willigenburg APP, Volkerts ER: Acute and subchronic effects of nefazodone and imipramine on highway driving, cognitive functions, and daytime sleepiness in healthy adult and elderly subjects. J Clin Psychopharmacol 15:30–40, 1995

Van Putten T, Shaffer I: Delirium associated with bupropion (letter). J Clin Psychopharmacol 10:234, 1990

van Zwieten PA: Inhibition of the central hypotensive effect of clonidine by trazodone, a novel antidepressant. Pharmacology 15:331–336, 1977

Voortman G, Paanakker JE: Bioavailability of mirtazapine from Remeron tablets after single and multiple oral dosing. Human Psychopharmacology 10 (suppl):S83–S96, 1995

Walker PW, Cole JO, Gardner EA, et al: Improvement in fluoxetine-associated sexual dysfunction in patients switched to bupropion. J Clin Psychiatry 54:459–465, 1993

Walters L: Unique aspects of the chemistry and pharmacokinetics of trazodone, in Trazodone—An Advance in Antidepressant Therapy. Edited by Stern M. South Africa, The Medicine SA Journal (Pty) Ltd, 1982, pp 10–12

Weisler RH, Johnston JA, Lineberry CG, et al: Comparison of bupropion and trazodone for the treatment of major depression. J Clin Psychopharmacol 14:170–179, 1994

Wender PH, Reimherr FW: Bupropion treatment of attention-deficit hyperactivity disorder in adults. Am J Psychiatry 147:1018–1020, 1990

Wheatley D: Evaluation of trazodone in the treatment of anxiety. Current Therapeutic Research 20:74–83, 1976

Yamatsu K, Kaneko T, Yamanishi Y: A possible mechanism of central action of trazodone in rats, in Proceedings of the First International Symposium on Trazodone, Montreal 1973. Edited by Ban T, Silvestrini B. Basel, Karger, 1974, pp 11–17

Yasui N, Otani K, Keneko S, et al: Inhibition of trazodone metabolism by thioridazine in humans. Ther Drug Monit 17:333–335, 1995

Zikov M, Roes KCR, Pols AG: Efficacy of Org 3770 (mirtazapine) vs amitriptyline in patients with major depressive disorder: a meta-analysis. Human Psychopharmacology 10 (suppl):S135–S145, 1995

Zimmer B, Daly F, Benjamin L: More on combination antidepressant therapy. Arch Gen Psychiatry 41:527–528, 1984

Zmitek A: Trazodone-induced mania. Br J Psychiatry 151:274–275, 1987

Zubieta JK, Alessi NE: Acute and chronic administration of trazodone in the treatment of disruptive behavior disorders in children. J Clin Psychopharmacol 12:346–351, 1992

Zubieta JK, Demitrack MA: Possible bupropion precipitation of mania and a mixed affective state (letter). J Clin Psychopharmacol 11:327–328, 1991

FOURTEEN

Benzodiazepines

James C. Ballenger, M.D.

HISTORY AND DISCOVERY

The development of the benzodiazepines began in the mid-1950s when Roche Laboratories began to investigate the potential therapeutic properties of myanesin. Myanesin had demonstrated sedative and muscle relaxant features when tested on animals, but when administered to humans, its effects were weak and only brief in duration (Randall 1982). However, this finding stimulated interest and subsequent investigation of two compounds that had been initially developed in 1955 by Roche chemists Leo Sternbach and Earl Reeder. In May 1957, when these compounds were submitted for pharmacological evaluation, laboratory tests indicated their superiority to meprobamate on all measures used and to chlorpromazine on some.

The first benzodiazepine was patented in 1959 and introduced as Librium in 1960. Known generically as methaminodiazepoxide, Librium's generic name was later changed to chlordiazepoxide (Sternbach 1982). Continued testing of related compounds led to the development and introduction in 1963 of diazepam, an antianxiety agent 3–10 times more potent than chlordiazepoxide, with a broader spectrum of activity and greater muscle relaxant properties. The study of benzodiazepine derivatives has continued, and now more than three dozen benzodiazepines are available on the market (Smith and Wesson 1985) derived from or related to these early compounds (Sternbach 1982). Alprazolam, a triazolobenzodiazepine, has received the most recent attention. In 1992, it was given the first U.S. Food and Drug Administration (FDA) approval for treatment of panic disorder.

STRUCTURE-ACTIVITY RELATIONS

Chemically, the benzodiazepines are made up of 2-amino-benzodiazepine 4-oxides (Sternbach 1982). The first benzodiazepine developed, chlordiazepoxide, was the result of a compound created by treating the quinazoline N-oxide with methylamine, a primary amine (Sternbach 1982). During early studies at Roche Laboratories, there was scientific concern regarding the chemical validity of this compound. Based on scientific knowledge of chemical interactions, the chemical process used to develop chlordiazepoxide did not result in the anticipated final product. Further investigation revealed that the development of chlordiazepoxide resulted from the expansion of an atypical ring in the benzodiazepine derivative, and the compound contained a seven-member diazepine ring rather than a six-member pyrimidine ring (Sternbach and Reeder 1961).

Continued laboratory study and attempts to develop other related but improved compounds led to the discovery that the features shared by these compounds were the 1,4-benzodiazepine ring system, a chlorine in the 7 position, and the phenyl group in the 5 position (Sternbach 1982) (Figure 14–1). This discovery ultimately led to the development of several related compounds, including diazepam. Most benzodiazepines have a 5-aryl and a 1,4-diazepine ring, and modification of the ring systems produces benzodiazepines with somewhat different properties. Also, increasing the electron-attracting ability of the attachment at the R_1 position (occupied by chlorine in Figure 14–1) increases the potency of the resultant benzodiazepine (e.g., NO_2 for the potent benzodiazepine nitrazepam)

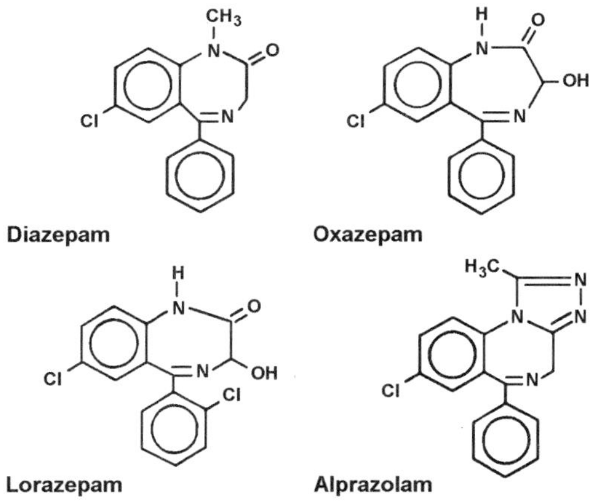

Figure 14–1. Chemical structures for benzodiazepines.
Source. Reprinted from Bernstein JG: *Handbook of Drug Therapy in Psychiatry,* 2nd Edition. Littleton, MA, PSG Publishing, 1988. Copyright 1988, Mosby-Year Book. Used with permission.

(Malizia and Nutt 1995). The benzodiazepine currently most often prescribed for the treatment of anxiety—alprazolam—is a triazolobenzodiazepine, formed by the addition of a heterocyclic ring that joins the 1 and 2 positions of the benzodiazepine ring system (Sternbach 1982).

PHARMACOLOGICAL PROFILE

Animal Studies

Numerous hypotheses regarding the mechanism by which the benzodiazepines reduce anxiety have undergone rigorous scientific investigation with animal experimentation. Most of the animal studies conducted to predict the ability of the benzodiazepines to reduce anxiety use an anticonflict or antipunishment effect, also known as a behavioral disinhibitory or behavioral antisuppressant action (Dantzer 1977; Gray 1982; Haefely 1978; Kilts et al. 1981; Sepinwall and Cook 1978; Simon and Soubrie 1979; Thiébot and Soubrié 1983).

The Geller-Seifter test (Geller and Seifter 1960) and the Vogel punished drinking test (Vogel et al. 1971), two of the most frequently used conflict tests, predict antianxiety efficacy of benzodiazepines (or other drugs) by their ability to increase responsivity in a conflict or punishment situation. In the Geller-Seifter test, the rat is rewarded with food for pressing a lever. However, the rat is alternately and variably given shocks when pressing the lever,

thereby decreasing its willingness to depress the lever. In the Vogel punished drinking test, thirsty rats are allowed to drink water but are given shocks through either the water spout or the bars on the floor of the cage. Again, shocks alternate with no shock in a variable way in the experimental setting. In both of these tests, when rats were administered benzodiazepines, their response rate during the potential shock situation increased, but the benzodiazepine had no effect on their responsivity in a nonshock situation. The effects of the benzodiazepines were also greater after they had been administered for several days (Cook and Sepinwall 1975; File and Hyde 1978; Margules and Stein 1968).

The punished locomotion test, which was developed more recently than the other two tests, administers shock to the rat as it moves from one metal plate to another, alternating shock with no shock on a variable schedule. Although this test is used less frequently, the effect of benzodiazepines in the punished locomotion test is again to enhance animal movement in the potential punishment situation (File 1990).

Other predictive tests have been developed that assess animal responses in social situations. Rats are placed in settings that are either unfamiliar or extremely well lit, and then the setting is alternated on a variable basis. Antianxiety potency is predicted by the amount of time rats spend engaged socially in these settings. As might be anticipated, rats spend the greatest amount of time in social interaction when placed in a familiar setting or without bright light. Benzodiazepines have been shown to be effective in increasing the amount of time spent in social interaction in the unfamiliar or bright conditions. These tests have been validated behaviorally by assessing anxiety through measures associated with decreased social interaction in animals (e.g., self-grooming, defecation). Also, physiological validation was accomplished by measuring changes in adrenocorticotropic hormone (ACTH), hypothalamic noradrenaline, and corticosterone (File 1980, 1985, 1990; File and Hyde 1978, 1979).

Anxiety in the social situation has also been assessed with the elevated plus-maze, a device shaped like a plus sign with two closed and two open arms. The benzodiazepines or other anxiolytics lead the rat to spend increased amounts of time on the open arms of the maze. This measure has also been validated physiologically and behaviorally with regard to anxiety (Pellow and File 1986; Pellow et al. 1985).

Pharmacological Properties

Almost all of the benzodiazepines have similar pharmacological profiles. All are sedating; in fact, it is difficult to separate the anxiety-reducing properties of the benzodiazepines from their sedating properties. Therefore, they have prominent hypnotic activity, and all have anticonvulsant and muscle relaxant activity. All these actions are thought to be secondary to effects on the central nervous system (CNS).

Muscle relaxation is thought to be mediated at the spinal cord level and antianxiety effects in cortical or, perhaps, limbic areas (Lader 1987). Anticonvulsant activity appears to occur through inhibition of seizure activity by potentiation of γ-aminobutyric acid (GABA)ergic neuronal circuits (see next section) at multiple levels of the CNS, including the brain stem. Ataxic side effects presumably are secondary to benzodiazepine actions in the cerebellum, hypnotic effects in the reticular formation, and amnestic effects in the hippocampus.

At routine doses, benzodiazepines have little effect on the cardiovascular and respiratory systems, which probably explains their wide margin of safety. Even in overdose situations, patients who have taken only a benzodiazepine rarely experience respiratory depression severe enough to require attention. More commonly, serious overdoses are the result of combining a benzodiazepine with another depressant drug, usually alcohol (Finkle et al. 1979; Greenblatt et al. 1977).

The effects of benzodiazepines on sleep have been well studied and include increases in total time asleep, reduction in sleep latency, decreased awakenings, and decreases in Stages 1, 2, 3, and 4 sleep (Greenblatt and Shader 1974; Mendelson et al. 1977). Benzodiazepines generally decrease time spent in rapid eye movement (REM) sleep but increase the number of REM cycles and, therefore, the number of dreams. When benzodiazepines are discontinued after chronic use, rebound increases in REM sleep often occur, and patients often report increases in nightmares or bizarre dreams.

PHARMACOKINETICS AND DISPOSITION

Administered orally, benzodiazepines are generally well absorbed from the gastrointestinal tract and reach peak levels within 30 minutes to 6–8 hours. Clorazepate is metabolized in the stomach to its active metabolite before absorption. Only lorazepam and midazolam are predictably absorbed after intramuscular injection. The high lipid solubility of most of the benzodiazepines (e.g., diazepam) allows for easy passage into the brain (DeVane et al. 1991). This also means, however, that activity of the benzodiazepines may be prolonged in extremely overweight people, who tend to have a higher ratio of fat to lean tissue

(Bernstein 1988; Harvey 1985). The benzodiazepines are predominantly bound to plasma proteins.

The benzodiazepines are metabolized primarily through the liver, and most are biotransformed by oxidation or Phase I metabolism. A few benzodiazepines, including lorazepam, temazepam, and lormetazepam, are biotransformed by conjugation to inactive glucuronides, sulfates, and acetylated substances; this process is also known as Phase II metabolism (Greenblatt et al. 1983). Some benzodiazepines, including diazepam, chlordiazepoxide, and flurazepam, are metabolized through both Phase I and II processes (Lader 1987).

The mechanism by which these drugs are metabolized (i.e., through the liver) is of significance in prescribing the benzodiazepines for certain groups of patients. Benzodiazepines that are metabolized by Phase II alone are better tolerated in patients with impaired liver function. Patients affected include elderly people, alcoholic individuals with cirrhotic livers, and people who smoke. Metabolism of Phase I drugs slows in the elderly, and the benzodiazepines metabolized by Phase II processes only are better tolerated in these individuals (Lader 1987). However, clinicians should use caution when prescribing any of the benzodiazepines for patients who have significant hepatic impairment or who are elderly, and these patients should be monitored regularly and carefully.

Duration of benzodiazepine action is, in part, related to lipid solubility, in that how quickly a benzodiazepine gets into the brain and how quickly it leaves the brain defines its duration of therapeutic action. Half-life is almost as important, and the benzodiazepines have widely divergent half-lives with different clinical effects (Table 14–1). Obviously, the shorter half-life benzodiazepines require multiple daily dosing. This clinical feature can be positive and reassuring for some patients but may have negative connotations for others. Specifically, the recurrence of anxiety symptoms with a rapid decline in blood level in those agents with short half-lives (e.g., alprazolam) can be a concern for some patients (e.g., those with panic disorder).

The duration of action of many of the benzodiazepines is much more dependent on the half-lives of the active metabolites than of the parent compounds. Perhaps the most clinically important example is the hypnotic flurazepam. Although its half-life is only 2–3 hours, the half-life of its primary metabolite, *N*-desalkylflurazepam, is more than 50 hours. In the case of flurazepam, this feature is often negative because it can cause unwanted daytime drowsiness. Diazepam and its metabolite desmethyldiazepam both have long half-lives. When diazepam is used for anxiety relief, this can be a positive factor by providing smooth

Table 14–1.   Benzodiazepines and their metabolites (including half-life)

Drug	Half-life	Active metabolites	Half-life
Triazolam	Short (<6 hours)	None	
Alprazolam	Intermediate (6–20 hours)	Not clinically important	
Lorazepam	Intermediate (6–20 hours)	None	
Oxazepam	Intermediate (6–20 hours)	None	
Temazepam	Intermediate (6–20 hours)	None	
Chlordiazepoxide	Intermediate (6–20 hours)	Desmethylchlordiazepoxide	Intermediate (6–20 hours)
		Demoxepam	Long (>20 hours)
		Nordiazepam	Long (>20 hours)
Diazepam	Long (>20 hours)	Nordiazepam	Long (>20 hours)
Clorazepate	Short (<6 hours)	Nordiazepam	Long (>20 hours)
Halazepam	Short (<6 hours)	Nordiazepam	Long (>20 hours)
Prazepam	Short (<6 hours)	Nordiazepam	Long (>20 hours)
Flurazepam	Short (<6 hours)	N-hydroxyethyl-flurazepam	Short (<6 hours)
		N-desalkylflurazepam	Long (>20 hours)

Source.   Adapted from Harvey SC: "Hypnotics and Sedatives," in *Goodman and Gilman's The Pharmacological Basis of Therapeutics*, 7th Edition. Edited by Gilman AG, Goodman LS, Rall TW. New York, Macmillan, 1985, pp. 339–371. Copyright 1985, the McGraw-Hill Companies. Used with permission.

relief of anxiety that does not depend on multiple daily dosing.

Other factors that affect elimination rate and half-life include the length of time that the drug is prescribed and the number of doses administered each day. For example, when an individual is prescribed diazepam for sleeping and takes it only once daily or infrequently as needed, the drug will have a much shorter half-life than that experienced by the patient who takes diazepam several times a day for an extended period (Bernstein 1988).

There are conflicting reports regarding the correlation between dose and plasma levels. Four early studies using benzodiazepines to treat anxiety, sleep difficulties, or a combination of symptoms showed no correlation between plasma concentrations and patient responsivity (Bond et al. 1977; Kangas et al. 1979; Tansella et al. 1975, 1978). However, other studies in which patients were treated for anxiety found a positive correlation between benzodiazepine plasma level and patient improvement (Bellantuono et al. 1980; Curry 1974; Dasberg et al. 1974).

Other studies have reported a positive correlation between alprazolam plasma levels and treatment response in patients with panic disorder. Lesser and colleagues (1992) studied plasma levels in 96 patients with panic disorder who were treated with either 2 or 6 mg of alprazolam or placebo. This study reported a significant correlation between plasma level of alprazolam and reduction in panic and phobic symptomatology and in side effects. Plasma level was definitely correlated with reduction in panic at-

tacks. However, plasma concentrations varied greatly among patients administered identical doses of alprazolam. This finding should underscore the need for individual dosing to achieve the maximum benefit with the fewest side effects.

The individual variation among patients regarding dose and plasma level in panic disorder was replicated by Greenblatt and colleagues (1993). This study also reported a greater reduction in spontaneous panic attacks in patients with higher plasma levels of alprazolam at week 3. Patients with higher plasma levels also had a decrease in situational panic attacks but not to a significant degree. Not surprisingly, an increase in side effects was also correlated with higher plasma levels. It is significant that by week 8 of the study, plasma level was no longer correlated with symptom reduction or side effects.

MECHANISM OF ACTION

The GABA Role

The elucidation of the mechanism of action for the benzodiazepines began with the discovery that GABA serves as the major inhibitory neurotransmitter in the CNS, with receptors located on approximately 30% of cortical and thalamic neurons (Costa et al. 1975; Haefely 1985; Olsen and Tobin 1990). Considerable evidence now indicates that the major pharmacological effects of the benzodiazepines are produced secondary to the binding of the benzodiazepines to GABA$_A$ receptors in the CNS. Extensive research has confirmed the critical interrelatedness of benzodiazepine actions and GABAergic mechanisms (Costa et al. 1975; Haefely et al. 1975; Polc et al. 1974). This relation can be clearly demonstrated by the ability of the benzodiazepines to prevent or extinguish seizures caused by agents that interfere with normal GABAergic function (Haefely 1985) or by the fact that pretreatment with antagonists of GABA (e.g., bicuculline) blocks benzodiazepine effects.

Knowledge of how benzodiazepines produce anxiolytic effects is evolving rapidly. GABA increases the propensity of the benzodiazepines to bind to specific receptor sites on the GABA-benzodiazepine receptor complex, and the converse is also true (i.e., both mutually enhance the binding of the other) (Paul and Skolnick 1982; Tallman et al. 1978, 1980). The principal action of GABA is to open the chloride ionophore on this complex. Although benzodiazepines appear to have no effect themselves on the GABA$_A$ complex or the ionophore, in the presence of GABA, benzodiazepines increase GABA's effects on the chloride ionophore. That is, they increase the number of openings of the chloride channel, which causes decreased cellular excitability (Bernstein 1988; Hsiao and Potter 1990; Study and Barker 1981).

Therefore, the primary action of the benzodiazepines is thought to be to increase the frequency of the openings of the chloride channel. Mechanisms other than enhancement of GABA inhibition have also been suggested, including increases in calcium-dependent potassium (K$^+$) conductance (Polc 1988). Although the evidence linking the benzodiazepines and GABA is strong, other potential mechanisms may be involved. Researchers have hypothesized that anxiety disorders are caused by abnormalities in both GABA and brain norepinephrine and that agents that correct these abnormalities are effective in reducing anxiety (Bernstein 1988). Oxazepam, a benzodiazepine often prescribed for anxiety, has been shown to decrease turnover of the two common transmitters serotonin and norepinephrine. Investigators believe that this characteristic is at least partially responsible for its sedative and anxiolytic effects (Harvey 1985).

Benzodiazepine Receptors

In the 1970s, several groups of researchers identified specific benzodiazepine binding sites in the brain (Bossman et al. 1977; Braestrup and Squires 1977; Möhler and Okada 1977a, 1977b; Squires and Braestrup 1977). The important discovery of high affinity, saturable, and stereospecific binding of benzodiazepine in the CNS provided the

basis for which to explain the diverse actions of benzodiazepines. Evidence that these benzodiazepine receptors are localized on neurons in the CNS and mediate the pharmacological actions of the benzodiazepines is principally provided by the strong correlation between anxiolytic potencies of various benzodiazepines and their ability to displace tritiated benzodiazepines from benzodiazepine receptors in vitro. This mediation is also shown by the benzodiazepines' potencies as anticonvulsants, anxiolytics, and muscle relaxants and in various animal models of inhibited behaviors (Young and Kuhar 1980). By convention, these receptors have been called the *benzodiazepine receptor* or the *benzodiazepine-GABA receptor*. However, it is important to remember that other substances also bind to this receptor complex (e.g., picrotoxin, alcohol, barbiturates, muscimol, penicillin, neurosteroids).

The GABA$_A$ receptor complex is an oligomeric glycoprotein. It was originally thought to have two subunits (α and β), each with 4 segments with 20 amino acids (Barnard et al. 1988). The GABA site is apparently associated with the β subunit and the benzodiazepine receptor with the α subunit (Thomas and Tallman 1981). It also appears that there are 4 membrane-spanning regions of approximately 20–30 hydrophobic amino acids in each subunit (Figure 14–2) (Zorumski and Isenberg 1991). However, cloning studies have defined 15 different proteins in this receptor in the mammalian CNS (Lüddens and Korpi 1995; Lüddens et al. 1995; Seeburg et al. 1990), and at least 5 subunits have multiple (1–6) variants within each. Although the possible number of variations in the benzodiazepine receptor probably exceeds 500, currently 6 α, 3 β, 2 (or 3) σ, and 1 δ subunits are known (Lüddens and Wisden 1991). Other studies suggest 5 subunits: 6 α, 4 β, 2 γ, 2 δ, and a retinal (rho) (Malizia and Nutt 1995). It is now known that the pharmacology of the benzodiazepine receptor varies principally according to the α subunit expressed. Expression of the σ_2 subunit is required for the GABA$_A$-chloride channels formed to respond consistently and robustly to benzodiazepines. If the σ_2 subunit is replaced by an σ_1 subunit, the benzodiazepine receptors are more reminiscent of the peripheral-type benzodiazepine receptors (Ymer et al. 1990).

Although most benzodiazepines bind to GABA$_A$-benzodiazepine receptors with similar affinities throughout the brain, there are some differences for certain benzodiazepines. Although controversy in this area remains (Malizia and Nutt 1995), benzodiazepine receptors have been characterized as either type I (with high affinity for triazolopyridazines and β-carbolines) (Nielsen and Braestrup 1980; Sieghart et al. 1985) or type II (with lower affinities for these compounds). Type I receptors are the

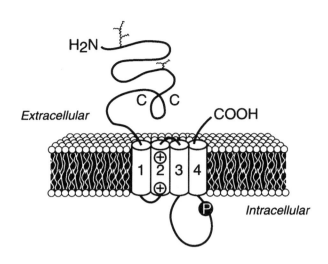

Figure 14–2. Model for γ-aminobutyric acid A (GABA$_A$) receptor subunits.
Source. Reprinted from Zorumski CF, Isenberg KE: "Insights Into the Structure and Function of GABA-Benzodiazepine Receptors: Ion Channels and Psychiatry." *American Journal of Psychiatry* 148:162–173, 1991. Used with permission.

most common GABA$_A$ receptor class in the CNS. The number of type II receptors is high in the hippocampus, striatum, and spinal cord (Lo et al. 1983; Sieghart et al. 1985), whereas the number of type I receptors is high in the cerebellum and low in the hippocampus. Numbers of both subtypes are equally high in cortical layers (Faull and Villiger 1988; Faull et al. 1987; Olsen et al. 1990). A third class of benzodiazepine receptor is primarily located in cerebellar granule cells, involves the α$_6$ subunit, and is relatively insensitive to benzodiazepines (Lüddens et al. 1990).

The functions of the β, σ, and δ subunits are less well known, but they do seem to be involved in agonist (GABA) binding (Lüddens and Wisden 1991). The GABA$_A$-benzodiazepine receptor complex is presumably a pentamer composed of α, β, and σ glycoprotein subunits, each with four regions that span the membrane (Figure 14–3) (Zorumski and Isenberg 1991). The actual functional characteristics of the receptor in terms of GABA or benzodiazepine binding would presumably result from whatever subunits were involved in the unit. Given the apparent and probably tremendous heterogeneity of these subunits, there appears to be a strong possibility that new and potentially more selective therapeutic agents can be synthesized because of this heterogeneity.

Benzodiazepine binding sites occur centrally or pe-

ripherally; however, there does not appear to be a receptor function for the peripheral type (Haefely 1985). This topic is discussed in more detail in a section later in this chapter (see "Peripheral-Type Benzodiazepine Receptors").

Ligands of the Benzodiazepine Receptor: Agonists, Antagonists, and Inverse Agonists

The benzodiazepines' action on the GABA receptor complex is mediated through the benzodiazepine receptor on this complex but in what appears to be a unique mechanism described as *positive allosteric modulation* (Haefely 1990). The binding site for the benzodiazepines operates differently from that for other neurotransmitter receptors; that is, the benzodiazepine receptor mediates the effects of different drugs that have directly opposing effects (i.e., either increasing or decreasing anxiety). To further investigate the benzodiazepine-GABAergic interaction, agents that have agonist, antagonist, and inverse agonist actions have been studied (for review, see Doble and Martin 1992; Gardner et al. 1993; Nutt 1989).

In addition to the benzodiazepines, zopiclone, triazolopyridazines, pyrazoloquinolinone derivatives, zolpidem, and some β-carboline derivatives have benzodiazepine agonist activity, reduce anxiety, and are sedating in a manner similar, but not identical, to the benzodiazepines. They do so by acting synergistically with GABA to increase the openings of the chloride channel (Blanchard et al. 1979; Klepner et al.

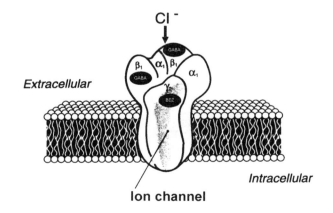

Figure 14–3. Model of the γ-aminobutyric acid (GABA)-benzodiazepine (BDZ) receptor complex.
Source. Reprinted from Zorumski CF, Isenberg KE: "Insights Into the Structure and Function of GABA-Benzodiazepine Receptors: Ion Channels and Psychiatry." *American Journal of Psychiatry* 148:162–173, 1991. Used with permission.

1979; Stephens et al. 1984; Yokoyama et al. 1982).

Benzodiazepine antagonists block the ability of benzodiazepine agonists to amplify the effects of GABA but have no intrinsic activity themselves. The imidazobenzodiazepine derivative Ro 15-1788 is one of the best studied benzodiazepine antagonists. In both animal and human studies, this antagonist has been found to have properties that enable it to totally negate all anxiety-reducing actions of benzodiazepines (Bonetti et al. 1982; Darragh et al. 1981a, 1981b, 1982a, 1982b; Haefely 1985; Hunkeler et al. 1981; Möhler et al. 1981; Polc et al. 1981). The action of Ro 15-1788 is accomplished by its ability to inhibit benzodiazepine binding to CNS neuronal binding sites (Möhler and Richards 1981; Richards et al. 1982).

The important discovery of an anxiogenic (i.e., anxiety-increasing) ligand utilized the social interaction test and found that ethyl-β-carboxylate (β-CCE), by acting on benzodiazepine binding sites, increased anxiety (File et al. 1982). The anxiogenic property attributed to β-CCE in animals was replicated in humans (Dorow et al. 1983) and was confirmed in animal experiments (Corda et al. 1983; File and Pellow 1984; File et al. 1984; Hindley et al. 1985; Pellow and File 1986; Petersen et al. 1982, 1983; Stephens and Kehr 1985). Although most β-carbolines are anxiogenic, others have been developed that have anxiolytic properties instead (File 1990).

Inverse agonists act directly to decrease the number of times that the chloride channel opens (Costa and Guidotti 1985; Zorumski and Isenberg 1991); thus, they have anxiogenic properties. These inverse agonists include β-carboline derivatives and the diazepam-binding inhibitor peptide (Breier and Paul 1988). Administration of inverse agonists is usually accompanied in animals (Hommer et al. 1987) and in humans (Dorow et al. 1983) by specific physiological effects indicative of stress (e.g., elevated heart rate, blood pressure, and certain stress hormones).

Partial agonists. Partial agonists are compounds that have less functional effect after occupying the receptor than do full agonists. Their ability to activate the receptor is low; therefore, a higher fraction of receptors must be occupied to match the action of a full agonist. A full response might not occur even with 100% receptor occupancy. The recent discovery that certain compounds can function as partial agonists at one receptor and full agonists at another complicates the issue (Knoflach et al. 1993; Wafford et al. 1993). Partial agonists along the entire spectrum of agonist, antagonist, and inverse agonist have now been synthesized (Cole et al. 1995).

There is considerable excitement, and clinical research is under way in this area, primarily based on the theoretical possibility that partial agonists have anxiolytic properties but would not be as sedating as or as prone to cause withdrawal symptoms as full agonists (Feely et al. 1989; Martin et al. 1990). The agent under most vigorous clinical study has been abecarnil (Ballenger 1991; Potokar and Nutt 1994). The data on partial agonist function that have been established recently have also led to an increased understanding of traditional benzodiazepines. For instance, identification of clonazepam's partial agonism (Gent et al. 1985) may explain why it is associated with less tolerance and fewer withdrawal difficulties than are other benzodiazepines that are full agonists.

Endogenous ligands. The presence of the benzodiazepine receptor argues for the existence of an endogenous ligand for this receptor (Paul et al. 1980). In theory, it could be an anxiolytic agonist or, in fact, an anxiogenic inverse agonist (see Haefely 1988 for review). However, no ligand in living humans has been found (Costa 1989). Perhaps the most likely candidate at this time is the diazepam-binding inhibitor, which is thought to have anxiogenic properties (DeRobertis et al. 1988).

Note that DeBlas and Sangameswaran (1986) isolated N-desmethyldiazepam (a metabolite of several benzodiazepines, including diazepam, chlordiazepoxide, and medazepam) from the brains of rats never exposed to benzodiazepines. Benzodiazepine metabolites were also found in human brains that were stored in the 1940s (long before development of the first benzodiazepine in the early 1960s) (File 1988). Investigators have hypothesized that the source of these naturally occurring benzodiazepine-like substances may come from the diet, based on evidence that benzodiazepine biosynthesis exists in fungi (Luckner 1984), and diazepam and lorazepam have been found in various foods (Unseld et al. 1988; Wildmann 1988).

Peripheral-Type Benzodiazepine Receptors

In determining exactly how the benzodiazepines affect certain behaviors and to pinpoint the specific benzodiazepine receptors in the brain, Braestrup and Squires (1977) made an unexpected and interesting discovery. They discovered another class of benzodiazepine binding sites—the *peripheral-type benzodiazepine receptors* (PBRs), so named because of their discovery in peripheral tissues, which were seen first in the kidney but were subsequently identified in all tissues including the CNS (Braestrup and Squires 1977).

Although very different from the GABA-benzodiazepine receptors, the PBRs do share some features, including their relatively high affinity for certain benzodiazepines. However, the two receptors have different binding specifications. In studies done on rodents, PBRs had high-affinity binding with 4'-chlorodiazepam (Krueger 1991). Conversely, GABA-benzodiazepine receptors have low affinity for this benzodiazepine derivative. Clonazepam and flumazenil have high affinity for GABA-benzodiazepine receptors but low affinity for PBRs. Multiple studies have found that GABA-benzodiazepine receptors interact with chloride channels at synaptic terminals, whereas PBRs are localized in mitochondria (Anholt et al. 1986). PBRs are found in the CNS at levels as great as and, in some cases, even higher than the GABA-benzodiazepine receptors (Marangos et al. 1982; Villiger 1985).

PBRs constitute more than 0.2% of the total mitochondrial protein (Antkiewicz-Michaluk et al. 1988). DeSouza and colleagues (1985) detected comparable receptor levels in other steroidogenic tissues. The conversion of cholesterol to pregnenolone, the initial step in the steroid synthetic pathway, takes place in the inner mitochondrial membrane. Steroid production is regulated by the transporting of cholesterol from the outer to the inner mitochondrial membranes. Hormones including adrenocorticotropin, luteinizing hormone, and follicle-stimulating hormone activate cholesterol transport from the outer to the inner mitochondrial membranes (Krueger 1991). Studies have confirmed that PBRs facilitate translocation of intramitochondrial cholesterol (Krueger and Papadopoulos 1990), supporting the hypothesis that PBRs are an important receptor site for certain previously unexplained physiological and behavioral actions attributed to benzodiazepines (Krueger 1991).

The work to date with PBRs indicates that benzodiazepines may bind to PBRs in the CNS, causing secondary behavioral effects (Krueger 1991). This line of reasoning and investigation is new but provides yet another hypothesis for the benzodiazepine mechanism of action. Knowing that PBRs have a primary role in steroid biosynthesis has shown, at least preliminarily, that agents that bind to PBRs regulate steroidogenesis, which may account for variation in pharmacological profiles and in tolerability among the benzodiazepines. Additional investigation is needed to determine how GABA-benzodiazepine receptors and PBRs are related in physiological regulation (Krueger 1991).

INDICATIONS

Benzodiazepines are generally well tolerated, with minimal side effects, and are efficacious for several conditions, most notably the treatment of anxiety and anxiety-related disorders. Indications for which benzodiazepines are used are similar to those for which barbiturates were once prescribed. However, the greater tolerability and safety profile of benzodiazepines have been responsible in large part for virtually eliminating barbiturates from being prescribed for anxiety conditions (Hollister 1982). In addition to their use as effective antianxiety agents, benzodiazepines have been proven to be effective hypnotics, an effect that is achieved through the same pharmacological actions that block or reduce anxiety (Hollister 1982).

Flurazepam has been one of the most frequently prescribed hypnotics in the United States, with confirmed efficacy supported by rigorous scientific and clinical studies. Flurazepam is effective in helping patients achieve and maintain sleep and does so with fewer of the troublesome side effects attributed to most other nonbenzodiazepine hypnotics and without the tolerance that develops to other drugs with long-term use (Kales et al. 1975). The short half-life benzodiazepine triazolam reached widespread popularity as a hypnotic largely because it was cleared from the system before morning and therefore was not associated with daytime drowsiness. However, concern and controversy surrounding triazolam's potential serious side effects (particularly at higher doses) have dampened enthusiasm and significantly reduced its use.

Benzodiazepines are also effective when used as muscle relaxants or as anticonvulsants, during alcohol withdrawal, and as intravenous anesthetics (Hollister 1982). Clonazepam is labeled as an anticonvulsant and is widely used for that indication, but it is also popular for treating anxiety conditions.

Benzodiazepines have become one of the most frequently used treatments for alcohol withdrawal. They are quite effective because of their cross-reactivity with alcohol as well as their anticonvulsant properties and anxiety-reducing efficacy. Benzodiazepines are traditionally given in a loading fashion and then rapidly tapered over the first 3–7 days of alcohol withdrawal.

The primary indications for benzodiazepines are certainly in the treatment of anxiety disorders. Eight benzodiazepines are labeled for anxiety (generalized anxiety disorder [GAD]), alprazolam is designated for panic disorder, and clonazepam is also widely used for these indications. Although benzodiazepines are used as ancillary medications in the management of obsessive-compulsive disorder, social phobias, and posttraumatic stress disorder (PTSD), their primary use has been in the treatment of GAD and more recently for panic disorder. Benzodiazepines have become the primary pharmacological treatment for GAD. Although certain psychotherapeutic techniques (e.g., support, meditation, relaxation) are effective and widely used, they are often relatively unavailable or unacceptable for various reasons. Thus, benzodiazepines have become the mainstay of treatment for GAD.

GAD is characterized by excessive anxiety and worry, accompanied by motoric symptoms of anxiety (e.g., tension, autonomic hyperactivity, and vigilance). Despite the seemingly simple nature of this disorder, GAD is often chronic (Angst and Vollrath 1991) and associated with considerable impairment and distress (Croft-Jeffreys and Wilkinson 1989).

Panic disorder is characterized by recurrent severe panic attacks and persistent worry that the panic attacks will recur or that they indicate serious medical or psychiatric consequences (Ballenger and Fyer 1993). Panic disorder is also a chronic condition in most clinical cases and is associated with even more morbidity than GAD. This includes frequent visits to the emergency room, family and occupational difficulties, financial dependency, abuse of alcohol, and even increased suicide attempts (Cowley 1992; Klerman et al. 1991; Markowitz et al. 1989; Weissman et al. 1989).

Because all benzodiazepines are apparently equally efficacious (Greenblatt and Shader 1974), the choice of a specific benzodiazepine is often influenced by physician or patient preference, side-effect differences (there are actually few), and marketplace issues. Diazepam was the most popular anxiolytic through the 1970s and early 1980s, when it was supplanted by alprazolam. In part, this change reflected a shift from one type of benzodiazepine to another. Diazepam has a long half-life and therefore has considerable accumulation over time. This feature results in the advantages of not needing multiple daily dosing and having less potential for withdrawal symptomatology when the drug is abruptly discontinued. However, these same characteristics can result in excess sedation and interference with optimal functioning. Alprazolam has a shorter half-life (6–20 hours), and its effective half-life is even shorter and therefore is associated with less accumulation, a multiple daily dosing requirement, and more potential for withdrawal symptoms when abruptly discontinued. More recently, clonazepam has become increasingly popular as a potent benzodiazepine with a longer half-life.

Early work with alprazolam in treating patients with panic disorder suggested it might have unique efficacy. Considerable research has established its efficacy for patients with panic disorder (Ballenger et al. 1988; Cross National Collaborative Panic Study, Second Phase Investigators 1992), leading to FDA approval for this indication. However, other benzodiazepines (e.g., diazepam, lorazepam, clonazepam) clearly are also effective when taken in sufficient doses (Charney and Woods 1989; Howell et al.

1987; Noyes et al. 1984; Schweizer et al. 1988), which also supports the theory that there are probably no specific indications for any one benzodiazepine.

Benzodiazepine treatment of GAD or panic disorder frequently proves to be long term, in keeping with the chronic nature of these disorders (Ballenger 1991; Romach et al. 1992; Schatzberg and Ballenger 1991). Most research experience with the benzodiazepines is short term, although longer-term treatment efficacy (i.e., up to 6 months) has been established in some trials (Cohn and Wilcox 1984; Fabre et al. 1981). In trials in which the benzodiazepine is discontinued blindly, original anxiety symptoms return in many patients (i.e., relapse), but this is not true for all patients (Rickels et al. 1980, 1983, 1990, 1991). Clinicians must periodically reassess the need for continued benzodiazepine therapy by tapering and discontinuing benzodiazepines if symptoms do not recur.

Benzodiazepines are also used to treat a number of conditions other than those previously described (Wesson 1985). The early use of benzodiazepines to treat schizophrenia-associated stress and/or anxiety proved ineffective. However, it was later postulated that the doses used were inadequate to achieve a therapeutic effect (Nestoros 1980). Because of clonazepam's rapid onset of action, it has been used as an adjunctive treatment with lithium to control the agitation seen during the acute manic phase of bipolar disorder (Chouinard et al. 1983). Benzodiazepines have also been used to treat night terrors as well as sleep or dream disturbances in patients with PTSD because benzodiazepines can decrease Stage 4 sleep (Friedman 1981; Kramer 1979). Clonazepam has also been used to treat nocturnal myoclonus (Boghew 1980; Matthews 1979) and tic douloureux when carbamazepine is ineffective (Court and Kase 1976).

Finally, the benzodiazepines have been used successfully in Third-World countries to treat tetanus, cerebral malaria, chloroquine toxicity, and maternal eclampsia (Ward 1985).

SIDE EFFECTS AND TOXICOLOGY

Benzodiazepines have proven efficacy for many conditions. Benzodiazepines that are used to treat anxiety disorders generally have a more favorable side-effect profile than the other pharmacological agents used for this indication (i.e., monoamine oxidase inhibitors and tricyclic antidepressants). Also, benzodiazepines begin to exert their therapeutic effects rapidly, with improvement generally seen in the first week of treatment.

As a class, benzodiazepines have remarkably few side

effects; the principal one is sedation. Patients report feeling sedated, drowsy, and slowed down and may fall asleep during daytime activities or have ataxia or slurred speech (Lader 1995; Linnoila et al. 1983). In laboratory settings, slowed psychomotor function has been observed (Hindmarch et al. 1991). Amnesia (anterograde) occurs with intravenous administration, and this effect is used widely in anesthesia induction (King 1992). However, amnesia has also been reported with oral dosing, especially with the hypnotic triazolam (Greenblatt et al. 1991). Amnesia is also present in less dramatic fashion in routine use, with some patients reporting relatively minor but demonstrable difficulties in learning new material (Barbee 1993; Ghoneim and Mewaldt 1990; Greenblatt et al. 1991; Hindmarch et al. 1991; King 1992; Lader 1995; Linnoila et al. 1983; L. G. Miller et al. 1988; Roth et al. 1984; Shader et al. 1986; Tönne et al. 1995). However, these side effects are generally transient and disappear quickly (usually within days) as tolerance to these effects develops in most patients (L. G. Miller et al. 1988).

Perhaps the greatest concern with the use of benzodiazepines is in elderly patients, in whom adverse events including falls from ataxia, hip fractures, and confusion are more common than in younger patients (Aiden et al. 1995; Lader 1995; Ray et al. 1987). In younger individuals, caution has always been suggested around benzodiazepine use and operation of heavy machinery. This advice is probably most important around the driving of automobiles, during which evidence of impairment could be significant in some individuals (O'Hanlon et al. 1995).

The controversy surrounding benzodiazepine administration and potential abuse or addiction in routine patient use is generally not supported by the available scientific evidence. (See Shader and Greenblatt 1993 for an excellent review of this complex area.) In a large community study of long-term alprazolam users, Romach and colleagues (1992) found that dosage did not escalate over prolonged use and that most patients used the benzodiazepines as prescribed. In fact, if deviations occurred, it was generally that a patient took less than the prescribed dosage. This area has been more controversial than warranted in part because of confusion over the meanings of addiction, dependence, and abuse. Recent efforts to clear up this confusion, especially differentiating abuse from withdrawal symptom liability, have been helpful (Ballenger 1993; Linsen et al. 1995; N. S. Miller 1995; N. S. Miller et al. 1995).

Evidence regarding the use of benzodiazepines during pregnancy is inconclusive. For this reason, pregnancy should be postponed until benzodiazepine treatment has been discontinued. In addition, because benzodiazepines are excreted through breast milk and place the nursing infant at risk for lethargy and inadequate temperature regulation, nursing mothers should also be cautioned against the use of benzodiazepines (Bernstein 1988).

Discontinuation

For the sake of thoroughness, a statement about discontinuation of the benzodiazepines is in order (see Ballenger et al. 1993; Shader and Greenblatt 1993). Numerous groups, including some medical professionals, have perpetuated the idea that if benzodiazepines are used long term, patients become "addicted" to the benzodiazepines, implying that they will abuse them or have an extreme withdrawal syndrome when the medication is discontinued. Actually, what occurs with benzodiazepines is similar to the effects of other medications used for long-term treatment of a medical and/or psychiatric condition and can be compared to what happens when a patient's cardiovascular medicine (e.g., propranolol, methyldopa) is suddenly discontinued (Garbus et al. 1979). In essence, the body goes through an adaptational process to the drug, and if medication is discontinued too abruptly, the patient can have withdrawal symptoms. The patient may also experience a transient recurrence of anxiety symptoms at levels more intense than those experienced before treatment; this is called *rebound*. The patient may also experience a return of symptoms that were present before treatment (relapse). However, if dosage is adjusted and gradually titrated downward, and if patients and their families are educated about what to expect during the discontinuation process, most patients can manage the transient withdrawal symptoms without much difficulty (see Ballenger et al. 1993 and Shader and Greenblatt 1993 for review), although this area remains somewhat controversial (Ashton 1995; Lader 1995).

DRUG-DRUG INTERACTIONS

Because benzodiazepines are frequently used for long-term treatment of conditions such as anxiety, the chances are high that at some point during treatment, the patient will receive another medication, either a prescription or an over-the-counter drug. It was originally believed that benzodiazepines did not interact with other drugs; however, it is now known that this is not the case. Cimetidine and disulfiram both slow the metabolism of benzodiazepines, causing them to have enhanced and prolonged effects. This is particularly true with the longer-acting benzodiazepines, including chlordiazepoxide and diazepam (Bernstein 1988; Glassman and Salzman 1987; Ruffalo and Thompson 1980). If a patient taking diazepam is also prescribed gallamine or succinylcholine, paralysis can result (Hansten 1985). Other drugs that can exacerbate the effects of benzodiazepines include isoniazid and estrogens, an effect produced by enzyme inhibition. Fluvoxamine inhibits the cytochrome P450 (CYP) 3A4 enzyme and can be associated with increased levels of alprazolam.

Other drugs act to reduce benzodiazepine effects. These drugs include antacids, which affect benzodiazepine metabolism by reduced gastrointestinal absorption, and tobacco and rifampin, which interfere with enzyme induction (Bernstein 1988). When digoxin is given to a patient taking benzodiazepines, the digoxin half-life increases; however, the mechanism by which this occurs is not known (Bernstein 1988).

At times, benzodiazepines, along with other sedative and anxiety-reducing medications, can cause significant sedation and CNS depression. When these drugs are taken at doses that are too high or when they are combined with alcohol or other sedating medications, they can cause significant sedation and occasionally respiratory depression as well (Bernstein 1988).

SUMMARY

Although the benzodiazepines continue to generate some controversy in the lay press and public, they are widely utilized because of their overall effectiveness in many common conditions (e.g., anxiety, alcoholism, stress, insomnia) and their favorable side-effect spectrum. Advances in the molecular neurobiology of the CNS benzodiazepine receptors hold considerable promise for better understanding of brain mechanisms underlying anxiety and for the possible development of even more specific and effective antianxiety agents.

REFERENCES

Aiden F, O'Connell D, Henry D, et al: Benzodiazepine use as a cause of cognitive impairment in elderly hospital inpatients. J Gerontol 50A (2):M99–M106, 1995

Angst J, Vollrath M: The natural history of anxiety disorders. Acta Psychiatr Scand 84:446–452, 1991

Anholt RRH, Pedersen PL, DeSouze EB, et al: The peripheral-type benzodiazepine receptor: localization to the mitochondrial outer membrane. J Biol Chem 261:576–583, 1986

Antkiewicz-Michaluk L, Guidotti A, Krueger KE: Molecular characterization and mitochondrial density of a recognition site for peripheral-type benzodiazepine ligands. Mol Pharmacol 34:272–278, 1988

Ashton H: Protracted withdrawal from benzodiazepines: the post-withdrawal syndrome. Psychiatric Annals 25: 174–179, 1995

Ballenger JC: Long-term pharmacologic treatment of panic disorder. J Clin Psychiatry 52:18–23, 1991

Ballenger JC, Fyer AJ: Examining criteria for panic disorder. Hosp Community Psychiatry 44:226–228, 1993

Ballenger JC, Burrows G, DuPont R, et al: Alprazolam in panic disorder and agoraphobia: results from a multicenter trial, I: efficacy in short-term treatment. Arch Gen Psychiatry 455:413–422, 1988

Ballenger JC, Pecknold J, Rickels K, et al: Medication discontinuation in panic disorder. J Clin Psychiatry 54 (10 suppl):15–21, 1993

Barbee JG: Memory, benzodiazepines, and anxiety: integration of theoretical and clinical perspectives. J Clin Psychiatry 54 (10 suppl):86–97, 1993

Barnard EA, Darlison MG, Fujita N, et al: Molecular biology of the GABA_A receptor. Adv Exp Med Biol 236:31–45, 1988

Bellantuono C, Reggi V, Tognoni G, et al: Benzodiazepines: clinical pharmacology and therapeutic use. Drugs 19: 195–219, 1980

Bernstein JG: Handbook of Drug Therapy in Psychiatry, 2nd Edition. Littleton, MA, PSG Publishing, 1988

Blanchard JC, Boireau A, Garret C, et al: In vitro and in vivo inhibition by zopiclone of benzodiazepine binding to rodent brain receptors. Life Sci 24:2417–2420, 1979

Boghew D: Successful treatment of restless legs with clonazepam (letter). Ann Neurol 8:341, 1980

Bond AJ, Hally DM, Lader MH: Plasma concentrations of benzodiazepines. British Journal of Clinical Psychopharmacology 4:51–56, 1977

Bonetti EP, Pieri L, Cumin R, et al: Benzodiazepine antagonist Ro 15-1788: neurological and behavioral effects. Psychopharmacology (Berl) 78:8–18, 1982

Bossman HB, Case KR, DiStefano P: Diazepam receptor characterization: specific binding of a benzodiazepine to macromolecules in various areas of rat brain. FEBS Lett 82:368–372, 1977

Braestrup C, Squires RF: Specific benzodiazepine receptors in rat brain characterized by high-affinity ^{3}H diazepam binding. Proc Natl Acad Sci U S A 74:3805–3809, 1977

Breier A, Paul SM: Anxiety and the benzodiazepine-GABA receptor complex, in Handbook of Anxiety, Vol 1. Edited by Roth M, Noyes R, Burrows GD. Amsterdam, Elsevier, 1988, pp 193–212

Charney DS, Woods SW: Benzodiazepine treatment of panic disorder: a comparison of alprazolam and lorazepam. J Clin Psychiatry 50:418–423, 1989

Chouinard G, Young SN, Annable L: Antimanic effects of clonazepam. Biol Psychiatry 18:451–466, 1983

Cohn JB, Wilcox CS: Long-term comparison of alprazolam, lorazepam and placebo in patients with an anxiety disorder. Pharmacotherapy 4:93–98, 1984

Cole BJ, Hellmann M, Seidelmann D, et al: Effects of benzodiazepine receptor partial inverse agonists in the elevated plus maze test of anxiety in the rat. Psychopharmacology (Berl) 12:118–126, 1995

Cook L, Sepinwall J: Behavioral analysis of the effects of and mechanisms of action of benzodiazepines, in Mechanism of Action of Benzodiazepines. Edited by Costa E, Grengard P. New York, Raven, 1975, pp 1–28

Corda MG, Blaker WD, Mendelson WB, et al: Beta-carbolines enhance shock-induced suppression of drinking rats. Proc Natl Acad Sci U S A 80:2072–2076, 1983

Costa E: Allosteric modulating centers of transmitter amino and receptors. Neuropsychopharmacology 2:167–174, 1989

Costa E, Guidotti A: Endogenous ligands for benzodiazepine recognition sites. Biochem Pharmacol 34:3399–3403, 1985

Costa E, Guidotti A, Mao CC, et al: New concepts in the mechanism of activity of BZs. Life Sci 17:167–185, 1975

Court JE, Kase CS: Treatment of tic douloureux with a new anticonvulsant (clonazepam). J Neurol Neurosurg Psychiatry 39:297–299, 1976

Cowley DS: Alcohol abuse, substance abuse, and panic disorder. Am J Med 92 (suppl 1A):41S–48S, 1992

Croft-Jeffreys C, Wilkinson G: Estimated costs of neurotic disorder in UK general practice 1985. Psychol Med 19:549–558, 1989

Cross National Collaborative Panic Study, Second Phase Investigators: Drug treatment of panic disorder: comparative efficacy of alprazolam, imipramine, and placebo. Br J Psychiatry 160:191–202, 1992

Curry SH: Concentration-effect relationship with major and minor tranquilizers. Clin Pharmacol Ther 16:192–197, 1974

Dantzer R: Behavioral effects of benzodiazepines: a review. Biobehavioral Reviews 1:71–86, 1977

Darragh A, Lambe R, Brick I, et al: Reversal of benzodiazepine-induced sedation by intravenous Ro 15-1788 (letter). Lancet 2:1042, 1981a

Darragh A, Lambe R, Scully M, et al: Investigation in man of the efficacy of a benzodiazepine antagonist, Ro 15-1788. Lancet 2:8–10, 1981b

Darragh A, Lambe R, Brick I, et al: Antagonism of the central effects of 3-methyl-clonazepam. Br J Clin Pharmacol 14:871–872, 1982a

Darragh A, Lambe R, Kenny M, et al: Ro 15-1788 antagonizes the central effects of diazepam in man without altering diazepam bioavailability. Br J Clin Pharmacol 14:677–682, 1982b

Dasberg HH, van der Klijn E, Guelen PJR, et al: Plasma concentrations of diazepam and its metabolite N-desmethyldiazepam in relation to anxiolytic effect. Clin Pharmacol Ther 15:473–483, 1974

DeBlas A, Sangameswaran L: Demonstration and purification of an endogenous benzodiazepine from the mammalian brain with a monoclonal antibody to benzodiazepines. Life Sci 39:1927–1936, 1986

DeRobertis E, Pena C, Paladini AC, et al: New developments in the search for the endogenous ligand(s) of central benzodiazepine receptors. Neurochem Int 13:1–11, 1988

DeSouza EB, Anholt RRH, Murphy KMM, et al: Peripheral-type benzodiazepine receptors in endocrine organs: autoradiographic localization in rat pituitary, adrenal and testis. Endocrinology 116:567–573, 1985

DeVane CL, Ware MR, Lydiard RB: Pharmacokinetics, pharmacodynamics, and treatment issues of benzodiazepines: alprazolam, adinazolam, and clonazepam. Psychopharmacol Bull 27:463–473, 1991

Doble A, Martin IL: Multiple benzodiazepine receptors: no reason for anxiety. Trends Pharmacol Sc 13:76–81, 1992

Dorow R, Horowski R, Paschelke G, et al: Severe anxiety induced by FG 7142, a beta-carboline ligand for benzodiazepine receptor function. Lancet 2:98–99, 1983

Fabre LF, McLendon DM, Stephens AG: Comparison of the therapeutic effect, tolerance and safety of ketazolam and diazepam administered for six months to outpatients with chronic anxiety neurosis. J Int Med Res 9:191–198, 1981

Faull RL, Villiger JW: Benzodiazepine receptors in the human hippocampal formation: a pharmacological and quantitative autoradiographic study. Neuroscience 26:783–790, 1988

Faull RL, Villiger JW, Holford NH: Benzodiazepine receptors in the human cerebellar cortex: a quantitative autoradiographic and pharmacological study demonstrating the predominance of type I receptors. Brain Res 411:379–385, 1987

Feely M, Boyland P, Picardo A, et al: Lack of anticonvulsant tolerance with RU 32698 and Ro 17-1812. Eur J Pharmacol 164:377–380, 1989

File SE: The use of social interaction as a method for detecting anxiolytic activity of chlordiazepoxide-like drugs. J Neurosci Methods 2:219–238, 1980

File SE: Animal models for predicting clinical efficacy of anxiolytic drugs: social behaviour. Neuropsychobiology 13:55–62, 1985

File SE: The benzodiazepine receptor and its role in anxiety. Br J Psychiatry 152:599–600, 1988

File SE: Preclinical studies of the mechanisms of anxiety and its treatment, in Neurobiology of Anxiety Disorders. Edited by Ballenger JC. New York, Wiley-Liss, 1990, pp 31–48

File SE, Hyde JRG: Can social interaction be used to measure anxiety? Br J Pharmacol 62:19–24, 1978

File SE, Hyde JRG: A test of anxiety that distinguishes between the actions of benzodiazepines and those of other minor tranquilizers and of stimulants. Pharmacol Biochem Behav 11:65–69, 1979

File SE, Pellow S: The anxiogenic action of PG 7142 in the social interaction test is reversed by chlordiazepoxide and Ro 15-1788 but not by CGS 8216. Arch Int Pharmacodyn Ther 271:198–205, 1984

File SE, Lister RG, Nutt DG: The anxiogenic action of benzodiazepine antagonists. Neuropharmacology 21:1033–1037, 1982

File SE, Lister RG, Maninov R, et al: Intrinsic behavioural actions of propyl beta-carboline-3-carboxylate. Neuropharmacology 23:463–466, 1984

Finkle BS, McCloskey KL, Goodman LS: Diazepam and drug associated deaths. JAMA 242:429–434, 1979

Friedman MJ: Post-Vietnam syndrome. Psychosomatics 22:931–941, 1981

Garbus SB, Weber MS, Priest RT, et al: The abrupt discontinuation of antihypertensive treatment. J Clin Pharmacol 19:476–486, 1979

Gardner CR, Tully WR, Hedgecock CJ: The rapidly expanding range of neuronal benzodiazepine receptor ligands. Prog Neurobiol 40:1–61, 1993

Geller I, Seifter J: The effects of meprobamate, barbiturates, D-amphetamine, and promazine on experimentally induced conflict in the rat. Psychopharmacologia 1:482–492, 1960

Gent JP, Feely MP, Haigh JRM: Differences between the tolerance characteristics of two anticonvulsant benzodiazepines. Life Sci 37:849–856, 1985

Ghoneim MM, Mewaldt SP: Benzodiazepines and human memory: a review. Anesthesiology 72:926–938, 1990

Glassman R, Salzman C: Interactions between psychotropic and other drugs: an update. Hosp Community Psychiatry 38:236–242, 1987

Gray JA: The Neuropsychology of Anxiety: An Enquiry into the Functions of the Septo-Hippocampal System. Oxford, England, Clarendon, 1982

Greenblatt DJ, Shader RI: Benzodiazepines in Clinical Practice. New York, Raven, 1974

Greenblatt DJ, Allen MD, Noel BJ, et al: Acute overdose with benzodiazepine derivatives. Clin Pharmacol Ther 21:497–514, 1977

Greenblatt DJ, Divoll M, Abernethy DR, et al: Clinical pharmacokinetics of the newer benzodiazepines. Clin Pharmacokinet 8:233–253, 1983

Greenblatt DJ, Harmatz JS, Shapiro L, et al: Sensitivity to triazolam in the elderly. N Engl J Med 324:1691–1698, 1991

Greenblatt DJ, Harmatz JS, Shader RI: Plasma alprazolam concentrations: relation to efficacy and side effects in the treatment of panic disorder. Arch Gen Psychiatry 50:715–722, 1993

Haefely W: Behavioral and neuropharmacological aspects of drugs used in anxiety and related states, in Psychopharmacology: A Generation of Progress. Edited by Lipton MA, DiMascio A, Killam KF. New York, Raven, 1978, pp 1359–1374

Haefely W: The biological basis of benzodiazepine actions, in The Benzodiazepines: Current Standards for Medical Practice. Edited by Smith DE, Wesson DR. Hingham, MA, MTP Press, 1985, pp 7–42

Haefely W: Endogenous ligands of the benzodiazepine receptor. Pharmacopsychiatry 21 (suppl 1):43–46, 1988

Haefely W: The GABA$_A$-benzodiazepine receptor: biology and pharmacology, in Handbook of Anxiety, Vol 3: The Neurobiology of Anxiety. Edited by Burrows GD, Roth M, Noyes R. Amsterdam, Elsevier Science, 1990, pp 165–188

Haefely W, Kuksar A, Möhler H, et al: Possible involvement of GABA in the central action of BZ derivatives. Adv Biochem Psychopharmacol 14:131–151, 1975

Hansten PD: Drug Interactions, 5th Edition. Philadelphia, PA, Lea & Febiger, 1985

Harvey SC: Hypnotics and sedatives, in Goodman and Gilman's The Pharmacological Basis of Therapeutics, 7th Edition. Edited by Gilman AG, Goodman LS, Rall TW. New York, Macmillan, 1985, pp 339–371

Hindley SW, Hobbs A, Paterson IA, et al: Microinjection of methyl-beta-carboline-3-carboxylate into nucleus raphe dorsalis reduces social interaction in the rat. Br J Pharmacol 86:753–761, 1985

Hindmarch I, Kerr JS, Sherwood N: The effects of alcohol and other drugs on psychomotor performance and cognitive function. Alcohol 26:71–79, 1991

Hollister LE: Pharmacology and clinical use of benzodiazepines, in Pharmacology of Benzodiazepines. Edited by Usdin E, Skolnick P, Tallman JF Jr, et al. London, Macmillan Press, 1982, pp 29–36

Hommer DW, Skolnick P, Paul SM: The benzodiazepine/GABA receptor complex and anxiety, in Psychopharmacology: The Third Generation of Progress. Edited by Meltzer HY. New York, Raven, 1987, pp 977–983

Howell EF, Laraia M, Ballenger JC, et al: Lorazepam treatment of panic disorder. Paper presented at the 140th annual meeting of the American Psychiatric Association, Chicago, IL, May 1987

Hsiao JK, Potter WZ: Mechanism of action of antipanic drugs, in Clinical Aspects of Panic Disorder. Edited by Ballenger JC. New York, Wiley-Liss, 1990, pp 297–317

Hunkeler W, Möhler H, Pieri L, et al: Selective antagonists of benzodiazepines. Nature 290:514–516, 1981

Kales A, Kales JD, Bixler EO, et al: Effectiveness of hypnotic drugs with prolonged use: flurazepam and pentobarbital. Clin Pharmacol Ther 18:356–364, 1975

Kangas L, Kanto J, Lehtinen V, et al: Long-term nitrazepam treatment in psychiatric outpatients with insomnia. Psychopharmacology (Berl) 63:63–66, 1979

Kilts CD, Commissaris RL, Rech RH: Comparison of anti-conflict drug effects in three experimental animal models of anxiety. Psychopharmacology (Berl) 74:290–296, 1981

King DJ: Benzodiazepines, amnesia, and sedation: theoretical and clinical issues and controversies. Human Psychopharmacology 7:79–87, 1992

Klepner CA, Lippa AS, Benson DI, et al: Resolution of two biochemically and pharmacologically distinct benzodiazepine receptors. Pharmacol Biochem Behav 11:457–462, 1979

Klerman GL, Weissman MM, Ouellette R, et al: Panic attacks in the community: social morbidity and health care utilization. JAMA 265:742–746, 1991

Knoflach F, Drescher U, Scheurer L, et al: Full and partial agonism displayed by benzodiazepine receptor ligands at recombinant γ-aminobutyric acid$_A$ receptor subtypes. J Pharmacol Exp Ther 266:385–391, 1993

Kramer M: Dream disturbances. Psychiatric Annals 9:50–68, 1979

Krueger KE: Peripheral-type benzodiazepine receptors: a second site of action for benzodiazepines. Neuropsychopharmacology 4:237–244, 1991

Krueger KE, Papadopoulos V: Peripheral-type benzodiazepine receptors mediate translocation of cholesterol from outer to inner mitochondrial membranes in adrenocortical cells. J Biol Chem 265:15015–15022, 1990

Lader M: Clinical pharmacology of benzodiazepines. Annu Rev Med 38:19–28, 1987

Lader M: Clinical pharmacology of anxiolytic drugs: past, present and future, in GABA Receptors and Anxiety: From Neurobiology to Treatment. Edited by Biggio G, Sanna E, Costa E. New York, Raven, 1995, pp 135–153

Lesser IM, Lydiard RB, Antal E, et al: Alprazolam plasma concentrations and treatment response in panic disorder and agoraphobia. Am J Psychiatry 149:1556–1562, 1992

Linnoila M, Erwin CW, Brendle A, et al: Psychomotor effects of diazepam in anxious patients and healthy volunteers. J Clin Psychopharmacol 3:988–996, 1983

Linsen SM, Zitman FG, Breteler MHM: Defining benzodiazepine dependence: the confusion persists. European Psychiatry 10:306–311, 1995

Lo MM, Niehoff DL, Kuhar MJ, et al: Differential localization of type I and type II benzodiazepine binding sites in substantia nigra. Nature 306:57–60, 1983

Luckner M: Secondary Metabolism in Microorganisms, Plants and Animals. Berlin, Springer-Verlag, 1984, pp 272–276

Lüddens H, Korpi ER: Biological functions of GABA$_A$ benzodiazepine receptor heterogeneity. J Psychiatr Res 29:77–94, 1995

Lüddens H, Wisden W: Function and pharmacology of multiple GABA$_A$ receptor subunits. Trends Pharmacol Sci 12:49–51, 1991

Lüddens H, Pritchett DB, Kohler M, et al: Cerebellar GABA$_A$ receptor selective for a behavioural alcohol antagonist. Nature 346:648–651, 1990

Lüddens H, Korpi ER, Seeburg PH: GABA$_A$/benzodiazepine receptor heterogeneity: neurophysiological implications. Neuropharmacology 34:245–254, 1995

Malizia A, Nutt DJ: Psychopharmacology of benzodiazepines—an update. Human Psychopharmacology 10:S1–S14, 1995

Marangos PJ, Patel J, Boulenger JP, et al: Characterization of peripheral-type benzodiazepine binding sites in brain using [^{3}H]Ro5-4864. Mol Pharmacol 22:26–32, 1982

Margules DL, Stein L: Increase of antianxiety activity and tolerance to behavioural depression during chronic administration of oxazepam. Psychopharmacology (Berl) 13:74–80, 1968

Markowitz JS, Weissman MM, Ouellette R, et al: Quality of life in panic disorder. Arch Gen Psychiatry 46:984–992, 1989

Martin JR, Kuwahara A, Horii I, et al: Evidence that benzodiazepine receptor partial agonist Ro 16-6028 has minimal abuse and physical dependence liability. Society for Neuroscience Abstracts 16:1104, 1990

Matthews WB: Treatment of restless legs syndrome with clonazepam (letter). BMJ 1:751, 1979

Mendelson WB, Gillin JC, Wyatt RJ: Human Sleep and Its Disorders. New York, Plenum, 1977

Miller LG, Greenblatt DJ, Barnhill JG, et al: Chronic benzodiazepine administration, I: tolerance is associated with benzodiazepine receptor down regulation and decreased γ-aminobutyric acid$_A$ receptor function. J Pharmacol Exp Ther 246:170–176, 1988

Miller NS: Liability and efficacy from long-term use of benzodiazepines: documentation and interpretation. Psychiatric Annals 25:166–173, 1995

Miller NS, Gold MS, Stennie K: Benzodiazepines: the dissociation of addiction from pharmacological dependence/withdrawal. Psychiatric Annals 25:149–152, 1995

Möhler H, Okada T: Benzodiazepine receptors: demonstration in the central nervous system. Science 198:849–851, 1977a

Möhler H, Okada T: Properties of ^{3}H diazepam binding to benzodiazepine receptors in rat cerebral cortex. Life Sci 20:2101–2110, 1977b

Möhler H, Richards JG: Agonist and antagonist benzodiazepine receptor interaction in vitro. Nature 294:763–764, 1981

Möhler H, Wu JY, Richards JG: Benzodiazepine receptors: autoradiographical and immunocytochemical evidence for their localization in regions of GABAergic synaptic contacts, in GABA and Benzodiazepine Receptors. Edited by Costa E, DiChaira G, Gessa GL. New York, Raven, 1981, pp 139–146

Nestoros JN: Benzodiazepines in schizophrenia: a need for reassessment. International Pharmacopsychiatry 15:171–179, 1980

Nielsen M, Braestrup C: Ethyl β-carboline 3-carboxylate shows differential benzodiazepine receptor interaction. Nature 286:606–607, 1980

Noyes R, Anderson DJ, Clancy J, et al: Diazepam and propranolol in panic disorder and agoraphobia. Arch Gen Psychiatry 41:287–292, 1984

Nutt D: Selective ligands for benzodiazepine receptors: recent developments, in Current Aspects of the Neurosciences. Edited by Osborne NN. New York, Macmillan, 1989, pp 259–293

O'Hanlon JF, Vermeeren A, Uiterwijk MMC, et al: Anxiolytics effects on the actual driving performance of patients and healthy volunteers in a standardized test: an integration of three studies. Neuropsychobiology 31:81–88, 1995

Olsen RW, Tobin AJ: Molecular biology of GABAA receptors. FASEB J 4:1469–1480, 1990

Olsen RW, McCabe RT, Wamsley JK: GABA$_A$ receptor subtypes: autoradiographic comparison of GABA, benzodiazepine, and convulsant binding sites in the rat central nervous system. J Chem Neuroanat 3:59–76, 1990

Paul SM, Skolnick P: Comparative neuropharmacology of antianxiety drugs. Pharmacol Biochem Behav 17 (suppl 1):37–41, 1982

Paul SM, Zatz M, Skolnick P: Demonstration of brain-specific benzodiazepine receptors in rat retina. Brain Res 187:243–246, 1980

Pellow S, File SE: Anxiolytic and anxiogenic drug effects in exploratory activity in an elevated plus-maze: a novel test of anxiety in the rat. Pharmacol Biochem Behav 24:525–529, 1986

Pellow S, Chopin P, File SE, et al: The validation of open/closed arm entries in an elevated plus-maze as a measure of anxiety in the rat. J Neurosci Methods 14:149–167, 1985

Petersen EN, Paschelke G, Kehr W, et al: Does the reversal of the anticonflict effect of phenobarbital by beta-CCE and FG 7142 indicate benzodiazepine receptor-mediated anxiogenic properties? Eur J Pharmacol 82:217–221, 1982

Petersen EN, Jensen LH, Honore T, et al: Differential pharmacological effects of benzodiazepine receptor inverse agonists, in Benzodiazepine Recognition Site Ligands: Biochemistry and Pharmacology. Edited by Biggio G, Costa E. New York, Raven, 1983, pp 57–64

Polc P: Electrophysiology of benzodiazepine receptor ligands: multiple mechanisms and sites of action. Prog Neurobiol 31:349–423, 1988

Polc P, Möhler H, Haefely W: The effect of diazepam on spinal cord activities: possible sites and mechanisms of action. Naunyn Schmiedebergs Arch Pharmacol 284:319–337, 1974

Polc P, Laurent JP, Scherschlicht R, et al: Electrophysiological studies on the specific benzodiazepine antagonist Ro 15-1788. Naunyn Schmiedebergs Arch Pharmacol 316:317–325, 1981

Potokar J, Nutt DJ: Anxiolytic potential of benzodiazepine receptor partial agonists. CNS Drugs 1:305–315, 1994

Randall LO: Discovery of benzodiazepines, in Pharmacology of Benzodiazepines. Edited by Usdin E, Skolnick P, Tallman JF Jr, et al. London, Macmillan Press, 1982, pp 15–22

Ray WA, Griffin MR, Schaffner W, et al: Psychotropic drug use and the risk of hip fracture. N Engl J Med 316:363–369, 1987

Richards JG, Möhler H, Haefely W: Benzodiazepine binding sites: receptors or acceptors? Trends Pharmacol Sci 3:233–235, 1982

Rickels K, Case WG, Diamond L: Relapse after short-term drug therapy in neurotic outpatients. International Pharmacopsychiatry 15:186–192, 1980

Rickels K, Case WG, Downing RW, et al: Long-term diazepam therapy and clinical outcome. JAMA 250:767–771, 1983

Rickels K, Schweizer E, Case WG, et al: Long-term therapeutic use of benzodiazepines, I: effects of abrupt discontinuation. Arch Gen Psychiatry 47:899–907, 1990

Rickels K, Case WG, Schweizer E, et al: Long-term benzodiazepine users 3 years after participation in a discontinuation program. Am J Psychiatry 148:757–761, 1991

Romach MK, Somer GR, Sobell LC, et al: Characteristics of long-term alprazolam users in the community. J Clin Psychopharmacol 12:316–332, 1992

Roth T, Roehrs T, Wittig R, et al: Benzodiazepines and memory. Br J Clin Pharmacol 18:45S–49S, 1984

Ruffalo RL, Thompson JF: Effect of cimetidine on the clearance of benzodiazepines. N Engl J Med 303:753–754, 1980

Schatzberg AF, Ballenger JC: Decisions for the clinician in the treatment of panic disorder: when to treat, which treatment to use, and how long to treat. J Clin Psychiatry 52:26–31, 1991

Schweizer E, Fox I, Case G, et al: Lorazepam vs alprazolam in the treatment of panic disorder. Psychopharmacol Bull 24:224–227, 1988

Seeburg PH, Wisden W, Verdoorn TA, et al: The GABA$_A$ receptor family: molecular and functional diversity. Cold Spring Harb Symp Quant Biol 55:29–44, 1990

Sepinwall J, Cook L: Behavioral pharmacology of anti-anxiety drugs, in Handbook of Psychopharmacology, Vol 13. Edited by Iversen LL, Iversen SD, Snyder SH. New York, Plenum, 1978, pp 345–393

Shader RI, Greenblatt DJ: Use of benzodiazepines in anxiety disorders. N Engl J Med 328:1398–1405, 1993

Shader RI, Dreyfuss D, Gerrein JR, et al: Sedative effects and impaired learning and recall following single oral doses of lorazepam. Clin Pharmacol Ther 39:526–529, 1986

Sieghart W, Eichinger A, Riederer P, et al: Comparison of benzodiazepine receptor binding in membranes from human or rat brain. Neuropharmacology 24:751–759, 1985

Simon P, Soubrie P: Behavioral studies to differentiate anxiolytic and sedative activity of the tranquilizing drugs, in Modern Problems in Pharmacopsychiatry, Vol 14. Edited by Boissier JR. Basel, Karger, 1979, pp 99–142

Smith DE, Wesson DR (eds): The Benzodiazepines: Current Standards for Medical Practice. Boston, MA, MTP Press Limited, 1985, pp 289–292

Squires RF, Braestrup CL: Benzodiazepine receptors in rat brain. Nature 266:732–734, 1977

often present at hypnotic doses. Phenobarbital and mephobarbital, which substitute a phenyl group at the 5 position, have anticonvulsant effects at doses that are not hypnotic. At increasingly higher doses, barbiturates induce anesthesia, coma, and ultimately death because the neurogenic- and hypoxic-driven respiratory drives are depressed. Simultaneous alcohol consumption reduces the lethal dose of barbiturates.

Tolerance and Dependence

With continued use, barbiturates result in the development of tolerance and dependence. Thus, sedative effects of barbiturates are largely lost by the third week of continuous fixed-dose treatment. The development of tolerance leads to the risk that the dose will be increased to obtain the same pharmacological effect. In addition, withdrawal symptoms can occur with abrupt discontinuation. Barbiturates have a higher abuse potential than other anxiolytics because of their powerful reinforcing effects and possible euphoriant effects. Alcohol and other sedative-hypnotics have additive CNS depressant effects when used with barbiturates.

Withdrawal symptoms from barbiturates may be minor (e.g., anxiety with somatic symptoms and orthostatic hypotension) or severe (e.g., delirium, convulsions, and possible death). Treatment of barbiturate withdrawal includes the reintroduction of the previous dose so that the drug can be tapered gradually. The use of a longer-acting barbiturate, such as phenobarbital, is appropriate for such a taper (Martin et al. 1979).

Pharmacokinetics

Barbiturates are metabolized by the 2C19 family of the cytochrome P450 system. Barbiturates induce their own metabolism, which results in a faster metabolism of the dose ingested and a reduced pharmacological effect. This is clinically relevant, because at maximal induction, the rate of metabolism is approximately doubled. Metabolism of barbiturates is slower in the elderly and infants. Other drugs metabolized by these enzymes, including dicumarol, exogenous corticosteroids and doxycycline, steroid hormones, cholesterol bisalts, and vitamins K and D, are also potentially affected by enzyme induction. Also, variable effects on other anticonvulsants such as phenytoin and valproate occur; therefore, close monitoring of the blood levels is indicated when these drugs are combined with barbiturates.

Mechanism of Action

Barbiturates allosterically modulate the γ-aminobutyric acid (GABA$_A$) receptor complex at a site different from the benzodiazepine site. Barbiturates increase the potency of GABA on the chloride ion channel (Haefely and Polc 1986). Electrophysiologically, barbiturates prolong the open configuration of the chloride channel, resulting in presynaptic (e.g., in the spinal cord) and postsynaptic (e.g., in the cortical and cerebellar pyramidal cells) inhibition. At higher concentrations, barbiturates increase chloride conductance even in the absence of GABA, an effect that contributes to their lethal potential. Phenobarbital and pentobarbital are weak in this respect and, therefore, have a higher therapeutic index.

Barbiturates have pharmacological effects other than through the GABA$_A$ receptor. At low doses, barbiturates depress voltage-dependent calcium currents in isolated hippocampal neurons and also inhibit the AMPA (α-amino-3-hydroxy-5-methyl-4-isoxazoleproprionate) subtype of glutamate receptors. At anesthestic doses, voltage-dependent sodium and potassium channels are also inhibited.

Indications

The use of barbiturates today in psychiatry is limited because their effects are not selective, and they have a low therapeutic index. Thus, they are used rarely to control anxiety, particularly given the availability of safer anxiolytics such as benzodiazepines (Koch-Weser and Greenblatt 1974). Likewise, the availability of safer sedative-hypnotics makes the use of barbiturates unnecessary. Barbiturates are used mainly in medicine as anticonvulsants and for intravenous anesthesia.

Intravenous amobarbitol was popular as a diagnostic and therapeutic aid in psychiatry for several years, although its use has waned considerably in the past decade. It was used in catatonia, mutism, and paralysis thought to be hysterical and also to facilitate recall of suppressed emotionally laden memories (Cole and Davis 1975). The use of a benzodiazepine instead might be safer because of the lower risk of respiratory depression.

CHLORAL HYDRATE

Chloral hydrate is occasionally prescribed as a sedative-hypnotic today. It is also used in children undergoing diagnostic and other procedures. With oral administration, chloral hydrate is rapidly metabolized to its active metabolite, trichloroethanol, by alcohol dehydrogenase in the liver, and the parent drug is largely undetectable in blood. Trichloroethanol is mostly conjugated with glucuronic acid and excreted in the urine. Chloral hydrate is an irritant to mucosal membranes and therefore can cause gastrointestinal distress unless it is diluted sufficiently or taken with food.

The pharmacological effect of trichloroethanol is through a barbiturate-like action on the GABA$_A$ receptor. Undesirable CNS effects include light-headedness, malaise, ataxia, and nightmares. Hangovers may also occur but are less common than with most barbiturates and benzodiazepines. Rare idiosyncratic reactions may occur, including disorientation, incoherence, and paranoia. Acute poisoning can cause hepatic and renal damage. Sudden withdrawal of chloral hydrate in habitual users can result in barbiturate-like withdrawal effects.

ANTIHISTAMINES

Antihistamines have not been adequately studied as anxiolytic agents and are probably less effective than appropriate benzodiazepines. Their antianxiety effects may be an aspect of their sedative effects. Hydroxyzine hydrochloride and hydroxyzine pamoate are both available by prescription. The pamoate form may cross the blood-brain barrier more efficiently than the hydrochloride form. Diphenhydramine is a more-sedating antihistamine that is often used as a hypnotic, but validating studies of its efficacy are lacking. It is available over the counter in the United States, with resulting unsupervised use. The disadvantages of antihistamines include their unpredictable effects, use in subtherapeutic doses, paradoxical agitation, rapid development of tolerance, and residual daytime sedation.

MEPROBAMATE

Meprobamate was the first nonbarbiturate antianxiety drug to become extensively used. It was synthesized in 1950 and initially drew attention because of its muscle relaxant properties (Berger 1970). It had a taming effect in monkeys and some selective action on the thalamus and the limbic system. Meprobamate does not closely resemble any other psychoactive drug currently in general use, except carisoprodol, a drug sold as a muscle relaxant with sedative properties (Elenbaas 1980).

The original approval of meprobamate by the FDA in 1955 was based on two positive open clinical trials in heterogeneous groups of anxious outpatients. In those days,

the FDA, by law, required only proof of safety not of efficacy. Meprobamate was marketed under the trade names of Miltown and Equanil. Meprobamate continued in wide general use through 1972, when the benzodiazepines generally replaced it. Meprobamate has a sedative antianxiety effect in anxious patients, but its effects in nonanxious volunteers are untested (Rall 1993; Roache and Griffiths 1987).

Pharmacological Profile

Meprobamate falls pharmacologically between the barbiturates and the benzodiazepines. It causes CNS depression but does not produce anesthesia. In animals, it releases behaviors suppressed by past adverse experiences, a property it shares with all other antianxiety drugs. Meprobamate depresses polysynaptic spinal reflexes more than monosynaptic reflexes; barbiturates are less selective in this regard. This action was originally believed to be the basis of meprobamate's muscle relaxant effects. In fact, such effects are very difficult to differentiate from sedation and decreased anxiety at the human clinical level (Rall 1993).

Meprobamate has anticonvulsant properties resembling those of ethosuximide. Clinically, it suppresses absence attacks but sometimes aggravates tonic-clinic seizures. Naloxone can block meprobamate's antianxiety effects in laboratory animals. Meprobamate may have a modest degree of analgesic action in patients with musculoskeletal pain.

Pharmacokinetics and Disposition

Meprobamate taken orally in humans reaches a peak blood concentration in 1–3 hours. It is not bound much to plasma proteins. Meprobamate is metabolized in the liver by hydroxylation and glucuronide formation, and a small proportion is excreted unchanged. Its half-life is 6–17 hours in studies of acute administration; with chronic administration, the half-life may increase to 24–48 hours. The exact hepatic microsomal enzymes involved and the degree to which meprobamate induces their activity are unclear.

In suicidal overdose, meprobamate tablets can form a lump (bezoar) in the stomach. As the patient emerges from coma, gastric activity will break up the bezoar and reinduce the coma if gastroscopy has not been used to identify and remove the undissolved tablet mass (Rall 1993). Otherwise, suicide attempts with meprobamate are treated as one would treat a barbiturate overdose. The lethal dose can be as low as 30 tablets (12,000 mg), but the average lethal dose is approximately 28,000 mg.

Proposed Mechanisms of Action

There is a presumption that meprobamate, because of its pharmacological effects, *should* work like the barbiturates or the benzodiazepines, through GABA; however, meprobamate does not bind to any of the relevant receptors (Paul et al. 1981; Rall 1993; Squires and Braestrup 1977). Three mechanisms have been proposed to explain meprobamate's action.

1. *Benzodiazepine-GABA-chloride ionophore complex:* Meprobamate is thought to exert its anxiolytic effect by interacting with the benzodiazepine-GABA-chloride ionophore complex (Paul et al. 1981). Initial studies on the benzodiazepine receptor showed that only clinically active benzodiazepines could displace ^{3}H-benzodiazepines from these receptors. Meprobamate competitively inhibits GABA-enhanced benzodiazepine binding at the benzodiazepine receptor at concentrations in the range of its clinical efficacy. Studies by Olsen (1981) and Leeb-Lundberg and Olsen (1983) suggested that the chloride ionophore may be the site of action. Squires and Braestrup (1977) and Polc et al. (1982) proposed that instead of acting through the benzodiazepine receptor, meprobamate may act through the barbiturate-recognition site in order to enhance benzodiazepine binding. However, GABAergic transmission is not affected by meprobamate (Ableitner and Herz 1987). Thus, the precise mechanism of anxiolytic action by meprobamate through the benzodiazepine-GABA-chloride ionophore complex is not clear.
2. *Role of adenosine:* The central actions of meprobamate are associated with the potentiation of endogenously released adenosine (Phillis and DeLong 1984). Meprobamate has been shown to be a potent inhibitor of adenosine uptake by rat cerebral cortical synaptosomes (Phillis and DeLong 1984). This inhibitory effect results in an increase in extracellular adenosine levels (DeLong et al. 1985). In addition, meprobamate potentiates the actions of adenosine in cerebral cortical neurons, which explains its depressant effects on spinal reflexes and cortical evoked potentials and, perhaps, its antianxiety effects (Hyman and Nestler 1993). Evidence for the role of adenosine in the clinical effects of meprobamate is supported by the potent sedative actions of adenosine as well as the sedative actions of other drugs that also increase endogenous adenosine levels (DeLong et al. 1985). Adenosine antagonists

(e.g., caffeine) can increase anxiety. Further evidence for the role of adenosine in the action of meprobamate is that adenosine competitively inhibits ^{3}H-diazepam binding to the benzodiazepine receptor (Paul et al. 1981).

3. *Effect on catecholamines:* Meprobamate has been found to decrease the stress-associated increase in norepinephrine turnover in the brain (Lidbrink et al. 1972). The stress-induced decrease in turnover of dopamine in the synapses of the neostriatum is decreased further by meprobamate, but in the median eminence, the dopamine turnover is increased by meprobamate. The latter finding has been difficult to interpret.

Abuse Liability

The human abuse liability of meprobamate (compared with lorazepam and placebo) was studied on a research ward by Roache and Griffiths (1987) with drug-free persons who had formerly been addicted to sedatives. These investigators found, surprisingly, that subjects preferred meprobamate to lorazepam based on well-tested measures of abuse liability. Meprobamate resembled a barbiturate more than a benzodiazepine in that subjects taking high single doses of meprobamate (or barbiturates) were aware of their deficits in psychomotor performance, whereas those taking lorazepam believed they were doing well when their performance was in fact impaired.

Indications

Meprobamate is available in 200-mg, 400-mg, and 600-mg tablets and in a sustained-release capsule form called Meprospan. The only FDA-approved indication for meprobamate is as an anxiolytic, but the drug was also widely used in the past, and even studied, as a hypnotic.

A review of efficacy studies of meprobamate concluded that its efficacy had not been adequately proven (Greenblatt and Shader 1971). However, many of those studies were done in the 1950s and 1960s before the methodology for such studies was well established. A well-done study with an adequate sample size would likely show meprobamate's efficacy in generalized anxiety disorder (GAD) to be comparable to that of a standard benzodiazepine.

The appropriate initial dose of meprobamate, if used as a hypnotic, is 400 mg at bedtime, increasing to 600 mg or decreasing to 200 mg if the 400-mg dose is too weak or too sedating, respectively. In studies of meprobamate in the treatment of chronic anxiety, typical initial dosages were 400 mg orally three times a day, but starting with 200 mg orally three times a day might be adequate. Physical dependence on meprobamate has been observed after doses as low as 3,200 mg/day. The equivalent dose in diazepam units is probably 1 mg of diazepam to 50–60 mg of meprobamate. In the past, a number of patients found 400 mg of meprobamate at bedtime useful as a hypnotic. Studies in the 1970s reported it to be as effective as flurazepam in insomnia (Vogel et al. 1990).

In a survey of elderly community residents (mean age 81 years; range 72–91), meprobamate was used regularly by 1.3% compared with 0.8% for chlordiazepoxide and 0.9% for lorazepam. Almost 90% of the patients taking meprobamate judged it "effective" or "very effective." One-half had been taking meprobamate for more than 10 years (Hale et al. 1988).

Conclusion

Meprobamate deserves to remain in the armamentarium of the clinical psychopharmacologist, although it has no clear advantages over benzodiazepines. It may be abusable, but it is not abused in the current drug culture. Occasional patients find meprobamate more effective or better tolerated than newer drugs. However, it is clearly, on the basis of present knowledge, a third- or fourth-line drug to be tried only when more obviously effective drugs have failed.

BUSPIRONE

History and Discovery

Buspirone was the first nonsedative, nonbenzodiazepine antianxiety drug to be developed and marketed. It was synthesized initially in 1968 in a search for a better neuroleptic (A. S. Eison 1990; M. S. Eison et al. 1987). Chemically, buspirone resembles a butyrophenone antipsychotic drug more than it does any previously developed antianxiety or antidepressant drug. Buspirone, like typical neuroleptics, blocks the conditioned avoidance response in rats. It does not cause catalepsy in animals; instead, it reverses neuroleptic-induced catalepsy. Buspirone appeared, therefore, to be potentially a clozapine-like drug—an antipsychotic with few neurological side effects. However, a Phase 2 clinical trial in 10 newly rehospitalized schizophrenic patients taking an average maximum daily dose of 1,470 mg showed little, if any, beneficial effects (Sathananthan et al. 1975). One patient showed tremor, rigidity, and akathisia.

Buspirone did show efficacy on some animal tests predictive of antianxiety drug actions (Riblet et al. 1982, 1984), such as inhibition of footshock-induced fighting in mice, decrease in aggression in rhesus monkeys, and attenuation of conflict behavior. It had no sedative-hypnotic or anticonvulsant effects.

The earliest study in patients with DSM-II (American Psychiatric Association 1968) anxiety disorder had clearly positive results (Goldberg and Finnerty 1979). A series of double-blind, placebo-controlled studies compared buspirone with several benzodiazepines and placebo and documented efficacy in anxiety without any suggestion of neuroleptic side effects or of abuse liability. On this basis, the drug received FDA approval and was marketed in 1986.

Structure-Activity Relations

In addition to buspirone, three other azaspirones entered clinical trials in depressed or anxious patients (M. S. Eison 1990). Gepirone, the second azaspirone, was studied more as an antidepressant than as an antianxiety agent even though its pharmacology is similar to that of buspirone (Cott et al. 1988). Ipsapirone (Heller et al. 1990) and tandospirone (Peroutka 1985) were other azaspirones. Published controlled studies indicated that the three newer azaspirones have efficacy similar to that of buspirone, but none of these newer agents has been marketed.

Although all three newer azaspirones share buspirone's serotonergic effects, they lack its dopaminergic effects, suggesting that the serotonergic actions are the crucial ones. Gepirone, but not buspirone, can cause a full serotonergic syndrome in mice. The newer azaspirones may have more serotonergic effects than does buspirone; however, until well-designed comparative studies are completed, it will be difficult to determine whether buspirone has an advantage over the others.

Pharmacological Profile

Buspirone is believed to exert its antianxiety effect through serotonin-1A (5-HT_{1A}) presynaptic and postsynaptic receptors. Evidence indicates that other specific 5-HT_{1A} or 5-HT_2 medications (e.g., gepirone, ritanserin) have antianxiety effects and that more broadly antiserotonergic drugs (e.g., methysergide, cyproheptadine) do not. Lesions in the brain serotonergic system will block the antianxiety effects of both benzodiazepines and buspirone (A. S. Eison and Eison 1994). Buspirone is a full agonist at presynaptic (dorsal raphe) 5-HT_{1A} receptors, with resulting inhibition of neuronal firing and a decrease in serotonin synthesis. Buspirone is also a partial agonist at postsynaptic (hippocampus, cortex) 5-HT_{1A} receptors. In the presence of functional serotonin excess, buspirone acts as an antagonist, but in serotonin deficit states, it functions as an agonist.

Buspirone also prevents the increase in dopamine-2 receptors caused by standard neuroleptics (the presumed mechanism causing tardive dyskinesia [TD]) and reverses the neuroleptics' catalepsy-inducing action in rodents. In neuroradiographic studies, radioactively labeled buspirone is found on dopamine receptors throughout the brain. This is more obvious than its parallel binding to 5-HT$_{1A}$ receptors. In some respects, buspirone's pharmacology early on resembled that of apomorphine—a dopamine agonist with claimed antianxiety effects—more than it did those of either the neuroleptics or the benzodiazepines (M. S. Eison et al. 1987; Ortiz et al. 1987).

Buspirone "passes" antianxiety drug tests in animals by reversing conditioned suppression of behavior, reversing learned helplessness, and being effective in the Porsolt behavioral despair model. It reverses inhibition of conflict behavior (antianxiety) but also blocks conditioned avoidance responding (antipsychotic) (A. S. Eison et al. 1991).

Buspirone has no major effects on the benzodiazepine-GABA-chloride ionophore complex, the major site of benzodiazepine action. Buspirone has been shown in vivo to enhance benzodiazepine binding, perhaps through a conformational change mediated by a picrotoxin-sensitive site (A. S. Eison and Eison 1984). Buspirone lacks the benzodiazepines' sedative, muscle relaxant, or anticonvulsant actions. Buspirone does not affect benzodiazepine withdrawal symptoms (Schweizer and Rickels 1986). However, a recent study of patients with DSM-III-R (American Psychiatric Association 1987) GAD who had been taking benzodiazepines for 3–9 weeks is of interest in this regard (Chiaie et al. 1995). Forty-four patients who met study criteria were stabilized on 3–5 mg of lorazepam for 5 weeks and then randomly assigned double-blind to 15 mg of buspirone or placebo. Lorazepam was openly tapered over 2 weeks. Buspirone significantly reduced the average degree of withdrawal symptoms compared with placebo. This study did not address longer-term use of benzodiazepines nor did it state that withdrawal symptoms were eliminated completely. It does not support the "cold-turkey" discontinuation of benzodiazepines, which may well be unpleasant or even dangerous.

Buspirone lacks abuse potential as judged by relevant animal and human studies (Cole et al. 1982; Griffith et al. 1986). In humans, it does not impair psychomotor performance or potentiate the performance-impairing effects of alcohol. Benzodiazepines tend to impair performance in the above paradigms (Smiley 1987); buspirone not only does not impair performance but also improves the subject's awareness of any alcohol-induced decrements in performance (Sussman and Chou 1988).

Pharmacokinetics

Buspirone, taken orally at usual doses, has a short half-life ranging from 1 to 10 hours in healthy volunteers. If the drug is taken with food, first-pass metabolism is decreased, and higher "area-under-the-curve" values for buspirone blood levels are achieved (Jann 1988).

Buspirone has multiple metabolites, mainly hydroxylated derivatives. The major metabolite is 1-pyrimidinylpiperazine (1-PP); brain levels of 1-PP can be several times higher than blood levels. 1-PP lacks buspirone's serotonergic effects but may block α_2-noradrenergic receptors and cause an increase in 3-methoxy-4-hydroxyphenylglycol (MHPG) production. This effect is of interest because one study found a strong correlation between 1-PP blood levels and buspirone's efficacy in alcoholic patients (Tollefson et al. 1991).

The lesser efficacy of buspirone in benzodiazepine withdrawal or panic attacks may be caused by the noradrenergic effects of 1-PP. If so, other azaspirones that do not form 1-PP may be better tolerated in such situations.

Buspirone's pharmacokinetics are not altered in elderly persons, in whom buspirone is probably effective both in depression and in GAD (Bohm et al. 1990; Napoliello 1986). Buspirone has favorable effects in agitated patients with dementia but may have a slow (up to 7 weeks) onset of action (Gelenberg 1994).

Neuroendocrine Effects

Buspirone in single doses of 30–90 mg elevates plasma levels of prolactin and probably growth hormone in nonanxious subjects (Meltzer et al. 1983). Other studies have shown less effect on prolactin levels. (For example, at 100 mg in a single dose, but not at 50 mg, prolactin levels were elevated; however, no effect on cortisol, aldosterone, or growth hormone levels occurred at either dose [Cohn et al. 1986].) A study of 20 anxious patients receiving clinically usual buspirone dosages found no changes in prolactin, cortisol, or growth hormone levels when the drug was given in 5- to 10-mg doses three times per day (Cohn et al. 1986).

Indications

Anxiety disorders.   In a meta-analysis of 8 placebo-controlled studies in 520 patients with GAD, buspirone was significantly effective over placebo (Gammans et al. 1992). Buspirone is superior to placebo in the treatment of GAD even when depressive symptoms are present (Gammans et al. 1992; Sramek et al. 1996b). Buspirone also is likely to be more effective in relieving coexisting depressive symptoms than are the benzodiazepines, except perhaps for alprazolam. At doses in the range of 30–90 mg/day, buspirone is effective in major depressive disorder and even in melancholic depression. Buspirone has even been suggested to induce mania (Liegghio and Yeragani 1988; McDaniel et al. 1990), a sign that it may really be an antidepressant.

Buspirone has been shown to have efficacy in GAD and has been available for use in that condition in the United States since 1986. Most large-scale (i.e., N > 60) double-blind, random-assignment clinical studies have shown that buspirone is equal in efficacy to that of standard benzodiazepines in GAD or in less clearly specified chronic anxiety states. Buspirone often fails to show efficacy in small short-term trials, especially those with a crossover feature (Olajide and Lader 1987), probably because patients with substantial experience with benzodiazepines tend to respond less well to buspirone. However, the original report describing this phenomenon (Schweizer et al. 1986) found that 22 of 37 patients with previous benzodiazepine exposure had improvement; 26 of 29 patients without prior benzodiazepine exposure had similar improvement. Thus, one cannot say that previous benzodiazepine exposure eliminates all response to buspirone.

Buspirone's efficacy may increase over time. In one large open study of patients with GAD, improvement rates increased from about 50% at 3 months to about 70% over 6 months (Feighner 1987). These numbers may be slightly deceptive because dropouts were fairly numerous in this study. However, the few studies that followed up patients taking buspirone compared with a benzodiazepine through improvement and subsequent drug withdrawal and then observed patients for several weeks after the drugs were stopped noted withdrawal agitation and relapse to benzodiazepine use in the benzodiazepine-treated patients, whereas the buspirone-treated patients seemed to continue to improve for several weeks after buspirone was stopped and did not require further medication (Rickels and Schweizer 1990; Rickels et al. 1988).

Buspirone seems in most ways to be the ideal antianxiety drug. It lacks the benzodiazepines' sedation, ataxia, tolerance, and withdrawal symptoms; abuse liability; and propensity to interfere with complex psychomotor tasks on driving simulators and related tests. In addition, benzodiazepines are linked by association to driving accidents and to falls and injuries in the elderly (Hemmelgarn et al. 1997; Smiley 1987; Sussman 1987; Sussman and Chou 1988). Buspirone does not impair performance; furthermore, it leaves the subject more aware of impairment resulting from alcohol ingestion than do the benzodiazepines (Sussman 1987).

Buspirone appears to improve respiratory functions and partial arterial carbon dioxide (Pa_{CO_2}) pressure in patients with anxiety and severe lung disease (Sussman and Chou 1988). Buspirone lacks the ability of benzodiazepines to depress respiration, making it potentially the preferred drug in anxious patients with pulmonary disease.

Several pilot studies have suggested that buspirone may decrease alcohol consumption in both animals and humans and may have a role in the detoxification and postdetoxification treatment of anxious alcoholic patients (Bruno 1989; Kranzler and Myers 1989; Schuckit 1993; Tollefson et al. 1991). Buspirone was compared with placebo in a 12-week trial of alcoholic subjects receiving weekly relapse prevention psychotherapy. Buspirone increased retention, reduced anxiety, delayed return to heavy drinking, and resulted in fewer drinking days compared with placebo (Kranzler et al. 1994). Tollefson and colleagues (1992) also reported positive effects. However, buspirone was not significantly different from placebo on a number of anxiety and alcohol use measures in highly anxious alcoholic patients over a 6-month treatment period (Malcolm et al. 1992).

Buspirone was found to be helpful in some injection drug users with anxiety who were receiving methadone maintenance and who had developed acquired immunodeficiency syndrome (AIDS) or AIDS-related complex (ARC) (Batki 1990). In this sample, no evidence of abuse of buspirone was found, and some evidence indicated that abuse of other drugs decreased. Buspirone was generally well tolerated and facilitated the tapering or discontinuation of benzodiazepines in most patients taking benzodiazepines at the start of the study. The patients, as a group, were dubious both about trying buspirone and about decreasing benzodiazepine use, so the positive effects of buspirone occurred despite this resistance. Unfortunately, the positive effects of buspirone faded after a few months in one-third of the patients.

Buspirone has few side effects, both absolutely and compared with placebo. The rates reported are 12% for dizziness, 6% for headache, 8% for nausea, 5% for nervousness, 3% for light-headedness, and 2% for agitation (Gelenberg 1994). Tolerance to these side effects probably develops. They may be handled by dosage reduction. If the dose is increased slowly, side effects may be minimized.

Buspirone dosage should be started at 5 mg three times a day for 1 week and then increased by 5 mg every 2–4 days as tolerated until the patient is receiving 10 mg orally three times a day. The patient should be encouraged to continue taking that dose for at least 6 weeks before deciding that the drug is ineffective. The drug customarily has been given three times per day because of its short half-life, but it is not known whether giving all or two-thirds of the dose at bedtime might work as well with better patient acceptance.

Most reviews of buspirone point out that psychiatrists do not widely prescribe it because it works so slowly and because it has no value in patients who have been taking benzodiazepines; however, it is certainly worth trying in some of these patients. Buspirone can ameliorate benzodiazepine withdrawal symptoms if it is administered as the benzodiazepine is being stopped (Chiaie et al. 1995); however, starting buspirone 2 weeks before beginning to terminate benzodiazepine use would be preferable (Udelman and Udelman 1990). Many clinicians suggest that the best way to shift from a benzodiazepine to buspirone is to stabilize the patient on both agents for several weeks before tapering the benzodiazepine (Sussman 1987).

A benzodiazepine combined with buspirone may be even more effective in GAD than either alone; the two agents certainly work by different mechanisms, and many patients taking long-term benzodiazepine medication have substantial degrees of residual symptomatology (Haskell et al. 1986). Udelman and Udelman (1990), in their review, identified several earlier small-sample reports suggesting improvement when buspirone was added to benzodiazepine treatment.

Nevertheless, buspirone has never been used clinically to the extent that its apparent safety and efficacy would support. Why? Observing the reduction in anxiety symptoms over weeks in reports of double-blind studies of buspirone compared with a benzodiazepine leaves one doubting that most patients' conditions improve much faster with a benzodiazepine. Both drugs show some improvement (on the average) after 1 week, a bit more after 2 weeks, and the most by 4 weeks. Although benzodiazepine-placebo differences are often statistically significant at week 1 or 2, and benzodiazepines and buspirone both achieve significance by weeks 3 and 4, buspirone-benzodiazepine differences are not significant early in these studies.

Buspirone is presumably ineffective when given as a single dose to relieve anxiety, whereas benzodiazepines may be effective in such circumstances. However, one suspects that benzodiazepines are better for insomnia early in treatment, whereas buspirone relieves insomnia later as part of a general improvement; benzodiazepines, as a group, are good hypnotics independent of their other effects.

Another part of the problem may be that psychiatrists, who can handle complicated drug regimens, rarely see drug-free patients with GAD or the medical patients with secondary anxiety who are the ideal candidates for buspirone, whereas primary care physicians may not have the time or motivation to explain buspirone's delayed re-sponse to their patients and then to adjust the dose carefully over several weeks until the patient's condition is clearly improved.

In other anxiety disorders, matters are less clear. In panic disorder, buspirone (mean dose, 61 mg) was no different from placebo and inferior to alprazolam in a double-blind study (Sheehan et al. 1993). However, in a 16-week placebo-controlled trial of buspirone in panic disorder with agoraphobia, in which all patients received cognitive-behavior therapy, buspirone had beneficial effects on generalized anxiety and agoraphobia (Cottraux et al. 1995). Two open trials of buspirone in treatment of social phobia at dosages generally in the 30- to 60-mg/day range showed substantial improvement rates (Bruns et al. 1989; Schneier et al. 1993). An open trial of buspirone reported significantly reduced posttraumatic stress disorder symptoms in 7 of 8 patients (Duffy and Malloy 1994).

In obsessive-compulsive disorder, one crossover study comparing buspirone and clomipramine seemed to show equal efficacy for obsessive-compulsive disorder, a condition with a low rate of placebo response (Murphy et al. 1990); however, subsequent open and blind studies did not support efficacy of buspirone in obsessive-compulsive disorder (Grady et al. 1993; Jenike and Baer 1988; McDougle et al. 1993). Pigott and colleagues (1992) reported that buspirone, as an augmenting agent, is not statistically better than placebo, although a subgroup of patients (29%) did obtain an additional greater than 25% benefit. None of the previous studies were properly statistically powered to be able to detect such an effect.

Thus, buspirone has advantages over benzodiazepines in GAD, especially among the elderly, in whom the cognitive and psychomotor impairment of benzodiazepines can be particularly problematic. It might also have a role in the management of alcoholism.

Depression. The assessment of buspirone's efficacy in depression began when multisite, controlled trials comparing buspirone with a benzodiazepine showed that buspirone was superior in relieving (or preventing the emergence of) depressive symptoms in patients selected initially as having an anxiety disorder. Then, Schweizer and colleagues (1986) conducted an open study of buspirone at doses between 30 and 60 mg/day in outpatients with nonmelancholic depression with favorable results. This was followed by a placebo-controlled, double-blind 8-week trial (Rickels et al. 1990), in which buspirone doses were permitted to increase to as high as 90 mg/day. The average dose by week 8 was, in fact, 57 mg/day. The study involved 143 evaluable patients. Side effects were similar in frequency and type to those attributed to buspirone in anxiety studies. Patients who completed the study had a 65% improvement after taking buspirone and a 28% improvement with placebo.

In a larger study that probably included the Rickels et al. (1990) sample, 418 patients with major depression from five sites were randomized to buspirone treatment or placebo and followed up for 8 weeks. About one-third had major depression with melancholia, and this group had improvement superior to that shown with placebo by the end of the first week. Patients with higher initial levels of depression or of anxiety had a better response compared with placebo than did patients with fewer symptoms. Buspirone was begun at 5 mg three times a day, but the dose was rapidly increased. Improvement occurred in 21 patients (out of 101 responders) when the dose was greater than 60 mg/day, the current upper dose recommended for use in GAD. Of the total sample of depressed patients, those who improved markedly did so at an average of 40 mg/day for initial response and of 50 mg at the end of the 8-week study. The patterns of symptom change were compatible with a full antidepressant effect, not a coincidental improvement in anxiety symptoms (Robinson et al. 1990).

Because buspirone is available in pharmacies, physicians can prescribe it as an antidepressant. Because no comparative studies are available contrasting buspirone with more widely used antidepressants, it is difficult to guess its ultimate place in a psychopharmacologist's armamentarium compared with the now-ubiquitous selective serotonin reuptake inhibitors (SSRIs), the older tricyclic antidepressants (TCAs), or the monoamine oxidase inhibitors (MAOIs). Buspirone is certainly worth a trial in patients whose symptoms have not responded to two or three prior antidepressants, although the clinician should keep in mind the need to increase the dose, the relative expense of the drug, and the relatively benign side-effect profile. The recent availability of the 15-mg unit dose is helpful.

A few open trials suggested that adding buspirone to an antidepressant, including an SSRI, will often produce a better antidepressant response (Bakish 1991; Jacobsen 1991; Joffe and Schuller 1993). More systematic and controlled studies are needed.

Neuropsychiatric disorders. There are two negative studies of buspirone in TD (Brown et al. 1991; Goff et al. 1991). Only a third study pushed the dose above 40 mg/day to an upper limit of 180 mg/day. Moss et al. (1993) studied buspirone treatment in eight patients who had persistent TD, with pretreatment Abnormal Involuntary Movement Scale (AIMS) scores of 10 ± 6. These scores declined to 6 ± 3 ($P < .02$) at 12 weeks at a mean dose of about 150 mg. The improvement in TD began at

60 mg/day and was accompanied by diminished neuroleptic-induced parkinsonian symptoms and akathisia. Goff et al. (1991) observed a similar reduction in extrapyramidal side effects (EPS) in their sample even though buspirone raised haloperidol blood levels. Jann and colleagues (1990), in their review of movement disorders and azaspirones, noted that buspirone does not aggravate Parkinson's disease and, at higher doses, can even suppress dyskinesias caused by drugs used in the treatment of this disease.

A placebo-controlled trial on smoking cessation (all subjects received cognitive-behavioral intervention) found buspirone to be beneficial in those who had high trait anxiety, with negative effects on abstinence in those with low anxiety. The effects of the drug lasted only as long as the medication was consumed (Cinciripini et al. 1995).

A series of case reports and several uncontrolled studies of buspirone in agitated patients with dementia, mental retardation, or brain damage have been done (Herrmann and Eryavec 1993). Positive effects occur in some patients—often fewer than half in the larger series—but the drug is sometimes quite helpful, and the potential alternative drugs (e.g., neuroleptics, β-blockers, carbamazepine, lithium, clonazepam, trazodone, and SSRIs) either have not been adequately studied (Schneider and Sobin 1991) or, as with the neuroleptics, have not been very effective (Schneider et al. 1990). Note that Ratey and colleagues (1991) used buspirone in aggressive and/or anxious mentally retarded patients and found very low doses (2.5–10 mg/day) to be more effective than larger doses, suggesting a window effect.

Smiley (1987), in a review of the effects of benzodiazepines and buspirone on psychomotor performance, found either that buspirone had no deleterious effect on a wide range of tasks or, when it impaired performance, that clinically equivalent benzodiazepine doses had substantially worse effects.

Drug-Drug Interactions

Buspirone is surprisingly free of significant drug-drug interactions. It is not a substrate for the cytochrome P450 enzymes nor does it inhibit them. When buspirone was first released, it was said to have caused hypertensive states when added to MAOIs. These symptoms now appear to have been mild to moderate elevations in blood pressure rather than serious hypertensive or serotonergic crises of the sort elicited by SSRI-MAOI combinations. However, it is too early to say that buspirone can be added to MAOIs with impunity. Ciraulo and Shader (1990), after reviewing all data available to Bristol-Myers on buspirone-MAOI interactions, found insufficient evidence for a total prohibition of combined buspirone-MAOI therapy; we concur.

In one study in which diazepam and buspirone were given concurrently for 2 weeks, only desmethyldiazepam levels had a 20% elevation (Gammans et al. 1986). Baughman (1994), quoted in Gelenberg's (1994) summary of a conference on buspirone, noted that buspirone does not adversely affect parkinsonism and does not interact with the more commonly used antiparkinsonian drugs. Baughman suggested that buspirone reduces EPS caused by neuroleptics in schizophrenic patients. Buspirone has been reported to elevate haloperidol blood levels somewhat; it may also elevate cyclosporin-A levels, a clinically more important effect, because elevation of these levels may increase the risk for adverse effects on the kidneys.

Gelenberg (1994) noted that buspirone may reverse sexual dysfunction caused by SSRIs. An earlier report by Othmer and Othmer (1987) found that buspirone improved sexual function in patients with GAD. One drug-drug interaction that fortunately does not exist is between SSRIs and buspirone. The combination of two serotonergic drugs could cause a serotonergic syndrome but in this case does not.

New Antianxiety Agents

Currently, none of the other well-known azaspirones—gepirone, ipsapirone, and tandospirone—is in development for release in the United States, and publications dealing with their clinical effects are few and far between (Borison et al. 1990; Cott et al. 1988; Harto et al. 1988; Heller et al. 1990). A new azaspirone, lesopitron, has been tested for tolerance in volunteers and patients with GAD (Sramek et al. 1996a), although details of its development plans are unclear. Flesinoxan, a phenylpiperazine derivative, is a potent 5-HT$_{1A}$ agonist (Schipper et al. 1991). It lacks active metabolites, including 1-PP. Preclinical studies support its efficacy in animal models of anxiety and depression. It is currently undergoing clinical studies in GAD and major depression.

Other newer drugs include those that are active at benzodiazepine receptors but that are not chemically describable as benzodiazepines. Abecarnil is a β-carboline-3-carboxylate that may be a partial agonist at the benzodiazepine receptor. It has side effects similar to those of the benzodiazepines but may be clinically effective at dosages free of most side effects (Ballenger et al. 1991).

Conclusion

Buspirone is a novel drug with unique probable mechanisms of action that, somehow, has never been as widely used as it probably deserves. It is effective in GAD and almost certainly in major depression. It seems likely that this drug may have efficacy in social phobia and in anxiety disorders accompanying various chronic medical disorders. Buspirone's side effects are mainly mildly bothersome, and its drug-drug interactions are benign. It is relatively safe in overdose and free from abuse liability and performance impairment. If the drug is started cautiously, with the dose raised as needed up to 60–90 mg in major disorders, it should be a major addition to the psychopharmacological armamentarium.

Researchers now should develop a drug—perhaps a buspirone analogue with some improvements (faster onset of action and better customer acceptance but no physical or psychic dependence)—or attain a better understanding of how to best use buspirone. It is clear that many patients with symptoms that meet DSM-IV criteria for GAD either have relatively lifelong anxiety symptoms of GAD or have waxing and waning symptoms that could be helped by prolonged intermittent pharmacotherapy (Feighner 1987). Anxiety associated with chronic medical conditions may be similarly prolonged, recurrent, episodic, or fully chronic. Social phobia can be equally chronic, as can dysthymia, with an admixture of anxiety symptoms (Dubovsky 1990; Rickels 1987).

Benzodiazepines do work, and tolerance to their antianxiety effects does not develop over weeks or months (Rickels 1987); however, in patients with chronic anxiety, it can prove difficult to test the patient's need for longer benzodiazepine therapy because withdrawal symptoms are likely to resemble or to reactivate the symptoms of the patient's original condition (Lader 1987). Buspirone—or our hypothetical "super-buspirone"—could be tapered and stopped periodically without the complication of anxiety-like withdrawal symptoms.

In this chapter, we considered various ideas as to why buspirone is less widely used than it might be. More research is needed on how to optimize physician and patient response to buspirone until an even better anxiolytic drug emerges. The relative paucity of clinical articles on newer anxiolytics makes one suspect that none of these agents is close to release in the United States or Europe.

REFERENCES

Ableitner A, Herz A: Influence of meprobamate and phenobarbital upon local cerebral glucose utilization: parallelism with effects of the anxiolytic diazepam. Brain Res 403: 82–88, 1987

American Psychiatric Association: Diagnostic and Statistical Manual of Mental Disorders, 2nd Edition. Washington, DC, American Psychiatric Association, 1968

American Psychiatric Association: Diagnostic and Statistical Manual of Mental Disorders, 3rd Edition, Revised. Washington, DC, American Psychiatric Association, 1987

American Psychiatric Association: Diagnostic and Statistical Manual of Mental Disorders, 4th Edition. Washington, DC, American Psychiatric Association, 1994

Bakish D: Fluoxetine potentiation by buspirone: three case histories. Can J Psychiatry 36:749–750, 1991

Ballenger JC, McDonald S, Noyes R, et al: The first double-blind, placebo-controlled trial of a partial benzodiazepine agonist abecarnil (ZK 112–119) in generalized anxiety disorder. Psychopharmacol Bull 27:171–179, 1991

Batki SL: Buspirone in drug users with AIDS or AIDS-related complex. J Clin Psychopharmacol 10 (suppl 3): 111S–115S, 1990

Baughman OL: The safety record of buspirone in generalized anxiety disorder (monograph). J Clin Psychiatry 12:37–45, 1994

Berger FM: The discovery of meprobamate, in Discoveries in Biological Psychiatry. Edited by Ayd F, Blackwell B. Philadelphia, PA, JB Lippincott, 1970, pp 115–129

Bohm C, Robinson DS, Gammans RE, et al: Buspirone therapy in anxious elderly patients: a controlled clinical trial. J Clin Psychopharmacol 10 (suppl 3):47S–51S, 1990

Borison RL, Albrecht JW, Diamond BI: Efficacy and safety of a putative anxiolytic agent: ipsapirone. Psychopharmacol Bull 26:207–210, 1990

Brown S, Fanstman W, Mone R, et al: An open-label trial of buspirone in the treatment of tardive dyskinesia (abstract). Biol Psychiatry 29:65A, 1991

Bruno F: Buspirone in the treatment of alcoholic patients. Psychopathology 22 (suppl l):49–50, 1989

Bruns JR, Munjack DJ, Baltazar PL, et al: Buspirone for the treatment of social phobia. Family Practice Recertification (Cl. 22 Selective Therapeutic Index) 11 (No 9, suppl): 46–52, 1989

Chiaie RD, Pancheri P, Casacchia M, et al: Assessment of the efficacy of buspirone in patients affected by generalized anxiety disorder, shifting to buspirone from prior treatment with lorazepam: a placebo-controlled, double-blind study. J Clin Psychopharmacol 15:12–19, 1995

Cinciripini PM, Lapitsky L, Seay S, et al: A placebo-controlled evaluation of the effects of buspirone on smoking cessation: differences between high- and low-anxiety smokers. JNClin Psychopharmacol 15:182–191, 1995

Ciraulo DA, Shader RL: Question the experts: safety of buspirone with an MAOI. J Clin Psychopharmacol 10:306, 1990

Cohn JB, Wilcox CS, Meltzer HY: Neuroendocrine effects in patients with generalized anxiety disorder. Am J Med 80 (suppl 3B):36–40, 1986

Cole JO, Davis JM: Narcotherapy, in Comprehensive Textbook of Psychiatry, 2nd Edition. Edited by Freedman AM, Kaplan HI. Baltimore, MD, Williams & Wilkins, 1975, pp 1968–1969

Cole JO, Orzack MH, Beake B, et al: Assessment of the abuse liability of buspirone in recreational sedative users. J Clin Psychiatry 43:69–74, 1982

Cott JM, Kurtz NM, Robinson DS, et al: A 5-HT$_{1A}$ ligand with both antidepressant and anxiolytic properties. Psychopharmacol Bull 24:164–167, 1988

Cottraux J, Note ID, Cungi C, et al: A controlled study of cognitive behavior therapy with buspirone or placebo in panic disorder with agoraphobia. Br J Psychiatry 167:635–641, 1995

DeLong RE, Phillis JW, Barraco RA: A possible role of endogenous adenosine in the sedative action of meprobamate. Eur J Pharmacol 118:359–362, 1985

Dubovsky SL: Generalized anxiety disorder: new concepts and psychopharmacologic therapies. J Clin Psychiatry 51 (suppl l):3–10, 1990

Duffy JD, Malloy PF: Efficacy of buspirone in the treatment of posttraumatic stress disorder: an open trial. Ann Clin Psychiatry 6:33–37, 1994

Eison AS: Azapirones: history of development. J Clin Psychopharmacol 10 (suppl 3):2S–5S, 1990

Eison AS, Eison MS: Buspirone as a midbrain modulator: anxiolysis unrelated to traditional benzodiazepine mechanisms. Drug Development Research 4:109–119, 1984

Eison AS, Eison MS: Serotonergic mechanisms in anxiety. Prog Neuropsychopharmacol Biol Psychiatry 18:47–62, 1994

Eison AS, Yocca FD, Taylor DP: Mechanism of Action of Buspirone: Current Perspectives. New York, Academic Press, 1991, pp 279–326

Eison MS: Azapirones: mechanism of action in anxiety and depression. Drug Therapy Supplement, August 1990, pp 3–8

Eison MS, Taylor DP, Riblet LA: Atypical psychotropic agents—trazodone and buspirone, in Drug Discovery and Development. Edited by William M, Malick JB. Clifton, NJ, Humana Press, 1987, pp 387–407

Elenbaas JK: Centrally acting oral skeletal muscle relaxants. Am J Hosp Pharm 37:1313–1323, 1980

Feighner JP: Buspirone in the long-term treatment of generalized anxiety disorder. J Clin Psychiatry 48 (No 12, suppl):3–6, 1987

Gammans RE, Mayol RF, LaBudde JA: Metabolism and disposition of buspirone. Am J Med 80 (suppl 3B):41–51, 1986

Gammans RE, Stringfellow JC, Hvizdos AJ, et al: Use of buspirone in patients with generalized anxiety disorder and coexisting depressive symptoms: a meta-analysis of eight randomized, controlled trials. Neuropsychbiology 25:193–201, 1992

Gelenberg AJ: Academic highlights—buspirone: seven year update. J Clin Psychiatry 55:222–229, 1994

Goff D, Midha K, Brotman A, et al: An open trial of buspirone added to neuroleptics in schizophrenic patients. J Clin Psychopharmacol 11:193–197, 1991

Goldberg HL, Finnerty RJ: The comparative efficacy of buspirone and diazepam in the treatment of anxiety. Am J Psychiatry 136:1184–1187, 1979

Goodman LS, Gilman A (eds): The Pharmacologic Basis of Therapeutics, 4th Edition. New York, Macmillan, 1970

Grady TA, Pigott TA, L'Heureux F, et al: Double-blind study of adjuvant buspirone for fluoxetine-treated patients with obsessive-compulsive disorder. Am J Psychiatry 150:819–821, 1993

Greenblatt D, Shader R: Meprobamate: a study of irrational drug use. Am J Psychiatry 127:1297–1303, 1971

Griffith JD, Jasinaski DR, Casten GP, et al: Investigation of the abuse liability of buspirone in alcohol-dependent patients. Am J Med 80:30–35, 1986

Haefely W, Polc P: Physiology of GABA enhancement by benzodiazepines and barbiturates, in Benzodiazepine-GABA Receptors and Chloride Channels: Structural and Functional Properties. Edited by Olsen RW, Venter JC. New York, Alan R Liss, 1986, pp 97–133

Hale WE, May FE, Moore MT, et al: Meprobamate use in the elderly: a report from the Dunedin program. J Am Geriatr Soc 36:1003–1005, 1988

Harto NE, Branconnier RJ, Spera KF, et al: Clinical profile of gepirone, a nonbenzodiazepine anxiolytic. Psychopharmacol Bull 24:154–160, 1988

Haskell D, Cole JO, Schniebolk BS, et al: A survey of diazepam patients. Psychopharmacol Bull 22:434–438, 1986

Heller AH, Beneke M, Kuemmel B, et al: Ipsapirone: evidence of efficacy in depression. Psychopharmacol Bull 26:219–222, 1990

Hemmelgarn B, Suissa S, Huang A, et al: Benzodiazepine use and the risk of motor vehicle crash in the elderly. JAMA 278:27–31, 1997

Herrmann N, Eryavec G: Buspirone in the management of agitation and aggression associated with dementia. American Journal of Geriatric Psychiatry l:249–253, 1993

Hyman SE, Nestler EJ: The Molecular Foundations of Psychiatry. Washington, DC, American Psychiatric Press, 1993

Jacobsen FM: Possible augmentation of antidepressant response by buspirone. J Clin Psychiatry 52:217–220, 1991

Jann MW: Buspirone: an update on a unique anxiolytic agent. Pharmacotherapy 8:100–116, 1988

Jann MW, Froemming JH, Borison RL: Movement disorders and the azapirone anxiolytic drugs. J Am Board Fam Pract 3:111–119, 1990

Jenike MA, Baer L: An open trial of buspirone in obsessive-compulsive disorder. Am J Psychiatry 145:1285–1286, 1988

Joffe RT, Schuller DR: An open study of buspirone augmentation of serotonin reuptake inhibitors in refractory depression. J Clin Psychiatry 54:269–271, 1993

Koch-Weser J, Greenblatt DJ: The archaic barbiturate hypnotics. N Engl J Med 291:790–791, 1974

Kranzler HR, Myers RE: An open trial of buspirone in alcoholics. J Clin Psychopharmacol 9:379–380, 1989

Kranzler HR, Burleson JA, Del Boca FK, et al: Buspirone treatment of anxious alcoholics: a placebo-controlled trial. Arch Gen Psychiatry 51:720–731, 1994

Lader M: Long-term anxiolytic therapy: the issue of drug withdrawal. J Clin Psychiatry 48 (No 12, suppl):12–16, 1987

Leeb-Lundberg LMF, Olsen RW: Heterogeneity of benzodiazepine receptor interactions with gamma-aminobutyric acid and barbiturate receptor sites. Mol Pharmacol 23: 315–325, 1983

Lidbrink P, Corrodi H, Fuxe K, et al: Barbiturates and meprobamate: decreases in catecholamine turnover of central dopamine and noradrenaline neuronal systems and the influence of immobilization stress. Brain Res 45:507–524, 1972

Liegghio NE, Yeragani VK: Buspirone-induced hypomania: a case report. J Clin Psychopharmacol 8:226–227, 1988

Malcolm R, Anton RF, Randall CL, et al: A placebo-controlled trial of buspirone in anxious inpatient alcoholics. Alcohol Clin Exp Res 16:1007–1013, 1992

Martin PR, Kapur BM, Whiteside EA, et al: Intravenous phenobarbital therapy in barbiturate and other hypnosedative withdrawal reactions: a kinetic approach. Clin Pharmacol Ther 26:256–264, 1979

McDaniel JS, Ninan PT, Magnuson JV: Possible induction of mania by buspirone (letter). Am J Psychiatry 147:125–126, 1990

McDougle CJ, Goodman WK, Leckman JF, et al: Limited therapeutic effect of addition of buspirone in fluvoxamine-refractory obsessive-compulsive disorder. Am J Psychiatry 150:647–649, 1993

Meltzer HY, Flemming R, Robertson A: The effect of buspirone on prolactin and growth hormone secretion in man. Arch Gen Psychiatry 40:1099–1102, 1983

Mendelson WB, Gillin JC, Wyatt RJ: Human Sleep and Its Disorders. New York, Plenum, 1977

Moss LE, Neppe VM, Drevets WC: Buspirone in the treatment of tardive dyskinesia. J Clin Psychopharmacol 13:204–209, 1993

Murphy DL, Pato MT, Pigott TA: Obsessive compulsive disorder: treatment with serotonin-selective uptake inhibitors, azapirones, and other agents. J Clin Psychopharmacol 10 (suppl 3):91S–100S, 1990

Napoliello MJ: An interim multicentre report on 677 anxious geriatric outpatients treated with buspirone. Br J Clin Pract 2:71–73, 1986

Olajide D, Lader M: A comparison of buspirone, diazepam, and placebo in patients with chronic anxiety states. J Clin Psychopharmacol 7:148–152, 1987

Olsen RW: The GABA postsynaptic membrane receptor-ionophore complex: site of action of convulsant and anticonvulsant drugs. Mol Cell Biochem 39:261–279, 1981

Ortiz A, Pohl R, Gershon S: Azaspirodecanediones in generalized anxiety disorder: buspirone. J Affect Disord 13:131–143, 1987

Othmer E, Othmer SC: Effect of buspirone on sexual dysfunction in patients with generalized anxiety disorder. J Clin Psychiatry 48:201–203, 1987

Paul S, Marangos P, Skolnick P: The benzodiazepine-GABA-chloride ionophore receptor complex: common site of minor tranquilizer action. Biol Psychiatry 16:213–229, 1981

Peroutka S: Selective interaction of novel anxiolytics with 5-HT$_{1A}$. Biol Psychiatry 20:971–979, 1985

Phillis JW, DeLong RE: A purinergic component in the central actions of meprobamate. Eur J Pharmacol 101:295–297, 1984

Pigott TA, L'Heureux F, Hill JL, et al: A double-blind study of adjuvant buspirone hydrochloride in clomipramine-treated patients with obsessive-compulsive disorder. J Clin Psychopharmacol 12:11–18, 1992

Polc P, Bonetti EP, Schaffner R, et al: A three-state model of the benzodiazepine receptor explains the interaction between the benzodiazepine antagonist to Ro 15-1788, benzodiazepine tranquilizers, β-carbolines, and phenobarbital. Naunyn Schmiedebergs Arch Pharmacol 321:256–260, 1982

Rall TW: Hypnotics and sedatives, in Goodman and Gilman's The Pharmacological Basis of Therapeutics, 8th Edition. Edited by Gilman AG, Rall TW, Nies AS, et al. New York, McGraw-Hill, 1993, pp 345–382

Ratey J, Sovner R, Park A, et al: Buspirone treatment of aggression and anxiety in mentally retarded patients: a multiple baseline placebo lead-in study. J Clin Psychiatry 52:159–162, 1991

Riblet LA, Taylor DP, Eison MS, et al: Pharmacology and neurochemistry of buspirone. J Clin Psychiatry 43:11–16, 1982

Riblet LA, Eison AS, Eison MS, et al: Neuropharmacology of buspirone. Psychopathology 17:69–78, 1984

Rickels K: Antianxiety therapy: potential value of long-term treatment. J Clin Psychiatry 48 (No 12, suppl):7–11, 1987

Rickels K, Schweizer E: The clinical course and long-term management of generalized anxiety disorder. J Clin Psychopharmacol 10 (suppl 3):101S–110S, 1990

Rickels K, Schweizer E, Csanalosi I, et al: Long-term treatment of anxiety and risk of withdrawal. Arch Gen Psychiatry 45:444–450, 1988

Rickels K, Amsterdam J, Clary C, et al: Buspirone in depressed outpatients: a controlled study. Psychopharmacol Bull 26:163–167, 1990

Roache J, Griffiths RR: Lorazepam and meprobamate dose effects in humans: behavioral effects and abuse liability. J Pharmacol Exp Ther 243:978–988, 1987

Robinson DS, Rickels R, Feighner J, et al: Clinical effects of the 5-HT$_{1A}$ partial agonists in depression: a composite analysis of buspirone in the treatment of depression. J Clin Psychopharmacol 10 (suppl 3):67S–76S, 1990

Sathananthan GL, Sanghvi I, Phillips N, et al: MJ 9022: correlation between neuroleptic potential and stereotypy. Curr Ther Res 18:701–705, 1975

Schipper J, Tulp MTM, Berkelmans J, et al: Preclinical pharmacology of flesinoxan: a potential anxiolytic and antidepressant drug. Human Psychopharmacology 6:S53–S61, 1991

Schneider LS, Sobin PB: Non-neuroleptic medications in the management of agitation in Alzheimer's disease and other dementia: a selective review. International Journal of Geriatric Psychiatry 6:691–708, 1991

Schneider LS, Pollock VE, Lyness SA: A meta-analysis of controlled trials of neuroleptic treatment in dementia. J Am Geriatr Soc 38:553–563, 1990

Schneier FR, Saoud JB, Campeas R, et al: Buspirone in social phobia. J Clin Psychopharmacol 18:251–256, 1993

Schuckit MA: Buspirone: is it an effective drug for alcohol rehabilitation? Drug Abuse and Alcoholism Newsletter 22(2), April 1993

Schweizer E, Rickels K: Failure of buspirone to manage benzodiazepine withdrawal. Am J Psychiatry 143:1590–1592, 1986

Schweizer E, Rickels K, Lucki I: Resistance to the antianxiety effect of buspirone in patients with a history of benzodiazepine use. N Engl J Med 314:719–720, 1986

Sheehan DV, Harnett-Sheehan K, Soto S, et al: The relative efficacy of high-dose buspirone and alprazolam in the treatment of panic disorder: a double-blind placebo-controlled study. Acta Psychiatr Scand 88:1–11, 1993

Smiley A: Effects of minor tranquilizers and antidepressants on psychomotor performance. J Clin Psychiatry 48 (suppl 12):22–28, 1987

Squires R, Braestrup C: Benzodiazepine receptors in rat brain. Nature 266:732–734, 1977

Sramek JJ, Fresquet A, Marion-Landais G, et al: Establishing the maximum tolerated dose of lesopitron in patients with generalized anxiety disorder: a bridging study. J Clin Psychopharmacol 16:454–458, 1996a

Sramek JJ, Tansman M, Suri A, et al: Efficacy of buspirone in generalized anxiety disorder with coexisting mild depressive symptoms. J Clin Psychiatry 57:287–291, 1996b

Sussman N: Treatment of anxiety with buspirone. Psychiatric Annals 17:114–118, 1987

Sussman N, Chou JCY: Current issues in benzodiazepine use of anxiety disorders. Psychiatric Annals 18:139–145, 1988

Tollefson GD, Lancaster SP, Montagne-Clouse J: The association of buspirone and its metabolic l-pyrimidinylpiperazine in the remission of co-morbid anxiety with depressive features and alcohol dependency. Psychopharmacol Bull 27:163–170, 1991

Tollefson GD, Montague-Clouse J, Tollefson SL: Treatment of comorbid generalized anxiety in a recently detoxified alcoholic population with a selective serotonergic drug buspirone. J Clin Psychopharmacol 12:199–226, 1992

Udelman HD, Udelman DL: Concurrent use of buspirone in anxious patients during withdrawal from alprazolam therapy. J Clin Psychiatry 51 (No 9, suppl):46–50, 1990

Vogel GW, Buffenstein A, Hennessey M, et al: Drug effects on REM sleep and on endogenous depression. Neurosci Biobehav Rev 14:49–63, 1990

SIXTEEN

Venlafaxine

Justine M. Kent, M.D., and Jack M. Gorman, M.D.

HISTORY AND DISCOVERY

Venlafaxine is a bicyclic phenylethylamine derivative with a structure and chemical profile that distinguish it from the tricyclic antidepressants (TCAs) and the selective serotonin reuptake inhibitors (SSRIs). Venlafaxine was first identified as having a neurochemical profile predictive of antidepressant activity in a search among novel compounds with the ability to displace [3H]imipramine from rat cortical binding receptors, an in vitro measure of ability to inhibit serotonin uptake. In vitro, it was found to block the reuptake of both norepinephrine and serotonin, leading to its description as a serotonin-norepinephrine reuptake inhibitor (SNRI). Venlafaxine was thus predicted to have antidepressant activity comparable to the TCAs, but without significant binding to neuroreceptors implicated in many of the adverse effects associated with the TCAs (Muth et al. 1986). Additional preclinical investigations showed that venlafaxine has in vivo activity consistent with models of antidepressant efficacy (Lloyd et al. 1992; Mitchell and Fletcher 1993). Clinical trials confirmed venlafaxine's antidepressant properties along with a benign side-effect profile. Venlafaxine was released for the treatment of depression in the United States in spring 1994.

STRUCTURE-ACTIVITY RELATIONS

Venlafaxine is a bicyclic compound (Figure 16–1). It has a novel biochemical structure that is unrelated to any of the heterocyclic antidepressants or SSRIs.

PHARMACOLOGICAL PROFILE

Venlafaxine and its active metabolite, O-desmethylvenlafaxine (ODV), are potent inhibitors of neuronal reuptake of serotonin, norepinephrine, and, more weakly, of dopamine in in vitro preparations (Bolden-Watson and Richelson 1993; Muth et al. 1986). Venlafaxine and ODV have no substantial affinity for muscarinic, cholinergic, histamine-H_1, or α-adrenergic receptors in vitro; they also have no monoamine oxidase A (MAO-A) or monoamine oxidase B (MAO-B) inhibitory activity (Muth et al. 1986). This selectivity appears to be an advantage when compared with the TCAs because venlafaxine is associated with fewer anticholinergic, central nervous system, and cardiac adverse effects. Venlafaxine had preclinical antidepressant activity in classic animal paradigms of antidepressant activity (Lloyd et al. 1992; Mitchell and Fletcher 1993; Moyer et al. 1984).

PHARMACOKINETICS AND DISPOSITION

After oral administration, venlafaxine is well absorbed from the gastrointestinal tract and undergoes extensive first-pass metabolism in the liver to its active metabolite, ODV. The primary route of excretion for venlafaxine, ODV, and its other minor metabolites is via the kidney (Howell et al. 1993). ODV's clearance (half-life = 10 hours) is slower than that of venlafaxine (half-life = 4 hours); therefore, steady-state ODV concentrations in plasma are higher than those of venlafaxine in most patients (Klamerus et al. 1992).

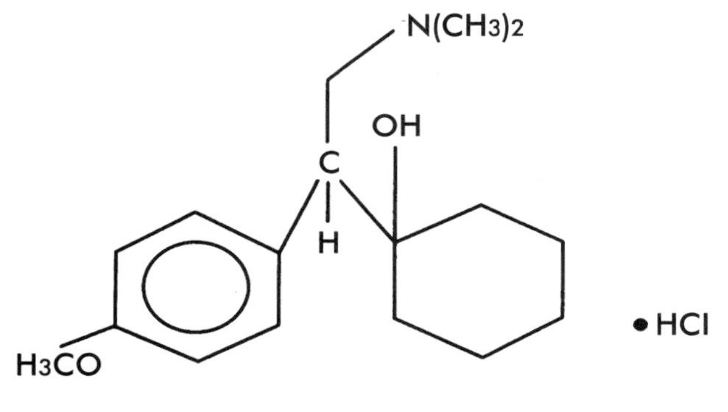

Figure 16–1. Chemical structure for venlafaxine.

In a randomized crossover study of the comparative bioavailability of venlafaxine and ODV, the investigators concluded that the same daily dose of venlafaxine can be given in either two or three divided doses to achieve equivalent total exposure and peak plasma concentrations (Troy et al. 1995b). Venlafaxine and its major metabolite, ODV, are 27% and 30%, respectively, bound to protein in human plasma (package insert). This relatively low degree of binding suggests that the probability of drug-drug interactions based on protein binding is remote.

Venlafaxine is available in immediate-release (IR) and extended-release (XR) formulations. The recommended starting dose of immediate-release venlafaxine is 75 mg/day, divided into two or three doses, but lower starting doses may be appropriate in patients with a history of sensitivity to medication side effects. The dose may be increased to the recommended maximum of 375 mg/day in three divided doses (package insert). The extended-release preparation is available in 37.5-, 75-, and 150-mg doses. Once-daily dosing with the extended-release formulation achieves bioavailability equivalent to that of twice-daily dosing with the immediate-release formulation. The extended-release preparation may be taken in the morning or evening, and bioavailability is not affected by coadministration with a meal (Troy et al. 1997). In a multicenter dose-response study of depressed outpatients treated with three different doses of immediate-release venlafaxine on a twice-a-day schedule, a trend analysis suggested that efficacy was dose-related (Mendels et al. 1993).

Clearance of venlafaxine and its metabolites may be significantly reduced in patients with cirrhosis and in patients with severe renal disease; therefore, dosing should be adjusted accordingly. In otherwise healthy elderly depressed patients, adjustments in dosing do not appear to be necessary. However, beginning with a low starting dose and increasing the dose slowly is a sensible approach in elderly patients.

MECHANISM OF ACTION

The mechanism of action of venlafaxine is believed to be related to its in vitro inhibition of serotonin and norepinephrine reuptake and therefore may be similar to that of the TCAs. It does not inhibit MAO, and its weak inhibition of dopamine reuptake may or may not be clinically significant (Muth et al. 1986).

INDICATIONS

Venlafaxine is currently approved by the U.S. Food and Drug Administration (FDA) for the treatment of depression, although its use in the treatment of other psychiatric disorders is being studied. Its efficacy in the treatment of depression has been established in several placebo-controlled noncomparative trials (Guelfi et al. 1995; Khan et al. 1991; Mendels et al. 1993; Schweizer et al. 1991; Shrivastava et al. 1994). In comparative studies, venlafaxine has been at least as effective as imipramine, clomipramine, fluoxetine, and trazodone (Clerc et al. 1994; Cunningham et al. 1994; Dierick et al. 1996; Samuelian et al. 1992; Schweizer et al. 1994). In doses up to 225 mg/day, venlafaxine's side-effect profile was superior to that of imipramine and clomipramine and comparable to that of trazodone and fluoxetine.

In two studies of severely depressed inpatients with melancholia, venlafaxine was shown to be an effective antidepressant when compared with placebo (Guelfi et al. 1995) and to be comparable or superior to fluoxetine (Clerc et al. 1994). The extended-release preparation was reported to be as safe and effective as the immediate-release preparation in the treatment of depressed outpatients in a premarketing, double-blind, placebo-controlled trial (Cunningham 1997).

Venlafaxine has the unique ability to induce a rapid desensitization of β-adrenoreceptors in the rat pineal gland, unlike other antidepressants that require repeated administration to induce noradrenergic subsensitivity (down-regulation of receptors). This finding raised the question of whether venlafaxine's effects correlate with a shorter latency to clinical antidepressant efficacy compared with other available antidepressants (Moyer et al. 1984, 1992). Most clinical studies to date appear to support the potential advantage of venlafaxine having a more rapid onset of action than do reference antidepressants. Several studies

(Guelfi et al. 1995; Khan et al. 1991; Rudolph et al. 1991; Schweizer et al. 1991; Shrivastava et al. 1994) found an earlier onset of action when compared with placebo in the first 2 weeks of treatment. However, none of these studies were designed as comparative trials to examine specifically latency of onset of clinical antidepressant effect. In support of an early onset of activity, two placebo-controlled clinical studies were reviewed in which the venlafaxine dose was rapidly escalated, and efficacy was measured frequently early in treatment of depressed outpatient populations. Three different statistical approaches were used to assess the onset of activity, and all three methodologies indicated that venlafaxine was superior to placebo by the time of the first efficacy measurements at day 7 of treatment. This superiority was maintained throughout the length of the clinical trials (Derivan et al. 1995). This supports the idea that aggressive dosing of venlafaxine may result in more rapid clinical improvement. However, rapid escalation of dose may also be associated with increased incidence of adverse effects (see section, "Side Effects and Toxicology," later in this chapter) and therefore may be best reserved for those patients requiring rapid treatment because of severe morbidity and mortality risks.

Long-term open-label trials of venlafaxine originally suggested that venlafaxine's efficacy is maintained over a 12-month period (Magni and Hackett 1992; Tiller et al. 1992). A meta-analysis of three double-blind, placebo-controlled extension studies confirmed that the 1-year relapse rate was significantly lower in the venlafaxine-treated group than in the placebo group (Mendlewicz 1995).

Although venlafaxine is currently approved only for the treatment of depression, several preliminary studies and case studies have been reported on the use of venlafaxine in the treatment of various anxiety disorders and childhood and adult attention-deficit/hyperactivity disorder. Two case reports (Ananth et al. 1995; Zajecka et al. 1990), an open-label study (Rauch et al. 1996), and an 8-week double-blind, placebo-controlled study (Yaryura-Tobias et al. 1994) suggested that venlafaxine may have potential use in the treatment of obsessive-compulsive disorder. In one case report, a patient with obsessive-compulsive disorder who was given venlafaxine had a reduction in obsessive-compulsive disorder symptoms but, interestingly, no significant reduction in concurrent depressive symptoms (Zajecka et al. 1990). In an open-label case series of four patients being treated with venlafaxine for panic disorder, preliminary results indicated that venlafaxine may be efficacious. However, Geracioti (1995) noted that in these patients with panic disorder, venlafaxine was better tolerated in lower doses than those recommended

for the treatment of depression. In an open-label chart review of eight cases of social phobia treated with venlafaxine, six of the patients had marked symptomatic improvement, suggesting a potential role in the treatment of this anxiety disorder (Kelsey 1995).

Three open-label clinical trials have reported positively on the potential usefulness of venlafaxine in the treatment of adult attention-deficit/hyperactivity disorder (Adler et al. 1995; Findling et al. 1996; Hedges et al. 1995). An additional preliminary clinical study of patients with dual diagnoses of attention-deficit/hyperactivity disorder and depression or dysthymia suggested that monotherapy with venlafaxine may be as effective as a combination of stimulants and antidepressants in this treatment group (Hornig-Rohan and Amsterdam 1995). In case reports, venlafaxine was also reported to be effective in two adult patients with attention-deficit/hyperactivity disorder, one with coexisting major depression and a second with coexisting major depression and generalized anxiety disorder (Wilens et al. 1995). In a case report of venlafaxine treatment in a child with attention-deficit/hyperactivity disorder and coexisting conduct and obsessive-compulsive disorders, after 6 weeks of treatment, the attention, organization, and obsessive-compulsive disorder symptoms were moderately to markedly reduced (Pleak and Gormly 1995). Further controlled clinical trials are needed to establish the potential role of venlafaxine in the treatment of these and other psychiatric disorders.

SIDE EFFECTS AND TOXICOLOGY

Venlafaxine inhibits the reuptake of serotonin and norepinephrine without significant effects on muscarinic, cholinergic, histaminic, or α-adrenergic receptors. Thus, its antidepressant activity appears to be equivalent to that of the TCAs and SSRIs but with a less adverse side-effect profile. Unlike the TCAs, venlafaxine administration results in minimal to no anticholinergic side effects, orthostatic hypotension, or sedation. In addition, venlafaxine appears to have no significant cardiac toxicity and does not affect the seizure threshold. In common with the SSRIs, nausea, headache, and insomnia are frequent complaints of patients taking venlafaxine. However, venlafaxine differs from the SSRIs in having lower incidences of anxiety and sexual dysfunction. The incidence of sexual dysfunction, including abnormal ejaculation/orgasm and impotence, ranges from 3% to 12% and appears to be dose related, with the incidence increasing at doses greater than 375 mg/day.

The most frequently reported adverse effect associated with venlafaxine is nausea, with an incidence of up to 37% found in placebo-controlled trials (package insert). It is the most common reason for discontinuation of venlafaxine and may be dose related (Khan et al. 1991). Nausea can reportedly be minimized with low starting doses and administration of the medication with meals (Fabre and Putman 1987). Absorption of venlafaxine is not affected by administration with food (package insert).

Other common side effects reported (>10% of subjects) in published pooled data include headache, insomnia, somnolence, dry mouth, dizziness, constipation, asthenia, sweating, and nervousness. Although venlafaxine has not been associated with adverse cardiovascular effects, modest increases in blood pressure have been reported in association with venlafaxine treatment (Cunningham et al. 1994; Fabre and Putman 1987; Schweizer et al. 1991). Sustained hypertension, manifest as an increase in supine diastolic blood pressure, has been reported in 3%–13% of patients taking venlafaxine and appears to be dose related (package insert). The manufacturer recommends regular monitoring of blood pressure for all patients taking venlafaxine.

During premarketing evaluation, there were 14 reports of acute overdose with venlafaxine, either alone or in combination with other drugs and/or alcohol. The dose ingested in all cases was estimated to be only several times the usual therapeutic dose. All 14 patients recovered without sequelae (data on file, Wyeth-Ayerst Laboratories, April 1994). Postmarketing spontaneous reports of overdoses involving venlafaxine alone or in combination with other drugs and/or alcohol, have included a variety of symptoms such as vomiting, tremor, agitation, diarrhea, lethargy, sinus tachycardia, bradycardia, prolonged Q-T interval, hypotension, and seizures (D. Albano, Wyeth-Ayerst Laboratories, December 1997). In postmarketing experience, venlafaxine has been associated with lethal overdoses, predominantly in combination with other drugs and/or alcohol. However, venlafaxine overdose alone has not been clearly linked with fatalities. In a published case report, a 41-year-old woman with severe central nervous system depression required intubation after ingesting a significant overdose of venlafaxine in combination with smaller amounts of two other central nervous system active medications (Fantaskey and Burkhart 1995).

DRUG-DRUG INTERACTIONS

Venlafaxine undergoes extensive hepatic metabolism by the cytochrome P450 (CYP) enzyme system, particularly the CYP2D6 isoenzyme. However, it appears to have a rather weak affinity for the CYP2D6 isoenzyme and, consequently, is a low-potency inhibitor of the isoenzyme. Because CYP2D6 is subject to genetic polymorphisms, patients' abilities to metabolize drugs via this system vary. In a study involving CYP2D6-poor and CYP2D6-extensive metabolizers, the total concentration of active compounds (venlafaxine and ODV) was comparable in the two groups (data on file, Wyeth-Ayerst Laboratories, April 1996). Therefore, dosage adjustment appears unnecessary when venlafaxine is coadministered with a CYP2D6 inhibitor.

In vitro and in vivo studies suggest that venlafaxine is a significantly weaker CYP2D6 inhibitor compared with fluoxetine and paroxetine (Amchin et al. 1996; Lam et al. 1997). Furthermore, in vitro and in vivo studies have shown venlafaxine to cause little or no inhibition of other cytochrome P450 isoenzymes, including CYP1A2, CYP2C9, CYP2C19, and CYP3A4 (Ball et al. 1997; data on file, Wyeth-Ayerst Laboratories, December 1997).

Cimetidine inhibits the first-pass hepatic metabolism of venlafaxine. However, because cimetidine causes only a minimal increase in overall pharmacological activity of venlafaxine and ODV, close monitoring and dose adjustment may only be necessary in cases of preexisting hypertension or hepatic disease or in elderly patients. Venlafaxine is not highly protein bound, so interactions resulting from displacement of a highly bound drug are not expected.

Venlafaxine is contraindicated in patients taking monoamine oxidase inhibitors (MAOIs) because of the risk of neuroleptic malignant-like syndrome, hypertensive crisis, or a serotonin-like syndrome. As with cyclic antidepressants and SSRIs, venlafaxine treatment should not be initiated until 2 weeks after discontinuation of an MAOI, and MAOI therapy should not be initiated until at least 7 days after discontinuation of venlafaxine. Limited data have been reported regarding the coadministration of venlafaxine with other central nervous system active drugs; therefore, caution should be used when combining these medications. Venlafaxine appears to have no clinically significant interactions with lithium (Troy et al. 1996), diazepam (Troy et al. 1995a), or alcohol (Troy et al. 1992).

SUMMARY

In summary, venlafaxine's clinical profile is similar to that of the SSRIs in terms of safety and tolerability, and its efficacy appears to be comparable to that of the heterocyclic antidepressants and the SSRIs. The extended-release preparation allows a once-daily dosing schedule, like the SSRIs, which increases medication compliance. Venlafaxine offers an advantage over other antidepressants in having a low potential for cytochrome P450–mediated drug-drug interactions, making it a good choice in patients taking other drugs utilizing the P450 system for metabolism.

REFERENCES

Adler LA, Resnick S, Kunz M, et al: Open-label trial of venlafaxine in adults with attention deficit disorder. Psychopharmacol Bull 31:785–788, 1995

Amchin JD, Ereshefsky L, Zaryaranski WM: Effect of venlafaxine versus fluoxetine on the metabolism of dextromethorphan, a CYP2D6 marker. American Psychiatric Association 1996 Annual Meeting New Research Program and Abstracts (NR362). Washington, DC, American Psychiatric Association, 1996, p 165

Ananth J, Burgoyne K, Smith M, et al: Venlafaxine for treatment of obsessive-compulsive disorder (letter). Am J Psychiatry 152:1832, 1995

Ball SE, Ahern D, Scatina J, et al: Venlafaxine: *in vitro* inhibition of CYP2D6 dependent imipramine and desipramine metabolism; comparative studies with selected SSRIs, and effects on human hepatic CYP3A4, CYP2C9 and CYP1A2. Br J Clin Pharmacol 43:619–626, 1997

Bolden-Watson C, Richelson E: Blockade by newly developed antidepressants of biogenic amine uptake into rat brain synaptosomes. Life Sci 52:1023–1029, 1993

Clerc GE, Ruimy P, Verdeau-Palles J: A double-blind comparison of venlafaxine and fluoxetine in patients hospitalized for major depression and melancholia. Int Clin Psychopharmacol 9:139–143, 1994

Cunningham LA (for the Venlafaxine XR 208 Study Group): Once-daily venlafaxine extended release (XR) and venlafaxine immediate release in outpatients with major depression. Ann Clin Psychiatry 9:157–164, 1997

Cunningham LA, Borison RL, Carman JS, et al: A comparison of venlafaxine, trazodone, and placebo in major depression. J Clin Psychopharmacol 14:99–106, 1994

Derivan A, Entsuah AR, Kikta D: Venlafaxine: measuring the onset of antidepressant action. Psychopharmacol Bull 31:439–447, 1995

Dierick M, Ravizza L, Realini R, et al: A double-blind comparison of venlafaxine and fluoxetine for treatment of major depression in outpatients. Prog Neuropsychopharmacol Biol Psychiatry 20:57–71, 1996

Fabre LF, Putman HP: An ascending single-dose tolerance study of Wy-45,030, a bicyclic antidepressant in healthy men. Current Therapeutic Research 42:901–909, 1987

Fantaskey A, Burkhart KK: A case report of venlafaxine toxicity. Clinical Toxicology 33:359–361, 1995

Findling RL, Schwartz MA, Flannery DJ, et al: Venlafaxine in adults with attention-deficit/hyperactivity disorder: an open clinical trial. J Clin Psychiatry 57:184–189, 1996

Geracioti TD: Venlafaxine treatment of panic disorder: a case series. J Clin Psychiatry 56:408–410, 1995

Guelfi JD, White C, Hackett D, et al: Effectiveness of venlafaxine in patients hospitalized for major depression and melancholia. J Clin Psychiatry 56:450–458, 1995

Hedges D, Reimherr FW, Rogers A, et al: An open trial of venlafaxine in adult patients with attention deficit hyperactivity disorder. Psychopharmacol Bull 31:779–783, 1995

Hornig-Rohan M, Amsterdam JD: Venlafaxine versus stimulant therapy in patients with dual diagnoses of attention-deficit disorder and depression (abstract). Psychopharmacol Bull 31:580, 1995

Howell SR, Husbands GE, Scatina JA, et al: Metabolic disposition of 14C-venlafaxine in mouse, rat, dog, rhesus monkey and man. Xenobiotica 23:349–359, 1993

Kelsey JE: Venlafaxine in social phobia. Psychopharmacol Bull 31:767–771, 1995

Khan A, Fabre LF, Rudolph R: Venlafaxine in depressed outpatients. Psychopharmacol Bull 27:141–144, 1991

Klamerus KJ, Maloney K, Rudoph RL, et al: Introduction of a composite parameter to the pharmacokinetics of venlafaxine and its active O-desmethyl metabolite. J Clin Pharmacol 32:716–724, 1992

Lam YWF, Alfaro CL, Ereshefsky L, et al: Cross-over comparison of CYP2D6 inhibition: insignificant effect of venlafaxine compared to sertraline, paroxetine and fluoxetine. American Psychiatric Association 1997 Annual Meeting New Research Program and Abstracts (NR267). Washington, DC, American Psychiatric Association, 1997, p 139

Lloyd GK, Cronin S, Fletcher A, et al: The profile of venlafaxine, a novel antidepressant agent, in behavioral antidepressant drug models (abstract). Clin Neuropharmacol 15 (suppl 1):428B, 1992

Magni G, Hackett D: An open-label evaluation of the long-term safety and clinical acceptability of venlafaxine in depressed patients (abstract). Clin Neuropharmacol 15 (suppl 1): 323, 1992

Mendels J, Johnston R, Mattes J, et al: Efficacy and safety of b.i.d. doses of venlafaxine in a dose-response study. Psychopharmacol Bull 29:169–174, 1993

Mendlewicz J: Pharmacologic profile and efficacy of venlafaxine. Int Clin Psychopharmacol 10 (suppl 2):5–13, 1995

Mitchell PJ, Fletcher A: Venlafaxine exhibits pre-clinical antidepressant activity in the resident-intruder social interaction paradigm. Neuropharmacology 32:1001–1009, 1993

Moyer JA, Muth EA, Haskins JT, et al: *In vivo* antidepressant profiles of the novel bicyclic compounds Wy-45,030 and Wy-45,881 (abstract no 76.12). Society for Neuroscience Abstracts 10:261, 1984

Moyer JA, Andree TH, Haskins JT, et al: The preclinical pharmacological profile of venlafaxine: a novel antidepressant agent (abstract). Clin Neuropharmacol 15 (suppl 1):435B, 1992

Muth EA, Haskins JT, Moyer JA, et al: Antidepressant biochemical profile of the novel bicyclic compound Wy-45,030, an ethyl cyclohexanol derivative. Biochem Pharmacol 35:4493–4497, 1986

Pleak RR, Gormly LJ: Effects of venlafaxine treatment for ADHD in a child (letter). Am J Psychiatry 152:1099, 1995

Rauch SL, O'Sullivan RL, Jenike MA: Open treatment of obsessive-compulsive disorder with venlafaxine: a series of ten cases. J Clin Psychopharmacol 16:81–83, 1996

Rudolph R, Entsuah R, Derivan A: Early clinical response in depression to venlafaxine hydrochloride (abstract no P-26–12). Biol Psychiatry 29:630S, 1991

Samuelian JC, Tatossian A, Hackett D: A randomized, double-blind, parallel group comparison of venlafaxine and clomipramine in outpatients with major depression (abstract). Clin Neuropharmacol 15 (suppl 1):324B, 1992

Schweizer E, Weise C, Clary C, et al: Placebo-controlled trial of venlafaxine for the treatment of major depression. J Clin Psychopharmacol 11:233–236, 1991

Schweizer E, Feighner J, Mandos LA, et al: Comparison of venlafaxine and imipramine in the acute treatment of major depression in outpatients. J Clin Psychiatry 55:104–108, 1994

Shrivastava R, Patrick R, Scherer N, et al: A dose-response study of venlafaxine (abstract). Neuropharmacology 10 (suppl 3):221, 1994

Tiller J, Johnson G, O'Sullivan B, et al: Venlafaxine: a long term study (abstract). Clin Neuropharmacol 14 (suppl):342B, 1992

Troy S, Piergies A, Lucki I, et al: Venlafaxine pharmacokinetics and pharmacodynamics (abstract). Clin Neuropharmacol 15 (suppl 1):324B, 1992

Troy SM, Lucki I, Peirgies AA, et al: Pharmacokinetic and pharmacodynamic evaluation of the potential drug interaction between venlafaxine and diazepam. J Clin Pharmacol 35:410–419, 1995a

Troy SM, Parker VD, Fruncillo RJ, et al: The pharmacokinetics of venlafaxine when given in a twice-daily regimen. J Clin Pharmacol 35:404–409, 1995b

Troy SM, Parker VD, Hicks DR, et al: Pharmacokinetic interaction between multiple-dose venlafaxine and single-dose lithium. J Clin Pharmacol 36:175–181, 1996

Troy SM, DiLea C, Martin PT, et al: Pharmacokinetics of once daily venlafaxine extended release (XR) in healthy volunteers. Current Therapeutic Research 58:504–514, 1997

Wilens TE, Biederman J, Spencer TJ: Venlafaxine for adult ADHD. Am J Psychiatry 152:1099–1100, 1995

Yaryura-Tobias JA, Neziroglu FA, McKay DR: The action of venlafaxine on obsessive-compulsive disorder (abstract). Biol Psychiatry 35:737, 1994

Zajecka JM, Fawcett J, Guy C: Coexisting major depression and obsessive-compulsive disorder treated with venlafaxine. J Clin Psychopharmacol 10:152–153, 1990

Antipsychotics

SEVENTEEN

Antipsychotic Medications

Stephen R. Marder, M.D.

Antipsychotic drugs are used to treat nearly all forms of psychosis, including schizophrenia, schizoaffective disorder, affective disorders with psychosis, and psychoses associated with organic mental disorders. Although these drugs have become standard treatments in psychiatry and medicine, they have important limitations: they are not effective for all patients, they have several serious adverse effects, and even patients who respond well often continue to have serious signs and symptoms of illness. These limitations have led to a search for newer drugs that have fewer adverse effects and similar or improved effectiveness. In this chapter, I discuss the conventional antipsychotics that were discovered during the early 1950s and that have defined antipsychotic treatment until recently. Owens and Risch, in Chapter 18 of this volume, focus on newer antipsychotics, including clozapine, risperidone, sertindole, olanzapine, and quetiapine.

All of the conventional antipsychotics produce significant neurological side effects and, for this reason, are often referred to as neuroleptics. However, the discovery of newer drugs with fewer motor side effects indicates that defining this group by a particular side effect is probably inaccurate. Thus, the term *antipsychotic* is preferable for describing these drugs. In this chapter, I use the terms *traditional* or *conventional antipsychotic* to describe drugs that were previously termed *neuroleptic*.

HISTORY AND DISCOVERY

Henri Laborit, a French surgeon with an interest in drugs that would decrease preoperative anxiety, convinced the Rhone-Poulenc laboratories of the importance of identifying compounds that would relax patients and make surgical shock less likely. Chlorpromazine, a compound synthesized by Paul Charpentier in 1950, clearly fulfilled Laborit's goals. Patients who received intravenous doses of 50–100 mg had some drowsiness, but, more important, they appeared relatively indifferent to the surgical procedure. Laborit realized the potential of chlorpromazine and succeeded in convincing several psychiatrists to administer the drug to patients with psychosis and agitation. Although Delay and Deniker were not the first to observe the antipsychotic effects of chlorpromazine, their report in 1952 to the Société Medico-Psychologique is often cited as the first public report of an effective drug for the treatment of a major mental disorder.

Within a year of chlorpromazine's introduction, the mental hospitals of Paris had changed. Restraint devices, seclusion, and the need for locked units became relatively uncommon, as they are today. The major factor that contributed to the rapid acceptance of chlorpromazine in France and subsequently in nearly every corner of the world was the absence of any other effective treatment for schizophrenia or other forms of psychosis. Chlorpromazine was relatively inexpensive to administer to large numbers of patients. Despite its side effects, it was very safe. Because chlorpromazine was effective for a large proportion of patients to whom it was administered, its advantages became apparent to clinicians who used it in appropriate patients. Chlorpromazine also stimulated the pharmaceutical industry to develop other phenothiazines during the first years after its discovery. Thioridazine and fluphenazine, as well as newer classes of drugs such as the butyrophenones (e.g., haloperidol) and the thioxanthenes (e.g., thiothixene), were developed during this time. Reserpine was also found to be an effective antipsychotic drug in the United States at about the same time that chlorpromazine was gaining acceptance. Reserpine initially became a popular alternative to chlorpromazine and other antipsychotics but then faded from use, probably because of its side effects and the perception that it was less effective than chlorpromazine.

The side effects of chlorpromazine, particularly drug-induced parkinsonism and other extrapyramidal side effects (EPS), were reported shortly after its introduction in 1952 (Lehmann and Hanrahan 1954). The early observations of the effectiveness of chlorpromazine and other antipsychotics may have resulted in a tendency to underestimate the seriousness of their side effects. Although Delay and other early researchers of chlorpromazine found that patients usually responded to doses in the range of 200–400 mg/day, later researchers found that many individuals tolerated much higher doses. When more potent drugs such as haloperidol and fluphenazine became available, doses comparable to 2,000 mg or more of chlorpromazine (or 40 mg of haloperidol or fluphenazine) were commonly prescribed. Several carefully designed studies showed that these higher doses resulted in more side effects but seldom in greater efficacy (Baldessarini et al. 1988). As a result, the recent trend has been directed at treating patients with the lowest effective antipsychotic dose.

STRUCTURE-ACTIVITY RELATIONS

Phenothiazines

The phenothiazine antipsychotics are characterized by a three-ring structure with a six-member central ring (Table 17–1). The activity of the group can be affected by substitutions at positions 2 or 10. The phenothiazines are usually categorized into three classes based on substitutions at position 10.

1. The *aliphatic class*—represented by chlorpromazine—consists of drugs that have relatively low potency at D_2 receptors compared with other antipsychotics, more antimuscarinic activity, more sympathetic and parasympathetic activity, and more sedation.
2. The *piperidine class*—represented by thioridazine—has the third carbon of the side chain and the basic nitrogen incorporated into a piperidine ring. This class has a clinical profile similar to that of the aliphatic class, with somewhat reduced potency at D_2 sites.

3. The *piperazine class*—represented by trifluoperazine and fluphenazine—has a piperazine ring substituted in the side chain. These drugs have fewer antimuscarinic and autonomic effects but greater affinity for D_2 sites when compared with aliphatic and piperidine phenothiazines. As a result, they produce more EPS.

For all three groups, substitutions at the 2 position can affect the drug's potency. Increasing the electron-withdrawing tendency at this position by substituting a trifluromethyl group, for example, will increase antipsychotic potency.

Thioxanthenes

Thioxanthene antipsychotics have a three-ring structure that is similar to that of the phenothiazines, but with a carbon substituted for a nitrogen atom in the middle ring. Substitutions in the comparable areas of the molecule have similar effects on activity. Thioxanthenes are characterized by geometric isomerism, with the *cis* isomers having greater potency than the *trans*. Thiothixene—the most commonly prescribed thioxanthene in the United States—has a piperazine substitution at position 10, whereas chlorprothixene has an aliphatic side chain. Clopenthixol and flupentixol, which are commonly used outside of the United States, have piperazine side chains.

Butyrophenones

Butyrophenone antipsychotics are characterized by a substituted phenyl ring, which is attached to a carbonyl group attached by a 3-carbon chain to a tertiary amino group. Most of the clinically useful butyrophenones have a piperidine ring attached to the tertiary amino group. Drugs in this class tend to be potent D_2 antagonists and have minimal anticholinergic and autonomic effects. Haloperidol, a substituted piperidine, is the most commonly used drug from this class.

Dibenzoxazepines

Dibenzoxazepine antipsychotics have a three-ring structure with a seven-member center ring. Loxapine, a dibenzoxazepine, is the only drug from this class that is available in the United States. Clozapine, a dibenzodiazepine, differs from loxapine in having a nitrogen instead of an oxygen atom in the middle ring, as well as differences in side chains. These differences have a substantial influence on clozapine's affinity for various receptors (including the D_2 receptors), which may explain its atypical antipsychotic activity.

Table 17–1.   Selected antipsychotic drugs

Drug	Routes of administration	Usual daily oral dose (mg)	Sedation	Autonomic effects	Extra-pyramidal side effects	Structure
Phenothiazines						
Chlorpromazine	Oral, intramuscular, depot	200–600	+++	+++	++	
Fluphenazine	Oral, intramuscular, depot	2–20	+	+	+++	
Trifluoperazine	Oral, intramuscular	5–30	++	+	+++	
Perphenazine	Oral, intramuscular	8–64	++	+	+++	
Thioridazine	Oral	200–600	+++	+++	++	
Butyrophenones						
Haloperidol	Oral, intramuscular, depot	5–20	+	+	+++	
Thioxanthenes						
Thiothixene	Oral, intramuscular	5–30	+	+	+++	
Dihydroindolones						
Molindone	Oral	20–100	++	+	++	
Dibenzoxazepines						
Loxapine	Oral, intramuscular	20–100	++	+	++	

Note.   + = mild; ++ = moderate; +++ = severe.
Source.   Adapted from Silver et al. 1994, pp. 901–903.

Others Classes of Antipsychotics

The diphenylbutylpiperidines include pimozide, which is approved for use in the United States only for the treatment of Tourette's disorder but is used elsewhere as an antipsychotic. Fluspirilene and penfluridol are other compounds of this class that are prescribed as antipsychotics in Europe. Relatively little is understood about structure-activity relations in the other classes of antipsychotic compounds (Baldessarini 1990).

PHARMACOLOGICAL PROFILE

Behavioral Effects

Antipsychotic drugs produce a wide spectrum of physiological actions, only some of which are essential to their antipsychotic action. Some of these effects differ among the various classes of antipsychotics. For example, aliphatic phenothiazines have potent antimuscarinic and autonomic effects, whereas others have more potent effects on dopaminergic or serotonergic systems. The effect that is common to all conventional antipsychotic agents is a high affinity for dopamine receptors, particularly D_2 receptors. These effects are useful for defining this class of compounds.

As mentioned in the earlier section, "History and Discovery," chlorpromazine has the unusual property of inducing a state of relative indifference to stressful situations. All of the traditional antipsychotics share this property, which has been called *ataraxia*. The effect differs from sedation in that the individual may not be drowsy but is instead calm and relatively uninterested in the environment. Individuals who are taking antipsychotics appear to have a decrease in their emotional responsiveness and have been described as lacking initiative. When patients are agitated or excited, these drugs may calm them without causing excessive sedation.

The calming effect of antipsychotics in humans is paralleled by their effect on the conditioned avoidance response in animals. In this research paradigm, animals are trained to make a conditioned response (e.g., moving to a safer place) following a sensory cue such as the ringing of a bell that precedes the onset of a shock. The response to the sensory cue is blocked by the antipsychotic drug. As a result, the animal will not move to a safer place until after the shock is administered (Baldessarini 1990).

In rodents, traditional antipsychotics also block responses such as stereotypies and hyperactivity, which are induced by dopamine agonists such as apomorphine. This effect has been found to be a reasonably reliable predictor of antipsychotic activity in patients. Moreover, the dose-response relationship in animals provides information about the likely clinical dose range for patients. It is commonly used as a screening device to identify compounds that are likely to have clinical efficacy as antipsychotics (Gerlach 1991).

Antipsychotic drugs have other effects on animal behavior. They reduce responses to a variety of stimuli, and they reduce exploratory behavior. Antipsychotics also block self-stimulation to reward centers in the brain such as the medial forebrain bundle, and they reduce some feeding behaviors.

Motor Effects

When animals are administered a traditional antipsychotic in relatively high doses, they develop a syndrome with immobility, increased muscle tone, and abnormal postures called *catalepsy*. In addition, these agents decrease spontaneous motor activity. These motor effects in animals and humans are caused by dopamine-receptor blockade in the striatum and inactivation of dopamine neurons in the substantia nigra (Gerlach 1991).

In humans, all of the traditional antipsychotic medications produce EPS, including parkinsonism (i.e., stiffness, tremor, and shuffling gait), dystonia (i.e., abrupt onset, sometimes bizarre muscular spasms affecting mainly the musculature of the head and neck), and akathisia (with objective and subjective restlessness). These effects are described in greater detail in the section, "Side Effects and Toxicology."

Endocrine Effects

Antipsychotic drugs influence the secretion of hormones in the pituitary and elsewhere mainly as a result of their blockade of dopamine receptors. All traditional antipsychotics increase serum prolactin concentration in the usual clinical dose range (Meltzer 1985). This increase occurs because prolactin secretion by the anterior pituitary is tonically inhibited by dopamine. Therefore, blockade of dopamine receptors in the tuberoinfundibular pathway results in prolactin elevation. This sometimes produces gynecomastia and galactorrhea. Antipsychotics also suppress levels of luteinizing hormone (LH) and follicle-stimulating hormone (FSH) (Reichlin 1992). These changes can lead to amenorrhea and inhibition of orgasms in women. Other changes in sexual functioning are described in the section, "Side Effects and Toxicology."

PHARMACOKINETICS AND DISPOSITION

All of the antipsychotics are well absorbed when they are administered orally or parenterally. Oral administration leads to less predictable absorption than parenteral administration. Liquid concentrates are absorbed slightly more rapidly than pills. In general, intramuscular preparations reach their peak concentrations sooner than oral drugs and, as a result, have an earlier onset of action. For example, intramuscular administration of most antipsychotics results in peak plasma levels in about 30 minutes, with clinical effects emerging within 15–30 minutes. Oral administration of most antipsychotics results in peak plasma levels 1–4 hours after administration. Steady-state levels are reached in 4–7 days. However, an optimal clinical response to these agents may emerge within the first week or may be delayed for 6 weeks or longer.

The bioavailability (i.e., the amount of drug reaching the site of action in the brain) is substantially greater when antipsychotics are administered parenterally than when they are administered orally. This difference may result from the incomplete absorption of the drug in the gastrointestinal tract and from extensive metabolism of oral drugs during the first pass through liver and gut. Several factors can interfere with the gastrointestinal absorption of these drugs, including antacids, coffee, smoking, and food. The metabolism of antipsychotic drugs is largely hepatic and occurs through conjugation with glucuronic acid, hydroxylation, oxidation, demethylation, and sulfoxide formation. The metabolism of the phenothiazines and thioxanthenes is particularly complex. For example, chlorpromazine has more than 100 different potential metabolites, with some metabolites having significant amounts of pharmacological activity. Although most phenothiazine metabolites are inactive, some such as 7-hydroxychlorpromazine and 7-hydroxyfluphenazine may contribute to the therapeutic activity of the parent drug (Midha et al. 1993).

In the case of thioridazine, a substantial amount of the drug's activity is from metabolites that may be more active than thioridazine itself. One metabolite, mesoridazine, is also marketed as an antipsychotic. On the other hand, haloperidol has only one major metabolite, reduced haloperidol, which has substantially less antidopaminergic activity than the parent compound. However, a study found that reduced haloperidol is converted back to the parent compound and may contribute to antipsychotic activity (Chakraborty et al. 1989).

Most antipsychotics are metabolized by the cytochrome P450 (CYP) 2D6 and CYP3A subfamilies (Preskorn 1996). These isoenzymes also metabolize a number of drugs that are commonly combined with antipsychotics, resulting in important drug-drug interactions. These interactions are discussed in a later section (see "Drug-Drug Interactions") and in Table 17–2.

The systemic clearance of antipsychotics is high as the result of a high hepatic extraction ratio. As a result, only negligible amounts of the unchanged drug are excreted by the kidneys. Most antipsychotics have elimination half-lives of about 10–30 hours, partially because of the high lipid solubility of antipsychotics, which results in large amounts of drug being stored in tissues such as fat, lung, and brain. This may explain the high concentrations of antipsychotic drugs—about twice the plasma concentration—that have been found in human and animal brain. Note that the biological activity of antipsychotics may per-

Table 17–2. Antipsychotic drugs and cytochrome P450 (CYP) isoenzymes

Isoenzyme	Antipsychotic drugs	Other drugs
CYP1A2	Clozapine	**Substrates:** amitriptyline, clomipramine, imipramine, propranolol, theophylline, warfarin, caffeine **Inhibitors:** fluvoxamine, paroxetine
CYP2D6	Haloperidol, perphenazine, risperidone, thioridazine, sertindole, olanzapine, clozapine	**Substrates:** fluoxetine, paroxetine, sertraline, venlafaxine, amitriptyline, clomipramine, desipramine, imipramine, nortriptyline, propranolol, metoprolol, timolol, codeine, encainide, flecainide, propafenone **Inhibitors:** paroxetine, sertraline, fluoxetine
CYP3A3/4	Clozapine, sertindole, quetiapine	**Substrates:** amitriptyline, clomipramine, imipramine, nefazodone, sertraline, carbamazepine, ethosuximide, terfenadine, alprazolam, clonazepam, diazepam, midazolam, triazolam, diltiazem, nifedipine, verapamil, erythromycin, cyclosporine, lidocaine, acetaminophen, quinidine, cisapride **Inhibitors:** ketoconazole, nefazodone, fluvoxamine, fluoxetine

Source. Adapted from Preskorn 1996 and Ereshefsky et al. 1996.

sist for periods of time that would not be predicted from their terminal half-lives. The pharmacokinetics of antipsychotics in plasma may not accurately reflect the kinetics at receptor sites in the brain (Campbell and Baldessarini 1985; Hubbard et al. 1987).

Most antipsychotics are highly protein bound. For example, more than 90% of a drug such as fluphenazine or haloperidol is bound to plasma protein. The remaining unbound portion is the drug that is available for passing through the blood-brain barrier. In theory, conditions that alter the amount of plasma protein will alter the amount of bioavailable antipsychotic drug.

The pharmacokinetics of long-acting injectable antipsychotics differ markedly from those of short-acting oral and injectable drugs. Long-acting fluphenazine and haloperidol are administered as esters dissolved in sesame oil. The oil is injected into a muscle, and the drug gradually diffuses from the oily vehicle into the surrounding tissues. The rate-limiting step appears to be the rate of diffusion, because once the drug enters the tissue, it is rapidly hydrolyzed, and the parent compound is released. Plasma concentrations of short-acting drugs rise rather rapidly during the absorption phase and then decline during a distribution and elimination phase. Long-acting compounds, on the other hand, are absorbed continually during the interval between injections. Moreover, for patients who have received multiple injections, the drug will be absorbed from multiple injection sites simultaneously. As a result, long-acting compounds need a much longer time to reach steady state, and they are eliminated much more slowly than short-acting compounds. For example, the decanoate forms of haloperidol and fluphenazine require about 3 months to reach steady state, and substantial plasma concentrations can be detected months after therapy has been discontinued (Marder et al. 1989).

MECHANISM OF ACTION

The discovery of drugs that were effective against psychosis was an important event in biological psychiatry; understanding the mechanism of action of these drugs could provide valuable information about the biology of psychosis. The important breakthrough came in 1963 when Carlsson and Lindquist reported that administering chlorpromazine or haloperidol to mice resulted in an accumulation of dopamine metabolites in dopamine-rich brain areas. They hypothesized that the drugs blocked receptors for dopamine and that feedback mechanisms resulted in an increase in dopamine release. Since that time, others have found that all of the effective antipsychotics bind to

dopamine receptors. In 1976, Seeman and colleagues and Creese and colleagues reported that the affinity of the traditional antipsychotics for D_2 receptors is highly correlated with their effective clinical dose. In contrast, a similar relationship does not exist between affinity for other receptors (e.g., muscarinic or adrenergic) and clinical effectiveness. This observation has led to the conclusion that the traditional antipsychotic drugs exert their effects against psychosis by blocking D_2 receptors.

Others have proposed that schizophrenia and other psychotic illnesses are related to an overactive dopamine system. This dopamine hypothesis of schizophrenia has resulted in an exhaustive search for abnormalities in the dopamine systems of schizophrenic individuals. For the most part, this search has had mixed results and remains unproven (Marder et al. 1991). The fact that antipsychotic medications relieve schizophrenic psychosis by decreasing dopamine activity does not mean that schizophrenia is caused by increased dopamine activity. It is common in medicine for illnesses to be treated through mechanisms that are unrelated to the actual cause of the illness. For example, hypertension can be treated by drugs with different biological activities that are far removed from the actual cause of hypertension. In a similar manner, schizophrenic psychosis—or any psychosis—may be attenuated by methods that are unrelated to the cause of schizophrenia.

Studies using positron-emission tomography have improved the understanding of the importance of D_2 receptors in the clinical effects of traditional antipsychotics. Investigators used highly selective D_2 receptor ligands and found that EPS tend to occur when a drug occupies a high proportion of D_2 receptor sites, usually more than 80%. Occupancy rates that were somewhat lower resulted in antipsychotic responses without obvious EPS (Farde et al. 1992). Clozapine, a nontraditional antipsychotic, was effective when D_2 occupancy was 20%–60%; thus, other transmitters, particularly serotonin, may contribute to clozapine's effectiveness (Sedvall 1996).

Recent information indicates that the theory that antipsychotic drugs work by blocking D_2 receptors is an oversimplification. An antipsychotic will occupy dopamine receptor sites within hours after a patient receives an adequate dose of drug (Farde et al. 1992). However, the clinical response to the medication may require days or weeks. Studies monitoring plasma homovanillic acid (HVA), a metabolite of dopamine, are consistent with the hypothesis that the delayed response may be caused by a decrease in dopamine turnover. When drug-free patients receive an antipsychotic, plasma HVA levels increase during the first few days and then decline in some patients (Bowers 1984). Some (but not all) studies indicate that the decline in HVA levels is correlated with the amount of reduction in psychosis. Furthermore, patients who have high plasma HVA levels prior to treatment appear to be more likely to respond to antipsychotics. These observations are supported by studies on the firing rates of midbrain dopamine neurons of rats. Treatment with haloperidol results in a short-term increase in the firing of these neurons followed by a prolonged decrease in firing that has been referred to as *depolarization inactivation* (Chiodo and Bunney 1987). It has been proposed that the antipsychotic effects of these drugs are associated with the decrease in firing. Taken together, these findings suggest that for an antipsychotic response to occur, the blockade of D_2 receptors is an initial response that must be followed by a decrease in dopamine activity.

INDICATIONS

Antipsychotic medications are effective for nearly every medical and psychiatric condition that results in psychosis. In this regard, this group of drugs is antipsychotic rather than antischizophrenic. The effectiveness of these drugs is often limited by their neurological side effects. For this reason, clinicians may choose not to treat certain psychotic conditions that are either mild or transitory.

Acute Schizophrenia and Schizoaffective Disorder

Numerous clinical studies have found that antipsychotic medications are effective for reducing psychotic symptoms in acute schizophrenia and schizoaffective disorders. The effectiveness of these agents was recently confirmed by a systematic review carried out by a Schizophrenia Patient Outcome Research Team (Dixon et al. 1995).

Antipsychotic medications are effective for treating nearly all of the symptoms associated with schizophrenia, although the extent of their effectiveness is highly variable in specific patients. Symptoms such as hallucinations, delusions, and disorganized thoughts—also called *positive symptoms* because they were attributed to reflect abnormal function—are more likely to decrease with drugs than are symptoms such as blunted affect, emotional withdrawal, and lack of social interest—also called *negative symptoms* because they were attributed to the absence of normal brain function. For many patients, antipsychotics will result in substantial reduction, or even remission, of positive symptoms, but negative symptoms will be minimally affected and will continue to impair the patient's social recovery.

Antipsychotics may also cause what has been referred

to as *secondary negative symptoms* (Buchanan and Gold 1996). That is, both EPS and sedation from antipsychotics can either worsen negative symptoms or cause new symptoms to arise. Akinesia, a manifestation of antipsychotic-induced parkinsonism, can lead to decreased gestures, masked facies, decreased speech, and reduced interest in social activities. These symptoms may decline if EPS are adequately treated.

All of the traditional antipsychotic medications are equally effective. Clinicians and researchers who prescribed these drugs during the years immediately following their discovery reported that certain forms or subtypes of schizophrenia improved more with particular antipsychotics. These observations have not withstood careful study. In other words, all of the traditional antipsychotic drugs are equally effective for all subtypes of schizophrenia.

A small population of patients with schizophrenia should probably not be treated with antipsychotic medications. The possible justifications for withholding medications are that 1) the illness is unaffected or worsened by medications, 2) the patient has a history of complete recovery in a brief time without drugs, or 3) the adverse effects are too severe in proportion to the improvement that results from drug treatment. If a patient's clinical history indicates that he or she belongs to one of these three groups, the clinician could make a rational decision to withhold antipsychotic medications.

In certain conditions, antipsychotic drug treatment becomes problematic, and the risk-benefit ratio shifts. Antipsychotics should be prescribed cautiously for patients with seriously impaired hepatic function because these drugs are primarily metabolized in the liver. Patients with Parkinson's disease may have difficulty tolerating traditional antipsychotics because of EPS.

In the past, some senior psychotherapists reported that patients who were able to engage in intensive psychotherapy appeared to do better without antipsychotic medications. Clinicians are often impressed by an occasional patient who does extremely well without antipsychotics and sustains a complete or nearly complete recovery while receiving skilled psychotherapy. It is important not to generalize from experience with these rather rare individuals to the vastly greater number of patients with schizophrenia who will be helped to a substantial degree by medication. Moreover, an extensive literature indicates that psychosocial treatments are most effective when they are administered to patients who are also receiving antipsychotics.

A review by Wyatt (1991) concluded that early intervention with antipsychotics reduced long-term morbidity and decreased the number of rehospitalizations. In other words, even if a patient eventually recovers without drugs, the amount of time spent in a psychotic state may be related to a worse long-term outcome.

Investigators have also claimed that patients with a very poor prognosis or whose psychosis persists while taking drugs should not receive them. For example, patients with "Kraepelinian schizophrenia" appear to have poor drug responses, severe negative symptoms, a greater risk for schizophrenia in their first-degree relatives, and poor premorbid sociosexual adjustment (Keefe et al. 1990). Others have suggested that schizophrenic patients with enlarged cerebral ventricles (Weinberger et al. 1980) or other evidence of structural abnormalities of the brain (Crow 1980) are likely to respond poorly to antipsychotics. However, the fact that these patients respond to a limited extent to antipsychotics should not be viewed as evidence that these patients are not helped by their medications. The evidence that structural abnormalities limit the amount of improvement is far from convincing. In my clinical experience, when antipsychotic medications are discontinued in severely ill, treatment-refractory patients in chronic care hospitals, their conditions deteriorate. Many of these patients may also respond to clozapine (Kane et al. 1988; Meltzer et al. 1990).

Maintenance Therapy in Schizophrenia

Antipsychotics have been reliably shown to decrease the frequency of relapse in schizophrenic patients who have recovered from a psychotic episode (Dixon et al. 1995). Kissling (1992) used placebo-controlled studies to estimate that approximately 72% of patients will have a relapse in a year without an antipsychotic, whereas treated patients are likely to have relapse rates of approximately 23%. These findings support the practice of continuing antipsychotic treatment in patients after they have recovered from a psychotic episode. Some clinicians are often tempted to discontinue medications in patients who have been well and stable for a prolonged period. Unfortunately, these patients also have high relapse rates when their medications are discontinued (Hogarty et al. 1976).

The value of long-term antipsychotic drug treatment for well-stabilized patients has also been clarified by a series of studies by Johnson and colleagues (1983). Patients who relapsed while receiving antipsychotic medications had episodes that were less severe than those in patients who discontinued their drugs. Drug-maintained patients were less likely to have episodes with self-destructive behavior, violence, and antisocial acts. In addition, patients who relapsed while not taking medications were more likely to require involuntary hospitalization. Patients who

discontinued their medications actually ended up, on average, receiving more total medication, because the drug dose needed to treat relapses was much higher than the dose for relapse prevention.

In 1989, an international group of experts reached a consensus on the indications for neuroleptic relapse prevention: 1–2 years of maintenance antipsychotic therapy was recommended for patients following a first episode. Although this may be somewhat longer than current practice in many settings, this recommendation was made because individuals at this stage of their illness often have the most to lose. Patients may be working or involved in educational programs, both of which can be jeopardized by a second psychotic episode. Moreover, the self-image of patients and their personal relationships may be permanently altered by their illness. The experts at the consensus conference also recommended that patients who have had multiple episodes receive maintenance neuroleptic treatment for at least 5 years. For patients with a history of serious suicide attempts or violent, aggressive behavior, maintenance treatment with neuroleptics may be indicated for longer periods—perhaps indefinitely (Kissling et al. 1991).

Mania

All of the traditional antipsychotic drugs are effective in reducing manic excitement. In comparison with lithium, valproic acid, and carbamazepine, antipsychotic drugs often have a more rapid onset of action. Therefore, an antipsychotic may be combined with an antimanic drug during the first days of treatment of severe excited states, before the antimanic compound has its onset of action. Once lithium or another antimanic compound becomes effective, the dose of antipsychotic may be reduced and eventually discontinued. In most cases, antimanic drugs are more effective and are associated with fewer side effects than antipsychotic drugs for mania. Some studies indicate that patients with mood disorders are more vulnerable to developing tardive dyskinesia than are patients with schizophrenia; thus, these drugs should be used for as short a time as possible.

Depression With Psychotic Features

Patients with major depressive episodes with psychotic features will often benefit from a combination of antipsychotic and antidepressant medications. The added benefits of antipsychotic medications are most apparent for those patients with severe delusions. When the psychotic component of the episode has responded to treatment, the antipsychotic medications should be withdrawn.

Other Indications

Antipsychotic drugs are effective for reducing psychotic symptoms in a number of organic mental syndromes, including dementia and psychotic states due to stimulant drugs. They can be useful for controlling agitation and chorea in Huntington's disease. Both haloperidol and pimozide have been shown to be helpful in treating symptoms of Tourette's disorder. Antipsychotics are occasionally useful for patients with pervasive developmental disorder and mental retardation, but there is some concern that these drugs are overprescribed for these conditions. Prochlorperazine is commonly prescribed for nausea and vomiting. Chlorpromazine is sometimes useful for intractable hiccups.

SIDE EFFECTS AND TOXICOLOGY

Acute Extrapyramidal Side Effects

EPS, including akathisia, dystonia, tremor, akinesia, bradykinesia, and rigidity, are the major problems in prescribing traditional antipsychotics. The most common EPS is akathisia, which is a subjective feeling of restlessness. Patients who experience severe akathisia will often pace continuously or move their feet restlessly while sitting. Some patients complain that they are unable to feel comfortable, regardless of what they do. Severe akathisia can cause patients to feel anxious or irritable, and some reports suggest that severe akathisia can result in aggressive or suicidal acts. One study found that as many as 75% of patients treated with a conventional dose of haloperidol will experience some degree of akathisia (Van Putten et al. 1984). Other studies reported that 25% of patients experience akathisia (Braude et al. 1983). Akathisias can be difficult to assess and are frequently misdiagnosed as anxiety or agitation (Weiden et al. 1987).

Acute dystonic reactions are abrupt-onset, sometimes bizarre muscular spasms affecting mainly the musculature of the head and neck. Sometimes, however, dystonias of the trunk and lower extremities lead to gait disturbances that may be confused with hysteria. Dystonia usually appears within the first few days of therapy and when patients are treated with large doses of high-potency neuroleptics such as haloperidol or fluphenazine. Dystonia almost always responds rapidly to antiparkinsonian medications and can usually be prevented by either pretreatment with these drugs or limiting the neuroleptic dosage prescribed. Younger patients and males are more prone than other patients to develop acute dystonia (Lavin and Rifkin 1992). One study found that 21% of male subjects younger than 30 developed acute dystonic reactions (Swett 1975).

Parkinsonism, which includes symptoms such as stiffness, tremor, and shuffling gait, affects about 30% of patients who receive chronic treatment with traditional antipsychotics. Patients with parkinsonism may also experience akinesia, a side effect that causes difficulty in initiating movement. In some cases, drug-induced parkinsonism can be nearly identical to Parkinson's disease (Lavin and Rifkin 1992).

For most patients, EPS are treatable. The anticholinergic antiparkinsonian drugs such as benztropine or trihexyphenidyl are by far the most commonly used drugs for EPS. Many clinicians prescribe these drugs routinely for patients who are taking antipsychotics, particularly potent antipsychotics. Several studies indicate that prescribing antiparkinsonian medications before patients have EPS can prevent dystonias (Lavin and Rifkin 1992; Winslow et al. 1986). Unfortunately, these drugs also have their own side effects, including dry mouth, constipation, urinary retention, and blurry vision. Other studies indicate that anticholinergic antiparkinsonian drugs can also cause some loss of memory (Gelenberg et al. 1989). This side effect is dose dependent and remits when the drug is stopped.

Other drugs for treating EPS include amantadine (which is effective against parkinsonism) and propranolol (which is effective in managing akathisia). Both of these drugs can be added to anticholinergic antiparkinsonian drugs.

Some unfortunate people are highly sensitive to EPS—particularly akathisia—at the dose that is necessary to control their psychoses. Some of these patients may agree to tolerate these side effects, at least temporarily, while their most troublesome psychotic symptoms are being treated. For others, the discomfort brought on by medication side effects may seem worse than the illness itself. These patients may be good candidates for newer agents such as clozapine, sertindole, olanzapine, or risperidone.

Tardive Dyskinesia

Tardive dyskinesia is a movement disorder that may occur after chronic treatment with antipsychotic medications. Patients with tardive dyskinesia may have any or all of a number of abnormal movements, such as mouth and tongue movements (e.g., lip smacking, sucking, and puckering) and facial grimacing. Other movements may include irregular movements of the limbs, particularly choreoathetoid-like movements of the fingers and toes, and slow, writhing movements of the trunk. Younger patients tend to develop slower athetoid movements of the trunk, extremities, and neck. The movements of tardive dyskinesia tend to increase when a patient is aroused and tend to decrease when he or she is relaxed. They are typically absent during sleep. Diagnostic criteria for tardive dyskinesia developed by Schooler and Kane (1982) require that patients have at least 3 months of antipsychotic drug exposure and that the movements persist for at least 4 weeks. Seriously disabling dyskinesia is uncommon, but a small proportion of patients may have tardive dyskinesia that affects walking, breathing, eating, and talking.

At least 10%–20% of patients treated with antipsychotics for more than 1 year develop tardive dyskinesia. In chronically institutionalized patients, the prevalence is 15%–20% (Kane et al. 1986). Prospective studies indicate that the cumulative incidence of tardive dyskinesia is 5% at 1 year, 10% at 2 years, 15% at 3 years, and 19% at 4 years (Kane et al. 1986). Certain populations are at greater risk than others for developing tardive dyskinesia. Older patients are at increased risk, and elderly women are particularly vulnerable. Moreover, tardive dyskinesia in elderly patients is less likely to remit when antipsychotics are discontinued. Patients with affective disorders may also be at a greater risk for developing tardive dyskinesia when they are treated with antipsychotics. Other possible risk factors for tardive dyskinesia are the dose of antipsychotic medications and the length of time taking these drugs (Kane and Lieberman 1992).

Early observations of the course of tardive dyskinesia suggested that the disorder was inevitably progressive and irreversible. In other words, once patients developed even mild dyskinesias, they would likely progress toward severe tardive dyskinesia. More recent evidence indicates otherwise. Tardive dyskinesia does not appear to be a progressive disorder for most patients. It seems to develop rapidly and then to stabilize and often to improve. Several studies have followed the course of tardive dyskinesia in patients who continued taking antipsychotic drugs for several years. The consensus was that most patients had a reduction in the severity of tardive dyskinesia, even if their antipsychotic drugs were continued. Moreover, this reduction can be clinically meaningful in some patients.

The American Psychiatric Association Task Force on Tardive Dyskinesia (1992) issued a report that included many recommendations for preventing and managing tardive dyskinesia. These recommendations include the following:

1. Establishing objective evidence that antipsychotic medications are effective for an individual
2. Using the lowest effective dose of antipsychotic

3. Prescribing cautiously to children, elderly people, and individuals with mood disorders
4. Examining patients on a regular basis for evidence of tardive dyskinesia
5. When tardive dyskinesia is diagnosed, considering alternatives to antipsychotics, obtaining informed consent, and also considering dosage reduction
6. If the tardive dyskinesia worsens, considering a number of options, including discontinuing the antipsychotic, switching to a different drug, or considering a trial of clozapine

Neuroleptic Malignant Syndrome

The clinical characteristics of neuroleptic malignant syndrome (NMS) include 1) severe muscular rigidity; 2) autonomic instability, including hyperthermia, tachycardia, increased blood pressure, tachypnea, and diaphoresis; and 3) changing levels of consciousness. A patient with NMS usually presents with muscular rigidity, and the condition progresses to elevated temperature, fluctuating consciousness, and unstable vital signs. These symptoms are often associated with elevations in creatine phosphokinase (CPK). Elevations in liver transaminases, leukocytosis, myoglobinemia, and myoglobinuria are less frequent. Acute renal failure may also occur. Mortality in well-developed cases has been reported to range from 20% to 30% and may be higher when depot forms are used. More recent studies indicate that mortality from NMS has been reduced (Shalev et al. 1989).

NMS is more common when high-potency antipsychotics are prescribed in high doses and when dose is escalated rapidly. The syndrome is twice as common in males as in females and is more likely to be present in younger patients. Clinicians should be concerned about any patient who has severe muscular rigidity and a rising body temperature, because early diagnosis and treatment can be life-saving. The most effective means for preventing NMS probably involves the early diagnosis and management of severe muscular rigidity.

When NMS is diagnosed or suspected, antipsychotics should be discontinued and supportive and symptomatic treatment begun. This treatment may include reducing EPS with antiparkinsonian medications, correcting fluid and electrolyte imbalances, reducing fevers, and managing cardiovascular symptoms such as hyper- or hypotension. Gratz and colleagues (1992) suggested that when patients have fevers higher than 101°F, antipsychotics and anticholinergics should be discontinued. At that time, treatment with dopamine agonists such as bromocriptine should be considered, along with intensive medical monitoring if the fever exceeds 103°F. If these treatments are inadequate, dantrolene or benzodiazepines should be considered. After patients recover from NMS, they can usually be treated with a different antipsychotic drug or even with the same drug that caused NMS.

Neuroendocrine Side Effects

The most significant and consistent neuroendocrine effect of antipsychotics is hyperprolactinemia. Some patients develop tolerance to the prolactin-elevating effects of these drugs after several weeks (Meltzer 1985). In women, elevated prolactin can lead to menstrual abnormalities, including anovulatory cycles and infertility, menses with abnormal luteal phases, or frank amenorrhea and hypoestrogenemia (Reichlin 1992). Galactorrhea is a relatively common side effect that results from the direct effect of prolactin on the breast tissue. It may be uncomfortable but is seldom of any medical significance. Female patients have also reported decreased libido and anorgasmia.

In men, elevated prolactin levels can lower testosterone levels and result in impotence. Male patients frequently report ejaculatory and erectile disturbances that are probably related to the autonomic effects of the antipsychotic. These problems tend to be most prominent with low-potency drugs and are usually dose related.

Cardiovascular Side Effects

Low-potency antipsychotic medications such as chlorpromazine or thioridazine can cause orthostatic hypotension through α_1-adrenergic blockade. The more potent dopamine blockers such as haloperidol or fluphenazine are less likely to cause autonomic effects. Chlorpromazine may cause prolongation of the Q-T and P-R intervals, ST depression, and T-wave blunting, and thioridazine may cause Q-T and T-wave changes. Both should be used cautiously in patients with increases in their Q-T intervals.

Other Side Effects

Low-potency antipsychotics, particularly chlorpromazine, may cause photosensitivity reactions consisting of severe sunburn or rash. As a result, patients should be instructed to use sunscreens. These drugs may also be associated with an uncommon discoloration of the skin. Skin areas that are exposed to sunlight, particularly the face and neck, develop blue-gray metallic discoloration. This skin reaction is usually associated with long-term treatment involving high drug doses.

Patients receiving long-term treatment with chlorpromazine may develop granular deposits in the anterior lens and posterior cornea. These deposits (visualized on slit lamp examination) seldom affect the patient's vision. Changing the drug given to the patient will usually result in a gradual improvement in the condition.

High doses of thioridazine (i.e., >1,000 mg/day) can result in retinal pigmentation. This condition can lead to serious visual impairment or blindness. Moreover, the condition may not remit when thioridazine is discontinued. Therefore, thioridazine should not be prescribed in doses higher than 800 mg/day.

Coexisting Medical Conditions

Pregnancy. No clear evidence indicates that antipsychotic drugs are associated with congenital malformations. These drugs do cross the placenta, and there are suggestions from animal studies that prenatal exposure may affect the development of the dopamine system. Altshuler et al. (1996) recently performed a meta-analysis on the effects of first-trimester exposure to low-potency antipsychotics. These investigators found that these agents resulted in a very small increase in the relative risk for congenital anomalies. (The baseline incidence was 2.0%, and the incidence with antipsychotics was 2.4%.) No evidence suggests that high-potency drugs increase the risk to the fetus.

Clinicians should attempt to discontinue antipsychotic drugs during the first trimester if this is feasible and should consider carefully whether the risks of prescribing these drugs during the remainder of a patient's pregnancy are justified by the likely benefits. If patients have a history of relapse when antipsychotics are discontinued, the drugs are relatively safe. When an antipsychotic is prescribed, high-potency compounds are probably safer than low-potency compounds.

Antipsychotics are secreted with lactation. Mothers who are being treated with these drugs should not breastfeed.

Seizure disorders. Antipsychotics lower seizure thresholds and should be prescribed with caution to patients with seizure disorders. This adverse effect is more likely to occur with low-potency drugs than with high-potency drugs.

DRUG-DRUG INTERACTIONS

Several drugs, including certain heterocyclic antidepressants, selective serotonin reuptake inhibitors (SSRIs), β-blockers, and anticonvulsants, can affect the metabolism of antipsychotics. As noted in Table 17–2, a number of traditional antipsychotics are metabolized by the CYP2D6 isoenzyme. Thus, drugs such as fluoxetine can lead to an increase in plasma levels and a resultant worsening of EPS. This also explains the observation that chlorpromazine and thioridazine levels are increased when propranolol is added. Conversely, barbiturates and carbamazepine may decrease plasma levels by enhancing metabolism of the antipsychotic. Many studies have found that anticholinergic antiparkinsonian medications decrease antipsychotic blood levels, but more recent and better controlled studies have concluded that antipsychotic levels are unaffected (Leipzig and Mendelowitz 1992). Antacids can decrease the absorption of antipsychotic.

Antipsychotic drugs antagonize the effects of dopamine agonists or L-dopa when these drugs are used to treat parkinsonism. Chlorpromazine, haloperidol, and thiothixene can block the antihypertensive effects of guanethidine (Janowsky et al. 1973). Antipsychotics may also enhance the effects of central nervous system depressants such as analgesics, anxiolytics, and hypnotics (Leipzig and Mendelowitz 1992).

CONCLUSION

Antipsychotic drugs are effective agents for treating psychosis that results from schizophrenia or other illnesses. In treating schizophrenia, these agents are also effective in preventing relapse in stabilized individuals. However, antipsychotic medications have some important limitations. They have serious side effects (particularly neurological effects) that can result in severe discomfort on the one hand and prolonged abnormal movement disorders on the other. In addition, not every patient's psychosis responds well to these agents. Newer antipsychotic drugs such as clozapine, olanzapine, sertindole, and risperidone appear to have milder side effects without compromising effectiveness. In the near future, these drugs may replace the traditional antipsychotic agents.

REFERENCES

Altshuler LL, Cohen L, Szuba MP, et al: Pharmacologic management of psychiatric illness during pregnancy: dilemmas and guidelines. Am J Psychiatry 153:592–606, 1966

American Psychiatric Association Task Force on Tardive Dyskinesia: Tardive Dyskinesia: A Task Force Report of the American Psychiatric Association. Washington, DC, American Psychiatric Press, 1992

Baldessarini RJ: Drugs and the treatment of psychiatric disorders, in The Pharmacological Basis of Therapeutics, 8th Edition. Edited by Gilman AG, Rall TW, Nies AS, et al. New York, Pergamon, 1990, pp 383–435

Baldessarini RJ, Cohen BM, Teicher MH: Significance of neuroleptic dose and plasma level in the pharmacological treatment of psychoses. Arch Gen Psychiatry 45:79–90, 1988

Bowers MB Jr: Homovanillic acid in caudate and prefrontal cortex following neuroleptics. Eur J Pharmacol 99:103–105, 1984

Braude WM, Barnes TRE, Gore SM, et al: Clinical characteristics of akathisia: a systematic investigation of acute psychiatric inpatient admissions. Br J Psychiatry 143:139–150, 1983

Buchanan RW, Gold JM: Negative symptoms: diagnosis, treatment and prognosis. Int Clin Psychopharmacol 11 (suppl 2):3–11, 1996

Campbell A, Baldessarini RJ: Prolonged pharmacologic activity of neuroleptics (letter). Arch Gen Psychiatry 42:637, 1985

Carlsson A, Lindquist M: Effect of chlorpromazine or haloperidol on the formation of 3-methoxytyramine and normetanephrine in mouse brain. Acta Pharmacologica et Toxicologica 20:140–144, 1963

Chakraborty BS, Hubbard JW, Hawes EM, et al: Interconversion between haloperidol and reduced haloperidol in healthy volunteers. Eur J Clin Pharmacol 37:45–48, 1989

Chiodo LA, Bunney BS: Population response of midbrain dopaminergic neurons to neuroleptics: further studies on time course and nondopaminergic neuronal influences. J Neurosci 7:629–633, 1987

Creese I, Burt DR, Snyder SH: Dopamine receptor binding predicts clinical and pharmacologic potencies of antischizophrenic drugs. Science 192:481–483, 1976

Crow TJ: Molecular pathology of schizophrenia: more than one disease process? BMJ 280:66–68, 1980

Dixon LB, Lehman AF, Levine J: Conventional antipsychotic medications for schizophrenia. Schizophr Bull 21:567–577, 1995

Ereshefsky L, Riesenman C, Lam YWF: Serotonin selective reuptake inhibitor drug interactions and cytochrome P450 system. J Clin Psychiatry 57 (suppl 8):17–25, 1996

Farde L, Nordstrom AL, Wiesel FA, et al: Positron emission tomographic analysis of central D_1 and D_2 dopamine receptor occupancy in patients treated with classical neuroleptics and clozapine. Arch Gen Psychiatry 49:538–544, 1992

Gelenberg AJ, Van Putten T, Lavori PW, et al: Anticholinergic effects on memory: benztropine versus amantadine. J Clin Psychiatry 9:180–185, 1989

Gerlach J: New antipsychotics classification, efficacy, and adverse effects. Schizophr Bull 17:289–309, 1991

Gratz SS, Levinson DF, Simpson GM: Neuroleptic malignant syndrome, in Adverse Effects of Psychotropic Drugs. Edited by Kane JM, Lieberman JA. New York, Guilford, 1992, pp 266–284

Hogarty GE, Ulrich RF, Mussare F, et al: Drug discontinuation among long term, successfully maintained schizophrenic outpatients. Disorders of the Nervous System 37: 494–500, 1976

Hubbard JW, Ganes DA, Midha KK: Prolonged pharmacologic activity of neuroleptic drugs. Arch Gen Psychiatry 44: 99–100, 1987

Janowsky DS, El-Yousef MK, Davis JM, et al: Antagonism of guanethidine by chlorpromazine. Am J Psychiatry 130:808–812, 1973

Johnson DAW, Pasterski JM, Ludlow JM, et al: The discontinuance of maintenance neuroleptic therapy in chronic schizophrenic patients: drug and social consequences. Acta Psychiatr Scand 67:339–352, 1983

Kane JM, Lieberman J: Tardive dyskinesia, in Adverse Effects of Psychotropic Drugs. Edited by Kane JM, Lieberman JA. New York, Guilford, 1992, pp 235–245

Kane JM, Woerner M, Borenstein M: Integrating incidence and prevalence of tardive dyskinesia. Psychopharmacol Bull 22:254–258, 1986

Kane JM, Honigfeld G, Singer J, et al: Clozapine for the treatment-resistant schizophrenic: a double-blind comparison versus chlorpromazine/benztropine. Arch Gen Psychiatry 45:789–796, 1988

Keefe RSE, Mohs RC, Silverman JM, et al: Characteristics of Kraepelinian schizophrenia and their relation to premorbid sociosexual functioning, in The Neuroleptic Nonresponsive Patient: Characterization and Treatment. Edited by Angrist B, Schulz SC. Washington, DC, American Psychiatric Press, 1990, pp 1–21

Kissling W: Ideal and reality of neuroleptic relapse prevention. Br J Psychiatry 161 (suppl):133–139, 1992

Kissling W, Kane JM, Barnes TRE, et al: Guidelines for neuroleptic relapse prevention in schizophrenia: towards a consensus view, in Guidelines for Neuroleptic Relapse Prevention in Schizophrenia. Edited by Kissling W. Berlin, Springer-Verlag, 1991, pp 155–163

Lavin MR, Rifkin A: Neuroleptic-induced parkinsonism, in Adverse Effects of Psychotropic Drugs. Edited by Kane JM, Lieberman JA. New York, Guilford, 1992, pp 175–188

Lehmann HE, Hanrahan AE: CPZ: new inhibiting agent for psychomotor excitement and manic states. Archives of Neurology and Psychiatry 71:227–237, 1954

Leipzig RM, Mendelowitz A: Adverse psychotropic drug-drug interactions, in Adverse Effects of Psychotropic Drugs. Edited by Kane JM, Lieberman JA. New York, Guilford, 1992, pp 13–76

Marder SR, Hubbard JW, Van Putten T, et al: The pharmacokinetics of long-acting injectable neuroleptic drugs: clinical implications. Psychopharmacology (Berl) 98:433–439, 1989

Marder SR, Wirshing W, Van Putten T: Drug treatment of schizophrenia: overview of recent research. Schizophr Res 4:81–90, 1991

Meltzer HY: Long-term effects of neuroleptic drugs on the neuroendocrine system. Biochem Psychopharmacol 40:50–68, 1985

Meltzer HY, Bernett S, Bastani B, et al: Effects of six months of clozapine treatment on the quality of life of chronic schizophrenic patients. Hosp Community Psychiatry 41: 892–897, 1990

Midha KK, Marder SR, Jaworski TJ, et al: Clinical perspectives of some neuroleptics through development and application of their assays. Ther Drug Monit 15:179–189, 1993

Preskorn SH: Clinical Pharmacology of Selective Serotonin Reuptake Inhibitors. Caddo, OK, Professional Communications, 1996, p 158

Reichlin S: Neuroendocrinology, in Williams Textbook of Endocrinology, 8th Edition. Edited by Williams RH. Orlando, FL, WB Saunders, 1992, pp 135–219

Schooler NR, Kane JM: Research diagnoses for tardive dyskinesia. Arch Gen Psychiatry 39:486–487, 1982

Sedvall GC: Neurobiological correlates of acute neuroleptic treatment. Int Clin Psychopharmacol 11 (suppl 2):41–46, 1996

Seeman P, Lee T, Chau-Wong M, et al: Antipsychotic drug doses and neuroleptic/dopamine receptors. Nature 261: 717–719, 1976

Shalev A, Hermesh H, Munitz H: Mortality from neuroleptic malignant syndrome. J Clin Psychiatry 51:18–25, 1989

Silver JM, Yudofsky SC, Hurowitz GI: Psychopharmacology and electroconvulsive therapy, in The American Psychiatric Press Textbook of Psychiatry, 2nd Edition. Edited by Hales RE, Yudofsky SC, Talbott JA. Washington, DC, American Psychiatric Press, 1994, pp 897–1007

Swett C: Drug-induced dystonia. Am J Psychiatry 132:532–534, 1975

Van Putten T, May PRA, Marder SR: Akathisia with haloperidol and thiothixene. Arch Gen Psychiatry 41:1036–1039, 1984

Weiden PJ, Mann JJ, Haas G, et al: Clinical nonrecognition of neuroleptic-induced movement disorders: a cautionary study. Am J Psychiatry 144:1148–1153, 1987

Weinberger DR, Bigelow LB, Kleinman JE, et al: Cerebral ventricular enlargement in chronic schizophrenia. Arch Gen Psychiatry 37:11–13, 1980

Winslow RS, Stiller V, Coons DJ, et al: Prevention of acute dystonic reactions in patients beginning high potency neuroleptics. Am J Psychiatry 143:707–710, 1986

Wyatt RJ: Neuroleptics and the natural course of schizophrenia. Schizophr Bull 17:325–351, 1991

EIGHTEEN

Atypical Antipsychotics

Michael J. Owens, Ph.D., and S. Craig Risch, M.D.

The widely held dopamine hypothesis regarding the pathophysiology of schizophrenia is based on two main lines of evidence. First, almost all clinically useful antipsychotic drugs are dopamine receptor antagonists. Second, dopamine agonists (i.e., drugs such as dextroamphetamine, which increase the synaptic availability of dopamine) can produce positive symptoms of psychosis (i.e., hallucinations, delusions, and thought disorders) that are indistinguishable from those produced by paranoid schizophrenia. Indeed, the ability of antipsychotic drugs to produce an antipsychotic action, as well as extrapyramidal side effects (EPS), has been primarily attributed to their ability to block the dopamine, subtype 2 (D_2), receptor in the mesolimbocortical and nigrostriatal dopamine systems, respectively. Although the inhibitory effects of these antipsychotics on classical D_2 receptors appear to correlate superbly with their clinical antipsychotic potency, this neurochemical effect alone cannot explain all of the clinically relevant differences between these drugs.

Since the advent of antipsychotic use in the treatment of schizophrenia, there has been a search for superior drugs because the "typical," "classical," or "traditional" D_2 blocking antipsychotics often do not result in a full remission of symptoms or, in many cases, even a significant reduction. This search has focused on compounds with an improved therapeutic profile (i.e., improved efficacy on both positive and negative symptoms and decreased side effects). These compounds, of which clozapine is considered the prototypical agent, have been termed *atypical antipsychotics*. Indeed, clozapine differs from typical antipsychotics (i.e., haloperidol and chlorpromazine) in

producing minimal or no EPS in humans or catalepsy (defined as immobility for 20 seconds) in rodents at therapeutic doses. Perhaps more important is that clozapine, unlike typical antipsychotics, reduces both the positive and the negative symptoms of schizophrenia. The fact that clozapine differs clinically from typical antipsychotics, together with the data showing that clozapine is a relatively weak D_2 antagonist and that the efficacy of all antipsychotics increases over time, has made up the dominant impetus suggesting that the original dopamine hypothesis of schizophrenia needs revising.

Unlike other chapters in Section II of this volume, "Classes of Psychiatric Treatments: Animal and Human Pharmacology," in which many different compounds are reviewed, only clozapine, risperidone, and olanzapine are routinely used as atypical antipsychotics at this time, although several others will soon be available. Therefore, we begin this chapter by reviewing several hypotheses, based primarily on animal studies of clozapine and recent advances in molecular neuropharmacology (i.e., the cloning of a number of receptors that bind antipsychotic drugs), that have been promulgated to explain the differences between typical and atypical antipsychotics. This portion of the chapter summarizing preclinical data falls under the categories "Mechanism of Action" and "Pharmacological Profile." It is beyond the scope of this chapter to review in detail all the atypical antipsychotics currently under clinical investigation. Therefore, we focus primarily on the clinical pharmacology and therapeutics of clozapine, risperidone, and olanzapine, the only atypical antipsychotics currently approved for use in the United States. We also review, to the extent available, those atypical antipsychotics that are likely to be approved for use in the near future (quetiapine, ziprasidone, and sertindole).

MECHANISM OF ACTION

On the basis of clozapine's activity, the mechanism of action of atypical antipsychotics is thought to be based on either the drugs' differential actions in various subpopulations of dopamine neurons, their binding to different dopamine receptor subtypes, or additional binding to other neurotransmitter receptors. First, we compare and contrast the neurophysiological effects of clozapine with those of typical antipsychotics. Some of these differences possibly give clozapine an atypical profile. Second, we describe the receptor binding profile of several putative atypical antipsychotic agents. Note that these differences in receptor binding are probably responsible for the neurophysiological differences between clozapine and other typical antipsychotics.

It has been suggested that clozapine, unlike other typical antipsychotics, has mesolimbic dopaminergic specificity relative to its actions on nigrostriatal dopamine neurons and that this may underlie its relative lack of EPS and tardive dyskinesia liability. Much of this evidence has come from electrophysiological studies of midbrain dopamine neurons. In general, dopamine neurons originating in the ventral tegmental area (VTA; A10 cell group) project to the nucleus accumbens, amygdala, and neocortex and make up the mesolimbocortical dopamine system. These projections are thought to be responsible for most symptoms associated with schizophrenia, although data to confirm this are limited. In contrast, the dopamine cells of the substantia nigra (SN; A9 cell group) project primarily to the caudate-putamen and make up the nigrostriatal dopamine system. This pathway is thought to be involved in the motor disturbances associated with EPS and tardive dyskinesia, although recent evidence suggests that this pathway also may be involved in the behavioral manifestations of schizophrenia.

The pioneering work of Bunney et al. (1987, 1991) showed that acute administration of haloperidol increases the firing rate of VTA and SN dopamine neurons. This response is probably the result of a lack of local and distant negative feedback on dopamine cells after D_2 receptor blockade. In contrast, acute clozapine administration only increases the firing rate of VTA neurons.

Of more physiological significance are the changes observed after chronic administration of these compounds. On a time scale similar to that in which antipsychotics exert their clinical effects, typical antipsychotics such as

haloperidol significantly decrease the number of spontaneously active dopamine neurons encountered in the VTA and SN. Subsequent examination reveals that these cells enter into a state of depolarization-induced block (inactivation) and decreased dopaminergic function. Clozapine differs from typical antipsychotics in that chronic administration does not induce depolarization block of SN dopamine neurons but does induce inactivation in dopamine neurons of the VTA (Chiodo and Bunney 1983, 1985; Hand et al. 1987). The delayed onset of depolarization block in the VTA is thought to be related to the increased efficacy observed over time with all antipsychotic drugs, including clozapine, whereas the lack of EPS with clozapine is hypothesized to be the result of preservation of the activity of the SN neurons.

Very similar results are observed after olanzapine administration (Stockton and Rasmussen 1996). Although all efficacious antipsychotics produce depolarization block, the selective inactivation of VTA neurons is not observed with all putative atypical antipsychotics (Skarsfeldt 1995). Although depolarization block is a primary consequence of chronic antipsychotic treatment, other findings have questioned somewhat the functional importance of depolarization block in the mechanism of action of antipsychotics—clozapine included—because the release of dopamine from nerve terminals may be more independent of cell firing than previously thought.

In addition to the differential effects of typical and atypical antipsychotics on dopamine neuronal firing, clozapine and haloperidol produce different patterns of electrotonic coupling (i.e., passive flow of current between neurons) that can occur in the absence of an action potential in neurons of the striatum or nucleus accumbens (Onn and Grace 1995). Excellent, up-to-date reviews on the actions of antipsychotics on dopamine neuronal activity and the neurophysiology of dopaminergic terminal fields can be found in O'Donnell and Grace (1996) and Grace et al. (1997).

The electrophysiological actions just described are thought to result in neurochemical differences as well. Studies have shown that acute administration of typical antipsychotic drugs results in more prominent effects on dopamine metabolism in the striatum than in mesolimbocortical areas; in contrast, clozapine appears to augment dopamine turnover to a relatively greater degree in mesolimbic areas (Deutch et al. 1991). Based on the electrophysiological findings suggesting that increased firing of dopamine neurons after acute antipsychotic drug administration is secondary to a lack of negative feedback caused by D_2 receptor blockade, the data suggest that clozapine preferentially alters mesolimbocortical dopamine neurons.

Using in vivo voltammetry, which can measure local catecholamine release over very short epochs, researchers have reported that clozapine preferentially blocked dopamine release in the nucleus accumbens compared with the striatum. However, this finding was not replicated by others (see Meltzer 1991). Additional studies have been reported using in vivo microdialysis, another technique that can measure local dopamine release in specific brain regions. Ichikawa and Meltzer (1991) found evidence that chronically administered clozapine does not interfere with either mesolimbic (nucleus accumbens) or nigrostriatal dopamine metabolism. These findings also suggest that dopamine release from nerve terminals may not be significantly affected by the presence of depolarization block. Because microdialysis measures synaptic overflow of a neurotransmitter, however, it cannot accurately measure synaptic dopamine concentrations that may be more than sufficient to alter synaptic transmission without being sufficient to cause synaptic overflow. Moreover, local tissue damage inherent in microdialysis experiments can release dopamine neurons from depolarization block.

There is also evidence that clozapine may preferentially increase dopamine release in the prefrontal cortex (Moghaddam 1994; Moghaddam and Bunney 1990). This finding, together with the relatively weaker D_2 receptor blockade produced by clozapine in relation to that produced by typical antipsychotics, may lead to a net increase in mesocortical dopamine activity. Indeed, the "hypofrontality" theory that has been postulated states that the negative symptoms of schizophrenia may be the result of a cortical dopamine deficit. Thus, one could speculate that clozapine may reduce both the negative and the positive symptoms of schizophrenia because of its ability to increase cortical and decrease nucleus accumbens dopamine activity, respectively. Moreover, the relative lack of effect on nigrostriatal dopamine systems may be responsible for the lack of EPS associated with clozapine.

Although it appears that there is indeed some regional specificity for clozapine compared with typical antipsychotics, logic and physical chemistry dictate that this must have some basis in the selective binding of clozapine to certain dopamine receptor populations and/or other additional receptors. These findings are explored in the following section.

PHARMACOLOGICAL PROFILE

D_2, D_3, and D_4 Receptors

Although, as we stated at the outset of this chapter, recent findings have suggested that the dopamine hypothesis of schizophrenia needs revision, findings from positron-emission tomography (PET) studies have provided further proof that the D_2 receptor is involved in the pathophysiology of schizophrenia and the mechanism of action of antipsychotics. Seeman and colleagues have reported that drug-naive schizophrenic patients have increased numbers of D_2 receptors in the putamen (Seeman 1987, 1992b; Seeman et al. 1989a). These increases in D_2 receptor binding may actually represent increases in D_4 receptors and not D_2 receptors. Moreover, chemically distinct antipsychotic agents occupy from 65% to—in the case of haloperidol—upward of 90% of D_2 receptors in the putamen at clinically relevant doses (Farde et al. 1986, 1988, 1993). Of special significance is the finding that, unlike typical antipsychotics, clozapine occupies only 40%–50% of D_2 receptors in the striatum, whereas 80%–90% occupancy is observed in limbic areas (Farde et al. 1989).

Although it is generally thought that the high affinity for D_2 receptors in the striatum is responsible for the EPS associated with typical antipsychotics, selective D_2 antagonists may possess some atypical antipsychotic activity. Before describing some of these findings, it is helpful to briefly characterize some properties of the D_2 receptor.

The cloning of the D_2 receptor (Bunzow et al. 1988; Grandy et al. 1989) has enabled the simultaneous visualization and distribution of D_2 receptors and messenger ribonucleic acid (mRNA) in the brains of rats (Mansour et al. 1990; Meador-Woodruff et al. 1989; Mengod et al. 1989), primates (Lidow et al. 1989; Meador-Woodruff et al. 1991), and humans (Meador-Woodruff et al. 1996) (Figure 18–1). Along with the anterior pituitary, the highest concentrations are observed in the nigrostriatal and mesolimbic dopamine systems, and somewhat less is observed in primate cortex. D_2 receptors are located both postsynaptically and presynaptically, where they probably act as autoreceptors. Increases in D_2 receptor binding are observed after antipsychotic treatment through unclear mechanisms that are thought to include both transcriptional (i.e., increased mRNA synthesis) and posttranscriptional (i.e., not related to changes in receptor synthesis) processes (Seeman 1992b; Srivastava et al. 1990; Van Tol et al. 1990; Xu et al. 1992).

Shortly after the initial cloning of the D_2 receptor, it was found that different isoforms of the same receptor are synthesized through alternative RNA splicing (Chio et al. 1990; Giros et al. 1989; Monsma et al. 1989). The two different isoforms vary by 29 amino acids in the third cytoplasmic loop near the guanine nucleotide binding protein (G protein) recognition site. Although this difference does not appear to result in binding differences between D_2 ligands, its location near the G protein regulatory site may

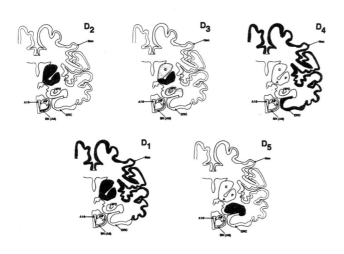

Figure 18–1. Brain region location of mRNA for human dopamine receptors (grey stippled regions). Abbreviations: 3 = third ventricle; AC = nucleus accumbens; AM = amygdala; C = caudate nucleus; Cx = cerebral cortex; G = globus pallidus; H = hypothalamus; Hipp = hippocampus; ICJ = islands of Calleja; L = lateral ventricle; O = olfactory tubercle; P = putamen; SN = substantia nigra; VTA = ventral tegmental area.

Source. Reprinted from Meador-Woodruff JH, Mansour A, Civelli O, et al: "Dopamine Receptor mRNA Expression in Human Striatum and Neocortex." *Neuropsychopharmacology* 15:17–29, 1996. Copyright 1996, the American College of Neuropsychopharmacology; and Seeman P: "Dopamine Receptor Sequences: Therapeutic Levels of Neuroleptics Occupy D$_2$ Receptors, Clozapine Occupies D$_4$." *Neuropsychopharmacology* 7:261–284, 1992. Copyright 1992, the American College of Neuropsychopharmacology. Used with permission of Elsevier Science Publishing Co., Inc.

result in differences in intracellular transduction mechanisms and receptor regulation (Zhang et al. 1994).

The apparent selectivity and demonstrated efficacy of clozapine have spawned increased research efforts to develop selective mesolimbic D$_2$ antagonists. Such compounds may prove to have superior clinical utility by possessing good antipsychotic activity (mesolimbic D$_2$ blockade) and little liability for EPS (relative sparing of striatal D$_2$ receptors). The substituted benzamides sulpiride, raclopride, and remoxipride are the prototypical agents of this class (Ögren and Hall 1992; Wadworth and Heel 1990). These compounds show clear in vivo differences in their potency to block D$_2$-mediated behaviors. Thus, these compounds possess a wide separation between

doses that cause catalepsy in preclinical studies and doses that block dopamine agonist–induced behaviors, indicative of antipsychotic activity. Although it has been postulated that the substituted benzamides and clozapine might possess some mesolimbic specificity, there has not been an unequivocal description as to how this might occur. It should also be noted that the substituted benzamides can bind to other receptors as well and that D$_2$ selectivity is a relative term. Nevertheless, some clinical trials have provided evidence of clinical efficacy with reduced propensity, but not absence, of EPS (Lewander et al. 1992).

As mentioned earlier in this chapter, D$_2$ receptors can act presynaptically as autoreceptors located either on the somatodendritic portion of the neuron or on presynaptic terminals. Those located on presynaptic terminals inhibit the release of dopamine into the synaptic cleft when activated. Utilizing low doses of the dopamine agonist apomorphine, Tamminga and others have investigated its antipsychotic potential (Tamminga and Gerlach 1987). The main effect of apomorphine at low doses is stimulation of presynaptic dopamine autoreceptors and diminishment of dopaminergic function, whereas at higher doses postsynaptic agonistic actions predominate. Pursuing this line of research, medicinal chemists and pharmacologists have synthesized compounds purported to have higher affinity for autoreceptors than apomorphine does and reduced postsynaptic affinity. These compounds have been reported in preclinical studies to produce fewer EPS than do typical antipsychotic agents (Carlsson 1988a, 1988b; Heffner et al. 1992; Wiedemann et al. 1992). Although these compounds are hoped to primarily decrease transmission in the mesolimbic dopamine system, it is not clear whether this can be achieved, because some dopaminergic neurons do not have autoreceptors (Kilts et al. 1987).

A somewhat similar, related strategy is represented by partial dopamine agonists. These compounds, by definition, have a high affinity for the D$_2$ receptor but limited intrinsic activity to produce a full agonist effect. Thus, in the presence of normal or increased dopaminergic stimulation (mesolimbic system; positive symptoms), such compounds would compete with endogenous dopamine and act as functional antagonists. Conversely, under conditions of low dopaminergic tone (mesocortical system; negative symptoms), partial agonists would be expected to augment dopaminergic function. For example, the $S(+)$-N-n-propylnoraporphines act as functional dopamine antagonists and also show an apparent limbic selectivity (Baldessarini et al. 1991; Campbell et al. 1991). Partial agonists with relatively high intrinsic activity, such as B-HT-920, do not induce catalepsy in laboratory studies. Partial agonists such as SDZ 208-912 display a clear separation of doses between those producing catalepsy and those antagonizing dopamine-mediated behaviors (Coward et al. 1990; Meltzer 1991; Naber et al. 1992), although SDZ 208-912 was removed from clinical trials because it produced EPS.

The D_3 receptor has also been cloned and studied (Sokoloff et al. 1990, 1992a). This receptor has considerable homology with the D_2 receptor but has 10–100 times higher affinity for dopamine than do D_2 receptors. Thus, the effects of dopaminergic agonists and autoreceptor-selective agonists may be attributable to their actions primarily on D_3 receptors. The D_3 receptor appears to be expressed predominantly in the mesolimbic dopaminergic system and substantially less in the nigrostriatal system, hippocampus, and entorhinal cortex (Bouthenet et al. 1991; Buckland et al. 1992; Diaz et al. 1994; Meador-Woodruff et al. 1996; Sokoloff et al. 1990) (Figure 18–1). A small amount of D_3 mRNA is expressed in human cortex, as Schmauss et al. (1993) reported an absence of D_3 mRNA in postmortem motor and parietal cortex from 16 of 18 schizophrenic patients compared with control subjects. The diagnostic specificity—and relationship to schizophrenia compared with antipsychotic drug treatment—of this finding is unclear because similar alterations were observed in samples from long-term hospitalized patients with affective disorders.

Like the D_2 receptor, the D_3 receptor has a high affinity for antipsychotic drugs in vitro. Typical antipsychotics such as haloperidol are 10–20 times more potent at D_2 receptors than at D_3 receptors. However, atypical antipsychotics such as clozapine and several substituted benzamides are only 2–3 times more potent at the D_2 receptor (Schwartz et al. 1992; Sokoloff et al. 1990, 1992b). Thus, the ratio of binding in vitro to the D_3 receptor compared with the D_2 receptor is higher for several atypical antipsychotics compared with typical antipsychotics. This, combined with the localization of D_3 receptors primarily in the mesolimbic system, might represent the ability of atypical antipsychotics such as clozapine to treat schizophrenia while sparing the nigrostriatal dopamine system (Snyder 1990).

There are shortcomings, however, of relying on drug affinities derived from in vitro binding studies. Only free drug in the extracellular water compartment is available in vivo for binding to a given receptor. This fraction of total drug is dependent on several bioavailability and pharmacokinetic considerations. Therefore, selectivity based on in vitro binding affinities may not be apparent in vivo. For example, at commonly used clinical doses, the D_2 receptors are blocked by about 80%, whereas D_3 receptors would be blocked by only 2%–40% (Seeman 1992a,

1992b). As Seeman has pointed out, no neuroleptics block D_3 receptors more readily than D_2. Moreover, no agonists discriminate between these receptors because the affinities of agonists at the D_3 receptor are similar to those at the high-affinity state of the D_2 receptor.

Although a selective D_3 antagonist would be of considerable interest as an antipsychotic, preliminary genetic linkage studies have not found evidence for a link between D_3 receptor abnormalities and schizophrenia (Sokoloff et al. 1992c). Indeed, numerous linkage studies have led to consistent and incontrovertible results that there is no significant linkage between schizophrenia and D_1, D_2, D_3, D_4, or D_5 receptors.

The D_4 receptor is the latest receptor in the D_2 receptor family to be cloned (Van Tol et al. 1991). The D_4 receptor has homology similar to both the D_2 and the D_3 receptor. In general, the D_4 receptor has less or equal affinity for dopamine agonists and antagonists than does the D_2 receptor. The finding that clozapine has greater than 10-fold higher affinity for the D_4 receptor than for the D_2 receptor is of considerable interest. Moreover, the affinity constant of clozapine for the D_4 receptor is similar to the free concentration of clozapine observed during antipsychotic treatment (Figure 18–2) (Seeman 1992a, 1992b; Van Tol et al. 1991). However, Roth et al. (1995) examined a series of typical and atypical antipsychotics and determined that the ratio of D_4 to D_2 binding could not be used to differentiate the two classes of antipsychotics.

Several variants of the D_4 receptor have been found in the human population and have different antipsychotic binding properties, although the importance of this finding is not known (Van Tol et al. 1992). Recently, Seeman et al. (1993, 1995) and others (Murray et al. 1995; Sumiyoshi et al. 1995) have reported increases in D_4 receptors in schizophrenic striatal and nucleus accumbens tissue. D_4 receptors were determined by a somewhat controversial method wherein binding of radioligands that label D_2 and D_3 receptors was subtracted from binding of radioligands that label D_2, D_3, and D_4 receptors. This increase in D_4 receptors may actually represent the increases in D_2 receptors reported in the past (see section, "Pharmacological Profile," earlier in this chapter). Reynolds and Mason (1994) were unable to discriminate D_4 from D_2 and D_3 receptors using raclopride (D_2 and D_3) to competitively inhibit [^{3}H]nemonapride (D_2, D_3, and D_4) binding in schizophrenic tissue; however, Seeman and Van Tol (1995) presented evidence to suggest that this is a methodological issue. It is not known whether this apparent increase in D_4 receptors is related to the pathophysiology of schizophrenia or is a consequence of antipsychotic treatment, because chronic haloperidol administration in-

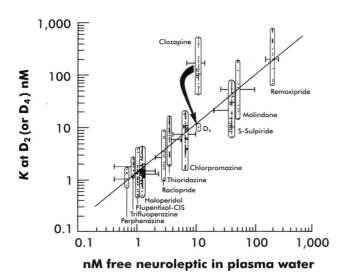

Figure 18–2. The neuroleptic dissociation constants (K) at the D_2 receptor closely match the free neuroleptic concentrations in the patients' plasma water. Each point indicates a K value. Clozapine is the only drug that does not fit the D_2 correlate, but its affinity at D_4 (arrow) does. The plasma molarities for *cis*-flupentixol and for *S*-sulpiride are half those published for the racemates that are used clinically.
Source. Reprinted from Seeman P: "Dopamine Receptor Sequences: Therapeutic Levels of Neuroleptics Occupy D_2 Receptors, Clozapine Occupies D_4." *Neuropsychopharmacology* 7:261–284, 1992. Copyright 1992, the American College of Neuropsychopharmacology. Used with permission of Elsevier Science Publishing Co., Inc.

creases striatal D_4 mRNA expression and receptor protein concentrations in laboratory animals (Schoots et al. 1995).

Areas of high D_4 receptor mRNA expression include the frontal and entorhinal cortex and hippocampus (Figure 18–1). However, D_4 receptor binding, using the subtraction method, is observed in cortex, striatum, and nucleus accumbens (Lahti et al. 1995; Murray et al. 1995). This distribution differs from the D_2 and D_3 receptors and may partly explain the lack of EPS with clozapine. Additionally, the D_4 receptor may represent frontal cortical labeling observed with ^{11}C-clozapine in a PET study reported by Lundberg et al. (1989).

D_1 and D_5 Receptors

Although the existence of the D_1 receptor has been known since the late 1970s, it was not until 1990 before the receptor was cloned from rat and human tissue by four groups simultaneously (Dearry et al. 1990; Monsma et al.

1990; Sunahara et al. 1990; Zhou et al. 1990). D_1 mRNA expression is highest in caudate, putamen, and nucleus accumbens and is somewhat lower in neocortex (Meador-Woodruff et al. 1996) (Figure 18–1). The D_1 receptor, unlike the D_2 receptor, stimulates the production of cyclic adenosine monophosphate (cAMP) and is distributed similarly to D_2 receptors (Clark and White 1987; Cortés et al. 1989; Mansour et al. 1991) (Figure 18–1). Of particular interest to this review is the finding that selective D_1 antagonists are effective in preclinical tests predictive of antipsychotic activity just like D_2 antagonists (Clark and White 1987; Waddington and Daly 1992). It has since been shown that these two receptors can interact either synergistically or antagonistically through G proteins and/or second-messenger generation (Bertorello et al. 1990; Piomelli et al. 1991; Seeman et al. 1989b, 1994; Wachtel et al. 1989). Indeed, Seeman et al. (1989b) found this link uncoupled in the brains of schizophrenic patients. These authors have suggested that a consequence of this might be excessive D_2 activity and the possible inability of antipsychotics to bind efficiently to their receptors. These investigators reported that this uncoupling is not the result of an altered amino acid sequence of the D_1 receptor, as deduced from the D_1 gene (Ohara et al. 1993).

In general, most antipsychotics currently in use bind to both D_2 and D_1 receptors. No correlation has been found between the atypical nature of an antipsychotic and its D_1 affinity, although as a group, atypical antipsychotics are less potent at the D_1 receptor (Meltzer et al. 1989). However, Farde et al. (1989) reported that clozapine displaces the D_1 PET ligand ^{11}C-SCH-23390 more efficiently than do typical antipsychotic drugs.

In addition to preclinical antipsychotic activity, D_1 antagonists can produce catalepsy in rodents and EPS in primates. Therefore, an atypical nature assigned to these compounds is certainly not due to D_1 selectivity alone but may be the result of the combination of low subclinical doses of a D_1 antagonist and a D_2 antagonist, which may potentiate each other, resulting in an antipsychotic effect without producing EPS.

The D_5 receptor, a second member of the D_1 receptor subfamily that has homology similar to the D_1 receptor, has been isolated and cloned from human (Sunahara et al. 1991) and rat (Tiberi et al. 1991) tissue. Like the D_1 receptor, the D_5 receptor is linked to adenylate cyclase and cAMP production and has affinities for various agonists and antagonists—much like the D_1 receptor—with the notable exception of dopamine itself, which is about 10 times more potent at the D_5 receptor. This suggests that the D_5 receptor may be important in maintaining dopaminergic tone. The D_5 receptor is expressed at much lower concentrations than the D_1 receptor, and its highest expression is observed in the hippocampus and entorhinal cortex (Meador-Woodruff et al. 1996) (Figure 18–1). Until a selective antagonist can be found, the clinical utility of D_5 ligands as antipsychotics remains unknown.

Serotonin Receptors

In recent years, it has been hypothesized that clozapine's atypical actions may at least partly result from its actions at other neurotransmitter receptors, such as certain serotonin (5-hydroxytryptamine [5-HT]) receptor subtypes. The involvement of serotonin neural circuits in the mechanism of action of atypical antipsychotic drugs was postulated partly because serotonin is known to exert a regulatory action on dopamine neurons. Neurochemical studies suggest that serotonin projections tonically inhibit mesolimbic and nigrostriatal dopaminergic activity. Moreover, serotonin may directly inhibit dopamine release from striatal nerve terminals (Dray et al. 1976; Soubrie et al. 1984). These findings led to the hypothesis that 5-HT_{2A} antagonists might decrease the inhibition of dopamine activity produced by chronic antipsychotics (i.e., depolarization block, postsynaptic D_2 antagonism), functionally increasing dopaminergic activity in certain areas. This hypothesis is supported by recent PET studies examining the effects of 5-HT_{2A} antagonists on [^{11}C]raclopride binding (Dewey et al. 1995). This also suggests that there may be relative differences in the optimal magnitude of dopaminergic blockade needed in different brain areas. Moreover, complete dopaminergic blockade may not be beneficial for negative symptoms and may result in EPS.

Much of the data suggesting the involvement of the 5-HT_{2A} receptor has come from Meltzer and colleagues (Meltzer 1995; Meltzer et al. 1989), who examined the receptor-binding profile of a large series of antipsychotic drugs. They noted that typical and atypical antipsychotics can be distinguished by lower D_2 and higher 5-HT_{2A} pK_i values (a logarithmic measure of drug affinity for its receptor) of atypical compounds. Absolute potency at the 5-HT_{2A} receptor alone is not the determining factor, but atypical antipsychotics appear to have 5-HT_{2A}-to-D_2 pK_i ratios of at least 1.1 (>13-fold higher affinity). Likewise, Seeman (1992a) reported that those antipsychotics with less propensity to cause rigidity have higher 5-HT_{2A}-to-D_2 ratios. 5-HT_{2A} blockade, however, cannot account for the atypical actions of all purported atypical antipsychotics, such as remoxipride and raclopride, because their 5-HT_{2A}/D_2 blocking profile is similar to that of classical antipsychotics.

The suggestion has been made to coadminister 5-HT_{2A} antagonists with a typical antipsychotic to determine whether this would produce a clozapine-like profile. Even low doses of typical antipsychotics, however, produce 80%–90% D_2 receptor blockade, which makes it difficult to produce the relatively greater 5-HT_{2A} to D_2 receptor occupancy rates as that observed with clozapine (40%–50% D_2 occupancy [Farde et al. 1989, 1993] and 80%–90% frontal cortical 5-HT_{2A} receptor occupancy [Nordstrom et al. 1993]) determined by PET studies.

In addition to the 5-HT_{2A} receptor, there is evidence that other serotonin receptor subtypes may play a role in the action of atypical antipsychotics. The 5-HT_{2C} receptor has been implicated in the mechanism of action of atypical antipsychotics because clozapine has a higher affinity for 5-HT_{2C} receptors than for D_2 receptors (Canton et al. 1990). Also, in situ hybridization studies have shown that there are high densities of 5-HT_{2C} mRNA in the SN and nucleus accumbens, whereas the striatum and VTA have lower densities (Molineaux et al. 1989). However, chlorpromazine has a higher affinity for 5-HT_{2C} receptors than for D_2 receptors. Indeed, most typical and atypical antipsychotics bind weakly to 5-HT_{2C} receptors labeled with ^{3}H-mesulergine.

5-HT_3 antagonists have also been proposed to be potential antipsychotics. Unlike other serotonin receptors, the 5-HT_3 receptor is a component of a ligand-gated cation channel. After binding, serotonin rapidly increases membrane sodium and potassium conductance, resulting in depolarization. 5-HT_3 receptors are found in the area postrema, where they are probably responsible for the antiemetic properties of these compounds. Receptors are also found in the nucleus of the solitary tract, entorhinal cortex, and limbic regions (Kilpatrick et al. 1987). Activation of these receptors leads to an increase in dopamine release in the mesolimbic and perhaps the nigrostriatal pathway. It is also known that clozapine binds with moderate affinity (dissociation constant [K_d] ≈ 100 nmol/L) to the 5-HT_3 receptor, whereas the typical antipsychotics spiperone, haloperidol, fluphenazine, and (–)sulpiride are inactive (Bolanos et al. 1990; Watling et al. 1990). However, loxapine, also a typical antipsychotic, binds to 5-HT_3 receptors with the same affinity as clozapine (Hoyer et al. 1989).

Conflicting evidence has also been generated from electrophysiological studies examining the effect of 5-HT_3 antagonists on dopamine neuron firing rates. In a study by Sorensen et al. (1989) comparing MDL 73,147EF (dolasetron) (a 5-HT_3 antagonist) and haloperidol, acute haloperidol administration increased dopamine firing rates in the SN and the VTA, whereas acute MDL 73,147EF had no effect. However, chronic treatment with both haloperidol and MDL 73,147EF decreased the firing rate of neurons in both the SN and the VTA, results consistent with evidence of depolarization block and likely antipsychotic efficacy. However, in vivo studies (Ashby et al. 1990) using the 5-HT$_3$ antagonist BRL 43694 (granisetron) showed no effect on the firing rate of dopamine neurons acutely or chronically in either brain region. In contrast, the potent and selective 5-HT$_3$ antagonist BRL 46470A selectively reduced the number of spontaneously active dopamine neurons in the VTA of the rat brain while having no effect on the SN region, an action shared by clozapine. This finding suggests that BRL 46470A may possess an atypical antipsychotic profile.

Similar selective inhibition of VTA dopamine neurons has been reported for the 5-HT$_3$ antagonists zatosetron (Rasmussen et al. 1991) and granisetron (Minabe et al. 1992). However, based on the clinical findings or lack thereof (see next paragraph), the model of selective VTA inactivation may produce false-positive results.

In a review by Reynolds (1992), and the lack of data since then, he concluded that in several clinical trials the 5-HT$_3$ antagonist ondansetron was not clinically effective in the treatment of schizophrenia. However, this finding may have resulted from the nature of the experimental design of these studies and the pharmacokinetic properties of the drug more than a lack of intrinsic efficacy.

Monsma et al. (1993) reported the cloning of a novel serotonin receptor linked to the stimulation of adenylate cyclase, tentatively identified as the 5-HT$_6$ receptor. This receptor is localized exclusively in the central nervous system, predominantly in the striatum, limbic, and cortical regions (Monsma et al. 1993; Ward et al. 1995). The pharmacological profile of this receptor is of interest because clozapine, olanzapine, and some other atypical antipsychotics display relatively high affinity for this site ($K_i < 20$ nmol/L), unlike dopamine or spiperone (both > 10 μmol/L). However, some typical antipsychotics, such as loxapine, chlorpromazine, and fluphenazine, also display relative high affinity for this site (Monsma et al. 1993; Roth et al. 1994). The recently cloned 5-HT$_7$ receptor also binds several antipsychotic drugs (Roth et al. 1994; Shen et al. 1993) but does not discriminate atypical from typical antipsychotics.

Sigma (σ) receptors have been implicated in schizophrenia because a stereoisomer of certain related benzomorphans (opiates) possesses profound psychotomimetic properties and antagonists might therefore possess antipsychotic properties. Indeed, several drugs possessing preclinical antipsychotic activity, including haloperidol, bind to the receptor. These drugs (it is unclear whether they are agonists or antagonists), some of which bind only weakly to the D$_2$ receptor, can also alter dopaminergic firing rates (Largent et al. 1988; Snyder and Largent 1989; Steinfels et al. 1989; Taylor and Schlemmer 1992; Wachtel and White 1988).

Critical review of the literature has shown that the psychotomimetic and dysphoric effects of these opiates have been attributed to the wrong stereoisomer—that is, the psychotomimetic effects are produced by the levo-enantiomer, but the dextro-enantiomer is what is defined as the site (Itzhak and Stein 1990; Musacchio 1990; Walker et al. 1990). Additionally, classic ligands, such as pentazocine, dextromethorphan, (+)3-PPP [(+)-3-(3-hydroxyphenyl)-N-propylpiperidine hydrochloride], and 1,3-di-o-tolylguanidine, do not block or cause psychotomimetic behaviors. Finally, clozapine is essentially devoid of activity at the receptor, and ligands possessing preclinical antipsychotic activity may cause motor disturbances (see Walker et al. 1990).

There is increasing evidence that cortical glutamatergic neurons can regulate dopaminergic function, particularly in projection fields of the mesolimbocortical and nigrostriatal systems. Although there are both ionotropic and metabotropic glutamate receptors, we focus on the ionotropic class.

The ionotropic glutamate receptors (N-methyl-D-aspartate [NMDA], α-amino-3-hydroxy-5-methylisoxazole-4-propionic acid [AMPA], and kainate) are oligomers composed of individual subunits: NMDA (NMDAR1 and NMDAR2A–D); AMPA (GluR1–GluR4); and kainate (GluR5–GluR7, KA1, and KA2). This important new development in neuropsychopharmacology (i.e., glutamate receptors; excitatory amino acid receptors) has been reviewed in various detail by Hyman and Nestler (1993), Hollmann and Heinemann (1994), and Owens et al. (1996). Phencyclidine acts as an antagonist at the NMDA subtype of the glutamate receptor and can cause profound schizophrenia-like symptoms. This implies that mechanisms that decrease NMDA receptor (glutamatergic) function may produce psychosis and that the glutamatergic system might be hypofunctional in schizophrenia. Based on known glutamatergic neurobiology (see reviews above), this is not inconsistent with the dopamine hypothesis of schizophrenia (Olney and Farber 1995), although there is little pharmacological evidence of effective antipsychotic actions of glutamate agonists (Kalivas et al. 1989; Olney 1992; Tamminga et al. 1992). However, Goff and colleagues (1995) recently reported that D-cycloserine, a partial agonist at the glycine recognition site of the NMDA receptor, at a dose of 50 mg/day produced a significant reduction in negative symptoms when added to conventional antipsychotic therapy in patients who have schizophrenia with prominent negative symptoms.

This observation, coupled with increasingly compelling data for glutamatergic abnormalities in schizophrenia (Tsai et al. 1995), has led to increasing interest in the glutamatergic properties of atypical antipsychotic medications. For example, preclinical studies have found that chronic antipsychotic treatment can alter glutamatergic activity. Both chronic haloperidol and raclopride administration increase NMDAR1 subunit immunoreactivity in the striatum. This effect is not observed for clozapine (Fitzgerald et al. 1995). In this study, both haloperidol and clozapine increased GluR1 immunoreactivity in the prefrontal cortex, and clozapine alone increased GluR2 immunoreactivity in the frontal/parietal cortex, nucleus accumbens, and hippocampus.

In the past decade, there has been an explosion of information about the neurotransmitter role of neuropeptides. Indeed, opioid peptides, cholecystokinin, and neurotensin can regulate dopaminergic activity in laboratory animals. For example, haloperidol increases neurotensin and neurotensin mRNA concentrations in the mesolimbic (nucleus accumbens) and nigrostriatal (dorsolateral striatum) dopamine systems, whereas the atypical antipsychotics clozapine and sertindole only increase neurotensin activity in the mesolimbic system (Kinkead et al. 1993). Interestingly, Diaz et al. (1994) observed that in the nucleus accumbens, antipsychotic blockade of D_2 receptors increases neurotensin expression, whereas D_3 blockade decreases it. These actions occur in distinct subnuclei of the nucleus accumbens, but the effects of D_2 blockade predominate. Thus, there is ample evidence that neuropeptide-based drugs would alter dopaminergic activity. Unfortunately, few peptidergic ligands are available for detailed preclinical studies predictive of antipsychotic activity, although peptide-based drugs may hold great promise in the future.

Neuronal expression of Fos, a nuclear transcription factor and the protein product of the immediate-early gene *c-fos*, is increased by several physiological and pharmacological treatments that activate neuronal function. As such, Fos immunoreactivity or *c-fos* mRNA expression has been used to map functional pathways in the central nervous system. Of interest is the finding that clozapine and haloperidol produce different induction patterns after acute administration; haloperidol increases expression in the striatum, nucleus accumbens, and septum, and clozapine increases it in the nucleus accumbens, septum, and prefrontal cortex. Moreover, all antipsychotics referred to as atypical produce a greater increase in expression in the nucleus accumbens than in the dorsolateral striatum (Guo et al. 1995; Robertson and Fibiger 1996; Robertson et al.

1994). Deutch et al. (1995) observed that clozapine, but not risperidone, induces Fos expression in the paraventricular nucleus of the thalamus. Although the functional significance of these findings is unclear, they further support a neuroanatomically selective or different pattern of effects produced by clozapine. Because transcription factors such as Fos are required for alterations in gene transcription, it can be assumed that clozapine and haloperidol, for example, do produce distinct differences in the expression of various genes in the striatum. It will be of great interest to determine what these gene products are.

To summarize, we use the known pharmacology of clozapine to review those biological characteristics that may confer an atypical nature on an antipsychotic. Clozapine may be able to decrease mesolimbic dopamine activity while sparing nigrostriatal function and possibly even increasing cortical dopamine activity. The mechanisms as to how this selectivity occurs are unknown but are certainly based on preferential binding to certain populations of dopamine receptors (i.e., mesolimbic) and/or dopamine receptor subtypes (i.e., D_4), perhaps along with relatively greater $5\text{-HT}_{2A}/D_2$ blockade than that observed with typical antipsychotics. Although these types of mechanisms are certain to exist, the ultimate therapeutic efficacy almost certainly derives from adaptive changes in neuronal structure (e.g., synaptic arborization patterns) and function (e.g., persistent changes in the levels of neurotransmitter, receptors, and/or intracellular signaling messengers) induced by chronic exposure to antipsychotics. Indeed, for most classes of psychotherapeutic agents, understanding this neuronal plasticity is what will define the mechanism of action of a given drug.

CLOZAPINE

History and Discovery

As elaborated above, over the past several decades animal and molecular studies have begun to further elucidate the neuroanatomical and neurotransmitter circuits involved in cognition and behavior. This increased understanding of brain neurobiology has led to the development of newer hypotheses regarding the pathophysiology of psychosis and innovative approaches to psychopharmacological treatments. Specifically, putative medications exploiting differential potencies on D_1, D_2, D_3, and D_4 receptors; partial dopamine receptor agonists; sigma receptor antagonists; NMDA receptor antagonists; serotonin receptor antagonists (5-HT_{2A}, 5-HT_3, 5-HT_6, and 5-HT_7); muscarinic receptor antagonists; and α-adrenergic agonists and antagonists have been developed and are being studied in early clinical trials. Unfortunately, some of these agents have not proved efficacious or have had unacceptable adverse side effects and have not undergone further clinical development. However, others, including risperidone, olanzapine, sertindole, quetiapine, and ziprasidone, have proven efficacious and well tolerated in recent clinical studies. Excellent reviews of ongoing research on a wide variety of novel atypical antipsychotic medications have been produced by Gerlach (1991), Meltzer (1992a), Lieberman (1993), Pickar (1995), and Jibson and Tandon (1996).

Currently, only clozapine and risperidone (discussed later in this chapter, following the discussion of clozapine) among new atypical antipsychotic agents have had widespread clinical use in the United States, although the use of olanzapine has grown quickly since its introduction in the fall of 1996. Clozapine received approval from the U.S. Food and Drug Administration (FDA) for clinical use in the United States in 1990; however, it has been extensively used outside of the United States since the 1970s.

As reviewed by Hippius (1989), clozapine was first reported to be an effective antipsychotic medication by Austrian and German clinicians in the mid-1960s. Its use was controversial even then because it was dogma that EPS were "necessary" for antipsychotic efficacy. Although clozapine was clearly an effective antipsychotic, it lacked EPS, causing some clinicians to questions its inclusion as a "real neuroleptic." Unfortunately, in 1974, as clozapine's popularity was growing in Europe, eight patients in Finland died from clozapine-associated agranulocytosis, and the routine use of clozapine was discontinued in many parts of the world. However, clozapine remained available in some countries, and its remarkable efficacy in otherwise refractory patients eventuated in its reemergence in the late 1980s for use in selected (treatment-resistant or medication-intolerant) patients with the current laboratory monitoring system.

Structure-Activity Relations

As reviewed in detail by Baldessarini and Frankenburg (1991), clozapine is 8-chloro-11-(4-methyl-1-piperazinyl)-5H-dibenzo[b,e][1,4]diazepine (Figure 18–3). It was originally developed in 1960 by Hünziker et al. (1963). No alternative has yet been developed with the same degree

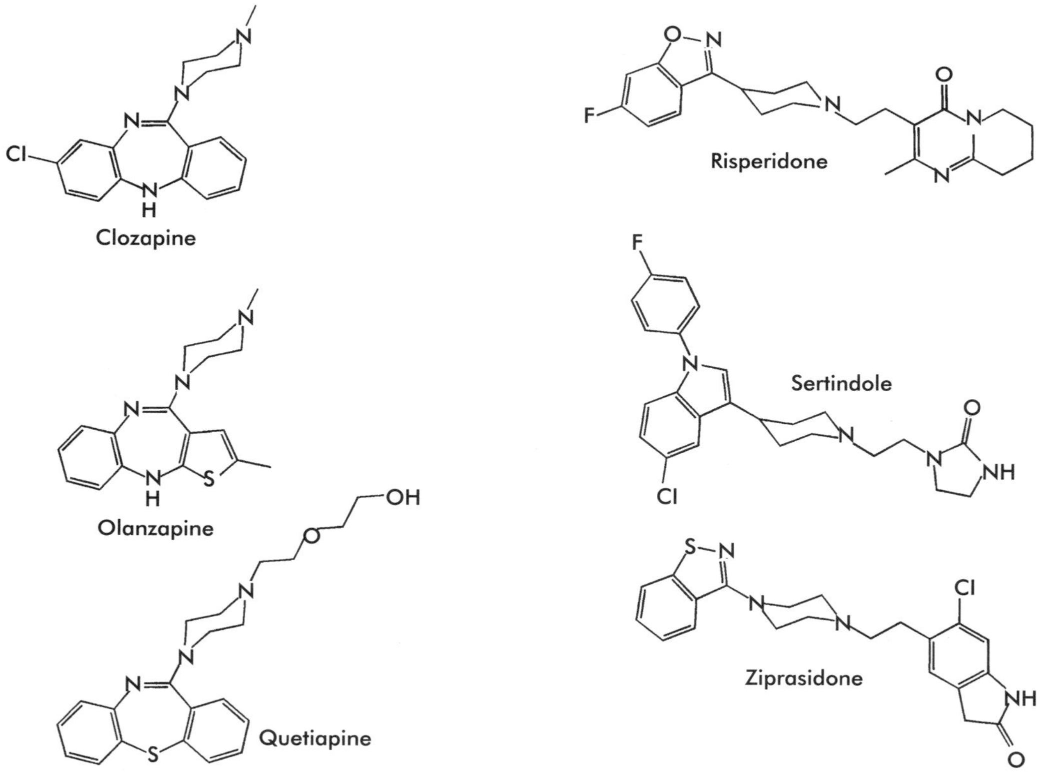

Figure 18–3. Chemical structures for the atypical antipsychotics described in the text.

of antipsychotic efficacy and lack of EPS but with an absence of bone marrow toxicity, although olanzapine (Figure 18–3) is being developed as such. Clozapine is structurally similar, but not identical, to loxapine, an antipsychotic that does not have atypical antipsychotic properties. Clozapine's principal metabolites are believed to be *N*-desmethyl and *N*-oxide metabolites with low pharmacological activity (Baldessarini and Frankenburg 1991).

Indications and Pharmacotherapeutics

Clozapine is currently approved for use in 1) "treatment-refractory" schizophrenic patients (i.e., those in whom adequate trials of several different classes of typical D_2-blocking antipsychotic medications have failed), 2) patients with unmanageable EPS from typical D_2-blocking antipsychotic medications, and/or 3) patients with tardive dyskinesia. However, ongoing clinical research investigations suggest the clinical utility of clozapine, alone or in combination with other psychotropics, in patients with schizoaffective disorder and refractory bipolar disorder (manic or depressed), as well as during the early stages (i.e., first and second episodes) of schizophrenia.

The major reason for the current restrictions on clozapine's clinical indications has been the occurrence of clozapine-induced agranulocytosis in approximately 1%–2% of patients, with reports of occasional fatalities. Because clozapine-induced agranulocytosis occurs in approximately 1%–2% of patients, weekly laboratory monitoring of a patient's complete and differential blood count is required for the pharmaceutical dispensing of clozapine in the United States. Several ongoing studies are attempting to elucidate both the mechanisms and the predictors of clozapine-associated agranulocytosis in attempts to reduce or eliminate this potentially fatal side effect.

Clozapine has received approval for use in human subjects, despite its infrequent but potentially fatal adverse side effects, because 1) an increasing number of studies has suggested its antipsychotic efficacy in otherwise treatment-refractory or unresponsive schizophrenic patients, and 2) it has a markedly reduced incidence of EPS and tardive dyskinesia as compared with typical antipsychotic medications.

Many open studies, and several randomized, parallel-design, short-term (4–6 weeks) studies (Kane et al. 1988) and crossover studies (Pickar et al. 1992b), have shown the superior antipsychotic efficacy of clozapine over standard D_2-blocking antipsychotic reductions (i.e., chlorpromazine and fluphenazine) in approximately one-third of treatment-refractory schizophrenic patients. The superior antipsychotic efficacy of clozapine in these studies has been confirmed for both the positive symptoms of psychosis (i.e., hallucinations, delusions, thought disorder) and the negative symptoms of psychosis (i.e., anhedonia, asociality, blunted affect). Other preliminary studies suggest that an additional 15%–30% of patients who are unresponsive to clozapine in the first few months may show significant improvement after 6 months to 2 years of continued clozapine pharmacotherapy (Meltzer 1992b).

Chronic treatment with clozapine has also been associated with improvement in "functionality," including increased vocational, social, and interpersonal adaptation in otherwise chronically impaired, treatment-refractory patients. This improvement has resulted in diminished frequency and duration of hospitalizations and an increased ability of disabled patients to increase their educational level and to reenter the workplace. Consequently, several studies throughout the world have indicated that clozapine therapy, despite a higher cost of medication to the individual, has resulted in significant savings to society, as evidenced by reduced hospital costs (Meltzer et al. 1993), and in potentially improved economic productivity of otherwise chronically ill patients. In addition to significant clinical improvement in a large minority of otherwise treatment-resistant schizophrenic patients, an apparent complete remission of illness has been noted in a smaller subset of patients.

Unlike traditional antipsychotic medications, clozapine monotherapy is only rarely associated with EPS or tardive dyskinesia (Lieberman et al. 1991). Furthermore, some investigators have observed a marked attenuation or complete elimination of EPS and tardive dyskinesia in affected patients. Although it is not yet known whether these findings are the result of withdrawal from traditional antipsychotics or a specific therapeutic effect, we have noted the disappearance of tardive dyskinesia with clozapine treatment and its reappearance with the withdrawal of clozapine prior to reinstitution of other pharmacotherapy. Finally, although a few cases of neuroleptic malignant syndrome have been reported to be associated with clozapine monotherapy, the incidence of clozapine-associated neuroleptic malignant syndrome would be expected to be less than that occurring with typical antipsychotics. It is of interest that clozapine has been used successfully in the antipsychotic treatment of patients who have experienced neuroleptic malignant syndrome associated with typical antipsychotic pharmacotherapy.

Despite its increasingly widespread clinical use, there is still a great deal of disparity in clinical practice in the administration of clozapine pharmacotherapy. When clozapine was first introduced, it was recommended that candidates for clozapine pharmacotherapy have antipsychotic medication "washouts" for up to 1 week prior to the initiation of clozapine. However, the withdrawal of typical antipsychotic medication prior to the initiation of clozapine may sometimes be associated with significant clinical deterioration. Withdrawal should therefore be individualized. Starting clozapine in drug-withdrawn patients is preferable, but if necessary, low doses of a high-potency agent may be used until clozapine pharmacotherapy is established. Typically, clozapine is begun at 12.5–25 mg/day and increased in 25-mg increments each day, as tolerated (see section, "Side Effects and Toxicology," later in this chapter). When patients begin to show appreciable clinical improvement, their previous D_2-blocking, typical antipsychotic therapy may then be titrated downward and discontinued. Rarely, patients need or benefit from continued combined treatment with clozapine and a high-potency typical antipsychotic medication (e.g., haloperidol, fluphenazine). The continued use of "combination therapy," however, puts the patient at increased and continued risk for EPS, tardive dyskinesia, and neuroleptic malignant syndrome.

As noted earlier in this chapter, in addition to the antipsychotic efficacy of clozapine, preliminary studies suggest that it has significant antimanic and antidepressant effects in patients with schizoaffective and bipolar disorders in whom traditional psychopharmacological regimens have failed. Conversely, patients with schizoaffective or bipolar disorder unresponsive to clozapine monotherapy may benefit from the addition of lithium, valproic acid, or antidepressants when clozapine monotherapy does not adequately control the affective symptoms. Lithium plus clozapine has been associated with a higher rate of neurological side effects, including neuroleptic malignant syndrome. Although any antidepressant may be used, the serotonin-specific reuptake inhibitors have fewer synergistic side effects (i.e., decreased anticholinergic, hypotensive, sedative, and cardiac conduction effects). Fluoxetine administration has been reported to increase clozapine plasma levels markedly and produce toxicity via pharmacokinetic interactions (displacing serum-bound proteins and competing for hepatic microsomal enzyme metabolism). These same pharmacokinetic interactions may also occur with tricyclic and other antidepressant agents metabolized by the hepatic P450 microsomal system. The antidepressant bupropion probably should not be used in patients receiving clozapine because both medications are associated with a significantly increased incidence of seizures. Although benzodiazepines have been used concurrently with clozapine, there have been

occasional reports of severe respiratory depression or arrests with their combined use. Thus their concomitant use is discouraged, especially, but not exclusively, with their concurrent initiation.

There is no universal agreement as to the "optimal" daily dose of clozapine pharmacotherapy. Although doses in the range of 200–400 mg/day have occasionally been associated with significant improvement and efficacy, greater improvement in otherwise unresponsive or partially responsive patients may occur with doses in the range of 500–900 mg/day. Seizures occur with an increased incidence in clozapine-treated patients. The occurrence of seizures appears to be dose related, possibly occurring at a rate of 0.7% per 100-mg dose. Patients experiencing seizures may be treated with concurrent anticonvulsants, but carbamazepine should be avoided because of its occasional propensity to suppress bone marrow (aplastic anemia). Although both agents (carbamazepine and clozapine) can cause bone marrow toxicity, carbamazepine is thought to be directly toxic to bone marrow, and clozapine may represent an immunological mechanism. Valproate may be the safest and best tolerated anticonvulsant in clozapine-treated patients who experience seizures. It is emphasized that clozapine-associated seizures do not necessarily contradict its continued use. If a patient experiences a clozapine-associated seizure, the clozapine dose may be temporarily reduced or stopped and anticonvulsants initiated. When therapeutic levels of anticonvulsants are achieved, the clozapine dose may be titrated upward to its previous therapeutic levels.

Confounding the determination of a particular patients' most effective daily dose is the observation that some patients appear to need increased time taking medication, rather than increased doses of medication, for an optimal therapeutic response. Thus, some patients who experience little or no improvement during the first 3–4 months of therapy will go on to improve significantly after 6 months to 2 years of continued pharmacotherapy.

There is currently no consensus as to the optimal daily dose or adequacy of duration of a trial of clozapine pharmacotherapy. Some centers recommend the titration of a patient's dose up to approximately 450–650 mg/day during the first few months unless significant improvement occurs at lower doses. If a patient has had no appreciable improvement at 450–650 mg/day for 6 months, then titration up to a maximum of 900 mg/day with concurrent anticonvulsant administration may be considered, with a continued trial for an additional 6 months to 1 year. Other clinicians are less or more aggressive in dose titration. However, it does appear that approximately one-third of patients will not experience significant benefits from clozapine pharmacotherapy, regardless of the dose or the duration of the trial.

Side Effects and Toxicology

In addition to an approximately 1% incidence of potentially life-threatening agranulocytosis and the above-described dose-related seizures, clozapine has a few other undesirable but usually manageable side effects. Clozapine may frequently produce profound and often prolonged sedation, hypersalivation, enuresis (daytime and nighttime), and anticholinergic side effects (i.e., dry mouth, blurred vision, urinary retention, and constipation). Elderly patients and patients taking other medications with significant anticholinergic properties may rarely experience anticholinergic delirium. These side effects are usually time limited, although they may persist for months. They are often dose related and may respond to a temporary reduction in dose or to treatment with other medications with pharmacological properties opposite to the problematic side effects (i.e., caffeine for sedation, bulk-increasing agents for constipation, cholinomimetic drugs for anticholinergic side effects, and anticholinergic medications for hypersalivation). Occasional patients may also experience urinary incontinence, either nighttime or daytime, which may also respond to anticholinergic agents. In almost all cases, these side effects eventually remit or are manageable with continued clozapine administration.

Orthostatic hypotension and tachycardia, not necessarily interrelated, occur frequently during clozapine pharmacotherapy and may respond to a temporary dose reduction or adjunctive pharmacological interventions. Both of these side effects are potentially dangerous and need careful clinical monitoring and attention to the side effects of concurrently administered medications that may be synergistic in toxicity.

During the first few months of clozapine pharmacotherapy, some patients experience high "benign" fevers (100–103°F). These temperature elevations are usually not related to neuroleptic malignant syndrome or sepsis, nor are they anticholinergically mediated, although these etiologies must be ruled out. These temperature elevations usually remit with continued clozapine administration. When they occur, they may be managed with antipyretic agents.

As discussed earlier in this chapter, 1% of clozapine-treated patients develop clinically significant suppression of bone marrow blood precursors, particularly the granulocyte series, but rarely also the erythropoid and platelet progenitors. Consequently, weekly monitoring of complete blood count and differential is recommended throughout the duration of clozapine pharmacotherapy. Although agranulocytosis can occur at any time, its incidence peaks between 2 and 6 months of pharmacotherapy. In some cases, even more frequent monitoring may be indicated during this time in high-risk patients (i.e., those who are older, medically ill, receiving potentially toxic concurrent medications, or experiencing large fluctuations in white blood cell count). It is important to note, however, that significant fluctuations—both increases and decreases—in white blood cell count occur frequently early in clozapine pharmacotherapy and do not necessarily indicate agranulocytosis or sepsis. Current laboratory monitoring recommendations include temporarily discontinuing clozapine if the white blood cell count drops to 3,000/mm^3 or the granulocyte count falls to 1,500/mm^3. Subsequently, clozapine may be carefully reinstituted after complete recovery of white blood cell and granulocyte counts. Clozapine should be permanently discontinued if the white blood cell count drops to 2,000/mm^3 or the granulocyte count falls to 1,000/mm^3. Patients experiencing agranulocytosis should be seen and monitored by a hematologist and usually need immediate hospital admission to a medical service for reverse isolation and aggressive monitoring and treatment.

Because clozapine most frequently suppresses the granulocyte series of white blood cells, a differential cell count is recommended. Theoretically, the total white blood cell count could remain within normal limits despite the presence of agranulocytosis. Clozapine, like any medication, may also affect other organ systems, and other laboratory indices, including liver function tests, should also be monitored, although less frequently if they remain normal. More in-depth, comprehensive reviews of the clinical use of clozapine have been produced by Kane et al. (1988), Lieberman et al. (1989), and Baldessarini and Frankenburg (1991).

Mechanism of Action

Despite the abundance of side effects mentioned above, the increasingly widespread use of clozapine pharmacotherapy has generated excitement and hope in the treatment of chronically ill psychotic patients. A great deal of interest has been generated in understanding what pharmacological properties of clozapine contribute to its increased efficacy in some otherwise medication-refractory patients.

As reviewed in the beginning of this chapter, several hypotheses have been generated to explain the increased the efficacy of certain atypical antipsychotics. Clozapine appears to have many of these properties, including an increased ratio of D_1 to D_2 blockade, greater D_3 and D_4 antagonism, 5-HT$_{2A}$ and 5-HT$_{2C}$ antagonistic properties, anticholinergic and antiadrenergic properties, and increased mesolimbic specificity with relative sparing of nigrostriatal dopaminergic neurons.

In addition to its greater effectiveness in the treatment of positive symptoms, clozapine has also been associated with relatively greater effectiveness in the treatment of the negative, or deficit, symptoms of psychosis. Many investigators have noted the association of prominent negative symptoms with relative reductions in prefrontal cortical blood flow and glucose metabolism seen during PET or single photon emission computerized tomography (SPECT) scanning of schizophrenic patients (Andreasen et al. 1992; Berman et al. 1992; Buchsbaum et al. 1992; Wolkin et al. 1992). Several preliminary studies (Pickar et al. 1992a) have reported the ability of clozapine pharmacotherapy to improve, or at least not worsen, this relative "hypofrontality" as compared with traditional D_2-blocking antipsychotics. This effect, as shown in functional brain imaging, has been proffered as a possible explanation for clozapine's reduction of the negative symptoms of psychosis.

Which, if any, of clozapine's pharmacological properties described above, or combinations thereof, contribute to the increased therapeutic efficacy of clozapine awaits further elucidation. However, such insights could potentially aid in the development of newer, alternative atypical antipsychotic agents with fewer adverse side effects.

Current experience suggests that at least one-third of typical antipsychotic-refractory schizophrenic patients will not show appreciable benefit from clozapine pharmacotherapy. Given the considerable expense and adverse side effects associated with clozapine pharmacotherapy, it would be of considerable clinical utility to predict a priori potential responders and nonresponders to clozapine. In this regard, Pickar et al. (1992b) and Risch and Lewine (1993, 1995) have reported preliminary data suggesting that schizophrenic patients with relatively low ratios of homovanillic acid (HVA) to 5-hydroxyindoleacetic acid (5-HIAA) in cerebrospinal fluid may experience significantly greater benefit with clozapine pharmacotherapy than patients with relatively higher HVA-to-5-HIAA ratios. These observations have involved only a small number of subjects and require replications in larger groups of patients. They add support, however, to the theoretical hy-

potheses elaborated by Meltzer (1992a) and others of the potential importance of central nervous system dopaminergic and serotonergic interactions in the pathogenesis and pharmacotherapy of schizophrenia.

RISPERIDONE

Risperidone was introduced in 1993 in the United States. Chemically it is 3-[2-[4-(6-fluoro-1,2-benzisoxazol-3-yl)-1piperidinyl]ethyl]-6,7,8,9-tetrahydro-2-methyl-4H-pyrido[1,2-a]pyrimidin-4-one (Figure 18–3).

Pharmacokinetics[1]

Risperidone is well absorbed. Total recovery of radioactivity at 1 week from a single 1-mg oral dose is 85%, including 70% in the urine and 15% in the feces. Risperidone is extensively metabolized in the liver by cytochrome P450 (CYP) 2D6, to a major active metabolite, 9-hydroxyrisperidone, which is the predominant circulating species, and appears approximately of equal efficacy with risperidone with respect to receptor-binding activity and some effects in animals (a second minor pathway is N-dealkylation). Consequently, the clinical effect of the drug probably results from the combined concentrations of risperidone plus 9-hydroxyrisperidone, which are dose proportional over the dosing range of 1–16 mg daily (0.5–8 mg twice daily).

The relative oral bioavailability of risperidone from a tablet is 94% (coefficient of variation [CV] = 10%) as compared with a solution. Because food does not affect either the rate or the extent of absorption of risperidone, the drug can be given with or without meals. The enzyme that catalyzes the hydroxylation of risperidone to 9-hydroxyrisperidone is CYP2D6, also called debrisoquin hydroxylase. It is also the enzyme responsible for the metabolism of many neuroleptics, antidepressants, antiarrhythmics, and other drugs. CYP2D6 is subject to genetic polymorphism (about 6%–8% of whites and a very low percentage of Asians have little or no activity and are "poor metabolizers") and to inhibition by a variety of substrates and some nonsubstrates, notably quinidine. Extensive metabolizers convert risperidone rapidly into 9-hydroxyrisperidone, whereas poor metabolizers convert it much more slowly. Extensive metabolizers, therefore, have lower risperidone

---

[1] Information in this section was abstracted from the *Physicians' Desk Reference*, 1996, and package insert.

and higher 9-hydroxyrisperidone concentrations than do poor metabolizers.

After oral administration of solution or tablet, mean peak plasma concentrations occur at about 1 hour. Peak 9-hydroxyrisperidone concentrations occur at about 3 hours in extensive metabolizers and 17 hours in poor metabolizers. The apparent half-life of risperidone is 3 hours (CV = 30%) in extensive metabolizers and 20 hours (CV = 40%) in poor metabolizers. The apparent half-life of 9-hydroxyrisperidone is about 21 hours (CV = 20%) in extensive metabolizers and 30 hours (CV = 25%) in poor metabolizers. Steady-state concentrations of risperidone are reached in 1 day in extensive metabolizers and would be expected to be reached in about 5 days in poor metabolizers. Steady-state concentrations of 9-hydroxy-risperidone are reached in 5–6 days (measured in extensive metabolizers).

Because risperidone and 9-hydroxyrisperidone are approximately of equal efficacy, the sum of their concentrations is pertinent. The pharmacokinetics of the sum of risperidone and 9-hydroxyrisperidone after single and multiple doses are similar in extensive and poor metabolizers; overall mean elimination half-life is about 20 hours. In analyses comparing adverse reaction rates in extensive and poor metabolizers in controlled and open studies, no important differences were seen.

Risperidone could be subject to two kinds of drug-drug interactions. First, inhibitors of CYP2D6 could interfere with the conversion of risperidone to 9-hydroxy-risperidone. This in fact occurs with quinidine, giving essentially all recipients a risperidone pharmacokinetic profile that is typical of poor metabolizers. The plasma protein binding of risperidone is about 90% over the in vitro concentration range of 0.5–200 ng/mL and increases with increasing concentrations of α_1-acid glycoprotein. The plasma binding of 9-hydroxyrisperidone is about 77%. Neither the parent nor the metabolite displace each other from the plasma binding sites (Medical Economics 1996).

Clinical Studies

Multicenter clinical trials that led to the FDA approval of risperidone found that risperidone had an efficacy that was at least equal to that of haloperidol and produced significantly fewer EPS (Borison et al. 1987; Chouinard et al. 1993; Marder and Meibach 1994; Peuskens 1995). Combined results from several trials showed risperidone at 6 mg/day to have greater efficacy than haloperidol at 20 mg/day with respect to reduced positive and negative symptoms.

Since risperidone's introduction in 1993, there has been a great deal of clinical experience, which is summa-rized below. In fact, at the time of this writing, risperidone has surpassed haloperidol as the antipsychotic most frequently prescribed by psychiatrists in the United States.

Pharmacologically, risperidone is a D_2 antagonist that also has potent 5-HT$_{2A}$, as well as α_1 and α_2, antagonistic effects. It is essentially devoid of anticholinergic effects. As noted above, the parent compound risperidone has a pharmacologically active metabolite, 9-OH-risperidone, which is believed to be essentially equipotent with the parent drug. Risperidone itself has a half-life of approximately 4–6 hours, whereas its metabolite has a half-life of approximately 22 hours.

A recent United States multicenter study and an international multicenter study have indicated that risperidone can be given once daily with equal efficacy and with no significant increase in adverse side effects because of the long half-life of its active metabolite. Side effects accompanying risperidone that occur at a level of greater than 5% and twice that of placebo include somnolence, fatigue, orthostatic dizziness, tachycardia, nausea, dyspepsia, diarrhea, weight gain, sexual dysfunction (including ejaculatory problems, dysmenorrhea, priapism, erectile dysfunction, and diminished desire), and rhinitis. Many of these side effects also appear to occur with other atypical antipsychotics. However, in premarketing studies, discontinuation because of adverse side effects when placebo adjusted was remarkably low: discontinuation due to EPS was 2.1%, dizziness 0.7%, hypotension 0.6%, somnolence 0.5%, and nausea 0.3%. At present, no true estimate of the prevalence of tardive dyskinesia accompanying risperidone is known. However, case reports in the literature have described possible risperidone-induced tardive dyskinesia.

Risperidone has also been reported to be rarely associated with neuroleptic malignant syndrome (Tarsy 1996; Webster and Wijeratne 1994). However, for theoretical reasons, such as its 5-HT$_{2A}$ blocking actions, which potentiate its nigrostriatal dopamine transmission, as well as the numbers of patients with 3–4 years of exposure, it would appear that the prevalence of tardive dyskinesia may be substantially lower with risperidone than with typical antipsychotics. Confirmation of this possibility awaits larger numbers of patients with longer periods of exposure to this medication.

In neuroleptic-naive patients, risperidone is typically begun at 1 mg twice a day and increased as tolerated to a target dose of 3–6 mg/day. Recent experience suggests that the initially recommended target dose of 6 mg/day is unnecessarily high and that at least 70% of patients can be optimally treated at daily doses of 3 mg/day or less and approximately 90% at doses below 6 mg/day. Of note is that at this dose the incidence of EPS produced by risperidone is indistinguishable from that of placebo.

When risperidone was first introduced into the United States market, it was suggested that risperidone could be given at 1 mg twice a day on day 1, 2 mg twice a day on day 2, and 3 mg twice a day on day 3. However, clinical experience suggests that this titration was too rapid for some patients. Consequently, patients should be monitored for tolerance of risperidone in relation to side effects (e.g., sedation, hypotension) and the titration performed as clinically tolerated.

For patients already taking other antipsychotics with risperidone, it is suggested, as previously described for clozapine in this chapter, that the medications be overlapped. Specifically, 1) for patients taking high doses of high-potency antipsychotics, the high-potency antipsychotic dose should be reduced by approximately one-third as risperidone is added at 1–2 mg/day and titrated upward; and 2) for patients taking relatively low doses of high-potency antipsychotics, a dose reduction of approximately two-thirds of the high-potency antipsychotics is recommended as risperidone is added in an identical manner. Typical antipsychotics should be tapered as the risperidone is adjusted upward, again to a target dose of 3–6 mg/day. In premarketing studies, a dosage of 6 mg/day was associated with the greatest efficacy with fewest EPS. However, in postmarketing studies, most patients' conditions can be managed at approximately 3 mg/day.

Some investigators believe that the onset of risperidone's efficacy may be delayed in a subgroup of patients, much like that of clozapine as described earlier in this chapter, and consequently, it is not clear what the optimal dose titration with respect to time should be in any given individual. However, our experience indicates that some patients may need several months of risperidone trial before an optimal response is achieved; therefore, it should not be discontinued before this time of exposure simply because of an apparent lack of efficacy. This is another reason for overlapping of the typical and atypical antipsychotics to allow the full benefit from the atypical profile. However, as noted previously, Meltzer and others argue that, optimally, the typical antipsychotics should be discontinued as soon as clinically appropriate because they may 1) predispose subjects to tardive dyskinesia, 2) complicate the pharmacokinetics and pharmacodynamics of dosage titration, and 3) potentially attenuate the full efficacy of the atypical medication.

A number of reports have emerged suggesting that risperidone, like clozapine, is associated with continued improvement over several years in quality-of-life scales, social functioning, reductions in length of hospital stays, and overall reductions in lifetime cost of illness (Addington et al. 1993; Bouchard et al. 1994; Chouinard et al.

1993; Lindstrom et al. 1994; Polsker 1994). Most recently, risperidone was compared with haloperidol in a randomized, double-blind study of 59 treatment-resistant schizophrenic patients (Green et al. 1997). Risperidone was shown to have significantly greater benefit than haloperidol on verbal working memory. The results of this study suggest that risperidone, in addition to reducing symptoms, may improve cognitive deficits in treatment-resistant schizophrenic patients and thus potentially further diminish disability.

Several recent studies, as reviewed by Mendelowitz and Lieberman (1995), have suggested risperidone's utility in patients whose symptoms are refractory to treatment with typical antipsychotics. Although clozapine remains the most studied of the antipsychotics in treatment-refractory patients, several studies have suggested that risperidone may sometimes be efficacious in true clozapine nonresponders. It is of particular note, however, that clozapine should not be discontinued in patients who are currently responding beneficially because severe withdrawal psychoses have emerged that may subsequently be treatment refractory to the reinitiation of clozapine.

Because of risperidone's relative safety and fewer adverse side effects as compared with typical antipsychotics, preliminary case reports and open studies, as reviewed by Mendelowitz and Lieberman (1995), have suggested its utility in the treatment of other psychotic disorders, including psychotic depression, mania, psychotic dementias, and psychosis in children and adolescents. Children, adolescents, and elderly patients have been successfully treated with as little as 0.5–1.5 mg/day. It has recently been reported (D. Jeste, personal communication, 1997) that risperidone may actually be cognitively enhancing in elderly patients with dementia, increasing Mini-Mental State Exam (Folstein et al. 1975) scores by an average of 3 points. Thus, given its lack of EPS at low doses, lack of anticholinergic side effects, and apparent cognitive enhancing effects, risperidone may be particularly useful in the treatment of delirium and dementia in elderly patients. However, these preliminary reports await confirmation in controlled studies of larger subject populations. In this regard, it is emphasized that there have been, at the time of this writing, no double-blind, placebo-controlled studies of risperidone's efficacy in patients with any of these syndromes and that there are currently no labeling indications in these areas.

OLANZAPINE

Olanzapine is of particular note because it is structurally related to clozapine. Chemically, olanzapine is 2-methyl-

4-(4-methyl-1-piperazinyl)-10*H*-thieno[2,3-*b*][1,5]benzodiazepine. It is a potent antipsychotic agent with nanomolar receptor affinity in vitro at serotonin 5-HT$_{2A/2C}$, 5-HT$_3$, and 5-HT$_6$; D$_4$/D$_3$/D$_1$/D$_2$; and muscarinic cholinergic (M$_1$–M$_5$), α_1-adrenergic, and histamine H$_1$ receptors (Bymaster et al. 1996). Although some structural and distinct metabolic differences are apparent, the compound has a pharmacological profile of activity similar to that of the atypical agent clozapine (Figure 18–3). This profile is especially distinct from that of the typical antipsychotic agents (e.g., haloperidol). On the basis of these findings, it could be predicted that olanzapine would have a unique profile highlighted by a wider range of efficacy than typical agents and a much lower incidence of undesirable side effects, such as EPS and hematoxicity, than either class.

In preclinical pharmacological studies, olanzapine had a range of receptor affinities distinct from those of traditional drugs and generally comparable to those of clozapine (Bymaster et al. 1996). The compound shows a greater affinity for serotonin (5-HT$_{2A}$) than for dopamine (D$_1$, D$_2$) receptors. In addition, the compound has affinity at the binding sites of D$_4$, D$_3$, 5-HT$_3$, 5-HT$_6$, H$_1$, α_1-adrenergic, and muscarinic M$_{1-5}$ receptors. There is no significant binding at 5-HT$_{1A}$, 5-HT$_{1B}$, 5-HT$_{1D}$, 5-HT$_7$, β-adrenoceptors, γ-aminobutyric acid (GABA)$_A$, GABA$_B$, sigma, opioid, or benzodiazepine receptors.

Electrophysiological studies corroborate the desirable property of olanzapine to selectively reduce dopamine activity in the mesolimbic (A$_{10}$) pathways thought to mediate psychosis while sparing striatal (A$_9$) pathways involved in extrapyramidal signs and symptoms. In addition, olanzapine blocks the NMDA receptor-mediated excitotoxicity induced by phencyclidine.

Behavioral studies with olanzapine have been consistent with the compound's receptor-binding profile. Olanzapine blocks 5-hydroxytryptophan-induced head twitches and increases quipazine-induced secretion of corticosterone, demonstrating 5-HT$_{2A}$ receptor antagonism in vivo. These actions occur at doses lower than those required to block dopamine-mediated behaviors. Inhibition of conditioned avoidance response has been widely used to predict the antipsychotic potential of a compound, whereas the induction of catalepsy is associated with the occurrence of EPS. The ratio of the dose required to interfere with conditioned avoidance to that required to induce catalepsy suggests antipsychotic activity with relatively low potential for EPS.

Olanzapine also increased punished responding in an animal conflict test predictive of a compound's anxiolytic potential. Similar to clozapine, olanzapine selectively antagonizes cocaine-induced hyperactivity compared with dextroamphetamine-induced hyperactivity in rats and also low-dose compared with high-dose *d*-amphetamine-induced hyperactivity. Olanzapine selectively antagonizes NMDA antagonist-induced activities, similar to clozapine.

Overall, the toxicological profile of olanzapine in animal studies has been quite unremarkable. Especially noteworthy has been the absence of evidence of bone marrow cytotoxicity in any of the species examined in these toxicology studies.

On the basis of these findings, olanzapine would be predicted to reduce both positive and negative symptomatology as well as the secondary depressive mood features seen in patients with schizophrenia. Furthermore, olanzapine would be expected to substantially lower the incidence of EPS without agranulocytosis, as seen with clozapine.

Both United States and international multicenter studies comparing olanzapine with haloperidol have suggested that olanzapine is effective in doses of 5.5–20 mg/day (Beasley et al. 1996; Tollefson et al. 1997). Its efficacy with respect to positive symptoms is equivalent to that of haloperidol and superior to that of haloperidol with respect to negative symptoms (Tollefson and Sanger 1997). In addition, these studies suggest that long-term treatment with olanzapine is associated with fewer relapses and higher achievement on a quality-of-life scale. In the studies reported to date, olanzapine has few, if any, significant EPS, especially as compared in blinded studies with haloperidol (Tran et al. 1997). In this regard, however, a recent animal study (Robertson and Fibiger 1996) indicated that olanzapine may increase *c-fos* activity in striatal areas in a dose-dependent manner, which may be an indication of potential EPS activity. In addition, akathisia was observed in premarketing trials at an incidence of greater than 5% and at least twice that of placebo. Akathisia occurs in a dose-dependent manner. Because the receptor pharmacology of olanzapine is similar to that of clozapine, it is anticipated that the side effects (and potentially their management) will be similar to clozapine's, as described above. However, of particular note is that there has been no evidence of leukopenia or agranulocytosis associated with olanzapine in either animal or human studies. Although a 10-mg starting dose is recommended, current data suggest that approximately 25% of patients will respond to 5 mg/day, 25% will require up to 10 mg/day, 25% will require up to 15 mg/day, and approximately 25% will require 20 mg/day. Incidentally, olanzapine has also been given to some patients in 25-mg doses; however, labeling suggests that doses of greater than 20 mg/day have not yet been studied.

SERTINDOLE[2]

Sertindole is an antipsychotic drug candidate discovered and patented by H. Lundbeck A.S. (Copenhagen, Denmark). Sertindole has been licensed to Abbott Laboratories (Abbott Park, Illinois) and is being developed by the Psychopharmacology Venture of Abbott Laboratories in the United States and Canada. Chemically, sertindole is 1-[2-[4-[5-chloro-1-(4-fluorophenyl)-1H-indol-3-yl]-1piperidinyl]ethyl]-2-imidazolidinone (Figure 18–3).

Sertindole combines a selective antagonistic effect on mesolimbic dopaminergic neurons with a serotonin-antagonistic effect and an α-adrenergic-antagonistic effect. It is anticipated that with such a profile, sertindole should be able to reduce the symptoms of schizophrenia at doses that cause minimal neurological side effects.

In in vitro receptor-binding studies using rat brain–derived membranes, sertindole had a pharmacological profile with nanomolar affinities for D_1, D_2, D_4, 5-HT_{2A}, and α_1-adrenergic receptors. Sertindole has a low affinity for α_2-adrenergic, histamine H_1, and sigma receptors. It shows no affinity for 5-HT_{1A}, phencyclidine, muscarinic, β-adrenergic, GABA, and excitatory amino acid receptors. Studies of the in vivo activity of sertindole also indicate potent 5-HT_{2A} antagonism, moderate α_1 antagonism, and weak D_2 antagonism.

Sertindole showed high selectivity for limbic dopamine neurons in a neurophysiological test model measuring spontaneously active dopamine neurons in VTA and SN pars compacta (SNC) after 3 weeks of oral treatment in rats. Oral administration of sertindole suppressed the spontaneous firing of dopamine neurons measured by a microelectrode recording technique in rat brain VTA. A 3-week oral administration was required for suppression of the dopamine neurons, and the median effective dose (ED_{50}) was determined to be 0.015 μmol/kg, approximately 100 times more potent than clozapine, which also induced a selective inhibition of the active dopamine neurons in the VTA. Sertindole was approximately 100 times less potent in suppressing dopamine neurons in rat brain SNC than in rat brain VTA. In contrast, haloperidol produced a nonselective inhibition of dopamine neurons in both VTA and SNC.

At the time of this writing, sertindole is under FDA review for marketing approval in the United States. Premarketing trials suggest that sertindole is an effective antipsychotic in doses of 12–24 mg/day. When compared with placebo and haloperidol at doses of 4, 8, and 16 mg, sertindole was at least as effective as haloperidol in reducing positive symptoms, and only sertindole (20 mg/day) was more effective than placebo in the treatment of negative symptoms (Zimbroff et al. 1997). The prevalence of EPS with sertindole is indistinguishable from that of placebo, even at very high doses (Casey 1996; Zimbroff et al. 1997). Side effects with sertindole include a mild increase, reversible with discontinuation, in Q-T interval of approximately 15–25 milliseconds (Jibson and Tandon 1996) and tachycardia, weight gain, decreased ejaculatory volume, nasal congestion, and occasional nausea. Of particular note, however, is the absence of anticholinergic activity and very little, if any, sedation. In addition, serum prolactin levels do not remain elevated during sertindole administration. Premarketing clinical trials have also shown the superiority of sertindole over haloperidol with respect to improvements on a quality-of-life scale, fewer relapses, and significant reductions in hospital days.

QUETIAPINE

Chemically, quetiapine is 2-[2-(4-dibenzo[b,f][1,4]-thiazepin-11-yl-1-piperazinyl)ethoxy]ethanol fumarate (Figure 18–3) and is structurally related to clozapine and olanzapine. Quetiapine was previously referred to as ICI 204,636 and as Seroquel, which has now become the trade name under which it is potentially to be marketed.

Quetiapine[3] is a novel antipsychotic agent that has high affinity for brain serotonin 5-HT_{2A} receptors and markedly lower affinity for D_2 and D_1 receptors as compared with standard antipsychotic agents. Quetiapine also has considerably less muscarinic cholinergic and α_1-

---

[2] The discussion of the pharmacology of sertindole was abstracted from the investigator's brochures associated with premarketing trials of sertindole.

[3] The information in this section was abstracted from investigator's brochures and other literature of premarketing studies of quetiapine.

adrenergic receptor antagonist activity than standard antipsychotic agents.

Quetiapine is active orally in classical tests for antipsychotic activity (i.e., conditioned avoidance tests and behavioral or electrophysiological tests measuring the reversing actions of dopamine agonists) and has substantial selectivity for the limbic system. Additionally, quetiapine, unlike standard antipsychotic agents, has little or no depolarization inactivation of nigrostriatal dopamine neurons, paradigms considered predictive of EPS liability.

Quetiapine has been studied in healthy volunteers or subjects with schizophrenia at daily doses of 25–450 mg. Quetiapine was well tolerated in clinical pharmacology studies. After oral administration, the absorption of quetiapine is rapid (mean time to maximum concentration $[T_{max}] = 1.2–1.8$ hours) and complete. The steady-state pharmacokinetics are dose proportional when quetiapine is given three times daily over a dose range of 25–150 mg. Steady-state plasma concentrations are within the limits predicted from single-dose data. Food has a variable, clinically insignificant effect on the bioavailability of quetiapine. The largest fractions of quetiapine-related material circulating in plasma are unchanged quetiapine (11%) and the inactive sulfoxide metabolite (10%). The elimination of quetiapine is relatively rapid (mean half-life of 2.2–3.2 hours) and primarily by metabolism. Less than 1% of the administered oral dose is excreted unchanged in urine and feces. Approximately 73% and 21% of the dose are quetiapine-related material excreted in the urine and feces, respectively.

Quetiapine's half-life is approximately 3 hours, so that two- or three-times-a-day dosing may be initially indicated.

Quetiapine has been shown to be effective in the treatment of both positive and negative symptoms of schizophrenia in doses of 150–800 mg/day. It is comparable to typical neuroleptics in this regard (Jibson and Tandon 1996). Quetiapine is notable for having a very low incidence of EPS, no sustained elevations of plasma prolactin, and no anticholinergic side effects.

ZIPRASIDONE[4]

Ziprasidone, formerly CP-88,059, is chemically 5-[2-[4-(1,2-benzisothiazol-3-yl)-1-piperazinyl]ethyl]-6-chloro-1,3-dihydro-2*H*-indol-2-one monohydrochloride (Figure 18–3). Ziprasidone was developed within a structure-activity investigation intended to find a compound that potently blocks D_2 receptors but that binds with even greater affinity to central $5-HT_{2A}$ receptors (Seeger et al. 1995).

Ziprasidone hydrochloride binds with high affinity to $5-HT_{2A}$, D_2, $5-HT_{1A}$, $5-HT_{2C}$, $5-HT_{1D}$, α_1-adrenergic, and D_1 receptors. Its affinity for $5-HT_2$ receptors is 11 times greater than its affinity for D_2 receptors.

In behavioral studies, an oral dose of ziprasidone hydrochloride of 1.5 mg/kg was required to decrease by 50% the locomotor stimulation elicited in rats by dextroamphetamine given subcutaneously in a dose of 1 mg/kg. The potency of ziprasidone hydrochloride in this respect is thus approximately one-tenth that of haloperidol. Similarly, an oral dose of ziprasidone hydrochloride of 2.4 mg/kg was required to antagonize by 50% the behavioral stereotypies elicited by apomorphine in rats. Blockade of the behavioral actions of apomorphine, as of amphetamine, is characteristic of dopamine receptor antagonists.

Perhaps the clearest reflection in animals of severe extrapyramidal dysfunction is catalepsy, which is seen in rats after treatment with typical antipsychotic drugs. Catalepsy is not observed after administration of ziprasidone hydrochloride at doses less than 12.1 mg/kg orally but is seen at that and higher doses. The dose of haloperidol at which catalepsy is observed is 0.8 mg/kg orally.

The firing rate of serotonergic neurons located in the dorsal raphe nucleus is known to be inhibited in vivo by $5-HT_{1A}$ agonists such as 8-hydroxy-dipropylaminotetralin (8-OH-DPAT) and buspirone. Ziprasidone hydrochloride at a dose of 100–200 μg/kg inhibits the spontaneous firing rate by 50%. Although the potency of ziprasidone hydrochloride is weak, when compared with that of established $5-HT_{1A}$ agonists such as 8-OH-DPAT, the data suggest that ziprasidone hydrochloride exerts $5-HT_{1A}$ agonist activity. Ziprasidone hydrochloride also antagonizes α_1 receptors, however, and unit activity of serotonergic neurons in this experimental preparation has also been reported to be decreased by α_1-adrenoceptor agonists. Regardless of mechanism, the effect of ziprasidone hydrochloride on serotonergic neuron firing appears to be weak. Ziprasidone also has been reported to block synaptic noradrenergic and serotonergic reuptake in a manner similar to that of venlafaxine and thus, although this has not yet been con-

---

[4] Information in this section was abstracted from investigator's brochures and other literature of premarketing trials of ziprasidone.

firmed, to have potent antidepressant properties.

Absorption, metabolism, and excretion of ziprasidone were studied in four healthy male subjects after oral administration of 20 mg of a mixture of ^{3}H- and ^{14}C-labeled ziprasidone. Total recovery of the administered dose was 88% ± 3.9% over a period of 11 days. The percentages of the dose excreted in urine and feces were 20% ± 1% and 66% ± 5%, respectively.

The absorption of ziprasidone is rapid, and the maximum concentration of drug in serum (C_{max}) for ziprasidone and metabolites occurs at 4–6 hours. On the basis of a preliminary analysis, approximately 60% of the total radioactivity in human serum is attributable to unchanged drug and the remaining 40% is largely accounted for by the sulfoxide and sulfone metabolites. The affinities of the sulfoxide and sulfone metabolites for 5-HT$_2$ and D$_2$ receptors are low with respect to ziprasidone and are thus unlikely to contribute to its antipsychotic effects.

Ziprasidone is extensively metabolized, and only a small amount of the drug is excreted in urine as unchanged drug. Seven metabolites in human urine are identified by ion spray gas chromatography/mass spectroscopy (GC/MS). These metabolites are similar to those found in rats, mice, and dogs. The major urinary metabolites are due to N-dealkylation of the ethyl side chain attached to the piperazinyl nitrogen and oxidation at the sulfur resulting in the formation of sulfoxide and sulfone. Preliminary data obtained from in vitro studies using human liver microsomes indicate that the formation of the major metabolites (sulfoxide and sulfone) is not mediated by CYP2D6.

Ziprasidone has recently been submitted to the FDA for marketing approval in the United States, and it is anticipated that it will be available in the near future. Premarketing studies suggest that ziprasidone in doses of 80–120 and 120–160 mg/day is effective in reducing both positive and negative psychotic symptoms; doses of 120–160 mg/day may be most appropriate for acute treatment, whereas doses of 80–120 mg/day may be sufficient for maintenance studies, although this remains to be confirmed in controlled studies.

Ziprasidone has very few, if any, EPS and very little, if any, anticholinergic activity (Jibson and Tandon 1996). Premarketing studies suggest that ziprasidone is associated with sexual dysfunction similar to that of placebo and that ziprasidone does not increase prolactin levels. Of interest is that weight gain was only comparable to that of typical neuroleptics, which would place it as producing the least weight gain among the atypical antipsychotics; however, "head-to-head" studies have not yet been performed. In premarketing studies, ziprasidone has been studied as a mesylate salt for intramuscular injection in doses of 5, 10,

or 20 mg two or four times daily and was reported to have rapid antipsychotic actions without EPS, tachycardia, postural hypotension, or electrocardiographic abnormalities. However, these observations must be verified in placebo-controlled studies. Nevertheless, this preparation is of interest because at the time of this writing no injectable atypical antipsychotics are available, and the clinical need for these agents is significant.

OTHER ATYPICAL ANTIPSYCHOTICS UNDER DEVELOPMENT

Other antipsychotics, including iloperidone, mazapertine, aripiprazole, and others, are undergoing Phase 2 study and, if trials prove successful, may undergo Phase 3 and Phase 4 premarketing study. However, not enough information from clinical trials is available at this time to warrant further discussion.

SUMMARY

The increasingly sophisticated understanding of neurobiology has led to significant advances in the understanding of the pathophysiology of schizophrenia. These insights have led to the development of new-generation atypical antipsychotic medications with potentially fewer adverse side effects and improved therapeutic efficacy. The prototype atypical antipsychotic agent, clozapine, has generated a new era of excitement and hope for the pharmacotherapy of treatment-resistant schizophrenic patients. An entire series of newer atypical antipsychotic agents, currently undergoing clinical trials, may further increase the understanding of the pathogenesis of schizophrenia and expand treatment alternatives.

REFERENCES

Addington DE, Jones B, Bloom D, et al: Reduction of hospital days in chronic schizophrenic patients with risperidone: a retrospective study. Clin Ther 15:917–926, 1993

Andreasen NC, Rezai K, Alliger R, et al: Hypofrontality in neuroleptic-naive patients and in patients with chronic schizophrenia: assessment with xenon 133 single-photon emission computed tomography and the Tower of London. Arch Gen Psychiatry 49:943–958, 1992

Ashby CR, Jiang LH, Kasser RJ, et al: Electrophysiological characterization of 5-hydroxytryptamine$_3$ receptors in rat medial prefrontal cortex. J Pharmacol Exp Ther 251:171–178, 1990

Baldessarini RJ, Frankenburg FR: Clozapine—a novel antipsychotic agent. N Engl J Med 324:746–754, 1991

Baldessarini RJ, Campbell A, Yeghiayan S, et al: Limbic-selective antidopaminergic effects of S(+)-aporphines compared to typical and atypical antipsychotic agents in the rat, in Biological Psychiatry, Vol 2. Edited by Racagni G, Brunello N, Fukuda T. Amsterdam, Elsevier Science Publishers, 1991, pp 837–840

Beasley CM, Tollefson G, Tran P, et al: Olanzapine versus placebo and haloperidol: acute phase results of the North American doubleblind olanzapine trial. Neuropsychopharmacology 14:111–124, 1996

Berman KF, Torrey EF, Daniel AG, et al: Regional cerebral blood flow in monozygotic twins discordant and concordant for schizophrenia. Arch Gen Psychiatry 49:927–934, 1992

Bertorello AM, Hopfield JF, Aperia A, et al: Inhibition by dopamine of $(Na^+ + K^+)$ ATPase activity in neostriatal neurons through D_1 and D_2 dopamine receptor synergism. Nature 347:386–388, 1990

Bolanos FJ, Schechter LE, Miquel MC, et al: Common pharmacological and physicochemical properties of 5-HT$_3$ binding sites in the rat cerebral cortex and NG 108-15 clonal cells. Biochem Pharmacol 40:1541–1550, 1990

Borison RL, Pathiraja AP, Diamond BL, et al. Risperidone: clinical safety and efficacy in schizophrenia. Psychopharmacol Bull 13:261–276, 1987

Bouchard RH, Pourcher E, et al: Multidimensional evaluation of risperidone efficacy in an institutional setting. Abstracts of the Annual Meeting of Collegium Internationale Neuro-Psychopharmacologicum, 1994, p 174

Bouthenet ML, Souil E, Martres MP, et al: Localization of dopamine D_3 receptor mRNA in the rat brain using in situ hybridization histochemistry: comparison with dopamine D_2 receptor mRNA. Brain Res 564:203–219, 1991

Buchsbaum MS, Haier RJ, Potkin SG, et al: Frontostriatal disorder of cerebral metabolism in never-medicated schizophrenics. Arch Gen Psychiatry 49:935–942, 1992

Buckland PR, O'Donovan MC, McGuffin P: Changes in dopamine D_1 and D_3 receptor mRNA levels in rat brain following antipsychotic treatment. Psychopharmacology 106:479–483, 1992

Bunney BS, Sesack SR, Silva NL: Midbrain dopamine systems: neurophysiology and electrophysiological pharmacology, in Psychopharmacology: The Third Generation of Progress. Edited by Meltzer HY. New York, Raven, 1987, pp 113–126

Bunney BS, Chiodo LA, Grace AA: Midbrain dopamine system electrophysiological functioning: a review and new hypothesis. Synapse 9:79–94, 1991

Bunzow JR, Van Tol HHM, Grandy DK: Cloning and expression of a rat D_2 dopamine receptor cDNA. Nature 336:783–787, 1988

Bymaster FP, Calligaro DO, Falcone JF, et al: Radioreceptor binding profile of the atypical antipsychotic olanzapine. Neuropsychopharmacology 14:87–96, 1996

Campbell A, Yeghiayan S, Baldessarini RJ, et al: Selective antidopaminergic effects of S(+)N-n-propylnoraporphine in limbic versus extrapyramidal sites in rat brain: comparisons with typical and atypical antipsychotic agents. Psychopharmacology 103:323–329, 1991

Canton H, Verriele L, Colpaert FC: Binding of typical and atypical antipsychotics to 5-HT$_{1C}$ and 5-HT$_2$ sites: clozapine potently interacts with 5-HT$_{1C}$ sites. Eur J Pharmacol 191:93–96, 1990

Carlsson A: The current status of the dopamine hypothesis of schizophrenia. Neuropsychopharmacology 1:179–186, 1988a

Carlsson A: Dopamine autoreceptors and schizophrenia, in Receptors and Ligands in Psychiatry. Edited by Sen AK, Lee T. Cambridge, England, Cambridge University Press, 1988b, pp 1–10

Casey DE: Behavioral effects of sertindole, risperidone, clozapine, and haloperidol in Cebus monkeys. Psychopharmacology 124:134–140, 1996

Chio CL, Hess GF, Graham RS, et al: A second molecular form of D_2 dopamine receptor in rat and bovine caudate nucleus. Nature 343:266–269, 1990

Chiodo LA, Bunney BS: Typical and atypical neuroleptics: differential effects of chronic administration on the activity of A9 and A10 midbrain dopaminergic neurons. J Neurosci 3:1607–1619, 1983

Chiodo LA, Bunney BS: Possible mechanisms by which repeated clozapine administration differentially affects the activity of two subpopulations of midbrain dopamine neurons. J Neurosci 5:2539–2544, 1985

Chouinard G, Jones B, Remington G, et al: A Canadian multicenter placebo-controlled study of fixed doses of risperidone and haloperidol in the treatment of chronic schizophrenic patients. J Clin Psychopharmacol 13:25–40, 1993

Clark D, White FJ: Review: D_1 dopamine receptor—the search for a function: a critical evaluation of the D_1/D_2 dopamine receptor classification and its functional implications. Synapse 1:347–388, 1987

Cortés R, Gueye B, Pazos A, et al: Dopamine receptors in human brain: autoradiographic distribution of D_1 sites. Neuroscience 28:263–273, 1989

Coward DM, Dixon AK, Urwyler S, et al: Partial dopamine-agonistic and atypical neuroleptic properties of the amino-erolines SDZ 208-911 and SDZ 208-912. J Pharmacol Exp Ther 252:279–285, 1990

Dearry A, Gingrich JA, Falardeau P, et al: Molecular cloning and expression of the gene for a human D_1 dopamine receptor. Nature 247:71–76, 1990

Deutch AY, Moghaddam B, Innis RB, et al: Mechanisms of action of atypical antipsychotic drugs: implications for novel therapeutic strategies for schizophrenia. Schizophr Res 4:121–156, 1991

Deutch AY, Öngür D, Duman RS: Antipsychotic drugs induce fos protein in the thalamic paraventricular nucleus: a novel locus of antipsychotic action. Neuroscience 66:337–346, 1995

Dewey SL, Smith GS, Logan J, et al: Serotonergic modulation of striatal dopamine measured with positron emission tomography (PET) and in vivo microdialysis. J Neurosci 15:821–829, 1995

Diaz J, Lévesque D, Griffon N, Lammers CH, et al: Opposing roles for dopamine D_2 and D_3 receptors on neurotensin mRNA expression in nucleus accumbens. Eur J Neurosci 6:1384–1387, 1994

Dray A, Gonye TJ, Oakley NR, et al: Evidence for the existence of a raphe projection to the substantia nigra in rat. Brain Res 113:45–57, 1976

Farde L, Hall H, Ehrin E, et al: Quantitative analysis of D_2 dopamine receptor binding in the living human brain by PET. Science 231:258–260, 1986

Farde L, Wiesel FA, Halldin C, et al: Central D_2-dopamine receptor occupancy in schizophrenic patients treated with antipsychotic drugs. Arch Gen Psychiatry 45:71–76, 1988

Farde L, Nordstrom AL, Weisel FA, et al: D_1 and D_2 dopamine occupancy during treatment with conventional and atypical neuroleptics. Psychopharmacology 99 (suppl): S28–S31, 1989

Farde L, Nordstrom AL, Weisel FA, et al: Positron emission tomographic analysis of central D_1 and D_2 dopamine receptor occupancy in patients treated with classical neuroleptics and clozapine: relation to extrapyramidal side effects. Arch Gen Psychiatry 49:538–544, 1993

Fitzgerald LW, Deutch AY, Gasic G, et al: Regulation of cortical and subcortical glutamate receptor subunit expression by antipsychotic drugs. J Neurosci 15:2453–2464, 1995

Folstein MF, Folstein SE, McHugh PR: Mini-Mental State: a practical method for grading the cognitive state of patients for the clinician. J Psychiatr Res 12:189–198, 1975

Gerlach J: New antipsychotics: classification, efficacy, and adverse effects. Schizophr Bull 17:289–309, 1991

Giros B, Sokoloff P, Martres MP, et al: Alternative splicing directs the expression of two D_2 dopamine receptor isoforms. Nature 342:923–926, 1989

Goff DC, Guschaun G, Manaach DS, et al: Dose-finding study of D-cycloserine added to neuroleptics for negative symptoms of schizophrenia. Am J Psychiatry 152:1213–1215, 1995

Grace AA, Bunney BS, Moore H, Todd CL: Dopamine cell depolarization block as a model for the actions of antipsychotic drugs. Trends Neurosci 20:31–37, 1997

Grandy DK, Marchionni MA, Makam H, et al: Cloning of the cDNA and gene for a human D_2 dopamine receptor. Proc Natl Acad Sci U S A 86:9762–9766, 1989

Green MF, Marshall BD, Wirshing WC, et al: Does risperidone improve verbal working memory in treatment resistant schizophrenia? Am J Psychiatry 154:797–804, 1997

Guo N, Klitenick MA, Tham C-S, Fibiger HC: Receptor mechanisms mediating clozapine-induced *c-fos* expression in the forebrain. Neuroscience 65:747–756, 1995

Hand TH, Hu XT, Wang RY: Differential effects of acute clozapine and haloperidol in the activity of ventral tegmental (A10) and nigrostriatal (A9) dopamine neurons. Brain Res 415:257–269, 1987

Heffner TG, Caprathe B, Davis M, et al: Effects of PD 128482, a novel dopamine autoreceptor agonist in preclinical antipsychotic tests, in Novel Antipsychotic Drugs. Edited by Meltzer HY. New York, Raven, 1992, pp 79–90

Hippius H: The history of clozapine. Psychopharmacology 99:53–55, 1989

Hollmann M, Heinemann S: Cloned glutamate receptors. Annu Rev Neurosci 17:31–108, 1994

Hoyer D, Gozlan H, Bolanos F, et al: Interaction of psychotropic drugs with central 5-HT_3 recognition sites: fact or fiction? Eur J Pharmacol 171:137–139, 1989

Hünziker F, Künzle F, Schmutz J: Uber ein 5-Stellung basisch substituierte 5-H Dibenzo [b,e]-1,4-diazepine. Helv Chir Acta 46:2337–2346, 1963

Hyman SE, Nestler EJ: The Molecular Foundations of Psychiatry. Washington, DC, American Psychiatric Press, 1993

Ichikawa J, Meltzer HY: Differential effects of repeated treatment with haloperidol and clozapine on dopamine release and metabolism in the striatum and the nucleus accumbens. J Pharmacol Exp Ther 256:248–357, 1991

Itzhak Y, Stein I: Sigma binding sites in the brain: an emerging concept for multiple sites and their relevance for psychiatric disorders. Life Sci 47:1073–1081, 1990

Jibson MD, Tandon R: A summary of research findings on the new antipsychotic drugs. Essential Psychopharmacology 1:27–37, 1996

Kalivas PW, Duffy P, Barrow J: Regulation of the mesocorticolimbic dopamine system by glutamic acid receptor subtypes. J Pharmacol Exp Ther 251:378–387, 1989

Kane J, Honigfeld G, Singer J, et al: Collaborative study group: clozapine for the treatment-resistant schizophrenic: a double-blind comparison with chlorpromazine. Arch Gen Psychiatry 45:789–796, 1988

Kilpatrick GJ, Jones BJ, Tyers MB: Identification and distribution of 5-HT_3 receptors in rat brain using radioligand binding. Nature 330:746–748, 1987

Kilts CD, Anderson CM, Ely TD, et al: Absence of synthesis-modulating nerve terminal autoreceptors on mesamygdaloid and other mesolimbic dopamine neuronal populations. J Neurosci 7:3961–3975, 1987

Kinkead BL, Owens MJ, Nemeroff CB: Serotonin antagonists as antipsychotics, in Serotonin: From Cell Biology to Pharmacology and Therapeutics. Edited by Vanhooutte PM, Saxena PR, Paoletti R, et al. Dordrecht, The Netherlands, Kluwer, 1993, pp 289–296

Lahti RA, Roberts RC, Tamminga CA: D_2-family receptor distribution in human postmortem tissue: an autoradiographic study. NeuroReport 6:2505–2512, 1995

Largent BL, Wikström H, Snowman AM, et al: Novel antipsychotic drugs share high affinity for receptors. Eur J Pharmacol 155:345–347, 1988

Lewander T, Uppfeldt G, Köhler C, et al: Remoxipride and raclopride: pharmacological background and clinical outcome, in Novel Antipsychotic Drugs. Edited by Meltzer HY. New York, Raven, 1992, pp 67–78

Lidow MS, Goldman-Rakic PS, Rakic P, et al: Dopamine D_2 receptors in the cerebral cortex: distribution and pharmacological characterization with [^{3}H]raclopride. Proc Natl Acad Sci U S A 86:6412–6416, 1989

Lieberman JA: Understanding the mechanism of action of atypical antipsychotic drugs. Br J Psychiatry 163 (suppl 22):7–18, 1993

Lieberman JA, Kane JM, Johns CA: Clozapine: guidelines for clinical management. J Clin Psychiatry 50:329–338, 1989

Lieberman JA, Saltz BL, Johns CA, et al: The effects of clozapine on tardive dyskinesia. Br J Psychiatry 158:503–510, 1991

Lindstrom E, Knorring L, Eberhard G: Studies of selected outcome-related clinical parameters following short-term and long-term treatment with risperidone. Annual Meeting of Collegium International, NeuroPsychopharmacologicum P-58–223, 1994

Lundberg T, Lindström LH, Hartvig P, et al: Striatal and frontal cortex binding of 11-C-labelled clozapine visualized by positron emission tomography (PET) in drug-free schizophrenics and healthy volunteers. Psychopharmacology 99:8–12, 1989

Mansour A, Meador-Woodruff JH, Bunzow JR, et al: Localization of dopamine D_2 receptor mRNA and D_1 and D_2 receptor binding in the rat brain and pituitary: an in situ hybridization-receptor autoradiographic analysis. J Neurosci 10:2587–2600, 1990

Mansour A, Meador-Woodruff JH, Zhou QY, et al: A comparison of D_1 receptor binding and mRNA in rat brain using receptor autoradiographic and in situ hybridization techniques. Neuroscience 45:359–371, 1991

Marder SR, Meibach RC: Risperidone in the treatment of schizophrenia. Am J Psychiatry 151:825–835, 1994

Meador-Woodruff JH, Mansour A, Bunzow JR, et al: Distribution of D_2 dopamine receptor mRNA in rat brain. Proc Natl Acad Sci U S A 86:7625–7628, 1989

Meador-Woodruff JH, Mansour A, Civelli O, et al: Distribution of D_2 dopamine receptor mRNA in the primate brain. Prog Neuropsychopharmacol Biol Psychiatry 15:885–893, 1991

Meador-Woodruff JH, Damask SP, Wang J, et al: Dopamine receptor mRNA expression in human striatum and neocortex. Neuropsychopharmacology 15:17–29, 1996

Medical Economics Company: Physicians' Desk Reference, 50th Edition. Montvale, NJ, Medical Economics, 1996

Meltzer HY: The mechanism of action of novel antipsychotic drugs. Schizophr Bull 17:263–287, 1991

Meltzer HY: Novel Antipsychotic Drugs. New York, Raven, 1992a

Meltzer HY: Dimensions of outcome with clozapine. Br J Psychiatry 160 (suppl 17):46–53, 1992b

Meltzer HY: Role of serotonin in the action of atypical antipsychotic drugs. Clin Neurosci 3:64–75, 1995

Meltzer HY, Matsubara S, Lee JC: Classification of typical and atypical drugs on the basis of dopamine D_1, D_2 and serotonin$_2$ pK_i values. J Pharmacol Exp Ther 251:238–246, 1989

Meltzer HY, Cole P, Way L, et al: Cost-effectiveness of clozapine in neuroleptic resistant schizophrenia. Am J Psychiatry 150:1630–1638, 1993

Mendelowitz AJ, Lieberman SA: New findings in the use of atypical antipsychotics: focus on risperidone. J Clin Psychiatry Case Comment Series 2:1–12, 1995

Mengod G, Martinez-Mir MI, Vilaró MT, et al: Localization of the mRNA for the dopamine D_2 receptor in the rat brain by in situ hybridization histochemistry. Proc Natl Acad Sci U S A 86:8560–8564, 1989

Minabe Y, Ashby CR, Wang RY: Effects produced by acute and chronic treatment with granisetron alone or in combination with haloperidol on midbrain dopamine neurons. Eur Neuropsychopharmacol 2:127–133, 1992

Moghaddam B: Preferential activation of cortical dopamine neurotransmission by clozapine: functional significance. J Clin Psychiatry 55 (suppl B):27–29, 1994

Moghaddam B, Bunney BS: Acute effects of typical and atypical antipsychotic drugs on the release of dopamine from prefrontal cortex, nucleus accumbens, and striatum of the rat: an in vivo microdialysis study. J Neurochem 54:1755–1760, 1990

Molineaux SM, Jessell TM, Axel R, et al: 5-HT$_{1C}$ receptor is a prominent serotonin receptor subtype in the central nervous system. Proc Natl Acad Sci U S A 86:6793–6797, 1989

Monsma FJ, McVittie LD, Gerfen CR, et al: Multiple D_2 dopamine receptors produced by alternative RNA splicing. Nature 342:926–929, 1989

Monsma FJ, Mahan LC, McVittie LD, et al: Molecular cloning and expression of a D_1 dopamine receptor linked to adenylyl cyclase activation. Proc Natl Acad Sci U S A 87:6723–6727, 1990

Monsma FJ, Shen Y, Ward RP, et al: Cloning and expression of a novel serotonin receptor with high affinity for tricyclic psychotropic drugs. Mol Pharmacol 43:320–327, 1993

Murray AM, Hyde TM, Knable MB, et al: Distribution of putative D_4 dopamine receptors in postmortem striatum from patients with schizophrenia. J Neurosci 15:2186–2191, 1995

Musacchio JM: The psychotomimetic effects of opiates and the receptor. Neuropsychopharmacology 3:191–199, 1990

Naber D, Gaussares C, Moeglen JM, et al: Efficacy and tolerability of SDZ HDC 912, a partial dopamine D_2 agonist, in the treatment of schizophrenia, in Novel Antipsychotic Drugs. Edited by Meltzer HY. New York, Raven, 1992, pp 99–107

Nordstrom AL, Farde L, Halldin C: High 5-HT$_2$ receptor occupancy in clozapine treated patients demonstrated by PET. Psychopharmacology 110:365–367, 1993

O'Donnell PO, Grace AA: Basic neurophysiology of antipsychotic drug action, in Handbook of Experimental Pharmacology: Antipsychotics. Edited by Csernansky JC. New York, Springer-Verlag, 1996, pp 163–202

Ögren SO, Hall H: Comparison of the effects of different substituted benzamides on dopamine receptor function in the rat, in Novel Antipsychotic Drugs. Edited by Meltzer HY. New York, Raven, 1992, pp 59–66

Ohara K, Ulpian C, Seeman P, et al: Schizophrenia: dopamine D_1receptor sequence is normal, but has DNA polymorphisms. Neuropsychopharmacology 8:131–135, 1993

Olney JW: Glutamatergic mechanisms in neuropsychiatry, in Novel Antipsychotic Drugs. Edited by Meltzer HY. New York, Raven, 1992, pp 155–169

Olney JW, Farber NB: Glutamate receptor dysfunction and schizophrenia. Arch Gen Psychiatry 52:998–1007, 1995

Onn S-P, Grace AA: Repeated treatment with haloperidol and clozapine exerts differential effects on dye coupling between neurons in subregions of striatum and nucleus accumbens. J Neurosci 15:7024–7036, 1995

Owens MJ, Mulchahey JJ, Stout SC, et al: Molecular and neurobiological mechanisms in the treatment of psychiatric disorders, in Psychiatry. Edited by Tasman A, Kay J, Lieberman JA. Philadelphia, PA, WB Saunders, 1997, pp 210–257

Peuskens J, Risperidone Study Group: Risperidone in the treatment of chronic schizophrenic patients: a multi-national, multi-centre, double-blind, parallel-group study versus haloperidol. Br J Psychiatry 166:712–726, 1995

Pickar D: Prospects for the pharmacotherapy of schizophrenia. Lancet 345:557–562, 1995

Pickar D, Litman RE, Owen RR, et al: Response to clozapine predictors. Abstracts of the 31st Annual Meeting of the American College of Neuropsychopharmacology, San Juan, Puerto Rico, December 1992a, p 48

Pickar D, Woen RR, Litman RE, et al: Clinical and biologic response to clozapine in patients with schizophrenia. Arch Gen Psychiatry 49:345–353, 1992b

Piomelli D, Pilon C, Giros B, et al: Dopamine activation of the arachidonic acid cascade as a basis for D_1/D_2 receptor synergism. Nature 353:164–167, 1991

Polsker GL: Risperidone: does it give "enough bang for the buck"? Inpharma 16:7–8, 1994

Rasmussen K, Stockton ME, Czachura JF: The 5-HT$_3$ receptor antagonist zatosetron decreases the number of spontaneously active A10 dopamine neurons. Eur J Pharmacol 205:113–116, 1991

Reynolds GP: Developments in the drug treatment of schizophrenia. Trends Pharmacol Sci 13:116–121, 1992

Reynolds GP, Mason SL: Are striatal dopamine D_4 receptors increased in schizophrenia? J Neurochem 63:1576–1577, 1994

Risch SC, Lewine RJ: Low cerebrospinal fluid homovanillic acid/5-hydroxyindoleacetic acid ratio predicts clozapine efficacy: a replication (letter). Arch Gen Psychiatry 50:670, 1993

Risch SC, Lewine RRJ: CSF HVA:5-HIAA ratio increases accompanying clozapine efficacy (letter). Arch Gen Psychiatry 52:244, 1995

Robertson GS, Fibiger HC: Effects of olanzapine on regional *c-fos* expression in rat forebrain. Neuropsychopharmacology 14:105–110, 1996

Robertson GS, Matsumura H, Fibiger HC: Induction patterns of fos-like immunoreactivity in the forebrain as predictors of atypical antipsychotic activity. J Pharmacol Exp Ther 271:1058–1066, 1994

Roth BL, Craigo SC, Choudhary MS, et al: Binding of typical and atypical antipsychotic agents to 5-hydroxytryptamine-6 and 5hydroxytryptamine-7 receptors. J Pharmacol Exp Ther 268:1403–1410, 1994

Roth BL, Tandra S, Burgess LH, et al: D_4 dopamine receptor binding affinity does not distinguish between typical and atypical antipsychotic drugs. Psychopharmacology 120:365–368, 1995

Schmauss C, Haroutunian V, Davis KL, et al: Selective loss of dopamine D_3-type receptor mRNA expression in parietal and motor cortices of patients with chronic schizophrenia. Proc Natl Acad Sci U S A 90:8942–8946, 1993

Schoots O, Seeman P, Guan H-C, et al: Long-term haloperidol elevates dopamine D_4 receptors by 2-fold in rats. Eur J Pharmacol 289:67–72, 1995

Schwartz JC, Sokoloff P, Giros B, et al: The dopamine D_3 receptor as a target for antipsychotics, in Novel Antipsychotic Drugs. Edited by Meltzer HY. New York, Raven, 1992, pp 135–144

Seeger TF, Seymour PA, Schmidt AW, et al: Ziprasidone (CP-88,059): a new antipsychotic with combined dopamine and serotonin receptor antagonist activity. J Pharmacol Exp Ther 275:101–113, 1995

Seeman P: Dopamine receptors and the dopamine hypothesis of schizophrenia. Synapse 1:133–152, 1987

Seeman P: Receptor selectivities of atypical neuroleptics, in Novel Antipsychotic Drugs. Edited by Meltzer HY. New York, Raven, 1992a, pp 145–154

Seeman P: Dopamine receptor sequences: therapeutic levels of neuroleptics occupy D_2 receptors, clozapine occupies D_4. Neuropsychopharmacology 7:261–284, 1992b

Seeman P, Van Tol HHM: Dopamine D_4-like receptor elevation in schizophrenia: cloned D_2 and D_4 receptors cannot be discriminated by raclopride competition against [^{3}H] nemonapride. J Neurochem 64:1413–1415, 1995

Seeman P, Guan HC, Niznik HB: Endogenous dopamine lowers the dopamine D_2 receptor density as measured by [^{3}H]raclopride: implications for positron emission tomography of the human brain. Synapse 3:96–97, 1989a

Seeman P, Niznik HB, Guan HC, et al: Link between D_1 and D_2 dopamine receptors is reduced in schizophrenia and Huntington diseased brain. Proc Natl Acad Sci U S A 86:10156–10160, 1989b

Seeman P, Hong-Chang G, Van Tol HHM: Dopamine D_4 receptors elevated in schizophrenia. Nature 365:441–445, 1993

Seeman P, Sunahara RK, Niznik HB: Receptor-receptor link in membranes revealed by ligand competition: example for dopamine D_1 and D_2 receptors. Synapse 17:62–64, 1994

Seeman P, Guan H-C, Van Tol HHM: Schizophrenia: elevation of dopamine D_4-like sites, using [^{3}H]nemonapride and [^{125}I]epidepride. Eur J Pharmacol 286:R3–R5, 1995

Shen Y, Monsma FJ, Metcalf MA, et al: Molecular cloning and expression of a 5-hydroxytryptamine$_7$ serotonin receptor subtype. J Biol Chem 268:18200–18204, 1993

Skarsfeldt T: Differential effects of repeated administration of novel antipsychotic drugs on the activity of midbrain dopamine neurons in the rat. Eur J Pharmacol 281:289–294, 1995

Snyder SH: The dopamine connection. Nature 247:121–122, 1990

Snyder SH, Largent BL: Receptor mechanisms in antipsychotic drugs action: focus on sigma receptors. J Neuropsychiatry 1:7–15, 1989

Sokoloff P, Giros B, Martres MP, et al: Molecular cloning and characterization of a novel dopamine receptor (D_3) as a target for neuroleptics. Nature 247:146–151, 1990

Sokoloff P, Martres MP, Giros B, et al: The third dopamine receptor (D_3) as a novel target for antipsychotics. Biochem Pharmacol 43:656–666, 1992a

Sokoloff P, Andrieux M, Besancon R, et al: Pharmacology of human dopamine D_3 receptor expressed in a mammalian cell line: comparison with D_2 receptor. Eur J Pharmacol 225:331–337, 1992b

Sokoloff P, Levesque D, Martres MP, et al: The dopamine D_3 receptor as a key target for antipsychotics. Clin Neuropharmacol 15 (suppl 1):456A–457A, 1992c

Sorensen SM, Humphreys TM, Palfreyman MF: Effects of acute and chronic MDL 73,147, a 5-HT$_3$ receptor antagonist, on A9 and A10 dopamine neurons. Eur J Pharmacol 163:115–120, 1989

Soubrie P, Reisine TD, Glowinski J: Functional aspects of serotonin transmission in the basal ganglia: a review and an in vivo approach using the push-pull cannula technique. Neuroscience 131:615–624, 1984

Srivastava LK, Morency MA, Bajwa SB, et al: Effect of haloperidol on expression of dopamine D_2 receptor mRNAs in rat brain. J Mol Neurosci 2:155–161, 1990

Steinfels GF, Tam SW, Cook L: Electrophysiological effects of selective σ-receptor agonists, antagonists, and the selective phencyclidine receptor agonist MK-801 on midbrain dopamine neurons. Neuropsychopharmacology 2:201–207, 1989

Stockton ME, Rasmussen K: Electrophysiological effects of olanzapine, a novel atypical antipsychotic, on A9 and A10 dopamine neurons. Neuropsychopharmacology 14:97–104, 1996

Sumiyoshi T, Stockmeier CA, Overholser JC, et al: Dopamine D_4 receptors and effects of guanine nucleotides on [^{3}H]raclopride binding in postmortem caudate nucleus of subjects with schizophrenia or major depression. Brain Res 681:109–116, 1995

Sunahara RK, Niznik HB, Weiner DM, et al: Human dopamine D_1 receptor encoded by an intronless gene on chromosome 5. Nature 247:80–83, 1990

Sunahara RK, Guan HC, O'Dowd BF, et al: Cloning of the gene for a human dopamine D_5 receptor with higher affinity for dopamine than D_1. Nature 350:614–619, 1991

Tamminga CA, Gerlach J: New neuroleptics and experimental antipsychotics in schizophrenia, in Psychopharmacology: The Third Generation of Progress. Edited by Meltzer HY. New York, Raven, 1987, pp 1129–1140

Tamminga CA, Cascella N, Fakouhi TD, et al: Enhancement of NMDA-mediated transmission in schizophrenia: effects of milacemide, in Novel Antipsychotic Drugs. Edited by Meltzer HY. New York, Raven, 1992, pp 171–177

Tarsy D: Risperidone and neuroleptic malignant syndrome (letter). JAMA 275:446, 1996

Taylor DP, Schlemmer RF: Sigma "antagonists": potential antipsychotics? in Novel Antipsychotic Drugs. Edited by Meltzer HY. New York, Raven, 1992, pp 189–201

Tiberi M, Jarvie KR, Silvia C, et al: Cloning, molecular characterization, and chromosomal assignment of a gene encoding a second D_1 dopamine receptor subtype: differential expression pattern in rat brain compared with the D_{1A} receptor. Proc Natl Acad Sci U S A 88:7491–7495, 1991

Tollefson GD, Sanger JR: Negative symptoms: a path analytic approach to a double-blind placebo and haloperidol-controlled clinical trial with olanzapine. Am J Psychiatry 154:466–474, 1997

Tollefson GD, Beasley CM, Tran PV, et al: Olanzapine versus haloperidol in the treatment of schizophrenia and schizoaffective and schizophreniform disorders: results of an international collaborative study. Am J Psychiatry 154:457–465, 1997

Tran PV, Dellva MA, Tollefson GD, et al: Extrapyramidal symptoms and tolerability of olanzapine versus haloperidol in the acute treatment of schizophrenia. J Clin Psychiatry 58:205–211, 1997

Tsai G, Passani LA, Slusher BS, et al: Abnormal excitatory neurotransmitter metabolism in schizophrenic brain. Arch Gen Psychiatry 52:829–836, 1995

Van Tol HHM, Riva M, Civelli O, et al: Lack of effect of chronic dopamine receptor blockade on D_2 dopamine receptor mRNA level. Neurosci Lett 111:303–308, 1990

Van Tol HHM, Bunzow JR, Guan H, et al: Cloning of the gene for a human dopamine D_4 receptor with high affinity for the antipsychotic clozapine. Nature 350:610–614, 1991

Van Tol HH, Wu CM, Guan HC, et al: Multiple dopamine D_4 receptor variants in the human population. Nature 358:149–152, 1992

Wachtel SR, White FJ: Electrophysiological effects of BMY 14802, a new potential antipsychotic drug, on midbrain dopamine neurons in the rat: acute and chronic studies. J Pharmacol Exp Ther 244:410–416, 1988

Wachtel SR, Hu XT, Gallaway MP, et al: D_1 dopamine receptor stimulation enables the postsynaptic, but not autoreceptor, effects of D_2 dopamine agonists in nigrostriatal and mesoaccumbens dopamine systems. Synapse 4:327–346, 1989

Waddington JL, Daly SA: The status of "second generation" selective D_1 dopamine receptor antagonists as putative atypical antipsychotic agents, in Novel Antipsychotic Drugs. Edited by Meltzer HY. New York, Raven, 1992, pp 109–115

Wadworth AN, Heel RC: Remoxipride: a review of its pharmacodynamic and pharmacokinetic properties, and therapeutic potential in schizophrenia. Drugs 40:863–879, 1990

Walker JM, Bowen WD, Walker FD, et al: Sigma receptors: biology and function. Pharmacol Rev 42:355–402, 1990

Ward RP, Hamblin MW, Lachowicz JE, et al: Localization of serotonin subtype 6 receptor messenger RNA in the rat brain by in situ hybridization histochemistry. Neuroscience 64:1105–1111, 1995

Watling KJ, Beer MS, Stanton JA, et al: Interaction of the atypical neuroleptic clozapine with 5-HT_3 receptors in the cerebral cortex and superior ganglion of the rat. Eur J Pharmacol 182:465–472, 1990

Webster P, Wijeratne C: Risperidone-induced neuroleptic malignant syndrome. Lancet 334:1228–1229, 1994

Wiedemann K, Krieg JC, Loycke A: Novel dopamine autoreceptor agonists B-HT 920 and EMD 49980 in the treatment of patients with schizophrenia, in Novel Antipsychotic Drugs. Edited by Meltzer HY. New York, Raven, 1992, pp 91–98

Wolkin A, Sanfilipo M, Wolf AP, et al: Negative symptoms and hypofrontality in chronic schizophrenia. Arch Gen Psychiatry 49:959–965, 1992

Xu S, Monsma FJ, Sibley DR, et al: Regulation of D_{1A} and D_2 dopamine receptor mRNA during ontogenesis, lesion and chronin antagonist treatment. Life Sci 50:383–396, 1992

Zhang L-J, Lachowicz JE, Sibley DR: The D_{2S} and D_{2L} dopamine receptor isoforms are differentially regulated in Chinese hamster ovary cells. Mol Pharmacol 45:878–889, 1994

Zhou QY, Grandy DK, Thambi L, et al: Cloning and expression of human and rat D_1 dopamine receptors. Nature 347:76–80, 1990

Zimbroff DL, Kane JM, Tamminga CA, et al: Controlled, dose-response study of sertindole and haloperidol in the treatment of schizophrenia. Am J Psychiatry 154:782–791, 1997

NINETEEN

Treatment of
Extrapyramidal Side Effects

Joseph K. Stanilla, M.D., and
George M. Simpson, M.D.

HISTORY OF
EXTRAPYRAMIDAL SIDE EFFECTS

The description of chlorpromazine's therapeutic proper-ties (Delay and Deniker 1952; Laborit et al. 1952) was soon followed by the description of its tendency to pro-duce extrapyramidal side effects (EPS), which were indis-tinguishable from classic Parkinson's disease. A debate soon arose regarding the relationship between EPS and therapeutic efficacy. Flügel (1953) suggested that a thera-peutic response from chlorpromazine required the devel-opment of EPS. Haase (1954) postulated that the dose of antipsychotic medication that produced minimal sub-clinical rigidity and hypokinesia—the "neuroleptic threshold"—was the minimal dose necessary for thera-peutic antipsychotic effect and was manifested by micro-graphic handwriting changes. Other investigators also re-ported that EPS were necessary for therapeutic efficacy (Denham and Carrick 1960; Karn and Kasper 1959).

Brooks (1956), on the other hand, suggested that "signs of parkinsonism heralded the particular effect being sought" (p. 1122), but "the therapeutic effects were not dependent on extrapyramidal dysfunction. On the con-trary, alleviation of such dysfunction, as soon as it oc-curred, sped the progress of recovery" (p. 1122). The need to develop EPS for therapeutic efficacy was questioned by others as well. The differences in opinion regarding EPS and antipsychotic efficacy were partially attributable to differences in definitions of EPS and in methodologies of the studies (Chien and DiMascio 1967).

Haase's concept that mild, subclinical EPS manifested by handwriting changes was an indicator of a therapeutic dose was investigated in studies that found no difference in therapeutic response at doses beyond the neuroleptic threshold (Angus and Simpson 1970a; G. M. Simpson et al. 1970). Patients treated with doses beyond the neuro-leptic threshold received significantly larger doses of medication without further therapeutic benefit. This find-ing has been discussed more fully (Baldessarini et al. 1988) and replicated (McEvoy et al. 1991). When clozapine was first developed in 1960, it sparked little interest as a poten-tial antipsychotic. Many investigators believed EPS were necessary for antipsychotic effect, and clozapine appeared not to produce EPS. Even after studies showed that clo-zapine had antipsychotic activity, interest regarding com-mercial development was still limited. The hesitancy on the part of the pharmaceutical company was related to the belief held by many members of the psychiatric commu-nity that a drug could not have antipsychotic effect with-out producing EPS (Hippius 1989).

In contrast, the current goal in the development of new antipsychotic medications is to replicate the EPS pro-file of clozapine and to develop antipsychotics that do not produce EPS. This situation essentially brings the story of EPS full circle (Hippius 1989).

The terms used to name and characterize antipsy-chotic medications have also evolved. The term *tranquil-*

izer was initially introduced to characterize the psychic effects of reserpine. The term *neuroleptic*, derived from Greek and meaning *to clasp the neuron*, was introduced to describe chlorpromazine and the extrapyramidal effects it produced (Delay et al. 1952). Until clozapine was approved for use, all commercially available drugs with antipsychotic properties had the *neuroleptic* properties of 1) blocking apomorphine- and amphetamine-induced stereotypy; 2) antagonizing the conditioned avoidance response; and 3) producing catalepsy, elevated serum prolactin levels, and EPS. For that reason, all antipsychotic drugs were referred to as *neuroleptics*.

With the subsequent development of clozapine and other antipsychotic drugs that have reduced EPS profiles, the term *neuroleptic* no longer correctly categorizes all drugs with antipsychotic effects, so that the term *antipsychotic* is more accurate and preferable.

Severe EPS can have a significantly negative effect on treatment outcome by contributing to poor compliance and exacerbation of psychiatric symptoms (Van Putten et al. 1981). Akathisia, in particular, is associated with a poor clinical outcome (Levinson et al. 1990; Van Putten et al. 1984), increased violence (Keckich 1978), and even suicide (Shear et al. 1983). The presence of EPS early in treatment may place a patient at increased risk for developing tardive dyskinesia (Saltz et al. 1991). Orofacial tardive dyskinesia may have a negative effect on the social acceptability of patients, even though they are often unaware of the movements (Boumans et al. 1994). Laryngeal dystonia can adversely affect speech, breathing, and swallowing (Feve et al. 1995; Khan et al. 1994) and potentially can be life-threatening (Koek and Pi 1989). Clearly, EPS are significant, need to be assessed, and should be minimized so that the overall treatment and health of patients may be optimized.

TYPES OF EXTRAPYRAMIDAL SIDE EFFECTS

Four types of EPS have been delineated. The treatment of each should be individualized.

Acute dystonic reactions (ADRs) generally are the first EPS to appear and are often the most dramatic (Angus and Simpson 1970b). Dystonias are involuntary sustained or spasmodic muscle contractions that cause abnormal twisting or rhythmical movements and/or postures. ADRs tend to occur suddenly and generally involve muscles of the head and neck (i.e., torticollis, facial grimacing, oculogyric crisis). Almost 90% of all ADRs occur within 4 days of antipsychotic initiation or dosage increase, and virtually

100% occur by day 10 (Singh et al. 1990; Sramek et al. 1986). Although tardive dystonia can occur, movements beyond this time frame are much less likely to be ADRs, and other conditions, including seizures, should be considered.

Akathisia is the next type of EPS to appear. Akathisia, meaning "inability to sit," comprises both an objective, restless movement and a subjective feeling of restlessness that the patient experiences as the need to move. Because it may be difficult for a patient to explain the sensation of akathisia, the diagnosis can be overlooked. At times, patients may show the classic movements of akathisia but not have the subjective distress. This condition has been termed *pseudoakathisia* and may be a type of tardive syndrome (Barnes 1990).

The third type of EPS, *(pseudo)parkinsonism*, is virtually indistinguishable from classic Parkinson's disease. The symptoms include a generalized slowing of movement (akinesia), masked facies, cogwheeling, rigidity, resting tremor, and hypersalivation. Parkinsonism generally occurs after a few weeks or more of antipsychotic treatment. Akinesia must be differentiated from primary depression and the blunted affect of schizophrenia (Rifkin et al. 1975).

Tardive syndromes constitute the fourth type of EPS; tardive dyskinesia and tardive dystonia are the two most common tardive syndromes. Tardive dyskinesia consists of irregular, stereotypical movements of the mouth, face, and tongue and choreoathetoid movements of the fingers, arms, legs, and trunk. Patients frequently have no awareness of the abnormal movements, which may be related to frontal-lobe dysfunction (Sandyk et al. 1993).

PREVALENCE OF EXTRAPYRAMIDAL SIDE EFFECTS

Ayd (1961) first reported the prevalence of EPS: the overall prevalence was 39%, and 21% had akathisia, 15% had parkinsonism, and only 2% had ADRs. Varying rates of occurrence have been reported since then, including much more frequent rates for ADRs. A prospective study found the prevalence of ADR to range from 17% to 38%, with the higher rate occurring with haloperidol (Sramek et al. 1986). In general, higher prevalence rates for all types of EPS occur with higher doses and higher-potency antipsychotics. In a series of surveys of 721 schizophrenic patients conducted over 10 years, McCreadie (1992) reported a point prevalence of 23% for akathisia or pseudoakathisia, 27% for parkinsonism, and 29% for tardive dyskinesia. Forty-four percent had no movement disorder. A 10-year prospective study found that the overall prevalence of tardive dyskinesia within a group remained fairly stable—30% at baseline, 37% at 5 years, and 32% at 10 years (Gardos et al. 1994).

Extrapyramidal movements have also been reported to occur in 17%–29% of neuroleptic-naive patients with schizophrenia (Caligiuri et al. 1993; Chatterjee et al. 1995). This finding raises questions about the role of antipsychotics in the etiology of tardive dyskinesia (G. M. Simpson et al. 1981).

ETIOLOGY OF EXTRAPYRAMIDAL SIDE EFFECTS

The exact mechanisms involved in the production of EPS are not known. Control of motor activity appears to involve an interaction between nigrostriatal dopaminergic, intrastriatal cholinergic, and γ-aminobutyric acid (GABA)ergic neurons (Côté and Crutcher 1991).

Extrapyramidal movements classically have been thought to result from blockade of nigrostriatal dopaminergic tracts by antipsychotic medications, resulting in a relative increase in cholinergic activity (Snyder et al. 1974). Drugs that decrease cholinergic activity or increase dopaminergic activity reduce EPS, presumably by restoring the two systems to their previous equilibrium. This effect has been observed in ADRs in monkeys (Casey et al. 1980).

Increased EPS have been associated with decreased serum calcium levels. Calcium is involved in the function of the cholinergic system and the metabolism of dopamine (Kuny and Binswanger 1989), and antipsychotic drugs bind to the calcium-dependent activator of several enzyme systems (calmodulin [el-Defrawi and Craig 1984]).

GABA may have an effect on EPS through inhibitory feedback on the dopamine system. Reduced GABA synthesis and reduced GABA levels have been detected with tardive dyskinesia (Gunne et al. 1984; Thaker et al. 1987). The effect of GABA on ADR is not as clear. In baboons, ADRs were increased by drugs that increased GABA as well as by drugs that decreased GABA (Casey et al. 1980).

Metabolites of antipsychotics may contribute to EPS. Haloperidol used intravenously has a much lower incidence of EPS than when it is used orally or intramuscularly, even extremely high doses are used. Haldol is metabolized in the liver to reduced haloperidol. When administered intravenously, haloperidol enters the central nervous system (CNS) before metabolites are produced. Investigators have proposed that dopamine D_2 receptor saturation by

haloperidol rather than reduced haloperidol could account for the difference in EPS production (Menza et al. 1987).

Ethnic differences in metabolism of medications have been suggested to account for differences in the rates of EPS and tardive dyskinesia. An evaluation of the prevalence of tardive dyskinesia among Chinese patients in Beijing and Hong Kong found significant differences in the rates (8% vs. 19%). Significant differences were also found in rates of tardive dyskinesia for Korean patients in Seoul and Yanji, China (15.8% vs. 20.3%). The authors suggested that the differences in prevalence that have been reported among ethnic groups may more likely be a result of prescribing practices and other factors than genetic and ethnic differences in metabolism (Pi et al. 1993).

Investigations of clozapine and its novel effect on dopamine and serotonin receptors have led to additional theories of the development of EPS. Typical antipsychotics initially increase dopamine synthesis, turnover, and release in the striatum of baboons (Meldrum et al. 1977). This increased dopamine production reaches a maximum 1–5 hours after a single antipsychotic injection, which corresponds in time with the development of ADRs in baboons. During chronic antipsychotic treatment (up to 11 days), the capacity of the antipsychotics to provoke an increased turnover of dopamine is markedly diminished. Chronic haloperidol treatment causes decreased striatal dopaminergic neurotransmission and upregulation of postsynaptic D_2 receptors (Ichikawa and Meltzer 1991). In contrast, chronic clozapine treatment causes a slight *increase* in striatal dopaminergic neurotransmission and no changes in D_2 receptors. These differences may partly explain the lack of EPS and tardive dyskinesia with use of clozapine.

D_1 receptor antagonists have a lower EPS potential than traditional D_2 antipsychotics in nonhuman primates (Coffin et al. 1989). Patients who were clinical responders to antipsychotics and who had lower D_2 receptor occupancy by positron-emission tomography (PET) analysis had a lower incidence of EPS. Patients treated with clozapine had significantly lower D_2 receptor occupancy than patients treated with typical antipsychotics (Farde et al. 1992). The balanced D_1/D_2 receptor function may help prevent development of EPS and tardive dyskinesia (Gerlach and Hansen 1992).

The high ratio of serotonin-2 (5-HT_2) receptor blockade to striatal D_2 receptor blockade, which is found with clozapine, may also contribute to clozapine's lack of EPS (Meltzer et al. 1989). Catalepsy in animal models correlates with EPS. Blockade of serotonergic neurotransmission appears to reverse or prevent catalepsy induced by D_2 receptor blockade (Meltzer and Nash 1991).

Clozapine also has a high affinity for D_3 and D_4 receptors (Sokoloff et al. 1990; Van Tol et al. 1991). The binding of clozapine to these receptors has been proposed as a possible factor involved in clozapine's favorable EPS profile (Meltzer 1992).

The existence of a noradrenergic pathway from the locus coeruleus to the limbic system has been proposed as a modulator involved in symptoms of tardive dyskinesia, akathisia, and tremor (Wilbur et al. 1988). Clozapine is a potent α_1-adrenergic receptor antagonist in the brain, causing α_1 receptor upregulation and increased noradrenaline metabolism, factors that may affect clozapine's EPS profile (Baldessarini et al. 1992).

It has been proposed that free radicals, possibly produced by chronic antipsychotic use, contribute to neuropathic damage and development of tardive dyskinesia and that vitamin E, as an antioxidant, can limit the process (Cadet et al. 1986). However, levels of lipid peroxides, theoretically produced by free radicals, do not correlate with tardive dyskinesia (McCreadie et al. 1995), and changes in levels are not correlated with treatment with vitamin E. Nonetheless, these changes could be occurring centrally and not be apparent in the periphery (Corrigan et al. 1993).

A somewhat related theory suggested that increased iron levels in the basal ganglia may contribute to tardive dyskinesia because iron is involved in the production of free radicals (Ben-Shachar and Youdim 1987). Neuroimaging and pathological studies have not identified increased iron levels on a consistent basis, though (Elkashef et al. 1994).

RATING EXTRAPYRAMIDAL SIDE EFFECTS

Investigations of treatment for EPS led to the need to develop instruments to evaluate and quantify EPS. An initial EPS scale had both clinical validity and high interrater reliability, but it did not adequately assess tremor and salivation (G. M. Simpson et al. 1964). Scores were low despite obvious and disabling tremor or salivation, which required treatment with antiparkinsonian medication. Therefore, the scale was expanded to 10 items rated on a 5-point scale, including tremor and salivation (G. M. Simpson and Angus 1970). The Simpson-Angus Scale has good psychometric properties and is simple to use and score. It has been modified for outpatient use by elimination of the leg rigidity item and by replacing head dropping with head rotation. Studies using this scale have shown that scores correlate with dosages and plasma levels of an antipsychotic. The scale is widely used in clinical trials and can be completed by nurses for the routine monitoring of antipsychotic treatment.

The Simpson-Angus Scale does not include a direct rating for bradykinesia or akinesia. Mindham (1976) modified this scale to include an item for lack of facial expression. Additional rating scales for EPS have since been developed, including the Chouinard Extrapyramidal Rating Scale (Chouinard et al. 1980), the Targeting of Abnormal Kinetic Effects (TAKE) Scale (Wojcik et al. 1980), the St. Hans Rating Scale for Extrapyramidal Syndromes (Gerlach et al. 1993), and the Dyskinesia Identification System Condensed User Scale (DISCUS) (Kalachnik and Sprague 1993).

The modified Simpson-Angus Scale includes a single item for rating akathisia. More comprehensive scales have been devised specifically to rate akathisia, including the Barnes Akathisia Rating Scale (Barnes 1989), the Hillside Akathisia Scale (Fleischhacker et al. 1989), and the Prince Henry Hospital Akathisia Rating Scale (PHH Scale; Sachdev 1994).

Scales have also been developed to assess dyskinetic movements. These scales include the Abnormal Involuntary Movement Scale (AIMS; Guy 1976) and the Simpson/Rockland Scale (G. M. Simpson et al. 1979).

Instrumental devices have been developed to assess EPS, and several correlate well with clinical scales (Büchel et al. 1995). Instrumental devices have the advantage of increased reliability of quantitative measures, primarily through the elimination of subjective error associated with clinical raters. These devices have disadvantages, however, such as that 1) greater patient cooperation is often needed than with clinical scales; 2) physical contact with the subject may be necessary, which can affect measurements; and 3) evaluation of an anatomical area is often limited, unlike clinical scales, which usually evaluate a patient in many specific anatomical areas and globally. At present, clinical scales generally can be considered to have better global clinical validity with greater ease of use, whereas instrumental measures provide greater reliability.

ANTICHOLINERGIC MEDICATIONS

Antiparkinsonian medications, including anticholinergic, antihistaminic, and dopaminergic agents, primarily have been used to treat EPS (Table 19–1).

Trihexyphenidyl

History and Discovery

Trihexyphenidyl, a synthetic analogue of atropine, was introduced in 1949 (as benzhexol hydrochloride) and was

Table 19–1. Pharmacological agents used for the treatment of neuroleptic-induced parkinsonism and acute dystonic reactions

Compound	Type	Relative equivalence (mg)[a]	Route	Availability	Dosing	Therapeutic dosage used in studies (mg)
Benztropine (Cogentin)	Anticholinergic	1	Oral	Tablets (0.5, 1, 2 mg)	Once to twice a day	1–12
			Injectable	Ampules (1 mg/mL [2 mL])	Every 30 minutes until symptom relief	2–8
Trihexyphenidyl (Artane)	Anticholinergic	2.5	Oral	Tablets (2 or 5 mg) Elixir (2 mg/mL) Sequels (5 mg [sustained release])	Once to twice a day	2–30
Procyclidine (Kemadrin)	Anticholinergic	2[b]	Oral	Tablets (5 mg, scored)	Two to three times a day	5–55
Diphenhydramine (Benadryl)	Antihistaminic	50	Oral	Tablets (25 or 50 mg)	Two to four times a day	50–400
			Injectable	Ampules (10 mg/mL [10 or 30 mL]) or (50 mg/mL [10 mL])	Every 30 minutes until symptom relief	
Biperiden (Akineton)	Anticholinergic	1	Oral	Tablets (2 mg)	Two to three times a day	2–24
			Injectable	Ampules (5 mg/mL [1 mL])	Every 30 minutes until symptom relief	2–8
Amantadine (Symmetrel)	Dopaminergic	N/A	Oral	Tablets (100 mg)	Once to twice a day	100–300

Source. [a]de Leon et al. 1994; [b]Timberlake et al. 1961.

found to be effective in the treatment of Parkinson's disease in a study of 411 patients (Doshay et al. 1954). Thereafter, it was also used to treat neuroleptic-induced parkinsonism (NIP) (Rashkis and Smarr 1957).

Structure-Activity Relations

Trihexyphenidyl, a tertiary amine analogue of atropine, is a competitive antagonist of acetylcholine and other muscarinic agonists that competes for a common binding site on muscarinic receptors (Yamamura and Snyder 1974). It exerts little blockade at nicotinic receptors (Timberlake et al. 1961). Trihexyphenidyl and all drugs in this class are referred to as anticholinergic, antimuscarinic, or atropine-like drugs.

Pharmacological Profile

The pharmacological properties of trihexyphenidyl are qualitatively similar to those of atropine and other anticholinergic drugs, although trihexyphenidyl acts primarily centrally with few peripheral effects and little sedation. In the eye, anticholinergic drugs block both the sphincter muscle of the iris, which leads to pupil dilation (mydriasis), and the ciliary muscle of the lens, which pre-

vents accommodation and causes cycloplegia. In the heart, anticholinergics usually produce a mild tachycardia through vagal blockade at the sinoatrial (S-A) node pacemaker, although a mild slowing can occur. In the gastrointestinal tract, anticholinergics reduce gut motility and salivary and gastric secretions. Salivary secretion is particularly sensitive and can be completely abolished. In the respiratory system, anticholinergics reduce secretions and can produce mild bronchodilatation. Anticholinergics inhibit the activity of sweat glands and mildly decrease contractions in the urinary and biliary tracts (Brown and Taylor 1996).

Pharmacokinetics and Disposition

Peak concentration for trihexyphenidyl is reached 1–2 hours after oral administration, and its half-life is 10–12 hours (Cedarbaum and McDowell 1987). As a tertiary amine, it readily crosses the blood-brain barrier to enter the CNS (Brown and Taylor 1996).

Mechanism of Action

The presumed mechanism of action of trihexyphenidyl for treatment of EPS is the blockade of intrastriatal cholinergic activity, which is relatively increased compared with nigrostriatal dopaminergic activity, which is decreased by antipsychotic blockade. The blockade of cholinergic activity returns the system to its previous equilibrium.

Indications

Anticholinergic agents were reported to be effective treatment for NIP from open empiric trials (Medina et al. 1962; Rashkis and Smarr 1957). Eventually, controlled trials were conducted, but most only involved comparisons with other anticholinergics and not with placebo. Despite the limited evidence of efficacy compared with placebo, anticholinergic agents became the mainstay of treatment for NIP and remain so today.

Trihexyphenidyl has U.S. Food and Drug Administration (FDA) approval for the treatment of all forms of parkinsonism, including NIP. Daily doses of 5–30 mg have been used in studies of trihexyphenidyl in treatment of Parkinson's disease and NIP. The individual therapeutic dose must be determined empirically, though, and can vary widely.

Side Effects and Toxicology

Peripheral side effects. Peripheral side effects of trihexyphenidyl result from parasympathetic muscarinic blockade and occur in a consistent hierarchy among different organs. They are qualitatively similar to the side effects of atropine and other anticholinergic drugs but are quantitatively fewer because of trihexyphenidyl's reduced peripheral activity (Brown 1990).

Anticholinergic drugs initially reduce salivary and bronchial secretions and sweat production. Reduced salivation produces dry mouth and contributes to the high incidence of dental caries among chronically ill psychiatric patients (Winer and Bahn 1967). Treatment for this condition is basically nonexistent. Activities that stimulate salivation, such as chewing sugar-free gum or sucking hard candy, are limited by the need for constant use. Reduced sweating can contribute to heat prostration and heat stroke, particularly in warmer ambient temperatures.

The next physiological effects occur in the eyes and heart. Pupillary dilation and inhibition of accommodation in the eye lead to photophobia and blurred vision. Attacks of acute glaucoma can occur in susceptible subjects with narrow-angle glaucoma, although this is relatively uncommon. The next effect, vagus nerve blockade, leads to increased heart rate and is more apparent in patients with high vagal tone (usually younger males). Subsequent effects are inhibition of urinary bladder function and bowel

motility, which can produce urinary retention, constipation, and obstipation. Sufficiently high doses of anticholinergics will inhibit gastric secretion and motility (Brown 1990).

Central side effects. Memory disturbance is the most common central side effect of anticholinergic medications, because memory is dependent on the cholinergic system (Drachman 1977). Patients with underlying brain disorders are more susceptible to memory disturbance (Fayen et al. 1988). Patients with chronic psychiatric disorders often have a decreased ability to express themselves, so evaluation of memory is more difficult, and subtle memory changes may be overlooked or attributed to the underlying illness. Memory disturbances were identified in patients with Parkinson's disease treated with anticholinergics (Yahr and Duvoisin 1968), even in some patients receiving only small doses (Stephens 1967).

Anticholinergic toxicity produces restlessness, irritability, disorientation, hallucinations, and delirium. Elderly patients are at increased risk for both memory loss and toxic delirium, even at very low anticholinergic doses, because of the natural loss of cholinergic neurons with aging (Perry et al. 1977). Toxic levels can produce a clinical situation identical to that of atropine poisoning, including fixed, dilated pupils; flushed face; sinus tachycardia; urinary retention; dry mouth; and fever. This condition can proceed to coma, cardiorespiratory collapse, and death.

Drug-Drug Interactions

Anticholinergic effects, including side effects, may increase when trihexyphenidyl or any anticholinergic is combined with amantadine.

Anticholinergic effect on antipsychotic blood levels. Some investigators have suggested that anticholinergic medications can affect antipsychotic blood levels. A review of this subject indicated that the available data were too limited to reach a definite conclusion on this matter (McEvoy 1983). The best studies indicate that anticholinergic drugs do not affect antipsychotic blood levels or, at most, lower levels only transiently.

Anticholinergic effect on antipsychotic activity. Haase and Janssen (1965) reported from open studies that if anticholinergic drugs were added to antipsychotic drugs given at the neuroleptic threshold, rigidity, hypokinesia, and therapeutic effects would disappear. Other studies have found no change or an improvement in scores of psychopathology with the addition of anticholinergics (Hanlon et al. 1966; G. M. Simpson et al. 1980).

Anticholinergic Abuse

Anticholinergic drugs may be abused for their euphoriant and hallucinogenic effects and may be combined with street drugs for enhanced effect. Trihexyphenidyl reportedly is the anticholinergic most likely to be abused (MacVicar 1977). Theoretically, one anticholinergic should be as effective as another, although idiosyncratic responses are possible. The potential for abuse must be considered, particularly in patients with a history of substance abuse.

Benztropine

History and Discovery

Benztropine was found to be effective in the treatment of 302 patients with Parkinson's disease (Doshay 1956). The best results in the control of rigidity, contracture, and tremor were obtained at doses of 1–4 mg/day for older patients and 2–8 mg/day for younger ones. Doses of 15–30 mg/day caused excessive flaccidity in some patients, who became unable to lift their arms or raise their heads off the bed. Subsequently, benztropine was found to be effective for treatment of NIP (Karn and Kasper 1959).

Structure-Activity Relations

Benztropine was synthesized by uniting the tropine portion of atropine with the benzohydryl portion of diphenhydramine hydrochloride. Benztropine is a tertiary amine with activity similar to that of trihexyphenidyl. As a tertiary amine, it enters the CNS.

Pharmacological Profile

Benztropine has the pharmacological properties of an anticholinergic and an antihistaminic. It produces less sedation (in experimental animals) than does diphenhydramine, however.

Pharmacokinetics and Disposition

Little is known about the pharmacokinetics of benztropine. A correlation between serum anticholinergic levels and the presence of EPS has been found (Tune and Coyle 1980). There is little correlation between the total daily dose of benztropine and the serum anticholinergic level, with the serum activity for a given dose varying 100-fold among subjects. When treated with increased doses of benztropine, patients with EPS had increased serum anticholinergic activity and decreased EPS. Relatively small increments in the oral dose of all anticholinergic drugs can result in significant nonlinear increases in serum anticholinergic activity levels. Benztropine has a long-acting effect and can be given once or twice a day.

Indications

Benztropine has FDA approval for the treatment of all forms of parkinsonism, including NIP. Daily doses of 1–8 mg have generally been used to treat NIP.

Mechanism of Action, Side Effects, and Drug Interactions

The mechanism of action, side effects, and drug interactions of benztropine are similar to those of trihexyphenidyl. Benztropine was reported to be less stimulating and more sedating than trihexyphenidyl and other anticholinergic agents when used to treat patients with Parkinson's disease (Doshay 1956; England and Schwab 1959). Although this finding has not been tested in double-blind studies, these properties might account for the fact that trihexyphenidyl is reportedly the anticholinergic drug more likely to be abused.

Biperiden

Biperiden is an analogue of trihexyphenidyl. It has greater peripheral anticholinergic activity than trihexyphenidyl and greater activity against nicotinic receptors (Timberlake et al. 1961). Biperiden is well absorbed from the gastrointestinal tract. Its metabolism is not completely understood but involves hydroxylation in the liver. Its activity, pharmacological profile, and side effects are similar to those of other anticholinergics. It has FDA approval for the treatment of all forms of parkinsonism, including NIP. Daily doses of 2–24 mg have been used in studies of biperiden for treatment of parkinsonism and NIP.

Procyclidine

Procyclidine is an analogue of trihexyphenidyl (Schwab and Chafetz 1955). Its activity, pharmacology, and side effects are similar to those of other anticholinergics. Little information is available on its pharmacokinetics. It has FDA approval for the treatment of all forms of parkinsonism, including NIP. Daily doses of 5–55 mg have been used in studies of procyclidine for treatment of parkinsonism and NIP (Timberlake et al. 1961).

ANTIHISTAMINIC MEDICATIONS

Diphenhydramine

History and Discovery

Antihistaminic agents have been used to treat Parkinson's disease. Diphenhydramine, one of the first antihistamines developed and used clinically (Bovet 1950), has been the primary antihistamine studied in the treatment of EPS. Other antihistamines have not been systematically studied for the treatment of EPS, but those with central anticholinergic activity may be effective for the treatment of EPS.

Structure-Activity Relations

All drugs referred to as antihistamines are reversible, competitive inhibitors of histamine at the H_1 receptor. Some antihistamines also inhibit the action of acetylcholine at the muscarinic receptor. Central muscarinic blockade rather than histaminic blockade is believed to be responsible for the therapeutic effect of antihistamines for EPS. Ethanolamine antihistamines (diphenhydramine, dimenhydrinate, carbinoxamine maleate) have the greatest anticholinergic activity, and ethylenediamines have the least. Antihistamines, such as terfenadine and astemizole, have no anticholinergic activity, whereas many of the remaining antihistamines have very mild anticholinergic activity (Babe and Serafin 1996).

Pharmacological Profile

Antihistamines inhibit the constrictor action of histamine on respiratory smooth muscle. They restrict the vasoconstrictor and vasodilatory effects of histamine on vascular smooth muscle and block histamine-induced capillary permeability. Antihistamines with CNS activity are depressants, producing diminished alertness, slowed reaction times, and somnolence. They can also block motion sickness. Antihistaminic drugs with anticholinergic activity also have mild antimuscarinic pharmacological properties similar to other atropine-like drugs (Babe and Serafin 1996).

Pharmacokinetics and Disposition

Diphenhydramine is well absorbed from the gastrointestinal tract. Peak concentrations occur 2–3 hours after oral administration. Its therapeutic effects usually last 4–6 hours, and it has a half-life of 3–9 hours. Diphenhydramine is widely distributed throughout the body, and as a tertiary amine, it enters the CNS. Age does not affect its pharmacokinetics. It undergoes demethylations in the liver and is then oxidized to carboxylic acid (Paton and Webster 1985).

Mechanism of Action

Diphenhydramine has some anticholinergic activity. Central anticholinergic activity is believed to be the basis for its effect in diminishing EPS.

Indications

Diphenhydramine has FDA approval for the treatment of all forms of parkinsonism, including NIP, in the elderly and for mild cases in other age groups. It is probably not as efficacious for treating EPS as pure anticholinergic drugs, but it may be better tolerated in patients bothered by anticholinergic side effects, such as geriatric patients. Diphenhydramine also tends to be more sedating than anticholinergics, which can also be beneficial for some patients. Dosages generally range from 50 to 400 mg/day given in divided doses.

Diphenhydramine also has indications for multiple other conditions unrelated to EPS.

Side Effects and Toxicology

The primary side effect of diphenhydramine is sedation. Although other antihistamines may cause gastrointestinal distress, diphenhydramine has a low incidence of this effect. Dry mouth and dry respiratory passages may occur. In general, the toxic effects are similar to those of trihexyphenidyl and other anticholinergics.

Drug-Drug Interactions

Diphenhydramine has no reported interactions with other drugs. It has an additive depressant effect when used in combination with alcohol or other CNS depressants.

DOPAMINERGIC MEDICATIONS

Anticholinergic side effects and inadequate treatment response eventually led to the investigation of other agents to treat EPS. Initially, both methylphenidate and intravenous caffeine were investigated as treatments of NIP. Neither achieved general use despite apparent efficacy (Brooks 1956; Freyhan 1959).

Amantadine

History and Discovery

Amantadine is an antiviral agent that is effective against A2 (Asian) influenza (Wingfield et al. 1969). It was unexpectedly found to reduce symptoms in patients with Parkinson's disease (Parkes et al. 1970; Schwab et al. 1969). Soon after, amantadine was reported to be effective for NIP (Kelly and Abuzzahab 1971).

Structure-Activity Relations

Amantadine is a water-soluble tricyclic amine. It binds to the M2 protein, a membrane protein that functions as an ion channel on the influenza A virus (Hay 1992). Its activity in reducing EPS is not known.

Pharmacological Profile

Amantadine is effective in preventing and treating illness from influenza A virus. It also reduces the symptoms of parkinsonism.

Pharmacokinetics and Disposition

In young, healthy subjects, amantadine is slowly and well absorbed from the gastrointestinal tract, with unchanged oral bioavailability over the dose range of 50–300 mg. It reaches steady state in 4–7 days. Plasma concentrations (0.12–1.12 μg/mL) appear to correlate with decline in EPS (Greenblatt et al. 1977; Pacifici et al. 1976). It has relatively constant blood levels, has a long duration of action (Aoki et al. 1979), and is excreted unchanged by the kidneys. Its elimination half-life is about 16 hours, which is prolonged in elderly patients and those with impaired renal function (Hayden et al. 1985).

Mechanism of Action

Amantadine produces antiviral activity by binding to the M2 protein on the viral membrane and inhibiting replication (Hay 1992). Its mechanism of action as an antiparkinsonian agent is less clear. It has no anticholinergic activity in tests on animals and is only 1/209,000th as potent as atropine (Grelak et al. 1970). It appears to cause the release of dopamine and other catecholamines from intraneuronal storage sites in an amphetamine-like mechanism. It also has activity at glutamate receptors, which may contribute to its antiparkinsonian effect (Stoof et al. 1992). Amantadine has preferential selectivity for central catecholamine neurons (Grelak et al. 1970; Strömberg et al. 1970).

Indications

Amantadine was investigated more extensively than anticholinergic agents with respect to efficacy for EPS. Most, but not all, studies found that amantadine was effective and equivalent to benztropine for treatment of parkinsonism (DiMascio et al. 1976; Fann and Lake 1976; Stenson et al. 1976). Some found that amantadine was more effective than benztropine (Merrick and Schmitt 1973) or effective in EPS refractory to benztropine (Gelenberg 1978). Some studies, though, found that amantadine was inferior to benztropine (Kelly et al. 1974), no more effective than placebo (Mindham et al. 1972), or unable to control EPS when used to replace an anticholinergic agent

(McEvoy et al. 1987). The different results can be attributed to inconsistent methodologies and patient populations. The conclusion that can be drawn from these studies is that amantadine is an effective drug for treating parkinsonism, but no clear data support its use prior to using anticholinergic agents.

Most of the studies of treatment of EPS have been of short duration. In patients who have Parkinson's disease, amantadine appears to lose efficacy after several weeks (Mawdsley et al. 1972; Schwab et al. 1972). Similar studies evaluating the long-term efficacy of amantadine for EPS have not been conducted.

Amantadine has also been evaluated for the specific treatment of akathisia but in only a small number of patients. The conclusion from these studies was that amantadine is probably not effective for the specific treatment of akathisia (Fleischhacker et al. 1990).

Amantadine has FDA approval for the treatment of NIP and Parkinson's disease as well as for the treatment and prophylaxis of influenza A respiratory illness. Doses of 100–300 mg/day are used for treatment of NIP, and plasma concentrations appear to correlate with improvement.

Side Effects and Toxicology

At 100–300 mg/day, amantadine does not produce adverse effects as readily as anticholinergic medications do. Side effects result from CNS stimulation, with symptoms including irritability, tremor, dysarthria, ataxia, vertigo, agitation, reduced concentration, hallucinations, and delirium (Postma and Tilburg 1975). Hallucinations often are visual. Side effects are more likely to occur in elderly patients and those with reduced renal function (Borison 1979; Ing et al. 1979). Toxic effects are directly related to elevated amantadine serum levels (>1.5 μg/mL). Resolution of toxic symptoms is dependent on renal clearance and may require dialysis in extreme cases, although less than 5% of amantadine is removed by dialysis.

Patients with congestive heart failure or peripheral edema should be monitored because of amantadine's ability to increase availability of catecholamines. Long-term use of amantadine may produce livedo reticularis in the lower extremities from the local release of catecholamines and resulting vasoconstriction (Cedarbaum and Schleifer 1990). Amantadine should be used with caution in patients with seizures because of possible increased seizure activity. Amantadine is embryotoxic and teratogenic in animals, but no well-controlled studies of teratogenicity have been done in women.

Drug-Drug Interactions

Amantadine has no reported interactions with other drugs. Anticholinergic side effects may be increased when amantadine is used in combination with an anticholinergic agent.

β-Adrenergic Receptor Antagonists

History and Discovery

Propranolol was reported to be effective for the treatment of restless legs syndrome (Ekbom's syndrome; Ekbom 1965), which resembles the physical movements of akathisia (Strang 1967). Later it was reported to be effective in treatment of neuroleptic-induced akathisia (Kulik and Wilbur 1983; Lipinski et al. 1983). Subsequently, other β-blockers have been investigated for treatment of akathisia (Table 19–2).

Structure-Activity Relations

Competitive β-adrenergic receptor antagonism is the property common to all β-blockers. β-Blockers are distinguished by the additional properties of their relative affinity for β_1 and β_2 receptors (selectivity), lipid solubility, intrinsic β-adrenergic receptor *agonist* activity, blockade of α-receptors, capacity to induce vasodilation, and general pharmacokinetic properties (Hoffman and Lefkowitz 1996). β-Blockers with high lipid solubility readily cross the blood-brain barrier.

Pharmacological Profile

The major pharmacological effects of β-blockers involve the cardiovascular system. They slow the heart rate and decrease cardiac contractility, although these effects are modest in a normal heart. In the lung, they can cause bronchospasm, but, again, there is little effect in normal lungs. They block glycogenolysis, which prevents production of glucose during hypoglycemia (Hoffman and Lefkowitz 1996). They affect lipid metabolism by preventing release of free fatty acids while elevating triglyceride levels (Miller 1987). In the CNS, they produce fatigue, sleep disturbance (insomnia and nightmares), and CNS depression (Drayer 1987; Gengo et al. 1987).

Pharmacokinetics and Disposition

All β-blockers, except atenolol and nadolol, are well absorbed from the gastrointestinal tract. All are metabolized in the liver. Propranolol and metoprolol undergo significant first-pass effect with bioavailability as low as 25%. Large interindividual variation (as much as 20-fold) leads to wide variation in clinically therapeutic doses (Hoffman and Lefkowitz 1996). Metabolites appear to have limited β-receptor antagonistic activity. The degree to which a particular β-blocker enters the CNS is related directly to its lipid solubility (see Table 19–2).

Table 19–2.   β-Blockers investigated in the treatment of akathisia

Compound	Relative lipid solubility[a]	Relative potency of β-receptor blockade[b]	Bioavailability (% of dose)	Selectivity of β-receptor blockade	Effective for akathisia?	Therapeutic dosage used in studies (mg)
Propranolol (Inderal)	20.2	1	~30	$\beta_1 = \beta_2$	Yes	20–120
Betaxolol (Kerlone)	3.89	4	~80–90	β_1	Yes	5–20
Metoprolol (Lopressor)	0.98	1	~40–50	$\beta_1 > \beta_2$	Yes	~300
Pindolol (Visken)	0.82	6	~90	$\beta_1 = \beta_2$	Yes	5
Nadolol (Corgard)	0.066	2.9	~30	$\beta_1 = \beta_2$	Yes	40–80
Sotalol (Betapace)	0.039	0.3	~100	$\beta_1 = \beta_2$	No	40–80
Atenolol (Tenormin)	0.015	1	~40–50	β_1	No	50–100

[a]Relative extent to which the drug partitions between an organic solvent and an aqueous buffer; in this case, η-octanol/aqueous phosphate.
[b]Extent of inhibition of isoprenaline-induced tachycardia.
Source.   Pharmacological properties from Drayer 1987; McDevitt 1987.

Mechanism of Action

The exact mechanism of action of β-blockers in the treatment of EPS is unclear. The existence of a noradrenergic pathway from the locus coeruleus to the limbic system has been proposed as a modulator involved in symptoms of tardive dyskinesia, akathisia, and tremor (Wilbur et al. 1988). Lipid solubility and the corresponding ability to enter the CNS appear to be the most important factors determining the efficacy of a β-blocker in treating akathisia and perhaps other types of EPS (Adler et al. 1991).

Indications

β-Blockers have FDA approval primarily for cardiovascular indications, and propranolol is also indicated for familial essential tremor, but there are no FDA-approved indications for the treatment of any type of EPS.

β-Blockers primarily have been studied for the treatment of akathisia. Both nonselective (β₁ and β₂ antagonism) and selective (β₁ antagonism) β-blockers have been reported to be efficacious. The studies generally have been done for short periods and have involved small numbers of patients who were often receiving varying combinations of additional antiparkinsonian agents or benzodiazepines to which β-blockers were added (Fleischhacker et al. 1990). Based on these studies, it is difficult to draw any firm conclusions, but β-blockers probably have some efficacy in the treatment of akathisia.

The maximum benefit for propranolol occurred at 5 days (Fleischhacker et al. 1990). Betaxolol may be the β-blocker of choice in patients with lung disease and smokers because of its β₁ selectivity at lower doses (5–10 mg/day).

β-Blockers have been reported to be beneficial for tremor of Parkinson's disease (Foster et al. 1984) and lithium-induced tremor (Gelenberg and Jefferson 1995) in addition to essential tremor. However, for neuroleptic-induced tremor, propranolol was no better than placebo (Metzer et al. 1993), which could indicate a difference in etiologies for the different tremors.

Side Effects and Toxicology

Side effects of β-blockers result from β-receptor blockade. β₂ blockade of bronchial smooth muscle causes bronchospasm. Individuals with normal lung function are unlikely to be affected, but smokers and patients with lung disease can develop serious breathing difficulties. β-Blockers can contribute to heart failure in susceptible individuals, such as those with compensated heart failure, acute myocardial infarction, or cardiomegaly. Abrupt cessation of β-blockers can also exacerbate coronary heart disease in susceptible patients and produce angina or, potentially, myocardial infarction (Hoffman and Lefkowitz 1996).

In individuals with normal heart function, bradycardia produced by β-blockers is insignificant. However, in patients with conduction defects or when β-blockers are combined with other drugs that impair cardiac conduction, β-blockers can contribute to serious conduction problems.

β-Blockers can block the tachycardia associated with hypoglycemia, eliminating this warning sign in diabetic patients. β₂ blockade also can inhibit glycogenolysis and glucose mobilization, interfering with recovery from hypoglycemia (Hoffman and Lefkowitz 1996).

β-Blockers can impair exercise performance and produce fatigue, insomnia, and major depression. The development of major depression probably only occurs in individuals with a predisposition to developing depression, though.

Drug-Drug Interactions

β-Blockers can have significant interactions with other drugs. Chlorpromazine in combination with propranolol may increase blood levels of both drugs. Additive effects on cardiac conduction and blood pressure may occur when β-blockers are combined with drugs with similar effects (e.g., calcium channel blockers). Phenytoin, phenobarbital, and rifampin increase the clearance of propranolol. Cimetidine increases propranolol blood levels by decreasing hepatic metabolism. Propranolol reduces theophylline clearance. Aluminum salts (antacids), cholestyramine, and colestipol may decrease absorption of β-blockers (Hoffman and Lefkowitz 1996).

BENZODIAZEPINES

History and Discovery

Diazepam was initially shown to be effective in the treatment of restless legs syndrome (Ekbom 1965). Subsequently, diazepam, lorazepam, and clonazepam were reported to be beneficial for neuroleptic-induced akathisia (Adler et al. 1985; Donlon 1973; Kutcher et al. 1987). Clonazepam has also been reported to be beneficial for drug-induced dystonia (O'Flanagan 1975).

Structure-Activity Relations

The benzodiazepines have a benzene ring fused to a seven-membered diazepine ring. All benzodiazepines promote the binding of GABA to GABA receptors, magnifying the effects of GABA. Benzodiazepines require the presence of GABA to exert their effects, unlike barbiturates, which can directly affect the GABA receptor (Hobbs et al. 1996).

Pharmacological Profile

All benzodiazepines have similar effects qualitatively but differ quantitatively. Nearly all the effects occur in the CNS, including sedation, hypnosis, decreased anxiety, anterograde amnesia, and anticonvulsant activity. Two peripheral effects are coronary vasodilatation after intravenous administration of certain benzodiazepines and neuromuscular blockade, which occurs only with very high doses (Hobbs et al. 1996).

Benzodiazepines are not general neuronal depressants, unlike barbiturates. Increasing doses produce sedation, hypnosis, and then stupor. At standard doses, benzodiazepines cause only muscle relaxation in animals but not in humans, except for clonazepam, but at only very high doses. Benzodiazepines inhibit seizures but do not stop the seizure focus. Clonazepam is a more selective anticonvulsant than most benzodiazepines, but tolerance develops to the anticonvulsant effect. All benzodiazepines decrease sleep latency, decrease rapid eye movement (REM) and Stage 4 sleep, and increase total sleep time. During chronic use, the effect on various stages of sleep usually declines. Cardiac effects are minor except in severe intoxication. No direct gastrointestinal effects are apparent (Hobbs et al. 1996).

Pharmacokinetics and Disposition

All benzodiazepines are rapidly absorbed orally, except for clorazepate, which is first decarboxylated in gastric juice and then absorbed. Benzodiazepines are characterized by their elimination half-lives as ultrashort-, short-, intermediate-, and long-acting. They are bound to protein in direct proportion to their lipid solubility.

Benzodiazepines have an initial rapid uptake into the brain, directly correlated with the degree of lipid solubility, followed by a redistribution into other organs. The duration of CNS effects is probably affected more by the rate of redistribution than by any other property (Dettli 1986). This contributes to the fact that the clinical duration of action is frequently much shorter than the half-life.

All benzodiazepines but three are extensively metabolized to produce active by-products, which generally have half-lives much longer than the parent compound. The active metabolites are generally of little therapeutic benefit and frequently are responsible for side effects and toxicity. Only temazepam, oxazepam, and lorazepam have no active metabolites and instead directly undergo glucuronic conjugation and then renal elimination.

Mechanism of Action

Benzodiazepines are thought to enhance GABA-induced increases in conductance of the chloride ion (Cl^-) at the GABA receptor, augmenting the inhibitory effects of GABAergic pathways. The mechanism of action of reduction in EPS is unknown, but it may be related to augmentation of inhibitory GABAergic effect (Hobbs et al. 1996).

Indications

Benzodiazepines have FDA approval for the treatment of anxiety disorders, agoraphobia, insomnia, and seizure disorders; the management of alcohol withdrawal; anesthetic premedication; and skeletal muscle relaxation; however, they have not been approved for any type of EPS. As noted above, a few initial reports indicated that benzodiazepines were beneficial for the treatment of akathisia. Other studies have also reported similar benefit (Bartels et al. 1987; Braude et al. 1983; Director and Muniz 1982; Gagrat et al. 1978; Horiguchi and Nishimatsu 1992; Kutcher et al. 1989; Pujalte et al. 1994).

Clonazepam has been reported to be effective in the treatment of tardive dyskinesia (Bobruff et al. 1981; Thaker et al. 1990). Doses of 1–10 mg were used in the first study; the optimal dose was reported to be 4 mg/day, and many patients were unable to tolerate higher doses. In the second study, 2–4.5 mg/day were used, and tolerance developed after 5–8 months.

Although some of the studies were limited by short duration and small numbers of subjects who were also receiving other antiparkinsonian agents, the overall conclusion was that benzodiazepines probably have some efficacy in the treatment of akathisia and tardive dyskinesia. The potential problems associated with chronic use of benzodiazepines—tolerance and abuse—must be kept in mind, however.

Lorazepam (intermediate-acting) and clonazepam (long-acting) are the two primary benzodiazepines that have been studied in the treatment of EPS. Because clonazepam has a long duration of action, it can often be given once a day. Lorazepam has the advantage of no active metabolites, so potential side effects and toxicity are avoided.

Side Effects and Toxicology

The side effects of benzodiazepines at low doses are relatively mild. As dosages increase, benzodiazepines cause increased reaction time, motor incoordination, impairment of mental and motor function, somnolence, lethargy, confusion, and anterograde amnesia. Cognition appears to be less affected than motor performance, and patients are often unaware of these effects (Hobbs et al. 1996).

Hypnotic doses of benzodiazepines do not affect respiration in healthy adults. At higher doses, alveolar respiration is suppressed from depression of the hypoxic drive, which is exaggerated in patients with chronic obstructive pulmonary disease. Benzodiazepines can cause apnea when given with anesthesia or opiates. Apnea can also occur when benzodiazepine intoxication occurs in combination with another CNS depressant, such as alcohol (Hobbs et al. 1996).

Dizziness, ataxia, vomiting, and slurred speech have also been reported (Bobruff et al. 1981). The incidence of side effects increases with age (Meyer 1982; Monane 1992).

Benzodiazepine withdrawal is a potential serious occurrence, with symptoms generally beginning 1–3 days after the last dose. Symptoms are similar to those of acute alcohol withdrawal and include anxiety, tremulousness, autonomic irregularities (including blood pressure and heart rate fluctuations), gastrointestinal symptoms, agitation, hallucinations (particularly visual), delirium, and seizures. Withdrawal seizures can occur without the appearance of any other significant withdrawal symptoms. Withdrawal symptoms are more likely to occur with higher doses, although we have witnessed grand mal seizures and acute persecutory delusions following withdrawal of daily doses of only 1–2 mg of clonazepam.

Although not an actual side effect, benzodiazepine abuse should always be considered, particularly in patients with a history of abuse of drugs and other medications.

Drug-Drug Interactions

Benzodiazepines produce increased CNS depression when administered with other CNS depressants, but otherwise there are no known drug interactions.

BOTULINUM TOXIN

History and Discovery

Botulinum toxin, produced by *Clostridium botulinum*, causes botulism when ingested. The first clinical use of the toxin was to treat childhood strabismus (Scott 1980). The first focal dystonia treated was blepharospasm (Elston 1988). Since then, botulinum toxin has been used to treat several other conditions associated with excessive muscle activity, including neuroleptic-induced dystonias (Hughes 1994).

Structure-Activity Relations

There are seven immunologically distinct botulinum toxins (L. L. Simpson 1981). Type A is the primary type used

clinically (Hambleton 1992). Type F and possibly B also have clinical utility but have much shorter durations of action—3 weeks or fewer compared with 3 months or more (Borodic et al. 1996). The toxin is quantified by bioassay, expressed as mouse units, which refers to the dose that is lethal to 50% of animals following intraperitoneal injection (Quinn and Hallet 1989).

Pharmacological Profile

Botulinum toxin binds to cholinergic motor nerve terminals, preventing release of acetylcholine and producing a functionally denervated muscle. The prevention of acetylcholine release occurs within a few hours, but the clinical effect does not occur for 1–3 days. The innervation gradually becomes restored, although the number or size of active muscle fibers is reduced (Odergren et al. 1994).

Pharmacokinetics and Disposition

After binding to the presynaptic nerve terminal, the toxin is taken into the nerve cell and metabolized. When antibodies are present, the toxin is metabolized by immunological processes.

Mechanism of Action

Botulinum toxin acts presynaptically to block the release of acetylcholine at the neuromuscular junction. This produces a functional chemical denervation and paralysis of the muscle. Clinical use of the toxin aims to reduce the excessive muscle activity without producing significant weakness (Hughes 1994).

Indications

The FDA has approved the use of botulinum toxin for strabismus, blepharospasm, and other facial nerve disorders (Jankovic and Brin 1991). Botulinum toxin has also been used to treat focal neuroleptic-induced dystonias that may occur as part of tardive dyskinesia, including laryngeal dystonia (Blitzer and Brin 1991) and refractory torticollis (Kaufman 1994). For laryngeal dystonia, toxin is injected percutaneously through the cricothyroid membrane into the thyroarytenoid muscle bilaterally. Eighty percent to 90% of patients respond, and the effect lasts 3–4 months and sometimes longer.

Side Effects and Toxicology

The major potential side effect is focal weakness in the muscle group injected, which is usually dose dependent. This effect generally is temporary, given the mechanism of action. Transient weakness can occur through diffusion of the toxin into surrounding noninjected muscles (Hughes 1994).

Antibodies to the toxin can develop, which can prevent a therapeutic response, particularly during subsequent treatments. The two main factors that apparently contribute to the development of antibodies are an early age at first receiving toxin and total cumulative dose (Jankovic and Schwartz 1995). Some patients with antibodies will respond to other botulin serotypes, such as type F (Greene and Fahn 1993). Local skin reactions can also occur. Some degree of muscle atrophy can occur in injected muscles (Hughes 1994). Reinnervation usually takes place over 3–4 months (Odergren et al. 1994).

No contraindications are known. The effect on the fetus is unknown, so its use is not recommended during pregnancy. When neuromuscular junction disorders, such as myasthenia gravis, are present, patients could theoretically experience increased weakness. The long-term effects are unknown (Hughes 1994).

Drug-Drug Interactions

Botulinum toxin has no reported interactions with other drugs.

VITAMIN E (α-TOCOPHEROL)

History and Discovery

The existence of vitamin E was postulated in 1922 when it appeared that rats required an unknown dietary supplement to sustain pregnancy. That supplement, vitamin E, or α-tocopherol, was eventually isolated from wheat germ oil (Evans et al. 1936). Vitamin E deficiency in animals leads to several specific diseases, but in humans, there is little evidence for any specific metabolic effects or illnesses. Despite the paucity of evidence for its benefit, vitamin E has been used over the years to treat multiple conditions, including infertility, various menstrual disorders, neurological and muscular disorders, and anemias (Marcus and Coulston 1996).

Vitamin E was proposed as a treatment for tardive dyskinesia after it was noted that a neurotoxin in rats induced an irreversible movement disorder and axonal damage similar to that caused by vitamin E deficiency. Investigators proposed that chronic antipsychotic use might produce free radicals, which would contribute to neurological damage and tardive dyskinesia, and that the antioxidant effect of vitamin E could attenuate the damage (Cadet et al. 1986).

Structure-Activity Relations

Eight tocopherols have vitamin E activity, and α-tocopherol constitutes 90% of all activity. It is similar in structure to coenzyme Q_4 (Marcus and Coulston 1996).

Pharmacological Profile

Vitamin E is an antioxidant, which is thought to account for its physiological activity. In animals, vitamin E is involved in fatty acid metabolism and, as an antioxidant, presumably prevents oxidation of cellular components or prevents formation of toxic oxidation products (Witting 1972). It also increases the absorption and cellular levels of vitamin A while protecting against elevated levels of vitamin A (Underwood 1984).

In humans, symptoms of vitamin E deficiency are rare and almost always result from malabsorption (Bieri and Farrell 1976). The only consistent laboratory finding is that subjects with low serum vitamin E levels have increased hemolysis of erythrocytes exposed to oxidizing agents (Leonard and Losowsky 1967). Also, patients with glucose-6-phosphate dehydrogenase deficiency may have improved erythrocyte survival when treated with large doses of vitamin E (Corash et al. 1980).

Pharmacokinetics and Disposition

Vitamin E, being a fat-soluble vitamin, is absorbed from the gut into the lymphatic system in chylomicrons (MacMahon and Neale 1970). It is secreted by the liver in very-low-density lipoproteins. It becomes associated with plasma β-lipoproteins, is distributed to all tissues, and is stored extensively in the liver and adipose. A possible binding protein has been isolated (Wolf 1994). Plasma concentrations vary widely and fluctuate with concentrations of lipids. The ratio of vitamin E to total lipids has been used to determine vitamin E status. Values below 0.8 mg/g are thought to indicate a deficiency (Horwitt et al. 1972).

Mechanism of Action

Vitamin E is believed to be a reducing agent, or antioxidant, similar to coenzyme Q_4. A reducing agent is capable of accepting an electron from an oxidizing agent, or a "free radical." Researchers believe that free radicals are toxic to various cellular components and metabolic activities and that antioxidants provide protection to cells by "neutralizing" free radicals.

Indications

Currently, the only known indication is treatment of vitamin E deficiency, which almost always results from malabsorption syndromes or abnormal transport, such as with abetalipoproteinemia. In most cases, other vitamins and nutrients are also deficient, so that symptoms may not be a result of only vitamin E deficiency. Supplementation in children has been shown to be effective for the neurological symptoms resulting from malabsorption and vitamin E deficiency in chronic cholestasis (Sokol et al. 1993). A rare condition of spinocerebellar degeneration appears to be caused by deficiency without malabsorption (Sokol 1988).

Studies of vitamin E treatment of tardive dyskinesia have reported a range of results from general benefit (Adler et al. 1993; Dabiri et al. 1994; Lohr et al. 1988), to benefit only in subjects with tardive dyskinesia of less than 5 years (Egan et al. 1992; Lohr and Caligiuri 1996), to no benefit (Schmidt et al. 1991; Shriqui et al. 1992). Based on the studies currently published, definite conclusions regarding the efficacy of vitamin E in the treatment of tardive dyskinesia are not yet determined.

At the time of publication, a major double-blind study using vitamin E to treat tardive dyskinesia had just been completed. A preliminary analysis of the effect of vitamin E on the entire group had been made. The complete evaluation of the data might ultimately show that particular populations of patients benefited, but the preliminary evaluation of the data indicates that, for the group as a whole, vitamin E did not provide any benefit in the treatment of tardive dyskinesia. The complete analysis of the results of this study may eventually help reach a definite conclusion regarding the use of vitamin E for treatment of tardive dyskinesia.

One milligram of *dl*-α-tocopheryl acetate is equivalent to the activity of one international unit (IU) of vitamin E. The minimum daily requirement of vitamin E is estimated to be 10–30 mg (Marcus and Coulston 1996). In studies of tardive dyskinesia, doses up to 1,600 mg/day have been used.

Side Effects and Toxicology

Side effects are minimal when vitamin E is given orally. Infant deaths occurred when vitamin E was given intravenously. This was believed to be the result of polysorbates used in preparation rather than vitamin E itself (Mino 1992). Vitamin E should not be given intravenously, but, if necessary, it can be given intramuscularly.

High levels of vitamin E can interfere with bleeding abnormalities associated with vitamin K deficiency; otherwise, no significant side effects are known. Doses up to 3,200 mg/day in studies for conditions other than tardive dyskinesia have been used without significant adverse effects (Kappus and Diplock 1992).

Drug-Drug Interactions

The only known drug interactions are with vitamin K, when it is being given for a deficiency and bleeding abnormalities, and possibly with oral anticoagulants. High doses of vitamin E can exacerbate the coagulation abnormalities in both cases, so high doses are contraindicated in these two conditions (Kappus and Diplock 1992).

TREATMENT OF EXTRAPYRAMIDAL SIDE EFFECTS

Treatment of Acute Dystonic Reactions

Intramuscular anticholinergics are the treatment of choice for ADRs. Benztropine (2 mg) or diphenhydramine (50–100 mg) generally will produce complete resolution within 20–30 minutes. The dose should be repeated after 30 minutes if complete recovery does not occur. Starting a standing dose of an antiparkinsonian agent afterward is generally not necessary. ADRs do not recur unless large doses of high-potency antipsychotics are being used or the dose is increased. Prophylaxis is discussed more completely later in this chapter (see section, "Prophylaxis of EPS").

Treatment of Akathisia and Parkinsonism

The initial treatment of akathisia and parkinsonism (referred to here as EPS) is identical—evaluating the dose and type of antipsychotic (Table 19–3). An increase in dose beyond the neuroleptic threshold will *not* produce any greater therapeutic benefit but will increase EPS (Angus and Simpson 1970a; Baldessarini et al. 1988; McEvoy et al. 1991). Studies have found that EPS frequently can be eliminated with a reduction in dose or change to a

Table 19–3. Treatment of akathisia and parkinsonism

Step	Action
1	Reduce dose of antipsychotic, if clinically possible
2	Substitute lower-potency antipsychotic
3	Add anticholinergic agent
4	Titrate anticholinergic to maximum dose tolerable
5	Add amantadine in combination with anticholinergic or substitute as a single agent
6	Add benzodiazepine or β-blocker
7	In cases of severe extrapyramidal side effects, stop antipsychotic temporarily and repeat process, beginning with Step 3
8	Substitute antipsychotic with clozapine or another atypical antipsychotic

lower-potency antipsychotic (Braude et al. 1983; Stratas et al. 1963).

If the above steps do not resolve EPS or cannot be accomplished, the addition of an anticholinergic drug would be the next step. Maximum therapeutic response occurs in 3–10 days; more severe EPS take a longer time to respond (DiMascio et al. 1976; Fann and Lake 1976). The anticholinergic dose should be increased until EPS are alleviated or an unacceptable degree of anticholinergic side effects is obtained.

Akathisia frequently does not respond as well to anticholinergic medications as do parkinsonism and ADRs (DiMascio et al. 1976). Akathisia is more likely to respond if symptoms of parkinsonism are also present (Fleischhacker et al. 1990).

If EPS remain uncontrolled, amantadine can be either added to the regimen or substituted as a single agent. The next step would be the addition of a benzodiazepine or a β-blocker, although fewer data support both of these treatments.

In cases of severe EPS, the antipsychotic should be stopped temporarily because severe EPS may be a risk factor for development of neuroleptic malignant syndrome (Levinson and Simpson 1986).

Additional drugs have been studied or suggested as treatments for akathisia. Limited data support use of amantadine for treatment of akathisia. Clonidine has been studied in a small number of patients, but its limited benefit was further affected by sedation and hypotension (Fleischhacker et al. 1990). Sodium valproate was reported to have no significant effect on akathisia and to increase parkinsonism (Friis et al. 1983).

Iron supplementation has been suggested as a possible treatment for akathisia (Blake et al. 1986). Gold and Lenox (1995) reviewed the evidence and concluded that iron supplements at best would have no effect on akathisia, but they could potentially worsen the condition and promote further long-term damage. Therefore, iron supplementation should not be considered a treatment for akathisia or be given indiscriminantly.

For patients who have severe, refractory EPS that have not responded to standard treatments, the use of clozapine specifically to treat the EPS is indicated (Casey 1989). This can even be true for patients who do not have any psychotic symptoms, if the EPS are judged to be severe enough to be disabling or potentially life-threatening, such as a laryngeal dystonia.

Patients treated with clozapine were found to have significantly less parkinsonism than patients treated with the combination of chlorpromazine and an antiparkinsonian agent (benztropine) (Kane et al. 1988). The prevalence

and incidence of akathisia have also been shown to be lower in patients treated with clozapine than in patients treated with typical antipsychotics (Chengappa et al. 1994; Kurz et al. 1995). A double-blind prospective study of clozapine found that after 16 weeks of clozapine treatment, no patient had definite akathisia, and only 2 of 47 patients had possible akathisia. Both of those patients had akathisia at baseline (Stanilla et al. 1995). Given the significant negative effect that akathisia has on the outcome of schizophrenia, the use of clozapine in refractory akathisia should also be considered a definite treatment option.

Like clozapine, other antipsychotics with atypical properties are less likely to produce EPS than are typical antipsychotics. Their use in the prevention and treatment of EPS is discussed later in this chapter (see section, "Atypical Antipsychotics").

Treatment of Tardive Dyskinesia

Historically, tardive dyskinesia has been refractory to treatment, which helps explain the large number of drugs that have been used in attempts to alleviate the condition. Treatments investigated have included, but are not limited to, noradrenergic antagonists (propranolol, clonidine), dopamine and other catecholamine antagonists, dopaminergic drugs, catecholamine-depleting drugs (reserpine, tetrabenazine), GABAergic drugs, cholinergic drugs (deanol, choline, lecithin), catecholaminergic drugs (Kane et al. 1992), calcium channel blockers (Cates et al. 1993), and selective monoamine oxidase inhibitors (selegiline; Goff et al. 1993). Based on the investigations of the above drugs, the American Psychiatric Association Task Force on Tardive Dyskinesia concluded that no consistently effective treatment for tardive dyskinesia was available (Kane et al. 1992).

The variability of clinical raters (Bergen et al. 1984), the placebo response of patients (Sommer et al. 1994), and the diurnal and longitudinal variability of tardive dyskinesia (Hyde et al. 1995; Stanilla et al. 1996) contribute to difficulty in evaluating the effects of any treatment of tardive dyskinesia. The degree of improvement would need to be greater than the sum of the above variations to show an actual benefit.

Several drugs have been shown or have been suggested to have some benefit for treatment of tardive dyskinesia, although most have limitations. These drugs include botulinum toxin, clonazepam, vitamin E, and clozapine. Other atypical antipsychotics may also have a benefit in the prevention and treatment of tardive dyskinesia and are discussed below.

Botulinum toxin is beneficial for treating specific tardive dystonias, and laryngeal dystonia is probably the one that is most commonly associated with tardive dyskinesia (Hughes 1994). The injections must be repeated every 3–6 months, and botulinum toxin is not a general treatment for all movements of tardive dyskinesia.

Clonazepam was reported to reduce the movements of tardive dyskinesia for up to 9 months, although tolerance developed to the benefits. Thaker et al. (1990) reported that when the drug was weaned and stopped for 2 weeks and then resumed, the benefits returned. Potential limitations are the inherent problems associated with chronic use of a benzodiazepine.

Vitamin E has not been consistently shown to be beneficial in all studies. Larger long-term studies are needed to determine its effect on tardive dyskinesia.

Clozapine decreases symptoms of tardive dyskinesia (G. M. Simpson et al. 1978), with the greatest reduction occurring in cases of severe tardive dyskinesia and tardive dystonia (Lieberman et al. 1991). Unlike studies of the other drugs described above, these findings have been replicated in large studies and suggest that clozapine is unlikely to cause tardive dyskinesia (Chengappa et al. 1994; Kane et al. 1993). The disadvantages of clozapine are the potential side effects of agranulocytosis and seizures and the need for weekly blood monitoring.

Three possible mechanisms for clozapine's benefit have been proposed. First, clozapine may suppress the tardive dyskinesia movements in a fashion similar to that of typical antipsychotics. Second, tardive dyskinesia may improve spontaneously, because the typical antipsychotics are no longer present to cause or sustain tardive dyskinesia. This result occurs in a percentage of patients when antipsychotics are withdrawn. Third, clozapine may have an active therapeutic effect on tardive dyskinesia (Lieberman et al. 1991). This issue remains to be clarified. In some patients, tardive dyskinesia movements have recurred on withdrawal of clozapine, but long-term follow-up studies have not been reported.

Based on the above information, clozapine is the only drug that could be considered a definite treatment of tardive dyskinesia, with the potential for complete resolution. Before changing to clozapine, however, a trial of clonazepam, risperidone, and olanzapine or, perhaps, vitamin E should be considered, keeping in mind that the current data regarding their benefit in tardive dyskinesia are limited or inconsistent.

Atypical Antipsychotics

In many cases, the development of EPS is the rate-limiting step in the antipsychotic treatment of psychosis. Cloza-pine demonstrated that this side effect was not necessary for antipsychotic activity. The significance of clozapine's favorable EPS profile and beneficial effect on negative symptoms and in treatment-refractory patients has led to the investigation of multiple additional "atypical" antipsychotics in an attempt to reproduce clozapine's benefits while eliminating its more serious side effects of agranulocytosis and seizures.

Risperidone has an antipsychotic effect at doses that do not produce parkinsonism. Unlike clozapine, though, higher doses are associated with EPS (Chouinard et al. 1993). Risperidone has an advantage over clozapine of not producing agranulocytosis or requiring continual blood count monitoring.

The mean changes in the Extrapyramidal Symptom Rating Scale (ESRS) scores from baseline to worst score were significantly lower for all doses of risperidone (2–16 mg/day) than for haloperidol (20 mg/day). At 6 mg/day, there was no difference in the mean change score between risperidone and placebo. There was a linear relationship between the mean change scores and the dose of risperidone on 4 of 12 ESRS scores and between the dose of risperidone and the use of antiparkinsonian medication. Both risperidone and haloperidol caused acute dystonic reactions. Patients with severe EPS at baseline were more likely to develop EPS while taking risperidone (Simpson and Lindermayer 1997).

Fewer data are available regarding risperidone's production of akathisia or effect on tardive dyskinesia. One study found that the occurrence of akathisia was the same for risperidone as it was for haloperidol (Marder and Meibach 1994). There have been anecdotal reports of risperidone's improvement of tardive dyskinesia in some patients, but controlled data regarding its effectiveness in the treatment of tardive dyskinesia are limited (Chouinard 1995; Meco et al. 1989).

Risperidone can cause serum prolactin levels to increase above the normal range (Dickson et al. 1995). This is one of the classic attributes of a neuroleptic medication and a finding that does not occur with therapeutic doses of clozapine.

Although risperidone produces fewer EPS than haloperidol does, there are few data comparing risperidone directly with clozapine in this regard. In one study involving 20 patients treated with risperidone and clozapine in a crossover design, 7 patients required benztropine for EPS during the risperidone phase, whereas none did during the clozapine phase. Also, during the risperidone phase, 2 patients were unable to complete the study because of poor response compared with no dropouts during the clozapine phase.

over time without treatment. Potential cholinergic sensitization leading to subsequent EPS would be a reason to limit the routine use of prophylactic anticholinergic agents.

It needs to be emphasized that antiparkinsonian agents should be withdrawn slowly and gradually over weeks or months, not abruptly as has been done in the reported studies. Patients should be evaluated for recurrence of EPS following a partial dose reduction of the antiparkinsonian agent. This process should be continued until the antiparkinsonian agent is completely withdrawn or the lowest dose for maintenance control is achieved.

CONCLUSION

The unique properties of chlorpromazine and other similarly active agents to ameliorate psychotic symptoms and to produce parkinsonian-like side effects were described in the early 1950s by French psychiatrists. Theories soon arose regarding the relationship between these two properties. The recognition of the benefits of reducing parkinsonian side effects led to investigations of methods to reduce EPS and to the development of instruments to measure EPS. The debate over the routine and prophylactic use of antiparkinsonian agents has continued since that time. It appears that prophylactic antiparkinsonian agents need to be used in some situations but probably less frequently and for briefer periods than has generally been the practice. The trend toward the use of lower dosages of antipsychotics should also lead to decreased need for use of antiparkinsonian agents. Finally, the advent of atypical antipsychotic agents has opened a new chapter in both the treatment and the prevention of EPS and suggests that, in the future, EPS will be less of a problem than they have been in the past.

A summary of an American Psychiatric Association Task Force report on tardive dyskinesia suggested that "[a] deliberate and sustained effort must be made to maintain patients on the lowest effective amount of drug and to keep the treatment regimen as simple as possible" (Baldessarini et al. 1980, p. 1168) and to discontinue anticholinergic drugs as soon as possible. Apart from a greater emphasis on avoiding the initial use of antiparkinsonian agents, this statement remains valid.

REFERENCES

Adler L, Angrist B, Peselow E, et al: Efficacy of propranolol in neuroleptic-induced akathisia. J Clin Psychopharmacol 5:164–166, 1985

Adler LA, Angrist B, Weinreb H, et al: Studies on the time course and efficacy of β-blockers in neuroleptic-induced akathisia and the akathisia of idiopathic Parkinson's disease. Psychopharmacol Bull 27:107–111, 1991

Adler LA, Peselow E, Rotrosen J, et al: Vitamin E treatment of tardive dyskinesia. Am J Psychiatry 150:1405–1407, 1993

Ananth JV, Horodesky S, Lehmann HE, et al: Effect of withdrawal of antiparkinsonian medication on chronically hospitalized psychiatric patients. Laval Médical 41:934–938, 1970

Angus JWS, Simpson GM: Handwriting changes and response to drugs—a controlled study. Acta Psychiatr Scand Suppl 21:28–37, 1970a

Angus JWS, Simpson GM: Hysteria and drug-induced dystonia. Acta Psychiatr Scand Suppl 21:52–58, 1970b

Aoki FY, Sitar DS, Ogilvie RI: Amantadine kinetics in healthy young subjects after long-term dosing. Clin Pharmacol Ther 26:729–736, 1979

Arvanitis LA, Miller BG, and the Seroquel Trial 13 Study Group: Multiple fixed doses of "Seroquel" (quetiapine) in patients with acute exacerbation of schizophrenia: a comparison with haloperidol and placebo. Biol Psychiatry 42:233–246, 1997

Ayd FJ: A survey of drug-induced extrapyramidal reactions. JAMA 175:1054–1060, 1961

Babe KS, Serafin WE: Histamine, bradykinin, and their antagonists, in Goodman and Gilman's The Pharmacological Basis of Therapeutics, 9th Edition. Edited by Hardman JG, Limbird LE, Molinoff PB, et al. New York, McGraw-Hill, 1996, pp 581–600

Baker LA, Cheng LY, Amara IB: The withdrawal of benztropine mesylate in chronic schizophrenic patients. Br J Psychiatry 143:584–590, 1983

Baldessarini RJ, Cole JO, Davis JM, et al: Tardive dyskinesia: summary of a task force report of the American Psychiatric Association. Am J Psychiatry 137:1163–1172, 1980

Baldessarini RJ, Cohen BM, Teicher MH: Significance of neuroleptic dose and plasma level in the pharmacological treatment of psychoses. Arch Gen Psychiatry 45:79–91, 1988

Baldessarini RJ, Huston-Lyons D, Campbell A, et al: Do central antiadrenergic actions contribute to the atypical properties of clozapine? Br J Psychiatry 160 (suppl 17):12–16, 1992

Barnes TRE: A rating scale for drug-induced akathisia. Br J Psychiatry 1564:672–676, 1989

Barnes TR: Movement disorder associated with antipsychotic drugs: the tardive syndromes. International Review of Psychiatry 2:355–366, 1990

Bartels M, Heide K, Mann K, et al: Treatment of akathisia with lorazepam: an open clinical trial. Pharmacopsychiatry 20:51–53, 1987

Beasley CM Jr, Tollefson G, Tran P, et al: Olanzapine versus placebo and haloperidol: acute phase results of the North American double-blind olanzapine trial. Neuropsychopharmacology 14:111–123, 1996

Beasley CM Jr, Tollefson G, Tran P: Safety of olanzapine. J Clin Psychiatry 58 (suppl 10):13–17, 1997

Ben-Shachar D, Youdim MBH: Neuroleptic induced dopamine receptor supersensitivity and tardive dyskinesia may involve altered brain iron metabolism. Abstract presented at the proceedings of the British Pharmacological Society, December 17–19, 1986. Br J Pharmacol 90 (suppl):95, 1987

Bergen JA, Griffiths DA, Rey JM, et al: Tardive dyskinesia: fluctuating patient or fluctuating rater. Br J Psychiatry 144:498–502, 1984

Bieri JG, Farrell PM: Vitamin E. Vitam Horm 34:31–75, 1976

Blake DR, William AC, Pall H, et al: Iron and akathisia (letter). BMJ 292:1393, 1986

Blitzer A, Brin MF: Laryngeal dystonia: a series with botulinum toxin therapy. Ann Otol Rhinol Laryngol 100:85–89, 1991

Bobruff A, Gardos G, Tarsy D, et al: Clonazepam and phenobarbital in tardive dyskinesia. Am J Psychiatry 138:189–193, 1981

Borison RL: Amantadine-induced psychosis in a geriatric patient with renal disease. Am J Psychiatry 136:111–112, 1979

Borodic G, Johnson E, Goodnough M, et al: Botulinum toxin therapy, immunologic resistance, and problems with available materials. Neurology 46:26–29, 1996

Boumans CE, de Mooij KJ, Koch PA, et al: Is the social acceptability of psychiatric patients decreased by orofacial dyskinesia: Schizophr Bull 20:339–344, 1994

Bovet D: Introduction to antihistamine agents and antergan derivatives. Ann N Y Acad Sci 50:1089–1126, 1950

Braude WM, Barnes TR, Gore SM: Clinical characteristics of akathisia: a systematic investigation of acute psychiatric inpatient admissions. Br J Psychiatry 143:139–150, 1983

Brooks GW: Experience with use of chlorpromazine and reserpine in psychiatry with special reference to the significance and management of extrapyramidal dysfunction. N Engl J Med 254:1119–1123, 1956

Brown JH: Atropine, scopolamine, and related antimuscarinic drugs, in Goodman and Gilman's The Pharmacological Basis of Therapeutics, 8th Edition. Edited by Gilman AG, Rall TW, Nies AS, et al. New York, Pergamon, 1990, pp 150–165

Brown JH, Taylor P: Muscarinic receptor agonists and antagonists, in Goodman and Gilman's The Pharmacological Basis of Therapeutics, 9th Edition. Edited by Hardman JG, Limbird LE, Molinoff PB, et al. New York, McGraw-Hill, 1996, pp 141–160

Büchel C, de Leon J, Simpson GM, et al: Oral tardive dyskinesia: validation of a measuring device using digital image processing. Psychopharmacology (Berl) 117:162–165, 1995

Cadet JL, Lohr J, Jeste D: Free radicals and tardive dyskinesia (letter). Trends Neurosci 9:107–108, 1986

Cahan RB, Parrish DD: Reversibility of drug-induced parkinsonism. Am J Psychiatry 116:1022–1023, 1960

Caligiuri MP, Lohr JB, Jeste DV: Parkinsonism in neuroleptic-naive schizophrenic patients. Am J Psychiatry 150:1343–1348, 1993

Casey DE: Clozapine: neuroleptic-induced EPS and tardive dyskinesia. Psychopharmacology (Berl) 99:S47–S53, 1989

Casey DE, Gerlach J, Christensson E: Dopamine, acetylcholine, and GABA effects in acute dystonia in primates. Psychopharmacologia 70:83–87, 1980

Cates M, Lusk K, Wells BG: Are calcium-channel blockers effective in the treatment of tardive dyskinesia? Ann Pharmacother 27:191–196, 1993

Cedarbaum JM, McDowell FH: Sixteen-year follow-up of 100 patients begun on levodopa in 1968: emerging problems, in Advances in Neurology, Vol 45: Parkinson's Disease. Edited by Yahr MD, Bergmann KJ. New York, Raven, 1987, pp 469–472

Cedarbaum JM, Schleifer LS: Drugs for Parkinson's disease, spasticity, and acute muscle spasms, in Goodman and Gilman's The Pharmacological Basis of Therapeutics, 8th Edition. Edited by Gilman AG, Rall TW, Nies AS, et al. New York, Pergamon, 1990, pp 463–484

Chatterjee A, Chakos M, Koreen A, et al: Prevalence and clinical correlates of extrapyramidal signs and spontaneous dyskinesia in never-medicated schizophrenic patients. Am J Psychiatry 152:1724–1729, 1995

Chengappa KN, Shelton MD, Baker RW, et al: The prevalence of akathisia in patients receiving stable doses of clozapine. J Clin Psychiatry 55:142–145, 1994

Chien CP, DiMascio A: Drug-induced extrapyramidal symptoms and their relations to clinical efficacy. Am J Psychiatry 123:1490–1498, 1967

Chouinard G: Effects of risperidone in tardive dyskinesia: an analysis of the Canadian multicenter risperidone study. J Clin Psychopharmacol 15 (suppl):36S–44S, 1995

Chouinard G, Ross-Chouinard A, Annable L, et al: Extrapyramidal Symptom Rating Scale (Poster presented at the 3rd annual meeting of the Canadian College of Neuropsychopharmacology, Edmonton, Alberta, Canada, May 12–13, 1980). Can J Neurol Sci 7:233, 1980

Chouinard G, Jones B, Remington G, et al: A Canadian multicenter placebo-controlled study of fixed doses of risperidone and haloperidol in the treatment of chronic schizophrenic patients (published erratum appears in J Clin Psychopharmacol 13:149, 1993). J Clin Psychopharmacol 13:25–40, 1993

Coffin VL, Latranyi MB, Chipkin RE: Acute extrapyramidal syndrome in Cebus monkeys: development medicated by dopamine D_2 but not D_1 receptors. J Pharmacol Exp Ther 249:769–774, 1989

Corash L, Spielberg S, Bartsocas C, et al: Reduced chronic hemolysis during high-dose vitamin E administration in Mediterranean-type glucose-6-phosphate dehydrogenase deficiency. N Engl J Med 303:416–420, 1980

Corrigan FM, van Rhijn AG, MacKay AVP, et al: Vitamin E treatment of tardive dyskinesia (letter). Am J Psychiatry 150:991–992, 1993

Côté L, Crutcher MD: The basal ganglia, in Principles of Neural Science, 3rd Edition. Edited by Kandel ER, Schwartz JH, Jessell TM. New York, Elsevier, 1991, pp 647–659

Dabiri LM, Pasta D, Darby JK, et al: Effectiveness of vitamin E for treatment of long-term tardive dyskinesia. Am J Psychiatry 151:925–926, 1994

Delay J, Deniker P: Trente-huit cas de psychoses traitées par la cure prolongée et continue de 4560 RP. Léme Congrès des Alién. et Neurol de Langue Française, Luxembourg, 21–27 juillet 1952 [Thirty-eight cases of psychoses treated with a long and continued course of 4560 RP. The Congress of the French Language for Alienists and Neurologists, Luxembourg, 21–27 July 1952]. Paris, Masson et Cie, 1952, pp 503–513

Delay J, Deniker P, Harl JM: Traitement des états d'excitation et d'agitation par une méthode médicamenteuse dérivée de l'hibernothérapie [Therapeutic method derived from hiberno-therapy in excitation and agitation states]. Annales Medico-Psychologiques (Paris) 110:267–273, 1952

de Leon J, Canuso C, White AO, et al: A pilot effort to determine benztropine equivalents of anticholinergic medications. Hosp Community Psychiatry 45:606–607, 1994

Denham J, Carrick JEL: Therapeutic importance of extrapyramidal phenomena evoked by a new phenothiazine. Am J Psychiatry 116:927–928, 1960

Dettli L: Benzodiazepines in the treatment of sleep disorders: pharmacokinetic aspects. Acta Psychiatr Scand Suppl 332:9–19, 1986

Dickson RA, Dalby JT, Williams R, et al: Risperidone-induced prolactin elevations in premenopausal women with schizophrenia (letter). Am J Psychiatry 152:7–8, 1995

DiMascio A, Bernardo DL, Greenblatt DJ, et al: A controlled trial of amantadine in drug-induced extrapyramidal disorders. Arch Gen Psychiatry 33:599–602, 1976

Director KL, Muniz CE: Diazepam in the treatment of extrapyramidal symptoms: a case report. J Clin Psychiatry 43:160–161, 1982

Donlon PT: The therapeutic use of diazepam for akathisia. Psychosomatics 14:222–225, 1973

Doshay LJ: Five-year study of benztropine (Cogentin) methanesulfonate: outcome in three hundred two cases of paralysis agitans. JAMA 162:1031–1034, 1956

Doshay LJ, Constable K, Zier A: Five year follow-up of treatment with trihexyphenidyl (Artane): outcome in four hundred and eleven cases of paralysis agitans. JAMA 154:1334–1336, 1954

Drachman DA: Memory and cognitive function in man: does the cholinergic system have a specific role? Neurology 27:783–790, 1977

Drayer DE: Lipophilicity, hydrophilicity, and the central nervous system side effects of beta blocker. Pharmacotherapy 7:87–91, 1987

Egan MF, Hyde TM, Albers GW, et al: Treatment of tardive dyskinesia with vitamin E. Am J Psychiatry 149:773–777, 1992

Ekbom KA: Restless legs. Swedish Medical Journal 62:2376–2378, 1965

Ekdawi MY, Fowke R: A controlled trial of anti-Parkinson drugs in drug-induced parkinsonism. Br J Psychiatry 112:633–636, 1966

el-Defrawi MH, Craig TJ: Neuroleptics, extrapyramidal symptoms, and serum-calcium levels. Compr Psychiatry 25:539–545, 1984

Elkashef AM, Egan MF, Frank JA, et al: Basal ganglia iron in tardive dyskinesia: an MRI study. Biol Psychiatry 35:16–21, 1994

Elston J: Botulinum toxin treatment of blepharospasm. Adv Neurol 50:579–581, 1988

England AC Jr, Schwab RS: Treatment in internal medicine: the management of Parkinson's disease. AMA Archives of Internal Medicine 104:439–468, 1959

Evans HM, Emerson OH, Emerson GA: The isolation from wheat germ oil of an alcohol, α-tocopherol, having properties of vitamin E. J Biol Chem 113:329–332, 1936

Fann WE, Lake CR: Amantadine versus trihexyphenidyl in the treatment of neuroleptic-induced parkinsonism. Am J Psychiatry 133:940–943, 1976

Farde L, Nordström AL, Wiesel FA, et al: Positron emission tomographic analysis of central D_1 and D_2 dopamine receptor occupancy in patients treated with classical neuroleptics and clozapine: relation to extrapyramidal side effects. Arch Gen Psychiatry 49:538–544, 1992

Fayen M, Goldman MB, Moulthrop MA, et al: Differential memory function with dopaminergic versus anticholinergic treatment of drug-induced extrapyramidal symptoms. Am J Psychiatry 145:483–486, 1988

Feve A, Angelard B, Lacau St Guily J: Laryngeal tardive dyskinesia. J Neurol 242:455–459, 1995

Fleischhacker W, Bergmann KJ, Perovich R, et al: The Hillside Akathisia Scale: a new rating instrument for neuroleptic-induced akathisia, parkinsonism and hyperkinesia. Psychopharmacol Bull 25:222–226, 1989

Fleischhacker WW, Roth SD, Kane JM: The pharmacologic treatment of neuroleptic-induced akathisia. J Clin Psychopharmacol 10:12–21, 1990

Flügel F: Neue klinische Beobachtungen zur Wirkung des Phenothiazinkorpers Megaphen auf psychische Krankheitsbidler [Clinical observations on the effect of the phenothiazine derivative megaphen on psychic disorders in children]. Med Klin 48:1027–1029, 1953

Foster NL, Newman RP, LeWitt, et al: Peripheral beta-adrenergic blockade treatment of parkinsonian tremor. Ann Neurol 16:505–508, 1984

Freyhan FA: Therapeutic implications of differential effects of new phenothiazine compounds. Am J Psychiatry 115:577–585, 1959

Friis T, Christensen TR, Gerlach J: Sodium valproate and biperiden in neuroleptic-induced akathisia, parkinsonism and hyperkinesia: a double-blind cross-over study with placebo. Acta Psychiatr Scand 67:178–187, 1983

Gagrat D, Hamilton J, Belmaker RH: Intravenous diazepam in the treatment of neuroleptic-induced acute dystonia and akathisia. Am J Psychiatry 135:1232–1233, 1978

Gardos G, Case DE, Cole JO, et al: Ten-year outcome of tardive dyskinesia. Am J Psychiatry 151:836–841, 1994

Gelenberg AJ: Amantadine in the treatment of benztropine-refractory extrapyramidal disorders induced by antipsychotic drugs. Current Therapeutic Research, Clinical and Experimental 23:375–380, 1978

Gelenberg AJ, Jefferson JW: Lithium tremor. J Clin Psychiatry 56:283–287, 1995

Gengo FM, Huntoon L, McHugh WB: Lipid-soluble and water-soluble beta-blockers: comparison of the central nervous system depressant effect. Arch Intern Med 147:39–43, 1987

Gerlach J, Hansen L: Clozapine and D_1/D_2 antagonism in extrapyramidal functions. Br J Psychiatry 160 (suppl 17):34–37, 1992

Gerlach J, Korsgaard S, Clemmesen P, et al: The St. Hans Rating Scale for Extrapyramidal Syndromes: reliability and validity. Acta Psychiatr Scand 87:244–252, 1993

Goff DC, Renshaw PF, Sarid-Segal O, et al: A placebo-controlled trial of selegiline (L-deprenyl) in the treatment of tardive dyskinesia. Biol Psychiatry 33:700–706, 1993

Gold R, Lenox RH: Is there a rationale for iron supplementation in the treatment of akathisia? A review of the evidence. J Clin Psychiatry 56:476–483, 1995

Greenblatt DJ, DiMascio A, Harmatz JS, et al: Pharmacokinetics and clinical effects of amantadine in drug-induced extrapyramidal symptoms. J Clin Pharmacol 17:704–708, 1977

Greene PE, Fahn S: Use of botulinum toxin type F injections to treat torticollis in patients with immunity to botulinum toxin type A. Mov Disord 8:479–483, 1993

Grelak RP, Clark R, Stump JM, et al: Amantadine-dopamine interaction: possible mode of action in parkinsonism. Science 169:203–204, 1970

Gunn KP: Ziprasidone: safety and efficacy. Schizophr Res 18:132–139, 1996

Gunne LM, Häggström JE, Sjöquist B: Association with persistent neuroleptic-induced dyskinesia of regional changes in brain GABA synthesis. Nature 309:347–349, 1984

Guy W: ECDEU Assessment Manual for Psychopharmacology, Revised Edition. Washington, DC, U.S. Department of Health, Education and Welfare, 1976

Haase HJ: Über Vorkommen und Deutung des psychomotorischen Parkinson-symdroms bei Megaphen-bzw, Largactil Dauer-behandlung [The presentation and meaning of the psychomotor Parkinson syndrome during long-term treatment with megaphen, also know as Largactil]. Nervenarzt 25:486–492, 1954

Haase HJ, Janssen PAJ: The Action of Neuroleptic Drugs. Chicago, IL, Year Book, 1965

Hambleton P: Clostridium botulinum toxins: a general review of involvement in disease, structure, mode of action and preparation for clinical use. J Neurol 239:16–20, 1992

Hanlon TE, Schoenrich C, Freinek W, et al: Perphenazine-benztropine mesylate treatment of newly admitted psychiatric patients. Psychopharmacologia 9:328–339, 1966

Hay AJ: The action of amantadine against influenza A viruses: inhibition of the M2 ion channel protein. Seminars in Virology 3:21–30, 1992

Hayden FG, Minocha A, Spyker DA, et al: Comparative single-dose pharmacokinetics of amantadine hydrochloride and rimantadine hydrochloride in young and elderly adults. Antimicrob Agents Chemother 28:216–221, 1985

Hippius H: The history of clozapine. Psychopharmacology (Berl) 99 (suppl):S3–S5, 1989

Hobbs WR, Rall TW, Verdoorn TA: Hypnotics and sedatives; ethanol, in Goodman and Gilman's The Pharmacological Basis of Therapeutics, 9th Edition. Edited by Hardman JG, Limbird LE, Molinoff PB, et al. New York, McGraw-Hill, 1996, pp 361–396

Hoffman BB, Lefkowitz RJ: Catecholamines, sympathomimetic drugs, and adrenergic receptor antagonists, in Goodman and Gilman's The Pharmacological Basis of Therapeutics, 9th Edition. Edited by Hardman JG, Limbird LE, Molinoff PB, et al. New York, McGraw-Hill, 1996, pp 199–248

Horiguchi J, Nishimatsu O: Usefulness of antiparkinsonian drugs during neuroleptic treatment and the effect of clonazepam on akathisia and parkinsonism occurred after antiparkinsonian drug withdrawal: a double-blind study. Jpn J Psychiatry Neurol 46:733–739, 1992

Horwitt MK, Harvey CC, Dahm CH Jr, et al: Relationship between tocopherol and serum lipid levels for determination of nutritional adequacy. Ann N Y Acad Sci 203:223–236, 1972

Hughes AJ: Botulinum toxin in clinical practice. Drugs 48:888–893, 1994

Hyde TM, Egan MF, Brown RJ, et al: Diurnal variation in tardive dyskinesia. Psychiatry Res. 56:53–57, 1995

Ichikawa J, Meltzer HY: Differential effects of repeated treatment with haloperidol and clozapine on dopamine release and metabolism in the striatum and the nucleus accumbens. J Pharmacol Exp Ther 256:348–357, 1991

Idzorek S: Antiparkinsonian agents and fluphenazine decanoate. Am J Psychiatry 133:80–82, 1976

Ing TS, Daugirdas JT, Soung LS, et al: Toxic effects of amantadine in patients with renal failure. Can Med Assoc J 120:695–698, 1979

Jankovic J, Brin MF: Therapeutic uses of botulinum toxin. N Engl J Med 324:1186–1194, 1991

Jankovic J, Schwartz K: Response and immunoresistance to botulinum toxin injections. Neurology 45:1743–1746, 1995

Kalachnik JE, Sprague RL: The Dyskinesia Identification System Condensed User Scale (DISCUS): reliability, validity, and a total score cut-off for mentally ill and mentally retarded populations. J Clin Psychol 49:177–189, 1993

Kane J, Honigfeld G, Singer J, et al: Clozapine for the treatment-resistant schizophrenic, double-blind comparison with chlorpromazine. Arch Gen Psychiatry 45: 789–796, 1988

Kane JM, Jeste DV, Barnes TRE, et al: Treatment of tardive dyskinesia, in Tardive Dyskinesia: A Task Force Report of the American Psychiatric Association. Washington, DC, American Psychiatric Association, 1992, pp 103–120

Kane JM, Werner MG, Pollack S, et al: Does clozapine cause tardive dyskinesia? J Clin Psychiatry 54:327–330, 1993

Kappus H, Diplock AT: Tolerance and safety of vitamin E: a toxicological position report. Free Radic Biol Med 13:55–74, 1992

Karn WN, Kasper S: Pharmacologically induced Parkinson-like signs as index of the therapeutic potential. Diseases of the Nervous System 20:119–122, 1959

Kaufman DM: Use of botulinum toxin injections for spasmodic torticollis of tardive dystonia. J Neuropsychiatry Clin Neurosci 6:50–53, 1994

Keckich WA: Violence as a manifestation of akathisia. JAMA 240:2185, 1978

Keepers GA, Casey DE: Use of neuroleptic-induced extrapyramidal symptoms to predict future vulnerability to side effects. Am J Psychiatry 148:85–89, 1991

Keepers GA, Clappison VJ, Casey DE: Initial anticholinergic prophylaxis for neuroleptic-induced extrapyramidal syndromes. Arch Gen Psychiatry 40:1113–1117, 1983

Kelly JT, Abuzzahab FS: The antiparkinson properties of amantadine in drug-induced parkinsonism. J Clin Pharmacol 11:211–214, 1971

Kelly JT, Zimmermann RL, Abuzzahab FS Sr, et al: A double-blind study of amantadine hydrochloride versus benztropine mesylate in drug-induced parkinsonism. Pharmacology 12:65–73, 1974

Khan R, Jampala VC, Dong K, et al: Speech abnormalities in tardive dyskinesia. Am J Psychiatry 151:760–762, 1994

Klett CJ, Caffey E: Evaluating the long-term need for antiparkinson drugs by chronic schizophrenics. Arch Gen Psychiatry 26:374–379, 1972

Koek RJ, Pi EH: Acute laryngeal dystonic reactions to neuroleptics. Psychosomatics 30:359–364, 1989

Kulik AV, Wilbur R: Case report of propranolol (Inderal) pharmacotherapy for neuroleptic-induced akathisia and tremor. Prog Neuropsychopharmacol Biol Psychiatry 7:223–225, 1983

Kuny S, Binswanger U: Neuroleptic-induced extrapyramidal symptoms and serum calcium levels. Pharmacopsychiatry 21:67–70, 1989

Kurz M, Hummer M, Oberbauer H, et al: Extrapyramidal side effects of clozapine and haloperidol. Psychopharmacology (Berl) 118:52–56, 1995

Kutcher SP, Mackenzie S, Galarraga W, et al: Clonazepam treatment of adolescents with neuroleptic-induced akathisia (letter). Am J Psychiatry 144:823–824, 1987

Kutcher S, Williamson P, MacKenzie S, et al: Successful clonazepam treatment of neuroleptic-induced akathisia in older adolescents and young adults: a double-blind, placebo-controlled study. J Clin Psychopharmacol 9: 403–406, 1989

Laborit H, Huguenard P, Alluaume R: Un nouveau stabilisateur vegetatif (le 4560 RP) [A new vegetative stabilizer (4560 RP)]. Presse Med 60:206–208, 1952

Leonard PJ, Losowsky MS: Relationship between plasma vitamin E level and peroxide hemolysis test in human subjects. Am J Clin Nutr 20:795–798, 1967

Levinson DF, Simpson GM: Neuroleptic-induced extrapyramidal symptoms with fever: heterogeneity of the "neuroleptic malignant syndrome." Arch Gen Psychiatry 43: 839–848, 1986

Levinson DF, Simpson GM, Singh H, et al: Fluphenazine dose, clinical response, and extrapyramidal symptoms during acute treatment. Arch Gen Psychiatry 47:761–768, 1990

Lieberman JA, Saltz BL, Johns CA, et al: The effects of clozapine on tardive dyskinesia. Br J Psychiatry 158:503–510, 1991

Lipinski JF, Zubenko GS, Barreira P, et al: Propranolol in the treatment of neuroleptic-induced akathisia. Lancet 1:685–686, 1983

Lohr JB, Caligiuri MP: A double-blind placebo-controlled study of vitamin E treatment of tardive dyskinesia. J Clin Psychiatry 57:167–173, 1996

Lohr JB, Cadet JL, Lohr MA, et al: Vitamin E in the treatment of tardive dyskinesia: the possible involvement of free radical mechanisms. Schizophr Bull 14:291–296, 1988

Luchins DJ, Freed WJ, Wyatt RJ: The role of cholinergic supersensitivity in the medical symptoms associated with the withdrawal of antipsychotic drugs. Am J Psychiatry 137:1395–1398, 1980

MacMahon MT, Neale E: The absorption of α-tocopherol in control subjects and in patients with intestinal malabsorption. Clin Sci 38: 197–210, 1970

MacVicar K: Abuse of antiparkinsonian drugs by psychiatric patients. Am J Psychiatry 134:809–811, 1977

Manos N, Gkiouzepas J, Tzotzoras T, et al: Gradual withdrawal of antiparkinson medication in chronic schizophrenics: any better than the abrupt? J Nerv Ment Dis 169:659–661, 1981

Marcus R, Coulston AM: Fat-soluble vitamins: vitamins A, K, and E, in Goodman and Gilman's The Pharmacological Basis of Therapeutics, 9th Edition. Edited by Hardman JG, Limbird LE, Molinoff PB, et al. New York, McGraw-Hill, 1996, pp 1573–1590

Marder SR, Meibach RC: Risperidone in the treatment of schizophrenia. Am J Psychiatry 151:825–835, 1994

Mawdsley C, Williams IR, Pullar IA, et al: Treatment of parkinsonism by amantadine and levodopa. Clin Pharmacol Ther 13:575–583, 1972

McClelland HA, Blessed G, Bhate S, et al: The abrupt withdrawal of antiparkinsonian drugs in schizophrenic patients. Br J Psychiatry 124:151–159, 1974

McCreadie RG: The Nithsdale schizophrenia surveys: an overview. Soc Psychiatry Psychiatr Epidemiol 27:40–45, 1992

McCreadie RG, MacDonald E, Wiles D, et al: The Nithsdale schizophrenia surveys, XIV: plasma lipid peroxide and serum vitamin E levels in patients with and without tardive dyskinesia, and in normal subjects. Br J Psychiatry 167:610–617, 1995

McDevitt DG: Comparison of pharmacokinetic properties of beta-adrenoceptor blocking drugs. Eur Heart J 8 (suppl M):9–14, 1987

McEvoy JP: The clinical use of anticholinergic drugs as treatment for extrapyramidal side effects of neuroleptic drugs. J Clin Psychopharmacol 3:288–302, 1983

McEvoy JP, McCue M, Freter S: Replacement of chronically administered anticholinergic drugs by amantadine in outpatient management of chronic schizophrenia. Clin Ther 9:429–433, 1987

McEvoy JP, Hogarty GE, Steingard S: Optimal dose of neuroleptic in acute schizophrenia: a controlled study of the neuroleptic threshold and higher haloperidol dose. Arch Gen Psychiatry 48:739–745, 1991

Meco G, Bedini L, Bonifati V, et al: Risperidone in the treatment of chronic schizophrenia with tardive dyskinesia: a single-blind crossover study vs. placebo. Current Therapeutic Research 46:876–883, 1989

Medina C, Kramer MD, Kurland AA: Biperiden in the treatment of phenothiazine-induced extrapyramidal reactions. JAMA 182:1127–1129, 1962

Meldrum BS, Anlezark GM, Marsden CD: Acute dystonia as an idiosyncratic response to neuroleptics in baboons. Brain 100:313–326, 1977

Meltzer HY: The importance of serotonin-dopamine interactions in the action of clozapine. Br J Psychiatry 160 (suppl 17):22–29, 1992

Meltzer HY, Nash JF: Effects of antipsychotic drugs on serotonin receptors. Pharmacol Rev 43:587–604, 1991

Meltzer HY, Matsubara S, Lee JC: Classification of typical and atypical antipsychotic drugs on the basis of dopamine D-1, D-2 and serotonin$_2$ pKi values. J Pharmacol Exp Ther 251:238–246, 1989

Menza MA, Murray GB, Holmes VF, et al: Decreased extrapyramidal symptoms with intravenous haloperidol. J Clin Psychiatry 48:278–280, 1987

Merrick EM, Schmitt P: A controlled study of the clinical effects of amantadine hydrochloride (Symmetrel). Current Therapeutic Research 15:552–558, 1973

Metzer WS, Paige SR, Newton JE: Inefficacy of propranolol in attenuation of drug-induced parkinsonian tremor. Mov Disord 8:43–46, 1993

Meyer BR: Benzodiazepines in the elderly. Med Clin North Am 66:1017–1035, 1982

Miller NE: Effects of adrenoceptor-blocking drugs on plasma lipoprotein concentrations. Am J Cardiol 60:17E–23E, 1987

Mindham RHS: Assessment of drugs in schizophrenia: assessment of drug-induced extrapyramidal reactions and of drugs given for their control. Br J Clin Pharmacol 3 (suppl):395–400, 1976

Mindham RHS, Gaind R, Anstee BH, et al: Comparison of amantadine, orphenadrine, and placebo in the control of phenothiazine-induced parkinsonism. Psychol Med 2:406–413, 1972

Mino M: Clinical uses and abuses of vitamin E in children. Proc Soc Exp Biol Med 200:266–270, 1992

Moleman P, Schmitz PJM, Ladee GA: Extrapyramidal side effects and oral haloperidol: an analysis of explanatory patient and treatment characteristics. J Clin Psychiatry 43:492–496, 1982

Monane M: Insomnia in the elderly. J Clin Psychiatry 53 (suppl 6):23–28, 1992

Odergren T, Tollback A, Borg J: Electromyographic single motor unit potentials after repeated botulinum toxin treatments in cervical dystonia. Electroencephalogr Clin Neurophysiol 93:325–329, 1994

O'Flanagan PM: Clonazepam in the treatment of drug-induced dyskinesia. BMJ 1(5952):269–270, 1975

Pacifici GM, Nardini M, Ferrari P, et al: Effect of amantadine on drug-induced parkinsonism: relationship between plasma levels and effect. Br J Clin Pharmacol 3:883–889, 1976

Parkes JD, Zilkha KJ, Calver DM, et al: Controlled trial of amantadine hydrochloride in Parkinson's disease. Lancet 1:259–262, 1970

Paton DM, Webster DR: Clinical pharmacokinetics of H$_1$-receptor antagonists (the antihistamines). Clin Pharmacokinet 10:477–497, 1985

Perry EK, Perry RH, Blessed G, et al: Necropsy evidence of central cholinergic deficits in senile dementia (letter). Lancet 1(8004):189, 1977

Petit M, Raniwalla J, Tweed J, et al: A comparison of an atypical and typical antipsychotic, zotepine versus haloperidol in patients with acute exacerbation of schizophrenia: a parallel-group double-blind trial. Psychopharmacol Bull 32:81–87, 1996

Pi EH, Gutierrez MA, Gray GE: Cross-cultural studies in tardive dyskinesia (letter). Am J Psychiatry 150:991, 1993

Postma JU, Tilburg VW: Visual hallucinations and delirium during treatment with amantadine (Symmetrel). J Am Geriatr Soc 23:212–215, 1975

Pujalte D, Bottaï T, Huë B, et al: A double-blind comparison of clonazepam and placebo in the treatment of neuroleptic-induced akathisia. Clin Neuropharmacol 17:236–242, 1994

Quinn N, Hallet M: Dose standardisation of botulinum toxin (letter) (published erratum appears in Lancet 1[8646]:1092, 1989). Lancet 1(8644):964, 1989

Rashkis HA, Smarr ER: Protection against reserpine-induced "parkinsonism." Am J Psychiatry 113:1116, 1957

Reeves K, Harrigan EP: The efficacy and safety of two fixed doses of ziprasidone in schizophrenia and schizoaffective disorder. Poster presented at the 149th annual meeting of the American Psychiatric Association, New York, NY, May 4–9, 1996

Rifkin A, Quitkin F, Klein DF: Akinesia, a poorly recognized drug-induced extrapyramidal behavioral disorder. Arch Gen Psychiatry 32:672–674, 1975

Sachdev P: A rating scale for acute drug-induced akathisia: development, reliability, and validity. Biol Psychiatry 35:263–271, 1994

Saltz BL, Woerner MG, Kane JM, et al: Prospective study of tardive dyskinesia incidence in the elderly. JAMA 266:2402–2406, 1991

Sandyk R, Kay SR, Awerbuch GI: Subjective awareness of abnormal involuntary movements in schizophrenia. Int J Neurosci 69:1–20, 1993

Schmidt M, Meister P, Baumann P: Treatment of tardive dyskinesias with vitamin E. European Psychiatry 6:201–207, 1991

Schwab RS, Chafetz ME: Kemadrin in the treatment of parkinsonism. Neurology 5:273–277, 1955

Schwab RS, England AC, Poskanzer DC, et al: Amantadine in the treatment of Parkinson's disease. JAMA 208: 1160–1170, 1969

Schwab RS, Poskanzer DC, England AC Jr, et al: Amantadine in Parkinson's disease: review of more than two years' experience. JAMA 222:792–795, 1972

Scott AB: Botulinum toxin injections into extra ocular muscles as an alternative to strabismus surgery. Ophthalmology 87:1044–1049, 1980

Shear MK, Frances A, Weiden P: Suicide associated with akathisia and depot fluphenazine treatment. J Clin Psychopharmacol 3:235–236, 1983

Shriqui CL, Bradwejn J, Annable L, et al: Vitamin E in the treatment of tardive dyskinesia: a double-blind placebo-controlled study. Am J Psychiatry 149:391–393, 1992

Simpson GM: Long-acting, antipsychotic agents and extrapyramidal side effects. Diseases of the Nervous System 31 (suppl):12–14, 1970

Simpson GM, Angus JWS: A rating scale for extrapyramidal side effects. Acta Psychiatr Scand 212:11–19, 1970

Simpson GM, Lindermayer JP: Extrapyramidal symptoms in patients treated with risperidone. J Clin Psychopharmacol 17:194–201, 1997

Simpson GM, Amuso D, Blair JH, et al: Phenothiazine-produced extrapyramidal system disturbance. Arch Gen Psychiatry 10:199–208, 1964

Simpson GM, Amin M, Kunz E: Withdrawal effects of phenothiazines. Compr Psychiatry 6:347–351, 1965

Simpson GM, Krakov L, Mattke D, et al: A controlled comparison of the treatment of schizophrenic patients when treated according to the neuroleptic threshold or by clinical judgement. Acta Psychiatr Scand Suppl 212:38–43, 1970

Simpson GM, Beckles D, Isalski Z, et al: Some methodological considerations in the evaluation of drug-induced extrapyramidal disorders: a study of X10-029, a new morphanthridine derivative. J Clin Pharmacol 12:142–152, 1972

Simpson GM, Lee JH, Shrivastava RK: Clozapine in tardive dyskinesia. Psychopharmacologia 56:75–80, 1978

Simpson GM, Lee JH, Zoubok B, et al: A rating scale for tardive dyskinesia. Psychopharmacologia 64:171–179, 1979

Simpson GM, Cooper TB, Bark N, et al: Effect of antiparkinsonian medications on plasma levels of chlorpromazine. Arch Gen Psychiatry 37:205–208, 1980

Simpson GM, Pi EH, Sramek JJ Jr: Adverse effects of antipsychotic agents. Drugs 21:138–151, 1981

Simpson LL: The origin, structure, and pharmacologic activity of botulinum toxin. Pharmacol Rev 33:155–188, 1981

Singh H, Levinson DF, Simpson GM, et al: Acute dystonia during fixed-dose neuroleptic treatment. J Clin Psychopharmacol 10:389–396, 1990

Small JG, Hirsch SR, Arvanitis LA, et al: Quetiapine in patients with schizophrenia: a high- and low-dose double-blind comparison with placebo. Arch Gen Psychiatry 54: 549–557, 1997

Snyder S, Greenberg D, Yamamura HI: Antischizophrenic drugs and brain cholinergic receptors. Arch Gen Psychiatry 31:58–61, 1974

Sokol RJ: Vitamin E deficiency and neurologic disease. Annu Rev Nutr 8:351–373, 1988

Sokol RJ, Butler-Simon N, Conner C, et al: Multicenter trial of d-alpha-tocopheryl polyethylene glycol 1000 succinate for treatment of vitamin E deficiency in children with chronic cholestasis. Gastroenterology 104:1727–1735, 1993

Sokoloff P, Giros B, Martres MP, et al: Molecular cloning and characterization of a novel dopamine receptor (D_3) as a target for neuroleptics. Nature 347:146–151, 1990

Sommer BR, Cohen BM, Satlin A, et al: Changes in tardive dyskinesia symptoms in elderly patients treated with ganglioside GM1 or placebo. J Geriatr Psychiatry Neurol 7:234–237, 1994

Sramek JJ, Simpson GM, Morrison RL, et al: Anticholinergic agents for prophylaxis of neuroleptic-induced dystonic reactions: a prospective study. J Clin Psychiatry 47:305–309, 1986

St. Jean A, Donald MW, Ban TA: Uses and abuses of antiparkinsonian medication. Am J Psychiatry 120:801–803, 1964

Stanilla JK, Nair C, de Leon J, et al: Clozapine does not produce akathisia or parkinsonism. Poster presented at the 34th annual meeting of the American College of Neuropsychopharmacology, San Juan, Puerto Rico, December 11–15, 1995

Stanilla JK, Büchel C, Alarcon J, et al: Diurnal and weekly variation of tardive dyskinesia measured by digital image processing. Psychopharmacology (Berl) 124:373–376, 1996

Stanilla JK, de Leon J, Simpson GM: Clozapine withdrawal resulting in delirium with psychosis: a report of three cases. J Clin Psychiatry 58:252–255, 1997

Stenson RL, Donlon PT, Meyer JE: Comparison of benztropine mesylate and amantadine HCL in neuroleptic-induced extrapyramidal symptoms. Compr Psychiatry 17:763–768, 1976

Stephens DA: Psychotoxic effects of benzhexol hydrochloride (Artane). Br J Psychiatry 113:213–218, 1967

Stern TA, Anderson WH: Benztropine prophylaxis of dystonic reactions. Psychopharmacologia 61:261–262, 1979

Stoof JC, Booij J, Drukarch B: Amantadine as N-methyl-D-aspartic acid receptor antagonist: new possibilities for therapeutic applications? Clin Neurol Neurosurg 94: S4–S6, 1992

Strang RR: The syndrome of restless legs. Med J Aust 24:1211–1213, 1967

Stratas NE, Phillips RD, Walker PA, et al: A study of drug induced parkinsonism. Diseases of the Nervous System 24:180, 1963

Strömberg U, Svensson TH, Waldeck B: On the mode of action of amantadine. J Pharm Pharmacol 22:959–962, 1970

Swett C, Cole JO, Shapiro S, et al: Extrapyramidal side effects in chlorpromazine recipients. Arch Gen Psychiatry 34:942–943, 1977

Thaker GK, Tamminga CA, Alphs LD, et al: Brain gamma-aminobutyric acid abnormality in tardive dyskinesia: reduction in cerebrospinal fluid GABA levels and therapeutic response to GABA agonist treatment. Arch Gen Psychiatry 44:522–529, 1987

Thaker GK, Nguyen JA, Strauss ME, et al: Clonazepam treatment of tardive dyskinesia: a practical GABAmimetic strategy. Am J Psychiatry 147:445–451, 1990

Timberlake WH, Schwab RS, England AC Jr: Biperiden (Akineton) in parkinsonism. Arch Neurol 5:560–564, 1961

Tollefson GD, Beasley CM Jr, Tamura RN, et al: Blind, controlled, long-term study of the comparative incidence of treatment-emergent tardive dyskinesia with olanzapine or haloperidol. Am J Psychiatry 154:1248–1254, 1997a

Tollefson GD, Beasley CM Jr, Tran PV, et al: Olanzapine versus haloperidol in the treatment of schizophrenia and schizoaffective and schizophreniform disorders: results of an international collaborative trial. Arch Gen Psychiatry 54: 457–465, 1997b

Tune L, Coyle JT: Serum levels of anticholinergic drugs in treatment of acute extrapyramidal side effects. Arch Gen Psychiatry 37:293–297, 1980

Underwood BA: Vitamin A in animal and human nutrition, in The Retinoids, Vol I. Edited by Sporn MB, Roberts AB, Goodman DS. New York, Academic Press, 1984, pp 263–374

Van Putten T, May PR, Marder SR, et al: Subjective response to antipsychotic drugs. Arch Gen Psychiatry 38:187–190, 1981

Van Putten TR, May PR, Marder SR: Response to antipsychotic medication: the doctor's and the consumer's view. Am J Psychiatry 141:16–19, 1984

Van Tol H, Bunzow J, Guan H, et al: Cloning of the gene for a human dopamine D_4 receptor with high affinity for the antipsychotic clozapine. Nature 350:610–614, 1991

Wilbur R, Kulik FA, Kulik AV: Noradrenergic effects in tardive dyskinesia, akathisia and pseudoparkinsonism via the limbic system and basal ganglia. Prog Neuropsychopharmacol Biol Psychiatry 12:849–864, 1988

Winer JA, Bahn S: Loss of teeth with antidepressant drug therapy. Arch Gen Psychiatry 16:239–240, 1967

Wingfield WL, Pollack D, Grunert RR: Therapeutic efficacy of amantadine HCl and rimantadine HCl in naturally occurring influenza A2 respiratory illness in man. N Engl J Med 281:579–584, 1969

Witting LA: The role of polyunsaturated fatty acids in determining vitamin E requirements. Ann N Y Acad Sci 203: 192–198, 1972

Wojcik J, Gelenberg A, La Brie RA, et al: Prevalence of tardive dyskinesia in an outpatient population. Compr Psychiatry 21:370–379, 1980

Wolf G: Structure and possible function of an alpha-tocopherol-binding protein. Nutr Rev 52:97–98, 1994

Yahr MD, Duvoisin RC: Medical therapy of parkinsonism. Modern Treatment 5:283–300, 1968

Yamamura HI, Snyder SH: Muscarinic cholinergic receptor binding in the longitudinal muscle of the guinea pig ileum with [^{3}H] quinuclidinyl benzilate. Mol Pharmacol 10:861–867, 1974

Zimbroff DL, Kane JM, Tamminga CA, et al: Controlled, dose-response study of sertindole and haloperidol in the treatment of schizophrenia. Am J Psychiatry 154:782–791, 1997

Drugs for Treatment of Bipolar Disorder

in cells throughout the body, especially the brain, have provided fertile ground for research over the years.

It is worth noting that there exist in nature two stable isotopes of lithium (^{6}Li and ^{7}Li) that can readily be detected by nuclear magnetic resonance (NMR) spectroscopy (Detellier 1983). The isotope most commonly visualized with NMR spectroscopy is ^{7}Li, which constitutes almost 93% of natural lithium. Because reports indicate that these two isotopes may have small differences in biological activity, formulations of one or the other stable isotope might prove interesting in light of its relatively narrow therapeutic index as a psychotropic medication (Sherman et al. 1984). The introduction of ^{7}Li NMR techniques and magnetic resonance imaging (MRI) in vivo has permitted the determination of lithium transport and distribution in living organ or tissue, as well as the capability to differentiate free from membrane-bound intracellular lithium pools in intact cell systems (i.e., erythrocytes [red blood cells; RBCs] and liposomes) and in brain (Detellier 1983; Renshaw and Wicklund 1988; Renshaw et al. 1986).

In a study of 14 patients with bipolar disorder who underwent ^{7}Li NMR 1 month after initiation of lithium treatment for acute mania, the reduction in manic symptoms correlated significantly ($r = .64$) with the lithium concentration in the brain but not with that in serum ($r = .33$) (Kato et al. 1994). In a recent study, using ^{7}Li NMR in psychiatric patients, long-term lithium treatment resulted in a brain-to-serum concentration ratio of 0.76, as well as a significant correlation between lithium brain concentration and both serum concentration and daily dose (Riedl et al. 1997). Other studies using ^{7}Li NMR suggest that lithium is eliminated more slowly from brain and that the brain-to-serum concentration ratio varies with the circadian cycle (Komoroski et al. 1993; Plenge et al. 1994).

It is interesting that the lithium concentration in brain at 12 hours was independent of the lithium dosing schedule, despite the fact that the risk of relapse in bipolar patients taking lithium doses on alternate days is threefold greater than that in patients taking daily doses (Jensen et al. 1995, 1996). ^{1}H-NMR studies of RBCs in bipolar patients showed an elevation of proton spin lattice (T_1) relaxation times that returns to a normal level relative to control subjects after a week of lithium treatment (Rosenthal et al. 1986). Similar observations have been noted in MRI studies in frontal and temporal areas of the brain in bipolar patients (Rangel-Guerra et al. 1983). These studies may be indicative of lithium's effects on intracellular hydration and water transport (Ballast et al. 1986). Studies using these MRI techniques are under way to determine whether lithium concentrations in brain regions are associated with changes in myoinositol and with dimensional

(e.g., cognitive, psychological, motoric, neurovegetative) features of treatment response.

Lithium and Membrane Transport

It has been known for at least 40 years that lithium undergoes active transport across cell membranes (Zerahn 1955). Both membrane transport systems and ion channels play roles in the regulation of intracellular lithium. Transport systems may be either adenosine triphosphate (ATP) driven, like the sodium potassium ATPase pump, or driven by the net free energy of transmembrane concentration gradients, like the sodium-calcium exchange pump. These transport systems are likely to be relevant to the regulation of lithium in the cell body because they essentially regulate all steady-state intracellular ion concentration. Numerous studies have characterized the membrane transport of lithium and its interaction with other cations in both brain and peripheral tissues in an effort to address a potential mode of action of lithium in the treatment of bipolar disorder (Bach and Gallicchio 1990; Mota de Freitas et al. 1991; Riddell 1991).

Early evidence suggested that, in excitable cells, lithium influx occurred primarily through the voltage-sensitive Na$^+$ channel (Carmiliet 1964; El-Mallakh 1990; Keynes and Swan 1959). Lithium entry has been shown to occur on activation of the channel, especially during the depolarization phase, wherein lithium rushes into the cells at the expense of Na$^+$. This property of lithium may be reflected in the increase in plasma levels of lithium that occur as a patient becomes euthymic after treatment for an acute manic episode (Degkwitz et al. 1979). Additional evidence in neuroblastoma-glioma hybrid cells has indicated that lithium may also use the ouabain-sensitive Na,K-ATPase, but this was not observed in neurons in primary culture (Gorkin and Richelson 1981; Richelson 1977). Extrusion of lithium from the cell appears to depend on the gradient-dependent Na$^+$-Li$^+$ exchange process, wherein intracellular lithium substitutes for intracellular Na$^+$ (Hitzemann et al. 1989; Sarkadi et al. 1978). However, although evidence indicates that lithium enters the cell equally displacing Na$^+$ in excitable cells, lithium does have a tendency to accumulate in the cell because the removal of lithium is less efficient than that of Na$^+$ (Coppen and Shaw 1967; El-Mallakh 1990). Na,K-ATPase may play an indirect role because it establishes the Na$^+$ gradient in neurons: the greater is the Na$^+$ gradient, the greater is the rate of Na$^+$ efflux through the Na$^+$-Li$^+$ exchange.

Over the years, clinical studies of patients with manic-depressive disorder have revealed evidence for an increase in Na$^+$ retention and intracellular Na$^+$ (Coppen and Shaw 1963; Coppen et al. 1966; Naylor et al. 1970, 1971); a decrease in Na,K-ATPase activity (Hokin-Neaverson and Jefferson 1989a, 1989b; Naylor and Smith 1981; Naylor et al. 1980; Nurnberger et al. 1982); and, more recently, an increase in intracellular calcium in peripheral blood cells in both mania and depression (Dubovsky et al. 1991a, 1992). Lithium treatment has resulted in a reduction in intra-RBC Na$^+$ (Hermoni et al. 1987; Hitzemann et al. 1989), and studies using Fura 2-acetomethoxy ester (Fura 2-AM) fluorescence have identified a lithium-induced reduction of Ca^{2+} in platelets of bipolar patients (Dubovsky et al. 1991b). The fact that free calcium ion concentration tends to parallel free sodium concentration may account for the lithium-induced reduction in free Ca^{2+} ion concentrations noted previously (Mullins and Brinley 1977; Torok 1989).

Studies have suggested that an alteration in the activity of the Na,K-ATPase pump could result in significant changes in neuronal excitability and may represent a pathogenesis for mood disorders (El-Mallakh 1983; Hokin-Neaverson et al. 1974; Naylor and Smith 1981). However, clinical studies in RBCs over the years have reported conflicting data in patients with bipolar disorder, and a reduction in Na,K-ATPase activity has been noted predominantly in the depressed phase of both unipolar and bipolar patients (Akagawa et al. 1980; Alexander et al. 1986; Choi et al. 1977; Dagher et al. 1984; El-Mallakh 1983; Glen and Reading 1973; Hokin-Neaverson and Jefferson 1989b; Hokin-Neaverson et al. 1974; Naylor et al. 1974a; Nurnberger et al. 1982; Reddy et al. 1989; Sengupta et al. 1980; Strzyzewski et al. 1984). Multiple factors, such as psychotropic drugs, circulating hormones, and diet, have probably contributed to much of this variability (Swann 1984, 1988; A. J. Wood et al. 1989b).

Early studies in frog muscle found that lithium is a poor substrate for Na,K-ATPase (Keynes and Swan 1959). Studies in whole brain of animals revealed an acute inhibition of lithium on Na,K-ATPase activity. Evidence indicated that chronic lithium treatment resulted in an inhibition of the Na,K-ATPase enzyme in synaptosomal membrane fractions from brain that appeared to be regionally specific to the hippocampus (Guerri et al. 1981; Swann et al. 1980). Furthermore, this inhibition represented a reduction in the maximum rate of metabolism (V_{max}) of the enzyme, with no apparent change in affinity (K_m [a dissociation constant that provides a measure of the affinity of the substrate(s) for the enzyme]), and was selective for neurons that have the enzyme subtype with high affinity for ouabain binding. Similar observations of lithium inhibition of Na,K-ATPase have been made in peripheral neurons and have been attributed to an action of lith-

ium competing for the intracellular Na$^+$ activation site of the enzyme (Ritchie and Straub 1980).

On the other hand, studies of RBC membranes in patients treated with lithium have revealed evidence for increased activity of Na,K-ATPase (Bunney and Garland-Bunney 1987; Dick et al. 1978; Hokin-Neaverson et al. 1976; B. B. Johnson et al. 1980; Mallinger et al. 1987; Naylor et al. 1974b, 1980; Reddy et al. 1989; Swann 1988; A. J. Wood et al. 1989a). These data have been accounted for in part by a concomitant lithium-induced inhibition, mediated through intracellular interaction with the Na$^+$ binding site, and activation, mediated through an extracellular K site (Collard 1986; Lazarus and Muston 1978). However, although the flux of lithium through voltage-dependent sodium channels may contribute to the regulation of steady-state lithium homeostasis within the cell, the gating of lithium via ion channels is likely to be more physiologically relevant at the synapse. In the local environment of a dendritic spine, where the surface-to-volume ratio becomes relatively large, the lithium component of a synaptic current can theoretically cause very significant increases in the local lithium concentration after a train of synaptic stimuli (Kabakob et al., in press). This remains a fertile area for future investigation.

RBCs have served as a cell model for a series of clinical investigations over the years because they share lithium transport properties with neurons and are easily accessible (Bach and Gallicchio 1990; Mota de Freitas et al. 1991). At therapeutic levels, influx of lithium into RBCs occurs predominantly through passage as a cation through the "leak," or passive diffusion, pathway. Additional routes of entry for lithium include an Na$^+$ (Li$^+$)–K$^+$ cotransport pathway and the anion exchange pathway, wherein its small size and high charge density permit its anionic transport in complex with bicarbonate. Efflux of lithium occurs primarily through the Na$^+$-Li$^+$ countertransport pathway, and additional routes are through the passive leak pathway and (to a lesser extent) the Na,K-ATPase pump. There is no evidence that lithium treatment alters the transport properties of either the leak or the Na$^+$ (Li$^+$)–K$^+$ cotransport pathway.

Although early studies suggested that the RBC-to-plasma lithium concentration ratio was related to a history of bipolar disorder, and that a higher ratio was associated with a clinical response to lithium treatment, it was soon evident that a large interindividual variation precluded adequate replication of these findings (Mendels and Frazer 1973; Ramsey et al. 1979; Richelson et al. 1986; Szentistvanyi and Janka 1979). These investigations, however, led to the hypothesis that the pathogenesis of affective disorders was related to membrane dysfunction (Ehrlich and

Diamond 1980). This hypothesis was followed by a series of studies using lithium transport properties in RBCs as a genetic marker and reporting a reduction in Na^+-Li^+ transport rates in a subgroup of bipolar patients and some family members (Ehrlich and Diamond 1979, 1980; Frazer et al. 1978; Ostrow et al. 1978; Pandey et al. 1977, 1978; Ramsey et al. 1979; Sarkadi et al. 1978; Shaughnessy et al. 1985; Szentistvanyi and Janka 1979). Here again, variability of data both within and between patients contributed to the failure to replicate these findings in other studies (Dagher et al. 1984; Egeland et al. 1984; Greil et al. 1977; Mallinger et al. 1983; Richelson et al. 1986). These data were also confounded by the fact that lithium treatment results in a progressive inhibition of Na^+-Li^+ countertransport (Ehrlich et al. 1981, 1983) and a history of hypertension is associated with elevated rates of Na^+-Li^+ transport (Canessa et al. 1980, 1987). In a recent study of 22 bipolar patients in which the RBC apparent rate constant for lithium efflux (K_{exch}) was used, the investigators suggested that this index may serve to predict the risk of failure of maintenance therapy at 1 year (Mallinger et al. 1997).

Over the years, investigators have observed that chronic administration of lithium increases choline concentration in RBCs by more than 10-fold (Jope et al. 1978, 1980; Lee et al. 1974; Lingsch and Martin 1976; Meltzer et al. 1982; Rybakowski et al. 1978; Stoll et al. 1991; Uney et al. 1985). This appears to be the result of not only an inhibition of choline transport but also an enhanced phospholipase D–mediated degradation of choline-containing phospholipids (Chapman et al. 1982; B. L. Miller et al. 1989, 1990). The latter effect of chronic lithium use may be mediated by its action on protein kinase C (PKC), which is discussed later in this chapter.

Because lithium also has been shown to inhibit choline transport in the human brain (Ehrlich et al. 1980), this effect of lithium may account for a lithium-induced increase in cholinergic tone in the brain, which accounts for its therapeutic effects (Jope 1979; Uney and Marchbanks 1987; Uney et al. 1986). However, unlike in RBCs, in which choline transport inhibition is irreversible, choline in the brain can be readily metabolized to acetylcholine or incorporated into lipids. The effect of this effect of lithium is currently unknown (Diamond et al. 1982/1983; Lingsch and Martin 1976; Uney et al. 1986). Although studies have attempted to use intra-RBC choline concentration before and after lithium administration as a predictor of clinical response, the data are conflicting and need further study (Haag et al. 1984, 1987; Kuchel et al. 1984; Stoll et al. 1991).

It is of interest that lithium efflux appears to be inhibited by approximately 50% in patients after treatment with lithium for at least 1 week and is associated with a threefold increase in the apparent K_m for the Na^+-Li^+ pathway, with no change in the countertransport rate V_{max} (Ehrlich et al. 1981). NMR studies have found that the intracellular uptake of lithium is rather slow and have confirmed the increased accumulation of intra-RBC lithium after several days of chronic exposure to lithium (Riddell 1991). Similarly, as we have noted, chronic use of lithium results in a significantly elevated intracellular concentration of choline that persists long after lithium levels in both plasma and RBCs are no longer detectable (Lee et al. 1974; Lingsch and Martin 1976; Meltzer et al. 1982; Rybakowski et al. 1978). These effects of lithium appear to correspond to the time course of the clinical efficacy of lithium treatment and have led to suggestions that chronic lithium use may induce an evolving change in membrane structure or interaction with membrane-bound enzymes (Ehrlich et al. 1983).

Although these data are of considerable interest, caution must be used in direct extrapolation from a nonnucleated peripheral cell model to one involving excitable nucleated neuronal cells within the brain. Moreover, recent data, such as those on Na,K-ATPase, support the evolution of specific gene products expressed and posttranslationally regulated uniquely, not only to neurons but also among brain regions (Arystarkhoua and Sweadner 1996; Grillo et al. 1994; Lecuona et al. 1996; Malik et al. 1996; Munzer et al. 1994; Sahin-Erdemli et al. 1995). Thus, although the RBC may be used as a peripheral model for lithium transport, extrapolations to lithium homeostasis in the brain or as a potential genetic marker for variations in ionic homeostatic processes in the brain underlying the pathophysiology of a disease such as bipolar disorder remain highly speculative. On the other hand, a better understanding of activity-dependent mechanisms via ligand-gated ion channels for creating localized increases of intracellular lithium at sites of high synaptic activity may be critical for lithium's therapeutic specificity and ability to regulate synaptic function in the brain.

MECHANISM OF ACTION

Unlike most psychotropic drugs, which primarily treat symptomatology, lithium is effective in prophylactically stabilizing the underlying disease process by reducing the frequency and severity of the profound mood cycling associated with bipolar disorder. Thus, identification of the molecular target(s) for the long-term action of lithium in the brain may lead to new psychopharmacological strategies and, in concert with the discovery of susceptibility genes, will improve the understanding of the pathophysiology of the disorder (Lenox and Watson 1994; Lenox et al., in press).

Lithium and Circadian Rhythms

Although studies of circadian rhythms in patients with affective disorders have often been limited by their cross-sectional design and heterogeneous patient populations and have been confounded by significant variability, disturbance in biological rhythms has remained a viable hypothesis underlying the (episodic) dysregulation observed in bipolar illness (Goodwin and Jamison 1990). The alteration in circadian rhythms appears to be manifested in an overall reduction in amplitude, possibly attributable to phase instability, and the tendency to phase advance that is observed in rapid eye movement (REM) sleep and core temperature relative to the sleep-wake cycle. Lithium has been shown to slow circadian oscillators in a wide variety of species ranging from plants to humans (Klemfuss and Kripke 1989). Note that deuterium shares this property. Because both lithium and deuterium increase the density of tissue water, both compounds may exert their chronotropic effects by virtue of their action on membrane processes (Hallonquist et al. 1986).

Various studies in animals have reported that lithium appears to lengthen the endogenous period of several circadian rhythms under free-running conditions. In the presence of environmental cues (zeitgebers) for entrainment, this lengthening of the circadian rhythm by chronic lithium administration is reflected in a delay in rhythms associated with wheel-running, sleep-wake cycle, and photoperiodic reproductive response, as well as several endocrine and biochemical variables.

In a study of squirrel monkeys, chronic lithium administration at "therapeutic" concentrations significantly lengthened the period of free-running circadian activity rhythms (Welsh and Moore-Ede 1990). However, the effects of lithium on the regulation of hormones and neurotransmitter receptors in the brain have not consistently shown a phase delay (Kafka et al. 1983; McEachron et al. 1982; Wirz-Justice 1983; Wirz-Justice et al. 1982). Although this may reflect the ability of lithium to differentially dissociate circadian rhythms, similar to findings observed with antidepressants, supportive data remain weak.

Comparable studies in humans have been less convincing, undoubtedly because of the previously noted limitations associated with clinical investigations (Johnsson et al. 1983; Welsh et al. 1986; Wever 1979). It has been observed in various studies that lithium can phase-delay circadian rhythms in human subjects entrained to a 24-hour-day schedule, consistent with its ability to lengthen the intrinsic period of a circadian oscillator (Kripke et al. 1979; Kupfer et al. 1970; Mendels and Chernik 1973). Although few studies have examined the effects of lithium on circadian rhythms in bipolar patients, one study of a bipolar patient studied in depth revealed evidence for a significant and sustained lithium-induced delay in circadian core temperature and onset of REM, with a reduction in percentage of REM during total sleep time (Campbell et al. 1989). These data were consistent with earlier electroencephalographic findings in a series of patients with bipolar disorder (Kupfer et al. 1970, 1974). However, it has been difficult to indicate a clinical correlation of change in affective state with a lithium-induced resynchronization of circadian rhythms (Campbell et al. 1989; Kripke et al. 1978; Wehr and Goodwin 1979).

It is also of interest that data from earlier studies by Lewy et al. (1987) reported that bipolar patients appear to be supersensitive to light-induced reduction of nocturnal plasma melatonin levels. Wever (1979) suggested that a pacemaker with increased sensitivity to zeitgebers might become phase-advanced relative to the slower intrinsic period of the human circadian oscillator. This observation is also of interest because melatonin has been reported to promote internal and external synchronization in both animals and humans. An alteration in relative melatonin concentrations might therefore be instrumental in dissociation between different circadian rhythms (Arendt et al. 1986; Gwinner and Benzinger 1978; Rao and Mager 1987). Furthermore, studies by Seggie et al. (1989) examining dark adaptation threshold documented an increased sensitivity to light in bipolar patients that appears to be reduced in male patients receiving chronic lithium administration. Such a lithium-induced increase in dark adaptation threshold appears to be related to the effects of lithium on the adenylate cyclase second-messenger system (Carney et al. 1988; Kaschka et al. 1987).

In a recent study, Williams and Jope (1995) determined that there is a circadian rhythm for the DNA-binding activity for the transcription factor family AP-1 by the cholinergic agonist pilocarpine (see section, "Lithium and Gene Expression," later in this chapter) and sought to investigate the potential effect of lithium on this circadian rhythm. After acute lithium treatment, pilocarpine administration induced generalized seizures after about 20 minutes and stimulated AP-1 DNA binding activity, which increased (to 900% of basal) within 4.5 hours. Interestingly, a circadian variation was apparent in AP-1 DNA-binding activity, and stimulation at 8:00 A.M. was 1.5 times that at 4:00 P.M. However, although pilocarpine induced seizures in the presence of lithium, there was no circadian variation in pilocarpine-stimulated AP-1 DNA-binding activity. These findings suggest that lithium exerts a complex action on the circadian rhythm of many biochemical mediators that are known to exert both short- and long-term effects on neuronal function.

It remains a working hypothesis that the therapeutic action of lithium can be attributed to its efficacy in correcting a putative phase advance and/or internal desynchronization of these biological rhythms in patients with bipolar disorder. It has yet to be determined to what extent this hypothesis is related to lithium's action in directly altering the sensitivity of the intrinsic pacemaker to environmental cues and/or the coupling process between internal oscillators, through either the suprachiasmatic nucleus or melatonin secretion.

Lithium and Neurotransmission

Serotonin

Extensive research has been devoted to the effect of lithium on brain monoaminergic systems. A leading current theory hypothesizes that the antidepressant effects of lithium are the result of an augmentation of serotonin (5-hydroxytryptamine [5-HT]) function in the central nervous system (CNS) (de Montigny et al. 1983, 1988; Meltzer and Lowy 1987; Price et al. 1990). Preclinical studies show that lithium's effects on serotonin function may occur at a variety of levels, including precursor uptake, synthesis, storage, catabolism, release, receptors, and receptor-effector interaction (Bunney and Garland 1984; Bunney and Garland-Bunney 1987; Goodnick and Gershon 1985; Knapp and Mandell 1975; Price et al. 1990). Overall, reasonable evidence from preclinical studies suggests that lithium enhances serotonergic neurotransmission, although its effects on serotonin appear to vary depending on brain region, length of treatment, and serotonin receptor subtype (Bunney and Garland 1984; Bunney and Garland-Bunney 1987; Goodnick and Gershon 1985; Price et al. 1990; A. J. Wood and Goodwin 1987). Several preclinical studies show that tryptophan uptake and/or content are increased in synaptosomes and brain tissue after short-term and long-term treatment, whereas a single dose is without effect (Berggren 1987; Goodnick and Gershon 1985; Laakso and Oja 1979; Price et al. 1990; Swann et al. 1981; Tagliamonte et al. 1971). Studies of the effects of short-term lithium treatment on brain concentrations of serotonin or 5-hydroxy-indoleacetic acid (5-HIAA) have yielded conflicting results, although most tend to show increases in one or both (Berggren 1987; Goodnick and Gershon 1985; Price et al.

1990; Swann et al. 1981; Tagliamonte et al. 1971). In contrast, most long-term studies tend to show that serotonin and 5-HIAA levels decrease with lithium treatment (Ahluwalia and Singhal 1980; Bunney and Garland 1984; Collard 1978; Collard and Roberts 1977; Shukla 1985; Treiser et al. 1981). Treiser et al. (1981) found that long-term lithium treatment increased basal and K^+-stimulated serotonin release in the hippocampus but not in the cortex. Another study also reported that lithium increased serotonin release in the parietal cortex, hypothalamus, and hippocampus after 2–3 weeks but not after a single injection or 1 week of treatment (Friedman and Wang 1988).

Studies on receptor binding have shown complex, regionally specific effects of acute or chronic lithium treatment on the density of 5-HT$_1$ or 5-HT$_2$ receptors, although most suggest decreases in both sites, at least in the hippocampus (Godfrey et al. 1989; Goodnick and Gershon 1985; Goodwin et al. 1986b; Hotta and Yamawaki 1988; Maggi and Enna 1980; Mizuta and Segawa 1989; Newman et al. 1990; Odagaki et al. 1990; Tanimoto et al. 1983; Treiser and Kellar 1980; Treiser et al. 1981). Similarly, the reported effects of both short- and long-term lithium treatment on 5-HT$_2$-mediated head twitch behavior and hyperactivity responses to the serotonin precursor 5-hydroxytryptophan (5-HTP) have been inconsistent (Friedman et al. 1979a; Goodwin et al. 1986b; Grahame-Smith and Green 1974; Harrison-Read 1979). However, the prolactin response to serotonin is more consistently reported to be increased after short-term lithium administration (Koenig et al. 1984; Meltzer and Lowy 1987; Meltzer et al. 1981). Recent studies have attempted to clarify the roles of pre- and postsynaptic receptors in mediating the effects of lithium on serotonin function. Investigators used a variety of methodologies to provide evidence that lithium produces a subsensitivity of presynaptic inhibitory 5-HT$_{1A}$ receptors (Friedman and Wang 1988; Goodwin et al. 1986a; Hotta and Yamawaki 1988; Mork and Geisler 1989a; Newman et al. 1990; Wang and Friedman 1988), which might result in a net increase of the amount of serotonin released per impulse.

In a series of important preclinical investigations, Blier, de Montigny, and others (Blier and de Montigny 1985; Blier et al. 1987) used electrophysiological recordings to measure the effects of lithium on the serotonin system. Short-term lithium did not affect the responsiveness of the postsynaptic neuron to serotonin or the electrical activity of the serotonin neurons, but it enhanced the efficacy of the ascending (presynaptic) serotonin system (Blier and de Montigny 1985; Blier et al. 1987). These observations led the investigators to propose that lithium might increase the efficacy of other antidepressant treatments (Blier and de Montigny 1985; Blier et al. 1987). Several open and double-blind clinical investigations have reported that approximately 50% of nonresponders are converted to responders with lithium administration within 2 weeks (de Montigny et al. 1981, 1983; Heninger et al. 1983). Although these effects have been attributed to the net effect of presynaptic facilitation of serotonin release onto "sensitized" receptors, convincing direct evidence of enhanced serotonin function in humans has been difficult to obtain (Cowen et al. 1989; Manji et al. 1991b).

Many early studies in cerebrospinal fluid (CSF) of human subjects are difficult to interpret because of their methodology and study design, and they are most often confounded by concomitant alterations in mood state and neurovegetative symptomatology. Small increases in 5-HIAA levels in CSF have been reported after subchronic lithium treatment in bipolar patients (Berrettini et al. 1985b; Bowers and Heninger 1977; Fyro et al. 1975; Goodnick 1990; Goodnick and Gershon 1985; Linnoila et al. 1984; Price et al. 1990; Swann et al. 1987), and some studies have found a significant positive correlation between pretreatment levels of 5-HIAA in CSF and lithium response (Bowers and Heninger 1977; Goodnick 1990; Goodnick and Gershon 1985). Although several studies have suggested that long-term lithium treatment "normalizes" a previously low platelet serotonin uptake in bipolar patients, an effect that may persist for several weeks after discontinuation (Born et al. 1980; Coppen et al. 1980; Meltzer et al. 1983; Poirier et al. 1988), the effects of lithium treatment on [^{3}H]imipramine binding in platelets remain inconclusive (Meltzer and Lowy 1987; Poirier et al. 1988; Price et al. 1990; K. Wood et al. 1983). Neuroendocrine studies in patients have been more consistent, showing that acute or subacute lithium treatment results in augmented prolactin and/or cortisol responses to various challenges (e.g., fenfluramine, tryptophan, 5-HTP) in affectively ill patients (Cowen et al. 1989; Glue et al. 1986; McCance et al. 1989; Meltzer et al. 1984; Muhlbauer 1984; Muhlbauer and Muller-Oerlinghausen 1985; Price et al. 1989). However, studies in healthy volunteer subjects after 2 weeks of "therapeutic" lithium did not have increased neuroendocrine responses, suggesting that lithium's effect on the serotonergic system may depend on its underlying activity (Manji et al. 1991a).

Overall, current evidence from both preclinical and clinical studies supports a role for lithium in enhancing presynaptic activity in the serotonergic system in the brain. Direct studies of lithium's effects on serotonergic neurotransmission in humans have previously been limited by several factors: the complexity of the widespread distribution of serotonergic fibers throughout the brain, the multiple receptor subtypes (which have only been recently recognized), the relative lack of serotonin-specific pharmacological agents and outcome variables reflecting selective serotonergic responses, and inadequate attention to effects dependent on duration of treatment and affective or physiological state of the patient. With the current understanding of the molecular neurobiology of both receptor subtypes and the transporter in the serotonergic system, we anticipate newer and more specific pharmacological probes for future preclinical and clinical investigations.

Dopamine

The effect of lithium on dopamine synthesis and transmission has been investigated extensively in preclinical studies by directly determining changes in dopamine or homovanillic acid and indirectly examining lithium-induced changes in dopamine-linked behaviors (Bunney and Garland 1984; Bunney and Garland-Bunney 1987; Goodnick and Gershon 1985). Studies in animals suggest that lithium may differentially affect dopamine pathways, increasing dopamine turnover in hypothalamic-tuberoinfundibular dopamine neurons, with conflicting reports about changes in brain stem areas (Corrodi et al. 1967; Goodnick and Gershon 1985; Murphy 1976). Lithium administration has also been found to cause a dose-dependent decrease of dopamine formation (Ahluwalia and Singhal 1980; Ahluwalia et al. 1981; Engel and Berggren 1980; Eroglu et al. 1981; Frances et al. 1981; Friedman and Gershon 1973; Hesketh et al. 1978), which occurs at doses that are 25% lower in the striatum than in the limbic forebrain (Laakso and Oja 1979; Poitou and Bohuon 1975; Segal et al. 1975).

In an effort to assess the effects of chronic lithium treatment on dopamine receptors and their coupling to guanine nucleotide binding proteins (G proteins), Carli et al. (1994) found that chronic lithium treatment did not modify the antagonist saturation binding to either dopamine, subtype 1 (D_1), or D_2 receptors. However, competition studies of the same antagonists by dopamine revealed biphasic curves, and the inhibition constant of the high-affinity site was significantly increased after chronic Li$^+$, suggesting an alteration in the coupling efficacy between G proteins and dopamine receptors. Furthermore, chronic but not acute lithium administration led to a reduction of guanosine triphosphate (GTP)-induced and dopamine-sensitive adenylate cyclase activity, without changes in the basal activity or in forskolin (colforsin)-induced cyclic adenosine monophosphate (cAMP) production.

Overall, these results suggest that chronic lithium treatment diminishes neostriatal dopaminergic activity, probably through an alteration in both the coupling process and the capacity of the G proteins, once activated, to stimulate adenylate cyclase. In a more recent study (Acquas and Fibiger 1996), the effects of chronic lithium treatment on methylphenidate, D_1 receptor agonist (A-77636), and tactile stimulation-induced increases in frontal cortical acetylcholine release were studied in the rat using in vivo brain microdialysis. Although chronic lithium administration did not influence normal arousal-related increases in cortical acetylcholine release, it did reduce dopamine-mediated increases in acetylcholine, which may have relevance for its efficacy in preventing large affective excursions from the norm.

Based on the heuristic hypothesis that supersensitive dopamine receptors underlie the development of manic episodes, it has been postulated that lithium would prevent dopamine receptor supersensitivity (Bunney and Garland 1984; Bunney and Garland-Bunney 1987; Goodnick and Gershon 1985). In a series of studies, lithium prevented haloperidol-induced dopamine receptor upregulation (Bunney 1981; Rosenblatt et al. 1980; Verimer et al. 1980) and supersensitivity to iontophoretically applied dopamine or intravenous apomorphine (Gallager et al. 1978). Lithium treatment also partially prevented the development of electrical intracranial self-stimulation usually produced by haloperidol in rats (Bunney and Garland-Bunney 1987; Goodnick and Gershon 1985; Staunton et al. 1982a, 1982b). Thus, lithium appears to be effective in blocking both the behavioral and the biochemical manifestations of supersensitive dopamine receptors induced by receptor blockade. Interestingly, there is significantly less evidence that lithium is effective in blocking dopamine receptor supersensitivity induced by other methods (i.e., tyrosine hydroxylase inhibitors, reserpine, or lesions of the dopamine pathways) (Beckmann et al. 1975; Bloom et al. 1981; Bunney 1981; Pert et al. 1978; Rosenblatt et al. 1980; Tanimoto et al. 1983; Verimer et al. 1980).

A proposed site of action for lithium's ability to block behavioral supersensitivity is the postsynaptic receptor and the prevention of haloperidol-induced increases in dopamine receptors. Although this theory is consistent with the observation that lithium can decrease locomotor activity even in the absence of presynaptic dopamine terminals (Swerdlow et al. 1985), lithium treatment does not result in any consistent effects on the density of D_1 or D_2 receptors. Reports purporting to show its ability to block the increase in dopamine receptor density after receptor blockade are conflicting. However, a study designed to examine lithium's effects on both pre- and post-synaptic dopamine receptors using different doses of apomorphine suggested that the drug was equally effective at both sites (Verimer et al. 1980). Indeed, electrophysiological data examining the effects of lithium on presynaptic dopamine receptors in the substantia nigra are also compatible with a blockade of dopamine receptor supersensitivity (Gallager et al. 1978). Thus, despite significant functional evidence, dopamine receptor binding studies remain inconclusive, suggesting a possible post-receptor site of lithium action that may be related to receptor-effector coupling. Interestingly, some studies have reported a lack of effect when lithium is administered after the induction of dopamine supersensitivity (Bloom et al. 1983; Klawans et al. 1976; Staunton et al. 1982a, 1982b), suggesting that in this model lithium exerts its greatest effects prophylactically.

Among the numerous behavioral effects of lithium in animals, perhaps the best studied are those on stimulant-induced activity. Lithium's ability to antagonize increases in locomotor activity produced by amphetamine has gained much attention, perhaps because this model has been postulated to be a better representation of lithium's effects on manic behavior (Allikmets et al. 1979; Bunney and Garland-Bunney 1987; Goodnick and Gershon 1985; Klawans et al. 1976; Pert et al. 1978; Staunton et al. 1982a). It is also of interest that lithium has been reported to attenuate the euphoriant and motor-activating effects of oral amphetamine in depressed patients, although equivocal results have been observed with methylphenidate challenge (Huey et al. 1981; van Kammen et al. 1985). Lithium has been shown to exert an inhibitory effect on intracranial self-stimulation subacutely. However, this effect does not persist with chronic administration, suggesting a possible lack of relevance to its long-term mood-stabilizing effects (Seeger et al. 1981).

Studies of dopamine and its metabolites in the CSF of patients before and after lithium treatment have produced conflicting results (Berrettini et al. 1985b; Bowers and Heninger 1977; Fyro et al. 1975; Goodnick and Gershon 1985; Linnoila et al. 1983; Swann et al. 1987). A longitudinal study of one unipolar and seven bipolar female patients found that lithium reduced the levels of 3,4-dihydroxyphenylacetic acid (DOPAC), dopamine, and homovanillic acid in all patients (Linnoila et al. 1983). However, the possible role of alterations in mood state and motor activity remains a confounding variable, as it does for all clinical investigations in which this research strategy has been used. The administration of lithium to bipolar patients or control subjects does not significantly affect serum prolactin levels (Brown et al. 1981; Lal et al.

1978; Manji et al. 1991a; Rosenblatt et al. 1979) nor does it alter prolactin response to thyrotropin-releasing hormone in control subjects. However, in patients with mania, lithium does appear to enhance thyrotropin-releasing-hormone-stimulated prolactin response, which is once again suggestive of a differential response in patients compared with control subjects (Tanimoto et al. 1981). Although data from human investigations are sparse, lithium's postulated ability to reduce both pre- and postsynaptic aspects of dopamine transmission represents an attractive mechanism for its antimanic therapeutic action.

Norepinephrine

Lithium's effects on norepinephrine have been reported to be specific for both time points and brain regions (Ahluwalia and Singhal 1981; Bliss and Ailion 1970; Cameron and Smith 1980; Colburn et al. 1967; Goodnick and Gershon 1985; Katz and Kopin 1969; Katz et al. 1968; Kuriyama and Speken 1970; Poitou and Bohuon 1975; Schildkraut et al. 1969; Stern et al. 1969; K. Wood et al. 1985). Most early studies conducted at single time points found no alterations in the levels of norepinephrine or the rate of synthesis. Subsequent investigations revealed biphasic effects, with early increases in labeled norepinephrine uptake into rat brain synaptosomes and increases in the rate of norepinephrine synthesis, followed by a return to baseline values after chronic treatment (Ahluwalia and Singhal 1980; Cameron and Smith 1980; Colburn et al. 1967; Kuriyama and Speken 1970; Tanimoto et al. 1981). Both acute and chronic lithium treatment have been reported to increase (Schildkraut et al. 1966, 1969) or not to change the turnover of norepinephrine in some regions of the brain (Ahluwalia and Singhal 1980; Ho et al. 1970). Although these results suggested that lithium may increase the activity of the enzyme monoamine oxidase, subsequent data remain conflicting (Berrettini et al. 1979; Dawood and Welch 1979; Murphy 1976; Poitou and Bohuon 1975; Segal et al. 1975).

As is the case with the other neurotransmitters, the effects of lithium on norepinephrine receptor binding studies in rodent brain have been generally inconclusive (Maggi and Enna 1980; Schultz et al. 1981; Treiser and Kellar 1979). However, significant effects have been consistently observed on β-adrenergic receptor-mediated cAMP accumulation, lithium inhibiting the response both in vivo and in vitro (discussed in detail later in this chapter). Studies have also investigated the effects of chronic lithium on drug-induced changes in β receptor sensitivity. Lithium was unable to block antidepressant-induced downregulation (Rosenblatt et al. 1979) and in fact produced a greater

subsensitivity (i.e., cAMP response) (Mork et al. 1990), but it prevented reserpine or 6-hydroxydopamine-induced β-adrenergic receptor supersensitivity (Hermoni et al. 1980; Pert et al. 1979; Treiser and Kellar 1979). Additional data from preclinical and clinical studies suggest that lithium treatment results in subsensitive α_2 receptors (Catalano et al. 1984; Goodnick and Meltzer 1984a; Goodwin et al. 1986a; Huey et al. 1981; Murphy et al. 1974). In preclinical studies, long-term lithium attenuates α_2-adrenergic-mediated behavioral effects (Goodwin et al. 1986a; Smith 1988) and presynaptic α_2 inhibition of norepinephrine release (Spengler et al. 1986) while enhancing K^+-evoked norepinephrine release (Ebstein et al. 1983).

Although lithium has been reported to reduce high-affinity platelet [^3H]clonidine binding (Garcia-Sevilla et al. 1986; Pandey et al. 1989; K. Wood and Coppen 1983), compatible with a functional "uncoupling" of the receptor from the G protein (Kim and Neubig 1987; Neubig et al. 1988), interpretation of these data is confounded by the coexistence of a newly discovered imidazoline-binding site. Additional clinical investigations of lithium reported a decrease in growth hormone response to clonidine (an α_2 partial agonist) in control subjects (Brambilla et al. 1988; Catalano et al. 1984). Lithium also appears to reverse the blunted growth hormone response observed in depressed patients (Brambilla et al. 1988). These bidirectional effects should serve to remind us that lithium's effects may depend in part on the preexisting set point of the neural substrate—an attractive notion in view of lithium's efficacy in the treatment of manic as well as depressive episodes.

In clinical investigations, both increases and decreases in plasma and urinary norepinephrine metabolite levels have been reported after lithium treatment (Beckmann et al. 1975; Corona et al. 1982; Goodnick 1990; Greenspan et al. 1970; Grof et al. 1986; Linnoila et al. 1983; Murphy et al. 1979; Schildkraut 1973, 1974; Swann et al. 1987). Lithium has been reported to reduce the excretion of norepinephrine and its metabolites in manic patients while increasing its excretion in depressed patients, an effect associated with higher plasma norepinephrine concentrations in some patients (Beckmann et al. 1975; Bowers and Heninger 1977; Greenspan et al. 1970; Schildkraut 1973). However, there is also evidence that urinary excretion of 3-methoxy-4-hydroxyphenylglycol is low during bipolar depression and elevated during mania-hypomania (Bond et al. 1972; Jones et al. 1973; Post et al. 1977; Schildkraut et al. 1973; Wehr 1977). In part, these inconsistencies may be related to the inability to control adequately for state-dependent changes in affective states, with associated changes in activity level, arousal, and sympathetic outflow.

Studies have found that 2 weeks of lithium administration in control subjects resulted in increases in urinary norepinephrine and normetanephrine, and an increase in fractional norepinephrine release, and a trend toward significantly increased plasma norepinephrine, suggesting an enhanced neuronal release of norepinephrine (Manji et al. 1991a). These data are compatible with similar observations of increased plasma levels of dihydroxyphenylglycol, a major extraneuronal norepinephrine metabolite (Poirier-Littre et al. 1993). Thus, current evidence supports an action of lithium in facilitating the release of norepinephrine, possibly through effects on the presynaptic α_2 "autoreceptor," and reducing the β-adrenergic–stimulated adenylate cyclase response, which may contribute to lithium's attenuation of the euphorigenic effects of amphetamine.

Acetylcholine

Neurochemical, behavioral, and physiological studies suggest that the cholinergic system is involved in affective illness (Dilsaver and Coffman 1989) and that lithium alters the synaptic processing of acetylcholine in rat brain. Early studies reporting an inhibitory effect on cholinergic activity utilized toxic concentrations of lithium (Krell and Goldberg 1973; Marchbanks 1982; Miyauchi et al. 1980), which replaced sodium and interfered with the high-affinity transport of choline into cholinergic terminals that is required for the synthesis of acetylcholine (Jope 1979; Simon and Kuhar 1976). The addition of up to 1 mM lithium in vitro has no effect on acetylcholine synthesis or release, but chronic in vivo lithium treatment appears to increase acetylcholine synthesis, choline transport, and acetylcholine release in rat brain (Jope 1979; Simon and Kuhar 1976). Although some investigators have reported reductions in acetylcholine levels in rat brain after subchronic administration (Ho and Tsai 1975; Krell and Goldberg 1973; Ronai and Vizi 1975), Jope (1979) reported increased synthesis of acetylcholine in cortex, hippocampus, and striatum after 10 days of lithium administration.

Several laboratories have investigated lithium's effects on the density of muscarinic receptors, with conflicting results (Kafka et al. 1982; Lerer and Stanley 1985; Levy et al. 1983; Maggi and Enna 1980; Tollefson and Senogles 1982). Chronic lithium has been reported to increase (Kafka et al. 1982; Lerer and Stanley 1985; Levy et al. 1983), decrease (Tollefson and Senogles 1982), or have no effect on (Maggi and Enna 1980) the binding of [³H]quinuclidinyl benzilate in various areas of rat brain,

whereas in human caudate nucleus, lithium is reported to reduce the affinity of [³H]quinuclidinyl benzilate binding. The effects of lithium on both up- and downregulation of muscarinic receptors in the brain have also been investigated. Although there have been reports that lithium can abolish the increase in [³H]quinuclidinyl benzilate binding produced by atropine but is without effect on the downregulation induced by the cholinesterase inhibitor diisopropylfluorophosphonate, these data vary and are inconclusive (Lerer and Stanley 1985; Levy et al. 1983).

We examined both receptor binding and muscarinic receptor-coupled phosphoinositide (PI) response in rat hippocampus during atropine-induced upregulation (Ellis and Lenox 1990) and found that chronic treatment with atropine results in an upregulation of muscarinic receptors and a supersensitivity of the PI response in the hippocampus. Coadministration of chronic lithium prevented the development of the supersensitivity of the muscarinic receptor PI response without significantly affecting the extent of upregulation of receptor binding sites. These findings are consistent with an effect of chronic lithium on upregulation of neuronal muscarinic receptors observed by Liles and Nathanson (1988) in neuroblastoma cells. Those authors suggested that lithium's actions are exerted at a point beyond the receptor binding site, possibly affecting the coupling of the newly upregulated receptors at the level of the signal-transducing G proteins. Thus, similar to the case for dopaminergic and β-adrenergic receptors, it has been suggested that lithium can block the development of cholinergic receptor supersensitivity.

In behavioral studies, chronic lithium is reported to enhance some cholinergically mediated responses, including catalepsy and hypothermia. The effect of lithium on pilocarpine-induced catalepsy and hypothermia was of the same order of magnitude as the enhancement induced by chronic scopolamine pretreatment. Combined administration of both pretreatments resulted in additive effects, suggesting that different mechanisms may be involved (Dilsaver and Hariharan 1988; Lerer and Stanley 1985; Russell et al. 1981). Of interest in this regard is a study by Dilsaver and Hariharan (1989), which reported that chronic lithium treatment results in a supersensitivity of nicotine-induced hypothermia in rats.

Perhaps the most striking example of lithium's ability to potentiate muscarinic responses comes from the lithium-pilocarpine seizure model (Hirvonen et al. 1990; Honchar et al. 1983; Jope et al. 1986; Ormandy and Jope 1991; Persinger et al. 1988; Terry et al. 1990). In large doses, pilocarpine and other muscarinic agonists cause prolonged and usually lethal seizures in rats. Although lithium alone is not a convulsant, pretreatment with lithium increases the sensitivity of pilocarpine by almost 20-fold (Hirvonen et al. 1990; Honchar et al. 1983; Jope et al. 1986; Ormandy and Jope 1991; Persinger et al. 1988; Terry et al. 1990). Significantly, this behavioral effect of lithium is markedly attenuated by intracerebroventricular administration of myoinositol in both rats and mice (Kofman et al. 1991; Tricklebank et al. 1991), representing perhaps the best correlation between a biochemical and a behavioral effect of lithium (see subsection, "Phosphoinositide Turnover," under "Lithium and Signal Transduction" later in this chapter).

A synergism with the cholinergic system also occurs in electrophysiological studies in hippocampal slices, in which pilocarpine and lithium together (but neither alone) produce spontaneous epileptiform bursting (Jope et al. 1986; Ormandy and Jope 1991). Elegant studies of rat hippocampus have shown that lithium can reverse muscarinic agonist–induced desensitization, an effect that is mediated through PI hydrolysis and can be reversed by inositol (Pontzer and Crews 1990). Studies by Evans et al. (1990) have suggested that lithium's role in lithium-pilocarpine seizures is to increase excitatory transmission through a presynaptic facilitatory effect. Lithium alone also augmented synaptic responses, and this effect of lithium could be blocked by a PKC inhibitor. These results suggest that lithium's effects in this model may occur through a PKC-mediated presynaptic facilitation of neurotransmitter release. Biochemical, electrophysiological, and behavioral data suggest that chronic lithium administration stimulates acetylcholine synthesis and release in rat brain and potentiates some cholinergic-mediated physiological events. Interestingly, similar to the situation observed with the catecholaminergic system, pharmacological studies indicate that chronic lithium prevents muscarinic receptor supersensitivity, most likely through postreceptor mechanisms.

γ-Aminobutyric Acid and Neuropeptides

In contrast with the abundant literature on lithium's effects on monoamine neurotransmitters, much less work has been conducted on the amino acid neurotransmitters and neuropeptides (Bernasconi 1982; Lloyd et al. 1987; Nemeroff 1991). Studies have suggested that previously low levels of γ-aminobutyric acid (GABA) in plasma and CSF are normalized in bipolar patients treated with lithium (Berrettini et al. 1983, 1986), paralleling reported GABA changes observed in several regions of rat brain (Ahluwalia et al. 1981; Gottesfeld et al. 1971; Maggi and Enna 1980). It is worth noting that, after withdrawal of chronic lithium, GABA levels return to normal in the stria-

tum and the midbrain but remain elevated in the pons-medulla (Ahluwalia et al. 1981), possibly because of reportedly elevated levels of the GABA-synthesizing enzyme glutamic acid decarboxylase. Lithium has also been postulated to prevent GABA uptake, and chronic lithium administration was shown to significantly decrease low-affinity [^{3}H]GABA sites in the corpus striatum and the hypothalamus (Maggi and Enna 1980). Because lithium has no effect on in vitro [^{3}H]GABA binding, these receptor changes have been interpreted as downregulation secondary to activation of the GABAergic system (Maggi and Enna 1980). Although the clinical relevance of these findings remains unclear, it is significant that decreases in GABA levels in CSF have been reported in depressed patients (Berrettini et al. 1982; Post et al. 1980a).

Among the peptides, the opioid system has been the most extensively studied. Lithium administration has been reported to produce time- and dose-dependent increases in Met-enkephalin and Leu-enkephalin levels in the basal ganglia and the nucleus accumbens and to increase dynorphin levels (as determined by immunoreactive dynorphin A [1–8] peptide) in the striatum (Sivam et al. 1986, 1988). The lithium-induced increase in dynorphin was accompanied by an increase in the abundance of prodynorphin messenger ribonucleic acid (mRNA) (Sivam et al. 1988), suggesting that the effects on the dynorphin levels are at least partially mediated through increased transcription and translation (see "Conclusion" section in this chapter). Acute studies with lithium have identified the enhanced release of several opioid peptides from hypothalamic slices and have suggested an effect at the inhibitory presynaptic opioid autoreceptor (Burns et al. 1990). Chronic lithium administration did not affect the basal hypothalamic release of any of the opioids, but it prevented the naloxone-stimulated release of the peptides in vitro, a finding compatible with lithium-induced autoreceptor subsensitivity (Burns et al. 1990).

Lithium is reported to decrease the affinity of opiate receptors in vitro, whereas subchronic lithium administration is reported in some, but not all, studies to decrease the number of opioid-binding sites in rat forebrain structures (Goodnick and Gershon 1985). Additional support for effects on the opioidergic system comes from behavioral studies in which lithium produced aversive states in rats that could be blocked by the depletion of central pools of β-endorphin or by the blockade of μ-opioid receptors (Mucha and Herz 1985). It has also been demonstrated that chronic lithium administration abolishes both the secondary reinforcing effects of morphine and the aversive effects of the opioid antagonist naloxone (Blancquaert et al. 1987; Lieblich and Yirmiya 1987; Mucha and Herz 1985;

Shippenberg and Herz 1991; Shippenberg et al. 1988).

Lithium has been shown to increase the substance P content of striatum when it is chronically administered to rats, an effect that is antagonized by the concurrent administration of haloperidol (Hong et al. 1983). More recent studies have found a lithium-induced increase in tachykinin levels that appears to be associated with an increase in transcription of the rat preprotachykinin gene (Sivam et al. 1989). Studies of the effects of subchronic lithium on regional brain concentrations of substance P, neurokinin A, calcitonin gene-related peptide, and neuropeptide Y have demonstrated a regionally specific increase in the immunoreactivity of all the peptides except calcitonin gene-related peptide, which was significantly decreased in the pituitary gland (Mathe et al. 1990). In one of the few applicable clinical studies, CSF levels of various proopiomelanocortin peptides were examined in euthymic bipolar patients before and during lithium treatment. Lithium had no significant effects on the CSF levels of any of the peptides (Berrettini et al. 1985a, 1987).

Similarly to carbamazepine and valproic acid, lithium may facilitate certain aspects of GABAergic neurotransmission through several mechanisms. The clinical relevance of these findings at this point remains largely unknown. However, as one of the few systems likewise affected by the other commonly used mood stabilizers, the GABAergic system is worthy of more carefully controlled investigation. With respect to the peptides, only the opioidergic system has been studied to any extent. The bulk of the evidence suggests that lithium facilitates presynaptic opioidergic function while antagonizing certain opioid-mediated effects. The preliminary reports of effects of alterations in the levels of tachykinins in the striatum may be intriguing in view of the commonly observed lithium-induced side effects of tremor.

Lithium and Signal Transduction

Phosphoinositide Turnover

In recent years, research on the molecular mechanisms underlying the therapeutic effects of lithium has focused on intracellular second-messenger generating systems and in particular on receptor-coupled hydrolysis of phosphatidylinositol-4,5-bisphosphate (PIP_2) (Baraban et al. 1989; Manji et al. 1995b). At therapeutically relevant concentrations in humans, lithium is a potent inhibitor of the intracellular enzyme inositol monophosphatase (the concentration at which 50% of the enzyme's activity was inhibited [K_i] = 0.8 mM) within the hydrolytic pathway of PIP_2, which results in an accumulation of inositol mono-phosphate (IP) and a reduction in the generation of free inositol (Allison and Stewart 1971; Hallcher and Sherman 1980; Sherman et al. 1986). Lithium has also been shown to have additional potential sites of action in the PI cycle, where it has been reported to inhibit the inositol polyphosphatase that dephosphorylates certain forms of inositol triphosphate [$I(1,3,4)P$] and inositol bisphosphate [$I(1,4)P$].

Because the brain has limited access to inositol other than that derived from the recycling of inositol phosphates, the ability of a cell to maintain sufficient supplies of myoinositol can be crucial to the resynthesis of the PIs and the maintenance and efficiency of signaling (Sherman 1991). Furthermore, because the mode of enzyme inhibition is uncompetitive, lithium's effects have been postulated to be most pronounced in systems undergoing the highest rate of PIP_2 hydrolysis (see reviews in Nahorski et al. 1991, 1992).

Thus, Berridge et al. (1982) first proposed that the physiological consequence of lithium's action is derived through the relative depletion of free inositol. Its selectivity could be attributed to its preferential action in the brain, resulting in suppression of PI hydrolysis in the most overactive receptor-mediated neuronal pathways (Berridge 1989; Berridge et al. 1989). Because several subtypes of adrenergic (e.g., α_1), cholinergic (e.g., m_1, m_3, m_5), serotonergic (e.g., $5\text{-}HT_2$, $5\text{-}HT_1$), and dopaminergic (e.g., D_1) receptors are coupled to PIP_2 turnover in the CNS (Fisher et al. 1992; Mahan et al. 1990; Rana and Hokin 1990; Vallar et al. 1990), this hypothesis offers a plausible explanation for lithium's therapeutic efficacy in treating both poles of bipolar disorder by the compensatory stabilization of an inherent biogenic amine imbalance in critical regions of the brain (Lenox 1987).

Studies have examined the effects of lithium on receptor-mediated PI response in brain in a few neurotransmitter systems (e.g., cholinergic, serotonergic, noradrenergic, and histaminergic). Although some investigators have found a reduction in agonist-stimulated PIP_2 hydrolysis in brain slices from rats exposed acutely and chronically to lithium, these findings have often been small, inconsistent, and subject to methodological differences (Casebolt and Jope 1989; Ellis and Lenox 1990; Godfrey et al. 1989; Kendall and Nahorski 1987; Whitworth and Kendall 1989). Muscarinic receptor–mediated PIP_2 turnover appears to be a major site of action exerted by lithium in vivo. Early studies that were later replicated indicated that the increase in IP and the reduction in brain myoinositol content induced by lithium are significantly enhanced by the coadministration of the cholinergic agonist pilocarpine and are blocked by pretreatment with cholinergic antagonists (i.e., atropine and scopolamine) (Allison 1978; Allison et al. 1976; Sherman et al. 1986). In addition, studies of rat and mouse cerebral cortical slices have reported potent inhibitory effects of lithium on muscarinic-stimulated IP_3 and IP_4 accumulation (Kennedy et al. 1989, 1990; Whitworth and Kendall 1988). In these cases, the effects of lithium occur after a characteristic lag of 5–10 minutes, suggesting an indirect mechanism consistent with the inositol depletion hypothesis noted previously. Furthermore, as we have noted, studies from our laboratory have provided data supporting an indirect effect of chronic lithium in rat brain on the coupling of newly upregulated muscarinic receptor sites to the PI response (Ellis and Lenox 1990; Lenox and Ellis 1990; Lenox et al. 1991).

Several lines of evidence suggest that the action of chronic lithium may not simply be directly manifested in receptor-mediated activity coupled to this second-messenger pathway. Although investigators have observed that levels of inositol in brain remain reduced in rats receiving chronic lithium (Sherman et al. 1985), it has been difficult to confirm that the reduction in inositol levels results in a reduction in the resynthesis of PIP_2, which is the substrate for agonist-induced PI turnover. However, the inability to consistently demonstrate a lithium-induced reduction in levels of PIP_2 may be attributable to a small, rapidly turned over, signal-related pool of PIP_2 and/or recent evidence that the resynthesis of inositol phospholipids may also occur through base exchange reactions from other larger pools of phospholipids, such as phosphatidylcholine. Initial attempts to verify this hypothesis at this level of the PI cycle by examining the effects of lithium on muscarinic-stimulated accumulation of IP_1 in brain slices in the presence of exogenously added inositol were unsuccessful (Kendall and Nahorski 1987). More recently, studies examining the effects of chronic lithium on $I(1,4,5)P_3$ mass in cortical slices have shown a time-dependent decline that is attenuated in the presence of high concentrations of inositol (Kennedy et al. 1990; Varney et al. 1992). Further evidence in support of the inositol depletion hypothesis of lithium action has been observed in studies examining the diacylglycerol (DAG) arm of the PIP_2 resynthesis pathway (see subsection, "Protein Kinase C," later in this chapter).

Although pharmacological concentrations of extracellular inositol have been reported to attenuate some of lithium's biochemical, behavioral, and toxic effects, in animal studies, the addition of inositol appeared to prevent but did not reverse the effects of lithium on the PI system (Kennedy et al. 1990; Kofman and Belmaker 1993; Maslanski et al. 1992; Tricklebank et al. 1991). Further-

more, the therapeutic actions of lithium occur only after chronic treatment and remain in evidence long after discontinuation—actions that cannot be attributed only to inositol reductions evident in the presence of lithium. Indeed, in a study using proton magnetic resonance spectroscopy ([1]H-labeled magnetic resonance spectroscopy), lithium administration to a small sample of bipolar depressed and manic patients produced a significant reduction in the levels of myoinositol in frontal (but not occipital) cortex. Although these changes persisted for at least 3–4 weeks, they were observed as early as after 5 days of treatment, when the clinical state was largely unchanged (Moore et al. 1997). Thus, overall, both the preclinical and the clinical data suggest that, although lithium causes a relative depletion of myoinositol in the brain, the effects of chronic lithium administration may be mediated via a secondary cascade of signaling changes (Jope and Williams 1994; Lenox and Manji 1995; Manji et al. 1995b). The possible role of G proteins and, in particular, the PKC signaling cascade as sites for the action of chronic lithium in brain is discussed later in this chapter.

Adenylate Cyclase

The other major receptor-coupled second-messenger system in which lithium has been shown to have significant effects is adenylate cyclase, which generates cAMP (Belmaker 1981). cAMP accumulation by various neurotransmitters and hormones is reported to be inhibited by lithium at therapeutic concentrations both in vivo and in vitro, but the sensitivity appears to be less than that observed in the PI system (Andersen and Geisler 1984; Ebstein et al. 1980; Forn and Valdecasas 1971; Geisler and Klysner 1985; Geisler et al. 1985; Mork and Geisler 1987, 1989a, 1989b, 1989c, 1995; Newman and Belmaker 1987). Norepinephrine- and adenosine-stimulated cAMP accumulation in rat cortical slices are inhibited significantly by 1–2 mM Li; in human brain tissue, the 50% inhibitory concentration (IC_{50}) for lithium inhibition of norepinephrine-stimulated cAMP accumulation is approximately 5 mM (Newman et al. 1983). Studies in humans have reported that lithium treatment at therapeutic levels results in an attenuation of the plasma cAMP increase in response to epinephrine (Ebstein et al. 1976; Friedman et al. 1979b) and have produced evidence for an attenuation in adrenergic receptor coupling to adenylate cyclase in peripheral cells (Risby et al. 1991). In fact, lithium inhibition of vasopressin-sensitive or thyroid-stimulating hormone (TSH)–sensitive adenylate cyclase is thought to contribute to the commonly observed side effects of nephrogenic diabetes insipidus and hypothyroidism seen in patients being treated with lithium over an extended period (Dousa 1974; Wolff et al. 1970).

Lithium attenuation of β-adrenoceptor-stimulated adenylate cyclase activity has also been shown in membrane, slice, and synaptosomal preparations from rat brain both in vitro and ex vivo (Andersen and Geisler 1984; Ebstein et al. 1980; Geisler and Klysner 1985; Geisler et al. 1985; Mork and Geisler 1987, 1989a, 1989b, 1989c; Newman and Belmaker 1987). However, Godfrey (1989) reported no change in isoproterenol-stimulated adenylate cyclase response in rat cortical slices after 3 days of lithium treatment. Most recently, our laboratory had similar results using in vivo microdialysis in cortex of rats exposed to chronic lithium administration (Manji et al. 1991b; Masana et al. 1992). Postreceptor stimulation of adenylate cyclase (e.g., with forskolin, fluoride, or nonhydrolyzable analogues of GTP) has also been shown to be inhibited by lithium in slices and membranes from rat cerebral cortices (Andersen and Geisler 1984; Geisler et al. 1985; Mork and Geisler 1987; Newman and Belmaker 1987), and several studies have also revealed lithium-induced increases in basal cAMP. These data are of interest in the light of findings that chronic lithium increases the mRNA for adenylate cyclase with downstream enhancement of protein kinase A (PKA) activity and increased levels of brain-derived neurotrophic factor in the hippocampus (Nibuya et al. 1996). Because alterations in brain-derived neurotrophic factor have been hypothesized to contribute to antidepressant properties, these findings may account in part for the clinical action of lithium in the presence of antidepressants in the treatment of refractory depression.

In contradistinction, Mori et al. (1996) reported that lithium, but not rubidium, significantly decreased the cAMP-stimulated microtubule-associated protein (MAP2) endogenous phosphorylation in microtubule fraction, which appeared to be related to a direct inhibitory effect of lithium on cAMP-dependent phosphorylation (PKA). This same group of investigators (Zanardi et al. 1997) examined the cAMP-dependent phosphorylation system in platelets of euthymic bipolar patients and healthy volunteers before and after 15 days of lithium treatment. They found that 15 days of lithium treatment enhanced the basal and the cAMP-stimulated ^{32}P incorporation in the 22- and 38-kilodalton phosphoproteins in bipolar patients, but not in healthy subjects. Although the effect of chronic lithium on cAMP-dependent phosphorylation remains of interest, results to date appear inconsistent.

Lithium in vitro inhibits the stimulation of adenylate cyclase by guanyl imidodiphosphate, or Gpp(NH)p (a poorly hydrolyzable analogue of GTP), and calcium-calmodulin, both of which can be overcome by Mg^{2+} (An-

dersen and Geisler 1984; Mork and Geisler 1989c; Newman and Belmaker 1987). Lithium also competes with both Mg^{2+} and Ca^{2+} for membrane binding sites, and lithium's inhibition of the solubilized catalytic unit of adenylate cyclase can also be overcome by Mg^{2+}. These findings suggest that lithium's inhibition of adenylate cyclase in vitro may be caused by competition with Mg^{2+} on a site on the catalytic unit of adenylate cyclase (Andersen and Geisler 1984; Newman and Belmaker 1987). However, the inhibitory effects of chronic lithium treatment on adenylate cyclase in rat brain are not reversed by Mg^{2+}, and these effects persist after washing of the membranes but are reversed by increasing concentrations of GTP (Mork and Geisler 1989c). These results suggest that the physiologically relevant effects of lithium (i.e., those seen on chronic drug administration and not reversed immediately with drug discontinuation) may be exerted at the level of signal-transducing G proteins at a GTP-responsive step.

G Proteins

Because lithium has been shown to affect both PI turnover and adenylate cyclase activity, recent research has focused on mechanisms shared by these two major second-messenger-generating systems, namely the signal-transducing G proteins. Thus, neurotransmitter function might be modulated through alterations in intracellular signaling. Lithium might be effective because it alters the postsynaptic signal generated in response to several endogenous neurotransmitters (see review in Manji 1992). Multiple receptors converge onto a single G protein, but individual receptors may also "talk" to more than one G protein. Likewise, single G proteins may modulate more than one effector, and several G proteins may also converge on a single effector. Thus, the G proteins are in a position to coordinate receptor-effector activity that is critical to the regulation of neuronal function, thereby maintaining a functional balance between neurotransmitter systems in brain. In addition, these signaling proteins may represent attractive targets to explain lithium's efficacy in treating both poles of bipolar disorder.

As we have noted, experimental evidence has shown that lithium may alter receptor coupling to PI turnover in the absence of consistent changes in the density of the receptor sites themselves. Because fluoride ion will directly activate G-protein-coupled second-messenger response, efforts have been made to examine the effect of lithium on sodium fluoride–stimulated PI response in brain. Although Godfrey et al. (1989) reported a 21% reduction of fluoride-stimulated PI response in cortical membranes of rats treated with lithium for 3 days, no change in response was observed in cortical slices from rats that were given lithium for 30 days.

In a more recent study of chronic lithium administration in rats, Song and Jope (1992) reported an attenuation of PI turnover in response to GTP analogues, even in the presence of labeled PI as a substrate. Avissar et al. (1988) reported that lithium dramatically eliminated isoproterenol- and carbachol-induced increases in [³H]GTP binding in rat cerebral cortical membranes in the presence of 0.6 mM lithium chloride and in washed cortical membranes from rats treated with lithium carbonate for 2–3 weeks. In animals withdrawn from lithium for 2 days, the agonist-stimulated response returned.

Follow-up studies in humans have reported a normalization of previously elevated agonist-induced [³H]GTPγS binding in leukocytes from lithium-treated euthymic bipolar patients (Schreiber et al. 1991). These studies have been of heuristic interest, and considerable data suggest an action of lithium at the level of G protein. However, such a direct action of lithium on G-protein function has been difficult to replicate in the light of several methodological problems.

First, similar studies in other laboratories have been difficult in the light of an inability to identify reliable agonist-induced binding of labeled GTP in the brain because of significant nonspecific binding and variable hydrolysis of the GTP. Attempts to replicate these effects of both acute and chronic lithium, not only in brain but also in other tissues such as platelets and heart, using agonist-induced release of labeled nonhydrolyzable GTP analogues were unsuccessful (Ellis and Lenox 1991). If there existed such marked sensitivity of G-protein activation to the lithium ion, routine assays of coupled second-messenger responses such as agonist-stimulated hydrolysis of PI in brain slices in the presence of 10 mM lithium chloride would be impossible. Furthermore, standard preparations of GTP salts are compounded with lithium and have been used for years to study G-protein function.

Investigations have also addressed the role of G proteins in the action of lithium-induced attenuation of receptor-mediated adenylate cyclase activity in both rodents and humans. In a series of studies in which in vivo microdialysis measurements of cAMP were used to assess lithium's effects on G proteins in the intact animal, chronic lithium treatment produced a significant increase in basal and postreceptor-stimulated (cholera toxin or forskolin) adenylate cyclase activity while attenuating the β-adrenergic-mediated effect in rat frontal cortex or hippocampus. In addition, pertussis toxin–catalyzed [³²P]adenosine 5′diphosphate (ADP)-ribosylation in membranes from these brain regions of lithium-treated

animals was significantly increased (Manji et al. 1991b; Masana et al. 1992). Because pertussis toxin selectively catalyzes ADP ribosylation of the undissociated, inactive αβγ-heterotrimeric form of G_i, these results suggest that chronic lithium administration may reduce activation of G_i through a stabilization of the inactive conformation (Manji et al. 1991b; Masana et al. 1992). If dissociation of G-protein subunits was inhibited by lithium, this could decrease β-adrenergic-stimulated adenylate cyclase activity while simultaneously producing a relative stabilization of the receptor in a high-affinity state.

These observations in animals are supported by data from a clinical investigation of control subjects who had 2 weeks of lithium administration. Basal- and postreceptor-stimulated adenylate cyclase activity was increased in platelets, associated with a 40% increase in pertussis toxin–catalyzed [³²P]ADP-ribosylation in platelet membranes (Hsiao et al. 1992). Once again, these data suggest a stabilization of the inactive undissociated αβγ heterotrimeric form of G_i. Such a contention is also supported by the recent demonstration that chronic in vivo lithium administration reduces the subsequent in vitro sensitivity of rat cortical membranes to guanine nucleotide–induced reductions in pertussis toxin–catalyzed [³²P]ADP ribosylation (Manji et al., in press a).

More recently, it has been shown that lithium promotes calpain-mediated proteolytic cleavage of G_o, effects that have been postulated to occur via a stabilization of the G protein in its αβγ heterotrimeric conformation (Greenwood and Jope 1994). Moreover, these investigators also found that the addition of GTPγS was able to overcome lithium's effects. Taken together, the results suggest that, although chronic lithium administration leads to the stabilization of G_i (and possibly G_o) in the undissociated αβγ conformation, the application of high concentrations of exogenous guanine nucleotides can overcome these effects, similar to findings on rat brain adenylate cyclase activity noted earlier in this chapter. At present, the possible effects of chronic lithium administration on the absolute levels of $G\alpha_s$ and $G\alpha_i$ remain unclear; that is, two independent laboratories have not observed any alterations (P. P. Li et al. 1991; Manji et al. 1991a; Masana et al. 1992), whereas another has reported small but significant decreases in the levels of the α_s, α_{i1}, and α_{i2} in rat frontal cortex (Colin et al. 1991). However, chronic lithium administration in rats has been shown to reduce the levels of mRNA for various G proteins in brain, including $G\alpha_{i1}$, $G\alpha_{i2}$, and $G\alpha_s$ (Colin et al. 1991; P. P. Li et al. 1991).

Currently, the molecular mechanisms underlying lithium's effects on G proteins remain to be fully established. Although data indicate that competition with mag-

ministration may lead to an increased membrane translocation and subsequent degradation and downregulation of PKC isozymes (K. P. Huang 1989; Kishimoto et al. 1989; Nishizuka 1992). Such a mechanism would be consistent with data indicating that lithium acutely activates PKC, whereas prolonged treatment is associated with reduced phorbol ester–mediated responses, including neurotransmitter release (Anderson et al. 1988; Bitran et al. 1990; Evans et al. 1990; Lenox et al. 1992b; Manji et al. 1993; Reisine and Zatz 1987; Sharp et al. 1991; Wang and Friedman 1989; Zatz and Reisine 1985). On the other hand, there is evidence that membrane translocation, degradation, and conversion of PKC to a constitutively active phorbol-insensitive form (i.e., PKM) may play a role in at least some of the PKC-mediated events observed after chronic lithium exposure (Manji and Lenox 1994). PKC isozymes involved in such a process may account for regulation of the expression of MARCKS observed in cells exposed to either long-term phorbol ester or chronic lithium, and they may ultimately play a role in the action of lithium at a nuclear level.

Glycogen Synthase Kinase-3β and Its Role in Development

It is well known that lithium ion can have a significant effect on the development of a variety of organisms (Stachel et al. 1993). In particular, in *Xenopus*, lithium significantly alters the ventral-dorsal axis of the developing embryo (Kao et al. 1986). One hypothesis regarding this action of lithium stemmed from its inhibition of inositol monophosphatase and alteration in the dorsal-ventral balance of PI signaling in the embryo (Ault et al. 1996; Berridge et al. 1989). Support for this hypothesis was derived by the observation that exposure to high concentrations of myo-inositol could reverse the effect of lithium (Busa and Gimlich 1989). In an interesting series of studies in *Xenopus*, however, inhibition of inositol monophosphatase by another inhibitor did not result in similar alteration in morphogenesis, suggesting that lithium may be acting in an alternative pathway (Klein and Melton 1996). These studies revealed that lithium inhibits glycogen synthase kinase-3β activity ($K_i = 2.1$ mM), which antagonizes the *wnt* signaling pathway associated with normal dorsal-ventral axis development in the *Xenopus* embryo. Studies using an embryo expressing a dominant negative form of glycogen synthase kinase-3 suggest that myoinositol reversal of dorsalization of the embryonic axis by lithium may be mediated by events independent of inositol monophosphatase inhibition (Hedgepeth et al. 1997). It has yet to be determined to what extent this effect of lithium on

glycogen synthase kinase-3β is relevant to its mood-stabilizing properties in the brain.

Lithium and Gene Expression

As discussed earlier in this chapter, in recent years, it has become increasingly appreciated that any relevant biochemical models of lithium's actions must attempt to account for its special clinical profile (prophylactic efficacy against both mania and depression), which normally requires several weeks to develop, and the maximum benefit may not be even seen for several months (Goodwin and Jamison 1990; Schou 1991) and is not immediately reversible on drug discontinuation (Faedda et al. 1993; Suppes et al. 1991). Patterns of effects requiring such prolonged administration of the drug suggest alterations at the genomic level. Neuronal plasticity clearly depends on making long-term adjustments to changing physiological and pharmacological stimuli and is mediated in large part by the activation and inactivation of the expression of subsets of genes with temporal specificity.

In recent years, it has become clear that long-term changes in neuronal synaptic function are correlated with, and in some cases have been shown to be dependent on, the induction of new programs of gene expression (Sheng and Greenberg 1990). Substantial progress has been made both in identifying the genes responsive to transsynaptic stimulation and in elucidating the processes that convert ephemeral second-messenger-mediated events into long-term cellular phenotypic alterations. This has been particularly important for neurobiology, wherein we attempt to understand the mechanism(s) by which short-lived events (e.g., stressors) can have profound, long-term (perhaps lifelong) behavioral consequences (Kandel 1983; Post 1992) and, more importantly for the present discussion, may help to unravel the processes by which a simple monovalent cation such as lithium may produce a long-term stabilization of mood in individuals vulnerable to bipolar illness.

Until recently, little has been known about the transcriptional and posttranscriptional factors regulated by chronic drug treatment, although it has long been appreciated that both the diversity of neuronal responses and the long-term changes in plasticity are dependent on the selective regulation of gene expression. As articulated by Morgan and Curran (1991), the nucleus can be viewed as a complex arena in which multiple signal transduction pathways converge and thus is a likely downstream target of drugs such as lithium and valproic acid, which require chronic administration to manifest clinical efficacy. Although gene expression can be regulated by a variety of processes, several lines of evidence suggest that phosphorylation is used most frequently to regulate long-term neuronal responsiveness. In view of the effects of lithium on PKC described above, we reviewed the effects of lithium on PKC-mediated gene expression. We found that this mood-stabilizing agent exerts major effects at the level of gene expression and that these effects are largely mediated via PKC-induced alterations in the nuclear transcription regulatory factors that are responsible for modulating the expression of specific genes of functional importance with the potential for long-term and enduring changes in the CNS.

Several studies have found that lithium alters *fos* expression in different cell systems, including the brain, through a PKC-mediated mechanism (Kalasapudi et al. 1990; Weiner et al. 1991). Thus, preincubation of cultured PC12 cells (a rat pheochromocytoma cell line) with lithium for 16 hours markedly potentiates *fos* expression in response to the muscarinic agonist carbachol. That lithium's effects are mediated via PKC is supported by the observation that lithium pretreatment also potentiates *fos* expression in response to phorbol esters (Kalasapudi et al. 1990). Moreover, lithium's effects appear be selective for the PKC signal transduction pathway and do not appear to be the result of a nonspecific alteration in mRNA stability, because the *fos* expression in response to adenylate cyclase activation is unaffected under identical conditions (Divish et al. 1991).

Interestingly, paralleling the results observed in cell culture, a single intraperitoneal injection of lithium results in an augmentation of pilocarpine-induced *fos* gene expression in rat brain, which can be antagonized by the m_1/m_3 muscarinic antagonist pirenzepine (Weiner et al. 1991). Studies of chronic lithium in rats have also reported brain region–specific effects on both basal and inducible *fos* expression (Mathe et al. 1995). Recent studies in cloned cell lines have also reported that chronic lithium (1 mM) resulted in a significant increase in AP-1–binding activity (Chen et al. 1997). These results are similar to earlier findings from studies in which valproate was used. Using a luciferase reporter gene system and site-directed mutagenesis, the same laboratory (Manji et al. 1996b; Yuan et al. 1997) confirmed the ability of lithium or valproate to alter the expression of genes driven by an AP-1–containing promoter. These lithium-induced effects on the expression of cfos mRNA and AP-1–binding activity, generally thought to mediate a "second wave" of specific neuronal genes of functional importance, suggest the potential for long-term and enduring changes in the CNS.

Long-term regulation of synaptic function could result from a modification in receptors, G proteins, effectors, proteins involved in neurotransmitter release, cytoskeletal remodeling, and enzymes involved in neurotransmitter biosynthesis. Providing an example of this is a recent study showing that incubation of cerebellar granule cells with 1.5 mM lithium results in biphasic effects on the levels of both *fos* mRNA and muscarinic m_3 receptor mRNA—early increases in the expression of both, followed by a decline after several days of incubation, both of which occur in the absence of toxic effects (Gao et al. 1993). This would be entirely consistent with our suggestion of a biphasic effect of lithium on PKC-mediated responses. Crucial to the present discussion is the fact that chronic, "therapeutic," in vivo administration of lithium also significantly modulates the expression of many genes in rat brain, several of which are known to contain PKC-responsive elements. It is also of interest that chronic lithium is reported to significantly affect the expression of various components of second-messenger-generating systems. Thus, chronic lithium reduces the levels of $G\alpha_{i1}$ mRNA and $G\alpha_{i2}$ mRNA in brain while also reducing the levels of $G\alpha_s$ mRNA in the latter.

The possibility that these intriguing effects of lithium on G-protein mRNA are mediated via PKC is suggested by a recent study reporting that PKC activation produces a similar decrease in $G\alpha_s$ mRNA and $G\alpha_{i2}$ levels in vitro (Thiele and Eipper 1990). Chronic lithium administration in rats also increases the expression of adenylate cyclase type I and type II rat cortex, as noted previously. These effects on adenylate cyclase gene expression are accompanied by increased levels of the protein, consistent with increases in basal cortical adenylate cyclase activity observed after chronic lithium administration (Manji et al. 1996b).

With evidence for a role of neuropeptides in both the pathogenesis and the treatment of affective illness (Nemeroff 1991), it is noteworthy that lithium administration (both acute and chronic) also regulates the expression of various neuromodulatory peptide hormones and receptors. Thus, acute lithium administration is reported to increase the levels of neuropeptide Y mRNA in the hippocampus (Weiner et al. 1992) and to increase the levels of striatal preprotachykinin mRNA in the striatum. Interestingly, the expression of both neuropeptide Y and proenkephalin are directly regulated by PKC (Giraud et al. 1991; Kislauskis and Dobner 1990). The effects of lithium on neuropeptide gene expression are also observed after more prolonged administration; increases in the expression of both prodynorphin and preprotachykinin in striatal tissue, as well as similar increases in glucocorticoid type II mRNA, have been reported.

In a more recent study, Zachrisson et al. (1995) examined the effects of 4 weeks of lithium administration (via food supplementation) on the expression of several neuropeptide mRNAs in rat brain. Using in situ hybridization, they observed increases in neuropeptide Y mRNA levels in the hippocampus, layers II–III of the entorhinal cortex, nucleus accumbens shell, and medial caudate-putamen. Somatostatin mRNA expression increased in layers IV–VI of the entorhinal cortex and in the lateral caudate putamen. By using in situ hybridization, it appears that chronic lithium administration can affect discrete populations of neuropeptide Y– and somatostatin mRNA–expressing neurons in the brain. These complex effects on the gene expression of multiple neuromodulators and on various components of second-messenger-generating systems may serve to explain the role of lithium in the long-term restoration of the functional balance of neurotransmitter activity in the CNS and thereby to restabilize mood and dampen periodic neurobiological oscillations of mood in bipolar patients and depression in unipolar patients (Lenox and Manji 1995; Manji et al. 1995b).

Lithium and Neuroanatomical Site of Action

Although data related to the neuroanatomical localization of lesions in the brains of bipolar patients are only now being accumulated by using structural and functional neuroimaging strategies, alterations in the right hemisphere related to limbic and frontal association areas have been of particular interest (Manji et al., in press b). Additional evidence implicating temporal-lobe dysfunction associated with epileptic disorders remains of considerable interest (Drezniak and Lenox, unpublished data). The premise that lithium exerts its therapeutic actions by acting at such specific neuroanatomical sites and/or their cells of projection is supported by several lines of evidence.

First, atomic absorption spectrophotometric, radiographic dielectric track registration, and NMR studies indicate that lithium does not distribute evenly throughout the brain after either acute or chronic administration. There is evidence for preferential accumulation in the forebrain diencephalon, that is, the hypothalamus, and telencephalon structures, namely, caudate and hippocampus (Bond et al. 1972; Ebadi et al. 1974; Edelfors 1975; Heurteaux et al. 1986; Lam and Christensen 1992; Mukherjee et al. 1976; Nelson et al. 1980; Ramaprasad et al. 1992; Sander et al. 1994; Savolainen et al. 1990; Smith and Amdisen 1981; Spirtes 1976; Thellier et al. 1980a, 1980b). Second, as noted previously, preclinical studies of lithium's effects on neurotransmitter systems have revealed changes, particularly in the serotonin system, that are brain region specific. Third, the relative regional and cell distribution of overactive ligand-gated ion channels in the brains of bipolar patients may be important in dictating relative rates of lithium transport. Fourth, studies in which PI turnover was assessed after lithium administration indicate regional differences in inositol depletion and agonist-stimulated [^{3}H]IP accumulation, primarily between forebrain structures and hindbrain structures (Allison et al. 1980; R. D. Johnson and Minneman 1985; Rooney and Nahorski 1986; Savolainen et al. 1990; Sherman et al. 1986; Song and Jope 1992). Moreover, the effects of lithium are most apparent in cells in which inositol is not only limiting but also undergoing the greatest activation of receptor-mediated PI hydrolysis (Gani et al. 1993; Heacock et al. 1993; Sarri et al. 1995; Watson and Lenox 1996). Finally, regional brain—namely, hippocampal—distribution of PKC isozymes and alterations in MARCKS expression after chronic lithium administration may confer even further specificity of action. Collectively, these studies indicate that the long-term therapeutic action of lithium may indeed possess cell and regional brain specificity that underlies its prophylactic efficacy in the treatment of bipolar disorder.

INDICATIONS

Psychiatric Indications

Affective Disorders

As discussed elsewhere in this book, lithium is the most widely used treatment for bipolar disorder. Although it is far from the perfect drug, it has clearly revolutionized treatment of this disorder. Lithium has proved useful in the treatment of acute episodes of mania and depression and, perhaps most important, in the long-term prophylaxis of the illness.

Acute mania.   Lithium was approved by the U.S. Food and Drug Administration (FDA) in 1970 for the treatment of acute mania. Results of early uncontrolled, single-blind studies, when combined, indicate that approximately 81% (334 of 413) of manic patients show at least a partial response to lithium monotherapy. Subsequently, controlled, double-blind studies similarly revealed a 70%–80% response rate of lithium monotherapy in the treatment of acute manic episodes (reviewed in Goodwin and Jamison 1990; Goodwin et al. 1969; Maggs 1963; Schou et al. 1954). Despite this impressive response rate and the evidence that lithium is the drug of choice for long-term prophylaxis (see below), its 5- to 10-day latency of response has limited its use as the sole agent in the treatment of acute manic episodes in everyday clinical practice.

In several double-blind studies (Goodnick and Meltzer 1984b; Post et al. 1980b; Prien et al. 1972; Shopsin et al. 1971), lithium has been compared with neuroleptic drugs in the treatment of acute mania. The results suggested that the neuroleptics are superior only in the initial management of acutely manic patients. More recent clinical studies have clearly verified the efficacy of benzodiazepines, such as lorazepam, as an adjunct to lithium in the acute manic phase of the illness to control hyperactivity, agitation, and insomnia (Lenox et al. 1992a). This strategy affords the practical advantage of parenteral administration and limits unnecessary exposure to neuroleptics in this patient population. Thus, most clinicians currently prescribe either a benzodiazepine or (when necessary) a neuroleptic in combination with lithium during the early stages of the treatment of mania, and then gradually taper the neuroleptic or benzodiazepine after stabilization of the patient's acute symptomatology. As discussed in the dosing section, clinicians frequently observe an increase in plasma lithium levels (which often necessitates a lowering of the lithium dose) after the manic episode has subsided. At present, it is unclear whether this is a result of increased uptake of lithium into excitable tissue during mania (as we have discussed), an increase in renal blood flow and glomerular filtration rate, or a combination thereof.

The use of anticonvulsants in the treatment of patients with bipolar disorder has increased significantly over the past 5 years, leading to FDA approval of valproate for the treatment of acute mania. In earlier observations and a recent double-blind, placebo-controlled investigation in which valproate was compared with lithium in the 3-week treatment of acute mania, it was evident that lithium was particularly effective for a subpopulation of patients, whereas valproate appeared to have efficacy for a broader spectrum of patients (Bowden et al. 1994; Calabrese and Delucchi 1990; Gerner and Stanton 1992; McElroy et al. 1992). Carbamazepine has less consistent supporting data but remains actively used in clinical practice (Keck et al. 1992). With the enhanced clinical recognition of the anticonvulsants, treatment strategies have more readily shifted to combining lithium with an anticonvulsant when mood stabilization proves to be more refractory with monotherapy. Lithium remains the treatment of choice for adolescent or adult patients presenting for the first time with classical bipolar acute mania.

Long-term prophylaxis of bipolar disorder. Numerous placebo-controlled studies have unequivocally documented the efficacy of lithium in the long-term pro-

phylactic treatment of bipolar disorder (reviewed in Goodwin and Jamison 1990). Lithium's beneficial effects appear to involve a reduction in both the number of episodes and their intensity; approximately 70%–80% of all bipolar patients have at least a partial response to lithium. The cumulative data from 10 major double-blind studies in which lithium prophylaxis was compared with placebo showed that approximately 34% of patients receiving lithium had relapses, whereas 81% of patients receiving placebo had relapses.

Additional evidence for lithium prophylaxis is found in studies in which successful lithium treatment was discontinued. In at least 14 studies, an average of 50% of patients relapsed within 5 months of abrupt termination of treatment (Suppes et al. 1991). It is of interest that the relative risk of mania appeared to be fivefold greater than that of depression. Additional reports have supported the appearance of an increased risk for precipitation of an affective episode during the period of discontinuation, but this risk is significantly reduced if the lithium is tapered slowly (Faedda et al. 1993). Although there is evidence that patients maintained at standard serum lithium concentrations (0.8–1.0 mM) not only significantly reduced the risk of relapse but also decreased the risk of subsyndromal symptomatology, the role of compliance has not been thoroughly addressed (Gelenberg et al. 1989; Keller et al. 1992; Solomon et al. 1996).

Adequate lithium treatment, particularly in the context of a lithium clinic, is also reported to reduce the excessive mortality observed in patients with the illness (Coppen and Abou-Saleh 1988; Coppen et al. 1991; Muller-Oerlinghausen et al. 1991; Vestergaard and Aagaard 1991). Debate continues as to the relative efficacy of lithium in preventing manic and depressive episodes. After careful analysis of the controlled studies, Goodwin and Jamison (1990) concluded that despite common clinical opinion, little support exists for the idea that lithium has greater prophylaxis against mania than against major depression. Nevertheless, patients do seem to report mild breakthrough depressive symptoms more commonly than hypomanic symptoms, although it is difficult to rule out the selective reporting of aversive symptoms by the patients. However (as is discussed in Bowden, Chapter 35, in this volume), data are accumulating that perhaps as many as half of all bipolar patients show an inadequate long-term response to lithium monotherapy, necessitating the addition or substitution of another agent, most commonly an anticonvulsant or an antidepressant. Issues related to the widened spectrum of patients being treated with lithium, as well as lack of compliance and potential increased risk of relapse during lithium discontinuation (see below), may have contributed to this apparent reduction in the efficacy of the monotherapy (Grof et al. 1993). These questions deserve further attention in future investigations.

Reports over the past several years have suggested that certain features of bipolar disorder are predictive of a poor response to lithium. Patients who experience mixed states, severe stage III mania, and/or rapid cycling are all likely to show a poor response to lithium. In addition, the type and sequence of episodes may also be important—for example, patients with a sequence of mania-depression-normal intervals do better with lithium than do those with a sequence of depression-mania-normalcy. The greater is the number of interepisode symptoms resulting from concomitant personality disorder or substance abuse, the less effective lithium response is likely to be. The potential phenomenon of "lithium discontinuation refractoriness" in certain individuals has been identified (Post et al. 1992), but more extensive study is required to assess the generalizability of the phenomenon. However, lithium is frequently discontinued for pregnant patients. Although controlled studies are lacking, refractoriness to lithium reinstitution does not appear to be a common occurrence in this population. As noted earlier, it is more clear that abrupt lithium discontinuation after long-term maintenance treatment often results in the emergence of a manic episode, and the rate of exacerbation can be modified by using a gradual discontinuation strategy (Faedda et al. 1993; Suppes et al. 1993).

Investigators studying the mechanism(s) of action of the drug and the neurobiology of bipolar affective disorder must be cognizant of the clinical features associated with lithium response and discontinuation. These may provide clues not only about the targets of lithium's actions but also about long-term homeostatic processes occurring during long-term lithium administration (Lenox et al., in press).

Acute treatment of depression.   In addition to the well-established efficacy of lithium as a potentiating agent in the treatment of refractory depression (de Montigny et al. 1983; Heninger et al. 1983; Price 1989) (as discussed in the next section), there is now considerable evidence for the antidepressant efficacy of lithium monotherapy, particularly in the treatment of bipolar depression. However, the antidepressant effects (shown in placebo-controlled studies) often do not become evident until the third or fourth weeks of treatment, perhaps explaining the negative results noted in earlier studies of shorter duration (see Goodwin and Jamison 1990). Interestingly, an average of 79% of bipolar patients are reported to respond to the drug, compared with only 36% of unipolar patients. Also,

in several controlled studies, the antidepressant efficacy of lithium has been compared with that of standard antidepressants. In four of five studies, lithium had efficacy equal to that of tricyclic antidepressants, albeit with a slower onset of action in two of the studies (Goodwin and Jamison 1990). The clinical observation of breakthrough depressions in bipolar patients despite maintenance of therapeutic lithium suggests that some patients may experience only modest antidepressant effects. Nevertheless, given the now well-documented ability of antidepressants to induce rapid cycling and precipitate manic episodes (Goodwin and Jamison 1990; Wehr and Goodwin 1987), lithium monotherapy is recommended for treatment of bipolar depression.

Potentiation of antidepressant response.   One of the major advances in psychopharmacology in the last decade has been the recognition of lithium augmentation as a strategy in treating depression that is refractory to monotherapy with conventional antidepressants (both tricyclic antidepressants and monoamine oxidase inhibitors). It has been established in open studies (and subsequently in controlled studies) that about half of all treatment-refractory depressed patients respond to the addition of lithium to their ongoing antidepressant regimen (with a higher response rate in bipolar subjects), usually within 1–2 weeks (de Montigny et al. 1983; Heninger et al. 1983; Price 1989). Although lithium potentiation is more efficacious in patients with bipolar disorder, it also has clear efficacy in the treatment of those with unipolar depression. The relative safety of this strategy and the short time needed to assess its efficacy suggest that a trial of lithium augmentation should be considered before switching antidepressants in patients with nonresponding depression. The lithium augmentation strategy derived from de Montigny's heuristic proposal that the enhancement of ascending presynaptic serotonergic function would translate into potentiation of antidepressant efficacy (de Montigny et al. 1983). However, considerable data have shown that lithium can affect PKC, which may regulate the function of multiple neurotransmitter systems (Manji and Lenox 1994). It is tempting to speculate that it is this effect on multiple interacting neurotransmitter systems that underlies its remarkable efficacy in treating refractory depression.

Schizophrenia

Given some degree of similarity in the acute symptomatology of mania and certain forms of schizophrenia (particularly paranoid schizophrenia), it is not surprising that the efficacy of lithium has been investigated in these disorders. The results of the double-blind studies of lithium in patients with schizophrenia have generally been disappointing; greater efficacy has been observed for neuroleptics. Lithium shows some efficacy in the treatment of the affective symptoms but is generally without benefit on the "core schizophrenic" symptoms (Atre-Vaidya and Taylor 1989; Collins et al. 1991). There is considerably more evidence for the efficacy of lithium in the treatment of schizoaffective disorder: a meta-analysis of published findings suggested an improvement in 77% of lithium-treated schizoaffective individuals (Delva and Letemendia 1982). Although lithium appears to be useful for patients with this condition, treatment with neuroleptics and other agents is usually necessary (Goodnick and Meltzer 1984b).

Aggression

The antiaggressive effect of lithium has been investigated in animal studies and in clinical studies over the past 20 years, and the preponderance of data has suggested that lithium reduces impulsive aggression (see Nilsson 1993 for an excellent review). Indeed, Schou (1987) described lithium's antiaggressive effects as one of its best-documented effects outside of the treatment of bipolar illness. At serum levels similar to those used in the treatment of bipolar illness, lithium has generally been reported to exert antiaggressive effects in psychiatric populations, in children with behavior problems, in individuals with mental retardation, and in prisoners with "uncontrolled rage outbursts" (Nilsson 1993). Note that most studies have been conducted in institutions, and there is little research on the antiaggressive effects of lithium in the outpatient setting. In view of the reported association between serotonergic function and aggressive and impulsive disorders, it is not surprising that the antiaggressive properties of lithium have generally been ascribed to an enhancement of serotonergic function (Coccaro et al. 1989). Although it is not approved by the FDA for treatment of aggression, it is clear that additional studies of lithium for this purpose are warranted, not only with respect to defining the range of clinically responsive conditions, but also regarding the neurobiological mechanisms underlying its efficacy.

Other Psychiatric Conditions

The efficacy of lithium has been investigated in the treatment of obsessive-compulsive disorder, attention-deficit/hyperactivity disorder, late luteal phase dysphoric disorder, borderline personality disorder, alcoholism, Tourette's disorder, anxiety disorders, and eating disorders. However, there is little convincing evidence for lithi-

um's efficacy in treating these disorders (Jefferson et al. 1983; F. N. Johnson 1987).

Nonpsychiatric Indications

Cluster Headache

The best-established nonpsychiatric use of lithium is in the long-term prophylactic treatment of cluster headache (Bussone et al. 1990). The cyclic, recurrent nature of the illness was the original impetus for investigating lithium's efficacy. Indeed, there is general agreement that lithium not only is an effective treatment but also should be regarded as a first-line agent in this disorder. Interestingly, the therapeutic efficacy of lithium in cluster headache requires similar plasma levels and generally shows a 3-week latency to response (F. N. Johnson and Minnai 1993). The most interesting mechanistic studies have focused on alterations in both membrane phospholipids and receptor-effector coupling by lithium (de Belleroche et al. 1984, 1986). Finally, it is noteworthy that there appear to be differences in human leukocyte antigen in patients with responses to lithium (Giacovazzo et al. 1985, 1986). Whether the mood-stabilizing properties of lithium show a similar human leukocyte antigen association remains unclear.

Effects of Lithium on Blood Cells and the Function of Granulocytes

After the administration of therapeutic doses of lithium, fairly reproducible hematopoietic effects have been documented, especially on granulocyte leukocytes. The observation that lithium stimulation of leukocytosis involves a true proliferative response, rather than just a shift of cell populations from the marginating to the circulatory pool of cells, led investigators to examine bone marrow for changes in miotic cell proliferation. These studies showed that lithium increases the number of pluripotential hematopoietic stem cells (colony-forming unit [CFU]–stem cells), granulocyte-macrophage progenitors (CFU–granulocyte macrophages), and megakaryocyte progenitors (CFU-megakaryocytes) in several species, including humans. These now-well-documented effects of lithium on blood cell formation have led to an investigation of this monovalent cation in the treatment of various hematopoietic disorders (particularly after anticancer or anti-AIDS chemotherapy) to ameliorate the bone marrow toxicity associated with these treatments. Although Lyman and Williams (1991) concluded, after a detailed review of the literature, that lithium is clearly effective in reducing both the severity and the duration of chemotherapy- or radiotherapy-associated neutropenia, lithium is not routinely used as an adjunct in these conditions. Nevertheless, given the extensive clinical use of lithium worldwide and its lack of toxicity when administered at therapeutic doses, the use of lithium to ameliorate bone marrow suppression remains an area worthy of further long-term clinical investigation.

Most recently, "hematological" studies of lithium have highlighted its potential role in modulating the hematopoietic toxicity associated with zidovudine. Despite the reported efficacy of the drug in producing immunological improvement, decreasing the incidence of opportunistic infections, and reducing AIDS mortality, its use has been associated with hematopoietic suppression, manifested by anemia, neutropenia, and overall bone marrow suppression (Fischl et al. 1987). Studies have confirmed the efficacy of concentrations similar to those attained clinically (i.e., 1.0 mM) in attenuating the toxicity of zidovudine on CFU–granulocyte macrophages; CFU-megakaryocytes; and burst-forming unit, erythroid progenitor stem cells obtained from mice infected with Rauscher leukemia virus (Gallicchio and Hughes 1992; Gallicchio et al. 1992).

The clinical studies of lithium in HIV-infected patients are much more preliminary but offer promise. In a pilot study, Roberts et al. (1988) showed that three of five zidovudine-treated AIDS patients receiving doses of lithium sufficient to attain therapeutic plasma levels showed significant neutrophilia. Interestingly, three of five patients receiving lithium tolerated higher doses of zidovudine. Other small studies have shown similar (albeit modest) benefit of concomitant lithium administration.

Antiviral Effects of Lithium

The use of lithium as an antiviral agent is receiving growing consideration following the demonstration about 15 years ago that lithium inhibited the replication of certain viruses under particular experimental conditions (Skinner et al. 1980). Several studies have since reported that lithium inhibits the replication of several DNA viruses (see Cernescu et al. 1988). There is less agreement on RNA viruses; two RNA virus groups are not inhibited by lithium, whereas inhibition of paramyxoviruses are reported. The mechanisms by which lithium inhibits DNA replication through DNA polymerase in herpesvirus are presently unknown but are thought to occur through modification of intracellular second-messenger systems.

In this context, it is noteworthy that the enhancement of tumor necrosis factor cytotoxicity by lithium has been shown to be mediated by alterations in the PI second-messenger system (Beyaert et al. 1993). In particular, treatment of the transformed cell line L929 with the combination of tumor necrosis factor and lithium induced an increase in cytidine diphosphate–DAG that preceded the onset of cell killing by approximately 1 hour. Moreover, the cytotoxic effects of lithium were sensitive to the PKC inhibitor staurosporine. In vitro studies have revealed the positive effects of lithium on HIV in MT4 (a transformed lymphocyte cell line) and CEM cells (an acute lymphoblastic leukemia T cell line). Gallicchio et al. (1993) investigated the effect of lithium in animals infected with murine immunodeficiency virus, demonstrating a marked reduction in the development of lymphadenopathy and splenomegaly. These investigators suggested that lithium may be effective in modulating murine immunodeficiency virus infection. They raised important questions related to the potential role of lithium in the pathophysiological processes associated with retroviral infections.

To date, virtually all of the relevant detailed clinical studies on the potential antiviral efficacy of lithium have been directed to the treatment of herpes simplex virus infections. A large study of 177 subjects found that chronic lithium administration resulted in a significant reduction in the recurrence rate of these infections, and most patients reported a reduction to less than half the pretreatment rate (Amsterdam et al. 1990a, 1990b). Other double-blind prospective studies have identified a similar beneficial effect of lithium, which appears to be independent of any modulation of affective symptoms.

SIDE EFFECTS AND TOXICOLOGY

General Considerations

Lithium has a narrow therapeutic index in humans; its currently recommended therapeutic serum concentration range is 0.8–1.2 mEq/L (Gelenberg et al. 1989; Schatzberg and Cole 1991). Side effects and toxicity become increasingly more evident at doses that result in higher serum levels (Jefferson et al. 1987). A recent review of the literature reveals that 35%–93% of patients complain about adverse side effects of lithium treatment. The most common side effects reported are noted in Table 20–1, which presents pooled data from 12 individual studies of 1,094 patients (Goodwin and Jamison 1990). It is of interest that when patients are asked about the most troublesome side effects that often lead to noncompliance with long-term lithium treatment, the most common are related to cognitive dysfunction (i.e., mental confusion, poor concentration, mental slowness, and memory problems).

The major physiological systems predisposed to lithium-induced symptomatology and toxicity include the gastrointestinal, renal, endocrine, and nervous systems, as

Table 20–1. Lithium side effects

Side effect	Percentage with subjective complaint[a]	Relative importance in noncompliance[b]
Excessive thirst	35.9	
Polyuria	30.4	4
Memory problems	28.2	1
Tremor	26.6	3[c]
Weight gain	18.9	2
Drowsiness/tiredness	12.4	5
Diarrhea	8.7	
Any complaint	73.8	
No complaints	26.2	

[a]Pooled percentages from 12 studies including 1,094 patients.
[b]Relative ranking of importance of side effects for lithium noncompliance in 71 patients (Goodwin and Jamison 1990).
[c]Included incoordination.

well as the teratogenicity affecting the developing fetus. Most of the side effects appear to be dose related and transient in nature (Jefferson 1990; Schou 1989; Vestergaard et al. 1988). Although sustained-release formulations of lithium may be useful in ameliorating some lithium-induced side effects, enhanced gastrointestinal symptomatology may preclude this treatment strategy. Thus, risk factors that predispose to side effects and toxicity of lithium include reduced renal clearance with age or renal disease, organic brain disorder, physical illness with vomiting and/or diarrhea, diuretic and/or other concomitant pharmacotherapy, low sodium intake and/or high sodium excretion, and pregnancy.

The vulnerability of certain organ systems to lithium-induced effects may be due not only to a preferential accumulation of lithium but also to its action as outlined above on the various ion transport, second-messenger, and receptor-signaling systems shared in both the brain and periphery. The CNS, which is the apparent site of its therapeutic action, is particularly sensitive to side effects and toxicity. Studies have even reported that lithium distribution throughout brain regions can be nonuniform, resulting in relatively greater potential effects in selected regions of the brain (Sansone and Ziegler 1985). Clinical manifestations of a fine hand tremor is one of the most common reported side effects in 31%–65% of patients. This can be associated with reduced motor coordination, nystagmus, and muscular weakness most notable in the early phases of treatment (Goodwin and Jamison 1990). Evidence for cogwheel rigidity has been reported with long-term treatment with lithium alone and has been attributed to the antidopaminergic effects of lithium, although this observation has been most apparent during concomitant neuroleptic exposure (Asnis et al. 1979).

Central Nervous System

The cognitive effects of lithium appear to be some of the most problematic for patients, yet they remain the least studied. Clinical reports of noncompliance with lithium over the years have attributed difficulty with both creativity and productivity and a lack of drive to lithium treatment. Yet two noted studies carried out in artists, writers, and business executives ($N = 30$) being treated with lithium found that more than 75% of these patients believed that lithium either enhanced or did not change their creative productivity (Marshall et al. 1970; Schou 1979a). In addition, it has been difficult to find convincing evidence for cognitive effects of lithium in animal studies. Studies of lithium-induced effects on intellectual functioning such as memory, associative processing, semantic reasoning, and rate of psychomotor and cognitive performance in bipolar patients remain contradictory (see review in Goodwin and Jamison 1990). Judd et al. (1987) reported data demonstrating a "slowing of the rate of central information processing" (pp. 1467–1468) in a series of control subjects administered therapeutic doses of lithium, a finding that supported earlier observations by Schou (1968). However, these studies were relatively short term, and there is evidence that accommodation to some of the cognitive effects of lithium occurs. Further research in this area is warranted because lithium appears to have profound effects on PKC-mediated events in the brain (as noted previously), PKC has been implicated in long-term potentiation in the hippocampus (Manji and Lenox 1994), and the subjective effects of lithium on cognition remain such an important clinical issue in compliance.

The neurotoxic effects of lithium that generally occur at higher serum concentrations or in patients with the risk factors we have noted are associated with increasing signs of cognitive impairment, lassitude, restlessness, and irritability (Jefferson et al. 1987). Although this symptomatology is reversible within 5–10 days, neurotoxicity can progress to frank delirium, ataxia, coarse tremors, seizures, and ultimately to coma and death. It is of interest that recent behavioral models of lithium's action in the brain, as well as its neurotoxic effect on seizure threshold, have reported reversibility with inositol administration, thus implicating lithium's action on the PI signaling pathway in these neurobehavioral and neurotoxic events (Kofman and Belmaker 1993). Consistent with our earlier observations, these data may also implicate the PI system as a target for lithium action on a continuum from its therapeutic to its neurotoxic effects.

Endocrine Systems

Lithium has been shown to exert effects on various endocrine systems; interested readers are directed to excellent recent reviews of the subject (F. N. Johnson 1988; Lazarus 1986). In a study of 330 bipolar patients treated with lithium for 5 months to 3 years, Schou (1968) first reported that lithium therapy induced goiter at an overall rate of 3.6%. Lithium appears to exert antithyroid effects at different levels of thyroid function, including inhibition of hormone synthesis and release, inhibition of the action of TSH, and peripheral metabolism of thyroxine.

Although reports of lithium-induced hypothyroidism range from 5% to 35% because of variability in the criteria for diagnosis and the sensitivity of laboratory tests, the prevalence of clinical hypothyroidism is estimated more likely to be 5% and more common in women (Jefferson 1990). It is generally accepted that approximately 30% of patients have elevated levels of TSH, although most do not have statistically significant decreases in the levels of circulating thyroid hormones. This suggests that a compromised substrate may be necessary for the development of overt hypothyroidism (Amdisen and Andersen 1982; Lindstedt et al. 1977; Rogers and Whybrow 1971). Such a suggestion is supported by studies showing an increased likelihood of elevations in TSH and decreases in thyroid hormones during lithium therapy in individuals with serum antithyroid antibodies (Calabrese et al. 1985; Myers et al. 1985).

Patients taking lithium manifest a high prevalence of thyroid autoantibodies (15%–30%), suggesting a relative induction by lithium (Deniker et al. 1978; Lazarus 1986). Furthermore, low-normal thyronine levels have been associated with lethargy and cognitive impairment in patients treated with lithium for at least 6 months, and triiodothy-

ronine was in the low-normal range in patients who relapsed (Hatterer et al. 1989). Because lithium has been shown to suppress the cAMP formation induced by TSH stimulation, lithium-induced hypothyroidism may occur by an "uncoupling" of the TSH receptor from adenylate cyclase, resulting in a compensatory increased secretion of TSH (McHenry et al. 1990; Mori et al. 1989; Tseng et al. 1989). Although this is an attractive hypothesis and is likely to play some role in the reduced sensitivity to the effects of TSH, lithium also inhibits forskolin-stimulated iodine uptake in thyroid cells, suggesting that additional effects distal to cAMP formation (e.g., protein kinase) are involved (Mori et al. 1989; Urabe et al. 1991). In this context, it is noteworthy that lithium's effects are mimicked by PKC activators and blocked by PKC inhibitors in cultured thyroid tissue, suggesting that lithium's action on both adenylate cyclase and PKC contributes to the observed thyroid dysfunction.

Another possible endocrine complication of lithium treatment, hyperparathyroidism, was first reported by Garfinkel et al. (1973) and is much less common (Nordenstrom et al. 1992; Taylor and Bell 1993). Although the clinical significance of lithium-induced primary hyperparathyroidism has remained controversial, studies have reported increased parathyroid hormone secretion in at least a subset of patients (Christiansen et al. 1978), and there is accompanying evidence for modest increases in serum calcium and parathyroid hyperplasia in several reports (Lazarus 1986; Mannisto 1980). Since then, hyperparathyroidism associated with lithium therapy has been reported in more than 20 cases. However, the effect of lithium on parathyroid hormone secretion during clinical treatment remains controversial, at least in part because of the lack of pretreatment parathyroid hormone levels in most of the cases and the inability to demonstrate an alteration in the set point for parathyroid hormone secretion in healthy subjects undergoing subacute lithium administration (Spiegel et al. 1984). Nevertheless, the longitudinal studies, together with the reports of parathyroid hyperplasia and elevations of serum calcium, suggest that abnormal parathyroid hormone secretion may occur in at least a subset of individuals treated with lithium.

Of interest is that in vitro data in parathyroid cells exposed to lithium indicate an action on both parathyroid hormone release and mitogenic properties similar to that observed with PKC activation (Saxe and Gibson 1991, 1993). Lithium at therapeutic levels appears to have diverse effects on the parathyroid gland, causing a rightward shift in the calcium-sensing set point and thereby abnormally releasing parathyroid hormone. In cases of preexisting parathyroid abnormalities, lithium may serve to unmask an incipient adenoma and cause hyperplasia of the gland (Mallette et al. 1989; McHenry et al. 1991).

Renal Function

Lithium is excreted from the body almost entirely from the kidney, and there is no evidence for any significant protein binding. Lithium reversibly reduces the kidney's ability to concentrate urine primarily through effects on renal tubular function, resulting in the clinical manifestation of polyuria (>3 L/24 hours) (E. Walker and Green 1982). This impairment of renal tubular concentrating ability has been associated with a reversible acute epithelial swelling and glycogen disposition in the distal nephron. It is related to both the dose and the duration of lithium treatment and occurs in 20%–30% of patients treated with lithium (Goodwin and Jamison 1990; R. G. Walker 1993). Studies have indicated that once-daily dosing of lithium may result in relatively less renal symptomatology than a multiple-dosing treatment strategy, but further confirmation is needed (Lauritsen et al. 1981; Schou et al. 1982). Lithium appears to inhibit vasopressin (V_2 receptor)-stimulated cAMP production, reducing water reabsorption in the distal tubules and collecting ducts and resulting in nephrogenic diabetes insipidus (Dousa and Hechter 1970a, 1970b; Jefferson 1990).

There is also evidence for a dipsogenic effect of lithium through interaction with the renin-angiotensin system in the brain (Jefferson 1990). The mechanism for the inhibition of cAMP generation probably involves an effect at the level of G proteins, and more recent studies have suggested additional mechanisms involving prostaglandin pathways and PKC (Anger et al. 1990; Yamaki et al. 1991). A more progressive development of impairment of urinary concentrating ability has been observed in patients taking long-term lithium treatment, especially in those exposed to periods of lithium toxicity or concomitant exposure treatment with neuroleptics (R. G. Walker 1993). Although such patients on renal biopsy may have chronic focal interstitial nephropathy, similar lesions have been noted in psychiatric patients with no exposure to lithium. There is little evidence for lithium-induced chronic glomerular toxicity, although there are case reports of a reversible minimal lesion nephrotic syndrome (R. G. Walker 1993). In a recent review, Gitlin (1993) cited evidence that up to 5% of lithium-treated patients may develop signs of renal insufficiency, and in two reported cases progressive renal failure was diagnosed. However, such data lack comparable statistics for rate of renal insufficiency in the general population or in untreated bipolar patients and may be related to an increased risk of renal effects of lith-ium observed in patients exposed to periods of acute toxicity (Schou et al. 1989; R. G. Walker 1993).

Less Common Side Effects

The cardiovascular effects of orally administered lithium are rather benign. Most commonly, electrocardiogram recordings show a flattening and inversion of the T wave (Tilkian et al. 1976). Lithium has been shown to prolong sinus node recovery time. Caution is recommended in patients with bradycardia or sinus node dysfunction, as well as in those being treated concomitantly with drugs affecting sinus node conduction (Jefferson 1991; Mitchell and MacKenzie 1982; Roose et al. 1979). Because weight gain can be a significant side effect of long-term lithium treatment, the action of lithium on glucose metabolism has been examined over the years with rather conflicting results (Garland et al. 1988; Mellerup et al. 1983; Peselow et al. 1980). Consistent with lithium's ability to inhibit cAMP formation, there appears to be more consistent evidence for an insulin-like action resulting in a relative hypoglycemia (Jefferson 1991). Other lesser side effects of lithium treatment include an exacerbation of existing psoriasis, hair loss, leukocytosis, decreased libido, and altered taste sensation (Schou 1989).

Teratogenic Effects

Lithium treatment in humans has been associated with teratogenic properties predominantly affecting the cardiovascular development during the first trimester of pregnancy. Earlier studies based on the original work of Schou et al. (1973), which led to the development of the International Register of Lithium Babies, revealed an increased rate of Ebstein's anomaly that was 400 times higher than that observed in the general population (Nora et al. 1974). More recent controlled epidemiological studies have reported an apparently reduced rate of Ebstein's anomaly in the range of 0.1%–0.7%, approximately 20–140 times greater than in the general population (Elia et al. 1987; Jacobson et al. 1992; Zalstein et al. 1990). The risk of major congenital malformations with lithium treatment in the first trimester is now thought to be in the range of 4%–12%, whereas the prevalence in an untreated comparison cohort is in the range of 2%–4% (L. S. Cohen et al. 1994). Lithium is currently indicated as a category D drug in the current edition of *Drugs in Pregnancy and Lactation* (Briggs et al. 1990), which states that "there is positive evidence of human fetal risk, but benefits from use in pregnant women may be acceptable despite the risk" (pp. 357–358).

In a recent review, L. S. Cohen et al. (1994) recommended a reconsideration of the relative risks associated with discontinuation compared with maintenance of lithium treatment during pregnancy. They outlined new guidelines for patients continuing lithium during the first trimester of pregnancy, suggesting prenatal diagnosis by fetal echocardiogram and high-resolution ultrasound examination at 16–18 weeks of gestation. Lithium passes through the placental barrier in the latter months of pregnancy and is present in breast milk, which can result in toxicity to the neonate manifesting in lethargy, hypotonia, and cyanosis.

DRUG-DRUG INTERACTIONS

Psychotropic Drugs

Overall, lithium has surprisingly few clinically significant interactions with most routinely prescribed psychotropic drugs. This perhaps explains in part why (despite its relatively low therapeutic index) a trial of adjunctive lithium therapy has been investigated in the treatment of numerous psychiatric conditions (see previous section; Table 20–2).

Table 20–2. Potentially clinically significant drug interactions with lithium

Drug	Potential manifestations
Diuretics	Affect lithium clearance
Thiazides	Alter (usually raise) plasma lithium levels
Aldosterone antagonists	
Xanthine derivatives	
Loop diuretics and potassium-sparing diuretics	Cause fewer problems than other diuretics
Nonsteroidal anti-inflammatory drugs (NSAIDs)	Decrease lithium clearance and raise plasma lithium levels
Diclofenac	May cause fewer problems than other NSAIDs
Indomethacin	
Ibuprofen	
Naproxen	
Phenylbutazone	
Sulindac	
Neuroleptics	Worsen extrapyramidal side effects
	May result in neurotoxicity (high-potency agents appear to carry greater risk)
Antiarrhythmics	May potentiate cardiac conduction effects

Benzodiazepines

Few clinically relevant interactions between lithium and benzodiazepines occur, although certain individuals may be at greater risk for CNS depressant effects when the combination of the two drugs is used. In this context, the lithium-benzodiazepine combination has been suggested to produce an idiosyncratic reaction manifested by profound hypothermia in one individual (Naylor and McHarg 1977). Nevertheless, a combination of benzodiazepines and lithium has been used extensively in the clinical setting, and few major adverse effects have been noted (Jefferson et al. 1981; Lenox et al. 1992a). Indeed, in view of the potential for sleep deprivation to induce manic episodes (Wehr et al. 1987), the judicious use of a benzodiazepine is recommended in the treatment of bipolar patients experiencing sleep disruption.

Neuroleptics

The practice of combining neuroleptics with lithium is generally considered safe and efficacious (Goodwin and Jamison 1990), but caution is recommended, particularly with the high-potency neuroleptics. There are reports of pharmacokinetic interactions between lithium and neuroleptics, but these are generally regarded as not clinically significant (Jefferson et al. 1983). Although lithium-neuroleptic neurotoxicity is a relatively rare phenomenon, it has been most widely associated with haloperidol (W. J. Cohen and Cohen 1974), and more than 40 cases are reported in the literature (see Ross and Coffey 1987; Werstiuk and Steiner 1987). This syndrome is characterized by altered mental status, cerebellar signs and symptoms, tremor, and extrapyramidal symptoms. Some patients also have fever and elevations in serum liver enzymes, raising the possibility that these may represent atypical cases of neuroleptic malignant syndrome.

In contrast, a chart review of 425 patients treated with lithium and haloperidol revealed that side effects occurred with no greater incidence with the two drugs combined than with either drug alone (F. N. Johnson 1984). Similarly, a study examining the prevalence of electroencephalogram abnormalities in patients treated with a combination of lithium and haloperidol found that the incidence of such abnormalities was not greater with the two drugs combined than with either drug alone (or with no drug) (Abrams and Taylor 1979). Thus, overall, it appears that this potential interaction is relatively rare. Nevertheless, given the abundant preclinical data supporting an effect of lithium on the dopaminergic system and the severity of the neurotoxicity, it seems prudent for clinicians to be aware of this interaction and to discontinue both drugs if toxicity develops.

Clozapine, an atypical antipsychotic that has been approved by the FDA for treatment-resistant schizophrenia (Baldessarini and Frankenburg 1991), has proven superior efficacy over traditional antipsychotics in patients with this condition (Baldessarini and Frankenburg 1991; Kane 1990; Kane et al. 1988). A growing body of literature suggests that clozapine may be a useful and well-tolerated agent in the treatment of excited manic-psychotic phases of bipolar and schizoaffective disorders, even in patients who have failed to respond to, or do not tolerate, conventional somatic therapies (reviewed in Tohen, in press). More recently, controlled studies have indicated that clozapine appears to be effective and well-tolerated in the short-term and maintenance treatment of severe or psychotic mood disorders, particularly in the manic-excited phases of schizoaffective and bipolar disorders, even in patients who have not responded well to conventional pharmacotherapies (Tohen, in press). Thus, it is not surprising that clinicians have coadministered clozapine and lithium. Seizures were reported in two patients shortly after the addition of lithium to clozapine (Guadalupe et al. 1994).

In addition, other adverse effects have been reported in the literature with the combination of clozapine and lithium; four patients developed reversible neurological symptoms (i.e., involuntary jerking of limbs, hand tremor, tongue twitching, agitation, confusion, and bizarre nihilistic delusions). Two of these patients were rechallenged, and only one had a recurrence of symptoms. Currently, the exact frequency with which the combination of lithium and clozapine (or the more recently introduced, structurally similar, atypical antipsychotic, olanzapine) lowers seizure threshold or results in other neurological sequelae remains unknown.

Also reported in the literature were two cases of diabetic ketoacidosis associated with concomitant clozapine and lithium treatment (Koval et al. 1994; Peterson and Byrd 1996). Although there were only two cases, some of the clinical similarities include the fact that both patients were African Americans who had been taking both clozapine and lithium at the time they first presented with diabetic ketoacidosis. Neither had a toxic level of lithium, and both had taken lithium for extended periods. Furthermore, in both cases, the complication occurred early (within 5–6 weeks) in the course of clozapine treatment. Interestingly, neither patient had a history of diabetes or hyperglycemia (although one patient had a family history of diabetes and continued to manifest insulin-dependent diabetes 2 years after clozapine treatment was discontinued). To date, the frequency of such a potential interaction is unknown and warrants further study.

Anticonvulsants

As noted earlier and more fully discussed in Chapter 35, several anticonvulsants—most notably, valproate and carbamazepine—are being extensively used in the treatment of bipolar disorder. Increasingly, these agents (in particular valproate) are being coadministered with lithium, and a recent study evaluated the pharmacokinetic effects and safety of coadministration of lithium and valproate in 16 healthy volunteers. In a randomized, placebo-controlled, two-period (12 days each), crossover trial (Granneman et al. 1996), valproate or placebo was given twice daily. The investigators found that lithium pharmacokinetics were unchanged by valproate but that some of valproate's pharmacokinetic measures (maximum drug concentration in serum [C_{max}], minimum drug concentration in serum [C_{min}], and area under the concentration-time curve) rose slightly during lithium coadministration. Overall, however, adverse events did not change significantly, suggesting that the concomitant administration of lithium and valproate appears to be safe in patients with bipolar disorder.

Antidepressants

The combination of lithium and various classes of antidepressants has been used extensively in many patients. The preponderance of the data suggest that, although minor side effects are common, major adverse effects are relatively uncommon (Price 1987). There are reports of increased incidence of myoclonic jerks in patients receiving a combination of lithium and monoamine oxidase inhibitors, but this has not been extensively investigated. In view of the enhancement of serotonergic function by lithium, there is the potential for an increased risk of the so-called serotonin syndrome in individuals receiving a combination of lithium and selective serotonin reuptake inhibitors or monoamine oxidase inhibitors, but the clinical data to date are sparse.

Electroconvulsive Therapy

Although not a true drug-drug interaction, the use of lithium during a course of electroconvulsive therapy (ECT) warrants discussion. In recent years, ECT has emerged as a remarkably efficacious, potentially life-saving treatment for many psychiatric conditions for which lithium is also used, including severe depression and mania (Crowe 1984). There is thus a clear need to establish the safety and potential efficacy of lithium treatment during ECT. Despite this clinical need, however, there is a dearth of adequate studies addressing this important issue (Rudorfer and Linnoila 1987).

Several case reports have suggested that the combination of lithium and ECT may be associated with a neurotoxic syndrome characterized by confusion, disorientation, and decreased responsiveness (reviewed in Rudorfer and Linnoila 1987). However, a comprehensive retrospective review (Perry and Tsuang 1979) and a prospective, controlled, double-blind study (Coppen et al. 1981) both reported no increased morbidity for lithium-ECT. In fact, the well-known need to continue maintenance medication after ECT and lithium's latency of onset of action prompted Coppen et al. (1981) to suggest that lithium might be introduced early during the course of ECT to minimize the likelihood of relapse after ECT termination. This suggestion has not been generally accepted in routine clinical practice. Despite the lack of clear-cut evidence of neurotoxicity in general, it does appear that some patients are more susceptible to neurotoxic manifestations. Additionally, given the lack of obvious benefit of combining lithium and ECT in most patients, it seems prudent to discontinue lithium during the course of ECT. In cases of established lack of adequate response to either treatment alone, or in cases of known rapid relapse after ECT discontinuation, the lithium-ECT combination treatment can be conducted judiciously, by using "low therapeutic" lithium levels, avoiding other medications, and monitoring for any symptoms that are suggestive of neurotoxicity.

Nonpsychotropic Drugs

The largest single class of drugs producing a clinically significant interaction with lithium are the diuretics, several types of which can elevate lithium levels and produce toxicity. It is now well established that diuretics decrease renal lithium clearance, which frequently necessitates a reduction of the lithium dose to avoid toxicity. Any drug capable of altering renal function should be used judiciously in patients receiving lithium, and more frequent plasma level determinations and a reduction of the dose should be performed if necessary. However, perhaps because of their more proximal site of action, thiazide diuretics are also sometimes used to treat lithium-induced nephrogenic diabetes insipidus (discussed previously). Other classes of diuretics have been less well studied. The present data suggest, however, that a careful monitoring of lithium levels is warranted when using osmotic diuretics, loop diuretics, aldosterone antagonists, or other potassium-sparing diuretics.

The effects of cardiac drugs that alter sinus node conduction (e.g., quinidine and digoxin) could be potentiated by lithium. It is clear that the combination of lithium with cardiac drugs requires careful monitoring, including regular electrocardiograms. Several nonsteroidal antiinflammatory drugs can also increase plasma lithium levels, perhaps by an inhibition of renal tubular prostaglandin synthesis. Almost all of the older nonsteroidal antiinflammatory drugs (including diclofenac, ibuprofen, indomethacin, naproxen, and phenylbutazone) have been shown to interact with lithium and often result in toxicity, although preliminary studies suggest that sulindac may be less frequently associated with toxicity. Lithium is also known to prolong the action of neuromuscular agents, necessitating a reduction in dose or, in the case of patients undergoing certain surgical procedures or ECT, complete cessation.

It has been recognized that methylxanthines (such as caffeine) may significantly interfere with the clearance of some psychotropic drugs, such as lithium, that are mainly excreted by the kidneys. Early studies (reviewed in Finley et al. 1995) found mixed effects of caffeine ingestion on lithium clearance. Jefferson (1988) described two case reports of enhanced lithium-induced tremor after elimination of caffeine from the diet and concluded that marked reduction in caffeine intake may cause lithium retention, increased lithium levels, and thus aggravation of lithium-induced tremor. Most recently, it has been shown that in lithium-maintained patients with high daily caffeine intake, abrupt cessation of caffeine results in a significant (24%) increase in lithium blood levels (Mester et al. 1995). Irrespective of the potential role of caffeine withdrawal in triggering affective episodes, this study suggests that the marked reduction of caffeine from the diet (as is frequently done in controlled inpatient settings) of lithium-treated patients should be done cautiously in patients with high baseline levels of lithium in blood.

CONCLUSION

Lithium is a monovalent cation with complex physiological and pharmacological effects within the brain. By virtue of the ionic properties it shares with other important monovalent and divalent cations, such as sodium, magnesium, and calcium, its transport into cells provides ready access to a host of intracellular enzymatic events affecting short- and long-term cell processes. It may be that, in part, the therapeutic efficacy of lithium in the treatment of both poles of bipolar disorder may rely on the "dirty" characteristics of its multiple sites of pharmacological interaction.

Strategic models to further delineate the mechanism(s) of action of lithium that are relevant to its therapeutic effects must account for several critical variables in experimental design. Lithium has a relatively low therapeutic index, requiring careful attention to the tissue concentrations at which effects of the drug are being observed in light of the known toxicity of lithium within the CNS. Although such a poor therapeutic index may suggest a continuum between some of the biological processes underlying therapeutic efficacy and toxicity, it may also account in part for the variability of effects of lithium observed in animal and in vitro studies. The therapeutic action of lithium is delayed, requiring more long-term administration to establish efficacy for both its treatment of acute mania and its prophylaxis of the recurrent affective episodes associated with bipolar disorder. Although its therapeutic effects are not reversed immediately with abrupt discontinuation, there is accumulating evidence that abrupt withdrawal of lithium may sensitize the patient's system to an episode of mania (Klein et al. 1992; Suppes et al. 1991).

The ability of lithium to stabilize an underlying dysregulation of limbic and limbic-associated function is critical to understanding its mechanism of action. The biological processes in the brain that are responsible for the episodic clinical manifestation of mania and depression may be caused by an inability to mount the appropriate compensatory responses necessary to maintain homeostatic regulation, thereby resulting in sudden oscillations beyond immediate adaptive control (Depue et al. 1987; Goodwin and Jamison 1990; Mandell et al. 1984). The resultant clinical picture is reflected in disruptions of behavior, circadian rhythms, neurophysiology of sleep, and neuroendocrine and biochemical regulation within the brain. Regulation of signal transduction within critical regions of the brain remains an attractive target for psychopharmacological interventions. The behavioral and physiological manifestations of the illness are complex and are mediated by a network of interconnected neurotransmitter pathways. The biogenic amines have been strongly implicated in the regulation of these physiological processes by virtue of their pharmacological actions and predominant neuroanatomical distribution within limbic-related brain regions. Thus, lithium's ability to modulate the release of serotonin at presynaptic sites and modulate receptor-mediated supersensitivity in the brain remains a relevant line of investigation into the respective action of lithium in altering the clinical manifestation of depression and mania in patients with bipolar disorder.

However, it is at the molecular level that some of the most exciting advances in the understanding of the long-term therapeutic action of lithium will continue in the coming years. The lithium cation possesses the selective ability, at clinically relevant concentrations, to alter the PI second-messenger system, potentially altering the activity and dynamic regulation of receptors that are coupled to this intracellular response. Subtypes of muscarinic receptors in the limbic system may represent particularly sensitive targets in this regard, especially in light of the putative role of cholinergic neurotransmission in both lithium action and affective state.

Finally, it would appear that the current studies of the long-term lithium-induced changes in PKC and potentially other kinase-mediated events in the brain offer a most promising avenue for future investigation. Critical phosphoprotein substrates that play a role in the neuroplastic processes involved in cytoskeletal restructuring provide an opportunity for long-term dynamic regulation of signaling involving ion transport, neurotransmitter release, and the receptor-response complex. Furthermore, downstream alterations in gene expression through phosphoproteins acting as transcription factors can have a significant long-term effect on the precise profile of proteins that are available for the regulation of signal transduction in specific regions of the brain. It remains to be determined whether forthcoming research identifying the molecular targets for lithium in the brain will lead to elucidation of the pathophysiology of bipolar disorder and the discovery of a new generation of mood stabilizers.

REFERENCES

Abrams R, Taylor MA: EEG observations during combined lithium and neuroleptic treatment. Am J Psychiatry 136: 336–337, 1979

Acquas E, Fibiger HC: Chronic lithium attenuates dopamine D1-receptor mediated increases in acetylcholine in rat frontal cortex. Psychopharmacology 125:162–167, 1996

Aderem A: The MARCKS brothers: a family of protein kinase C substrates. Cell 71:713–716, 1992

Ahluwalia P, Singhal RL: Effect of low-dose lithium administration and subsequent withdrawal on biogenic amines in rat brain. Br J Pharmacol 71:601–607, 1980

Ahluwalia P, Singhal RL: Monoamine uptake into synaptosomes from various regions of rat brain following lithium administration and withdrawal. Neuropharmacology 20: 483–487, 1981

Ahluwalia P, Grewaal DS, Singhal RL: Brain GABAergic and dopaminergic systems following lithium treatment and withdrawal. Progress in Neuro-Psychopharmacology 5:527–530, 1981

Akagawa K, Watanabe M, Tsukada Y: Activity of Na-K-ATPase in manic patients. J Neurochem 35:258–260, 1980

Alexander DR, Deeb M, Bitar F, et al: Sodium-potassium, magnesium, and calcium ATPase activities in erythrocyte membranes from manic-depressive patients responding to lithium. Biol Psychiatry 21:997–1007, 1986

Allikmets LH, Stanley M, Gershon S: The effect of lithium on chronic haloperidol enhanced apomorphine aggression in rats. Life Sci 25:165–170, 1979

Allison JH: Lithium and brain *myo*-inositol metabolism, in Cyclitols and Phosphoinositides. Edited by Wells WW, Eisenberg F Jr. New York, Academic Press, 1978, pp 507–519

Allison JH, Stewart MA: Reduced brain inositol in lithium treated rats. Nature: New Biology 233:267–268, 1971

Allison JH, Blisner MW, Holland WH, et al: Increased brain *myo*-inositol 1-phosphate in lithium-treated rats. Biochem Biophys Res Commun 71:664–670, 1976

Allison JH, Boshans RL, Hallcher LM, et al: The effects of lithium on myo-inositol levels in layers of frontal cerebral cortex, in cerebellum, and in corpus callosum of the rat. J Neurochem 34:456–458, 1980

Amdisen A, Andersen C: Lithium treatment of thyroid function: a survey of 237 patients in long term lithium treatment. Pharmacopsychiatria 15:149–155, 1982

Amsterdam JD, Maislin G, Potter L, et al: Reduced rate of recurrent genital herpes infections with lithium carbonate. Psychopharmacol Bull 26:343–347, 1990a

Amsterdam JD, Maislin G, Rybakowski J: A possible antiviral action of lithium carbonate in herpes simplex virus infections. Biol Psychiatry 27:447–453, 1990b

Andersen PH, Geisler A: Lithium inhibition of forskolin-stimulated adenylate cyclase. Neuropsychobiology 12:1–3, 1984

Anderson SMP, Godfrey PP, Grahame-Smith DG: The effects of phorbol esters and lithium on 5-HT release in rat hippocampal slices (abstract). Br J Pharmacol 93:96P, 1988

Anger MS, Shanley P, Mansour J, et al: Effects of lithium on cAMP generation in cultured rat inner medullary collecting tubule cells. Kidney Int 37:1211–1218, 1990

Arendt J, Aldhous M, Marks V: Alleviation of jet lag by melatonin: preliminary results of controlled double blind trial. BMJ 292:1170–1174, 1986

Arystarkhoua E, Sweadner KJ: Isoform-specific monoclonal antibodies to Na, K-ATPase alpha subunits: evidence for a tissue-specific post-translational modification of the alpha subunit. J Biol Chem 271:23407–23417, 1996

Asnis GM, Asnis D, Dunner DL, et al: Cogwheel rigidity during chronic lithium therapy. Am J Psychiatry 136:1225–1226, 1979

Atre-Vaidya N, Taylor MA: Effectiveness of lithium in schizophrenia: do we really have an answer? J Clin Psychiatry 50:170–173, 1989

Aulde J: The use of lithium bromide in combination with solution of potassium citrate. Medical Bulletin (Philadelphia) 9:35–39, 69–72, 228–233, 1887

Ault KT, Durmwicz G, Galione A, et al: Modulation of *Xenopus* embryo mesoderm-specific gene expression and dorsoanterior patterning by receptors that activate the phosphatidylinositol cycle signal transduction pathway. Development 122:2033–2041, 1996

Avissar S, Schreiber G, Danon A, et al: Lithium inhibits adrenergic and cholinergic increases in GTP binding in rat cortex. Nature 331:440–442, 1988

Bach RO, Gallicchio VS: Lithium and Cell Physiology. New York, Springer-Verlag, 1990

Baldessarini RJ, Frankenburg FR: Clozapine: a novel antipsychotic agent. N Engl J Med 324:746–754, 1991

Ballast CL, Sharp PR, Domino EF: Effect of lithium on RBC water permeability. Biol Psychiatry 21:426–427, 1986

Baraban JM, Worley PF, Snyder SH: Second messenger systems and psychoactive drug focus on the phosphoinositide system and lithium. Am J Psychiatry 146:1251–1260, 1989

Bebchuk JM, Arfken C, Dolan-Manji S, et al.: A preliminary investigation of a PKC inhibitor (Tamoxifen) in the treatment of acute mania (abstract). Abstracts of the American College of Neuropsychopharmacology Annual Meeting, Hawaii, December 1997

Beckmann H, St-Laurent J, Goodwin FK: The effect of lithium on urinary MHPG in unipolar and bipolar depressed patients. Psychopharmacologia 42:277–282, 1975

Belmaker RH: Receptors, adenylate cyclase, depression, and lithium. Biol Psychiatry 16:333–350, 1981

Berggren U: Effects of short-term lithium administration on tryptophan levels and 5-hydroxytryptamine synthesis in whole brain and brain regions in rats. J Neural Transm 69:115–121, 1987

Bernasconi R: The GABA hypothesis of affective illness: influence of clinically effective antimanic drugs on GABA turnover, in Basic Mechanisms in the Action of Lithium. Edited by Emrich HM, Adenhoff JB, Lux HM. Amsterdam, Excerpta Medica, 1982, pp 183–192

Berrettini WH, Vogel WH, Ladman RK: Effects of lithium therapy on MAO in manic-depressive illness. Am J Psychiatry 136:836–838, 1979

Berrettini WH, Nurnberger JI Jr, Hare T, et al: Plasma and CSF GABA in affective illness. Br J Psychiatry 141:483–487, 1982

Berrettini WH, Nurnberger JI Jr, Hare TA, et al: Reduced plasma and CSF gamma-aminobutyric acid in affective illness. Biol Psychiatry 18:185–194, 1983

Berrettini WH, Nurnberger JI Jr, Chan JS, et al: Pro-opiomelanocortin-related peptides in cerebrospinal fluid: a study of manic-depressive disorder. Psychiatry Res 16:287–302, 1985a

Berrettini WH, Nurnberger JI, Scheinin M, et al: Cerebrospinal fluid and plasma monoamines and their metabolites in euthymic bipolar patients. Biol Psychiatry 20:257–269, 1985b

Berrettini WH, Nurnberger JI Jr, Hare TA, et al: CSF GABA in euthymic manic-depressive patients and controls. Biol Psychiatry 21:844–846, 1986

Berrettini WH, Nurnberger JI Jr, Zerbe RL, et al: CSF neuropeptides in euthymic bipolar patients and controls. Br J Psychiatry 150:208–212, 1987

Berridge MJ: Inositol triphosphate, calcium, lithium, and cell signaling. JAMA 262:1834–1841, 1989

Berridge MJ, Downes CP, Hanley MR: Lithium amplifies agonist-dependent phosphatidylinositol responses in brain and salivary glands. Biochem J 206:587–595, 1982

Berridge MJ, Downes CP, Hanley MR: Neural and developmental actions of lithium: a unifying hypothesis. Cell 59:411–419, 1989

Beyaert R, Heyninck K, De Valck D, et al.: Enhancement of tumor necrosis factor cytotoxicity by lithium chloride is associated with increased inositol phosphate accumulation. J Immunol 151:291–300, 1993

Bitran JA, Potter WZ, Manji HK, et al: Chronic Li^+ attenuates agonist- and phorbol ester-mediated Na^+/Ha^+ antiporter activity in HL-60 cells. Eur J Pharmacol 188:193–202, 1990

Bitran JA, Manji HK, Potter WZ, et al: Down-regulation of PKC alpha by lithium in vitro. Psychopharmacol Bull 31:449–452, 1995

Blackshear PJ: The MARCKS family of cellular protein kinase C substrates. J Biol Chem 268:1501–1504, 1993

Blancquaert JP, Lefebvre RA, Willems JL: Antiaversive properties of opioids in the conditioned taste aversion test in the rat. Pharmacol Biochem Behav 27:437–441, 1987

Blier P, de Montigny C: Short-term lithium administration enhances serotonergic neurotransmission: electrophysiological evidence in the rat CNS. Psychopharmacology (Berl) 113:69–77, 1985

Blier P, de Montigny C, Tardif D: Short-term lithium treatment enhances responsiveness of postsynaptic 5-HT$_{1A}$ receptors without altering 5-HT autoreceptor sensitivity: an electrophysiological study in the rat brain. Synapse 1:225–232, 1987

Bliss EL, Ailion J: The effect of lithium upon brain neuroamines. Brain Res 24:305–310, 1970

Bloom FE, Rogers J, Schulman JA, et al: Receptor plasticity: inferential changes after chronic treatment with lithium desmethylimipramine or ethanol detected by electrophysiological correlates, in Neuroreceptors: Basic and Clinical Aspects. Edited by Usdin E, Bunney WE Jr, Davis JM. New York, Wiley, 1981, pp 37–53

Bloom FE, Baetge G, Deyo S, et al: Chemical and physiological aspects of the actions of lithium and antidepressant drugs. Neuropharmacology 22:359–365, 1983

Bond PA, Jenner JA, Sampson DA: Daily variation of the urine content of 3-methoxy-4-hydroxyphenylglycol in two manic-depressive patients. Psychol Med 2:81–85, 1972

Born GVR, Grignani G, Martin K: Long-term effect of lithium on the uptake of 5-hydroxytryptamine by human platelets. Br J Clin Pharmacol 9:321–325, 1980

Borner C, Guadagno SN, Fabbro D, et al: Expression of four protein kinase C isoforms in rat fibroblasts: distinct subcellular distribution and regulation by calcium and phorbol esters. J Biol Chem 267:12892–12899, 1992

Bowden CL, Brugger AM, Swann AC, et al: Efficacy of divalproex vs. lithium and placebo in the treatment of mania. JAMA 271:918–924, 1994

Bowers MB, Heninger GR: Lithium: clinical effects and cerebrospinal fluid acid monoamine metabolites. Communications in Psychopharmacology 1:135–145, 1977

Brambilla F, Catalano M, Lucca A, et al: Effect of lithium treatment on the GH-clonidine test in affective disorders. Eur J Clin Pharmacol 35:601–605, 1988

Brami BA, Leli U, Hauser G: Influence of lithium on second messenger accumulation in NG108-15 cells. Biochem Biophys Res Commun 174:606–612, 1991a

Brami BA, Leli U, Hauser G: Origin of the diacylglycerol produced in excess of inositol phosphates by lithium in NG108-15 cells (abstract). J Neurochem 57 (suppl):S9, 1991b

Briggs GG, Freeman RK, Yaffe SJ: Drugs in Pregnancy and Lactation, 3rd Edition. Baltimore, MD, Williams & Wilkins, 1990

Brown GM, Grof E, Grof P: Neuroendocrinology of depression—a discussion. Psychopharmacol Bull 17:10–12, 1981

Bunney WE Jr: Neuronal receptor function in psychiatry: strategy and theory, in Neuroreceptors: Basic and Clinical Aspects. Edited by Usdin E, Bunney WE Jr, Davis JM. New York, Wiley, 1981, pp 241–255

Bunney WE, Garland BL: Lithium and its possible modes of action, in Neurobiology of Mood Disorders. Edited by Post RM, Ballenger J. Baltimore, MD, Williams & Wilkins, 1984, pp 731–743

Bunney WE, Garland-Bunney BL: Mechanism of action of lithium in affective illness: basic and clinical implications, in Psychopharmacology: The Third Generation of Progress. Edited by Meltzer HY. New York, Raven, 1987, pp 553–565

Burns G, Herz A, Nikolarakis KE: Stimulation of hypothalamic opioid peptide release by lithium is mediated by opioid autoreceptors: evidence from a combined in vitro, ex vivo study. Neuroscience 36:691–697, 1990

Busa WB, Gimlich RL: Lithium-induced teratogenesis in frog embryos prevented by a polyphosphoinositide cycle intermediate or a diacylglycerol analog. Dev Biol 132:315–324, 1989

Bussone G, Leone M, Peccarisi C, et al: Double blind comparison of lithium and verapamil in cluster headache prophylaxis. Headache 30:411–417, 1990

Cade JFJ: Lithium salts in the treatment of psychotic excitement. Med J Aust 36:349–352, 1949

Calabrese JR, Delucchi GA: Spectrum of efficacy of valproate in 55 patients with rapid-cycling bipolar disorder. Am J Psychiatry 147:431–434, 1990

Calabrese JR, Gulledge AD, Hahn K, et al: Autoimmune thyroiditis in manic-depressive patients treated with lithium. Am J Psychiatry 142:1318–1321, 1985

Cameron OG, Smith CB: Comparison of acute and chronic lithium treatment on ^{3}H-norepinephrine uptake by rat brain slices. Psychopharmacology (Berl) 67:81–85, 1980

Campbell SS, Gillin JC, Kripke DF, et al: Lithium delays circadian phase of temperature and REM sleep in a bipolar depressive: a case report. Psychiatry Res 27:23–29, 1989

Canessa M, Adragna N, Solomon HS, et al: Increased sodium-lithium countertransport in red cells of patients with essential hypertension. N Engl J Med 302:772–776, 1980

Canessa M, Brugnara C, Escobales N: The Li$^+$-Na$^+$ exchange and Na$^+$-K$^+$-Cl$^+$ cotransport systems in essential hypertension. Hypertension 10 (suppl I):4–10, 1987

Carli M, Anand-Srivastava MB, Molina-Holgado E, et al: Effects of chronic lithium treatments on central dopaminergic receptor systems: G proteins as possible targets. Neurochem Int 24:13–22, 1994

Carmiliet EE: Influence of lithium ions on the transmembrane potential and cation content of cardiac cells. J Gen Physiol 47:501–530, 1964

Carney PA, Fitzgerald CT, Monaghan CE: Influence of climate on the prevalence of mania. Br J Psychiatry 152:820–823, 1988

Casebolt TL, Jope RS: Long-term lithium treatment selectively reduces receptor-coupled inositol phospholipid hydrolysis in rat brain. Biol Psychiatry 25:329–340, 1989

Catalano M, Bellodi L, Lucca A, et al: Lithium and alpha-2-adrenergic receptors: effects of lithium ion on clonidine-induced growth hormone release. Neuroendocrinology Letters 6:61–66, 1984

Cernescu C, Popescu L, Constantinescu S, et al: Antiviral effect of lithium chloride. Virologie 39:93–101, 1988

Chapman BE, Beilharz GR, York MJ, et al: Endogenous phospholipase and choline release in human erythrocytes: a study using ^{1}H NMR spectroscopy. Biochem Biophys Res Commun 105:1280–1287, 1982

Chen G, Manji HK, Hawver DB, et al: Chronic sodium valproate selectively decreases protein kinase C alpha and epsilon in vitro. J Neurochem 63:2361–2364, 1994

Chen G, Yuan P, Hawver DB, et al: Increase in AP-1 transcription factor DNA binding activity by valproic acid. Neuropsychopharmacology 16:238–245, 1997

Choi SJ, Taylor MA, Abrams R: Depression, ECT, and erythrocyte adenosine triphosphatase activity. Biol Psychiatry 12:75–81, 1977

Christiansen C, Baastrup PC, Lindgren P, et al: Endocrine effects of lithium, II: "primary" hyperparathyroidism. Acta Endocrinol (Copen) 88:528–534, 1978

Coccaro EF, Siever LJ, Klar HM, et al: Serotonergic studies in patients with affective and personality disorders: correlates with suicidal and impulsive aggressive behavior. Arch Gen Psychiatry 46:587–599, 1989

Cohen LS, Friedman JM, Jefferson JW, et al: A reevaluation of risk of in utero exposure to lithium. JAMA 271:146–150, 1994

Cohen WJ, Cohen NJ: Lithium carbonate, haloperidol and irreversible brain damage. JAMA 230:1283–1287, 1974

Colburn RW, Goodwin FK, Bunney WE Jr, et al: Effect of lithium on the uptake of noradrenaline by synaptosomes. Nature 215:1395–1397, 1967

Colin SF, Chang HC, Mollner S, et al: Chronic lithium regulates the expression of adenylate cyclase and G$_i$-protein alpha subunit in rat cerebral cortex. Proc Natl Acad Sci U S A 88:10634–10637, 1991

Collard KJ: Lithium effects on brain 5-HT metabolism, in Lithium in Medical Practice. Edited by Johnson FN, Johnson S. Lancaster, England, MTP Press, 1978, pp 123–133

Collard KJ: Effects of lithium on brain metabolism, in Endocrine and Metabolic Effects of Lithium. Edited by Lazarus JH. New York, Plenum, 1986, pp 55–98

Collard KJ, Roberts MHT: Effects of lithium on the elevation of forebrain 5-hydroxyindoles by tryptophan. Neuropharmacology 16:671–673, 1977

Collins PJ, Larkin EP, Shubsachs AP: Lithium carbonate in chronic schizophrenia: a brief trial of lithium carbonate added to neuroleptics for treatment of resistant schizophrenic patients. Acta Psychiatr Scand 84:150–154, 1991

Coppen A, Abou-Saleh MT: Lithium therapy: from clinical trials to practical management. Acta Psychiatr Scand 78:754–762, 1988

Coppen A, Shaw DM: Mineral metabolism in melancholia. BMJ 2:1439–1444, 1963

Coppen A, Shaw DM: The distribution of electrolytes and water in patients after taking lithium carbonate. Lancet 2:805–806, 1967

Coppen A, Shaw DM, Malleson A, et al: Mineral metabolism in mania. BMJ 1:71–75, 1966

Coppen A, Swade C, Wood K: Lithium restores abnormal platelet 5-HT transport in patients with affective disorders. Br J Psychiatry 136:235–238, 1980

Coppen A, Abou-Saleh MT, Milln P, et al: Lithium continuation therapy following electroconvulsive therapy. Br J Psychiatry 139:284–287, 1981

Coppen A, Standish-Barry H, Bailey J, et al: Does lithium reduce the mortality of recurrent mood disorders? J Affect Disord 23:1–7, 1991

Corona GL, Cucchi ML, Santagostino G, et al: Blood noradrenaline and 5-HT levels in depressed women during amitriptyline or lithium treatment. Psychopharmacology (Berl) 77:236–241, 1982

Corrodi H, Fuxe K, Hokfelt T, et al: The effect of lithium on cerebral monoamine neurons. Psychopharmacologia 11:345–353, 1967

Cowen PJ, McCance SL, Cohen PR, et al: Lithium increases 5-HT-mediated neuroendocrine responses in tricyclic resistant depression. Psychopharmacology (Berl) 99:230–232, 1989

Crowe RR: Current concepts: electroconvulsive therapy—a current perspective. N Engl J Med 311:163–167, 1984

Dagher G, Gay C, Brossard M, et al: Lithium, sodium and potassium transport in erythrocytes of manic-depressive patients. Acta Psychiatr Scand 69:24–36, 1984

Davis JM: Overview: maintenance therapy in psychiatry, II: affective disorders. Am J Psychiatry 133:1–13, 1976

Dawood I, Welch W Jr: The stimulation of rat brain monoamine oxidase by dietary lithium chloride. Experientia 35:991–992, 1979

de Belleroche J, Cook GE, Das I, et al: Erythrocyte choline concentrations and cluster headache. BMJ (Clinical Research Edition) 288:268–270, 1984

de Belleroche J, Kilfeather S, Das I, et al: Abnormal membrane composition and membrane-dependent transduction mechanisms in cluster headache. Cephalalgia 6:147–153, 1986

Degkwitz R, Koufen H, Consbruch U, et al: Untersuchungen zur lithiumbilanz wahrend der manie [Investigation on lithium levels during mania]. International Pharmacopsychiatry 14:199–212, 1979

Delva NJ, Letemendia FJ: Lithium treatment in schizophrenia and schizo-affective disorders. Br J Psychiatry 141:387–400, 1982

de Montigny C, Grunberg F, Mayer A, et al: Lithium induces rapid relief of depression in tricyclic antidepressant drug non-responders. Br J Psychiatry 138:252–256, 1981

de Montigny C, Cournoyer G, Morissette R, et al: Lithium carbonate addition in tricyclic antidepressant-resistant unipolar depression: correlations with the neurobiological actions of tricyclic antidepressant drugs and lithium ion on the serotonin system. Arch Gen Psychiatry 40:1327–1334, 1983

de Montigny C, Chaput Y, Blier P: Lithium augmentation of antidepressant treatments: evidence for the involvement of the 5-HT system?, in New Concepts in Depression. Edited by Briley M, Fillion G. Basingstoke, England, Macmillan, 1988, pp 144–160

Deniker P, Eygiem A, Bernheim R, et al: Thyroid antibody levels during lithium therapy. Neuropsychobiology 4:270–275, 1978

Depue RA, Karuss SP, Spoont MR: A two-dimensional threshold model of seasonal bipolar affective disorder, in Psychopathology: An Interactional Perspective. Edited by Magnusson D, Ohman A. Orlando, FL, Academic Press, 1987, pp 95–123

Detellier C: Alkali metals, in NMR of Newly Accessible Nuclei. Edited by Laszlo P. New York, Academic Press, 1983, pp 105–151

Diamond JM, Meier K, Gosenfeld LF, et al: Recovery of erythrocyte Li^+/Na^+ countertransport and choline transport from lithium therapy. J Psychiatr Res 17:385–393, 1982/1983

Dick DAT, Naylor GJ, Dick EG: Effects of lithium on sodium transport across membranes, in Lithium in Medical Practice. Edited by Johnson FN, Johnson S. Lancaster, England, MTP Press, 1978, pp 183–192

Dilsaver SC, Coffman JA: Cholinergic hypothesis of depression: a reappraisal. J Clin Psychopharmacol 9:173–179, 1989

Dilsaver SC, Hariharan M: Amitriptyline-induced supersensitivity of a central muscarinic mechanism: lithium blocks amitriptyline-induced supersensitivity. Psychiatry Res 25:181–186, 1988

Dilsaver SC, Hariharan M: Chronic treatment with lithium produces supersensitivity to nicotine. Biol Psychiatry 25:792–795, 1989

Divish MM, Sheftel G, Boyle A, et al: Differential effect of lithium on fos protooncogene expression mediated by receptor and postreceptor activators of protein kinase C and cyclic adenosine monophosphate: model for its antimanic action. J Neurosci Res 28:40–48, 1991

Dousa TP: Interaction of lithium with vasopressin-sensitive cyclic AMP system of human renal medulla. Endocrinology 95:1359–1366, 1974

Dousa T, Hechter O: Lithium and brain adenylyl cyclase. Lancet 1:834–835, 1970a

Dousa T, Hechter O: The effect of NaCl and LiCl on vasopressin-sensitive adenyl cyclase. Life Sci 9:765–770, 1970b

Downes CP, Stone MA: Lithium-induced reduction in intracellular inositol supply in cholinergically stimulated parotid gland. Biochem J 234:199–204, 1986

Drummond AH, Raeburn CA: The interaction of lithium with thyrotropin releasing hormone-stimulated lipid metabolism in GH_3 pituitary tumor cells. Biochem J 224:129–136, 1984

Dubovsky SL, Lee C, Christiano J, et al: Elevated platelet intracellular calcium concentration in bipolar depression. Biol Psychiatry 29:441–450, 1991a

Dubovsky SL, Lee C, Christiano J, et al: Lithium lowers platelet intracellular ion concentration in bipolar patients. Lithium 2:167–174, 1991b

Dubovsky SL, Murphy J, Thomas M, et al: Abnormal intracellular calcium ion concentration in platelets and lymphocytes of bipolar patients. Am J Psychiatry 149:118–120, 1992

Ebadi MS, Simmons VJ, Hendrickson MJ, et al: Pharmacokinetics of lithium and its regional distribution in rat brain. Eur J Pharmacol 27:324–329, 1974

Ebstein R, Belmaker R, Grunhaus L, et al: Lithium inhibition of adrenaline-stimulated adenylate cyclase in humans. Nature 259:411–413, 1976

Ebstein RP, Hermoni M, Belmaker RH: The effect of lithium on noradrenaline-induced cyclic AMP accumulation in rat brain: inhibition after chronic treatment and absence of supersensitivity. J Pharmacol Exp Ther 213:161–167, 1980

Ebstein RP, Lerer B, Shlaufman M, et al: The effect of repeated electroconvulsive shock treatment and chronic lithium feeding on the release of norepinephrine from rat cortical vesicular preparations. Cell Mol Neurobiol 3:191–201, 1983

Edelfors S: Distribution of sodium, potassium and lithium in the brain of lithium-treated rats. Acta Pharmacologica et Toxicologica 37:387–392, 1975

Egeland JA, Kidd JR, Frazer A, et al: Amish study V: lithium-sodium countertransport and catechol-O-methyl-transferase in pedigrees of bipolar probands. Am J Psychiatry 141:1049–1054, 1984

Ehrlich BE, Diamond JM: Lithium fluxes in human erythrocytes. Am J Physiol 237:C102–C110, 1979

Ehrlich BE, Diamond JM: Lithium, membranes, and manic-depressive illness. J Membr Biol 52:187–200, 1980

Ehrlich BE, Diamond JM, Braun LD, et al: Effects of lithium on blood-brain barrier transport of the neurotransmitter precursors choline, tyrosine and tryptophan. Brain Res 193:604–607, 1980

Ehrlich BE, Diamond JM, Gosenfeld L: Lithium-induced changes in sodium-lithium countertransport. Biochem Pharmacol 30:2539–2543, 1981

Ehrlich BE, Diamond JM, Fry V, et al: Lithium's inhibition of erythrocyte cation countertransport involves a slow process in the erythrocyte. J Membr Biol 75:233–240, 1983

Elia J, Katz IR, Simpson GM: Teratogenicity of psychotherapeutic medications. Psychopharmacol Bull 23:531–586, 1987

Ellis J, Lenox RH: Chronic lithium treatment prevents atropine-induced supersensitivity of the muscarinic phosphoinositide response in rat hippocampus. Biol Psychiatry 28:609–619, 1990

Ellis J, Lenox RH: Receptor coupling to G proteins: interactions not affected by lithium. Lithium 2:141–147, 1991

El-Mallakh RS: The Na,K-ATPase hypothesis for manic depression. Med Hypotheses 12:253–282, 1983

El-Mallakh RS: The ionic mechanism of lithium action. Lithium 1:87–92, 1990

Engel J, Berggren U: Effects of lithium on behaviour and central monoamines. Acta Psychiatr Scand 61 (suppl 280): 133–143, 1980

Eroglu L, Hizal A, Koyuncuoglu H: The effect of long-term concurrent administration of chlorpromazine and lithium on the striatal and frontal cortical dopamine metabolism in rats. Psychopharmacology (Berl) 73:84–86, 1981

Evans MS, Zorumski CF, Clifford DB: Lithium enhances neuronal muscarinic excitation by presynaptic facilitation. Neuroscience 38:457–468, 1990

Faedda GL, Tondo L, Baldessarini RJ: Outcome after rapid vs gradual discontinuation of lithium treatment in bipolar disorders. Arch Gen Psychiatry 50:448–455, 1993

Finley PR, Warner MD, Peabody CA: Clinical relevance of drug interactions with lithium. Clin Pharmacokinet 29:172–191, 1995

Fischl MA, Richman DD, Grieco MH, et al: The efficacy of azidothymidine (AZT) in the treatment of patients with AIDS and AIDS-related complex: a double-blind, placebo-controlled trial. N Engl J Med 317:185–191, 1987

Fisher SK, Heacock AM, Agranoff BW: Inositol lipids and signal transduction in the nervous system: an update. J Neurochem 58:18–38, 1992

Forn J, Valdecasas FG: Effects of lithium on brain adenylyl cyclase activity. Biochem Pharmacol 20:2773–2779, 1971

Frances H, Maurin Y, Lecrubier Y, et al: Effect of chronic lithium treatment on isolation-induced behavioral and biochemical effects in mice. Eur J Pharmacol 72:337–341, 1981

Frazer A, Mendels J, Brunswick D, et al: Erythrocyte concentrations of the lithium ion: clinical correlates and mechanisms of action. Am J Psychiatry 135:1065–1069, 1978

Friedman E, Gershon S: Effect of lithium on brain dopamine. Nature 243:520–521, 1973

Friedman E, Wang HY: Effect of chronic lithium treatment on 5-hydroxytryptamine autoreceptors and release of 5-[³H]hydroxytryptamine from rat brain cortical, hippocampal, and hypothalamic slices. J Neurochem 50: 195–201, 1988

Friedman E, Dallob A, Levine G: The effect of long-term lithium treatment on reserpine-induced supersensitivity in dopaminergic and serotonergic transmission. Life Sci 25:1263–1266, 1979a

Friedman E, Oleshansky MA, Moy P, et al: Lithium and catecholamine-induced plasma cyclic AMP elevation, in Lithium Controversies and Unresolved Issues. Edited by Cooper TB, Gershon S, Kline NS, et al. Amsterdam, Excerpta Medica, 1979b, pp 730–736

Fyro B, Petterson U, Sedvall G: The effect of lithium treatment on manic symptoms and levels of monoamine metabolites in cerebrospinal fluid of manic depressive patients. Psychopharmacologia 44:99–103, 1975

Gallager DW, Pert A, Bunney WE Jr: Haloperidol-induced presynaptic dopamine supersensitivity is blocked by chronic lithium. Nature 273:309–312, 1978

Gallicchio VS, Hughes NK: Effective modulation of the haematopoietic toxicity associated with zidovudine exposure to murine and human haematopoietic progenitor stem cells in vitro with lithium chloride. J Intern Med 231:219–226, 1992

Gallicchio VS, Messino MJ, Hulette BC, et al: Lithium and hematopoiesis: effective experimental use of lithium as an agent to improve bone marrow transplantation. J Med 23:195–216, 1992

Gallicchio VS, Cibull ML, Hughes NK, et al: Effect of lithium in murine immunodeficiency virus infected animals. Pathobiology 61:216–221, 1993

Gani D, Downes CP, Bramham J: Lithium and myo-inositol homeostasis. Biochemica Biophysica Acta 1177:253–269, 1993

Gao XM, Fukamauchi F, Chuang DM: Long-term biphasic effects of lithium treatment on phospholipase C-coupled M3muscarinic acetylcholine receptors in cultured cerebellar granule cells. Neurochem Int 22:395–403, 1993

Garcia-Sainz JA, Gutierrez VG: Activation of protein kinase C alters the interaction of alpha$_2$ adrenoceptors and the inhibitory G protein (Gi) in human platelets. FEBS Lett 257:427–430, 1989

Garcia-Sevilla JA, Guimon J, Garcia-Vallejo P, et al: Biochemical and functional evidence of supersensitive platelet alpha-2-adrenoceptors in major affective disorder: effect of long-term lithium carbonate treatment. Arch Gen Psychiatry 43:51–57, 1986

Garfinkel PE, Ezrin C, Stancer HC: Hypothyroidism and hyperparathyroidism associated with lithium. Lancet 2:331–332, 1973

Garland EJ, Remick RA, Zis AP: Weight gain with antidepressants and lithium. J Clin Psychopharmacol 8:323–330, 1988

Garrod AB: The Nature and Treatment of Gout and Rheumatic Gout. London, Walton & Maberly, 1859

Geisler A, Klysner R: The effect of lithium in vitro and in vivo on dopamine-sensitive adenylate cyclase activity in dopaminergic areas of the rat brain. Acta Pharmacologica et Toxicologica (Copenhagen) 56:1–5, 1985

Geisler A, Klysner R, Andersen PH: Influence of lithium in vitro and in vivo on the catecholamine-sensitive cerebral adenylate cyclase systems. Acta Pharmacologica et Toxicologica (Copenhagen) 56:80–97, 1985

Gelenberg AJ, Kane JM, Keller MB, et al: Comparison of standard and low serum levels of lithium for maintenance treatment of bipolar disorder. N Engl J Med 321:1489–1493, 1989

Gerner RH, Stanton A: Algorithm for patient management of acute manic states: lithium, valproate or carbamazepine? J Clin Psychopharmacol 12:57S–63S, 1992

Giacovazzo M, Martelletti P, Romiti A, et al: Relationship between HLA antigen subtypes and lithium response in cluster headache. Headache 25:268–270, 1985

Giacovazzo M, Martelletti P, Romiti A, et al: Genetic markers of cluster headache and the links with the lithium salts therapy. Int J Clin Pharmacol Res 61:19–22, 1986

Giraud P, Kowalski C, Barthel F, et al: Striatal proenkephalin turnover and gene transcription are regulated by cyclic AMP and protein kinase C-related pathways. Neuroscience 43:67–79, 1991

Gitlin MJ: Lithium-induced renal insufficiency. J Clin Psychopharmacol 13:276–279, 1993

Glen AIM, Reading HW: Regulatory action of lithium in manic-depressive illness. Lancet 2:1239–1241, 1973

Glue PW, Cowen PJ, Nutt DJ, et al: The effect of lithium on 5-HT mediated neuroendocrine response and platelet 5-HT receptors. Psychopharmacology (Berl) 90:398–402, 1986

Godfrey PP: Potentiation by lithium of CMP-phosphatidate formation in carbachol-stimulated rat cerebral-cortical slices and its reversal by myo-inositol. Biochem J 258:621–624, 1989

Godfrey PP, McClue SJ, White AM, et al: Subacute and chronic in vivo lithium treatment inhibits agonist- and sodium fluoride-stimulated inositol phosphate production in rat cortex. J Neurochem 52:498–506, 1989

Goodnick P: Effects of lithium on indices of 5-HT and catecholamines in the clinical content: a review. Lithium 1:65–73, 1990

Goodnick PJ, Gershon ES: Lithium, in Handbook of Neurochemistry. Edited by Lajtha A. New York, Plenum, 1985, pp 103–149

Goodnick PJ, Meltzer HY: Neurochemical changes during discontinuation of lithium prophylaxis, I: increases in clonidine-induced hypotension. Biol Psychiatry 19:883–889, 1984a

Goodnick PJ, Meltzer HY: Treatment of schizoaffective disorders. Schizophr Bull 10:30–48, 1984b

Goodwin FK, Jamison KR: Manic-Depressive Illness. New York, Oxford University Press, 1990

Goodwin FK, Murphy DL, Bunney WE: Lithium-carbonate treatment in depression and mania. Arch Gen Psychiatry 21:486–496, 1969

Goodwin GM, DeSouza RJ, Wood AJ, et al: Lithium decreases 5-HT1A and 5-HT2 receptor and alpha-2 adrenoceptor mediated function in mice. Psychopharmacology (Berl) 90:482–487, 1986a

Goodwin GM, DeSouza RJ, Wood AJ, et al: The enhancement by lithium of the 5-HT1A mediated serotonin syndrome produced by 8-OH-DPAT in the rat: evidence for a postsynaptic mechanism. Psychopharmacology (Berl) 90:488–493, 1986b

Gorkin RA, Richelson E: Lithium transport by mouse neuroblastoma cells. Neuropharmacology 20:791–801, 1981

Gottesfeld Z, Ebstein BS, Samuel D: Effect of lithium on concentrations of glutamate and GABA levels in amygdala and hypothalamus of rat. Nature 234:124–125, 1971

Grahame-Smith DG, Green AR: The role of brain 5-hydroxytryptamine in the hyperactivity produced in rats by lithium and monoamine oxidase inhibition. Br J Pharmacol 52:19–26, 1974

Granneman GR, Schneck DW, Cavanaugh JH, et al: Pharmacokinetic interactions and side effects resulting from concomitant administration of lithium and divalproex sodium. J Clin Psychiatry 57:204–206, 1996

Greenspan K, Schildkraut JJ, Gordon EK, et al: Catecholamine metabolism in affective disorders, 3: MHPG and other catecholamine metabolites in patients treated with lithium carbonate. J Psychiatr Res 7:171–183, 1970

Greenwood AF, Jope RS: Brain G-protein proteolysis by calpain: enhancement by lithium. Brain Res 636:320–326, 1994

Greil W, Eisenreid F, Becker BF, et al: Interindividual differences in the Na⁺-dependent Li⁺ countertransport system and in the Li⁺ distribution ratio across the red cell membrane among Li⁺-treated patients. Psychopharmacology (Berl) 53:19–26, 1977

Grillo C, Piroli G, Gonzalez SL, et al: Glucocorticoid regulation of mRNA encoding (Na⁺K) ATPase alpha 3 and beta 1 subunits in rat brain measured by in situ hybridization. Brain Res 657:83–91, 1994

Grof E, Brown GM, Grof P, et al: Effects of lithium administration on plasma catecholamines. Psychiatry Res 19:87–92, 1986

Grof P, Alda M, Grof E, et al: The challenge of predicting response to stabilizing lithium treatment: the importance of patient selection. Br J Psychiatry 163 (suppl 21):16–19, 1993

Guadalupe G, Crismon ML, Dorson PG: Seizures in two patients after the addition of lithium to a clozapine regimen. J Clin Pharmacol 14:426–428, 1994

Guerri C, Ribelles M, Grisolia S: Effect of lithium and lithium and alcohol administration on Na⁺-K⁺ ATPase. Biochem Pharmacol 30:25–30, 1981

Gwinner E, Benzinger J: Synchronization of a circadian rhythm in pinealectomized European starlings by daily injections of melatonin. J Comp Physiol [A] 127:209–213, 1978

Haag M, Haag H, Eisenried F, et al: RBC-choline: changes by lithium and relation to prophylactic response. Acta Psychiatr Scand 70:389–399, 1984

Haag M, Granzow L, Greil W, et al: RBC-choline: a biological marker of the outcome of lithium prophylaxis? Prog Neuropsychopharmacol Biol Psychiatry 11:209–212, 1987

Halenda SP, Volpi M, Zavoico GB, et al: Effects of thrombin, phorbol myristate acetate, and prostaglandin D2 on 40–41 kDa protein that is ADP ribosylated by pertussis toxin in platelets. FEBS Lett 204:341–346, 1986

Hallcher LM, Sherman WR: The effects of lithium ion and other agents on the activity of myoinositol-1-phosphatase from bovine brain. J Biol Chem 255:10896–10901, 1980

Hallonquist JD, Goldberg MA, Brandes JS: Affective disorders and circadian rhythms. Can J Psychiatry 31:259–272, 1986

Harrison-Read PE: Evidence from behavioural reactions to fenfluramine, 5-hydroxyptryptophan, and 5-methoxy-N,N-dimethyltryptamine for differential effects of short-term and long-term lithium on indoleaminergic mechanisms in rats. Br J Pharmacol 66:144–145, 1979

Hatterer JA, Kocsis JH, Stokes PE: Thyroid function in patients maintained on lithium. Psychiatry Res 26:249–258, 1989

Heacock AM, Seguin EB, Agranoff BW: Measurement of receptor-activated phosphoinositide turnover in rat brain: nonequivalence of inositol phosphate and CDP-diacylglycerol formation. J Neurosci 60:1087–1092, 1993

Hedgepeth CM, Conrad LJ, Zhang J, et al: Activation of the Wnt signaling pathway: a molecular mechanism for lithium action. Dev Biol 185:82–91, 1997

Heninger GR, Charney DS, Sternberg DE: Lithium carbonate augmentation of antidepressant treatment: an effective prescription for treatment-refractory depression. Arch Gen Psychiatry 40:1335–1342, 1983

Hermoni M, Lerer B, Ebstein RP, et al: Chronic lithium prevents reserpine-induced supersensitivity of adenylate cyclase. J Pharm Pharmacol 32:510–511, 1980

Hermoni M, Barzilai A, Rahamimoff H: Modulation of the Na⁺-Ca²⁺ antiport by its ionic environment: the effect of lithium. Isr J Med Sci 23:44–48, 1987

Hesketh JE, Nicolaou NM, Arbuthnott GW, et al: The effect of chronic lithium administration on dopamine metabolism in rat striatum. Psychopharmacology (Berl) 56:163–166, 1978

Heurteaux C, Baumann N, Lachapelle F, et al: Lithium distribution in the brain of normal mice and of "quaking" dysmelinating mutants. J Neurochem 46:1317–1321, 1986

Hirvonen MR, Paljarri L, Naukkarinen A, et al: Potentiation of malaoxon-induced convulsions by lithium: early neuronal injury, phosphoinositide signaling and calcium. Toxicol Appl Pharmacol 104:276–289, 1990

Hitzemann R, Mark C, Hirschowitz J, et al: RBC lithium transport in the psychoses. Biol Psychiatry 25:296–304, 1989

Ho AKS, Tsai CS: Lithium and ethanol preference. J Pharm Pharmacol 27:58–60, 1975

Ho AKS, Loh HH, Craves F, et al: The effect of prolonged lithium treatment on the synthesis rate and turnover of monoamines in brain regions of rats. Eur J Pharmacol 10:72–78, 1970

Hokin-Neaverson M, Jefferson JW: Deficient erythrocyte Na,K-ATPase activity in different affective states in bipolar affective states in bipolar affective disorder and normalization by lithium therapy. Neuropsychobiology 22:18–25, 1989a

Hokin-Neaverson M, Jefferson JW: Erythrocyte sodium pump activity in bipolar affective disorder and other psychiatric disorders. Neuropsychobiology 22:1–7, 1989b

Hokin-Neaverson M, Spiegel DA, Lewis WC: Deficiency of erythrocyte sodium pump activity in bipolar manic-depressive psychosis. Life Sci 15:1739–1748, 1974

Hokin-Neaverson M, Burckhardt WA, Jefferson JW: Increased erythrocyte Na⁺ pump and NaK-ATPase activity during lithium therapy. Res Commun Mol Pathol Pharmacol 14:117–126, 1976

Honchar MP, Olney JW, Sherman WR: Systemic cholinergic agents induce seizures and brain damage in lithium-treated rats. Science 220:323–325, 1983

Hong JS, Tilson HA, Yoshikawa K: Effects of lithium and haloperidol administration on the rat brain levels of substance P. J Pharmacol Exp Ther 224:590–597, 1983

Hotta I, Yamawaki S: Possible involvement of presynaptic 5-HT autoreceptors in effect of lithium on 5-HT release in hippocampus of rat. Neuropharmacology 27:987–992, 1988

Hsiao JK, Manji HK, Chen GA, et al: Lithium administration modulates platelet G_i in humans. Life Sci 50:227–233, 1992

Huang F, Yoshida Y, Cunha-Melo JR, et al: Differential down-regulation of protein kinase C isozymes. J Biol Chem 264:4238–4243, 1989

Huang KP: The mechanism of protein kinase C activation. Trends Neurosci 12:425–432, 1989

Huey LY, Janowsky DS, Judd LL, et al: Effects of lithium carbonate on methylphenidate-induced mood, behaviour, and cognitive processes. Psychopharmacology (Berl) 73:161–164, 1981

Huganir RL, Greengard P: Regulation of neurotransmitter receptor desensitization by protein phosphorylation. Neuron 5:555–567, 1990

Hunter T, Karin M: The regulation of transcription by phosphorylation. Cell 70:375–387, 1992

Isakov N, McMahon P, Altman A: Selective post-transcriptional down-regulation of protein kinase C isoenzymes in leukemic T cells chronically treated with phorbol ester. J Biol Chem 265:2091–2097, 1990

Jacobson SJ, Jones K, Johnson K, et al: Prospective multicentre study of pregnancy outcome after lithium exposure during first trimester. Lancet 339:530–533, 1992

Jakobs KH, Bauer S, Watanabe Y: Modulation of adenylate cyclase of human platelets by phorbol ester: impairment of the hormone-sensitive inhibitory pathway. Eur J Biochem 151:425–430, 1985

Jefferson JW: Lithium tremor and caffeine intake: two cases of drinking less and shaking more. J Clin Psychiatry 49:72–73, 1988

Jefferson JW: Lithium: the present and the future. J Clin Psychiatry 51 (suppl 8):4–19, 1990

Jefferson JW: Update on lithium in clinical practice: an interview with James W. Jefferson, M.D. Currents in Affective Illness 10:5–14, 1991

Jefferson JW, Greist JH, Baudhiun M: Lithium: interactions with other drugs. J Clin Psychopharmacol 1:124–134, 1981

Jefferson JW, Greist JH, Ackerman DL: Lithium Encyclopedia for Clinical Practice. Washington, DC, American Psychiatric Press, 1983

Jefferson JW, Greist JH, Ackerman DL, et al: Lithium Encyclopedia for Clinical Practice, 2nd Edition. Washington, DC, American Psychiatric Press, 1987

Jensen HV, Plenge P, Mellerup ET, et al: Lithium prophylaxis of manic-depressive disorder: daily lithium dosing schedule versus every second day. Acta Psychiatr Scand 92:69–74, 1995

Jensen HV, Plenge P, Stensgaard A, et al: Twelve-hour brain lithium concentration in lithium maintenance treatment of manic-depressive disorder: daily versus alternate-day dosing schedule. Psychopharmacology 124:275–278, 1996

Johnson BB, Naylor GJ, Dick EG, et al: Prediction of clinical course of bipolar manic depressive illness treated with lithium. Psychol Med 10:329–334, 1980

Johnson FN: The History of Lithium Therapy. Basingstoke, England, Macmillan, 1984

Johnson FN: Depression and Mania: Modern Lithium Therapy. Oxford, England, IRL Press, 1987

Johnson FN: Lithium treatment of aggression, self-mutilation, and affective disorders in the context of mental handicap. Reviews in Contemporary Pharmacotherapy 1:9–18, 1988

Johnson FN, Minnai G: Potential alternative applications of oral lithium. Reviews in Contemporary Pharmacotherapy 4:237–250, 1993

Johnson G, Gershon S, Burdock EI, et al: Comparative effects of lithium and chlorpromazine in the treatment of acute manic states. Br J Psychiatry 119:267–276, 1971

Johnson RD, Minneman KP: Alpha 1-adrenergic receptors and stimulation of [3H] inositol metabolism in rat brain: regional distribution and parallel inactivation. Brain Res 341:7–15, 1985

Johnsson A, Engelmann W, Pflug B, et al: Period lengthening of human circadian rhythms by lithium carbonate, a prophylactic for depressive disorders. International Journal of Chronobiology (London) 8:129–147, 1983

Jones FD, Maas JW, Dekirmenjian M, et al: Urinary catecholamine metabolites during behavioural changes in a patient with manic-depressive cycles. Science 179:300–302, 1973

Jope RS: Effects of lithium treatment in vitro and in vivo on acetylcholine metabolism in rat brain. J Neurochem 33:487–495, 1979

Jope RS, Williams MB: Lithium and brain signal transduction systems. Biochem Pharmacol 47:429–434, 1994

Jope RS, Jenden DJ, Ehrlich BE, et al: Choline accumulates in erythrocytes during lithium therapy. N Engl J Med 299:833–834, 1978

Jope RS, Jenden DJ, Ehrlich BE, et al: Erythrocyte choline concentrations are elevated in manic patients. Proc Natl Acad Sci U S A 77:6144–6146, 1980

Jope RS, Morrisett RA, Snead OC: Characterization of lithium potentiation of pilocarpine induced status epilepticus in rats. Exp Neurol 91:471–480, 1986

Judd LL, Squire LR, Butters N, et al: Effects of psychotropic drugs on cognition and memory in normal humans and animals, in Psychopharmacology: The Third Generation of Progress. Edited by Meltzer HY. New York, Raven, 1987, pp 1467–1475

Kabakob AY, Karkanias NB, Lenox RL, et al: Synapse specific accumulation of lithium in intracellular microdomains: a model for uncoupling coincidence detection in the brain. Synapse (in press)

Kafka M, Wirz-Justice A, Naber D, et al: Effect of lithium on circadian neurotransmitter receptor rhythms. Neuropsychobiology 8:41–50, 1982

Kafka MS, Wirz-Justice A, Naber D, et al: Circadian rhythms in rat brain neurotransmitter receptors. Federation Proceedings 42:2796–2801, 1983

Kalasapudi VD, Sheftel G, Divish MM, et al: Lithium augments fos protoonocogene expression in PC12 pheochromocytoma cells: implications for therapeutic action of lithium. Brain Res 521:47–54, 1990

Kandel ER: From metapsychology to molecular biology: explorations into the nature of anxiety. Am J Psychiatry 140:1277–1293, 1983

Kane JM: The efficacy of clozapine in the treatment of schizophrenia: a long-term perspective. J Clin Psychiatry 8:9–14, 1990

Kane JM, Honigfeld G, Singer J, et al: Clozapine for the treatment-resistant schizophrenic: a double-blind comparison with chlorpromazine. Arch Gen Psychiatry 45:789–796, 1988

Kao KR, Masui U, Elinson RP, et al: Lithium-induced respecification of pattern in *Xenopus laevic* embryos. Nature 322:371–373, 1986

Kaschka WP, Mokrusch T, Korth M: Early physiological effects of lithium treatment: electrooculographic and adaptometric findings in patients with affective and schizoaffective psychoses. Pharmacopsychiatry 20:203–207, 1987

Katada T, Gillman AG, Watanabe Y, et al: Protein C phosphorylates the inhibitory guanine-nucleotide-binding regulatory component and apparently suppresses its function in hormonal inhibition of adenylate cyclase. Eur J Biochem 151:431–437, 1985

Kato T, Inubushi I, Takahashi S: Relationship of lithium concentrations in the brain measured by lithium-7 magnetic resonance spectroscopy to treatment response in mania. J Clin Psychopharmacol 14:330–335, 1994

Katz RI, Kopin KJ: Release of ^{3}H-norepinephrine and ^{3}H-serotonin evoked from brain slices by electric field stimulation: calcium dependence and the effects of lithium and tetrodotoxin. Biochem Pharmacol 18:1935–1939, 1969

Katz RI, Chase TN, Kopin IJ: Evoked release of norepinephrine and serotonin from brain slices: inhibition by lithium. Science 162:466–467, 1968

Keck PE, McElroy SL, Nemeroff CB: Anticonvulsants in the treatment of bipolar disorder. J Neuropsychiatry Clin Neurosci 4:395–405, 1992

Keller MB, Lavori PW, Kane JM, et al: Subsyndromal symptoms in bipolar disorder: a comparison of standard and low serum levels of lithium. Arch Gen Psychiatry 49:317–376, 1992

Kendall DA, Nahorski SR: Acute and chronic lithium treatments influence agonist- and depolarization-stimulated inositol phospholipid hydrolysis in rat cerebral cortex. J Pharmacol Exp Ther 241:1023–1027, 1987

Kennedy ED, Challiss RJ, Nahorski SR: Lithium reduces the accumulation of inositol polyphosphate second messengers following cholinergic stimulation of cerebral cortex slices. J Neurochem 53:1652–1655, 1989

Kennedy ED, Challiss RAJ, Ragan CI, et al: Reduced inositol polyphosphate accumulation and inositol supply induced by lithium in stimulated cerebral cortex slices. Biochem J 267:781–786, 1990

Keynes RS, Swan RC: The permeability of frog muscle fibers to lithium ions. J Physiol (Lond) 147:626–638, 1959

Kim MH, Neubig RR: Membrane reconstitution of high affinity alpha-2-adrenergic agonist binding with guanine nucleotide regulatory proteins. Biochemistry 26:3664–3672, 1987

Kishimoto A, Mikawa K, Hashimoto K, et al: Limited proteolysis of protein kinase C subspecies by calcium-dependent neutral protease (calpain). J Biol Chem 264:4088–4092, 1989

Kislauskis E, Dobner PR: Mutually dependent response elements in the cis-regulatory region of the neurotensin/neuromedin N gene integrate environmental stimuli in PC12 cells. Neuron 4:783–795, 1990

Klawans HL, Weiner WJ, Nausieda PA: The effect of lithium on an animal model of tardive dyskinesia. Prog Neuropsychopharmacol Biol Psychiatry 1:53–60, 1976

Klein E, Lavie P, Meiraz R, et al: Increased motor activity and recurrent manic episodes: risk factors that predict rapid relapse in remitted bipolar disorder patients after lithium discontinuation—a double blind study. Biol Psychiatry 31:279–284, 1992

Klein PS, Melton DA: A molecular mechanism for the effect of lithium on development. Proc Natl Acad Sci U S A 93:8455–8459, 1996

Klemfuss H, Kripke DF: Effects of lithium on circadian rhythms, in Chronopharmacology, Cellular and Biochemical Interactions. Edited by Lemmer B. New York, Marcel Dekker, 1989, pp 281–297

Knapp S, Mandell AJ: Effects of lithium chloride on parameters of biosynthetic capacity for 5-hydroxytryptamine in rat brain. J Pharmacol Exp Ther 193:812–823, 1975

Koenig JI, Meltzer HY, Gudelsky GA: Alterations of hormonal responses following lithium treatment in the rat. Proceedings of the Eighth International Congress of Endocrinology, 1984, p 1037

Kofman O, Belmaker RH: Biochemical, behavioral and clinical studies of the role of inositol in lithium treatment and depression. Biol Psychiatry 34:839–852, 1993

Kofman O, Belmaker RH, Grisaru N, et al: Myo-inositol attenuates two specific behavioral effects of acute lithium in rats. Psychopharmacol Bull 27:185–190, 1991

Komoroski RA, Newton JEO, Sprigg JR, et al: In vivo ^{7}Li nuclear magnetic resonance study of lithium pharmacokinetics and chemical shift imaging in psychiatric patients. Psychiatry Res 50:67–76, 1993

Koval MS, Rames LJ, Christie S: Diabetic ketoacidosis associated with clozapine treatment (letter). Am J Psychiatry 151:1520--1521, 1994

Krell RD, Goldberg AM: Effect of acute and chronic administration of lithium on steady-state levels of mouse brain choline and acetylcholine. Biochem Pharmacol 22:3289–3291, 1973

Kripke DF, Mullaney DJ, Atkinson M, et al: Circadian rhythm disorders in manic-depressives. Biol Psychiatry 13:335–351, 1978

Kripke DF, Judd LL, Hubbard B, et al: The effect of lithium carbonate on the circadian rhythm of sleep in normal human subjects. Biol Psychiatry 14:545–548, 1979

Krupinski J, Rajaram R, Lakonishok M, et al: Insulin-dependent phosphorylation of GTP-binding proteins in phospholipid vesicles. J Biol Chem 63:12333–12341, 1988

Kuchel PW, Hunt GE, Johnson GFS, et al: Lithium, red blood cell choline and clinical state: a prospective study in manic-depressive patients. J Affect Disord 6:83–94, 1984

Kupfer DJ, Wyatt RJ, Greenspan K, et al: Lithium carbonate and sleep in affective illness. Arch Gen Psychiatry 23:35–40, 1970

Kupfer DJ, Reynolds CF III, Weiss BL, et al: Lithium carbonate and sleep in affective disorders. Arch Gen Psychiatry 30:79–84, 1974

Kuriyama K, Speken R: Effect of lithium on content and uptake of norepinephrine and 5-hydroxytryptamine in mouse brain synaptosomes and mitochondria. Life Sci 9:1213–1220, 1970

Kuroda T, Nishizuka Y: Limited proteolysis of protein kinase C subspecies by calcium-dependent neural protease (calpain). J Biol Chem 264:4088–4092, 1989

Laakso ML, Oja SS: Transport of tryptophan and tyrosine in rat brain slices in the presence of lithium. Neurochem Res 4:411–423, 1979

Lal S, Nair NPV, Guyda H: Effect of lithium on hypothalamic-pituitary dopaminergic function. Acta Psychiatr Scand 57:91–96, 1978

Lam RH, Christensen S: Regional and subcellular localization of Li+ and other cations in the rat brain following long-term lithium administration. J Neurochem 59:1372–1380, 1992

Lange C: Om Periodiske Depressionstilstande og deres Patogenese [About periodic depression and its pathogenesis]. Copenhagen, Jacob Lunds Forlag, 1886

Lauritsen BJ, Mellerup ET, Plenge P, et al: Serum lithium concentrations around the clock with different treatment regimens and the diurnal variation of the renal lithium clearance. Acta Psychiatr Scand 64:314–319, 1981

Lazarus JH: Endocrine and Metabolic Effects of Lithium. New York, Plenum, 1986

Lazarus JH, Muston LJ: The effect of lithium on the iodide concentrating mechanism in mouse salivary gland. Acta Pharmacologica et Toxicologica (Copenhagen) 43:55–58, 1978

Lecuona E, Luquin S, Avila J, et al: Expression of the beta 1 and beta 2 (AMOG) subunits of the Na, K-ATPase in neural tissues: cellular and developmental distribution patterns. Brain Res Bull 40:167–174, 1996

Lee G, Lingsch C, Lyle PT, et al: Lithium treatment strongly inhibits choline transport in human erythrocytes. Br J Clin Pharmacol 1:365–370, 1974

Leli U, Hauser G: Lithium modifies diacylglycerol levels and protein kinase C in neuroblastoma cells. Abstract presented at the 8th International Conference on Second Messengers and Phosphoproteins, Z187F, Glasgow, Scotland, August 3–6, 1992

Lenox RH: Role of receptor coupling to phosphoinositide metabolism in the therapeutic action of lithium, in Molecular Mechanisms of Neuronal Responsiveness (Adv Exp Biol Med). Edited by Ehrlich YH. New York, Plenum, 1987, pp 515–530

Lenox RH, Ellis J: Potential targets for the action of lithium in the brain: muscarinic receptor regulation. Clin Neuropharmacol 13 (suppl):215–216, 1990

Lenox RH, Manji HK: Lithium, in American Psychiatric Press Textbook of Psychopharmacology. Edited by Nemeroff CB, Schatzberg AF. Washington, DC, American Psychiatric Press, 1995, pp 303–350

Lenox RH, Watson DG: Targets for lithium action in the brain: protein kinase C substrates and muscarinic receptor regulation. Clin Neuropharmacol 15:612A–614A, 1992

Lenox RH, Watson DG: Lithium and the brain: a psychopharmacological strategy to a molecular basis for manic depressive illness. Clin Chem 40:309–314, 1994

Lenox RH, Watson DG, Ellis J: Muscarinic receptor regulation and protein kinase C: sites for the action of chronic lithium in the hippocampus. Psychopharmacol Bull 27:191–199, 1991

Lenox RH, Newhouse PA, Creelman WL, et al: Adjunctive treatment of manic agitation with lorazepam versus haloperidol: a double-blind study. J Clin Psychiatry 53:47–52, 1992a

Lenox RH, Watson DG, Patel J, et al: Chronic lithium administration alters a prominent PKC substrate in rat hippocampus. Brain Res 570:333–340, 1992b

Lenox RH, McNamara RK, Watterson JM, et al: Myristoylated Alanine-Rich C Kinase Substrate (MARCKS): a molecular target for the therapeutic action of mood stabilizers in the brain? J Clin Psychiatry 57 (suppl 13):23–31, 1996

Lenox RH, McNamara RK, Papke RL, et al: Neurobiology of lithium: an update. J Clin Psychiatry (in press)

Lerer B, Stanley M: Effect of chronic lithium on cholinergically mediated responses and [³H]QNB binding in rat brain. Brain Res 344:211–219, 1985

Levy A, Zohar J, Belmaker RH: The effect of chronic lithium pretreatment on rat brain muscarinic receptor regulation. Neuropharmacology 21:1199–1201, 1983

Lewy AJ, Sack RL, Miller LS, et al: Antidepressant and circadian phase-shifting effects of light. Science 235: 352–354, 1987

Li PP, Tam YK, Young LT, et al: Lithium decreases Gs, Gi-$_1$ and Gi-$_2$ alpha-subunit mRNA levels in rat cortex. Eur J Pharmacol 206:165–166, 1991

Li X, Jope RS: Selective inhibition of the expression of signal transduction proteins by lithium in nerve growth factor-differentiated PC12 cells. J Neurochem 65:2500–2508, 1995

Lieblich I, Yirmiya R: Naltrexone reverses a long term depressive effect of a toxic lithium injection on saccharin preference. Physiol Behav 39:547–550, 1987

Liles WC, Nathanson NM: Alteration in the regulation of neuronal muscarinic acetylcholine receptor number induces by chronic lithium in neuroblastoma cells. Brain Res 439:88–94, 1988

Linder D, Gschwendt M, Marks F: Phorbol ester-induced down-regulation of the 80-kDa myristoylated alanine-rich C-kinase substrate-related protein in Swiss 3T3 fibroblasts. J Biol Chem 267:24–26, 1992

Lindstedt G, Nilsson L, Walinder J, et al: On the prevalence, diagnosis and management of lithium-induced hypothyroidism in psychiatric patients. Br J Psychiatry 130:452–458, 1977

Lingsch C, Martin K: An irreversible effect of lithium administration to patients. Br J Pharmacol 57:323–327, 1976

Linnoila M, Karoum F, Rosenthal N, et al: Electroconvulsive treatment and lithium carbonate. Arch Gen Psychiatry 40:677–680, 1983

Linnoila M, Miller TL, Barko J, et al: Five antidepressant treatments in depressed patients. Arch Gen Psychiatry 41:688–692, 1984

Lloyd KG, Morselli PL, Bartholini G: GABA and affective disorders. Medical Biology (Helsinki) 65:159–165, 1987

Lyman GH, Williams CC: Lithium attenuation of leukopenia associated with cancer chemotherapy, in Lithium and the Blood. Edited by Gallicchio VS. Basel, Switzerland, Karger, 1991, pp 30–45

Maggi A, Enna SJ: Regional alterations in rat brain neurotransmitter systems following chronic lithium treatment. J Neurochem 34:888–892, 1980

Maggs R: Treatment of manic illness with lithium carbonate. Br J Psychiatry 109:56–65, 1963

Mahan LC, Burch RM, Monsma FJ Jr, et al: Expression of striatal D$_1$ dopamine receptors coupled to inositol phosphate production and Ca^{2+} mobilization in Xenopus oocytes. Proc Natl Acad Sci U S A 87:2196–2200, 1990

Malik N, Canfield VA, Beckers MC, et al: Identification of the mammalian Na,K-ATPase subunit. J Biol Chem 271: 22754–22758, 1996

Mallette LE, Khouri K, Zengotita H, et al: Lithium treatment increases intact and midregion parathyroid hormone and parathyroid volume. J Clin Endocrinol Metab 68:654–660, 1989

Mallinger AG, Mallinger J, Himmelhoch JM, et al: Essential hypertension and membrane lithium transport in depressed patients. Psychiatry Res 10:11–16, 1983

Mallinger AG, Hanin I, Himmelhoch JM, et al: Stimulation of cell membrane sodium transport activity by lithium: possible relationship to therapeutic action. Psychiatry Res 22:49–59, 1987

Mallinger AG, Frank E, Thase ME, et al: Low rate of membrane lithium transport during treatment correlates with outcome of maintenance pharmacotherapy in bipolar disorder. Neuropsychopharmacology 16:325–332, 1997

Mandell AJ, Knapp S, Ehlers C, et al: The stability of constrained randomness: lithium prophylaxis at several neurobiological levels, in Neurobiology of Mood Disorders. Edited by Post RM, Ballenger JC. Baltimore, MD, Williams & Wilkins, 1984, pp 744–776

Manji HK: G proteins: implications for psychiatry. Am J Psychiatry 149:746–760, 1992

Manji HK, Lenox RH: Long-term action of lithium: a role for transcriptional and posttranscriptional factors regulated by protein kinase C. Synapse 16:11–28, 1994

Manji HK, Bitran JA, Masana MI, et al: Signal transduction modulation by lithium: cell culture, cerebral microdialysis and human studies. Psychopharmacol Bull 27:199–208, 1991a

Manji HK, Hsiao JK, Risby ED, et al: The mechanisms of action of lithium. Arch Gen Psychiatry 48:505–512, 1991b

Manji HK, Etcheberrigaray R, Chen G, et al: Lithium dramatically decreases membrane-associated PKC in the hippocampus: selectivity for the alpha isozyme. J Neurochem 61:2303–2310, 1993

Manji HK, Chen G, Shimon H, et al: Guanine nucleotide-binding proteins in bipolar affective disorder: effects of long-term lithium treatment. Arch Gen Psychiatry 52: 135–144, 1995a

Manji HK, Potter WZ, Lenox RH: Signal transduction pathways: molecular targets for lithium's actions. Arch Gen Psychiatry 52:531–543, 1995b

Manji HK, Bersudsky Y, Chen G, et al: Modulation of protein kinase C isozymes and substrates by lithium: the role of myo-inositol. Neuropsychopharmacology 15:370–381, 1996a

Manji HK, Chen G, Hsiao JK, et al: Regulation of signal transduction pathways by mood-stabilizing agents: implications for the delayed onset of therapeutic efficacy. J Clin Psychiatry 13 (suppl 57):34–46, 1996b

Manji HK, Chen G, Hsiao JK, et al: Regulation of signal transduction pathways by mood stabilizing agents: implications for the pathophysiology and treatment of bipolar affective disorder, in Mechanisms of Antibipolar Treatments. Edited by Manji HK, Bowden CL, Belmaker RH. Washington, DC, American Psychiatric Press (in press a)

Manji HK, McNamara RK, Lenox RH: Mechanisms of action of lithium in bipolar illness, in Hormones, Neurotransmitters and Affective Disorders. Edited by Halbreich U. (in press b)

Mannisto PT: Endocrine side-effects of lithium, in Handbook of Lithium Therapy. Edited by Johnson FN. Baltimore, MD, University Park Press, 1980, pp 310–322

Marchbanks RM: The activation of presynaptic choline uptake by acetylcholine release. J Physiol (Paris) 78:373–378, 1982

Marshall MH, Neumann CP, Robinson M: Lithium, creativity, and manic-depressive illness: review and prospectus. Psychosomatics 11:406–488, 1970

Masana MI, Bitran JA, Hsiao JK, et al: In vivo evidence that lithium inactivates G_i modulation of adenylate cyclase in brain. J Neurochem 59:200–205, 1992

Maslanski JA, Leshko L, Busa WB: Lithium-sensitive production of inositol phosphates during amphibian embryonic mesoderm induction. Science 256:243–245, 1992

Mathe AA, Jousisto-Hanson J, Stenfors C, et al: Effect of lithium on tachykinins, calcitonin gene-related peptide, and neuropeptide Y in rat brain. J Neurosci Res 26:233–237, 1990

Mathe AA, Miller JC, Stenfors C: Chronic dietary lithium inhibits basal c-fos mRNA expression in rat brain. Prog Neuropsychopharmacol Biol Psychiatry 19:1177–1187, 1995

McCance SL, Cohen PR, Cowen PJ: Lithium increases 5-HT-mediated prolactin release. Psychopharmacology (Berl) 99:276–281, 1989

McEachron DL, Kripke DF, Hawkins R, et al: Lithium delays biochemical circadian rhythms in rats. Neuropsychobiology 8:12–29, 1982

McElroy SL, Keck PE, Pope HG, et al: Valproate in the treatment of bipolar disorder: literature review and clinical guidelines. J Clin Psychopharmacol 12:42S–52S, 1992

McHenry CR, Rosen IB, Rotstein LE, et al: Lithiumogenic disorders of the thyroid and parathyroid glands as surgical disease. Surgery 108:1001–1005, 1990

McHenry CR, Racke F, Meister M, et al: Lithium effects on dispersed bovine parathyroid cells grown in tissue culture. Surgery 110:1061–1066, 1991

Mellerup ET, Dam H, Wildschiotz G, et al: Diurnal variation of blood glucose during lithium treatment. J Affect Disord 5:341–347, 1983

Meltzer HY, Lowy MT: The serotonin hypothesis of depression, in Psychopharmacology: The Third Generation of Progress. Edited by Meltzer HY. New York, Raven, 1987, pp 513–526

Meltzer HY, Simonovic M, Sturgeon RD, et al: Effect of antidepressants, lithium and electroconvulsive treatment on rat serum prolactin levels. Acta Psychiatr Scand 63 (suppl 290):100–121, 1981

Meltzer HL, Kassir S, Dunner DL, et al: Repression of a lithium pump as a consequence of lithium ingestion by manic-depressive subjects. Psychopharmacology (Berl) 54:113–118, 1982

Meltzer HY, Arora RC, Goodnick P: Effect of lithium carbonate on serotonin uptake in blood platelets of patients with affective disorders. J Affect Disord 5:215–221, 1983

Meltzer HY, Lowy M, Robertson A, et al: Effect of 5-hydroxytryptophan on serum cortisol levels in major affective disorders, III: effect of antidepressants and lithium carbonate. Arch Gen Psychiatry 41:391–397, 1984

Mendels J, Chernik DA: The effect of lithium carbonate on the sleep of depressed patients. International Pharmacopsychiatry 8:184–192, 1973

Mendels J, Frazer A: Intracellular lithium concentration and clinical response: towards a membrane theory of depression. J Psychiatr Res 10:9–18, 1973

Mester R, Toren P, Mizrachi I, et al: Caffeine withdrawal increases lithium blood levels. Biol Psychiatry 37:348–350, 1995

Miller BL, Jenden DJ, Tang C, et al: Factors influencing erythrocyte choline concentrations. Life Sci 44:477–482, 1989

Miller BL, Lin KM, Djenderedjian A, et al: Changes in red blood cell choline and choline-bound lipids with oral lithium. Experientia 46:454–456, 1990

Miller JC, Mathe AA: Basal and stimulated C-fos mRNA expression in the rat brain: effect of chronic dietary lithium. Neuropsychopharmacology 16:408–418, 1997

Mitchell JE, MacKenzie TB: Cardiac effects of lithium therapy in man: a review. J Clin Psychiatry 43:47–51, 1982

Miyauchi T, Okiawa S, Kitada Y: Effects of lithium chloride on the cholinergic system in different brain regions in mice. Biochem Pharmacol 29:654–657, 1980

Mizuta T, Segawa T: Chronic effects of imipramine and lithium on 5-HT receptor subtypes in rat frontal cortex, hippocampus and choroid plexus: quantitative receptor autoradiographic analysis. Jpn J Pharmacol 50:315–326, 1989

Moore GJ, Bebchuk JM, Manji HK: Proton MRS in manic depressive illness: monitoring of lithium-induced brain myoinositol (abstract). Abstracts of the Society of Neuroscience 27th Annual Meeting. New Orleans, LA, October 1997

Morgan JI, Curran T: Stimulus-transcription coupling in the nervous system: involvement of the inducible proto-oncogenes fos and jun. Annu Rev Neurosci 14:421–451, 1991

Mori M, Tajima K, Oda Y, et al: Inhibitory effect of lithium on the release of thyroid hormones from thyrotropin-stimulated mouse thyroids in a perifusion system. Endocrinology 124:1365–1369, 1989

Mori S, Zanardi R, Popoli M, et al: Inhibitory effect of lithium on cAMP dependent phosphorylation system. Life Sci 59:PL99–PL104, 1996

Mork A, Geisler A: Mode of action of lithium on the catalytic unit of adenylate cyclase from rat brain. Pharmacol Toxicol 60:241–248, 1987

Mork A, Geisler A: Effects of GTP on hormone-stimulated adenylate cyclase activity in cerebral cortex, striatum, and hippocampus from rats treated chronically with lithium. Biol Psychiatry 26:279–288, 1989a

Mork A, Geisler A: Effects of lithium ex vivo on the GTP-mediated inhibition of calcium-stimulated adenylate cyclase activity in rat brain. Eur J Pharmacol 168:347–354, 1989b

Mork A, Geisler A: The effects of lithium in vitro and ex vivo on adenylate cyclase in brain are exerted by distinct mechanisms. Neuropharmacology 28:307–311, 1989c

Mork A, Geisler A: Effects of chronic lithium treatment on agonist-enhanced extracellular concentrations of cyclic AMP in the dorsal hippocampus of freely moving rats. J Neurochem 65:134–139, 1995

Mork A, Klysner R, Geisler A: Effects of treatment with a lithium-imipramine combination on components of adenylate cyclase in the cerebral cortex of the rat. Neuropharmacology 29:261–267, 1990

Mota de Freitas DE, Espanol MT, Dorus E: Lithium transport in red blood cells of bipolar patients, in Lithium and the Blood. Edited by Gallicchio VS. Farmington, CT, Karger, 1991, pp 96–120

Mucha RF, Herz A: Motivational properties of kappa and mu opioid receptor agonists studied with place and taste preference conditioning. Psychopharmacology (Berl) 86:274–280, 1985

Muhlbauer HD: The influence of fenfluramine stimulation on prolactin plasma levels in lithium long-term-treated manic-depressive patients and healthy subjects. Pharmacopsychiatry 17:191–193, 1984

Muhlbauer HD, Muller-Oerlinghausen B: Fenfluramine stimulation of serum cortisol in patients with major affective disorders and healthy controls: further evidence for a central serotonergic action of lithium in man. J Neural Transm 61:81–94, 1985

Mukherjee BP, Bailey PT, Pradhan SN: Temporal and regional differences in brain concentrations of lithium in rats. Psychopharmacology 48:119–121, 1976

Muller-Oerlinghausen B, Ahrens B, Volk J, et al: Reduced mortality of manic-depressive patients in long-term lithium treatment: an international collaborative study by IGSLI. Psychiatry Res 36:329–331, 1991

Mullins LJ, Brinley FJ: Calcium binding and regulation in nerve fibers, in Calcium Binding Protein and Calcium Function. Edited by Wasserman RH, Corradino RA, Carafoli E. New York, North-Holland, 1977, pp 87–95

Munzer JS, Daly SE, Jewell-Motz EA, et al: Tissue- and isoform-specific kinetic behavior of the Na,K-ATPase. J Biol Chem 269:16668–16676, 1994

Murphy DL: Effects of lithium on catecholamines and other brain neurotransmitters. Neuroscience Research Progress Bulletin 14:165–169, 1976

Murphy DL, Donnelly C, Moskowitz J: Inhibition by lithium of prostaglandin E1 and norepinephrine effects on cyclic adenosine monophosphate production in human platelets. Clin Pharmacol Ther 14:810–814, 1974

Murphy DL, Lake CR, Slater S, et al: Psychoactive drug effects on plasma norepinephrine and plasma dopamine beta-hydroxylase in man, in Catecholamines: Basic and Clinical Frontiers. Edited by Usdin E, Kopin IJ, Barchas J. New York, Pergamon, 1979, pp 918–920

Myers DH, Carter RA, Burns BH, et al: A prospective study of the effects of lithium on thyroid function and on the prevalence of antithyroid antibodies. Psychol Med 15:55–61, 1985

Nahorski SR, Ragan CI, Challiss RAJ: Lithium and the phosphoinositide cycle: an example of uncompetitive inhibition and its pharmacological consequences. Trends Pharmacol Sci 12:297–303, 1991

Nahorski SR, Jenkinson S, Challiss RA: Disruption of phosphoinositide signalling by lithium. Biochem Soc Trans 20:430–434, 1992

Naylor GJ, McHarg A: Profound hypothermia on combined lithium carbonate and diazepam treatment (letter). BMJ 2:22, 1977

Naylor GJ, Smith AHW: Defective genetic control of sodium-pump density in manic depressive psychosis. Psychol Med 11:257–263, 1981

Naylor GJ, McNamee HB, Moody JP: Erythrocyte sodium and potassium in depressive illness. J Psychosom Res 14:173–177, 1970

Naylor GJ, McNamee HB, Moody JP: Changes in erythrocyte sodium and potassium on recovery from depressive illness. Br J Psychiatry 118:219–223, 1971

Naylor GJ, Dick DAT, Dick EG, et al: Erythrocyte membrane cation carrier in mania. Psychol Med 6:659–663, 1974a

Naylor GJ, Dick DAT, Dick EG, et al: Lithium therapy and erythrocyte membrane cation carrier. Psychopharmacologia 37:81–86, 1974b

Naylor GJ, Smith AHW, Dick EG, et al: Erythrocyte membrane cation carrier in manic-depressive psychosis. Psychol Med 10:521–525, 1980

Nelson SC, Herman MM, Bensch KG, et al: Localization and quantitation of lithium in rat tissue following intraperitoneal injections of lithium chloride, II: brain. J Pharmacol Exp Ther 212:11–15, 1980

Nemeroff CB: Neuropeptides and Psychiatric Disorders. Washington, DC, American Psychiatric Press, 1991

Nestler EJ, Terwilliger RZ, Duman RS: Regulation of endogenous ADP-ribosylation by acute and chronic lithium in rat brain. J Neurochem 64:2319–2324, 1995

Neubig RR, Gantzos RD, Thomsen WJ: Mechanism of agonist and antagonist binding to alpha-2-adrenergic receptors: evidence for a precoupled receptor-guanine nucleotide protein complex. Biochemistry 27:2374–2384, 1988

Newman ME, Belmaker RH: Effects of lithium in vitro and ex vivo on components of the adenylate cyclase system in membranes from the cerebral cortex of the rat. Neuropharmacology 26:211–217, 1987

Newman M, Klein E, Birmaher B, et al: Lithium at therapeutic concentrations inhibits human brain noradrenaline sensitive cyclic AMP accumulation. Brain Res 278:380–381, 1983

Newman ME, Drummer D, Lerer B: Single and combined effects of desipramine and lithium on serotonergic receptor number and second messenger function in rat brain. J Pharmacol Exp Ther 252:826–831, 1990

Nibuya M, Jung A, Nester EJ, et al: Chronic administration of lithium increases the expression of CREB and BDNF in rat hippocampus. Society for Neuroscience Abstracts 22 (part 1):182, 1996

Nilsson A: The anti-aggressive actions of lithium. Reviews in Contemporary Pharmacotherapy 4:269–285, 1993

Nishizuka Y: Intracellular signaling by hydrolysis of phospholipids and activation of protein kinase C. Science 258:607–614, 1992

Nishizuka Y: Protein kinase C and lipid signaling for sustained cellular responses. FASEB J 17:484–496, 1995

Nora JJ, Nora AH, Toews WH: Lithium, Ebstein's anomaly and other congenital heart defects. Lancet 1:594–595, 1974

Nordenstrom J, Strigard K, Perbeck L, et al: Hyperparathyroidism associated with treatment of manic-depressive disorders by lithium. Eur J Surg 158:207–211, 1992

Nurnberger J Jr, Jimerson DC, Allen JR, et al: Red cell ouabain-sensitive Na+-K+-adenosine triphosphatase: a state marker in affective disorder inversely related to plasma cortisol. Biol Psychiatry 17:981–992, 1982

Odagaki Y, Koyama T, Matsubara S, et al: Effects of chronic lithium treatment on serotonin binding sites in rat brain. J Psychiatr Res 24:271–277, 1990

Olianas MC, Onali P: Phorbol esters increase GTP-dependent adenylate cyclase activity in rat brain striatal membranes. J Neurochem 7:890–897, 1986

Ormandy G, Jope RS: Analysis of the convulsant-potentiating effects of lithium in rats. Exp Neurol 111:356–361, 1991

Ostrow DG, Pandey GN, Davis JM, et al: A heritable disorder of lithium transport in erythrocytes of a subpopulation of manic-depressive patients. Am J Psychiatry 135:1070–1078, 1978

Pandey GN, Ostrow DG, Haas M, et al: Abnormal lithium and sodium transport in erythrocytes of a manic patient and some members of his family. Proc Natl Acad Sci U S A 74:3607–3611, 1977

Pandey GN, Sarkadi M, Haas M, et al: Lithium transport pathways in human red blood cells. J Gen Physiol 72:233–247, 1978

Pandey GN, Janicak PG, Javaid JI, et al: Increased 3H-clonidine binding in the platelets of patients with depressive and schizophrenic disorders. Psychiatry Res 28:73–88, 1989

Perry P, Tsuang MT: Treatment of unipolar depression following electroconvulsive therapy: relapse rate comparisons between lithium and tricyclics therapies following ECT. J Affect Disord 1:123–129, 1979

Persinger MA, Makarec K, Bradley JC: Characteristics of limbic seizures evoked by peripheral injections of lithium and pilocarpine. Physiol Behav 44:27–37, 1988

Pert A, Rosenblatt JE, Sivit C, et al: Long-term treatment with lithium prevents the development of dopamine receptor supersensitivity. Science 201:171–173, 1978

Pert CB, Pert A, Rosenblatt JE, et al: Catecholamine receptor stabilization: a possible mode of lithium's antimanic action, in Catecholamines: Basic and Clinical Frontiers. Edited by Usdin E, Kopin IJ, Barchas JD. New York, Pergamon, 1979, pp 583–585

Peselow ED, Dunner DL, Fieve RR, et al: Lithium carbonate and weight gain. J Affect Disord 2:303–310, 1980

Peterson GA, Byrd SL: Diabetic ketoacidosis from clozapine and lithium cotreatment (letter). Am J Psychiatry 153:737–738, 1996

Plenge P, Stensgaard A, Jensen HV, et al: 24-Hour lithium concentration in human brain studied by Li-7 magnetic resonance spectroscopy. Biol Psychiatry 36:511–516, 1994

Poirier MF, Galzin AM, Pimoule C, et al: Short-term lithium administration to healthy volunteers produces long-lasting pronounced changes in platelet serotonin uptake but not imipramine binding. Psychopharmacology (Berl) 94:521–526, 1988

Poirier-Littre MF, Loo H, Dennis T, et al: Lithium treatment increases norepinephrine turnover in the plasma of healthy subjects (letter). Arch Gen Psychiatry 50:72–73, 1993

Poitou P, Bohuon C: Catecholamine metabolism in the rat brain after short and long term lithium administration. J Neurochem 25:535–537, 1975

Pontzer NJ, Crews FT: Desensitization of muscarinic stimulated hippocampal cell firing is related to phosphoinositide hydrolysis and inhibited by lithium. J Pharmacol Exp Ther 253:921–929, 1990

Post RM: Transduction of psychosocial stress into the neurobiology of recurrent affective disorder. Am J Psychiatry 149:999–1010, 1992

Post RM, Stoddard FJ, Gillin JC, et al: Alterations in motor activity, sleep, and biochemistry in a cycling manic-depressive patient. Arch Gen Psychiatry 34:470–477, 1977

Post RM, Ballenger JC, Hare TA, et al: Cerebrospinal fluid GABA in normals and patients with affective disorders. Brain Res Bull 5 (suppl 2):755–759, 1980a

Post RM, Jimerson DC, Bunney WE Jr, et al: Dopamine and mania: behavioral and biochemical effects of the dopamine receptor blocker pimozide. Psychopharmacology (Berl) 67:297–305, 1980b

Post RM, Leverich GS, Altshuler L, et al: Lithium-discontinuation-induced refractoriness: preliminary observations. Am J Psychiatry 149:1727–1729, 1992

Price LH: Antidepressants, in Depression and Mania: Modern Lithium Therapy. Edited by Johnson FN. Oxford, England, IRL Press, 1987, pp 161–166

Price LH: Lithium augmentation in tricyclic-resistant depression, in Treatment of Tricyclic-Resistant Depression. Edited by Extein IL. Washington, DC, American Psychiatric Press, 1989, pp 49–79

Price LH, Charney DS, Delgado PL, et al: Lithium treatment and serotoninergic function. Arch Gen Psychiatry 46:13–19, 1989

Price LH, Charney DS, Delgado PL, et al: Lithium and serotonin function: implications for the serotonin hypothesis of depression. Psychopharmacology (Berl) 100:3–12, 1990

Prien RF, Caffey EM Jr, Klett CJ: Comparison of lithium carbonate and chlorpromazine in the treatment of mania: report of the Veterans Administration and National Institute of Mental Health Collaborative Study Group. Arch Gen Psychiatry 26:146–153, 1972

Ramaprasad S, Newton JE, Cardwell D, et al: In vivo ^{7}Li NMR imaging and localized spectroscopy of rat brain. Magn Reson Med 25:308–318, 1992

Ramsey TA, Frazer A, Mendels J, et al: The erythrocyte lithium-plasma lithium ratio in patients with primary affective disorder. Arch Gen Psychiatry 36:457–461, 1979

Rana RS, Hokin LE: Role of phosphoinositides in transmembrane signaling. Physiol Rev 70:115–164, 1990

Rangel-Guerra RA, Perez-Payan H, Minkoff L, et al: Nuclear magnetic resonance in bipolar disorders. AJNR Am J Neuroradiol 4:229–231, 1983

Rao ML, Mager T: Influence of the pineal gland on the pituitary function in humans. Psychoendocrinology 12:141–147, 1987

Reddy PL, Khanna S, Subhash MN, et al: Erythrocyte membrane Na-K ATPase activity in affective disorder. Biol Psychiatry 26:533–537, 1989

Reisine T, Zatz M: Interactions between lithium, calcium, diacylglycerides and phorbol esters in the regulation of ACTH release from AtT-20 cells. J Neurochem 49:884–889, 1987

Renshaw PF, Wicklund S: In vivo measurement of lithium in humans by nuclear magnetic resonance spectroscopy. Biol Psychiatry 23:465–475, 1988

Renshaw PF, Haselgrove JC, Bolinger L, et al: Relaxation and imaging of lithium in vivo. Magn Reson Imaging 4:193–198, 1986

Richelson E: Lithium ion entry through the sodium channel of cultured mouse neuroblastoma cells: a biochemical study. Science 196:1001–1002, 1977

Richelson E, Snyder K, Carlson J, et al: Lithium ion transport in erythrocytes of randomly selected blood donors and manic-depressive patients: lack of association with affective illness. Am J Psychiatry 143:457–462, 1986

Riddell FG: Studies on Li$^+$ transport using ^{7}Li and ^{6}Li nuclear magnetic resonance, in Lithium and the Cell. Edited by Birch NJ. San Diego, CA, Academic Press, 1991, pp 85–98

Riedl U, Barocka A, Kolem H, et al: Duration of lithium treatment and brain lithium concentration in patients with unipolar and schizoaffective disorder—a study with magnetic resonance spectroscopy. Biol Psychiatry 41:844–850, 1997

Risby ED, Hsiao JK, Manji HK, et al: The mechanisms of action of lithium. Arch Gen Psychiatry 48:513–524, 1991

Ritchie JM, Straub RW: Observations on the mechanism for the active extrusion of lithium in mammalian non-myelinated nerve fibres. J Physiol 304:123–124, 1980

Roberts DE, Berman SM, Nakasato S, et al: Effect of lithium carbonate on zidovudine-associated neutropenia in the acquired immunodeficiency syndrome. Am J Med 85:428–431, 1988

Rogers M, Whybrow P: Clinical hypothyroidism occurring during lithium treatment: two case histories and a review of thyroid function in 19 patients. Am J Psychiatry 128:150–155, 1971

Ronai AZ, Vizi SE: The effect of lithium treatment on the acetylcholine content of rat brain. Biochem Pharmacol 24:1819–1820, 1975

Rooney TA, Nahorski SR: Regional characterization of agonist and depolarization-induced phosphoinositide hydrolysis in rat brain. J Pharmacol Exp Ther 239:873–880, 1986

Roose SP, Bone S, Haidorfer C, et al: Lithium treatment in older patients. Am J Psychiatry 136:843–844, 1979

Rosenblatt JE, Pert CB, Tallman JF, et al: The effect of imipramine and lithium on alpha- and beta-receptor binding in rat brain. Brain Res 160:186–191, 1979

Rosenblatt JE, Pert A, Layton B, et al: Chronic lithium reduced ^{3}H-spiroperidol binding in rat striatum. Eur J Pharmacol 67:321–322, 1980

Rosenthal J, Strauss A, Minkoff L, et al: Identifying lithium-responsive bipolar depressed patients using nuclear magnetic resonance. Am J Psychiatry 143:779–780, 1986

Ross DR, Coffey CE: Neuroleptics and anxiolytics, in Depression and Mania: Modern Lithium Therapy. Edited by Johnson FN. Oxford, England, IRL Press, 1987, pp 167–171

Rudorfer MV, Linnoila M: Electroconvulsive therapy, in Lithium Combination Treatment. Edited by Johnson FN. Basel, Switzerland, Karger, 1987, pp 164–178

Russell RW, Pechnick R, Jope RS: Effects of lithium on behavioral reactivity: relation to increases in brain cholinergic activity. Psychopharmacology (Berl) 73:120–125, 1981

Rybakowski J, Frazer A, Mendels J: Lithium efflux from erythrocytes incubated in vitro during lithium carbonate administration. Communications in Psychopharmacology 2:105–112, 1978

Sagi-Eisenberg R: GTP-binding proteins as possible targets for protein kinase C action. Trends Biochem Sci 14:355–357, 1989

Sahin-Erdemli I, Medford RM, Songu-Mize E: Regulation of Na$^+$,K($+$)-ATPase alpha-subunit isoforms in rat tissues during hypertension. Eur J Pharmacol 292:163–171, 1995

Sander G, Di Scala G, Oberling P, et al: Distribution of lithium in the rat brain after a single administration known to elicit aversive effects. Neurosci Lett 166:1–4, 1994

Sansone MEG, Ziegler DK: Lithium toxicity: a review of neurologic complications. Clin Neuropharmacol 8:242–248, 1985

Sarkadi B, Alifimoff JK, Gunn RB, et al: Kinetics and stoichiometry of Na-dependent Li transport in human red blood cells. J Gen Physiol 72:249–265, 1978

Sarri E, Picatoste F, Claro E: Neurotransmitter specific profiles of inositol phosphates in rat brain cortex: relation to the mode of receptor activation of phosphoinositide phospholipase C. J Pharmacol Exp Ther 272:77–84, 1995

Savolainen KM, Hirvonen MR, Tarhanen J, et al: Changes in cerebral inosito-1-phosphate concentrations in LiCl-treated rats: regional and strain differences. Neurochem Res 15:541–545, 1990

Saxe AW, Gibson G: Lithium increases tritiated thymidine uptake by abnormal human parathyroid tissue. Surgery 110:1067–1076, 1991

Saxe A, Gibson G: Effect of lithium on incorporation of bromodeoxyuridine and tritiated thymidine into human parathyroid cells. Arch Surg 128:865–869, 1993

Schatzberg AF, Cole JO: Manual of Clinical Psychopharmacology, 2nd Edition. Washington, DC, American Psychiatric Press, 1991

Schildkraut JJ: The effects of lithium on norepinephrine turnover and metabolism: basic and clinical studies, in Lithium: Its Role in Psychiatric Research and Treatment. Edited by Gershon S, Shopsin B. New York, Plenum, 1973, pp 51–73

Schildkraut JJ: The effects of lithium on norepinephrine turnover and metabolism: basic and clinical studies. J Nerv Ment Dis 158:348–360, 1974

Schildkraut JJ, Schanberg SM, Kopin IJ: The effects of lithium ion on ^{3}H-norepinephrine metabolism in brain. Life Sci 16:1479–1483, 1966

Schildkraut JJ, Logue MA, Dodge GA: The effect of lithium salts on the turnover and metabolism of norepinephrine in rat brain. Psychopharmacologia 14:135–141, 1969

Schildkraut JJ, Keeler BA, Grob EL, et al: MHPG excretion and clinical classification in depressive disorders. Lancet 1:1251–1252, 1973

Schou M: Lithium in psychiatric therapy and prophylaxis. J Psychiatr Res 6:67–95, 1968

Schou M: Artistic productivity and lithium prophylaxis in manic-depressive illness. Br J Psychiatry 135:97–103, 1979a

Schou M: Lithium research at the Psychopharmacology Research Unit, Risskov, Denmark: a historical account, in Origin, Prevention and Treatment of Affective Disorders. Edited by Schou M, Stromgren E. London, Academic Press, 1979b, pp 1–8

Schou M: Use in other psychiatric conditions, in Depression and Mania: Modern Lithium Therapy. Edited by Johnson FN. Oxford, England, IRL Press, 1987, pp 44–50

Schou M: Lithium Treatment of Manic-Depressive Illness, 4th Edition, Revised. Basel, Switzerland, Karger, 1989

Schou M: Clinical aspects of lithium in psychiatry, in Lithium and the Cell. Edited by Birch NJ. London, Academic Press, 1991, pp 1–6

Schou M, Juel-Neilsen N, Stromberg E, et al: The treatment of manic psychoses by the administration of lithium salts. J Neurol Neurosurg Psychiatry 17:250–260, 1954

Schou M, Goldfield MD, Weinstein MR, et al: Lithium and pregnancy, I: report from the Register of Lithium Babies. BMJ 2:135–136, 1973

Schou M, Amdisen A, Thomsen K, et al: Lithium treatment regimen and renal water handling: the significance of dosage pattern and tablet type examined through comparison of results from two clinics with different treatment regimens. Psychopharmacology (Berl) 77:387–390, 1982

Schou M, Hansen HE, Thomsen K, et al: Lithium treatment in Aarhus, 2: risk of renal failure and of intoxication. Pharmacopsychiatry 22:101–103, 1989

Schreiber G, Avissar S, Danon A, et al: Hyperfunctional G proteins in mononuclear leukocytes of patients with mania. Biol Psychiatry 29:273–280, 1991

Schultz JE, Siggins GR, Schocker FW, et al: Effects of prolonged treatment with lithium and tricyclic antidepressants on discharge frequency, norepinephrine responses and beta receptor binding in rat cerebellum: electrophysiological and biochemical comparison. J Pharmacol Exp Ther 216:28–38, 1981

Seeger TF, Gardner EL, Bridger WF: Increase in mesolimbic electrical self-stimulation after chronic haloperidol: reversal by L-dopa or lithium. Brain Res 215:404–409, 1981

Segal DS, Callaghan M, Mandell AJ: Alterations in behaviour and catecholamine biosynthesis induced by lithium. Nature 254:58–59, 1975

Seggie J, Carney PA, Parker J, et al: Effect of chronic lithium on sensitivity to light in male and female bipolar patients. Prog Neuropsychopharmacol Biol Psychiatry 13:543–549, 1989

Sengupta N, Datta SC, Sengupta D, et al: Platelet and erythrocyte membrane ATPase activity in depression and mania. Psychiatry Res 3:337–344, 1980

Sharp T, Bramwell SR, Lambert P, et al: Effect of short- and long-term administration of lithium on the release of endogenous 5-HT in the hippocampus of the rat in vivo and in vitro. Neuropharmacology 30:977–984, 1991

Shaughnessy R, Greene SC, Pandey GN, et al: Red-cell lithium transport and affective disorders in a multigeneration pedigree: evidence for genetic transmission of affective disorders. Biol Psychiatry 20:451–460, 1985

Sheng M, Greenberg ME: The regulation and function of c-fos and other immediate early genes in the nervous system. Neuron 4:477–485, 1990

Sherman WR: Lithium and the phosphoinositide signalling system, in Lithium and the Cell. Edited by Birch NJ. London, Academic Press, 1991, pp 121–157

Sherman WR, Munsell LY, Wong YHH: Differential uptake of lithium isotopes by rat cerebral cortex and its effect on inositol phosphate metabolism. J Neurochem 42:880–882, 1984

Sherman WR, Munsell LY, Gish BG, et al: Effects of systemically administered lithium on phosphoinositide metabolism in rat brain, kidney, and testis. J Neurochem 44:798–807, 1985

Sherman WR, Gish BG, Honchar MP, et al: Effects of lithium on phosphoinositide metabolism in vivo. Federation Proceedings 45:2639–2646, 1986

Shippenberg TS, Herz A: Influence of chronic lithium treatment upon the motivational effects of opioids: alteration in the effects of mu- but not kappa-opioid receptor ligands. J Pharmacol Exp Ther 256:1101–1106, 1991

Shippenberg TS, Millan MJ, Mucha RF, et al: Involvement of beta-endorphin and mu-opioid receptors in mediating the aversive effect of lithium in the rat. Eur J Pharmacol 154:135–144, 1988

Shopsin B, Kim SS, Gershon S: A controlled study of lithium vs. chlorpromazine in acute schizophrenics. Br J Psychiatry 119:435–440, 1971

Shukla GS: Combined lithium and valproate treatment and subsequent withdrawal: serotonergic mechanism of their interaction in discrete brain regions. Prog Neuropsychopharmacol Biol Psychiatry 9:153–156, 1985

Simon JR, Kuhar MJ: High affinity choline uptake: ionic and energy requirement. J Neurochem 27:93–99, 1976

Sivam SP, Strunk C, Smith DR, et al: Proenkephalin-A gene regulation in the rat striatum: influence of lithium and haloperidol. Mol Pharmacol 30:186–191, 1986

Sivam SP, Takeuchi K, Li S, et al: Lithium increases dynorphin A(1–8) and prodynorphin mRNA levels in the basal ganglia of rats. Brain Res 427:155–163, 1988

Sivam SP, Krause JE, Takeuchi K, et al: Lithium increases rat striatal beta- and gamma-preprotachykinin messenger FNAs. J Pharmacol Exp Ther 248:1297–1301, 1989

Skinner GR, Hartley C, Buchan A, et al: The effect of lithium chloride on the replication of herpes simplex virus. Med Microbiol Immunol (Berl) 168:139–148, 1980

Smith DF: Lithium attenuates clonidine-induced hypoactivity: further studies in inbred mouse strains. Psychopharmacology (Berl) 94:428–430, 1988

Smith DF, Amdisen A: Lithium distribution in rat brain after long-term central administration by minipump. J Pharm Pharmacol 33:805–806, 1981

Solomon DA, Ristow WR, Keller MB, et al: Serum lithium levels and psychosocial function in patients with bipolar I disorder. Am J Psychiatry 153:1301–1307, 1996

Song L, Jope R: Chronic lithium treatment impairs phosphatidylinositol hydrolysis in membranes from rat brain regions. J Neurochem 58:2200–2206, 1992

Spengler RN, Hollingsworth PJ, Smith CB: Effects of long-term lithium and desipramine treatment upon clonidine-induced inhibition of ^{3}H-norepinephrine release from rat hippocampal slices (abstract). Federation Proceedings 45:681, 1986

Spiegel AM, Rudorfer MV, Marx SJ, et al: The effect of short term lithium administration on suppressibility of parathyroid hormone secretion by calcium in vivo. J Clin Endocrinol Metab 59:354–357, 1984

Spirtes MA: Lithium levels in monkey and human brain after chronic, therapeutic oral dosage. Pharmacol Biochem Behav 5:143–147, 1976

Stabel S, Parker PJ: Protein kinase C. Pharmacol Ther 51:71–95, 1991

Stachel SE, Grunwald DJ, Myers PZ, et al: Lithium perturbation and goosecoid expression identify a dorsal specification pathway in the pregastrula zebrafish. Development 117:1261–1274, 1993

Staunton DA, Magistretti PJ, Shoemaker WJ, et al: Effects of chronic lithium treatment on dopamine receptors in the rat corpus striatum, I: locomotor activity and behavioral supersensitivity. Brain Res 232:391–400, 1982a

Staunton DA, Magistretti PJ, Shoemaker WJ, et al: Effects of chronic lithium treatment on dopamine receptors in the rat corpus striatum, II: no effect on denervation or neuroleptic-induced supersensitivity. Brain Res 232:401–412, 1982b

Stern DN, Fieve RR, Neff NH, et al: The effect of lithium chloride administration on brain and heart norepinephrine turnover rates. Psychopharmacologia 14:315–322, 1969

Stoll AL, Cohen BM, Snyder MB, et al: Erythrocyte choline concentration in bipolar disorder: a predictor of clinical course and medication response. Biol Psychiatry 29:1171–1180, 1991

Strassheim D, Palmer T, Milligan G, et al: Alterations in G-protein expression and the hormonal regulation of adenylate cyclase in the adipocytes of obese (fa/fa) Zuker rats. J Biochem 276:197–202, 1991

Strzyzewski W, Rybakowski J, Potok E, et al: Erythrocyte cation transport in endogenous depression: clinical and psychophysiological correlates. Acta Psychiatr Scand 70:248–253, 1984

Suppes T, Baldessarini RJ, Faedda GL, et al: Risk of recurrence following discontinuation of lithium treatment in bipolar disorder. Arch Gen Psychiatry 48:1082–1088, 1991

Suppes T, Baldessarini RJ, Faedda GL, et al: Discontinuation of maintenance treatment in bipolar disorder: risks and implications. Harvard Reviews in Psychiatry 1:131–144, 1993

Swann AC: Caloric intake and (Na$^+$,K$^+$)-ATPase: differential regulation by alpha-1 and beta noradrenergic receptors. Am J Physiol 247:R449–R455, 1984

Swann AC: Norepinephrine and (Na$^+$,K$^+$)-ATPase: evidence for stabilization by lithium or imipramine. Neuropharmacology 27:261–267, 1988

Swann AC, Marini JL, Sheard MH, et al: Effects of chronic dietary lithium on activity and regulation of [Na$^+$,K$^+$]-adenosine triphosphatase in rat brain. Biochem Pharmacol 29:2819–2823, 1980

Swann AC, Heninger GR, Roth RH, et al: Differential effects of short and long term lithium on tryptophan uptake and serotonergic function in cat brain. Life Sci 28:347–354, 1981

Swann AC, Koslow SH, Katz MM, et al: Lithium carbonate treatment of mania. Arch Gen Psychiatry 44:345–354, 1987

Swerdlow NR, Lee D, Koob GF, et al: Effects of chronic dietary lithium on behavioral indices of dopamine denervation supersensitivity in the rat. J Pharmacol Exp Ther 235:324–329, 1985

Szentistvanyi I, Janka Z: Correlation between lithium ratio and Na-dependent Li transport in red blood cells during lithium prophylaxis. Biol Psychiatry 14:973–977, 1979

Tagliamonte A, Tagliamonte P, Perez-Cruet J, et al: Effect of psychotropic drugs on tryptophan concentration in the rat brain. J Pharmacol Exp Ther 177:475–480, 1971

Tanaka C, Nishizuka Y: The protein kinase C family for neuronal signaling. Annu Rev Neurosci 17:551–567, 1994

Tanimoto K, Maeda K, Yamaguchi N, et al: Effect of lithium on prolactin responses to thyrotropin releasing hormone in patients with manic state. Psychopharmacology (Berl) 72:129–133, 1981

Tanimoto K, Maeda K, Terada T: Inhibitory effect of lithium on neuroleptic and serotonin receptors in rat brain. Brain Res 265:148–151, 1983

Taylor JW, Bell AJ: Lithium-induced parathyroid dysfunction: a case report and review of the literature. Ann Pharmacother 27:1040–1043, 1993

Terry JB, Padzernik TL, Nelson SR: Effect of LiCl pretreatment on cholinomimetic-induced seizures and seizure-induced brain edema in rats. Neurosci Lett 114:123–127, 1990

Thellier M, Heurteaux C, Wissocq JC: Quantitative study of the distribution of lithium in the mouse brain for various doses of lithium given to the animal. Brain Res 199:175–197, 1980a

Thellier M, Wissocq JC, Heurteaux C: Quantitative microlocation of lithium in the brain by a (n,alpha) nuclear reaction. Nature 283:299–302, 1980b

Thiele EA, Eipper BA: Effect of secretogogues on components of the secretory system in AtT-20 cells. Endocrinology 126:809–817, 1990

Tilkian AG, Schroder JS, Kao J, et al: Effect of lithium on cardiovascular performance: report on extended ambulatory monitoring and exercise testing before and during lithium therapy. Am J Cardiol 38:701–708, 1976

Tohen M: Atypical antipsychotic agents in mania-clinical studies, in Mechanisms of Antipolar Treatments: Focus on Lithium, Carbamazepine and Valproate. Edited by Manji HK, Bowden CL, Belmaker RH. Washington, DC, American Psychiatric Press (in press)

Tollefson GD, Senogles S: A cholinergic role in the mechanism of lithium in mania. Biol Psychiatry 18:467–479, 1982

Torok TL: Neurochemical transmission and the sodium pump. Prog Neurobiol 32:11–76, 1989

Treiser S, Kellar KJ: Lithium effects on adrenergic receptor supersensitivity in rat brain. Eur J Pharmacol 58:85–86, 1979

Treiser S, Kellar KJ: Lithium: effects on serotonin receptors in rat brain. Eur J Pharmacol 64:183–185, 1980

Treiser SL, Cascio CS, O'Donohue TL, et al: Lithium increases serotonin release and decreases serotonin receptors in the hippocampus. Science 213:1529–1531, 1981

Tricklebank MD, Singh L, Jackson A, et al: Evidence that a proconvulsant action of lithium is mediated by inhibition of myo-inositol phosphatase in mouse brain. Brain Res 558:145–148, 1991

Trousseau A: Clinique Medicale de l'Hôtel-Dieu de Paris, 3rd Edition. Paris, France, JB Balliere et Fils, 1868

Tseng FY, Pasquali D, Field JB: Effects of lithium on stimulated metabolic parameters in dog thyroid slices. Acta Endocrinol (Copenh) 121:615–620, 1989

Uney JB, Marchbanks RM: Inhibition of choline transport in human brain by lithium treatment, in Cellular and Molecular Basis of Cholinergic Function. Edited by Dowdall MJ, Hawthorne JN. New York, VCH Publishers, 1987, pp 774–780

Uney JB, Marchbanks RM, Marsh A: The effect of lithium on choline transport in human erythrocytes. J Neurol Neurosurg Psychiatry 48:229–233, 1985

Uney JB, Marchbanks RM, Reynolds GP, et al: Lithium prophylaxis inhibits choline transport in post-mortem brain (letter). Lancet 2:458, 1986

Urabe M, Hershman JM, Pang XP, et al: Effect of lithium on function and growth of thyroid cells in vitro. Endocrinology 129:807–814, 1991

Ure A: Researches on gout. Medical Times 11:145, 1844/1845

Vallar L, Muca C, Magni M, et al: Differential coupling of dopaminergic receptors expressed in different cell types: stimulation of phosphatidylinositol 4,5-bisphosphate hydrolysis in LtK-fibroblasts, hyperpolarization, and cytosolic-free Ca^{2+} concentration decrease in GH$_4$Cl cells. J Biol Chem 265:10320–10326, 1990

van Kammen DP, Docherty JP, Marder SR, et al: Lithium attenuates the activation-euphoria but not the psychosis induced by d-amphetamine in schizophrenia. Psychopharmacology (Berl) 87:111–115, 1985

Varney MA, Godfrey PP, Drummond AH, et al: Chronic lithium treatment inhibits basal and agonist-stimulated responses in rat cerebral cortex and GH$_3$ pituitary cells. Mol Pharmacol 4:671–678, 1992

Verimer T, Goodale DB, Long JP, et al: Lithium effects on haloperidol-induced pre- and postsynaptic dopamine receptor supersensitivity. J Pharm Pharmacol 32:665–666, 1980

Vestergaard P, Aagaard J: Five-year mortality in lithium-treated manic-depressive patients. J Affect Disord 21:33–38, 1991

Vestergaard P, Poulstrup I, Schou M: Prospective studies on a lithium cohort, 3: tremor, weight gain, diarrhea, psychological complaints. Acta Psychiatr Scand 78:434–441, 1988

Walker E, Green M: Soft signs of neurological dysfunction in schizophrenia: an investigation of lateral performance. Biol Psychiatry 17:381–386, 1982

Walker RG: Lithium nephrotoxicity. Kidney Int 44 (suppl 42):S93–S98, 1993

Wang HY, Friedman E: Chronic lithium: desensitization of autoreceptors mediating serotonin release. Psychopharmacology (Berl) 94:312–314, 1988

Wang HY, Friedman E: Lithium inhibition of protein kinase C activation-induced serotonin release. Psychopharmacology (Berl) 99:213–218, 1989

Watanabe Y, Horn F, Bauer S, et al: Protein kinase C interferes with Ni-mediated inhibition of human platelet adenylate cyclase. FEBS Lett 192:23–27, 1985

Watson DG, Lenox RH: Chronic lithium-induced down-regulation of MARCKS in immortalized hippocampal cells: potentiation by muscarinic receptor activation. J Neurochem 67:767–777, 1996

Watson SP, Shipman L, Godfrey PP: Lithium potentiates agonist formation of [^{3}H]CDP-diacylglycerol in human platelets. Eur J Pharmacol 188:273–276, 1990

Wehr TA: Phase and biorhythm studies in affective illness. Ann Intern Med 87:319–335, 1977

Wehr TA, Goodwin FK: Rapid cycling in manic-depressives induced by tricyclic antidepressants. Arch Gen Psychiatry 36:555–559, 1979

Wehr TA, Goodwin FK: Can antidepressants cause mania and worsen the course of affective illness? Am J Psychiatry 144:1403–1411, 1987

Wehr TA, Sack DA, Rosenthal NE: Sleep reduction as a final common pathway in the genesis of mania. Am J Psychiatry 144:201–204, 1987

Weiner ED, Kalaaspudi VD, Papolos DF, et al: Lithium augments pilocarpine-induced fos gene expression in brain. Brain Res 553:117–122, 1991

Weiner ED, Mallat AM, Papolos DF, et al: Acute lithium treatment enhances neuropeptide Y gene expression in rat hippocampus. Brain Res Mol Brain Res 12:209–214, 1992

Welsh DK, Moore-Ede MC: Lithium lengthens circadian period in a diurnal primate, Saimiri sciureus. Biol Psychiatry 28:117–126, 1990

Welsh DK, Nino-Murcia G, Gander PH, et al: Regular 48-hour cycling of sleep duration and mood in a 35-year-old woman: use of lithium in time isolation. Biol Psychiatry 21:527–537, 1986

Werstiuk ES, Steiner M: Anti-psychotics, II: butyrophenones, in Lithium Combination Treatment. Edited by Johnson FN. Basel, Switzerland, Karger, 1987, pp 84–104

Wever RA: The Circadian System of Man. New York, Springer-Verlag, 1979

Whitworth P, Kendall DA: Lithium selectively inhibits muscarinic receptor-stimulated inositol tetrakisphosphate accumulation in mouse cerebral cortex slices. J Neurochem 51:258–265, 1988

Whitworth P, Kendall DA: Effects of lithium on inositol phospholipid hydrolysis and inhibition of dopamine D_1 receptor-mediated cyclic AMP formation by carbachol in rat brain slices. J Neurochem 53:536–541, 1989

Williams MB, Jope RS: Circadian variation in rat brain AP-1 DNA binding activity after cholinergic stimulation: modulation by lithium. Psychopharmacology 122:363–368, 1995

Wirz-Justice A: Antidepressant drugs: effects on the circadian system, in Circadian Rhythms in Psychiatry. Edited by Wehr TA, Goodwin FK. Pacific Grove, CA, Boxwood, 1983, pp 235–264

Wirz-Justice A, Groos GA, Wehr TA: The neuropharmacology of circadian timekeeping in mammals, in Vertebrate Circadian Systems: Structure and Physiology. Edited by Aschoff J, Daan S, Groos GA. New York, Springer-Verlag, 1982, pp 1–26

Wolff J, Berens SC, Jones AB: Inhibition of thyrotropin-stimulated adenylyl cyclase activity of beef thyroid membranes by low concentration of lithium ion. Biochem Biophys Res Commun 39:77–82, 1970

Wood AJ, Goodwin GM: A review of the biochemical and neuropharmacological actions of lithium. Psychol Med 17:579–600, 1987

Wood AJ, Elphick M, Aronson JK, et al: The effect of lithium on cation transport measured in vivo in patients suffering from bipolar affective illness. Br J Psychiatry 155:504–510, 1989a

Wood AJ, Elphick M, Grahame-Smith DG: Effect of lithium and of other drugs used in the treatment of manic illness on the cation-transporting properties of Na^+,K^+-ATPase in mouse brain synaptosomes. J Neurochem 52:1042–1049, 1989b

Wood K, Coppen A: Prophylactic lithium treatment of patients with affective disorder is associated with decreased platelet ^{3}H-dihydroergocryptine binding. J Affect Disord 5:253–258, 1983

Wood K, Swade C, Abou-Saleh M, et al: Drug plasma levels and platelet 5-HT uptake inhibition during long-term treatment with fluvoxamine or lithium in patients with affective disorder. Br J Clin Pharmacol 15:365S–368S, 1983

Wood K, Swade C, Abou-Saleh MT, et al: Apparent supersensitivity of platelet 5-HT receptors in lithium-treated patients. J Affect Disord 8:69–72, 1985

Yamaki M, Kusano E, Tetsuka T, et al: Cellular mechanism of lithium-induced nephrogenic diabetes insipidus in rats. Am J Physiol 261:F505–F511, 1991

Young LT, Woods CM: Mood stabilizers have differential effects on endogenous ADP ribosylation in C6 glioma cells. Eur J Pharmacol 309:215–218, 1996

Young S, Parker PJ, Ullrich A, et al: Down-regulation of protein kinase C is due to an increased rate of degradation. Biochem J 24:775–779, 1987

Yuan PX, Chen G, Granneman GJ, et al: Increase in the expression of AP-1 regulated genes in brain by the mood stabilizing agents lithium and valproic acid (abstract). Abstracts of the Society of Neuroscience 27th Annual Meeting. New Orleans, LA, October 1997

Zachrisson O, Mathe AA, Stenfors C, et al: Region-specific effects of chronic lithium administration on neuropeptide Y and somatostatin mRNA expression in the rat brain. Neurosci Lett 194:89–92, 1995

Zalstein E, Koren G, Einarson T, et al: A case-control study on the association between first trimester exposure to lithium and Ebstein's anomaly. Am J Cardiol 65:817–818, 1990

Zanardi R, Racagni G, Smeraldi E, et al: Differential effects of lithium on platelet protein phosphorylation in bipolar patients and healthy subjects. Psychopharmacology (Berl) 129:44–47, 1997

Zatz M, Reisine TD: Lithium induces corticotropin secretion and desensitization in cultured anterior pituitary cells. Proc Natl Acad Sci U S A 82:1286–1290, 1985

Zerahn K: Studies on the active transport of lithium in the isolated frog skin. Acta Physiol Scand 33:347–358, 1955

than 6 years, and in 1987 as an antiepileptic without age limitations. Carbamazepine is currently considered a major antiepileptic and continues to be increasingly prescribed because it produces less psychological and neurological toxicity than either phenytoin or phenobarbital (Loiseau and Duche 1989).

Structure-Activity Relations

Carbamazepine (5-carbamyl-5*H*-dibenz[*b,f*]azepine or 5*H*-dibenz[*b,f*]azepine-5-carboxamide) is an iminostilbene derivative with a tricyclic structure similar to that of the tricyclic antidepressant (TCA) imipramine (Kutt 1989; Levy et al. 1989; Rall and Schleifer 1985) (Figure 21–1). Iminodibenzyl (a precursor of carbamazepine) and a number of iminodibenzyl derivatives possess local anesthetic as well as antihistaminic properties but only modest antiepileptic activity. When a carbamyl (carboxamide) group is added at the 5 position of iminodibenzyl, considerable antiepileptic activity is conferred. However, the strongest antiepileptic effects occur when the carbamyl side chain is combined with iminostilbene to make carbamazepine, the structure of which is similar to iminodibenzyl except for a double bond between the 10 and 11 positions (Figure 21–1).

Pharmacological Profile

The antiepileptic profile of carbamazepine is similar to that of phenytoin. The drug is effective against maximal electroshock seizures at nontoxic doses but is ineffective against pentylenetetrazole-induced seizures (Macdonald 1989). However, carbamazepine is more effective than

phenytoin in reducing stimulus-induced discharges in the amygdala of kindled rats (Albright and Burnham 1980). In addition, it has antidiuretic effects that may be associated with reduced serum antidiuretic hormone (ADH) concentrations and (with chronic administration) is associated with decreases in peripheral thyroid function indices, increased urinary free cortisol secretion, and a high incidence of escape from dexamethasone suppression (Post et al. 1991).

In humans, carbamazepine has been shown to be effective in the treatment of simple-partial, complex-partial, and generalized tonic-clonic seizures. Carbamazepine is ineffective against and may even exacerbate absence seizures. It is also effective in the treatment of paroxysmal pain syndromes such as trigeminal neuralgia (Blom 1963).

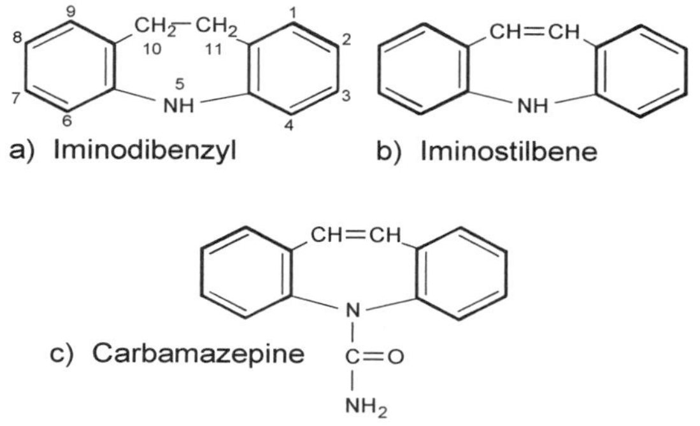

Pharmacokinetics and Disposition

After oral ingestion, the absorption of carbamazepine is slow, erratic, and unpredictable, although absorption in patients with epilepsy may be more rapid than in healthy volunteer subjects, and first-pass metabolism is minimal (Morselli 1989). Peak plasma concentrations are generally attained 4–8 hours after ingestion, but peaks as late as 26 hours have been reported (Table 21–1). The time of administration may have a significant effect on the absorption rate; absorption is slower with evening than with morning doses. The irregular absorption of carbamazepine has been attributed to a very slow dissolution rate in gastrointestinal fluid and to modification of gastrointestinal transit time by the anticholinergic properties of the drug.

Precise data on the absolute bioavailability of carbamazepine do not exist (because of the lack of an injectable formulation), but ranges of 75%–85% have been estimated from studies in which the ^{14}C-labeled molecule has been used (Ketter and Post 1994). Solutions, suspensions, syrups, and the newly developed chewable and slow-release formulations of carbamazepine seem to have similar bioavailabilities. The slow-release formulations, however, produce more stable plasma concentrations. It is worth noting that, in cases of massive overdose, peak plasma carbamazepine concentrations have been reached during the second or third day after ingestion.

Carbamazepine is distributed rapidly into all tissues; 75%–78% is bound to plasma proteins, including proteins other than albumin. Concentrations of carbamazepine in cerebrospinal fluid (CSF) correspond with concentrations of free drug in plasma and range from 17% to 31% of those in plasma.

Figure 21–1. Carbamazepine and its precursors.
Source. Reprinted from Kutt H: "Carbamazepine: Chemistry and Methods of Determination," in *Antiepileptic Drugs,* 3rd Edition. Edited by Levy RH, Dreifuss FE, Mattson RH, et al. New York, Raven, 1989, pp. 457–471. Used with permission.

Table 21–1. Population data for valproate and carbamazepine

	Peak absorption (hours)	Elimination half-life (hours)	Time to steady state (days)	Protein binding (%)	Therapeutic range (μg/mL)
Carbamazepine	2–8	2–17	2–4	73–88	3–14
Valproate	1–4	5–20	2–4	70–95	50–150

Source. Reprinted from Wilder BJ: "Pharmacokinetics of Valproate and Carbamazepine." *Journal of Clinical Psychopharmacology* 12:64S–68S, 1992. Used with permission.

Carbamazepine undergoes almost complete biotransformation in humans and is metabolized in the liver by the cytochrome P450 system to a wide number of metabolites, many of which have antiepileptic activity (Figure 21–2). The predominant pathway of metabolism in humans involves conversion to the 10,11-epoxide (Figure 21–3). This metabolite is as active as carbamazepine and has neurotoxic side effects. Its concentrations in plasma and brain may reach 50% of those of carbamazepine. The 10,11-epoxide is metabolized further to inactive compounds that are excreted in the urine, principally as glucuronides. Carbamazepine is also inactivated by conjugation and hydroxylation. Less than 3% of the drug is excreted in the urine as the parent compound or the epoxide.

Carbamazepine's elimination half-life ranges from 18 to 55 hours. During long-term treatment, carbamazepine may induce its own metabolism (a phenomenon called *autoinduction*), and its half-life may be decreased to 2–17 hours (Figure 21–4). The half-life of the 10,11-epoxide is much shorter than that of the parent compound (6–7 hours).

Treatment with carbamazepine for epilepsy, trigeminal neuralgia, and mania is usually started at a dose of 100–200 mg taken either once or twice daily. The dose is increased (usually by 100 or 200 mg every few days) according to the patient's response and side effects, usually to serum concentrations ranging from 4 to 15 μg/mL. Although there is no clear relationship between carbamazepine serum concentration and response, therapeutic concentrations for epilepsy, paroxysmal pain syndromes, and mania are reported to be 4–15 μg/mL. Significantly, neurological side effects become more frequent at serum concentrations above 9 μg/mL. In one study in which low (15–25 μmol/L) and high (28–40 μmol/L) serum concentrations of carbamazepine were compared in the maintenance treatment of patients with bipolar disorder, no difference in efficacy was found between the two concentrations (Simhandl et al. 1993).

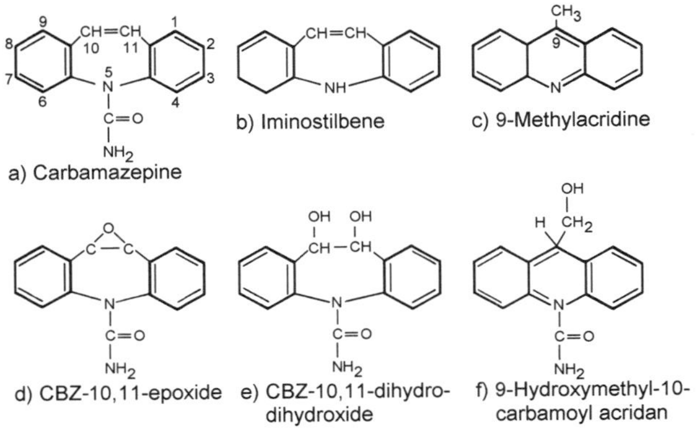

Figure 21–2. Carbamazepine (CBZ) and its metabolites and breakdown products.
Source. Reprinted from Kutt H: "Carbamazepine: Chemistry and Methods of Determination," in *Antiepileptic Drugs*, 3rd Edition. Edited by Levy RH, Dreifuss FE, Mattson RH, et al. New York, Raven, 1989, pp. 457–471. Used with permission.

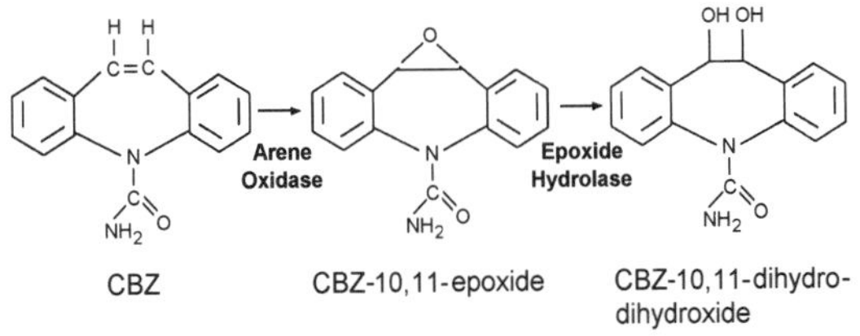

Figure 21–3. Major pathway of carbamazepine (CBZ) metabolism. This pathway of CBZ metabolism produces a CBZ-10,11-epoxide, a compound that has both anticonvulsant and toxic properties. The CBZ-10,11-epoxide is further metabolized by epoxide hydrolase. The action of epoxide hydrolase is blocked by valproate (VPA); therefore, when VPA is administered concurrently with CBZ, the CBZ-10,11-epoxide metabolite accumulates.
Source. Reprinted from Wilder BJ: "Pharmacokinetics of Valproate and Carbamazepine." *Journal of Clinical Psychopharmacology* 12:64S–68S, 1992. Used with permission.

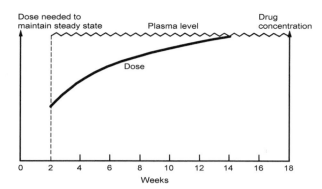

Figure 21–4. Carbamazepine (CBZ) dosage adjustments versus time to compensate for autoinduction. The clearance of CBZ approximately doubles in the first 2–3 months of therapy. To maintain therapeutic plasma levels, the daily dose must be increased, often by 100%.
Source. Reprinted from Wilder BJ: "Pharmacokinetics of Valproate and Carbamazepine." *Journal of Clinical Psychopharmacology* 12:64S–68S, 1992. Used with permission.

Mechanism of Action

Carbamazepine's many actions can be divided into two basic mechanisms (reviewed in Levy et al. 1989; Macdonald 1989; Post et al. 1984a, 1991, 1992; Rall and Schleifer 1985): 1) effects on neuronal ion channels to reduce high-frequency repetitive firing of action potentials and 2) effects on synaptic and postsynaptic transmission. The weight of evidence suggests that carbamazepine's antiepileptic action can be attributed to the reduction of high-frequency neuronal discharge through binding to and inactivating voltage-sensitive sodium channels and decreasing sodium influx in a voltage-, frequency-, and use-dependent fashion (Macdonald 1989; Post et al. 1992). Because carbamazepine's effects on sodium channels are acute, and because its antiepileptic and antinociceptive effects are more rapid in onset than its antimanic or antidepressant effects, Post et al. (1992) speculated that the drug's sodium channel effects do not account for its mood-stabilizing properties. Noteworthy studies (Post et al. 1992; Zona et al. 1990) suggested that carbamazepine may also act on potassium channels to increase potassium conductance, thereby providing another possible mechanism for its antiepileptic effects.

Regarding synaptic and postsynaptic actions, carbamazepine has been reported to alter neurotransmitter concentrations, metabolism, receptors, and second-messenger systems. Indeed, the drug affects multiple neurotransmitter systems implicated in the pathophysiology of mood disorders. The primary neurotransmitters thus far shown to be altered by carbamazepine include adenosine, norepinephrine, dopamine, serotonin, acetylcholine, γ-aminobutyric acid (GABA), glutamate, substance P, and aspartate (Macdonald 1989; Post et al. 1991, 1992). Carbamazepine binds to adenosine receptors and acts as an adenosine receptor antagonist. However, studies suggest that this property of carbamazepine is not responsible for its antiepileptic effects. Carbamazepine acutely increases locus coeruleus firing and decreases glutamate release; subchronic treatment decreases norepinephrine, dopamine, and GABA turnover and blocks adenylate cyclase activity stimulated by norepinephrine, dopamine, and adenosine. Chronic carbamazepine administration is associated with increases in adenosine receptors, substance P sensitivity and levels, and plasma free tryptophan; decreases in CSF somatostatin; and greater decreases in GABA turnover (Post et al. 1991, 1992).

It is unclear whether carbamazepine's activities on these systems play a role in its antiepileptic properties. However, the ability of the drug to decrease release of the excitatory amino acid aspartate and its effects on α_2-adrenergic receptors have been implicated in its antiepileptic activity (Post et al. 1992). Additionally, although carbamazepine is not active at the central-type benzodiazepine receptor (which is linked to chloride channels and related to the antiepileptic effects of diazepam, clonazepam, and lorazepam), it may exert some of its antiepileptic effects by acutely binding to and acting as an antagonist at the "peripheral-type" benzodiazepine receptor, which appears to be linked to calcium channels (Post et al. 1992). Carbamazepine does not modify $GABA_A$ receptors, but it may have effects at the $GABA_B$ receptor. Although these effects probably do not contribute to the drug's antiepileptic properties, they may contribute to its antinociceptive effects. Finally, some of carbamazepine's effects on second-messenger systems include decreased activity of adenylate and guanylate cyclase and reductions of some aspects of phosphoinositide turnover (Post et al. 1992).

Thus far, none of these mechanisms has been linked to the psychotropic effects of carbamazepine, and it remains unknown whether the actions underlying the drug's antiepileptic effects are also responsible for its mood-stabilizing properties. Indeed, Post et al. (1992) have speculated that different biochemical effects of carbamazepine may underlie its efficacy in different seizure types. It is noteworthy that carbamazepine does not block either stimulant-induced hyperactivity in animals or dopamine receptors in vitro. Thus, it exerts its antimanic effects through a mechanism other than dopamine receptor antagonism (Post et al. 1991).

Indications

Carbamazepine is currently approved in the United States for the treatment of complex-partial seizures, generalized tonic-clonic seizures, and other minor or partial seizure disorders (reviewed in Levy et al. 1989; Loiseau and Duche 1989; Mattson et al. 1992). Controlled studies have shown that carbamazepine has the following characteristics:

1. It is as effective as phenytoin and valproate in the treatment of primary tonic-clonic and secondarily generalized tonic-clonic seizures.
2. It is comparable to or better than phenobarbital and primidone in suppressing primary tonic-clonic and secondarily generalized tonic-clonic seizures.
3. It is comparable to or better than all of these drugs in controlling the entire range of partial seizures (i.e., simple- and complex-partial seizures with or without secondary generalization). Indeed, it is a drug of first choice in symptomatic location-related (partial) epilepsy with partial or secondary generalized tonic-clonic seizures. However, carbamazepine is ineffective in, and may even exacerbate, absence seizures.

Carbamazepine is also approved for treatment of a variety of paroxysmal pain syndromes, including trigeminal neuralgia. Although not formally approved for treatment of bipolar disorder, carbamazepine is frequently used as an alternative or adjunct to lithium in lithium-resistant or -intolerant patients. Research supporting its efficacy in patients with bipolar disorder is summarized later in this chapter.

Acute mania. To date, at least 12 double-blind studies have shown that carbamazepine is superior to placebo and comparable to lithium and antipsychotics in the short-term treatment of acute mania; approximately two-thirds of patients in these studies have shown significant improvement (Ballenger and Post 1978; Brown et al. 1987; Desai et al. 1987; Grossi et al. 1984; Keck et al. 1992a; Lenzi et al. 1986; Lerer et al. 1987; Lusznat et al. 1988; Möller et al. 1989; Müller and Stoll 1984; Okuma et al. 1979, 1990; Post 1990; Post et al. 1984a; Small 1990; Small et al. 1991) (Table 21–2). However, only seven studies (Ballenger and Post 1978; Grossi et al. 1984; Hernandez-Avila et al. 1996; Lerer et al. 1987; Okuma et al. 1979; Post et al. 1984a; Small et al. 1991) are unconfounded by concurrent lithium and neuroleptic administration and thus allow for more meaningful interpretation.

Pooled data from the studies just mentioned reveal that the overall response rate to carbamazepine in patients with acute mania was 50%, compared with 56% for lithium monotherapy and 61% for neuroleptic monotherapy (differences that are not significant) (Keck et al. 1992a). These studies further indicate that carbamazepine's onset of acute antimanic action is comparable to that of neuroleptics and is perhaps slightly more rapid than that of lithium (significant antimanic effects are usually evident within 1–2 weeks of treatment). They also indicate that carbamazepine is generally better tolerated than neuroleptics and lithium (with fewer extrapyramidal side effects [EPS]). Moreover, carbamazepine's antimanic effects may be augmented by or synergistic with concurrent administration of other mood-stabilizing agents (including lithium and valproate) and neuroleptics (Keck et al. 1992b; Ketter et al. 1992; Tohen et al. 1994). In patients whose symptoms respond to carbamazepine, therapeutic serum concentrations are similar to those in epileptic patients, generally 4–15 µg/mL with carbamazepine dosages of 200–2,000 mg/day.

Acute major depression. Only three controlled studies have examined the efficacy of carbamazepine in the treatment of patients with unipolar or bipolar major depression (Table 21–3). In the first study (Neumann et al. 1984), 10 patients (bipolar and unipolar) were randomly assigned to treatment with carbamazepine ($n = 5$) or trimipramine ($n = 5$). Both treatments were associated with significant antidepressant effects, and no significant differences were found between the two groups.

In the second study (Post et al. 1985), 12 (34%) of 35 bipolar and unipolar patients with treatment-resistant depression had a marked antidepressant response to treatment with carbamazepine alone. Fifty-four percent (19) of the patients had at least a mild degree of improvement. Substitution of carbamazepine with placebo was associated with loss of response in some patients whose depression had responded to carbamazepine. Also, the time course of antidepressant response to carbamazepine in responders was longer than that in patients with mania and comparable to that of standard antidepressants: patients began to show antidepressant effects after 2–3 weeks of treatment and had maximal antidepressant effects after 4–6 weeks.

In the third study (Small 1990), patients with treatment-resistant unipolar or bipolar depression were randomly assigned to a 4-week trial of lithium, carbamazepine, or a combination of both drugs. Of patients randomized to carbamazepine or to the combination, 32% had moderate or marked improvement, whereas 13% of

Table 21–2.   Controlled studies of carbamazepine in treatment of acute mania

Study	N	Design	Concomitant medications	Duration (days)	Outcome
Placebo-controlled					
Ballenger and Post 1978; Post et al. 1984a	19	B-A-B-A; CBZ v. P	None	11–56	63% response to CBZ; significant relapse on P
Placebo + neuroleptic					
Klein et al. 1984	14	CBZ + HAL v. P + HAL; CBZ + HAL	HAL, 15–45 mg/day; HAL	35	71% response to CBZ + HAL; 54% response to P + HAL; both groups improved, but CBZ + HAL group's improvement was greater
Müller and Stoll 1984	6	P + HAL		21	
Möller et al. 1989	11 CBZ; 9 P	CBZ + HAL v. P + HAL	HAL 24 mg/day; levomepromazine prn	21	No significant difference
Placebo + lithium					
Desai et al. 1987	5	CBZ + L v. P + L	L; ND	28	CBZ + L response > P + L response by 14
Lithium-controlled					
Lerer et al. 1987	14 CBZ; 14 L	CBZ v. L	None	28	79% response to L > 29% response to CBZ
Small et al. 1991	24 CBZ; 24 L	CBZ v. L	None	56	33% response for both groups
Neuroleptic-controlled					
Grossi et al. 1984	18 CBZ; 19 CPZ	CBZ v. CPZ	ND	21	67% response to CPZ; 59% response to CBZ
Okuma et al. 1979	32 CBZ; 28 CPZ	CBZ v. CPZ	None	21–35	66% response to CBZ; 54% response to CPZ
Hernandez-Avila et al. 1996	10 CBZ; 10 HAL	CBZ v. HAL	ND	35	71% response to CBZ; 67% response to HAL
Neuroleptic + neuroleptic					
Brown et al. 1987	8 CBZ; 9 HAL	CBZ + CPZ; HAL + CPZ	CPZ	28	HAL group had higher dropout rate because of EPS
Lithium + neuroleptic					
Lusznat et al. 1988	22	CBZ + CPZ; HAL v. L + CPZ, HAL	HAL, CPZ	42	No significant difference
Lenzi et al. 1986	22	CBZ + CPZ v. L + CPZ	CPZ	19	73% response for both groups
Okuma et al. 1990	101	CBZ + neuroleptics (80%); neuro-leptics	Neuroleptics	28	62% response to CBZ; 59% response to mean level 0.46 mEq/L

Note.   CBZ = carbamazepine; P = placebo; HAL = haloperidol; L = lithium; ND = not documented; EPS = extrapyramidal side effects; CPZ = chlorpromazine.
Source.   Adapted from Keck PE Jr, McElroy SL, Nemeroff CB: "Anticonvulsants in the Treatment of Bipolar Disorder." *Journal of Neuropsychiatry and Clinical Neuroscience* 4:395–405, 1992. Used with permission.

Table 21–3. Controlled studies of carbamazepine in treatment of acute depression

Study	N	Design	Concomitant medications	Duration (days)	Outcome
Neumann et al. 1984	10 (bipolar and unipolar)	CBZ v. TRI	None	28	CBZ and TRI equally effective
Post et al. 1985	24 bipolar				
	11 unipolar	B-A-B-A	None	Median 45	34% marked response to CBZ; 54% response overall
Small 1990	4 bipolar	L v. CBZ v. L + CBZ	None	28, then L + CBZ for 28	32% response to CBZ, L + CBZ; 13% response to L
	24 unipolar				

Note. CBZ = carbamazepine; L = lithium; TRI = trimipramine.
Source. Adapted from Keck PE Jr, McElroy SL, Nemeroff CB: "Anticonvulsants in the Treatment of Bipolar Disorder." *Journal of Neuropsychiatry and Clinical Neuroscience* 4:395–405, 1992. Used with permission.

the lithium-treated patients showed improvement.

Significantly, one small controlled study suggested that carbamazepine's acute antidepressant effects may be augmented by lithium. Of 15 patients with major depression refractory to carbamazepine alone, 8 (53%) had a rapid onset of antidepressant response (within a mean of 4 days) after the blind addition of lithium (Kramlinger and Post 1989). Finally, open studies indicated that carbamazepine may be effective in treatment-resistant depression. For instance, in a retrospective review of 16 patients with treatment-resistant melancholic depression who were treated with carbamazepine either alone or in conjunction with other psychotropics, 7 (44%) had moderate or marked improvement (Cullen et al. 1991).

Prophylactic treatment of bipolar disorder. Six controlled studies have examined the efficacy of carbamazepine in the long-term treatment of patients with bipolar disorder. Approximately one-half to two-thirds of patients had a significant prophylactic response over 1–2 years (Bellaire et al. 1988; Denicoff et al. 1997; Lusznat et al. 1988; Okuma et al. 1981; Placidi et al. 1986; Watkins et al. 1987). In the only placebo-controlled study (Okuma et al. 1981), 60% of patients had not relapsed with carbamazepine treatment at 1-year follow-up, as compared with 22% of patients receiving placebo. In the other four controlled studies, carbamazepine appeared comparable to lithium in reducing affective episodes and prolonging euthymic intervals. Also, carbamazepine's mood-stabilizing effects have been reported to be augmented by the concurrent administration of lithium, valproate, thyroid hormone, antipsychotics, and antidepressants.

The prophylactic effects of carbamazepine, however, may be better for mania than for depression, are often incomplete even in responders, and may produce tachyphylaxis in some patients (Frankenburg et al. 1988; Post et al. 1990). For example, of 24 lithium-refractory, affectively ill patients who showed a marked acute response to carbamazepine and were followed up for a mean of 4 years, 50% had significant breakthrough episodes during the second or third year of treatment despite adequate serum concentrations (Post et al. 1990). This apparent loss of efficacy has been hypothesized to be due to the development of contingent tolerance or to the progression of the underlying illness. On the other hand, Murphy et al. (1989) suggested that the methodological limitations of the controlled trials cast doubt on the prophylactic efficacy of carbamazepine.

Predictors of treatment response. Early studies suggested that certain factors associated with poor response to lithium might be associated with a favorable antimanic response to carbamazepine. These factors included more severe mania, rapid cycling (the occurrence of four or more mood episodes within 1 year), greater dysphoria or depression during mania (so-called *mixed* or *dysphoric* mania), and a lower incidence of familial bipolar disorder (Goodwin 1990; Kishimoto et al. 1983; McElroy et al. 1992a; Post et al. 1987, 1991). However, studies indicate that decreasing or stable frequencies of episodes (Denicoff et al. 1997; Post et al. 1990), course of illness marked predominantly by manic episodes (Okuma 1993), and decreasing severity of mania (Small et al. 1991) correlate with a favorable response to carbamazepine. Factors not associated with antimanic response to carbamazepine include the presence of psychosensory symptoms and response to other antiepileptics (Post et al.

1991). For instance, patients whose mania did not respond to valproate and phenytoin has been reported to respond to carbamazepine (Post et al. 1984b).

Factors possibly associated with a favorable antidepressant response to carbamazepine in one study included more severe depression at the time of treatment, a history of more discrete episodes of depression, and a history of less chronicity (Post et al. 1985, 1991). In this study (Post et al. 1991), the patients with the greatest degree of thyroid hormone decrement (either thyroxine [T_4] or free T_4) while receiving carbamazepine had the best antidepressant response. A trend toward greater improvement was observed in bipolar rather than in unipolar patients. Factors such as family history, mild electroencephalogram (EEG) abnormalities, and psychosensory symptoms, however, did not predict antidepressant response.

Side Effects and Toxicology

Carbamazepine has a favorable side-effect profile compared with lithium, antipsychotics, and other antiepileptics (Andrews et al. 1990; Gram and Jensen 1989; Levy et al. 1989; Mattson et al. 1992; Pellock 1987; Pellock and Willmore 1991; Post et al. 1991; Rall and Schleifer 1985; Smith and Bleck 1991). Notably, the drug rarely causes EPS or renal side effects. It is associated with less cognitive and neurological toxicity than are phenytoin and phenobarbital; was associated with less weight gain, hair changes, and tremor than was valproate in one study of a large group of patients with epilepsy (Mattson et al. 1992); and in another study was associated with less memory impairment than was lithium in a group of patients with mood disorders (Andrews et al. 1990). However, 33%–50% of patients receiving carbamazepine experience side effects. These most commonly include neurological symptoms such as diplopia, blurred vision, fatigue, nausea, vertigo, nystagmus, and ataxia. These neurological side effects are dose related, usually transient, and reversible with dose reduction. Elderly patients, however, may be more sensitive to them.

Less frequent side effects of carbamazepine include transient leukopenia, which occurs in approximately 10%–12% of patients with epilepsy and in approximately 2.1% of patients with major affective disorders (Tohen et al. 1995); transient thrombocytopenia; rash in up to 10%–12% of patients; hyponatremia and, less commonly, hypoosmolality; liver enzyme elevations in 5%–15% of patients; and other central nervous system (CNS) toxicities, such as mild peripheral polyneuropathies and involuntary movement disorders.

The leukopenia associated with carbamazepine primarily involves granulocytes but does not predispose patients to infection, is not related to the serious idiopathic dyscrasias agranulocytosis and aplastic anemia, and usually resolves spontaneously despite continuation of medication. In the event of asymptomatic leukopenia, thrombocytopenia, or elevated liver enzymes, the carbamazepine dose can be reduced, or (in cases with severe changes) the drug can be discontinued. Once the abnormalities normalize, carbamazepine may be increased or restarted at a lower dose. If rash develops, carbamazepine may be continued as long as there is no associated fever, bleeding, exfoliative skin lesions, or other signs or symptoms of hypersensitivity. Carbamazepine-induced rash can be successfully treated with steroids.

Hyponatremia is most likely the result of water retention resulting from carbamazepine's antidiuretic effect. It occurs in 6%–31% of patients, is rare in children but probably more common in elderly people, occasionally occurs many months after the initiation of carbamazepine treatment, and often necessitates withdrawal from the drug. Carbamazepine may also decrease total and free T_4 levels and increase free cortisol levels, but these effects are rarely clinically relevant.

Rare, non-dose-related, idiosyncratic, and unpredictable but serious and potentially fatal side effects of carbamazepine include blood dyscrasias (agranulocytosis and aplastic anemia), hepatic failure, exfoliative dermatitis (e.g., Stevens-Johnson syndrome), and pancreatitis. Other rare side effects include systemic hypersensitivity reactions, conduction disturbances (sometimes resulting in bradycardia or Stokes-Adams syndrome), psychological disturbances (e.g., sporadic cases of psychosis and mania), and (very rarely) renal effects (e.g., renal failure, oliguria, hematuria, and proteinuria). The development of a severe blood dyscrasia caused by carbamazepine occurs in 2 of 575,000 treated patients per year, with a mortality of approximately 1 in 575,000 (Seetharam and Pellock 1991). Although most cases occur within the first 3–6 months of treatment, some have occurred after more extended periods of exposure. Note that transient leukopenia, thrombocytopenia, or hepatic enzyme elevations are not related to these life-threatening reactions. Routine blood monitoring does not permit anticipation of blood dyscrasias, hepatic failure, or exfoliative dermatitis (Pellock and Willmore 1991). Thus, educating the patient about the signs and symptoms of hepatic, hematological, or dermatological reactions and instructing him or her to report these signs and symptoms if they occur, along with careful monitoring of the patient's clinical status, are probably better than routine laboratory screening for detecting these serious side effects.

Carbamazepine has teratogenic effects (Jones et al. 1989; Levy et al. 1989; Rosa 1991). First-trimester exposure is associated with an increased risk of neural tube defects, craniofacial defects, fingernail hypoplasia, and developmental delay. Fortunately, the frequency of neural tube defects in general, as well as those associated with in utero antiepileptic exposure, may be reduced by prophylactic treatment with high doses of folate—ideally begun well before conception occurs (Centers for Disease Control 1991; Delcado-Escveta and Janz 1992).

Early signs of carbamazepine toxicity typically develop several hours after a given dose and include dizziness, ataxia, sedation, and diplopia. Higher concentrations are associated with nystagmus and obtundation. Acute intoxication can result in hyperirritability, stupor, or coma. Carbamazepine can be fatal in overdose: of 311 reported overdoses, 9 resulted in death, and the lethal doses of carbamazepine were 4–60 g (Gram and Jensen 1989). The most common symptoms of carbamazepine overdose are nystagmus, ophthalmoplegia, cerebellar signs and EPS, impaired consciousness, convulsions, and respiratory dysfunction. Cardiac symptoms include tachycardia, arrhythmia, conduction disturbances, and hypotension. Gastrointestinal and anticholinergic symptoms may also occur. Coma may develop with serum carbamazepine concentrations as low as 80 µmol/L.

In the presence of carbamazepine intoxication, the concentration of the 10,11-epoxide may exceed that of the parent compound. Indeed, it has been suggested that the course of intoxication correlates more closely with the course of the 10,11-epoxide serum concentrations than with the concentrations of carbamazepine itself. Treatment of carbamazepine intoxication includes symptomatic treatment, gastric lavage (which should be undertaken up to 12 hours after ingestion), and hemoperfusion, which may accelerate carbamazepine's elimination. Forced diuresis, peritoneal dialysis, and hemodialysis, however, are not recommended (Gram and Jensen 1989).

Drug-Drug Interactions

Carbamazepine has important interactions with a variety of other drugs (Ketter et al. 1991a, 1991b; Levy et al. 1989). First, because carbamazepine is a potent inducer of catabolic enzymes, it stimulates the metabolism and decreases the plasma levels of many other metabolized medications, including haloperidol and other antipsychotics, methadone, antiasthmatics (e.g., prednisone, methylprednisolone, and theophylline), warfarin, valproate, TCAs, benzodiazepines, and hormonal contraceptives. Indeed, although failure of oral contraceptives is more common in women using phenytoin and/or phenobarbital, instances in patients receiving carbamazepine have also been reported (Mattson et al. 1986).

Second, because the metabolism of carbamazepine is exclusively hepatic, certain enzyme inhibitors can inhibit carbamazepine metabolism, increase serum carbamazepine concentrations, and precipitate carbamazepine toxicity. These medications include acetazolamide, the calcium channel blockers diltiazem and verapamil (but not nifedipine), danazol, dextropropoxyphene, propoxyphene, erythromycin, isoniazid, and valproate.

Third, combinations of carbamazepine with other enzyme-inducing agents, including antiepileptics, can increase carbamazepine 10,11-epoxide concentrations and result in signs of toxicity at normally tolerable serum concentrations. Indeed, some studies indicate a connection between plasma 10,11-epoxide concentrations and side effects; neurological side effects are also more frequent in patients receiving carbamazepine with other antiepileptics (Gram and Jensen 1989).

Finally, the potential exists for pharmacodynamic interactions with other neurotoxic drugs. Thus, although most patients tolerate carbamazepine when it is given in conjunction with lithium or antipsychotics, cases of enhanced neurotoxicity have been reported with both combinations (Fogel 1988). In one study, the combination of carbamazepine and lithium caused greater memory impairment than either drug alone (Andrews et al. 1990).

VALPROATE

History and Discovery

Valproic acid was first synthesized by Burton in the United States in 1882 and subsequently was used as an organic solvent. The drug's antiepileptic properties were discovered serendipitously by Meunier in 1963 in France. Meunier used valproic acid as a vehicle for other compounds that were being screened for antiepileptic activity and found that compounds that did not have antiepileptic properties when administered alone inhibited seizure activity when dissolved in valproic acid and concluded that the antiepileptic activity was due to the solvent, valproic acid, rather than to the test drugs (Fariello and Smith 1989; Levy et al. 1989; Penry and Dean 1989).

Initial clinical trials confirming valproate's efficacy in the treatment of epilepsy were conducted in Europe in the mid-1960s with the sodium salt of the drug. Valproate was first introduced as an antiepileptic in France in 1967. It has been used in Holland and Germany since 1968 and in the United Kingdom since 1973, and it became available in the

United States in 1978. An enteric-coated formulation, divalproex sodium, was introduced to the United States market in 1983, and a formulation consisting of a capsule containing coated particles of divalproex sodium was introduced in 1989. Interestingly, the first report of valproate having therapeutic effects in patients with bipolar disorder appeared in France in 1966 (Lambert et al. 1966).

Structure-Activity Relations

Valproic acid (dipropylacetic acid) is a simple branched-chain carboxylic acid that is structurally distinct from other antiepileptic and psychotropic compounds (Figure 21–5) (Levy et al. 1989; Rimmer and Richens 1985). Although straight-chain acids have little or no antiepileptic activity, other branched-chain carboxylic acids have potencies similar to that of valproate in antagonizing pentylenetetrazole-induced seizures. However, increasing the number of carbon atoms to nine introduces marked sedative properties. The primary amide of valproic acid (valpromide, which is available in Europe but not the United States) has been reported to be about twice as potent as the parent compound.

Pharmacological Profile

Valproate blocks pentylenetetrazole-induced and maximal electroshock seizures in a variety of animals (with somewhat better efficacy in the former than in the latter) and suppresses secondarily generalized seizures without affecting focal activity in cortical cobalt- and alumina-lesioned animals (Fariello and Smith 1989). Valproate also has antikindling properties—preventing the spread of epileptiform activity in cats without affecting focal seizures (Leveil and Nanquet 1977). In humans, valproate has activity against a wide variety of epilepsy types while causing only minimal sedation and other CNS side effects.

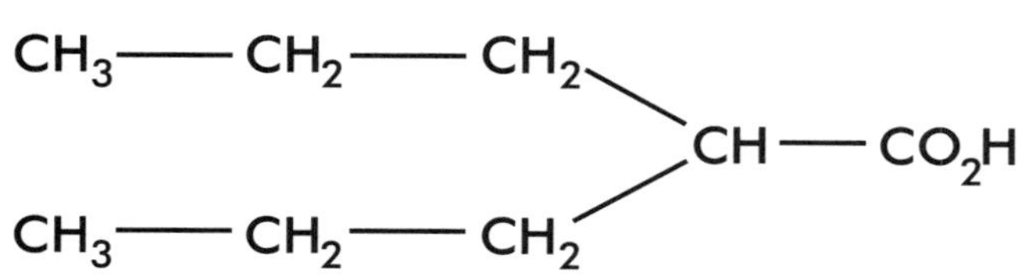

$$CH_3 \!-\! CH_2 \!-\! CH_2$$
$$CH \!-\! CO_2H$$
$$CH_3 \!-\! CH_2 \!-\! CH_2$$

Figure 21–5. Chemical structure for valproic acid (2-propyl-pentanoic acid).
Source. Reprinted from Kupferberg AJ: "Valproate: Chemistry and Methods of Determination," in *Antiepileptic Drugs,* 3rd Edition. Edited by Levy RH, Dreifuss FE, Mattson RH, et al. New York, Raven, 1989, pp. 577–582. Used with permission.

Pharmacokinetics and Disposition

Valproate is commercially available in the United States in four oral preparations: divalproex sodium, an enteric-coated, stable coordination compound containing equal proportions of valproic acid and sodium valproate in a 1:1 molar ratio; valproic acid; sodium valproate; and divalproex sodium sprinkle capsules containing coated particles of divalproex sodium that can be ingested intact or pulled apart and sprinkled on food. Valproate is also available in suppository form for rectal administration, and an intravenous preparation is now available. As mentioned, valpromide, the amide of valproic acid, is available in Europe. There are only minor differences in the pharmacokinetics of these preparations, and valproic acid is the common compound in plasma (Table 21–1).

The bioavailability of valproate approaches 100% with all preparations (Levy et al. 1989; Penry and Dean 1989; Wilder 1992). All preparations taken orally, except divalproex sodium, are rapidly absorbed after oral ingestion, attaining peak serum concentrations within 2 hours (see Table 21–1). Divalproex sodium reaches peak serum concentrations within 3–8 hours. The divalproex sodium sprinkle formulation has an earlier onset of absorption but a slower rate of absorption than divalproex sodium tablets (Figure 21–6). Absorption can also be delayed if the drug is taken with food.

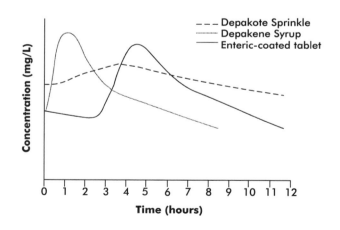

Figure 21–6. Absorption of three valproate (VPA) formulations after oral dosing in patients taking chronic VPA therapy: valproic acid (Depakene Syrup) versus enteric-coated divalproex sodium tablets versus divalproex sodium sprinkle capsules.
Source. Reprinted from Wilder BJ: "Pharmacokinetics of Valproate and Carbamazepine." *Journal of Clinical Psychopharmacology* 12:64S–68S, 1992. Used with permission.

Valproate is highly protein bound, predominantly to serum albumin and proportional to the albumin concentration. Although patients with low levels of albumin have a higher fraction of unbound drug, the steady-state level of total drug is not altered. Only the unbound drug crosses the blood-brain barrier and is bioactive. Thus, when valproate is displaced from protein-binding sites through drug interactions, the total drug concentration may not change; however, the pharmacologically active unbound drug does increase and may produce signs and symptoms of toxicity. Moreover, when the plasma concentration of valproate increases in response to increased dosing, the amount of unbound (active) valproate increases disproportionately and is metabolized with an apparent increase in clearance of total drug, yielding lower-than-expected total plasma concentrations (Levy et al. 1989; Wilder 1992) (Figures 21–7 and 21–8). In addition, valproate protein binding is increased by low-fat diets and decreased by high-fat diets.

The correlation between valproate serum concentration and both its antiepileptic and its antimanic effects is poor, but the concentration range generally required for good clinical effect is approximately 50–125 or 150 μg/mL. There appears to be a response threshold at 50 μg/mL—the approximate valproate serum concentration at which plasma albumin sites begin to become saturated—because valproate concentrations of equal to or greater than 50 μg/mL are more often associated with response than are lower concentrations (Rimmer and Richens 1985). However, some patients with epilepsy or mania have clinical response only with serum concentrations well above 100 μg/mL and, in some cases, with serum concentrations approaching 200 μg/mL (McElroy et al. 1992b). Conversely, patients with cyclothymia may respond to serum valproate concentrations of less than 50 μg/mL (Jacobsen 1993).

Valproate is metabolized primarily in the liver by two metabolic pathways to a large number of metabolites, some of which have antiepileptic and/or toxic effects (Levy et al. 1989; Penry and Dean 1989; Rimmer and Richens 1985; Wilder 1992) (Figure 21–9). These two metabolic pathways are 1) mitochondrial β-oxidation to 3-OH-valproate, 3-oxo-valproate, and 2-en-valproate; and 2) P450 microsomal metabolism to the toxic 4-en- and 2,4-en- metabolites and to a number of inactive metabolites that are conjugated with glucuronide. Of note, the 2-en-valproate metabolite is considered an active antiepileptic with a long half-life (Wilder 1992). Less than 3% of valproate is excreted unchanged in the urine and feces. Valproate's elimination half-life is typically 5–20 hours and can be altered by agents that affect the mitochondrial and/or microsomal enzymes systems responsible for its metabolism. Mitochondrial β-oxidation

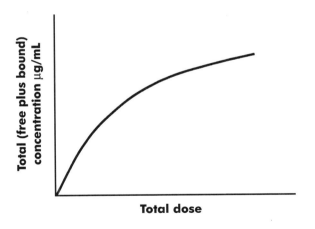

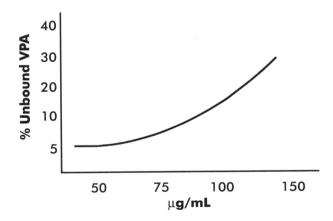

Figure 21–7. Accelerated metabolism of valproate (VPA). As the plasma concentration of VPA increases, clearance of VPA also increases. This increased clearance is secondary to the disproportionate concentration of unbound VPA produced at high levels that becomes available for metabolism (see Figure 21–8).
Source. Reprinted from Wilder BJ: "Pharmacokinetics of Valproate and Carbamazepine." *Journal of Clinical Psychopharmacology* 12:64S–68S, 1992. Used with permission.

Figure 21–8. Total valproate (VPA) concentrations. As the total concentration of VPA increases, protein-binding sites become saturated, and the percentage of unbound to bound VPA increases.
Source. Reprinted from Wilder BJ: "Pharmacokinetics of Valproate and Carbamazepine." *Journal of Clinical Psychopharmacology* 12:64S–68S, 1992. Used with permission.

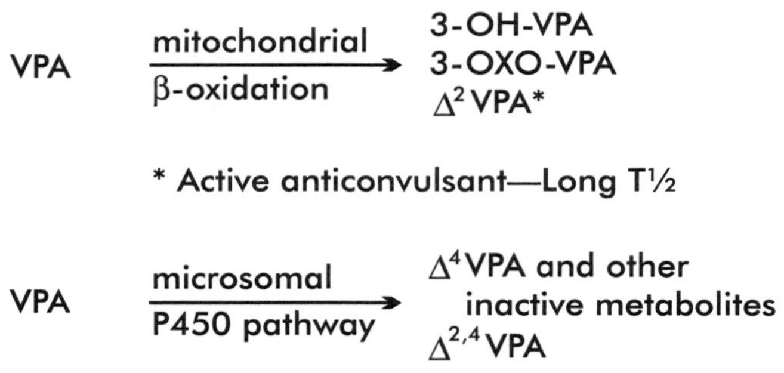

VPA $\xrightarrow[\beta\text{-oxidation}]{\text{mitochondrial}}$ 3-OH-VPA
3-OXO-VPA
Δ^2 VPA*

* Active anticonvulsant—Long T½

VPA $\xrightarrow[\text{P450 pathway}]{\text{microsomal}}$ Δ^4 VPA and other inactive metabolites
$\Delta^{2,4}$ VPA

Figure 21–9. Two pathways for metabolism of valproate (VPA). VPA is metabolized within the mitochondria by the β-oxidative pathway, which metabolizes medium- and long-chain fatty acids. This is the major metabolic pathway used by patients taking VPA as monotherapy. VPA is also metabolized by the microsomal P450 pathway, which occurs outside the mitochondria and is increased when VPA is administered in combination with enzyme-inducing drugs (i.e., carbamazepine).
Source. Reprinted from Wilder BJ: "Pharmacokinetics of Valproate and Carbamazepine." *Journal of Clinical Psychopharmacology* 12:64S–68S, 1992. Used with permission.

(the pathway used extensively for processing fatty acids) is the more important pathway for valproate's metabolism, especially when valproate is administered alone. However, P450 microsomal metabolism is increased (along with the toxic metabolites it generates) when valproate is administered with other drugs that induce the P450 system, thereby increasing chances of adverse effects, including (extremely rarely and primarily in children) liver necrosis.

Treatment with valproate for epilepsy or bipolar disorder is usually begun at a dosage of 15 mg/kg/day (usually 500–1,000 mg/day in two to four divided doses). The drug can be "orally loaded" at 20 mg/kg/day in patients with status epilepticus and acute mania to induce more rapid response. As with carbamazepine, the valproate dose is increased according to the patient's response and side effects, usually by 250–500 mg/day every 1–3 days and to serum concentrations of 50–150 µg/mL. Of note, neurological side effects become more frequent at serum concentrations above 100 µg/mL. Once the patient is stabilized, the entire valproate dosage may be taken as one daily dose before sleep to enhance convenience and compliance.

Mechanism of Action

Like carbamazepine, valproate has many effects, and the mechanisms underlying its antiepileptic and mood-stabilizing actions are unknown. One theory is that valproate induces its antiepileptic and possibly its mood-stabilizing effects by changes in the metabolism of GABA, the major inhibitory neurotransmitter in the mammalian CNS (Emrich et al. 1981; Fariello and Smith 1989; Post et al. 1992; Rimmer and Richens 1985). Valproate inhibits the catabolism of GABA, increases its release, decreases GABA turnover, increases GABA$_B$ receptor density, and may also enhance neuronal responsiveness to GABA. Studies have suggested that valproate-induced increases in brain levels of GABA and improved neuronal responsiveness to GABA are associated with seizure control. Other research, however, suggests that valproate exerts its antiepileptic effects by direct neuronal effects (i.e., reducing sodium influx and increasing potassium efflux). Yet other effects of valproate include decreased dopamine turnover, decreased N-methyl-D-aspartate (NMDA)-mediated currents, decreased release of aspartate, and decreased CSF somatostatin concentrations. Note that, unlike carbamazepine, valproate does not bind to the peripheral-type benzodiazepine receptor (except at high concentrations) (Post et al. 1992).

Indications

The indications for valproate that are currently recognized by the FDA are for the treatment of the manic episodes associated with bipolar disorder, for sole and adjunctive therapy in the treatment of simple and complex absence seizures, and for adjunctive therapy in multiple seizure types that include absence seizures. Controlled studies have also shown that valproate is highly effective in other primarily generalized epilepsies, including generalized tonic-clonic and myoclonic seizures, as well as in secondarily generalized tonic-clonic seizures, infantile spasms, photosensitive epilepsy, and febrile seizures (Anonymous 1988; Bourgeois 1989; Rimmer and Richens 1985).

Acute mania. Numerous open studies and seven controlled trials (four placebo-controlled, one haloperidol-controlled, one lithium-controlled, and one placebo- and lithium-controlled) indicate that valproate is effective in the treatment of acute mania (Bowden et al. 1994; McElroy et al. 1992b). In the controlled trials (Bowden et al. 1994; Brennan et al. 1984; Emrich et al. 1985; Freeman et al. 1992; McElroy et al. 1996; Pope et al. 1991; Post et al. 1984b), valproate was superior to placebo and comparable to lithium and haloperidol in the short-term treatment of acute mania; 71 (53%) of 134 patients who received valproate had a moderate or marked reduction in acute manic symptoms (Table 21–4). In these studies, the antimanic response to valproate occurred within several days to

Table 21–4. Controlled studies of valproate in treatment of acute mania

Study	N	Design	Concomitant medications	Duration (days)	Outcome
Emrich et al. 1985	5	A-B-A	None	Variable	4/5 marked response; 1/5 no response
Brennan et al. 1984	8	A-B-A	None	14	6/8 marked response; 2/8 no response
Post et al. 1984b	1	Crossover to P, CBZ, VPA; Phenytoin	None	Variable	Marked response to CBZ only
Pope et al. 1991	36	VPA v. P	Lorazepam	21	VPA > P on all scales
Freeman et al. 1992	27	VPA v. L	None	21	92% response to L; 63% response to VPA
Bowden et al. 1994	179	VPA v. L v. P	Lorazepam, chloral hydrate	21	VPA > P, L > P, VPA = L
McElroy et al. 1996	36	VPA v. HAL	Lorazepam	6	VPA = HAL

Note. VPA = valproate; P = placebo; CBZ = carbamazepine; L = lithium; HAL = haloperidol.
Source. Adapted from Keck PE Jr, McElroy SL, Nemeroff CB: "Anticonvulsants in the Treatment of Bipolar Disorder." *Journal of Neuropsychiatry and Clinical Neuroscience* 4:395–405, 1992. Used with permission.

2 weeks of achieving a serum valproate concentration equal to or greater than 50 µg/mL.

Indeed, in an open-label, rater-blind study of valproate administration via an oral loading dosage of 20 mg/kg/day to 19 patients with acute mania, 10 (53%) of the patients had a significant response within 5 days of treatment with minimal side effects (Keck et al. 1993). Similarly, in a controlled comparison study with haloperidol, divalproex administered at 20 mg/kg/day produced rapid antimanic and antipsychotic effects comparable to those of haloperidol (McElroy et al. 1996). In contrast, preliminary open data indicate that the hypomanic episodes of cyclothymia and possibly bipolar II disorder may respond to lower valproate doses and serum concentrations (i.e., doses of 125–500 mg/day and serum concentrations of 20–45 µg/mL) (Jacobsen 1993). Open reports also suggest that the acute antimanic effects of valproate may be augmented by lithium, carbamazepine, and antipsychotics, including clozapine (Keck et al. 1992b; Ketter et al. 1992; McElroy et al. 1988a; Suppes et al. 1992).

Acute major depression. No controlled studies of valproate in the treatment of acute unipolar or bipolar major depression have been done. Open studies suggest that valproate is less effective in the treatment of acute depression than in the treatment of acute mania. Of 195 acutely depressed patients receiving valproate in four open trials, 58 (30%) had a significant acute antidepressant response (McElroy et al. 1992b). However, open data also suggest that valproate may be more effective in ameliorating depression when administered over longer periods (Hayes 1989); that its prophylactic antidepressant effects may be superior to its acute antidepressant effects (Calabrese and Delucchi 1990; Calabrese et al. 1992); and/or that it may be more likely to exert antidepressant effects in certain subtypes of bipolar patients—including, for example, those with bipolar II disorder (Puzynski and Klosiewicz 1984).

Prophylactic treatment of bipolar disorder. One controlled study has tested the efficacy of valproate in the long-term treatment of bipolar disorder. In this study, 83 patients with bipolar disorder (according to DSM-III criteria [American Psychiatric Association 1980]) were randomly assigned to treatment with lithium or valpromide (a formulation of valproate not available in the United States) and followed up for up to 2 years (Lambert and Venaud 1994). The mean number of recurrent affective episodes per patient during the maintenance period was comparable in the lithium-treated (0.61 per patient) and the valpromide-treated (0.51 per patient) groups. Other open studies suggested that the drug reduces the frequency and intensity of manic and depressive episodes over extended periods in some patients, including those with rapid cycling, mixed bipolar disorder, bipolar II disorder, and schizoaffective disorder (Calabrese and Delucchi 1990; Calabrese et al. 1992; Emrich and Wolf 1992; Guscott 1992; Hayes 1989; McElroy et al. 1992b; Puzynski and Klosiewicz 1984; Suppes et al. 1992). These studies also indicated that valproate may be more effective in the prevention of manic and mixed episodes than depressive episodes. The drug's mood-stabilizing effects may also be augmented by concurrent treatment with lithium, carbamazepine, standard antipsychotics, antidepressants, thyroid hormone, and clozapine.

Predictors of treatment response.   Although inconsistencies exist, various factors are emerging as possibly being associated with a favorable antimanic or mood-stabilizing response to valproate. These factors include rapid cycling, dysphoric or mixed mania, later age at onset and/or shorter duration of illness, and possibly mania due to or associated with medical or neurological illness (McElroy et al. 1988a, 1988b, 1992a, 1992b; Stoll et al. 1994). For instance, in an open-label prospective study of valproate in 101 patients with rapid-cycling bipolar I and II disorder who were followed up for a mean of 17.2 months, 52 of 58 (90%) had a marked or moderate antimanic response, 88 of 94 (94%) had a prophylactic antimanic response, 13 of 15 (87%) had an acute anti–mixed state response, and 17 of 18 (94%) had a prophylactic anti–mixed state response (Calabrese et al. 1993). Moreover, among these patients, antimanic response was associated with decreasing or stable frequencies of episodes and nonpsychotic mania; antidepressant response was associated with worsening nonpsychotic mania and the absence of borderline personality disorder.

In a controlled comparison of valproate and lithium in 27 patients with bipolar disorder and acute mania, high depression scores during episodes of acute mania were associated with a favorable antimanic response to valproate (Clothier et al. 1992; Freeman et al. 1992). However, in a double-blind, placebo-controlled trial of valproate in acutely manic bipolar patients, Pope et al. (1991) found that the 12 patients whose symptoms responded to valproate did not differ with respect to frequency of rapid cycling from the 5 valproate-treated patients who showed no response (McElroy et al. 1991). Also, antimanic response to valproate was not correlated with the degree of depression during mania. Similarly, in a double-blind, placebo-controlled trial conducted by Bowden et al. (1994), valproate was as effective in patients with rapid-cycling mania (defined in this study as four manic episodes within the past year) as in those with non-rapid-cycling mania. Therefore, whether valproate is more effective in mixed mania and rapid cycling than it is in pure mania or nonrapid cycling or whether it is more effective than lithium in these variants is currently unclear.

Evidence suggesting that secondary or complicated mania responds well to valproate is similarly mixed. In an open study of 56 valproate-treated patients with mania, response was associated with the presence of nonparoxysmal abnormalities on EEG but not with neurological soft signs or abnormalities on computed axial tomography scans of brain (McElroy et al. 1988b). Nevertheless, there was a trend for responders to have histories of closed head trauma antedating the onset of their affective symptoms (Pope et al. 1988). Furthermore, case reports described successful valproate treatment of organic brain syndromes with affective features (Kahn et al. 1988) and mental retardation in patients with bipolar disorder or symptoms (Kastner et al. 1993; Sovner 1989).

In primarily open and retrospective studies, factors such as sex, presence of psychotic symptoms, family history of mood or neurological disorder, and response to lithium and other antiepileptics showed no significant association with antimanic response to valproate. However, the diagnosis of schizoaffective disorder, bipolar type, has been associated with a less favorable valproate response than has the diagnosis of bipolar disorder (McElroy et al. 1992b; Tohen et al. 1994).

Side Effects and Toxicology

Valproate is generally well tolerated and has a low incidence of adverse effects and a favorable side-effect profile compared with other antiepileptics, lithium, and antipsychotics (Anonymous 1988; Beghi et al. 1986; Dreifuss 1989; Smith and Bleck 1991). For instance, valproate is less likely to cause cognitive impairment than are other antiepileptics (Beghi et al. 1986; Vining 1987) and has been associated with a lower incidence of side effects than has lithium in bipolar patients (Vencovsky et al. 1983). In a double-blind, placebo-controlled trial of valproate versus lithium, Bowden et al. (1994) found the rate of premature termination for intolerance to be 11% in the lithium-treated group, whereas it was 6% for valproate and 3% for placebo. Like carbamazepine, valproate rarely causes renal side effects or EPS. Unlike carbamazepine, it rarely causes thyroid, cardiac, dermatological, or allergic effects. However, the drug is associated with both benign and potentially fatal side effects (for thorough reviews, see Beghi et al. 1986; Pellock and Willmore 1991; Rimmer and Richens 1985; Smith and Bleck 1991). Common dose-related side effects are gastrointestinal distress (e.g., anorexia, nausea, dyspepsia, indigestion, vomiting, and diarrhea), benign elevations in hepatic transaminase, and neurological symptoms (most commonly, tremor and sedation). Gastrointestinal complaints, benign hepatic transaminase elevations, and sedation are more likely to occur at the initiation of treatment and usually subside with dose reduction and/or over time.

Of significance is that gastrointestinal complaints are more frequent with valproic acid and sodium valproate than with the enteric-coated divalproex sodium formulation (Wilder et al. 1983). However, gastrointestinal complaints that persist despite dose reduction may be relieved by using divalproex sprinkle capsules or by the addition of a histamine-2 receptor antagonist (e.g., famotidine or cimetidine) (Stoll et al. 1991). Tremor can be managed with dose reduction or treatment with β-blockers. Coagulopathies, impaired platelet function, and transient thrombocytopenia (which are reversible with drug discontinuation) occur less frequently. Fairly frequent side effects that are often bothersome to patients include hair loss (which is usually transient), increased appetite, and weight gain. Hair loss may be minimized by cotreatment with a multivitamin containing zinc and selenium (Hurd et al. 1984).

Rare, idiosyncratic adverse effects that are not dose related but could be fatal include irreversible hepatic failure, acute hemorrhagic pancreatitis, and (extremely rarely) agranulocytosis. The risk of pancreatitis may be greater in mentally retarded adults treated with valproate (Buzan et al. 1995). Clear-cut risk factors for the development of valproate-associated irreversible hepatic failure have been identified in patients with epilepsy and include 1) young age (especially 2 years or younger), 2) administration of valproate in conjunction with other antiepileptics, and 3) presence of other medical or neurological abnormalities in addition to epilepsy. Since these factors were identified, the rate of valproate-associated fatal hepatic toxicity has decreased despite increased use of the drug. Thus, the overall rate of fatal hepatic toxicity decreased from 1 in 10,000 between 1978 and 1984 to 1 in 49,000 in 1985 and 1986. Furthermore, no hepatic fatalities have been reported to date in patients older than 10 years receiving valproate as antiepileptic monotherapy (Dreifuss et al. 1989).

Other serious side effects of valproate include teratogenicity (particularly neural tube defects with first-trimester exposure) and coma and death when taken in overdose. Offspring of mothers taking valproate have been reported to have an incidence of neural tube defects of 1%–1.5%. Minor dysmorphic syndromes have also been reported. Although the mechanism of valproate's teratogenicity is unknown, the formation of free radicals during the microsomal metabolism of valproate has been implicated. Valproate depletes selenium, a necessary component for the synthesis of glutathione peroxidase, which is an important free radical scavenger and antioxidant (Wilder 1992). Thus, multivitamins with trace metals (as well as folinic acid) have been recommended for women of childbearing potential who are taking valproate (and other antiepileptics) (Wilder 1992).

Regarding overdose, recovery from coma has occurred with serum valproate concentrations of greater than 2,000 µg/mL. In addition, serum valproate concentrations have been reduced by hemodialysis and hemoperfusion, and valproate-induced coma has been reversed with naloxone (Rimmer and Richens 1985). Because transient hepatic enzyme elevations, leukopenia, and thrombocytopenia are not predictive of life-threatening reactions (and thus, routine blood monitoring does not permit anticipation of hepatic failure or blood dyscrasias), it is generally not necessary to perform routine blood monitoring of hematological and hepatic function in epileptic patients receiving chronic antiepileptic medication (Pellock and Willmore 1991). Superior to routine laboratory screening is education of patients about the signs and symptoms of hepatic or hematological dysfunction and instructing them to report these symptoms if they occur, in conjunction with careful monitoring of the patient's clinical status. Nevertheless, because clinical experience with valproate in the treatment of psychiatric patients is not as extensive as it is for epileptic patients, many authorities recommend that hepatic and hematological parameters be monitored periodically when using valproate to treat psychiatric illness. In general, our group monitors these tests several times during the initiation of treatment and, once the patient is stable, every 6–24 months thereafter as long as the patient continues taking the drug.

Drug-Drug Interactions

Because valproate is highly protein bound and extensively metabolized by the liver, a number of potential drug-drug interactions may occur with other protein-bound or metabolized drugs (Fogel 1988; Levy et al. 1989; Rall and Schleifer 1985; Rimmer and Richens 1985). Thus, free fraction concentrations of valproate in serum can be increased and valproate toxicity precipitated by coadministration of other highly protein-bound drugs (e.g., aspirin) that can displace valproate from its protein-binding sites. Because valproate tends to inhibit drug oxidation—it is the only major antiepileptic that does not induce hepatic microsomal enzymes—serum concentrations of a number of metabolized drugs can be increased by the coadministration of valproate. Thus, valproate has been reported to increase serum concentrations of phenobarbital, phenytoin, and TCAs. Conversely, the metabolism of valproate can be increased, and valproate serum concentrations subsequently decreased, by coadministration of microsomal enzyme-inducing drugs such as carbamazepine; drugs that inhibit metabolism may increase valproate concentrations in serum. Fluoxetine, for instance, has been reported to boost valproate concentrations (Sovner and Davis 1991).

Finally, neurological reactions may occur when valproate is administered with other neurotoxic drugs. For example, increased sedation and (extremely rarely) delirium have been reported when valproate is administered with antipsychotics (Costello and Suppes 1995). However, an initial report of the combination of valproate and clonazepam inducing absence status in three patients with absence epilepsy has not been replicated. Indeed, in our experience, patients in general tolerate the combination of valproate with antipsychotics and benzodiazepines, including clonazepam, very well.

BENZODIAZEPINES

The benzodiazepines as a class are discussed in detail in Ballenger, Chapter 14, in this volume. Because these drugs have antiepileptic properties (i.e., diazepam in status epilepticus and clonazepam in absence epilepsy), their use in the treatment of bipolar disorder is briefly reviewed here.

In general, studies examining the efficacy of benzodiazepines in patients with bipolar disorder are inconsistent. Of four controlled studies evaluating clonazepam in the treatment of acute mania (Table 21–5), clonazepam was found to be superior to placebo in one, superior to lithium in another, and comparable to haloperidol in a third (Chouinard 1987; Chouinard et al. 1983; Edwards et al. 1991). In the fourth study (Bradwejn et al. 1990), lorazepam was found to be superior to clonazepam, which had no significant antimanic effects.

All of these studies were confounded by small sample sizes, short durations of treatment, and difficulties in distinguishing putative specific antimanic effects from non-specific sedative effects. Moreover, the first two studies were further confounded by the coadministration of neuroleptics. However, in a controlled study comparing lorazepam with haloperidol as adjuncts to lithium in the treatment of acute manic agitation, the two treatments appeared to be comparable (Lenox et al. 1992). This suggests that lorazepam (and perhaps other benzodiazepines) may be safe, effective alternatives to neuroleptics in the initial or early management of manic agitation until the effects of the primary mood-stabilizing agent become apparent. Also, open studies suggest that lorazepam may have beneficial effects in the short-term treatment of catatonia, which is often a manifestation of the manic phase of bipolar disorder (Bodken 1990; Rosebush et al. 1990).

Although there are no controlled studies of benzodiazepines in the treatment of bipolar depression, one open study reported the successful treatment of 21 (84%) of 25 depressed patients with open-label clonazepam (maximum daily doses of 1.5–6.0 mg) (Kishimoto et al. 1983). Of this group, 18 had major depression and 9 had bipolar depression, including 8 who had failed to respond to previous treatment with two or more antidepressants. However, treatment of panic disorder with various benzodiazepines has been associated with treatment-emergent depression (Tesar 1990).

Two studies have examined the prophylactic efficacy of benzodiazepines in patients with bipolar disorder. In the first, bipolar patients requiring combined maintenance treatment with lithium and haloperidol did equally well when their regimens were changed to lithium and clonazepam (Sachs et al. 1990). However, the second study (the only study to date attempting to assess the efficacy of clonazepam alone as a maintenance treatment) had to be prematurely terminated after the first five patients who were enrolled relapsed within the first 2–15 weeks of treatment (Aronson et al. 1989). Of note, the poor results observed in this study may have been due in part to the inclusion of lithium-refractory patients and to rapid tapering of antipsychotics before the initiation of clonazepam treatment (Chouinard 1989).

In summary, available studies have not yet definitively proven that benzodiazepines have specific antimanic, antidepressant, or long-term mood-stabilizing properties

Table 21–5. Controlled studies of clonazepam and lorazepam in treatment of acute mania

Study	N	Design	Concomitant medications	Duration (days)	Outcome
Chouinard et al. 1983	12	Crossover with L	HAL	10	CPM > L
Edwards et al. 1991	40	CPM v. P	CPZ	5	CPM > P
Chouinard 1987	12	CPM v. HAL	None	7	CPM, HAL comparable
Bradwejn et al. 1990	24	CPM v. LPM	None	14	61% response to LPM; 18% response to CPM

Note.   CPM = clonazepam; LPM = lorazepam; HAL = haloperidol; L = lithium.
Source.   Adapted from Keck PE Jr, McElroy SL, Nemeroff CB: "Anticonvulsants in the Treatment of Bipolar Disorder." *Journal of Neuropsychiatry and Clinical Neuroscience* 4:395–405, 1992. Used with permission.

apart from their nonspecific sedative effects. However, benzodiazepines may be extremely useful in the treatment of acute manic agitation either in place of or in conjunction with antipsychotics 1) until the effects of other primary mood-stabilizing agents become apparent; 2) in the short-term treatment of insomnia, anxiety, or catatonia associated with either mania or depression; and perhaps 3) as adjunctive maintenance agents in combination with lithium, carbamazepine, or valproate.

OTHER ANTIEPILEPTICS

Oxcarbazepine

Available in Europe but not yet available in the United States, oxcarbazepine (10,11-dihydro-10-oxo-carbamazepine), the 10-keto analogue of carbamazepine, has a chemical structure and antiepileptic profile similar to that of carbamazepine (Anonymous 1989; Dam and Jensen 1989). Oxcarbazepine has been shown to be as effective as carbamazepine in suppressing generalized tonic-clonic seizures and partial seizures, with and without secondary generalization. Preliminary reports also suggest that it may have antineuralgic effects.

Oxcarbazepine and carbamazepine, however, have significantly different pharmacokinetic profiles. Unlike carbamazepine, oxcarbazepine does not appear to induce the hepatic microsomal P450 enzyme system, and it is not metabolized to an epoxide with neurotoxic effects. Rather, oxcarbazepine is rapidly and extensively converted to the 10-hydroxy metabolite, an active metabolite responsible for most of the drug's antiepileptic effects. These differ-

ences suggest that oxcarbazepine may be an easier drug to administer, with fewer drug-drug interactions, and easier to tolerate with less neurotoxicity. Nevertheless, oxcarbazepine's most common side effects are tiredness, headache, dizziness, and ataxia. Also, it has been reported to cause allergic reactions and hyponatremia, although less frequently than does carbamazepine.

Four controlled studies assessing the efficacy of oxcarbazepine in the treatment of acute mania have shown that oxcarbazepine is superior to placebo and comparable to haloperidol and lithium after 14 days of treatment (Emrich 1990; Emrich et al. 1985; Müller and Stoll 1984) (Table 21–6). In these studies, the tolerability of oxcarbazepine was better than that of haloperidol and comparable to that of lithium. These results are limited, however, by the concomitant use of haloperidol (and in some cases lithium) in both treatment groups in the two largest studies (Emrich 1990). In addition, although the average oxcarbazepine dosage used in these studies was 1,400–2,400 mg/day, the optimal dosage range for the antimanic effects of oxcarbazepine has not yet been established.

Oxcarbazepine has not been tested in the treatment of acute major depression. However, two controlled studies have compared the prophylactic efficacy of oxcarbazepine with that of lithium in patients with bipolar disorder (Table 21–7). In the first study, Cabrera et al. (1986), using an oxcarbazepine dosage of only 900 mg/day, found significant decreases in the rates of recurrent manic and depressive episodes in both the oxcarbazepine- and the lithium-treated groups. In the second study, Wildgrube (1990) found a higher rate of relapse in patients maintained on ox-

Table 21–6. Controlled studies of oxcarbazepine in treatment of acute mania

Study	N	Design	Concomitant medications	Duration (days)	Outcome
Emrich et al. 1985	6	A-B-A	None	Variable	4/6 (67% had > 50% decrease in IMPS scores)
Müller and Stoll 1984	10 OX; 10 HAL	OX v. HAL	None	14	Mean decrease of 55% in BRMAS scores in both groups
Emrich 1990	19 OX; 19 HAL	OX v. HAL	HAL, L	14	Mean decrease of 64% in BRMAS scores in both groups
Emrich 1990	28 OX; 24 L	OX v. L	HAL	14	Mean decrease of 63% in BRMAS scores in both groups

Note. OX = oxcarbazepine; IMPS = Inpatient Multidimensional Psychiatric Scale (Lorr et al. 1962); BRMAS = Bech-Raefelson Mania Scale (Bech et al. 1986); HAL = haloperidol; L = lithium.
Source. Adapted from Keck PE Jr, McElroy SL, Nemeroff CB: "Anticonvulsants in the Treatment of Bipolar Disorder." *Journal of Neuropsychiatry and Clinical Neuroscience* 4:395–405, 1992. Used with permission.

Table 21–7.   Controlled studies of carbamazepine and oxcarbazepine as preventive therapy in patients with bipolar disorder

Study	N	Design	Concomitant medications	Duration (years)	Outcome
Okuma et al. 1981	12 CBZ; 10 P	CBZ v. P	Not specified, but permitted for breakthrough episodes	1	40% relapse on CBZ; 78% relapse on P
Placidi et al. 1986	20 CBZ; 16 L	CBZ v. L	TCAs, CPZ for breakthrough episodes	to 3	67% response rate for both groups
Watkins et al. 1987	19 CBZ; 18 L	CBZ v. L	Neuroleptics, antidepressants for breakthrough episodes	1.5	Mean time in remission: CBZ 16 months, L 9.4 months
Lusznat et al. 1988	20 CBZ; 21 L	CBZ v. L	Neuroleptics, antidepressants for breakthrough episodes	to 1	45% CBZ patients at 12 months, 25% L patients at 12 months, 25% CBZ rehospitalized, 50% L rehospitalized
Bellaire et al. 1988	46 CBZ; 52 L	CBZ v. L	ND	1	Mean reduction in number of episodes comparable: 1.8/year to 0.67/year CBZ, 1.7/year to 0.7/year L
Cabrera et al. 1986	4 OX; 6 L	OX v. L	Neuroleptics (1 OX, 2 L)	Up to 22	3/4 OX, 6/6 L had significant decrease in affective episodes
Wildgrube 1990	8 OX; 7 L	OX v. L	ND	Up to 33	6/8 OX, 3/7 L treatment failures

Note.   CBZ = carbamazepine; OX = oxcarbazepine; ND = not described; TCAs = tricyclic antidepressants; CPZ = chlorpromazine; L = lithium.
Source.   Reprinted from Keck PE Jr, McElroy SL, Nemeroff CB: "Anticonvulsants in the Treatment of Bipolar Disorder." *Journal of Neuropsychiatry and Clinical Neuroscience* 4:395–405, 1992. Used with permission.

carbazepine than in those receiving lithium. However, the subjects in the oxcarbazepine-treated group were significantly older and more severely ill at the initiation of treatment than those in the group randomly assigned to lithium treatment. The small sample size in each study makes further interpretation of their data difficult, and larger studies are needed to establish the optimal dosage and therapeutic efficacy of oxcarbazepine as a maintenance agent for the treatment of bipolar disorder.

Phenytoin

Although there are no controlled studies of phenytoin in the treatment of bipolar disorder, open studies performed in the late 1940s and early 1950s indicated that phenytoin may be helpful in the treatment of psychiatric patients with acute mania or maniclike presentations (e.g., "excited psychoses") (Gutierrez-Esteinou and Cole 1988). For instance, in an open-label study of phenytoin in 60 state hospital psychiatric patients, the best results were observed in the "excited" group, and improvement was shown in 73% of 16 patients

with "excited schizophrenia" (n = 22) and 89% of 8 patients with mania (n = 9) (Kalinowsky and Putnam 1943). In a similar open-label trial of phenytoin in 73 psychotic patients, 11 of whom had manic-depressive illness, 5 of 9 patients in the manic phase and 1 of 2 in the depressive phase showed improvement (Kubanek and Rowell 1946). The authors concluded that phenytoin was useful in the treatment of "excited chronic psychoses." In yet another one-label study of 45 chronic patients with a wide range of diagnoses, 1 patient with mania and some patients with schizophrenia (only those with catatonia) showed improvement (Freyhan 1945). In short, although these studies are methodologically flawed and no controlled data yet indicate that phenytoin is effective in the treatment of mania, it may be considered as a treatment alternative for some patients resistant to lithium, carbamazepine, and valproate.

Lamotrigine

Lamotrigine, an anticonvulsant with established efficacy (mainly as adjunctive therapy) in partial seizures, is believed to act by inhibiting the stimulated presynaptic release of glutamate and may have antidepressant and/or mood-stabilizing effects. In a 6-month, open-label trial of 67 patients with treatment-refractory bipolar I and II disorders, lamotrigine was administered as monotherapy in 17 (25%) and as adjunctive therapy in 50 (75%) (Calabrese et al. 1995). Of 39 (58%) patients who presented in the depressed phase, 9 (23%) had moderate improvement in reduction of depressive symptoms and 18 (46%) showed marked improvement. Of 25 patients who presented in hypomanic, manic, or mixed states, 4 (16%) had moderate improvement in manic symptoms and 15 (60%) showed marked improvement. In a second open trial (Sporn and Sachs 1997), 16 patients with treatment-resistant bipolar I or II disorder received lamotrigine as adjunctive treatment for affective episodes. Eight (50%) of 16 patients were rated as responders, and lamotrigine appeared to exert antidepressant and mood-stabilizing effects in these patients. These preliminary results are being followed up in a double-blind study.

Gabapentin

Gabapentin is a new anticonvulsant that is effective as adjunctive therapy in the treatment of partial seizures with and without secondary generalization. Four reports have described its effects in the treatment of psychiatric disorders (McElroy et al. 1997; Ryback and Ryback 1995; Short and Cooke 1995; Stanton et al. 1996). In one report (Stanton et al. 1996), gabapentin monotherapy appeared to ameliorate manic symptoms in patients with bipolar disorder. In a second report (Ryback and Ryback 1995), gabapentin produced improvement in behavioral dyscontrol in an adolescent with intermittent explosive disorder, organic mood disorder (secondary to closed head injury), and attention-deficit/hyperactivity disorder. Conversely, hypomanic symptoms were described in a patient with epilepsy when gabapentin was added to carbamazepine and lamotrigine (Short and Cooke 1995). Finally, McElroy et al. (1997) used open-label, adjunctive gabapentin to treat nine patients with bipolar I or II disorder who were experiencing hypomanic, manic, or mixed states inadequately responsive to mood stabilizers. Of the nine patients, seven had a moderate or marked reduction in manic symptoms by 1 month of gabapentin treatment. Another patient had moderate improvement after 3 months. Of these eight patients, six continued to have antimanic responses for follow-up periods ranging from 1 to 7 months. A double-blind, placebo-controlled study of gabapentin as adjunctive therapy in patients with bipolar disorder is under way and should clarify the potential usefulness of this agent in bipolar disorder.

Progabide

Open studies and one controlled comparison with imipramine suggest that progabide and its congeners (effective antiepileptics that act as indirect potentiators of GABA) may have acute antidepressant effects (Post et al. 1991). Although these antiepileptics have not yet been studied in the treatment of mania, studies of these drugs in patients with bipolar disorder appear warranted in the light of GABA's potential role in the pathogenesis of mood disorder.

Barbiturate Antiepileptics

Barbiturate antiepileptics have not been well studied in the treatment of bipolar disorder. However, in an open study of primidone and/or mephobarbital in 27 patients with mood disorders refractory to lithium, carbamazepine, valproate, and phenytoin, 9 patients had sustained positive effects with primidone and 3 had positive effects with mephobarbital after failure of primidone treatment (Hayes 1993).

Acetazolamide

Inoue et al. (1984) in Japan reported that acetazolamide (a diuretic with antiepileptic properties) was effective in patients with atypical psychoses characterized by dreamy or confusional states and often associated with the premenstrual or puerperal period. Testing of this drug in bipolar patients—especially those with associated confusion or perimenstrual or puerperal exacerbation of their symptoms—would therefore appear to be warranted.

CONCLUSION

Growing evidence indicates that a variety of antiepileptic drugs have beneficial effects in the treatment of bipolar disorder. To date, the antiepileptics best studied in the treatment of bipolar disorder are carbamazepine and valproate. These drugs have acute antimanic and long-term mood-stabilizing effects (and possibly acute antidepressant effects) in some bipolar patients, including those inadequately responsive to or intolerant of lithium. Despite the lack of formal FDA indications for bipolar disorder, carbamazepine and valproate are considered by many authorities to be second-line agents to lithium for lithium-refractory or lithium-intolerant patients. Moreover, in light of preliminary data indicating that carbamazepine and valproate may be effective in rapid-cycling and dysphoric mania (bipolar variants known to be poorly responsive to lithium), some clinicians use these antiepileptics as first-line treatments for such patients. Indeed, our group considers carbamazepine and valproate, along with lithium, as first-line treatments for bipolar disorder. Other, less well-studied antiepileptic compounds, including oxcarbazepine and phenytoin, may also have mood-stabilizing effects. Although it is unclear whether benzodiazepines have specific mood-stabilizing effects, they are useful adjuncts to primary mood stabilizers in the treatment of acute manic agitation and catatonia.

It is important to remember that the antiepileptics may be synergistic with other mood-stabilizing agents—including one another—in the treatment of bipolar disorder that responds inadequately to monotherapy. Indeed, although viewed together as a class of drugs, the antiepileptics are in fact very different agents, possessing different chemical structures, pharmacological properties, pharmacokinetics, side effects, and efficacies in the treatment of epilepsy. Thus, even though carbamazepine and valproate may share similar predictors of response for bipolar disorder (e.g., dysphoric mania), different bipolar patients may respond to one agent but not to the other or may tolerate one agent better than the other, as is the case for patients with epilepsy. Clinicians therefore have a wide range of medications and combinations of medications to choose from when treating bipolar disorder. Furthermore, although the actions underlying the antiepileptic properties of these drugs may or may not be responsible for their mood-stabilizing effects, any future drugs with antiepileptic activity should be screened as putative antimanic, mood-stabilizing, or antidepressant agents.

REFERENCES

Albright PS, Burnham WM: Development of a new pharmacological seizure model: effects of anti-convulsants on cortical and amygdala-kindled seizures in the rat. Epilepsia 21:681–689, 1980

American Psychiatric Association: Diagnostic and Statistical Manual of Mental Disorders, 3rd Edition. Washington, DC, American Psychiatric Association, 1980

Andrews DG, Schweitzer I, Marshall N: The comparative side effects of lithium, carbamazepine and combined lithium-carbamazepine in patients treated for affective disorders. Human Psychopharmacology 5:41–45, 1990

Anonymous: Sodium valproate. Lancet 2:1229–1231, 1988

Anonymous: Oxcarbazepine. Lancet 2:196–198, 1989

Aronson TA, Skukla S, Hirschowitz J: Clonazepam treatment of five lithium-refractory patients with bipolar disorder. Am J Psychiatry 146:77–80, 1989

Ballenger JC, Post RM: Therapeutic effects of carbamazepine in affective illness: a preliminary report. Communications in Psychopharmacology 2:159–175, 1978

Bech P, Kastrup M, Rafaelsen OJ: Mini-compendium of rating scales for anxiety, depression, mania, schizophrenia, with corresponding DSM-III syndromes. Acta Psychiatr Scand 73(S236):29–31, 1986

Beghi E, DiMascio R, Sasanelli F, et al: Adverse reactions to antiepileptic drugs: a multicenter survey of clinical practice. Epilepsia 27:323–330, 1986

Bellaire W, Demish K, Stoll KD: Carbamazepine versus lithium in prophylaxis of recurrent affective disorders. Psychopharmacology (Berl) 96:2875, 1988

Blom S: Tic douloureux treated with a new anticonvulsant: experiences with G 32883. Arch Neurol 2:357–366, 1963

Bodken JA: Emerging uses for high-potency benzodiazepines in psychotic disorders. J Clin Psychiatry 51:41S–46S, 1990

Bourgeois BFD: Valproate: clinical use, in Antiepileptic Drugs, 3rd Edition. Edited by Levy RH, Dreifuss FE, Mattson RH, et al. New York, Raven, 1989, pp 633–642

Bowden CL, Brugger AM, Swann AC, et al: Efficacy of divalproex vs. lithium and placebo in the treatment of mania. JAMA 271:918–924, 1994

Bradwejn J, Shriqui C, Koszycki D, et al: Double-blind comparison of the effects of clonazepam and lorazepam in mania. J Clin Psychopharmacol 10:403–408, 1990

Brennan MJW, Sandyk R, Borsook D: Use of sodium valproate in the management of affective disorders: basic and clinical aspects, in Anticonvulsants in Affective Disorders. Edited by Emrich HM, Okuma T, Müller AA. Amsterdam, Excerpta Medica, 1984, pp 56–65

Brown D, Silverstone T, Cookson J: Carbamazepine compared to haloperidol in acute mania. International Journal of Clinical Psychopharmacology 48:89–93, 1987

Buzan RD, Firestone D, Thomas M, et al: Valproate-associated pancreatitis and cholecystitis in six mentally retarded adults. J Clin Psychiatry 56:529–532, 1995

Cabrera JF, Muhlbauer HD, Schley J, et al: Long-term randomized clinical trial of oxcarbazepine vs. lithium in bipolar and schizoaffective disorders: preliminary results. Pharmacopsychiatry 19:282–283, 1986

Calabrese JR, Delucchi GA: Spectrum of efficacy of valproate in 55 rapid-cycling manic depressives. Am J Psychiatry 147:431–434, 1990

Calabrese JR, Markovitz PJ, Kimmel SE, et al: Spectrum of efficacy of valproate in 78 rapid-cycling bipolar patients. J Clin Psychopharmacol 12:53S–56S, 1992

Calabrese JR, Woyshville MJ, Kimmel SE, et al: Predictors of valproate response in bipolar rapid cycling. J Clin Psychopharmacol 13:280–283, 1993

Calabrese JR, Woyshville MJ, Bowden CL, et al: Spectrum of efficacy of lamotrigine in treatment-refractory manic depression. Second International Conference on Affective Disorders. Jerusalem, Israel, September 1995

Centers for Disease Control: Use of folic acid for prevention of spina bifida and other neural tube defects. JAMA 266:1190–1191, 1991

Chouinard G: Clonazepam in acute and maintenance treatment of bipolar affective disorder. J Clin Psychiatry 48: 29S–36S, 1987

Chouinard G: Clonazepam in treatment of bipolar psychotic patients after discontinuation of neuroleptics (letter). Am J Psychiatry 146:1642, 1989

Chouinard G, Young SN, Annable L: Antimanic effect of clonazepam. Biol Psychiatry 18:451–486, 1983

Clothier J, Swann AC, Freeman T: Dysphoric mania. J Clin Psychopharmacol 12:13S–16S, 1992

Costello LE, Suppes T: A clinically significant interaction between clozapine and valproate. J Clin Psychopharmacol 15:139–140, 1995

Cullen M, Mitchell P, Brodaty H, et al: Carbamazepine for treatment-resistant melancholia. J Clin Psychiatry 52: 472–476, 1991

Dalby MA: Antiepileptic and psychotropic effect of carbamazepine (Tegretol) in the treatment of psychomotor epilepsy. Epilepsia 12:325–334, 1971

Dam M, Jensen PK: Potential antiepileptic drugs: oxcarbazepine, in Antiepileptic Drugs, 3rd Edition. Edited by Levy RH, Dreifuss FE, Mattson RH, et al. New York, Raven, 1989, pp 913–924

Delcado-Escveta AV, Janz D: Consensus guidelines: preconception counseling management, and care of the pregnant woman with epilepsy. Neurology 42:149–160, 1992

Denicoff KD, Smith-Jackson EE, Disney ER, et al: Comparative prophylactic efficacy of lithium, carbamazepine, and the combination in bipolar disorder. J Clin Psychiatry 58:470–478, 1997

Desai NG, Gangadhar BN, Channabasavanna SM, et al: Carbamazepine hastens therapeutic action of lithium in mania, in Proceedings of the International Conference of New Directions in Affective Disorders, Jerusalem, Israel, September 1987

Dreifuss FE: Valproate toxicity, in Antiepileptic Drugs, 3rd Edition. Edited by Levy RH, Dreifuss FE, Mattson RH, et al. New York, Raven, 1989, pp 643–651

Dreifuss FE, Langer DH, Moline KA, et al: Valproic acid hepatic fatalities, II: U.S. experience since 1984. Neurology 39:201–207, 1989

Edwards R, Stephenson U, Flewett T: Clonazepam in acute mania: a double-blind trial. Aust N Z J Psychiatry 25:238–242, 1991

Emrich HM: Studies with oxcarbazepine (Trileptal) in acute mania. Int Clin Psychopharmacol 5:83S–88S, 1990

Emrich HM, Wolf R: Valproate treatment of mania. Prog Neuropsychopharmacol Biol Psychiatry 16:691–701, 1992

Emrich HM, von Zerssen D, Kissling W, et al: On a possible role of GABA in mania: therapeutic efficacy of sodium valproate, in GABA and Benzodiazepine Receptors. Edited by Costa E, Dicharia G, Gessa GL. New York, Raven, 1981, pp 287–296

Emrich HM, Dose M, von Zerssen D: The use of sodium valproate, carbamazepine, and oxcarbazepine in patients with affective disorders. J Affect Disord 8:243–250, 1985

Fariello R, Smith MC: Valproate: mechanisms of action, in Antiepileptic Drugs, 3rd Edition. Edited by Levy RH, Dreifuss FE, Mattson RH, et al. New York, Raven, 1989, pp 567–575

Fogel BS: Combining anticonvulsants with conventional psychopharmacologic agents, in Use of Anticonvulsants in Psychiatry: Recent Advances. Edited by McElroy SL, Pope HG Jr. Clifton, NJ, Oxford Health Care, 1988, pp 77–94

Frankenburg FR, Tohen M, Cohen BM, et al: Long-term response to carbamazepine: a retrospective study. J Clin Psychopharmacol 8:130–132, 1988

Freeman TW, Clothier JL, Pazzaglia P, et al: A double-blind comparison of valproate and lithium in the treatment of acute mania. Am J Psychiatry 149:108–111, 1992

Freyhan FA: Effectiveness of diphenylhydantoin in management of nonepileptic psychomotor excitement states. Arch Neurol Psychiatry 53:370–374, 1945

Gerner RH, Stanton A: Algorithm for patient management of acute manic states: lithium, valproate, or carbamazepine? J Clin Psychopharmacol 12:57S–63S, 1992

Goodwin FK: Medical treatment of manic episodes, in Manic-Depressive Illness. Edited by Goodwin FK, Jamison KR. New York, Oxford University Press, 1990, pp 603–629

Gram L, Jensen PK: Carbamazepine toxicity, in Antiepileptic Drugs, 3rd Edition. Edited by Levy RH, Dreifuss FE, Mattson RH, et al. New York, Raven, 1989, pp 555–565

Grossi E, Sacchetti E, Vita A, et al: Carbamazepine vs. chlorpromazine in mania: a double-blind trial, in Anticonvulsants in Affective Disorders. Edited by Emrich HM, Okuma T, Müller AA. Amsterdam, Excerpta Medica, 1984, pp 177–187

Guscott R: Clinical experience with valproic acid in 22 patients with refractory bipolar mood disorder. Can J Psychiatry 37:590, 1992

Gutierrez-Esteinou R, Cole JO: Psychiatric effects of phenytoin and ethosuximide, in Use of Anticonvulsants in Psychiatry: Recent Advances. Edited by McElroy SL, Pope HG Jr. Clifton, NJ, Oxford Health Care, 1988, pp 59–76

Hayes SG: Long-term use of valproate in primary psychiatric disorders. J Clin Psychiatry 50:35S–39S, 1989

Hayes SG: Barbiturate anticonvulsants in refractory affective disorders. Ann Clin Psychiatry 5:35–44, 1993

Hernandez-Avila CA, Ortega-Soto HA, Jasso A, et al: Carbamazepine versus haloperidol for the treatment of acute manic episodes. Abstract presented at the 149th annual meeting of the American Psychiatric Association, New York, May 1996

Hurd RW, Van Rinsvelt HA, Wilder BJ, et al: Selenium, zinc, and copper changes with valproic acid: possible relation to drug side effects. Neurology 34:1394–1395, 1984

Inoue H, Hazama H, Hamazoe K, et al: Antipsychotic and prophylactic effects of acetazolamide (Diamox) on atypical psychosis. Folia Psychiatrica et Neurologica Japonica 38:425–436, 1984

Jacobsen FM: Low-dose valproate: a new treatment for cyclothymia, mild rapid-cycling disorders, and premenstrual syndrome. J Clin Psychiatry 54:229–234, 1993

Jones KL, Lacro RV, Johnson KA, et al: Pattern of malformations in the children of women treated with carbamazepine during pregnancy. N Engl J Med 320:186–188, 1989

Kahn D, Stevenson E, Douglas CJ: Effect of sodium valproate in three patients with organic brain syndromes. Am J Psychiatry 145:1010–1011, 1988

Kalinowsky LB, Putnam TJ: Attempts at treatment of schizophrenia and other non-epileptic psychoses with Dilantin. Archives of Neurology and Psychiatry 49:414–420, 1943

Kastner T, Finesmith R, Walsh K: Brief report: long-term administration of valproic acid in the treatment of affective symptoms in people with mental retardation. J Clin Psychopharmacol 13:448–451, 1993

Keck PE Jr, McElroy SL, Nemeroff CB: Anticonvulsants in the treatment of bipolar disorder. J Neuropsychiatry Clin Neurosci 4:395–405, 1992a

Keck PE Jr, McElroy SL, Vuckovic A, et al: Combined valproate and carbamazepine treatment of bipolar disorder. J Neuropsychiatry Clin Neurosci 4:319–322, 1992b

Keck PE Jr, McElroy SL, Tugrul KC, et al: Valproate oral loading in the treatment of acute mania. J Clin Psychiatry 54:305–308, 1993

Ketter TA, Post RM: Clinical pharmacology and pharmacokinetics of carbamazepine, in Anticonvulsants in Mood Disorders. Edited by Joffe RT, Calabrese JR. New York, Marcel Dekker, 1994, pp 147–188

Ketter TA, Post RM, Worthington K: Principles of clinically important drug interactions with carbamazepine, part I. J Clin Psychopharmacol 11:198–203, 1991a

Ketter TA, Post RM, Worthington K: Principles of clinically important drug interactions with carbamazepine, part II. J Clin Psychopharmacol 11:306–313, 1991b

Ketter TA, Pazzaglia PJ, Post RM: Synergy of carbamazepine and valproate in affective illness: case report and review of the literature. J Clin Psychopharmacol 12:276–281, 1992

Kishimoto A, Ogura C, Hazama H, et al: Long-term prophylactic effects of carbamazepine in affective disorder. Br J Psychiatry 143:327–331, 1983

Klein E, Bental E, Lerer B, et al: Carbamazepine and haloperidol in excited psychoses. Arch Gen Psychiatry 41:165–170, 1984

Kramlinger KG, Post RM: The addition of lithium to carbamazepine: antidepressant efficacy in treatment-resistant depression. Arch Gen Psychiatry 46:794–800, 1989

Kubanek JL, Rowell RC: The use of Dilantin in the treatment of psychotic patients unresponsive to other treatments. Diseases of the Nervous System 7:47–50, 1946

Kupferberg AJ: Valproate: chemistry and methods of determination, in Antiepileptic Drugs, 3rd Edition. Edited by Levy RH, Dreifuss FE, Mattson RH, et al. New York, Raven, 1989, pp 577–582

Kutt H: Carbamazepine: chemistry and methods of determination, in Antiepileptic Drugs, 3rd Edition. Edited by Levy RH, Dreifuss FE, Mattson RH, et al. New York, Raven, 1989, pp 457–471

Lambert PA, Venaud G: Comparative study of valpromide versus lithium as prophylactic treatment in affective disorders. Nervure 17:1–9, 1994

Lambert PA, Cavaz G, Borselli S, et al: Action neuropsychotrope d'un nouvel anti-épileptique: le Dépamide. Ann Med Psychol (Paris) 1:707–710, 1966

Lenox RH, Newhouse PA, Creelman WL, et al: Adjunctive treatment of manic agitation with lorazepam vs. haloperidol: a double-blind study. J Clin Psychiatry 53:47–52, 1992

Lenzi A, Lazzerini F, Grossi E, et al: Use of carbamazepine in acute psychosis: a controlled study. J Int Med Res 14:78–84, 1986

Lerer B, Moore N, Meyendorff E, et al: Carbamazepine versus lithium in mania: a double-blind study. J Clin Psychiatry 48:89–93, 1987

Leveil V, Nanquet R: A study of the action of valproic acid on the kindling effect. Epilepsia 18:229–234, 1977

Levy RH, Dreifuss FE, Mattson RH, et al (eds): Antiepileptic Drugs, 3rd Edition. New York, Raven, 1989

Loiseau P, Duche B: Carbamazepine: clinical use, in Antiepileptic Drugs, 3rd Edition. Edited by Levy RH, Dreifuss FE, Mattson RH, et al. New York, Raven, 1989, pp 533–554

Lorr M, Klett CJ, McNair DM, et al: Inpatient Multidimensional Psychiatric Scale. Palo Alto, CA, Consulting Psychologists Press, 1962

Lusznat RM, Murphy DP, Nunn CMH: Carbamazepine vs. lithium in the treatment of prophylaxis of mania. Br J Psychiatry 153:198–204, 1988

Macdonald RL: Carbamazepine: mechanisms of action, in Antiepileptic Drugs, 3rd Edition. Edited by Levy RH, Dreifuss FH, Mattson RH, et al. New York, Raven, 1989, pp 447–455

Mattson RH, Cramer JA, Damey PD, et al: Use of oral contraceptives by women with epilepsy. JAMA 2556:238–240, 1986

Mattson RH, Cramer JA, Collins JF, et al: A comparison of valproate with carbamazepine for the treatment of complex partial seizures and secondarily generalized tonic-clonic seizures in adult. N Engl J Med 327:765–771, 1992

McElroy SL, Keck PE Jr: Valproate treatment of bipolar and schizoaffective disorder. Can J Psychiatry 38:62S–66S, 1993

McElroy SL, Pope HG Jr (eds): Use of Anticonvulsants in Psychiatry: Recent Advances. Clifton, NJ, Oxford Health Care, 1988

McElroy SL, Keck PE Jr, Pope HG Jr, et al: Valproate in the treatment of rapid-cycling, bipolar disorder. J Clin Psychopharmacol 8:275–279, 1988a

McElroy SL, Pope HG Jr, Keck PE Jr, et al: Treatment of psychiatric disorders with valproate: a series of 73 cases. Psychiatrie Psychobiologie 3:81–85, 1988b

McElroy SL, Keck PE Jr, Pope HG Jr, et al: Correlates of antimanic response to valproate. Psychopharmacol Bull 27:127–133, 1991

McElroy SL, Keck PE Jr, Pope HG Jr, et al: Clinical and research implications of the diagnosis of dysphoric or mixed mania or hypomania. Am J Psychiatry 149:1633–1644, 1992a

McElroy SL, Keck PE Jr, Pope HG Jr, et al: Valproate in bipolar disorder: literature review and treatment guidelines. J Clin Psychopharmacol 12:42S–52S, 1992b

McElroy SL, Keck PE Jr, Stanton SP, et al: A randomized comparison of divalproex oral loading versus haloperidol in the initial treatment of acute psychotic mania. J Clin Psychiatry 57:142–146, 1996

McElroy SL, Soutullo CA, Keck PE Jr, et al: A pilot trial of gabapentin in the treatment of bipolar disorder. Ann Clin Psychiatry 9:99–103, 1997

Möller MJ, Kissling W, Riehl T, et al: Double-blind evaluation of the antimanic properties of carbamazepine as a comedication to haloperidol. Prog Neuropsychopharmacol Biol Psychiatry 13:127–136, 1989

Morselli PL: Carbamazepine: absorption, distribution, and excretion, in Antiepileptic Drugs, 3rd Edition. Edited by Levy RH, Dreifuss FE, Mattson RH, et al. New York, Raven, 1989, pp 473–490

Müller AA, Stoll KD: Carbamazepine and oxcarbazepine in the treatment of manic syndromes: studies in Germany, in Anticonvulsants in Affective Disorders. Edited by Emrich HM, Okuma T, Müller AA. Amsterdam, Excerpta Medica, 1984, pp 134–147

Murphy DJ, Gannon MA, McGennis A: Carbamazepine in bipolar affective disorder. Lancet 2:1151–1152, 1989

Neumann J, Seidel K, Wunderlich BP: Comparative studies of the effect of carbamazepine and trimipramine in depression, in Anticonvulsants in Affective Disorders. Edited by Emrich HM, Okuma T, Müller AA. Amsterdam, Excerpta Medica, 1984, pp 160–166

Okuma T: Effects of carbamazepine and lithium on affective disorders. Neuropsychobiology 27:138–145, 1993

Okuma T, Inanaga K, Otsuki S, et al: Comparison of the antimanic efficacy of carbamazepine and chlorpromazine. Psychopharmacology (Berl) 66:211–217, 1979

Okuma T, Inanaga K, Otsuki S, et al: A preliminary doubleblind study on the efficacy in prophylaxis of manic depressive illness. Psychopharmacology (Berl) 73:95–96, 1981

Okuma T, Yamashita I, Takahasi R, et al: Comparison of the antimanic efficacy of carbamazepine and lithium carbonate by double-blind controlled study. Pharmacopsychiatry 23:143–150, 1990

Pellock JM: Carbamazepine side effects in children and adults. Epilepsia 28:564S–570S, 1987

Pellock JM, Willmore LJ: A rational guide to routine blood monitoring in patients receiving antiepileptic drugs. Neurology 41:961–964, 1991

Penry JK, Dean JC: The scope and use of valproate in epilepsy. J Clin Psychiatry 40:17S–22S, 1989

Placidi GF, Lenzi A, Lazzerini F, et al: The comparative efficacy and safety of carbamazepine versus lithium: a randomized, double-blind 3 year trial in 83 patients. J Clin Psychiatry 47:490–494, 1986

Pope HG Jr, McElroy SL, Satlin A, et al: Head injury, bipolar disorder, and response to valproate. Compr Psychiatry 29:34–38, 1988

Pope HG Jr, McElroy SL, Keck PE Jr, et al: Valproate in the treatment of acute mania: a placebo-controlled study. Arch Gen Psychiatry 48:62–68, 1991

Post RM: Approaches to treatment-resistant bipolar affectively ill patients. Clin Neuropharmacol 11:93–104, 1988

Post RM: Non-lithium treatment for bipolar disorder. J Clin Psychiatry 51:9S–16S, 1990

Post RM, Ballenger JC, Uhde TW, et al: Efficacy of carbamazepine in manic-depressive illness: implications for underlying mechanisms, in Neurobiology of Mood Disorders. Edited by Post RM, Ballenger JC. Baltimore, MD, Williams & Wilkins, 1984a, pp 77–816

Post RM, Berettini W, Uhde TW, et al: Selective response to the anticonvulsant carbamazepine in manic depressive illness: a case study. J Clin Psychopharmacol 4:178–185, 1984b

Post RM, Uhde TW, Roy-Byrne PP, et al: Antidepressant effects of carbamazepine. Am J Psychiatry 143:29–34, 1985

Post RM, Uhde TW, Roy-Byrne PP, et al: Correlates of antimanic response to carbamazepine. Psychiatry Res 21:71–83, 1987

Post RM, Leverich GS, Rosoff AS, et al: Carbamazepine prophylaxis in refractory affective disorders: a focus on longterm follow-up. J Clin Psychopharmacol 10:318–327, 1990

Post RM, Altshuler LL, Ketter TA, et al: Antiepileptic drugs in affective illness: clinical and theoretical implications, in Advances in Neurology, Vol 55. Edited by Smith D, Treiman D, Trimble M. New York, Raven, 1991, pp 239–277

Post RM, Weiss SRB, Chuang DM: Mechanisms of action of anticonvulsants in affective disorders: comparison with lithium. J Clin Psychopharmacol 12:23S–35S, 1992

Prien RF, Gelenberg AJ: Alternatives to lithium for preventive treatment of bipolar disorder. Am J Psychiatry 146:840–848, 1989

Puzynski S, Klosiewicz L: Valproic Acid amid as a prophylactic agent in affective and schizoaffective disorders. Psychopharmacol Bull 20:151–159, 1984

Rall TW, Schleifer LS: Drugs effective in the therapy of the epilepsies, in The Pharmacological Basis of Therapeutics. Edited by Gilman AG, Goodman LS, Rall TW, et al. New York, Macmillan, 1985, pp 446–472

Rimmer E, Richens A: An update on sodium valproate. Pharmacotherapy 5:171–184, 1985

Rosa FWL: Spina bifida in infants of women treated with carbamazepine during pregnancy. N Engl J Med 324:674–677, 1991

Rosebush PI, Hildeband AM, Furlong BG, et al: Catatonic syndrome in a general psychiatric inpatient population: frequency, clinical presentation, and response to lorazepam. J Clin Psychiatry 51:357–362, 1990

Ryback R, Ryback L: Gabapentin for behavioral dyscontrol. Am J Psychiatry 152:1319, 1995

Sachs GS, Weilburg JB, Rosebaum JF: Clonazepam vs. neuroleptics as adjuncts to lithium maintenance. Psychopharmacol Bull 26:137–143, 1990

Seetharam MN, Pellock JM: Risk-benefit assessment of carbamazepine in children. Drug Saf 6:148–158, 1991

Short C, Cooke L: Hypomania induced by gabapentin. Br J Psychiatry 166:679–680, 1995

Simhandl CH, Denke E, Thau K: The comparative efficacy of carbamazepine low and high serum level and lithium carbonate in the prophylaxis of affective disorders. J Affect Disord 28:221–231, 1993

Small JG: Anticonvulsants in affective disorders. Psychopharmacol Bull 26:25–36, 1990

Small JG, Klapper MH, Milstein V, et al: Carbamazepine compared with lithium in the treatment of mania. Arch Gen Psychiatry 48:915–921, 1991

Smith MC, Bleck TP: Convulsive disorders: toxicity of anticonvulsants. Clin Neuropharmacol 14:97–115, 1991

Sovner R: The use of valproate in the treatment of mentally retarded persons with typical and atypical bipolar disorders. J Clin Psychiatry 50:40S–43S, 1989

Sovner R, Davis JM: A potential drug interaction between fluoxetine and valproic acid. J Clin Psychopharmacol 11:389, 1991

Sporn J, Sachs G: The anticonvulsant lamotrigine in treatment-resistant manic-depressive illness. J Clin Psychopharmacol 17:185–189, 1997

Stanton SP, Keck PE Jr, McElroy SL: Treatment of acute mania with gabapentin (letter). Am J Psychiatry 154:287, 1996

Stoll AL, Vuckovic A, McElroy SL: Histamine 2-receptor antagonists for the treatment of valproate-induced gastrointestinal distress. Ann Clin Psychiatry 3:301–304, 1991

Stoll AL, Banov M, Kolbrener M, et al: Neurologic factors predict a favorable valproate response in bipolar and schizoaffective disorder. J Clin Psychopharmacol 14:311–313, 1994

Suppes T, McElroy SL, Gilbert J, et al: Clozapine in the treatment of dysphoric mania. Biol Psychiatry 32:270–280, 1992

Takezaki H, Hanaoka M: The use of carbamazepine (Tegretol) in the control of manic-depressive psychosis and other manic, depressive states. Clinical Psychiatry 13:173–182, 1971

Tesar GE: High potency benzodiazepines for short-term management of panic disorder: the U.S. experience. J Clin Psychiatry 51:4S–10S, 1990

Tohen M, Castillo J, Pope HG Jr, et al: Concomitant use of valproate and carbamazepine in bipolar and schizoaffective disorders. J Clin Psychopharmacol 14:67–70, 1994

Tohen M, Castillo J, Baldessarini RJ, et al: Blood dyscrasias with carbamazepine and valproate: a pharmacoepidemiological study of 2,228 patients at risk. Am J Psychiatry 152:413–418, 1995

Vencovsky E, Soucek K, Zatecká I: Comparison of side effects of lithium and dipropylacetamide (Depamide). Ceskoslovensk Psychiatrie 79:223–227, 1983

Vining EPG: Cognitive dysfunction associated with antiepileptic drug therapy. Epilepsia 28:18S–22S, 1987

Watkins SE, Callender K, Thomas DR, et al: The effect of carbamazepine and lithium on remission from affective illness. Br J Psychiatry 150:180–182, 1987

Wilder BJ: Pharmacokinetics of valproate and carbamazepine. J Clin Psychopharmacol 12:64S–68S, 1992

Wilder BJ, Karas BJ, Penry JK, et al: Gastrointestinal tolerance of divalproex sodium. Neurology 33:808–811, 1983

Wildgrube C: Case studies on prophylactic long-term effects of oxcarbazepine in recurrent affective disorders. Int Clin Psychopharmacol 5:89S–94S, 1990

Zona C, Tancredi V, Palma E, et al: Potassium currents in rat cortical neurons in culture are enhanced by the antiepileptic drug carbamazepine. Can J Physiol Pharmacol 68:545–547, 1990

TWENTY-TWO

Calcium Channel Antagonists as Novel Agents for the Treatment of Bipolar Disorder

Steven L. Dubovsky, M.D.

The introduction of the anticonvulsants carbamazepine and divalproex sodium has greatly expanded psychiatric treatment options for bipolar illness (see Keck and McElroy, Chapter 21, in this volume). However, the anticonvulsants are not always effective for the 25%–33% of bipolar patients who are at least partially unresponsive to lithium (Aronson et al. 1989; Post 1988; Prien and Gelenberg 1989). Because many patients cannot tolerate lithium side effects or the regular monitoring that taking the drug requires, up to 50% of them discontinue or reduce the dose of the drug even if it is effective (Prien and Gelenberg 1989). The anticonvulsants are also not without significant side effects, and they require routine blood tests, which can reduce compliance. In addition, lithium, carbamazepine, and valproate are all problematic medications for pregnant patients.

The calcium channel antagonists, or calcium channel blockers (CCBs), a novel class of medications that has been studied as possible antimanic agents, have a favorable side-effect profile, do not require routine blood level monitoring, and may be safer during pregnancy. In addition, some of these medications could prove to be effective in subtypes of bipolar disorder that do not respond completely to standard treatments; they could also be especially useful for medically ill bipolar patients. Studying the spectrum of response to CCBs could reveal phenotypic (e.g., rapid cycling) or biological (e.g., alterations of intracellular calcium ion concentration) markers of preferential response to these medications. Conversely, commonalities of action of CCBs, lithium, and anticonvulsants could provide new insights into the pathophysiology of bipolar illness.

Many clinicians are relatively unfamiliar with the CCBs as alternatives or supplements to lithium. One reason for this lack of awareness may be related to an increasing reliance on industry support for investigation of possible new applications of medications in an era of minimal federal funding for innovative drug research and severely reduced capacity of clinical facilities to fund clinical investigations. Whereas industry support has been an important factor in the study and popularization of the antimanic potential of the anticonvulsants, manufacturers of the CCBs have largely been uninterested in this application (Dubovsky 1994).

Despite slower research into the uses of CCBs as potential antimanic drugs, there is mounting evidence that they may have important psychiatric applications. In this chapter, I review the pharmacology of the CCBs and the evidence supporting their efficacy in the treatment of bipolar illness. Clinical guidelines for the use of CCBs and a critical discussion of recent concerns about this class of medications are also offered.

HISTORY AND DISCOVERY

Verapamil, the first calcium channel antagonist to be introduced, was synthesized in 1962 (Morris et al. 1992).

A derivative of papaverine (Bigger and Hoffman 1991), verapamil was found to have negative inotropic effects that in 1967 were postulated to be a result of the reduction of excitation-contraction coupling caused by inhibition of calcium influx into cardiac cells (Fleckenstein et al. 1967). In addition to blocking calcium influx, the intracellular action of the calcium ion (Ca^{2+}) may be inhibited by substances that enhance efflux, intracellular storage, or binding of Ca^{2+} to inactivating proteins or that activate second messengers that counteract the intracellular actions of the calcium ion. However, aside from dantrolene, which blocks the release of intracellular stored Ca^{2+} and which is used to treat malignant hyperthermia, the CCBs are the only drugs in widespread clinical use specifically for their calcium antagonist activities.

Four additional classes of CCBs have been developed since the introduction of the phenylalkylamine verapamil (Cohan 1990; Freedman and Waters 1987; Materson 1995; Morris et al. 1992; Murad 1991; Nayler 1994) (Table 22–1). These medications are heterogeneous in their structure and actions and are not interchangeable (Triggle 1992). However, they all have the capacity to reduce excessive excitability of diverse cellular systems. As a result, many of the CCBs have been used to treat various forms of angina, hypertension, migraine headaches, Raynaud's phenomenon, esophageal spasm, premature labor, and epilepsy (Bigger and Hoffman 1991; Kim 1991; Murad 1991).

Verapamil and diltiazem, but not the 1,4-dihydropyridines (DHPs), have Class IV antiarrhythmic activity and are used to treat supraventricular arrhythmias (Triggle 1992). Several CCBs have been found to retard the development of atherosclerosis in animals (Freedman and Waters 1987) and humans (Lichtlen et al. 1990). The DHP nimodipine, which is used to block cerebral arteriospasm after subarachnoid hemorrhage, was thought to slow the deteriorating effects of Alzheimer's disease (Bigger and Hoffman 1991; Ikeda et al. 1992), but a multicenter study found it to be ineffective for most patients (Bayer Pharmaceuticals, personal communication, November 1995). The role of elevated free intracellular calcium ion concentration ($[Ca^{2+}]_i$) in neuronal death could make the CCBs useful in reducing brain damage after anoxia or other injuries if they are administered quickly enough (Cohan 1990). The use of nifedipine (chewed up and placed under the tongue) to treat hypertensive crises associated with monoamine oxidase inhibitors (Clary and Schweizer 1987; Kim 1991) has been criticized on the grounds that absorption of nifedipine from the buccal mucosa is inadequate (Gerber and Nies 1991). CCBs have been found to potentiate antimalarial treatment and to reduce toxicity caused by gentamicin, amphotericin B, and cyclosporine (Nayler 1994). Nimodipine reduces morphine requirements in patients with cancer pain, possibly by interfering with down-regulation of opioid receptors (Santillan et al. 1994).

The first type of calcium antagonist used in psychiatry was calcitonin, which lowers $[Ca^{2+}]_i$ by driving Ca^{2+} into intracellular storage sites. Carman and Wyatt (1979) found that three manic patients had a temporary reduction of agitation after injections of subcutaneous salmon calcitonin but not of placebo. After receiving an unstated dose of salmon calcitonin for 20 days, a group of nine patients with chronic "psychopathological suffering" (Mussini et al. 1984), a state accompanied by depression or anxiety but no formal diagnoses, felt tranquilized and had reduced scores on the Brief Psychiatric Rating Scale (Overall and Gorham 1962).

The first report of the use of a CCB in the treatment of mania was a double-blind, placebo-controlled trial of verapamil in a single manic patient (Dubovsky et al. 1982). The decision to investigate this use of a CCB was based on observations that the intracellular calcium ion is involved in the regulation of many processes implicated in bipolar affective disorders and that lithium might interfere with the intracellular action of Ca^{2+} (Dubovsky and Franks 1983). Verapamil was chosen because its cardiovascular effects were being studied by a colleague and the manufacturer was willing to make it available to the investigators at a time at which none of the CCBs had yet been approved for use in the United States.

Subsequently, case reports and open and double-blind studies involving approximately 200 patients with bipolar disorder (reviewed in Dubovsky 1993) have suggested the antimanic efficacy of verapamil compared with placebo or with no treatment. Two studies have reported equivalent antimanic efficacy with lithium (Garza-Trevino et al. 1992; Hoschl and Kozemy 1989). However, with the exception of a few studies (Dubovsky et al. 1986; Garza-Trevino et al. 1992; Hoschl and Kozemy 1989; Hoschl et

Table 22–1.   Calcium channel blocker classes

Class	Examples
Phenylalkylamine	Verapamil, norverapamil, D600, gallopamil
1,4-Dihydropyridine	Nifedipine, nicardipine, nimodipine, amlodipine, nisoldipine, felodipine, nitrendipine
Benzothiazepine	Diltiazem, TA3090
Diphenylpiperazine	Flunarizine, cinnarizine
Dihydrodibenzothiepin (benzothiepine)	Monatepil

al. 1986), patients in most studies have been only moderately ill, trials have been brief, and additional medications (especially neuroleptics) have been used as needed. Applications of other CCBs as antimanic drugs and mood stabilizers have been suggested by the results of a 2-week open trial of diltiazem in 7 manic patients (Caillard 1985), a 3-year follow-up study of a bipolar patient for whom flunarizine was successfully substituted for lithium (Lindelius and Nilsson 1992), a 1-week trial of nimodipine (Brunet et al. 1990), and an extended double-blind follow-up study of 11 patients with bipolar disorder and 1 patient with recurrent brief depression receiving high doses of nimodipine (Pazzaglia et al. 1993; Post et al. 1993).

As is true of lithium, the usefulness of CCBs in the treatment of depression is not as clear as their applications in mania. Nifedipine reduces immobility in the behavioral despair test, which is thought to be an animal model of antidepressant activity (Mogilnicka et al. 1987). Flunarizine was thought to reduce depressive recurrences in one patient (Lindelius and Nilsson 1992), and one patient with recurrent brief depression responded to blind trials of both nimodipine and verapamil (Post et al. 1993). Verapamil may have acute antidepressant properties in some bipolar depressed patients (J. Berlant, unpublished data, April 1994; Deicken 1990; Dubovsky et al. 1992a) and in psychotically depressed patients (Jacques and Cox 1991). Hoschl and Kozemy (1989) found that, overall, verapamil was no more effective than placebo and was inferior to amitriptyline in the treatment of depression. However, a few patients did seem to have a genuine antidepressant response to verapamil in this study and in a previous report by the same authors (Hoschl et al. 1986). Because the investigators did not differentiate between bipolar and unipolar depression, it is possible that—as would be expected with lithium—those subjects with bipolar depression were more likely to respond to verapamil. Verapamil appeared to augment the antidepressant action of imipramine in a patient with unipolar depression who had previously responded to lithium augmentation. When imipramine was discontinued 6 months later, the patient remained euthymic while taking verapamil alone (Pollack and Rosenbaum 1987). Conversely, Eccleston and Cole (1990) thought that nifedipine gave rise either to depression itself or to resistance to antidepressants in five patients with unipolar depression.

STRUCTURE-ACTIVITY RELATIONS

Different classes of calcium channel antagonists have significantly different structures (Figure 22–1), leading to differential activity in various tissues. This differential activity depends on interactions with ion-specific calcium channels in the cell membrane. A consideration of the structure of calcium channels is therefore central to an understanding of the structural specificity of the medications that act on them.

Extracellular calcium ions enter the cytosol through receptor-operated channels that are gated by receptors for hormones and transmitters such as the excitatory amino acids, as well as through potential-dependent channels (PDCs) that are gated by membrane potential. Additional pathways for calcium entry include a "leak" through an ungated channel and exchange of extracellular calcium ions for intracellular sodium ions (Na^+) (Cohan 1990; Rosenberg 1991; Triggle 1992). Under physiological conditions, PDCs can be regulated by receptor-mediated events, such as the production of inositol triphosphate (Bergamaschi et al. 1990; Janis and Triggle 1991), and receptor-operated channels can be gated by voltage-dependent events (Bergamaschi et al. 1990). In addition, extracellular Ca^{2+} entering the cell may release calcium ions from intracellular

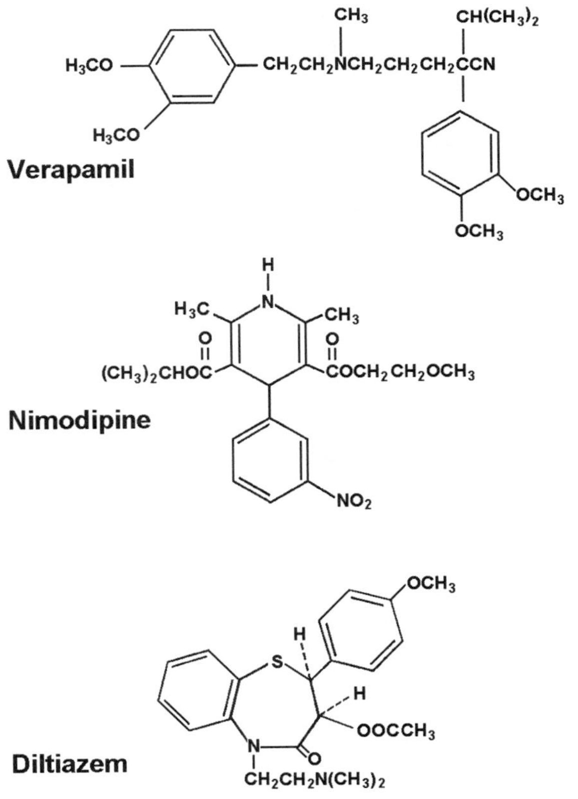

Figure 22–1. Chemical structures for some calcium channel blockers.

stores, and "trigger" amounts of calcium ions released from intracellular stores may facilitate calcium channel opening (Dubovsky and Franks 1983; Murad 1991). Even subtle alterations of the function of one kind of calcium channel may therefore have significant effects on the overall balance of calcium-dependent cellular activity.

CCBs interact with the PDC. This type of channel consists of five allosterically linked subunits, α_1, α_2, β, γ, and δ. The α_1 channel has a hydrophobic region that spans the cell membrane and outlines the actual calcium pore (Figure 22–2). In the brain, PDCs for calcium are localized in regions that are rich in synapses, perhaps because high $[Ca^{2+}]_i$ must be produced rapidly in order to regulate the release of neurotransmitters (Fox et al. 1991). Endogenous regulators that are unrelated to neurotransmitters appear to modulate PDC gating and CCB binding (Janis and Triggle 1991) and may be altered in disease states (Triggle 1992).

Four subtypes of PDCs have been identified (Fox et al. 1991; Janis and Triggle 1991; Kenny et al. 1991; Murad 1991; Siesjo 1990; Triggle 1992):

1. The L (or long-lasting) channel, the only PDC shown definitely to bind CCBs, requires significant depolarization for Ca^{2+} entry and inactivates slowly.
2. The T (or transient) channel is activated by a small depolarization and inactivates rapidly.
3. The N (neither L nor T) channel, which is primarily found on central nervous system neurons, is unresponsive to CCBs.
4. The rapidly inactivating P (Purkinje cell) channel identified in cerebellar Purkinje cells is insensitive to the DHP CCBs.

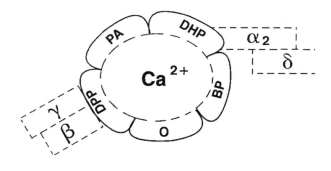

Figure 22–2. Structure of the calcium channel blocker (CCB) binding site.
PA = phenylalkylamine binding site; DHP = 1,4-dihydropyridine binding site; BP = benzothiazepine binding site; DPP = diphenylpiperazine binding site; O = other binding sites.

N and P channels may participate in the release of neurotransmitters in response to the action potential, whereas the role of L channels is less certain. Studies of the actions of specific CCBs on L channels may be complicated by differential binding of CCBs by the same channels in different tissues, alteration of findings by slight changes in experimental conditions, and confusion of N and L channels (Janis and Triggle 1991; Kenny et al. 1991).

CCBs bind primarily to L channels (Bigger and Hoffman 1991). Nimodipine, nicardipine, methoxyverapamil, flunarizine, and cinnarizine may also antagonize T channels (Cohan 1990; Janis and Triggle 1991), and a phenylalkylamine-binding site exists on the inner mitochondrial membrane (Zernig 1992).

At least four, and possibly seven or more, distinct binding sites for different classes of CCBs exist on the L channel α_1 subunit (Kenny et al. 1991; Murad 1991), allosterically linked to one another and to the Ca^{2+} gating site and capable of regulation by circulating factors (Janis and Triggle 1991) (Figure 22–2). The other subunits may allosterically modify the CCB affinity of the α_1 subunit (Kenny et al. 1991). For example, occupation of the DHP receptor increases binding to the benzothiazepine receptor and vice versa (Materson 1995). However, phenylalkylamine and DHP receptors do not enhance each other's binding (Materson 1995). These differences may predict differences in the effect of combining two classes of CCBs. The conformation of the α_1 subunit and therefore the affinity of the L channel for a given CCB can be altered by guanine nucleotide binding protein (G-protein) activity; cyclic adenosine monophosphate (cAMP)-dependent phosphorylation, actions of Ca^{2+} mediated by calmodulin and protein kinase C, and Ca^{2+} binding to the α_1 subunit (Bergamaschi et al. 1990).

Thus far, four separate genes coding for the α_1 subunit have been identified, producing different versions of CCB-binding sites (Triggle 1992). Depending on the distribution of binding sites for a given chemical class of CCBs, that class may be more or less active in a particular tissue or region. Variations in CCB structure produce changes in potency at different L channels in several tissues (Janis and Triggle 1991). For example, DHPs are more selective for vascular tissue, whereas verapamil and diltiazem have more prominent antiarrhythmic properties (Triggle 1992).

Several additional features of the calcium channel contribute to the activity profiles of CCBs of different structures (Janis and Triggle 1991; Triggle 1992). In addition to allosteric regulation by other sites and the influence of circulating modulators, membrane potential determines the conformation (and thus the affinity) of CCB-binding sites. DHP binding is enhanced by membrane depolarization, the CCB stabilizing the channel in an inactivated state. Most DHPs are uncharged at physiological pH and easily gain access to the receptor through the cell membrane if it is sufficiently depolarized. Charged DHPs such as amlodipine have a slower onset of action because of interactions with negatively charged phosphate headgroups in the cell membrane. Verapamil and diltiazem, which are also charged at physiological pH, gain access to the receptor through open channels and are therefore more active when channel openings are more frequent. The activity dependence of both charged and uncharged CCBs makes these drugs much more potent in hyperactive than in normal tissue. Actions measured in normal cell preparations may not reflect activity in pathological states.

Most of the currently available CCBs share a rapid onset and short duration of action (Nayler 1994). The only important exception is amlodipine, a nifedipine derivative, which has a long elimination half-life and a slow rate of dissociation from binding sites on calcium channels (Nayler 1994). Monatepil, an experimental CCB that is structurally dissimilar from amlodipine, also has a long plasma half-life and is highly lipophilic (Nayler 1994). Although there are a number of differences among the DHPs, as a group these CCBs share more properties with one another than they do with the phenylalkylamines and benzothiazepines (Materson 1995). For example, verapamil and diltiazem have negative chronotropic effects, whereas the DHPs tend to increase heart rate. In contrast, DHPs are more likely to cause pedal edema.

Figure 22–3 further describes structure-activity relations that have been defined for the DHP CCBs (Janis and Triggle 1991). The activity of the (–) enantiomer of verapamil is greater than the activity of the (+) enantiomer. Micromolar concentrations of Ca^{2+} are required for binding of the DHPs, whereas the same Ca^{2+} concentrations inhibit receptor binding of phenylalkylamines and diltiazem (Janis and Triggle 1991). The structure-activity relations that have been defined for the CCBs apply to activity at L channels in various tissues and have not been specifically correlated with clinical effects.

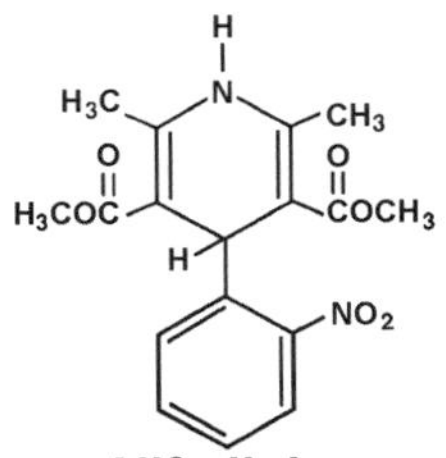

PHARMACOLOGICAL PROFILE

Table 22–2 presents a summary of the absorption, distribution, and excretion of some CCBs compared with those of lithium, carbamazepine, and valproate (Benet and Williams 1991; Kim 1991; Morris et al. 1992). The CCBs are almost completely absorbed after oral administration, but

Nifedipine

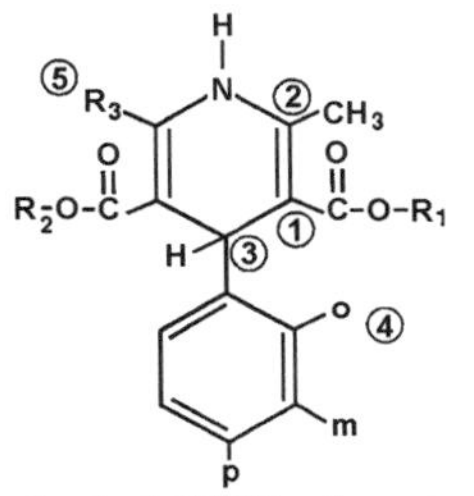

Basic 1,4 DHP structure

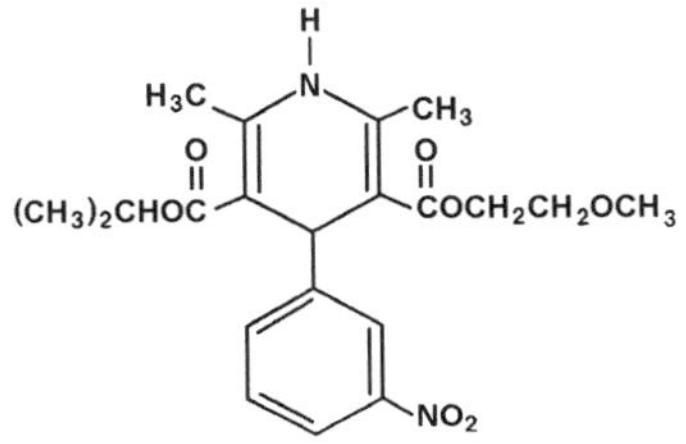

Nimodipine

Figure 22–3. Structure-activity relations for 1,4-dihydropyridines (DHPs).
1. $CO_2R > COCH_3 > CN > H$.
2. Basic substituent in this position (e.g., amlodipine) results in slow onset, long duration of action, and high stereoselectivity.
3. Torsion angle of aryl ring influences activity.
4. $o \geq m > p$.
5. Greater activity with R = small alkyl, amine, or aminoalkyl.
Source. Adapted from Janis and Triggle 1991; Triggle 1992.

their bioavailability is decreased by extensive first-pass hepatic metabolism (Murad 1991). First-pass metabolism also results in considerable interindividual variability in blood level at a given dose (Morris et al. 1992). Oral bioavailability of the CCBs is less than that of other drugs used to treat mania, but effective concentrations are an order of magnitude lower (Table 22–2).

Peak plasma levels of most CCBs are achieved within 30 minutes to 3 hours after oral administration, but amlodipine does not reach peak plasma concentrations for 6 hours (Morris et al. 1992). Most CCBs have elimination half-lives in the range of 1.3–6 hours (Kim 1991; Murad 1991) except for amlodipine, which has a half-life of

Table 22–2. Profiles of some calcium channel blockers and antimanic drugs

Drug	Oral availability (%)	Plasma protein binding (%)	Volume of distribution (L/kg)	Half-life (hours)	Effective concentration
Verapamil	22 ± 8	90	5 ± 2.1	4 ± 1.5	40–120 ng/mL
Diltiazem	44 ± 10	78	3.1 ± 1.2	3.7 ± 1.2	Unknown
Nifedipine	50 ± 13	96	0.78 ± 0.22	2.5 ± 1.3	27–67 ng/mL
Lithium	100	0	0.79 ± 0.34	22 ± 8	0.5–1.5 mEq/L
Carbamazepine	70	74	1.4 ± 0.4	15 ± 5	4–10 µg/mL
Valproate	100	93	0.22 ± 0.07	14 ± 3	50–125 µg/mL

35–50 hours (Benet and Williams 1991). Although amlodipine can be given once daily, the short half-lives of most CCBs require multiple dosing. However, because repeated administration saturates hepatic metabolizing enzymes, bioavailability and half-life increase with chronic administration, and the dosing interval can be increased (Benet et al. 1991; Morris et al. 1992). All CCBs are extensively bound to plasma proteins.

Verapamil is metabolized by dealkylation and demethylation to at least 12 metabolites. One of these, norverapamil, has about 20% as much cardiovascular activity as verapamil in animal models and an elimination half-life of 10 hours (Morris et al. 1992; Murad 1991). After oral administration, verapamil and norverapamil can be recovered from human cerebrospinal fluid (Doran et al. 1985), although penetration of the more lipophilic nimodipine across the blood-brain barrier is better (Freedman and Waters 1987). One piece of experimental evidence that the concentration of phenylalkylamines in the brain is sufficient for a therapeutic effect is the protective effect of this class after cerebral ischemia in rats (Rosenberg 1991).

Diltiazem, which is metabolized by deacetylation or demethylation, has active metabolites that do not appear to be clinically important (Morris et al. 1992). Nifedipine, nicardipine, and most of the other DHPs have inactive metabolites. Most people are rapid metabolizers of nifedipine and possibly other DHPs; about 17% are slow metabolizers.

MECHANISM OF ACTION

Free intracellular Ca^{2+} concentration is normally regulated very tightly at around 100 nM, or one-ten thousandth the Ca^{2+} concentration in extracellular fluid (Fox et al. 1991). The regulation of $[Ca^{2+}]_i$ is complex, depending on calcium influx pathways (described previously) as well as extrusion of Ca^{2+} from the cell by a calcium–adenosine triphosphatase (ATPase) membrane pump, up-

take of Ca^{2+} into intracellular stores, and complexing with intracellular inactivating proteins. Calcium influx in the brain is determined by the membrane potential, receptor activity, availability of excitatory amino acids, and intracellular Na^+ concentration (Rosenberg 1991; Triggle 1992). Elevations of $[Ca^{2+}]_i$ produced by increased Ca^{2+} influx from the extracellular space and/or release of Ca^{2+} from intracellular stores provide a bidirectional intracellular signal that may stimulate cellular processes at moderate elevations and inhibit the same processes at further elevations or at different phases of the cell cycle (Dubovsky et al. 1992a).

Significant elevations of $[Ca^{2+}]_i$ have been found in blood platelets (Dubovsky et al. 1989, 1991a, 1991b, 1992b; Tan et al. 1990) and lymphocytes (Dubovsky et al. 1992b) of manic and bipolar depressed patients who are affectively ill but not in platelets of unipolar depressed patients, control subjects, or bipolar patients who are euthymic after treatment with various medications or electroconvulsive therapy. Elevated $[Ca^{2+}]_i$ could reflect a primary alteration in intracellular Ca^{2+} homeostasis, or it could be a downstream result of elevated activity of G proteins linked to influx or release mechanisms. Consistent with the latter possibility are observations of hyperactive receptor-linked G proteins in mononuclear leukocyte membrane preparations of untreated manic patients (but not lithium-treated euthymic bipolar patients) (van Calker et al. 1993) and heightened activation of the platelet phosphatidylinositol system, which is linked to G proteins and mobilizes the influx and release of Ca^{2+} (Brown et al. 1993). Whether produced by excessive receptor activation of G proteins or some other mechanism, excess elevations of $[Ca^{2+}]_i$ could be the effector arm that produces the mixtures and alternations of elevated and inhibited cellular activity that are characteristic of bipolar illness (Dubovsky et al. 1992a).

Lithium treatment normalizes platelet $[Ca^{2+}]_i$ (Dubovsky et al. 1989, 1991a), leukocyte G-protein response to agonists (van Calker et al. 1993), and agonist-induced accumulation of inositol phosphates (Greil et al.

1991). In addition, in vitro incubation with lithium inhibited the coupling of muscarinic cholinergic and β-adrenergic receptors to their G proteins (Avissar and Schreiber 1992) and lowers platelet $[Ca^{2+}]_i$ significantly in ill bipolar patients but not in control subjects (Dubovsky et al. 1991b). Lithium had no effect on platelet $[Ca^{2+}]_i$ in another study (Tan et al. 1990), but patients were euthymic and the action of lithium on intracellular Ca^{2+} dynamics may differ between the ill and well states (Dubovsky et al. 1992a). Carbamazepine inhibits Ca^{2+} currents in a variety of models, and the time course of suppression of calcium-dependent potentials is comparable to that produced by verapamil (Messing et al. 1985; Schirrmacher et al. 1993; Walden et al. 1992). This anticonvulsant may alter influx through *N*-methyl-D-aspartate (NMDA) receptor–gated channels (Post et al. 1993). Lithium, carbamazepine, and CCBs could all correct elevated Ca^{2+} influx. Reduction of Ca^{2+} influx produced by CCBs could also alter intracellular Ca^{2+} homeostasis sufficiently to compensate for dysregulated intracellular signaling associated with other mechanisms.

Several objections can be raised to the hypothesis that attenuation of excessive rises in $[Ca^{2+}]_i$ produced by stimulation of neurons with hypersensitivity of this or a related messenger system is a mechanism of action of CCBs in bipolar illness. First, L channels do not appear to be involved in the action potential–dependent release of neurotransmitters (Janis and Triggle 1991). However, neurotransmitters activate L channels, making them an important component of neuronal signaling (Fox et al. 1991). Another problem is that low concentrations of CCBs do not affect neurotransmitter release or neuronal Ca^{2+} currents because depolarization in these cells is normally too brief to permit sufficient binding of the CCBs (Triggle 1992). A response to this objection is that higher concentrations of CCBs may alter neuronal activity, and some negative reports may be the result of confusing L channels with other channels that do not respond to CCBs. CCBs do have significant effects on neurons with prolonged or marked depolarization (Janis and Triggle 1991). This may be why the effects of antimanic drugs such as lithium on $[Ca^{2+}]_i$ are evident in hyperactive peripheral cells from bipolar patients but not in normally active cells from control subjects (Dubovsky et al. 1992a).

It could also be argued that it is the anticonvulsant property of CCBs (Janis and Triggle 1991) and not their effect on Ca^{2+} currents that accounts for their antimanic activity (Post et al. 1993). Although reduction of neuronal excitability does convey anticonvulsant effects to the CCBs, these effects do not appear to be in proportion to their antimanic potential. In addition, the anticonvulsant potency of many of the CCBs is manifested mainly in animal models and is not apparent in humans with epilepsy or electrically induced seizures.

INDICATIONS

The available data suggest that CCBs are most useful for the treatment of mania that responds to lithium, but patients cannot tolerate the medication, whereas mania that does not respond to lithium seems less likely to respond to verapamil (Barton and Gitlin 1987; Kennedy et al. 1986). In the few reported cases in which verapamil (Dubovsky et al. 1982, 1986) or diltiazem (Caillard 1985) was administered to manic patients with brain damage, the CCBs were well tolerated. CCBs might be considered for the treatment of patients with physical conditions for which other medications would be more dangerous (e.g., pregnancy) or for which a CCB might be helpful (Amery et al. 1981; Leys et al. 1988; Litzinger et al. 1985; Reiter et al. 1989; Walsh et al. 1986; Yamawaki and Yanagawa 1986). Possibly because of compensatory changes in calcium channels or CCB receptors, tachyphylaxis and withdrawal do not occur (Murad 1991). CCBs do not alter exercise tolerance (Gerber and Nies 1991).

CCBs have been studied in randomized trials during pregnancy for the treatment of maternal hypertension, premature labor, and fetal arrhythmias without evidence of teratogenicity and without significant effects on uteroplacental blood flow (Byerly et al. 1991; Carbonne et al. 1993; Ulmsten et al. 1980; Wide-Swensson et al. 1996). However, an insufficient number of patients have been studied during the first trimester to be certain that CCBs have no adverse effects on the fetus, and there are no data about the later development of children who were exposed to CCBs during pregnancy. Although verapamil might be a viable alternative to lithium, carbamazepine, and valproate in the treatment of pregnant bipolar patients, so far there has been only one published report in which sustained-release verapamil was administered to three pregnant patients with mania with good control of mania and uneventful delivery of normal babies (Goodnick 1993).

Most manic patients enrolled in studies of verapamil either have responded to lithium or have not received lithium, so they cannot be said to have been unresponsive to it. A few rapid-cycling patients have benefited from verapamil (Wehr et al. 1988), and addition of verapamil to lithium has been helpful to some patients who did not respond to lithium alone (Brotman et al. 1986). However, most patients with complex or treatment-refractory bipolar illness should probably be treated first with anticonvulsants with or without lithium, because there has been much more published positive experience with these drug combinations in such situations.

Verapamil has been noted to prevent antidepressant-induced hypomania (Barton and Gitlin 1987; Dubovsky et al. 1986; Gitlin and Weiss 1984; Solomon and Williamson 1986). Extended follow-up studies of several patients demonstrated the usefulness of nimodipine in maintenance therapy for bipolar illness (Manna 1991; Post et al. 1993), and verapamil also has been found to be effective in the clinical setting in preventing affective recurrence. As noted previously, CCBs do not have impressive antidepressant properties, but they may be helpful in some cases of bipolar or highly recurrent depression (Hoschl et al. 1986; Jacques and Cox 1991; Lindelius and Nilsson 1992; Post et al. 1993).

The heterogeneity of CCB-binding sites provides for different spectra of action of the various CCBs, and patients whose symptoms do not respond to one class of drug may have a good response to another (Post et al. 1993). Combinations of CCBs with one another and with other antimanic drugs could also produce additive effects on Ca^{2+}-dependent mechanisms that could make such combinations useful in treatment-refractory states. However, such possibilities have not been investigated formally.

The CCBs do not appear to be helpful for the treatment of chronic, treatment-refractory schizophrenia (Grebb et al. 1986; Pickar et al. 1987; Uhr et al. 1988), although they may reduce signs of tardive dyskinesia (Leys et al. 1988; Reiter et al. 1989). Verapamil in doses of 240–480 mg/day produced modest improvement in panic disorder in 11 patients and marked improvement in 4 (Klein and Uhde 1988). Although further studies for this indication have not been reported, clinicians sometimes find that adding verapamil to antidepressants and/or benzodiazepines enhances the antipanic efficacy of these drugs.

The available preparations and recommended maximum doses of some CCBs are summarized in Table 22–3 (Murad 1991). The usual daily doses of verapamil in the treatment of mania have been 240–480 mg, although some patients may need higher doses. The sustained-release preparation often is not as effective as standard preparations, possibly because blood levels are inadequate. The reported daily dose of nimodipine in the treatment of bipolar illness has ranged from 360 mg (Brunet et al. 1990) to 720 mg (Post et al. 1993), twice the maximum dose approved by the U.S. Food and Drug Administration (Table 22–3).

SIDE EFFECTS AND TOXICOLOGY

The most common side effects of CCBs are consequences of excessive vasodilatation (e.g., dizziness, headache, skin flushing, tachycardia, nausea, and digital dysesthesia); in addition, aggravation of myocardial ischemia may rarely occur (Bigger and Hoffman 1991; Gerber and Nies 1991; Murad 1991). Precapillary dilatation with reflex postcapillary constriction can increase capillary hydrostatic pressure and cause peripheral edema (Gerber and Nies 1991). The highest incidence of vascular side effects occurs with the DHPs (Gerber and Nies 1991). Verapamil and diltiazem are more likely than other preparations to produce sinus bradycardia and atrioventricular block and may aggravate heart failure. Coughing, wheezing, rashes, somnolence, constipation, and (very rarely) psychosis may be caused by the CCBs (Bigger and Hoffman 1991; Freedman and Waters 1987; Gerber and Nies 1991; Kim 1991; Murad 1991). Akathisia (Jacobs 1983), parkinsonism (Chouza et al. 1986), and delirium (Jacobsen et al. 1987) have occasionally been associated with use of calcium channel antagonists. Toxic serum concentrations of CCBs have not been defined as they have for lithium and anticonvulsants (Benet and Williams 1991).

Verapamil has usually been considered to be safe for long-term administration (Mauritson et al. 1982). However, two concerns have recently been raised about the

Table 22–3. Some calcium channel blocker preparations and doses

Drug	Trade name	Size supplied (mg)	Usual daily dose, mg (maximum)
Verapamil	Calan, Isoptin	40, 80, 120, 240 SR	120–480 (480)
Nimodipine	Nimotop	30	60–120 (180)
Nifedipine	Procardia, Adalat	10, 20	30–120 (180)
Nicardipine	Cardene	20, 30	60–120 (120)
Diltiazem	Cardizem	30	30–120 (360)

Note. SR = sustained release.

safety of chronic use of CCBs. The first question emerged from a 1995 retrospective comparison of automated charts (supplemented by telephone interviews of some subjects) of a group of hypertensive patients in a Seattle health maintenance organization who were treated with either the β-adrenergic blockers propranolol, metoprolol, nadolol, or atenolol or one of the CCBs nifedipine, diltiazem, or verapamil (Psaty et al. 1995). Records of patients who did not have obvious cardiac disease at the time they began treatment for hypertension were considered, and 384 patients who had had a fatal or nonfatal myocardial infarction between July 1989 and December 1993 were matched for age and sex with 1,108 treated hypertensive patients who had not had a myocardial infarction during the same period. Compared with patients taking a β-blocker, the relative risk of myocardial infarction for patients taking a CCB was 1.60 (95% confidence interval [CI] = 1.121–2.270). The risk, which increased with increasing doses, was similar for all three CCBs. The authors proposed as possible mechanisms of this apparent increased coronary risk of CCBs in hypertensive patients a proarrhythmic effect, ischemia from coronary steal, reflex-increased sympathetic nervous system activity, or poorer compliance with the more frequent dosing that is necessary with CCBs.

This study had a number of important limitations in addition to its retrospective, open design and the limited data that were available from chart review. First, the uncontrolled nature of the treatment made it impossible to determine whether patients with more severe hypertension or with hypertension complicated by other factors that increase coronary risk were more likely to be selected for CCB therapy (Buring et al. 1995). Second, even though the results were statistically significant, the total number of patients who had had a myocardial infarction was too small to be confident that the risk was actually increased by CCBs (Buring et al. 1995). The capacity of CCBs such as nifedipine, verapamil, and monatepil to slow the growth of newly formed atherosclerotic lesions in humans and animals (Nayler 1994) should reduce rather than increase the risk of reinfarction.

In a meta-analysis of 16 randomized trials of 8,350 patients treated with nifedipine for secondary prevention after myocardial infarction, Furberg et al. (1995) found a somewhat increased risk of death (relative risk = 1.16; 95% CI = 1.01–1.33) in nifedipine-treated patients; higher doses were associated with higher mortality. The authors speculated that, in patients without vasospasm, peripheral and coronary vasodilatation could worsen cardiac ischemia or that intermittent reflex increases in sympathetic activity might rupture atherosclerotic plaques or

provoke tachyarrhythmias. These speculations are contradicted by the observation that CCBs dampen the increase in $[Ca^{2+}]_i$ that occurs in ischemic cardiac muscle and that may contribute to tachyarrhythmias, which should make these drugs capable of protecting against arrhythmia (Nayler 1991).

In a prospective, randomized, 3-year, multicenter comparison of the DHP CCB isradipine with the diuretic hydrochlorothiazide in 883 hypertensive patients, Borhani et al. (1996) found that the increase in intimal medial thickening of the carotid artery over time, as measured by B-mode ultrasound, was less with the CCB than with the diuretic. Both groups of patients had the same number of fatal and nonfatal major vascular events (e.g., stroke and myocardial infarction), and the mortality in the two groups was identical. There were significantly more reports of angina pectoris during hospitalization and of nonmajor events and procedures (defined as transient ischemic attacks, dysrhythmia, premature ventricular contractions, aortic valve replacement, or femoral/popliteal bypass grafts), in the CCB group. However, the 95% CI for minor events was quite wide, and the significance was not substantial ($P = .02–.03$ for various events), especially when the multiple comparisons were considered. No test of significance reached the a priori P value of .01 (.00625 after Bonferroni adjustment) that was set for intimal thickening, and because the study was not designed to detect differences in adverse clinical events between the CCB and diuretic groups, no a priori P value was set for these events. Despite these weaknesses, an accompanying editorial suggests that DHP CCBs should be avoided in patients with hypertension and other forms of cardiovascular disease (Chobanian 1996).

The finding of increased coronary risk with CCBs is contradicted by prospective, randomized, controlled trials in patients who already have coronary disease. For example, the Danish Verapamil Infarction Trials (DAVIT I and II) found a statistically significant reduction (by 25%–36%) in the rates of reinfarction and mortality over 6 months in patients taking verapamil compared with placebo beginning within 2 weeks of a myocardial infarction (Hansen 1994; Jespersen 1994; Vaage-Nilsen et al. 1995). On 18-month follow-up of 869 DAVIT II patients, verapamil was associated with significant reductions in relation to placebo in the overall incidence of angina, reinfarction, and mortality (Jespersen et al. 1994). A post hoc analysis of the DAVIT II data indicated that verapamil had the greatest effect in reducing mortality (by 60% over 18 months) in post–myocardial infarction patients with ventricular or atrial tachycardia or fibrillation (Vaage-Nilsen et al. 1995).

In another study of 1,073 patients randomly assigned to groups receiving verapamil or placebo 7–21 days after an acute myocardial infarction, a significant reduction in angina occurred with verapamil, but only a nonsignificant decrease in reinfarction and no reduction in mortality were found (Rengo et al. 1996). Combining data with those of a second prospective trial made the reduction in reinfarction rates reach statistical significance (Rengo et al. 1996).

Although large case-controlled studies can provide suggestive information about the potential risks of new medications like the CCBs, no randomized, controlled trial has supported the hypothesis that CCBs pose a cardiovascular risk to hypertensive patients. Until such evidence emerges, there seems little justification for withholding these drugs, especially in patients who are not hypertensive or who are not vulnerable to coronary steal resulting from medication-induced vasodilatation.

Another recent naturalistic study of geriatric patients, the data of which were reported for all subjects (Pahor et al. 1996a) as well as for hypertensive patients only (Pahor et al. 1996b), raised concerns about the possibility that CCBs might promote cancer in some elderly individuals. Between 1982 and 1983, 10,000 people age 65 years and older received comprehensive interviews that included assessment of the use of various medications, after which they received periodic telephone follow-up and assessment of medical records (Pahor et al. 1996a). Information about whether cancer was diagnosed between the sixth follow-up in 1988 and the seventh follow-up in 1992 was obtained prospectively from Medicare review files of hospital discharges, death certificates, interviews with relatives, and examination of newspaper obituaries and the National Death Index. After excluding patients who had had cancer in 1988 or were not available for thorough follow-up, 5,052 participants were followed up between 1988 and 1992.

Within this subgroup, 420 people were observed to develop cancer, most frequently of the colon, prostate, lung, lymphatics, blood, urinary tract, and breast. Of these patients, 169 died of their cancers (Pahor et al. 1996a). When cancer risk factors such as cigarette smoking and alcohol use were controlled for, investigators found that patients who reported taking CCBs (diltiazem, nifedipine, or verapamil) for any reason at the onset of the original study were more likely to develop cancer than were all other study participants (relative risk = 1.72; $P = .0005$). This association was significant for verapamil and nifedipine but not diltiazem. Use of other antihypertensive agents, nitrates, digoxin, corticosteroids, and anticoagulants was not associated with an increased cancer risk.

In their second analysis, Pahor et al. (1996b) examined the 750 patients (mean age 78 years) in the sample who were taking β-adrenergic blockers, angiotensin-converting enzyme inhibitors, or CCBs for hypertension. Patients taking CCBs were significantly more likely than those taking β-blockers to develop cancer.

Both of these analyses have serious shortcomings. First, because the use of CCBs was assessed only at entry into the study and not throughout the follow-up, it is impossible to state that these medications were taken for a sufficient period to promote carcinogenesis or even that patients were taking CCBs at all in any proximity to the development of cancer. Second, the authors tallied only those cancers that led to hospitalization or death, and given the small number of cancer cases relative to the total sample size, a few unrecognized or outpatient cancers in subjects who were not taking CCBs (as well as a few patients who developed cancer after switching from a CCB to another antihypertensive) would change the results significantly.

The authors (Pahor et al. 1996b) and two editorialists (Alderman 1996; Daling 1996) argued that CCBs could promote cancer by interfering with programmed cell death (apoptosis), an intracellular calcium-dependent process that destroys cancer cells. However, an increase in $[Ca^{2+}]_i$ is also necessary for the proliferation of a number of human cancer cells, including breast cancer, ovarian cancer, and promyelocytic leukemia (Popper and Batra 1993; Saporiti et al. 1995; Taylor and Simpson 1992). In vitro, verapamil inhibits tumor proliferation (Saporiti et al. 1995), and verapamil and diltiazem block the mitogenic action of calcium on human HT-39 breast cancer cells (Taylor and Simpson 1992). When breast cancer cells were transplanted onto athymic mice, amlodipine reduced tumor growth by 106% and verapamil by 68%, and both drugs also significantly reduced tumor size (Taylor and Simpson 1992).

CCBs have also been found to be useful as adjuncts to cancer chemotherapy, albeit by a mechanism unrelated to calcium channel antagonism. Resistance to anticancer drugs is associated with overexpression of a gene called MDRI, which codes for a P glycoprotein that serves as an energy-dependent drug extrusion pump. Although the clinical significance of this observation has been disputed (Harris and Hochhauser 1992), hyperactivity of P glycoprotein increases anticancer drug efflux, reducing intracellular accumulation of the medication (Gupta et al. 1994; Harris and Hochhauser 1992; Pereira et al. 1995). In vitro, verapamil antagonizes P glycoprotein and increases intracellular concentrations of antineoplastic agents (Pereira et al. 1995). Verapamil did not potentiate a 3-day trial of doxorubicin (Adriamycin) in superficial bladder cancer (Tsushima et al. 1994), but this may be because P glycoprotein is not strongly expressed in this type of cancer (Tsushima et al. 1994) or because the overall response rate was too good to show significant improvement with the addition of verapamil. Verapamil has been found to increase the action of tamoxifen against breast cancer in vitro, possibly through an action on an estrogen receptor (Gupta et al. 1994). Only a prospective, randomized trial of a sufficiently large number of patients over a sufficiently long period in which medication use is controlled could provide adequate evidence of a cancer promoting effect of CCBs or any other medication.

DRUG-DRUG INTERACTIONS

Adding CCBs to β-adrenergic blocking agents can depress ventricular function and produce cardiac slowing and atrioventricular block (Murad 1991), whereas additive effects with α-adrenergic blocking agents may produce hypotension (Morris et al. 1992). Verapamil and nitrendipine increase plasma concentrations of digoxin and produce bradycardia, hypotension, or atrioventricular block (Bigger and Hoffman 1991; Gerber and Nies 1991). Pharmacokinetic and pharmacodynamic interactions with other drugs used to treat mania are noted in Table 22–4 (Brodie and MacPhee 1986; Chouza et al. 1986; Dubovsky et al. 1987; Jacobs 1983; Kumana and Mahon 1981; Kupersmith and Slater 1985; MacPhee et al. 1986; Morris et al. 1992; Valdiserri 1985; Weinrauch et al. 1984).

CONCLUSION

Possibly because of the differential interest of pharmaceutical companies in supporting research and educational programs (Dubovsky 1994), the efficacy of the CCBs as alternatives to lithium in the treatment of bipolar affec-

tive disorder has not been as widely appreciated as has that of the anticonvulsants. The CCBs may be particularly useful for patients who cannot tolerate other antimanic drugs, those who have brain damage, and those who are pregnant. The use of these medications in maintenance therapy and in complicated illnesses such as rapid cycling has not been the subject of extended, prospective, double-blind studies, but the same is true of the anticonvulsants. As with the latter medications, clinical experience suggests that combining a CCB with another antimanic drug may be helpful for some treatment-refractory patients, but this application has not been studied formally and has the potential for drug interactions. In view of differences in CCB-binding sites as well as in the pharmacology of the CCBs, it seems likely that different preparations will have different spectra of action, at least in some cases. However, until more research is available, the CCBs should be considered second- or third-line treatments for bipolar illness.

The CCBs were initially studied as antimanic drugs because investigators thought that intracellular Ca^{2+} signaling might be unstable in some patients with bipolar disorders. Patients who have peripheral evidence of increased $[Ca^{2+}]_i$ may be more likely to respond to this class of medication (Dubovsky et al. 1991b), whereas those who do not may have a better response to treatments acting on different signaling mechanisms.

Regardless of the specific clinical uses of the CCBs that will eventually be ascertained, studying them may be one of several new approaches to understanding intracellular mechanisms in mood disorders. As these mechanisms are better understood, treatments that act more specifically on one or another intracellular effector may accompany biological and clinical measurements that predict their efficacy in a given bipolar subtype.

REFERENCES

Alderman MH: More news about calcium antagonists. Am J Hypertens 9:710–712, 1996

Amery WK, Wauquier A, Van Neuten JM, et al: The antimigrainous pharmacology of flunarizine (R14 950), a calcium antagonist. Drugs Exp Clin Res 7:1–10, 1981

Aronson TA, Shukla S, Hirschowitz J: Clonazepam treatment of five lithium-refractory patients with bipolar disorder. Am J Psychiatry 146:77–80, 1989

Avissar S, Schreiber G: The involvement of guanine nucleotide binding proteins in the pathogenesis and treatment of affective disorders. Biol Psychiatry 31:435–459, 1992

Barton BM, Gitlin MJ: Verapamil in treatment-resistant mania: an open trial. J Clin Psychopharmacol 7:101–103, 1987

Table 22–4. Some calcium channel blocker interactions

Drug	Interaction effects
Lithium	Neurotoxicity
	Choreoathetosis
	Parkinsonism
	Cardiac slowing
	Decreased lithium levels (?)
Carbamazepine	Increased carbamazepine levels
	Neurotoxicity
Neuroleptics	Increased parkinsonism

Benet LZ, Williams RL: Design and optimization of dosage regimens: pharmacokinetic data, in Goodman and Gilman's The Pharmacological Basis of Therapeutics, 8th Edition. Edited by Gilman AG, Rall TW, Nies AS, et al. New York, Pergamon, 1991, pp 1650–1735

Benet LZ, Mitchell JR, Sheiner LB: Pharmacokinetics: the dynamics of drug absorption, distribution, and elimination, in Goodman and Gilman's The Pharmacological Basis of Therapeutics, 8th Edition. Edited by Gilman AG, Rall TW, Nies AS, et al. New York, Pergamon, 1991, pp 3–32

Bergamaschi S, Trabucchi M, Battaini F, et al: Modulation of dihydropyridine-sensitive calcium channels: a role for G proteins. Eur Neurol 30 (suppl 2):16–20, 1990

Bigger JT, Hoffman BF: Antiarrhythmic drugs, in Goodman and Gilman's The Pharmacological Basis of Therapeutics, 8th Edition. Edited by Gilman AG, Rall TW, Nies AS, et al. New York, Pergamon, 1991, pp 840–873

Borhani NO, Mercuri M, Borhani PA, et al: Final outcome results of the multicenter isradipine diuretic atherosclerosis study (MIDAS): a randomized controlled trial. JAMA 276:785–792, 1996

Brodie MJ, MacPhee GJA: Carbamazepine neurotoxicity precipitated by diltiazem. BMJ 292:1170–1171, 1986

Brotman AW, Farhadi AM, Gelenberg AJ: Verapamil treatment of acute mania. J Clin Psychiatry 47:136–138, 1986

Brown AS, Mallinger AG, Renbaum LC: Elevated platelet membrane phosphatidylinositol-4,5-biphosphate in bipolar mania. Am J Psychiatry 150:1252–1254, 1993

Brunet G, Cerlich B, Robert P, et al: Open trial of a calcium antagonist, nimodipine, in acute mania. Clin Neuropharmacol 13:224–228, 1990

Buring JE, Glynn RJ, Hennekens C: Calcium channel blockers and myocardial infarction: a hypothesis formulated but not yet tested. JAMA 274:654–655, 1995

Byerly WG, Hartmann A, Foster DE, et al: Verapamil in the treatment of maternal paroxysmal supraventricular tachycardia. Ann Emerg Med 20:552–554, 1991

Caillard V: Treatment of mania using a calcium antagonist—preliminary trial. Neuropsychobiology 14:23–26, 1985

Carbonne B, Jannet D, Touboul C, et al: Nicardipine treatment of hypertension during pregnancy. Obstet Gynecol 81:908–914, 1993

Carman JS, Wyatt RJ: Calcium: pacesetting the periodic psychoses. Am J Psychiatry 136:1035–1039, 1979

Chobanian AV: Calcium channel blockers: lessons learned from MIDAS and other clinical trials. JAMA 276:829–830, 1996

Chouza C, Scaramelli A, Carmano JL, et al: Parkinsonism, tardive dyskinesia, akathisia and depression induced by flunarizine. Lancet 1:1303–1304, 1986

Clary C, Schweizer E: Treatment of MAOI hypertensive crisis with sublingual nifedipine. J Clin Psychiatry 48:249–250, 1987

Cohan SL: Pharmacology of calcium antagonists: clinical relevance in neurology. Eur Neurol 30 (suppl 2):28–30, 1990

Daling JR: Calcium channel blockers and cancer: is an association biologically plausible? Am J Hypertens 9:713–714, 1996

Deicken RF: Verapamil treatment of bipolar depression (letter). J Clin Psychopharmacol 10:148–149, 1990

Doran AR, Narang PK, Meigs CY, et al: Verapamil concentrations in cerebrospinal fluid after oral administration (letter). N Engl J Med 312:1261–1262, 1985

Dubovsky SL: Calcium antagonists in manic-depressive illness. Neuropsychobiology 27:184–192, 1993

Dubovsky SL: Why don't we hear more about the calcium antagonists? Biol Psychiatry 35:149–150, 1994

Dubovsky SL, Franks RD: Intracellular calcium ions in affective disorders: a review and an hypothesis. Biol Psychiatry 18:781–797, 1983

Dubovsky SL, Franks RD, Lifschitz M, et al: Effectiveness of verapamil in the treatment of a manic patient. Am J Psychiatry 139:502–504, 1982

Dubovsky SL, Franks RD, Allen S, et al: Calcium antagonists in mania: a double-blind study of verapamil. Psychiatry Res 18:309–320, 1986

Dubovsky SL, Franks RD, Allen S: Verapamil: a new antimanic drug with potential interactions with lithium. J Clin Psychiatry 48:371–372, 1987

Dubovsky SL, Christiano J, Daniell LC, et al: Increased platelet intracellular calcium concentration in patients with bipolar affective disorders. Arch Gen Psychiatry 46:632–638, 1989

Dubovsky SL, Lee C, Christiano J, et al: Elevated intracellular calcium ion concentration in bipolar depression. Biol Psychiatry 29:441–450, 1991a

Dubovsky SL, Lee C, Christiano J, et al: Lithium decreases platelet intracellular calcium ion concentrations in bipolar patients. Lithium 2:167–174, 1991b

Dubovsky SL, Murphy J, Christiano J, et al: The calcium second messenger system in bipolar disorders: data supporting new research directions. J Neuropsychiatry Clin Neurosci 4:3–14, 1992a

Dubovsky SL, Murphy J, Thomas M, et al: Abnormal intracellular calcium ion concentration in platelets and lymphocytes in bipolar patients. Am J Psychiatry 149:118–120, 1992b

Eccleston D, Cole AJ: Calcium-channel blockade and depressive illness. Br J Psychiatry 156:889–891, 1990

Fleckenstein JA, Kammermeier H, Doring H, et al: Zum Wirkungs-Mechanismus neurartiger Koronardilatatoren mit gleichzeitig Sauerstoff-einsparenden, myokard-Effekten, Prenylamin und Iproveratril. Zeitschrift für Kreislaufforschung 56:716–744, 1967

Fox AP, Hirning LD, Mogul DJ, et al: Modulation of calcium channels by neurotransmitters, hormones and second messengers, in Calcium Channels: Their Properties, Functions, Regulation, and Clinical Relevance. Edited by Hurwitz L, Partridge LD, Leach JK. Boca Raton, FL, CRC Press, 1991, pp 251–263

Freedman DD, Waters DD: "Second generation" dihydropyridine calcium antagonists: greater vascular selectivity and some unique applications. Drugs 34:578–598, 1987

Furberg CD, Psaty BM, Meyer JV: Nifedipine: dose-related increase in mortality in patients with coronary heart disease. Circulation 92:1326–1331, 1995

Garza-Trevino ES, Overall JE, Hollister LE: Verapamil versus lithium in acute mania. Am J Psychiatry 149:121–122, 1992

Gerber JS, Nies AS: Antihypertensive agents and the drug therapy of hypertension, in Goodman and Gilman's The Pharmacological Basis of Therapeutics, 8th Edition. Edited by Gilman AG, Rall TW, Nies AS, et al. New York, Pergamon, 1991, pp 784–813

Gitlin MJ, Weiss J: Verapamil as maintenance treatment in bipolar illness: a case report. J Clin Psychopharmacol 4:341–343, 1984

Goodnick PJ: Verapamil prophylaxis in pregnant women with bipolar disorder (letter). Am J Psychiatry 150:1560, 1993

Grebb JA, Shelton RC, Taylor EH, et al: A negative, double-blind placebo-controlled clinical trial of verapamil in chronic schizophrenia. Biol Psychiatry 21:691–694, 1986

Greil W, Steber R, van Calker D: The agonist-stimulated accumulation of inositol phosphates is attenuated in neutrophils from male patients under chronic lithium therapy. Biol Psychiatry 30:443–451, 1991

Gupta V, Kamath N, Tkalcevic GT, et al: Potentiation of tamoxifen activity by verapamil in a human breast cancer cell line. Biochem Pharmacol 47:1701–1704, 1994

Hansen JF: Review of postinfarct treatment with verapamil: combined experience of early and late intervention studies with verapamil in patients with acute myocardial infarction. Danish Study Group on Verapamil in Myocardial Infarction. Cardiovasc Drugs Ther 8 (suppl 3):543–547, 1994

Harris AL, Hochhauser D: Mechanisms of multidrug resistance in cancer treatment. Acta Oncologica 31:205–213, 1992

Hoschl C, Kozemy J: Verapamil in affective disorders: a controlled, double-blind study. Biol Psychiatry 25:128–140, 1989

Hoschl C, Blahos J, Kabes J: The use of calcium channel blockers in psychiatry, in Biological Psychiatry, 1985. Edited by Shagass CE, Josiassen RC, Bridger WH, et al. New York, Elsevier, 1986, pp 330–332

Ikeda M, Dewar D, McCulloch J: A correlative study of calcium channel antagonist binding and local neuropathological features in the hippocampus in Alzheimer's disease. Brain Res 589:313–319, 1992

Jacobs MB: Diltiazem and akathisia. Ann Intern Med 99: 794–795, 1983

Jacobsen FM, Sack DA, James SP: Delirium induced by verapamil (letter). Am J Psychiatry 144:248, 1987

Jacques RM, Cox SJ: Verapamil in major (psychotic) depression. Br J Psychiatry 158:124–125, 1991

Janis RA, Triggle DJ: Drugs acting on calcium channels, in Calcium Channels: Their Properties, Functions, Regulation, and Clinical Relevance. Edited by Hurwitz L, Partridge LD, Leach JK. Boca Raton, FL, CRC Press, 1991, pp 195–249

Jespersen CM: Role of ischemia in postinfarction heart failure: hypothetical considerations based on use of verapamil in the DAVIT II Study. Danish Study Group on Verapamil in Myocardial Infarction. Cardiovasc Drugs Ther 8:823–828, 1994

Jespersen CM, Hansen JF, Mortensen LS: The prognostic significance of post-infarction angina pectoris and the effect of verapamil on the incidence of angina pectoris and prognosis. The Danish Study Group on Verapamil in Myocardial Infarction. Eur Heart J 15:270–276, 1994

Kennedy S, Ozersky S, Robillard M: Refractory bipolar illness may not respond to verapamil (letter). J Clin Psychopharmacol 6:316–317, 1986

Kenny BA, Kilpatrick AT, Spedding M: Quantification of the affinity of drugs acting at the calcium channel, in Cellular Calcium: A Practical Approach. Edited by McCormack JG, Cobbold PH. Oxford, England, IRL Press, 1991, pp 267–282

Kim KE: Comparative clinical pharmacology of calcium channel blockers. Am Fam Physician 43:583–588, 1991

Klein E, Uhde TW: Controlled study of verapamil for treatment of panic disorder. Am J Psychiatry 145:431–434, 1988

Kumana CR, Mahon WA: Bizarre perceptual disorder of extremities in patients taking verapamil (letter). Lancet 1:1324–1325, 1981

Kupersmith J, Slater W: Calcium channel blockers: pharmacologic basis for therapeutic properties. Hospital Formulary 20:184–195, 1985

Leys D, Vermersch P, Daniel T, et al: Diltiazem for tardive dyskinesia. Lancet 1:250–251, 1988

Lichtlen PR, Hugenholz PG, Rafflenbeul W: Retardation of angiographic progression of coronary artery disease by nifedipine: results of International Nifedipine Trial on Antiatherosclerotic Therapy. Lancet 335:1109–1113, 1990

Lindelius R, Nilsson CG: Flunarizine as maintenance treatment of a patient with bipolar disorder (letter). Am J Psychiatry 149:139, 1992

Litzinger M, Nelson PG, Pun RYK: Does nitrendipine block calcium channels in mammalian neurons? Implications for treatment of ischemic cell death. Neurology 35 (suppl 1):141, 1985

MacPhee G, McInnes GT, Thompson G, et al: Verapamil potentiates carbamazepine neurotoxicity: a clinically important inhibitory interaction. Lancet 1:700–703, 1986

Manna V: Disturbi affettivi bipolari e ruolo del calcio intraneuronale: effetti terapeutici del trattamento con sali di litio e/o calcio antagonista in pazienti con rapida inversione di polarita [Bipolar affective disorders and the role of intracellular calcium: therapeutic effects of treatment with lithium salts and/or calcium antagonists in patients with rapid cycling]. Minerva Med 82:757–763, 1991

Materson BJ: Calcium channel blockers: is it time to split the lump? Am J Hypertens 8:325–329, 1995

Mauritson DR, Winniford MD, Walker WS, et al: Oral verapamil for paroxysmal supraventricular tachycardia: a long-term double blind randomized trial. Ann Intern Med 96:409–412, 1982

Messing RO, Carpenter CL, Greenberg DA: Mechanism of calcium channel inhibition by phenytoin: comparison with classical calcium channel antagonists. J Pharmacol Exp Ther 235:407–411, 1985

Mogilnicka E, Czyzak A, Maj J: Dihydropyridine calcium channel antagonists reduce immobility in the mouse behavioral despair test; antidepressants facilitate nifedipine action. Eur J Pharmacol 138:413–416, 1987

Morris AD, Meredith PA, Reid JL: Pharmacokinetics of calcium antagonists: implications for therapy, in Calcium Antagonists in Clinical Medicine. Edited by Epstein M. Philadelphia, PA, Hanley & Belfus, 1992, pp 49–67

Murad F: Drugs used for the treatment of angina: organic nitrates, calcium-channel blockers, and β-adrenergic agents, in Goodman and Gilman's The Pharmacological Basis of Therapeutics, 8th Edition. Edited by Gilman AG, Rall TW, Nies AS, et al. New York, Pergamon, 1991, pp 764–783

Mussini M, Agricola R, Moia GC, et al: A preliminary study on the use of calcitonin in clinical psychopathology. J Int Med Res 12:23–29, 1984

Nayler WG: Cardioprotective aspects of calcium antagonists. J Cardiovasc Pharmacol 18 (suppl 6):S10–S14, 1991

Nayler WG: New trends in calcium antagonism: are they meaningful? Am J Hypertens 7:1265–1305, 1994

Overall JE, Gorham DR: The Brief Psychiatric Rating Scale. Psychol Rep 10:799–812, 1962

Pahor M, Guralnik JM, Ferrucci L, et al: Calcium-channel blockade and incidence of cancer in aged populations. Lancet 348:493–498, 1996a

Pahor M, Guralnik JM, Salive ME, et al: Do calcium channel blockers increase the risk of cancer? Am J Hypertens 9:695–699, 1996b

Pazzaglia PJ, Post RM, Ketter TA, et al: Preliminary controlled trial of nimodipine in ultra-rapid cycling affective dysregulation. Psychiatry Res 49:257–272, 1993

Pereira E, Teodori E, Dei S, et al: Reversal of multidrug resistance by verapamil analogues. Biochem Pharmacol 50(4):451–457, 1995

Pickar D, Wolkowitz O, Doran A: Clinical and biochemical effects of verapamil administration to schizophrenic patients. Arch Gen Psychiatry 44:113–119, 1987

Pollack MH, Rosenbaum JF: Verapamil in the treatment of recurrent unipolar depression. Biol Psychiatry 22:779–782, 1987

Popper LD, Batra S: Calcium mobilization and cell proliferation activated by extracellular ATP in human ovarian tumour cells. Cell Calcium 14:209–218,1993

Post RM: Approaches to treatment-resistant bipolar affectively ill patients. Clin Neuropharmacol 11:93–104, 1988

Post RM, Ketter TA, Pazzaglia PJ, et al: New developments in the use of anticonvulsants as mood stabilizers. Neuropsychobiology 27:132–137, 1993

Prien RF, Gelenberg AJ: Alternatives to lithium for preventive treatment of bipolar disorder. Am J Psychiatry 146:840–848, 1989

Psaty BM, Heckbert SR, Koepsell TD, et al: The risk of myocardial infarction associated with antihypertensive drug therapies. JAMA 274:620–625, 1995

Reiter S, Adler R, Angrist B: Effect of verapamil on tardive dyskinesia and psychosis in schizophrenic patients. J Clin Psychiatry 50:26–27, 1989

Rengo F, Carbonin P, Pahor M, et al: A controlled trial of verapamil in patients after acute myocardial infarction: results of the calcium antagonist reinfarction Italian study (CRIS). Am J Cardiol 77:365–369, 1996

Rosenberg GA: Calcium channel blockers in neurological disorders, in Calcium Channels: Their Properties, Functions, Regulation, and Clinical Relevance. Edited by Hurwitz L, Partridge LD, Leach JK. Boca Raton, FL, CRC Press, 1991, pp 377–384

Santillan R, Maestre JM, Hurle MA, et al: Enhancement of opiate analgesia by nimodipine in cancer patients chronically treated with morphine: a preliminary report. Pain 58:129–132, 1994

Saporiti A, Brocchieri A, Porta C, et al: Effect of different platelet agonists on intracellular free Ca++ concentrations in human tumor cells: possible role in tumor growth. Int J Cancer 62:291–296, 1995

Schirrmacher K, Mayer A, Walden J, et al: Effects of carbamazepine on action potentials and calcium currents in rat spinal ganglion cells in vitro. Neuropsychobiology 27:176–179, 1993

Siesjo BK: Calcium in the brain under physiological and pathological conditions. Eur Neurol 30 (suppl 2):3–9, 1990

Solomon L, Williamson P: Verapamil in bipolar illness. Can J Psychiatry 31:442–444, 1986

Tan CH, Javors MA, Seleshi E, et al: Effects of lithium on platelet ionic intracellular calcium concentration in patients with bipolar (manic-depressive) disorder and healthy controls. Life Sci 46:1175–1180, 1990

Taylor JM, Simpson RU: Inhibition of cancer cell growth by calcium channel antagonists in the athymic mouse. Cancer Res 52:2413–2418, 1992

Triggle DJ: Biochemical and pharmacologic differences among calcium channel antagonists: clinical implications, in Calcium Antagonists in Clinical Medicine. Edited by Epstein M. Philadelphia, PA, Hanley & Belfus, 1992, pp 1–27

Tsushima T, Ohmori H, Ohi Y, et al: Intravesical instillation chemotherapy of adriamycin with or without verapamil for the treatment of superficial bladder cancer: the final results of a collaborative randomized trial. Cancer Chemother Pharmacol 35 (suppl):S69–S75, 1994

Uhr SB, Jackson K, Berger PA: Effects of verapamil administration on negative symptoms of chronic schizophrenia. Psychiatry Res 23:351–352, 1988

Ulmsten U, Anderson KE, Wingerup I: Treatment of premature labor with the calcium antagonist nifedipine. Arch Gynecol 229:1–5, 1980

Vaage-Nilsen M, Hansen JF, Hagerup L, et al: Effect of verapamil on the prognosis of patients with early postinfarction electrical or mechanical complications. The Danish Verapamil Infarction Trial II (DAVIT II). Int J Cardiol 48:255–258, 1995

Valdiserri EV: A possible interaction between lithium and diltiazem: case report. J Clin Psychiatry 46:540–541, 1985

van Calker D, Forstner U, Bohus M, et al: Increased sensitivity to agonist stimulation of the Ca^{2+} response in neutrophils of manic-depressive patients: effect of lithium therapy. Neuropsychobiology 27:180–183, 1993

Walden J, Grunze H, Bingmann D, et al: Calcium antagonistic effects of carbamazepine as a mechanism of action in neuropsychiatric disorders: studies in calcium dependent model epilepsies. Eur Neuropsychopharmacol 2:455–462, 1992

Walsh TL, Lavenstein B, Licamele WL, et al: Calcium antagonists in the treatment of Tourette's disorder. Am J Psychiatry 143:1467–1468, 1986

Wehr T, Sack D, Rosenthal N, et al: Rapid cycling affective disorder: contributing factors and treatment responses in 51 patients. Am J Psychiatry 145:179–184, 1988

Weinrauch LA, Belok S, D'Elia JA: Decreased serum lithium during verapamil therapy. Am Heart J 108:1378–1380, 1984

Wide-Swensson DG, Ingemarsson I, Lunell N, et al: Calcium channel blockade (isradipine) in treatment of hypertension in pregnancy: a randomized placebo-controlled study. Am J Obstet Gynecol 173:872–878, 1996

Yamawaki S, Yanagawa K: Possible central effect of dantrolene sodium in neuroleptic malignant syndrome. J Clin Psychopharmacol 6:378–379, 1986

Zernig G: Photoaffinity labeling of the partially purified mitochondrial phenylalkylamine calcium antagonist receptor. Mol Pharmacol 42:1010–1013, 1992

Other Agents

TWENTY-THREE

Cognitive Enhancers

Deborah B. Marin, M.D., and Kenneth L. Davis, M.D.

Identification of neurotransmitter deficits in the brains of patients with Alzheimer's disease (AD) has fostered the development of pharmacological strategies to alleviate these deficits (Davies and Maloney 1976). Consistent demonstration of central cholinergic depletion in patients with AD, in conjunction with the cholinergic system's involvement in learning, generated many studies that focused on cholinergic enhancement. Although the cholinergic approach has yielded some promising findings, the results to date have not revealed a consistently robust treatment for the cognitive disturbances seen in patients with AD (Chatellier and Lacomblez 1990; Davis et al. 1992; Farlow et al. 1992; Tariot et al. 1987a). It can be hypothesized that the variable results with the cholinergic replacement strategy in AD may be due in part to deficiencies in other neurotransmitters. If so, correction of deficits in multiple neurotransmitters would be expected to be more efficacious than a purely cholinergic approach.

An alternative to the palliative treatment of AD with neurotransmitter replacement strategies is the development of treatments that could slow the neurodegenerative process of AD and consequent cognitive decline. In this chapter, we review the cholinergic and combined neurotransmitter approaches and discuss strategies designed to modify the course of AD through their presumed alteration of the fundamental pathophysiological processes in the disease.

CHOLINERGIC AGENTS

Multiple lines of evidence support a critical role for cholinergic mechanisms in AD, including the following:

1. Centrally active anticholinergic agents produce cognitive deficits in humans (Drachman and Leavitt 1974; Dundee and Pandit 1972).
2. Cholinergic neurotransmission modulates memory and learning (Deutsch 1971).
3. Lesions of the central cholinergic system create learning and memory impairments that can be reversed with cholinomimetic administration (Bartus et al. 1987; Collerton 1986; Olton and Wenk 1987).
4. Postmortem studies of patients with AD document cholinergic cell loss in the septum and nucleus basalis of Meynert, decreased concentrations of choline acetyltransferase and acetylcholinesterase, and a correlation between these changes and degree of cognitive impairment (Davies and Maloney 1976; Perry et al. 1978).

Improvement of the overall functioning of the central cholinergic system could theoretically result from prevention of neuronal degeneration, increasing acetylcholine availability, and activation of postsynaptic cholinergic receptors. Of the several possible methods that could achieve these goals, three strategies have been clinically used: acetylcholine precursors, cholinesterase inhibitors, and postsynaptic agonists.

It has been reasoned that enhancing the availability of acetylcholine precursors could increase acetylcholine synthesis, thereby providing an increased pool of neurotransmitter for cholinergic transmission. Acetylcholine precursor treatments with choline or lecithin represented early attempts to enhance cholinergic transmission in AD. Because the choline uptake system is saturated under normal conditions, increases in extracellular choline will not enhance acetylcholine synthesis or release. Nonetheless, increased extracellular choline availability may be beneficial during intense cholinergic activity and greater demand for precursor. Acetylcholine precursor therapy could therefore enhance cognitive performance in patients with AD if amounts of acetylcholine precursor are insufficient. However, little evidence supports the efficacy of the precursor loading approach (for review, see Bartus et al. 1985).

Cholinesterase Inhibitors

Physostigmine

History and discovery.   The use of physostigmine and other cholinesterase inhibitors is based on the goal of enhancing cholinergic neurotransmission through inhibiting the breakdown of acetylcholine.

Structure.   Physostigmine is a natural alkaloid that contains a tertiary amine.

Pharmacological profile.   Physostigmine is a reversible anticholinesterase that effectively increases the concentration of acetylcholine at the sites of cholinergic transmission.

Pharmacokinetics and disposition.   Physostigmine is absorbed in the gastrointestinal tract, subcutaneous tissue, and mucous membranes. It is hydrolyzed and inactivated within 2 hours, thus requiring multiple doses each day. Physostigmine readily crosses the blood-brain barrier.

Mechanism of action.   Physostigmine enhances cholinergic transmission through its increasing acetylcholine availability in the central nervous system (CNS).

Indications.   Most studies in which physostigmine is administered parenterally have reported transient cognitive improvement in at least a subgroup of patients with AD (Mohs and Davis 1987). Oral administration of the compound has also been shown to have some efficacy. Some have speculated that long-term treatment with physostigmine may delay deterioration in patients with AD. Two studies with small patient samples suggest that long-term treatment with the medication may attenuate the course of cognitive decline (Beller et al. 1988; Jenike et al. 1990).

The limited efficacy of physostigmine may reflect the biological heterogeneity of patients and the pharmacological properties of the medication. There is significant interindividual variability in the gastrointestinal absorption, hepatic catabolism, hydrolysis, and CNS penetration of this compound (Whelpton and Hurst 1985). The unpredictable concentrations in blood (and therefore in the CNS) that are achieved with a given dose necessitate individual titration of medication dosing. The peripheral-to-brain partitioning of physostigmine also hampers its clinical utility. Blood levels required to achieve CNS concentrations necessary for cognitive enhancement may be associated with significant adverse effects, including gastrointestinal distress, hypotension, and bradycardia. Therefore, ineffective CNS penetration may have led to the lack of response in some patients tested with this drug. Novel drug delivery systems that overcome the blood-brain barrier problem have yet to be systematically tested. The medication's short half-life is also problematic because this characteristic causes continuous fluctuations in blood levels. Because of the inverted-∪-shaped dose-response curve observed with physostigmine, nonoptimal blood levels could also limit the beneficial effects observed with this agent.

Side effects.   The side effects observed with physostigmine include depressed mood, anxiety, salivation, bradycardia, and gastrointestinal distress.

Drug-drug interactions.   Physostigmine has been used primarily as a single agent for treating AD. As we describe later in this chapter, physostigmine has been shown to be safely administered in conjunction with selegiline (L-deprenyl).

Tetrahydroaminoacridine

History and discovery.   Two pilot studies in patients with a diagnosis of AD suggested that 9-amino-1,2,3,4,-tetrahydroacridine (THA), administered alone or in combination with lecithin, was associated with improvement in performances on psychometric tests and global assessments (Kaye et al. 1982; Summers et al. 1981). Summers et al. (1986) documented significant improvement in global status and psychometric performance in 16 subjects treated with THA. These earlier studies led to several multicenter trials to evaluate the efficacy of THA in patients with AD.

Structure. THA is an aminoacridine compound that is a reversible synthetic acetylcholinesterase inhibitor. It has an empirical formula of $C_{13}H_{14}N_2 \times HCl \times H_2O$.

Pharmacological profile. In vitro studies indicate that THA inhibits plasma and tissue acetylcholinesterase (Adem 1992). Unlike physostigmine, which interacts with the catalytic site of acetylcholinesterase, THA produces allosteric inhibition by binding to a hydrophobic region on the active surface of the enzyme (Adem 1992). THA has also been shown to interact with muscarinic and nicotinic receptors (Adem 1992). THA increases presynaptic acetylcholine release by blocking slow potassium channels and increases postsynaptic monoaminergic stimulation by interfering with the uptake of noradrenaline and serotonin (Drukarch et al. 1987, 1988). These latter characteristics of THA occur at concentrations higher than those required for acetylcholinesterase inhibition and therefore probably do not contribute to the drug's clinical effects.

Pharmacokinetics and disposition. THA is rapidly absorbed after oral administration; maximum concentrations in plasma are reached within 1–2 hours. THA is about 55% bound by plasma proteins and is metabolized by the cytochrome P450 system to multiple metabolites. After aromatic ring hydroxylation, the metabolites of THA undergo glucuronidation. The elimination half-life is 2–4 hours. THA is concentrated 10-fold in the brain, in part because of its high lipid solubility (Nielsen et al. 1989).

Mechanism of action. THA enhances cholinergic transmission through its increasing acetylcholine availability in the CNS.

Indications. Several double-blind, placebo-controlled studies have assessed the therapeutic efficacy of THA in larger patient samples. THA and lecithin administration produced minimal cognitive improvement in a study of 67 subjects (Chatellier and Lacomblez 1990). Statistically significant improvement was shown in Mini-Mental State Exam scores (Folstein et al. 1975) in another investigation of 39 patients (Gauthier et al. 1990). In a 6-week crossover trial, using an enriched-population design with 215 patients, Davis et al. (1992) found that the THA-treated group had significantly less decline in cognitive function than did the placebo-treated group, as assessed by the cognitive subscale of the Alzheimer's Disease Assessment Scale (ADAS-cog; Rosen et al. 1984). A 12-week parallel-group design study of 273 patients reported a significant dose-related improvement in cognition with THA treatment (Farlow et al. 1992). A double-blind, crossover study of 89 subjects showed that THA was superior to placebo in its effect on Mini-Mental State Exam scores (Sahakian and Coull 1993). A 30-week, double-blind, placebo-controlled, parallel-group trial with 653 patients showed the efficacy of THA when compared with placebo, and significant dose-response trends favored higher doses of the compound (Knapp et al. 1994).

In reviewing THA's efficacy, the different doses used across studies must be considered. Efficacy does seem to be dose dependent, and many of the early studies used low doses of the medication. The outcome measures used to assess medication response also must be considered. For example, use of the Clinical Global Assessment Scale (Guy 1976) does not necessarily identify whether improvement with THA was the result of cognitive enhancement (Davis et al. 1992; Farlow et al. 1992). Different methods of administration of the Clinical Global Assessment Scale could also lead to discrepant results (Davis et al. 1992; Farlow et al. 1992).

Side effects and toxicology. Side effects most often associated with THA include nausea, abdominal distress, tachycardia, and liver toxicity. Despite earlier reports of significant hepatic toxicity, THA is relatively safe (Summers et al. 1989). Hepatic toxicity is dose dependent and reversible.

Drug-drug interactions. Because THA undergoes extensive hepatic metabolism by the P450 system, drug-drug interactions may occur when this agent is given concurrently with others that undergo extensive metabolism through cytochrome P450. Coadministration of THA with theophylline has been shown to double theophylline's elimination half-life and plasma concentration.

Velnacrine

History and discovery. Velnacrine (HP 029) is a cholinesterase inhibitor for the treatment of AD. Animal studies determined that velnacrine significantly enhances long-term potentiation (considered an electrophysiological model for memory formation within the hippocampus) (Tanaka et al. 1989). The drug reverses scopolamine- or lesion-induced memory impairment in rodents

(Fielding et al. 1989). Velnacrine has been shown to ameliorate the decline in short-term memory associated with aging in nonhuman primates (Jackson et al. 1995).

Structure.   Velnacrine maleate is the maleate salt of an alcohol derivative of THA (Puri et al. 1990).

Pharmacological profile.   Velnacrine inhibits both true cholinesterase and pseudocholinesterase and does not cause release of acetylcholine or act as a muscarinic agonist.

Pharmacokinetics and disposition.   Velnacrine is well absorbed after oral administration. Mean peak plasma levels are attained 0.75–1.2 hours after dosing. The mean half-life range is 1.6–2.0 hours. Most of the drug is conjugated before excretion (Puri et al. 1990).

Indications.   Patients with AD show marked intersubject variability in drug tolerance within the therapeutic dose range of velnacrine (Cutler et al. 1990). Double-blind, placebo-controlled studies have reported modest clinical improvement in patients with AD (Antuono 1995; Clipp and Moore 1995; Murphy et al. 1991; Zemlan et al. 1996). A 6-week dose-ranging study revealed that subjects who received velnacrine scored significantly better than placebo on the ADAS-cog (Zemlan et al. 1996). A 24-week dose-ranging study that included 301 patients with AD found that the cognitive scores of the placebo-treated group deteriorated significantly more than those of the active medication group, and the results were dose dependent (Antuono 1995).

Side effects and toxicology.   Side effects of velnacrine include dizziness, diarrhea, and headache. Reversible liver toxicity is observed in a dose-dependent manner with this compound (Murphy et al. 1991).

Drug-drug interactions.   No specific drug-drug interactions have been observed with velnacrine, which is still undergoing clinical evaluation.

Donepezil

History and discovery.   Donepezil (E2020) is a cholinesterase inhibitor that has been developed for the treatment of AD.

Structure.   The chemical structure for donepezil is (*R,S*)-1-benzyl-4[(5,6-dimethoxy-1-indanon)-2-yl]methyl-piperidine hydrochloride (Ohnishi et al. 1993).

Pharmacological profile.   Donepezil inhibits acetylcholinesterase in a mixed competitive-noncompetitive manner (Galli et al. 1994). Donepezil produces dose-dependent increases in extracellular acetylcholine concentration in the brain (Kawashima et al. 1994).

Pharmacokinetics and disposition.   Donepezil is well absorbed after oral administration. In elderly subjects, the mean time to maximum peak plasma concentration is 5.2 ± 2.8 hours, and the mean half-life is 103.8 ± 40.6 hours (Mihara et al. 1993; Ohnishi et al. 1993). The time to maximum plasma concentration and the half-life both increase with age (Ohnishi et al. 1993). The inhibitor dissociation constant for donepezil is lower than that for THA (Nochi et al. 1995). Donepezil is mainly metabolized by the liver (Ohnishi et al. 1993).

Indications.   A 12-week double-blind, placebo-controlled study with 161 patients demonstrated cognitive improvement on the ADAS-cog in individuals treated with 5 mg/day of donepezil.

Side effects and toxicology.   In healthy elderly subjects, single oral dosing of the compound was tolerated (Ohnishi et al. 1993). Donepezil is not associated with liver toxicity in subjects with AD (S. L. Rogers et al. 1996).

Drug-drug interactions.   No specific drug-drug interactions have been observed with donepezil.

Galanthamine

History and discovery.   Galanthamine has been used clinically since the early 1960s in the treatment of paresis, paralysis, and myasthenia gravis (Mihailova et al. 1989). It has also been shown to reverse spatial memory deficits in hypocholinergic mice (Sweeney et al. 1988).

Structure.   Galanthamine is a tertiary amine of the phenthrene group.

Pharmacological profile.   Galanthamine is a potent inhibitor of acetylcholinesterase. In vivo, maximal inhibition of acetylcholinesterase is approached 30 minutes after oral administration (Thomsen et al. 1990).

Pharmacokinetics and disposition.   Galanthamine is rapidly absorbed after oral administration. Cerebral concentrations that are three times higher than its plasma level are observed after its administration. Galanthamine's half-life of 7 hours is longer than that of THA or physostigmine (Thomsen et al. 1990). Metabolites include epigalanthamine and galanthaminone (Mihailova et al. 1989).

Indications. Eighteen patients with possible AD who received galanthamine for up to 6 months showed no statistically significant improvement on neuropsychological measures (Dal-Bianco et al. 1991).

Side effects and toxicology. Administration of galanthamine has been associated with agitation, sleeplessness, and irritability (Thomsen et al. 1990).

Summary

Several methodological issues must be considered in interpreting studies of cholinesterase inhibitors. Intersubject variability in bioavailability and inadequate dosing could attenuate response patterns. For example, a given dosing regimen may be less than optimal for one patient yet therapeutic for another. Crossover designs may include carryover effects that detract from a drug's effect in comparison with placebo. Repeated assessments lead to learning effects that can erroneously inflate a patient's response to medication and can produce carryover effects on discontinuation of the drug. A perfect test would be free of such effects and would involve multiple ways of asking the relevant questions. Most outcome measures used in therapeutic trials assess memory, yet AD is also a disease of learning. Finally, another problem is the shifting baseline resulting from the progression of the severity of AD. The longer the study, the more this becomes a factor that needs to be addressed. Overall, double-blind, placebo-controlled studies suggest some therapeutic efficacy with these agents. These findings suggest that anticholinesterase therapy is likely to benefit a subgroup of patients with AD.

Cholinergic Agonists

The use of muscarinic agonists for cognitive enhancement is supported by their beneficial effects on memory and learning in hypocholinergic animals (Haroutunian et al. 1985). The use of postsynaptic agonists is of interest because of the observed depletion of presynaptic (M2) receptors in conjunction with the relative preservation of postsynaptic (M1) sites in AD (Whitehouse and Kellar 1987).

Significant advances have been made in identifying muscarinic receptor subtypes. Research using molecular biology techniques has identified the presence of five mus-

carinic receptor subtypes, m1 through m5 (Ashkenazi et al. 1989; Birdsall et al. 1989; Bonner 1989; Bonner et al. 1987; Fukada et al. 1989). Studies with pharmacological antagonists have identified three classes of muscarinic receptors, M1, M2, and M3. The m1–m5 and M1–M3 systems overlap. Activation of the m1, m3, and m5 receptors causes cellular excitation, whereas activation of the m2 and m4 subtypes produces inhibitory effects (Ashkenazi et al. 1989; Bonner 1989). Although the exact locations of the m1–m5 receptors are not known, the distribution of messenger ribonucleic acid (mRNA) for these sites has been determined (Buckley et al. 1988). For example, most mRNA located in the cerebral cortex and hippocampus is for m1 and m3 receptors, making these sites potentially the most important for the pharmacological enhancement of cognition.

Although muscarinic receptors play a significant role in memory, evidence suggests involvement of the nicotinic system in AD. The nicotinic receptors can be divided into super-high-, high-, and low-affinity subtypes (Nordberg et al. 1992). Brains of patients with AD show decrements in the high-affinity nicotinic sites (Nordberg et al. 1992). In animal studies, the nicotinic antagonist mecamylamine produces a dose-dependent impairment of memory comparable to that observed with scopolamine (Elrod and Buccafusco 1991). The nicotinic and muscarinic systems appear to modulate performance jointly in learning and memory (Riekkinen et al. 1990). Data from animal studies suggest that presynaptic nicotinic receptors mediate a positive feedback mechanism that modulates cholinergic activity (Elrod and Buccafusco 1991).

Incomplete information exists regarding the contributions of different nicotinic and muscarinic subtypes in cognition and the pathophysiology of AD. To date, the development and implementation of pharmacological treatments for patients with AD have not approached the basic science findings.

RS-86

RS-86 (2-ethyl-8-methyl-2,8-diazospiro-4,5-decan-1,3-dionhydrobromide) is a muscarinic receptor agonist that has a relatively higher affinity for M1 than for M2 sites. The postsynaptic effects of RS-86 are hypothesized to enhance cholinergic neurotransmission. Oral administration of RS-86 produced minimal (Wettstein and Spiegal 1984) or no (Bruno et al. 1985; Mouradian et al. 1988) effects in patients with AD. A 2-week, double-blind, placebo-controlled trial including a best-dose finding phase also demonstrated no therapeutic drug effects in AD (Hollander et al. 1987).

Bethanechol

Bethanechol is a synthetic β-methyl analogue of acetylcholine. The agonist effects of bethanechol on M1 and M2 cholinergic receptors are believed to enhance cholinergic neurotransmission. Studies in patients with AD have reported modest improvement with this agent (Harbaugh et al. 1989; Penn et al. 1988; Read et al. 1990). Variable dose responses may contribute to the heterogeneous response patterns (Read et al. 1990).

Bethanechol must be administered by an intracerebroventricular route because it does not cross the blood-brain barrier. This route of administration has substantial risks, including perioperative complications, pneumocephalus, seizures, and chronic subdural hematoma (Gauthier et al. 1986; Penn et al. 1988). Thus, intracerebroventricular treatment with bethanechol is not a viable option for cholinergic enhancement in patients with AD.

Arecoline

Arecoline is a natural alkaloid that has both muscarinic and nicotinic agonist properties. Its cholinergic agonist properties are thought to be responsible for its enhancement of cholinergic transmission. Arecoline has been shown to improve learning in healthy volunteer subjects (Sitaram et al. 1978). Modest improvement in picture recognition, verbal memory, and visuospatial construction after arecoline infusion has been observed in patients with AD (Christie et al. 1981; Raffaele et al. 1991; Tariot et al. 1988a).

Oxotremorine

Oxotremorine is a synthetic cholinergic agonist with a half-life of several hours. Oxotremorine administered to patients with AD produced no cognitive-enhancing effects and significant side effects, including panic and depression (Davis et al. 1987).

AF102B

AF102B [(±)cis-2-methylspiro(1,3-oxathiolane-5,3′-quinuclidine] is a structurally rigid analogue of acetylcholine. Unlike most of the cholinergic agents described previously, AF102B is a selective M1 agonist (Potter 1987). This characteristic is desirable because activation of the M2 autoreceptors can result in decreased acetylcholine release. In addition, M1 receptors are present in the hippocampus and cerebral cortex and may play a significant role in cognitive processes (Potter 1987). Like other cholinergic agonists, AF102B effectively reverses the cognitive impairments observed in hypocholinergic animals (Dawson et al. 1994; Nakahara et al. 1988).

Indications. A 10-week double-blind, placebo-controlled study demonstrated cognitive improvement in patients with AD treated with AF102B (Fischer et al. 1996).

Xanomeline

Xanomeline, 3-[4-(hexyloxy)-1,2,5-thiadiazol-3-yl]-1,2,5,6-tetrahydro-1-methylpyridine, is a selective partial M1 agonist (Sauerberg et al. 1992). Xanomeline is extensively biotransformed to a number of metabolites (Kasper et al. 1995). Safety trials in human subjects demonstrate cholinergic symptoms with increased doses, including gastrointestinal symptoms and hypotension (Sramek et al. 1995).

ENA 713

History and discovery. ENA 713 is an acetylcholinesterase inhibitor that was developed for the treatment of AD. ENA 713 has been shown to ameliorate learning deficits in basal forebrain–lesioned rats (Niigawa et al. 1995).

Structure. ENA 713 is a carbamate-type acetylcholinesterase inhibitor. The structure is (+)(s)-N-Ethyl-3-[l-dimethylamino ethyl]-N-methylphenyl-carbonate hydrogentartate.

Pharmacological profile. ENA 713 is a pseudo irreversible acetylcholinesterase inhibitor. This characteristic causes it to provide prolonged inhibition of acetylcholinesterase after the drug has been cleared from the plasma. ENA 713 shows selectivity for brain acetylcholinesterase, particularly in the hippocampus and cortex. A single 3-mg dose of ENA 713 produces 30%–40% inhibition of central acetylcholinesterase, with minimal inhibition of peripheral acetyl- or butylcholinesterase (Anand and Gharabawi 1996). Inhibition of acetylcholinesterase activity occurs within 30 minutes of administration. Phase 1 and 2 trials suggest that the therapeutic dose is 6–12 mg/day.

Pharmacokinetics and disposition. ENA 713 is rapidly absorbed, reaching peak plasma levels within 30 minutes, and lasting up to 6 hours (Niigawa et al. 1995).

Indications. A 13-week placebo-controlled study with 402 patients reported that 3 mg of ENA 713 twice a day improved cognition. Another double-blind, placebo-controlled study of 8 weeks' duration with 114 patients with AD found that 6–12 mg/day of ENA 713 improved cognitive function. Long-term studies of ENA 713 are in progress (Anand and Gharabawi 1996).

Side effects and toxicology. ENA 713 does not alter liver function, does not produce cardiac toxicity, and does not affect blood pressure. Side effects are cholinergic, with gastrointestinal symptoms being the most common adverse effects.

Drug-drug interactions. ENA 713 has no significant interactions with other drugs.

Nicotine

The reduction in nicotinic receptors in the brains of subjects with AD suggests the potential usefulness of strategies to provide additional stimulation of the remaining nicotinic receptors to enhance cognition in patients with AD (Sugaya et al. 1990). Nicotine administration has been shown both to improve the attentional component and to facilitate retention of the memory process (Warburton and Wesnes 1984). Intramuscular nicotine administration to primates improved performance on a delayed matching-to-sample task (Buccafusco and Jackson 1991). Intravenous nicotine administration to six patients with AD improved performance in recall (Newhouse et al. 1988). It is unfortunate that the anxiety and depressive symptoms associated with nicotine administration represent toxic effects that lessen the clinical utility of this compound.

Summary

None of the cholinergic agonist approaches tested to date has yielded the clinical benefit initially anticipated. Yet it may very well be that the potential benefits of postsynaptic enhancement have not been adequately tested. The diverse physiological effects of muscarinic and nicotinic activation limit the clinical usefulness of the agents currently used. Arecoline, RS-86, and bethanechol probably do not have much effect on the m1 and m3 receptor sites in the cortex (Potter et al. 1991). The importance of targeting the appropriate site is exemplified by the compound oxotremorine, which actually decreases acetylcholine release through its action on the presynaptic m2 receptor.

Development of therapies that are directed specifically at the receptors involved in cognition will enhance therapeutic efficacy and avoid undesirable side effects. Future directions in cholinergic enhancement may include manipulation of specific subtypes of both the muscarinic and the nicotinic receptors. Postsynaptic therapy is also limited by the fact that agonist administration provides a nonphysiological tonic stimulation, whereas the physiological state is characterized by phasic mechanisms.

OTHER NEUROTRANSMITTER SYSTEMS

The heterogeneous nature of the neurochemical deficits in AD may significantly contribute to variable response patterns observed with anticholinesterases. Studies in animals also indicate the involvement of multiple neurotransmitter systems in learning and memory. For example, noradrenergic brain lesions negate cholinomimetic enhancement of memory. Clonidine administration restores the efficacy of cholinomimetic treatment in animals with combined noradrenergic and cholinergic lesions (Haroutunian et al. 1990). Postmortem studies show major neurotransmitter losses of the noradrenergic and somatostatinergic systems in patients with AD. These findings suggest that anticholinesterase administration (in conjunction with an agent that augments another neurotransmitter system found to be deficient in AD) may be a more appropriate strategy for some patients.

Selegiline

History and Discovery

Selegiline has been used for the treatment of depression and Parkinson's disease. Use of selegiline for cognitive enhancement in AD is based on the following:

- The monoaminergic system is involved in cognitive behaviors and AD.
- Selegiline's antioxidant effect, through its inhibition of monoamine oxidase B, may prevent cell death.
- Selegiline interferes with the increased activity of monoamine oxidase B that is observed in patients with AD (Oreland and Gottfries 1986).

Structure

Selegiline [(−)-(R)-N,α-dimethyl-N-2-propynylphenthylamine hydrochloride] is a levorotatory acetylenic derivative of phenethylamine.

Pharmacological Profile

Selegiline is an irreversible monoamine oxidase inhibitor that selectively inhibits monoamine oxidase B at low doses.

Pharmacokinetics and Disposition

Selegiline is absorbed readily after oral administration. Three metabolites—N-desmethyl-deprenyl (mean half-life 2 hours), amphetamine (mean half-life 18 hours), and methamphetamine (mean half-life 21 hours)—are found in serum and urine.

Indications

The results of four double-blind, placebo-controlled trials with small patient samples suggest that subchronic treatment with selegiline at 10 mg/day improves performance on attention, memory, and learning tasks (Agnoli et al. 1990; Mangoni et al. 1991; Piccinin et al. 1990; Tariot et al. 1987a, 1987b). Higher doses of selegiline were not as efficacious and were associated with more side effects (Tariot et al. 1987b). The beneficial effects of selegiline do not appear to result from its antidepressant action, because the monoamine oxidase A inhibitor tranylcypromine does not improve cognitive performance (Tariot et al. 1988b). The results for selegiline need to be replicated with larger patient samples and longer treatment trials to determine whether this agent will have clinically significant effects on cognition in patients with AD.

Side Effects and Toxicology

At low doses (10 mg/day), selegiline administration is not associated with tyramine sensitivity. Selegiline is well tolerated at low doses. Side effects include nausea, dizziness, abdominal discomfort, and dry mouth.

Drug-Drug Interactions

Selegiline administration to patients taking levodopa may lead to an exacerbation of levodopa-associated side effects. These effects may be reduced by lowering the dose of levodopa.

Combined Treatment Approaches

Animal and postmortem human studies suggest that a treatment approach using cholinergic-noradrenergic combinations may be more efficacious than cholinomimetic or monoaminergic agents alone. A pilot study with clonidine and physostigmine treatment in nine patients confirmed the safety of combining these agents in patients with AD (Davidson et al. 1989). One study noted that the combination of selegiline and a cholinesterase inhibitor was superior to administration of a cholinesterase alone, whereas two other investigations did not demonstrate significant cognitive improvement with the combination of a cholinesterase inhibitor and selegiline (Marin et al. 1995; Schneider et al. 1993; Sunderland et al. 1992). Inadequate physostigmine levels achieved in the latter trial may have led to spuriously poor results. Future studies are needed to determine the potential efficacy of combination treatments.

NEW APPROACHES

The approaches described here generally offer palliative treatment to augment the functioning of deficient neurotransmitter systems in patients with AD. Advances in the understanding of the biology of AD permit the development of strategies that may alter its underlying pathophysiology.

Glutamatergic Agents

Glutamatergic agents have not been systematically used for the treatment of AD. However, in this section, we review the rationale for and provide examples of potential glutamatergic agents for the treatment of AD.

History and Discovery

Glutamate is the major excitatory neurotransmitter of pyramidal neurons (Fonnum 1984). The postsynaptic effects of glutamate are mediated via several different receptor subtypes. These receptors can be classified according to their prototypic agonists (i.e., N-methyl-D-aspartate [NMDA], quisqualate, and kainate) (Foster and Fagg 1987).

Different receptor subtypes of the glutamatergic system have been implicated in memory processing. NMDA receptor blockade with aminophosphonopentanoic acid in the CA_1 region of the hippocampus prevents long-term potentiation (Collingridge and Bliss 1987). Binding of aminophosphonopentanoic acid to NMDA receptors disrupts spatial learning in a manner similar to that observed with hippocampal lesions (Morris et al. 1986). Antagonist binding to quisqualate and kainate receptors interferes with passive avoidance training in rodents (Danysz et al. 1988). Extensive loss of NMDA sites has been detected in the brains of patients with AD (Greenamyre et al. 1985). Increased kainate receptor binding has been observed in postmortem studies (Geddes et al. 1985). Glutamate can induce neurotoxicity (Rothman and Olney 1987). The excitatory and neurotoxic effects of glutamate can occur through both NMDA and non-NMDA receptors (Greenamyre and Young 1989). NMDA and non-NMDA antagonists protect against injury caused by ischemia (Greenamyre and Young 1989; Rothman and Olney 1987). Thus, glutamate's wide CNS distribution and its neurotoxic properties implicate it as a potential contributor to the pathogenesis of several CNS neurodegenerative disorders.

Given that glutamate can enhance learning as well as produce neurotoxicity, determination of the optimal glutamatergic strategy must take into consideration the complex functions of glutamate and the various glutamatergic receptors. Both NMDA and non-NMDA sites could be potential targets for therapeutic approaches. A strategy that enhances glutamatergic transmission is supported by the presynaptic glutamatergic losses observed in AD and glutamate's role in cognition. However, excessive augmentation of glutamatergic functioning could be neurotoxic. Glutamatergic blockade could protect against neurotoxic effects but may potentially interfere with memory processing.

Glycine Site Inhibitors

Antagonism of the glycine modulatory site of the NMDA receptor could decrease neurotoxicity mediated by glutamate. 1-Hydroxy-3-amino-2-pyrrolidone (HA-966) and L-aminocyclobutane appear to inhibit NMDA-specific binding and to block NMDA responses (Hood et al. 1989; Watson et al. 1989). The glycine antagonists kynurenic acid and 7-chloro-kynurenic acid do not interfere with passive avoidance in mice. These findings indicate that antagonism at the glycine site may interfere with glutamate's neurotoxicity without causing cognitive impairment (Chiamulera et al. 1991), a finding whose relevance to altering the course of AD depends on glutainate's involvement in cell death in patients with AD.

Non-NMDA Antagonists

Non-NMDA antagonism may provide a potential therapeutic strategy to decrease glutamatergic functioning and neurotoxicity. Antagonists of the non-NMDA receptors include 2,3-dihydroxy-6-nitro-7-sulfamoyl-benzo(F)quinoxaline (NBQX), 6,7-dinitroquinoxaline-2,3-dione (DNQX), and 6-cyano-7-nitroquioxaline-2,3-dione (CNQX) (Honore et al. 1988; Sheardon et al. 1990). These agents have been shown to protect against the effects of ischemia by blocking non-NMDA sites (Sheardon et al. 1990). Clinical trials are necessary to determine whether these agents can interfere with cell death and alter the course of AD.

Partial Agonists

Given the complex sequelae of glutamatergic activation, a partial agonist approach is optimal. The glycine agonist milacemide enhances learning in normal and amnestic rodents (Handelmann et al. 1989). One clinical trial of this drug, however, did not enhance cognition and was accompanied by significant liver toxicity (Pomara et al. 1991). The partial glycine agonist D-cycloserine has also been shown to reverse memory impairments caused by scopolamine in healthy subjects (Jones et al. 1992). A 2-week, placebo-controlled, crossover study with 12 patients with AD did not find that D-cycloserine improved cognition

when compared with placebo (Randolph et al. 1994). As with other glutamatergic-modulating agents, further clinical studies are necessary to test their potential efficacy.

Summary

Modulation of the glutamatergic system may provide several therapeutic strategies to enhance cognition and diminish the neuronal toxicity observed in patients with AD. No large-scale clinical trials yet conducted with glutamatergic modulators have found these agents to prevent neuronal damage, enhance memory, and have acceptable side-effect profiles.

Antiinflammatory Agents

History and Discovery

As with glutamatergic strategies, antiinflammatory agents have not been widely tested in the treatment of AD. However, basic science and epidemiological findings suggest the utility of these agents for AD treatment.

Several lines of evidence indicate the involvement of the immune system and inflammation in AD. Involvement of the immune system in AD and other CNS disorders refutes the long-held belief that the brain is immunologically privileged. Histochemical studies document the presence of several markers of inflammation in the brains of subjects with AD (Bauer et al. 1991; McGeer et al. 1989b; Styren et al. 1990). Furthermore, the immune response in the CNS has been shown to colocalize with senile plaques, suggesting a role for an immune response in the pathophysiology of AD (McGeer et al. 1989a).

Increased numbers of reactive glia and microglia (believed to be related to macrophages) have been observed in several postmortem studies of brains of AD subjects (Styren et al. 1990). Activated T lymphocytes, a hallmark of the cell-mediated response observed in chronic inflammatory states, has also been observed in postmortem studies of subjects with AD (McGeer et al. 1989b; J. Rogers et al. 1988). Complement proteins (including the membrane attack components) associated with the classical pathway have also been identified in senile plaques and tangles (McGeer et al. 1989a). The implications of the presence of complement proteins is that host cells can be inadvertently attacked and destroyed by these molecules.

Elevated concentrations of interleukins, agents that signal cell proliferation and the production of mediators of the inflammatory response, have also been noted in patients with AD. Specifically, concentrations of tumor necrosis factor, interleukin-1 (IL-1), and interleukin-6 (IL-6) have been elevated in patients with AD (Altstiel and

Sperber 1991; Bauer et al. 1991; Fillit et al. 1991). The role of cytokines in amyloidogenesis is supported by their ability to stimulate amyloid precursor protein synthesis (Goldgaber et al. 1989). Acute-phase proteins—inflammatory response molecules that are induced by interleukins—have also been elevated in AD (Heinrich et al. 1990). C-reactive protein, α_2-macroglobulin, and α_1-antichymotrypsin concentrations are increased in patients with AD compared with age-matched control subjects (Abraham et al. 1988; Bauer et al. 1991; Matsubara et al. 1990; Rozmuller et al. 1990). Increased α_1-antichymotrypsin concentrations are particularly intriguing because the α_1-antichymotrypsin molecule is a component of senile plaques (Bauer et al. 1991). α_1-Antichymotrypsin may contribute to abnormal processing of amyloid precursor protein, leading to β-amyloid deposition (Bauer et al. 1991). It has been suggested that the immune system response in AD originates in the CNS. Evidence to support this hypothesis includes the following:

- Astrocyte expression of IL-1 and IL-6 receptors has been shown (Frei et al. 1989; Guilian et al. 1986).
- IL-6 induces neurite formation in pheochromocytoma cell lines (Satoh et al. 1988), suggesting the presence of IL-6 receptors on neurons.
- Microglia and astrocytes can secrete IL-1 and IL-6, respectively (Frei et al. 1989).

The question that needs to be answered is what CNS events cause cytokine production. Whether local brain injury, an immunological process, or an autoimmune phenomenon induces the acute-phase response is unknown. Nonetheless, a definite immune response in AD could lead to cell death and enhance β-amyloid deposition. These data suggest that antiinflammatory therapy may slow progression of the illness. Evidence suggests that chronic exposure to antiinflammatory agents is protective against the development of AD. The prevalence of AD among patients at rheumatoid arthritis clinics—a population likely to have received chronic antiinflammatory therapy—was significantly less than that observed in the general population older than 64 years (McGeer et al. 1992a). Elderly patients with leprosy who had been treated with the antiinflammatory agent dapsone had significantly lower rates of dementia than did drug-free patients (McGeer et al. 1992b). A 6-month double-blind trial with the nonsteroidal antiinflammatory agent indomethacin documented that the conditions of patients with AD who received active drug declined significantly less than did those of patients who received placebo (J. Rogers et al. 1988). An open-label safety study that included 20 subjects with AD

reported that prednisone was well tolerated and affected serum concentrations in the acute phase in moderate doses (Aisen et al. 1996). Future studies with antiinflammatory agents in patients with AD are necessary to determine the usefulness of antiinflammatory strategies.

CONCLUSION

Several strategies for cognitive enhancement have been attempted in patients with AD. An adequate acetylcholinesterase inhibitor has not yet been tested with all the necessary parameters. Combined neurotransmitter therapies have also not been adequately tested to determine the level of efficacy that could be achieved with this approach. Strategies to delay the progression of AD are now being explored and may provide the most effective means to treat the cognitive deterioration observed in patients who have AD.

REFERENCES

Abraham CR, Selkoe DJ, Potter H: Immunohistochemical identification of the serine protease inhibitor alpha-1 antichymotrypsin in the brain amyloid deposits of Alzheimer's disease. Cell 52:487–501, 1988

Adem A: Putative mechanisms of action of tacrine in Alzheimer's disease. Acta Neurol Scand 139:69–74, 1992

Agnoli A, Martucci N, Fabbrini G, et al: Monoamine oxidase and dementia: treatment with an inhibitor of MAO-B activity. Dementia 1:109–114, 1990

Aisen PS, Marin DB, Altstiel L, et al: A pilot study of prednisone in Alzheimer's disease. Dementia 7:201–206, 1996

Altstiel LD, Sperber K: Cytokines in Alzheimer's disease. Prog Neuropsychopharmacol Biol Psychiatry 15:481–495, 1991

Anand R, Gharabawi G: Efficacy and safety results of the early phase studies with exelon (ENA 713) in Alzheimer's disease: an overview. J Drug Dev Clin Pract 8:109–116, 1996

Antuono PG: Effectiveness and safety of velnacrine for the treatment of Alzheimer's disease: a double-blind, placebo-controlled study. Mentane Study Group. Arch Intern Med 155:1766–1772, 1995

Ashkenazi A, Peralta EG, Winslow JW, et al: Functional diversity of muscarinic receptor subtypes in cellular signal transduction and growth. Trends Pharmacol Sci Suppl 10:16–22, 1989

Bartus RT, Dean RL, Pontecorvo MJ, et al: The cholinergic hypothesis: a historical overview, current perspective and future directions. Ann N Y Acad Sci 444:332–358, 1985

Bartus RT, Dean RL, Flicker C: Cholinergic psychopharmacology: an integration of human and animal research on memory, in Psychopharmacology: The Third Generation of Progress. Edited by Meltzer HY. New York, Raven, 1987, pp 219–232

Bauer J, Strauss S, Schreiter-Gasser U, et al: Interleukin-6 and alpha-2-macroglobulin indicate an acute phase response in the Alzheimer's disease cortices. FEBS Lett 285:111–114, 1991

Beller SA, Overall JE, Rhoades HM, et al: Long term outpatient treatment of senile dementia with oral physostigmine. J Clin Psychiatry 49:400–404, 1988

Birdsall N, Buckley N, Doods H: Nomenclature for muscarinic receptor subtypes recommended by symposium. Trends Pharmacol Sci Suppl 10:7–9, 1989

Bonner TI: New subtypes of muscarinic acetylcholine receptors. Trends Pharmacol Sci Suppl 10:11–15, 1989

Bonner TI, Buckley A, Young AC, et al: Identification of a family of muscarinic acetylcholine receptor genes. Science 237:527–532, 1987

Bruno G, Mohr E, Gillepsie M, et al: RS-86 therapy of Alzheimer's disease. Arch Neurol 43:659–661, 1985

Buccafusco JJ, Jackson W: Beneficial effects of nicotine administered prior to a delayed matching-to-sample task in young and aged monkeys. Neurobiol Aging 12:233–238, 1991

Buckley NJ, Bonner TI, Brann MR: Localization of a family of muscarinic receptor mRNAs in rat brain. J Neurosci 8:4646–4652, 1988

Chatellier G, Lacomblez L: Tacrine (tetrahydroaminoacridine; THA) and lecithin in senile dementia of the Alzheimer's type: a multi-center trial. BMJ 300:495–499, 1990

Chiamulera C, Costa S, Reggiani A: Effect of NMDA and strychnine-insensitive glycine site antagonist on NMDA-mediated convulsions and learning. Psychopharmacology 102:551–552, 1991

Christie JE, Shering A, Ferguson J, et al: Physostigmine and arecoline: effects of intravenous infusions in Alzheimer's presenile dementia. Br J Psychiatry 138:46–50, 1981

Clipp EC, Moore MJ: Caregiver time use: an outcome measure in clinical trial research on Alzheimer's disease. Clin Pharmacol Ther 58:228–236, 1995

Collerton D: Cholinergic function and intellectual decline in Alzheimer's disease. Neuroscience 19:1–28, 1986

Collingridge GL, Bliss TVP: NNMA receptors—their role in long-term potentiation. Trends Neurosci 10:288–293, 1987

Cutler NR, Murphy MF, Nash RJ, et al: Clinical safety, tolerance and plasma levels of the oral anticholinesterase 1,2,3,4-tetrahydro-9-aminoacradin-I-olmaleate (HP 029) in Alzheimer's disease: preliminary findings. J Clin Pharmacol 39:556–561, 1990

Dal-Bianco P, Maly J, Wober C, et al: Galanthamine treatment in Alzheimer's disease. J Neural Transm Suppl 33:59–63, 1991

Danysz W, Wroblewski JT, Costa E: Learning impairment in rats by N-methyl-D-aspartate receptor antagonist. Neuropharmacology 27:653–656, 1988

Davidson M, Bierer LM, Kaminsky R, et al: Combined administration of physostigmine and clonidine to patients with dementia of the Alzheimer type: a pilot safety study. Alzheimer Dis Assoc Disord 1:1–4, 1989

Davies P, Maloney AJ: Selective loss of central cholinergic neurons in Alzheimer's disease. Lancet 2:1403–1405, 1976

Davis KL, Hollander E, Davidson M, et al: Induction of depression with oxotremorine in Alzheimer's disease patients. Am J Psychiatry 144:468–471, 1987

Davis KL, Thal LJ, Gamzu ER, et al: A double-blind, placebo-controlled multicenter study of tacrine in Alzheimer's disease. N Engl J Med 327:1253–1259, 1992

Dawson GR, Bayley P, Channell S, et al: A comparison of the effects of the novel muscarinic receptor agonists L-689,660 and AF102B in tests of reference and working memory. Psychopharmacology 113:361–368, 1994

Deutsch JA: The cholinergic synapse and the site of memory. Science 174:788–794, 1971

Drachman DA, Leavitt J: Human memory and the cholinergic system. Arch Neurol 30:113–121, 1974

Drukarch B, Kits S, Van der Meer EG, et al: 9-Amino-1,2,3,4-tetrahydroacridine (THA), an alleged drug for the treatment of Alzheimer's disease, inhibits acetylcholinesterase activity and slows outward K^+ current. Eur J Pharmacol 141:153–157, 1987

Drukarch B, Leysen JE, Stoof JC: Further analysis of the neuropharmacological profile of 9-amino-1,2,3,4-tetrahydroacridine (THA), an alleged drug for the treatment of Alzheimer's disease. Life Sci 42:1011–1017, 1988

Dundee JW, Pandit SK: Anterograde amnesic effects of pethidine, hyoscine, and diazepam in adults. Br J Pharmacol 44:140–144, 1972

Elrod K, Buccafusco JJ: Correlation of the amnestic effects of nicotinic antagonists with inhibition of regional brain acetylcholine synthesis in rats. J Pharmacol Exp Ther 258:403–409, 1991

Farlow M, Gracon SI, Hershey LA, et al: A controlled trial of tacrine in Alzheimer's disease. JAMA 268:2523–2529, 1992

Fielding S, Cornfeldt ML, Szewczak MR, et al: HP-029, a new drug for the treatment of Alzheimer's disease: its pharmacological profile. Paper presented at the 4th World Conference on Clinical Pharmacology and Therapeutics, West Berlin, Germany, July 28–30, 1989

Fillit H, Ding W, Buee L, et al: Elevated circulating tumor necrosis factor levels in Alzheimer's disease. Neurosci Lett 129:318–320, 1991

Fischer A, Heldman E, Gurwitz D, et al: M1 agonist for the treatment of Alzheimer's disease: novel properties and clinical update. Ann N Y Acad Sci 77:189–196, 1996

Folstein MF, Folstein SE, McHugh PR: Mini-Mental State: a practical method for grading the cognitive state of patients for the clinician. J Psychiatr Res 12:189–198, 1975

Fonnum F: Glutamate: a neurotransmitter in mammalian brain. J Neurochem 42:1–11, 1984

Foster AC, Fagg GE: Taking apart the NMDA receptor. Nature 329:395–396, 1987

Frei K, Malipiero UV, Leist TP, et al: On the cellular source and function of interleukin 6 produced in the central nervous system in viral diseases. Eur J Immunol 19:689–694, 1989

Fukada K, Kubo T, Maeda A, et al: Selective effector coupling of muscarinic acetylcholine receptor subtypes. Trends Pharmacol Sci Suppl 10:4–10, 1989

Galli A, Nori F, Benini L, et al: Acetylcholinesterase protection and the anti-diisopropylfluorophosphate efficacy of E2020. Eur J Pharmacol 270:189–193, 1994

Gauthier S, Leblanc R, Quirion R, et al: Transmitter-replacement therapy in Alzheimer's disease using intracerebroventricular infusions of receptor agonists. Can J Neurol Sci 13:394–402, 1986

Gauthier S, Bouchard R, Lamontagne A, et al: Tetrahydro-aminoacridine-lecithin combination treatment in patients with intermediate-stage Alzheimer's disease. N Engl J Med 322:1272–1276, 1990

Geddes JW, Monaghan DT, Cotman CW, et al: Plasticity of hippocampal circuitry in Alzheimer's disease. Science 230:1179–1181, 1985

Goldgaber D, Harris H, Hal T, et al: Interleukin-1 regulates synthesis of amyloid beta protein precursor mRNA in human endothelial cells. Proc Natl Acad Sci U S A 86:7606–7610, 1989

Greenamyre JT, Young AB: Excitatory amino acids and Alzheimer's disease. Neurobiol Aging 10:593–602, 1989

Greenamyre JT, Penney JB, Young AB: Alterations in L-glutamate binding in Alzheimer's and Huntington's diseases. Science 227:1496–1498, 1985

Guilian D, Baker TJ, Shin LN, et al: Interleukin-1 of the central nervous system is produced by ameboid microglia. J Exp Med 164:594–604, 1986

Guy W (ed): Clinical Global Assessment Scale (CGI), in ECDEU Assessment Manual for Psychopharmacology (DHEW Publ No ADM-76-338). Washington, DC, U.S. Government Printing Office, 1976, pp 218–222

Handelmann GE, Nevins ME, Mueller LL, et al: Milacemide, a glycine prodrug, enhances performance of learning tasks in normal and amnestic rodents. Pharmacol Biochem Behav 34:823–838, 1989

Harbaugh RE, Reeder TM, Senter HJ, et al: Intracerebroventricular bethanechol chloride administration in Alzheimer's disease: results of a collaborative double-blind study. J Neurosurg 71:481–486, 1989

Haroutunian V, Kanof PD, Davis KL: Pharmacological alleviation of cholinergic lesion induced memory deficits in rats. Life Sci 37:945–952, 1985

Haroutunian V, Kanof PD, Tsuboyama G, et al: Restoration of cholinomimetic activity by clonidine in cholinergic plus adrenergic lesioned rats. Brain Res 507:261–266, 1990

Heinrich PC, Castell JV, Andus T: Interleukin-6 and the acute phase response. Biochem J 265:621–636, 1990

Hollander E, Davidson M, Mohs RC, et al: RS-86 in the treatment of Alzheimer's disease: cognitive and biological effects. Biol Psychiatry 22:1067–1078, 1987

Honore T, Davies SN, Drejer J, et al: Quinoxalinediones: potent competitive non-NMDA glutamate receptor antagonist. Science 241:701–703, 1988

Hood WF, Sun ET, Cornpton RP, et al: 1-Aminocyclo-butane-1-carboxylate (ACBC): a specific antagonist of the N-methyl-D-aspartate receptor coupled glycine receptor. Eur J Pharmacol 161:281–282, 1989

Jackson WJ, Buccafusco JJ, Terry AV, et al: Velnacrine maleate improves delayed matching performance by aged monkeys. Psychopharmacology 119:391–398, 1995

Jenike MA, Albert MS, Baer L: Oral physostigmine as treatment for Alzheimer's disease: a long-term outpatient trial. Alzheimer Dis Assoc Disord 4:226–231, 1990

Jones RW, Wesnes KA, Kirby J: Effects of NMDA modulation in scopolamine dementia. Ann N Y Acad Sci 64:241–244, 1992

Kasper SC, Bonate PL, DeLong AF: High performance liquid chromatographic assay for xanomeline, a specific M-1 agonist, and its metabolite in human plasma. J Chromatogr B Biomed Appl 669:397–404, 1995

Kawashima K, Sato A, Yoshizawa M, Fjii T, et al: Effects of the centrally acting cholinesterase inhibitors tetrahydroaminoacrine and E2020 on the basal concentration of extracellular acetylcholine in the hippocampus of freely moving rats. Naunyn Schmiedebergs Arch Pharmacol 350:523–528, 1994

Kaye WH, Sitaram H, Weingartner H, et al: Modest facilitation of memory in dementia with combined lecithin and anticholinesterase treatment. Biol Psychiatry 17:275–280, 1982

Knapp MJ, Knopman DS, Solomon PR, et al: A 30-week randomized controlled trial of high-dose tacrine in patients with Alzheimer's disease. The Tacrine Study Group. JAMA 271:985–991, 1994

Mangoni A, Grassi MP, Frattola L, et al: Effects of a MAO-B inhibitor in the treatment of Alzheimer disease. Eur Neurol 31:100–107, 1991

Marin DB, Bierer LB, Ryan TM, et al: Physostigmine and deprenyl combination therapy for Alzheimer's disease. Psychiatry Res 58:181–189,1995

Matsubara E, Hirai S, Amari M, et al: Alpha-1 antichymotrypsin as a possible biochemical marker for Alzheimer-type dementia. Ann Neurol 28:561–567, 1990

McGeer PL, Akiyama H, Itagaki S, et al: Activation of the classical complement pathway in brain tissue of Alzheimer patients. Neurosci Lett 107:341–346, 1989a

McGeer PL, Akiyama H, Itagaki S, et al: Immune system response in Alzheimer's disease. Can J Neurol Sci 16:516–527, 1989b

McGeer PL, McGeer EG, Rogers J, et al: Does antiinflammatory treatment protect against Alzheimer's disease? in Alzheimer's Disease: New Treatment Strategies. Edited by Khachaturian ZS, Blass JP. New York, Marcel Dekker, 1992a, pp 165–171

McGeer PL, Harada N, Kimura H, et al: Prevalence of dementia amongst elderly Japanese with leprosy: apparent effect of chronic drug therapy. Dementia 3:146–149, 1992b

Mihailova D, Yamboliev I, Zhivkova Z, et al: Pharmacokinetics of galanthamine hydrobromide after single subcutaneous and oral dosage in humans. Pharmacology 39:50–58, 1989

Mihara M, Ohnishi A, Tomono Y, et al: Pharmacokinetics of E2020, a new compound for Alzheimer's disease, in healthy male volunteers. Int J Clin Pharmacol Ther Toxicol 31:223–229, 1993

Mohs RC, Davis KL: The experimental pharmacology of Alzheimer's disease and related dementias, in Psychopharmacology: The Third Generation of Progress. Edited by Meltzer HY. New York, Raven, 1987, pp 921–928

Morris RGM, Anderson E, Lynch GS, et al: Selective impairment of learning and blockade of long-term potentiation by an N-methyl-D-aspartate receptor antagonist, AP5. Nature 319:774–776, 1986

Mouradian MM, Mohr E, Williams AJ, et al: No response to high dose muscarinic agonist therapy in Alzheimer's disease. Neurology 38:606–608, 1988

Murphy MF, Hardiman ST, Nash RJ, et al: Evaluation of HP 029 (velnacrine maleate) in Alzheimer's disease. Ann N Y Acad Sci 640:253–262, 1991

Nakahara N, Iga Y, Mizobe F, et al: Amelioration of experimental amnesia (passive avoidance failure) in rodents by selective M_1 agonist AF102B. Jpn J Pharmacol 48:502–505, 1988

Newhouse PA, Sunderland T, Tariot PN, et al: Intravenous nicotine in Alzheimer's disease: a pilot study. Psychopharmacology (Berl) 95:171–175, 1988

Nielsen JA, Mena JEE, Williams IH, et al: Correlation of brain levels of 9-amino-1,2,3,4-tetrahydro-aminoacridine (THA) with neurochemical and behavioral changes. Eur J Pharmacol 173:53–64, 1989

Niigawa H, Tanimukai S, Takeda M, et al: Effects of SDZ ENA 713, novel acetylcholinesterase inhibitor, on learning of rats with basal forebrain lesions. Prog Neuropsychopharmacol Biol Psychiatry 19:171–186, 1995

Nochi S, Asakawa N, Sato T: Kinetic study on the inhibition of acetycholinesterase by 1-benzyl-4-[5,6-dimethoxy-1-indanon)-2-yl]methylpiperidine hydrocholoride (E2020). Biol Pharm Bull 18:1145–1147, 1995

Nordberg A, Alafuzoff I, Winblad B: Nicotinic and muscarinic subtypes in the human brain: changes with aging and dementia. J Neurosci Res 31:103–111, 1992

Ohnishi A, Mihara M, Kamakura H, et al: Comparison of pharmacokinetics of E2020, a new compound for Alzheimer's disease, in healthy young and elderly subjects. J Clin Pharmacol 33:1086–1091, 1993

Olton DS, Wenk GL: Dementia: animal models of the cognitive impairments produced by degeneration of the basal forebrain cholinergic system, in Psychopharmacology: The Third Generation of Progress. Edited by Meltzer HY. New York, Raven, 1987, pp 941–953

Oreland L, Gottfries CG: Brain and monoamine oxidase in aging and in dementia of Alzheimer's type. Prog Neuropsychopharmacol Biol Psychiatry 10:533–540, 1986

Penn RD, Martin EM, Wilson RS, et al: Intraventricular bethanechol infusion in Alzheimer's disease: results of double-blind and escalating dose trials. Neurology 38:219–222, 1988

Perry EK, Tomlinson BE, Blessed G, et al: Correlation of cholinergic abnormalities with senile plaques and mental test scores in senile dementia. BMJ 2:1457–1459, 1978

Piccinin FL, Finali G, Piccirilli M: Neuropsychological effects of L-deprenyl in Alzheimer's type dementia. Clin Neuropharmacol 13:147–163, 1990

Pomara N, Mendels J, Lewitt PA, et al: Multicenter trial of milacemide in the treatment of Alzheimer's disease. Biol Psychiatry 29 (suppl):718, 1991

Potter LT: Muscarinic receptors in the cortex and hippocampus in relation to the treatment of Alzheimer's disease, in International Symposium on Muscarinic Cholinergic Mechanisms. Edited by Cohen S, Sokolovsky M. London, Freud Publishing, 1987, pp 294–301

Potter LT, Ballesteros LA, Bichajian LH, et al: Evidence of paired M2 muscarinic receptors. Mol Pharmacol 39:211–212, 1991

Puri SK, Hsu R, Ho I: Multiple dose pharmacokinetics, safety, and tolerance of velnacrine maleate in healthy elderly subjects: a potential therapeutic agent for Alzheimer's disease. J Clin Pharmacol 30:948–955, 1990

Raffaele KC, Berardi A, Morris P, et al: Effects of acute infusion of the muscarinic cholinergic agonist arecoline on verbal and visuo-spatial function in dementia of the Alzheimer type. Prog Neuropsychopharmacol Biol Psychiatry 15:643–648, 1991

Randolph C, Roberts JW, Tierney MC, et al: D-Cycloserine treatment of Alzheimer's disease. Alzheimer Dis Assoc Dis 8:198–205, 1994

Read SL, Frazee J, Shapira J, et al: Intracerebroventricular bethanechol for Alzheimer's disease: variable dose-related responses. Arch Neurol 47:1025–1030, 1990

Riekkinen P Jr, Sirvio J, Aaltonen M, et al: Effects of concurrent manipulations of nicotinic and muscarinic receptors on spatial and passive avoidance learning. Pharmacol Biochem Behav 54:405–410, 1990

Rogers J, Luber-Narod J, Styren SD, et al: Expression of immune-system-associated antigens by cells of the human central nervous system: relationship to the pathology of Alzheimer's disease. Neurobiol Aging 9:339–349, 1988

Rogers SL, Friedhoff LT, and the Donepezil Study Group: The efficacy and safety of donepezil in patients with Alzheimer's disease: results of a US multicentre, randomized, double blind, placebo controlled trial. Dementia 7:293–303, 1996

Rosen WG, Mohs RC, Davis K: A new rating scale for Alzheimer's disease. Am J Psychiatry 141:1356–1364, 1984

Rothman SM, Olney JW: Excitoxicity and the NMDA receptor. Trends Neurosci 7:299–302, 1987

Rozmuller JM, Stam FC, Eikelenboom P: Acute phase proteins are present in amorphous plaques in the cerebral but not in the cerebellar cortex of patients with Alzheimer's disease. Neurosci Lett 109:75–78, 1990

Sahakian BJ, Coull JT: Tetrahydroaminoacridine (THA) in Alzheimer's disease: an assessment of attentional and mnemonic function using CANTAB. Acta Neurol Scand Suppl 149:29–35, 1993

Satoh T, Makamura S, Taga T, et al: Induction of neuronal differentiation in PC12 cells by B-cell stimulatory factor 2/interleukin 6. Mol Cell Biol 8:3546–3549, 1988

Sauerberg P, Olesen S, Nielson S, et al: Novel functional M1 selective muscarinic agonists, synthesis and structure-activity relationships of 3-C1,2,5-thiadiazolyl)-methylpyridines. J Med Chem 35:2275, 1992

Schneider LS, Olin JT, Pawluczyk S: A double-blind crossover pilot study of L-deprenyl (selegiline) combined with cholinesterase inhibitors in Alzheimer's disease. Am J Psychiatry 150:321–323, 1993

Sheardon MJ, Nielsoen EO, Hansen AJ, et al: 2,3-Dihydroxy-6-nitro-7-sulfamoyl-benzo(F)quinoxaline: a neuroprotectant for cerebral ischemia. Science 247:571–574, 1990

Sitaram N, Weingartner H, Gillin JC: Human serial learning: enhancement with arecoline and impairment with scopolamine correlated with performance on placebo. Science 201:274–276, 1978

Sramek JJ, Hurley DJ, Wardle TS, et al: The safety and tolerance of xanomeline tartrate in patients with Alzheimer's disease. J Clin Pharmacol 35:800–806, 1995

Styren SD, Civin WH, Rogers J: Molecular cellular and pathologic characterization of HLA-DR immunoreactivity in normal elderly and Alzheimer's disease brain. Exp Neurol 110:93–104, 1990

Sugaya K, Giacobini E, Chiappinelli VA: Nicotinic acetylcholine receptor subtypes in human frontal cortex: changes in Alzheimer's disease. J Neurosci Res 27:349–359, 1990

Summers WK, Viesselman JO, Marsh GM, et al: Use of THA in treatment of Alzheimer-like dementia: pilot study in twelve patients. Biol Psychiatry 16:145–153, 1981

Summers WK, Majovski LV, Marsh GM, et al: Oral tetrahydroaminoacridine in long-term treatment of senile dementia of the Alzheimer type. N Engl J Med 315:1241–1245, 1986

Summers WK, Koehler AL, Marsh GM, et al: Long-term hepatoxicity of tacrine. Lancet 1:729, 1989

Sunderland T, Molchan S, Lawlor B, et al: A strategy of "combination chemotherapy" in Alzheimer's disease: rationale and preliminary results with physostigmine plus deprenyl. Int Psychogeriatr 4 (suppl 2):291–309, 1992

Sweeney JE, Hohmann CF, Moran TM, et al: A long-acting cholinesterase inhibitor reverses spatial memory deficits in mice. Pharmacol Biochem Behav 31:141–147, 1988

Tanaka Y, Sakurai M, Hayashi S: Effect of scopolamine and HP 029, a cholinesterase inhibitor, on long term potentiation in hippocampal slices of the guinea pig. Neurosci Lett 98:179–183, 1989

Tariot PN, Cohen RM, Sunderland T, et al: L-Deprenyl in Alzheimer's disease. Arch Gen Psychiatry 44:427–433, 1987a

Tariot PN, Sunderland T, Weingartner H, et al: Cognitive effects of L-deprenyl in Alzheimer's disease. Psychopharmacology (Berl) 91:489–495, 1987b

Tariot PN, Cohen RM, Welkowitz JA, et al: Multiple-dose arecoline infusions in Alzheimer's disease. Arch Gen Psychiatry 45:901–905, 1988a

Tariot PN, Sunderland T, Cohen RM, et al: Tranylcypromine compared with L-deprenyl in Alzheimer's disease. J Clin Psychopharmacol 8:23–27, 1988b

Thomsen T, Bickel U, Fischer JP, et al: Stereoselectivity of cholinesterase inhibition by galanthamine and tolerance in humans. Eur J Clin Pharmacol 39:603–605, 1990

Warburton DM, Wesnes K: Drugs as research tools in psychology: cholinergic drugs and information processing. Neuropsychobiology 11:121–132, 1984

Watson GB, Bolanowski MA, Baganoff MP, et al: Glycine antagonist action of 1-aminocyclobutane-1-carboxylate (ACBC) in Xenopus oocytes injected with rat brain mRNA. Eur J Pharmacol 167:291–294, 1989

Wettstein A, Spiegal R: Clinical studies with the cholinergic drug RS-86 in Alzheimer's disease (AD) and senile dementia of the Alzheimer type (SDAT). Psychopharmacology (Berl) 84:572–573, 1984

Whelpton R, Hurst P: Bioavailability of oral physostigmine (letter). N Engl J Med 313:1293–1294, 1985

Whitehouse PJ, Kellar KJ: Nicotinic and muscarinic cholinergic receptors in Alzheimer's disease and related disorders. J Neural Transm Suppl 24:175–182, 1987

Zemlan FP, Keys M, Richter RW, et al: Double blind, placebo controlled study of velnacrine in Alzheimer's disease. Life Sci 586:1823–1832, 1996

TWENTY-FOUR

Sedative-Hypnotics

Seiji Nishino, M.D., Ph.D.,
Emmanuel Mignot, M.D., Ph.D., and
William C. Dement, M.D., Ph.D.

In this chapter, we examine some of the pharmacological properties of barbiturates, benzodiazepines, and other sedative-hypnotic compounds. Sedative drugs moderate excitement, decrease activity, and induce calmness, whereas hypnotic drugs produce drowsiness and facilitate the onset and maintenance of a state that resembles normal sleep in its electroencephalographical characteristics. Although these agents are central nervous system (CNS) depressants, they usually produce therapeutic effects at far lower doses than those that cause generalized depression of the CNS and coma.

Some sedative-hypnotic drugs retain other therapeutic uses, as muscle relaxants (especially benzodiazepines), antiepileptic agents, or preanesthetic medications. Although the benzodiazepines are used widely as antianxiety drugs, whether their effect on anxiety is truly distinct from their effect on sleepiness remains unconfirmed.

Sedative-hypnotics are important drugs to the neuroscientist. These substances modulate basic behaviors such as arousal and response to stress. Understanding their mode of action could thus help to elucidate neurochemical and neurophysiological control of these behaviors.

BARBITURATES

History

Before 1900, a few agents, such as bromide, chloral hydrate, paraldehyde, urethane, and sulfonal, were used as sedatives and hypnotics. Barbital, one of the derivatives of barbituric acid, was introduced in 1903 and soon became extremely popular in clinical medicine because of its sleep-inducing and anxiolytic effects (Maynert 1965). In 1912, phenobarbital was introduced. In addition to its use as a sedative-hypnotic, phenobarbital has become one of the most important pharmacological treatments for epilepsy. Since then, more than 2,500 barbiturate analogues have been synthesized, of which about 50 have been made commercially available and only 20 of which are still on the market.

The success of the partial separation of anticonvulsant from sedative-hypnotic properties led to the development of nonsedative anticonvulsants such as phenytoin in the late 1930s and trimethadione in the early 1940s. The success of barbiturates as sedative-hypnotics was largely overshadowed by the discovery of benzodiazepines in the late 1960s. With pharmacological properties very similar to those of barbiturates, these compounds have a much safer pharmacological profile. Thus, benzodiazepines have replaced barbiturates in many indications, especially for psychiatric conditions in which suicide is a possibility.

Structure-Activity Relations

Barbituric acid (2,4,6-trihexahydroxypyrimidine) is the parent compound of all barbiturates. This basic structure lacks central depressant activity, and the addition of two alkyl groups at position 5 is needed to confer sedative activity (Figure 24–1).

The barbituric acid derivatives do not dissolve readily in water but are quite soluble in nonpolar solvents, a feature shared with most other organic compounds that de-

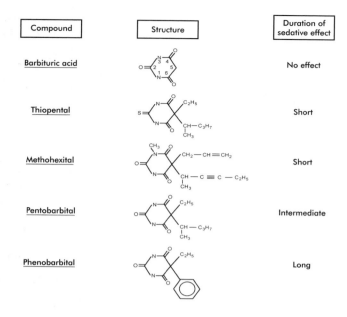

Figure 24–1. Structure-activity relations among barbiturates.

press the CNS. In general, structural changes that increase liposolubility also decrease their duration of action, decrease latency to onset of activity, accelerate metabolic degradation, and often increase hypnotic potency.

Derivatives with large aliphatic groups at position 5 have greater activity than those with methyl groups but shorter duration of action. However, groups larger than seven carbons lose their hypnotic activity and tend to confer convulsant activity. Methylation of the 1-*N* atom increases liposolubility and shortens duration of action, and desmethylation may increase the duration of action (Rall 1990).

Pharmacological Profile

The main effects of barbiturates are sedation, sleep induction, and anesthesia. Some of the barbiturates, such as phenobarbital, also have selective anticonvulsant properties. The mechanisms of action of barbiturates are complex and still not fully understood. Nonanesthetic doses of barbiturates preferentially suppress polysynaptic responses. Pertinent to their sedative-hypnotic effects is the fact that the mesencephalic reticular activating system is extremely sensitive to these drugs (Killam 1962). The synaptic site of inhibition is either postsynaptic (e.g., at the level of cortical and cerebellar pyramidal cells and in the cuneate nucleus, substantia nigra, and thalamus relay neurons) or presynaptic (e.g., in the spinal cord). This inhibition occurs only at synapses where physiological inhi-

bition is γ-aminobutyric acid (GABA)ergic and not glycinergic or monoaminergic. Thus, barbiturates, like benzodiazepines, potentiate GABA-mediated inhibitory processes in the brain. However, it remains unclear whether all of the effects of barbiturates are entirely mediated by GABAergic mechanisms.

Barbiturates do not displace benzodiazepines from their binding sites; instead, barbiturates enhance benzodiazepine binding by increasing the affinity of the receptor for benzodiazepines (Leeb-Lumberg et al. 1980). They also enhance the binding of GABA and its agonists to specific binding sites (Asano and Ogasawara 1981). These effects are almost completely dependent on the presence of chloride or other anions that are known to permeate the chloride channels associated with the GABA receptor complex, and they are competitively antagonized by picrotoxin (a convulsant) (Olsen et al. 1978). Taken together, these observations suggest that the macromolecular complex composed of GABA$_A$-ergic receptors, chloride ionophores, and binding sites for benzodiazepines (ω-site) is an important site of action for depressant barbiturates (see Figure 24–4 later in this chapter).

Although both barbiturates and benzodiazepines can potentiate the GABA-induced increase in chloride conductance, barbiturates appear to increase the duration of the open state of chloride channels that are regulated by GABA$_A$-ergic receptors. In contrast, benzodiazepines increase the frequency of channel openings with little effect on the duration. Barbiturates may prolong the activation of the channel by acting directly on the ion channel (Enna and Möhler 1987; Richter and Holman 1982).

Effects on stages of sleep. Barbiturates decrease sleep latency; however, they slightly increase fast electroencephalogram (EEG) activity during sleep. Barbiturates decrease body movement during sleep. Stage 2 sleep increases, whereas Stages 3 and 4 slow-wave sleep (SWS) generally decrease, except in some patients with anxiety and in patients who are addicted to barbiturates. Rapid eye movement (REM) sleep latency is prolonged, and both the total time spent in REM sleep and the number of REM cycles are diminished. With repeated nighttime administration, drug tolerance to the effects on sleep occurs in a few days. Discontinuation of barbiturates may lead to insomnia and disrupted sleep patterns (with a decrease in Stage 2 sleep) and increases in REM sleep (Kay et al. 1976).

Pharmacokinetics and Disposition

For hypnotic use, barbiturates are usually administered orally. Barbiturates are rapidly absorbed in the stomach, and their absorption decreases when the stomach is full. Because the sodium salts are rapidly dissolved, they are more rapidly absorbed than free acids.

Barbiturates are metabolized mainly in the liver. Oxidation of the larger of the two side chains at position 5 is a major catabolic pathway. It generally produces inactive polar metabolites that are rapidly excreted in the urine (Rall 1990). Changes in liver function can markedly alter the rate at which these compounds are inactivated. Chronic administration leads to pharmacokinetic tolerance even when low or infrequent doses of barbiturates are used (see section, "Drug-Drug Interactions," later in this chapter).

The rate of penetration of barbiturates into the CNS varies according to their lipophilicity. In general, liposolubility decreases latency to onset of action and duration of action. Thiopental, for example, enters the CNS rapidly and is used to rapidly induce anesthesia; barbitone crosses into the brain so slowly that it is inappropriate as a hypnotic drug.

Indications

Although clinical trials have shown that the barbiturates have sedative and hypnotic properties, they generally compare poorly with benzodiazepines. The patient feels "drugged" the next day, and there is always the risk of fatal overdose because of the depressant effect on respiration. Barbiturates suppress respiration, and the therapeutic dose of barbiturates may cause fatal respiratory depression in patients with sleep apnea. Patients with sleep apnea should therefore avoid taking barbiturates. Because of these risks, many clinicians have stopped using barbiturates as hypnotics and sedatives (one exception is the treatment of severe psychomotor excitation) and prescribe them only as anticonvulsants.

Barbiturates have also been administered intravenously to facilitate interviewing patients (i.e., amobarbital interview). This technique is also helpful in 1) mobilizing the stuporous catatonic patient, 2) aiding the diagnosis of intellectual impairment, and 3) lessening disturbance associated with previous negative experiences (i.e., abreactions).

The drugs are contraindicated in patients with porphyria because barbiturates enhance porphyrin synthesis. Liver function should be checked before and during drug administration. Liver dysfunction can significantly prolong the sedative effects of these drugs and may lead to fatal overdose.

Side Effects and Toxicology

In treating many patients who are prescribed barbiturates, it is difficult to control symptoms without producing oversedation. Patients typically oscillate between anxiety and torpor. Mental performance is often impaired, and patients should not drive or operate dangerous machinery.

Patients whose conditions have been stabilized for years with barbiturates must be considered drug dependent. Withdrawal leads to anxiety, agitation, trembling, and, frequently, convulsions. Substitution of a benzodiazepine that can be withdrawn more easily later is often successful.

In some patients, barbiturates repeatedly produce excitement rather than depression (paradoxical excitement), and the patients may appear to be intoxicated.

Hypersensitive reactions (especially of the skin) may occur, and instances of megaloblastic anemia have been reported.

Overdosage. An overdose of barbiturates leads to fatal respiratory and cardiovascular depression. Suicide attempts frequently involve overdoses of barbiturates, either taken alone or taken in combination with alcohol or other psychotropic drugs, particularly tricyclic antidepressants. These suicide attempts unfortunately are often successful. Depending on local factors such as proximity to a hospital and expertise of staff for intensive emergency care, death occurs in 0.5%–10% of these cases. Severe poisoning results at 10 times the hypnotic dose, and twice that amount may be fatal.

Tolerance and dependence. Tolerance to barbiturates occurs rapidly and is a result of both pharmacokinetic factors (e.g., liver-enzyme induction) and pharmacodynamic factors (e.g., neuronal adaptation to chronic drug administration). Cross-tolerance develops to alcohol, gas anesthetics, and other sedatives, including benzodiazepines.

Psychological dependence (i.e., drug-seeking behavior) is common. Patients typically visit several physicians to obtain more barbiturates. Physical dependence may be induced by doses of 500 mg/day. Intoxication may occur, as evidenced by impaired mental functioning, emotional instability, and neurological signs. Abrupt discontinuation after high dosage is likely to induce convulsions and delirium. After normal dosage, withdrawal phenomena include anxiety, insomnia, restlessness, agitation, tremor, muscle twitching, nausea and vomiting, orthostatic hypotension, and weight loss.

Drug-Drug Interactions

Barbiturates used with other CNS depressants can cause severe depression. Ethanol is the drug most frequently used, and interactions with antihistaminic compounds are also common. Monoamine oxidase inhibitors and methylphenidate also increase the CNS depressant effect of barbiturates.

Barbiturates may increase the activity of hepatic microsomal enzymes two- to threefold. Clinically, this change is particularly important for patients who are also receiving metabolic competitors such as warfarin or digitoxin, for which careful control of plasma concentrations is vital (Rall 1990).

BENZODIAZEPINES

History

Benzodiazepines were first synthesized in the 1930s but were not systematically evaluated until 20 years later. The introduction in the early 1950s of chlorpromazine and meprobamate, which had sedative effects in animals, led to the decade of increasingly sophisticated in vivo pharmacological screening methods that were used to identify the sedative properties of benzodiazepines. Since the introduction of chlordiazepoxide, which was synthesized by Sternbach in 1957, into clinical medicine, more than 3,000 benzodiazepines have been synthesized. About 40 are in clinical use.

Several drugs chemically unrelated to the benzodiazepines have been shown to have sedative-hypnotic effects with a benzodiazepine-like profile, and it has been determined that these drugs act via the benzodiazepine receptor.

Most of the benzodiazepines on the market were selected for their high anxiolytic potential relative to CNS depression. Nevertheless, all benzodiazepines have sedative-hypnotic properties to various degrees, and some compounds that facilitate sleep have been used as hypnotics.

Mainly because of their remarkably low capacity to produce fatal CNS depression, benzodiazepines have displaced barbiturates as sedative-hypnotic agents.

Structure-Activity Relations

The term *benzodiazepine* refers to the portion of the structure composed of benzene rings (A) fused to a seven-membered diazepine ring (Figure 24–2). However, most of the older benzodiazepines contain a 5-aryl substituent (ring C) and a 1,4-diazepine ring, and the term has come to mean 1,4-benzodiazepines.

A substituent (most often chloride) at position 7 is essential for biological activity. A carbonyl at position 2 enhances activity and is generally present. Most of the newest products also substitute the 2 position, as with

flurazepam. These general features are important for the metabolic fate of the compounds. Because the 7 and 2 positions of the molecule are resistant to all major degradative pathways, many of the metabolites retain substantial pharmacological activity.

Pharmacological Profile

The benzodiazepines share with the barbiturates anticonvulsant and sedative-hypnotic effects. In addition, they have the remarkable ability to reduce anxiety and aggression (Cook and Sepinwall 1975). Several lines of evidence indicate that benzodiazepines are powerful potentiators of GABA. Although this hypothesis is generally accepted, other neurotransmitters may also be involved in these actions.

Schmidt and colleagues in 1967 first reported that diazepam could potentiate the inhibitory effects of GABA on the spinal cords in cats. Later, it was shown that the effect of diazepam could be abolished if the endogenous content of GABA was depleted. This finding established that diazepam (and related benzodiazepines) did not act directly through GABA but modulated inhibitory transmission through GABA in some other way. It was subsequently reported that benzodiazepines bind specifically to neural elements in the mammalian brain with high affinity and that an excellent correlation exists between drug affinities for these specific binding sites and in vivo pharmacological potencies (Möhler and Okada 1977; Squires and Braestrup 1977). The binding of a benzodiazepine to this

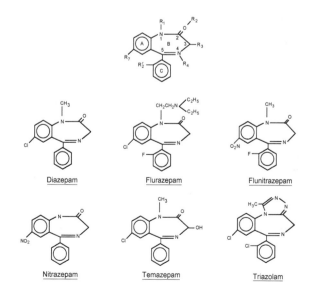

Figure 24–2. Chemical structures for some commonly used benzodiazepines.

receptor site is enhanced in the presence of GABA or a GABA agonist, thereby suggesting that a functional (but independent) relationship exists between the GABA receptor and the benzodiazepine receptor (Tallman et al. 1978).

Barbiturates (and to some extent alcohol) also seem to produce anxiolytic and sedative effects at least partly by facilitating GABAergic transmission (see the earlier section, "Barbiturates"). This common action for chemically unrelated compounds can be explained by their ability to stimulate specific sites on the $GABA_A$ receptor complex.

The benzodiazepines bind with high affinity to the benzodiazepine receptor so that the action of GABA on its receptor is allosterically enhanced. Thus, GABA can produce stronger postsynaptic inhibition in the presence of a benzodiazepine.

The inhibitory effect of GABA is mediated by chloride ion channels. When the $GABA_A$ receptor is occupied by GABA or GABA agonists, such as muscimol, the chloride channels open, and chloride ions diffuse into the cell. One of the binding sites on the chloride ion channel is activated by barbiturates. As was described earlier in this chapter, barbiturates appear to increase the duration of the open state of the chloride channel, whereas benzodiazepines increase the frequency of channel openings with little effect on duration. Note that selective $GABA_A$ agonists, such as muscimol, have no sedative or anxiolytic properties; thus, the whole $GABA_A$ receptor complex (GABA/BZ-Cl⁻ channel) must be involved to show sedative-hypnotic properties.

Thus, it may be concluded that ω benzodiazepine agonists act as sedative-hypnotics by activating a specific benzodiazepine receptor that facilitates inhibitory GABAergic transmission. Other sedative-hypnotics, such as barbiturates and alcohol, also facilitate GABAergic transmission by acting on sites associated more directly with the chloride channel (Figure 24–3). Therefore, ω benzodiazepine agonists are assumed to potentiate only the ongoing, physiologically initiated action of GABA (at $GABA_A$ receptors), whereas barbiturates can cause inhibition at all GABAergic synapses regardless of whether these synapses are physiologically active. This fundamental difference between the allosteric effects of benzodiazepines within the $GABA_A$ receptor complex and the conducive effects of barbiturates on the chloride ion channel may explain why low doses of barbiturates have a pharmacological profile similar to that of benzodiazepines, whereas high doses of barbiturates cause a profound and sometimes fatal suppression of brain synaptic transmission.

In the mammalian CNS, two subtypes of ω receptors have been recognized. Benzodiazepine ω1 (or BZ1) receptors are sensitive to β-carbolines, imidazopyridines (e.g., zolpidem), and triazolopyridazines. Benzodiazepine ω2 (or BZ2) receptors have low affinity for these ligands and relatively high affinity for benzodiazepines. Benzodiazepine ω1 sites are enriched in the cerebellum, while ω2 sites are mostly present in the spinal cord, and both receptor subtypes are found in the cerebral cortex and hippocampus. Benzodiazepine ω1 and ω2 receptor subtypes are also located peripherally in adrenal chromaffin cells. Another subtype, ω3, was identified and commonly labeled the *peripheral benzodiazepine receptor subtype* because of its distribution on glial cell membranes in nonnervous tissues, such as adrenal, testis, liver, and kidney. It was later detected in the CNS, especially on the mitochondrial membrane and not in association with $GABA_A$ receptors. The ω3 subtype has high affinity for benzodiazepines and isoquinoline carboxamides. The functional role of this receptor is not known but may be involved in the sedative-hypnotic effects of some neuroactive steroids (pregnenolone, dehydroepiandrosterone, allopregnanolone, tetrahydrodeoxycorticosterone) (Edgar et al. 1997; Friess et al. 1996). These compounds are indeed metabolized through the mitochondrial benzodiazepine receptor and may also act directly on the $GABA_A$/BZ-Cl⁻ to express their sedative-hypnotic effects (Rupprecht et al. 1996).

Ligand-gated ion channels mediate fast synaptic neurotransmission in the CNS. These ion channels include the molecularly related nicotinic acetylcholine receptors, glycine receptors, the serotonin-3 receptor (5-hydroxytryptamine-3, 5-HT_3), and $GABA_A$ receptors. The structural feature common to all these receptors is a four-membrane-spanning domain. Four or five subunits with

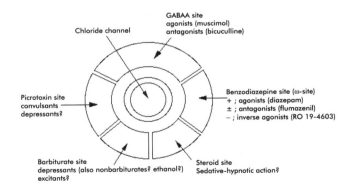

Figure 24–3. Diagrammatic representation of the complex macromolecular components of the γ-aminobutyric acid (GABA)ergic receptor, chloride ionophores, and benzodiazepine binding sites.
Source. Adapted from Olsen et al. 1991.

this structure are assembled around a central channel pore, the gating of which is controlled by the respective neurotransmitters.

Regarding the structure of the GABA$_A$ receptor, molecular cloning studies have reported that many unrelated genes (α_{1-6}, β_{1-3}, γ_{1-3}, δ, and ρ) exist and contain a truly astonishing variety of GABA$_A$ receptor subtypes (Lüddens and Wisden 1991). The functional significance of these multiple subtypes is not entirely clear at present and must be studied further to better understand how the site of drug action affects various physiological functions (e.g., sleep, anxiety, muscle relation) and possibly the pathology of some psychiatric and sleep disorders.

Nonbenzodiazepine hypnotics (acting on the benzodiazepine receptor). Until about 1980, it was widely accepted that the benzodiazepine structure was a prerequisite for the anxiolytic profile and for recognition of and binding to the benzodiazepine receptor. However, more recently, two chemically unrelated drugs—the imidazopyridine zolpidem and the cyclopyrrolone zopiclone—have been shown to be useful sedative-hypnotics with benzodiazepine-like profiles (Figure 24–4). Other chemical classes of drugs that are structurally dissimilar to the benzodiazepines (e.g., tri-

azolopyridazines) but act through the benzodiazepine receptor have also been developed and have anxiolytic activity in humans.

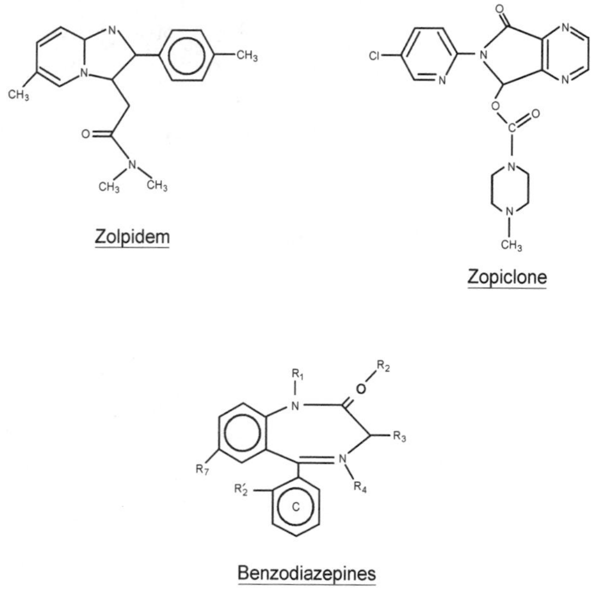

Nonbenzodiazepine hypnotics have a pharmacological profile slightly different from that of classic benzodiazepines. Zolpidem, for example, binds selectively to ω1 (BZ1) and has sedative-hypnotic properties when compared with other properties such as anxiolytic activity or muscle relaxation. Zolpidem and zopiclone have short half-lives—3 hours and 6 hours, respectively. These drugs were originally thought to not appreciably affect the REM sleep pattern, whereas the quality of SWS may be slightly increased (Jovanovic and Dreyfus 1983; Shlarf 1992). Rebound effects (insomnia, anxiety), which are commonly seen following withdrawal of short-acting benzodiazepines, are minimal. These compounds also induce little respiratory depression and have less abuse potential than do clinical benzodiazepine hypnotics. However, much longer clinical trials are needed to show whether the imidazopyridine or cyclopyrrolones have any significant advantages over the short to medium half-life benzodiazepines in the treatment of insomnia.

Benzodiazepine antagonists, partial agonists, and inverse agonists. As knowledge of the relation between the structure of benzodiazepine receptor ligands and their pharmacological properties has increased, potent receptor agonists that stimulate the receptor and produce pharmacological effects qualitatively similar to those of classic benzodiazepines have been developed. *Antagonists*, which block the effects of the agonists without having any effects themselves, and *partial agonists*, drugs that have a mixture of agonistic and antagonistic properties, have also been introduced (Haefley 1988). Partial agonists may be particularly important to develop in the future as sedative-hypnotics that lack common side effects such as ataxia and amnesia.

At the molecular level, *benzodiazepine agonists* are defined as drugs that induce a conformational change in the receptor that produces functional consequences in terms of cellular changes, whereas antagonists occupy only the binding site. Braestup and Nielsen (1986) found that a group of nonbenzodiazepine compounds, the β-carbolines, not only antagonized the action of the full agonists but also had intrinsic activity themselves. These compounds are called *benzodiazepine inverse agonists* because they have biological effects exactly opposite to those of the pure agonists while also having intrinsic activity like agonists. Their effects are blocked by antagonists; thus, the benzodiazepine receptor is particularly unique in that it has a bidirectional function (Figure 24–5).

Figure 24–4. Two nonbenzodiazepine hypnotics—zolpidem (an imidazopyridine) and zopiclone (a cyclopyrrolone)—have been shown to be useful sedative-hypnotics with benzodiazepine-like profiles.

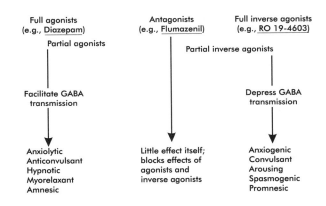

Figure 24–5. Properties of the various types of benzodiazepine receptor ligands. GABA = γ-aminobutyric acid.

Natural ligands for benzodiazepine receptor in the brain.

The presence of benzodiazepine receptors in the brain suggests that natural ligands modulate GABAergic transmission through these sites. Small amounts of benzodiazepines, such as diazepam and desmethyldiazepam, can be detected in human and animal tissues. This finding was confirmed with human brain tissue samples stored since the 1940s before the first synthesis of benzodiazepines (Sangameswaran et al. 1986). These benzodiazepines most likely originate from plants, such as wheat, corn, potatoes, or rice, and the levels detected are too low to be pharmacologically active (i.e., diazepam, <1 ng/g; desmethyldiazepam, 0.5 ng/g).

Other endogenous benzodiazepine-like substances with neuromodulatory effects probably exist in mammals. Endogenous ligands named *diazepam-binding inhibitors* or *endozepines* that bind to the benzodiazepine site on the GABA$_A$-ergic receptor complex have been identified and are being isolated by using biochemical purification protocols (Costa and Guidotti 1991; Marquardt et al. 1986; Rothstein et al. 1992). Their intrinsic action, like that of diazepam, is to potentiate GABA$_A$-receptor-mediated neurotransmission by acting as positive allosteric modulators of this receptor. Endozepines are present in the brain at pharmacologically active concentrations and may play a role both physiologically (e.g., regulation of memory, sleep, and learning) and pathologically (e.g., in panic attacks or hepatic encephalopathy) (Mullen et al. 1990; Nutt et al. 1990). Finally, endozepines have been involved in a newly described neurological condition, *idiopathic recurring stupor*, which is characterized by recurrent episodes of stupor or coma in the absence of any known toxic, metabolic, or structural brain damage. In this condition, the concentrations of endozepines are greatly increased in the plasma of affected individuals, and stupor can be interrupted by flumazenil injections, a benzodiazepine antagonist. Thus, further knowledge of the roles of endozepines in physiological and pathological processes should be forthcoming once these endogenous ligands have been isolated and characterized (Rothstein et al. 1992).

Pharmacokinetics and Disposition

Benzodiazepines are generally absorbed rapidly and completely. Plasma binding is high (i.e., about 98% for diazepam). Benzodiazepines are very lipophilic (except for oxazepam), and penetration into the brain is rapid. For rapid onset of action, diazepam is available as an emulsion, which is administered intravenously for rapid control of epilepsy; midazolam is a water-soluble benzodiazepine suitable for intravenous injection.

The major metabolic pathways for the 1,4-benzodiazepines are shown in Figure 24–6. Medazepam is metabolized to diazepam, which is *N*-desmethylated to desmethyldiazepam. Chlordiazepoxide is also partly converted to desmethyldiazepam. Clorazepate is transformed to desmethyldiazepam.

Desmethyldiazepam is a critically important metabolite for biological activity because of its long half-life of more than 72 hours. Because diazepam's half-life is about 36 hours, the concentration of its desmethyl derivative soon exceeds that of diazepam during chronic administra-

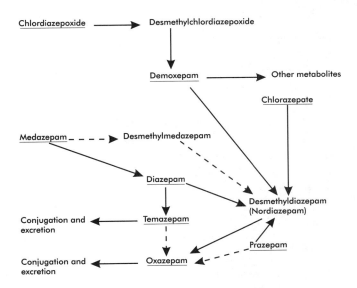

Figure 24–6. Metabolic pathways for the principal 1,4-benzodiazepines (solid and broken arrows denote major and minor pathways, respectively; commercially available drugs are underscored). Flurazepam, flunitrazepam, nitrazepam, and triazolam have separate metabolic pathways.

tion. Desmethyldiazepam undergoes oxidation to oxazepam, which (like its 3-hydroxy analogue temazepam) is rapidly conjugated with glucuronic acid and excreted.

Among the various benzodiazepines, triazolam has a particularly short half-life (<4 hours), and flurazepam and nitrazepam both have long half-lives (see Table 24–2 later in this chapter). A major active metabolite of flurazepam, N-desalkylflurazepam, has a very long half-life of about 100 hours.

Because benzodiazepines are often prescribed for long periods, their long-term pharmacokinetics are important. Diazepam and desmethyldiazepam reach plateau levels after a few weeks. Diazepam concentrations may then decline somewhat without much change in the concentration of the desmethyl metabolite.

Although benzodiazepines can stimulate liver metabolism in some animals, induction is of little clinical significance in humans.

Effects on Stages of Sleep

The hypnotic effects of benzodiazepines have been suggested to result from the modulatory effects of the GABAergic system on the raphe and locus coeruleus monoaminergic projections, but this hypothesis only partially explains their action. Magnocellular regions of the basal forebrain are now recognized as important sites for sleep-wake regulation and are likely to be involved (Szymusiak 1995). Neurons that are selectively active during SWS have been described in this structure, and GABAergic-cholinergic interactions at this level are believed to be involved in the initiation of sleep.

Another important site of action for benzodiazepines might be the suprachiasmatic nucleus (SCN). In SCN-lesioned animals, benzodiazepine treatment does not induce sleep (Edgar et al. 1993), but the hypnotic effect is restored if the SCN-lesioned animal is sleep deprived before drug administration. Benzodiazepines thus may facilitate the release of a sleep debt accumulated during wakefulness rather than produce de novo sleep (Mignot et al. 1992).

The effects of benzodiazepines on sleep architectures are well known. Most benzodiazepines decrease sleep latency, especially when first used, and diminish the number of awakenings (Table 24–1). All benzodiazepines increase time spent in Stage 2 sleep. Benzodiazepines also affect the quality of the SWS pattern. Thus, Stages 3 and 4 sleep are suppressed and remain so during the period of drug administration. The decrease in Stage 4 sleep is accompanied by a reduction in nightmares.

Most benzodiazepines increase REM latency. The time spent in REM sleep is usually shortened; however, the

Table 24–1. Comparative properties of benzodiazepines and barbiturates on sleep parameters

	Benzodiazepines	Barbiturates
Total sleep time	↑ tolerance with short-acting agents	↑ rapid tolerance
Stage 2 %	↑	↑
Slow-wave sleep (Stages 3 and 4) %	↓	↓ (slight)
REM latency	↑	↑
REM %	↓ (slight)	↓
Withdrawal	Rebound insomnia with short-acting agents Carryover effectiveness with long-acting agents REM rebound (slight)	Rebound decrease in Stage 2 and total sleep time REM rebound

Note. REM = rapid eye movement sleep.

reduction in percentage of REM sleep is minimal because the number of cycles of REM sleep usually increases late in the sleep time. Despite the shortening of SWS and REM sleep, the net effect of administration of benzodiazepines is usually an increase in total sleep time, so that the individual feels that the quality of sleep has improved. Furthermore, the hypnotic effect is greatest in subjects with the shortest baseline total sleep time.

If the benzodiazepine is discontinued after 3–4 weeks of nightly use, a considerable rebound in the amount and density of REM sleep and SWS may occur. However, this is not a consistent finding.

Because long-acting benzodiazepine hypnotics impair daytime performance and increase the risk of falls in geriatric patients, several shorter-acting compounds have been introduced and are the preferred choice for elderly patients (see section on the management of insomnia in the elderly) (Figure 24–7). However, it has since been found that short-acting benzodiazepines induce rebound insomnia (a worsening of sleep difficulty beyond baseline levels on discontinuation of a hypnotic) (Kales et al. 1979), rebound anxiety, anterograde amnesia, and even paradoxical rage. Many other factors, such as the subtype of insomnia being treated and the dosage and duration of treatment, are also important to explain the occurrence of these specific side effects that may also be observed with other benzodiazepines. Nevertheless, enthusiasm for the shorter-acting compounds has been tempered.

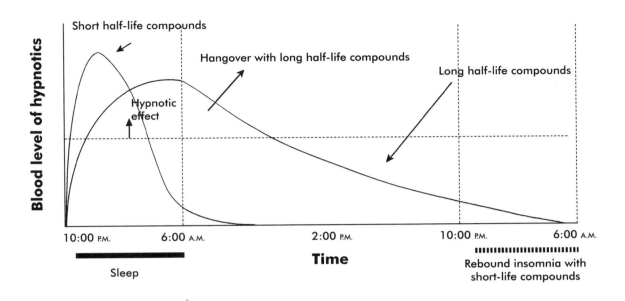

Figure 24–7.   Duration of action of hypnotics and hangover and rebound insomnia. Hypnotics with long half-lives may impair daytime performance the day after drug administration, whereas short-acting compounds may induce rebound insomnia on discontinuation.

Indications

Benzodiazepines are the drug treatment of choice in the management of anxiety, insomnia, and stress-related conditions. Although none of the currently available compounds has any significant advantage over the others, some drugs can be selected to match the patient's symptom patterns to the pharmacokinetics of the various drugs. If a patient has a persistent high level of anxiety, one of the precursors of desmethyldiazepam such as diazepam or clorazepate is most appropriate. Patients with fluctuating anxiety may prefer to take shorter-acting compounds, such as oxazepam or lorazepam, when stressful circumstances occur or are expected.

An ideal hypnotic should induce sleep rapidly without producing sedation the next day. Both flurazepam and nitrazepam are inappropriately long as hypnotics unless a persistent anxiolytic effect is desired the next day (see Figure 24–7). Even in such situations, diazepam given as one dose at night may be preferable. Oxazepam penetrates too slowly for a dependable hypnotic effect (slow onset of action). Both lorazepam and temazepam are appropriate treatments for insomnia, but the dosages available are quite high (Table 24–2). Triazolam is the shortest-acting hypnotic available. When very small doses of benzodiazepines (which were assumed to have no significant hypnotic action) are administered to patients with insomnia,

sleep quality often improves greatly, and usually it is not necessary to use a benzodiazepine at a hypnotic dose as a first-choice treatment.

Benzodiazepines can increase the frequency of apnea and exacerbate oxygen desaturation in healthy subjects and in subjects with chronic bronchitis (Geddes et al. 1976). Although many reports suggest that benzodiazepines are safe in patients with obstructive sleep apnea, other authors disagree, and it seems wise to avoid hypnotics in patients with severe sleep apnea. One of the only other contraindications is myasthenia gravis, a condition in which muscle relaxation with benzodiazepines can exacerbate muscle atonia.

Benzodiazepines have many indications other than sleep induction and anxiolysis, such as epilepsy (see Keck and McElroy, Chapter 21, in this volume). Lorazepam and diazepam can be used for relaxation procedures, preoperative medication, and sedation during minor operations and investigations, often causing retrograde amnesia, a side effect that is sometimes desirable in this indication. Benzodiazepines have been used to manage alcohol withdrawal because cross-tolerance usually exists with alcohol, but large doses are often needed to suppress the withdrawal syndrome. Finally, benzodiazepines, especially clonazepam, are indicated in the treatment of many sleep disorders in adults and infants (see Reite, Chapter 48, in this volume).

Table 24–2. Pharmacokinetic properties of most commonly used hypnotic compounds acting on the benzodiazepine receptors (in the United States)

Hypnotic compounds	Usual dose (mg)	T_{max}/Half-life (hours)	Active metabolites
Flurazepam (Dalmane)	15–30	0.5–1.0/48–150	N-desalkyl-flurazepam
Quazepam (Doral)	7.5–15	2/48–120	2-oxoquazepam, N-dealkyl-2-oxoquazepam
Estazolam (ProSom)	1–2	4.9/18–30	L-oxyestazolam
Temazepam (Restoril)	15–30	1.5/8–20	None
Triazolam (Halcion)	0.125–0.25	1.3/2–6	None
Nonbenzodiapines			
Zolpidem (Ambien)	5–10	2.8/1.5–2.4	None
Zopiclone	3.75–7.5	1.5/5–6	None

Note. T_{max} is the time required to reach the maximal plasma concentration. Half-life is the time required by the body to metabolize or inactivate half the amount of a substrate taken.

Side Effects and Toxicology

When a benzodiazepine is taken at high doses, tiredness, drowsiness, and profound feelings of detachment are common but can be minimized by a careful dose adjustment. Headache, dizziness, ataxia, confusion, and disorientation are less common except in the elderly. A marked potentiation of the depressant effect of alcohol occurs. Other less common side effects include weight gain, skin rash, menstrual irregularities, impairment of sexual function, and, very rarely, agranulocytosis.

Although otherwise asymptomatic subjects clearly show mental impairment with benzodiazepines, the situation with anxious patients is more complex. Because anxiety itself interferes with mental performance, alleviation of anxiety may result in improved functioning, which more than compensates for the direct drug-related decrement. The effects in some patients may be complicated and unpredictable, even at low dosages.

Because the safety of benzodiazepines in early pregnancy is not established, they should be avoided unless absolutely necessary. Diazepam is secreted in breast milk and may make the baby sleepy, unresponsive, and slow to feed.

Overdosage. The benzodiazepines are extremely widely prescribed, so it is not surprising that they are used in many suicide attempts. For adults, overdoses of benzodiazepines reportedly are not fatal unless alcohol or other psychotropic drugs are taken simultaneously. Typically, the patient falls asleep but is arousable and wakes after 24–48 hours. Treatment is supportive. A stomach pump is usually more punitive than therapeutic, and dialysis is usually useless because of high plasma binding.

Tolerance and dependence. Dependence, both psychological and physical, occurs with benzodiazepines as with other sedative-hypnotics. Abrupt discontinuation results in withdrawal phenomena such as anxiety, agitation, restlessness, and tension, which are usually delayed for several days because of the long half-life of the major metabolite, desmethyldiazepam. Even with the normal dosage, some patients have withdrawal effects. The fact that some patients gradually increase the dose suggests tolerance, but increases in dose are sometimes related to particularly stressful crises.

Psychological dependence is also common, based on the high incidence of repeat prescriptions, but it is mild, and the drug-seeking behavior is much less persistent than with barbiturates.

ALCOHOL-TYPE HYPNOTICS AND GAMMA-HYDROXYBUTYRATE

The alcohol type of hypnotics include the chloral derivatives, of which chloral hydrate, clomethiazole, and ethchlorvynol are still used occasionally in the elderly. Chloral hydrate is metabolized to another active sedative-hypnotic—trichloroethanol. These drugs have short half-lives (about 4–6 hours) and decrease sleep latency and number of awakenings; SWS is slightly depressed, but overall REM sleep time is largely unaffected. Chloral hydrate and its metabolite have an unpleasant taste and frequently cause epigastric distress and nausea. Undesirable side effects include light-headedness, ataxia, and nightmares. The chronic use of these drugs can lead to tolerance and occasionally to physical dependence. As with barbiturates, overdosage can lead to respiratory and cardiovascular depression, and therapeutic use of these drugs has largely been superseded by benzodiazepines.

γ-Hydroxybutyrate is a hypnotic agent that has been

used mostly in the treatment of insomnia in narcoleptic patients (Scrima et al. 1990). Although the compound is structurally related to GABA, its mode of action involves specific non-GABAergic binding sites and a potent inhibitory effect on dopaminergic transmission (Vayer et al. 1987). The compound promotes SWS and REM sleep (Lapierre et al. 1990), but its effects on sleep architecture are short lasting, and repeated administration is usually necessary during the night. It is rarely used in other indications and is frequently abused by athletes because of its SWS-promoting effects, with resulting increases in growth hormone secretion (Chin et al. 1992). γ-Hydroxybutyrate is also commonly abused because of its euphoric effects (Chin et al. 1992).

ANTIHISTAMINES

Antihistamines, such as promethazine, diphenhydramine, and doxylamine, are sometimes prescribed as sleep inducers. They decrease sleep latency but do not increase total sleep time (Reite et al. 1997). These compounds are especially useful for patients who cannot sleep well because of acute allergic reactions or itching. Sedative antihistamines may also be prescribed in people who tend to abuse psychoactive drugs, because sedative antihistamines have not been shown to have abuse potential.

MELATONIN

Melatonin is a neurohormone produced by the pineal gland during the dark phase of the day-night cycle. In animals, melatonin has been implicated in the circadian regulation of sleep and in the seasonal control of reproduction. Studies suggest that melatonin administration may have some therapeutic effects in various disturbances of circadian rhythmicity such as jet lag (Arendt et al. 1987), shift work (Folkard et al. 1993), non-24-hour sleep-wake cycle in blind subjects (Arendt et al. 1988), and delayed sleep phase insomnia (Dahlitz et al. 1991), an effect associated with few side effects (e.g., headaches or nausea). High doses of melatonin (3–100 mg), which increase serum melatonin levels far beyond the normal nocturnal range, have been suggested to produce hypnotic effects in humans, especially in the elderly (Haimov et al. 1995). Lower, more physiological doses of melatonin (e.g., 0.3 mg) might also be active, but the data available to date are less convincing.

In humans, the production of melatonin during the dark period declines with age; this effect parallels declines in sleep quantity and quality (Van Coevorden et al. 1991). In one report, older patients with insomnia had a lower secretion of 6-sulphatoxymelatonin (the main melatonin metabolite) than did younger people or older subjects without insomnia (Haimov et al. 1994). These results suggest that deficiency in nocturnal melatonin secretion might contribute to disrupted sleep in the elderly; thus, in this population, insomnia is a particularly attractive indication for melatonin.

One of the difficulties in establishing therapeutic efficacy of melatonin is its short half-life (20–30 minutes). Bedtime melatonin administration reduces sleep latency but has few objective effects on sleep architecture. It is also unclear whether the hypnotic effect of a physiological or pharmacological dose is a direct effect on sleep or an indirect effect on circadian timing that subsequently gates the release of sleep or both. Finally, very few double-blind, placebo-controlled studies have been done, and most current reports are confounded by strong placebo effects in the context of a melatonin fad. Melatonin might be an effective hypnotic in some indications, but better controlled studies are needed to establish efficacy in specific indications. The purity of the products sold in health food stores is also a problem, and the long-term effects of melatonin administration in humans are unknown.

THALIDOMIDE

Thalidomide is a unique hypnotic compound that deserves special mention. The compound was first introduced as a sleep-inducing agent in the 1950s but was rapidly withdrawn after accumulating reports of secondary fetal malformations. In the 1960s, thalidomide was found to be surprisingly effective in the treatment of severe granulomatous skin complications associated with leprosy (e.g., erythema nodosum). Since then, thalidomide has been reintroduced to treat various conditions that involve pathological immune reactions (e.g., graft-versus-host disease, lupus) and pharyngeal ulcerations in patients with acquired immunodeficiency syndrome (AIDS) (see Kaplan 1994). In patients with leprosy and AIDS, thalidomide inhibited the production of tumor necrosis factor alpha (TNFα).

Together with γ-hydroxybutyrate, thalidomide is one of the few hypnotics that increases REM sleep and SWS (Frederickson et al. 1977; Kaitin 1985) (benzodiazepines and barbiturates decrease REM sleep and deep SWS). Thalidomide does not bind to or enzymatically modify any neurotransmitter systems known to be involved in the regulation of sleep (e.g., histamine, serotonin, benzodiazepine, excitatory amino acids, and GABA) (Kanbayashi et al. 1996). Thalidomide thus may affect sleep through neuroimmune interactions in the brain, because TNFα and other cytokines secreted by the microglia in the brain have been reported to be endogenous sleep-modulating substances (Krueger et al. 1995). Thalidomide analogues with hypnotic effects and/or immunomodulatory effects without any teratogenic effects in animals are available experimentally but have never been developed for clinical use. Thalidomide thus remains a unique and powerful pharmacological tool to study the regulation of normal and abnormal sleep that could lead to the development of new hypnotic agents.

GENERAL CONSIDERATIONS IN THE PHARMACOLOGICAL TREATMENT OF INSOMNIA

Insomnia is a subjective complaint of insufficient, inadequate, or nonrestrictive sleep (see Buysse and Reynolds 1990). Disturbances in daytime functioning, such as fatigue, mood disturbances, and impaired performance, result from inadequate sleep. Insomnia is a common symptom. In 1983, a survey indicated that 35% of the general population reported having trouble sleeping in the past year, and 17% considered their problem serious (Mellinger et al. 1985). In the same survey, 7.1% of the population had used a hypnotic in the past year (Mellinger et al. 1985).

Insomnia is a symptom that must be explored clinically before treatment is initiated. Sleep disturbances often indicate a larger psychiatric problem, such as depression. As mentioned above, a complaint of insomnia is also common with old age, especially in an institutional setting. In other cases, environmental factors (e.g., noise) and associated sleep disorders (periodic leg movements, sleep apneas, parasomnias) may be involved.

A useful initial approach to the patient with insomnia is to consider the duration of the complaint. Insomnia can occur as a transient (1–2 days), short-term (more than a few days to a few months), or chronic disturbance (several months or even years). The duration of insomnia not only suggests its cause (see Table 24–3) but also provides some guidance on how to use hypnotics.

Transient insomnias are typically caused by an environmental acute stressor or jet lag and shift work. In this indication, pharmacotherapy with benzodiazepine hypnotics or other hypnotics has no risks because dependence on the treatment is unlikely to develop if the therapy lasts less than a week to 10 days.

Short-term (a few days to a few months) insomnias are

particularly important to recognize because they may evolve into chronic, psychophysiological insomnia if not or inadequately treated. Typically, patients develop insomnia during a stressful period of their lives (e.g., work or personal difficulties). The condition frequently worsens if untreated, and the patient worries excessively about his or her sleep, which evolves toward a behaviorally learned, chronic insomnia that does not resolve once the stressful period is over. In this indication, the use of benzodiazepine hypnotics on a daily basis is also dangerous because it may lead to tolerance and dependence. Reassurance regarding the favorable resolution of the stressful event is important, and the patient should be instructed to use hypnotic medications intermittently (e.g., every few days, as needed) to avoid the development of tolerance. An education in sleep hygiene (not taking naps even when very tired, having regular wake-up times, avoiding caffeine and alcohol) is also important to reduce the possibility of evolution into a chronic problem.

Chronic insomnia first should be evaluated with a sleep log for a 2-week period. Most commonly, some degree of sleep state misperception is present, and patients with insomnia greatly exaggerate the complaint (i.e., they sleep more than they claim and take less time to fall asleep than they report). In most cases, insomnia has developed as the result of psychological factors and negative conditioning, as mentioned above. In rare cases, insomnia began in childhood and has persisted in adulthood (idiopathic insomnia). In chronic insomnia, improved sleep hygiene and various behavioral techniques that aim to reduce negative conditioning (stimulus control therapy), sleep restriction, and phototherapy are often helpful on a long-term basis, but these methods are only successful if the patient is motivated and if specialized clinical supervision is available. The most appropriate use of drugs is in patients in whom sleep disturbance is clearly causing some daytime dysfunction. If the clinician decides to use pharmacotherapy, it is always helpful to start with the lowest dose of hypnotic possible (hypnotic medications are frequently overdosed) to reduce the risk of tolerance and dependence and to try to avoid daily use.

Insomnia can also be classified on the basis of individual clinical features—that is, as sleep initiation, sleep maintenance, or termination (early-morning awakening). In this context, the most important pharmacological properties to consider when selecting a hypnotic for treatment are how quickly it acts and how long the effects last (see Table 24–2 for commonly used compounds). The rate of absorption is the most critical factor determining onset of action. T_{max} (time required to reach the maximal plasma concentration) is the pharmacological parameter that best

Table 24–3. Nosological classification of insomnia (International Classification of Sleep Disorders Diagnostic Criteria)

Category	% of patients with corresponding diagnosis[a]	Description
Psychophysiological	15	Transient or persistent insomnia that develops as a result of psychological factors, physiological tension/arousal, and negative conditioning
Idiopathic insomnia	<5	Insomnia and daytime dysfunction, which begin in childhood and continue into adulthood
Associated with sleep-induced respiratory impairment	5–10	Frequent respiratory pauses or hypoxia (e.g., sleep apnea, alveolar hypoventilation) that lead to brief arousals during the night
Associated with periodic leg movements and restless legs	12	Repetitive, stereotyped jerking leg movements or unpleasant dysesthesias in legs on falling asleep, which frequently interrupt sleep
Associated with psychiatric disorders	35	Insomnia associated with behavioral symptoms and underlying biological disturbances of psychiatric disorders (including affective, anxiety, psychotic, and personality disorders)
Associated with neurological disorders	~5	Insomnia associated with neurological disorders, such as cerebral degenerative disorders, dementia, and parkinsonism
Associated with other medical disorders	~5	Insomnia associated with other medical disorders, such as nocturnal cardiac ischemia, chronic obstructive pulmonary disease, and sleep-related asthma; sleep is expected to improve when the underlying condition is treated
Associated with chronic drugs and alcohol	12	Insomnia associated with use of, tolerance to, or withdrawal from CNS-active agents, including stimulants, sedative-hypnotics, and alcohol
Sleep state misperception	5–10	Subjective insomnia complaint that is not substantiated by polysomnography
Transient sleep-wake disorders[b]	NA	Rapid time-zone change (jet lag) or schedule or work shift change results in symptoms of insomnia during new, desired sleep hours, and sleepiness during new, desired wake hours
Persistent sleep-wake disorders[b]	NA	A frequently changing sleep-wake schedule, delayed or advanced sleep phase syndrome, non-24-hour sleep-wake pattern, or irregular sleep-wake pattern results in symptoms of insomnia during desired sleep hours and sleepiness during desired wake hours

Note.   CNS = central nervous system; NA = not available.
[a]Estimated from approximately 2,000 patients with a diagnosed disorder of initiating and maintaining sleep by 20 centers; contributed by the Association of Sleep Disorders Centers National Case Series (Coleman 1983).
[b]These diagnoses are classified as disorders of the circadian rhythm sleep disorders in the *International Classification of Sleep Disorders* diagnostic criteria (American Sleep Disorders Association 1990).
Source.   Adapted from Buysse and Reynolds 1990.

predicts onset of action. After absorption, hypnotics are distributed to various organs; distribution and drug elimination influence the duration of action. The elimination half-life (see Table 24–2) usually provides a good first estimate of the duration of action for drugs that have comparable absorption and distribution profiles. Hypnotics with long durations of action are helpful for patients who have difficulty both initiating and maintaining sleep. One advantage of these long-acting compounds is that rebound insomnia is often delayed and milder if the drug has to be

withdrawn (see Figure 24–7). Patients who have difficulty initiating sleep might prefer short-acting compounds; however, for these compounds, it may be necessary, paradoxically, to switch to longer-acting hypnotics before withdrawal of all hypnotic treatment.

The importance of determining whether insomnia is the symptom of an underlying neuropsychiatric condition must be emphasized (see Table 24–3). For depression, trazodone (25–50 mg), amitriptyline (10 mg), trimipramine (25–50 mg), or doxepin (25–50 mg) can be used as hypnotics or in combination with other hypnotics. Most schizophrenic patients also have persistent insomnia (initiation and maintenance of sleep), and phenothiazines, such as chlorpromazine, thioridazine, and levomepromazine, are effective therapies. When psychotic symptoms are associated with insomnia, butyrophenones, such as haloperidol, also can be used. For insomnia associated with anxiety disorders, hypnotics supplemented with anxiolytics can be used, and this treatment may prevent rebound insomnia and its related anxiety.

Sleep disturbances are very frequent complaints in old age, and treatment must be initiated carefully in this population (see also Salzman et al., Chapter 46, in this volume). About 12% of the United States population is older than 60 years, and this population receives 35%–40% of all sedative-hypnotic prescriptions (Gottlieb 1990).

Before starting pharmacological therapy, all possible causes of insomnia should be examined (i.e., psycho-physiological, associated with drugs and alcohol, disturbance of the sleep-wake cycle, associated with periodic leg movements, sleep apnea, or other physical or psychiatric conditions). Before selecting a specific hypnotic, the clinician should consider the pharmacological properties, side-effect profiles, patients' medical health and histories, and patients' histories of sedative-hypnotic use. The special case of melatonin has been discussed earlier in this chapter. Hypnotics or their active metabolites often accumulate during chronic use in elderly patients, and this accumulation may cause cognition problems, disorientation, confusion, and, occasionally, falls. Hypnotics with short or intermediate half-lives are thus recommended, and the lowest dose possible should be used. Compounds with a short half-life, such as triazolam or zolpidem, may be effective for problems with sleep initiation and sleep fragmentation. Zolpidem has little muscle relaxant effect and may be preferable. Compounds with an intermediate hypnotic profile, such as estazolam and temazepam, are also reported to be effective in elderly patients. Hypnotics with intermediate half-lives may alter less daytime performance and memory and are less likely to induce rebound insomnia after withdrawal compared with regular hypnotics.

CONCLUSION

The mechanism of action of most currently available hypnotics (barbiturates, alcohol, benzodiazepines, zolpidem, and zopiclone) involves a modulatory effect of GABAergic activity. These compounds stimulate GABAergic transmission by acting on the $GABA_A/BZ-Cl^-$ macromolecular complex, known to contain multiple modulatory binding sites and many receptor subtypes. This recently discovered molecular diversity suggests that new GABAergic hypnotic compounds with better side-effect profiles will be developed in the future.

Other non-GABAegic hypnotics, including mostly sedative antidepressants, antihistamines, and melatonin, are viable strategies in the treatment of insomnia. Their prescription, as for other regular benzodiazepine-like hypnotic compounds, should be guided by the knowledge that insomnia is a heterogeneous condition that should be explored clinically before any pharmacological treatment is initiated.

REFERENCES

American Sleep Disorders Association: The International Classification of Sleep Disorders: Diagnostic and Coding Manual. Rochester, MN, American Sleep Disorders Association, 1990

Arendt J, Aldhous M, Marks V, et al: Some effects of jet-lag and their alleviation by melatonin. Ergonomics 30:1379–1393, 1987

Arendt J, Aldhous M, Wright J: Synchronisation of a disturbed sleep-wake cycle in a blind man by melatonin treatment. Lancet i:772–773, 1988

Asano T, Ogasawara N: Chloride-dependent stimulation of GABA and benzodiazepine receptor binding by pentobarbital. Brain Res 225:212–216, 1981

Braestrup C, Nielsen M: Benzodiazepine binding in vivo and efficacy, in Benzodiazepine/GABA Receptors and Chloride Channels: Structural and Functional Properties. Edited by Olsen RW, Venter JC. New York, Alan R Liss, 1986, pp 167–184

Buysse DJ, Reynolds III CF: Insomnia, in Handbook of Sleep Disorders. Edited by Thorpy MJ. New York, Marcel Dekker, 1990, pp 375–433

Chin M, Kreutzer RA, Dyer JL: Acute poisoning from γ-hydroxybutyrate in California. West J Med 156:380–384, 1992

Coleman RM: Diagnosis, treatment, and follow-up of about 8,000 sleep/wake disorder patients, in Sleep/Wake Disorders; National History, Epidemiology, and Long Term Evolution. Edited by Guilleminault C, Lugaresi E. New York, Raven, 1983, pp 29–35

Cook L, Sepinwall J: Behavioral analysis of the effects and mechanisms of action of benzodiazepines. Adv Biochem Psychopharmacol 14:1–28, 1975

Costa E, Guidotti A: Diazepam binding inhibitor (DBI): a peptide with multiple biological actions. Life Sci 49:325–344, 1991

Dahlitz M, Alvarez B, Vignan J, et al: Delayed sleep phase syndrome response to melatonin. Lancet 337:1121–1124, 1991

Edgar DM, Dement WC, Fuller CA: Effect of SCN-lesions on sleep in squirrel monkeys: evidence for opponent processes in sleep-wake regulation. J Neurosci 13:1065–1079, 1993

Edgar DM, Seidel WF, Gee KW, et al: CCD-3693: an orally bioavailable analog of the endogenous neuroactive steroid, pregnanolone, demonstrates potent sedative hypnotic action in the rat. J Pharmacol Exp Ther 282:420–429, 1997

Enna SJ, Möhler H: γ-aminobutyric acid (GABA) receptors and their association with benzodiazepine recognition sites, in Psychopharmacology: The Third Generation of Progress. Edited by Meltzer HY. New York, Raven, 1987, pp 265–272

Folkard S, Arendt J, Clark M: Can melatonin improve shift workers' tolerance of the night shift? Some preliminary findings. Chronobiol Int 10:315–320, 1993

Frederickson RC, Slater IH, Dusenberrry WE: A comparison of thalidomide and pentobarbital—new methods for identifying novel hypnotic drugs. J Pharmacol Exp Ther 203:240–251, 1977

Friess E, Lance M, Holster F: The effects of 'neuroactive' steroids upon sleep in human and rats (abstract). J Sleep Res 5:S69, 1996

Geddes DM, Rudorf M, Saunders KB: Effect of nitrazepam and flurazepam on the ventilatory response to carbon dioxide. Thorax 31:548–551, 1976

Gottlieb GL: Sleep disorders and their management: special considerations in the elderly. Am J Med 88:29S–33S, 1990

Haefley W: Partial agonists of the benzodiazepine receptor: from animal data to results in patients, in Chloride Channels and Their Modulation by Neurotransmission and Drugs. Edited by Biggio G, Costa E. New York, Raven, 1988, pp 275–292

Haimov I, Laudon M, Zisapel N, et al: Sleep disorders and melatonin rhythms in elderly people. BMJ 309:167, 1994

Haimov I, Lavie P, Lauden M, et al: Melatonin treatment of sleep onset insomnia in the elderly. Sleep 18:598–603, 1995

Jovanovic UJ, Dreyfus JF: Polygraphical sleep recording in insomniac patients under zopiclone or nitrazepam. Pharmacology 27 (suppl 2):136–145, 1983

Kaitin KI: Effects of thalidomide and pentobarbital on neuronal activity in the preoptic area during sleep and wakefulness in the cat. Psychopharmacology (Berl) 85:47–50, 1985

Kales A, Shlarf MB, Kales JD, et al: Rebound insomnia: a potential hazard following withdrawal of certain benzodiazepines. JAMA 241:1691–1695, 1979

Kanbayashi T, Nishino S, Tafti M, et al: Thalidomide, a hypnotic with immune modulating properties, increases cataplexy in canine narcolepsy. Neuroreport 12:1881–1886, 1996

Kaplan G: Cytokine regulation of disease progression in leprosy and tuberculosis. Immunobiology 191:564–568, 1994

Kay DC, Blackburn AB, Buckingham JA, et al: Human pharmacology of sleep, in Pharmacology of Sleep. Edited by Williams RL, Karakan I. New York, Wiley, 1976, pp 83–210

Killam K: Drug action on the brainstem reticular formation. Pharmacol Rev 14:175–224, 1962

Krueger JM, Takahashi S, Kapas L: Cytokines in sleep regulation. Adv Neuroimmunol 5:171–188, 1995

Lapierre O, Montplaisir J, Lamarre M, et al: The effect of gamma-hydroxybutyrate on nocturnal and diurnal sleep of normal subjects: further consideration on REM sleep-triggering mechanisms. Sleep 13:24–30, 1990

Leeb-Lumberg F, Snowman A, Olsen RW: Barbiturate receptor sites are coupled to benzodiazepine receptors. Proc Natl Acad Sci U S A 77:7467–7472, 1980

Lüddens H, Wisden W: Function and pharmacology of multiple GABA$_A$ receptor subunit. Trends Pharmacol Sci 12:49–51, 1991

Marquardt H, Todaro GJ, Shoyab M: Complete amino acid sequences of bovine and human endozepines: homology with rat diazepam binding inhibitor. J Biol Chem 261: 9727–9731, 1986

Maynert EW: Sedative and hypnotics, II: barbiturates, in Drill's Pharmacology in Medicine. Edited by DiPalma IR. New York, McGraw-Hill, 1965, pp 188–209

Mellinger GD, Balter MB, Uhlenhuth EH: Insomnia and its treatment: prevalence and correlates. Arch Gen Psychiatry 42:225–232, 1985

Mignot E, Edgar DM, Miller JD, et al: Strategies for the development of new treatments in sleep disorders medicine, in Target Receptors for Anxiolytics and Hypnotics: From Molecular Pharmacology to Therapeutics. Edited by Mendelewicz J, Racagni G, Karger AG. Basel, Karger, 1992, pp 129–150

Möhler H, Okada T: Benzodiazepine receptor: demonstration in the central nervous system. Science 198:849–851, 1977

Mullen KD, Szauter KM, Kaminsky-Russ K: "Endogenous" benzodiazepine activity in physiological fluids of patients with hepatic encephalopathy. Lancet 336:81–83, 1990

Nutt DJ, Glue P, Lawson C, et al: Flumazenil provocation of panic attacks. Arch Gen Psychiatry 47:917–925, 1990

Olsen RW, Tick MK, Miller T: Dihydropicotoxine binding to crayfish muscle sites possibly related to γ-aminobutyric acid receptor-ionophores. Mol Pharmacol 14:381–390, 1978

Olsen RW, Bureau MH, Endo S, et al: The GABA$_A$ receptor family in the mammalian brain. Neurochem Res 16:317–325, 1991

Rall TR: Hypnotics and sedatives; ethanol, in The Pharmacological Basis of Therapeutics, 8th Edition. Edited by Gilman AG, Rall TW, Niles AS, et al. New York, Pergamon, 1990, pp 345–382

Reite M, Ruddy J, Nagel K: Concise Guide to Evaluation and Management of Sleep Disorders, 2nd Edition. Washington, DC, American Psychiatric Press, 1997

Richter JA, Holman JR Jr: Barbiturates: their in vivo effects and potential biochemical mechanisms. Prog Neurobiol 18:275–319, 1982

Rothstein JD, Guidotti A, Tinuper P, et al: Endogenous benzo-diazepine receptor ligands in ideopathic recurring stupor. Lancet 340:1002–1004, 1992

Rupprecht R, Hauser CAE, Trapp T, et al: Neurosteroids: molecular mechanisms of action and psychopharmacological significance. J Steroid Biochem Mol Biol 56:163–168, 1996

Sangameswaren L, Fales HM, Friedrich P, et al: Purification of a benzodiazepine from bovine brain and detection of benzo-diazepine like immunoreactivity in human brain. Proc Natl Acad Sci U S A 83:9236–9240, 1986

Schmidt RF, Vogel ME, Zimmermann M: Effect of diazepam on presynaptic inhibition and other spinal reflexes. Naunyn Schmiedebergs Arch Pharmacol 258:69–82, 1967

Scrima L, Hartman PG, Johnson FH, et al: The effects of gamma-hydroxybutyrate on the sleep of narcolepsy patients: a double-blind study. Sleep 13:479–490, 1990

Shlarf MB: Pharmacology of classic and novel hypnotic drugs, in Target Receptors for Anxiolytics and Hypnotics: From Molecular Pharmacology to Therapeutics. Edited by Mendelwicz J, Racagni G. Basel, Karger, 1992, pp 109–116

Squires RF, Braestrup C: Benzodiazepine receptors in rat brain. Nature 266:732–734, 1977

Szymusiak R: Magnocellular nuclei of the basal forebrain: substrates of sleep and arousal regulation. Sleep 18:478–500, 1995

Tallman JF, Thomas JW, Gllager DW: GABAergic modulation of benzodiazepine binding site sensitivity. Nature 274:383–385, 1978

Van Coevorden A, Mockel J, Laurent E, et al: Neuroendocrine rhythms and sleep in aging men. Am J Physiol 260:651–661, 1991

Vayer P, Mandel P, Maitre M: Gamma-hydroxybutyrate, a possible neurotransmitter. Life Sci 41:1547–1557, 1987

TWENTY-FIVE

Stimulants in Psychiatry

Jan Fawcett, M.D., and Katie A. Busch, M.D.

The colorful history of stimulants began with the discovery of the psychoactive effects of cocaine, which has pharmacological properties remarkably similar to those of amphetamine despite their dissimilar chemical structures. Amphetamine, like cocaine, was introduced in medicine because of its ability to alleviate fatigue temporarily and to enhance mental and physical performance. The marked and varied effects of amphetamine, despite its relatively simple structure and its potential for abuse and dependence, have made it a topic of interest and controversy since it was first synthesized in 1887.

Today, the major areas of medical use of stimulants are the treatment of narcolepsy, for which amphetamine or methylphenidate (MPH) is used to relieve the symptoms of sleepiness and involuntary sleeping without affecting the etiology of the illness, and in the treatment of attention-deficit/hyperactivity disorder (ADHD) in children, which continues to generate scientific, medical, and public controversy. Stimulants are also of possible value in treating adult attention-deficit disorder or residual ADHD, and they are still used in the treatment of obesity despite significant medical and scientific doubts as to their long-term benefits in maintaining weight loss and concerns about abuse and dependence. This latter use has recently increased with the introduction of the famous and more recently controversial combination of the relatively weak stimulant phentermine with the serotonin (5-hydroxytryptamine [5-HT])-releasing forms of fenfluramine, known as "Phen-Fen," which are reviewed here. Interestingly, just as this chapter was going to press, fenfluramine was voluntarily withdrawn from the market because of concerns regarding its use, which are reviewed in this chapter. Other proposed uses of stimulants include the treatment of affective disorders and certain organic brain disorders and their use in cancer patients receiving high doses of opiates for pain. These uses are discussed later in this chapter.

Studies stating that stimulants had no place in general psychiatry were based on work in the 1960s, which is considered flawed by some (Chiarello and Cole 1987) and valid by others (Satel and Nelson 1989). In contrast, however, there exist open case reports of the effectiveness of stimulants in medically ill patients, poststroke patients, and acquired immunodeficiency syndrome (AIDS) patients with depression. There have also been recent reports of stimulant use to augment antidepressant medications in treatment-resistant patients (i.e., partial responders) and treatment-refractory patients (i.e., total nonresponders), as well as evidence that certain patients may require more dopaminergic effects for effective antidepressant treatment. These reports leave open the question of the usefulness of stimulants in these and other areas of psychiatry.

Dextroamphetamine (DAMPH) and MPH are the two most commonly used stimulants in psychiatry and medicine. They have both similarities and differences in effect. In this chapter, we focus on these two compounds as primary examples of stimulant medications. We consider their mechanisms of action and the current evidence concerning their therapeutic and adverse effects and the hazards associated with their use. Other weaker but clinically used stimulants, such as phentermine and pemoline, will be discussed in their clinical contexts.

HISTORY AND DISCOVERY

The first known stimulant, cocaine, was isolated in the mid-eighteenth century. In 1884, cocaine was given to Bavarian soldiers, who reported that it decreased fatigue (R. L. Patrick 1977). Amphetamine was first synthesized in 1887 and has certain similarities to cocaine in its potent psychomotor stimulant activity. Amphetamine was studied by Alles (1933), who wanted to find a synthetic substitute for ephedrine after Chen and Schmidt (1930) had rediscovered ephedrine, which had been isolated from the *Ephedra vulgaris* plant in 1925. Alles and Leake developed techniques for evaluating the toxicity and activity of phenylalkylamines (Alles 1933). The most active of these compounds was *d,l*-phenylisopropylamine, or amphetamine, the dextro isomer of which was found to increase alertness and wakefulness and to promote improved physical and mental performance in people who are fatigued or bored, as well as to suppress appetite (R. L. Patrick 1977).

Amphetamines were used by both sides in World War II. It has been contended that Japan had large supplies of amphetamines that were placed on the open market after the war, leading to an epidemic of amphetamine abuse and cases of amphetamine psychosis, first in Japan in the 1950s and then in the United States in the 1960s (Fischman 1987). R. L. Patrick (1977) mentioned that it is "one of the ironies in history of psychopharmacology that the Haight-Ashbury amphetamine epidemic took place less than a mile from the University of California San Francisco Medical Center, where Alles and Leake had synthesized amphetamines more than 40 years earlier" (p. 335). In 1958, the piperazine derivative of amphetamine, MPH, was first introduced to treat hyperactivity in children (Anders and Ciaranello 1977).

In an excellent historical review, Connell (1968) observed that there were more than 50 preparations of "amphetamine substances," either alone as derivatives or in combination with other drugs (notably barbiturates), on the market. At that time, Connell reviewed the status of the clinical uses of amphetamines for a wide range of medical conditions. Narcolepsy was probably the first disorder for which amphetamine was used clinically (Prinzmetal and Bloomberg 1935). Amphetamine revolutionized therapy for this condition and, although its use was not curative, it was noted that "the drug may enable the patient to become symptom free" (Connell 1968, p. 235). The effec-

tive dose ranged as high as 30–50 mg, taken in divided doses two or three times daily.

The use of amphetamine in the treatment of parkinsonism dates back to 1937, when it was used for muscular rigidity and postencephalitic parkinsonism. By 1968, its use in the treatment of this condition had been largely superseded by more effective agents (Connell 1968). Connell observed that amphetamine was first used in treating epilepsy because of its action in antagonizing the sedative effect of narcotics. It was later found that amphetamine itself may have beneficial effects, particularly in the milder epileptic states, and it has been used as the sole method of medication for epilepsy, with varying results. Connell pointed out that in 1968, it was more common for amphetamine to be used in combination with other anticonvulsant drugs than by itself. This is in accordance with the observations of Hoffman and Lefkowitz (1993), who noted that amphetamine "can obtund the maximal electroshock seizure discharge" (p. 211).

Connell (1968) also noted that the role of amphetamine in the treatment of barbiturate poisoning had changed over the previous 25 years and observed that Riishede (1950) found a lower mortality in patients treated with amphetamine than in those treated with nikethamide. Methylamphetamine was often preferred because of its greater vasoconstricting action, together with a more marked stimulating effect on respiration and muscle tone. Connell (1968) observed that the use of amphetamines in barbiturate poisoning had "been superseded by other drugs and other methods of treatment" (p. 235).

Amphetamines were also widely used in the treatment of drug addiction and alcoholism to offset sleepiness and lethargy. This continued until the recognition of the dangers of amphetamine dependence and abuse of amphetamines, "together with the vicious cycle of amphetamine to counteract effect of sedatives, followed by sedatives to counteract the use of amphetamines (e.g., insomnia)" (Connell 1968, p. 235). This realization led to the discontinuation of amphetamine use in the treatment of these conditions.

Amphetamines were used to treat "psychopathic states," based on their effects on electroencephalogram tracings and the clinical state of adults with aggressive psychopathology (Hill 1947; Hill and Watterson 1942). Researchers described these states as including very deep sleep, excessive sexual appetite, a history of long-continuing nocturnal enuresis, epilepsy, and occasional convulsive seizures in the patient. Connell (1968) noted that the "paradoxical" effect of "quieting the emotional behavior, in which the patient tolerated high doses without disturbance of sleep" (p. 235), was of great interest. He concluded that using amphetamines to treat psychopathic states and delinquency produced results that were "variable and somewhat unpredictable" (p. 235). Connell also mentioned that Bradley and Bowen (1941) had reported the use of amphetamines to modify antisocial behavior in children. He summarized clinical observations of the effects of amphetamine as showing that "when children are withdrawn or lethargic, the amphetamines tended to make them more alert, more accessible to persons and the environment" (Connell 1968, p. 236).

The "paradoxical" effect of amphetamine noted in psychopathic adults was also seen in aggressive, noisy children; children who were hyperactive tended to move more quietly, to be calmer, and to quarrel less when taking amphetamines. These observations appear to precede those of the effect of amphetamine and MPH in hyperkinetic children with a diagnosis of what is now called ADHD. Amphetamines were also used to treat enuresis, based on observations that some enuretic patients slept very deeply (Connell 1968). In a regimen developed by Hodge and Hutchings (1952), a starting dose of 2.5 mg is used at bedtime for 1 week, and the dose is then increased to 5 mg/week and subsequently raised every week until the patient is sleeping more lightly. Connell (1968) commented that this method of treatment may result in failure as often as success.

The next historical use of amphetamines, and perhaps one of its most common uses, was in the treatment of obesity. Connell (1968) commented that there was "an increasing body of opinion suggesting that the contribution of amphetamines to the long-term treatment of obesity is small or nonexistent and does not justify their use now that the dangers of dependency and abuse are so much better known" (p. 236). He mentioned the possibility that diethylpropion and fenfluramine have fewer reports of abuse potential and of side effects such as stimulation of the nervous system. Connell (1968) noted that

> the value of amphetamines in the treatment of depressive disorder has been the subject of considerable controversy, but it would seem that there is an increasing number of psychiatrists who maintain that it has no use at all in the treatment of depression and that the dangers of dependence and abuse prohibit its use not only in depression but in psychiatric practice. (p. 237)

This view is very similar to the position taken by Wheatley (1969) based on the use of amphetamines prescribed by general practitioners to treat depression. Shaw (1964) stated that the "amphetamine drugs hold a very doubtful place in the treatment of depression" (p. 28).

Connell (1968) also observed that methamphetamine was being used increasingly less frequently in psychiatric practice as an abreactive agent to treat neurotic conditions and as an aid in the diagnosis of psychiatric disorders.

The epidemic of amphetamine abuse peaked in the United States in the 1960s and 1970s and was in decline by 1978, when the cocaine epidemic was well under way (Foltin and Fischman 1991). In 1970, amphetamine and its derivatives were scheduled under the Controlled Substances Act.

From the perspective of the history of stimulants, the indications for their use has considerably narrowed over the years. The reasons for this probably include the realization of the risks of abuse and dependence on these agents, that newer and more effective agents have been shown to work in treating some of these conditions, and that the stimulants have simply been shown to be ineffective and have thus fallen into disuse. At the same time, an interest in the clinical use of stimulants in psychiatry remains, as evidenced by case reports of positive treatment responses in patients with particular types of affective disorders and some other psychiatric conditions. These areas of possible effectiveness for the stimulants are reviewed in the "Indications" section of this chapter.

STRUCTURE-ACTIVITY RELATIONS

Phenylisopropylamine (amphetamine) is a relatively simple structure and forms the template for a wide variety of pharmacologically active substances. Although amphetamine is a central nervous system (CNS) stimulant, minor modifications of it result in agents that can produce a broad spectrum of effects, including decongestant, anorectic, antidepressant (bupropion and the monoamine oxidase inhibitor [MAOI] tranylcypromine), and hallucinogenic (Glennon 1987). As noted by Glennon (1987), although health professionals and the lay public may assume that all amphetamine derivatives could possess amphetamine-like characteristics, this is not necessarily the case. Although amphetamine itself has (most notably) CNS stimulant, anorectic, and vasoconstrictor properties, a review of its structure-activity relations shows that its major properties (plus psychomimetic, MAO inhibition, and neurotransmitter uptake effects) can be enhanced by structural modification at the expense of other effects.

With respect to the behavioral properties of the simple phenylisopropylamines, two general groups, the CNS stimulant and the hallucinogenic properties, can be considered. The phenylisopropylamine molecule can be arbitrarily divided into three structural components: 1) the aromatic nucleus, 2) the terminal amine, and 3) the isopropyl side chain. In general, substitution on the aromatic nucleus of amphetamine results in agents that are less potent or inactive as CNS stimulants (Glennon 1987). The substitution of two or more methoxy groups plus ethyl, methyl, or bromine groups on the aromatic nucleus creates hallucinogens of various potencies.

Several popular hallucinogens of abuse result from the substitution of methylenedioxy substitutions on two carbons of the aromatic ring. This results in 2,3-methylenedioxyamphetamine (MDA) or 3,4-MDA, known as the "love drug," which has behavioral properties distinct from those of either amphetamine or other typical hallucinogens. The end monomethyl analogue of 3,4-MDA, *N*-methyl-3,4-methylenedioxymethamphetamine (MDMA) or "XTC" ("Ecstasy"), is perhaps one of the best-known contemporary stimulant hallucinogens of abuse (Glennon 1987). These compounds have often been called "designer drugs" because their structure-activity relations have been used to design new derivatives of a known agent, the resulting drugs not yet being covered under the Controlled Substances Act of 1970.

Substitution on the terminal amine group of amphetamine tends to reduce the hallucinogenic potency of phenylisopropylamines. Methamphetamine may have stronger CNS stimulant properties than does amphetamine. The *d*-isomer of amphetamine has been generally found to have far more potent CNS stimulant effects than does the *l*-isomer. In contrast, the *l*-isomers of the hallucinogenic phenylisopropylamines have more potent hallucinogenic effects (Glennon 1987). Removal of an α-methyl group of amphetamine leads to the formation of phenylethylamine, which has little CNS-stimulating effect because of its rapid breakdown by MAO-B. The removal of an α-methyl group of a hallucinogenic phenylisopropylamine usually results in retention of activity but a decrease in potency. In contrast, 3,4-MDA is unique because it seems to have both stimulant and hallucinogenic effects and may produce effects that are distinct from these properties. However, it is also unique in that it possesses a methylenedioxy group on the aromatic ring in the 3,4 position. The addition of a methyl group to the terminal chain to produce MDMA appears to increase the potency of its CNS stimulant effects while somewhat decreasing its hallucinogenic activity (Glennon 1987).

There have been contradictory reports in the literature about the relative effects of *d*- and *l*-isomers of amphetamine on mood activation and neurohormone responses and effects that are presumed to result from increases in norepinephrine and dopamine systems. Smith and Davis (1977) showed in control subjects that DAMPH was more efficacious than MPH, which was more efficacious than *l*-amphetamine, in increasing euphoric and activating moods; this result presumably reflects the potency of dopamine actions. In contrast, Janowsky and Davis (1976) found that MPH had 1.5 times the ability of DAMPH to increase activation of psychosis in schizophrenic patients. In both studies, DAMPH was about twice as effective as *l*-amphetamine. The drugs were given orally in the former study and intravenously in the latter, which could explain the difference.

Studies of the effects of the *d*- and *l*-isomers on growth hormone, adrenocorticotropic hormone, cortisol, and prolactin secretion have varied in both animals and humans and are therefore inconclusive. Older reports (Arnold et al. 1972, 1976) suggested that levoamphetamine or *d,l*-amphetamine might have clinical superiority in the treatment of hyperkinetic children. This claim, together with the short half-life of DAMPH, has led to the marketing of a preparation containing four salts of levo- and DAMPH (DAMPH saccharate, amphetamine aspartate, DAMPH sulfate, and amphetamine sulfate). Studies comparing this formulati on (Adderal) with MPH have not yet been published but will be useful in estimating any clinical advantages of this combination.

MPH piperazine–substituted phenylisopropylamine containing a methyl ester has "two chiral centers that give rise to four optical isomers: *d*-threo, *l*-threo, *d*-erythro, and *l*-erythro" (K. S. Patrick et al. 1987, p. 1387). The present pharmaceutical product of MPH contains only the threo racemate in the *d-l* form. The *d*-threo enantiomer of MPH is believed to be responsible for the therapeutic activity. K. S. Patrick et al. (1981) synthesized pure *d-l* threo-*p*-hydroxy MPH and found that the locomotor-inducing activity in the rat after intracerebroventricular administration was nearly twice that of the parent compound. In a review of the pharmacokinetics of MPH, the researchers suggested that "it is possible that the individual therapeutic response to racemic MPH may in part depend on the enantiomeric disposition of circulating MPH (i.e., responders may metabolize MPH with enantioselectivity differing from nonresponders, thereby producing a different profile of effects)" (K. S. Patrick et al. 1987, p. 1394). The example provided by MPH suggests how enantioselective metabolism may alter enantiomorphic structure-activity relations and produce different response patterns in individual patients.

PHARMACOLOGICAL PROFILE

Amphetamine produces stimulating effects on the CNS such as arousal, wakefulness, euphoria, lessening of fatigue, and increased energy and self-confidence. Another central action is the inhibition of appetite. In humans, both cocaine and amphetamine produce behaviors characterized by repetitious arrangement of objects. Such behaviors may be analogous to stereotyped behaviors induced by amphetamines in animals (K. S. Patrick et al. 1981). Amphetamine is a weak base; one theory for its mechanism of action is its dissipation of the pH gradient intracellularly (see next section, "Mechanism of Action").

Amphetamine can be metabolized by either aromatic or aliphatic hydroxylation, yielding parahydroxyamphetamine or norephedrine, respectively, both of which are biologically active (Williams et al. 1973). Amphetamine is excreted unchanged in the urine (34% in human control subjects). It is also metabolized to benzoic acid (23%), which is subsequently converted to hippuric acid or to parahydroxyamphetamine (2%). This is, in turn, converted to parahydroxynorefedron (0.4%) (Figure 25–1).

Because of the basic nature of amphetamine and its excretion pattern, both hydration and the use of ammonium chloride, 500 mg every 3–4 hours, to acidify the urine accelerate its excretion and possibly shorten the duration of the amphetamine reaction. Urine pH should be kept below 5 (Tinklenburg and Berger 1977). The metabolism of MPH is shown in Figure 25–2. The major metabolite of MPH is ritalinic acid, which is inactive. Thin-layer chromatographic analysis of human plasma collected 2 hours after administration of labeled MPH indicates that more than 75% of the total radioactivity is ritalinic acid, whereas compounds appearing to be parahydroxyritalinic acid and 6-oxoritalinic acid make up approximately 1%–2% of the activity, respectively (K. S. Patrick et al. 1987).

"Since MPH is a basic drug, plasma protein binding would be expected to be associated with α-acid glycoprotein and lipoprotein fractions, not primarily with albumin, which generally binds acidic drugs" (K. S. Patrick et al. 1987, p. 1388). Twelve percent of MPH is bound in an albumin solution of pH 7.4, which is comparable to the 15% that is bound in whole plasma. Clinical concentrations of MPH in blood are 2–20 ng/mL, which is below that of most psychotherapeutic agents. Such a minute amount requires sensitive analytical methodology for therapeutic drug monitoring, often requiring gas chromatography–mass spectrometry methods. Like amphetamine, MPH accumulates in highly perfused tissues and accumulates rapidly in the brain within 1–5 minutes after intravenous administration. Although typical doses of amphetamine result in significantly higher plasma concentrations than do typical doses of MPH, it appears that the pharmacological actions of MPH in humans can be attributed solely to the parent compound (K. S. Patrick et al. 1987).

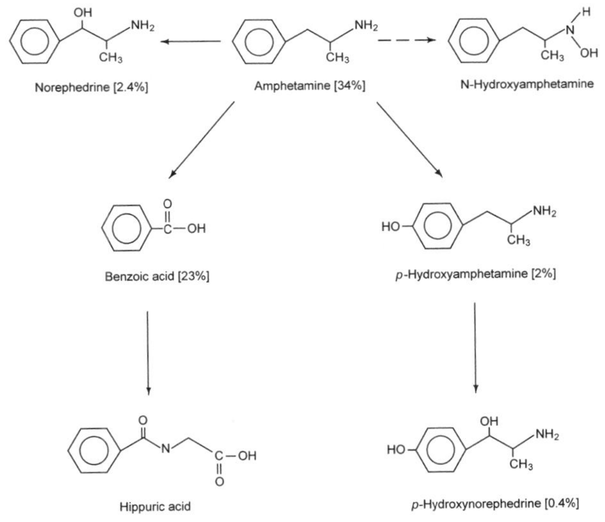

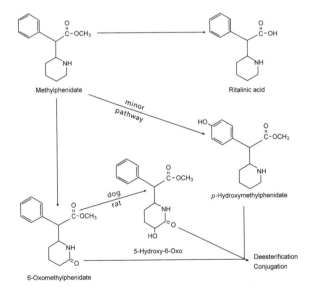

Figure 25–1. Metabolic pathway for amphetamine in humans.
Source. Reprinted from Patrick RL: "Amphetamine and Cocaine: Biological Mechanisms," in *Psychopharmacology: From Theory to Practice.* Edited by Barchas JD, Berger PA, Ciaranello RD, et al. New York, Oxford University Press, 1977, pp. 331–340. Used with permission.

Figure 25–2. Metabolic pathway for methylphenidate.
Source. Reprinted from Patrick KS, Mueller RA, Gualtieri CT, et al: "Pharmacokinetics and Actions of Methylphenidate," in *Psychopharmacology: The Third Generation of Progress.* Edited by Meltzer H. New York, Raven, 1987, pp. 1387–1395. Used with permission.

MECHANISM OF ACTION

The two prototypic stimulants amphetamine and MPH, although they have some similar net effects, also have differences in structure-activity relations and mechanisms of action. As noted by Seiden et al. (1993), "both the releasing and uptake-inhibiting actions of [amphetamine] are mediated by the catecholamine uptake transporter" (p. 640). In 1959, Axelrod et al. demonstrated that epinephrine could be rapidly and selectively taken up by the heart, spleen, and glandular organs, each of which has sympathetic innervation. It was subsequently discovered that norepinephrine-containing neurons could bind or take up norepinephrine against a concentration gradient; later, it was found that the uptake transporter could release catecholamines (CAs) as well as reclaim them back into the nerve terminals.

Further investigation found that amphetamine apparently inhibits the uptake and release of dopamine or norepinephrine or both. The catecholamine transporter normally moves dopamine from the outside to the inside of the cell. However, in the presence of some drugs, such as amphetamine, the direction of transport appears to be reversed, and dopamine is moved from the inside to the outside of the cell through a mechanism called *exchange diffusion*, which occurs at low doses (1–5 mg/kg) of amphetamine. Moderate to high doses of amphetamine (>5 mg/kg) cause the release of dopamine through exchange diffusion across the cell membrane, passive diffusion of amphetamine into the cell, and an interaction between amphetamine and the vesicle membrane transporter. A passive diffusion of amphetamine into the storage vesicle, causing alkalization of the vesicle, results in the release of dopamine from the vesicles as well, which is then subject to release by the cell membrane. These mechanisms, as well as a blocking of reuptake of dopamine by amphetamine, all lead to an increase in synaptic norepinephrine and dopamine. Other antidepressant medications acting on catecholamines, including both dopamine and norepinephrine, tend to exert their action by simply blocking the reuptake mechanism.

MPH appears to release dopamine stored in the vesicles alone, whereas amphetamine releases dopamine from newly synthesized pools and increases dopamine diffusion from the vesicles into the cell. This mechanism appears to distinguish amphetamine from antidepressant medication in terms of its rapidity of onset of effect and from MPH in terms of its potency. Further support for these differentiations include the findings that blocking catecholamine synthesis by α-methyl-*p*-tyrosine interferes with dopamine

release by both amphetamine and MPH, whereas reserpine, which releases dopamine from storage sites in vesicles, interferes significantly only with MPH effects and does not totally inhibit amphetamine effects. This again differentiates the two dopamine storage pools—1) vesicular storage, which is dependent on an inward proton pump and the maintenance of low intravesicular pH, and 2) cytoplasmic storage, which has neither of these requirements (Seiden et al. 1993).

The structure of amphetamine is similar to that of both norepinephrine and dopamine. Part of the mechanism related to the vesicular action of amphetamine is that it is a weak base and causes alkalinization of the storage vesicles. Amphetamine also induces the release of [^{3}H]serotonin from chromaffin granules from the adrenal medulla (Sulzer and Rayport 1990). Although amphetamine competitively inhibits MAO in vitro, it appears to be a weak MAOI in moderate doses in vivo. Evidence suggests that amphetamine in high doses may act as a competitive inhibitor for MAO-A (Mantle et al. 1976; Miller et al. 1980). This effect seems to be less significant physiologically than the catecholamine-releasing effects of the drugs.

Brown et al. (1978) showed that, although amphetamine given in doses of 20 mg to control subjects causes stimulation of both growth hormone and cortisol, MPH in the same dose causes stimulation of only growth hormone. The elation caused by MPH was found to be correlated with elevation of growth hormone. This led Brown et al. (1978) to suggest that the elation response may be related to the dopamine effects of both stimulants, whereas the cortisol response may be related to the norepinephrine effects of amphetamine alone. The norepinephrine effects of amphetamine may explain its higher incidence of increased pulse and hypertension.

In studies with human subjects, Nurnberger et al. (1984) showed that DAMPH-induced excitation is due to stimulation of the CNS by dopamine, whereas cardiovascular effects, increased blood pressure, and increased norepinephrine levels in serum result from noradrenergic effects that can be blocked by propranolol. In a recent report, Kuczenski and Segal (1997) compared the potency of MPH with amphetamine in the rat brain, showing "considerably lower" levels of dopamine and norepinephrine release and no effect on serotonin release with MPH, in contrast to amphetamine.

Nicola et al. (1996) used specific dopamine, subtype 1 (D_1), and D_2 receptor blockers in mice and found that "dopamine and amphetamine [by increasing endogenous extracellular dopamine levels] reduce excitatory synaptic transmission in the nucleus accumbens by activating presynaptic dopamine receptors with D_1-like properties" (p. 1602). Sloviter et al. (1978) first noticed the similarity between the effects of high doses of DAMPH in rats and the behavioral syndrome caused by intense activation of the serotonin receptor. Those researchers pursued studies showing that responsiveness of the amphetamine syndrome could be blocked by either serotonin synthesis inhibition or receptor blockade. This finding suggests that amphetamine acts indirectly through the serotonin system by activating serotonin receptors, possibly through the displacement of endogenous serotonin.

Recently, Weisenberg et al. (1997) reported that the combination of phentermine with fenfluramine produced greater sustained serotonin reductions in selected regions of rat brain than either drug alone. Baumann et al. (1996) did not find a similar effect in the mouse forebrain. The importance of this question is considered later in this chapter with a discussion of the possible risks of serotonergic neurotoxicity with a phentermine-fenfluramine combination used widely for appetite suppression and weight loss. Recent data published by Colado et al. (1997) provide evidence that the hallucinogenic stimulant MDMA ("Ecstasy") produces serotonergic neurotoxicity by the formation of free radicals, whereas fenfluramine produces similar effects by some other unidentified mechanism.

INDICATIONS

The *Physicians' Desk Reference* (PDR; 1998) lists two indications approved by the U.S. Food and Drug Administration for DAMPH: 1) narcolepsy and 2) ADHD. The indications listed for MPH are 1) attention-deficit disorders in children and 2) narcolepsy. Other therapeutic uses of stimulant medications are controversial, principally because they have become drugs of abuse when sold illicitly or prescribed irresponsibly. As a result, amphetamine is a Schedule II and MPH a Schedule III substance under the Controlled Substances Act of 1970. Moreover, certain states (e.g., Wisconsin) have passed even more restrictive legislation limiting the use of stimulants to specific indications. Stimulants are prohibited in some European countries.

Are stimulants ineffective in relation to their risks and thus without a place in psychiatric practice? Or has concern over the abuse potential of these drugs in certain vulnerable populations led to a suppression of their use in cases in which they could be medically useful (and even possibly lifesaving), as in severe, treatment-refractory depression?

Since 1987, there have been three published reviews of the use of psychostimulants and several reviews prelimi-

nary to case reports. Of the major reviews, Chiarello and Cole (1987) dealt with the use of stimulants in general psychiatry, Satel and Nelson (1989) focused on the use of psychostimulants in the treatment of affective disorders, and Ayd and Zohar (1987) emphasized the role of stimulants in treatment-resistant affective disorders. Based on these reviews, the efficacy of DAMPH alone in treating patients with affective disorders is controversial. This is based on the fact that no double-blind studies have been done since 1962. Many of the studies that have been reported have shown high rates of response to placebo that were not exceeded by DAMPH response rates and were done on a short-term basis. Chiarello and Cole (1987) pointed out that the studies were not adequate to conclude whether DAMPH did in fact have therapeutic effects for some patients, and data may have been analyzed in such a way that the authors missed positive effects. However, Satel and Nelson (1989) observed that studies of imipramine (IMI) compared with placebo carried out at approximately the same time, presumably with similar methodology and interpretation, showed that IMI was superior to placebo in 15 of 24 studies. This was a more robust outcome than could be drawn from the three or four double-blind, placebo-controlled studies in which DAMPH was used in doses ranging from 10 to 30 mg/day.

MPH was studied in four reported double-blind trials in the late 1960s and early 1970s, in doses of up to 30–40 mg/day, showing modest responses in comparison to placebo. Clinical effects were evident in some patients. Pemoline was also studied in double-blind, placebo-controlled trials in the mid- to late 1970s and was shown to have modest effects when given as a sole treatment. The studies of these three major stimulants and critical reviews of these studies seem to echo the conclusion that, although some effects might be noted in some patients, the evidence as to whether these responses will persist over time is mixed. No good evidence would establish stimulants as a responsible first-line treatment in patients with depressive illness when the benefits of these drugs in placebo-controlled studies are compared with those of other available antidepressant medications.

Open studies have a significant disadvantage compared with placebo-controlled studies in that they do not account for placebo response. (These studies also tend to be published more often if they are positive than if they turn out to have negative results.) On the other hand, open studies tend to have more flexible dose ranges and may provide useful information about the type of clinical responses seen and in what type of patients they are seen, because they may not treat groups of more highly selected patients.

Five open studies of amphetamine, benzedrine, or

DAMPH have been completed and have involved 185 subjects, ranging from hospitalized patients with retardation or agitation to those with neurotic depressions. According to various criteria, improvement was seen in 30%–76% of the subjects. In two open studies of MPH used to treat various types of depressive disorders at doses of 30–60 mg/day, improvement was reported in 76%–82% of subjects.

In addition, a number of uncontrolled studies and case reports have been reported in which stimulants, most frequently MPH, have been used for the treatment of depression in various types of medically ill patients. Between 1956 and 1991, studies of 159 medically ill patients were reported and showed positive responses in 68%–98% of patients (Kraus and Burch 1992). One study in adult patients with cancer showed a response in 23 of 30 patients (77%), whereas another similar study showed response in 14 of 17 patients (82%) (Fernandez et al. 1987). From 1988 to 1992, four studies (Angrist et al. 1992; Fernandez et al. 1988a, 1988b; Holmes et al. 1989) presented 38 case reports of patients with human immunodeficiency virus (HIV)-related neuropsychiatric symptoms, including depression; 86% (33) of the subjects showed some improvement, and 65% (25) showed moderate to marked improvement.

Two studies (Johnson et al. 1992; Lazarus et al. 1992) described case reports of response to MPH in poststroke patients with depression. One showed that 70% of subjects improved, and the other showed that 80% improved with doses ranging from 5 mg twice daily to total doses of 40 mg/day. In a subsequent study, Lazarus et al. (1994) showed a more rapid onset of response with MPH compared with nortriptyline therapy. The average response time for MPH responders was 2.4 days compared with 27 days for the nortriptyline group. Gwirtsman et al. (1994) reported the results of a study in which MPH was given in one or two doses of 5–15 mg in addition to tricyclic antidepressants (TCAs). Improvement was seen at 1 week in 30% of the patients and at 2 weeks in 63% of the patients starting the trial, suggesting that the combination produced an accelerated response. A report by Fernandez et al. (1995) found that MPH in a dosage of 30 mg/day produced a response and an onset of response that were equivalent to those produced by desipramine (DMI) given at 150 mg/day in depressed AIDS patients. In an open trial of DAMPH at a median dose of 10 mg/day, Wagner et al. (1997) found a rapid onset of improvement of depression and low energy in 18 of 19 AIDS patients. Olin and Masand (1996) reported a chart review of 59 cancer patients treated for depression with either DAMPH or MPH over 5 years at Massachusetts General Hospital. Those authors

noted some improvement in 83% of patients, substantial improvement in 73%, and no differences in efficacy between stimulants or across diagnostic categories for depression.

A review of open series and case reports of medically ill patients with various diagnoses showed that stimulants had two important advantages. The first advantage was the rapidity of response; most authors agreed that a response was evident within 2–3 days—much earlier than the average time for other antidepressants. The second advantage often cited was the dearth of side effects compared with other antidepressant medications, especially in medically ill patients. (The question of side effects and hazards is reviewed in the "Side Effects and Toxicology" section later in this chapter.)

Stimulants as Potentiators for Antidepressant Medications

The literature has supported the use of stimulants as augmenters of antidepressant medications in treatment-resistant patients. In 1971, Wharton et al. published a paper that had been read at the annual meeting of the American Psychiatric Association in 1969. The researchers reported on seven patients with recurrent refractory psychotic depressive illness, five of whom had had repeated courses of electroconvulsive therapy. Five of the patients recovered within 2 weeks of receiving IMI at 150 mg/day and MPH 10 mg twice daily (Wharton et al. 1971). The other two patients recovered more gradually without requiring electroconvulsive therapy. Wharton et al. (1971) documented a rise in serum IMI levels after the addition of MPH, and they hypothesized that this rapid increase in blood levels might be related to the enhanced response. Five of the patients who could be followed up maintained their response for 2–3 years. Subsequently, in a letter to the *American Journal of Psychiatry*, Flemenbaum (1971) reported on "six to ten" patients (p. 239) treated with MPH-IMI combinations and noted a rapid onset of effect and correction of hypotension associated with TCA medication. However, Flemenbaum did note three cases of young patients with labile hypertension who had hypertensive episodes associated with the MPH-IMI combination.

Cooper and Simpson (1973) reported another case, that of a 61-year-old patient with a 19-year history of depressive disorder. The patient had not benefited from various treatment modalities and sustained a partial response with 300 mg/day of IMI but still required hospitalization; however, marked improvement occurred with the addition of a maximum dose of 40 mg of MPH. Cooper and

Simpson reported an almost 20-fold increase in IMI levels and a 50% increase in DMI levels. In this case, within 2 weeks after MPH was withdrawn, plasma IMI and DMI levels had returned to baseline values, and the patient apparently relapsed. The authors presented this as a confirmation of the observation by Perel et al. (1969) that IMI metabolism was inhibited by MPH.

Drimmer et al. (1983) presented the case of a patient with a diagnosis of bipolar depression with hypomania who had had a depressive episode and was not helped by up to 350 mg/day of amoxapine. The patient was then treated with DMI at a dose of 200 mg/day and sustained marked improvement in mood and agitation within 3 days of the addition of MPH at a dose of 10 mg twice daily (Drimmer et al. 1983). The patient experienced a relapse after MPH was gradually withdrawn and again responded to its reinstatement at a dose of up to 40 mg/day. No significant increases in DMI levels were noted in this patient. The authors believed that the rapidity of response when MPH was added to DMI, as well as the lack of DMI increase, argued against the hypothesis that a mechanism of enhancement of TCA levels was responsible for the potentiating effect of MPH. Rather, they argued that the dopaminergic effects of MPH were more likely to be the basis for its potentiating effects on IMI and DMI treatment.

Myers and Stewart (1989) further commented on the rapidity of onset of a DMI-MPH combination in the case of a 69-year-old male patient admitted for the treatment of transitional cell carcinoma of the bladder. The patient had developed suicidal ideation and was threatening to jump out of his fourth-floor hospital window. However, within 2 days of administration of this combination, he was no longer suicidal and was able to enjoy watching television. He relapsed within 4 days of discontinuation of MPH but then responded to 400 mg/day of DMI (Myers and Stewart 1989).

Although the mechanism of action of the combination of IMI or DMI plus MPH is unclear, the available case reports suggest that it may be an effective combination for patients with treatment-resistant depression. This combination has the advantage of rapid response and relatively few hazards, except for the possibility of elevated blood pressure in patients with histories of labile hypertension.

Linet (1989) reported on a 36-year-old male patient whose condition did not improve after administration of 300 mg/day of IMI, despite potentiation with triiodothyronine; tryptophan, 8,000 mg/day; and L-thyroxine, 0.15 mg/day, as well as DAMPH augmentation up to a dosage of 45 mg three times daily. The patient's IMI dosage was discontinued, and he subsequently had no particular response to 60 mg/day of fluoxetine until the addition of 45 mg of DAMPH three times daily, which resulted in "significant and sustained clinical improvement" (p. 804) after 2.5 years of depression. His response was maintained for 5 months, and he relapsed on four subsequent occasions when attempts were made to taper DAMPH and increase the dose of fluoxetine.

Metz and Shader (1991) reported four cases of patients refractory to TCAs, three of whom either had partial responses to fluoxetine or relapsed on fluoxetine under stress but improved when 9.375–18.750 mg/day of pemoline was added. These responses were monitored and observed to last for 9–23 months. The addition of either DAMPH or pemoline to fluoxetine is suggested by these case reports as a way of treating partial responses in patients taking fluoxetine or in those who have relapsed in treatment. Although the use of stimulants with other antidepressants has not been documented in a double-blind study (which is not surprising, considering the expense of double-blind, placebo-controlled studies, the lack of commercial interest in these older stimulants, and the relatively small percentage of patients treated with antidepressants who require stimulant potentiation), published case reports suggest the efficacy and probable safety of this combination in patients with depression that has been resistant to successful treatment with existing antidepressant agents.

MAOIs are currently used mainly to treat depression that has proven refractory to other antidepressant medications, some cases of "atypical depression," and severe panic or anxiety disorders that are unresponsive to other pharmacological therapies. Because of their potential for interactions with dietary substances and other medications, as well as their frequent side effects, MAOIs are usually not used until after treatment with other medications has failed. However, clinicians who treat depressive illnesses that are resistant to conventional pharmacological treatment still encounter patients who not only require MAOIs but also may have failed to respond to these agents and to electroconvulsive therapy. In patients with highly resistant depression, the stakes become higher in many cases because hopelessness induced by the depressive illness is augmented by the reality of a lack of response and a further increased risk of suicide.

Feighner et al. (1985) reported on the use of a combination of MAOI, TCA, and stimulant therapy for treatment-resistant depression. The researchers cited 16 subjects, 13 of whom improved when various MAOIs were potentiated by either DAMPH or MPH. Fawcett et al. (1991) presented 32 cases of patients who were refractory to long series of trials with TCAs, selective serotonin reuptake inhibitors (SSRIs) (in some cases), and (in 14 cases) electroconvulsive therapy without a response to treatment. Seventy-eight percent of these patients responded with the addition of either pemoline or DAMPH to one to four different MAOIs in their maximum tolerated doses. DAMPH was given in dosages of 10–40 mg four times daily and pemoline in dosages of 18.75–37.50 mg three times daily to patients receiving maximum tolerated doses of 40–120 mg of MAOIs. The patients' ages ranged from 20 to the early 80s (Fawcett et al. 1991). Neither of these two reports of stimulant potentiation of MAOIs reported any serious side effects except for the possible switching of several patients into hypomania or mania in the series conducted by Fawcett et al. (1991). Both studies reviewed older literature in which three cases of death had ensued after the administration of MAOIs potentiated with DAMPH (Dally 1962; Krisko et al. 1969; Lloyd and Walker 1965; Mason 1962; Smilkstein et al. 1987; Stockley 1973; Zeck 1961). Two of these three cases involved elevated blood pressure, hyperpyrexia, seizures, and death; one case did not show elevation of blood pressure but did show hyperpyrexia, seizures, and death. These cases were reported in the literature in the early to late 1960s.

Although the use of stimulants with MAOIs is contraindicated in PDR, in addition to the observations of Feighner et al. (1985), in some patients with high-risk depression for whom all other treatments have failed, the use of stimulants to potentiate MAOIs has proved helpful and even lifesaving.

The decision to prescribe stimulants should be based on a clinical history of treatment-resistant or treatment-refractory illness. This is true of other uses of stimulants in treating depression (such as their use in treating medically ill stroke patients, elderly patients, or treatment-resistant patients), as well as the use of stimulants to potentiate MAOIs in patients with highly treatment-resistant depressive illness. The patient's medical status and his or her capacity for careful compliance with the prescribed regimen should be evaluated. In making these clinical decisions, careful judgment should be used in evaluating the risks and benefits and determining what is best for an individual patient.

The use of stimulants may not be necessary in the average patient; however, we believe that although the continual emergence of new antidepressant medications may increase patients' chances of treatment response, a significant percentage of patients, because of idiosyncratic differences or medical conditions, do not respond at all to these medications or cannot tolerate their effects. These patients may find themselves in severe states of impairment or even at risk for death by suicide. These patients may benefit from the use of stimulants alone or in combination to potentiate other available antidepressant medi-

cations. The clinical literature on the possible usefulness of stimulants must be available to psychiatrists, as well as to those who legislate the use of these substances. The latter group may be motivated more by their concern for potential danger and may not be fully aware of the potential benefits of psychostimulants to patients who may not otherwise recover and regain control of their lives.

Fawcett and Siomopoulos (1971) reported the use of DAMPH to predict antidepressant response and showed data suggesting that patients who were responsive to 10 mg of DAMPH were more likely to respond to DMI. This predictive effect of DAMPH was confirmed by van Kammen and Murphy (1978). Sabelli et al. (1983) reported the use of MPH to predict DMI response as opposed to nortriptyline response in patients with major depression. In a paper entitled "Challenging the Amphetamine Challenge Test," Kravitz et al. (1990) reviewed this issue based on new data. These data suggested that, although DAMPH challenge did tend to predict DMI response about 70% of the time, the degree of correct prediction might not be powerful enough in the individual patient to justify the use of the stimulant challenge test as a routine procedure.

Summary of the Use of Stimulants in Depression

Although double-blind studies performed in the 1960s did not produce data strongly supporting the efficacy of stimulants in treating a broad range of depressed patients, it is important to recognize that the designs of these studies were highly flawed. Placebo response rates were extremely high, making it difficult for stimulants to show a higher rate of effectiveness. Although these studies do not offer support for the efficacy of stimulants used alone in the treatment of depression, they certainly do not convincingly rule out the possibility that stimulants may be effective for some patients.

Open studies point in a slightly different direction, emphasizing the value of stimulants in treating patients with severe medical illnesses, poststroke patients, elderly patients, patients with severe heart disease, and AIDS patients, all of whom had concurrent depression and increased risks associated with side effects to antidepressant medications. Three recent reports (Hornstein et al. 1996; Mooney and Haas 1993; Plenger et al. 1996) continue to support a possible role for stimulants in the treatment of 88 patients recovering from moderate brain injury. Low to moderate doses of MPH and DAMPH reduced depression and apathy and improved cognitive functions. One study of 38 patients also showed a reduction in anger and temper outbursts compared with patients given placebo, whereas an open study of MPH (0.3 mg/kg twice a day) in 12 patients with chronic closed head injury found no benefit (Speech et al. 1993). The effectiveness of MPH in the treatment of negative symptoms in dementia has been reported (Galynker et al. 1997).

A case report noted improvement of prominent apathy secondary to multiple subcortical infarcts, and single photon emission computed tomography and reaction time showed selective improvement of frontal system function. Wroblewski et al. (1992) reported a trend toward a lesser incidence of seizures in 30 patients with active seizure disorders taking MPH. Their results provide some reassurance that giving MPH to brain-injured patients is not likely to increase the risk of seizure.

In general, these case reports were positive, showing a high rate of improvement in patients with a relatively low rate of side effects and a rapid response time of 2–3 days. It has been noted that case reports are generally published when they are positive; thus, the efficacy of stimulants in these patients may be overestimated.

The use of stimulants to potentiate other antidepressant medications in patients with either treatment-resistant depression or partial response has been raised in several studies—including their use with MAOIs, despite the PDR's warnings against this practice. The use of stimulants to predict TCA response showed some theoretical interest, but the movement to more widespread use of SSRIs diminishes the significance and value of this early research.

Some studies have reviewed the hypothesis that dopamine hypofunction may play a significant role in depressive illness. D'haenen and Bossuyt (1994) reported an increase in D_2 receptor density in depressed patients. These studies, viewed in the context of antidepressant effects reported with the use of the dopamine agonists bromocriptine, piribedil, and pergolide, further strengthen the hypothesis that the dopamine system is an important mechanism in at least some depressed patients (Bouckoms and Mangini 1993; Post et al. 1978; Theohar et al. 1981). The therapeutic use of stimulants in selected patients appears to have a growing theoretical and empirical basis, particularly in view of the limited dopaminergic effects of most standard antidepressant medications.

Other Uses of Stimulants in Psychiatry and Medicine

ADHD in children has been a continually accepted indication for the use of psychostimulants. This use has not been without some social controversy concerning the use of drugs in children and the possibilities of adverse side effects. Possible effects include growth retardation, which has not been substantiated, and possible negative cognitive effects that seem to result from overdose in some children, as well as overuse or inappropriate use as the result of poor clinical diagnosis.

Barkley (1977) reviewed 15 studies of the use of amphetamines in children with ADHD, involving a total of 915 patients. The studies had various designs, including the use of hospital staff, teachers, clinicians, and parents as judges of response. The studies reviewed showed that, on average, symptoms improved in 74% of subjects and were unchanged or worsened in 26%. Fourteen of these reports were studies of MPH that involved a total of 866 patients and used clinicians, parents, and teachers as judges of outcome. These studies showed that, on average, symptoms improved in 77% of subjects and were unchanged or worsened in 23%. Pemoline was used in two studies of 105 subjects. In these studies, clinicians and teachers judged outcome, and symptoms improved in 73% of subjects and were unchanged or worsened in 27%. In another eight studies, 417 children had a mean improvement rate of 39% compared with a mean rate of unchanged or worsening symptoms of 61%.

Barkley (1977) concluded in this review that most children taking psychostimulant medications are judged as improved, whereas a small percentage are not. The author also concluded that follow-up studies find the long-term psychosocial adjustment of these children to be essentially unaffected by stimulant treatment. Barkley then noted that the search needed to consider specific variables for measures of improvement rather than just general improvement, as many studies up until that time had tended to do.

More recently, Schachar and Tannock (1993) looked for evidence of a sustained effect of stimulant treatment in children with ADHD. Eighteen studies were identified with a duration of at least 3 months. Seventeen were studies of MPH, and one was a study of DAMPH; none involved pemoline or slow-release stimulants. Eleven of these studies were randomized, controlled trials, whereas seven used quasi-experimental designs without randomization. The results of the randomized, controlled trials showed the psychostimulants to provide a greater benefit than did the nonrandomized trials. This finding suggested to the researchers that the "efficacy of extended treatment may have been underestimated because more seriously disturbed children were assigned to medication treatment than to control treatments in nonrandomized trials" (p. 81). Reviewing 11 randomized, controlled studies that collectively involved 271 children medicated for an average of 6 months, the authors found that "results of 8 out of the 11 randomized controlled trials indicate clear beneficial effects of prolonged treatment with MPH on the core behavioral features of ADHD, that is, poor sustained attention, impulsiveness, and excessive motor activity" (p. 89).

Of the three studies that failed to find extended stimulant treatment to be efficacious, one was discounted because of an attrition rate of more than 50%. The results of a second study indicated that prolonged MPH treatment did reduce the severity of poor symptoms, but the improvements were comparable in magnitude to those obtained with IMI. Another study found that behavioral improvements obtained with MPH were no longer discernible when medication was discontinued. Schachar and Tannock (1993) concluded that there is no evidence that

> longer term benefits of MPH are greater than those of treatment with the TCA IMI, nor are they potentiated by adjunctive pharmacological treatment with thioridazine or nonpharmacological therapy such as cognitive training, educational tutoring or the combination of parent training and self-control training. (p. 90)

It was also shown that the beneficial effects of treatment dissipate rapidly when treatment is terminated. Stimulant treatment did not appear to reduce symptoms to a level considered to be in the range of normal behavior. It was concluded that few children made sufficient progress to become symptom free at the end of the trial. In addition, although short-term treatment had a significant effect on social and academic symptoms, extended treatment produced a far less clear result. Schachar and Tannock (1993) further concluded that future studies of extended treatment must address questions about the development of drug tolerance, as well as concerns about long-term adverse effects, such as abnormal movement and dysphoria.

The modest effectiveness of MPH indicated by these studies suggests a need to combine medication with educational interventions and psychological therapies. Satterfield et al. (1987) showed indirect evidence for the superior effectiveness of combining intensive multimodal therapy and MPH over medication alone. However, no direct evidence exists in longer-term studies to support this contention (Satterfield et al. 1981, 1987; Schachar and Tannock 1993).

Psychostimulants have been shown to be helpful in treating the core symptoms of ADHD in children, both acutely and over at least a 6-month period. It is also clear that the effect of psychostimulants is toward improvement and not total suppression of symptoms—the symptoms return when medications are discontinued. There is

still concern about the long-term effects of these medications and of ADHD itself in terms of delinquency and other conduct disturbances.

Klein and Wender (1995) reviewed the use of MPH in children with ADHD, concluding that "at appropriately high doses of MPH, a large proportion of children are not only better, many are well. "In addition to having the cardinal features of their disorder eliminated, appropriately medicated children experience improvement in other important functional domains, such as in social interactions with parents, teachers, and peers, in academic performance, and in self-esteem" (p. 429). Spencer et al. (1996b) found "155 studies of 5,778 children, adolescents, and adults documenting the efficacy of stimulants in an estimated 70% of subjects" (p. 409). They further found that "the literature clearly documents that stimulants not only improve abnormal behaviors of ADHD, but also self-esteem, cognition, and social and family function" (p. 409).

Wender et al. (1985) described the use of stimulants in adults with similar problems of attention, concentration, and focus, terming this syndrome *adult attention deficit disorder*. Their study involved patients meeting the Utah criteria for residual ADHD, which included a history of core symptoms of childhood ADHD having been reported by a parent using the Conners Teacher Rating Scale (Sprague et al. 1974). Wender et al. (1985) found that, although pemoline was not more effective than placebo, MPH reduced core symptoms. This reduction occurred (sometimes dramatically) in 57% of subjects taking MPH and in 11% taking placebo.

Spencer et al. (1995) replicated the results of Wender et al. (1985) in a randomized, 7-week, placebo-controlled, crossover study of 23 adults with ADHD, using standardized instruments for the diagnosis of ADHD and separate assessments of ADHD. With a "robust" dose of MPH (1.0 mg/kg/day), Spencer et al. (1995) found "a marked therapeutic response for methylphenidate treatment of ADHD symptoms that exceeded the placebo response (78% vs 4%, $P < .0001$)" (p. 434).

Of particular interest is a report by Castellanos et al. (1996) based on the measurement of homovanillic acid levels in cerebrospinal fluid. In this study, 45 boys met DSM-III (American Psychiatric Association 1980) criteria for ADHD before beginning double-blind trials of MPH, DAMPH, or placebo. This study replicated the results of a prior study that found a significant correlation between homovanillic acid levels in cerebrospinal fluid and ratings of hyperactivity in subjects taking placebo. It also showed that, after baseline symptom severity was controlled for, higher homovanillic acid levels in cerebrospinal fluid predicted better response, whereas lower homovanillic acid levels were associated with worsening on some measures.

Spencer et al. (1996a) described another interesting finding in a study of 124 children and adolescents who were compared with 109 control subjects. Using appropriate correction by age and parental height, the authors found small but significant height differences that were evident in early- but not in late-adolescent children with ADHD. The height differences were unrelated to the use of psychotropic medications. The investigators concluded that "ADHD may be associated with temporary deficits in growth in height in mid-adolescence that may normalize by late adolescence. This effect appears to be mediated by ADHD and not its treatment" (p. 1460).

Stimulants have long been accepted as valuable in treating narcolepsy, which is often treated by psychiatrists as well as by neurologists and general physicians. The chronic use of stimulants in many cases reduces episodes of daytime sleepiness, which can cause impairment and danger, especially if the sleepiness occurs while the patient is driving. Stimulants do not reverse the cataplexy that some narcoleptic patients experience, but either TCAs or SSRIs in combination with stimulants may be helpful for this condition.

Although several studies have suggested that stimulants may improve negative symptoms in schizophrenic patients, others have shown that stimulants may worsen positive symptoms of schizophrenia, such as delusions and hallucinations (Lieberman et al. 1990). There is also evidence that schizophrenic patients have high rates of comorbid substance abuse, perhaps as a consequence of the blunted affectivity associated with negative symptoms of the disease.

In one report, Insel et al. (1983) reported positive effects of DAMPH given to patients with obsessive-compulsive disorder. The experience of these authors suggests that these patients also had lower levels of anxiety when DAMPH was used.

Khantzian et al. (1984) presented three cases of cocaine abuse in which patients were treated with MPH, all three of whom demonstrated improvement. This experience led to the hypothesis that cocaine abuse may be associated with the presence of dysthymic disorder or chronic depression without the full neurovegetative symptomatology of major depression. It was further hypothesized that the "normalizing effect of MPH with the pilot cases makes a compelling argument for more extensive clinical study to test the possibility that a minimal brain dysfunction syndrome or attention deficit disorder or a variant contributes to cocaine dependence" (pp. 110–111). This hypothesis was also based on the fact that the patients did not develop

tolerance to MPH. It was also mentioned that the authors had treated four other subjects who had abused cocaine and who did not have symptoms of attention-deficit disorder. Khantzian et al. (1984) observed dose escalations without prolonged facilitation of cocaine abstinence. Hence, initial observations indicated that only a subpopulation of abusers respond favorably to MPH treatment of cocaine abuse. This has led to a proposal for further study of the use of MPH in cocaine abusers with symptoms of ADHD (H. D. Kleber, personal communication, May 1993).

SIDE EFFECTS AND TOXICOLOGY

The effects of amphetamine include the alpha and beta actions that are common to indirectly acting sympathomimetic drugs. Amphetamine given orally raises both systolic and diastolic blood pressure. Heart rate is often reflexively slowed, and, with large doses, cardiac arrhythmias may occur. Cardiac output is not enhanced by therapeutic doses, and cerebral blood flow is little changed (Hoffman and Lefkowitz 1993). Smooth muscles respond to amphetamine in general as they do to other sympathomimetic drugs. There is a contractile effect on the urinary bladder sphincter, an effect that has been used in treating enuresis and incontinence. Pain and difficulty in micturition can therefore occur. Amphetamine may cause relaxation of the intestine and may delay the movement of intestinal contents, but the opposite effect may also be seen. The response of the human uterus varies, but usually an increase in tone occurs. Contraindications for amphetamine include advanced arteriosclerosis, symptomatic cardiovascular disease, moderate to severe hypertension, hyperthyroidism, as well as a history of drug abuse (PDR 1998).

Side effects noted with therapeutic doses of amphetamine also include mild gastrointestinal disturbance, anorexia, dry mouth, tachycardia, cardiac arrhythmias, insomnia, and restlessness (Meyler 1966). Headache, palpitations, dizziness, vasomotor disturbances, agitation, confusion, dysphoria, apprehension, and delirium have also been also mentioned. Other side effects that have been documented include flushing, pallor, a swaying sensation, excessive sweating, and muscular pains. Tiredness and sleepiness, as well as lethargy and listlessness, together with a mild depression of mood, may occur when the effect wears off.

The unsupervised use of amphetamine or the abuse of this substance involves taking doses in excess of therapeutic doses to experience the psychological effects of the drug, such as euphoria. This excess use also leads to a tendency to loquaciousness and diminution of inhibitions. Tolerance is progressive in some individuals, and drug dependence may occur.

The effects of large doses of amphetamine include marked euphoria and overcheerfulness, restlessness, rapid and slurred speech, and tension, anxiety, and irritability. Other effects may include excessively dry mouth, producing a tendency to rub the tongue along the inside of the lower lip; tachycardia and cardiac arrhythmias; brisk reflexes, dilation of the pupils, and occasionally, a sluggish response to light; fine tremor of the limbs; and weight loss. Amphetamine psychosis, which has been described in detail elsewhere (Connell 1968), presents as a paranoid psychosis in a setting of clear consciousness. A rare confusional state may occur for a short time, but this is usually short lived. After withdrawal in a patient who has taken large quantities of amphetamine, excessive tiredness and sleepiness may be noted. More important, however, the patient may experience severe depression with suicidal ideation and the danger of suicide attempts.

Although most studies of stimulants in general psychiatry have emphasized the lack of side effects or adverse events associated with their use, some reports have suggested caution and careful monitoring in prescribing stimulant medications for psychiatric patients. Several reports have suggested the possibility of hypertension as a side effect, particularly in patients with hypertension illness or labile hypertension. There have been an increasing number of reports of cerebral hemorrhage and cerebral angiitis with the use of intravenous stimulants or the ingestion of large amounts. However, it appears that in these cases, either self-administered overdoses were being taken by individuals who were abusing drugs or the medications were not being given under medical supervision (Bergstrom and Keller 1992; Brust 1992; Carson et al. 1987; Citron et al. 1970; Harrington et al. 1983; Imanse and Vanneste 1990; Kalant and Kalant 1975; Lazarus et al. 1992; Ragland et al. 1993; C. L. Rumbaugh et al. 1971; D. L. Rumbaugh 1971; Trugman 1988). In addition, increasing reports of cardiomyopathy and myocardial infarction have been noted in patients who had abused stimulants intravenously and, less commonly, in those taking high oral doses (Call et al. 1982; O'Neill et al. 1983; Packe et al. 1990).

The increasingly widespread use of the stimulant phentermine in combination with the serotonin-releasing drug fenfluramine as an anorexigenic combination ("Phen-Fen") has focused increasing attention on the hazards of this combination. McCann et al. (1997), reporting on the increased incidence of primary pulmonary hypertension arising in populations using this combination,

stated that "whether concomitant use of other drugs that share certain pharmacological actions with fenfluramine (e.g., phentermine, selective serotonin reuptake inhibitors, and tricyclic antidepressants) influence the risk of developing PPH has not been determined" (p. 670). However, Connolly et al. (1997), reporting on 24 cases of valvular heart disease associated with phentermine-fenfluramine, stated that pulmonary hypertension has been associated with phentermine alone, based on a study by Heuer (1978), and further pointed out that phentermine interferes with the pulmonary clearance of serotonin (Morita and Mehendale 1983).

Graham and Green (1997) reported on another 28 cases of valvular disease associated with the use of the phentermine-fenfluramine combination. The mean duration of treatment was 10 months (range 2–36 months) when symptoms first developed. The average dose of phentermine was 30 mg (range 15–60 mg), and the average dose of fenfluramine was 60 mg (range 10–120 mg). A dose of phentermine of more than 30 mg/day was significantly ($P = .02$) associated with multivalvular disease. Because fenfluramine is not a true stimulant in that its actions are primarily serotonergic, a review of its pharmacology other than as it is affected by stimulants such as phentermine, which often are coadministered with it, is beyond the scope of this chapter. However, the information reviewed here, including the possible potentiation of serotonin-depleting properties, raises the caution that the combination of phentermine, a mild stimulant, with fenfluramine may increase the risk of primary pulmonary hypertension or valvular heart disease. This concern may be academic, however, and is further narrowed to the use of phentermine alone or with other agents since fenfluramine was voluntarily withdrawn from the market for the above-described reasons at the time this chapter was written.

Recently, attention has been drawn to the possible association of liver toxicity with the use of pemoline (PDR 1998). Thirteen cases of acute hepatic failure have been reported since pemoline was first marketed in 1973. The rate of reported cases (which could be an underestimate) is 4–17 times that expected in the general population. Of the 13 cases reported since May 1996, 11 resulted in death or transplantation, usually within 4 weeks of the onset of signs or symptoms of liver failure. The earliest onset of hepatic abnormalities occurred within 6 months after initiation of treatment. This resulted in a labeling warning that pemoline should not be "ordinarily considered as first line drug therapy for ADHD" (Pemoline—Abbott Laboratories package insert).

Sterling et al. (1996) presented a case of pemoline-induced autoimmune hepatitis in a 46-year-old woman receiving the drug for the management of multiple sclerosis. That the hepatitis was autoimmune in nature was based on elevations of antinuclear antibodies, antithyroid antibodies, and immunoglobulins A and M. These features disappeared after normalization of the patient's liver enzymes and remained absent for 6 months after prednisone therapy.

Berkovitch et al. (1995) reported a case of fatal fulminant failure after transplantation failure and, calculating the relative risk, found a significant association suggesting causation. However, Shevell and Schreiber (1997), in a descriptive meta-analysis of the literature, concluded that current assumptions about the risk of acute hepatic failure posed by pemoline use alone are overestimates; those authors recommend monitoring of hepatic function during pemoline therapy.

Risk of Abuse or Addiction

The epidemic of amphetamine abuse during the 1960s gave rise to the subsequent abuse of stimulants both orally and intravenously, as well as to the development of "designer drugs" with both stimulant and hallucinogenic potency. These phenomena have underscored the risks of stimulant abuse and dependence and have focused attention on the availability and possible misuse of psychostimulant drugs.

Findings of high rates of coexisting abuse of alcohol, cocaine, opiates, and (in some cases) stimulants in patients with Axis I disorders were reported in the Epidemiologic Catchment Area study sampled in 1980–1984 by Regier et al. (1990). That survey found the prevalence of amphetamine abuse or dependence within the 6 months preceding the survey (6-month prevalence) to be 0.2%, whereas the prevalence of abuse or dependence at any time during the respondents' lifetime (lifetime prevalence) was 1.7%. Sixty-six percent of patients who had amphetamine abuse or dependence had a comorbid mental disorder; 33% had a comorbid affective disorder and 33% a comorbid anxiety disorder.

Blumberg et al. (1971) reported the findings of a chromatographic examination of urine samples in 332 young psychiatric patients: 24.1% had at least one positive test for amphetamines. Robinson and Wolkind (1970) reported that 16 of 54 (29.6%) patients in a psychiatric hospital had evidence of nonprescribed amphetamines in their urine.

These studies (although they are from a period when stimulant abuse was close to its peak, in the late 1960s) demonstrated the high rate of abuse of stimulant medications among psychiatric patients. On the other hand, we are aware of few, if any, reports of stimulant abuse among patients who have no histories of drug or alcohol abuse and whose use of psychostimulants for the treatment of psychiatric disorders such as major depression is medically supervised.

The classifications of stimulants as Class II or III narcotic substances requiring regulation (and in some cases, triplicate prescription) are based on the recognition of the addictive potential of these stimulants. The concern about addictive potential is also reflected in some state laws contraindicating the use of stimulants for any treatment indication, such as depression or other psychiatric indications, other than those specifically spelled out in that state's laws. However, reports of the use of stimulants in clinical practice have described very few incidents of diagnosed patients increasing the dose, becoming dependent, or abusing stimulant medications. Metz and Shader (1991) described the case of a patient with a history of stimulant abuse who abused MPH. Several authors and reviewers of the literature on stimulants have stated that there simply are no studies showing that patients being treated for depression or other specific psychiatric syndromes are prone to abuse or to become addicted to stimulants.

It is increasingly recognized that comorbidity exists between affective disorders, personality disorders, and even addictive disorders such as alcoholism. Clinical discretion in the treatment of patients with comorbid addictive disorders with stimulants is certainly always indicated. It has yet to be confirmed, however, that patients with depression or other specific medical or psychiatric indications for the use of stimulants are at any higher risk for abuse of or addiction to these agents than are patients without these conditions. It therefore seems that concerns about the abuse or addictive potential of stimulants need not automatically be interpreted as constituting a risk for patients who might benefit from their use under the care of a skilled psychiatrist. This question needs to be examined in terms of the risks and benefits related to the clinical state of each patient. It should be recognized that in a significant percentage of patients, their severe, debilitating, and even life-threatening depressive illnesses do not respond to available antidepressant medications. In the discussion that follows, we consider some theoretical reasons that stimulants may add an ingredient of response in these patients when other medications fail.

A report from the Drug Abuse Warning Network (DAWN) (Carabillo 1978) presented a collection of episodic reports obtained from hospital emergency rooms, medical examiners, and crisis intervention centers in the continental United States. These reports documented incidents conforming to the definition of *drug abuse*, or the nonmedical use of a substance for psychic effects, dependence, or self-destruction. *Drug abuse* was further defined as the use of prescription drugs in a manner inconsistent with accepted medical practice. DAWN surveys of incidents from July 1, 1973, through September 30, 1976, showed a marked difference in the reporting of abuse of various stimulants in the anorectic class. Amphetamine, methamphetamine, and phenmetrazine were ranked highest, whereas phentermine was in the middle ranges, and mazindol and chlorphentermine were ranked at the bottom of the list.

The relation of cumulative DAWN incidents of anorectic drug abuse to dosage units prescribed for these drugs was tabulated for the period from July 1, 1973, to December 30, 1975. Amphetamine and methamphetamine were still ranked highest, by rate as well as by mention, whereas phentermine and chlorphentermine were in the middle range, and diethylpropion, fenfluramine, mazindol, and benzphetamine were at the low end. A comparison of DAWN-reported incidents and total prescriptions for various anorexiants from July 1973 to December 1975 again showed reports involving amphetamine preparations to be five times those involving phenmetrazine, which was five times those of diethylpropion, phentermine, benzphetamine, and mazindol. Some of the anorexiants, such as diethylpropion, may be less often abused because of patterns of metabolic conversion of limited capacity to form the primary metabolites seen with modest doses. It is considered unlikely, in view of this, that the rapid incremental effects seen with increasing doses of DAMPH would be obtainable with diethylpropion, according to this report. More recent DAWN (1994) emergency room reports found that 1.9% reported amphetamine, 3.4% reported methedrine, 0.1% reported unspecified stimulants, and 0.2% reported MPH use, suggesting a similar liability among stimulants to that reported in more detail in 1973.

When tested for self-administration and "liking," amphetamine and cocaine score at the top of all such measures. Phenmetrazine and diethylpropion are also chosen above placebo 60%–80% of the time, and 40%–60% of subjects exclusively choose active drug. Phenylpropanolamine and mazindol were chosen at placebo levels despite their identification as stimulants by subjects discriminating between them and placebo. Caffeine, despite its widespread consumption in caffeinated beverages, resulted in experimentally low doses being chosen above placebo levels by about half of the subjects tested. High doses of caffeine (i.e., the equivalent of more than three cups of coffee) were avoided by most of the subjects tested (Foltin and Fischman 1991).

It can therefore be readily seen that stimulant drugs do present hazards of abuse and dependence. However, patients with specific psychiatric disorders, such as major depression and adult attention hyperactivity disorder, may have a decreased risk of abuse, particularly in medically supervised environments.

DRUG-DRUG INTERACTIONS

Burrell et al. (1969) reported that MPH may interfere with the metabolism of drugs such as IMI. Their findings were supported by Cooper and Simpson (1973), as well as by an original report by Wharton et al. (1971). This might indicate that the mechanism for this effect on DMI metabolism may be the inhibition of cytochrome P450 enzyme systems, suggesting a possible increase of other drugs metabolized by various subfamilies of this system. A second possible drug interaction is the use of stimulants with other potential stimulant drugs taken for other purposes, such as phenylpropanolamine used as a decongestant and other over-the-counter medicines that might produce significant hypertension. Cerebral hemorrhage has been reported in a few cases of patients taking phenylpropanolamine alone, and its combination with psychostimulants might prove hazardous for some patients via this mechanism.

Although we have reported on the use of stimulants with MAOIs and found no apparent interactions (Fawcett et al. 1991), any such use should be carefully monitored for the possibility of hypertensive reactions or hyperpyrexia. Three or four cases of severe interactions producing hypertension, hyperpyrexia, convulsions, and death have been reported. The use of psychostimulants in significant doses may overwhelm the effect of antihypertensive medications and produce clinically significant hypertension in some individuals.

CONCLUSION

Psychostimulants are potent substances that should be used only after careful clinical diagnosis (both psychiatric and medical). This use should be followed with great clinical care in selected patients. The informed and careful use of these substances may produce benefits for individuals with significant psychiatric disorders who are not responsive to currently available treatment. Stimulants should be prescribed by skilled clinicians who are familiar with their potential clinical (e.g., behavior, nervousness, mania) and medical (e.g., tachycardia, elevated blood pressure, sweats) side effects, toxic effects, and drug-drug interactions.

REFERENCES

Alles GA: The comparative physiological actions of *dl*-beta-phenylisopropylamines. J Pharmacol Exp Ther 47: 339–354, 1933

American Psychiatric Press: Diagnostic and Statistical Manual of Mental Disorders, 3rd Edition. Washington, DC, American Psychiatric Association, 1980

Anders TF, Ciaranello RD: Pharmacologic treatment of minimal brain dysfunction syndrome, in Psychopharmacology: From Theory to Practice. Edited by Barchas JD, Berger PA, Ciaranello RD, et al. New York, Oxford University Press, 1977, pp 425–435

Angrist B, D'Hollosy M, Sanfilipo M, et al: Central nervous system stimulants as symptomatic treatments for AIDS-related neuropsychiatric impairment. J Clin Psychopharmacol 12:268–272, 1992

Arnold LE, Wender PH, McCloskey K, et al: Levoamphetamine and dextroamphetamine: comparative efficacy in the hyperkinetic syndrome. Arch Gen Psychiatry 27:816–822, 1972

Arnold LE, Huestis RD, Smeltzer DJ, et al: Levoamphetamine vs dextroamphetamine in minimal brain dysfunction. Arch Gen Psychiatry 33:292–301, 1976

Axelrod J, Weil-Malherbe H, Tomchick R: The physiological disposition of ³H-epinephrine and its metabolite metanephrine. J Pharmacol Exp Ther 127:251–256, 1959

Ayd FJ, Zohar J: Psychostimulant (amphetamine or methylphenidate) therapy for chronic and treatment-resistant depression, in Treating Resistant Depression. Edited by Zohar J, Belmaker RH. New York, PMA Publishing, 1987, pp 343–355

Barkley RA: A review of stimulant drug research with hyperactive children. J Child Psychol Psychiatry 18:137–165, 1977

Baumann MH, Schuster CR, Rothman RB: Effects of phentermine and cocaine on fenfluramine-induced depletion of serotonin in mouse brain. Drug Alcohol Depend 41(1):71–74, 1996

Bergstrom DL, Keller C: Drug-induced myocardial ischemia and acute myocardial infarction. Critical Care Nursing Clinics of North America 4(2):273–278, 1992

Berkovitch M, Pope E, Phillips J, et al: Pemoline-associated fulminant liver failure: testing the evidence for causation. Clin Pharmacol Ther 57:696–698, 1995

Blumberg AG, Cohen M, Heaton AM, et al: Covert drug abuse among voluntary hospitalized psychiatric patients. JAMA 217:1659–1661, 1971

Bouckoms A, Mangini L: Pergolide: an antidepressant adjuvant for mood disorders? Psychopharmacol Bull 29:207–211, 1993

Bradley C, Bowen M: Amphetamine (benzedrine) therapy of children's behavior disorders. Am J Orthopsychiatry 11:92–103, 1941

Brown WA, Corriveau DP, Ebert MH: Acute psychologic and neuroendocrine effects of dextro-amphetamine and methylphenidate. Psychopharmacology (Berl) 58:189–195, 1978

Brust JCM: Stroke and substance abuse, in Stroke: Pathophysiology, Diagnosis, and Management, 2nd Edition. Edited by Barnett HJM, Mohr JP, Stein BM, et al. New York, Churchill Livingstone, 1992, pp 875–893

Burrell JM, Black M, Wharton RN, et al: Inhibition of imipramine metabolism by methylphenidate (abstract). Federation Proceedings 28:418, 1969

Call TD, Hartneck J, Dickinson WA, et al: Acute cardiomyopathy secondary to intravenous amphetamine abuse. Ann Intern Med 97:559–560, 1982

Carabillo EA: U.S.A. Drug Abuse Warning Network, in Central Mechanisms of Anorectic Drugs. Edited by Garattini S, Samanin R. New York, Raven, 1978, pp 461–471

Carson P, Oldroyd K, Phadke K: Myocardial infarction due to amphetamine. BMJ 294:1525–1526, 1987

Castellanos FX, Elia J, Kruesi MJ, et al: Cerebrospinal fluid homovanillic acid predicts behavioral response to stimulants in 45 boys with attention deficit/hyperactivity disorder. Neuropsychopharmacology 14:125–137, 1996

Chen KK, Schmidt CF: Ephedrine and related substances. Medicine (Baltimore) 9:1–117, 1930

Chiarello RJ, Cole JO: The use of psychostimulants in general psychiatry. Arch Gen Psychiatry 44:286–295, 1987

Citron BP, Halpert M, McCarron M, et al: Necrotizing angiitis associated with drug abuse. N Engl J Med 283:1003–1011, 1970

Colado MI, O'Shea E, Granados R, et al: In vivo evidence for free radical involvement in the degeneration of rat brain 5-HT following administration of MDMA ("Ecstasy") and *p*-chloramphetamine but not the degeneration following fenfluramine. Br J Pharmacol 121:889–900, 1997

Connell PH: The use and abuse of amphetamines. Practitioner 200:234–243, 1968

Connolly HM, Crary JL, McGoon MD, et al: Valvular heart disease associated with fenfluramine-phentermine. N Engl J Med 337:581–588, 1997

Cooper TB, Simpson GM: Concomitant imipramine and methylphenidate administration: a case report. Am J Psychiatry 130:6, 1973

Dally PJ: Fatal reaction associated with tranylcypromine and methylamphetamine. Lancet 1:1235–1236, 1962

D'haenen HA, Bossuyt A: Dopamine D₂ receptor density in depression measured with single photon emission computed tomography. Biol Psychiatry 35:128–132, 1994

Drimmer EJ, Gitlin MJ, Gwirtsman HE: Desipramine and methylphenidate combination treatment for depression: case report. Am J Psychiatry 140:241–242, 1983

Drug Abuse Warning Network: Annual E.R. Department Data (DAWN Series No 14–17). U.S. Department of Health and Human Services, 1994

Fawcett J, Siomopoulos V: Dextroamphetamine response as a possible predictor of improvement with tricyclic therapy in depression. Arch Gen Psychiatry 25:247–255, 1971

Fawcett J, Kravitz HM, Zajecka JM, et al: CNS stimulant potentiation of monoamine oxidase inhibitors in treatment-refractory depression. J Clin Psychopharmacol 11:127–132, 1991

Feighner JP, Herbstein J, Damlouji N: Combined MAOI, TCA and direct stimulant therapy of treatment resistant depression. J Clin Psychiatry 46:206–209, 1985

Fernandez F, Adams F, Holmes VF, et al: Methylphenidate for depressive disorders in cancer patients. Psychosomatics 28:455–459, 1987

Fernandez F, Adams F, Levy JK, et al: Cognitive impairment due to AIDS-related complex and its response to psychostimulants. Psychosomatics 29:38–46, 1988a

Fernandez F, Levy JK, Galizzi H: Response of HIV-related depression to psychostimulants: case reports. Hosp Community Psychiatry 39:628–631, 1988b

Fernandez F, Levy JK, Samley HR, et al: Effects of methylphenidate in HIV-related depression: a comparative trial with desipramine. Int J Psychiatry Med 25:53–67, 1995

Fischman MW: Cocaine and the amphetamines, in Psychopharmacology: The Third Generation of Progress. Edited by Meltzer HY. New York, Raven, 1987, pp 1543–1553

Flemenbaum A: Methylphenidate: a catalyst for the tricyclic antidepressants? Am J Psychiatry 128:239, 1971

Foltin RW, Fischman MW: Assessment of abuse liability of stimulant drugs in humans: a methodological survey. Drug Alcohol Depend 28:3–48, 1991

Galynker I, Ieronimo C, Miner C, et al: Methylphenidate treatment of negative symptoms in patients with dementia. J Neuropsychiatry Clin Neurosci 9:231–239, 1997

Glennon RA: Psychoactive phenylisopropylamines, in Psychopharmacology: The Third Generation of Progress. Edited by Meltzer HY. New York, Raven, 1987, pp 1627–1634

Graham DJ, Green L: Further cases of valvular heart disease associated with fenfluramine-phentermine (letter). N Engl J Med 337:635, 1997

Gwirtsman HE, Szuba MP, Toren L, et al: The antidepressant response to tricyclics in major depressives is accelerated with adjunctive use of methylphenidate. Psychopharmacol Bull 39:157–164, 1994

Harrington H, Heller HA, Dawson D, et al: Intracerebral hemorrhage and oral amphetamine. Arch Neurol 40:503–507, 1983

Heuer L: Pulmonary hypertension. Cher Prax 23:497, 1978

Hill D: Amphetamine in psychopathic states. British Journal of Addiction 44:50–54, 1947

Hill D, Watterson D: Electro-encephalographic studies of psychopathic personalities. Journal of Neurology and Psychiatry 5:47–65, 1942

Hodge RS, Hutchings HM: Enuresis: a brief review, a tentative theory and a suggested treatment. Arch Dis Child 27:498–504, 1952

Hoffman BB, Lefkowitz RJ: Catecholamines and sympathomimetic drugs, in The Pharmacological Basis of Therapeutics, 8th Edition. Edited by Gilman AG, Goodman LS, Rall TW, et al. New York, Macmillan, 1993, pp 187–220

Holmes VF, Fernandez F, Levy JK: Psychostimulant response in AIDS-related complex patients. J Clin Psychiatry 50:5–8, 1989

Hornstein A, Lennihan L, Seliger G, et al: Amphetamine in recovery from brain injury. Brain Inj 10:145–148, 1996

Imanse J, Vanneste J: Intraventricular hemorrhage following amphetamine abuse. Neurology 40:1318–1319, 1990

Insel TR, Hamilton JA, Guttmacher LB, et al: d-Amphetamine in obsessive-compulsive disorder. Psychopharmacology (Berl) 80:231–235, 1983

Janowsky D, Davis JM: Methylphenidate, dextroamphetamine, and levoamphetamine. Arch Gen Psychiatry 33:304–308, 1976

Johnson ML, Roberts MD, Rossa R, et al: Methylphenidate in stroke patients with depression. Am J Phys Med Rehabil 71:239–241, 1992

Kalant H, Kalant OJ: Death in amphetamine users: causes and rates. Can Med Assoc J 112:299–304, 1975

Khantzian EJ, Gawin F, Kleber HD, et al: Methylphenidate (Ritalin®) treatment of cocaine dependence—a preliminary report. J Subst Abuse Treat 1:107–112, 1984

Klein RG, Wender P: The role of methylphenidate in psychiatry. Arch Gen Psychiatry 52:429–433, 1995

Kraus MF, Burch EA: Methylphenidate hydrochloride as an antidepressant: controversy, case studies and review. South Med J 85:985–991, 1992

Kravitz HM, Edwards JH, Fawcett J, et al: Challenging the amphetamine challenge test: report of an antidepressant study. J Affect Disord 20:121–128, 1990

Krisko I, Lewis E, Johnston JE: Severe hyperpyrexia due to tranylcypromine-amphetamine toxicity. Ann Intern Med 70:559–564, 1969

Kuczenski R, Segal D: Effects of methylphenidate on extracellular dopamine, serotonin and norepinephrine: comparison with amphetamine. J Neurochem 68:2032–2037, 1997

Lazarus LW, Winemiller DR, Lingam VR, et al: Efficacy and side effects of methylphenidate for post-stroke depression. J Clin Psychiatry 53:447–449, 1992

Lazarus L, Moberg P, Langsley PR, et al: Methylphenidate and nortriptyline in the treatment of poststroke depression. Arch Phys Med Rehabil 75:403–406, 1994

Lieberman JA, Kinon BJ, Loebel AD: Dopaminergic mechanisms in idiopathic and drug-induced psychoses. Schizophr Bull 16:97–110, 1990

Linet LS: Treatment of a refractory depression with a combination of fluoxetine and d-amphetamine. Am J Psychiatry 146:803–804, 1989

Lloyd JTA, Walker DRH: Death after combined dexamphetamine and phenelzine. BMJ 2:168–169, 1965

Mantle TJ, Tipton KF, Garrett NJ: Inhibition of monoamine oxidase by amphetamine and related compounds. Biochem Pharmacol 25:2073–2077, 1976

Mason A: Fatal reaction associated with tranylcypromine and methylamphetamine. Lancet 1:1073, 1962

McCann UD, Seiden LS, Rubin LJ, et al: Brain serotonin neurotoxicity and primary pulmonary hypertension from fenfluramine and dexfenfluramine. JAMA 278:666–672, 1997

Metz A, Shader RI: Combination of fluoxetine with pemoline in the treatment of major depressive disorder. Int Clin Psychopharmacol 6:93–96, 1991

Meyler L: The Side Effects of Drugs. Amsterdam, Excerpta Medica Foundation, 1966

Miller HH, Shore PA, Clarke DE: In vivo monoamine oxidase inhibition by *d*-amphetamine. Biochem Pharmacol 29:1347–1354, 1980

Mooney GF, Haas LF: Effect of methylphenidate on brain injury-related anger. Arch Phys Med Rehabil 74:153–160, 1993

Morita T, Mehendale HM: Effects of chlorphentermine and phentermine on the pulmonary disposition of 5-hydroxytryptamine in the rat in vivo. Am Rev Respir Dis 127:747–750, 1983

Myers WC, Stewart JT: Use of methylphenidate. Hosp Community Psychiatry 40:754, 1989

Nicola SM, Kombian SB, Malenka RC: Psychostimulants depress excitatory synaptic transmission in the nucleus accumbens via presynaptic D1-like dopamine receptors. J Neurosci 26:1591–1604, 1996

Nurnberger JI, Simmons-Alling S, Kessler L, et al: Separate mechanisms for behavioral, cardiovascular, and hormonal responses to dextroamphetamine in man. Psychopharmacology (Berl) 84:200–204, 1984

Olin J, Masand P: Psychostimulants for depression in hospitalized cancer patients. Psychosomatics 37:57–62, 1996

O'Neill ME, Arnolda LF, Coles DM, et al: Acute amphetamine cardiomyopathy in a drug addict. Clin Cardiol 6:189–191, 1983

Packe GE, Garton MJ, Jennings K: Acute myocardial infarction caused by intravenous amphetamine abuse. Br Heart J 64:23–24, 1990

Patrick KS, Kilts CD, Breese GR: Synthesis and pharmacology of hydroxylated metabolites of methylphenidate. J Med Chem 24:1237–1240, 1981

Patrick KS, Mueller RA, Gualtieri CT, et al: Pharmacokinetics and actions of methyl-phenidate, in Psychopharmacology: The Third Generation of Progress. Edited by Meltzer H. New York, Raven, 1987, pp 1387–1395

Patrick RL: Amphetamine and cocaine: biological mechanisms, in Psychopharmacology: From Theory to Practice. Edited by Barchas JD, Berger PA, Ciaranello RD, et al. New York, Oxford University Press, 1977, pp 331–340

Perel JM, Black N, Wharton RN, et al: Inhibition of imipramine metabolism by methylphenidate (abstract). Federation Proceedings 28:418, 1969

Physicians' Desk Reference, 52nd Edition. Montvale, NJ, Medical Economics, 1998

Plenger PM, Dixon CE, Castillo RM, et al: Subacute methylphenidate treatment for moderate to moderately severe traumatic brain injury: a preliminary double-blind placebo-controlled study. Arch Phys Med Rehabil 77:536–540, 1996

Post RM, Gerner RH, Carman JS: Effects of a dopamine agonist piribedil in depressed patients. Arch Gen Psychiatry 35:609–615, 1978

Prinzmetal M, Bloomberg W: The use of benzedrine for the treatment of narcolepsy. JAMA 105:2051–2054, 1935

Ragland AS, Ismail Y, Arsura EL: Myocardial infarction after amphetamine use. Am Heart J 125:247–249, 1993

Regier DA, Farmer ME, Rae DS, et al: Comorbidity of mental disorders with alcohol and other drug abuse: results from the Epidemiologic Catchment Area (ECA) study. JAMA 264:2511–2518, 1990

Riishede J: Treatment of acute barbiturate poisoning; a comparison of nikethamide and amphetamine. Lancet 2:789–792, 1950

Robinson AE, Wolkind SN: Amphetamine abuse amongst psychiatric inpatients: the use of gas chromatography. Br J Psychiatry 116:643–644, 1970

Rumbaugh CL, Bergeron RT, Fang HCH, et al: Cerebral angiographic changes in the drug abuse patient. Radiology 101:335–344, 1971

Rumbaugh DL, Bergeron RT, Scanlan RL, et al: Cerebral vascular changes secondary to amphetamine abuse in the experimental animal. Radiology 101:345–351, 1971

Sabelli HC, Fawcett J, Javaid JI, et al: The methylphenidate test for differentiating desipramine-responsive from nortriptyline-responsive depression. Am J Psychiatry 140:212–214, 1983

Satel SL, Nelson JC: Stimulants in the treatment of depression: a critical overview. J Clin Psychiatry 59:241–249, 1989

Satterfield JH, Satterfield BT, Cantwell DP: Three multimodal treatment of 100 hyperactive boys. Behavioral Pediatrics 98:650–655, 1981

Satterfield JH, Satterfield BT, Shell AM: Therapeutic interventions to prevent delinquency in hyperactive boys. J Am Acad Child Adolesc Psychiatry 26:56–64, 1987

Schachar R, Tannock R: Childhood hyperactivity and psychostimulants: a review of extended treatment studies. Journal of Child and Adolescent Psychopharmacology 3:81–97, 1993

Seiden LS, Sabol KE, Ricaurte GA: Amphetamine: effects on catecholamine systems and behavior. Annu Rev Pharmacol Toxicol 32:639–677, 1993

Shaw DM: Antidepressant drugs. Practitioner 192:28–32, 1964

Shevell M, Schreiber R: Pemoline-associated hepatic failure: a critical analysis of the literature. Pediatr Neurol 16(1):14–16, 1997

Sloviter E, Drust EG, Connor JD: Evidence that serotonin mediates some behavioral effects of amphetamine. J Pharmacol Exp Ther 6:348–352, 1978

Smilkstein MJ, Smolinske SC, Rumack BH: A case of MAO inhibitor/MDMA interaction: agony after ecstasy. Clinical Toxicology 25:149–152, 1987

Smith RC, Davis JM: Comparative effects of d-amphetamine/amphetamine and methylphenidate on mood in man. Psychopharmacology (Berl) 53:1–12, 1977

Speech TH, Rao SM, Osmon DC, et al: A double-blind controlled study of methylphenidate treatment in closed head injury. Brain Inj 7:333–338, 1993

Spencer T, Wilens T, Biederman J, et al: A double-blind, crossover comparison of methylphenidate and placebo in adults with childhood-onset attention-deficit hyperactivity disorder. Arch Gen Psychiatry 52:434–443, 1995

Spencer T, Biederman J, Harding M, et al: Growth deficits in ADHD children revisited: evidence for disorder-associated growth delays? J Am Acad Child Adolesc Psychiatry 35:1460–1469, 1996a

Spencer T, Biederman J, Wilens T, et al: Pharmacotherapy of attention-deficit hyperactivity disorder across the life cycle. J Am Acad Child Adolesc Psychiatry 35:409–432, 1996b

Sprague RL, Cohen M, Werry JS: Normative data on the Conners Teacher's Rating Scale and Abbreviated Scale (technical report). Urbana-Champaign, University of Illinois Children's Research Center, 1974

Sterling MJ, Kane M, Grace ND: Pemoline-induced autoimmune hepatitis. Am J Gastroenterol 91:2233–2234, 1996

Stockley IH: Drug interactions: monoamine oxidase inhibitors, I: interactions with sympathomimetic amines. The Pharmaceutical Journal 210:590–594, 1973

Sulzer D, Rayport S: Amphetamine and other psychostimulants reduce pH gradients in midbrain dopaminergic neurons and chromaffin granules: a mechanism of action. Neuron 5:797–808, 1990

Theohar C, Fischer-Cornelssen K, Akesson H, et al: Bromocriptine as antidepressant: double-blind comparative study with imipramine in psychogenic and endogenous depression. Current Therapeutic Research 30:830–842, 1981

Tinklenburg JR, Berger PA: Treatment of abusers of non-addictive drugs, in Psychopharmacology: From Theory to Practice. Edited by Barchas JD, Berger PA, Ciaranello RD, et al. New York, Oxford University Press, 1977, pp 386–403

Trugman JM: Cerebral arteritis and oral methylphenidate. Lancet 1:584–585, 1988

van Kammen DP, Murphy DL: Prediction of antidepressant response by a one day d-amphetamine trial. Am J Psychiatry 135:1179–1184, 1978

Wagner GH, Rabkin JG, Rabkin R: Dextroamphetamine as a treatment for depression and low energy in AIDS patients: a pilot study. J Psychosom Res 42:407–411, 1997

Weisenberg B, Vosmer G, Seiden LS: Combined phentermine/fenfluramine administration enhances depletion of serotonin from central terminal fields. Synapse 26:36–45, 1997

Wender PH, Reimherr FW, Wood D, et al: A controlled study of methylphenidate in the treatment of attention deficit disorder, residual type, in adults. Am J Psychiatry 142:547–552, 1985

Wharton RN, Perel JM, Dayton PG, et al: A potential clinical use for methylphenidate with tricyclic antidepressants. Am J Psychiatry 127:1619–1625, 1971

Wheatley D: Amphetamines in general practice: their use in depression and anxiety. Seminars in Psychiatry 1:163–173, 1969

Williams RT, Caldwell RJ, Dreng LG: Comparative metabolism of some amphetamine in various species, in Frontiers of Catecholamine Research. Edited by Schneider SH, Esdin E. Oxford, England, Pergamon, 1973, pp 927–932

Wroblewski BA, Leary JM, Phelan AM, et al: Methylphenidate and seizure frequency in brain injured patients with seizure disorders. J Clin Psychiatry 53:86–89, 1992

Zeck P: The dangers of some antidepressant drugs. Med J Aust 2:607–608, 1961

TWENTY-SIX

Electroconvulsive Therapy

Gary S. Figiel, M.D., William M. McDonald, M.D.,
W. Vaughn McCall, M.D., and Charles Zorumpski, M.D.

The clinical practice of electroconvulsive therapy (ECT) developed from the work of Ladhaus von Meduna (1985) on the therapeutic benefits of camphor monobromide-induced convulsions in patients with schizophrenia. Following his lead, in 1938 Cerletti and Bini (1940) reported that convulsions could be safely induced in humans by an electrical stimulus. Since that time, ECT has been found to be consistently effective in the treatment of depression, mania, and schizophrenia (Abrams 1992).

Led by the growing awareness of the limitations of pharmacological options in treating psychiatric disorders, a surge of new research in ECT began in the 1970s and has continued through today (Cerletti 1940). This work has displayed more rigorous scientific methodology than previously was used and has primarily examined the clinical indications for the use of ECT, optimal treatment techniques, methods to minimize the cognitive and cardiac side effects from ECT, and ECT's mechanisms of action.

In this chapter, we review the use of ECT in the treatment of psychiatric disorders, most notably depression but also including mania, schizophrenia, and Parkinson's disease. The mechanism of action of ECT is discussed within the context of its anticonvulsant and amnestic effects and in relation to the supplemental use of rapid-rate transcranial magnetic stimulation (rTMS). Finally, we provide an overview of the literature on the potential side effects and complications of ECT and discuss recommendations for its use in clinical practice.

USE OF ELECTROCONVULSIVE THERAPY

The use of ECT declined from the 1960s to the 1980s, but since then its use has steadily increased. ECT is most commonly administered to patients with depression, followed by those with schizophrenia and mania. Probably because of the increased incidence of depression in women, they are more likely to receive ECT than are men. Middle and upper socioeconomic groups are more frequently administered ECT. Consistent with this finding, ECT is much more commonly used in private hospitals than in public facilities. No doubt reflecting the safe and effective way that ECT can now be administered, recent studies have shown a significant increase in the number of elderly patients receiving ECT. Unfortunately, there may be still a significant lack of access to ECT in many metropolitan areas. It is hoped that ongoing education of physicians and the public will ensure the availability of ECT to all who might benefit from it (Sackeim et al. 1995).

EFFICACY OF ELECTROCONVULSIVE THERAPY

Major Depression

ECT is most commonly used for the treatment of depression. An American Psychiatric Association (APA) Task Force reported that ECT is an effective treatment in up to

80% of patients with either unipolar or bipolar major depression (American Psychiatric Association 1990). ECT should no longer be considered a treatment of last resort but may be considered as a treatment of first choice when a rapid clinical response is essential in severely ill patients, when a history of a positive response to ECT or of medication refractoriness or intolerance is present, and finally, when patients and family request ECT over other treatment options. Although the short-term therapeutic benefits of ECT are clearly established, the 6-month relapse rate after ECT during antidepressant therapy remains particularly high (Sackeim et al. 1995).

ECT Compared With Antidepressants and Predictors of Response

Although ECT has commonly been reported to be more effective when compared with antidepressants, the literature from which this conclusion is drawn has major methodological flaws. In most studies, subtherapeutic doses of antidepressants were used. Nonetheless, ECT has been found to be equal to or superior to all pharmacological agents with which it has been compared.

Clinical predictors of response to ECT remain elusive. Potential positive predictors of response include increasing age and the presence of psychotic and catatonic symptoms. Several studies have reported that patients with longer current episodes of depression are less likely to respond to ECT. Surprisingly, the presence of the endogenous or melancholic subtypes of depression has not been able to predict a positive response to ECT.

Prudic et al. (1996) recently reported that patients in whom one or more tricyclic antidepressants trials had failed before ECT responded less favorably to ECT than did patients in whom adequate antidepressant trials had not failed before ECT. More recent work from the same group suggests that these findings may not pertain to newer second-generation antidepressants (Prudic et al. 1996; Sackeim et al. 1995).

To date, no biological marker has been found that can consistently predict patients' response to ECT. Scott et al. (1990) reported that the release of oxytocin-associated neurophysin after ECT is associated with a positive clinical response from ECT. In addition, a large number of preexisting structural abnormalities observed on brain magnetic resonance imaging (MRI) scans appear in many elderly depressed patients referred for ECT. Preliminary observations suggest that these preexisting structural brain changes may predispose some elderly depressed patients to a less favorable response from ECT and to an increased risk for developing ECT-induced interictal delirium

(Hickie et al. 1995). Clearly, these research areas are of tremendous potential clinical significance and require further study.

Stimulus Dosing in Electroconvulsive Therapy for Treatment of Depression

Questions about the proper management of the electrical stimulus have been central to the science and practice of ECT since the inception of the treatment. Cerletti and Bini modeled their expectations for ECT on the success of pharmacologically induced convulsive therapy. Therefore, these pioneers assumed that the ECT stimulus should be convulsive. Interestingly, the first ECT session, in 1938 in Rome, involved two subconvulsive stimulations before Cerletti and Bini increased the stimulus intensity to produce a convulsion (Endler 1988). Thus, the first ECT session was a "titrated" ECT session involving the serial application of increasing stimulus intensities passing from the subconvulsive range through the convulsive threshold. Issues in stimulus dosing that have been considered since that time have included 1) whether the stimulus should be subconvulsive or convulsive; 2) what is the optimal stimulus waveform; 3) if a convulsive stimulus is desired, to what degree the stimulus intensity should be in excess of the convulsive threshold; and 4) which physiological parameters provide useful feedback to continuously refine stimulus dosing throughout the ECT course.

Convulsive, subconvulsive, and sham stimulation.

The use of nonconvulsive electrical stimulation to treat psychological problems preceded the introduction of ECT by decades. Most of the treatments involved administering static electricity to parts of the body not limited to the head (Grover 1924). Diagnostic indications included neurasthenia. The availability of commercial ECT devices did not mean the immediate replacement of subconvulsive with convulsive stimulation. Instead, some practitioners used the devices to deliver lengthy (several minutes long) subconvulsive cranial stimulation. This practice faded from American psychiatry as it became clear that subconvulsive stimulation was associated with a *poorer* outcome than conventional psychotherapy in psychoneurotic patients (Hargrove et al. 1953).

The elements of *modified* ECT (including muscle relaxation and general anesthesia) were described early in the history of ECT. The wide-scale adoption of these modifications raised new questions as to whether the seizure was central to the antidepressant efficacy of ECT or whether anesthesia alone would be just as effective. The Northwick Park trial (Crow et al. 1982) and the Leicestershire trial (Brandon et al. 1984) are examples of two "sham" ECT studies in which anesthesia alone was compared with real ECT. It was convincingly demonstrated that real ECT was more effective, especially for the most severe forms of depression (Brandon et al. 1984; Crow et al. 1982).

Thus, the effectiveness of ECT was clearly linked to the production of a seizure. Neither anesthesia alone without the electrical stimulus nor the use of subconvulsive stimuli appears to have real merit in the treatment of depression.

Stimulus waveform.   Given that a convulsive stimulus is necessary for the antidepressant effects of ECT, a nearly infinite number of variations were available for formulating the stimulus waveform. The earliest ECT devices delivered a sinusoidal stimulus, probably because that was the standard waveform for domestic use. Other waveforms available on early ECT devices included the "chopped" sine wave, the unidirectional pulse square wave, and the alternating brief pulse square wave. Although some investigators had a suspicion that sine wave stimuli may have produced slightly better antidepressant effects than did brief pulse stimuli, these suspicions were overwhelmed by convincing data that sine wave ECT produced more memory side effects than brief pulse ECT, irrespective of the placement of the stimulating electrode (Weiner et al. 1986). The more severe memory side effects produced by sinusoidal stimuli may be explained by the slower rise time for each sine wave cycle as compared with the brief pulse cycle. Consequent to its slower rise time, much of the sine wave stimulus is subconvulsive and thus presumably adds nothing to the therapeutic effect of ECT, adding only to its side effects. The abrupt rise in the brief pulse waveform allows for the entire stimulus to be above the convulsive threshold (suprathreshold). Because much of the sine wave stimulus is "wasted" in the subconvulsive range, it would be predicted that brief pulse stimuli would be more efficient, requiring a stimulus of smaller magnitude to produce a seizure.

These expectations were borne out in the studies of Weiner (1980), which showed that brief pulse stimuli could provoke a seizure with only one-third of the energy required with sine wave stimuli. Brief pulse ECT devices now dominate the American scene, virtually replacing the sine wave devices for the reasons described above (Farah and McCall 1993).

Magnitude of the stimulus dose.   The consensus regarding the need for convulsive (as opposed to subconvulsive) stimuli and brief pulse waveforms would seem to make stimulus dosing in ECT a straightforward process, except for the question of by how much the stimulus should exceed the convulsive threshold. For years, ECT practitioners were satisfied that the answer to this question was found in the work of Ottosson (1962), who compared routine ECT with ECT modified by pretreatment with intravenous lidocaine. He found that seizures induced by lidocaine-modified ECT were shorter than those induced by routine ECT, and an inverse relation was found between seizure duration and antidepressant effect. From this work it was widely accepted that stimulus doses producing seizures longer than 25–30 seconds had an antidepressant effect (American Psychiatric Association 1978).

This clinical wisdom was shattered with the groundbreaking work of Sackeim in the late 1980s. Sackeim et al. (1993) showed that if the magnitude of the electrical stimulus was just barely above the convulsive threshold, then ECT was ineffective with right-unilateral-stimulating electrode placement, despite the production of electrographic seizures typically in excess of 25 seconds. In contrast, bilateral ECT was fully effective with stimuli minimally above or 2.5 times above the seizure threshold, but excess memory side effects accrued only at the higher stimulus dose (Sackeim et al. 1993). These dose-response relationships are true to the extent that the stimulus exceeded the convulsive threshold for a given patient, and they are not related to the absolute magnitude of the stimulus dose. This situation is analogous to the pharmacological treatment of depression with tricyclic antidepressants: serum blood levels are more important than the absolute oral dose in determining both efficacy and side effects.

These findings led to the following conclusions: 1) with right-unilateral electrode placement, the stimulus should be substantially ($\geq$2.5 times) above the convulsive threshold to ensure the efficacy of ECT, and 2) with bilateral electrode placement, the stimulus should not be excessively above the convulsive threshold to avoid undue memory side effects. The APA Task Force on ECT (1990) responded to these discoveries by recommending that the ECT stimulus should be "moderately" suprathreshold, without exactly defining *moderate*. This recommendation assumes that the convulsive threshold is known for each patient. The APA Task Force recommendation was further complicated by the uncertainty regarding how best to determine the convulsive threshold for each patient. The convulsive threshold varies by a factor of at least 40-fold in large patient samples, thus making the mean threshold for a group of patients useless for individual cases (Sackeim et al. 1991). It is clear that the convulsive threshold is related to age, sex, race, choice of stimulating electrode placement, and, perhaps, cranial dimensions (Colenda and McCall 1996; McCall et al. 1993b; Sackeim et al. 1991). Still, these factors predict only a small amount of the variance in the convulsive threshold. Statistical models to predict the convulsive threshold fare poorly, especially in patients with high thresholds (Colenda and McCall 1996).

The bulk of the evidence thus suggests that it is important to determine the dose of the stimulus as a proportion of the convulsive threshold and that the convulsive threshold of each patient should be known, preferably by measuring convulsive threshold early in the ECT course. The most accurate means of measuring the convulsive threshold for a given patient is empirical observation: giving intentionally subconvulsive stimuli at the first treatment and, in the same session, following with successively larger stimuli until a seizure is produced. This stimulus "titration" technique defines the convulsive threshold for each patient.

If ECT practitioners follow the above reasoning and the stimulus dosing recommendations of the APA Task Force, then most practitioners should titrate the convulsive threshold at the first ECT session. In fact, a recent survey of ECT practitioners showed that a minority performs titration of the stimulus dose (Farah and McCall 1993). The reasons for this are unclear, but possible explanations include concerns that 1) the subconvulsive stimulations inherent in stimulus titration might be medically dangerous, 2) subconvulsive stimulation might add to memory side effects, or 3) producing a barely suprathreshold seizure with right-unilateral placement is an ineffective treatment, thus "wasting" the first treatment.

It is true that subconvulsive stimulation transiently slows the heart rate, and if subconvulsive stimulation is given in the presence of β-blockers and no anticholinergic drug, there is risk of substantial asystole (McCall 1996; McCall et al. 1994). On the other hand, atropine pretreatment eliminates this risk. The possibility of excess acute cognitive side effects with subconvulsive stimuli has been examined and discounted (Prudic et al. 1994). The possibility of a sluggish antidepressant response when a titrated, "moderately" suprathreshold approach is combined with right-unilateral placement, however, is a real concern. A prospective, randomized trial of a titrated, moderately suprathreshold dosing strategy with right-unilateral electrode placement in older depressed subjects was found to produce a slower antidepressant response than did a fixed, high-dose stimulus with right-unilateral electrode placement (McCall et al. 1995). Interpretation of this study is made more difficult because of differences between treatment assignments (titrated vs. fixed dose; moderate vs.

high dose). At the very least, however, it is clear that different dosing strategies affect the antidepressant outcome of right-unilateral ECT, even when both of the doses being compared are substantially above the convulsive threshold.

Refinement of stimulus dosing during electroconvulsive therapy.   The report of Sackeim et al. (1993) that threshold right-unilateral ECT produced seizures of ≥25 seconds without antidepressant efficacy cast into doubt the clinical wisdom that the stimulus dose was therapeutic if the electrographic seizure lasted 25 seconds. Investigators have scrambled to find a physiological marker of treatment adequacy to replace seizure duration. The most promising candidate is seizure morphology. Ottosson (1962) reported that lidocaine changed the shape of ECT seizures and affected duration, although the first finding is largely overlooked. Lidocaine-modified seizures, in addition to being less efficacious than standard ECT seizures, were characterized by loss of spike activity and poor postictal suppression (Ottosson 1962).

This finding is now extended by new evidence that seizure morphology indeed varies with ECT techniques of different efficacies. In general, greater seizure intensity is apparent as ECT techniques progress from lower (right-unilateral, low stimulus intensity) to higher (bilateral, high stimulus intensity) efficacy (Krystal et al. 1993). Electrode placement and stimulus intensity have independent and additive effects on seizure morphology. Seizures of greater intensity are characterized by higher peak ictal amplitudes, greater stereotypy of the ictal discharge, greater symmetry and coherence between the left and right cerebral hemispheres, and more profound postictal suppression. Preliminary evidence suggests that greater seizure intensity is predictive of greater likelihood of response and/or faster response (McCall and Farah 1994; Nobler et al. 1993).

The natural extension of this reasoning leads to the hope that seizure morphology could guide decisions about stimulus intensity as the course of ECT progresses. For example, if seizure intensity is poor in the middle of the treatment course, then treatment technique should be changed (by switching electrode placement and/or increasing the stimulus intensity) to optimize clinical outcome. At least one manufacturer of ECT devices now incorporates automated measures of seizure intensity into its ECT chart recorder, and the accompanying owner's manual instructs the practitioner to increase the stimulus intensity if the seizure morphology appears to be degraded (Swartz and Abrams 1994). The unstated implication is that poor seizure morphology is a problem and that increasing the stimulus intensity will fix the problem. This instruction might have merit if stimulus intensity is the primary determinant of seizure morphology, but other factors, such as age and baseline convulsive threshold, likely play an equal role in determining seizure shape (McCall et al. 1996).

Our impression is that poor seizure morphology (i.e., in older patients with high thresholds) is little influenced by increasing the stimulus intensity. Therefore, we believe it is premature to recommend stimulus dosing on the basis of seizure morphology. The importance of seizure morphology in predicting clinical outcome is far from being understood, and more work is needed to make it a practical tool for governing ECT technique.

Recommendations for stimulus dosing. Our recommendations for stimulus dosing are made with the following two caveats: 1) recommendations can be made only in regard to major depression; it is unknown whether dosing strategies for other diagnoses should be the same or different; and 2) dosing recommendations can be made only in the context of the chosen electrode placement and the patient's clinical condition. It is clear that a supraconvulsive stimulus is necessary to obtain ECT's antidepressant effect. It is likely that any supraconvulsive stimulus will have antidepressant efficacy with bilateral electrode placement, but a stimulus at least 2.5 times the convulsive threshold is required for right-unilateral ECT in most patients. Those patients with the most serious complications of major depression (i.e., active suicidal behavior in the hospital, catatonia, or food refusal) merit an approach most likely to yield quick antidepressant results. In such circumstances, bilateral ECT with a relatively high, fixed dose could be justified; stimulus dose titration would not be required because concern about cognitive side effects becomes a purely secondary issue, based on the severity of the patient's clinical status. However, whether fixed, high-dose right-unilateral ECT could provide an equally fast and effective response needs to be examined.

In contrast, there is the depressed outpatient in whom medication has failed but who is otherwise nonurgent. If this patient pursued the entire index course of ECT as an outpatient, then ECT using an right-unilateral technique, with the dose titrated to 2.5 times the convulsive threshold, may improve the patient's chances of completing the course as an outpatient with minimal supervision. Other special situations favoring titrated right-unilateral ECT include depressed patients with comorbid borderline personality disorder and depressed patients with comorbid dementia. These examples share a poorer risk-benefit ratio and a corresponding need to minimize even transient memory side effects. Other dosing strategies, such as ti-

trated bilateral or high, fixed-dose right-unilateral ECT, occupy the strategic middle ground between titrated right-unilateral and fixed-dose bilateral ECT for patients whose condition is of intermediate acuity. Finally, although seizure morphology may eventually prove a useful guide to stimulus dosing, evidence is now insufficient to recommend it.

Mania

Early anecdotal reports suggested that ECT was beneficial in the treatment of mania. Since 1970, several retrospective studies have consistently confirmed these earlier observations (Mukherjee et al. 1994). Small et al. (1988) conducted a major prospective controlled trial in which the efficacy of ECT was compared with that of lithium in the treatment of mania. The results of this study showed that patients who received ECT improved more during the first 8 weeks of treatment than did patients who received lithium. After 8 weeks of treatment, ECT and lithium were comparable in efficacy. In addition, the authors observed that patients who had mixed symptoms of depression and mania responded particularly well to ECT.

Controversy persists over whether unilateral ECT is as effective as bilateral ECT in the treatment of mania. Unfortunately, in most studies of ECT in which unilateral ECT was found not to be as effective as bilateral ECT in the treatment of mania, either the amount of electrical charge used or the percentage by which the electrical stimulus exceeded the seizure threshold was not reported. At Emory University, we have found that fixed, high-dose unilateral ECT is effective in the treatment of many patients with severe mania. In addition, most patients are significantly improved by the sixth session of ECT, although some patients may require a greater number of treatments before they respond.

Schizophrenia

Fink and Sackeim (1996) recently provided an excellent review on the use of ECT in the treatment of schizophrenia. The authors cautiously noted that most studies examining the efficacy of ECT in treating schizophrenia do not meet present standards for scientific methodology. Nonetheless, the authors concluded that ECT is a highly effective treatment for psychosis and that ECT should be considered particularly in patients with first episodes of schizophrenia, especially when they have symptoms of agitation, increased psychomotor activity, delirium, or delusions. The authors also concluded that ECT was effective in treating schizophrenia when catatonia or positive symptoms of psychosis were present. They speculated that by using ECT early in the course of schizophrenia, the progressive, debilitating effects of the illness may be avoided.

Of interest is that the literature to date suggests that ECT combined with neuroleptics is probably more effective than ECT or neuroleptics alone in treating schizophrenia. In general, the conclusions of the authors are consistent with the recommendations of the APA Task Force report, which stated that "ECT is an effective treatment for schizophrenia in the following clinical conditions: 1) patients with catatonia; or 2) when affective symptoms are present; or 3) when there is a history of a previous favorable response to ECT" (American Psychiatric Association 1990, p. 8). Clearly, there is a need for further research in this area.

Parkinson's Disease

For the past two decades, ECT has been reported to be effective in the treatment of patients with Parkinson's disease (Rasmussen and Abrams 1991). These reports have included patients with and without psychiatric illnesses. Favorable predictors of response include advanced age, severe disability ("on-off" syndromes), and painful dyskinesias. Reduction in symptoms of Parkinson's disease tends to occur during the first several sessions of ECT. However, the effects from ECT are not permanent and usually last from several days to several months, although prolonged improvement has been reported in a few patients. Although maintenance ECT studies in patients with Parkinson's disease are lacking, our clinical experience has suggested that the therapeutic benefits of ECT in these patients can be sustained with maintenance ECT.

Unilateral ECT appears to be as effective as bilateral ECT in treating Parkinson's disease. However, because of the increased risk for ECT-induced interictal delirium in patients with Parkinson's disease, careful consideration must be given to the amount of electrical charge administered, the type of electrode placement used, and the frequency of treatments (Figiel et al. 1991). At Emory University, we have found that the delirium from ECT observed in Parkinson's patients can be significantly reduced without losing the treatment's efficacy by 1) using exclusively right-unilateral ECT with an initial electrical stimulus approximately 250% above the seizure threshold, 2) administering ECT treatments every 3–4 days, 3) withholding the dose of levodopa on the morning of ECT, and 4) discontinuing ECT until the cognitive impairment completely resolves if any impairment in attention or orientation develops and then restarting ECT at a lower electrical charge.

Other Psychiatric Illnesses

In one small study, ECT was effective in treating panic disorder in patients with coexisting panic disorder and depression (Figiel et al. 1992). Whether ECT is effective in treating panic disorder alone is unknown. Although, in general, ECT alone is not believed to have a significant therapeutic effect on obsessive-compulsive disorder, some preliminary reports have been positive. Whether selective serotonin reuptake inhibitors can be used safely in combination with ECT to treat obsessive-compulsive disorder requires examination. ECT has not been directly examined in the treatment of either posttraumatic stress disorder or generalized anxiety disorder.

Although ECT has been reported to be effective in treating neuroleptic malignant syndrome, some cardiac complications have been reported in patients with neuroleptic malignant syndrome treated with ECT. Until more clinical studies are completed, however, we agree with the APA Task Force's recommendations that ECT should be reserved for patients with neuroleptic malignant syndrome who are refractory to or intolerant of standard medical treatments (American Psychiatric Association 1990).

One small study reported that ECT did not appear to be effective in the treatment of elderly patients with late-onset psychoses (paraphrenia) (Figiel et al. 1992). This is of interest given ECT's efficacy for most other psychotic disorders. The authors speculated that the high incidence of severe preexisting structural brain changes may explain the poor response from ECT in patients with these disorders.

CONTRAINDICATIONS TO ELECTROCONVULSIVE THERAPY

Although there are no absolute contraindications for ECT, several clinical conditions may increase the risk of complications from ECT:

- Recent myocardial infarction
- Any illness that increases intracranial pressure
- Medical conditions that may disrupt the blood-brain barrier (e.g., multiple sclerosis, recent cerebrovascular accident)
- Aneurysm
- Bleeding disorders

When treating high-risk patients with ECT, clinicians must understand the effects of ECT on cerebral and cardiac physiology and combine this information with data from the extant ECT literature to help develop individual risk-benefit ratios.

PRETREATMENT MEDICAL EVALUATION FOR ELECTROCONVULSIVE THERAPY

All patients should be given a thorough medical and neuropsychiatric evaluation before beginning ECT. Particular emphasis should be placed on diseases affecting the central nervous system (CNS) and the cardiovascular system. The pre-ECT evaluation should include a physical examination, a mental status examination, a medical history, and a review of systems. The patient's mental status should be evaluated before ECT is begun and monitored closely before the administration of all ECT sessions.

Along with the physical examination, some basic laboratory tests (blood count and electrolytes) and an electrocardiogram should be done in all patients before ECT. Clinicians should obtain a chest X ray in patients with a history of cardiac or pulmonary disease. Finally, spine films should be considered in patients with a history of back pain, positive findings on physical examination, or medical conditions that may affect the skeletal system.

Information obtained from the patient's neuropsychiatric history must include the following:

- History of prior ECT and any complications
- History of dementia
- History of any other neurological illnesses
- Any symptoms or signs on neurological examination suggestive of increased intracranial pressure
- Any other medical conditions that may affect the CNS

Based on the patient's examination, some may need a brain imaging scan before ECT. Whether all patients referred for ECT should routinely receive brain scans needs to be reevaluated.

From a cardiac standpoint, the clinician must determine the patient's cardiovascular risk factors and whether the patient has angina. The patient's exercise tolerance should also be estimated. On the basis of this information, the clinician can decide whether a cardiology consult is needed before ECT. One of the best means to reduce the incidence of ECT-induced cardiac complications is to ensure that the patient has received optimum medical management before undergoing ECT.

In general, patients are given their cardiac (except lidocaine), pulmonary (except theophylline), and glaucoma (except anticholinesterases) medications 1–2 hours before a treatment. Theophylline has been associated with status epilepticus during ECT. As a result, we recommend discontinuing theophylline during ECT, if clinically feasible. If not, blood levels of theophylline should be closely monitored and patients maintained on the lowest clinically effective dose. Patients with glaucoma who are receiving echothiophate should be switched to another medication because echothiophate can adversely interact with succinylcholine. In diabetic patients, hypoglycemic medications are usually withheld on the morning of treatment to minimize the risk of hypoglycemia. In general, patients with epilepsy should continue taking their anticonvulsants during ECT. If difficulty arises in eliciting seizures, a decrease in dose of the anticonvulsant can be considered.

The APA Task Force on ECT recommends that, in general, all psychotropic medications should be discontinued before ECT (American Psychiatric Association 1990). When neuroleptics are necessary to control agitation or psychotic symptoms, a high-potency neuroleptic is probably preferable to minimize any hypotension that may develop during ECT. There is no convincing evidence that antidepressants administered during ECT either augment the antidepressant properties of ECT or increase the speed of response.

Concerns have been raised over whether monoamine oxidase inhibitors can be used safely with anesthesia. At Emory University, we require a 48-hour washout of monoamine oxidase inhibitors before ECT. Lithium is also usually discontinued at least 48 hours before ECT because of a potentially increased risk of delirium during ECT.

Benzodiazepines can interfere with the induction of a seizure during ECT, thereby resulting in a decreased efficacy from the treatments. As a result, benzodiazepines should be reduced to the lowest possible dose or stopped before ECT. Patients taking benzodiazepines should be on a stable dose for 24–48 hours before ECT to reduce the risk of prolonged seizures or status epilepticus during ECT. Finally, informed consent should be obtained from all patients before ECT. Patients deemed to be incompetent may require the appointment of a legal guardian for consent (Sackeim et al. 1995).

TREATMENT TECHNIQUE

ECT sessions are usually scheduled for the morning. The patient's bladder and rectum should be emptied before treatment. Patients should have nothing to eat or drink for at least 6–8 hours before receiving a treatment. The ECT treatment team consists of a psychiatrist, an anesthesiologist (or nurse anesthetist), and a nursing team specially trained in ECT. The ECT treatment area should have resuscitative equipment available in case a medical emergency arises.

The standard anesthetic agent used is methohexital, a short-acting barbiturate. Methohexital is given in a dose of approximately 1 mg/kg. Immediately after the onset of methohexital's effect, a muscle relaxant is administered intravenously. Succinylcholine, in doses of 0.75–1.50 mg/kg, is a widely used depolarizing blocking agent. In patients with musculoskeletal disease, a nondepolarizing agent can be considered. Anticholinergic agents, such as atropine or glycopyrrolate, have often been used to prevent ECT-induced bradycardia and to minimize airway secretions. An anticholinergic agent should always be used if a β-blocker is used to control the ECT-induced rise in blood pressure and heart rate. Atropine (0.4–1.0 mg) or glycopyrrolate (0.2–0.4 mg) can be given either intramuscularly 30 minutes before the treatment or intravenously at the time of the treatment. At Emory University, we prefer to administer atropine intravenously at the time of the treatment because of its potent vagolytic effects.

Caffeine sodium benzoate (usual dose = 120–140 mg) may be administered intravenously during ECT to maintain adequate seizure duration. Caffeine appears to lengthen seizure duration during ECT without lowering the seizure threshold. At present, it is not known whether caffeine either augments ECT's antidepressant effects or increases the speed of response during a course of ECT. Thus, it seems the use of caffeine during ECT should be reserved for patients who are having short seizures during ECT and who do not require or cannot tolerate higher stimulus doses.

The patient is oxygenated by positive-pressure ventilation from the onset of anesthesia until spontaneous respiration is resumed. In addition, the patient is monitored with a pulse oximeter and should likewise have blood pressure and heart rate continuously monitored. Before the electrical stimulus is administered, a rubber bite block is inserted into the patient's mouth.

Regardless of the electrode placement selected, meticulous care should ensure that the electrodes are properly applied. The hair should be removed or parted, and the scalp should be cleansed and prepared with a saline or conductive gel. The electrodes should be adequately spaced to prevent excess shunting of the electrical stimulus and to prevent skin burns.

In bilateral ECT, electrodes are placed frontotemporally, with the center of each electrode approximately 1 inch (2.54 cm) above the center of an imaginary line whose endpoints are the tragus of the ear and the external canthus of the eye.

With unilateral ECT, d'Elia electrode placement is believed to be the safest and most effective (Weiner and Coffey 1986). In this technique, one electrode is placed over the nondominant frontotemporal area, and the other electrode is placed high on the nondominant centroparietal scalp, just lateral to the midline vertex. Weiner and Coffey (1986) elegantly described in depth the potential clinical benefits from the d'Elia electrode placement when using unilateral ECT.

Typically, a seizure lasting 30–90 seconds occurs during treatment. The seizure is monitored by electroencephalography. Seizures lasting longer than 3 minutes should be terminated. This can easily be done by administering a second dose of methohexital. The motor manifestations of the seizure can be monitored by inflating a blood pressure cuff on the right ankle before the muscle relaxant is administered. By placing the blood pressure cuff on the right ankle, it is possible to monitor a generalized seizure when nondominant (right) unilateral ECT is used because the isolated limb is contralateral to the stimulated hemisphere. Patients are usually alert and oriented 20–45 minutes after receiving a treatment.

CARDIAC COMPLICATIONS IN PATIENTS RECEIVING ELECTROCONVULSIVE THERAPY

Studies have consistently shown ECT to be a highly effective treatment for medication-resistant affective illness among geriatric patients. Despite its high efficacy, however, ECT appears to be associated with an increased risk of cardiovascular complications in certain elderly patients who have or who are at risk for cardiovascular disease.

Prior studies have found vastly different rates of cardiac complications in the elderly receiving ECT. Results have ranged from 0% to 55%. The wide discrepancy in these results is probably influenced by the retrospective design of these studies, lack of continuous cardiovascular monitoring, and different definitions of what constitutes a cardiac complication. Despite these inconsistencies, most studies have found a correlation between increased cardiac complications and age. ECT often produces transient systemic hypertension and abrupt transitions in cardiac rate, which can result in myocardial ischemia or arrhythmias. The increased incidence of cardiac complications among elderly patients is probably associated with the increased rate of preexisting cardiac illnesses such as hypertension, coronary artery disease, and arrhythmias. On the basis of these observations, several authors have recommended the use of prophylactic cardiac medications to dampen cardiovascular responses during ECT in elderly patients with cardiovascular disease.

Research has now documented that labetalol (a short-acting drug with both α- and β-blocking activity), nifedipine (a calcium channel–blocking agent with vasodilating effects), and several other cardiac medications can be safely used to attenuate the cardiac response during ECT (Figiel et al. 1993). However, the number of elderly patients examined in these studies is small. In addition, the question of whether the prophylactic use of cardiac medications during ECT results in a decreased incidence of cardiac complications has not been examined.

Only four studies to date (Cattan et al. 1990; Figiel et al. 1993, 1994; Zielinski et al. 1993) have used continuous cardiac monitoring during ECT and also have used a rigorous definition of what constitutes a cardiac complication during ECT. Particular attention should be given to these four studies because they are the only published articles in the ECT literature that meet both of these important criteria. Two of these studies used ECT without cardiac medications (noncardiac-modified ECT), and the other two used ECT modified with labetalol and nifedipine (cardiac-modified ECT). As a result, we can begin to compare the safety and efficacy of the two ECT techniques.

In the first study, using noncardiac-modified ECT, Cattan et al. (1990) retrospectively found that 23% (17) of 81 patients older than 65 who were receiving ECT had cardiac complications. The rate of cardiac complications was significantly higher among the 39 patients older than 80 (14 patients, or 36%) than among the 42 patients ages 65–80 (5 patients, or 12%).

Zielinski et al. (1993) prospectively examined the type and incidence of ECT-induced cardiac complications in 40 elderly patients with preexisting cardiac disease who received noncardiac-modified ECT. They observed that, of these 40 patients, 8 (20%) experienced major cardiac complications during ECT, and 14 (35%) had minor cardiac complications during ECT (mainly transient reversible arrhythmias). Not surprisingly, the authors found a higher incidence of ECT-induced cardiac complications in patients with preexisting cardiac disease. No deaths occurred, and 38 of the 40 cardiac patients were able to complete their course of ECT.

Two prospective studies using cardiac-modified ECT (Figiel et al. 1993, 1994) were completed at Emory University. Neither study used a control group. The cardiac protocol for these two studies was identical. At the first treatment, the dose of labetalol was determined on the basis of the patient's age and cardiac status. In general, a starting dose of 10 mg was used. Whenever the maximum heart rate during ECT exceeded 100 beats/minute, the dose of labetalol was increased by 5 mg at subsequent treatments (the maximum dose of labetalol administered at any one treatment was 20 mg). In addition, whenever a patient experienced two successive recordings of systolic blood pressures exceeding 210 mm Hg, 10 mg of nifedipine in addition was given sublingually before induction with anesthesia at all subsequent treatments. Nifedipine has been shown to decrease systolic blood pressure during ECT without significantly affecting the heart rate. Continuous electrocardiogram and blood pressure monitoring were performed during all treatments. Any bradycardias, arrhythmias, hypotension, sustained hypertension, or ischemic changes on the electrocardiogram were documented. Patients were monitored in the recovery room for sustained hypertension or orthostatic blood pressure changes for approximately 60 minutes. In addition, patients were carefully monitored for shortness of breath or the development of chest pain.

A total of 38 elderly patients (mean age 70 years) participated in the first study (Figiel et al. 1993). Preexisting cardiac disease was common in these patients (26 patients, or 68%). We used the same criteria for cardiac complications as those used by Cattan et al. (1990) and Zielinski et al. (1993), and we observed no cardiac complications at any ECT treatment of these 38 patients (Figiel et al. 1993).

In addition, we recently completed a second prospective, cardiac-modified ECT study in which we used the identical cardiac protocol described above (labetalol and nifedipine). A total of 57 consecutive elderly patients (mean age 75 years) participated in this study. Of these patients, 44 (77%) had preexisting cardiac disease. Only 2 patients (4%) developed minor ECT-induced cardiac complications. Two patients developed brief episodes of orthostatic hypotension in the recovery room. Neither of these patients had any clinical symptoms, and both were treated by 15 additional minutes of bed rest and intravenous fluids (Figiel et al. 1994).

Despite findings that ECT can be a highly effective treatment for depression, numerous prior studies have found that elderly patients with preexisting cardiac disease are at increased risk for developing cardiac complications associated with ECT. On the basis of these observations, Maneksha (1991) recommended that patients with a history of "hypertension, coronary artery disease, valvular heart disease and congestive heart failure" should routinely be prophylactically treated with medications to attenuate the transient hypertension and tachycardia associated with ECT (p. 30).

Two investigations (McCall et all. 1991; Stoudemire et al. 1990) found labetalol to be successful in reducing the tachycardia associated with ECT. McCall et al. (1991) examined the effects of 10 mg of labetalol administered before ECT in 12 healthy, young subjects (mean age 40). They found that labetalol was effective in reducing the maximal heart rate and the rate pressure product during ECT. However, labetalol did not consistently control the systolic and diastolic pressure in these patients (McCall et al. 1991). In a second report, Stoudemire et al. (1990) also examined the effects of labetalol in 11 elderly (mean age 70.3) patients. They found that labetalol significantly reduced the maximal heart rate, mean arterial pressure, and frequency of arrhythmias during ECT. Labetalol did not interfere with seizure duration or therapeutic efficacy in these studies.

These observations are of potential import given that esmolol, a short-acting β-blocker, has been associated with shortened seizure duration during ECT. Our clinical experience with labetalol is similar to that of others. We have found labetalol to be particularly effective in controlling heart rate during ECT. However, some elderly patients pretreated with labetalol alone still have significant transient increases in blood pressure. In such instances, we have found that nifedipine can be used safely and effectively with labetalol to control the ECT-induced increase in blood pressure when labetalol alone is not effective.

Early anecdotal reports suggested that β-blockers might not be safe for use during ECT without the concomitant use of anticholinergic medications. On the basis of these earlier observations, we strongly urge that adequate doses of an anticholinergic medication (intravenous atropine, 0.4–0.8 mg, or glycopyrrolate, 0.2 mg) be used to prevent bradycardias whenever β-blockers are used during ECT. To help prevent ECT-induced hypotension, we additionally strongly recommend that all patients be adequately hydrated before undergoing ECT and that psychotropic medications be discontinued whenever possible. Given these caveats, however, the results of the two cardiac-modified ECT studies (Figiel et al. 1993, 1994) suggest that labetalol and nifedipine can be used safely in elderly patients during ECT.

The incidence of ECT-induced cardiac complications in the two cardiac-modified ECT studies (Figiel et al. 1993, 1994) appeared to be significantly lower than those observed in the noncardiac-modified ECT studies (Cattan et al. 1990; Zielinski et al. 1993). Clearly, similar studies are needed that attempt to replicate the findings of these cardiac-modified ECT studies and that examine whether other cardiac medications can be used as safely and effectively as labetalol and nifedipine during ECT. However, whether future studies should randomly assign elderly patients to receive placebo is a difficult question to answer,

particularly because a growing body of data suggests that cardiac-modified ECT can be done safely and effectively in the elderly.

Although ECT in general is safe and effective for elderly patients, significant ECT-induced cardiac complications are not uncommon. It seems reasonable to suggest that, by attenuating the cardiovascular response during ECT, one might expect a decrease in the incidence of cardiac complications during ECT in the elderly. This belief is supported by the two cardiac-modified ECT studies described earlier (Figiel et al. 1993, 1994). In the absence of contraindications to the use of β-adrenergic blocking agents, and after appropriate consultation with an anesthesiologist and a cardiologist, we and others recommend consideration of cardiac-modified ECT in elderly patients referred for ECT, particularly those who have preexisting cardiac disease.

FREQUENCY AND NUMBER OF TREATMENTS

We agree with the APA Task Force's recommendations that an ECT course should be completed when a plateau in response occurs (American Psychiatric Association 1990). There are no convincing data to support that additional treatments beyond this point reduce the rate of relapse after ECT (Barton et al. 1973). In addition, these recommendations also imply that, rather than giving a predetermined number of ECT sessions, the patient's clinical status during the course of ECT should dictate the number of treatments given.

The elegant work of Lerer et al. (1995) has shown that ECT administered twice weekly is no less effective than treatments administered three times a week. One advantage of a more frequent treatment schedule is a faster rate of response. On the other hand, a disadvantage is the potential development of more cognitive side effects from ECT. Given these observations, we believe that the frequency of ECT treatments should be tailored to the individual patient's needs. For example, a patient with a severe, life-threatening illness will benefit from a faster rate of response and should be given more frequent treatments. In patients for whom the risk of cognitive side effects from ECT is a concern (i.e., those with Alzheimer's disease, Parkinson's disease, or severe frontal lobe and caudate hyperintensities on brain MRI scan, as well as those receiving outpatient ECT), a less frequent ECT treatment schedule is certainly a reasonable choice.

COGNITIVE SIDE EFFECTS OF ELECTROCONVULSIVE THERAPY

The greatest area of concern with ECT has to do with the potential development of adverse cerebral and cognitive changes. The technique by which ECT is administered determines the incidence and severity of cognitive side effects that may develop during a course of ECT. Specifically, the type and severity of cognitive side effects from ECT are determined by electrode placement, the type of electrical waveform used, the intensity of the electrical stimulus, and the frequency of ECT sessions. Preexisting structural brain changes and medical illness, advancing age, and concomitant administration of certain psychotropic medications may also be involved (Sackeim et al. 1993).

Clearly, the degree of amnesia incurred during a course of ECT is greater with bilateral ECT than with unilateral ECT. In the area of ECT-induced memory loss, one of the most important findings in recent years has been the mild effects on memory when right-unilateral ECT is administered with a brief pulse stimulation. Many patients who receive bilateral ECT treatments do not complain of significant memory problems. However, some patients receiving bilateral ECT may report memory deficits lasting for as long as 6 months to several years after receiving ECT. Research is currently under way comparing the nature and severity of cognitive impairment from ECT that may occur in patients receiving minimally suprathreshold bilateral ECT with high-charge (>250% to suprathreshold) right-unilateral ECT. The results of these studies will help the clinician select the appropriate ECT technique to use in individual cases.

It has been clearly shown that a sine wave stimulus produces greater amnestic deficits than does a brief and ultrabrief stimulus pulse. In addition, Sackeim et al. (1991, 1993) reported that, within a specific waveform, the magnitude by which an electrical dose exceeds the seizure threshold (rather than the absolute electrical dose) may be related to the severity of cognitive defects that develop during ECT. Finally, Lerer et al. (1995) consistently reported that twice-weekly treatments produced less cognitive impairment than did treatments administered three times a week.

Interictal ECT-induced delirium is not an uncommon side effect in the elderly (Figiel and Coffey 1990). Interictal ECT-induced delirium is defined as a delirium meeting DSM-IV criteria (American Psychiatric Association 1994) that develops during a course of ECT and persists on days when the patient does not receive a treatment. This side effect is primarily observed in the elderly receiving ECT and increases in incidence with advancing age. ECT-induced interictal delirium is associated with prolonged hospitalizations and an increased risk of falls. Among the elderly, additional risk factors for interictal delirium are 1) Parkinson's disease, 2) Alzheimer's disease, 3) one or more cardiovascular risk factors, and 4) preexisting structural changes in the caudate nucleus observed on brain scans.

The incidence of delirium during ECT can vary dramatically depending on the ECT technique used. At Emory University, the incidence of delirium during ECT has been reduced to less than 5% in the elderly by initially administering suprathreshold (2.5 above threshold) right-unilateral ECT twice a week in patients at risk.

As a rule, an ECT-induced interictal delirium is a short-lived, reversible side effect if identified early. Once it has been identified, treatments should be held until the delirium resolves. Subsequent treatments should be administered less frequently at a lower electrical charge.

Does Electroconvulsive Therapy Cause Brain Damage?

Human autopsy studies of patients who have received ECT have shown no convincing evidence of irreversible brain damage when ECT is administered with current techniques. These findings are supported by a recent brain MRI study in which no significant structural brain changes were found immediately and 6 months after the completion of ECT. The reader is referred to excellent review articles on these areas of research (Devanand et al. 1994; Weiner 1984).

Effects of Electroconvulsive Therapy on Cerebral Physiology

Immediately after an ECT treatment, the electroencephalogram shows generalized slowing. This slowing tends to increase and persist longer after successive treatments. After a course of ECT is completed, slow-wave activity gradually decreases, and the electroencephalogram reverts to baseline activity within 3 months (Weiner et al. 1986). Rarely, electroencephalogram abnormalities may persist for more than 3 months. Prior electroencephalogram abnormalities may increase the risk for developing prolonged abnormalities after ECT, but the clinical significance of these abnormalities is unknown.

Electrically induced seizures in animals and humans have been shown to produce transient increases in permeability of the blood-brain barrier (Laursen et al. 1991). These findings are consistent with a brain MRI study in which increased T-1 relaxation times were observed after

ECT (Scott et al. 1990). Laursen et al. (1991) reported that the ECT-induced increase in blood-brain barrier permeability is associated with an increased stimulus intensity and an increased number of ECT treatments. In addition, Bolwig et al. (1977) was able to decrease changes in blood-brain barrier permeability during ECT by blocking ECT-induced hypertensive response with high-spinal anesthesia. Because a disturbed blood-brain barrier may predispose some patients toward ECT-induced neurological complications, work is needed to examine the ways by which ECT-induced changes in blood-brain barrier permeability can be minimized, such as by attenuating the ECT-induced cardiovascular response or by reducing the amount of the stimulus charge.

The combination of increased CO_2 production, decreased pH, and systemic hypertension leads to a doubling of cerebral blood flow during ECT (Broderston et al. 1973; Posner et al. 1969). The transiently increased cerebral blood flow results in a sharp rise in both intracranial and intraocular pressure (Maltbie et al. 1980). Methods that limit the accumulation of CO_2, such as forced hyperventilation, or that attenuate the increase in blood pressure tend to decrease the rise in intracranial pressure associated with ECT.

PROPHYLACTIC SOMATIC TREATMENT OF PATIENTS WITH ACUTE RESPONSE TO ELECTROCONVULSIVE THERAPY

The debate over appropriate prophylactic treatment for patients with an acute response to ECT has focused on the clinical decision to continue either antidepressant therapy or maintenance ECT. Confusion in this area persists because of the lack of controlled studies comparing the efficacy of antidepressants with that of maintenance ECT. Harold Sackeim and his colleagues are conducting a multicenter trial to investigate the relapse rate of patients who have responded to ECT and are randomly assigned to either placebo or antidepressant therapy. In the review presented here, we summarize the extant literature on maintenance ECT and post-ECT pharmacology.

Two studies (Aronson et al. 1987; Spiker et al. 1985) evaluated adult patients after an acute course of ECT for psychotic depression and found a relapse rate of 68% ($n = 53$ patients) at 1 year. Spiker et al. (1985) found a 1-year relapse rate of 50% in patients with delusional depression who initially responded to an acute course of ECT. Aronson et al. (1987) followed up patients with delusional depression who responded to either medication or ECT and found that 80% of the medication-responsive group

and 95% of the ECT-responsive patients relapsed in the first year after hospitalization. These studies did not compare the adequacy of either the initial (pre-ECT) or the continuation medication trial.

Sackeim et al. (1990) followed up 58 patients for 1 year after ECT and found a differential relapse rate of 64% in those with major depression (with and without psychotic features) in whom an adequate pre-ECT medication trial had failed. In contrast, the relapse rate in patients who did not receive an adequate pre-ECT antidepressant trial was only 32%. Other clinical and demographic factors were not significant in predicting relapse. Significantly, the adequacy of the post-ECT maintenance medication was not correlated with relapse. However, as in the studies cited above, the maintenance medications post-ECT were not standardized, and the evaluation of the pre-ECT medication trial was retrospective. The conclusion of this study is intuitively appealing: Patients whose symptoms do not respond to antidepressant medication before ECT are those most likely to relapse during maintenance medication. As is true of depressed patients with psychotic features, the relapse rates of almost two-thirds of patients in 1 year remain alarmingly high.

In a prospective study, Shapira et al. (1995) studied patients who responded to an acute course of ECT and subsequently received maintenance lithium for 6 months. Of the total 22 patients, 8 (36%) who relapsed did so in the first 13 weeks. Several clinical factors were associated with relapse, including shorter duration of index depressive episode, additional depressive episode in the previous 12 months, and again, failure of an adequate trial of antidepressant therapy before the ECT course.

The elderly are particularly prone to increased disability from depression and form a substantial proportion of patients in an acute ECT program. Data from naturalistic studies confirm that the relapse rates for elderly patients treated with ECT are also quite high. These rates have varied from 67% in 6 months (Karlinsky and Shulman 1984) to 75% in 1 year (Murphy 1983). The elderly may therefore be at increased risk for relapse after acute ECT.

Continuation/Maintenance Electroconvulsive Therapy in Major Depression

The high relapse rates of depressed patients receiving antidepressants after ECT have led clinicians to use alternative therapies, such as continuation/maintenance ECT, in patients who are at high risk for recurrence of their mood disorder. *Continuation ECT* is defined as ECT that continues for up to 6 months after the acute ECT course. Continuation ECT is differentiated from *maintenance ECT*, which is defined as ECT that continues for more than 6 months after the index course. In this chapter, the term *prophylactic ECT* is used to refer to any ECT treatments given as continuation or maintenance. Many of the studies reviewed here do not differentiate patients receiving continuation ECT from those receiving maintenance ECT, although treatment indications, side effects, and outcomes may be different for these two types of prophylactic ECT.

APA clinical guidelines (American Psychiatric Association 1990) for candidates for prophylactic ECT include patients who have recurring affective episodes that are responsive to ECT and/or who are resistant or intolerant to, or noncompliant with, antidepressant medications. Prophylactic ECT strategies are increasingly being used to treat major depression and bipolar disorder in patients thought to be at high risk for relapse. In a 1985 survey of private hospitals, 64% of the hospitals that provided ECT also provided prophylactic ECT (Levy and Albrecht 1985). Kramer (1987) found a similar use pattern, with 59% of respondents using continuation/maintenance ECT primarily for recurrent depression.

Several theories have been advanced to explain the potential therapeutic efficacy of prophylactic ECT over medication. First, Bourne (1954) suggested that patients with psychotic depression may become "convulsion dependent" such that they need to be tapered from ECT to prevent relapse. Recent studies support the concept that abruptly stopping medication may worsen the course of affective disorders (Klein et al. 1981; Murray 1994), and the same may be seen in ECT patients. Second, prophylactic ECT has a different mechanism of action than antidepressants, and patients in whom medication fails respond to an acute course of ECT. The corollary is that patients who respond preferentially to ECT may have lower relapse rates with prophylactic ECT than with medication. Third, prophylactic ECT may not provide an increased therapeutic benefit over medication at all. Rather, the benefit may be the result of solely better treatment compliance in the groups receiving ECT than in those receiving maintenance medication. Most reports of relapse rates in patients receiving prophylactic ECT include only those patients who were compliant and presented for their treatments. As Clarke et al. (1989) pointed out, when patients receiving continuation ECT do not complete 6 months of treatment, then relapse rates approach the 50% seen in patients receiving maintenance medication. Thus, future studies of ECT need to include both compliant and noncompliant patients in their outcome measures.

Most of the studies examining maintenance ECT are case reports (Thienhaus et al. 1990). The more recent reports follow a naturalistic design with relatively few subjects but generally describe a marked decrease in the number of hospitalizations, hospital days, and depressive symptoms; increased functional status; and stable cognitive functioning for the period of continuation ECT (Clarke et al. 1989; Decina et al. 1987; Loo et al. 1991; Thienhaus et al. 1990; Thornton et al. 1990). These positive results have been extended primarily to elderly populations (Jaffe et al. 1989; Loo et al. 1991; Thienhaus et al. 1990).

In a prospective study, Clarke et al. (1989) used continuation ECT in 27 patients who received an acute course of ECT because of a history of medication intolerance or resistance. The rate of rehospitalization was six times lower (8%) in patients who completed a 5-month course of continuation ECT than in patients who did not complete the protocol (47%). There are few other prospective studies, and no controlled trials, of continuation/maintenance ECT. Guidelines for the use of prophylactic ECT therefore remain vague primarily because of the paucity of data on which to base these guidelines. Monroe (1991) has delineated the contradiction of the increasing use of continuation/maintenance ECT and the lack of research defining the parameters of administering the treatments and potential side effects and contraindications. At the time of Monroe's review, the available studies of continuation/maintenance ECT included only 325 patients with depression (including 85 with bipolar disorder and 121 with psychotic depression).

TREATMENT RECOMMENDATIONS

Patients who receive an acute course of ECT usually fall into three categories: 1) patients who have failed previous trials of medication and are therefore relatively medication resistant; 2) patients who are severely ill (e.g., psychotic or suicidal); and 3) patients who cannot tolerate the side effects of antidepressant medication, because of either concomitant medical illness or a personal sensitivity to antidepressant side effects, or who are noncompliant with their medication trial. These groups overlap and include a number of patients who, because of their own experience or that of acquaintances or relatives, prefer ECT to traditional somatic treatment

1. Patients who have failed previous trials of medication and are therefore relatively medication resistant.
A significant minority of patients with major depression are relatively medication resistant despite adequate medication trials. Sackeim et al. (1990) found that

the most important factor in relapse after an acute course of ECT is whether the patient received an adequate pretreatment medication trial. In patients who had undergone an adequate pretreatment medication trial, the relapse rate after ECT was found to be twofold higher (64% vs. 32%) (Sackeim et al. 1990). Shapira et al. (1995) also found that patients who had received an adequate pretreatment pharmacotherapy trial relapsed at a significantly higher rate when they received lithium maintenance therapy. Interestingly, Grunhaus et al. (1990) reported a relapse rate of only 17% in patients in whom a previous medication trial had failed and who received up to 12 weeks of maintenance ECT.

Patients in whom an adequate medication trial has failed before ECT should be informed of the risk of relapse and given the option of continuation ECT for 6 months, followed by maintenance medication. The clinical decision of whether to continue ECT beyond 6 months should be made on an individual basis, weighing the risks (primarily cognitive effects vs. the risk of suicide or recurrent psychosis) and benefits (long-term effects of a period of mood stability).

2. Patients who are severely ill.   Some researchers have found that the 1-year relapse rate in patients with psychotic depression treated with medication alone may be as high as 95% (Aronson et al. 1987; Spiker et al. 1985). Petrides et al. (1994) retrospectively examined the records of patients with delusional depression treated with prophylactic ECT and found the relapse rate at 1 year to be only 42%. They compared their findings with those from the study by Aronson et al. (1987). Both patient groups were drawn from the same institution, although prophylactic ECT was not available at the time that Aronson et al. (1987) reported relapse rates of 95% in patients with delusional depression who were taking antidepressants. Vanelle et al. (1994) prospectively administered maintenance ECT (defined as ECT for more than 6 months after the index course), often with concomitant antipsychotic medication, approximately once a month for 1 year to a group of patients with psychotic depression and found full or partial remission in 80% of patients. Grunhaus et al. (1990) also found an excellent clinical response in patients with psychotic depression who were administered prophylactic ECT. Prophylactic ECT may therefore be a viable option in patients with delusional depression and should be discussed with these patients and their families.

3. Patients who cannot tolerate the side effects of antidepressant medication, because of either con- **comitant medical illness or a personal sensitivity to antidepressant side effects, or who are noncompliant with their medication trial.**   Most of the patients who cannot tolerate the side effects of antidepressant medication, because of either concomitant medical illness or a personal sensitivity to antidepressant side effects, can be tried on maintenance medication after a successful course of ECT. Many patients who are acutely ill may be extremely sensitive to the side effects of medications but may tolerate the same medication once they have responded to acute treatment. Conditions associated with depression, such as malnutrition and dehydration, may worsen the orthostatic hypotension from tricyclic antidepressants. In a patient with agitated depression, minimal activation from the selective serotonin reuptake inhibitors may be experienced as extreme agitation. Once the depressive episode has remitted, patients can usually tolerate an additional medication trial. Patients who are noncompliant with their antidepressant medication should be evaluated on an individual basis, and, after discussions with the patient and the family, the risks and benefits of prophylactic ECT should be weighed against an additional medication trial.

PROCEDURAL GUIDELINES FOR CONTINUATION ELECTROCONVULSIVE THERAPY

Treatment Parameters

At Emory University, the electrode placement and dose parameters used in the index course are maintained during maintenance ECT. Retrospective reviews have not found stimulus placement to affect outcome (Petrides et al. 1994), although no systematic studies have compared unilateral and bilateral placement in prophylactic ECT.

Treatment Intervals, Frequency, and Duration

There are few guidelines on what frequency of continuation ECT is optimal to maintain mood stability. The intervals between courses of prophylactic continuation ECT in the studies reviewed vary from 3–5 weeks (Loo et al. 1991) to 4–8 weeks (Thienhaus et al. 1990). Other clinicians argue that treatments should be gradually tapered from once a week to once a month, depending on clinical response (Aronson et al. 1987; Clarke et al. 1989; Matzen et al. 1988). Kramer (1987) surveyed 51 clinicians in 24 states and found the frequency and duration of maintenance ECT to vary from two treatments per week extending to once every 3–4 weeks over 30 months, to one treatment every 6 months over 60 months, to as long as 48 years. In Kramer's survey, clinicians described continuing ECT until the patient was asymptomatic for a predetermined period ranging from 1 month to 2 years.

Grunhaus et al. (1990) assessed individual patients' clinical histories and assigned them to either abbreviated maintenance ECT (i.e., once or twice a week for 4–12 weeks) or full maintenance ECT (i.e., gradually tapering ECT to once a month over 3 months and continuing once a month for 6 months). Abbreviated maintenance was used when symptoms were unresponsive to medication after the index episode and lasted more than 12 months or when the patient relapsed after a successful course of ECT or had difficulties tolerating continuation pharmacotherapy. Full maintenance was used in patients who relapsed after a successful course of ECT despite adequate pharmacotherapy. Among 10 patients, these authors found an excellent response in 6 (5 of 6 receiving abbreviated maintenance; 1 of 4 receiving full maintenance), particularly in those with delusional depression.

In a prospective study, Vanelle et al. (1994) administered maintenance ECT with an average frequency of once every 3.5–3.9 weeks for 1 year and found that 64% of patients needed shorter intervals to prevent a recurrence of their depressive disorders. The patients who required a shorter interval were older and had a longer duration of illness. Vanelle et al. (1994) posited that the older patients may have had a shorter time to relapse, a suggestion that is consistent with data showing that older patients tend to have accelerated mood cycles (Zis et al. 1980).

To further examine this area, at Emory University we recently retrospectively reviewed the treatment course of all patients receiving continuation/maintenance ECT from 1993 to 1994 to determine optimal treatment intervals for prophylactic ECT. All of these patients met the criteria set forth in the APA guidelines for maintenance ECT. After an acute course of ECT, patients were gradually tapered according to a schedule of prophylactic ECT treatments once every week for four treatments, then every 10 days for three treatments, then every 2 weeks for two treatments, then every 3 weeks for two treatments, and then once a month. In the 51 patients who had an ECT course lasting at least 3 months, 29 (57%) relapsed each time the treatments were extended beyond 2 weeks. The other 22 patients had treatment intervals of 17–28 days, and only 6 of the 22 patients (10% of the total of 59 patients) did not relapse when the treatment intervals were extended to an interval of one ECT treatment per month.

Recommendations for Treatment

The greatest risk of relapse after ECT is within the first few months after acute treatment (Clarke et al. 1989; Sackeim et al. 1990; Shapira et al. 1995). During this crucial period, many patients and their families describe a recurrence of symptoms of depression when treatment intervals are extended by even a few days. This pattern of response has resulted in the development of a continuation ECT protocol at Emory University in which treatment intervals between continuation ECT are extended in increments—from once a week for the first four treatments, to every 10 days for the next three treatments, then every 2 weeks for the final 4 months. During the 6 months of continuation ECT, treatments are not extended beyond every 2 weeks, because a high relapse rate (57%) is seen during the 6 months when continuation ECT treatments are extended beyond every 2 weeks. If a patient becomes symptomatic, the treatment interval is again shortened for additional treatments until the patient is clinically stable. The patient is then returned to the longest ECT treatment interval during which he or she remained healthy. Patients are encouraged to continue in ECT for at least 6 months. In the final month of continuation ECT, treatment with an antidepressant is initiated. However, which antidepressant drug can be safely and effectively used during continuation ECT requires further study. Patients who relapse quickly after discontinuation of continuation ECT should be considered for maintenance ECT.

Informed Consent

Individual hospital policies and state laws dictate the procedure for obtaining informed consent. Patients in outpatient ECT usually are subject to the same guidelines as are applicable to the ambulatory surgery service in the treating hospital. In general, the same policies governing consent for the index ECT course apply to the prophylactic course of ECT. The consent procedures have been reviewed extensively elsewhere (Abrams 1992; American Psychiatric Association 1978, 1990; Greenberg et al. 1993). A new consent should be obtained before each course of prophylactic ECT, when a patient changes from inpatient and outpatient status, and at least every 6 months. The patient's primary physician should also document at the beginning of each ECT course (i.e., at the time of the consent) the justification for the prophylactic ECT.

Cognitive Complications

There are few data on the cognitive changes of patients receiving repeated ECT over a period of months to years.

Most reports have focused on acute ECT and have shown either transient changes in memory or no neuroanatomical changes on MRI (Coffey et al. 1988). Most of the available reports in which prophylactic ECT has been used describe only minor subjective complaints, and few studies report objective neuropsychological testing. Grunhaus et al. (1990) reported that the patients in their study experienced minor memory difficulties (recent recall and names) that returned to normal with 6–8 months. Patients in a study by Vanelle et al. (1994) (mean age 70 ± 13 years) described either no subjective memory problems ($n = 8$) or minor subjective cognitive complaints ($n = 14$). Petrides et al. (1994) noted only minor subjective memory problems in 30 patients (mean age 52 ± 15 years) receiving an average of seven continuation ECT treatments over 2 months. Thienhaus et al. (1990) found stable cognitive function (as measured on the Mini-Mental State Exam [Folstein et al. 1975]) in six elderly patients (mean age 71 ± 5 years) over 1–5 years of prophylactic ECT.

Cost-Effectiveness

Several retrospective studies have reported a marked decrease in the number and length of hospital stays and in depressive symptoms, increased functional status, and stable cognitive functioning in patients who are compliant with prophylactic ECT (Clarke et al. 1989; Decina et al. 1987; Loo et al. 1991; Thienhaus et al. 1990; Thornton et al. 1990).

Summary

Prophylactic ECT is an effective and cost-efficient alternative to medication in a selected subgroup of patients with recurrent depression, particularly in elderly patients and those with a history of medication resistance and delusional depression. Patients in these subgroups may benefit from a period of mood stabilization with continuation ECT that is followed by maintenance medication. There is, however, a paucity of prospective research on prophylactic ECT, despite the increasing use of this treatment in clinical practice. Future research should focus on identification of selected subpopulations who may benefit from prophylactic medication compared with ECT, standardization of the techniques for administering the treatments, potential cardiac and cognitive side effects of repeated treatments, and cost-effectiveness of prophylactic ECT.

MECHANISMS OF ACTION

Despite having clear efficacy in the treatment of a variety of neuropsychiatric disorders, ECT remains a much mis-understood and maligned treatment. In part, this results from the invasiveness of the procedure and the lack of information about the mechanisms by which the treatment works. It is not surprising, however, that the mechanisms responsible for the therapeutic and adverse effects of ECT are uncertain, given that information about the pathophysiology of most major psychiatric disorders and of many neurological disorders is incomplete. As noted years ago by Seymour Kety (1974), a major problem in determining the mechanisms involved in ECT is that the treatment affects numerous processes of the CNS, and it is extremely difficult to determine which of these effects are important and which are irrelevant.

More than 100 theories have been proposed to explain the therapeutic effects of ECT. These range from hypotheses about psychological and psychodynamic processes to neurotransmitter changes, neuroendocrine effects, and alterations in second-messenger systems and gene expression (Sackeim 1994). On the basis of current information, it seems that certain theories about ECT can be discarded. For example, there is little evidence that anesthetics or muscle relaxants produce sustained clinical benefits in CNS disorders. Similarly, there is no convincing evidence that ECT produces structural brain damage or that the memory-impairing effects of ECT are necessary for clinical improvement (Devanand et al. 1994; Weiner 1984). The latter is particularly important because memory loss has been a popular lay theory. Current ECT practice, which includes the use of vigorous oxygenation, brief electrical pulses, titrated electrical dosing, and unilateral electrode placement, is largely directed toward diminishing memory impairment to the extent possible. Other psychological explanations for the effects of ECT are equally implausible.

Most serious efforts to understand the mechanisms of ECT's effects have centered on changes in CNS neurotransmitter systems and/or biochemical processes. For useful reviews of the biochemical effects of electrically induced seizures, the reader is referred to excellent papers by D. J. Nutt and Glue (1993) and Fochtmann (1994). The problem in identifying these mechanisms lies in the fact that ECT affects many CNS systems, and it is difficult to have confidence in mechanisms of action in illnesses that are poorly defined at a neurochemical level. Furthermore, much of the neurochemical information about ECT comes from studies of electroconvulsive shock (ECS) in animals, in which the assumption is made that the effects of repeated seizures in presumably normal animals are relevant to actions in patients with psychiatric disorders (Lerer et al. 1984).

Faced with these issues, investigators are left with several options. These include measuring changes in CNS systems of interest and making guesses about their relevance to neuropsychiatric disorders. Alternatively, it is possible to follow leads in psychopharmacology and to concentrate on processes that are altered by clinically useful medications. This assumes that the changes evoked by ECT are similar to drug effects, although this need not necessarily be the case (Sackeim 1994). An alternative strategy is to examine effects of ECT on CNS processes for which there is more detailed basic science information. The assumption here is that the effects of ECT on those CNS systems that are involved in the better-understood disorders have a higher likelihood of being related to clinical effects. Although none of these strategies is entirely satisfactory, in this chapter we concentrate on the latter approach and discuss specific examples in which ECT mechanisms may be closer to being understood.

Anticonvulsant Effects

The anticonvulsant effects of ECT include increases in seizure threshold and decreases in seizure duration (Sackeim et al. 1991). There is now considerable information about the cellular correlates of seizures (McNamara 1994), and it is of interest to determine whether these insights are relevant to the anticonvulsant effects of ECT. Given the role of γ-aminobutyric acid (GABA) as the major fast inhibitory transmitter in the CNS and as a target for several antiepileptic drugs (e.g., barbiturates, benzodiazepines, loreclezole) (Macdonald and Olsen 1994), it seems reasonable to expect changes in this transmitter system over a course of ECT. Indeed, data from studies in animals have demonstrated increases in the threshold for convulsant drugs that act via $GABA_A$ receptors (bicuculline and pentylenetetrazol) after ECS (D. H. Nutt et al. 1981; Plaznik et al. 1989). Furthermore, GABA levels have been shown to increase in certain CNS regions after ECS (Green et al. 1982), suggesting an increase in tonic inhibition in these regions after several seizures. At the receptor level, there is evidence for increases in the $GABA_B$ receptors that mediate pre- and postsynaptic inhibition in the CNS (Lloyd et al. 1985). Changes in the $GABA_A$ receptor–chloride channels that are the primary postsynaptic GABA receptors are less clear (Fochtmann 1994). A confusing observation is that repeated ECS may cause acute decreases in GABA synthesis and release (Green and Vincent 1987).

An intriguing finding in rodents is that repeated seizures cause the release of an anticonvulsant substance into cerebrospinal fluid. Anticonvulsant activity can be transferred to naive animals by intracerebroventricular injections of cerebrospinal fluid from animals who have experienced seizures (Tortella and Long 1985, 1988). Tortella et al. (1989) provided evidence that the anticonvulsant is an endogenous opioid and that treatment with naloxone, a broad-spectrum opiate receptor antagonist, blocks the anticonvulsant effects of ECS in animals. There is also evidence for upregulation of specific δ opiate binding sites (e.g., sites for D-alanine-D-leucine enkephalin [DADLE]) after repeated seizures (Hitzemann et al. 1987). Whether similar changes occur in humans remains speculative.

Efforts to identify the anticonvulsant mechanisms in ECT need to take into account changes in both seizure threshold and duration, because different mechanisms may govern the two phenomena. Of particular interest is the finding that adenosine is released extracellularly during periods of repeated CNS excitatory synaptic activation (such as that occurring during seizures). Adenosine acts at several receptor types and is a powerful local inhibitory modulator in certain CNS regions (Greene and Haas 1991; Palmer and Stiles 1995). Additionally, adenosine A1 receptors are upregulated by ECS in the cortex, but not the hippocampus or striatum, in animals (Gleiter et al. 1989). Clinically, the use of caffeine, an adenosine receptor antagonist, prolongs ECT-induced seizures (Hinkle et al. 1987; Shapira et al. 1987) with less effect on seizure threshold (McCall et al. 1993a). Furthermore, theophylline, another adenosine antagonist, has been associated with status epilepticus during ECT (Rasmussen and Zorumski 1993). This finding suggests that the release of adenosine, and perhaps increased sensitivity of certain adenosine receptors, may contribute to decreases in seizure duration during ECT. However, caffeine and theophylline have other effects that could influence CNS excitability, including phosphodiesterase inhibition, release of Ca^{2+} from intracellular stores, and possible effects on $GABA_A$ receptors (Sawynok and Yaksh 1993).

Much of the information about possible anticonvulsant effects of ECT has centered on enhanced inhibition after seizures. It is also important to consider how ECT influences major CNS excitatory systems, particularly the glutamatergic system. Seizures cause the acute release of glutamate, but there is less information about the effects of repeated seizures on glutamate release, uptake, and receptors. Of importance is the observation that the brain damage that accompanies prolonged status epilepticus appears to result, in large part, from excessive activation of the N-methyl-D-aspartate (NMDA) class of glutamate receptors (Clifford et al. 1989). However, seizure-related brain damage typically requires more than 20 minutes of continuous activity and is therefore unlikely to be relevant to ECT (Devanand et al. 1994; Gruenthal et al. 1986).

Amnestic Effects

An unfortunate aspect of ECT is that the treatment produces retrograde and anterograde amnesia. The causes of these memory disturbances are likely to be multifactorial and include the effects of anesthetic drugs, electrode placement, stimulus waveform, electrical dose, and generalized seizures (Calev et al. 1993). Progress in understanding the neural mechanisms involved in certain forms of memory makes it possible to consider how neurotransmitter changes could contribute to ECT-induced memory dysfunction. There is evidence that muscarinic cholinergic receptors contribute to some forms of memory, and in humans, antimuscarinic agents are associated with memory impairment (Krueger et al. 1992). In animals, the effects of ECS on central muscarinic systems have been variable (Fochtmann 1994). However, some studies suggest that ECT diminishes muscarinic binding in the cortex and hippocampus. There is also evidence for diminished behavioral responses to muscarinic agonists, decreases in brain choline acetyltransferase, and decreases in brain acetylcholine levels (D. J. Nutt and Glue 1993). Taken together, these findings suggest that alterations in CNS muscarinic systems may contribute to memory impairment.

Investigators believe that long-term potentiation is a synaptic mechanism that may be involved in memory processing and that disruption of this process could contribute to anterograde amnesia. The term *long-term potentiation* typically refers to a persistent enhancement of glutamate-mediated excitatory synaptic transmission that follows repeated synaptic use. ECS and generalized seizures disrupt the formation of long-term potentiation in animals and also produce memory impairment (Anwyl et al. 1987; Stewart and Reid 1993).

Several ECS-induced changes, including effects on muscarinic and adrenergic neurotransmission, could contribute to the inhibition of long-term potentiation. Furthermore, the enhanced inhibition that may contribute to the anticonvulsant effects of ECT could also play a role because these inhibitory systems can modulate efficacy at excitatory synapses (Kuba and Kumamoto 1990). Finally, the release of glutamate during a seizure may be involved in memory impairment. In many CNS regions, the induction of long-term potentiation depends on activation of the NMDA type of glutamate receptors. However, several groups have shown that untimely activation of NMDA receptors before delivery of a stimulus that induces long-term potentiation inhibits, rather than promotes, the induction of long-term potentiation. This effect may result from the release of certain second messengers, such as ni-

tric oxide, or from the activation of phosphatases that alter the phosphorylation status of important synaptic proteins (Zorumski and Izumi 1993). To date, there is little convincing evidence that any of the above mechanisms contribute to ECT-induced memory impairment in patients, although several avenues seem worth pursuing (Krueger et al. 1992).

Parkinson's Disease

ECT can be helpful in treating the motor symptoms of Parkinson's disease independent of its effects on affective symptoms. The effectiveness of antimuscarinic drugs in treating parkinsonian symptoms suggests that the effects of ECT on central muscarinic systems may be relevant (Fochtmann 1988). However, ECT also alters central dopaminergic systems that are more fundamentally involved in Parkinson's disease (Fochtmann 1994). Acutely, ECS increases dopamine levels in the frontal cortex and striatum and has variable effects on basal dopamine levels. Furthermore, dopamine autoreceptor sensitivity is diminished after ECS, an effect that would tend to augment dopamine release. There is also evidence that dopamine, subtype 1 (D_1), receptor agonists cause increased stimulation of adenylate cyclase after ECS. However, D_1 dopamine receptor binding is increased in the substantia nigra (Fochtmann et al. 1989), but not in the striatum (Nowak and Zak 1989), after ECS.

Phencyclidine-Induced Psychosis

Some evidence indicates that ECT can be an effective treatment in patients with phencyclidine-induced psychosis, producing benefit with a small number of treatments (Dinwiddie et al. 1988). It appears that a major effect of phencyclidine in the CNS occurs via open channel block of NMDA-type glutamate receptors. Of importance is the observation that phencyclidine-induced block shows voltage dependence and the block is long-lived, the ion channel closing around the phencyclidine molecule (MacDonald et al. 1991). Relief of NMDA channel block requires that NMDA ion channels open at depolarized membrane potentials (Huettner and Bean 1988). Thus, neuronal membrane depolarization and receptor agonist exposure are required for phencyclidine to exit the channel. Although it is not certain that blocking of NMDA ion channels is critical for phencyclidine psychosis, it is interesting that ECT-induced seizures would be expected to relieve phencyclidine block. That is, during a seizure, neurons depolarize (caused by synaptic excitation and action potential firing), and glutamate is released at synapses. These events would work in conjunction to rapidly relieve phencyclidine-induced block and could provide a rationale for the effectiveness of ECT.

Major Psychiatric Disorders

Much of the above discussion of ECT mechanisms has been highly speculative. Until more information about the cellular and synaptic pathophysiology of psychiatric disorders is available, it seems unlikely that the beneficial effects of ECT will be well understood. Certainly many of the effects outlined above could contribute, including effects on central dopaminergic and cholinergic systems. Furthermore, the usefulness of anticonvulsants as mood stabilizers makes it possible that the anticonvulsant effects of ECT could be important in the management of affective disorders. This latter hypothesis is attractive in that it could explain ECT's therapeutic effects in both mania and depression (Sackeim 1994). However, data directly indicating a therapeutic requirement for the anticonvulsant effects of ECT are lacking.

Because of the efficacy of psychotropic medications, there has been considerable interest in determining how the effects of ECT compare with known drug effects. Particular emphasis has been placed on examining the effects on biogenic amines. Of interest is that certain antidepressants cause β_1-adrenergic receptor subsensitivity, and similar effects occur with ECT (D. J. Nutt and Glue 1993). ECT has multiple other effects on the adrenergic system, including increases in norepinephrine turnover and α_1-adrenergic receptor sensitivity and possibly decreases in presynaptic α_2-adrenergic receptors. ECT also appears to enhance the function of the serotonergic transmitter system, producing increased behavioral sensitivity to serotonin receptor agonists and possibly increases in 5-hydroxytryptamine, subtype 2, receptor binding in the cerebral cortex (Fochtmann 1994; D. J. Nutt and Glue 1993; Sackeim 1994). The latter effect differs from changes induced by chronic antidepressant drug treatment.

RAPID-RATE TRANSCRANIAL MAGNETIC STIMULATION

Often asked is the question "What new treatment will eventually replace ECT?" Since its initial use, numerous other treatments have come and gone in psychiatry, but the use of ECT has persisted. Most recently, rTMS has yielded exciting preliminary results in the treatment of depression. However, given the highly safe and effective manner in which ECT can now be administered, the question asked should no longer be whether rTMS will replace ECT, but how rTMS can complement ECT in the treatment of psychiatric disorders (Pascual-Leone et al. 1996).

rTMS allows magnetic stimuli to stimulate the cerebral cortex noninvasively (Pascual-Leone et al. 1996). Lesion and imaging studies suggest that left prefrontal lobe dysfunction is pathophysiologically linked to depression. On the basis of these observations, several groups have begun to examine whether rTMS administered to the left prefrontal lobe may be of benefit in treating some patients with depression. In a recent randomized, placebo-controlled study, rTMS was found to be effective in treating 11 of 17 patients with psychotic depression (Pascual-Leone et al. 1996). The authors found that rTMS was most effective when applied over the left frontal lobe anterior to the motor cortex. However, the therapeutic benefits of rTMS were transient, lasting less than 1 month. Potential benefits of rTMS include the absence of anesthesia and absent or minimal cardiac and cognitive side effects. Potential side effects from rTMS are headaches and a small risk for developing a seizure during treatment.

The fact that rTMS uses subconvulsive stimuli challenges the long-held belief that a generalized seizure is required for ECT to be effective. We hope that continued study of the mechanism of action of rTMS will further the understanding of ECT and in turn allow clinicians to better understand the pathophysiology of depression and to provide the safest and most effective care to patients.

CONCLUSION

Nearly 60 years have passed since ECT was first used in the treatment of psychiatric disorders. The lack of rigorous scientific studies during the early use of ECT in part allowed controversy to develop over the use of ECT. Despite this ongoing controversy, ECT continues to be an extremely important tool in the treatment of several psychiatric disorders. This no doubt reflects the highly safe and effective manner in which ECT can now be administered. It is hoped that adequate research funding will be available in the future to further advance the study of ECT and to ensure that ECT will be adequately available to all patients who might benefit from it.

REFERENCES

Abrams R: Electroconvulsive Therapy, 2nd Edition. New York, Oxford University Press, 1992, pp 3–9

American Psychiatric Association: Report of the Task Force on Electroconvulsive Therapy of the American Psychiatric Association. Washington, DC, American Psychiatric Association, 1978

American Psychiatric Association: The Practice of Electroconvulsive Therapy: Recommendations for Practice, Training, and Privileging. Task Force Report on ECT. Washington, DC, American Psychiatric Association, 1990

American Psychiatric Association: Diagnostic and Statistical Manual of Mental Disorders, 4th Edition. Washington, DC, American Psychiatric Association, 1994

Anwyl R, Walshe J, Rowan M: Electroconvulsive treatment reduces long-term potentiation in rat hippocampus. Brain Res 435:377–379, 1987

Aronson TA, Shukla S, Hoff A: Continuation therapy after ECT for delusional depression: a naturalistic study of prophylactic treatments and relapse. Convuls Ther 3:241–259, 1987

Barton JL, Mehta S, Snaith RP: The prophylactic value of extra ECT in depressive illness. Acta Psychiatr Scand 49:386–392, 1973

Bolwig TG, Hertz MM, Westergaard E: Acute hypertension causing blood-brain barrier breakdown during epileptic seizures. Acta Neurol Scand 56:335–342, 1977

Bourne H, Long MB: Convulsion dependence. Lancet 2:1193–1196, 1954

Brandon S, Cowley P, McDonald C, et al: Electroconvulsive therapy: results in depressive illness from the Leicestershire trial. BMJ 288:22–25, 1984

Broderston P, Paulson OB, Bolwig TG, et al: Cerebral hyperemia in electrically induced epileptic seizures. Arch Neurol 28:334–338, 1973

Calev A, Pass HL, Shapira B, et al: ECT and memory, in The Clinical Science of Electroconvulsive Therapy. Edited by Coffey CE. Washington, DC, American Psychiatric Association, 1993, pp 125–142

Cattan RA, Barry PP, Mead G, et al: Electroconvulsive therapy in octogenarians. J Am Geriatr Soc 38:753–758, 1990

Cerletti U: L'elettroshock. Rivista Sperimentale Freniatria 64:209–310, 1940

Clarke TB, Coffey CE, Hoffman GW, et al: Continuation therapy for depression using outpatient electroconvulsive therapy. Convuls Ther 5:330–337, 1989

Clifford DB, Zorumski CF, Olney JW: Ketamine and MK-801 prevent degeneration of thalamic neurons induced by focal cortical seizures. Exp Neurol 105:272–279, 1989

Coffey CE, Figiel GS, Djang WT, et al: Effects of ECT on brain structure: a pilot prospective magnetic resonance imaging study. Am J Psychiatry 145:701–706, 1988

Colenda CC, McCall WV: A statistical model predicting the seizure threshold for right unilateral electroconvulsive therapy in 106 patients. Convuls Ther 12:3–12, 1996

Crow TJ, Deakin JFW, Johnstone EC, et al: Mechanism of action of ECT: relevance of clinical evidence. Paper presented at the 13th Congress of the Collegium Internationale Neuro-Psychologicum, Jerusalem, Israel, June 1982

Decina P, Guthrie EB, Sackheim HA, et al: Continuation ECT in the management of relapses of major affective episodes. Acta Psychiatr Scand 75:559–562, 1987

Devanand DP, Dwork AJ, Hutchinson ER, et al: Does ECT alter brain structure? Am J Psychiatry 151:957–970, 1994

Dinwiddie SH, Drevets WC, Smith DR: Treatment of phencyclidine-associated psychosis with ECT. Convuls Ther 4:230–235, 1988

Endler NS: The origins of electroconvulsive therapy (ECT). Convuls Ther 4:5–23, 1988

Farah A, McCall WV: Electroconvulsive therapy stimulus dosing: a survey of contemporary practices. Convuls Ther 9:90–94, 1993

Figiel GS, Coffey CE: Brain magnetic resonance imaging findings in ECT-induced delirium. J Neuropsychiatry Clin Neurosci 2:53–58, 1990

Figiel GS, Hassen M, Krishnan KRR, et al: ECT induced delirium in depressed patients with Parkinson's disease. J Neuropsychiatry Clin Neurosci 3:405–411, 1991

Figiel GS, Zorumski CF, Doraiswamy PM, et al: Simultaneous major depression and panic disorder: treatment with electroconvulsive therapy. J Clin Psychiatry 53:12–15, 1992

Figiel GS, DeLeo B, Zorumski CF, et al: Combined use of labetalol and nifedipine in controlling the cardiovascular response from ECT. J Geriatr Psychiatry Neurol 6:20–24, 1993

Figiel GS, McDonald L, LaPlante R: Cardiac modified ECT in the elderly (letter). Am J Psychiatry 151:790–791, 1994

Fink M, Sackeim HA: Convulsive therapy in schizophrenia? Schizophr Bull 22:27–39, 1996

Fochtmann LJ: A mechanism for the efficacy of ECT in Parkinson's disease. Convuls Ther 4:321–327, 1988

Fochtmann LJ: Animal studies of electroconvulsive therapy: foundations for future research. Psychopharm Bull 30:321–444, 1994

Fochtmann LJ, Cruciani R, Aiso M, et al: Chronic electroconvulsive shock increases D1 receptor binding in rat substantia nigra. Eur J Pharmacol 167:305–306, 1989

Folstein MF, Folstein SE, McHugh PR: Mini-Mental State: a practical method for grading the cognitive state of patients for the clinician. J Psychiatr Res 12:189–198, 1975

Gleiter CH, Deckett J, Nutt DJ, et al: Electroconvulsive shock (ECS) and the adenosine neuromodulatory system: effect of single and repeated ECS on the adenosine A1 and A2 receptors, adenylate cyclase and the adenosine uptake site. J Neurochem 52:641–646, 1989

Green AR, Vincent ND: The effect of repeated electroconvulsive shock on GABA synthesis and release in regions of rat brain. Br J Pharmacol 92:19–24, 1987

Green AR, Sant K, Bowdler JM, et al: Further evidence for a relationship between changes in GABA concentration in rat brain and enhanced monoamine mediated behavioral responses following repeated electroconvulsive shock. Neuropharmacology 21:981–984, 1982

Greenberg PE, Stiglin LE, Finkelstein SN, et al: Depression: a neglected major illness. J Clin Psychiatry 54:419–424, 1993

Greene RW, Haas HL: The electrophysiology of adenosine in the mammalian central nervous system. Prog Neurobiol 36:329–341, 1991

Grover BB: Handbook of Electrotherapy. Philadelphia, PA, Davis, 1924

Gruenthal M, Armstrong DR, Ault B, et al: Comparison of seizures and brain lesions produced by intracerebroventricular kainic acid and bicuculline methiodide. Exp Neurol 93:621–630, 1986

Grunhaus L, Pande AC, Hasket RF: Full and abbreviated courses of maintenance electroconvulsive therapy. Convuls Ther 6:130–138, 1990

Hargrove EA, Bennett AE, Ford FR: The value of subconvulsive electrostimulation in the treatment of some emotional disorders. Am J Psychiatry 8:612–616, 1953

Hickie I, Scott E, Mitchell P, et al: Subcortical hyperintensities on magnetic resonance imaging: clinical correlates and prognostic significance in patients with severe depression. Biol Psychiatry 37:151–160, 1995

Hinkle PE, Coffey CE, Weiner RD, et al: Use of caffeine to lengthen seizures in ECT. Am J Psychiatry 144: 1143–1148, 1987

Hitzemann RJ, Hitzemann BA, Blatt S, et al: Repeated electroconvulsive shock: effect on sodium dependency and regional distribution of opioid binding sites. Mol Pharmacol 31:562–566, 1987

Huettner JE, Bean BP: Block of N-methyl-D-aspartate-activated current by the anticonvulsant MK-801: selective binding to open channels. Proc Natl Acad Sci U S A 85:1307–1311, 1988

Jaffe R, Dubin WR, Roemer R, et al: Continuation and maintenance ECT—efficacy and safety. Paper presented at the 142nd annual meeting of the American Psychiatric Association, San Francisco, CA, May 1989

Karlinsky H, Shulman KI: The clinical use of electroconvulsive therapy in old age. J Am Geriatr Soc 32:183–186, 1984

Kety S: Effects of repeated electroconvulsive shock on brain catecholamines, in Psychobiology of Convulsive Therapy. Edited by Fink M, Kety S, McGaugh J, et al. Washington, DC, H. J. Winston and Sons, 1974, pp 285–294

Klein HE, Broucek B, Greil W: Lithium withdrawal triggers psychotic states. Br J Psychiatry 139:255–256, 1981

Kramer BA: Maintenance ECT: a survey of practice. Convuls Ther 3:260–268, 1987

Krueger RB, Sackeim HA, Gamzu ER: Pharmacological treatment of the cognitive side effects of ECT: a review. Psychopharm Bull 28:409–424, 1992

Krystal AD, Wiener RD, McCall WV, et al: The effects of ECT stimulus dose and electrode placement on the ictal electroencephalogram: an intraindividual cross-over study. Biol Psychiatry 24:759–767, 1993

Kuba K, Kumamoto E: Long-term potentiation in vertebrate synapses: a variety of cascades with common subprocesses. Prog Neurobiol 34:197–269, 1990

Laursen H, Gjerris A, Bolwig TG, et al: Cerebral edema and vascular permeability to serum proteins following electroconvulsive shock in rats. Convuls Ther 7:237–244, 1991

Lerer B, Weiner RD, Belmaker RH (eds): ECT: Basic Mechanisms. Washington, DC, American Psychiatric Association, 1984

Lerer B, Shapira B, Calev A, et al: Antidepressant and cognitive effects of twice- versus three-times weekly ECT. Am J Psychiatry 152:564–570, 1995

Levy SD, Albrecht E: Electroconvulsive therapy: a survey of use in the private psychiatric hospital. J Clin Psychiatry 46:125–127, 1985

Lloyd KG, Thuret F, Pilc A: Upregulation of gamma-aminobutyric acid (GABA)$_B$ binding sites in rat frontal cortex: a common action of repeated administration of different classes of antidepressants and electroshock. J Pharmacol Exp Ther 235:191–199, 1985

Loo H, Galinowski A, de Carvalho W, et al: The clonidine test in posttraumatic stress disorder. Am J Psychiatry 148:810, 1991

Macdonald RL, Olsen RW: GABA$_A$ receptor channels. Annu Rev Neurosci 17:569–602, 1994

MacDonald JF, Bartlett MC, Mody I, et al: Actions of ketamine, phencyclidine and MK-801 on NMDA receptor currents in cultured mouse hippocampal neurons. J Physiol Lond 432:483–508, 1991

Maltbie AA, Wingfield MS, Volow MR, et al: Electroconvulsive therapy in the presence of brain tumor. J Nerv Ment Dis 168:400–405, 1980

Maneksha FR: Hypertension and tachycardia during electroconvulsive therapy: to treat or not to treat? Convuls Ther 70:28–35, 1991

Matzen TA, Martin RL, Watt TJ, et al: The use of maintenance electroconvulsive therapy for relapsing depression. Jefferson Journal of Psychiatry 6:52–58, 1988

McCall WV: Asystole in electroconvulsive therapy: report of four cases. J Clin Psychiatry 57:199–203, 1996

McCall WV, Farah BA: Greater ictal EEG regularity during RUL ECT is associated with greater treatment efficiency (abstract). Convuls Ther 11:69, 1994

McCall WV, Shelp FE, Weiner RD, et al: Effects of labetalol on hemodynamics and seizure duration during ECT. Convuls Ther 7:5–14, 1991

McCall WV, Reid S, Rosenquist P, et al: A reappraisal of the role of caffeine in ECT. Am J Psychiatry 150:1543–1545, 1993a

McCall WV, Shelp FE, Weiner RD, et al: Convulsive threshold differences in right unilateral and bilateral ECT. Biol Psychiatry 24:759–767, 1993b

McCall WV, Reid S, Ford M: Electrocardiographic and cardiovascular effects of subconvulsive stimulation during titrated right unilateral ECT. Convuls Ther 10:25–33, 1994

McCall WV, Farah BA, Reboussin D, et al: Comparison of the efficacy of titrated, moderate dose and fixed, high dose RUL ET in the elderly. Am J Geriatr Psychiatry 3: 317–324, 1995

McCall WV, Robinette GD, Hardesty D: Relationship of seizure morphology to the convulsive threshold. Convuls Ther 12:147–151, 1996

McNamara JO: Cellular and molecular basis of epilepsy. J Neurosci 14:3413–3425, 1994

Meduna L: Autobiography, part 1. Convuls Ther 1:43–57, 1985

Monroe RRJ: Maintenance electroconvulsive therapy. Psychiatr Clin North Am 14:947–960, 1991

Mukherjee S, Sackeim HA, Schnur DB: Electroconvulsive therapy of acute mania episodes: a review of 50 years' experience. Am J Psychiatry 151:169–176, 1994

Murphy E: The prognosis of depression in old age. Br J Psychiatry 142:111–119, 1983

Murray JB: Lithium maintenance therapy for bipolar I patients: possible refractoriness to reinstitution after discontinuation. Psychol Rep 74:355–361, 1994

Nobler MS, Sackeim HA, Solomou M, et al: EEG manifestations during ECT: effects of electrode placement and stimulus intensity. Biol Psychiatry 34:321–330, 1993

Nowak G, Zak J: Repeated electroconvulsive shock (ECS) enhances striatal D1 dopamine receptor turnover in rats. Eur J Pharmacol 167:307–308, 1989

Nutt DJ, Glue P: The neurobiology of ECT: animal studies, in The Clinical Science of Electroconvulsive Therapy. Edited by Coffey CE. Washington, DC, American Psychiatric Association, 1993, pp 213–234

Nutt DH, Cowen PJ, Green AR: Studies of the postictal rise in seizure threshold. Eur J Pharmacol 71:287–295, 1981

Ottosson JO: Seizure characteristics and therapeutic efficiency in electroconvulsive therapy: an analysis of the antidepressant efficiency of grand mal and lidocaine-modified seizures. J Nerv Ment Dis 135:239–251, 1962

Palmer TM, Stiles GL: Adenosine receptors. Neuropharmacology 34:683–694, 1995

Pascual-Leone A, Rubio B, Pallardo F, et al: Rapid-rate transcranial magnetic stimulation of left dorsolateral prefrontal cortex in drug-resistant depression. Lancet 348:233–237, 1996

Petrides G, Dhossche D, Fink M, et al: Continuation ECT: relapse prevention in affective disorders. Convuls Ther 10:189–194, 1994

Plaznik A, Kostowski W, Stefanski R: The influence of antidepressive treatment on GABA related mechanisms in the rat hippocampus: behavioral studies. Pharmacol Biochem Behav 33:749–753, 1989

Posner JB, Plum F, Van Poznak A: Cerebral metabolism during electrically induced seizures in man. Arch Neurol 28: 388–395, 1969

Prudic J, Sackeim HA, Devanand DP, et al: Acute cognitive effects of subconvulsive electrical stimulation. Convuls Ther 10:4–24, 1994

Prudic J, Haskett RF, Mulsant B, et al: Resistance to antidepressant medications and short-term clinical response to ECT. Am J Psychiatry 153:985–992, 1996

Rasmussen K, Abrams R: Treatment of Parkinson's disease with electroconvulsive therapy. Psychiatr Clin North Am 14:925–934, 1991

Rasmussen KG, Zorumski CF: ECT in patients taking theophylline. J Clin Psychiatry 54:427–431, 1993

Sackeim HA: Central issues regarding the mechanism of action of electroconvulsive therapy: directions for future research. Psychopharm Bull 30:281–308, 1994

Sackeim HA, Prudic J, Devanad DP, et al: The impact of medication resistance and continuation pharmacotherapy on relapse following response to electroconvulsive therapy in major depression. J Clin Psychopharmacol 10:96–104, 1990

Sackeim HA, Devanand DP, Prudic J: Stimulus intensity, seizure threshold and seizure duration: impact on the efficacy and safety of electroconvulsive therapy. Psychiatr Clin North Am 14:803–843, 1991

Sackeim HA, Prudic J, Devanand DP, et al: Effects of stimulus intensity and electrode placement on the efficacy and cognitive effects of electroconvulsive therapy. N Engl J Med 328:839–846, 1993

Sackeim HA, Devanand DP, Nobler MS: Electroconvulsive therapy, in Psychopharmacology: The Fourth Generation of Progress. Edited by Bloom FE, Kupfer DJ. New York, Raven, 1995, pp 1123–1141

Sawynok J, Yaksh T: Caffeine as an analgesic adjuvant: a review of pharmacology and mechanisms of action. Pharmacol Rev 45:43–85, 1993

Scott AIF, Douglass RHB, Whitfield A, et al: Time course of cerebral magnetic resonance changes after electroconvulsive therapy. Br J Psychiatry 156:551–553, 1990

Shapira B, Lerer B, Gilboa D, et al: Facilitation of ECT by caffeine pretreatment. Am J Psychiatry 144:1199–1202, 1987

Shapira B, Gorfine M, Lerer B: A prospective study of lithium continuation therapy in depressed patients who have responded to electroconvulsive therapy. Convuls Ther 11:80–85, 1995

Small JG, Klapper MH, Kellams JJ, et al: Electroconvulsive therapy compared with lithium in the management of manic states. Arch Gen Psychiatry 45:727–732, 1988

Spiker DG, Stein J, Rich CL: Delusional depression and electroconvulsive therapy: one year later. Convuls Ther 1:167–172, 1985

Stewart C, Reid I: Electroconvulsive stimulation and synaptic plasticity in the rat. Brain Res 620:139–141, 1993

Stoudemire A, Knos G, Gladson M, et al: Labetalol in the control of cardiovascular responses to electroconvulsive therapy in high-risk depressed medical patients. J Clin Psychiatry 51:508–512, 1990

Swartz CM, Abrams R: ECT Instruction Manual. Lake Bluff, IL, Somatics, 1994

Thienhaus OJ, Margletta S, Bennet JA: A study of the clinical efficacy of maintenance ECT. J Clin Psychiatry 51:141–144, 1990

Thornton JE, Mulsant BH, Dealy R, et al: A retrospective study of maintenance electroconvulsive therapy in a university-based psychiatric practice. Convuls Ther 2:121–129, 1990

Tortella FC, Long JB: Endogenous anticonvulsant substance in rat cerebrospinal fluid after a generalized seizure. Science 228:1106–1108, 1985

Tortella FC, Long JB: Characterization of opioid peptide-like anticonvulsant activity in rat cerebrospinal fluid. Brain Res 456:139–146, 1988

Tortella FC, Long JB, Hong J-S, et al: Modulation of endogenous opioid systems by electroconvulsive shock. Convuls Ther 5:261–273, 1989

Vanelle JM, Loo H, Galinowski A, et al: Maintenance ECT in intractable manic-depressive disorders. Convuls Ther 10:195–205, 1994

Weiner RD: ECT and seizure threshold: effects of stimulus wave form and electrode placement. Biol Psychiatry 15:225–241, 1980

Weiner RD: Does electroconvulsive therapy cause brain damage? Behavioral and Brain Sciences 7:1–53, 1984

Weiner RD, Coffey CE: Minimizing therapeutic differences between bilateral and unilateral nondominant ECT. Convuls Ther 2:261–265, 1986

Weiner RD, Rogers HJ, Davidson SR, et al: Effects of electroconvulsive therapy upon brain electrical activity. Ann N Y Acad Sci 462:270–281, 1986

Zielinski RJ, Roose SP, Devanand DP, et al: Cardiovascular complications of ECT in depressed patients with cardiac disease. Am J Psychiatry 150:904–909, 1993

Zis AP, Grof P, Webster M, et al: Prediction of relapse in recurrent affective disorder. Psychopharmacol Bull 16:47–49, 1980

Zorumski CF, Izumi Y: Nitric oxide and hippocampal synaptic plasticity. Biochem Pharmacol 46:777–785, 1993

SECTION III

Clinical Psychobiology and Psychiatric Syndromes

David J. Kupfer, M.D., Section Editor

TWENTY-SEVEN

Biology of Mood Disorders

Dominique L. Musselman, M.D., Charles DeBattista, D.M.H., M.D., Kalpana I. Nathan, M.D., Clinton D. Kilts, Ph.D., Alan F. Schatzberg, M.D., and Charles B. Nemeroff, M.D., Ph.D.

HISTORY

The intriguing search for the biological substrates of affective disorders spans many centuries. Indeed, Hippocrates (460–357 B.C.) speculated that melancholia emerged when environmental conditions, such as the alignment of the planets, caused the spleen to secrete black bile which then darkened the mood. During the next 2,000 years, few significant contributions to our understanding of mood disorders emerged until Robert Burton's *Anatomy of Melancholy* (1621). Positing that depressed people often "are born of melancholy parents," Burton identified the genetic underpinnings of melancholia as well as other factors in the pathogenesis of depression including alcohol, diet, and biological rhythms. Through his careful longitudinal observations, Emil Kraepelin (1856–1926) was subsequently able to detect a genetic contribution to manic-depressive illness. He also hypothesized that other constitutional factors resulted in specific brain abnormalities in manic-depressive patients, although postmortem tissue studies were unrevealing.

Adolf Meyer (1866–1950) at Johns Hopkins University attempted to integrate psychological and biological theories of mental illness. Coining the term *psychobiology*, he speculated that depression was the result of genetic or biological factors with additional effects of the environment after birth. Influenced by the work of Freud and other contemporaries, Meyer also emphasized the importance of current life stressors in the generation of depressive symptoms.

Pathophysiological investigation into psychiatric illness retreated with the preeminence of psychoanalytic theory and practice during the immediate post–World War II era. Biological theories reemerged in the 1950s after the introduction of the effective antipsychotic agent chlorpromazine and were further fostered by the introduction of effective antidepressants. Furthermore, the biogenic amine hypothesis (attributed to Joseph Schildkraut, John Davis, and William Bunney with additional contributions by Alec Coppen and I. P. Lapin) posited that major depression was caused by a deficiency in central nervous system (CNS) concentration or receptor function of the neurotransmitters norepinephrine, epinephrine, and dopamine or the indoleamine serotonin.

American investigators during the 1960s, including Schildkraut (1965) and Bunney and Davis (1965), developed a variation of the biogenic amine hypothesis, the catecholamine hypothesis. The catecholamine hypothesis of affective disorders proposes that some types of depression are associated with a relative deficiency of catecholamines, particularly norepinephrine, in the CNS, whereas mania is associated with a relative overabundance of catecholamines. Substantial data have accumulated, however, demonstrating the contributions of other putative neurotransmitters in the maintenance of mood.

As American investigators during the 1960s focused on the importance of norepinephrine in the pathogenesis of abnormal mood states, European researchers—Alec Coppen (1968) in England and Lapin and Oxenkrug (1969) in the Soviet Union—turned their attention to the CNS serotonergic system. They proposed that a deficiency in serotonergic neuronal function produced depressive symptoms. This hypothesis was bolstered by the observations of Asberg and colleagues (1976a) that a sizable subgroup of depressed patients had low cerebrospinal fluid (CSF) concentrations of 5-hydroxyindoleacetic acid (5-HIAA) and moreover that this subgroup was at greater risk for attempting or committing suicide, particularly by violent means. The association between indices of reduced serotonin turnover and impulsive violent behavior has been consistently replicated in several studies (Roy et al. 1989; Traskman et al. 1981; Van Praag 1982), although it does not appear to be specific to depression (V. M. Linnoila and Virkkunen 1992; Virkkunen et al. 1994).

In the 1970s, Janowsky and colleagues (1972) proposed a variation in the catecholamine hypothesis: they suggested that a relative increase in CNS cholinergic activity in comparison to norepinephrine activity is associated with depression, whereas the converse is associated with mania.

Concurrent with the aforementioned work, psychiatrists repeatedly observed disturbances in mood in patients with clinical endocrinopathies. Indeed, hypercortisolemia was first noted as a feature of major depression in the late 1950s. During the 1970s, great strides were made in the understanding of the neuroendocrine mechanisms underlying major depression, including perturbations of the hypothalamic-pituitary-adrenal (HPA) and the hypothalamic-pituitary-thyroid (HPT) axes. Carroll's group demonstrated that 40%–50% of patients with endogenous depression show resistance to dexamethasone-induced HPA axis suppression, in the now well-known dexamethasone suppression test (DST) (W. A. Brown et al. 1979; Carroll and Davies 1970). Meanwhile Prange and colleagues (1969, 1972) detected abnormalities in the HPT axis in patients with major depression and also reported that augmentation of antidepressant treatment with thyroid hormone, triiodothyronine (T_3), was effective.

The biogenic amine hypotheses also arose in part from pharmacological interventions and observation of their effects on mood. Reserpine, a rauwolfia alkaloid antihypertensive agent, produces depressive symptoms in many patients, presumably resulting from depletion of biogenic amines from CNS neurons. The mood-elevating action of monoamine oxidase inhibitors (MAOIs) was discovered by the chance observation of the effects of iproniazid, a drug originally developed to treat tuberculosis. Imipramine, a tricyclic compound related to chlorpromazine and designed to treat schizophrenia, also elevates mood. Tricyclic antidepressants (TCAs) not only block the reuptake of norepinephrine and serotonin into presynaptic neurons but also are cholinergic receptor antagonists. Shopsin and colleagues (1975, 1976) found that administration of p-chlorophenylalanine, an inhibitor of serotonin synthesis, reversed the antidepressant action of imipramine (a TCA) as well as tranylcypromine (an MAOI). Interest in the mechanistic role of serotonin systems in depression was further stimulated by the introduction of selective serotonin reuptake inhibitors (SSRIs) (e.g., fluoxetine) in the late 1980s. In the past decade, advances in molecular biology have made possible the structural characterization and cloning of several serotonin receptors as well as the serotonin transporter. In this chapter, we review the genetics of mood disorders as well as neurotransmitter, psychoneuroendocrine, and brain imaging alterations in patients with affective disorders.

NOSOLOGY

Standardized diagnostic criteria for mood disorders not only assist in the detection and recognition of disorders such as major depression and bipolar disorder, but also indicate their prevalence. Moreover, reliable diagnostic criteria can be used to systematically evaluate treatment modalities, identify risk factors leading to development of a mood disorder, and herald preventive measures. DSM-IV (American Psychiatric Association 1994) has updated the classification of mood disorders. We briefly review the DSM-IV section on mood disorders and focus on changes in the spectrum of depressive and manic syndromes that were previously defined in accordance with DSM-III-R criteria (American Psychiatric Association 1987).

The DSM-IV section on mood disorders is divided into three parts. The first part describes mood episodes, including major depressive, manic, mixed, and hypomanic episodes. The second part sets criteria for mood disorders, including depressive and bipolar disorders, mood disorder due to a general medical condition, and substance-induced mood disorder. The third part includes the specifiers that describe either the most recent mood episode or the course of recurrent episodes.

The major depressive disorders have severity, psychotic, and remission specifiers; additional categories include catatonic, melancholic, and atypical features (Kendler et al. 1996), as well as postpartum onset. The recurrent major depressive disorders have longitudinal course specifiers (with and without interepisode recovery), as well as specifications for seasonal pattern and rapid cycling.

Depressive disorder not otherwise specified has been expanded to include premenstrual dysphoric disorder, minor depressive disorder (depressive symptoms subthreshold in severity to major depression), recurrent brief depressive disorder (episodes that occur at least once a month for 12 months, lasting from 2 days to 2 weeks), postpsychotic depressive disorder of schizophrenia, and major depressive disorder superimposed on psychotic disorders. The inclusion of these disorders makes it possible to validate depressive syndromes that fall short of DSM-III-R thresholds for depressive disorders. Because patients with these disorders have clinically significant impairment as measured by health care utilization and functional disability (Broadhead et al. 1990; Johnson et al. 1992; Skodol et al. 1994; Wells et al. 1989), these affective syndromes have been included in DSM-IV. In fact, recurrent brief depressive disorder is currently included in the *International Statistical Classification of Diseases and Related Health Problems*, Tenth Revision (ICD-10; World Health Organization 1992; American Psychiatric Association Task Force on DSM-IV 1991).

Criteria for bipolar mood disorder spectrum have been substantially revised. There is now a clear specification of the period of abnormally elevated, expansive, or irritable mood, which should last at least 1 week, or of any duration if hospitalization is necessary. Six separate sets of criteria define bipolar disorder, including single manic episode, most recent episode hypomanic, most recent episode manic, most recent episode mixed, most recent episode depressed, and most recent episode unspecified. Bipolar II disorder has been included, which specifies recurrent depressive episodes with hypomanic episodes.

The DSM-III-R criteria for mixed subtype of bipolar disorder describe two very different types of presentations: depressive and manic symptoms that are "intermixed" and those "rapidly alternating every few days." DSM-IV differentiates between and describes these two different patient populations. A rapid-cycling course specifier describes those patients with rapidly alternating symptoms, whereas "intermixed" presentations are now reclassified as mixed episode.

The unipolar and bipolar mood syndromes have each subsumed the overinclusive and ambiguous diagnosis of organic mood disorder. This diagnosis was listed in two different sections of DSM-III-R (organic mental disorders associated with Axis III physical disorders or conditions and psychoactive substance-induced organic mental disorders). Because multiple factors (biological, psychological, and social) contribute to the presentation of most mental disorders, the dichotomy between "organic" and "nonorganic" has become obsolete. The term *organic* has been replaced by the term *mood disorder due to . . .* and the related nonpsychiatric medical condition is included as part of the name of the disorder and included on Axis I (e.g., "mood disorder due to autoimmune thyroiditis, with hypomanic episode"). This subtyping scheme allows the clinician to indicate whether the individual's condition has met specific diagnostic criteria for major depression or manic episode or for a subthreshold or mixed presentation (American Psychiatric Association 1994; American Psychiatric Association Task Force on DSM-IV 1991).

Organic mood disorder had been listed within yet another section of DSM-III-R, psychoactive substance-induced organic mental disorders. In DSM-IV, substance-induced mood disorder has been placed within the mood disorders section. The specific substance used, the context in which the substance-induced mood disorder has developed (i.e., during intoxication or withdrawal), and the specific mood disorder are described (e.g., "cocaine withdrawal mood disorder, with major depressive episode"). The categorization of substance-induced mood disorder and mood disorder due to a nonpsychiatric medical condition under the rubric of mood disorders facilitates differential diagnosis while eliminating the anachronistic "organic" classification.

The "course specifiers" offered by DSM-IV (e.g., "with seasonal pattern," "postpartum mood disturbance," "with/without full interepisode recovery") for both unipolar and bipolar mood syndromes provide further diagnostic refinements. With each successive edition of DSM, identification of phenomenologically defined subsets of patients progresses, in the hope of improving identification, treatment, and even prevention of chronic and disabling mood disorders.

EPIDEMIOLOGY AND GENETICS

Epidemiology

Over the past 30 years, epidemiological studies of the major mood disorders have reported considerable variation in the prevalence of depression and bipolar mood disorder. This variability may be explained by the differing methodology of these surveys: sampling of the populations at risk, the particular diagnostic system used, the method for obtaining information about symptoms, and the time when information was obtained (Weissman et al. 1992).

The most extensive survey completed after publication of DSM-III (American Psychiatric Association 1980) is the Epidemiologic Catchment Area study sponsored by the National Institute of Mental Health. Between 1980 and 1984, 20,291 adults aged 18 and older were interviewed with the Diagnostic Interview Schedule (DIS;

Robins et al. 1981) in a variety of settings: community households, long-term treatment mental hospitals, nursing homes, and correctional institutions. The Epidemiologic Catchment Area study (based on DSM-III criteria) indicated the following 1-month prevalence rates (a guide in determining the number in the population with a disorder at a given point in time) per 100 persons: major depression (1.8), dysthymia (3.3), bipolar I (0.4), and bipolar II disorder (0.2). Lifetime prevalence rates (or risk of acquiring the disorder over a lifetime) per 100 persons were: major depression (4.9), dysthymia (3.3), bipolar I (0.8), and bipolar II disorder (0.5) (Regier et al. 1988). Another comprehensive epidemiological project, the National Comorbidity Study, has been completed more recently (Kessler et al. 1994). Data were derived by interviewing 8,098 noninstitutionalized persons aged 15–54 years in the 48 coterminous states. In brief, 17% of the respondents reported a history of major depression, 1.6% a manic episode, and 6% dysthymia (lifetime prevalence rates based on DSM-III-R criteria).

Genetics of Affective Disorder

The probability that a person will develop an affective disorder is influenced by a number of factors, including premature parental loss, inadequate rearing by parents, a history of traumatic events, certain personality traits, personal history or family history of affective episodes, the extent of social support, and recent stressful life events (Kendler et al. 1993b). The scrutiny of major depression and bipolar disorder in family, twin, and adoption studies demonstrates that genetic influences undoubtedly play a preeminent role in their etiology. Understanding this genetic contribution may help provide genetic counseling, early identification of those at risk, and clues about the specific genetic defect(s) associated with or responsible for vulnerability to these disorders (Michels and Marzuk 1993). We briefly review the steps necessary to clarify the role of genetic factors in a particular psychiatric disorder and the multiple methods of evaluating the data.

Family studies can provide initial evidence of genetic contributions. Morbid risk (i.e., adjusted prevalence) of the disorder is determined within the affected families, and the rate for patients' relatives is compared with that for relatives of control groups or for the general population. First-degree relatives (i.e., parents, siblings, and offspring) of patients with bipolar affective disorder are reported to be at least 24 times more likely to develop bipolar affective disorder than relatives of control subjects (Weissman et al. 1984). However, family studies cannot establish that a disorder is hereditary. Familial aggregation

may reflect a shared environment—for example, common exposure to a particular culture or to a virus (Pardes et al. 1989).

Twin studies compare the concordance rate for illness in pairs of monozygotic (identical) twins with the rate in dizygotic (nonidentical) twins. The rationale is that monozygotic twins share identical genes, whereas dizygotic twins share only half their genes. It is also assumed that both types of twins are exposed to the same prenatal and postnatal environment. Thus, if monozygotic twins show a greater concordance rate for a particular psychiatric disorder than do dizygotic twins, this is believed to be firm evidence for a strong genetic contribution to development of the disorder. However, the extent to which environmental factors can be considered equal for monozygotic and dizygotic twins is arguable. In utero, monozygotic twins share the identical placental circulation; dizygotic twins do not. Moreover, monozygotic twins may also elicit similar treatment from the environment by virtue of their similar appearance. Therefore, monozygotic twins have different life experiences than do dizygotic twins. However, the marked difference in concordance rates between monozygotic and dizygotic twins strongly supports the hypothesis of a major genetic contribution to the development of both unipolar depression (Kendler et al. 1992, 1993a; McGuffin et al. 1991; 1996; Tsuang and Faraone 1990) and bipolar disorder (Bertelson et al. 1977; Mendlewicz 1988). Recent twin studies provide no evidence that a shared family environment exerts a major influence on the development of major depression. In fact genetic factors appear to be the sole source of similarity for major depression in monozygotic and dizygotic twins (McGuffin et al. 1996; Kendler et al. 1993c).

Adoption studies attempt to elucidate the contribution of environment ("nurture") and genetic contribution ("nature") by studying children raised away from their biological parents. Cases of adopted children developing the affective disorder of their biological parent and, conversely, of adoptive children *not* developing the mood disorder of the parents with the disorder support the paramount role of genetic factors. However, one of the limitations of adoption studies is the environmental factors (including the in utero environment) that have already influenced the adopted child. Nevertheless, adoption studies show a greater prevalence rate of bipolar disorder among biological relatives than adopted relatives of bipolar patients (Mendlewicz and Rainier 1977; Wender et al. 1986). Despite their respective limitations, family, twin, and adoption studies all demonstrate a significant contribution of hereditary factors in the pathogenesis of affective disorder.

There are three major models regarding the mode of inheritance (i.e., *how* an illness is genetically transmitted and *what* constitutes the factor that is inherited). About one-quarter of the more than 4,000 illnesses transmitted through *monogenic inheritance* (i.e., caused by defects in a single major gene and transmitted according to a Mendelian pattern: dominant, recessive, or sex-linked) affect mental functioning. However, the prevalence of any one of these diseases (e.g., Lesch-Nyhan syndrome and phenylketonuria) is quite low (McKusick 1992). In contrast, other illnesses (e.g., atherosclerosis and diabetes) are believed to be caused by combined defects of several genes, or *polygenic inheritance*. The other mode of inheritance is *multifactorial inheritance*, based on the combination of major and minor gene effects, as well as the interaction between genes and the environment.

Statistical analysis, including both segregation and linkage, is used to search for both the mode of inheritance and the chromosomal location of the genes predisposing to the particular disorder under study. Segregation analysis compares the observed frequency of an illness in a pedigree (ancestral relationships of individuals of a family over two or more generations) with the pattern that would occur if a hypothesized mode of inheritance (i.e., monogenic vs. polygenic transmission) were true (McKusick 1992).

Another mode of analysis is linkage analysis (Gershon and Goldin 1987), which tests whether the observed co-occurrence of a disease and a marker for a genetic locus within a given pedigree are compatible with that locus contributing to disease susceptibility (Kauffman and Malaspina 1993). Linkage analysis may proceed along one of three possible lines—identification of an abnormal protein, or a particular nucleic acid sequence, or a "biological marker" gene that is consistently transmitted or "linked" with the gene(s) responsible for the affective illness. The "protein-gene" approach posits that when an abnormal protein is found to accompany a particular illness, this abnormal protein can be used to track the accompanying abnormal gene. Unfortunately, such specific neurochemical disturbances associated with the major psychiatric illnesses remain to be discovered. Second, linkage analysis can proceed according to the "gene-protein" approach. If a specific DNA sequence of the genome is consistently transmitted, or "linked," with the disease, the approximate chromosomal location of the abnormal gene is revealed (this is discussed in more detail later in this chapter).

Finally, the third approach is to study "candidate" genes, which are already implicated in the pathogenesis or pathophysiology of a particular disease. If a disease has a particular "biological marker" or an associated biological abnormality, it may derive from either an abnormal gene or from a gene "linked" (in close proximity) to it (Pardes et al. 1989). If the genomic region that codes for the biological marker is known, it permits a more direct search for the gene causing the disease (Botstein et al. 1980). Clearly, researchers would prefer to study a trait marker rather than a state marker for the illness of interest. Unfortunately, most biological markers of affective disorders identified thus far are state markers.

Linkage analysis uses a variety of genetic markers. The advances in molecular genetics are exemplified by the landmark paper by Botstein and colleagues (1980), who proposed treating differences in DNA sequences like allelic variants of a gene, and using these variations in DNA as markers to mapping of the genome. These variations in the sequence of nucleotide base pairs between individuals are termed *polymorphisms*. These polymorphisms between individuals or interindividual differences in DNA can be detected by using restriction enzymes from bacteria that recognize and cut at specific nucleic acid sequences within a strand of DNA, thereby producing DNA "restriction fragments" of characteristic lengths.

Polymorphisms—the variations in nucleotide base pair sequences—cause restriction fragments to vary in length. Radiolabeled single strands of DNA ("probes") are then used to bind to homologous sequences of restriction fragment DNA. The radiolabeled probe-restriction fragment combination is known as a restriction fragment length polymorphism (RFLP). The size differences of the RFLPs lead to differential electrophoretic migration (Southern 1975) and are visible as different banding patterns on X-ray film. When an RFLP cosegregates with an illness in members of a family, it could represent a gene mutation or a marker linked to the gene causing the disorder. In this way, the general chromosomal location of a disease-associated gene can be established, and more specific localization can begin. If the messenger RNA derived from the gene has a disease-appropriate neuroanatomical distribution, this increases the likelihood that the gene is a contributor to the psychiatric illness. Putative RFLPs have been identified in bipolar disorder, and it is hoped that the gene defects will be elucidated in the near future.

RFLPs are based on single nucleotide changes. Another polymorphism is known as the variable number of tandem repeats (VNTRs) (also known as "minisatellites") of a relatively short oligonucleotide sequence (Nakamura et al. 1987). In these polymorphisms, the variation in length of the DNA restriction fragments stems from differences in the number of short oligonucleotide sequences found between two adjacent restriction fragment sites. For example, a sequence with 100 base pairs can be repeated multiple times between two adjacent restriction fragment sites. The number of tandem repeats is inherited in Mendelian fashion and typically has numerous alleles (each one defined by a unique number of the repeated sequence). A VNTR locus is genotyped using the identical techniques as for an RFLP locus. Because VNTRs cluster at the ends of chromosomes and are not evenly spaced throughout the human genome (Royle et al. 1988), researchers have used another polymorphism, simple sequence repeat markers.

Simple sequence repeat markers (also known as "microsatellites") are similar to VNTRs, because they are based on a variable number of a sequence of nucleotides repeated in tandem. Unlike VNTRs, microsatellites are abundant and evenly distributed across the human genome (Weber and May 1989). The repeated sequence usually consists of two to five nucleotides (often $—(CA)_n—$, $—(AG)_n—$, or $—(AAAT)_n—$). If this sequence, repeated in tandem, consists of at least 20 uninterrupted units, then the locus is likely to show 60%–70% heterozygosity, based on inherited differences in the number of units repeated in tandem. These short stretches of DNA can be synthesized using the polymerase chain reaction (PCR) technique. The "amplified" amount of microsatellite is then detected by autoradiography, allele size varying according to the number (n) of repeated nucleotide sequences (Berrettini 1992).

Segregation and linkage analysis have not yet produced definitive results in the study of the major affective disorders (Kelsoe 1997). Two teams of investigators have reported two different genes associated with manic-depressive disorder. In a Pennsylvania Amish community, the gene reported to produce manic-depressive disorder was found to be positioned on chromosome 11 and inherited by autosomal dominant transmission (Egeland et al. 1987). Unfortunately, subsequent analysis has not confirmed this finding in an expanded data set of the same population (Kelsoe et al. 1989). Moreover, multiple other groups reported that the chromosome 11 marker was not linked with bipolar disorder (Byerley et al. 1992; Curtis et al. 1993; De Bruyn et al. 1994; Detera-Wadleigh et al. 1987; Ewald et al. 1994; Ginns et al. 1992, 1996; Hodgkinson et al. 1987; Kelsoe et al. 1993; Pauls et al. 1991). In an Israeli population, Baron and colleagues (1987) localized another gene responsible for bipolar disorder on the long arm of the X chromosome; this finding was later retracted (Baron et al. 1993). Other investigators have reported linkage between bipolar disorder and loci (McInnis 1997) on the X chromosome (Bocchetta et al. 1994; Del Zumpo et al. 1984; Knorring et al. 1985; Mendlewicz et al. 1987; Reich et al. 1969), chromosome 6

(Turner and King 1983), chromosome 11 (Egeland et al. 1987), chromosome 5 (Coon et al. 1993), chromosome 12 (Craddock et al. 1994), chromosome 16 (Ewald et al. 1995), chromosome 18 (Berrettini et al. 1994; Freimer et al. 1996; Stine et al. 1995), chromosome 21 (Straub et al. 1994), and chromosome 4 (Blackwood et al. 1996). Taken together, these reports suggest that bipolar illness exhibits *nonallelic genetic heterogeneity*—different genes are affected in different individuals yet produce a similar clinical disorder (Baron et al. 1987, 1993; Detera-Wadleigh et al. 1987; Egeland et al. 1987; Hodgkinson et al. 1987).

Further puzzles arise when *nongenetic* cases of an illness occur in the disease spectrum of depression or bipolar disorder; these nongenetic cases are known as *phenocopies*. Phenocopies present a clinical picture similar to that of a hereditary form; they have been reported in cases of major depression, manic-depressive disorder (Price et al. 1987), and other psychiatric disorders. If nongenetic forms of an illness can be detected and excluded, linkage studies can determine the linked markers that cosegregate with a disease in the remaining pedigrees.

Another obstacle in determining the genetic contribution to an affective illness is the degree of *penetrance* (i.e., the likelihood that the genetic disturbance will be expressed). In monozygotic twins discordant for bipolar disorder, both twins are likely to be at genetic risk, even if bipolar disorder remains unexpressed in the unaffected twin (Pardes et al. 1989).

Yet another conundrum is *variable expressivity*. The gene conferring susceptibility to a major mood disorder may be capable of producing a spectrum of clinical manifestations. One research group has reported that major affective disorder and anorexia nervosa cosegregate in families (Gershon et al. 1983). In relatives of patients with anorexia nervosa, the rate of major affective illness is significantly higher than in the relatives of control subjects; thus, a genetic variant of affective illness may be anorexia nervosa. The statistical techniques of segregation and linkage analyses are limited by several factors. Nevertheless, diagnostic refinement of the subtypes of depression and bipolar mood disorder offers the hope that new biological markers associated with these syndromes may be identified. Phenomenologically defined subsets of patients (with clear-cut presentations such as characteristic age at onset, symptoms, and response to medication) will undoubtedly provide geneticists with more uniform populations with which to modify existing models or produce new, more accurate paradigms regarding the contribution of genetic factors to the development of mood disorders.

NEUROENDOCRINE AND NEUROPEPTIDE HYPOTHESES

Several psychiatric disorders, including the major mood disorders, are associated with specific, highly reproducible neuroendocrine alterations. Conversely, certain endocrine disorders (e.g., hypothyroidism and Cushing's disease) are associated with higher than expected rates of psychiatric morbidity. Neuroendocrine abnormalities have long been thought to provide a unique "window to the brain," revealing clues about the pathophysiology of specific CNS neurotransmitter systems in the particular psychiatric disorder under study. This so-called neuroendocrine window strategy is based on an extensive literature that indicates that the secretion of the peripheral endocrine organs is largely controlled by their respective pituitary trophic hormone. This, pituitary hormone secretion in turn, is controlled primarily by the secretion of the hypothalamic release and release-inhibiting hormones. Unipolar depression (and to a lesser extent bipolar disorder) is associated with multiple endocrine alterations, specifically of the HPA, HPT, and growth hormone axes.

There is now considerable evidence that the secretion of these hypothalamic hypophysiotropic hormones is controlled by many of the classical neurotransmitters such as serotonin, acetylcholine, and norepinephrine, all previously posited to be involved in the pathophysiology of mood as well as anxiety disorders. Also, there is mounting evidence that components of the neuroendocrine axes (e.g., corticotropin-releasing factor [CRF]) may themselves contribute to depressive symptomatology.

Hypothalamic-Pituitary-Adrenal Axis

The HPA axis is the most intensely studied neuroendocrine axis in patients with major depression. Discovered in 1981, CRF is a 41-amino acid-containing peptide that acts as the major physiological regulator of adrenocorticotropic hormone (ACTH) and β-endorphin secretion from the anterior pituitary (Vale et al. 1981), and as such controls HPA axis activity. Within the hypothalamus, CRF-containing neurons project from the paraventricular nucleus to the median eminence (Swanson et al. 1983). Activation of this CRF-containing neural circuit occurs in response to stress, resulting in an increase in synthesis and release of ACTH, β-endorphin, and other pro-opiomelanocortin products. CRF is also found in extrahypothalamic brain regions including the amygdala and cortex.

Numerous reports document HPA axis hyperactivity in drug-free depressed and bipolar depressed patients, in-

cluding CNS (CRF), pituitary (ACTH), and adrenal (glucocorticoid) involvement (Tables 27–1 and 27–2). There is considerable evidence that CRF-containing circuits throughout the nervous system coordinate the endocrine, behavioral, autonomic, and immune responses to stress in mammals.

The hypersecretion of CRF hypothesis of depression is supported by elevated CRF concentrations in CSF, which have been documented in multiple studies of drug-free patients with major depression (Arato et al. 1986; Banki et al. 1987, 1992; France et al. 1988; Nemeroff et al. 1984; Risch et al. 1992) as well as in suicide victims (Arato et al. 1989), although not all studies agree (Roy et al. 1987a). These elevations of CRF concentrations in CSF are believed to be due to central CRF hypersecretion (Post et al. 1982). Raadsheer and colleagues (1994, 1995) reported that depressed patients had increased numbers of hypothalamic CRF neurons and CRF messenger RNA in postmortem tissue when compared with control subjects. In depressed patients, the neuropeptides vasopressin and oxytocin both potentiate CRF-mediated ACTH release (Gillies and Lowry 1979; Yates and Maran 1974). Postmortem examination also found that depressed patients had increased numbers of vasopressin and oxytocin-expressing neurons in the paraventricular nucleus of the hypothalamus in comparison to nondepressed control subjects (Purba et al. 1996).

The increase in CSF CRF concentrations that occurs

Table 27–1. Alterations in the activity of the hypothalamic-pituitary-adrenal (HPA) axis in depression

Increased corticotropin-releasing factor (CRF) in cerebrospinal fluid[a,b]

Blunted adrenocorticotropic hormone (ACTH) and β-endorphin response to CRF stimulation[a]

Decreased density of CRF receptors in frontal cortex of suicide victims

Diminished hippocampal volume

Pituitary gland enlargement in depressed patients[b]

Adrenal gland enlargement in depressed patients[b] and suicide victims

Increased ACTH production during depression

Increased cortisol production during depression[a]

Plasma glucocorticoid, ACTH, and β-endorphin nonsuppression after dexamethasone administration[a]

Increased urinary free cortisol concentrations

[a]State-dependent.
[b]Significantly correlated to postdexamethasone cortisol concentrations.

Table 27–2. Alterations in the activity of the hypothalamic-pituitary-adrenal (HPA) axis in bipolar disorder

---

Increased plasma cortisol concentrations

Blunted diurnal variation of plasma cortisol concentrations

Increased cortisol in cerebrospinal fluid

Nonsuppression of plasma glucocorticoid concentrations after dexamethasone administration

---

during depression is reduced on recovery following electroconvulsive therapy (ECT) (Nemeroff et al. 1991) and treatment with fluoxetine (DeBellis et al. 1993a). Indeed, reduction of CRF concentrations has been reported in healthy volunteers following administration of desipramine (Veith et al. 1992). Thus, elevated CSF CRF concentrations may represent a state marker of depression (Nemeroff et al. 1991a). Furthermore, high or increasing CSF CRF concentrations despite symptomatic improvement of major depression during antidepressant treatment has been reported to be the harbinger of early relapse (Banki et al. 1992) as previously reported for DST nonsuppression (see below). These findings, taken together with a vast literature documenting the depressogenic effects of CRF after direct CNS injection into laboratory animals support the CRF hypersecretion hypothesis of depression.

One sensitive method to assess the activity of the HPA axis is the use of the CRF stimulation test. CRF is administered intravenously (usually in a 1-µg/kg or 100-µg dose), and the ensuing ACTH (or β-endorphin) and cortisol responses are measured at 30-minute intervals over a 2- to 3-hour period (Hermus et al. 1984; Watson et al. 1986). In drug-free depressed patients, the ACTH and β-endorphin response to exogenously administered ovine CRF (oCRF) is blunted compared with that of nondepressed subjects (Amsterdam et al. 1987; P. W. Gold et al. 1984, 1986; Holsboer et al. 1984a; Kathol et al. 1989; Young et al. 1990). This phenomenon has been shown to occur in depressed DST nonsuppressors but not in DST suppressors (Krishnan et al. 1993). The attenuated ACTH response to CRH is likely due, at least in part, to chronic hypersecretion of CRF from the nerve terminals in the median eminence. This results in downregulation of anterior pituitary CRF-receptor density with resultant decreased pituitary responsivity to CRF, as has previously been demonstrated in laboratory animals (Aguilera et al. 1986; Holmes et al. 1987; Wynn et al. 1983, 1984, 1988). Furthermore, decreased density of CRF receptors in the frontal cortex has been reported in postmortem studies of suicide victims (Nemeroff et al. 1988b).

One variant of the standard CRF stimulation test that has been studied in detail is the combined dexamethasone/CRF test. Patients receive dexamethasone orally (1.0 or 1.5 mg) at 11:00 P.M. followed by CRF (100 µg infused intravenously) the next day. Holsboer and his colleagues (Holsboer et al. 1987; Holsboer-Trachsler et al. 1991; Schmider et al. 1995; von Bardeleben and Holsboer 1989) have shown that depressed patients have markedly increased ACTH and cortisol responses to CRF after dexamethasone administration when compared with control subjects. This test is thought to reveal the impaired negative feedback of glucocorticoids on the HPA axis.

Not only do hormonal measures of the HPA axis show evidence of hyperactivity in depression, but structural changes have been reported as well. Perhaps at least partly in response to the hypersecretion of CRF, the pituitary gland enlarges in depressed patients (Krishnan et al. 1991); this response is significantly correlated to postdexamethasone cortisol concentrations (Axelson et al. 1992). Another morphological change, enlargement of the adrenal gland, has been reported in suicide victims postmortem (Zis and Zis 1987) and in depressed patients by use of computed tomography (CT) (Amsterdam et al. 1987; Nemeroff et al. 1992). This enlargement is most likely secondary to chronic ACTH hypersecretion. Indeed, ACTH plasma concentrations are significantly increased in depressed patients in comparison to age-matched nondepressed control subjects (Deuschle et al. 1997). The adrenal gland enlargement in depressed patients, like other measures of HPA axis hyperactivity, diminishes after recovery from depression as assessed with magnetic resonance imaging (MRI) (Rubin et al. 1995).

Adrenal hypertrophy probably explains the fact that, unlike the blunted ACTH and β-endorphin response to CRF, the plasma cortisol response in depressed patients and nondepressed control subjects does not differ (Amsterdam et al. 1987; P. W. Gold et al. 1984, 1986; Holsboer et al. 1984b; Kathol et al. 1989; Young et al. 1990). Thus, for each pulse of ACTH, depressed patients with an enlarged adrenal cortex would be expected to secrete greater quantities of cortisol than would nondepressed control subjects. Adrenocortical hypertrophy could also explain the heightened cortisol response to pharmacological doses of ACTH (Amsterdam et al. 1983; Jaeckle et al. 1987; Kalin et al. 1982; Krishnan et al. 1990b; Linkowski et al. 1985).

Another indication of HPA axis hyperactivity in depression is cortisol hypersecretion, which is reflected in elevated plasma corticosteroid concentrations (Carpenter and Bunney 1971; J. L. Gibbons and McHugh 1962), increased levels of cortisol metabolites (Sachar et al. 1970), elevated 24-hour urinary free cortisol concentrations, and nonsuppression of plasma hydroxycorticosteroid levels after the administration of dexamethasone (the DST). Since Carroll's initial report (1968) and subsequent claims for diagnostic utility (Carroll 1982), the DST has generated considerable controversy (Arana and Mossman 1988). The rate of cortisol nonsuppression after dexamethasone administration generally has been found to be correlated with the severity of the subtype of depression (i.e., nearly all patients with major depression with psychotic features show DST nonsuppression) (Arana et al. 1985; Evans and Nemeroff 1983a; Krishnan et al. 1985; Schatzberg et al. 1984). Moreover, DST nonsuppressors also have elevated CRF concentrations in CSF (Pitts et al. 1990; Roy et al. 1987a).

One factor that may partially contribute to DST nonsuppression is the more rapid metabolism of dexamethasone that occurs in depressed patients (Ritchie et al. 1990). In summary, the many reports of HPA hyperactivity in drug-free depressed patients could be explained by hypersecretion of CRF during and/or immediately preceding a depressive episode, with secondary pituitary and adrenal gland hypertrophy. The DST usually normalizes after recovery from depression (Carroll 1968; Nemeroff and Evans 1984), and this test may help predict early relapse or poor prognosis (Arana et al. 1985). DST nonsuppression, like hypercortisolemia (Sachar et al. 1970), hypersecretion of CRF (Nemeroff et al. 1991a), blunting of the ACTH response to CRF (Amsterdam et al. 1988), and adrenal gland hypertrophy (Rubin et al. 1995), appears to be state dependent. The CRF hypothesis of depression has led to the development of a number of CRF-receptor antagonists to be used as novel antidepressants.

Alterations of the HPA axis have also been documented in patients with bipolar affective disorder (Kiriike et al. 1988; Stokes and Sikes 1987). This increased HPA activity has been associated with mixed manic states (Evans and Nemeroff 1983b; Krishnan et al. 1983; Swann et al. 1992), mania (Godwin et al. 1984; Linkowski et al. 1994), and depression in rapid-cycling patients (Kennedy et al. 1989) (Table 27–2).

Investigation of other CNS peptides that affect the HPA axis has proceeded as well, including the neurohypophyseal hormone vasopressin. Arginine vasopressin, a nonapeptide that stimulates ACTH secretion (Landon et al. 1965), also potentiates release of ACTH stimulated by CRF (Von Bardeleben et al. 1985). Unlike the ACTH response to CRF, the ACTH response to arginine vasopressin is unchanged in depression (Carroll et al. 1993). (For a discussion of the interaction of the amines and the HPA axis, see the following sections on norepinephrine, acetylcholine, and serotonin.)

Hypothalamic-Pituitary-Thyroid Axis

The HPT axis has also been closely scrutinized in patients with mood disorders. Hypothyroidism has long been known to be frequently associated with a markedly depressed mood. Moreover, many patients with rapid-cycling bipolar disorder have evidence of hypothyroidism, with some responding to thyroid hormone treatment (Bauer and Whybrow 1990a, 1990b; Cowdry et al. 1983). Use of thyroid hormone supplementation (usually T_3) has been reported to increase the rapidity of action of TCAs (Prange et al. 1969, 1980) and is as effective as lithium in converting depressed TCA nonresponders into responders (Joffe et al. 1993).

Discovered in 1970, thyrotropin-releasing hormone (TRH) is a tripeptide (pGlu-His-Pro-NH_2) found in the hypothalamus, where it acts as a hypothalamic hypophysiotropic hormone. Released from the median eminence, TRH is transported in the vessels of the hypothalamo-hypophyseal portal system to the anterior pituitary. At the adenohypophysis, TRH binds to the TRH receptors on the pituitary thyrotrophs, increasing the synthesis and release of thyroid-stimulating hormone (TSH) by activation of the phosphatidylinositol hydrolysis second-messenger system. Released into the general circulation, TSH binds to TSH receptors in the thyroid gland and causes the release of the thyroid hormones T_3 and thyroxine (T_4). In turn, thyroid hormones act at the anterior pituitary to inhibit TSH release and at the hypothalamus to inhibit the synthesis and secretion of TRH. TRH is widely distributed in extrahypothalamic brain areas, where it likely functions as a CNS neurotransmitter. Thyroid hormone receptors are also widely distributed throughout the mammalian brain. Thyroid hormone is necessary for normal neuronal development, and its absence leads to permanent brain damage (Dussault and Ruel 1987). Depression has been conceptualized as a disorder consisting of, or including, relative hypothyroidism within the CNS (Bauer and Whybrow 1988) accompanied by systemic euthyroidism (Jackson 1996). The active thyroid hormone in the brain, T_3, is converted locally from T_4 by brain Type II 5´-deiodinase (Visser et al. 1982). Inhibition of brain Type II 5´-deiodinase by cortisol (Hindal and Kaplan 1988), as might occur in some depressed patients, would enhance T_4 conversion to reverse T_3 (rT_3) by Type III deiodinase (Kaplan 1984). Indeed, increased CSF concentrations of rT_3 have been reported (V. M. Linnoila et al. 1983a) in patients with unipolar depression. Furthermore, treatment with desipramine (Campos-Barros et al. 1994) or fluoxetine (Baumgartner 1994) markedly increases Type II 5´-deiodinase activity throughout the rat brain leading to an increase in T_3 tissue concentrations (Baumgartner 1994).

The initial report of elevated CSF concentrations of TRH in depressed patients was published almost 20 years ago (Kirkegaard et al. 1979) and was subsequently confirmed by Banki and colleagues (1988), although discordant results exist (Roy et al. 1994). Elevated CSF concentrations of TRH are believed to be a reflection of increased extracellular fluid concentrations of the tripeptide, probably the result of central TRH hypersecretion (Post et al. 1982). The increase in pituitary gland size reported in depressed patients (Krishnan et al. 1991) may be due in part to TRH hypersecretion. Hatterer and colleagues (1993) reported low CSF concentrations of the thyroid transport globulin, transthyretin, in treatment-refractory depressed patients, suggesting that this might be one factor in "CNS hypothyroidism" and high CNS TRH concentrations.

Considered one of the most sensitive measures of HPT function, the TSH response to TRH (200–500 µg intravenously) is greater than normal in patients with primary hypothyroidism and attenuated in patients with primary hyperthyroidism. More than 20 years ago, approximately 25% of patients with major depression were reported to have a blunted TSH response to TRH (Kastin et al. 1972; Prange et al. 1972; Takahashi et al. 1973). This response was not due to hypersecretion of somatostatin; in fact, depressed patients consistently have been shown to have reduced CSF concentrations of somatostatin compared with nondepressed control subjects (Bissette et al. 1986; Rubinow et al. 1983). The blunted TSH response to exogenously administered TRH has been posited to be caused by chronic hypersecretion of TRH from the median eminence (i.e., elevated TRH release from the hypothalamus, producing downregulation of anterior pituitary TRH receptors), with resultant diminished anterior pituitary responsiveness to TRH. Following chronic administration of TRH, blunting of the TSH response to TRH has been observed in rats (Nemeroff et al. 1980). Adinoff and colleagues (1991) found an inverse relationship between the blunted TSH response to TRH and CSF TRH concentrations in 13 drug-free male alcoholic subjects. Moreover, Maeda and colleagues (1993) reported that repeated TRH administration in humans produces the blunted TSH response to TRH observed in depressed patients. Interestingly, Marangell and colleagues (1997) reported rapid improvement in mood in five of eight patients with refractory depression following intrathecal injection of 500 µg of protirelin (TSH). Studies documenting TRH hypersecretion and TRH receptor downregulation in human postmortem tissue are needed.

The maximal circadian secretion of TSH by pituitary thyrotrophs between 11:00 P.M. and 1:00 A.M. (Patel et al. 1972; Vanhaelst et al. 1972) has been used to improve the sensitivity of HPT measures in depression when compared with the standard TRH stimulation test (Table 27–3). Duval and colleagues (1990) performed a standard TRH (200 µg) stimulation test on subjects at 8:00 A.M. and 11:00 P.M. The difference between the 11:00 P.M. ΔTSH and the 8:00 A.M. ΔTSH, designated the ΔΔTSH, is markedly lower in depressed patients when compared with control subjects, with a diagnostic specificity of 95% and a diagnostic sensitivity of 89%. In a recent study of 30 depressed euthyroid patients, Duval and colleagues (1996) reported that the depressed patients with the lowest pretreatment 11:00 P.M. basal and TRH-stimulated TSH plasma concentrations showed the lowest rate of clinical response to antidepressant treatment. Another purportedly more sensitive indicator of depression than the TRH stimulation test is diminished nocturnal plasma TSH concentrations (Bartalena et al. 1990; Goldstein et al. 1980; Weeke and Weeke 1980).

In contradistinction to the blunted TSH response to TRH, 15% of depressed patients have an exaggerated TSH response to TRH (Extein et al. 1981). Patients with normal levels of T_3, T_4, and TSH who have an exaggerated TSH response to TRH are defined as having grade III hypothyroidism (Table 27–4). (In grade I hypothyroidism, plasma concentrations of T_3 and T_4 are decreased, plasma TSH concentrations are elevated because of the loss of the negative feedback on the pituitary, and the TSH response to TRH is markedly exaggerated. In grade II hypothyroidism, plasma concentrations of thyroid hormones are normal, but basal plasma TSH concentration is elevated, and the TSH response to TRH is exaggerated.)

Depressed patients have also been repeatedly shown

Table 27–3. Alterations in the activity of the hypothalamic-pituitary-thyroid (HPT) axis in depression

Increased thyrotropin-releasing hormone (TRH) in cerebrospinal fluid

Decreased nocturnal plasma thyroid-stimulating hormone (TSH) concentrations

Blunted TSH response to TRH stimulation[a]

Exaggerated TSH response to TRH stimulation

Decreased ΔΔTSH (difference between 11:00 P.M. ΔTSH and 8:00 A.M. ΔTSH after TRH administration)

Presence of antimicrosomal thyroid and/or antithyroglobulin antibodies[b]

[a]State-dependent.
[b]Correlated to postdexamethasone cortisol concentrations.

Table 27–4. Grades of hypothyroidism

Grade	T_3, T_4	Basal TSH	TSH response to TRH	Antithyroid antibodies
I	Decreased	Increased	Increased	Often present
II	Normal	Increased	Increased	Often present
III	Normal	Normal	Increased	Often present
IV	Normal	Normal	Normal	Present

Note. T_3 = triiodothyronine; T_4 = thyroxine; TRH = thyrotropin-releasing hormone; TSH = thyroid-stimulating hormone.

to have a higher than expected occurrence of symptomless autoimmune thyroiditis, as defined by the abnormal presence of circulating antimicrosomal thyroid or antithyroglobulin antibodies (M. S. Gold et al. 1982; Nemeroff et al. 1985; Reus et al. 1986). Depressed women with symptomless autoimmune thyroiditis and diffuse nontoxic goiter were more likely to have a reduced response to TRH administration than were depressed women without thyroid disease (Bunevicius et al. 1996). Moreover, the incidence of symptomless autoimmune thyroiditis is higher (i.e., 50%) in depressed patients who are DST nonsuppressors (Haggerty et al. 1987; Reus et al. 1986). These patients may be designated as having grade IV hypothyroidism (Table 27–4)—i.e., they have positive antithyroid antibodies but normal T_3, T_4, TSH, and TRH-induced TSH response (Haggerty et al. 1990).

Abnormalities of the HPT axis (e.g., hypothyroidism) have also been reported in patients with bipolar disorder, as demonstrated by an exaggerated TSH response to TRH and elevated basal plasma concentrations of TSH (Haggerty et al. 1987; Loosen and Prange 1982). In fact, two groups have reported a higher prevalence rate of hypothyroidism (grades I, II, and III) in bipolar patients who experience rapid cycling of their mood than in bipolar patients who do not (Bauer et al. 1990a; Cowdry et al. 1983). Other abnormalities of the thyroid axis have been documented in bipolar patients, including a blunted TSH response to TRH, a blunted or absent nocturnal surge in concentrations of plasma TSH (Sack et al. 1988; Souetre et al. 1988), and a higher than expected prevalence of antithyroid microsomal or antithyroglobulin antibodies (Lazarus et al. 1986; Myers et al. 1985) (Table 27–5). The presence of antithyroid antibodies is apparently not a result of lithium treatment, but lithium can exacerbate the process (Calabrese et al. 1985).

Hypothalamic–Growth Hormone Axis

Mood disorders are also associated with alterations in the activity of the growth hormone axis. Growth hormone is synthesized and secreted from the somatotrophs of the anterior pituitary. Its secretion is modulated by two hypothalamic hypophysiotropic hormones, growth-hormone–releasing factor (GRF) and somatostatin, as well as by the classical neurotransmitters (e.g., dopamine, norepinephrine, and serotonin) that innervate the GRF-containing neurons. Located primarily in the arcuate nucleus of the hypothalamus, GRF stimulates the synthesis and release of growth hormone. Inhibition of growth hormone release is mediated primarily by somatostatin, which is found predominantly in the periventricular nucleus of the hypothalamus. Unlike GRF, somatostatin is also widely distributed in extrahypothalamic brain regions, including the cerebral cortex, hippocampus, and amygdala. Both GRF and somatostatin are released from nerve terminals in the median eminence and transported via the hypothalamic-pituitary portal system to act on the growth hormone–producing somatotrophs of the anterior pituitary.

Release of growth hormone is stimulated by L-dopa (Boyd et al. 1970), a dopamine precursor, and by apomorphine, a centrally active dopamine agonist (Lal et al. 1975). Growth hormone release also occurs following the administration of the serotonin precursors L-tryptophan and 5-hydroxytryptophan) (Imura et al. 1973; Muller et al. 1974). The serotonin receptor antagonists methysergide and cyproheptadine interfere with the growth hormone response to hypoglycemia (Toivola et al. 1972). Under normal basal conditions, growth hormone is secreted in pulses that are highest during the initial hours of the night

Table 27–5. Alterations in the activity of the hypothalamic-pituitary-thyroid (HPT) axis in bipolar disorder

Blunted plasma thyroid-stimulating hormone (TSH) response to thyrotropin-releasing hormone (TRH) stimulation

Exaggerated plasma TSH response to TRH stimulation

Blunted or absent nocturnal surge in plasma TSH concentration

Presence of antimicrosomal thyroid and/or antithyroglobulin antibodies

(Finkelstein et al. 1972). In depressed patients, multiple findings indicate dysregulation of the secretion of growth hormone (Table 27–6); nocturnal growth hormone secretion is diminished in these individuals (Schilkrut et al. 1975), whereas in unipolar and bipolar depressed patients, daylight growth hormone secretion is exaggerated (Mendlewicz et al. 1985). Furthermore, multiple studies have reported a marked attenuation of the growth hormone response to clonidine (and, to a lesser extent, apomorphine) in depressed patients (Charney et al. 1982; Checkley et al. 1981; Matussek et al. 1980; Siever et al. 1982). (For further discussion, see the section on adrenergic receptors.)

Growth hormone response to stimulation by GRF has been scrutinized in depressed patients in a limited number of studies, and the results are discordant. Three research groups have reported a diminished growth hormone response to GRF in depressed patients (Contreras et al. 1996; Lesch et al. 1987a, 1987b; Risch 1991). However, Krishnan and colleagues (1988) found minimal differences between depressed patients and nondepressed control subjects in the plasma concentrations of growth hormone following GRF stimulation. These discordant findings could be explained by various other factors that can influence the growth hormone response to GRF, including gender, age, menstrual cycle, plasma glucocorticoid or somatomedin concentrations, and body weight (Casanueva et al. 1988, 1990; Krishnan et al. 1988). Further studies using GRF will assist in the development of a standard GRF stimulation test and further clarify the response of growth hormone to GRF in depressed patients. Somatostatin, the tetradecapeptide hypothalamic growth hormone release–inhibiting hormone, inhibits secretion of both CRF and ACTH (M. R. Brown et al. 1984; Heisler et al. 1982; Richardson and Schonbrunn 1981). Remarkably, as noted above, in several studies CSF concentrations of

somatostatin have been reported to be reduced in depressed patients (Agren and Lundqvist 1984; Bissette et al. 1986; Gerner and Yamada 1982; Rubinow et al. 1983, 1984). These decreased CSF concentrations of somatostatin correlate inversely with postdexamethasone plasma cortisol concentrations (Rubinow 1986); in fact, exogenous glucocorticoids reduce CSF somatostatin concentrations (Wolkowitz et al. 1987). Glucocorticoids likely inhibit somatostatinergic neurons within the anterior and periventricular hypothalamus because dexamethasone administration stimulates growth hormone release in nondepressed control subjects (Casaneuva et al. 1990). Dexamethasone-induced growth hormone secretion is significantly decreased in depressed patients (Thakore and Dinan 1994).

In patients with bipolar disorder, blunting of noradrenergic-stimulated growth hormone secretion has been observed during mania (Dinan et al. 1991). Table 27–6 summarizes the alterations of the hypothalamic-growth hormone axis in depression.

Hypothalamic-Pituitary-Gonadal Axis

Despite the higher incidence of depression in women and the purportedly increased occurrence of depression during and after menopause, data are limited on hypothalamic-pituitary-gonadal (HPG) axis function in patients with mood disorders. As with the HPA and HPT axes, the HPG axis is organized in a "hierarchical" fashion. Driven by a pulse generator in the arcuate nucleus of the hypothalamus, gonadotropin-releasing hormone (GnRH) secretion occurs in a pulsatile fashion (Knobil 1990). GnRH causes secretion of luteinizing hormone and follicle-stimulating hormone from gonadotrophs in the anterior pituitary (Midgely and Jaffe 1971). The ebb and flow of luteinizing hormone concentration in the peripheral circulation are used as an indication of pulses of GnRH secretion (Clarke and Cummins 1982) because peripheral plasma concentrations of GnRH, like that of TRH and CRF, cannot be reliably assessed (Meller et al. 1997). In the follicular phase of the menstrual cycle, luteinizing hormone pulses of nearly constant amplitude occur with regular frequency (i.e., every 1–2 hours) (Reame et al. 1984). In the luteal phase, luteinizing hormone pulse amplitude (reflecting GnRH secretion) is more variable, with pulse frequency declining to one pulse every 2–6 hours (Jaffe et al. 1990). Through negative feedback, gonadal steroids inhibit the secretion of GnRH from the hypothalamus as well as the secretion of luteinizing hormone and follicle-stimulating hormone from the pituitary. GnRH secretion is also inhibited by CRF (Jaffe et al.

Table 27–6. Alterations in the activity of the growth hormone axis in depression

Decreased nocturnal growth hormone

Increased daylight growth hormone secretion (unipolar and bipolar)

Decreased growth hormone response to clonidine and apomorphine

? Decreased growth hormone response to growth-hormone–releasing factor

Decreased somatostatin in cerebrospinal fluid[a]

[a]Significantly correlated to postdexamethasone cortisol concentrations.

1990) and β-endorphin (Ferin and Van de Wiele 1984).

In early studies, no significant differences were reported in plasma concentrations of luteinizing hormone and follicle-stimulating hormone in depressed postmenopausal women compared with nondepressed matched control subjects (Sachar et al. 1972). However, in a later study, plasma luteinizing hormone concentrations were decreased in depressed postmenopausal women compared with matched control subjects (Brambilla et al. 1990). Furthermore, depressed *pre*menopausal women show increased amplitude pulses of luteinizing hormone in a nonrhythmic fashion in comparison to nondepressed women of similar age (Meller et al. 1997).

Rather than measure baseline plasma levels of the pituitary gonadotropins in depressed patients, other investigators have studied the response of the pituitary to exogenous administration of GnRH. Normal luteinizing hormone and follicle-stimulating hormone responses to a high dose of GnRH (i.e., 250 μg) have been reported in male depressed and female depressed (pre- and postmenopausal) patients (Winokur et al. 1982), whereas a decreased luteinizing hormone response to a lower dose of GnRH (150 μg) has been reported in pre- and postmenopausal depressed patients (Brambilla et al. 1990). In a depressed cohort including both sexes (analyses of men and premenopausal versus postmenopausal depressed women were not separately performed), Unden and colleagues (1988) observed no change in baseline or TRH/luteinizing hormone-releasing hormone (LHRH)-stimulated luteinizing hormone or follicle-stimulating hormone concentrations (200 μg TRH and 100 μg LHRH combined, intravenously). Notably, plasma luteinizing hormone concentrations are increased in those individuals who have recovered from a manic state—possibly a trait phenomenon (Whalley et al. 1987).

As reviewed by Leibenluft and colleagues (1994), many measures of HPA, HPT, and human growth hormone axis activity do not fluctuate predictably during the menstrual cycle. However, estrogen and progesterone do exert important actions on certain elements of the HPA axis in women. Estrogen stimulates production of corticosteroid-binding globulin, thereby decreasing concentrations of unbound and pharmacologically active cortisol, whereas progesterone functions as a glucocorticoid receptor antagonist. In postmenopausal depressed women, dexamethasone nonsuppression is more common and occurs with lower plasma cortisol concentrations in comparison to premenopausal depressed women. Thus, ovarian steroids may play a protective role in depressed premenopausal women against elevated circulating glucocorticoids as might be seen during episodes of major depression effects (Young 1995). Additional research on the HPG axis in depression is clearly warranted.

Pineal Function and Circadian Rhythm

The pineal gland, which is regulated by sympathetic adrenergic input, produces the hormone melatonin, a marker for human circadian rhythm. The light/dark cycle synchronizes circadian melatonin secretion, with light acting as a suppressant. Seasonal changes of the duration of light and dark throughout the year produce corresponding changes in melatonin regulation. Alterations in the circadian rhythms of sleep and body temperature as well as plasma melatonin, prolactin, and cortisol concentrations have been reported in depressed patients. These may occur because of desynchronization of rhythms or phase advancement of certain rhythms in affective disorders.

The nocturnal secretion of melatonin is primarily induced by increased noradrenergic neurotransmission, resulting in increased activity of N-acetyltransferase, the rate-limiting step in conversion of serotonin to melatonin. Several studies have found reduced nocturnal output of melatonin in depressed patients (Boyce 1985; Nair and Hariharasubramanian 1984). Beck-Friis and colleagues (1985) reported that depressed patients with abnormal DST results have lower melatonin levels than those with normal DST results. This suggests that low melatonin states in depression occur in conjunction with HPA axis hyperactivity, but these data have not yet been replicated. Indeed, in a study of 38 depressed patients, Rubin and colleagues (1992) reported a trend toward elevated average nocturnal melatonin secretion, primarily accounted for in the study by 14 premenopausal subjects. Melatonin measures were not consistently related to HPA axis measures.

ROLE OF NEUROTRANSMITTERS AND RECEPTORS

The basic neurobiology of various neurotransmitters is discussed in detail in Wilcox et al., Chapter 1, and Mansour et al., Chapter 3, in this volume. Various approaches have been taken to the study of neurotransmitter function in humans with affective illnesses. These techniques include measurement of levels of neurotransmitters and their metabolites in peripheral blood and CSF, as well as in postmortem brain tissue; direct study of neurotransmitter receptors in platelets, leukocytes, and cell cultures of fibroblasts, as well as in postmortem brain; neuroendocrine and intracellular responses to receptor agonists and antagonists; and in vivo assessment of neurotransmitter receptors via brain imaging.

Norepinephrine and Adrenergic Receptors

Two primary components central to the "fight or flight" stress response observed by Cannon in 1911 (Vingerhoets 1985) and the "general adaptation syndrome" described by Selye (1936) are the HPA axis and the sympathoadrenal system. As noted earlier in this chapter, the catecholamine hypothesis of affective disorders proposes that some forms of depression are associated with a deficiency of catecholamine activity (particularly norepinephrine) at functionally important adrenergic receptor sites in the brain, whereas mania is associated with a relative excess (Schildkraut 1965).

The adrenal medulla and the sympathetic nervous system (SNS) together constitute the sympathoadrenal system. Many patients with major depression show dysregulation of the sympathoadrenal system. Although the CNS regulation of the sympathoadrenal system is only partially understood, CRF-containing neurons within the hypothalamus provide stimulatory input to the several autonomic centers involved in regulating peripheral sympathetic activity (Cummings et al. 1983; Merchenthaler et al. 1982; Swanson et al. 1983). Nerve impulses from CNS regulatory centers control catecholamine release from the SNS *and* the adrenal medulla. Physiological and pathological conditions causing sympathoadrenal activation in vivo include physical activity, acute coronary ischemia and heart failure, insulin-induced hypoglycemia, and even mental stress. Epinephrine in plasma is derived from the adrenal medulla, whereas plasma norepinephrine concentrations reflect its secretion largely from sympathetic nerve terminals, with the remaining norepinephrine provided from the adrenal medulla and extra-adrenal chromaffin cells. Peripheral plasma norepinephrine concentrations are determined not only by its rate of release from SNS nerve terminals but also by its reuptake into presynaptic terminals, local metabolic degradation, and redistribution into multiple physiological compartments.

Elevated CSF concentrations of the major metabolite of CNS norepinephrine, 3-methoxy-4-hydroxyphenylglycol (MHPG) (Schildkraut 1965), have been observed in patients with depression, mania, and schizoaffective disorder but not in schizophrenic patients (Sharma et al. 1994). DeBellis and colleagues (1993b) reported that CSF MHPG levels for nine depressed patients, although no different from those of control subjects, decreased significantly after treatment with the serotonergic antidepressant fluoxetine. More recent studies have documented that fluvoxamine or fluoxetine treatment of depression is associated with significant reductions of CSF MHPG (as well as 5-HIAA) concentrations, confirming the notion that even selective serotonergic antidepressants ultimately affect the noradrenergic system (Sheline et al. 1997).

Hypersecretion of norepinephrine in unipolar depression has also been documented by elevated plasma norepinephrine and norepinephrine metabolite concentrations (Louis et al. 1975; Roy et al. 1988; Veith et al. 1994; Wyatt et al. 1971) and elevated urinary concentrations of norepinephrine and its metabolites. Depressed patients have higher basal plasma concentrations of norepinephrine; however, those with melancholia have even greater elevations in plasma norepinephrine levels when subjected to orthostatic challenge than do either nondepressed control subjects or depressed patients without melancholia (Roy et al. 1987b). Furthermore, depressed patients who are DST nonsuppressors have significantly higher basal and cold-stimulated levels of norepinephrine than do depressed patients who are DST suppressors (Roy et al. 1987b). Following treatment with TCAs, urinary excretion of norepinephrine and its metabolites diminishes with plasma norepinephrine concentrations (Charney et al. 1981; Golden et al. 1988; M. Linnoila et al. 1982, 1986; Scubee-Moreau and Dresse 1979; Sulser et al. 1978). Thus, sympathoadrenal hyperactivity appears to represent a state, rather than a trait, marker of depression, possibly secondary to increased CRF release from CNS neurons.

Bipolar patients have significantly elevated plasma norepinephrine and epinephrine concentrations during manic episodes than during depression or euthymia (Maj et al. 1984). Indeed, manic patients also exhibit significantly increased urinary concentrations of norepinephrine in comparison to depressed patients or control subjects (Swann et al. 1987). In a later study, Swann and colleagues (1990) noted that an individual's "environmental sensitivity" had a significant effect on urinary norepinephrine excretion. Manic patients whose episodes were environmentally sensitive demonstrated elevated norepinephrine excretion, compared with patients with manic episodes that were unrelated to external stressors.

Table 27–7 summarizes the known major alterations of the norepinephrine system reported in depression.

Much research has emphasized the quantitation of catecholamine metabolites to discriminate among subtypes of depressed patients. Overall, with regard to urinary excretion of MHPG, unipolar depressed patients are more heterogeneous than are bipolar I patients, in that unipolar patients exhibit MHPG urinary concentrations over a wide range of values (Maas et al. 1972). Plasma and urinary concentrations of MHPG were significantly elevated in bipolar patients when they were manic compared with the

Table 27–7. Alterations in the norepinephrine system in depression

Increased or decreased 3-methoxy-4-hydroxyphenylglycol (MHPG)

Increased α_2-adrenergic binding in platelets

Blunted growth hormone response to clonidine

Increased β-adrenergic receptors in postmortem brain of suicide victims

? Downregulation of β-adrenergic receptors after treatment

MHPG concentrations when these patients were depressed (Halaris 1978). Indeed, bipolar depressed patients demonstrated significantly more diminished urinary MHPG concentrations than did unipolar depressed patients or healthy control subjects (Schildkraut et al. 1978a). More recent studies indicate that reduced urinary MHPG concentrations are characteristic of bipolar I depressed patients but not of bipolar II depressed patients, with MHPG levels similar to those of patients with unipolar depression (Muscettola et al. 1984; Schatzberg et al. 1989). Patients with unipolar depression generally have greater urinary MHPG concentrations than do bipolar I patients. Plasma concentrations of MHPG have also been reported to be increased in unipolar depressed patients in comparison to those with bipolar depression (Roy et al. 1986). However, urinary MHPG concentrations are diminished in some unipolar patients. Preliminary data suggest that these patients may be more likely to develop hypomania or mania than unipolar patients with high MHPG concentrations (Schatzberg et al. 1989).

MHPG urinary concentrations may assist in biochemical classification of unipolar depressed patients (Schatzberg et al. 1982; Schildkraut et al. 1981). The subtype with reduced MHPG levels may have diminished norepinephrine output or release. These individuals appear to respond well to antidepressants (such as imipramine), which inhibit neuronal uptake of norepinephrine, in comparison to patients with high urinary MHPG concentrations (Hollister et al. 1980; Maas et al. 1972, 1984; Schatzberg et al. 1985b), but this finding has not always been replicated (Janicak et al. 1986).

Schildkraut and colleagues (1978b) reported that discriminant function analysis of urinary catecholamines and metabolites yielded a depression-type (D-type) score that more clearly separated unipolar nonendogenous depressions from bipolar depressions than did urinary MHPG levels alone. In a subsequent report (Schatzberg et al. 1989), D-type scores provided greater sensitivity and specificity in differentiating among depressed patients with bipolar or schizoaffective disorder and those indi-

viduals with unipolar depression and all other depressions than were seen using individual catecholamine and metabolite measures or the sum of the catecholamines and their metabolites. Specifically, bipolar I depressed patients demonstrated significantly lower D-type scores than did subjects with all other depressive subtypes, including those with bipolar type II depression. D-type scores in patients with bipolar II disorders were similar to those in individuals with unipolar depression. D-type scores also have been reported to provide more precise discrimination between responders and nonresponders than do urinary MHPG levels alone (Mooney et al. 1991).

The relationship between sympathoadrenal and HPA axis activity has also been an active area of investigation in patients with major depression. Investigators have reported significant positive correlations between urinary cortisol and urinary MHPG concentrations in depressed patients (Rosenbaum et al. 1983; Schatzberg et al. 1989; Stokes et al. 1981), although not all reports agree (Maes et al. 1987). A similar positive correlation has been reported for plasma cortisol and epinephrine concentrations (Stokes et al. 1981). Both manic and depressed patients with high urinary MHPG concentrations likely have high norepinephrine turnover. Such patients often demonstrate elevated cortisol levels and respond poorly to fluoxetine as well as to those TCAs with predominantly noradrenergic reuptake inhibition (Schildkraut et al. 1984). More recent studies indicate that urinary concentrations of MHPG may predict clinical response to treatment (Mooney et al. 1988; Rosenbaum et al. 1992; Schatzberg et al. 1992; Sharma et al. 1990).

In the noradrenergic system, α_2 receptors have been the subject of considerable investigation. α_2 Receptors exist on both pre- and postsynaptic elements that inhibit the adenylate cyclase system; conversely, the α_1 receptor is not coupled to the adenylate cyclase system but is linked to processes that regulate cellular calcium ion fluxes. The presynaptic α_2 receptor has an inhibitory effect on the release of norepinephrine in the brain. Increased numbers of α_2 receptor binding sites in platelets in depressed patients have been observed (Halaris and Piletz 1990) as well as increased α_2 receptor density in the brains of suicide victims (Meana et al. 1992). Treatment with antidepressants has been associated with decreases in the density and sensitivity of these receptors on platelets.

Several methods have been used to investigate the role of the α_2 receptor in depression. An indirect method for studying α_2 receptors is to challenge subjects with the α_2 receptor agonist clonidine. Administration of clonidine induces growth hormone secretion, primarily through postsynaptic α_2 receptors. Several abnormalities in growth hormone release in patients with major depression have been reported (see Table 27–6). Growth hormone response to clonidine is blunted in unipolar depressed patients (Matussek et al. 1980; Siever et al. 1984), supporting the concept of decreased responsiveness of postsynaptic α_2-adrenergic receptors in depressed patients. Siever and colleagues (1992) reported that the growth hormone response to clonidine was significantly blunted in both acute and remitted depressed patients compared with control subjects, suggesting that the blunted growth hormone response to clonidine may be a trait marker in some forms of depression. The significance of this finding vis-à-vis α_2 receptor activity is not entirely clear. Clonidine binds to a nonadrenergic imidazoline site on platelets, and growth hormone responses to clonidine may involve other neural systems as well (e.g., somatostatin).

Another method of examining the function of α_2 receptors is to measure intracellular response following α_2 receptor activation. Activation of the α_2 receptor inhibits adenylate cyclase and produces a decrease in cyclic adenosine monophosphate (cAMP) concentrations, which mediates several physiological responses, including platelet aggregation. Some depressed patients demonstrate decreased platelet responsivity to epinephrine (Mooney et al. 1988). Moreover, norepinephrine stimulation of prostaglandin E1-α_2 receptor-coupled adenylate cyclase activity is generally reduced in depressed patients (Siever et al. 1984). Garcia-Sevilla and colleagues (1990) measured the functional status of α_2 receptors in depressed patients by assessing both inhibition of adenylate cyclase activity and induction of platelet aggregation. They concluded that the latter measure was a better marker to assess changes in the α_2 receptor in depressed patients.

The β_1- and β_2-adrenergic receptor subtypes are found postsynaptically and also stimulate the intracellular adenylate cyclase system. Preclinical studies have shown that chronic antidepressant administration produces desensitization of the β-adrenergic receptor. The β-adrenergic receptor downregulation hypothesis posits that the mode of action of clinically effective antidepressants is by decreasing the number of β-adrenergic receptor sites. Initial measurements of these β-adrenergic receptors in depressed patients have yielded somewhat mixed results. Mann and colleagues (1986) reported increased β-adrenergic receptor density in postmortem brain tissue of suicide victims. However, Crow and colleagues (1984) demonstrated decreased density of hippocampal β receptors in the postmortem brain tissue of depressed patients who had been hospitalized. In this latter group of patients, previous antidepressant treatment may have induced β-adrenergic re-

ceptor downregulation. Similarly, contradictory results have been reported from studies determining the B_{max} (number of binding sites) for β receptors on leukocytes. Some investigators have reported reduced B_{max} for peripheral β receptors in depressed patients, but others have documented no difference between depressed patients and healthy control subjects (Extein et al. 1979; Healy et al. 1985). Two features of the β-adrenergic receptor hypothesis are attractive. First, a reduction in the availability of released norepinephrine should result in an increase in postsynaptic β-adrenergic receptor density. Second, there is a time lag both in the clinical response to antidepressants and in the downregulation of the β-adrenergic receptor after antidepressant treatment.

Dopamine and Dopamine β-Hydroxylase and Monoamine Oxidase

Although dopamine has not garnered as much scrutiny as have other monoamines in the pathophysiology of depression, evidence is substantial that enhanced dopaminergic activity may play a primary role in psychotic depression. Compared with nonpsychotic depressed patients, depressed patients with psychotic symptoms have been reported to have lower serum dopamine β-hydroxylase (which catalyzes the hydroxylation of dopamine to norepinephrine) activity and higher concentrations of plasma dopamine as well as increased concentrations of CSF and plasma homovanillic acid (Aberg-Wistedt et al. 1985; Devanand et al. 1985; Schatzberg et al. 1985a; Sweeney et al. 1978).

Several studies have measured dopamine β-hydroxylase activity in major psychiatric disorders, including schizophrenia and affective disorders. However, results generally have been consistent only for patients with unipolar psychotic depression, who have been reported to have reduced concentrations. Sapru and colleagues (1989) reported lower serum dopamine β-hydroxylase activity in patients with psychotic major depression compared with control subjects, with no differences between patients with schizophrenia, bipolar disorder manic phase, or nonpsychotic major depression. Indeed, diminished dopamine β-hydroxylase activity has been hypothesized to be a risk factor for developing psychotic depression.

Several recent studies suggest that increased dopamine activity may occur, at least in part, as a result of increased adrenocortical activity. Glucocorticoids induce tyrosine hydroxylase, the rate-limiting enzyme in the biosynthesis of dopamine and norepinephrine. The administration of dexamethasone can significantly increase plasma free dopamine and homovanillic acid in healthy control subjects (Rothschild et al. 1984; Wolkowitz et al. 1985), and the administration of corticosterone or dexamethasone to rats significantly increases central dopamine activity (Rothschild et al. 1985; Wolkowitz et al. 1986). Schatzberg and colleagues (1985a) hypothesized that the glucocorticoids' enhancement of dopaminergic activity may underlie the development of psychosis in depressed patients.

Platelet monoamine oxidase activity has been studied as a possible biological marker in mood disorders. Bipolar probands and their relatives have been reported to have decreased platelet monoamine oxidase activity in comparison with unipolar patients or control subjects (Gershon et al. 1980; Leckman et al. 1977; Samson et al. 1985). Reduced platelet monoamine oxidase activity is found primarily in bipolar I, not in bipolar II, subjects (Samson et al. 1985). Although studies have suggested that monoamine oxidase activity is under strong genetic control and is linked to affective pathology, these results have not been widely replicated (Maubach et al. 1981). Interestingly, Schatzberg and colleagues (1987) reported that monoamine oxidase activity was significantly higher in patients with psychotic depression than in those with nonpsychotic depression or in healthy control subjects.

High platelet monoamine oxidase activity has been found to correlate with elevated urinary free cortisol levels and DST nonsuppression (Agren and Oreland 1982; Schatzberg et al. 1985b). The association between high platelet monoamine oxidase activity and DST nonsuppression has been replicated by several groups (Meltzer et al. 1988; G. N. Pandey et al. 1992). Monoamine oxidase activity correlated with nonsuppression on the DST. Mean 4:00 P.M. postdexamethasone cortisol levels were significantly higher in patients with high platelet monoamine oxidase activity. Several hypotheses have been put forth concerning this finding. Monoamine oxidase could be a genetic marker for a risk for nonsuppression in the face of developing depression. If elevated platelet monoamine oxidase activity were correlated with a corresponding increase in hypothalamic monoamine oxidase activity, a decrease in central noradrenergic tonic inhibition of HPA axis activity could then result in nonsuppression to dexamethasone challenge. Increased central monoamine oxidase activity could also be associated with serotonergic supersensitivity and elevated HPA axis activity. Conversely, increased glucocorticoid secretion may be associated with elevated levels of catecholamines, which then results in an increase in platelet monoamine oxidase activity.

The importance of dopamine in mood disorders has also been supported by observations that drugs that in-

crease dopamine availability (such as amphetamine) induce euphoria, whereas dopamine receptor antagonists block this effect. Even though amphetamine also stimulates norepinephrine release, adrenergic antagonists do not block the euphorigenic effect of psychostimulants (Nurnberger et al. 1984). Moreover, improvement in mood to a test dose of amphetamine has been reported to predict antidepressant response (Little 1988).

Many of the more recently developed antidepressants—including bupropion, sertraline, and perhaps venlafaxine—are thought to inhibit presynaptic dopamine reuptake (Schatzberg et al. 1997). However, the antidepressant effects of these drugs may depend predominantly on their serotonergic and noradrenergic effects rather than on their dopaminergic properties. Pramipexole, a D_2 and D_3 receptor agonist approved for the treatment of Parkinson's disease, has been shown to be an effective treatment of patients with major depression (Piercey et al. 1996).

The development of radiolabeled ligands, such as [^{11}C]dopac and [^{11}C]raclopride, allows for the in vivo evaluation of the role of dopamine in affective disorders. The density of D_2 receptors has been reported in positron-emission tomography (PET) studies to be increased in manic, but not depressed, patients (Willner 1983a, 1983b, 1983c). In another PET study, uptake of dopamine precursors was diminished in depressed patients (Agren and Reibring 1994). In contrast to these findings is a recent single photon emission computed tomography (SPECT) study documenting increased D_2 receptor binding in a group of drug-free depressed patients (D'haenen and Bossuyt 1994). It is also of interest to note that nomifensine, a selective dopamine reuptake inhibitor, was an effective antidepressant but was removed from the market because of the appearance of a Guillain-Barré syndrome in some patients.

Acetylcholine

As noted earlier, Janowsky and colleagues (1972) postulated that an increased ratio of cholinergic to adrenergic activity may underlie depression, whereas the reverse occurs in mania. Although the adrenergic-cholinergic balance hypothesis appears incomplete in the face of increasing data on the preeminent role of alterations in serotonergic neurotransmission in major depression, the importance of cholinergic mechanisms in some forms of depression is supported by both preclinical and clinical observations.

Animal models of depression (e.g., the forced swim model) are exacerbated by the administration of cholinesterase inhibitors such as physostigmine (McKinney 1984), whereas muscarinic receptor antagonists reverse the effects of such "procholinergic" agents. More convincing evidence of the importance of acetylcholine in the maintenance of mood is the induction of depressed mood following administration of physostigmine or cholinergic agonists (e.g., arecoline) in euthymic control subjects (El-Yousef et al. 1973), unipolar depressed patients (Janowsky and Risch 1984), and bipolar manic patients (Janowsky and Risch 1984). Indeed, depressive symptoms, including psychomotor retardation and depressed mood, are often unwelcome sequelae of acetylcholinesterase inhibitor treatment of Alzheimer's disease. Such sensitivity to the mood-lowering effects of cholinergic drugs appears dependent on the presence of an underlying psychiatric disorder. Patients with an affective illness such as mania, depression, or schizoaffective disorder are more vulnerable to the depressogenic effects of physostigmine than are patients with schizophrenia (Steinberg et al. 1993).

If cholinergic mechanisms contribute in some manner to the pathophysiology of major depression, then anticholinergic drugs should be effective antidepressants. Although physostigmine-induced dysphoria may be reversed with atropine (El-Yousef et al. 1973), little evidence indicates that anticholinergic medications have significant antidepressant properties (Janowsky and Risch 1984). Moreover, the newer antidepressants, including the SSRIs, have little affinity for muscarinic cholinergic receptors, yet remain effective antidepressants. Sitaram and colleagues (1984) proposed that primary affective illness (specifically bipolar disorder) may be characterized by a state-independent cholinergic hypersensitivity in conjunction with a state-dependent noradrenergic supersensitivity (during late depression and early mania), which return to normal during remission. These researchers intravenously administered arecoline during the second non–rapid eye movement (NREM) sleep period of the night, which resulted in significantly more rapid onset of rapid eye movement (REM) sleep in currently depressed as well as in remitted depressive patients than was seen in control subjects. This research group has replicated this finding of supersensitive cholinergic responses in patients with major depressive disorder (Dube et al. 1985; Jones et al. 1985). These findings also suggest that cholinergic sensitivity may play a key role in the pathogenesis of depression.

Schatzberg and Mooney (1991) have offered a slightly different perspective on acetylcholine/catecholamine interactions in depression. Increased acetylcholine activity may result in increased catecholamine output as well as the commonly co-occurring elevation in cortisol activity in a subgroup of depressed patients. Therefore, acetylcholine activity may not be reciprocal to catecholamine activity, as postulated by the original norepinephrine-acetylcholine hypothesis. The role of acetylcholine in the pathogenesis of mood disorders awaits further clarification.

γ-Aminobutyric Acid (GABA)

GABA exerts inhibitory, hyperpolarizing effects in almost all areas of the CNS. GABA is a major regulator of many CNS functions, such as seizure threshold, and it also has inhibitory input into other neurotransmitter systems such as norepinephrine and dopamine. Clinical and pharmacological data suggest that GABA metabolism may be altered in affective disorders.

Two types of GABA receptors, $GABA_A$ and $GABA_B$, have been identified. $GABA_A$ receptors are coupled to chloride ion channels and are associated with benzodiazepine-binding sites, whereas $GABA_B$ receptors are associated with calcium ion transport. $GABA_B$ agonists, such as baclofen, enhance cAMP production during exposure to other neurotransmitters such as norepinephrine, although they themselves have little effect on the second-messenger response. A decrease in the activity of GABAergic systems may play a role in depression by regulating receptor responses to catecholamines. For example, with the addition of baclofen to imipramine, downregulation of β-adrenergic receptor number and activity occurs more rapidly (Enna et al. 1986).

The role of the GABA system in the pathophysiology of certain convulsive disorders has been extensively studied, as has its role in mechanism of action of antiepileptic drugs. The anticonvulsants valproic acid and carbamazepine were serendipitously noted to have a mood-stabilizing effect, decreasing the intensity and frequency of manic and perhaps depressive phases of bipolar disorder. All antimanic agents (including lithium) have been suggested to stabilize mood in part by increasing GABA-ergic transmission, leading to the hypothesis that a relative GABA deficiency plays a role in mania (Bernasconi 1982).

B. I. Gold and colleagues (1980) reported that CSF GABA concentrations in depressed patients are significantly lower than in nondepressed control subjects; this finding has been replicated in several studies and found with GABA plasma concentrations as well (Petty and Schlesser 1981; Petty and Sherman 1984). Honig and colleagues (1989) directly measured GABA in brain tissue from patients undergoing cingulotomy for intractable depression and found that GABA concentration was inversely correlated with severity of depression. Low levels of GABA are not specific to cases of depression or mania but are also seen in alcoholism (Petty 1994).

Serotonin

While American psychobiological investigators in the 1960s focused on the pathoetiological contribution of norepinephrine circuit dysfunction to depression, European scientists scrutinized serotonergic mechanisms (Coppen et al. 1972). The permissive hypothesis of serotonin function postulates that the deficit in central serotonergic neurotransmission permits the expression of bipolar affective disorder but is not sufficient to cause it (Prange et al. 1974). According to this theory, both the manic and the depressive phases of bipolar illness are characterized by low central serotonin function but differ in high versus low norepinephrine activity. The efficacy of the selective serotonin antidepressants is both a product of early research based on this hypothesis and a stimulus for the ensuing and ongoing research on serotonin systems.

The hypothesis that a deficiency in central serotonergic function predisposes patients to affective illness has evolved from a number of findings. Several studies have detected reduced CSF concentrations of 5-HIAA, the principal metabolite of serotonin, in some depressed patients (Asberg et al. 1976a, 1976b; R. D. Gibbons and Davis 1986; Roy et al. 1989). Most attention has been paid to the relationship between low concentrations of CSF 5-HIAA and suicidal behavior in depressed patients. Asberg and colleagues (1976a) suggested that low concentrations of 5-HIAA may be a marker for suicidal behavior and for suicide risk in depressed patients. Several subsequent studies have replicated these observations and have suggested that decreased CSF 5-HIAA may predict suicidal behavior (Banki et al. 1984; G. L. Brown et al. 1982; Traskman et al. 1981). Low CSF 5-HIAA concentrations appear to be associated with more impulsive or aggressive methods of suicide (Traskman-Bendz et al. 1992), suggesting an association between decreased levels of 5-HIAA and suicide, aggression, or poor impulse control. Indeed, such low levels of 5-HIAA have also been associated with aggression or poor impulse control in impulsive violent criminal offenders (V. M. Linnoila et al. 1983b) and arsonists (Virkkunen et al. 1987). V. M. Linnoila and Virkkunen (1992) described a low-serotonin syndrome model, with associations between low 5-HIAA, hypoglycemia, and early-onset alcoholism (type II) and impulsive violent behavior, which suggests that low 5-HIAA levels may describe a behavioral dimension that goes beyond depression. Recent data strengthen the association between central serotonergic deficit and impulsivity, alcoholism, and hypoglycemia (Virkkunen et al. 1994).

Drugs that target the serotonin transporter site, thereby selectively inhibiting reuptake of serotonin (e.g., fluoxetine, sertraline, paroxetine, citalopram, and fluvoxamine) have been shown to be effective antidepressants. In addition to SSRIs, there is growing interest in agents that specifically interact with one or more serotonin receptor subtypes.

Several different serotonin receptor subtypes have been identified in recent years, a reflection of increased sophistication regarding biochemical and molecular biological techniques. Subtyping is based in part on the characteristics of binding to serotonin, other agonists, or antagonists. Three main classes—5-HT_1, 5-HT_2, and 5-HT_3 receptors—are further subdivided into subtypes 5-HT_{1A}, 5-HT_{1B}, 5-HT_{1D}, 5-HT_{1E}, and 5-HT_{1F}. The 5-HT_2 receptor appears to be virtually identical to the 5-HT_{1C} receptor; this class may be divided into 5-HT_{2A} and 5-HT_{2B} subtypes. The 5-HT_{1A} receptor in particular has been implicated in the pathophysiology of depression and anxiety. This receptor has a high affinity for serotonin, and chronic treatment with antidepressants in rats results in reduction of 5-HT_{1A} receptor sensitivity.

Antidepressants decrease the number of the low-affinity 5-HT_2 receptors, yet ECT increases them (Gonzalez-Heydrich and Peroutka 1990). Mann and colleagues (1986) reported an increased number of postsynaptic 5-HT_2 receptors in the brains of depressed patients. This finding suggests that a functional deficiency of presynaptic serotonergic neurotransmitter activity in depression may lead to an increased number or upregulation of postsynaptic 5-HT_2 serotonergic receptors (Risch et al. 1992). Indeed, Mattsubara and colleagues (1991) documented an increase in the number of 5-HT_1 and 5-HT_2 receptors in the prefrontal cortex of suicide victims, although other groups have not replicated this finding (Cheetham et al. 1990; Stockmeier et al. 1997).

5-HT_2-receptor binding to platelet membranes and serotonin-induced shape change and aggregation have been used to study 5-HT_2 receptors in patients with mood disorders. Beigon and colleagues (1990) suggested that the increase in number of 5-HT_2 receptors on platelets may be viewed as a state-dependent marker in major depression. In their study of 15 depressed patients, 3 weeks of treatment with maprotiline was associated with significant decreases in 5-HT_2-receptor binding in responders; in contrast, receptor binding increased or remained the same in the nonresponders.

The human platelet concentrates serotonin from plasma via the serotonin transporter in a fashion similar to that seen in the brain, and it therefore has been posited as a model of central serotonin neurons. [³H]Imipramine binds to the serotonin transporter on the presynaptic nerve terminal and on the platelet. A reduction in the number of platelet [3H]imipramine binding sites in depressed patients has been reported by several groups (Briley et al. 1980; Langer and Raisman 1983; Lewis and McChesney 1985; Nemeroff et al. 1988a). Perry et al. (1983) reported decreased density of [3H]imipramine binding sites in the hippocampus and occipital cortex of depressed patients, confirming the original studies by Stanley and colleagues (1982).

In contrast to these findings, the report of a multicenter study of 154 depressed patients and 130 control subjects concluded that [3H]imipramine binding is not a valid biological marker of endogenous depression (World Health Organization Collaborative Study 1990). No significant difference was observed in [3H]imipramine binding kinetics between depressed patients and control subjects. Findings among different centers had marked discrepancies, perhaps reflecting different biochemical techniques used for platelet isolation and membrane preparation. However, a recent meta-analysis of all of the published platelet [3H]imipramine-binding data revealed a reduction in the density of serotonin transporter sites in drug-free depressed patients when compared with that of control subjects (Ellis and Salmond 1994). Recently, Malison and colleagues (1997), in collaboration with our group, observed decreased serotonin-transporter binding in the midbrain of depressed patients compared to control subjects using [123I]2 β-carbomethoxy-3 β-(4-iodophenyl)tropane ([123I] β-CIT) and SPECT imaging.

In recent years, [3H]imipramine has been found to have less specificity than [3H]paroxetine (Nemeroff et al. 1991b). Nemeroff and colleagues (1994) reported that [3H]paroxetine-binding sites are reduced in the platelets of drug-free depressed patients. This may ultimately prove a more useful tool than [3H]imipramine.

Serotonergic systems are ultimately involved in the regulation of a variety of hormones, including cortisol, prolactin, and growth hormone. Administration of the serotonin-releasing agent fenfluramine results in an increase in plasma concentrations of ACTH, cortisol, and prolactin, as well as an increase in body temperature. Stahl and colleagues (1992) reported that fenfluramine-induced hyperthermic responses were blunted in unmedicated patients with major depression.

As noted above, serotonin agonists are effective stimulants of prolactin release. In nondepressed subjects, administration of L-tryptophan, a serotonin precursor, produces a robust increase in plasma prolactin concentrations. The prolactin response to L-tryptophan and to the serotonin-releasing agent fenfluramine is blunted in depression (Cowen and Charig 1987; Siever et al. 1984). It is important to note that patients with other psychiatric disorders, including Axis II diagnoses, also show a blunted prolactin response to fenfluramine.

The cortisol response to 5-hydroxytryptophan administration has been found to be enhanced in unmedicated depressed patients and to decrease following treatment with antidepressants (Koyama and Meltzer 1986). Noting a significant negative correlation between baseline plasma cortisol levels and the cortisol response to 5-hydroxytryptophan in nondepressed control subjects, Koyama and Meltzer (1986) postulated that serotonin may play an important role in the stimulation of basal plasma cortisol secretion.

Other studies of L-tryptophan have lent further support to the serotonin hypothesis of depression. Depressed patients exhibit reduced plasma concentrations of 5-hydroxytryptophan after ingestion of test doses of oral L-tryptophan (Deakin et al. 1990), and depressed patients have reduced plasma concentrations of serotonin in comparison to nondepressed control subjects (Maes et al. 1990). Furthermore, dietary restriction of tryptophan in patients whose depression had remitted after SSRI treatment induces a rapid relapse in symptoms (Delgado et al. 1990; Neumeister et al. 1997; Smith et al. 1997).

Because serotonin activates the HPA axis, increased serotonin activity could play a role in the increased HPA axis activity and pathogenesis of psychotic depression. Indeed, in a review of the literature, Schatzberg and Rothschild (1992) noted that increased serotonin uptake into platelets and increased CSF levels of 5-HIAA have both been reported in patients with psychotic depression. These findings point to the need for further studies scrutinizing serotonergic activity in psychotic depression. Table 27–8 summarizes the alterations in the serotonin system in depression.

Chronic administration of effective antidepressant therapy, including ECT, induces an upregulation in the number of 5-HT$_{1A}$ postsynaptic receptors (Hayakawa et

Table 27–8.   Alterations in the serotonin (5-HT) system in depression

Decreased plasma tryptophan concentrations

Decreased 5-hydroxyindoleacetic acid (5-HIAA) in cerebrospinal fluid

Increased 5-HIAA in psychotic depression

Increased postsynaptic 5-HT$_2$ receptors

Decreased [3H]imipramine binding

Decreased [3H]paroxetine binding

Blunted prolactin response to fenfluramine

al. 1993). Even antidepressants, such as desipramine, that act primarily on norepinephrine neurons such as desipramine appear to exert potent effects on 5-HT$_{1A}$ receptors (Lund et al. 1992). Conversely, most antidepressants—including MAOIs, TCAs, SSRIs, nefazodone, and trazodone—induce a downregulation of postsynaptic 5-HT$_2$ receptors (Cowen 1990). As mentioned above, one notable exception is ECT, which results in an upregulation of 5-HT$_2$ receptors (Lerer 1987).

Although the serotonin hypothesis of depression is supported by many lines of evidence, key elements in the pathophysiology of depression may exist "downstream," that is, in response to serotonin-receptor activation (e.g., effects on intracellular second-messenger systems) or alterations of the neuroendocrine system.

Intracellular Signal Transduction and Neurotropic Factors

In the past decade, rapid advances in molecular biology have provided insights into the mechanisms of intracellular signal transduction pathways. There are at least two major types of signal transduction pathways. The most widely studied has been the so-called second-messenger pathway. Second-messenger systems couple a neurotransmitter receptor with an intracellular second messenger such as cAMP, inositol phosphate, and nitric oxide. Second-messenger pathways are most commonly linked with guanine nucleotide-binding proteins (G proteins), which couple the neurotransmitter receptor to the second messenger. Through their interaction with membrane-bound receptors, the monoamines and amino acid neurotransmitters indirectly activate these second-messenger systems. A second type of intracellular messenger system utilizes receptors coupled directly to tyrosine kinases that interact with mitogen-activated protein kinases. This second pathway is intimately involved in gene transcription of neurotropic factors. The reader is directed to Chapter 1 for a detailed discussion of signal transduction and second-messenger systems.

Second-Messenger Systems

Among the most scrutinized of the second-messenger pathways is the G-protein-linked cAMP system. Many antidepressant effects are believed to be mediated through the cAMP system. Most serotonin receptors, for example, are G proteins linked to cAMP. Activation of the serotonin receptor leads to a conformation change in the G protein, which leads to activation of cAMP-dependent protein kinases. Among the proteins phosphorylated by such cAMP-dependent protein kinases is the cAMP response element binding (CREB) protein, which is believed to be responsible for mediating the effects of antidepressants on receptor protein up- and downregulation. All chronic antidepressant treatments appear to increase intracellular concentrations of CREB protein as well as cAMP-dependent protein kinases (Menkes et al. 1983; Sleight et al. 1995). Treatment for 14–21 days is necessary for induction of CREB protein (Nestler et al. 1989), paralleling the time observed in which downregulation of adrenergic and serotonergic receptors occurs as well as the time necessary for clinical response to antidepressants. Thus various antidepressants and the neurotransmitter systems they act on may ultimately target the same intracellular messenger that in turn mediates the efficacy of these drugs (Duman et al. 1997). Avissar and Schreiber (1992) have proposed that hyperactivity of G proteins, either as a trait marker or as a state function, leads to an unstable dynamic system in bipolar disorder. Lithium treatment is hypothesized to attenuate G-protein function, thereby stabilizing both manic and depressed mood states.

Phosphoinositide system and calcium. The phosphoinositide system is another second-messenger system that may be an additional target for antidepressants and mood stabilizers. Interaction with a receptor by a neurotransmitter leads to activation of the phospholipase C enzyme. This enzyme catalyzes the formation of inositol triphosphate, as well as diacylglycerol. Inositol triphosphate binds to a unique receptor on the endoplasmic reticulum within the cell to trigger the release of calcium, which regulates a variety of cell functions including the synthesis and release of monoamine neurotransmitters. Calcium also plays an important role in regulation of neuronal processes, including synthesis and release of neurotransmitters and modulation of ion channels that influence cell excitability. Several studies have implicated a hyperactivity of intracellular calcium release in bipolar disorder. For example, intracellular calcium is significantly higher in untreated bipolar depressed patients than in untreated unipolar depressed patients (Dubovsky et al. 1991). Because the calcium concentrations were similar in euthymic-treated bipolar patients and control subjects, elevated intracellular calcium concentrations may be a state-dependent marker in bipolar patients.

Antidepressants and lithium alter the metabolism of the phosphoinositide system. For example, TCAs decrease thrombin-stimulated inositol phosphate formation and increase levels of [^{3}H]inositol-labeled phospholipids (S. C. Pandey et al. 1991), likely through inhibition of phospholipase C. Such findings suggest that antidepressants may cause changes in the phosphoinositide signaling system and that changes in receptors caused by antidepressants may be related to their effects on membrane phospholipids. Lithium also appears to alter phosphoinositide turnover and metabolism (Baraban et al. 1989) through inhibition of inositol monophosphatase, although some discrepant results have been obtained (Lenox and Watson 1994). The theory that lithium's diverse actions on multiple neurotransmitter system are mediated via second-messenger systems remains an attractive one, but further study is required.

The action of antidepressants and mood stabilizers on neurotropic elements within the cell is only beginning to be explored. One important neurotropic factor is brain-derived neurotropic factor (BDNF). BDNF appears to regulate the maintenance and survival of neurons in the brain and influences remodeling of synaptic architecture (Lindsay et al. 1994; Thoenen 1995). Stimulation of 5-HT_2 receptors and α_1-adrenergic receptors appears to functionally increase BDNF in the hippocampus (Duman et al. 1994). Furthermore, long-term administration of various antidepressants or repeated ECT treatments increase BDNF expression (Nibuya et al. 1995, 1996). BDNF expression may be mediated via activation of CREB protein or directly through specialized membrane-bound receptors.

The role of intracellular factors in the pathophysiology of affective illnesses and the actions of psychotropic agents on them is one of the burgeoning areas in the investigation of the neurobiology of mood disorders. Efforts are under way to move beyond traditional neurotransmitter-receptor pharmacology and to target directly the second-messenger systems and neurotropic factors in the development of new psychopharmacological agents.

BRAIN IMAGING STUDIES

A variety of approaches, including genetic and family studies, measurement of neurochemical and neuroendocrine parameters, electrophysiological studies, study of the actions of antidepressant drugs, and, most recently, brain imaging methods (see Potter et al., Chapter 10, in this volume), have been used to investigate the etiology of the major mood disorders. As early as 1937, Papez proposed the limbic system as the location of the "seat of human emotions." Early study of CNS morphology and its relationship to affective disorder was limited to animal models and postmortem studies of humans. With the advent first of CT imaging and subsequently MRI, invaluable tools emerged for investigating the neural system(s) thought to be involved in the regulation of affect and the pathophysiology of affective disorder.

Early assumptions underpinning the use of brain imaging in the investigation of psychiatric disorders include the following:

1. Dysfunction of the CNS contributes to the pathogenesis and pathophysiology of the major mood disorders.
2. This dysfunction is associated with specific structural brain abnormalities.
3. Those particular structural brain abnormalities reflect functional CNS alterations.

In this section, we review the controlled structural (CT and MRI) and functional (PET and SPECT) imaging studies of patients with affective disorder. Even though there are many reports of ventriculomegaly in patients with schizophrenia, the literature is replete with CT and MRI studies reporting increased ventricle size in patients with unipolar and bipolar mood disorders. However, these studies are confounded by numerous methodological problems. As extensively reviewed by Figiel and colleagues (in press), most of these studies estimate lateral ventricle size by using a ventricular brain ratio. Unfortunately, few conclusions can be drawn from the CT literature on ventricular enlargement in affective disorder. More consistent, however, are the CT and MRI studies of increased ventricular size in depression in geriatric patients (those individuals older than 65) (Tables 27–9 and 27–10). Recent meta-analyses confirm the ventricular enlargement and increased sulcal prominence in patients with mood disorders; however, ventricular enlargement is greater in patients with schizophrenia. Ventricular enlargement is believed to be a nonspecific structural brain alteration (Elkis et al. 1995).

Table 27–9. Alterations on brain computed tomography

Major depression

Increased lateral ventricular size (geriatric depression[a]) (Abas et. al. 1990; Jacoby and Levy 1980; Pearlson et al. 1989)

Increased third ventricle width (Iacono et al. 1988; Schlegel et al. 1989)

± Cortical atrophy

Bipolar disorder

± Cortical atrophy

No cerebral asymmetry

Cerebellar atrophy (also in schizophrenic patients) (Lippman et al. 1982)

---

[a]Geriatric depression = depression in patients older than 65 years.

Table 27–10. Alterations on brain magnetic resonance imaging

Major depression

Increased ventricular size (geriatric depression[a]) (Abas et al. 1990; Jacoby and Levy 1980; Pearlson et al. 1989; Rabins et al. 1991)

Increased prevalence of subcortical (gray and white matter) hyperintensities (geriatric depression[a]) (Coffey et al. 1990) (late-onset depression[b]) (Figiel et al. 1991c)

Increased prevalence of periventricular hyperintensities (geriatric depression[a]) (Coffey et al. 1990)

Increased prevalence of hyperintensities of the basal ganglia (late-onset depression[b]) (Figiel and Nemeroff 1993; Figiel et al. 1991c)

Decreased cerebellar volume and smaller cerebellar vermis (Shah et al. 1992)

Smaller brain stem and medulla (Shah et al. 1992)

Smaller temporal lobe (Hauser et al. 1989a)

No significant structural changes in corpus callosum (Husain et al. 1991a)

Decreased caudate volume (Figiel and Nemeroff 1993; Krishnan et al. 1992)

Increased prevalence of hyperintensities of the caudate (geriatric depression[a]) (Coffey et al. 1990; Rabins et al. 1991)

Smaller putamen volume (Husain et al. 1991b)

Larger pituitary gland volume (Krishnan et al. 1991)

Decreased hippocampal volume (Sheline et al. 1996)

Bipolar disorder

Smaller temporal lobe volume bilaterally (Altshuler et al. 1991)

No significant structural changes in corpus callosum (Hauser et al. 1989b)

Increased prevalence of subcortical hyperintensities (Dupont et al. 1990, 1995; Figiel et al. 1991d; Swayze et al. 1990)

Increased prevalence of periventricular hyperintensities (Altshuler et al. 1995)

[a]Geriatric depression = depression in patients older than 65 years.
[b]Late-onset depression = depression that first appears in a patient after age 60.

The hippocampus, a structure of paramount importance to learning and memory, and which has high concentrations of glucocorticoid receptors, appears particularly vulnerable to the effects of stress on the brain (Sapolsky 1996). This integral part of the limbic system contains a high concentration of type I and II corticosteroid receptors and is well documented to exert an inhibitory influence on HPA axis activity (Jacobson and Sapolsky et al. 1991). Pro-

longed exposure to large doses of corticosteroids adversely affects the rodent and primate brain, inducing permanent loss of hippocampal neurons (Magarinos et al. 1996; McEwen 1992; Sapolsky 1994; Sapolsky et al. 1990; Uno et al. 1989). Moreover, bilateral hippocampal atrophy has been observed in patients with Cushing's syndrome, in whom the extent of hippocampal atrophy correlates with the magnitude of corticosteroid hypersecretion (Starkman et al. 1992). Indeed, significant reductions of hippocampal volume (12% on the right and 15% on the left) per MRI have been found in individuals with a history of major depression (and normal glucocorticoid plasma concentrations) in comparison to age-, education-, gender-, and height-matched control subjects. Furthermore, the extent of hippocampal atrophy was significantly correlated to the duration of depression; there was no difference in whole brain volume between these two groups (Sheline et al. 1996). Hippocampal atrophy has also been documented in individuals with combat-induced (Bremner et al. 1995; Gurvits et al. 1996) and childhood-induced (Bremner et al. 1997) posttraumatic stress disorder.

The abnormal presence of hyperintensities of gray and white matter (Table 27–10) has been reported in multiple MRI studies of geriatric patients with affective disorder, particularly those with late-onset depression (i.e., elderly depressed patients who experience their first depression after age 60). Subcortical hyperintensities in the elderly are age dependent and may reflect pathological changes stemming from genetic, perinatal, posttraumatic, demyelinating, and infectious factors (Valk and van der Knaap 1989) or from pathophysiological processes related to cerebrovascular disease, including arteriosclerosis of the small lacunar arterioles that supply the basal ganglia and subcortical white matter (Chimowitz et al. 1989; Greenwald et al. 1996; Lesser et al. 1996; Roman 1987). Indeed, hypertension is associated with white matter hyperintensity in both depressed and nondepressed control individuals (Lesser et al. 1996). Study of nondepressed control subjects has also revealed that increasing age is associated with reduction of the size of the putamen (Husain et al. 1991b) and caudate nuclei (Krishnan et al. 1990a), as well as of the size of the midbrain (Shah et al. 1992) and pituitary gland (Krishnan et al. 1991; Lurie et al. 1990).

To assess whether abnormal brain structure is associated with abnormal brain function, investigators used CT and MRI studies in association with neuroendocrine stimulation tests and neuropsychological testing, monitoring of patients' clinical course, and response to treatment. For example, postdexamethasone cortisol levels are significantly correlated with ventricular brain ratio (Rao et al. 1989) and pituitary volume (Axelson et al. 1992). Furthermore, in depressed elderly patients, caudate hyperintensities are associated with an increased risk for the development of TCA- and ECT-induced delirium (Figiel et al. 1989, 1990, 1991a), as well as neuroleptic-induced parkinsonism (Figiel et al. 1991b). Depressed patients (as well as psychiatrically and physically healthy elderly subjects) with large amounts (>10 cm^2) of white matter hyperintensities exhibit declines in cognitive performance in comparison to individuals with minimal or no white matter hyperintensities (Boone et al. 1992; Lesser et al. 1996).

In recent years, imaging of in vivo brain function (or dysfunction) became possible with SPECT, PET, and magnetic resonance spectroscopy (MRS). Certain of these methods assume that brain function is reflected in neuronal activity and that such activity can be characterized by measurement of cerebral blood flow, oxygen uptake, or utilization of glucose. Through the use of radiopharmaceuticals such as [^{123}I]iofetamine (Spectamine) and [^{99m}Tc]HMPAO (Ceretec), SPECT provides measurement of cerebral blood flow and is quantified in relative (rather than absolute) terms. Image resolution is as precise as 12 mm. SPECT is available in almost all clinical nuclear medicine facilities. In contrast, PET has better image resolution (down to 5 mm) and measures not only cerebral blood flow but also glucose utilization. This can be quantified in absolute measurements reflecting neurochemical activity. In addition, the localization and density of a diverse array of neurotransmitter receptors and transporters can be measured with PET and SPECT. A nearby cyclotron must produce the short-lived isotopes, such as radioactively labeled oxygen and glucose analogues, that PET requires. Such tracers include [^{15}O]-labeled water (to measure cerebral blood flow) and [^{18}F]-fluorodeoxyglucose, to map regional glucose utilization. The cost of the isotopes, equipment, and trained technicians makes PET quite expensive, and it is usually found only in specialized research centers. A relatively new application of MRI technology, functional MRI (fMRI), has permitted the detection of changes in regional cerebral blood flow without the use of radioactive tracers. The fMRI methods provide functional brain imaging in difficult populations (e.g., pediatric patients) with greater ability, relative to PET and SPECT, to provide images of neuronal activity in a shorter period. MRS provides estimates of the concentration and turnover of functional and structural markers of neurons, including constituents of cellular metabolism such as phosphocreatine.

PET, fMRI, and SPECT can be used to localize brain sites of altered synaptic activity associated with long-term behavioral patterns as well as short-lived mental phenom-

ena. Compared with nondepressed individuals, patients with unipolar depression have had a lateralized decrease in activity in the left lateral prefrontal cortex repeatedly documented by PET and SPECT investigations (Baxter et al. 1985, 1989; Bench et al. 1992; Dolan et al. 1993; Hurwitz et al. 1990; Martinot et al. 1990) (see Table 27–11). Similar reduction in activity of the left frontal cortex has been observed in depression secondary to other CNS disorders including epilepsy, human immunodeficiency virus, Huntington's chorea, and Parkinson's disease (Dolan et al. 1993; Weinberger et al. 1986, 1988).

Of particular interest is the decreased neuronal activity of the caudate and putamen associated with unipolar and bipolar depression. This is consistent with the MRI-documented morphological abnormalities of the basal ganglia (i.e., reduced size and increased prevalence of hyperintensities within these structures). The subcortical structures that constitute the basal ganglia are the caudate, putamen, and globus pallidus; most investigators also include the amygdala. The basal ganglia can be visualized as the motor behavioral effector mechanism that underlies the cognitive expression of emotion. Vulnerability to affective dysfunction might derive from disruption of connections between the basal ganglia or from interruption of pathways connecting the basal ganglia to other parts of the brain, specifically the limbic system and prefrontal cortex (Alexander et al. 1986; Krishnan 1991). This speculation would be consistent with the findings of subcortical hyperintensities (deep white matter and periventricular) found on MRI and the abnormal cortical neuronal activity re-

Table 27–11.   Alterations on brain positron-emission tomography

Major depression

Diminished cerebral glucose metabolic rates in the basal ganglia (Baxter et al. 1985; Buchsbaum et al. 1986)

Diminished left dorsal anterolateral prefrontal cerebral activity (Baxter et al. 1985, 1989; Bench et al. 1992; Hurwitz et al. 1990; Martinot et al. 1990)

Increased left ventrolateral prefrontal cortex blood flow and increased left amygdala activity (Drevets et al. 1992)

Decreased left subgenual prefrontal cortex activity (Drevets et al. 1997)

Diminished global cerebral metabolism in older depressed patients (Kumar et al. 1992)

Bipolar disorder

Decreased global cerebral activity during depression (Baxter et al. 1989)

Increased global cerebral activity during depression (Kishimoto et al. 1987)

ported in patients with depression and mania. Also requiring further scrutiny are those brain structures rich with corticosteroid receptors or major neuroanatomical connections with elements of the HPA axis (e.g., the amygdala and the hippocampus) and relevant cortical areas such as the cingulate and medial prefrontal cortex.

Ongoing research will determine the diagnostic specificity of the functional abnormalities associated with the major mood disorders as well as the stability or "state" dependency of these alterations. The findings of recent PET neuroimaging studies support a distinction between the neural substrates of normal sad mood states and the pathophysiology of depression. While common sites of altered synaptic activity for both induced sad mood states and major depression have been noted (e.g., left amygdala), such physiological states do not mimic the influence of major depression on frontal cortical function. Using PET images, Drevets and colleagues (1997) localized abnormally decreased activity in the left prefrontal cortex ventral to the corpus callosum genu in both familial bipolar depressed patients and familial unipolar depressed patients (patients with a family history of bipolar and unipolar depression, respectively). This diminished activity was explained in part by a corresponding reduction in volume in this same area as demonstrated by MRI. Furthermore, PET and SPECT studies of depressed patients often reveal significant correlation between the severity of depressive symptoms and the reduction in left frontal cortical function. Clinical response of depressed patients to antidepressant treatment may be associated with increased blood flow or metabolism within the basal ganglia, cingulate, or prefrontal cortex (Baxter et al. 1985, 1989; Bench et al. 1995; Drevets et al. 1992; Goodwin et al. 1993; Hurwitz et al. 1990; Kumar et al. 1991; Martinot et al. 1990; Reischies et al. 1989). However, one group has documented reductions in cerebral blood flow, both global and in anterior cortical regions, in manic patients and depressed individuals who have shown clinical remission of their symptoms following ECT (Nobler et al. 1994a) or treatment with oral antidepressants (Nobler et al. 1994b). Interestingly, Mayberg et al. (1997) reported that the metabolic response of depressed patients' rostral anterior cingulate metabolism differentiated antidepressant treatment responders from nonresponders.

Functional neuroimaging studies may have future potential in identifying effective treatment strategies tailored to the individual depressed patient or to those with certain symptom complexes (Bench et al. 1993). Several recent PET and SPECT studies of depressed patients have found differences in regional brain activity evident in pre- and posttreatment scans that distinguish treatment responders from nonresponders. Hyperactivity in the cingulate region of the frontal cortex prior to overnight sleep deprivation was associated with a positive clinical response of depressive symptoms to sleep deprivation. Nonresponders exhibited normal cingulate gyrus activity before and after sleep deprivation (Wu et al. 1992). Undoubtedly, brain imaging will continue its invaluable contributions to further understanding of the pathophysiology and treatment of unipolar and bipolar mood disorder.

CONCLUSION

We have attempted to review several biological hypotheses of mood disorders and relevant findings from diverse research studies. Mood disorders are likely heterogeneous, with pathophysiological changes occurring at neuroendocrinological, neurochemical, and neuroanatomical levels and with manifestations occurring in multiple systems and at different levels in each system. Interpretation of seemingly disparate individual biological studies is challenging, but over time, integration of their findings will form an overarching understanding of these complex disorders. Future research in delineating specific and sensitive biological mechanisms in mood disorders will extend our current understanding of pathophysiology and lead to breakthroughs in improved treatment strategies and, ultimately, prevention.

REFERENCES

Abas MA, Sahakian BJ, Levy R, et al: Neuropsychological deficits and CT scan changes in elderly depressives. Psychol Med 20:507–520, 1990

Aberg-Wistedt A, Wistedt B, Bertilsson L: Higher CSF levels of HVA and 5-HIAA in delusional compared to nondelusional depression. Arch Gen Psychiatry 42:925–926, 1985

Adinoff B, Nemeroff CB, Bissette G, et al: Inverse relationship between CSF TRH concentrations and the TSH response to TRH in abstinent alcohol-dependent patients. Am J Psychiatry 148:1586–1588, 1991

Agren H, Lundqvist G: Low levels of somatostatin in human CSF mark depressive episodes. Psychoneuroendocrinology 9:233–248, 1984

Agren H, Oreland L: Early morning awakening in unipolar depressives with higher levels of platelet MAO activity. Psychiatry Res 7:245–254, 1982

Agren H, Reibring L: PET studies of presynaptic monoamine metabolism in depressed patients and healthy volunteers. Pharmacopsychiatry 27:2–6, 1994

Aguilera G, Wynn PC, Harwood JP, et al: Receptor-mediated actions of corticotropin-releasing factor in pituitary gland and nervous system. Neuroendocrinology 43:79–88, 1986

Alexander GE, Delong MR, Strick PL: Parallel organization of functionally segregated circuits linking basal ganglia and cortex. Annu Rev Neurosci 9:357–381, 1986

Altshuler LL, Conrad A, Hauser P, et al: Reduction of temporal lobe volume in bipolar disorder: a preliminary report of magnetic resonance imaging. Arch Gen Psychiatry 48:482–483, 1991

Altshuler LI, Curran JG, Hauser P, et al: T2 hyperintensities in bipolar disorder: magnetic resonance imaging comparison and literature meta-analysis. Am J Psychiatry 152:1139–1144, 1995

American Psychiatric Association: Diagnostic and Statistical Manual of Mental Disorders, 3rd Edition. Washington, DC, American Psychiatric Association, 1980

American Psychiatric Association: Diagnostic and Statistical Manual of Mental Disorders, 3rd Edition, Revised. Washington, DC, American Psychiatric Association, 1987

American Psychiatric Association: Task Force on DSM-IV Options Book: Work in Progress 9/1/91. Washington, DC, American Psychiatric Press, 1991

American Psychiatric Association: Diagnostic and Statistical Manual of Mental Disorders, 4th Edition. Washington, DC, American Psychiatric Association, 1994

Amsterdam JD, Winokur A, Abelman E, et al: Cosyntropin (ACTH) stimulation test in depressed patients and healthy subjects. Am J Psychiatry 140:907–909, 1983

Amsterdam JD, Marinelli DL, Arger P, et al: Assessment of adrenal gland volume by computed tomography in depressed patients and healthy volunteers: a pilot study. Psychiatry Res 21:189–197, 1987

Amsterdam JD, Maislin G, Winokur A, et al: The oCRF test before and after clinical recovery from depression. J Affect Disord 14:213–222, 1988

Arana GW, Mossman D: The DST and depression: approaches to the use of a laboratory test in psychiatry. Neurol Clin 6:21–39, 1988

Arana GW, Baldessarini RJ, Ornsteen M: The dexamethasone suppression test for diagnosis and prognosis in psychiatry. Arch Gen Psychiatry 42:1193–1204, 1985

Arato M, Banki CM, Nemeroff CB, et al: Hypothalamic-pituitary-adrenal axis and suicide. Ann N Y Acad Sci 487:263–270, 1986

Arato M, Banki CM, Bissette G, et al: Elevated CSF CRF in suicide victims. Biol Psychiatry 25:355–359, 1989

Asberg M, Traskman L, Thoren P: 5-HIAA in the cerebrospinal fluid: a biochemical suicide predictor? Arch Gen Psychiatry 33:1193–1197, 1976a

Asberg M, Thoren P, Traskman L, et al: "Serotonin depression"—a biochemical subgroup within the affective disorders? Science 191:478–483, 1976b

Avissar S, Schreiber G: The involvement of guanine nucleotide binding proteins in the pathogenesis and treatment of affective disorders. Biol Psychiatry 31:435–459, 1992

Axelson DA, Doraiswamy PM, Boyko OB, et al: In vivo assessment of pituitary volume using MRI and systemic stereology: relationship to dexamethasone suppression test results in patients with affective disorder. Psychiatry Res 46:63–70, 1992

Banki CM, Arato M, Papp Z, et al: Biochemical markers in suicidal patients: investigations with cerebrospinal fluid amine metabolites and neuroendocrine tests. J Affect Disord 6:341–350, 1984

Banki CM, Bissette G, Arato M, et al: Cerebrospinal fluid corticotropin-releasing factor-like immunoreactivity in depression and schizophrenia. Am J Psychiatry 144:873–877, 1987

Banki CM, Bissette G, Arato M, et al: Elevation of immunoreactive CSF TRH in depressed patients. Am J Psychiatry 145:1526–1531, 1988

Banki CB, Karmacsi L, Bissette G, et al: CSF corticotropin-releasing hormone and somatostatin in major depression: response to antidepressant treatment and relapse. Eur Neuropsychopharmacol 2:107–113, 1992

Baraban JM, Worley PF, Snyder SH: Second messenger systems and psychoactive drug action: focus on the phosphoinositide system and lithium. Am J Psychiatry 146:1251–1260, 1989

Baron M, Risch N, Hamburger R, et al: Genetic linkage between X-chromosome markers and bipolar affective illness. Nature 326:289–292, 1987

Baron M, Freimer NF, Risch N: Diminished support for linkage between manic depressive illness and X-chromosome markers in three Israeli pedigrees. Nat Genet 3:49–55, 1993

Bartalena L, Placidi GF, Martino E, et al: Nocturnal serum thyrotropin (TSH) surge and the TSH response to TSH-releasing hormone: dissociated behavior in untreated depressives. J Clin Endocrinol Metab 71:650–655, 1990

Bauer MS, Whybrow PC: Thyroid hormones and the central nervous system in affective illness: interactions that may have clinical significance. Integrative Psychiatry 6:75–100, 1988

Bauer MS, Whybrow PC: Rapid cycling bipolar affective disorder, I: association with grade I hypothyroidism. Arch Gen Psychiatry 47:427–432, 1990a

Bauer MS, Whybrow PC: Rapid cycling bipolar affective disorder, II: treatment of refractory rapid cycling with high-dose levothyroxine: a preliminary study. Arch Gen Psychiatry 47:435–447, 1990b

Baumgartner A: The influence of antidepressant (desipramine, fluoxetine), prophylactic drugs (lithium, carbamazepine), and sleep deprivation on thyroid hormone metabolism in rat brain (abstract). Neuropsychopharmacology 10:494S, 1994

Baxter LR, Phelps MC, Mazziotta JC, et al: Cerebral metabolic rates for glucose in mood disorders studied with positron emission tomography (PET) and (F-18)-fluoro-2- deoxyglucose (FDG). Arch Gen Psychiatry 42:441–447, 1985

Baxter LR, Schwartz JM, Phelps ME, et al: Reduction of prefrontal cortex glucose metabolism common to three types of depression. Arch Gen Psychiatry 46:243–250, 1989

Beck-Friis J, Kjellman BF, Ljunggren JG, et al: The pineal gland and melatonin in affective disorder, in The Pineal Gland: Endocrine Aspects (Advances in Bioscience, Vol 53). Edited by Brown GM, Wainwright SD. Oxford, England, Pergamon, 1985, pp 313–325

Beigon A, Essar N, Israeli M, et al: Serotonin 5-HT2 receptor binding on blood platelets as a state dependent marker in major affective disorder. Psychopharmacology (Berl) 102:73–75, 1990

Bench CJ, Friston KJ, Brown RG, et al: The anatomy of melancholia: focal abnormalities of cerebral blood flow in major depression. Psychol Med 22:607–615, 1992

Bench CJ, Friston KJ, Brown RG, et al: Regional cerebral blood flow in depression measured by positron emission tomography: the relationship with clinical dimension. Psychol Med 23:579–590, 1993

Bench CJ, Frackowiak RSJ, Dolan RJ: Changes in regional cerebral blood flow on recovery from depression. Psychol Med 25:247–251, 1995

Bernasconi R: The GABA hypothesis of affective illness: influence of clinically effective antimanic drugs on GABA turnover, in Basic Mechanisms in the Action of Lithium. Edited by Emrich HM, Aldenhoff JB, Lux HD. Amsterdam, Elsevier, 1982, pp 183–192

Berrettini WH: Genetics in psychiatry. Paper presented at the 145th annual meeting of the American Psychiatric Association, Washington, DC, May 2–7, 1992

Berrettini WH, Ferraro TN, Goldin LR, et al: Chromosome 18 DNA markers and manic-depressive illness: evidence for a susceptibility gene. Proc Natl Acad Sci U S A 91: 5918–5921, 1994

Bertelson A, Harvald B, Hauge M: A Danish twin study of manic depressive disorders. Br J Psychiatry 130:330–351, 1977

Bissette G, Widerlov E, Walleus H, et al: Alterations in cerebrospinal fluid concentrations of somatostatin-like immunoreactivity in neuropsychiatric disorders. Arch Gen Psychiatry 43:1148–1151, 1986

Blackwood DH, He L, Morris SW, et al: A locus for bipolar affective disorder on chromosome 4p. Nat Genet 12: 427–430, 1996

Bocchetta A, Piccardi MP, Del Zompo M: Is bipolar disorder linked to Xq28? (letter). Nat Genet 6:224, 1994

Boone KB, Miller BL, Lesser IM, et al: Neuropsychological correlates of white-matter lesions in healthy elderly subjects: a threshold effect. Arch Neurol 49:549–554, 1992

Botstein D, White RL, Skolnick M, et al: Construction of a genetic linkage map in man using restriction fragment length polymorphisms. Am J Hum Genet 32:314–331, 1980

Boyce PM: 6-Sulphatoxy melatonin in melancholia. Am J Psychiatry 142:125–127, 1985

Boyd AE, Levovitz HE, Pfeiffer JB: Stimulation of growth hormone secretion by L-dopa. N Engl J Med 283:1425–1429, 1970

Brambilla F, Maggioni M, Ferrari E, et al: Tonic and dynamic gonadotropin secretion in depressive and normothymic phases of affective disorders. Psychiatry Res 32:229–239, 1990

Bremner JD, Randall P, Scott TM, et al: MRI-based measurement of hippocampal volume in combat-related posttraumatic stress disorder. Am J Psychiatry 152:973–981, 1995

Bremner JD, Randall P, Vermetten E, et al: MRI-based measurement of hippocampal volume in posttraumatic stress disorder related to childhood physical and sexual abuse: a preliminary report. Biol Psychiatry 41:23–32, 1997

Briley M, Langer SZ, Raiseman R, et al: Tritiated imipramine binding sites are decreased in platelets of untreated depressed patients. Science 209:303–305, 1980

Broadhead WE, Blazer DG, George LK, et al: Depression, disability days, and days lost from work in a prospective epidemiologic survey. JAMA 264:2524–2528, 1990

Brown GL, Ebert MH, Goyer PF, et al: Aggression, suicide, and serotonin: relationships to CSF amine metabolites. Am J Psychiatry 139:741–746, 1982

Brown MR, Rivier C, Vale W, et al: Central nervous system regulation of adrenocorticotropin secretion: role of somatostatins. Endocrinology 114:1546–1549, 1984

Brown WA, Johnson R, Mayfield D: 24 hour dexamethasone suppression test in a clinical setting: relationship to diagnosis, symptoms and responses to treatment. Am J Psychiatry 136:543–547, 1979

Buchsbaum MS, Wu J, DeLisi LE, et al: Frontal cortex and basal ganglia metabolic rates assessed by positron emission tomography with F2-deoxyglucose in affective illness. J Affect Disord 10:137–152, 1986

Bunevicius R, Lasas L, Kazanavicius G, et al: Pituitary responses to thyrotropin releasing hormone stimulation in depressed women with thyroid gland disorders. Psychoneuroendocrinology 21:631–639, 1996

Bunney WE Jr, Davis M: Norepinephrine in depressive reactions. Arch Gen Psychiatry 13:483–494, 1965

Byerley W, Plaetke R, Hoff M, et al: Tyrosine hydroxylase gene not linked to manic-depression in seven of eight pedigrees. Hum Hered 42:259–263, 1992

Calabrese JR, Gulledge AD, Hahn K, et al: Autoimmune thyroiditis in manic-depressive patients treated with lithium. Am J Psychiatry 142:1318–1321, 1985

Campos-Barros A, Meinhold H, Stula M, et al: The influence of desipramine on thyroid hormone metabolism in rat brain. J Pharmacol Exp Ther 268:1143–1152, 1994

Carpenter W, Bunney W: Adrenal cortical activity in depressive illness. Am J Psychiatry 128:31–40, 1971

Carroll BJ: Pituitary-adrenal function in depression. Lancet 1:1373–1374, 1968

Carroll BJ: Use of the dexamethasone test in depression. J Clin Psychiatry 43:44–50, 1982

Carroll BJ, Davies B: Clinical associations of 11-hydroxy-corticosteroid suppression and non-suppression in severe depressive illness. BMJ 3:285–287, 1970

Carroll BJ, Meller WH, Kathol RG, et al: Pituitary-adrenal axis response to arginine vasopressin in patients with major depression. Psychiatry Res 46:119–126, 1993

Casanueva FF, Burguera S, Tome M, et al: Depending on the time of administration, dexamethasone potentiates or blocks growth hormone-releasing hormone-induced growth hormone release in man. Neuroendocrinology 47:46–49, 1988

Casanueva FF, Burguera S, Murais C, et al: Acute administration of corticoids: a new and peculiar stimulus of growth hormone secretion in man. J Clin Endocrinol Metab 70:234–237, 1990

Charney DS, Menkes DB, Henninger GR: Receptor sensitivity and the mechanism of action of antidepressant treatment. Arch Gen Psychiatry 38:1160–1180, 1981

Charney DS, Henninger GR, Steinberg DE, et al: Adrenergic receptor sensitivity in depression: effects of clonidine in depressed patients and healthy controls. Arch Gen Psychiatry 39:290–294, 1982

Checkley SA, Slade AP, Shur P: Growth hormone and other responses to clonidine in patients with endogenous depression. Br J Psychiatry 138:51–55, 1981

Cheetham SC, Crompton MR, Katona CLE, et al: Brain 5-HT1 binding sites in depressed suicides. Psychopharmacology (Berl) 102:544–548,1990

Chimowitz MI, Awad IA, Furlan AJ: Periventricular lesions on MRI: facts and theories. Stroke 20:963–967, 1989

Clarke IJ, Cummins JT: The temporal relationship between gonadotropin releasing hormone (GnRH) and luteinizing hormone (LH) secretion in ovariectomized ewes. Endocrinology 111:1737–1739, 1982

Coffey CE, Figiel GS, Djang WT, et al: Subcortical hyperintensity on magnetic resonance imaging: a comparison of normal and depressed elderly subjects. Am J Psychiatry 147:187–189, 1990

Contreras F, Navarro MA, Menchon JM, et al: Growth hormone response to growth hormone releasing hormone in non-delusional and delusional depression and healthy controls. Psychol Med 26:301–307, 1996

Coon H, Jensen S, Hoff M, et al: A genome-wide search for genes predisposing to manic-depression, assuming autosomal dominant inheritance. Am J Hum Genet 52:1234–1249, 1993

Coppen A: Depressive states and indolealkylamines, in Advances in Pharmacology, Vol 6. Edited by Garattini S, Shore PA. New York, Academic Press, 1968, pp 283–291

Coppen A, Prange AJ Jr, Whybrow PC, et al: Abnormalities of indoleamines in affective disorders. Arch Gen Psychiatry 26:474–478, 1972

Cowdry RW, Wehr TA, Zis AP, et al: Thyroid abnormalities associated with rapid-cycling bipolar illness. Arch Gen Psychiatry 40:414–420, 1983

Cowen PJ: A role for 5-HT in the action of antidepressant drugs. Pharmacol Ther 46:43–51, 1990

Cowen PJ, Charig EM: Neuroendocrine responses to tryptophan in major depression. Arch Gen Psychiatry 44:958–966, 1987

Craddock N, McGuffin P, Owen M: Darier's disease cosegregating with affective disorder (letter). Br J Psychiatry 165:272, 1994

Crow TJ, Cross AJ, Cooper SJ, et al: Neurotransmitter receptors and monoamine metabolites in the brains of patients with Alzheimer-type dementia and depression, and suicides. Neuropharmacology 23:1561–1569, 1984

Cummings S, Elde R, Ellis J, et al: Corticotropin-releasing factor immunoreactivity is widely distributed with the central nervous system of the rat: an immunohistochemical study. J Neurosci 8:1355–1368, 1983

Curtis D, Sherrington R, Brett P, et al: Genetic linkage analysis of manic depression in Iceland. J R Soc Med 86:506–510, 1993

Deakin JFW, Pennell I, Upadhyaya AJ, et al: A neuroendocrine study of 5-HT function in depression: evidence for biological mechanisms of endogenous and psychosocial causation. Psychopharmacology (Berl) 101:85–92, 1990

DeBellis MD, Geracioti TD Jr, Altemus M, et al: Cerebrospinal fluid monoamine metabolites in fluoxetine-treated patients with major depression and in healthy volunteers. Biol Psychiatry 33:636–641, 1993a

DeBellis MD, Gold PW, Geracioti TD, et al: Fluoxetine significantly reduces CSF CRH and AVP concentrations in patients with major depression. Am J Psychiatry 150:656–657, 1993b

De Bruyn A, Mendelbaum K, Sandkuijl LA, et al: Nonlinkage of bipolar illness to tyrosine hydroxylase, tyrosinase, and D2 and D4 dopamine receptor genes on chromosome 11. Am J Psychiatry 151:102–106, 1994

Delgado PL, Charney DS, Price LH, et al: Neuroendocrine and behavioral effects of dietary tryptophan restriction in healthy subjects. Life Sci 45:2323–2332, 1990

Del Zumpo M, Bocchetta A, Goldin LR, et al: Linkage between X chromosome markers and manic-depressive illness: two Sardinian pedigrees. Acta Psychiatr Scand 70:282–287, 1984

Detera-Wadleigh SD, Berrettini WH, Goldin LR, et al: Close linkage of c-Harvey-ras-1 and the insulin gene to affective disorder is ruled out in three North American pedigrees. Nature 325:806–808, 1987

Deuschle M, Schwieger U, Weber B, et al: Diurnal activity and pulsatility of the hypothalamus-pituitary-adrenal system in male depressed patients and healthy controls. J Clin Endocrinol Metab 82:234–238, 1997

Devanand DP, Bowers MB, Hoffman FJ, et al: Elevated plasma homovanillic acid in depressed females with melancholia and psychosis. Psychiatry Res 15:1–4, 1985

D'haenen H, Bossuyt A: Dopamine D2 receptors in the brain measured with SPECT. Biol Psychiatry 35:128–132, 1994

Dinan TG, Yatham LN, O'Keane VO, et al: Blunting of noradrenergic-stimulated growth hormone release in mania. Am J Psychiatry 148:936–938, 1991

Dolan RJ, Bench CJ, Liddle PF, et al: Dorsolateral prefrontal cortex dysfunction in the major psychoses: symptom or disease specificity? J Neurol Neurosurg Psychiatry 56:1290–1294, 1993

Drevets WC, Videen TO, Price JL, et al: A functional anatomical study of unipolar depression. J Neurosci 12:3628–3641, 1992

Drevets WC, Price JL, Simpson JR Jr, et al: Subgenual prefrontal cortex abnormalities in mood disorders (see comments). Nature 386:824–827, 1997

Dube S, Kumar N, Ettedgui E, et al: Cholinergic REM induction response: separation of anxiety and depression. Biol Psychiatry 20:408–418, 1985

Dubovsky SL, Lee C, Christiano J, et al: Elevated platelet intracellular calcium concentration in bipolar depression. Biol Psychiatry 29:441–450, 1991

Duman RS, Heninger GR, Nestler EJ: Molecular psychiatry: adaptations of receptor-coupled signal transduction pathways underlying stress- and drug-induced neural plasticity. J Nerv Ment Dis 182:692–700, 1994

Duman RS, Heninger GR, Nestler EJ: A molecular and cellular theory of depression. Arch Gen Psychiatry 54:597–606, 1997

Dupont RM, Jernigan TL, Butters N, et al: Subcortical abnormalities detected in bipolar affective disorder using magnetic resonance imaging: clinical and neuropsychological difference. Arch Gen Psychiatry 1:55–60, 1990

Dupont RM, Jernigan TL, Heindel W, et al: Magnetic resonance imaging and mood disorders: localization of white matter and other subcortical abnormalities. Arch Gen Psychiatry 52:747–755, 1995

Dussault JH, Ruel J: Thyroid hormones and brain development. Annu Rev Physiol 49:321–334, 1987

Duval F, Macher JP, Mokrani MC: Difference between evening and morning thyrotropin responses to protirelin in major depressive episode. Arch Gen Psychiatry 47:443–448, 1990

Duval F, Mokrani M-C, Crocq M-A, et al: Effect of antidepressant medication on morning and evening thyroid function tests during a major depressive episode. Arch Gen Psychiatry 53:833–840, 1996

Egeland JA, Gerhard DS, Pauls DL, et al: Bipolar affective disorders linked to DNA markers on chromosome 11. Nature 325:783–787, 1987

Elkis H, Friedman L, Wise A, et al: Meta-analyses of studies of ventricular enlargement and cortical sulcal prominence in mood disorders: comparisons with controls or patients with schizophrenia. Arch Gen Psychiatry 52:735–746, 1995

Ellis PM, Salmond C: Is platelet imipramine binding reduced in depression? A meta-analysis (see comments). Biol Psychiatry 36:292–299, 1994

El-Yousef M, Janowsky DS, Davis JM, et al: Induction of severe depression in marijuana intoxicated individuals. British Journal of Addiction 68:321–325, 1973

Enna SJ, Karbon EW, Duman RS: GABA-B agonist and imipramine-induced modifications in rat brain beta-adrenergic receptor binding and function, in GABA and Mood Disorders: Experimental and Clinical Research. Edited by Bartholini G, Lloyd KG, Morselli PL. New York, Raven, 1986, pp 23–49

Evans DL, Nemeroff CB: Use of dexamethasone suppression test using DSM III criteria on an inpatient psychiatric unit. Biol Psychiatry 18:505–511, 1983a

Evans DL, Nemeroff CB: The dexamethasone suppression test in mixed bipolar disorder. Am J Psychiatry 140:615–617, 1983b

Ewald H, Mors O, Friedrich U, et al: Exclusion of linkage between manic depressive illness and tyrosine hydroxylase and dopamine D2 receptor genes. Psychiatric Genetics 4:13–22, 1994

Ewald H, Mors O, Flint T, et al: A possible locus for manic depressive illness on chromosome 16p13. Psychiatric Genetics 5:71–81, 1995

Extein I, Tallman J, Smith CC, et al: Changes in lymphocyte beta-adrenergic receptors in depression and mania. Psychiatry Res 36:292–299, 1979

Extein I, Pottash ALC, Gold MS: The thyrotropin-releasing hormone test in the diagnosis of unipolar depression. Psychiatry Res 5:311–316, 1981

Ferin M, Van de Wiele R: Endogenous opioid peptides and the control of the menstrual cycle. Eur J Obstet Gynecol Reprod Biol 18:365–373, 1984

Figiel GS, Nemeroff CB: The mesolimbic motor circuit and its role in neuropsychiatric disorders, in Vol 4: Advances in Physiology. Edited by Kalivas PW, Barnes CD. Boca Raton, FL, CRC Press, 1993, pp 20351–20357

Figiel GS, Krishnan KRR, Brenner JC, et al: Radiologic correlates of antidepressant-induced delirium: the possible significance of basal ganglia lesions. J Neuropsychiatry Clin Neurosci 1:188–190, 1989

Figiel GS, Coffey CE, Djang WT, et al: Brain magnetic resonance imaging findings in ECT-induced delirium. J Neuropsychiatry Clin Neurosci 2:53–58, 1990

Figiel GS, Krishnan KRR, Doraiswamy PM: Subcortical structural changes in ECT-induced delirium. J Geriatr Psychiatry Neurol 3:172–176, 1991a

Figiel GS, Krishnan KRR, Doraiswamy PM, et al: Caudate hypertensities in elderly depressed patients with neuroleptic-induced parkinsonism. J Geriatr Psychiatry Neurol 4:86–89, 1991b

Figiel GS, Krishnan KRR, Doraiswamy PM, et al: Subcortical hyperintensities on brain magnetic resonance imaging: a comparison between late age onset and early onset elderly depressed subjects. Neurobiol Aging 12:245–247, 1991c

Figiel GS, Krishnan KRR, Rao VP, et al: Subcortical hyperintensities on brain magnetic resonance imaging: a comparison of normal and bipolar subjects. J Neuropsychiatry Clin Neurosci 3:18–22, 1991d

Figiel GS, Botteron KN, Doraiswamy PM, et al: Structural brain changes in affective disorder: a review. J Neuropsychiatry Clin Neurosci (in press)

Finkelstein JW, Roffwarg HP, Boyar RM, et al: Age-related changes in the twenty-four-hour spontaneous secretion of growth hormone. J Clin Endocrinol Metab 35:665–670, 1972

France RD, Urban B, Krishnan KRR, et al: CSF corticotropin-releasing factor-like immunoreactivity in chronic pain patients with and without major depression. Biol Psychiatry 23:86–88, 1988

Freimer NB, Reus VI, Escamilla MA, et al: Genetic mapping using haplotype association and linkage methods suggests a locus for severe bipolar disorder (BP I) at 18q22-q23. Nat Genet 12:436–441, 1996

Garcia-Sevilla JA, Padro D, Giralt T, et al: Alpha-2 adrenoceptor-mediated inhibition of platelet adenyl cyclase and induction of aggregation in major depression. Arch Gen Psychiatry 47:125–132, 1990

Gerner RH, Yamada T: Altered neuropeptide concentrations in cerebrospinal fluid of psychiatric patients. Brain Res 238:298–302, 1982

Gershon ES, Goldin LR: The outlook for linkage research in psychiatric disorders. J Psychiatr Res 21:541–550, 1987

Gershon ES, Goldin LR, Lake CR, et al: Genetics of plasma dopamine-β-hydroxylase, erythrocyte catechol-O-methyltransferase and platelet monoamine oxidase in pedigrees of patients with affective disorders, in Enzymes and Neurotransmitters in Mental Disease. Edited by Usdin E, Sourkes L, Young MBH. New York, Wiley, 1980, pp 281–299

Gershon ES, Hamovit JR, Schreiber JL: Anorexia nervosa and major affective disorders associated in families: a preliminary report, in Childhood Psychopathology and Development. Edited by Guze SB, Earls FJ, Barrett JE. New York, Raven, 1983

Gibbons JL, McHugh PR: Plasma cortisol in depressive illness. J Psychiatr Res 1:162–171, 1962

Gibbons RD, Davis JM: Consistent evidence for a biological subtype of depression characterized by low CSF monoamine levels. Acta Psychiatr Scand 74:8–12, 1986

Gillies G, Lowry P: Corticotropin releasing factor may be modulated by vasopressin. Nature 278:463–464, 1979

Ginns EI, Egeland JA, Allen CR, et al: Update on the search for DNA markers linked to manic-depressive illness in the Old Order Amish. J Psychiatr Res 26:305–308, 1992

Ginns EI, Oh J, Egeland JA, et al: A genome-wide search for chromosomal loci linked to the bipolar affective disorder in the Old Order Amish. Nat Genet 12:431–435, 1996

Godwin CD, Greenberg LB, Shukla S: Predictive value of the dexamethasone suppression test in mania. Am J Psychiatry 141:1610–1612, 1984

Gold BI, Bowers MB, Roth RH, et al: GABA levels in CSF of patients with psychiatric disorders. Am J Psychiatry 137:362–364, 1980

Gold MS, Pottash AC, Extein I: Symptomless autoimmune thyroiditis in depression. Psychiatry Res 6:261–269, 1982

Gold PW, Chrousos GP, Kellner C, et al: Psychiatric implications of basic and clinical studies with corticotropin-releasing factor. Am J Psychiatry 141:619–627, 1984

Gold PW, Loriaux DL, Roy A, et al: Responses to corticotropin releasing hormone in the hypercortisolism of depression and Cushing's disease: pathophysiologic and diagnostic implications. N Engl J Med 314:1329–1335, 1986

Golden RN, Markey SP, Risby E, et al: Antidepressants reduce whole-body NE turnover while enhancing 6-hydroxymelatonin output. Arch Gen Psychiatry 45:150–154, 1988

Goldstein J, Van Cauter E, Linkowski P, et al: Thyrotropin nyctohemeral pattern in primary depression: difference between unipolar and bipolar women. Life Sci 27:1695–1703, 1980

Gonzalez-Heydrich J, Peroutka SJ: Serotonin receptors and reuptake sites: pharmacologic significance. J Clin Psychiatry 51 (suppl):5–12, 1990

Goodwin GM, Austin MP, Dougall N, et al: State changes in brain activity shown by the uptake of 99m-Tc-exametazime with single photon emission tomography in major depression before and after treatment. J Affect Disord 29:243–253, 1993

Greenwald BS, Kramer-Ginsberg E, Krishnan KRR, et al: MRI signal hyperintensities in geriatric depression. Am J Psychiatry 153:1212–1215, 1996

Gurvits TG, Shenton MR, Hokama H, et al: Magnetic resonance imaging study of hippocampal volume in chronic, combat-related posttraumatic stress disorder. Biol Psychiatry 40:1091–1099, 1996

Haggerty JJ, Simon JS, Evans DL, et al: Relationship of serum TSH concentration and antithyroid antibodies to diagnosis and DST response in psychiatric inpatients. Am J Psychiatry 144:1491–1493, 1987

Haggerty JJ, Evans DL, Golden RN, et al: The presence of anti-thyroid antibodies in patients with affective and non-affective psychiatric disorders. Biol Psychiatry 27:51–60, 1990

Halaris AE: Plasma 3-methoxy-4-hydroxyphenylglycol in manic psychosis. Am J Psychiatry 135:493–494, 1978

Halaris A, Piletz J: Platelet adrenoceptor binding as a marker in neuropsychiatric disorders. Abstracts of 17th CINP Congress, 1990, p 28

Hatterer JA, Herbert J, Hidaka C, et al: CSF transthyretin in patients with depression. Am J Psychiatry 150:813–815, 1993

Hauser PH, Altshuler LL, Berrettini W, et al: Temporal lobe measurement in primary affective disorder by magnetic resonance imaging. J Neuropsychiatry Clin Neurosci 1:128–134, 1989a

Hauser PH, Dauphinais D, Berrettini W, et al: Corpus callosum dimensions measured by magnetic resonance imaging in bipolar affective disorder and schizophrenia. Biol Psychiatry 26:659–668, 1989b

Hayakawa H, Yokota N, Kawai K, et al: Effects of electroconvulsive shock on the serotonin metabolism and serotonin1A receptors in the rat brain. Jpn J Psychiatry Neurol 47:418–419, 1993

Healy D, Carney PA, O'Halloran A, et al: Peripheral adrenoceptors and serotonin receptors in depression: changes associated with response to treatment with trazodone or amitriptyline. J Affect Dis 9:285–296, 1985

Heisler S, Reisine T, Hook V, et al: Somatostatin inhibits multireceptor stimulation of cyclic AMP formation and adrenocorticotropin secretion in mouse pituitary tumor cells. Proc Natl Acad Sci U S A 79:6502–6507, 1982

Hermus AR, Pieters GF, Smals AG, et al: Plasma adrenocorticotropin, cortisol, and aldosterone responses to corticotropin-releasing factor: modulatory effect of basal cortisol levels. J Clin Endocrinol Metab 58:187–191, 1984

Hindal JT, Kaplan MM: Inhibition of thyroxine 5´-deiodination type II in cultured human placental cells by cortisol, insulin, 3,5´-cyclic adenosine monophosphate and butyrate. Metabolism, Clinical and Experimental 37:664–668, 1988

Hodgkinson S, Sherrington R, Gurlin H, et al: Molecular genetic evidence for heterogeneity in manic depression. Nature 325:805–806, 1987

Hollister LE, Davis KL, Berger PA: Subtypes of depression based on excretion of MHPG and response to nortriptyline. Arch Gen Psychiatry 37:1107–1110, 1980

Holmes MC, Catt KJ, Aguilera G: Involvement of vasopressin in the down-regulation of pituitary corticotropin-releasing factor receptors after adrenalectomy. Endocrinology 121:2093–2098, 1987

Holsboer F, Haack D, Gerken A, et al: Plasma dexamethasone concentrations and different suppression response of cortisol and corticosterone in depressives and controls. Biol Psychiatry 19:281–291, 1984a

Holsboer F, Von Bardeleben U, Gerken A, et al: Blunted corticotropin and normal cortisol response to human corticotropin-releasing factor in depression (letter). N Engl J Med 311:1127, 1984b

Holsboer F, Von Bardeleben U, Weidemann K, et al: Serial assessment of corticotropin-releasing hormone response after dexamethasone in depression—implications for pathophysiology of DST nonsuppression. Biol Psychiatry 22:228–234, 1987

Holsboer-Trachsler E, Stohler R, Hatzinger M: Repeated administration of the combined dexamethasone/hCRH stimulation test during treatment of depression. Psychiatry Res 38:32–38, 1991

Honig A, Bartlett JR, Bouras N, et al: Amino acid levels in depression: a preliminary investigation. J Psychiatr Res 22:159–164, 1989

Hurwitz TA, Clark C, Murphy E, et al: Regional cerebral glucose metabolism in major depressive disorder. Can J Psychiatry 35:684–688, 1990

Husain MM, Figiel GS, Lurie SN, et al: MRI of corpus callosum and septum pellucidum in depression. Biol Psychiatry 29:300–301, 1991a

Husain MM, McDonald WM, Doraiswamy PM, et al: A magnetic resonance imaging study of putamen nuclei in major depression. Psychiatry Res 40:95–99, 1991b

Iacono WG, Smith GN, Moreau M, et al: Ventricular and sulcal size at the onset of psychosis. Am J Psychiatry 145:820–824, 1988

Imura H, Nakai Y, Hoshimi T: Effect of 5-hydroxytryptophan (5-HTP) on growth hormone and ACTH release in man. J Clin Endocrinol Metab 36:204–206, 1973

Jackson IMD: Does thyroid hormone have a role as adjunctive therapy in depression? Thyroid 6:63–67, 1996

Jacobson L, Sapolsky R: The role of the hippocampus in feedback regulation of the hypothalamic-pituitary-adrenocortical axis. Endocr Rev 12:118–134, 1991

Jacoby RJ, Levy R: Computed tomography in the elderly: affective disorder. Br J Psychiatry 136:270–275, 1980

Jaeckle RS, Kathol RG, Lopez JF, et al: Enhanced adrenal sensitivity to exogenous ACTH stimulation in major depression. Arch Gen Psychiatry 44:233–240, 1987

Jaffe RB, Plosker S, Marshall L, et al: Neuromodulatory regulation of gonadotropin-releasing hormone pulsatile discharge in women. Am J Obstet Gynecol 163:1727–1731, 1990

Janicak PG, Davis JM, Chan C, et al: Failure of urinary MHPG levels to predict treatment response in patients with unipolar depression. Am J Psychiatry 143:1398–1402, 1986

Janowsky DS, Risch SC: Cholinomimetic and anticholinergic drugs used to investigate an acetylcholine hypothesis of affective disorder and stress. Drug Development Research 4:125–142, 1984

Janowsky DS, El-Yousef MK, Davis JM, et al: A cholinergic-adrenergic hypothesis of mania and depression. Lancet 2:573–577, 1972

Joffe RT, Singer W, Levitt AJ, et al: A placebo-controlled comparison of lithium and triiodothyronine augmentation of tricyclic antidepressants in unipolar refractory depression. Arch Gen Psychiatry 50:387–394, 1993

Johnson J, Weissman MM, Klerman GL: Service utilization and social morbidity associated with depressive symptoms in the community. JAMA 267:1478–1483, 1992

Jones D, Kelwala S, Bell J, et al: Cholinergic REM sleep induction response correlation with endogenous major depressive type. Psychiatry Res 14:99–110, 1985

Kalin NH, Risch SC, Janowsky DS, et al: Plasma ACTH and cortisol concentrations before and after dexamethasone. Psychiatry Res 7:87–92, 1982

Kaplan MM: The role of thyroid hormone deiodination in the regulation of hypothalamo-pituitary function. Neuroendocrinology 38:254–260, 1984

Kastin AJ, Ehrensing RH, Schalch DS, et al: Improvement in mental depression with decreased thyrotropin response after administration of thyrotropin-releasing hormone. Lancet 2:740–742, 1972

Kathol RG, Jaeckle RS, Lopez JR, et al: Consistent reduction of ACTH responses to stimulation with CRH, vasopressin and hypoglycaemia in patients with depression. Br J Psychiatry 155:468–478, 1989

Kauffman CA, Malaspina D: Molecular genetics of schizophrenia. Psychiatric Annals 23:111–122, 1993

Kelsoe JR: The genetics of bipolar disorder. Psychiatric Annals 27:285–292, 1997

Kelsoe JR, Ginns EI, Egeland JA, et al: Re-evaluation of the linkage relationship between chromosome 11p loci and the gene for bipolar affective disorder in the Old Order Amish. Nature 342:238–243, 1989

Kelsoe JR, Kristbjanarson HH, Bergesch P, et al: A genetic linkage study of bipolar disorder and 13 markers on chromosome 11 including the D2 dopamine receptor. Neuropsychopharmacology 9:293–301, 1993

Kendler KS, Neale MC, Kessler RC, et al: A population-based twin study of major depression in women: the impact of varying definitions of illness. Arch Gen Psychiatry 49:257–266, 1992

Kendler KS, Pedersen N, Johnson L, et al: A pilot Swedish twin study of affective illness, including hospital- and population-ascertained subsamples. Arch Gen Psychiatry 50:699–706, 1993a

Kendler KS, Kessler RC, Neale MC, et al: The prediction of major depression in women: toward an integrated etiologic model. Am J Psychiatry 150:1139–1148, 1993b

Kendler KS, Neale MC, Kessler RC, et al: The lifetime history of major depression in women: reliability of diagnosis and heritability. Arch Gen Psychiatry 50:863–870, 1993c

Kendler KS, Eaves LJ, Walters EE, et al: The identification and validation of distinct depressive syndromes in a population-based sample of female twins. Arch Gen Psychiatry 53:391–399, 1996

Kennedy SH, Tighe S, McVey G, et al: Melatonin and cortisol "switches" during mania, depression, and euthymia in a drug-free bipolar patient. J Nerv Ment Dis 177:300–303, 1989

Kessler RC, McGonagle KA, Zhao S, et al: Lifetime and 12-month prevalence of DSM-III-R psychiatric disorders in the United States. Arch Gen Psychiatry 51:8–19, 1994

Kiriike N, Izumiya Y, Nishiwaki S, et al: TRH test and DST in schizoaffective mania, mania, and schizophrenia. Biol Psychiatry 24:415–422, 1988

Kirkegaard CJ, Faber J, Hummer L, et al: Increased levels of TRH in cerebrospinal fluid from patients with endogenous depression. Psychoneuroendocrinology 4:227–235, 1979

Kishimoto H, Takazu O, Ohno S, et al: 11C-glucose metabolism in manic and depressed patients. Psychiatry Res 22:81–88, 1987

Knobil E: The GnRH pulse generator. Am J Obstet Gynecol 163:1721–1727, 1990

Knorring LV, Perris C, Oreland L, et al: Morbidity risk for psychiatric disorders in families of probands with affective disorders divided according to levels of platelet MAO activity. Psychiatry Res 15:271–279, 1985

Koyama T, Meltzer HY: A biochemical and neuroendocrine study of the serotonergic system in depression, in New Results in Depression Research. Edited by Hippius H, Klerman GL, Matussek N. New York, Springer-Verlag New York, 1986, pp 169–188

Krishnan KRR: Organic bases of depression in the elderly. Annu Rev Med 42:261–266, 1991

Krishnan KRR, Maltbie AA, Davidson JRT: Abnormal cortisol suppression in bipolar patients with simultaneous manic and depressive symptoms. Am J Psychiatry 140:203–205, 1983

Krishnan KRR, France RD, Pelton S, et al: What does the dexamethasone suppression test identify? Biol Psychiatry 20:957–964, 1985

Krishnan KR, Manepalli AN, Ritchie JC, et al: Growth hormone-releasing factor stimulation test in depression. Am J Psychiatry 145:190–192, 1988

Krishnan KRR, Husain MM, McDonald WM, et al: In vivo assessment of caudate volume in man: effect of normal aging. Life Sci 47:1325–1329, 1990a

Krishnan KRR, Ritchie JC, Saunders WB, et al: Adrenocortical sensitivity to low dose ACTH administration in depressed patients. Biol Psychiatry 27:930–933, 1990b

Krishnan KRR, Doraiswamy PM, Lurie SN, et al: Pituitary size in depression. J Clin Endocrinol Metab 72:256–259, 1991

Krishnan KRR, McDonald WM, Escalona PR, et al: Magnetic resonance imaging of the caudate nuclei in depression. Arch Gen Psychiatry 49:553–557, 1992

Krishnan KRR, Rayasam K, Reed D, et al: The CRF corticotropin-releasing factor stimulation test in patients with major depression: relationship to dexamethasone suppression test results. Depression 1:133–136, 1993

Kumar A, Mozley D, Dunham C, et al: Semi-quantitative I-123 IMP SPECT studies in late onset depression before and after treatment. International Journal of Geriatric Psychiatry 6:775–777, 1991

Kumar A, Nadel DM, Alavi A, et al: High resolution 18 FDG PET studies in late-life depression (abstract). J Nucl Med 33:1013, 1992

Lal S, Martin JB, de la Vega C, et al: Comparison of the effect of apomorphine and L-dopa on serum growth hormone levels in man. Clin Endocrinol (Oxf) 4:277–285, 1975

Landon J, James VHT, Stoker DJ: Plasma cortisol response to lysine-vasopressin in comparison with other tests of human pituitary-adrenocortical function. Lancet 2:1156–1159, 1965

Langer SZ, Raisman R: Binding of [3H]imipramine and [3H]desipramine as biochemical tools for studies in depression. Neuropharmacology 22:407–413, 1983

Lapin I, Oxenkrug G: Intensification of the central serotonergic process as a possible determinant of thymoleptic effect. Lancet 1:132–136, 1969

Lazarus JH, McGregor AM, Ludgate M, et al: Effect of lithium carbonate therapy on thyroid immune status in manic depressive patients: a prospective study. J Affect Disord 11:155–160, 1986

Leckman JF, Gershon ES, Nichols AS, et al: Reduced MAO activity in first-degree relatives of individuals with bipolar affective disorders: a preliminary report. Arch Gen Psychiatry 34:601–606, 1977

Leibenluft E, Fiero PL, Rubinow DR: Effects of the menstrual cycle on dependent variables in mood disorder research. Arch Gen Psychiatry 51:761–781, 1994

Lenox RH, Watson DG: Lithium and the brain: a psychopharmacological strategy to a molecular basis for manic depressive illness. Clin Chem 40:309–314, 1994

Lerer B: Neurochemical and other neurobiological consequences of ECT: implications for the pathogenesis and treatment of affective disorders, in Psychopharmacology: The Third Generation of Progress. Edited by Meltzer HY. New York, Raven, 1987, pp 577–588

Lesch KP, Laux G, Erb A, et al: Attenuated growth hormone response to growth hormone RH in major depressive disorder. Biol Psychiatry 22:1495–1499, 1987a

Lesch KP, Laux G, Pfuller H, et al: Growth hormone response to GH-releasing hormone in depression. J Clin Endocrinol Metab 65:1278–1281, 1987b

Lesser IM, Boone KB, Mehringer CM, et al: Cognition and white matter hyperintensities in older depressed patients. Am J Psychiatry 153:1280–1287, 1996

Lewis DA, McChesney C: Tritiated imipramine binding distinguishes among subtypes of depression. Arch Gen Psychiatry 42:485–488, 1985

Lindsay RM, Wiegand SJ, Altar CA, et al: Neurotrophic factors: from molecule to man. Trends Neurosci 17:182–190, 1994

Linkowski P, Mendlewicz J, LeClerq R, et al: The 24 hour profile of ACTH and cortisol in major depressive illness. J Clin Endocrinol Metab 61:429–438, 1985

Linkowski P, Kerkhofs M, Van Onderbergen A, et al: The 24-hour profiles of cortisol, prolactin, and growth hormone secretion in mania. Arch Gen Psychiatry 51:616–624, 1994

Linnoila M, Karoum F, Calil HM, et al: Alteration of NE metabolism with desipramine and zimelidine in depressed patients. Arch Gen Psychiatry 39:1025–1028, 1982

Linnoila M, Guthrie S, Lane EA, et al: Clinical studies on NE metabolism: how to interpret the numbers. Psychiatry Res 17:229–239, 1986

Linnoila VM, Virkkunen M: Aggression, suicidality and serotonin. J Clin Psychiatry 53 (suppl):46–51, 1992

Linnoila VM, Cowdry R, Lamberg B-A, et al: CSF triiodothyronine (rT3) levels in patients with affective disorders. Biol Psychiatry 18:1489–1492, 1983a

Linnoila VM, Virkkunen M, Scheinin M, et al: Low cerebrospinal fluid 5-hydroxyindoleacetic acid concentration differentiates impulsive from nonimpulsive violent behavior. Life Sci 33:2609–2614, 1983b

Lippman S, Manshadi M, Baldwin H, et al: Cerebellar vermis dimensions on computerized tomographic scans of schizophrenia and bipolar patients. Am J Psychiatry 139:667–668, 1982

Little KY: Amphetamine, but not methylphenidate, predicts antidepressant response. J Clin Psychopharmacol 8:177–183, 1988

Loosen PT, Prange AJ Jr: Serum thyrotropin response to thyrotropin-releasing hormone in psychiatric patients: a review. Am J Psychiatry 139:405–416, 1982

Louis WJ, Doyle AE, Anavekar SN: Plasma noradrenaline concentration and blood pressure in essential hypertension, phaeochromocytoma and depression. Clinical Science and Molecular Medicine 48:239s–242s, 1975

Lund A, Mjellem-Jolly N, Hole K: Desipramine, administered chronically, influences 5-hydroxytryptamine 1A-receptors, as measured by behavioral tests and receptor binding in rats. Neuropharmacology 31:25–32, 1992

Lurie SN, Doraiswamy PM, Figiel GS, et al: In vivo assessment of pituitary gland volume with MRI: effect of age. J Clin Endocrinol Metab 71:505–508, 1990

Maas JW, Fawcett JA, Dekirmenjian H: Catecholamine metabolism, depressive illness and drug response. Arch Gen Psychiatry 26:252–262, 1972

Maas JW, Koslow SH, Katz MM, et al: Pretreatment neurotransmitter metabolite levels and response to tricyclic antidepressant drugs. Am J Psychiatry 141:1159–1171, 1984

Maeda K, Yoshimoto Y, Yamadori A: Blunted TSH and unaltered PRL responses to TRH following repeated administration of TRH in neurologic patients: a replication of neuroendocrine features of major depression. Biol Psychiatry 33:277–283, 1993

Maes M, de Ruyter M, Suy E: Cortisol response to dexamethasone and noradrenergic function in depression. Acta Psychiatr Scand 75:171–175, 1987

Maes M, Jacobs M-P, Suy E, et al: Suppressant effects of dexamethasone on the availability of plasma L-tryptophan and tyrosine in healthy controls and in depressed patients. Acta Psychiatr Scand 81:19–23, 1990

Magarinos A, McEwen BS, Flugge G, et al: Chronic psychosocial stress causes apical dendritic atrophy of hippocampal CA3 pyramidal neurons in subordinate tree shrews. J Neurosci 16:3534–3540, 1996

Maj M, Ariano MG, Arena F, et al: Plasma cortisol, catecholamine and cyclic AMP levels, response to dexamethasone suppression test and platelet MAO activity in manic-depressive patients: a longitudinal study. Neuropsychobiology 11:168–173, 1984

Malison RT, Pelton G, Carpenter L, et al: Reduced midbrain serotonin transporter binding in depressed vs. healthy subjects as measured by [^{123}I] b-CIT SPECT. Society for Neuroscience Abstracts 23:1220, 1997

Mann JJ, Stanley M, McBride PA, et al: Increased serotonin 2 and b-adrenergic receptor binding in the frontal cortices of suicide victims. Arch Gen Psychiatry 43:954–959, 1986

Marangell LB, George MS, Callahan AM, et al: Effects of intrathecal thyrotropin-releasing hormone (protirelin) in refractory depressed patients. Arch Gen Psychiatry 54:214–222, 1997

Martinot JL, Hardy P, Feline A, et al: Left prefrontal glucose metabolism in the depressed state: a confirmation. Am J Psychiatry 147:1313–1317, 1990

Mattsubara S, Arora RC, Meltzer HY: Serotonergic measures in suicide brain: 5-HT1A binding sites in frontal cortex of suicide victims. J Neural Transm 85:181–194, 1991

Matussek N, Ackenheil M, Hippius H, et al: Effects of clonidine on growth hormone release in psychiatric patients and controls. Psychiatry Res 2:25–36, 1980

Maubach M, Dieblod K, Fried W, et al: Platelet MAO activity in patients with affective psychosis and their first-degree relatives. Pharmacopsychiatry 14:87–93, 1981

Mayberg MS, Brannan SK, Mahurin RK, et al: Cingulate function in depression: a potential predictor of treatment response. Neuroreport 8:1057–1061, 1997

McEwen BS: Re-examination of the glucocorticoid hypothesis of stress and aging. Prog Brain Res 93:365–383, 1992

McGuffin P, Katz R, Rutherford J: Nature, nurture and depression: a twin study. Psychol Med 21:329–335, 1991

McGuffin P, Katz R, Watkins S, et al: A hospital-based twin register of the heritability of DSM-IV unipolar depression. Arch Gen Psychiatry 53:129–136, 1996

McInnis M: Recent advances in the genetics of bipolar disorder. Psychiatric Annals 27:482–488, 1997

McKinney WT: Animal models of depression: an overview. Psychiatric Developments 2:77–96, 1984

McKusick V: Mendelian Inheritance in Man, 10th Edition. Baltimore, MD, Johns Hopkins University Press, 1992

Meana JJ, Barturen F, Garcia-Sevilla JA: Alpha$_2$-adrenoceptors in the brain of suicide victims: increased receptor density associated with major depression. Biol Psychiatry 31:471–490, 1992

Meller WH, Zander KM, Crosby RD, et al: Luteinizing hormone pulse characteristics in depressed women. Am J Psychiatry 154:1454–1455, 1997

Meltzer HY, Lowy MT, Locascio JJ: Platelet MAO activity and the cortisol response to dexamethasone in major depression. Biol Psychiatry 24:129–142, 1988

Mendlewicz J: Genetics of depression and mania, in Depression and Mania. Edited by Georgotas A, Cancro R. New York, Elsevier, 1988, pp 20197–20212

Mendlewicz J, Rainier J: Adoption study supporting genetic transmission in manic-depressive illness. Nature 268:326–329, 1977

Mendlewicz J, Linkowski P, Kerkhofs M, et al: Diurnal hypersecretion of growth hormone in depression. J Clin Endocrinol Metab 60:505–512, 1985

Mendlewicz J, Simon P, Sevy S, et al: Polymorphic DNA marker on X-chromosome and manic depression. Lancet 1:1230–1232, 1987

Menkes DB, Rasenick MM, Wheeler MA, et al: Guanosine triphosphate activation of brain adenylate cyclase: enhancement by long-term antidepressant treatment. Science 129:65–67, 1983

Merchenthaler I, Vigh S, Petrusz P, et al: Immunocytochemical localization of corticotropin-releasing factor (CRF) in the rat brain. American Journal of Anatomy 165:385–396, 1982

Michels R, Marzuk P: Progress in psychiatry, I. N Engl J Med 329:552–560, 1993

Midgely AR, Jaffe RB: Regulation of human gonadotropins: episodic fluctuation of LH during the menstrual cycle. J Clin Endocrinol Metab 33:962–969, 1971

Mooney JJ, Schatzberg AF, Cole JO, et al: Rapid antidepressant response to alprazolam in depressed patients with high catecholamine output and heterologous desensitization of platelet adenyl cyclase. Biol Psychiatry 23:543–559, 1988

Mooney JJ, Schatzberg AF, Cole JO, et al: Urinary 3-methoxy-4-hydroxyphenylglycol and the depression-type score as predictors of differential responses to antidepressants. J Clin Psychopharmacol 11:339–343, 1991

Muller EE, Brambilla F, Cavagnini F, et al: Slight effect of L-tryptophan on growth hormone release in normal human subjects. J Clin Endocrinol Metab 39:1–5, 1974

Muscettola G, Potter WZ, Pickar D, et al: Urinary 3-methoxy-4-hydroxyphenylglycol and major affective disorders: a replication and new findings. Arch Gen Psychiatry 41:337–342, 1984

Myers DH, Carter RA, Burns BH, et al: A prospective study of the effects of lithium on thyroid function and on the prevalence of antithyroid antibodies. Psychol Med 15:55–61, 1985

Nair PNV, Hariharasubramanian N: Pilapil circadian rhythm of melatonin in endogenous depression. Prog Neuropsychopharmacol Biol Psychiatry 19:1215–1228, 1984

Nakamura Y, Leppert M, O'Connell P, et al: Variable number of tandem repeat (VNTR) markers for human gene mapping. Science 235:1616–1622, 1987

Nemeroff CB, Evans DL: Correlation between the dexamethasone suppression test in depressed patients and clinical response. Am J Psychiatry 141:247–249, 1984

Nemeroff CB, Bissette G, Martin JB, et al: Effect of chronic treatment with thyrotropin-releasing hormone (TRH) or an analog of TRH (linear-beta-alanine TRH) on the hypothalamic-pituitary-thyroid axis. Neuroendocrinology 30:193–199, 1980

Nemeroff CB, Widerlov E, Bissette G, et al: Elevated concentrations of CSF corticotropin-releasing factor-like immunoreactivity in depressed patients. Science 226:1342–1344, 1984

Nemeroff CB, Simon JS, Haggerty JJ, et al: Antithyroid antibodies in depressed patients. Am J Psychiatry 142:840–843, 1985

Nemeroff CB, Knight DL, Krishnan KRR, et al: Marked reduction in the number of platelet [3H]imipramine binding sites in geriatric depression. Arch Gen Psychiatry 45:919–923, 1988a

Nemeroff CB, Owens MJ, Bissette G, et al: Reduced corticotropin-releasing factor (CRF) binding sites in the frontal cortex of suicides. Arch Gen Psychiatry 45:577–579, 1988b

Nemeroff CB, Bissette G, Akil H, et al: Neuropeptide concentrations in the cerebrospinal fluid of depressed patients treated with electroconvulsive therapy: corticotropin-releasing factor, beta-endorphin and somatostatin. Br J Psychiatry 158:59–63, 1991a

Nemeroff CB, Knight DL, Krishnan KRR: Reduced platelet [3H]-paroxetine and [3H]-imipramine binding in major depression. Society for Neuroscience Abstracts 17:1472, 1991b

Nemeroff CB, Krishnan KKR, Reed D, et al: Adrenal gland enlargement in major depression: a computed tomographic study. Arch Gen Psychiatry 49:384–387, 1992

Nemeroff CB, Knight DL, Franks J, et al: Further studies on platelet serotonin transporter binding in depression. Am J Psychiatry 151:1623–1625, 1994

Nestler EJ, Terwilliger RZ, Duman RS: Chronic antidepressant administration alters the subcellular distribution of cyclic AMP-dependent protein kinase in rat frontal cortex. J Neurochem 53:1644–1647, 1989

Neumeister A, Praschak-Rieder N, Hesselmann B, et al: Rapid tryptophan depletion in drug-free depressed patients with seasonal affective disorder. Am J Psychiatry 154:1153–1155, 1997

Nibuya M, Morinobu S, Duman RS: Regulation of BDNF and trkB mRNA in rat brain by chronic electroconvulsive seizure and antidepressant drug treatments. J Neurosci 15:7539–7547, 1995

Nibuya M, Nestler EJ, Duman RS: Chronic antidepressant administration increases the expression of cAMP response element-binding protein (CREB) in rat hippocampus. J Neurosci 16:2365–2372, 1996

Nobler MS, Sackheim HA, Prohovnik I, et al: Regional cerebral blood flow in mood disorders, III: treatment and clinical response. Arch Gen Psychiatry 51:884–897, 1994a

Nobler MS, Sackheim HA, Prohovnik I, et al: Effects of antidepressant medication on rCBF in late-life depression (abstract). Biol Psychiatry 35:712, 1994b

Nurnberger JJ Jr, Simmons-Alling S, Kessler L, et al: Separate mechanisms for behavioral, cardiovascular and hormonal responses to dextroamphetamine in man. Psychopharmacology 84:200–204, 1984

Pandey GN, Sharma RP, Janicak PG, et al: Monoamine oxidase and cortisol response in depression and schizophrenia. Psychiatry Res 44:1–8, 1992

Pandey SC, David JM, Schwertz DW, et al: Effect of antidepressants and neuroleptics on phosphoinositide metabolism in human platelets. J Pharmacol Exp Ther 256:1010–1018, 1991

Papez JW: A proposed mechanism of emotion. Archives of Neurology and Psychiatry 38:725–743, 1937

Pardes H, Kauffmann CA, Pincus HA, et al: Genetics and psychiatry: past discoveries, current dilemmas, and future directions. Am J Psychiatry 146:435–443, 1989

Patel YC, Alford FP, Burger HG: The 24-hour plasma thyrotropin profile. Clin Sci 43:71–77, 1972

Pauls DL, Gerhard DS, Lacy LG, et al: Linkage of bipolar affective disorders to markers on chromosome 11p is excluded in a second lateral extension of Amish pedigree 110. Genomics 11:730–736, 1991

Pearlson GD, Rabins PV, Kim WS, et al: Structural brain CT changes and cognitive deficits in elderly depressives with and without reversible dementia. Psychol Med 19:573–584, 1989

Perry EK, Marshall EF, Blessed G, et al: Decreased imipramine binding in the brains of patients with depressive illness. Br J Psychiatry 142:188–192, 1983

Petty F: Plasma concentrations of GABA and mood disorders: a blood test for manic depressive disease? Clin Chem 40:296–302, 1994

Petty F, Schlesser MA: Plasma GABA in affective illness. J Affect Disord 3:339–343, 1981

Petty F, Sherman AD: Plasma GABA levels in psychiatric illness. J Affect Disord 6:131–138, 1984

Piercey MF, Hoffmann WE, Smith MW, et al: Inhibition of dopamine neuron firing by pramipexole, a dopamine D3 receptor-preferring agonist: comparison to other dopamine receptor agonists. Eur J Pharmacol 312:35–44, 1996

Pitts AF, Kathol RG, Gehris TL, et al: Elevated cerebrospinal fluid corticotropin-releasing hormone and arginine vasopressin in depressed patients with dexamethasone nonsuppression. Society for Neuroscience Abstracts 16:454, 1990

Post RM, Gold P, Rubinow DR, et al: Peptides in cerebrospinal fluid of neuropsychiatric patients: an approach to central nervous system peptide function. Life Sci 31:1–15, 1982

Prange AJ, Wilson IC, Rabon AM, et al: Enhancement of imipramine antidepressant activity by thyroid hormone. Am J Psychiatry 126:457–469, 1969

Prange AJ Jr, Wilson IC, Lara PP, et al: Effects of thyrotropin-releasing hormone in depression. Lancet 2:999–1002, 1972

Prange AJ Jr, Wilson IC, Lynn CW, et al: L-Tryptophan in mania: contribution to a permissive hypothesis of affective disorders. Arch Gen Psychiatry 30:56–62, 1974

Prange AJ, Loosen PT, Wilson I, et al: The therapeutic use of hormones of the thyroid axis in depression, in Neurobiology of Mood Disorders. Edited by Post CR, Ballenger J. Baltimore, MD, Williams & Wilkins, 1980, pp 311–322

Price RA, Kidd KK, Weissman MM: Early onset (under age 30 years) and panic disorder as markers for etiologic homogeneity in major depression. Arch Gen Psychiatry 44:434–440, 1987

Purba JS, Hoogendijk WJG, Hofman MA, et al: Increased number of vasopressin- and oxytocin-expressing neurons in the paraventricular nucleus of the hypothalamus in depression. Arch Gen Psychiatry 53:137–143, 1996

Raadsheer FC, Hoogendijk WJG, Stam FC, et al: Increased number of corticotropin-releasing hormone neurons in the hypothalamic paraventricular nuclei of depressed patients. Neuroendocrinology 60:436–444, 1994

Raadsheer FC, Van Heerikhuize JJ, Lucassen PJ, et al: Increased corticotropin-releasing hormone (CRH) mRNA in paraventricular nucleus of patients with Alzheimer's disease or depression. Am J Psychiatry 152:1372–1376, 1995

Rabins PV, Pearlson GF, Aylward E, et al: Cortical magnetic resonance imaging changes in elderly inpatients with major depression. Am J Psychiatry 148:617–620, 1991

Rao VP, Krishnan KRR, Goli V, et al: Neuroanatomical changes and hypothalamo-pituitary-adrenal axis abnormalities. Biol Psychiatry 26:729–732, 1989

Reame N, Sauder SE, Kelch RP, et al: Pulsatile gonadotropin secretion during the human menstrual cycle: evidence for altered pulse frequency of gonadotropin releasing hormone secretion. J Clin Endocrinol Metab 59:328–337, 1984

Regier DA, Boyd JH, Burke JD Jr, et al: One-month prevalence of mental disorders in the United States: based on five Epidemiologic Catchment Area sites. Arch Gen Psychiatry 45:768–779, 1988

Reich T, Clayton PJ, Winokur G: Family history studies, V: the genetics of mania. Am J Psychiatry 125:1358–1369, 1969

Reischies FM, Hedde JP, Drochner R: Clinical correlates of cerebral blood flow in depression. Psychiatry Res 29:323–326, 1989

Reus VI, Berlant J, Galante M, et al: Proceedings of the 41st annual meeting of the Society of Biological Psychiatry, Washington, DC, May 1986

Richardson UI, Schonbrunn A: Inhibition of adrenocorticotropin secretion somatostatin in pituitary cells in culture. Endocrinology 108:281–284, 1981

Risch SC: Growth hormone-releasing factor and growth hormone, in Neuropeptides and Psychiatric Disorders. Edited by Nemeroff CB. Washington, DC, American Psychiatric Press, 1991, pp 93–108

Risch SC, Lewine RJ, Kalin NH, et al: Limbic-hypothalamic-pituitary-adrenal axis activity and ventricular-to-brain ratio in affective illness and schizophrenia. Neuropsychopharmacology 6:95–100, 1992

Ritchie J, Belkin BM, Krishnan KRR, et al: Plasma dexamethasone concentration and the dexamethasone suppression test. Biol Psychiatry 27:159–173, 1990

Robins LN, Helzer JE, Croughan J, et al: National Institute of Mental Health Diagnostic Interview Schedule: its history, characteristics, and validity. Arch Gen Psychiatry 38:381–389, 1981

Roman GC: Senile dementia of the Binswanger type: a vascular form of dementia in the elderly. JAMA 258:1782–1788, 1987

Rosenbaum AH, Maruta T, Schatzberg AF, et al: Toward a biochemical classification of depressive disorders, VII: urinary free cortisol and urinary MHPG in depressions. Am J Psychiatry 140:314–318, 1983

Rosenbaum AH, Schatzberg AF, Bowden CL, et al: MHPG as a predictor of clinical response to fluoxetine: proceedings of the 18th Collegium Internationale Neuro-Psychopharmacologicum Congress, Nice, France. Clin Neuropharmacol 15:209B, 1992

Rothschild AJ, Langlais PJ, Schatzberg AF, et al: Dexamethasone increases plasma free dopamine in man. J Psychiatr Res 18:217–223, 1984

Rothschild AJ, Langlais PJ, Schatzberg AF, et al: The effects of a single dose of dexamethasone on monoamine and metabolite levels in rat brain. Life Sci 36:2491–2501, 1985

Roy A, Jimerson DC, Pickar D: Plasma MHPG in depressive disorders and relationship to the dexamethasone suppression test. Am J Psychiatry 126:457–469, 1986

Roy A, Pickar D, Paul S, et al: CSF corticotropin-releasing hormone in depressed patients and normal control subjects. Am J Psychiatry 144:641–645, 1987a

Roy A, Guthrie S, Pickar D, et al: Plasma NE responses to cold challenge in depressed patients and normal controls. Psychiatry Res 21:161–168, 1987b

Roy A, Pickar D, DeJong J, et al: Norepinephrine and its metabolites in cerebrospinal fluid, plasma and urine: relationship to hypothalamic-pituitary-adrenal axis function in depression. Arch Gen Psychiatry 45:849–857, 1988

Roy A, De Jong J, Linnoila M: Cerebrospinal fluid monoamine metabolites and suicidal behavior in depressed patients. Arch Gen Psychiatry 46:609–612, 1989

Roy A, Wolkowitz OM, Bissette G, et al: Differences in CSF concentrations of thyrotropin-releasing hormone in depressed patients and normal subjects: negative findings. Am J Psychiatry 151:600–602, 1994

Royle NJ, Clarkson RE, Wong Z, et al: Clustering of hypervariable minisatellites in the proterminal regions of human autosomes. Genomics 3:352–360, 1988

Rubin RT, Heist K, McGeoy SS, et al: Neuroendocrine aspects of primary endogenous depression, XI: serum melatonin measures in patients and matched controls. Arch Gen Psychiatry 49:558–567, 1992

Rubin RT, Phillips JJ, Sadow TF, et al: Adrenal gland volume in major depression: increase during the depressive episode and decrease with successful treatment. Arch Gen Psychiatry 52:213–218, 1995

Rubinow DR: Cerebrospinal fluid somatostatin and psychiatric illness. Biol Psychiatry 21:341–365, 1986

Rubinow DR, Gold PW, Post RM, et al: CSF somatostatin in affective illness. Arch Gen Psychiatry 40:409–412, 1983

Rubinow DR, Gold PW, Post RM, et al: Somatostatin in patients with affective illness and in normal volunteers, in Neurobiology of Mood Disorders. Edited by Post RM, Ballenger JC. Baltimore, MD, Williams & Wilkins, 1984, pp 369–387

Sachar E, Hellman L, Fukushima D, et al: Cortisol production in depressive illness. Arch Gen Psychiatry 23:289–298, 1970

Sachar EJ, Schalch, DS, Reichlin S, et al: Plasma gonadotrophins in depressive illness: a preliminary report, in Recent Advances in the Psychobiology of the Depressive Illnesses. Edited by Williams TA, Katz MM, Shield JA Jr. Washington, DC, U.S. Department of Health and Welfare, 1972, pp 229–233

Sack DA, James SP, Rosenthal NE, et al: Deficient nocturnal surge of TSH secretion during sleep and sleep deprivation in rapid-cycling bipolar illness. Psychiatry Res 23:179–191, 1988

Samson JA, Gudeman JE, Schatzberg AF, et al: Toward a biochemical classification of depressive disorders, VIII: platelet monoamine oxidase activity in subtypes of depressions. J Psychiatr Res 19:547–555, 1985

Sapolsky RM: Glucocorticoids, stress and exacerbation of excitotoxic neuron death. Seminars in Neurosciences 6:323–331, 1994

Sapolsky RM: Why stress is bad for your brain. Science 273:749–750, 1996

Sapolsky RM, Uno H, Rebert CS, et al: Hippocampal damage associated with prolonged stress exposure in primates. J Neurosci 9:2897–2902, 1990

Sapru MK, Rao BSSR, Channabasavana SM: Serum dopamine-beta-hydroxylase activity in classical subtypes of depression. Acta Psychiatr Scand 80:474–478, 1989

Schatzberg AF, Mooney JJ: Noradrenergic and cholinergic mechanisms in depressive disorders: implications for future treatment strategies, in Current Practices and Future Developments in the Pharmacotherapy of Mental Disorders. Edited by Meltzer HY, Nerozzi D. New York, Elsevier, 1991, pp 91–97

Schatzberg AF, Rothschild AJ: Serotonin activity in psychotic (delusional) major depression. J Clin Psychiatry 53 (10 suppl):52–55, 1992

Schatzberg AF, Orsulak PJ, Rosenbaum AH, et al: Towards a biochemical classification of depressive disorders, V: biochemical heterogeneity of unipolar depression. Am J Psychiatry 139:471–475, 1982

Schatzberg AF, Rothschild AJ, Bond TC, et al: The DST in psychotic depression: diagnostic and pathophysiologic implications. Psychopharmacol Bull 20:362–364, 1984

Schatzberg AF, Rothschild AJ, Langlais PJ, et al: A corticosteroid/dopamine hypothesis for psychotic depression and related states. J Psychiatr Res 19:57–64, 1985a

Schatzberg AF, Rothschild AJ, Gerson B, et al: Toward a biochemical classification of depressive disorders, IX: DST results and platelet MAO activity. Br J Psychiatry 146:633–637, 1985b

Schatzberg AF, Rothschild AJ, Langlais PJ, et al: Psychotic and nonpsychotic depressions, II: platelet MAO activity, plasma catecholamines, cortisol, and specific symptoms. Psychiatry Res 20:155–164, 1987

Schatzberg AF, Samson JA, Bloomingdale KL, et al: Toward a biochemical classification of depressive disorders, X: urinary catecholamines, their metabolites, and D-type scores in subgroups of depressive disorders. Arch Gen Psychiatry 46:260–268, 1989

Schatzberg AF, Bowden CL, Rosenbaum AH, et al: Prediction of response to fluoxetine versus desipramine. CME Syllabus and Proceedings Summary. 145th Annual Meeting. Washington, DC, American Psychiatric Association, 44 (No. 25D), 1992

Schatzberg AF, Cole JO, DeBattista C: Manual of Clinical Psychopharmacology, 3rd Edition. Washington, DC, American Psychiatric Press, 1997

Schildkraut JJ: The catecholamine hypothesis of affective disorders: a review of supporting evidence. Am J Psychiatry 122:509–522, 1965

Schildkraut JJ, Orsulak PJ, Schatzberg AF, et al: Toward a biochemical classification of depressive disorders, I: differences in urinary excretion of MHPG and other catecholamine metabolites in clinically defined subtypes of depression. Arch Gen Psychiatry 35:1427–1433, 1978a

Schildkraut JJ, Orsulak PJ, LaBrie RA, et al: Toward a biochemical classification of depressive disorders, II: application of multivariate discriminant function analysis to data on urinary catecholamines and metabolites. Arch Gen Psychiatry 35:1436–1439, 1978b

Schildkraut JJ, Orsulak PJ, Schatzberg AF, et al: Possible patho-physiological mechanisms in subtypes of unipolar depressive disorders based on differences in urinary MHPG levels. Psychopharmacol Bull 17:90–91, 1981

Schildkraut JJ, Orsulak PJ, Schatzberg AF, et al: Urinary MHPG in affective disorders, in Neurobiology of Mood Disorders. Edited by Post RM, Ballenger JC. Baltimore, MD, Williams & Wilkins, 1984, pp 519–528

Schilkrut R, Chandra O, Osswald M, et al: Growth hormone during sleep and with thermal stimulation in depressed patients. Neuropsychobiology 1:70–79, 1975

Schlegel S, Maier W, Philipp M, et al: Computed tomography in depression: association between ventricular size and psychopathology. Psychiatry Res 29:221–230, 1989

Schmider J, Lammers C-H, Gotthardt U, et al: Combined dexamethasone/corticotropin-releasing hormone test in acute and remitted manic patients, in acute depression, and in normal controls: I. Biol Psychiatry 38:797–802, 1995

Scubee-Moreau JJ, Dresse AE: Effect of various antidepressant drugs on the spontaneous firing rate of locus coeruleus and raphe dorsalis neurons of the rat. Eur J Pharmacol 57:219–225, 1979

Selye H: A syndrome produced by diverse nocuous agents. Nature 138:32, 1936

Shah SA, Doraiswamy PM, Husain MM, et al: Posterior fossa abnormalities in major depression: a controlled MRI study. Acta Psychiatr Scand 85:474–479, 1992

Sharma RP, Janicak PG, Javaid JI, et al: Platelet MAO inhibition, urinary MHPG, and leucocyte beta-adrenergic receptors in depressed patients treated with phenelzine. Am J Psychiatry 147:1318–1321, 1990

Sharma RP, Javaid JI, Faull K, et al: CSF and plasma MHPG, and CSF MHPG index: pretreatment levels in diagnostic groups and response to somatic treatments. Psychiatry Res 51:51–60, 1994

Sheline YI, Wang PW, Gado MH, et al: Hippocampal atrophy in recurrent major depression. Proc Natl Acad Sci U S A 93:3908–3913, 1996

Sheline Y, Bardgett ME, Csernansky JG: Correlated reductions in cerebrospinal fluid 5-HIAA and MHPG concentrations after treatment with selective serotonin reuptake inhibitors. J Clin Psychopharmacol 17:11–14, 1997

Shopsin B, Gershon S, Goldstein M, et al: Use of synthesis inhibitors in defining a role for biogenic amines during imipramine treatment in depressed patients. Psychopharmacology Communications 1:239–249, 1975

Shopsin B, Friedman E, Gershon S: Parachlorophenylalanine reversal of tranylcypromine effects in depressed outpatients. Arch Gen Psychiatry 33:811–819, 1976

Siever LJ, Uhde TW, Silberman EK, et al: Growth hormone response to clonidine as a probe of noradrenergic receptor responsiveness in affective disorder patients and controls. Psychiatry Res 6:171–183, 1982

Siever LJ, Murphy DL, Slater S, et al: Plasma prolactin change following fenfluramine in depressed patients compared to controls: an evaluation of central serotonergic responsivity in depression. Life Sci 34:1029–1039, 1984

Siever LJ, Trestman RL, Coccaro EF, et al: The growth hormone response to clonidine in acute and remitted depressed male patients. Neuropsychopharmacology 6:165–177, 1992

Sitaram N, Gillin JC, Bunney WE Jr: Cholinergic and catecholaminergic receptor sensitivity in affective illness: strategy and theory, in Neurobiology of Mood Disorders. Edited by Post RM, Ballenger JC. Baltimore, MD, Williams & Wilkins, 1984, pp 519–528

Skodol AE, Schwartz S, Dohrenwend BP, et al: Minor depression in a cohort of young adults in Israel. Arch Gen Psychiatry 51:542–551, 1994

Sleight AJ, Carolo C, Petit N, et al: Identification of 5-hydroxytryptamine$_7$ receptor binding sites in rat hypothalamus: sensitivity to chronic antidepressant treatments. Mol Pharmacol 47:99–103, 1995

Smith KA, Fairburn CG, Cowen PJ: Relapse of depression after rapid depletion of tryptophan. Lancet 349:915–919, 1997

Souetre E, Salvati E, Wehr TA, et al: Twenty-four hour profiles of body temperature and plasma TSH in bipolar patients during depression and during remission and in normal control subjects. Am J Psychiatry 145:1133–1137, 1988

Southern EM: Detection of specific sequences among DNA fragments separated by gel electrophoresis. J Mol Biol 98:503–517, 1975

Stahl SM, Hauger RL, Rausch JL, et al: Down regulation of serotonin receptor subtypes by nortriptyline and adinazolam in major depressive disorder: neuroendocrine and platelet markers. Paper presented in part at the 18th Annual Collegium Internationale Neuro-Psychopharmacologicum Congress, Nice, France, June 1992

Stanley M, Virgilio J, Gershon S: Tritiated [^{3}H] imipramine binding sites are decreased in the frontal cortex of suicides. Science 216:1337–1339, 1982

Starkman MN, Gebarski SS, Berent S, et al: Hippocampal formation volume, memory dysfunction, and cortisol levels of inpatients with Cushing's syndrome. Biol Psychiatry 32:756–765, 1992

Steinberg BJ, Weston S, Trestman RL, et al: Mood response to cholinergics in personality disorder patients. Annual Meeting New Research Program and Abstracts (NR113). Washington, DC, American Psychiatric Association, 1993, p 88

Stine OC, Xu J, Koskela R, et al: Evidence for linkage of bipolar disorder to chromosome 18 with a parent-of-origin effect. Am J Hum Genet 57:1384–1394, 1995

Stockmeier CA, Dilley GE, Shapiro LA, et al: Serotonin receptors in suicide victims with major depression. Neuropsychopharmacology 16:162–173, 1997

Stokes PE, Sikes CR: Hypothalamic-pituitary-adrenal axis in affective disorders, in Psychopharmacology: The Third Generation of Progress. Edited by Meltzer HY. New York, Raven, 1987, pp 589–607

Stokes PE, Frazer A, Casper R: Unexpected neuroendocrine-transmitter relationships. Psychopharmacol Bull 17: 72–75, 1981

Straub RE, Lehner T, Luo Y, et al: A possible vulnerability locus for bipolar disorder on chromosome 21q22.3. Nat Genet 8:291–296, 1994

Sulser F, Vetulani J, Mobley PL: Mode of action on antidepressant drugs. Biochem Pharmacol 27:257–261, 1978

Swann AC, Koslow SH, Katz MM, et al: Lithium carbonate treatment of mania. Arch Gen Psychiatry 44:345–354, 1987

Swann AC, Secunda SK, Stokes PE, et al: Stress, depression and mania; relationship between perceived role of stressful events and clinical and biochemical characteristics. Acta Psychiatr Scand 81:389–397, 1990

Swann AC, Stokes PE, Casper R, et al: Hypothalamic-pituitary-adrenocortical function in mixed and pure mania. Acta Psychiatr Scand 85:270–274, 1992

Swanson LW, Sawchenko PE, Rivier J, et al: Organization of ovine corticotropin-releasing factor immunoreactive cells and fibers in the rat brain: an immunohistochemical study. Neuroendocrinology 36:165–186, 1983

Swayze VW, Andreasen NC, Alliger RJ: Structural brain abnormalities in bipolar affective disorder. Arch Gen Psychiatry 47:1054–1059, 1990

Sweeney D, Nelson C, Bowers M, et al: Delusional versus nondelusional depression: neurochemical differences. Lancet 2:100–101, 1978

Takahashi S, Kondo H, Yoshimura M, et al: Antidepressant effect of thyrotropin-releasing hormone (TRH) and the plasma thyrotropin levels in depression. Folia Psychiatrica et Neurologica Japonica 27:305–314, 1973

Thakore JH, Dinan TG: Subnormal growth hormone responses to acutely administered dexamethasone in depression. Clin Endocrinol (Oxf) 40:623–627, 1994

Thoenen H: Neurotrophins and neuronal plasticity. Science 270:593–598, 1995

Toivola PTK, Gale CC, Goodner CJ, et al: Central alpha-adrenergic regulation of growth hormone and insulin. Hormones 3:192–213, 1972

Traskman L, Asberg M, Bertilsson L, et al: Monoamine metabolites in CSF and suicidal behavior. Arch Gen Psychiatry 10:253–261, 1981

Traskman-Bendz L, Alling C, Oreland L, et al: Prediction of suicidal behavior from biologic tests. J Clin Psychopharmacol 12 (2 suppl):21S–26S, 1992

Tsuang MT, Faraone SV: The Genetics of Mood Disorders. Baltimore, MD, Johns Hopkins University Press, 1990

Turner WJ, King S: BPD2: an autosomal dominant form of bipolar affective disorder. Biol Psychiatry 18:63–87, 1983

Unden F, Ljunggren JG, Beck-Friis J, et al: Hypothalamic-pituitary-gonadal axis pulse detection. Am J Physiol 250:E486–E493, 1988

Uno H, Tarara R, Else JG, et al: Hippocampal damage associated with prolonged and fatal stress in primates. J Neurosci 9(5):1705–1711, 1989

Vale W, Spiess J, Rivier C, et al: Characterization of a 41 residue ovine hypothalamic peptide that stimulates secretion of corticotropin of b-endorphin. Science 213:1394–1397, 1981

Valk J, van der Knaap MS: Magnetic Resonance of Myelin, Myelination, and Myelin Disorders. Berlin, Springer Verlag, 1989

Vanhaelst L, Van Cauter E, Degaute S, et al: Circadian variations of serum thyrotropin in man. J Clin Endocrinol Metab 35:479–482, 1972

Van Praag HM: Depression, suicide, and the metabolites of serotonin in the brain. J Affect Disord 4:21–29, 1982

Veith RC, Lewis N, Langohr JI, et al: Effect of desipramine on cerebrospinal fluid concentrations of corticotropin-releasing factor in human subjects. Psychiatry Res 46:1–8, 1992

Veith RC, Lewis L, Linares OA, et al: Sympathetic nervous system activity in major depression: basal and desipramine-induced alterations in plasma NE kinetics. Arch Gen Psychiatry 51:411–422, 1994

Vingerhoets A: Psychosocial Stress: An Experimental Approach. Lissa, The Netherlands, Swets and Zetilinger, 1985, p 2

Virkkunen M, Nuutila A, Goodwin FK, et al: Cerebrospinal fluid monoamine metabolite levels in male arsonists. Arch Gen Psychiatry 44:241–247, 1987

Virkkunen M, Rawlings R, Tokola R, et al: CSF biochemistries, glucose metabolism, and diurnal activity rhythms in alcoholic, violent offenders, fire setters, and healthy volunteers. Arch Gen Psychiatry 51:20–27, 1994

Visser TJ, Leonard JL, Kaplan MM, et al: Kinetic evidence suggesting two mechanisms for iodothyronine 5´-deiodination in rat cerebral cortex. Proc Natl Acad Sci U S A 79:5080–5084, 1982

Von Bardeleben U, Holsboer F: Cortisol response to a combined dexamethasone/human corticotropin-releasing hormone challenge in patients with depression. J Neuroendocrinol 1:485–488, 1989

Von Bardeleben U, Holsboer F, Stalla GK, et al: Combined administration of human corticotrophin-releasing factor and lysine vasopressin induces escape from dexamethasone suppression in healthy subjects. Life Sci 37:1613–1618, 1985

Watson SJ, Lopez JF, Young EA, et al: Effects of low dose ovine corticotropin-releasing hormone in humans: endocrine relationships and beta-endorphin/beta-lipotropin responses. J Clin Endocrinol Metab 66:10–15, 1986

Weber JL, May PE: Abundant class of human DNA polymorphisms which can be typed using the polymerase chain reaction. Am J Hum Genet 44:388–396, 1989

Weeke A, Weeke J: The 24-hour pattern of serum TSH in patients with endogenous depression. Acta Psychiatr Scand 62:69–74, 1980

Weinberger DR, Berman KF, Zec RF: Physiologic dysfunction of dorsolateral prefrontal cortex in schizophrenia, I: regional cerebral blood flow evidence. Arch Gen Psychiatry 43:114–124, 1986

Weinberger DR, Berman KF, Illowsky BP: Physiological dysfunction of dorsolateral prefrontal cortex in schizophrenia, III: a new cohort and evidence for a monoaminergic mechanism. Arch Gen Psychiatry 45:609–615, 1988

Weissman MM, Gershon ES, Kidd KK, et al: Psychiatric disorders in the relatives of probands with affective disorders: the Yale University-National Institute of Mental Health Collaborative Study. Arch Gen Psychiatry 41:13–21, 1984

Weissman MM, Merikangas KR, Boyd JH: Epidemiology of affective disorders, in Psychiatry, Vol I. Edited by Michels R, Cavenar JO, Brodie HKH, et al. Philadelphia, PA, JB Lippincott, 1992, pp 1–14

Wells KB, Stewart A, Hayes RD: The functioning and well-being of depressed patients: results of the Medical Outcomes Study. JAMA 262:914–919, 1989

Wender PH, Kety SS, Rosenthal D, et al: Psychiatric disorders in the biological and adoptive families of adopted individuals with affective disorders. Arch Gen Psychiatry 43:923–929, 1986

Whalley LJ, Kutcher S, Blackwood DHR, et al: Increased plasma LH in manic-depressive illness: evidence of a state-independent abnormality. Br J Psychiatry 150:682–684, 1987

Willner P: Dopamine and depression: a review of recent evidence. I. Empirical studies. Brain Res 287:211–224, 1983a

Willner P: Dopamine and depression: a review of recent evidence. II. Theoretical approaches. Brain Res 287:225–236, 1983b

Willner P: Dopamine and depression: a review of recent evidence. III. The effects of antidepressant treatments. Brain Res 287:237–246, 1983c

Winokur A, Amsterdam J, Caroff S, et al: Variability of hormonal responses to a series of neuroendocrine challenges in depressed patients. Am J Psychiatry 139:39–44, 1982

Wolkowitz OM, Sutton ME, Doran AR, et al: Dexamethasone increases plasma HVA but not MHPG in normal humans. Psychiatry Res 16:101–109, 1985

Wolkowitz OM, Sutton ME, Koulu M, et al: Chronic corticosterone administration in rats: behavioral and biochemical evidence of increased central dopaminergic activity. European Journal of Psychopharmacology 122:329–338, 1986

Wolkowitz OM, Rubinow DR, Breier A, et al: Prednisone decreases CSF somatostatin in healthy humans: implications for neuropsychiatric illness. Life Sci 41:1929–1933, 1987

World Health Organization Collaborative Study: Validity of imipramine platelet binding sites as a biological marker for depression. Pharmacopsychiatry 23:113–117, 1990

World Health Organization: International Statistical Classification of Diseases and Related Health Problems, 10th Revision. Geneva, Switzerland, World Health Organization, 1992

Wu JC, Gillin JC, Buchsbaum MS, et al: Effect of sleep deprivation on brain metabolism of depressed patients. Am J Psychiatry 149:538–543, 1992

Wyatt RJ, Portnoy B, Kupfer DJ, et al: Resting plasma catecholamine concentrations in patients with depression and anxiety. Arch Gen Psychiatry 24:65–70, 1971

Wynn PC, Aguilera G, Morell J, et al: Properties and regulation of high-affinity pituitary receptors for corticotropin-releasing factor. Biochem Biophys Res Commun 110:602–608, 1983

Wynn PC, Hauger RL, Holmes MC, et al: Brain and pituitary receptors for corticotropin-releasing factor: localization and differential regulation after adrenalectomy. Peptides 5:1077–1084, 1984

Wynn PC, Harwood JP, Catt KJ, et al: Corticotropin-releasing factor (CRF) induces desensitization of the rat pituitary CRF receptor-adenylase cyclase complex. Endocrinology 122:351–358, 1988

Yates FE, Maran JW: Stimulation and inhibition of adrenocorticotropin release, in Handbook of Physiology, Vol 4. Edited by Knobil E, Sawyer WH. Washington, DC, American Physiology Society, 1974, pp 367–404

Young EA: Glucocorticoid cascade hypothesis revisited: role of gonadal steroids. Depression 3:20–27, 1995

Young EA, Watson SJ, Kotun J, et al: Beta-lipotropin-beta-endorphin response to low-dose ovine corticotropin releasing factor in endogenous depression. Arch Gen Psychiatry 47:449–457, 1990

Zis KD, Zis A: Increased adrenal weight in victims of violent suicide. Am J Psychiatry 144:1214–1215, 1987

TWENTY-EIGHT

Neurobiology of Schizophrenia

Michael B. Knable, D.O.,
Joel E. Kleinman, M.D., Ph.D., and
Daniel R. Weinberger, M.D.

Since the last edition of this textbook, several contributions to the neurobiological understanding of schizophrenia have been published. Therefore, we have reorganized the chapter in order to emphasize recent developments in the genetics, neuropathology, and neurochemistry of schizophrenia. Because molecular biological techniques have greatly expanded the study of inherited factors in schizophrenia in recent years, we begin the chapter with an expanded section on genetic studies of schizophrenia. In the section on neuropathological findings in schizophrenia, we review modern postmortem neuropathological and neuroimaging studies, which continue to implicate medial temporal-lobe structures, prefrontal cortex, and limbic portions of the neostriatum. Because the reported neuropathological findings in schizophrenia have tended to be subtle and have not always been consistently replicated, a long-held alternative conception of the illness is that biochemical aberrations, without specific neuroanatomical correlates, may underlie schizophrenic symptoms. Our review, therefore, concludes with a discussion of findings relevant to neurotransmitter systems proposed to be dysfunctional in schizophrenia. We propose that the pathological and biochemical abnormalities that are observed in schizophrenia cannot be explained completely by inheritance of a small number of genes but that environmental interaction with a complex genetic predisposition contributes to abnormal development of the nervous system.

GENETIC STUDIES

Family and Adoption Studies

Schizophrenia occurs more commonly in family members of affected individuals than in the general population. However, most cases of schizophrenia occur without an apparent family history, which raises the possibility that some cases arise sporadically. Although results from family, twin, and adoption studies provide compelling evidence for a genetic contribution to schizophrenia, the nature of the inherited defect and its degree of penetrance are unknown. Schizophrenia occurs at similar prevalence rates throughout most regions of the world, despite diversity of cultural, racial, and socioeconomic groups. This observation lends weight to the concept of an inherited vulnerability with a relatively stable gene frequency.

Family and twin studies estimate the risk of schizophrenia in first-degree relatives and dizygotic twins of schizophrenic patients to be 10–15 times that of the general population. Studies that used modern diagnostic tools postulated a risk for first-degree relatives that is somewhat less than that stated in older studies. (For reviews, see Schulz 1991; Tsuang et al. 1991.) In studies of the offspring of monozygotic twins discordant for schizophrenia, no difference in the prevalence of schizophrenia could be ascertained in the children of the affected compared with the unaffected twins (Fischer 1971; Gottesman and Bertelsen 1989). Monozygotic twins of schizophrenic patients have a concordance rate for schizophrenia of approximately 30%–80%, depending on ascertainment methods (Kendler 1983; McGue 1992; Torrey 1992). From these monozygotic twin data, it may be inferred that nongenetic factors contribute to pathogenesis of schizophrenia.

Further support for a genetic vulnerability in schizophrenia comes from the following observations in adoption studies: 1) children of schizophrenic mothers who are adopted by nonschizophrenic adults have an increased risk for schizophrenia (Heston 1966; Kety 1983; Rosenthal et al. 1971, 1975), and 2) children of nonschizophrenic adults who are adopted away and raised by schizophrenic parents do not have an increased risk for schizophrenia (Wender et al. 1977). Adoption studies have also reported that paternal half-siblings of proband schizophrenic patients have an increased risk for schizophrenia, presumably due to a genetic factor transmitted solely through the father. Because these half-siblings did not share the same intrauterine environment, the putative genetic factor may predispose to disease development independently of this variable (Rosenthal and Kety 1968).

Chromosomal Linkage Studies

Linkage analyses assume that if a putative disease locus is in proximity to a known genetic marker, then the two segments of genetic material will remain in proximity after meiosis, even if recombination occurs. Linkage analyses also assume that a gene of major effect is associated with the illness in question, that only one disease gene segregates within a pedigree (homogeneity), and that the mode of inheritance is known. For complex behavioral traits and disorders such as schizophrenia, these assumptions clearly are not met. Linkage studies are currently done with statistical modeling of these variables. Linkage analysis results are also highly dependent on phenotypic definition, and statistical results can be dramatically altered if pedigree members later change diagnostic status.

Early linkage studies tested for linkage to chromosomal areas thought to be relevant to the illness based on observed chromosomal aberrations in particular pedigrees or because a gene of interest was known to exist on the chromosomal region studied. The first of these studies to be reported involved chromosome 5. In 1988, Bassett and colleagues described a family with facial and extremity dysmorphisms and psychosis who were found to have trisomy of chromosome 5 that was partially translocated to chromosome 1. In this kindred, several members had structural brain disease, including temporal-lobe atrophy, cavum septum pellucidum, and cavum vergae (Honer et al.

1992). Subsequently, Sherrington et al. (1988) presented evidence linking two DNA polymorphisms from the long arm of chromosome 5 to schizophrenia in five Icelandic and two English pedigrees. Unfortunately, linkage of similar segments of chromosome 5 to the schizophrenic phenotype has not been replicated in a number of other kindreds (Aschauer et al. 1990; Detera-Wadleigh et al. 1989; Hallmayer et al. 1992b; Kaufman et al. 1989; Kennedy et al. 1988; Macciardi et al. 1992; McGuffin et al. 1990; St Clair et al. 1989).

In another family, a carrier with centromeric portions of chromosome 5 translocated to chromosome 14 produced offspring with partial trisomy of the short arm of chromosome 5 and schizophrenia (Malaspina et al. 1992). Linkage of schizophrenia to portions of the short arm of chromosome 5 has been observed in one study (Silverman et al. 1996); however, in other studies, linkage has been rejected in various loci from the short arm of chromosome 5 (Coon et al. 1994b; Kennedy et al. 1989).

Similar theories have emerged for chromosome 11. Interest in chromosome 11 was stimulated after St Clair et al. (1990) described several members of a large Scottish pedigree who had psychotic illnesses and a balanced translocation from chromosome 11 to chromosome 1. However, studies of pedigrees from many different parts of the world have excluded linkage to the 11q translocation area (C. L. Barr et al. 1991; Diehl et al. 1991; Gill et al. 1993; Kalsi et al. 1995b; Muir et al. 1991; Nanko et al. 1992).

Because of claims that pairs of siblings with schizophrenia were likely to be of the same sex (Crow 1988), linkage of the illness to markers on sex chromosomes has been studied. Some studies reported that pairs of siblings with psychosis were more likely to be sex-concordant if the illness had been inherited paternally (Crow et al. 1989; Gorwood et al. 1992). Therefore, a dominant locus on the pseudoautosomal region of the sex chromosomes was hypothesized (the trait would be transmitted from father to daughter on the X chromosome and from father to son on the Y chromosome). Collinge et al. (1991) found that the DXYS14 allele, at the pseudoautosomal region of the sex chromosomes, was shared in a higher-than-chance expectation in siblings with psychosis. This finding was supported by the work of D'Amato et al. (1992) and Gorwood et al. (1992) in that a nonrandom segregation of the DXYS14 allele was reported, albeit in rather small sample sizes. Studies that used the logarithm of odds (LOD) method did not detect linkage of DXYS14 alleles to schizophrenia (Asherson et al. 1992; C. L. Barr et al. 1991; Crow et al. 1994; Kalsi et al. 1995a).

Advances in molecular biological techniques have provided the means to scan large segments of the genome in the search for linkage rather than beginning linkage studies based on chromosomal abnormalities observed in particular pedigrees. Originally, genomic scans were generated with markers cut at specific points by restriction fragment length polymorphisms (RFLPs). Recently, genomic scans have been conducted with the polymerase chain reaction and microsatellite markers, or simple repeat sequences of nucleotide bases, which appear in noncoding regions of the genome. Wang et al. (1995) scanned approximately 10% of the genome with microsatellite markers in 186 multiplex schizophrenia families (i.e., families with more than one affected member) and found evidence for linkage to a marker on 6p23. This study also presented supporting data for linkage to this region with the affected sibling pair and the affected pedigree member methods, nonparametric techniques that do not require the assumptions made with the LOD score method. This work has been replicated by some groups (Antonarakis et al. 1995; Moises et al. 1995b; Schwab et al. 1995a; Straub et al. 1995) but not others (Gurling et al. 1995; Mowry et al. 1995). However, the number of groups reporting linkage to chromosome 6 in widely divergent pedigrees provides the strongest genetic linkage data yet obtained for schizophrenia.

Systematic genome scanning produced results suggestive of, although not strictly statistically significant for, linkage to chromosome 22q (Coon et al. 1994a; Pulver et al. 1994; Vallada et al. 1995). Studies that used the affected sibling method also produced results suggestive of linkage (Gill et al. 1996; Moises et al. 1995a; Schwab et al. 1995b). Karayiorgou et al. (1995) reported that 2 of 100 randomly selected schizophrenic patients had a microdeletion in the 22q11 region. These patients had facial dysmorphisms similar to those seen in patients with velocardiofacial syndrome, a disorder with known deletions in the 22q11 regions and an increased risk for psychosis.

Candidate Gene Studies

Because of hypothesized abnormalities in dopaminergic transmission in schizophrenia, genes for the five types of dopamine receptors were among the first to be studied. Linkage studies (Campion et al. 1994; Coon et al. 1993; Jensen et al. 1993) and studies that have sought evidence for mutations in the D_1 receptor gene (Cichon et al. 1994; Liu et al. 1995) have not identified a role for this gene in schizophrenia. Likewise, the pharmacologically similar D_5 receptor gene does not appear to be linked to schizophrenia (Coon et al. 1993) or to have polymorphisms associated with the disease (Kalsi et al. 1996; Sobell et al. 1995).

The dopamine D_2 receptor gene also does not appear to be linked to schizophrenia (Campion et al. 1994; Coon

et al. 1993; Hallmayer et al. 1994; Moises et al. 1991). In case-control studies, however, Arinami et al. (1994, 1996) and Shaikh et al. (1994a) described a molecular variant of the D_2 receptor, in which a substitution of cysteine for serine at codon 311 was observed more frequently in schizophrenic patients than in control subjects. Subsequent studies have not replicated this finding in other cohorts (Asherson et al. 1994; Hattori et al. 1994; Laurent et al. 1994a; Nanko et al. 1994; Nothen et al. 1994; Sasaki et al. 1996a; Sobell et al. 1994).

Crocq et al. (1992) reported an excess of homozygosity for a polymorphism in the first exon of the dopamine D_3 receptor gene in schizophrenic patients compared with control subjects. Some subsequent studies have supported a modest association between homozygosity of the Ser-9-Gly polymorphism and schizophrenia (Griffon et al. 1996; Mant et al. 1994; Shaikh et al. 1996), but many other studies have not replicated this association (DiBella et al. 1994; Jonsson et al. 1993; Laurent et al. 1994b; Nimgaonkar et al. 1993; Nothen et al. 1993; Sabate et al. 1994; Saha et al. 1994; Yang et al. 1993). Linkage studies with D_3 receptor gene polymorphisms have not supported a role for this gene in schizophrenia (Coon et al. 1993; Sabate et al. 1994; Wiese et al. 1993).

The dopamine D_4 receptor has been excluded from linkage to schizophrenia in a number of studies (C. L. Barr et al. 1993; Campion et al. 1994; Coon et al. 1993; Macciardi et al. 1994; Maier et al. 1994; Shaikh et al. 1994b). The dopamine D_4 receptor gene has a highly variable 48 base pair repeat polymorphism in exon 3 and a 12 base pair polymorphism in exon 1, which have not been found to have allelic associations with schizophrenia (Catalano et al. 1993; Nanko et al. 1993; Petronis et al. 1995).

The gene encoding the serotonin receptor 5-HT$_2$ subtype has been excluded from linkage to schizophrenia in a Swedish kindred by Hallmayer et al. (1992a). However, a polymorphism in the noncoding portion of the 5-HT$_{2A}$ gene has been reported to be found more commonly in schizophrenic patients than in control subjects (Erdmann et al. 1996; Inayama et al. 1996; J. Williams et al. 1996). This substitution of cytosine for thymine at codon 102 does not alter the amino acid sequence and, presumably, the pharmacological properties of the receptor protein but may be a gene segment in linkage disequilibrium with the schizophrenic phenotype. Several groups have been unable to replicate this association (Arranz et al. 1996; Jonsson et al. 1996; Malhotra et al. 1996; Sasaki et al. 1996b).

It is not entirely surprising that linkage and candidate gene studies have not generated more strikingly positive results. Molecular biological techniques have been applied

1993b), which may be consistent with a disturbance of neuronal migration preventing normal development of neocortical lamination.

In support of the postmortem findings in the medial temporal lobe of patients with schizophrenia, a complementary MRI literature has accumulated in recent years. A few groups have found bilateral reductions in amygdala-hippocampal or parahippocampal gyrus volume (Breier et al. 1992; DeLisi et al. 1988; Marsh et al. 1994; Suddath et al. 1989, 1990; Young et al. 1991). Others have found reduced volume of these structures, or temporal neocortical areas, primarily in the left hemisphere (Barta et al. 1990; Bogerts et al. 1990a; Shenton et al. 1992). Of note are studies that have described reduced volume of the hippocampal complex in the affected members of monozygotic twin pairs discordant for schizophrenia (Suddath et al. 1990) and in first-break patients (Bogerts et al. 1990a). Studies using MRI spectroscopy to measure brain concentrations of N-acetylaspartate, a neuron-specific chemical, also support the notion that subtle neuronal pathology exists in the medial temporal lobe (Bertolino et al. 1996; Fukuzako et al. 1995; Nasrallah et al. 1994; Renshaw et al. 1995).

Prefrontal Cortex

Patients with lesions of the prefrontal cortex have symptoms that bear some resemblance to the schizophrenic syndrome. The "negative symptoms" of schizophrenia—poor motivation and drive, social withdrawal, flat affect, and impaired insight and judgment—rarely accompany damage to the temporal lobe but are often seen in patients with frontal-lobe lesions. Because neuropathological and neuroimaging studies have reported generalized reductions in the volume of cerebral cortex and dilatation of frontal horns of the lateral ventricles and the third ventricle, neuronal tissues outside of the temporal lobe also seem likely to be affected. Furthermore, if the neuropathological process in schizophrenia occurs during cortical development, it is likely to affect at least several cortical areas simultaneously.

The most widely reported data regarding frontal cortical abnormalities in schizophrenia are from cerebral blood flow (CBF) studies with single photon emission computed tomography (SPECT) and positron-emission tomography (PET). The original reports of Ingvar and Frantzen (1974a, 1974b) of decreased frontal-lobe metabolic activity ("hypofrontality") at rest have been confirmed by some investigators but disputed by others (for a review, see Berman and Weinberger 1991).

The concept that "hypofrontality" may exist as a state-dependent phenomenon has been proposed re-

cently. When regional CBF is measured during cognitive tasks that require intact function of the prefrontal cortex, schizophrenic patients are consistently hypofrontal. Weinberger et al. (1986) demonstrated a lack of activation of dorsolateral prefrontal cortex in schizophrenic patients given an automated version of the Wisconsin Card Sorting Test (WCST) during xenon-133 CBF measurement.

In studies of monozygotic twins discordant for schizophrenia, diminished activation of the dorsolateral prefrontal cortex while taking the WCST is invariably associated with the disorder, does not occur in unaffected co-twins, and is not affected by long-term neuroleptic exposure (Berman et al. 1992). Furthermore, the severity of diminished dorsolateral prefrontal cortex activation is correlated with diminished hippocampal volume in the affected twins, which suggests that the normal communication between medial temporal and prefrontal cortical areas may be disrupted in schizophrenia (Weinberger et al. 1992).

The cellular basis for the reduced prefrontal activity seen in schizophrenia is as yet unknown. Relative prefrontal blood flow is correlated with cerebrospinal fluid (CSF) concentrations of homovanillic acid (HVA) (Weinberger et al. 1988) and can be improved with dopaminergic drugs (Daniel et al. 1989, 1991; Dolan et al. 1995). This finding suggests that dopaminergic innervation of frontal cortex is necessary for normal functional activation.

Decreased neuronal density in layer VI (Benes et al. 1986) and decreased density of small interneurons in layer II of prefrontal cortex (Benes et al. 1991) have been described in neuropathological studies. These findings were interpreted to be the result of a cortical developmental abnormality because increased glial density and neuronal shrinkage were not observed. In a larger study with 16 specimens of frontal area 9 from schizophrenic patients, Selemon et al. (1995) described increased density of pyramidal and nonpyramidal neurons in layers III to VI. The authors attributed the finding to decreased volume of neuropil rather than altered number of neurons. Increased neuronal density was also observed in occipital cortex, which suggests that abnormal cortical structure in schizophrenia may be widespread but only clinically relevant in certain brain areas.

As in the hippocampus, the dorsolateral prefrontal area has been found to have reduced numbers of neurons stained with NADPH-d and white matter greater than 3 mm deep to cerebral cortex with increased numbers of NADPH-d neurons (Akbarian et al. 1993a, 1996). A similar finding suggestive of abnormal neuronal migration from the subplate has been observed with immunohistochemical staining for microtubule-associated protein (Anderson et al. 1996).

MRI studies support evidence of subtle neuronal abnormalities in the prefrontal cortex of schizophrenic patients. Volumetric studies have reported reductions in frontal cortex volume (Andreasen et al. 1994a; Breier et al. 1992; Raine et al. 1992; Zipursky et al. 1992), but this has not been universally observed (Kelsoe et al. 1988; Wible et al. 1995). MRI spectroscopy has detected decreased levels of N-acetylaspartate (Bertolino et al. 1996; Buckley et al. 1994) and high-energy phosphate-containing compounds (Fujimoto et al. 1992; Pettegrew et al. 1991, 1993) in the frontal lobes.

Thalamus

The thalamic nuclei have not received much attention in schizophrenia research. However, further study is warranted because the thalamus is interconnected with limbic structures and prefrontal cortex and because the thalamic circuits contribute to attention and sensory functions. Decreased volume of the central nucleus (Lesch and Bogerts 1984), decreased neuronal numbers in the dorsomedial nucleus (Pakkenberg 1990), and decreased concentration of a synaptic vesicle protein (rab3a) in the left thalamus (Blennow et al. 1996) have been reported in postmortem studies. Andreasen et al. (1994b) reported reduced signal intensity in the right dorsolateral thalamus by using a novel approach that averaged MRI scans from schizophrenic subjects and control subjects. In previous work with volumetric MRI studies, this group also described decreased volume of the thalamus (reviewed in Andreasen et al. 1995).

Cerebellum

Reduced size of the cerebellar vermis in some schizophrenic patients has been identified with CT scans (Heath et al. 1979; Weinberger et al. 1979) and in a postmortem study (Weinberger et al. 1980). When Lohr and Jeste (1986) attempted to control for vermian atrophy from other causes, they were not able to replicate this finding in a postmortem sample. Moreover, Weinberger et al. (1982) did not observe reduced size of the cerebellar vermis in patients with first-break schizophrenia. Taken together, these results suggest that reduced cerebellar size is not a primary feature of schizophrenia.

In summary, several consistent abnormalities are observed in the brains of schizophrenic patients: increased size of the cerebral ventricles, decreased size of medial temporal-lobe structures, and aberrant function of prefrontal cortex. These changes usually do not appear to progress, and no gliosis is observed in the nervous system. Thus, these brain abnormalities may have a neurodevelopmental origin.

NEUROCHEMICAL ABNORMALITIES

Dopamine

The dopamine hypothesis of schizophrenia has been a major impetus for research throughout the past 30 years. Carlsson and Lindquist (1963) reported that dopamine turnover was increased in laboratory animals given neuroleptics. Subsequently, the clinical efficacy of neuroleptics was shown to be correlated with their ability to displace radioligands from dopamine D_2 receptors (Creese et al. 1976; Seeman et al. 1976). Pharmacological induction of dopamine hyperactivity in laboratory animals produces behavioral alterations that are thought to be similar to symptoms in schizophrenic patients (Braff and Geyer 1990; Mathysse 1977). Clinicians also observed psychotic symptoms in patients exposed to drugs such as amphetamine or L-dopa (Angrist et al. 1973; Ellinwood 1967), which corresponded to results of laboratory investigations.

Until recently, investigations of dopaminergic function in schizophrenic patients have been constrained by the methodological problems inherent in studies of metabolites in biological fluids and postmortem neurochemical measures. CSF dopamine and HVA levels in schizophrenic patients generally do not differ from those in control subjects (Widerlov 1988). In fact, some investigators have found lower-than-normal levels of CSF HVA that are inversely correlated with the severity of negative symptoms in schizophrenic patients (Bowers 1974; Lindstrom 1985).

Davis et al. (1991) reviewed studies of plasma HVA levels. Although some studies found that plasma HVA levels correlate with severity of symptoms and response to neuroleptic treatment, note that plasma HVA concentrations are affected substantially by changes in renal clearance; this issue was not adequately addressed in these studies. Likewise, the possibility that increased plasma concentrations of HVA in drug-free schizophrenic patients may simply reflect alterations in peripheral autonomic function that accompany psychosis has not been widely acknowledged (Potter et al. 1989).

Studies of dopamine and HVA in postmortem brain tissue have yielded inconsistent results (Davis et al. 1991). Three studies reported increased postmortem dopamine levels. Bird et al. (1979b) found increased concentrations of dopamine in the nucleus accumbens and anterior perforated substance in schizophrenic patients. Crow et al. (1979) found an increased concentration of dopamine that was restricted to the caudate nucleus. Reynolds (1983) reported increased concentrations of dopamine in the amygdala, which was more prominent on the left side, of schizophrenic patients.

Postmortem studies of dopamine receptor binding in brains from schizophrenic patients have shown an increased number of dopamine D_2 receptors in the caudate nucleus, putamen, and nucleus accumbens. These changes have been reported in more than 20 studies (for reviews, see Davis et al. 1991; Hyde et al. 1991) and seem to imply that a primary abnormality of the dopamine receptor may underlie dopaminergic dysfunction in schizophrenia. Although chronic neuroleptic treatment also increases the number of dopamine D_2 receptors, some studies reported increased D_2 receptor binding in patients who were drug free for extended periods (for review, see Hyde et al. 1991).

Attempts to quantitate D_2 receptor density in vivo with PET have produced inconclusive results. Wong et al. (1986) used ^{11}C-spiperone in 10 drug-naive schizophrenic patients and found increased binding in the caudate nucleus. Two studies that used ^{11}C-raclopride did not replicate this finding (Farde et al. 1987, 1990). No group differences between 12 schizophrenic patients and control subjects were detected with [76]Br-bromospiperone (Martinot et al. 1990). Interpretation of these results requires consideration of several problems. First, raclopride has a lower affinity for dopamine receptors than spiperone does and may be more easily displaced by endogenous ligand. Second, the studies used different mathematical models for data analysis that cannot be easily compared. Third, patients in the studies may have had different severity and/or lengths of illness.

The possibility that dopaminergic neurotransmission varies in a state-dependent manner with clinical symptomatology has been suggested by recent in vivo imaging studies. Laruelle et al. (1996) reported that schizophrenic patients who were given amphetamine displaced striatal ^{123}I-IBZM, a D_2 receptor antagonist, more readily than did nonschizophrenic control subjects and that the degree of radioligand displacement is related to severity of psychotic symptomatology. In a longitudinal study of drug-free schizophrenic patients, Knable et al. (1997) showed that worsening of deficit symptoms is related to increased binding of ^{123}I-IBZM, which suggests that decreased endogenous dopamine activity may underlie deficit symptoms.

Fewer studies of the dopamine D_1 receptor are available. Because the clinical efficacy of neuroleptics was not correlated with displacement of ligands from the D_1 receptor, there was little initial interest in this receptor. Cross et al. (1981) and Seeman et al. (1987) reported that D_1 receptor binding in schizophrenic striatum was not different from that in control subjects. Hess et al. (1989) reported

decreased D_1 binding in the caudate nucleus and putamen. In a study of frontal cortical D_1 receptors, Knable et al. (1996) found increases in some cortical laminae that appeared to be related to chronic neuroleptic treatment.

Recently described members of the D_2-like dopamine receptor family have also been of interest to schizophrenia researchers because these receptors have affinity for neuroleptic drugs and anatomical distribution in limbic brain regions. A pharmacological method quantitating the difference in binding between two radioligands as a measure of D_4 density has indicated a substantial elevation in the striatum of schizophrenic subjects (Murray et al. 1995; Seeman et al. 1993). However, the observed elevation in D_4 receptor binding seemed greater than the concentration of striatal D_4 receptors measured with molecular biological techniques, and another group was unable to replicate these results (Reynolds and Mason 1994).

Experiments with animals have supported the view that the regulation of dopamine release may be aberrant in schizophrenia. Damage to the prefrontal cortex in rats potentiates the behavioral effects of amphetamine (Iversen 1971) and apomorphine (Scatton et al. 1982). Ibotenic acid lesions of medial prefrontal cortex in rats increase behavioral and biochemical evidence of dopamine hyperactivity in the basal ganglia, especially when the animals are stressed (Jaskiw et al. 1990).

Cortical modulation of subcortical dopamine release, in turn, may depend on intact cortical dopaminergic innervation. If mesocortical projections to the frontal cortex are damaged with 6-hydroxydopamine in rodents, both dopamine turnover and dopamine binding sites in the striatum increase (Carter and Pycock 1980; Pycock et al. 1980a, 1980b). Thus, cortical hypodopaminergia may play a role in some aspects of schizophrenia.

Defective subcortical dopamine transmission may also be altered by aberrant input to dopaminergic neurons from the medial temporal structures that have been implicated in the neuropathological literature on schizophrenia. Ibotenic acid lesions of ventral hippocampus in rats cause increased amphetamine-induced locomotion, increased dopamine concentrations in the nucleus accumbens, and decreased dihydrophenylacetic acid (DOPAC) and HVA concentrations in the medial prefrontal cortex (Lipska et al. 1992). Thus, a medial temporal cortical defect, which has been proposed in schizophrenia, may differentially affect dopamine transmission in subcortical and cortical systems, in a manner consistent with current models of the illness.

Glutamate

Abnormal glutamate transmission has been suspected in schizophrenia for several reasons. In animal models, destruction of cortical glutaminergic fibers increases the animals' susceptibility to the behavioral effects of dopaminergic drugs (Scatton et al. 1982). Glutamate normally stimulates the inhibitory neurotransmitter γ-aminobutyric acid (GABA) in the striatum, whereas dopamine inhibits GABA release. Thus, similar behavioral effects could be produced by deficient corticostriatal glutamate activity and excessive mesostriatal dopamine activity (Zukin and Javitt 1991). In addition, the normal phasic depolarization of ventral tegmental neurons is dependent on the presence of glutamate activity at the N-methyl- D-aspartate (NMDA) receptor (Johnson et al. 1992).

Glutaminergic system dysfunction in schizophrenia is also predicted by the phencyclidine (PCP) model of psychosis. PCP binds to a receptor located within the ion channel formed by the NMDA receptor complex and prevents the normal neuronal events produced by binding of glutamate to the NMDA receptor (for review, see Zukin and Javitt 1991).

Kim et al. (1980) reported a decreased concentration of glutamate in the CSF of schizophrenic patients, but other studies (Gattaz et al. 1982, 1985; Perry 1982) have not replicated this finding. Perry (1982) was unable to demonstrate differences in glutamate levels measured in six regions of postmortem brain tissue from schizophrenic patients and control subjects. Toru et al. (1988) measured multiple brain areas and found a decreased glutamate concentration in the angular gyrus of schizophrenic patients. Sherman et al. (1991a, 1991b) used synaptosomal preparations in postmortem brain tissue from schizophrenic patients and found deficient glutamate release with veratridine-induced depolarization or after exposure to NMDA or kainic acid.

Deficient function of glutamatergic neurons in schizophrenia has been proposed with postmortem receptor binding and in situ hybridization studies. In the hippocampus, decreased concentrations of glutamate receptors (Kerwin et al. 1988, 1990), presumably on pyramidal neurons; decreased concentrations of the messenger RNA encoding these receptors (Eastwood et al. 1995; Harrison et al. 1991); and decreased concentrations of glutamatergic metabolites (Tsai et al. 1995) have been reported. These findings await replication by other studies; however, the theory that putative abnormal development or cell loss occurs in the hippocampal area has been advocated by other methodologies.

Several studies have indicated that the concentration of glutamate receptors is increased in the prefrontal cortex of schizophrenic patients (Deakin et al. 1989; Simpson et al. 1992a; Toru et al. 1988). It is unclear whether this find-

ing represents an upregulation of postsynaptic glutamate receptors as the result of deficient innervation or a secondary abnormality associated with increased neuronal density in the prefrontal area.

In the basal ganglia, glutamate reuptake site binding (Simpson et al. 1992b) has been shown to decrease in conjunction with decreased binding of MK-801 to NMDA receptors (Kornhuber et al. 1989). Thus, corticostriatal glutamatergic function in schizophrenia may be deficient, and abnormal regulation of dopamine neurotransmission may result.

Serotonin

Early theories implicating serotonin in the pathogenesis of schizophrenia were based on the observation that lysergic acid diethylamide (LSD), an agonist for serotonergic receptors, could produce a psychosis with some features similar to those of schizophrenia. Animal studies have provided evidence for modulation of dopamine activity by serotonin (Dickinson and Curzon 1983; Korsgaard et al. 1985), and interest in the serotonin system in schizophrenia has been rekindled because many atypical neuroleptics (clozapine, risperidone, ritanserin, and setoperone) have 5-HT$_2$ antagonist properties (Bleich et al. 1988).

Few abnormalities of serotonergic neurotransmission in schizophrenia have been consistently replicated despite a considerable number of studies. Studies of brain and CSF serotonin and 5-hydroxyindoleacetic acid (5-HIAA) levels have produced conflicting results. However, several studies have replicated a correlation between low CSF 5-HIAA levels and the presence of ventriculomegaly and cortical thinning in schizophrenic patients (for review, see Bleich et al. 1988). Postmortem studies of serotonin receptors have focused mainly on the 5-HT$_2$ receptor subtype. In the nucleus accumbens (Mackay et al. 1978) and striatum (F. Owen et al. 1981), no difference in 5-HT$_2$ receptor binding between schizophrenic patients and control subjects has been reported. Binding sites in the frontal cortex have been reported to be decreased (Arora and Meltzer 1991; Bennett et al. 1979; Laruelle et al. 1993; Mita et al. 1986) or unchanged (Dean et al. 1996; Reynolds et al. 1983; Whitaker et al. 1981). Decreased density of serotonin reuptake sites has been reported in the prefrontal cortex (Laruelle et al. 1993) and in the hippocampus (Dean et al. 1996).

Norepinephrine

The noradrenergic system is implicated in schizophrenia for several reasons. Neuroleptics may produce some therapeutic effects via adrenergic receptors (for a review, see Van Kammen 1991). Elevated levels of plasma and

CSF norepinephrine have been reported in some studies but are subject to the same methodological pitfalls for dopamine metabolites described earlier in this chapter (for a review, see Van Kammen and Kelley 1991). CSF concentrations of norepinephrine and 3-methoxy-4-hydroxyphenylglycol (MHPG) have been correlated with severity of negative symptoms (Pickar et al. 1990; Van Kammen et al. 1990). A few studies have found elevated levels of norepinephrine in limbic areas of postmortem schizophrenic brain tissue (Farley et al. 1978; Kleinman et al. 1982), but conflicting studies also exist (Bird et al. 1979a; Crow et al. 1979). No consistently replicated abnormality of adrenergic receptors has emerged.

GABA

GABA, the major inhibitory neurotransmitter of the central nervous system, is found mainly in small interneurons in the cerebral cortex. Investigators have hypothesized that GABAergic cortical interneuron activity may be aberrant in schizophrenia. Evidence for this theory includes findings of increased density of $GABA_A$ receptors in schizophrenic cingulate cortex, which may represent an upregulation of receptors on pyramidal neurons following the loss or decreased functioning of local circuit interneurons (Benes et al. 1992). The preliminary finding of decreased GABA uptake sites in the hippocampus supports the putative loss of small interneurons (Reynolds et al. 1990). Alternatively, the data of Akbarian et al. (1995) indicate a functional abnormality of small neurons, because messenger RNA for glutamic acid decarboxylase, the principal synthetic enzyme for GABA, is decreased in the absence of neuronal loss in the prefrontal cortex. Further research is necessary to explore potential abnormalities of the GABA system.

Although few consistent neurochemical abnormalities have been identified, the ability of dopamine D_2 antagonists to reduce the symptoms of psychosis is a reliable pharmacological observation. This finding suggests an inability in schizophrenia to regulate dopamine turnover, especially when stressed. Dysregulation of dopamine neurotransmission may well relate to aberrant connectivity between areas that have been reliably observed to have structural and functional abnormalities.

CONCLUSION

Investigators at the beginning of the twentieth century implicated dysfunction of frontal and temporal cortices in psychosis. Recent schizophrenia research has produced findings that support their suspicions, but the nature and etiology of frontal- and temporal-lobe dysfunction remain unknown. Although a genetic predisposition to schizophrenia is well established, recent research findings in schizophrenia lead to the conclusion that multifactorial and, in part, environmentally derived insults to the brain probably contribute to the pathology of schizophrenia. Monozygotic twins do not have uniformly high concordance rates for schizophrenia, and the unaffected members of monozygotic twin pairs who are discordant for schizophrenia do not share with their schizophrenic twins the markers of structural brain pathology described in this chapter. In addition, some evidence indicates that people with schizophrenia may have an increased incidence of obstetrical complications or may have been exposed to viral infections or malnutrition during fetal life that could have altered brain development.

As a result of the genetic and environmental factors that may have contributed to the development of schizophrenia, several reproducible structural and physiological abnormalities of the brain can be found in schizophrenic patients. These abnormalities include enlargement of the cerebral ventricles, dilatation of cortical sulci, reduction in the size of several anteromedial temporal-lobe structures, and hypometabolism of dorsolateral prefrontal cortex during cognitive tasks. Clinical and neuropathological evidence supports the idea that these abnormalities result from a fixed "lesion" that is acquired early in life and that results in a relatively nonprogressive psychotic syndrome. In neuropathological studies, a lack of gliosis supports the notion that the neuronal lesions of schizophrenia are acquired before birth. Psychotic symptoms may begin in adolescence or early adulthood when maturation of a frontotemporolimbic neural network does not occur during a critical period of development.

In light of the structural brain abnormalities observed in schizophrenia, alterations in neurotransmitter function may be regarded as secondary to neuronal loss or altered neuronal development. This hypothesis is supported by

- Findings in laboratory animals that cortical lesions can differentially affect dopamine neurotransmission in subcortical and in distant cortical areas
- The correlation between prefrontal regional CBF in schizophrenic patients during cognitive tasks and CSF metabolites of dopamine
- The correlation between hippocampal size and activation of prefrontal cortical blood flow in schizophrenic patients

However, primary dysfunction of dopaminergic or other neurotransmitter systems may underlie the schizophrenic syndrome. Future research with better clinical and postmortem samples is necessary before one can reliably conclude that increased concentrations of dopamine, altered dopamine receptor function, or alterations in other neurotransmitters occur in schizophrenic patients independently of drug treatment artifacts and structural brain abnormalities.

REFERENCES

Akbarian S, Bunney WE, Potkin S, et al: Altered distribution of nicotinamide-adenine dinucleotide phosphate-diaphorase cells in frontal lobe of schizophrenics implies disturbance of cortical development. Arch Gen Psychiatry 50: 169–177, 1993a

Akbarian S, Vinuela A, Kim JJ, et al: Distorted distribution of nicotinamide-adenine dinucleotide phosphate-diaphorase neurons in temporal lobe of schizophrenics implies anomalous cortical development. Arch Gen Psychiatry 50:178–187, 1993b

Akbarian S, Kim JJ, Potkin SG, et al: Gene expression for glutamic acid decarboxylase is reduced without loss of neurons in prefrontal cortex of schizophrenics. Arch Gen Psychiatry 52:258–266, 1995

Akbarian S, Kim JJ, Potkin SG, et al: Maldistribution of interstitial neurons in prefrontal white matter of the brains of schizophrenic patients. Arch Gen Psychiatry 53:425–436, 1996

Altshuler L, Conrad A, Kovelman JA, et al: Hippocampal cell disorientation in schizophrenia: a controlled neurohistologic study of the Yakovlev collection. Arch Gen Psychiatry 44:1094–1098, 1987

Anderson SA, Volk DW, Lewis DA: Increased density of microtubule associated protein 2-immunoreactive neurons in the prefrontal white matter of schizophrenic subjects. Schizophr Res 19:111–119, 1996

Andreasen NC, Flashman L, Flaum M, et al: Regional brain abnormalities in schizophrenia measured with magnetic resonance imaging. JAMA 272:1763–1769, 1994a

Andreasen NC, Arndt S, Swayze V, et al: Thalamic abnormalities visualized through magnetic resonance image averaging. Science 266:294–298, 1994b

Andreasen NC, Swayze V, O'Leary DS, et al: Abnormalities in midline attentional circuitry in schizophrenia: evidence from magnetic resonance and positron emission tomography. Eur Neuropsychopharmacol 5 (suppl):37–41, 1995

Angrist BM, Sathananthan G, Gershon S: Behavioral effects of L-dopa in schizophrenic patients. Psychopharmacology (Berl) 31:1–12, 1973

Antonarakis SE, Blouin J-L, Pulver AK, et al: Schizophrenia susceptibility and chromosome 6p24-22. Nat Genet 11:235–236, 1995

Arinami T, Itokawa M, Enguchi H, et al: Association of dopamine D2 receptor molecular variant with schizophrenia. Lancet 343:703–704, 1994

Arinami T, Itokawa M, Aoki J, et al: Further association study on dopamine D2 receptor variant S311C in schizophrenia and affective disorders. Am J Med Genet 67:133–138, 1996

Arnold SE, Hyman BT, Van Hoese GW, et al: Some cytoarchitectural abnormalities of the entorhinal cortex in schizophrenia. Arch Gen Psychiatry 48:625–632, 1991

Arnold SE, Franz BR, Gur RC, et al: Smaller neuron size in schizophrenia in hippocampal subfields that mediate cortical-hippocampal interactions. Am J Psychiatry 152:738–748, 1995

Arora RC, Meltzer HY: Serotonin 2 (5-HT2) receptor binding in the frontal cortex of schizophrenic patients. J Neural Transm 85:19–29, 1991

Arranz MJ, Lin M-W, Powell J, et al: 5HT$_{2A}$ receptor T102C polymorphism and schizophrenia. Lancet 347:1831–1832, 1996

Aschauer HN, Aschauer-Treiber G, Isenberg KE, et al: No evidence for linkage between chromosome 5 markers and schizophrenia. Hum Hered 40:109–115, 1990

Asherson P, Parfitt E, Sargeant M, et al: No evidence for a pseudoautosomal locus for schizophrenia from linkage analysis of multiply affected families. Br J Psychiatry 161:63–68, 1992

Asherson P, Williams N, Roberts E, et al: DRD2 Ser 311/Cys311 polymorphism in schizophrenia (letter). Lancet 343:1045, 1994

Barr CE, Mednick SA, Munk-Jorgensen P: Exposure to influenza epidemics during gestation and adult schizophrenia: a 40-year study. Arch Gen Psychiatry 47:869–874, 1990

Barr CL, Kennedy JL, Pakstis J, et al: Progress in genome scan for linkage in schizophrenia. Psychiatr Genet 12:199–219, 1991

Barr CL, Kennedy JL, Lichter JB, et al: Alleles at the dopamine D4 receptor locus do not contribute to schizophrenia in a large Swedish kindred. Am J Med Genet 48:218–222, 1993

Barta PE, Pearlson GD, Powers RE, et al: Auditory hallucinations and smaller superior temporal gyral volume in schizophrenia. Am J Psychiatry 147:1457–1462, 1990

Bassett AS, Jones B, McGullivray B, et al: Partial trisomy chromosome 5 cosegregating with schizophrenia. Lancet 1:799–801, 1988

Benes FM, Davidson J, Bird E: Quantitative cytoarchitectural studies of the cerebral cortex of schizophrenics. Arch Gen Psychiatry 43:31–35, 1986

Benes FM, Sorenson I, Bird E: Reduced neuronal size in posterior hippocampus of schizophrenic patients. Schizophr Bull 17:597–608, 1991

Benes FM, Vincent SL, Alsterberg G, et al: Increase GABA$_A$ receptor binding in superficial layers of cingulate cortex in schizophrenics. J Neurosci 12:924–929, 1992

Bennett JP, Enna SJ, Bylund DB, et al: Neurotransmitter receptors in frontal cortex of schizophrenics. Arch Gen Psychiatry 36:927–934, 1979

Berman KF, Weinberger DR: Functional localization in the brain in schizophrenia, in American Psychiatric Press Review of Psychiatry, Vol 10. Edited by Tasman A, Goldfinger SM. Washington, DC, American Psychiatric Press, 1991, pp 24–59

Berman KF, Torrey EF, Daniel DG, et al: Regional cerebral blood flow in monozygotic twins discordant and concordant for schizophrenia. Arch Gen Psychiatry 49:927–934, 1992

Bertolino A, Nawroz S, Mattay VS, et al: A regionally specific pattern of neurochemical pathology in schizophrenia as assessed by multislice proton magnetic resonance spectroscopic imaging. Am J Psychiatry 153:1554–1563, 1996

Bird ED, Spokes EG, Iversen LL: Brain norepinephrine and dopamine in schizophrenia. Science 204:93–94, 1979a

Bird ED, Spokes EGS, Iversen LL: Increased dopamine concentrations in limbic areas of brain from patients dying with schizophrenia. Brain 102:347–360, 1979b

Bleich A, Brown SL, Kahn R, et al: The role of serotonin in schizophrenia. Schizophr Bull 14:297–315, 1988

Blennow K, Davidsson P, Gottfries C-G, et al: Synaptic degeneration in thalamus in schizophrenia. Lancet 348:692–693, 1996

Bogerts B, Meertz E, Schonfeldt-Bausch R: Basal ganglia and limbic system pathology in schizophrenia. Arch Gen Psychiatry 42:784–791, 1985

Bogerts B, Ashtari M, Degreef G, et al: Reduced temporal limbic structure volume on magnetic resonance images in first episode schizophrenia. Psychiatry Res 35:1–13, 1990a

Bogerts B, Falkai P, Haupts M, et al: Post-mortem volume measurements of limbic system and basal ganglia structures in chronic schizophrenics. Schizophr Res 3:295–301, 1990b

Bowers MB: Cortical dopamine turnover in schizophrenic syndromes. Arch Gen Psychiatry 31:50–54, 1974

Braff DL, Geyer MA: Sensorimotor gating and schizophrenia: human and animal model studies. Arch Gen Psychiatry 47:181–188, 1990

Breier A, Buchanan RW, Elkashef A, et al: Brain morphology and schizophrenia: a magnetic resonance imaging study of limbic, prefrontal cortex and caudate structures. Arch Gen Psychiatry 49:921–926, 1992

Brown R, Colter N, Corsellis JAN, et al: Postmortem evidence of structural brain changes in schizophrenia. Arch Gen Psychiatry 43:36–42, 1986

Buckley PF, Moore C, Long H, et al: 1H-Magnetic resonance spectroscopy of the left temporal and frontal lobes in schizophrenia: clinical, neurodevelopmental, and cognitive correlates. Biol Psychiatry 36:792–800, 1994

Campion D, D'Amato T, Bastard C, et al: Genetic study of D1, D2, and D4 receptors in schizophrenia. Psychiatry Res 51:215–223, 1994

Cannon TD, Mednick SA, Parnas J: Genetic and perinatal determinants of structural brain deficits in schizophrenia. Arch Gen Psychiatry 46:883–889, 1989

Carlsson A, Lindquist M: Effect of chlorpromazine or haloperidol on formation of 3-methoxytyramine and normetanephrine in mouse brain. Acta Pharmacology and Toxicology 20:140–144, 1963

Carter CJ, Pycock CJ: Behavioral and biochemical effects of dopamine and noradrenaline depletion within medial prefrontal cortex of rat. Brain Res 192:163–176, 1980

Catalano M, Nobile M, Novelli E, et al: Distribution of a novel mutation in the first exon of the human dopamine D4 gene in psychotic patients. Biol Psychiatry 34:459–464, 1993

Chakos MH, Lieberman JA, Bilder RM, et al: Increase in caudate nuclei volume of first-episode schizophrenia patients taking antipsychotic drugs. Am J Psychiatry 151:1430–1436, 1994

Christison GW, Casanova MF, Weinberger DR, et al: A quantitative investigation of hippocampal pyramidal cell size, shape, and variability of orientation in schizophrenia. Arch Gen Psychiatry 46:1027–1032, 1989

Cichon S, Nothen MM, Rietschel M, et al: Single-strand conformation analysis of the dopamine D1 receptor gene reveals no significant mutation in patients with schizophrenia and manic depression. Biol Psychiatry 36:850–853, 1994

Cleghorn JM, Zipursky RB, List SJ: Structural and functional brain imaging in schizophrenia. J Psychiatry Neurosci 16:53–74, 1991

Collinge J, Delisi LE, Boccio A, et al: Evidence for a pseudo-autosomal locus for schizophrenia using the method of affected sibling pairs. Br J Psychiatry 158:624–629, 1991

Colter N, Battal S, Crow TJ, et al: White matter reduction in the parahippocampal gyrus of patients with schizophrenia (letter). Arch Gen Psychiatry 44:1023, 1987

Conrad AJ, Abebe T, Austin R, et al: Hippocampal pyramidal cell disarray in schizophrenia as a bilateral phenomenon. Arch Gen Psychiatry 48:413–417, 1991

Coon H, Byerley W, Holik J, et al: Linkage analysis of schizophrenia with five dopamine receptor genes in nine pedigrees. Am J Hum Genet 52:327–334, 1993

Coon H, Holik J, Hoff M, et al: Analysis of chromosome 22 markers in nine schizophrenic pedigrees. Am J Med Genet 54:72–79, 1994a

Coon H, Jensen S, Holik J, et al: Genomic scan for genes predisposing to schizophrenia. Am J Med Genet 54:59–71, 1994b

Creese I, Burt DR, Snyder SH: Dopamine receptor binding predicts clinical and pharmacological potencies of anti-schizophrenic drugs. Science 192:481–483, 1976

Crocq MA, Mant R, Asherson P, et al: Association between schizophrenia and homozygosity at the dopamine D3 receptor gene. J Med Genet 29:858–860, 1992

Cross AJ, Crow TJ, Owen F: 3H-fluphenthixol binding in post-mortem brains of schizophrenics: evidence for a selective increase in dopamine D2 receptors. Psychopharmacology (Berl) 74:122–124, 1981

Crow TJ: Sex chromosomes and psychosis: the case for a pseudoautosomal locus. Br J Psychiatry 153:675–683, 1988

Crow TJ, Baker HF, Cross AJ, et al: Monoamine mechanisms in chronic schizophrenia: postmortem neurochemical findings. Br J Psychiatry 134:249–256, 1979

Crow TJ, Delisi LE, Johnstone EC: Concordance by sex in sibling pairs with schizophrenia is paternally inherited: evidence for a pseudoautosomal locus. Br J Psychiatry 155:92–97, 1989

Crow TJ, Delisie LE, Lofthouse R, et al: An examination of linkage of schizophrenia and schizoaffective disorder to the pseudoautosomal region (Xp22.3). Br J Psychiatry 164:159–164, 1994

D'Amato T, Campion D, Gorwood P, et al: Evidence for a pseudoautosomal locus for schizophrenia, II: replication of a non-random segregation of alleles at the DXYS14 locus. Br J Psychiatry 161:59–62, 1992

Daniel DG, Berman KF, Weinberger DR: The effect of apomorphine on regional cerebral blood flow in schizophrenia. J Neuropsychiatry Clin Neurosci 1:377–384, 1989

Daniel DG, Weinberger DR, Jones DW, et al: The effect of amphetamine on regional cerebral blood flow during cognitive activation in schizophrenia. J Neurosci 11:1907–1917, 1991

Davis KL, Kahn RS, Ko G, et al: Dopamine in schizophrenia: a review and reconceptualization. Am J Psychiatry 148:1474–1486, 1991

Davison K, Bagley CR: Schizophrenia-like psychoses associated with organic disorders of the central nervous system. Br J Psychiatry 113 (suppl 1):18–69, 1969

Deakin J, Slater P, Simpson M, et al: Frontal cortical and left temporal glutamatergic dysfunction in schizophrenia. J Neurochem 52:1781–1786, 1989

Dean B, Hayes W, Opeskin K, et al: Serotonin 2 receptors and the serotonin transporter in the schizophrenic brain. Behav Brain Res 73:169–175, 1996

Degreef G, Ashtari M, Bogerts B, et al: Volumes of ventricular system subdivisions measured from magnetic resonance images in first episode schizophrenic patients. Arch Gen Psychiatry 49:531–537, 1992

DeLisi L, Dauphinais ID, Gershon ES: Perinatal complications and reduced size of brain limbic structures in familial schizophrenia. Schizophr Bull 14:185–191, 1988

DeLisi L, Hoff AL, Schwartz JE, et al: Brain morphology in first-episode schizophrenic-like psychotic patients: a quantitative magnetic resonance imaging study. Biol Psychiatry 29:159–175, 1991

Detera-Wadleigh SD, Goldin L, Sherrington R, et al: Exclusion of linkage to 5q11-13 in families with schizophrenia and other psychiatric disorders. Nature 340:391–392, 1989

DiBella D, Catalano M, Strukel M, et al: Distribution of the MscI polymorphism of the dopamine D3 receptor in an Italian psychotic population. Psychiatr Genet 4:39–42, 1994

Dickinson SL, Curzon G: Roles of dopamine and 5-hydroxytryptamine in stereotyped and non-stereotyped behavior. Neuropharmacology 22:805–812, 1983

Diehl S, Su Y, Bray J, et al: Linkage studies of schizophrenia: exclusion of candidate genes on chromosome 5q and 11q. Psychiatr Genet 2:14–15, 1991

Dolan RJ, Fletcher P, Frith CD, et al: Dopaminergic modulation of impaired cognitive activation in the anterior cingulate cortex in schizophrenia. Nature 378:180–182, 1995

Dom R, DeSaedeleer J, Bogerts B, et al: Quantitative cytometric analysis of basal ganglia in catatonic schizophrenics, in Biological Psychiatry. Edited by Perris C, Struwe G, Jansson B. Amsterdam, Elsevier, 1981, pp 723–726

Done DJ, Johnstone EC, Frith CD, et al: Complications of pregnancy and delivery in relation to psychosis in adult life: data from the British perinatal mortality survey sample. BMJ 302:1576–1580, 1991

Eastwood SL, McDonald B, Burnet PWJ, et al: Decreased expression of mRNAs encoding non-NMDA glutamate receptors GluR1 and GluR2 in medial temporal lobe neurons in schizophrenia. Molecular Brain Research 29:211–223, 1995

Elkashef AM, Buchanan RW, Gellad F, et al: Basal ganglia pathology in schizophrenia and tardive dyskinesia: an MRI quantitative study. Am J Psychiatry 151:752–755, 1994

Ellinwood EH: Amphetamine psychosis, I: description of the individuals and the process. J Nerv Ment Dis 144:274–283, 1967

Erdmann J, Shimron-Abarbanell D, Rietschel M, et al: Systematic screening for mutations in the human serotonin-2A receptor gene: identification of two naturally occurring receptor variants and association analysis in schizophrenia. Hum Genet 97:614–619, 1996

Falkai P, Bogerts B, Rozumek M: Limbic pathology in schizophrenia: the entorhinal region. Biol Psychiatry 24:515–521, 1988

Farde L, Wiesel F, Hall H, et al: No D2 receptor increase in PET study of schizophrenia (letter). Arch Gen Psychiatry 44:671, 1987

Farde L, Wiesel FA, Stone-Elander S, et al: D2 dopamine receptors in neuroleptic-naive schizophrenic patients. Arch Gen Psychiatry 47:213–219, 1990

Farley IJ, Price KS, McCullogh E, et al: Norepinephrine in chronic paranoid schizophrenia: above normal levels in limbic forebrain. Science 200:456–458, 1978

Farmer A, Jackson R, McGuffin P, et al: Cerebral ventricular enlargement in chronic schizophrenia: consistencies and contradictions. Br J Psychiatry 150:324–330, 1987

Fischer M: Psychosis in the offspring of schizophrenic monozygotic twins and their normal co-twins. Br J Psychiatry 118:43–52, 1971

Fujimoto T, Nakano T, Takano T, et al: Study of chronic schizophrenics using ^{31}P magnetic resonance chemical shift imaging. Acta Psychiatr Scand 86:455–462, 1992

Fukuzako H, Takeuchi K, Hokazono Y, et al: Proton magnetic resonance spectroscopy of the left medial temporal and frontal lobes in chronic schizophrenia: preliminary report. Psychiatry Res 61:193–200, 1995

Gattaz WF, Gatz D, Beckmann H: Glutamate in schizophrenics and healthy controls. Archiv Psychiatrie Nervenkraakheit 231:221–225, 1982

Gattaz WF, Gasser T, Beckmann H: Multidimensional analysis of the concentration of 17 substances in the CSF of schizophrenics and controls. Biol Psychiatry 20:360–366, 1985

Gill M, McGuffin P, Parfitt E, et al: A linkage study of schizophrenia with DNA markers from the long arm of chromosome 11. Psychol Med 23:27–44, 1993

Gill M, Vallada H, Collier D, et al: A combined analysis of D22S278 marker alleles in affected sib-pairs: support for a susceptibility locus for schizophrenia at chromosome 22q12. Am J Med Genet 67:40–45, 1996

Goldberg TE, Gold JM, Braff DL: Neuropsychological functioning and time-linked information processing in schizophrenia, in American Psychiatric Press Review of Psychiatry, Vol 10. Edited by Tasman A, Goldfinger SM. Washington, DC, American Psychiatric Press, 1991, pp 60–78

Gorwood P, LeBoyer M, D'Amato T, et al: Evidence for a pseudoautosomal locus for schizophrenia, I: a replication study using phenotype analysis. Br J Psychiatry 161:55–58, 1992

Gottesman II, Bertelsen A: Confirming unexpressed genotypes for schizophrenia: risks in the offspring of Fischer's Danish identical and fraternal discordant twins. Arch Gen Psychiatry 46:867–872, 1989

Griffon N, Crocq MA, Pilon C, et al: Dopamine D3 receptor gene: organization, transcript variants, and polymorphism associated with schizophrenia. Am J Med Genet 67:63–70, 1996

Gur RE, Mozley D, Resnick SM, et al: Magnetic resonance imaging in schizophrenia, I: volumetric analysis of brain and cerebrospinal fluid. Arch Gen Psychiatry 48:407–412, 1991

Gurling H, Kalsi G, Chen AH-S, et al: Schizophrenia susceptibility and chromosome 6p24-22. Nat Genet 11:234–235, 1995

Hallmayer J, Kennedy JL, Wetterberg L, et al: Exclusion of linkage between the serotonin 2 receptor and schizophrenia in a large Swedish kindred. Arch Gen Psychiatry 49:216–219, 1992a

Hallmayer J, Maier W, Ackenheil M, et al: Evidence against linkage of schizophrenia to chromosome 5q11-q13 markers in systematically ascertained families. Biol Psychiatry 31:83–94, 1992b

Hallmayer J, Maier W, Schwab S, et al: No evidence of linkage between the dopamine D2 receptor gene and schizophrenia. Psychiatry Res 53:203–215, 1994

Harrison PJ, McLaughlin D, Kerwin RW: Decreased hippocampal expression of a glutamate receptor gene in schizophrenia. Lancet 337:450–452, 1991

Hattori M, Nanko S, Dai XY, et al: Mismatch PCR RFLP detection of DRD2 SER311CYS polymorphism and schizophrenia. Biochem Biophys Res Commun 202:757–763, 1994

Heath RG, Franklin DE, Schraberg D, et al: Gross pathology of the cerebellum in patients diagnosed and treated as functional psychiatric disorders. J Nerv Ment Dis 167:585–592, 1979

Hecker E: Die Hebephrenie. Archiv Pathologie Anatomie Physiologie Klinik Medizi 52:394, 1871

Heckers S, Heinsen H, Heinsen Y, et al: Cortex, white matter, and basal ganglia in schizophrenia: a volumetric postmortem study. Biol Psychiatry 29:556–566, 1991

Hess EJ, Brancha HS, Kleinman JE, et al: Dopamine receptor subtype imbalance in schizophrenia. Life Sci 40:1487–1497, 1989

Heston LL: Psychiatric disorders in foster home reared children of schizophrenic mothers. Br J Psychiatry 112:819–825, 1966

Hokama H, Shenton ME, Nestor PG, et al: Caudate, putamen, and globus pallidus volume in schizophrenia: a quantitative study. Psychiatry Res 61:209–229, 1995

Honer WG, Bassett AS, MacEwan W, et al: Structural brain imaging abnormalities associated with schizophrenia and partial trisomy of chromosome 5. Psychol Med 22:519–524, 1992

Hyde TM, Casanova MF, Kleinman JE, et al: Neuroanatomical and neurochemical pathology in schizophrenia, in American Psychiatric Press Review of Psychiatry, Vol 10. Edited by Tasman A, Goldfinger SM. Washington, DC, American Psychiatric Press, 1991, pp 7–23

Illowsky BP, Juliano DM, Bigelow LB, et al: Stability of CT scan findings in schizophrenia: results of an 8 year follow-up study. J Neurol Neurosurg Psychiatry 51:209–213, 1988

Inayama Y, Yoneda H, Sakai T, et al: Positive association between a DNA sequence variant in the serotonin 2A receptor gene and schizophrenia. Am J Med Genet 67:103–105, 1996

Ingvar DH, Frantzen G: Abnormalities of cerebral blood flow distribution in patients with chronic schizophrenia. Acta Psychiatr Scand 50:425–462, 1974a

Ingvar DH, Frantzen G: Distribution of cerebral activity in chronic schizophrenia. Lancet 2:1484–1486, 1974b

Iversen SD: The effect of surgical lesions to frontal cortex and substantia nigra on amphetamine responses in rats. Brain Res 31:295–311, 1971

Jakob H, Beckmann H: Prenatal developmental disturbances in the limbic allocortex in schizophrenics. J Neural Transm 65:303–326, 1986

Jaskiw GE, Karoum F, Weinberger DR: Persistent elevations in dopamine and its metabolites in the nucleus accumbens after mild subchronic stress in rats with ibotenic acid lesions of the medial prefrontal cortex. Brain Res 534:321–323, 1990

Jensen S, Plaetke R, Holik J, et al: Linkage analysis of schizophrenia: the D1 dopamine receptor gene and several flanking DNA markers. Hum Hered 43:58–62, 1993

Jernigan TL, Zisook S, Heaton RK, et al: Magnetic resonance imaging abnormalities in lenticular nuclei and cerebral cortex in schizophrenia. Arch Gen Psychiatry 48:881–890, 1991

Jeste DV, Lohr JB: Hippocampal pathologic findings in schizophrenia. Arch Gen Psychiatry 46:1019–1024, 1989

Johnson SW, Seutin V, North RA: Burst firing in dopamine neurons induced by N-methyl-D-aspartate: role of electrogenic sodium pump. Science 258:665–667, 1992

Jonsson E, Lannfelt L, Sokoloff P, et al: Lack of association between schizophrenia and alleles at the D3 receptor gene. Acta Psychiatr Scand 87:345–349, 1993

Jonsson E, Nothen M, Bunzel R, et al: 5HT$_{2A}$ receptor T102C polymorphism and schizophrenia (letter). Lancet 347:1831, 1996

Kalsi G, Curtis D, Brynjolfsson J, et al: Investigation by linkage analysis of the XY pseudoautosomal region in the genetic susceptibility to schizophrenia. Br J Psychiatry 167:390–393, 1995a

Kalsi G, Mankoo BS, Curtis D, et al: Exclusion of linkage of schizophrenia to the gene for the dopamine D2 receptor and chromosome 11q translocation sites. Psychol Med 25:531–537, 1995b

Kalsi G, Sherrington R, Mankoo BS, et al: Linkage study of the dopamine D5 receptor gene in multiplex Icelandic and English schizophrenia pedigrees. Am J Psychiatry 153:107–109, 1996

Karayiorgou M, Morris MA, Morrow B, et al: Schizophrenia susceptibility associated with interstitial deletions of chromosome 22q11. Proc Natl Acad Sci U S A 92:7612–7616, 1995

Kaufman CA, DeLisi L, Lehner T, et al: Physical mapping linkage analysis of the putative schizophrenia locus on chromosome 5q. Schizophr Bull 15:441–452, 1989

Kelsoe JR, Cadet JL, Pickar D, et al: Quantitative neuroanatomy in schizophrenia. Arch Gen Psychiatry 45:533–541, 1988

Kendell RE, Kemp IW: Maternal influenza in the etiology of schizophrenia. Arch Gen Psychiatry 46:878–882, 1989

Kendler KS: Overview: a current perspective on twin studies of schizophrenia. Am J Psychiatry 140:1413–1425, 1983

Kennedy J, Giuffra L, Moises H, et al: Evidence against linkage of schizophrenia to markers on chromosome 5 in a northern Swedish pedigree. Nature 336:167–170, 1988

Kennedy J, Giuffra L, Moises H, et al: Molecular genetic studies in schizophrenia. Schizophr Bull 15:383–391, 1989

Kerwin RW, Patel S, Meldrum BS, et al: Asymmetrical loss of glutamate receptor subtype in left hippocampus in schizophrenia. Lancet 1:583–584, 1988

Kerwin R, Patel S, Meldrum B: Quantitative autoradiographic analysis of glutamate binding sites in the hippocampal formation in normal and schizophrenic brain post mortem. Neuroscience 39:25–32, 1990

Kety SS: Mental illness in the biological and adoptive relative of schizophrenic adoptees: findings relevant to genetic and environmental factors in etiology. Am J Psychiatry 140:720–727, 1983

Kim JS, Kornhuber HH, Schmid-Burgk W, et al: Low cerebrospinal fluid glutamate in schizophrenic patients and a new hypothesis on schizophrenia. Neurosci Lett 20:379–382, 1980

Kleinman JE, Karoum F, Rosenblatt JE, et al: Postmortem neurochemical studies in chronic schizophrenia, in Biological Markers in Psychiatry and Neurology. Edited by Usdin E, Hanin I. New York, Pergamon, 1982, pp 67–76

Knable M, Hyde TM, Murray AM, et al: A post-mortem study of frontal cortical dopamine D1 receptors in schizophrenics, psychiatric controls and normal controls. Biol Psychiatry 40:1191–1199, 1996

Knable M, Egan MF, Heinz A, et al: Evidence for a relationship between altered dopaminergic function and negative symptoms in drug free schizophrenic patients: an I-123 IBZM SPECT study. Br J Psychiatry 171:574–577, 1997

Kornhuber J, Mack-Burkhardt F, Riedere P, et al: ^{3}H-MK801 binding sites in postmortem brain regions of schizophrenic patients. J Neural Transm 77:231–236, 1989

Korsgaard S, Gerlach J, Christensson E: Behavioral aspects of serotonin-dopamine interaction in the monkey. Eur J Pharmacol 118:245–252, 1985

Kovelman JA, Scheibel AB: A neurohistological correlate of schizophrenia. Biol Psychiatry 19:1601–1621, 1984

Laruelle M, Toti R, Abi-Dargham A, et al: Selective abnormalities of prefrontal serotonergic markers in schizophrenia: a post-mortem study. Arch Gen Psychiatry 50:810–818, 1993

Laruelle M, Abi-Dargham A, Van Dyck CH, et al: Single photon emission computerized tomography imaging of amphetamine-induced dopamine release in drug-free schizophrenic subjects. Proc Natl Acad Sci U S A 93:9235–9240, 1996

Laurent C, Bodeau-Pean S, Campion D, et al: No major role for the dopamine D2 receptor Ser → Cys^{311} mutation in schizophrenia. Psychiatr Genet 4:229–230, 1994a

Laurent C, Savoye C, Samolyk D, et al: Homozygosity of the dopamine D3 receptor locus is not associated with schizophrenia (letter). J Med Genet 31:260, 1994b

Lesch A, Bogerts B: The diencephalon in schizophrenia: evidence of reduced thickness of the periventricular gray matter. Eur Arch Psychiatry Neurol Sci 234:212–219, 1984

Lewis SW, Murray RM: Obstetrical complications, neurodevelopmental deviance and risk of schizophrenia. J Psychiatr Res 21:413–422, 1987

Lindstrom LH: Low HVA and normal 5HIAA CSF levels in drug free schizophrenic patients compared to healthy volunteers: correlations to symptomatology and family history. Psychiatry Res 14:265–273, 1985

Lipska BK, Jaskiw GE, Chrapusta S, et al: Ibotenic acid lesions of ventral hippocampus differentially effect dopamine and its metabolites in the nucleus accumbens and prefrontal cortex in rat. Brain Res 585:1–6, 1992

Liu Q, Sobell JL, Heston LL, et al: Screening the dopamine D1 receptor gene in 131 schizophrenics and eight alcoholics: identification of polymorphisms but lack of functionally significant sequence changes. Am J Med Genet 60:165–171, 1995

Lohr JB, Jeste DV: Cerebellar pathology in schizophrenia, a neuronometric study. Biol Psychiatry 21:865–875, 1986

Macciardi F, Kennedy JL, Ruocco L, et al: A genetic linkage study of schizophrenia to chromosome 5 markers in a northern Italian population. Biol Psychiatry 31:720–728, 1992

Macciardi F, Petronis A, Van Tol HHM, et al: Genetic analysis of the dopamine D4 receptor gene variant in an Italian schizophrenia kindred. Arch Gen Psychiatry 51:288–293, 1994

Mackay AVP, Doble A, Bird ED, et al: ^{3}H-Spiperone binding in normal and schizophrenic post-mortem human brain. Life Sci 23:527–532, 1978

Maier W, Schwab S, Hallmayer J, et al: Absence of linkage between schizophrenia and the dopamine D4 receptor gene. Psychiatry Res 53:77–86, 1994

Malaspina D, Warburton D, Amador X, et al: Association of schizophrenia and partial trisomy of chromosome 5p: a case report. Schizophr Res 7:191–196, 1992

Malhotra A, Goldman D, Buchanan R, et al: 5HT$_{2A}$ receptor T102C polymorphism and schizophrenia. Lancet 347:1830–1831, 1996

Mant R, Williams J, Asherson P, et al: The relationship between homozygosity at the dopamine D3 receptor gene and schizophrenia. Am J Med Genet 54:21–26, 1994

Marsh L, Suddath RL, Higgins N, et al: Medial temporal lobe structures in schizophrenia: relationship of size to duration of illness. Schizophr Res 11:225–238, 1994

Martinot JL, Peron-Magna P, Huret JD, et al: Striatal D2 dopaminergic receptors assessed with positron emission tomography and 76-Br bromospiperone in untreated schizophrenic patients. Am J Psychiatry 147:44–50, 1990

Mathysse S: Role of dopamine in selective attention. Adv Biochem Psychopharmacol 16:667–669, 1977

McCreadie RG, Hall DJ, Berry IJ, et al: The Nithsdale schizophrenia surveys, X: obstetric complications, family history and abnormal movements. Br J Psychiatry 161:799–805, 1992

McGue M: When assessing twin concordance use the probandwise not the pairwise rate. Schizophr Bull 18:171–176, 1992

McGuffin P, Sargeant M, Hetti G, et al: Exclusion of schizophrenia susceptibility gene from chromosome 5q11-q13 region: new data and reanalysis of previous reports. Am J Hum Genet 47:524–535, 1990

Mednick SA, Machon RA, Huttunen MO, et al: Adult schizophrenia following prenatal exposure to an influenza epidemic. Arch Gen Psychiatry 45:189–192, 1988

Mita T, Hanada S, Nishimo N, et al: Decreased serotonin S2 and increased dopamine D2 receptors in chronic schizophrenics. Biol Psychiatry 21:1407–1414, 1986

Moises HW, Gelernter J, Giuffra LA, et al: No linkage between D2 dopamine receptor gene region and schizophrenia. Arch Gen Psychiatry 48:643–647, 1991

Moises HW, Yang L, Kristbjarnarson H, et al: An international two-stage genome-wide search for schizophrenia susceptibility genes. Nat Genet 11:321–324, 1995a

Moises HW, Yang L, Li T, et al: Potential linkage disequilibrium between schizophrenia and locus D22S278 on the long arm of chromosome 22. Am J Med Genet 60:465–467, 1995b

Mowry BJ, Nancarrow DJ, Lenno DP, et al: Schizophrenia susceptibility and chromosome 6p24-22. Nat Genet 11:233–234, 1995

Muir WJ, Blackwood D, St. Clair D, et al: Linkage studies of the long arm of chromosome 11 in schizophrenic families (letter). Pychiatr Genet 2:18, 1991

Murray AM, Hyde TM, Knable MB, et al: Distribution of putative D4 dopamine receptors in postmortem striatum from patients with schizophrenia. J Neurosci 15:2186–2191, 1995

Nanko S, Gill M, Owen M, et al: Linkage study of schizophrenia on chromosome 11 in 2 Japanese families. Jpn J Psychiatry Neurol 46:155–159, 1992

Nanko S, Hattori M, Ikeda K, et al: Dopamine D4 receptor polymorphism and schizophrenia. Lancet 341:689–690, 1993

Nanko S, Hattori M, Dai XY, et al: DRD2 Ser311/Cys311 polymorphism in schizophrenia (letter). Lancet 343:1044, 1994

Nasrallah HA, Charles GT, McCalley-Whitters M, et al: Cerebral ventricular enlargement in subtypes of chronic schizophrenia. Arch Gen Psychiatry 39:774–777, 1982

Nasrallah HA, Skinner TE, Scmalbrock P, et al: Proton magnetic resonance spectroscopy of the hippocampal formation in schizophrenia: a pilot study. Br J Psychiatry 165:481–485, 1994

Nimgaonkar VL, Wessely S, Murray RM: Prevalence of familiality, obstetric complications, and structural brain damage in schizophrenic patients. Br J Psychiatry 153:191–197, 1988

Nimgaonkar VL, Zhang XR, Caldwell JG, et al: Association study of schizophrenia with dopamine D3 receptor gene polymorphism: probable effect of family history of schizophrenia. Am J Med Genet 48:214–217, 1993

Nothen MM, Cichon S, Propping P, et al: Excess of homozygosity at the dopamine D3 receptor gene in schizophrenia not confirmed (letter). J Med Genet 30:708, 1993

Nothen MM, Wildenauer D, Cichon S, et al: Dopamine D2 receptor molecular variant and schizophrenia. Lancet 343:1301–1302, 1994

Nyback H, Wiesel FA, Berggren BM: Computed tomography of the brain in patients with acute psychosis and in healthy volunteers. Acta Psychiatr Scand 65:403–414, 1982

O'Callaghan E, Larkin C, Kinsella A, et al: Obstetric complications, the putative familial-sporadic distinction, and tardive dyskinesia in schizophrenia. Br J Psychiatry 157:578–584, 1990

O'Callaghan E, Sham P, Takei N, et al: Schizophrenia after prenatal exposure to 1957 A2 influenza epidemic. Lancet 337:1248–1250, 1991

Onstad S, Skre I, Torgersen S, et al: Birthweight and obstetric complications in schizophrenic twins. Acta Psychiatr Scand 85:70–73, 1992

Owen F, Cross AJ, Crow TJ, et al: Neurotransmitter receptors in brain in schizophrenia. Acta Psychiatr Scand 63:20–28, 1981

Owen MJ, Lewis SW, Murray RM: Obstetric complications and cerebral abnormalities in schizophrenia. Psychol Med 15:27–41, 1988

Pakkenberg B: Post-mortem study of chronic schizophrenic brains. Br J Psychiatry 151:744–752, 1987

Pakkenberg B: Pronounced reduction of total neuron number in mediodorsal thalamic nucleus and nucleus accumbens in schizophrenics. Arch Gen Psychiatry 47:1023–1028, 1990

Perry TL: Normal cerebrospinal fluid and brain glutamate levels in schizophrenia do not support the hypothesis of glutamatergic neuronal dysfunction. Neurosci Lett 28:81–85, 1982

Petronis A, Macciardi F, Athanassiades A, et al: Association study between the dopamine D4 receptor gene and schizophrenia. Am J Med Genet 60:452–455, 1995

Pettegrew JW, Keshavan MS, Panchalingam K, et al: Alterations in brain high-energy phosphate and membrane phospholipid metabolism in first-episode, drug naive schizophrenics: a pilot study of the dorsal prefrontal cortex by in vivo phosphorous 31 nuclear magnetic resonance spectroscopy. Arch Gen Psychiatry 48:563–568, 1991

Pettegrew JW, Keshavan MS, Minshew NJ: [31]P nuclear magnetic resonance spectroscopy: neurodevelopment and schizophrenia. Schizophr Bull 19:35–53, 1993

Pfefferbaum A, Zipursky RB: Neuroimaging studies of schizophrenia. Schizophr Res 4:193–208, 1991

Pickar D, Breier A, Hsiao J, et al: Cerebrospinal fluid and plasma monoamine metabolites and their relation to psychosis. Arch Gen Psychiatry 47:641–648, 1990

Potter WZ, Hsiao JK, Goldman SM: Effects of renal clearance on plasma concentrations of homovanillic acid: methodologic cautions. Arch Gen Psychiatry 46:558–562, 1989

Pulver AE, Karayiorgou M, Wolyniec PS, et al: Sequential strategy to identify a susceptible gene for schizophrenia: report of potential linkage on chromosome 22q12-q13.1: part 2. Am J Med Genet 54:36–43, 1994

Pycock CJ, Kerwin RW, Carter CJ: Effect of lesions of cortical dopamine terminals on subcortical dopamine in rats. Nature 286:74–77, 1980a

Pycock CJ, Kerwin RW, Carter CJ: Effect of 6-hydroxydopamine lesions of medial prefrontal cortex in rat. J Neurochem 34:91–99, 1980b

Raine A, Lencz T, Reynolds GP, et al: An evaluation of structural and functional prefrontal deficits in schizophrenia: MRI and neuropsychological measures. Psychiatry Research: Neuroimaging 45:123–137, 1992

Reddy R, Mukherjee S, Schnur DB, et al: History of obstetric complications, family history, and CT scan findings in schizophrenic patients. Schizophr Res 3:311–314, 1990

Renshaw PF, Yurgelun-Todd D, Tohen M, et al: Temporal lobe proton magnetic spectroscopy of patients with first-episode psychosis. Am J Psychiatry 152:444–446, 1995

Reveley AM, Reveley MA, Clifford CA, et al: Cerebral ventricular size in twins discordant for schizophrenia. Lancet 2:540–541, 1982

Reynolds GP: Increased concentration and lateral asymmetry of amygdala dopamine in schizophrenia. Nature 305:527–529, 1983

Reynolds GP, Mason SL: Are striatal dopamine D4 receptors increased in schizophrenia? J Neurochem 63:1576–1578, 1994

Reynolds GP, Rossor MN, Iversen LL: Preliminary studies of human cortical 5-HT2 receptors and their involvement in schizophrenia and neuroleptic drug action. J Neural Transm 18 (suppl):273–277, 1983

Reynolds GP, Czudek C, Andrews HB: Deficit and hemispheric asymmetry of GABA uptakes sites in the hippocampus in schizophrenia. Biol Psychiatry 27:1038–1044, 1990

Rosenthal D, Kety SS: The Transmission of Schizophrenia. Elmsford, NY, Pergamon, 1968

Rosenthal D, Wender PH, Kety SS, et al: The adopted away offspring of schizophrenics. Am J Psychiatry 128:307–311, 1971

Rosenthal D, Wender PH, Kety SS, et al: Parent-child relationships and psychopathological disorder in the child. Arch Gen Psychiatry 32:466–476, 1975

Sabate O, Campion D, d'Amato T, et al: Failure to find evidence for linkage or association between the dopamine D3 receptor gene and schizophrenia. Am J Psychiatry 151:107–111, 1994

Saha N, Tsoi WF, Low PS, et al: Lack of association of the dopamine D3 receptor gene polymorphism (BalI) in Chinese schizophrenic males. Psychiatr Genet 4:201–204, 1994

Sasaki T, Macciardi FM, Badri F, et al: No evidence for association of dopamine D2 receptor variant with major psychosis. Am J Med Genet 67:415–417, 1996a

Sasaki T, Hattori M, Fukuda R, et al: 5HT$_{2A}$ receptor T102C polymorphism and schizophrenia (letter). Lancet 347:1832, 1996b

Scatton B, Worms P, Lloyd KG, et al: Cortical modulation of striatal function. Brain Res 232:331–343, 1982

Scheibel AB, Kovelman JA: Disorientation of the hippocampal pyramidal cell and its processes in the schizophrenic patient. Biol Psychiatry 16:101–102, 1981

Schulz SC: Genetics of schizophrenia: a status report, in American Psychiatric Press Review of Psychiatry, Vol 10. Edited by Tasman A, Goldfinger SM. Washington, DC, American Psychiatric Press, 1991, pp 79–97

Schulz SC, Koller MM, Kishore PR, et al: Ventricular enlargement in teenage patients with schizophrenia spectrum disorders. Am J Psychiatry 140:1592–1595, 1983

Schwab SG, Albus M, Hallmayer J, et al: Evaluation of a susceptibility gene for schizophrenia on chromosome 6p by multipoint affected sib-pair linkage analysis. Nat Genet 11:325–327, 1995a

Schwab SG, Lerer B, Albus M, et al: Potential linkage for schizophrenia on chromosome 22q12-q13: a replication study. Am J Med Genet 60:436–443, 1995b

Seeman P, Lee T, Chau-Wong M, et al: Antipsychotic drug doses and neuroleptic/dopamine receptors. Nature 261: 717–719, 1976

Seeman P, Bzowej NH, Guan HC, et al: Human brain D1 and D2 dopamine receptors in schizophrenia, Alzheimer's, Parkinson's and Huntington's diseases. Neuropsychopharmacology 1:5–15, 1987

Seeman P, Guan HC, Van Tol HHM: Dopamine D4 receptors elevated in schizophrenia. Nature 261:717–718, 1993

Selemon LD, Rajkowska G, Goldman-Rakic PS: Abnormally high neuronal density in the schizophrenic cortex: a morphometric analysis of prefrontal area 9 and occipital area 17. Arch Gen Psychiatry 52:805–818, 1995

Shaikh S, Collier D, Arranz M, et al: DRD2 Ser 311/Cys311 polymorphism in schizophrenia (letter). Lancet 343:1046, 1994a

Shaikh S, Gill M, Owen M, et al: Failure to find linkage between functional polymorphism in the dopamine D4 receptor gene and schizophrenia. Am J Med Genet 54:8–11, 1994b

Shaikh S, Collier DA, Sham PC, et al: Allelic association between a Ser-9-Gly polymorphism in the dopamine D3 receptor gene and schizophrenia. Hum Genet 97:714–719, 1996

Shelton RC, Weinberger DR: X-ray computerized tomography studies in schizophrenia: a review and synthesis, in Handbook of Schizophrenia, Vol I: The Neurology of Schizophrenia. Edited by Nasrallah HA, Weinberger DR. Amsterdam, Elsevier, 1986, pp 207–250

Shenton ME, Kikinis R, Jolesz FA, et al: Abnormalities of the left temporal lobe and thought disorder in schizophrenia: a quantitative magnetic resonance imaging study. N Engl J Med 327:604–612, 1992

Sherman AD, Davidson AT, Baruah S, et al: Evidence of glutamatergic deficiency in schizophrenia. Neurosci Lett 121:77–80, 1991a

Sherman AD, Hegwood TS, Baruah S, et al: Deficient NMDA-mediated glutamate release from synaptosomes of schizophrenics. Biol Psychiatry 30:1191–1198, 1991b

Sherrington R, Brynjolfsson J, Peturson H, et al: Localization of a susceptibility locus for schizophrenia on chromosome 5. Nature 336:164–167, 1988

Silverman JM, Greenberg DA, Altstiel LD, et al: Evidence of a locus for schizophrenia and related disorders on the short arm of chromosome 5 in a large pedigree. Am J Med Genet 67:162–171, 1996

Simpson M, Slater P, Royston M, et al: Alterations in phencyclidine and sigma binding sites in schizophrenic brains. Schizophr Res 6:41–48, 1992a

Simpson M, Slater P, Royston M, et al: Regionally selective deficits in uptake sites for glutamate and gamma-aminobutyric acid in the basal ganglia in schizophrenia. Psychiatr Res 42:273–282, 1992b

Sobell J, Sigurdson DC, Heston L, et al: S311C DRD2 variant: no association with schizophrenia. Lancet 344:621–622, 1994

Sobell JL, Lind TJ, Sigurdson DC, et al: The D5 dopamine receptor gene in schizophrenia: identification of a nonsense change and multiple missense changes but lack of association with disease. Hum Mol Genet 4:507–514, 1995

Sponheim SR, Iacono WG, Beiser M: Stability of ventricular size after the onset of psychosis in schizophrenia. Psychiatry Res 40:21–29, 1991

St Clair D, Blackwood D, Muir W, et al: No linkage of chromosome 5q11-13 markers to schizophrenia in Scottish families. Nature 339:305–307, 1989

St Clair D, Blackwood D, Muir W, et al: Association of a balanced autosomal translocation with major mental illness. Lancet 336:13–16, 1990

Straub RE, McLean CJ, O'Neill FA, et al: A potential vulnerability locus for schizophrenia on chromosome 6p24-22: evidence for genetic heterogeneity. Nat Genet 11: 287–293, 1995

Suddath R, Casanova MF, Goldberg TE, et al: Temporal lobe pathology in schizophrenia: a quantitative magnetic resonance imaging study. Am J Psychiatry 146:464–472, 1989

Suddath R, Christison GW, Torrey EF, et al: Anatomical abnormalities in the brains of monozygotic twins discordant for schizophrenia. N Engl J Med 322:789–794, 1990

Susser ES, Lin SP: Schizophrenia after prenatal exposure to the Dutch Hunger Winter of 1944–1945. Arch Gen Psychiatry 49:983–988, 1992

Swayze VW, Andreasen NC, Alliger RJ, et al: Subcortical and temporal structures in affective disorder and schizophrenia: a magnetic resonance imaging study. Biol Psychiatry 31:21–24, 1992

Torrey EF: Are we overestimating the genetic contribution to schizophrenia? Schizophr Bull 18:159–169, 1992

Torrey EF, Rawlings R, Waldman IN: Schizophrenic births and viral diseases in two states. Schizophr Res 1:73–77, 1988

Toru M, Watanabe S, Shibuya H, et al: Neurotransmitters, receptors and neuropeptides in post-mortem brains of chronic schizophrenic patients. Acta Psychiatr Scand 78:121–137, 1988

Tsai G, Passani LA, Slusher BS, et al: Abnormal excitatory neurotransmitter metabolism in schizophrenia brains. Arch Gen Psychiatry 52:829–836, 1995

Tsuang MT, Gilbertson MW, Faraone SV: The genetics of schizophrenia: current knowledge and future directions. Schizophr Res 4:157–171, 1991

Vallada HP, Gill M, Sham P, et al: Linkage studies on chromosome 22 in familial schizophrenia. Am J Med Genet 60:139–146, 1995

Van Kammen D: The biochemical basis of relapse and drug response in schizophrenia: review and hypothesis. Psychol Med 21:881–895, 1991

Van Kammen D, Kelley M: Dopamine and norepinephrine activity in schizophrenia. Schizophr Res 4:173–191, 1991

Van Kammen D, Peters J, Yao J, et al: Norepinephrine in acute exacerbations of chronic schizophrenia. Arch Gen Psychiatry 47:161–168, 1990

Vogt C, Vogt O: Alterations anatomiques de la schizophrenie et d'autres psychoses dites functionelles, in Proceedings of the First International Congress of Neuropathology, Vol 1. Turin, Italy, Rosenberg & Sellier, 1952, pp 515–532

Wang S, Cui-e-Sun, Walcczak CA, et al: Evidence for a susceptibility locus for schizophrenia on chromosome 6pter-p22. Nat Genet 10:41–46, 1995

Weinberger DR, Kleinman JE, Luchins DJ, et al: Cerebellar atrophy in chronic schizophrenia. Lancet 1:718–719, 1979

Weinberger DR, Kleinman JE, Luchins DJ, et al: Cerebellar atrophy in schizophrenia: a controlled postmortem study. Am J Psychiatry 137:359–361, 1980

Weinberger DR, DeLisi L, Perman GP, et al: Computed tomography in schizophreniform disorder and other acute psychiatric disorders. Arch Gen Psychiatry 39:778–793, 1982

Weinberger DR, Berman KF, Zec RF: Physiologic dysfunction of dorsolateral prefrontal cortex in schizophrenia, I: regional cerebral blood flow evidence. Arch Gen Psychiatry 43:114–124, 1986

Weinberger DR, Berman KF, Illowsky BP: Physiologic dysfunction of dorsolateral prefrontal cortex in schizophrenia, III: a new cohort and evidence for a monoaminergic mechanism. Arch Gen Psychiatry 45:609–615, 1988

Weinberger DR, Berman KF, Suddath R, et al: Evidence of dysfunction of a prefrontal-limbic network in schizophrenia: a magnetic resonance imaging and regional cerebral blood flow study of discordant monozygotic twins. Am J Psychiatry 149:890–897, 1992

Wender PH, Rosenthal D, Rainer JD, et al: Schizophrenics' adopting parents: psychiatric status. Arch Gen Psychiatry 34:777–784, 1977

Whitaker PM, Crow TJ, Ferrier IN: Tritiated LSD binding in frontal cortex in schizophrenia. Arch Gen Psychiatry 38:278–280, 1981

Wible CG, Shenton ME, Hokama H, et al: Prefrontal cortex and schizophrenia: a quantitative magnetic resonance imaging study. Arch Gen Psychiatry 52:279–288, 1995

Widerlov E: A critical appraisal of CSF monoamine metabolite studies in schizophrenia. Ann N Y Acad Sci 537:309–323, 1988

Wiese C, Lannfelt L, Kristbjarnarson H, et al: No linkage between schizophrenia and D3 dopamine gene locus in Icelandic pedigrees. Psychiatry Res 46:253–259, 1993

Williams AO, Reveley MA, Kolakowska T, et al: Schizophrenia with good and poor outcome, II: cerebral ventricular size and its clinical significance. Br J Psychiatry 146:239–246, 1985

Williams J, Spurlock G, McGuffin P, et al: Association between schizophrenia and T102C polymorphism of the 5-hydroxytryptamine type 2a-receptor gene. Lancet 347:1294–1296, 1996

Wong DF, Wagner HN, Tune LE, et al: Positron emission tomography reveals elevated D2 dopamine receptors in drug naive schizophrenics. Science 244:1558–1563, 1986

Yakovlev PI, Hamlin H, Sweet WH: Frontal lobotomy neuroanatomical observations. J Neuropathol Exp Neurol 9:250–285, 1950

Yang L, Weise C, Lannfelt L, et al: No association between schizophrenia and homozygosity at the D3 dopamine receptor gene. Am J Med Genet 48:83–86, 1993

Young AH, Blackwood DHR, Roxborough H, et al: A magnetic resonance imaging study of schizophrenia: brain structure and clinical symptoms. Br J Psychiatry 158:158–164, 1991

Zipursky RB, Lim KO, Sullivan EV, et al: Widespread cerebral gray matter volume deficits in schizophrenia. Arch Gen Psychiatry 49:195–205, 1992

Zukin SR, Javitt DC: The brain NMDA receptor, psychotomimetic drug effects, and schizophrenia, in American Psychiatric Press Review of Psychiatry, Vol 10. Edited by Tasman A, Goldfinger SM. Washington, DC, American Psychiatric Press, 1991, pp 480–498

TWENTY-NINE

Biology of Anxiety Disorders

Murray B. Stein, M.D., F.R.C.P.C., and Thomas W. Uhde, M.D.

In the past 15 years, there has been a marked surge of interest in anxiety disorders, as evidenced by an explosion of publications in this area. In 1979–1980, 3.0% of the research articles published in the *Archives of General Psychiatry* and the *American Journal of Psychiatry* (psychiatry's two journals with the highest impact factor by Science Citation Indices) were devoted to anxiety and stress-related disorders. By 1989–1990, research articles on anxiety and stress-related disorders accounted for 16.1% of the publications in these two journals (Pincus et al. 1993). In 1994 through 1996 alone, nearly 1,800 publications on anxiety disorders were listed in MEDLINE. This dramatic increase in research has provided us with a wealth of information about biological aspects of anxiety disorders. In this chapter, we review current neurobiological knowledge of these disorders.

It will be apparent that there is great disparity in the amount of neurobiological research that has been conducted on the various DSM-IV (American Psychiatric Association 1994) anxiety disorders. Panic disorder and obsessive-compulsive disorder have been the most thoroughly investigated anxiety disorders; accordingly, the largest portions of this chapter are devoted to them. Posttraumatic stress disorder (PTSD) assumes third place in terms of the amount of neurobiological research conducted thus far, with social phobia, other phobic disorders, and generalized anxiety disorder coming in far behind. With the exception of social phobia, the neurobiology of phobic disorders and generalized anxiety disorder is not discussed in this chapter. Interested readers are referred elsewhere for reviews of the biology of simple phobias,

generalized anxiety disorder, and blood-illness-injury phobias (Hoehn-Saric and McLeod 1993; Westenberg et al. 1996).

We have not attempted to provide a comprehensive review of the biology of each anxiety disorder. Such a task is clearly beyond the scope of a single chapter; in fact, entire books have been devoted to the neurobiology of specific anxiety disorders (e.g., Ballenger 1990; Friedman et al. 1995). In addition to limiting our review to the best-studied anxiety disorders, we opted to address mainly those findings with the strongest empirical (and replicable) databases. We also have drawn attention to a few preliminary findings that represent promising avenues of investigation on the neurobiology of anxiety and anxiety disorders.

NEUROBIOLOGY OF PANIC DISORDER AND AGORAPHOBIA

Until the early 1960s, panic disorder was subsumed under the rubric of different syndromes such as "soldier's heart," "neurocirculatory asthenia," and "cardiac neurosis" and was relegated to backseat status as a minor psychiatric disorder. Panic disorder is now known to be a common illness (12-month prevalence is approximately 1%; Eaton et al. 1994) with often devastating socioeconomic consequences (e.g., job loss, financial dependence, excessive health care utilization; Markowitz et al. 1989) and a markedly adverse effect on quality of life (Sherbourne et al. 1996). Panic disorder is frequently complicated by agoraphobia (Goisman et al. 1995); therefore, for the purposes of this chapter, panic and agoraphobia are considered as a single diagnostic entity.

Theories of the nature and etiology of panic disorder range from the biological to the psychological (for review, see McNally 1994). Among the anxiety disorders, panic disorder was the first to be extensively studied from a biological perspective. Through over two decades of research, what emerges is a picture of panic disorder as an often inherited illness, but exactly what is inherited has not been elucidated. Rather than present data within the framework of a single "theory" of panic disorder, in this section we provide an update on current knowledge regarding the familial transmission of panic disorder and present an overview of different prevailing hypotheses regarding the pathophysiology of panic disorder, keeping in mind that the panic disorder "syndrome" probably represents a heterogeneous group of neuropathological diatheses.

Heritability of Panic Disorder

Twin studies in panic disorder uniformly report a higher concordance rate for monozygotic than for dizygotic twins (Torgersen 1990), thereby suggesting (but not proving) a genetic basis for panic disorder. An early study suggested a possible linkage of panic disorder with the α-haptoglobin locus on chromosome 16q22 (Crowe et al. 1987). However, this research team could not replicate this finding with the later addition of more pedigrees (Crowe et al. 1990). Other investigations have not found evidence of linkage to five adrenergic receptor genes (Wang et al. 1992) or alteration in the sequencing of two particular serotonin receptor subtypes in panic disorder (Ohara et al. 1996). A recent study failed to find an association between panic disorder and the neuronal nicotinic acetylcholine receptor α_4 subunit (CHRNA4), found on chromosome 20 (Steinlein et al. 1997). Thus, although a genetic basis for panic disorder in at least some families is now strongly suspected (Vieland et al. 1996), linkage to any particular gene has yet to be established.

Neurochemical Hypotheses for the Pathophysiology of Panic Disorder

Early theorists such as Da Costa (1871) were impressed by the prominent cardiac symptoms that occur during panic attacks and coined the term *irritable heart syndrome*. Many theories to explain the pathophysiology of panic disorder have since been advanced, several of which are reviewed here.

Lactate hypothesis. The lactate hypothesis arose from the clinical observation that chronically anxious pa-

tients had decreased exercise tolerance; thus, investigators postulated that these subjects had an abnormality in lactate metabolism (Pitts and McClure 1967). Subsequent studies consistently found that the intravenous administration of sodium lactate to patients with panic disorder elicited panic attacks in 50%–70% of these individuals but in fewer than 10% of healthy control subjects (Liebowitz et al. 1984; Pohl et al. 1988). Even though changes in acid-base status (Gorman et al. 1990), serum-ionized calcium or phosphate (Fyer et al. 1984; Gorman et al. 1986), intravascular volume, and cerebral blood flow (CBF) (Mathew et al. 1989; Reiman et al. 1989) have each been postulated as the mechanism for lactate-induced panic, the available data suggest that none of these is necessary to its panicogenic properties. In fact, a study (Coplan et al. 1992b) that failed to find alterations in cisternal lactate or carbon dioxide (CO_2) levels following intravenous administration of sodium lactate to nonhuman primates raises serious questions about a direct central nervous system (CNS) effect of lactate.

In contrast, sodium lactate has been recognized as a potent respiratory stimulant. The degree to which hyperventilation ensues following lactate administration appears to be a major determinant of which patients experience panic attacks following lactate infusion (Gorman et al. 1988b). These findings suggest that the mechanism by which lactate induces panic is through its effects on respiratory drive, and they provide a strong rationale for the detailed scrutiny of respiratory function in panic disorder. In fact, the idea that panic attacks may be somehow linked to abnormalities in respiration is among the most compelling theories presently being tested.

Respiratory hypotheses. A prominent hypothesis, with several variants thereof, proposes that panic attacks are a result of (or at least associated with) abnormalities in respiratory function (Klein 1993). Almost all patients with panic disorder complain of shortness of breath or of having trouble breathing during their attacks. It has been suggested that panic attacks are nothing more than the conglomeration of symptoms that are the direct consequence of chronic hyperventilation (Hibbert 1984), but chronic hyperventilation does not, in fact, appear to be a characteristic of most patients with panic disorder (Garssen et al. 1996). In contrast, voluntary acute hyperventilation of room air *has* been shown to reproduce the attacks in 30%–50% of patients with panic disorder (Gorman et al. 1988a; Rapee 1986), suggesting that decrements in carbon dioxide partial pressure (pCO_2) may be important in the pathophysiology of panic in at least a subgroup of individuals. One study (Dager et al. 1995) found that brain lactate levels (measured with proton magnetic spectroscopy) following controlled ventilation increased to a greater degree in patients with panic disorder than in healthy control subjects, suggesting a possible link between the lactate and the respiratory hypotheses of panic disorder.

In apparent contradiction to the findings from hyperventilation studies, the inhalation of CO_2-enriched (5%, 7.5%, or 35%) air—which *raises* pCO_2—provoked panic attacks in an even greater proportion (50%–80%) of patients with panic disorder (Gorman and Papp 1990), was specific to panic disorder as opposed to other anxiety disorders (Gorman et al. 1994; Perna et al. 1995; Verburg et al. 1995), and led to panic attacks at a higher rate among persons with greater familial loading for panic disorder (Perna et al. 1996). In contrast to the anxiogenic hypersensitivity of patients with panic disorder to the effects of inhaled CO_2-enriched air, evidence for *chemoreceptor supersensitivity* (as would be exemplified by augmented ventilatory drive in response to a given inhaled CO_2 concentration) has been less forthcoming (Gorman et al. 1988a; Papp et al. 1995). Along these lines, it remains unproven that the vulnerability to CO_2-induced panic depends on an individual's sensitivity to changes in systemic CO_2 (presumably at the brain-stem level; Gorman et al. 1989). A viable alternative explanation is that patients with panic disorder are hypersensitive to the somatic sensations (e.g., dyspnea) evoked by the CO_2 but not necessarily to the hypercapnia, per se. This is highly plausible, given that doxapram, a respiratory stimulant that provokes hyperventilation and resultant *hypocapnia*, is itself a potent panicogen (Abelson et al. 1996).

Nonetheless, the finding of heightened behavioral sensitivity to CO_2 in conjunction with the striking finding of *irregular respiratory rhythm* in response to CO_2 (Papp et al. 1995) led investigators to propose that patients with panic disorder have a biologically based hypersensitive respiratory control system believed to operate at the level of brain-stem chemoreceptors (Gorman and Papp 1990; Gorman et al. 1989; Klein 1993).

Many (if not all) of the stimuli that induce panic share an ability to stimulate respiration and/or induce a sense of breathlessness. Klein (1993) proposed that patients with panic disorder have an abnormally low threshold for sensing impending suffocation and that panic attacks result from the triggering of a "false suffocation alarm." McNally and Eke (1996) argued that in patients with panic disorder, attacks following respiratory provocations (e.g., CO_2) do not necessarily indicate a biological abnormality but can alternatively be conceptualized as a tendency (perhaps learned) for patients to be frightened by and intolerant of the physical sensations (i.e., shortness of breath) induced by these challenges. Two studies that found altered respiratory rhythm *during sleep* in patients with panic disorder (Martinez et al. 1996; Stein et al. 1995b) indicate that breathing abnormalities in panic may have a physiological basis that lies outside the realm of conscious awareness of breathing difficulties. Pending further research, this controversy is unresolved.

Noradrenergic hypothesis. Several groups of investigators (Charney and Heninger 1986; Charney et al. 1984, 1989; Nesse et al. 1984; Nutt 1989; Uhde et al. 1984a) have contemplated noradrenergic dysfunction in panic disorder. One of the major stimuli behind these studies was the work of Redmond (1979) and colleagues, who identified a relation between activity of the major noradrenergic site in the brain, the locus coeruleus, and anxiety-like behaviors in primates. Subsequently, researchers used various experimental techniques in an effort to confirm the presence and importance of noradrenergic dysfunction in panic disorder.

Several groups have used pharmacological probes of the noradrenergic system in this regard. Some research teams showed that patients with panic disorder were behaviorally and cardiovascularly hyperreactive to the anxiogenic effects of orally administered yohimbine (an α_2 antagonist; Charney et al. 1984, 1987; Uhde et al. 1984a), indicating that these patients might have α_2-adrenergic receptor supersensitivity. Some investigators (Charney and Heninger 1986; Nutt 1989) also found blunted cardiovascular responses to the α_2-agonist clonidine, although this finding has not been replicated consistently (Uhde et al. 1989). This finding would actually be suggestive of α_2-adrenergic receptor subsensitivity rather than supersensitivity, as suggested by the yohimbine studies. Charney and Heninger (1986) proposed use of the term *dysregulation* to describe this curious state of supersensitivity to an antagonist but subsensitivity to an agonist putatively acting at the same receptor site(s).

Subnormal or "blunted" growth hormone (GH) responses to clonidine administration have been well-replicated findings in patients with panic disorder (Abelson et al. 1992; Charney and Heninger 1986; Nutt 1989; Rapaport et al. 1989; Tancer et al. 1993a; Uhde et al. 1992). The blunted GH response to clonidine usually has been attributed to postsynaptic α_2-adrenergic downregulation, and it has accordingly been considered supportive of the noradrenergic hypothesis of panic. However, it must be recognized that the regulation of GH release is complex and includes stimulatory and/or inhibitory inputs from the noradrenergic, cholinergic, dopaminergic, γ-aminobutyric acid (GABA)ergic, and serotonergic systems. Furthermore, GH secretion is directly stimulated by the GH releasing factor (GRF) and inhibited both by somatostatin-release inhibiting factor (SRIF) and by GH itself via an ultrashort feedback loop. Thus, although a diminished GH response to clonidine is clearly among the best-replicated biological findings in panic disorder—and may be a stable finding even during remission (Coplan et al. 1995)—the pathophysiological significance of these findings (particularly with regard to noradrenergic dysfunction) has not been fully elucidated.

Serotonergic Dysfunction in Panic Disorder

Serotonin has been alluded to as "a neurotransmitter for all seasons" (van Kammen 1987, p. 1), in reference to the increasing propensity for psychiatric investigators to uncover serotonergic dysfunction in nearly all neuropsychiatric disorders (e.g., depression, schizophrenia, obsessive-compulsive disorder, alcoholism). As reviewed by Coplan et al. (1992a), several (but not all) studies have found that patients with panic disorder are sensitive to the anxiogenic effects of serotonin receptor agonists such as m-chlorophenylpiperazine (m-CPP) and the indirect agonist fenfluramine. However, most recent studies have not found evidence of altered serotonin transporter binding on platelets in patients with panic disorder (Maguire et al. 1995; Stein et al. 1995a). Nonetheless, taken together and in the context of the proven efficacy of the selective serotonin reuptake inhibitors (SSRIs) in panic disorder (see Tollefson and Rosenbaum, Chapter 11, in this volume), further attention to the serotonin system (including the use of serotonin subtype probes; e.g., Lesch et al. 1992) will probably lead to significant advances in understanding the pathophysiology of panic disorder.

Adenosinergic Dysfunction in Panic Disorder

As shown in controlled studies and reviewed by Uhde (1990), patients with panic disorder are hypersensitive to the anxiogenic effects of caffeine (Boulenger et al. 1984). Caffeine's behavioral (including anxiogenic) effects, like those of other methylxanthines, are thought to be attributable to its properties as an antagonist at the receptor level of one of the brain's major neuromodulators, adenosine (Fredholm and Persson 1982). Accordingly, dysfunction at the level of the adenosine receptor has been hypothesized to occur in patients with panic disorder.

Caffeine's ability to enhance taste sensitivity is believed to be a result of its antagonist actions at peripheral adenosine receptors within gustatory pathways (Schiffman et al. 1985). Two independent studies found that caffeine lowers the taste threshold for quinine detection to a greater degree in patients with panic disorder than in control subjects (Apfeldorf and Shear 1993; DeMet et al. 1989), thereby lending some credence to an adenosinergic dysfunction model of panic disorder. Accordingly, investigators predicted that chronic treatment with an indirect adenosine agonist (dipyridamole) would ameliorate panic symptoms, but this drug has since been proven ineffective in the treatment of panic disorder (Stein et al. 1993a). When subtype-specific (e.g., A1, A2) drugs with good CNS penetrability become available for use in humans, it will be of interest to examine the drugs' efficacy in the treatment of panic disorder.

Other Neurobiological Models

As can be seen, there is no shortage of neurobiological models for panic disorder. One might argue that the plethora of models reflects the fact that none has been especially satisfactory. Although it is not our intent to burden the reader with an exhaustive list, we would be remiss not to at least draw attention to three additional chemical models that have gained some well-deserved notoriety.

Isoproterenol. The intravenous infusion of the β-adrenergic agonist isoproterenol provokes panic attacks in susceptible individuals at approximately the same rate as sodium lactate does (Pohl et al. 1988). However, considering that β-blockers are generally regarded as inefficacious in the treatment of panic disorder, a β-supersensitivity model of panic disorder would appear difficult to support.

Benzodiazepine receptor sensitivity. The unequivocal role for benzodiazepines in the treatment of panic disorder (see Ballenger, Chapter 14, in this volume), along with the rich preclinical literature on the importance of the GABA-benzodiazepine receptor complex in the mediation of anxiety (Zorumski and Isenberg 1991), makes this system a prime candidate for involvement in the pathogenesis of panic disorder. Two groups have independently observed altered benzodiazepine receptor sensitivity in panic disorder (Nutt et al. 1990; Roy-Byrne et al. 1990), as assessed by reduced sensitivity to the benzodiazepine-induced disruption of saccadic eye movements. Recent research suggests that this finding may not be specific to patients with panic disorder but may be a more general finding in patients with anxiety disorders (Roy-Byrne et al. 1996). Plasma levels of GABA have been found to be normal in patients with panic disorder (Goddard et al. 1996).

Cholecystokinin tetrapeptide.

The panicogenic effects of cholecystokinin tetrapeptide (CCK_4) (Bradwejn et al. 1990, 1991, 1992; de Montigny 1989) represent an exciting addition to the cadre of known panicogenic agents. Notably, cerebrospinal fluid (CSF) CCK concentrations were lower in 25 patients with panic disorder than in 16 healthy comparison subjects (Lydiard et al. 1992), perhaps reflecting increased CNS CCK-receptor sensitivity in panic disorder. Although recent studies of CCK_B antagonists for the treatment of panic disorder have had disappointing results (Cowley et al. 1996; Kramer et al. 1995), it seems likely that investigations of this and related neuropeptides will provide valuable information about the neurobiology of panic attacks.

Autonomic Dysfunction in Panic Disorder

Panic disorder has been widely hypothesized to be associated with dysfunction of the autonomic nervous system. This hypothesis is genuinely attractive, given that panic attacks are characterized by the reporting of tachycardia, palpitations, sweating, and trembling, symptoms strongly suggestive of autonomic activation. Although the subjective experience of autonomic-like symptoms in panic disorder is incontestable, objective evidence of autonomic hyperreactivity in panic disorder has been difficult to document in controlled studies.

Ambulatory studies of patients with panic disorder (Woods and Charney 1990) have found that panic attacks are not necessarily associated with autonomic activation (i.e., tachycardia or tachypnea). In several well-controlled laboratory studies involving physiological challenges such as postural change, cold pressor testing, and isotonic exercise (Roth et al. 1992; Stein and Asmundson 1994), investigators did not detect autonomic dysfunction in patients with panic disorder. Although a recent investigation reported differences between patients with panic disorder and healthy comparison subjects in the middle artery CBF response (measured by Doppler ultrasound) to postural challenge, the differences were small and of doubtful physiological consequence (Faravelli et al. 1997). Most researchers would now agree that augmented physiological reactivity in patients with panic disorder may simply reflect the poorer cardiovascular fitness of these individuals, many of whom restrict their activity because of their agoraphobia and/or their fear of the physical symptoms associated with exertion (Reiss 1988).

At this juncture, then, it is reasonable to conclude that although autonomic activation is a feature of some (but clearly not all) panic attacks, autonomic dysfunction per se is unlikely to play a causative role in the etiopathology of panic disorder.

Neuroendocrine Function in Panic Disorder

Hypothalamic-pituitary-adrenal axis.

Although dysfunction within various elements of the hypothalamic-pituitary-adrenal (HPA) axis is a well-established component of the pathophysiology of affective disorders (Nemeroff 1991; see also Musselman et al., Chapter 27, in this volume), this factor has been more difficult to ascertain in the case of panic disorder. Several studies have reported high rates of dexamethasone nonsuppression or elevated urinary free cortisol in patients with panic disorder, but these findings usually have been in the context of panic disorder complicated by depression (or, in some studies, severe agoraphobia; reviewed in Stein and Uhde 1990). Adrenocorticotropic hormone (ACTH) responses to corticotropin-releasing hormone (CRH) administration, although abnormally low in depressed patients, are probably normal or slightly enhanced in nondepressed patients with panic disorder (Curtis et al. 1997). Twenty-four-hour blood sampling indicates considerable heterogeneity in plasma cortisol and corticotropin levels in patients with panic disorder (Abelson and Curtis 1996a); some patients in that study had overnight hypercortisolemia and increased activity in ultradian secretory episodes, but the findings were subtle. Patients with the most severe panic (and the worst prognosis for recovery in that regard) may have the most profound HPA axis dysregulation (Abelson and Curtis 1996b).

Hypothalamic-pituitary-thyroid axis.

The recognition of abnormal thyroid functioning in some patients with depression led to the investigation of the hypothalamic-pituitary-thyroid (HPT) axis in patients with panic disorder. With few exceptions, a convincing majority of studies of anxiety disorders confirmed normal peripheral thyroid hormone levels, normal thyroid hormone end organ responsivity, normal thyroid autoimmune status, and normal thyrotropin responses to thyrotropin-releasing hormone (TRH) (Stein and Uhde 1993).

Sleep in Panic Disorder

In contrast to the extensive literature on sleep in patients with affective illness, only a few controlled studies of the sleep in patients with panic disorder have been done (for review, see Uhde 1994). At this juncture, most polysomnographic studies concur that patients with panic disorder have remarkably normal sleep architecture (Arriaga et al. 1996; Hauri et al. 1989; Mellman and Uhde 1989a; Stein et al. 1993b); in particular, the absence of shortened rapid eye movement (REM) latency (as seen in depression) is notable. No satisfactory explanation has yet been advanced for the occurrence of sleep panic attacks (Mellman and Uhde 1989b). These attacks, which seem to arise preferentially out of the transition between Stage 2 and Stage 3 sleep (Mellman and Uhde 1989a; Uhde 1994), at a time when dreaming is absent and cognitions are minimal, provide a compelling argument for the biological (as opposed to psychological) nature of at least some panic attacks. Several groups of investigators are attempting to characterize further the pathophysiology of sleep panic in the hope that this will provide clues to the biological basis for waking panic as well.

Neuroimaging Studies of Panic Disorder

Reiman and colleagues (1984) generated considerable excitement with their positron-emission tomography (PET) finding of abnormal asymmetry of CBF (i.e., left less than right) in lactate-vulnerable patients with panic disorder. This abnormality was seen at rest (or as "at rest" as someone can be with his or her head in a PET scanner) in the nonpanic state. Nordahl and colleagues (1990) used a different PET technique (^{18}F-deoxyglucose) and found hippocampal region metabolic asymmetry (also left less than right).

Subsequently, the St. Louis group (Reiman et al. 1989) identified several brain regions—most notably, the temporopolar cortex bilaterally—where blood flow increased during a lactate-induced anxiety attack. Unfortunately, this marked increase in temporopolar blood flow was later determined to be artifactual and actually reflected increased blood flow to extracranial muscles that occurred during teeth clenching (Drevets et al. 1992). Therefore, although this latter finding has not been sustained, the finding of hippocampal asymmetric blood flow (and metabolism) seems, for now, to be a true observation that supports involvement of the limbic lobe in the genesis of panic (Gorman et al. 1989).

Summary of the Biology of Panic Disorder

The discovery that lactate infusions resulted in panic attacks in susceptible individuals (Pitts and McClure 1967) ushered in a whole era of investigations into the biology of panic disorder. Instead of merely knowing that lactate can induce panic, we now know that a host of other substances (e.g., caffeine, isoproterenol, yohimbine, carbon dioxide, m-CPP, doxapram, CCK_4; for review, see Uhde et al. 1990) may also do so, but there are exceptions such as TRH and hypoglycemia (Stein and Uhde 1991; Uhde et al. 1984b). Some critics have argued that perhaps there is nothing "biological" about the response to this array of panicogens. Rather, each of these substances induces a constellation of physical symptoms that are interpreted by the individual in a way that leads to the experience of panic (Margraf et al. 1986; McNally 1994).

Shear and colleagues (1991) reported that when patients with panic disorder are treated with an effective nonpharmacological modality—cognitive-behavior therapy (Barlow 1988)—they are less vulnerable to lactate-induced panic. These observations provide a powerful impetus for the development of research paradigms that can remove (or at least minimize) the effects of expectancy and cognitions and thus enable the study of the neurobiology of panic disorder in its purest form. Sleep studies (particularly the study of sleep panic attacks) promise to provide information about autonomic and neurochemical mechanisms that may be involved in the pathophysiology of truly spontaneous panic attacks. Finally, as suggested by Klein (1993), a closer look at the respiratory attributes of various panicogens may illuminate a set of properties needed to elicit panic.

BIOLOGY OF SOCIAL PHOBIA

Social phobia is a disorder marked by the intense fear and/or avoidance of situations in which the individual feels that he or she will be scrutinized by others. In its extreme form, known as the *generalized subtype* of social phobia (Hazen and Stein 1995; Mannuzza et al. 1995; Stein 1996), social phobia might be considered an extreme form of shyness or even a personality disorder (e.g., avoidant). In its more circumscribed form, known as the *discrete* or *specific subtype* of social phobia, fear and avoidance are limited to one (or perhaps several) phobic situations, most commonly, public speaking (Stein et al. 1996). Preliminary evidence indicates that the generalized subtype of social phobia runs in families (Stein et al., in press), but studies of heritability have not yet been conducted. It is anticipated that future studies will reveal that the neurobiology of these two subtypes differs, but at present this remains speculative. Nonetheless, to the extent that it is possible to do so, we note where subtype specificity has been indicated for the particular studies reviewed below.

Sympathetic Nervous System Function in Social Phobia

When placed in social phobic situations (or even in anticipation of such exposure), patients with social phobia complain of tachycardia, tremor, and blushing—symptoms highly suggestive of adrenergic overactivity. In fact, in some patients, these symptoms are amenable to treatment with β-blockers such as propranolol or atenolol (Liebowitz et al. 1985). These observations have led investigators to test the hypothesis that the sympathetic nervous system, particularly the β-adrenergic receptor system, might be overactive in patients with social phobia.

Papp and colleagues (1988) infused intravenous epinephrine (2 μg/kg) into 11 patients with social phobia. Although 8 of the patients noted some anxiety symptoms, none reported that the infusion reproduced the symptoms experienced in social phobic situations. Possible explanations for this finding include the poor CNS penetrability of intravenous epinephrine, as well as the experimental context that lacked a "performance" or other scrutiny component.

Two groups (Heimberg et al. 1990; Levin et al. 1993) measured cardiovascular responses to a public speaking challenge in patients with social phobia. Levin et al. (1993) found no differences in cardiovascular reactivity between patients and control subjects, but (like Heimberg et al. 1990) they noted that the generalized social phobic subjects had *less* cardiovascular activation than did the discrete (public speaking) social phobic subjects. These two studies underscore the importance of considering the possibility that these two subgroups may be distinct from a biological perspective.

Peripheral noradrenergic responsivity was assessed in 15 patients with social phobia with a "naturalistic" challenge of the autonomic nervous system, the response to postural (or orthostatic) change (Stein et al. 1992, 1994). Compared with 20 healthy control subjects, patients with social phobia had normal heart rate and blood pressure responses to the postural challenge. In contrast, patients with social phobia had an exaggerated blood pressure response to the pressor effects of intravenously administered TRH (Tancer et al. 1990b). Stein and colleagues (1993c) measured β-adrenoceptor density and affinity on lymphocytes from patients with generalized social phobia and found these individuals to be no different from healthy control subjects. At present, then, it appears safe to say that autonomic functioning is different between generalized and discrete subtypes of social phobia, but we are a long way from characterizing the precise role of autonomic nervous system dysfunction in these disorders.

Neuroendocrine Function in Social Phobia

Compared with the understanding of neuroendocrine functioning in depressive disorders or in panic disorder, less information is available about the neuroendocrinology of social phobia. The team from the National Institute of Mental Health (NIMH; Tancer et al. 1990a) reported normal peripheral thyroid indices and normal thyrotropin responses to TRH infusion. Several studies have examined HPA axis function in social phobia. Uhde and colleagues (1994) reported similar rates of cortisol nonsuppression to dexamethasone in 64 patients with social phobia (9%) and in 30 control subjects (7%). These investigators observed normal 24-hour urinary free cortisol levels in the patients with social phobia, a finding also noted by Potts and colleagues (1991). These observations suggest that HPT and HPA axis functioning are likely to be normal in patients with social phobia; however, again, the generalized versus discrete subtype differences have not yet been examined. Furthermore, more detailed examination of HPA axis functioning with techniques such as corticotropin-releasing factor stimulation is clearly warranted.

Monoaminergic Function in Social Phobia

We are aware of only two studies that have assessed any aspect of monoaminergic functioning in patients with social phobia. In the first, Tancer and colleagues (1993b) administered the α_2-agonist clonidine (2 μg/kg intravenously) to 16 patients with social phobia and 31 healthy control subjects. The patients with social phobia had a blunted GH response to intravenous clonidine, thereby providing the first putative evidence of noradrenergic dysregulation in this disorder. However, a recent investigation did not find a blunted GH response to oral clonidine in patients with social phobia (Tancer et al. 1994). As a result, it appears that when this neuroendocrine abnormality does occur in patients with social phobia, it tends to be modest in degree and less consistent than the blunted GH responses in patients with panic disorder.

The study by Tancer et al. (1994) also involved oral administration of the dopamine agonist L-dopa and the indirect serotonin agonist fenfluramine to medication-free patients with social phobia and to healthy comparison subjects. Most patients with social phobia had the generalized type. No differences in GH or eye-blink responses to L-dopa were found, arguing against the involvement of a general disturbance in dopaminergic function in this disorder. An augmented cortisol response to fenfluramine was detected in the patients with social phobia, increasing the possibility that a specific abnormality in serotonin-2C ($5-HT_{2C}$) receptor functioning might be involved.

Neuroimaging Studies of Social Phobia

Only a few neuroimaging studies of social phobia have been conducted to date. Davidson et al. (1993) used proton magnetic resonance spectroscopy to measure the concentration of certain brain metabolites in 20 patients with social phobia (subtype not specified) and 20 age- and sex-matched healthy comparison subjects. They found that patients with social phobia had a lower ratio of N-acetylaspartate to other metabolites than did the comparison subjects. Although the neurobiological significance of this finding has not been elucidated, the investigators pointed out that the findings suggest a promising direction for future research. Stein and Leslie (1996) used brain single photon emission computed tomography (SPECT) with the ligand HMPAO to study CBF in patients with DSM-IV generalized social phobia and healthy comparison subjects; no systematic differences were detected in the resting (i.e., unstimulated) state. By using a ligand that measures the density of dopamine reuptake sites, investigators recently found that patients with generalized social phobia had markedly lower striatal dopamine reuptake densities than did age- and sex-matched comparison subjects (Tiihonen et al. 1997). These results suggest that generalized social phobia may be associated with dysfunction of the striatal dopaminergic system. All three studies included fairly small sample sizes (all had <20 subjects with social phobia) and must be replicated. Furthermore, studies comparing cerebral functioning in a neutral and socially anxious state (e.g., using script-driven imagery) are needed to shed further light on neuronal systems that may be implicated in the generation of social anxiety and thus should be investigated further as candidate brain systems that may be abnormal in patients with social phobia.

Summary of the Biology of Social Phobia

The neurobiology of social phobia remains obscure (for review, see Coplan et al. 1996). Because many patients with generalized social phobia respond to treatment with monoamine oxidase inhibitors or SSRIs, the next logical step in this phase of research is to use pharmacological probes (e.g., serotonergic subtype-specific probes) to examine specific aspects of monoaminergic function in generalized social phobia. In concert, it will be of interest to examine the relation between drug response and serotonin and dopamine genotypes, particularly given early in-

dications that these may influence certain personality styles and attributes, including anxiety-related traits such as shyness (Benjamin et al. 1996; Ebstein et al. 1996; Lesch et al. 1996).

BIOLOGY OF POSTTRAUMATIC STRESS DISORDER

PTSD, the only psychiatric disorder whose definition demands that a particular stressor precede its appearance (Davidson and Foa 1993), serves as the case in point for the myriad ways in which severe, unexpected, and uncontrollable stress may produce a neurobiological disturbance. Only in the past 15 years, and primarily in the past decade, has the biology of PTSD come under scrutiny. Furthermore, although it is understood that PTSD can occur following various traumatic events (e.g., sexual abuse, criminal victimization, burn injury), the current literature on the biology of PTSD refers almost exclusively to combat-related PTSD. Consequently, our discussion focuses primarily on that sphere of observation, but we note where new findings in other areas are emerging.

Psychophysiology of Posttraumatic Stress Disorder

Several studies have documented elevated blood pressure and/or heart rate in combat veterans with PTSD both when they are at rest and when they are exposed to reminders of war (e.g., combat scenes in movies, visualization of combat imagery) (Orr 1990; Pitman et al. 1987, 1990). In addition, several investigators noted that patients with combat-related PTSD show exaggerated startle reactivity (usually measured as the eye-blink response to a loud acoustic pulse) (Butler et al. 1990; Morgan et al. 1995, 1996; Orr et al. 1995; Shalev et al. 1992). Given that the neural substrates for startle reactivity are relatively well understood (Davis et al. 1993), the further study of startle reactivity in patients with PTSD promises to help delineate the neural circuits integral to the pathophysiology of this disorder (or, at minimum, the physiological hyperreactivity component thereof).

Adrenergic Dysfunction in Posttraumatic Stress Disorder

In contrast to the robust signs of autonomic hyperfunction arising out of the psychophysiological studies, biochemical evidence of sympathetic hyperfunction has been less clear cut. Although Kosten and colleagues (1987) found elevated 24-hour urinary norepinephrine and epinephrine levels in patients with PTSD, Pitman and Orr (1990) could not replicate this finding. Similarly, McFall and colleagues (1992) reported normal resting plasma epinephrine and norepinephrine levels in patients with PTSD, and the latter finding was also noted by Blanchard and colleagues (1991). Murburg et al. (1995) used a radioisotope dilution technique to assess plasma norepinephrine kinetics and found that basal sympathetic nervous system activity was normal in patients with PTSD. On the whole, the available data only partially support a role for sympathetic nervous system hyperfunction in the pathophysiology of PTSD.

Sleep in Posttraumatic Stress Disorder

It should be no great surprise that patients with PTSD sleep poorly, considering that hyperarousal is a key feature of the disorder. In fact, disrupted sleep is so prominent in patients with PTSD that one author referred to sleep disturbance as the "hallmark" of PTSD (Ross et al. 1989).

Ross and colleagues (1989) implicated REM sleep dysregulation as a critical factor in the development of both daytime (i.e., flashbacks) and nighttime (i.e., posttraumatic anxiety dreams) symptomatology in PTSD. Based on the evidence for adrenergic dysfunction in PTSD (see earlier section) and in another REM sleep disorder, narcolepsy, it is indeed compelling to want to implicate REM sleep dysfunction in the pathophysiology of PTSD. Abnormal REM sleep function and, in particular, an increase in movements during REM sleep (which is normally associated with muscle atony) have been noted to be features of PTSD in some studies (Ross et al. 1994), although this finding has not been reported uniformly across studies (Dow et al. 1996). At present, it is clear that patients with PTSD have disturbed sleep and frequent sleep complaints (Mellman et al. 1995), but a definitive role for sleep dysregulation in the pathophysiology of PTSD is not yet established.

HPA Axis Functioning in Posttraumatic Stress Disorder

It has been shown repeatedly that male combat veterans with PTSD have differences in HPA axis functioning compared with healthy subjects (Yehuda et al. 1990, 1994, 1995b, 1996). Combat veterans with PTSD have *lower* plasma cortisol levels and lower 24-hour urinary cortisol excretion (Yehuda et al. 1990) than do healthy control subjects, and this finding was recently extended to Holocaust survivors with PTSD (Yehuda et al. 1995a). In a recent study of female survivors of childhood sexual abuse who have PTSD, however, 24-hour urinary cortisol levels

were elevated (Lemieux and Coe 1995); the reasons for this contradiction are unclear. Combat veterans with PTSD also have greater suppression of plasma cortisol in response to low doses (i.e., 0.5 mg) of dexamethasone than do control subjects, and this finding may be attributable to increased glucocorticoid sensitivity at the pituitary level (Yehuda et al. 1995b). This enhanced dexamethasone sensitivity has also been observed in a study of adult female survivors of childhood sexual abuse (Stein et al. 1997c) and in a large unselected sample of Vietnam veterans (Boscarino 1996).

Neuroanatomy and Neurocognition in Posttraumatic Stress Disorder

In light of the well-established deleterious effects of chronic stress on neurons within the hippocampus—a region important in explicit memory systems in humans and other primates (Sapolsky 1992; Schacter et al. 1996)—recent research efforts have focused on determining whether patients with PTSD have explicit memory problems and manifest corresponding neuroanatomical evidence of hippocampal pathology.

Most studies published to date have found some evidence of short-term explicit verbal memory dysfunction in patients with PTSD (for review, see Stein et al. 1997a). However, the nature and extent of memory dysfunction have varied widely among the studies, from extensive short-term memory deficits in some (Bremner et al. 1993) to normal memory function in another (Gurvits et al. 1993). Part of this variance may be explained on the basis of comorbidity with chronic alcohol abuse or major depression, either of which may influence the tests of cognitive functioning.

Moving from tests of neuropsychological functioning to actual studies of brain morphometry, Bremner and colleagues (1995) showed that 26 male combat veterans with PTSD had reduced magnetic resonance imaging (MRI)-derived right-sided hippocampal volume (8% smaller than 22 healthy comparison subjects) and, moreover, that short-term verbal memory deficits were associated with the reduction in hippocampal volume. Gurvits et al. (1996) studied 7 male combat veterans with PTSD, 7 combat veterans without PTSD, and 8 volunteers who were not veterans and did not have PTSD; the investigators found a bilateral reduction (26% on the left; 22% on the right) in hippocampal volume in the subjects with PTSD. Bremner et al. (1997) compared hippocampal volume in 17 adult survivors of childhood sexual abuse—who were inpatients or outpatients at a Veterans Affairs hospital—and in 17 healthy subjects and found a 12% smaller volume in left-sided hippocampal volume in the abuse survivors. Stein et al. (1997b) found a small (5%) but statistically significant reduction in left-sided hippocampal volume in 21 women with severe childhood sexual abuse compared with 20 nonabused comparison subjects. Taken together, these studies provide a strong rationale for further assessing hippocampal neuroanatomy in PTSD. They also pose several questions to be addressed. In particular, the possibility that alcohol abuse (a common comorbid condition in PTSD) is responsible for the findings has not been ruled out, even though researchers in most studies have attempted to use statistical approaches (e.g., covarying for years of alcohol abuse) to address this likelihood. If future studies with adequate controls replicate these findings, they will have paved the way for a host of investigations into the role of abnormalities in brain structures and brain circuitry in PTSD.

Summary of the Biology of Posttraumatic Stress Disorder

In contrast to psychophysiological studies in panic disorder, which have failed to identify a clear-cut autonomic abnormality, studies in PTSD paint a much more lucid portrait of a disorder characterized by autonomic hyperarousal. The findings of memory (and, not reviewed above, attentional) dysfunction in PTSD, in concert with the intriguing findings of reduced hippocampal volume in this disorder, highlight the likely involvement of specific brain loci in the pathophysiology of this disorder. In interpreting these findings, we must be cognizant of several caveats. First, many of the findings (e.g., sympathetic hyperarousal and attentional disturbance) may be caused by depression, which is common in patients with PTSD. These findings therefore require replication in nondepressed subjects. Second, whether these findings can be replicated when substance abuse is controlled for remains to be established. Finally, as mentioned earlier in this section, the current literature on the biology of PTSD is still narrowly focused on combat veterans, although this seems to be changing. It will be interesting to learn how these findings will generalize to those for PTSD in other populations (e.g., sexual abuse survivors, motor vehicle accident victims).

BIOLOGY OF OBSESSIVE-COMPULSIVE DISORDER

Obsessive-compulsive disorder is an excellent example of how new developments in treatment have helped to advance the understanding of the pathophysiology of an illness. (It is also probably the only known example of how

research in humans has led to an effective treatment for a disease in dogs; Rapoport et al. 1992.) When it became clear that obsessive-compulsive disorder was selectively responsive to antidepressant drugs that potently blocked serotonin reuptake (see Chapter 11), it raised the obvious question "Is there a central serotonergic abnormality in obsessive-compulsive disorder?" The vast majority of research into the neurobiology of obsessive-compulsive disorder has been conducted with this question in mind. The association between obsessive-compulsive disorder and various neurological disorders has also been a focus of study for several research teams, leading to an increasing number and sophistication of neuroimaging studies.

Heritability of Obsessive-Compulsive Disorder

The literature on the heritability of obsessive-compulsive disorder has been reviewed by Black and colleagues (1992). They pointed out that twin and family studies have not identified a specific familial component to obsessive-compulsive disorder, although some support exists for a nonspecific increased risk for anxiety disorders in general among family members of obsessive-compulsive disorder probands. They concluded that although a genetic diathesis for obsessive-compulsive disorder may be present in some individuals, nongenetic factors also must be important. Some authorities speculate that genetic factors may account for more of the variance in the expression of early-onset obsessive-compulsive disorder (Bellodi et al. 1992). Interestingly, obsessive-compulsive disorder and Tourette's disorder, which share clinical features in many patients, may also be genetically related (Pauls et al. 1991). In a large family study of 100 probands with obsessive-compulsive disorder, investigators found that some cases were familial and related to tic disorders, some cases were familial and unrelated to tics, and other cases showed no evidence of family history of either (Pauls et al. 1995). From these studies, it appears likely that obsessive-compulsive disorder is a heterogeneous condition, with different etiologies for different subtypes. In this regard, a major step in the delineation of potentially mechanistically based subtypes comes from recent studies of the relationship between streptococcal infection and obsessive-compulsive disorder (see below).

Hypotheses for the Pathophysiology of Some Forms of Obsessive-Compulsive Disorder

Following up on their observations that some children with Sydenham's chorea (a complication of rheumatic fever characterized by neurological dysfunction) had prominent obsessive-compulsive symptoms, Swedo and colleagues (1989) sought to determine whether certain forms of childhood obsessive-compulsive disorder were associated with a trait marker of rheumatic fever susceptibility (Swedo et al. 1997). Monoclonal antibodies identify a B-lymphocyte antigen known as D8/17, which has been shown to be a trait marker for susceptibility to rheumatic fever as a complication of group A streptococcal infection. In their study, Swedo et al. measured D8/17 reactivity in blood from 27 children with pediatric autoimmune neuropsychiatric disorders associated with streptococcal infection, 9 children with Sydenham's chorea, and 24 healthy children. They found that the two patient groups had markedly elevated numbers of D8/17-positive cells compared with the healthy comparison group (Swedo et al. 1997). They concluded that D8/17 positivity might confer susceptibility not only to rheumatic fever but also to a poststreptococcal CNS syndrome that could manifest as predominantly obsessional or choreiform in nature, depending, perhaps, on specifically which regions of the brain are affected and which are spared.

In another study, investigators found significantly higher rates of D8/17 positivity in 31 patients with childhood-onset obsessive-compulsive disorder or Tourette's or chronic tic disorders compared with 21 healthy control subjects (Murphy et al. 1997). Remarkably, there was no overlap in distribution of the percentage of D8/17-positive cells between the two groups of subjects.

Taken together, these studies provide powerful new evidence in favor of an autoimmune (specifically, poststreptococcal) etiology for some cases of childhood-onset obsessive-compulsive disorder. If further studies of D8/17 confirm its suitability as a marker for a distinct subtype of obsessive-compulsive disorder or Tourette's disorder, then studies might be undertaken to evaluate the efficacy of immunosuppressive agents as a treatment and/or an antibiotic prophylaxis for the prevention of these conditions. Moreover, this line of research promises to unveil secrets about the pathophysiology of some forms of obsessive-compulsive disorder.

Serotonergic Dysfunction in Obsessive-Compulsive Disorder

Several techniques have been used to document the presence of a central serotonin abnormality in obsessive-compulsive disorder. These include the measurement of peripheral markers of (optimistically) central serotonin function, the measurement of serotonin breakdown products in the CSF, and the administration of serotonin chemical probes.

Peripheral serotonin markers in obsessive-compulsive disorder.   Serotonin levels in the blood of patients with obsessive-compulsive disorder are, not surprisingly, normal (Flament et al. 1987). Platelet serotonin uptake and binding to platelets of [^{3}H]imipramine and [^{3}H]paroxetine have also been examined as putative indices of central serotonin activity. These studies are too numerous to review in detail here, but suffice it to say that they have been mixed, with some (but not others) finding reduced density of serotonin reuptake sites in obsessive-compulsive disorder. Given the questionable relationship between platelet and CNS serotonin reuptake sites (Moret and Briley 1991), the meaning of these findings is far from clear.

CSF studies in obsessive-compulsive disorder.   The serotonin metabolite 5-hydroxyindoleacetic acid (5-HIAA) has been measured in the CSF of patients with obsessive-compulsive disorder as a potential indicator of central serotonin turnover. Insel and colleagues (1985) reported a significant increase (30% greater than control subjects) in CSF 5-HIAA in a small group of patients with obsessive-compulsive disorder ($N = 8$), but this is at odds with an earlier study by Thoren and colleagues (1980).

Although not a measure of central serotonin function, it is intriguing that elevated CSF levels of arginine vasopressin (Altemus et al. 1992) and somatostatin (Altemus et al. 1993) have been reported in patients with obsessive-compulsive disorder. The functional significance of these findings is as yet unknown, but these observations serve as the basis for some interesting hypotheses about the role of altered attention and memory in obsessive-compulsive disorder (Altemus et al. 1992).

Neuropharmacological probes of serotonin systems in obsessive-compulsive disorder.   Zohar and colleagues (1987) first showed that obsessive-compulsive symptoms could be transiently exacerbated in some patients with obsessive-compulsive disorder by orally administering the serotonin agonist m-CPP and that this effect could be blocked by chronic pretreatment with the effective antiobsessional agent clomipramine (Zohar et al. 1988). Since then, the exacerbating effects of m-CPP on obsessive-compulsive symptoms have been replicated in some studies (Hollander et al. 1988, 1992) but not others (Goddard et al. 1994; Pigott et al. 1993; Smeraldi et al. 1996). Although these discrepancies may result from subtle differences in the various protocols used in each study or from heterogeneity within the obsessive-compulsive disorder diagnostic syndrome, other neurotransmitter systems may actually be involved. Even though a putative serotonin agonist (i.e., m-CPP) is being used, and its effects have been reliably blocked with the use of the $5\text{-}HT_1/5\text{-}HT_2$ antagonist metergoline (Pigott et al. 1991), this is no guarantee that serotonergic activation is only one component in a complex neurobiological cascade that ultimately results in the expression of obsessive-compulsive symptoms. In this regard, considerable headway has been made into understanding brain systems involved in obsessive-compulsive disorder through the application of neuroimaging techniques.

Neuroanatomical and Neuroimaging Studies of Obsessive-Compulsive Disorder

Neuroanatomical considerations.   Several different brain lesions in humans have been associated with the appearance of obsessive-compulsive behaviors or outright obsessive-compulsive disorder. Von Economo's encephalitis in the early 1930s was associated with the occurrence of obsessive-compulsive disorder in a number of cases. As noted earlier in this chapter, an association between some cases of childhood-onset obsessive-compulsive disorder, some forms of tic disorder, and poststreptococcal illness is strongly suspected (Murphy et al. 1997; Swedo et al. 1997), leading many investigators to speculate that these disorders may be etiologically related. In fact, several authorities have proposed that both Tourette's disorder and obsessive-compulsive disorder might be disorders of the striatum, and the precise area of damage within the striatum and the size of the lesion would determine clinical symptomatology (Baxter 1990; Goodman et al. 1990; Wise and Rapoport 1989).

This hypothesis could accommodate many of the theories that have preceded it. For example, serotonergic neurotransmission is an important component of striatothalamocortical communication (and probably maintains a tonic inhibitory influence on dopamine function in these circuits), increasing the possibility that SSRIs may ameliorate obsessive-compulsive symptoms through modulatory effects in these brain regions (Baxter 1990). This theory could also explain the ameliorative effects of stereotaxic psychosurgical interventions that selectively sever fiber bundles interconnecting the orbitofrontal cortex and the dorsomedial and related thalamic nuclei (Baer et al. 1995; Spangler et al. 1996). In the past few years, direct neuroimaging techniques have become available that have permitted the preliminary testing of some of these theoretical notions.

Brain imaging studies.   Several investigators have attempted to delineate a neuroanatomical abnormality in obsessive-compulsive disorder by measuring the size or assessing the structural integrity of presumptively critical CNS structures. In particular, the basal ganglia have been the focus of a series of computed tomographic (CT) (Luxenberg et al. 1988) and, more recently, structural MRI studies (Aylward et al. 1996; Jenike et al. 1996; Kellner et al. 1991; Robinson et al. 1995). These findings have been remarkably inconsistent and suggest that if there is a deficit in caudate volume in obsessive-compulsive disorder, it may be very subtle or may occur in only a subgroup of patients. One of the aforementioned studies, which incorporated volumetric assessment of several cortical and subcortical structures, did, however, find evidence of *increased* total cortical volume in patients with obsessive-compulsive disorder; thus, the possibility is increased that some forms of obsessive-compulsive disorder reflect a neurodevelopmental failure in neuronal pruning (Jenike et al. 1996).

Techniques such as CT and MRI can assess only brain structure, not function. An examination of the literature on other neuropsychiatric disorders, such as Parkinson's disease and Huntington's disease, reveals that neuroradiologically determinable changes in structure do not occur (or occur only very late in the illness), even though functional indices of regional brain dysfunction are apparent. By analogy, we should not be surprised that the CT and MRI studies have not convincingly detected a specific CNS lesion in obsessive-compulsive disorder.

Functional neuroimaging studies with PET (Baxter et al. 1987; Nordahl et al. 1989; Perani et al. 1995) and SPECT (Machlin et al. 1991; Rubin et al. 1992) have consistently reported differences in cerebral metabolism between patients with obsessive-compulsive disorder and control subjects in one or more regions that constitute components of a cortical-striatal-thalamic-cortical loop. In particular, the medial prefrontal cortex and the basal ganglia in patients with obsessive-compulsive disorder have consistently had abnormalities compared with those in control subjects. Repeat studies after treatment with either pharmacotherapy or behavior therapy indicate that these regional abnormalities normalize as a correlate of symptom reduction (Baxter et al. 1992), adding further credence to the functional significance of these brain regions in the disorder.

Summary of the Biology of Obsessive-Compulsive Disorder

In summary, functional brain imaging studies in obsessive-compulsive disorder are strongly suggestive of an abnormality in basal ganglia–thalamic–orbitofrontal–cortical circuitry in obsessive-compulsive disorder, which may "normalize" to some extent during treatment. How serotonin reuptake inhibitors (and, for that matter, behavior therapies) exert their therapeutic influence remains uncertain, although an effect on one or more components of these neuronal circuits is likely. The most exciting new development on this frontier is the finding of a possible susceptibility marker (D8/17) for obsessive-compulsive disorder and/or tic disorders, which, in the wake of group A streptococcal infection, may increase the risk for the development of childhood obsessive-compulsive disorder. This subgroup of patients likely will be studied intensively from a neurogenetic and neuroimaging perspective in the coming years, so that the neural substrates for obsessive-compulsive disorder probably will become more clearly delineated.

FUTURE DIRECTIONS

Many studies have been conducted in recent years to attempt to learn more about the biology of anxiety disorders. Much of this work has served to dispel long-held beliefs about the pathophysiology of these disorders. For example, it is now proven that panic disorder is neither synonymous with nor caused by hyperventilation. Furthermore, it is now clear that panic disorder is not a state of sympathetic hyperactivity. So, we know a lot about what panic disorder is not. Does this mean that we are much closer to knowing what panic disorder is? Unfortunately, we do not. Although many myths have been debunked in the past decade of research in this area, unequivocal "positive" findings have been few and truly enlightening findings even fewer.

A notable exception is the case of obsessive-compulsive disorder. Incontrovertible evidence now exists that obsessive-compulsive disorder is a disorder of brain circuitry that traverses the basal ganglia. This indication is suggested by imaging studies, consistent with pharmacological and psychosurgical interventions, supported by comorbidity with other basal ganglia disorders (e.g., Tourette's disorder), and confirmed by experiments of nature (e.g., increased obsessive-compulsive symptoms in patients with Sydenham's chorea). In the next few years, as imaging techniques are refined and immunological therapies are tested, an understanding of obsessive-compulsive disorder at the cytoarchitectural and molecular levels is expected to be much improved.

What does the future hold for progress in comprehending the biology of other anxiety disorders? The fact that serotonergically active antidepressants (i.e., SSRIs)

have a broad spectrum of anxiolytic actions across disorders should spawn a new generation of studies testing the hypothesis that serotonergic dysfunction is a common feature of anxiety disorders. If this proves true, then the challenge will be to determine what other factors influence the syndromal expression of the disorder. These factors may turn out to be neurobiological in nature but may be experiential. In fact, it would not be surprising to discover that specific genes influencing specific behavioral tendencies (e.g., impulsivity or sensation-seeking) increase exposure to certain inciting events (e.g., criminal victimization), which increase risk for particular anxiety disorders (e.g., PTSD). If these predictions come true, then we will be witness to a veritable disintegration of the mind-body dichotomy as it applies to the anxiety disorders.

In the next 3–5 years, molecular genetics and neuroimaging will prove to be popular tools for studying the biology of these disorders. In the case of molecular genetics, it is hoped that "gene fishing"—the current approach in most studies—identifies genes that are associated with particular disorders. If not, then geneticists may turn their attention more to genes that might predispose more broadly to anxiety and/or depressive disorders, bearing in mind that these disorders are so comorbid that expecting to find simple phenotype-genotype relationships in this field is probably naive. In the case of functional neuroimaging studies, which are becoming more prevalent because of the relatively low cost and low invasiveness of newer techniques such as functional MRI, we can expect to see an explosion of research. However, the relevance of these techniques for the anxiety disorders at this time is questionable. To interpret "function" in functional MRI, well-developed tasks that activate specific brain regions are required; ideally, these should correspond to hypothesized functional abnormalities in the disorder under consideration. In the case of anxiety disorders, such tasks are not yet developed but certainly will be in the next few years. When this occurs, we may see informative, disorder-relevant cognitive tasks (e.g., directed attentional tasks for PTSD) being used in conjunction with functional MRI and related techniques to bring us closer to understanding the biology of anxiety disorders at a neural cognitive and metacognitive level.

REFERENCES

Abelson JL, Curtis GC: Hypothalamic-pituitary-adrenal axis activity in panic disorder: 24-hour secretion of corticotropin and cortisol. Arch Gen Psychiatry 53:323–331, 1996a

Abelson JL, Curtis GC: Hypothalamic-pituitary-adrenal axis activity in panic disorder: prediction of long-term outcome by pretreatment cortisol levels. Am J Psychiatry 153:69–73, 1996b

Abelson JL, Glitz D, Cameron OG, et al: Endocrine, cardiovascular, and behavioral responses to clonidine in patients with panic disorder. Biol Psychiatry 32:18–25, 1992

Abelson JL, Nesse RM, Weg JG, et al: Respiratory psychophysiology and anxiety: cognitive intervention in the doxapram model of panic. Psychosom Med 58:302–313, 1996

Altemus M, Pigott T, Kalogeras KT, et al: Abnormalities in the regulation of vasopressin and corticotropin releasing factor secretion in obsessive-compulsive disorder. Arch Gen Psychiatry 49:9–20, 1992

Altemus M, Pigott T, L'Heureux F, et al: CSF somatostatin in obsessive-compulsive disorder. Am J Psychiatry 150:460–464, 1993

American Psychiatric Association: Diagnostic and Statistical Manual of Mental Disorders, 4th Edition. Washington, DC, American Psychiatric Association, 1994

Apfeldorf WJ, Shear MK: Caffeine potentiation of taste in panic disorder. Biol Psychiatry 33:217–219, 1993

Arriaga F, Paiva T, Matos-Pires A, et al: The sleep of nondepressed patients with panic disorder: a comparison with normal controls. Acta Psychiatr Scand 93:191–194, 1996

Aylward EH, Harris GJ, Hoehn-Saric R, et al: Normal caudate nucleus in obsessive-compulsive disorder assessed by quantitative neuroimaging. Arch Gen Psychiatry 53:577–584, 1996

Baer L, Rauch SL, Ballantine HTJ, et al: Cingulotomy for intractable obsessive-compulsive disorder: prospective long-term follow-up of 18 patients. Arch Gen Psychiatry 52:384–392, 1995

Ballenger JC (ed): Neurobiology of Panic Disorder. New York, Alan R Liss, 1990

Barlow DH: Anxiety and Its Disorders: The Nature and Treatment of Anxiety and Panic. New York, Guilford, 1988

Baxter LR: Brain imaging as a tool in establishing a theory of brain pathology in obsessive compulsive disorder. J Clin Psychiatry 51 (suppl):22–25, 1990

Baxter LR Jr, Phelps ME, Mazziota JC, et al: Local cerebral glucose metabolic rates in obsessive-compulsive disorder: a comparison with rates in unipolar depression and in normal controls. Arch Gen Psychiatry 44:211–218, 1987

Baxter LR, Schwartz JM, Bergman KS, et al: Caudate glucose metabolic rate changes with both drug and behavior therapy for obsessive-compulsive disorder. Arch Gen Psychiatry 49:681–689, 1992

Bellodi L, Sciuto G, Diaferia G, et al: Psychiatric disorders in the families of patients with obsessive-compulsive disorder. Psychiatry Res 42:111–120, 1992

Benjamin J, Li L, Patterson C, et al: Population and familial association between the D4 dopamine receptor gene and measures of novelty seeking. Nat Genet 12:81–84, 1996

Black DW, Noyes R Jr, Goldstein RB, et al: A family study of obsessive-compulsive disorder. Arch Gen Psychiatry 49:362–368, 1992

Blanchard EB, Kolb LC, Prins A, et al: Changes in plasma norepinephrine to combat-related stimuli among Vietnam veterans with posttraumatic stress disorder. J Nerv Ment Dis 179:371–373, 1991

Boscarino JA: Posttraumatic stress disorder, exposure to combat, and lower plasma cortisol among Vietnam veterans: findings and clinical implications. J Consult Clin Psychology 64:191–201, 1996

Boulenger JP, Uhde TW, Wolff EA, et al: Increased sensitivity to caffeine in patients with panic disorders: preliminary evidence. Arch Gen Psychiatry 41:1067–1071, 1984

Bradwejn J, Koszycki D, Meterissian G: Cholecystokinin-tetrapeptide induces panic attacks in patients with panic disorder. Can J Psychiatry 35:83–85, 1990

Bradwejn J, Koszycki D, Meterissian G: Enhanced sensitivity to cholecystokinin-tetrapeptide in panic disorder: clinical and behavioral findings. Arch Gen Psychiatry 48:603–610, 1991

Bradwejn J, Koszycki D, Payeur R, et al: Replication of action of cholecystokinin tetrapeptide in panic disorder: clinical and behavioral findings. Am J Psychiatry 149:962–964, 1992

Bremner JD, Scott TM, Delaney RC, et al: Deficits in short-term memory in posttraumatic stress disorder. Am J Psychiatry 150:1015–1019, 1993

Bremner JD, Randall P, Scott TM, et al: MRI-based measurement of hippocampal volume in patients with combat-related posttraumatic stress disorder. Am J Psychiatry 152:973–981, 1995

Bremner JD, Randall P, Vermetten E, et al: MRI-based measurement of hippocampal volume in PTSD related to childhood physical and sexual abuse: a preliminary report. Biol Psychiatry 41:23–32, 1997

Butler RW, Braff DL, Rausch J, et al: Physiological evidence of exaggerated startle response in a subgroup of Vietnam veterans with combat-related posttraumatic stress disorder. Am J Psychiatry 147:1308–1312, 1990

Charney DS, Heninger GR: Abnormal regulation of noradrenergic function in panic disorders: effects of clonidine in healthy subjects and patients with agoraphobia and panic disorder. Arch Gen Psychiatry 43:1042–1054, 1986

Charney DS, Heninger GR, Breier A: Noradrenergic function in panic anxiety: effects of yohimbine in healthy subjects and patients with agoraphobia and panic disorder. Arch Gen Psychiatry 41:751–763, 1984

Charney DS, Woods SW, Goodman WK, et al: Neurobiological mechanisms of panic anxiety: biochemical and behavioral correlates of yohimbine-induced panic attacks. Am J Psychiatry 144:1030–1036, 1987

Charney DS, Innis RB, Duman RS, et al: Platelet α_2-receptor binding and adenylate cyclase activity in panic disorder. Psychopharmacology 98:102–107, 1989

Coplan JD, Gorman JM, Klein DF: Serotonin related functions in panic-anxiety: a critical overview. Neuropsychopharmacology 6:189–200, 1992a

Coplan JD, Sharma R, Rosenblum LA, et al: Effects of sodium lactate infusion on cisternal lactate and carbon dioxide levels in nonhuman subjects. Am J Psychiatry 149:1369–1373, 1992b

Coplan JD, Papp LA, Martinez J, et al: Persistence of blunted human growth hormone response to clonidine in fluoxetine-treated patients with panic disorder. Am J Psychiatry 152:619–622, 1995

Coplan JD, Andrews MW, Rosenblum LA, et al: Persistent elevations of CSF concentrations of corticotropin-releasing factor in adult nonhuman primates exposed to early life stressors: implications for the pathophysiology of mood and anxiety disorders. Proc Natl Acad Sci U S A 93: 1619–1623, 1996

Cowley DS, Adams JB, Pyke RE, et al: Effect of CI-988, a cholecystokinin-B receptor antagonist, on lactate-induced panic. Am J Psychiatry 40:550–552, 1996

Crowe RR, Noyes R, Wilson F, et al: A linkage study of panic disorder. Arch Gen Psychiatry 44:933–937, 1987

Crowe RR, Noyes R Jr, Samuelson S, et al: Close linkage between panic disorder and α-haptoglobin excluded in 10 families. Arch Gen Psychiatry 47:377–380, 1990

Curtis GC, Abelson JL, Gold PW: Adrenocorticotrophic hormone and cortisol responses to corticotropin-releasing hormone: changes in panic disorder and effects of alprazolam treatment. Biol Psychiatry 41:76–85, 1997

Da Costa JM: On irritable heart: a clinical study of a form of functional cardiac disorder and its consequences. Am J Med Sci 61:17–52, 1871

Dager SR, Strauss WL, Marro KI, et al: Proton magnetic resonance spectroscopy investigation of hyperventilation in subjects with panic disorder and comparison subjects. Am J Psychiatry 152:666–672, 1995

Davidson JRT, Foa EB (eds): Posttraumatic Stress Disorder: DSM-IV and Beyond. Washington, DC, American Psychiatric Press, 1993

Davidson JR, Krishnan KR, Charles HC, et al: Magnetic resonance spectroscopy in social phobia: preliminary findings. J Clin Psychiatry 54 (suppl):19–25, 1993

Davis M, Falls WA, Campeau S, et al: Fear-potentiated startle: a neutral and pharmacological analysis. Behav Brain Res 58:175–198, 1993

DeMet E, Stein MK, Tran C, et al: Caffeine taste test for panic disorder: adenosine receptor supersensitivity. Psychiatry Res 30:231–242, 1989

de Montigny C: Cholecystokinin tetrapeptide induces panic-like attacks in healthy volunteers: preliminary findings. Arch Gen Psychiatry 46:511–517, 1989

Dow BM, Kelsoe JR Jr, Gillin JC: Sleep and dreams in Vietnam PTSD and depression. Biol Psychiatry 39:42–50, 1996

Drevets WC, Videen TQ, MacLeod AK, et al: PET images of blood flow changes during anxiety: correction (letter). Science 256:1696, 1992

Eaton WW, Kessler RC, Wittchen HU, et al: Panic and panic disorder in the United States. Am J Psychiatry 151:413–420, 1994

Ebstein RP, Novick O, Umansky R, et al: Dopamine D4 receptor (DRD4) exon III polymorphism associated with the human personality trait of novelty seeking. Nat Genet 12:78–80, 1996

Faravelli C, Marinoni M, Spiti R, et al: Abnormal brain hemodynamic responses during passive orthostatic challenge in panic disorder. Am J Psychiatry 154:378–383, 1997

Flament MF, Rapaport JL, Murphy DL, et al: Biochemical changes during clomipramine treatment of childhood obsessive-compulsive disorder. Arch Gen Psychiatry 44:219–225, 1987

Fredholm BB, Persson CGA: Xanthine derivatives as adenosine receptor antagonists. Eur J Pharmacol 81:673–676, 1982

Friedman MJ, Charney DS, Deutch AY (eds): Neurobiological and Clinical Consequences of Stress: From Normal Adaptation to Post-Traumatic Stress Disorder. Philadelphia, PA, Lippincott-Raven Publishers, 1995

Fyer AJ, Gorman JM, Liebowitz MJ, et al: Sodium lactate infusion, panic attacks, and ionized calcium. Biol Psychiatry 19:1437–1447, 1984

Garssen BG, Buikhuisen M, Van Dyck R: Hyperventilation and panic attacks. Am J Psychiatry 153:513–518, 1996

Goddard AW, Sholomskas DE, Walton KE, et al: Effects of tryptophan depletion in panic disorder. Biol Psychiatry 36:775–777, 1994

Goddard AW, Narayan M, Woods SW, et al: Plasma levels of gamma-aminobutyric acid and panic disorder. Psychiatry Res 63:223–225, 1996

Goisman RM, Warshaw MG, Steketee GS, et al: DSM-IV and the disappearance of agoraphobia without a history of panic disorder: new data on a controversial diagnosis. Am J Psychiatry 152:1438–1443, 1995

Goodman WK, McDougle CJ, Price LH, et al: Beyond the serotonin hypothesis: a role for dopamine in some forms of obsessive-compulsive disorder? J Clin Psychiatry 51 (suppl):36–43, 1990

Gorman JM, Papp LA: Respiratory physiology of panic, in Neurobiology of Panic Disorder. Edited by Ballenger JC. New York, Alan R Liss, 1990, pp 187–203

Gorman JM, Cohen BS, Liebowitz MR, et al: Blood gas changes and hypophosphatemia in lactate-induced panic. Arch Gen Psychiatry 43:1067–1075, 1986

Gorman JM, Fyer MR, Goetz R, et al: Ventilatory physiology of patients with panic disorder. Arch Gen Psychiatry 45:31–39, 1988a

Gorman JM, Goetz RR, Uy J, et al: Hyperventilation occurs during lactate-induced panic. Journal of Anxiety Disorders 2:193–202, 1988b

Gorman J, Liebowitz MR, Fyer AJ, et al: A neuroanatomical hypothesis for panic disorder. Am J Psychiatry 146:148–161, 1989

Gorman JM, Goetz RR, Dillon D, et al: Sodium D-lactate infusion of panic disorder patients. Neuropsychopharmacology 3:181–189, 1990

Gorman JM, Papp LA, Coplan JD, et al: Anxiogenic effects of CO2 and hyperventilation in patients with panic disorder. Am J Psychiatry 151:547–553, 1994

Gurvits TG, Lasko NB, Schachter SC, et al: Neurological status of Vietnam veterans with chronic post-traumatic stress disorder. J Neuropsychiatry Clin Neurosci 5:183–188, 1993

Gurvits TG, Shenton MR, Hokama H, et al: Magnetic resonance imaging study of hippocampal volume in chronic, combat-related PTSD. Biol Psychiatry 40:1091–1099, 1996

Hauri PJ, Friedman M, Ravaris CL: Sleep in patients with spontaneous panic attacks. Sleep 12:323–337, 1989

Hazen AL, Stein MB: Clinical phenomenology and comorbidity, in Social Phobia: Clinical and Research Perspectives. Edited by Stein MB. Washington, DC, American Psychiatric Press, 1995, pp 3–41

Heimberg RG, Hope DA, Dodge CS, et al: DSM-III-R subtypes of social phobia: comparison of generalized social phobics and public speaking phobics. J Nerv Ment Dis 173:172–179, 1990

Hibbert GA: Hyperventilation as a cause of panic attacks. BMJ 288:263–264, 1984

Hoehn-Saric R, McLeod DR: Somatic manifestations of normal and pathological anxiety, in Biology of Anxiety Disorders. Edited by Hoehn-Saric R, McLeod DR. Washington, DC, American Psychiatric Press, 1993, pp 177–222

Hollander E, Fay B, Cohen R, et al: Serotonergic and noradrenergic sensitivity in obsessive-compulsive disorder: behavioral findings. Am J Psychiatry 145:1015–1017, 1988

Hollander E, DeCaria CM, Nitescu A, et al: Serotonergic function in obsessive-compulsive disorder. Arch Gen Psychiatry 49:21–28, 1992

Insel TR, Mueller EA, Alterman I, et al: Obsessive-compulsive disorder and serotonin: is there a connection? Biol Psychiatry 20:1174–1185, 1985

Jenike MA, Breiter HC, Baer L, et al: Cerebral structural abnormalities in obsessive-compulsive disorder: a quantitative morphometric magnetic resonance imaging study. Arch Gen Psychiatry 53:625–632, 1996

Kellner CH, Jolley RR, Holgate RC, et al: Brain MRI in obsessive-compulsive disorder. Psychiatry Res 36:45–49, 1991

Klein DF: False suffocation alarms, spontaneous panics, and related conditions: an integrative hypothesis. Arch Gen Psychiatry 50:306–317, 1993

Kosten TR, Mason JW, Giller EL, et al: Sustained urinary norepinephrine and epinephrine elevation in post-traumatic stress disorder. Psychoneuroendocrinology 12:13–20, 1987

Kramer MS, Cutler NR, Ballenger JC, et al: A placebo-controlled trial of L-365,260, a CCKB antagonist, in panic disorder. Biol Psychiatry 37:462–466, 1995

Lemieux AM, Coe CL: Abuse-related posttraumatic stress disorder: evidence for chronic neuroendocrine activation in women. Psychosom Med 57:105–115, 1995

Lesch KP, Wiesmann M, Hoh A, et al: 5-HT1A receptor-effector system responsivity in panic disorder. Psychopharmacology (Berl) 106:111–117, 1992

Lesch KP, Bengel D, Heils A, et al: Association of anxiety-related traits with a polymorphism in the serotonin transporter gene regulatory region. Science 274:1527–1531, 1996

Levin AP, Saoud JB, Strauman T, et al: Responses of "generalized" and "discrete" social phobias during public speaking. Journal of Anxiety Disorders 7:207–221, 1993

Liebowitz MR, Fyer AJ, Gorman JM, et al: Lactate provocation of panic attacks, I: clinical and behavioral findings. Arch Gen Psychiatry 41:764–770, 1984

Liebowitz MR, Gorman JM, Fyer AJ, et al: Social phobia: a review of a neglected anxiety disorder. Arch Gen Psychiatry 42:729–736, 1985

Luxenberg JS, Swedo SE, Flament MM, et al: Neuroanatomical abnormalities in obsessive-compulsive disorder detected with quantitative X-ray computed tomography. Am J Psychiatry 145:1089–1093, 1988

Lydiard RB, Ballenger JC, Laraia MT, et al: CSF cholecystokinin concentrations in patients with panic disorder and in normal comparison subjects. Am J Psychiatry 149:691–693, 1992

Machlin SR, Harris GJ, Pearlson GD, et al: Elevated medial-cortical blood flow in obsessive-compulsive patients: a SPECT study. Am J Psychiatry 148:1240–1242, 1991

Maguire KP, Norman TR, Apostolopoulos M, et al: Platelet [³H]paroxetine binding in panic disorder. J Affect Disord 33:117–122, 1995

Mannuzza S, Schneier FR, Chapman TF, et al: Generalized social phobia: reliability and validity. Arch Gen Psychiatry 52:230–237, 1995

Margraf J, Ehlers A, Roth W: Sodium lactate infusions and panic attacks: a review and critique. Psychosom Med 48:23–51, 1986

Markowitz JS, Weissman MM, Ouelette R, et al: Quality of life in panic disorder. Arch Gen Psychiatry 46:984–992, 1989

Martinez JM, Papp LA, Coplan JD, et al: Ambulatory monitoring of respiration in anxiety. Anxiety 2:296–302, 1996

Mathew RJ, Wilson WH, Tant S: Responses to hypercarbia induced by acetazolamide in panic disorder patients. Am J Psychiatry 146:996–1000, 1989

McFall ME, Veith RC, Murburg MM: Basal sympathoadrenal function in posttraumatic stress disorder. Biol Psychiatry 31:1050–1056, 1992

McNally RJ: Panic Disorder: A Critical Analysis. New York, Guilford, 1994

McNally RJ, Eke M: Anxiety sensitivity, suffocation fear, and breath-holding duration as predictors of response to carbon dioxide challenge. J Abnorm Psychol 105:146–149, 1996

Mellman TA, Uhde TW: Electroencephalographic sleep in panic disorder: a focus on sleep-related panic attacks. Arch Gen Psychiatry 46:178–184, 1989a

Mellman TA, Uhde TW: Sleep panic attacks: new clinical findings and theoretical implications. Am J Psychiatry 146:1204–1207, 1989b

Mellman TA, Kulick-Bell R, Ashlock LE, et al: Sleep events among veterans with combat-related posttraumatic stress disorder. Am J Psychiatry 152:110–115, 1995

Moret C, Briley M: Platelet ^{3}H-paroxetine binding to the serotonin transporter is insensitive to changes in central serotonergic innervation in the rat. Psychiatry Res 38:97–104, 1991

Morgan CA, Grillon C, Southwick SM, et al: Fear-potentiated startle in posttraumatic stress disorder. Biol Psychiatry 38:378–385, 1995

Morgan CA, Grillon C, Southwick SM, et al: Exaggerated acoustic startle reflex in Gulf War veterans with posttraumatic stress disorder. Am J Psychiatry 153:64–68, 1996

Murburg MM, McFall ME, Lewis N, et al: Plasma norepinephrine kinetics in patients with posttraumatic stress disorder. Biol Psychiatry 38:819–825, 1995

Murphy TK, Goodman WK, Fudge MW, et al: B lymphocyte antigen d8/17: a peripheral marker for childhood-onset obsessive-compulsive disorder and Tourette's syndrome. Am J Psychiatry 154:402–407, 1997

Nemeroff CB: Corticotropin-releasing factor, in Neuropeptides and Psychiatric Disorders. Edited by Nemeroff CB. Washington, DC, American Psychiatric Press, 1991, pp 75–92

Nesse RM, Cameron OG, Curtis GC, et al: Adrenergic function in patients with panic anxiety. Arch Gen Psychiatry 41:771–776, 1984

Nordahl TE, Benkelfat C, Semple WE, et al: Cerebral glucose metabolic rates in obsessive-compulsive disorder. Neuropsychopharmacology 2:23–28, 1989

Nordahl TE, Semple WE, Gross M, et al: Cerebral glucose metabolic differences in patients with panic disorder. Neuropsychopharmacology 3:261–272, 1990

Nutt DJ: Altered central α_2-adrenoceptor sensitivity in panic disorder. Arch Gen Psychiatry 46:165–169, 1989

Nutt DJ, Glue P, Lawson C, et al: Flumazenil provocation of panic attacks: evidence for altered benzodiazepine receptor sensitivity in panic disorder. Arch Gen Psychiatry 47:917–925, 1990

Ohara K, Xie D, Ishigaki T, et al: The genes encoding the $5HT_{1Da}$ and $5HT_{1Db}$ receptors are unchanged in patients with panic disorder. Biol Psychiatry 39:5–10, 1996

Orr SP: Psychophysiologic studies of posttraumatic stress disorder, in Biological Assessment and Treatment of Posttraumatic Stress Disorder. Edited by Giller EL Jr. Washington, DC, American Psychiatric Press, 1990, pp 137–157

Orr SP, Lasko NB, Shalev AY, et al: Physiologic responses to loud tones in Vietnam veterans with posttraumatic stress disorder. J Abnorm Psychol 104:75–82, 1995

Papp LA, Gorman JM, Liebowitz MR, et al: Epinephrine infusions in patients with social phobia. Am J Psychiatry 145:733–736, 1988

Papp LA, Martinez JM, Klein DF, et al: Rebreathing tests in panic disorder. Biol Psychiatry 38:240–245, 1995

Pauls DL, Raymond CL, Stevenson JM, et al: A family study of Gilles de la Tourette syndrome. Am J Hum Genet 48:154–163, 1991

Pauls DL, Alsobrook JP, Goodman W, et al: A family study of obsessive-compulsive disorder. Am J Psychiatry 152:76–84, 1995

Perani D, Colombo C, Bressi S, et al: [18F]FDG PET study in obsessive-compulsive disorder: a clinical/metabolic correlation study after treatment. Br J Psychiatry 166:244–250, 1995

Perna G, Bertani A, Arancio C, et al: Laboratory response of patients with panic and obsessive-compulsive disorders to 35% CO2 challenges. Am J Psychiatry 152:85–89, 1995

Perna G, Bertani A, Caldirola D, et al: Family history of panic disorder and hypersensitivity to CO2 in patients with panic disorder. Am J Psychiatry 153:1060–1064, 1996

Pigott TA, Zohar J, Hill JL, et al: Metergoline blocks the behavioral and neuroendocrine effects of orally administered m-CPP in patients with obsessive-compulsive disorder. Biol Psychiatry 29:418–426, 1991

Pigott TA, Hill JL, Grady TA, et al: A comparison of the behavioral effects of oral versus intravenous mCPP administration in obsessive-compulsive disorder patients and the effect of metergoline prior to IV mCPP. Biol Psychiatry 33:3–14, 1993

Pincus HA, Henderson B, Blackwood D, et al: Trends in research in two general psychiatric journals in 1969–1990: research on research. Am J Psychiatry 150:135–142, 1993

Pitman RK, Orr SP: 24-Hour urinary cortisol and catecholamine excretion in combat-related post-traumatic stress disorder. Biol Psychiatry 27:245–247, 1990

Pitman RK, Orr SP, Forgue DF, et al: Psychophysiologic assessment of posttraumatic stress disorder imagery in Vietnam combat veterans. Arch Gen Psychiatry 44:970–975, 1987

Pitman RK, Orr SP, Forgue DF, et al: Psychophysiologic responses to combat imagery of Vietnam veterans with posttraumatic stress disorder versus other anxiety disorders. J Abnorm Psychol 99:49–54, 1990

Pitts FN Jr, McClure JN: Lactate metabolism in anxiety neurosis. N Engl J Med 277:1329–1336, 1967

Pohl R, Yeragani VK, Balon R, et al: Isoproterenol-induced panic attacks. Biol Psychiatry 24:891–902, 1988

Potts NL, Davidson JR, Krishnan KR, et al: Levels of urinary free cortisol in social phobia. J Clin Psychiatry 52 (suppl):41–42, 1991

Rapaport MH, Risch SC, Gillin JC, et al: Blunted growth hormone response to peripheral infusions of human growth hormone-releasing factor in patients with panic disorder. Am J Psychiatry 146:92–95, 1989

Rapee R: Differential response to hyperventilation in panic disorder and generalized anxiety disorder. J Abnorm Psychol 95:24–28, 1986

Rapoport JL, Ryland DH, Kriete M: Drug treatment of canine acral lick: an animal model of obsessive-compulsive disorder. Arch Gen Psychiatry 49:517–521, 1992

Redmond DE Jr: New and old evidence for the involvement of a brain norepinephrine system in anxiety, in The Phenomenology and Treatment of Anxiety. Edited by Fann WE. New York, Spectrum Press, 1979, pp 153–203

Reiman EM, Raichle ME, Butler FK, et al: A focal brain abnormality in panic disorder, a severe form of anxiety. Nature 310:683–685, 1984

Reiman EM, Raichle ME, Robins E, et al: Neuroanatomical correlates of a lactate-induced panic attack. Arch Gen Psychiatry 46:493–500, 1989

Reiss S: Interoceptive theory of the fear of anxiety. Behav Res Ther 7:84–85, 1988

Robinson D, Wu H, Ashtari M, et al: Reduced caudate nucleus volume in obsessive-compulsive disorder. Arch Gen Psychiatry 52:393–398, 1995

Ross RJ, Ball WA, Sullivan KA, et al: Sleep disturbance as the hallmark of posttraumatic stress disorder. Am J Psychiatry 146:697–707, 1989

Ross RJ, Ball WA, Dinges DF, et al: Motor dysfunction during sleep in posttraumatic stress disorder. Sleep 17:723–732, 1994

Roth WT, Margraf J, Ehlers A, et al: Stress test reactivity in panic disorder. Arch Gen Psychiatry 49:301–310, 1992

Roy-Byrne PP, Cowley DS, Greenblatt DJ, et al: Reduced benzodiazepine sensitivity in panic disorder. Arch Gen Psychiatry 47:534–538, 1990

Roy-Byrne P, Wingerson DK, Radant A, et al: Reduced benzodiazepine sensitivity in patients with panic disorder: comparison with patients with obsessive-compulsive disorder and normal subjects. Am J Psychiatry 153:1444–1449, 1996

Rubin RT, Villanueva-Meyer J, Ananth J, et al: Regional Xenon 133 cerebral blood flow and cerebral technetium 99m HMPAO uptake in unmedicated patients with obsessive-compulsive disorder and matched normal control subjects. Arch Gen Psychiatry 49:695–702, 1992

Sapolsky RM: Stress, the Aging Brain, and the Mechanisms of Neuron Death. Cambridge, MA, MIT Press, 1992

Schacter DL, Alpert NM, Savage CR, et al: Conscious recollection and the human hippocampal formation: evidence from positron emission tomography. Proc Natl Acad Sci U S A 93:321–325, 1996

Schiffman SS, Gill JM, Diaz C: Methylxanthines enhance taste: evidence for modulation of taste by adenosine receptors. Pharmacol Biochem Behav 22:195–203, 1985

Shalev AY, Orr SP, Peri T, et al: Physiologic responses to loud tones in Israeli patients with posttraumatic stress disorder. Arch Gen Psychiatry 49:870–875, 1992

Shear MK, Fyer AJ, Ball G, et al: Vulnerability to sodium lactate in panic disorder patients given cognitive-behavioral therapy. Am J Psychiatry 148:795–797, 1991

Sherbourne CD, Wells KB, Judd LL: Functioning and well-being of patients with panic disorder. Am J Psychiatry 153:213–218, 1996

Smeraldi E, Diaferia G, Erzegovesi S, et al: Tryptophan depletion in obsessive-compulsive patients. Biol Psychiatry 40:398–402, 1996

Spangler WJ, Cosgrove GR, Ballantine HTJ, et al: Magnetic resonance image-guided stereotactic cingulotomy for intractable psychiatric disease. Neurosurgery 38:1071–1076, 1996

Stein MB: How shy is too shy? Lancet 347:1131–1132, 1996

Stein MB, Asmundson GJG: Autonomic function in panic disorder: cardiorespiratory and plasma catecholamine responsivity to multiple challenges of the autonomic nervous system. Biol Psychiatry 36:548–558, 1994

Stein MB, Leslie WD: A brain single photon-emission computed tomography (SPECT) study of generalized social phobia. Biol Psychiatry 39:825–828, 1996

Stein MB, Uhde TW: Panic disorder and major depression: lifetime relationship and biological markers, in Clinical Aspects of Panic Disorder. Edited by Ballenger J. New York, Alan R Liss, 1990, pp 151–168

Stein MB, Uhde TW: Endocrine, cardiovascular, and behavioral effects of intravenous TRH in patients with panic disorder. Arch Gen Psychiatry 48:148–156, 1991

Stein MB, Uhde TW: The thyroid and anxiety disorders, in The Thyroid Axis and Psychiatric Illness. Edited by Joffe RT, Levitt AJ. Washington, DC, American Psychiatric Press, 1993, pp 255–278

Stein MB, Tancer ME, Uhde TW: Physiologic and plasma norepinephrine responses to orthostasis in patients with panic disorder and social phobia. Arch Gen Psychiatry 49:311–317, 1992

Stein MB, Black B, Uhde TW: Lack of efficacy of the adenosine reuptake inhibitor dipyridamole in the treatment of anxiety disorders. Biol Psychiatry 33:647–650, 1993a

Stein MB, Enns MW, Kryger MH: Sleep in nondepressed patients with panic disorder, II: polysomnographic assessment of sleep architecture and sleep continuity. J Affect Disord 28:1–6, 1993b

Stein MB, Huzel LL, Delaney SM: Lymphocyte β-adrenoceptors in social phobia. Biol Psychiatry 34:45–50, 1993c

Stein MB, Asmundson GJG, Chartier MJ: Autonomic responsivity in generalized social phobia. J Affect Disord 31:211–221, 1994

Stein MB, Delaney SM, Chartier MJ, et al: [³H] paroxetine binding to platelets of patients with social phobia: comparison to patients with panic disorder and healthy volunteers. Biol Psychiatry 37:224–228, 1995a

Stein MB, Millar TW, Larsen DK, et al: Irregular breathing during sleep in patients with panic disorder. Am J Psychiatry 152:1168–1173, 1995b

Stein MB, Walker JR, Forde DR: Public-speaking fears in a community sample: prevalence, impact on functioning, and diagnostic classification. Arch Gen Psychiatry 53:169–174, 1996

Stein MB, Hanna C, Koverola C, et al: Structural brain changes in PTSD: does trauma alter neuroanatomy? Ann N Y Acad Sci 821:76–82, 1997a

Stein MB, Koverola C, Hanna C, et al: Hippocampal volume in women victimized by childhood sexual abuse. Psychol Med 27:951–960, 1997b

Stein MB, Yehuda R, Koverola C, et al: Enhanced dexamethasone suppression of plasma cortisol in adult women traumatized by childhood sexual abuse. Biol Psychiatry 42:680–686, 1997c

Stein MB, Chartier MJ, Hazen AL, et al: A direct-interview family study of generalized social phobia. Am J Psychiatry (in press)

Steinlein OK, Deckert J, Nothen MM, et al: Neuronal nicotinic acetylcholine receptor α4 subunit (CHRNA4) and panic disorder: an association study. Am J Med Genet (Neuropsychiatric Genetics) 74:199–201, 1997

Swedo SE, Rapoport JL, Cheslow DL, et al: High prevalence of obsessive-compulsive symptoms in patients with Sydenham's chorea. Am J Psychiatry 146:246–249, 1989

Swedo SE, Leonard HL, Mittleman BB, et al: Identification of children with pediatric autoimmune neuropsychiatric disorders associated with streptococcal infections by a marker associated with rheumatic fever. Am J Psychiatry 154:110–112, 1997

Tancer ME, Stein MB, Gelernter CS, et al: The hypothalamic-pituitary-thyroid axis in social phobia. Am J Psychiatry 147:929–933, 1990a

Tancer ME, Stein MB, Uhde TW: Effects of thyrotropin-releasing hormone on blood pressure and heart rate in social phobic and panic patients: a pilot study. Biol Psychiatry 27:781–783, 1990b

Tancer ME, Stein MB, Black B, et al: Blunted growth hormone responses to growth hormone releasing factor and to clonidine in panic disorder. Am J Psychiatry 150:336–337, 1993a

Tancer ME, Stein MB, Uhde TW: Growth hormone response to intravenous clonidine in social phobia: comparison to patients with panic disorder and healthy volunteers. Biol Psychiatry 34:591–595, 1993b

Tancer ME, Mailman RB, Stein MB, et al: Neuroendocrine responsivity to monoaminergic system probes in generalized social phobia. Anxiety 12:16–23, 1994

Thoren P, Asberg M, Bertillson L, et al: Clomipramine treatment of obsessive-compulsive disorder, II: biochemical aspects. Arch Gen Psychiatry 37:1289–1294, 1980

Tiihonen J, Kuikka J, Bergstrom K, et al: Dopamine reuptake site densities in patients with social phobia. Am J Psychiatry 154:239–242, 1997

Torgersen S: Twin studies in panic disorder, in Neurobiology of Panic Disorder. Edited by Ballenger J. New York, Alan R Liss, 1990, pp 51–58

Uhde TW: Caffeine provocation of panic: a focus on biological mechanisms, in Clinical Aspects of Panic Disorder. Edited by Ballenger J. New York, Alan R Liss, 1990, pp 219–242

Uhde TW: The anxiety disorders, in Principles and Practice of Sleep Medicine, 2nd Edition. Edited by Kryger MH, Roth T, Dement W. Philadelphia, PA, WB Saunders, 1994, pp 871–898

Uhde TW, Boulenger JP, Post RM, et al: Fear and anxiety: relationship to noradrenergic function. Psychopathology 17:8–23, 1984a

Uhde TW, Vittone BJ, Post RM: Glucose tolerance testing in panic disorder. Am J Psychiatry 141:1461–1463, 1984b

Uhde TW, Stein MB, Vittone BJ, et al: Behavioral and physiologic effects of short-term and long-term administration of clonidine in panic disorder. Arch Gen Psychiatry 46:170–177, 1989

Uhde TW, Tancer ME, Gurguis GNM: Chemical models of anxiety: evidence for diagnostic and neurotransmitter specificity. International Review Journal of Psychiatry 2:367–384, 1990

Uhde TW, Tancer ME, Rubinow DR, et al: Evidence for hypothalamo-growth hormone dysfunction in panic disorder: profile of growth hormone (GH) responses to clonidine, yohimbine, caffeine, glucose, GRF and TRH in panic disorder patients versus healthy volunteers. Neuropsychopharmacology 6:101–118, 1992

Uhde TW, Tancer ME, Gelernter CS, et al: Normal urinary-free cortisol and post-dexamethasone cortisol in social phobia: comparison to normal controls. J Affect Disord 30:155–161, 1994

van Kammen DP: 5-HT, a neurotransmitter for all seasons? Biol Psychiatry 22:1–3, 1987

Verburg K, Griez E, Meijer J, et al: Discrimination between panic disorder and generalized anxiety disorder by 35% carbon dioxide challenge. Am J Psychiatry 152:1081–1083, 1995

Vieland VJ, Goodman DW, Chapman T, et al: A new segregation analysis of panic disorder. Am J Med Genet 67:146–153, 1996

Wang ZW, Crowe RR, Noyes R Jr: Adrenergic receptor genes as candidate genes for panic disorder: a linkage study. Am J Psychiatry 149:470–474, 1992

β-Amyloid deposits are far more frequent in AD than in normal aging. NFTs are present in many dementing disorders and thus appear to represent a common convergence point in dementia (Joachim et al. 1987). Similarly, degeneration of neuronal cells occurs in many disorders of the central nervous system (CNS). The anatomical distribution of NFTs and degenerating neurons, however, has a unique profile in AD as compared with that in other diseases, and this profile corresponds to the nature of functional loss (Braak and Braak 1991; Van Hoesen et al. 1995). The interrelationship between each of these three lesions is not well defined, but recent data provide preliminary information on this point.

β-Amyloid Deposition

The presence of numerous compact deposits of β-amyloid peptide, also referred to as senile plaques, defines AD (Khachaturian 1985). Deposits of β-amyloid are found in the neuropil; in addition, aggregates of this peptide are commonly found in the cerebral vasculature (Glenner and Wong 1984; Masters et al. 1985; Wong et al. 1985). The 39–44 amino acid β-amyloid peptide is derived from a precursor referred to as β-amyloid precursor protein, or β-APP (Kang et al. 1987). Alternative splicing of a primary β-APP transcript gives rise to three major β-APP isoforms of 695, 751, and 770 amino acids (Kitaguchi et al. 1988; Ponte et al. 1988; Tanzi et al. 1988). Expression of the 695 β-APP isoform is restricted to neurons, in contrast to the longer isoforms that are ubiquitously expressed (Ponte et al. 1988). In AD, there appears to be an imbalance in neuronal β-APP isoform expression weighted toward high levels of the 751 and 770 β-APP isoforms (Johnson et al. 1990).

The physiological role of β-APP is not well understood, but several different functions have been proposed based primarily on data from cultured cell systems. The secreted form of β-APP has been observed to regulate cell proliferation in nonneuronal cells (Saitoh et al. 1989) and to promote cell adhesion (Breen et al. 1991; Chen and Yankner 1991; Schubert et al. 1989). In neuronal cells, soluble β-APP promotes survival (Mattson et al. 1993b), protects against excitotoxic or ischemic insults (Mattson et al. 1993b), regulates intracellular Ca^{2+} levels (Mattson et al. 1993a, 1993b), and promotes neurite outgrowth (Milward et al. 1992). Because β-APP has some functions apparently relevant to neuronal maintenance and viability, alterations in the expression and/or processing of the precursor protein may contribute to the development of AD pathology.

The expression of β-APP during development and in the adult organism is not essential. Transgenic mice in which the β-APP gene has been inactivated by homologous recombination have a nearly normal phenotype (Zheng et al. 1995). Expression of related proteins from the β-APP multigene family (Slunt et al. 1994; Wasco et al. 1992, 1993) is presumed to compensate for the ablated β-APP. The other β-APP family members lack sequences homologous to the β-amyloid peptide and, therefore, do not participate directly in β-amyloid formation in AD.

The generation of β-amyloid has been a topic of intense investigation. The peptide is produced by a series of intracellular proteolytic cleavages by enzymes termed *secretases* acting on β-APP (reviewed in Evin et al. 1994). The first cleavage results in the formation of a fragment of the precursor, with the β-amyloid domain located at the amino-terminus. The second processing event produces the carboxyl-terminus of β-amyloid that releases the peptide from the β-APP backbone. Carboxyl-terminal β-amyloid processing has an additional complexity in that the cleavage sites reside within the transmembrane domain of the precursor. Membrane damage, therefore, is a likely prerequisite to this cleavage event. The precursor protein can be alternatively processed to produce secreted β-APP by a proteolytic cleavage within the β-amyloid domain (Esch et al. 1990; Sisodia 1992), precluding β-amyloid formation.

The processing steps to generate β-amyloid are influenced by both genetic and environmental factors. Mutations that have been identified in the gene encoding β-APP are linked to AD (see section, "Genetics of Alzheimer's Disease," later in this chapter). Each of these mutations has been shown to promote β-amyloid processing toward the pathogenic state. β-APP "Swedish" and "Flemish" mutations result in increased production of β-amyloid (Cai et al. 1993; Citron et al. 1992, 1994; Haass et al. 1994; Johnston et al. 1994), whereas "London" and "Dutch" mutations result in the generation of a form of the peptide that aggregates at a rapid rate (N. Suzuki et al. 1994; Tamaoka et al. 1994; T. Wisniewski et al. 1991).

The formation of β-amyloid is a normal physiological process. The peptide is naturally produced by cultured cells in vitro (Busciglio et al. 1993; Haass et al. 1992; Seubert et al. 1992; Shoji et al. 1992) and in vivo when it is present in cerebrospinal fluid (Seubert et al. 1992; Vigo-Pelfrey et al. 1993), brain (Tabaton et al. 1994; Teller et al. 1996), and presumably all other tissues. The β-amyloid peptide appears to be produced as a minor by-product of β-APP catabolism (Higaki et al. 1995). The increased peptide levels observed in association with β-APP mutations or with overexpression of the β-APP gene, as in Down's syndrome, may simply result from increased turnover of unwanted β-APP molecules (Zhong et al. 1994). Both β-APP mutations and Down's syndrome result in accelerated onset of AD.

Two recently identified genes, referred to as *presenilins*, may participate in β-APP transport and discard processes (L'Hernault and Arduengo 1992). Mutations in presenilin genes linked to early-onset AD may perturb this function and promote β-amyloid generation (see section, "Genetics of Alzheimer's Disease," later in this chapter).

After β-amyloid peptide is produced, it is rapidly released from the cell into the extracellular space (Busciglio et al. 1993; Haass et al. 1992; Seubert et al. 1992; Shoji et al. 1992). This observation provides a simple explanation for the extracellular deposition of the peptide in brains of patients with AD.

Another important component of the deposition process is aggregation. Because β-amyloid is a small protein, synthetic homologues have been used to characterize the physical parameters of its aggregation. In fact, synthetic β-amyloid can polymerize into fibrils that are morphologically identical to those isolated from the brains of patients with AD (Kirschner et al. 1987). The structural features of β-amyloid that promote seeding, exponential growth, and insolubility of the protein aggregate have been identified with such assays (reviewed in Jarrett and Lansbury 1993; Mattson 1995; Soto et al. 1994).

A clear consensus from many laboratories indicates that the hydrophobic carboxyl-terminus of the peptide is critical for establishing aggregates. β-Amyloid species extended at the carboxyl-terminus, such as the 42 or 43 amino acid forms, have been shown to nucleate and aggregate significantly more rapidly than the more common 40 amino acid β-amyloid species (Jarrett et al. 1993). The "London" β-APP mutation, which produces increased amounts of longer β-amyloid species and is linked to the development of AD, can be explained in this context.

The longer β-amyloid species is the first to be deposited in brains of patients with AD, and then the 40 residue species is incorporated (Iwatsubo et al. 1994). The mass concentration of soluble β-amyloid is another critical factor in nucleating polymers. Small increases in β-amyloid production and concentration, such as those seen with "Swedish" and "Flemish" familial β-APP mutations, can dramatically accelerate the exponential nucleation rate (Jarrett and Lansbury 1993). Polymerization can be enhanced by factors that interact with the β-amyloid peptide. Accessory factors identified with aggregation include apolipoprotein E (ApoE, the protein; *APOE*, the gene) (Ma et al. 1994; T. Wisniewski and Frangione 1992), which is a protein involved in lipid metabolism that is a modulating genetic component of AD (see section, "Genetics of

Alzheimer's Disease," later in this chapter), zinc metal ions (Bush et al. 1994), and sulfated proteoglycans (Snow et al. 1987). Each of these β-amyloid aggregation promoting factors is believed to position the peptide in a structural conformation conducive to self-polymerization.

Once the β-amyloid peptide aggregate is formed, it can mediate several untoward activities, all of which are similar to the pathological processes in AD. The fact that β-amyloid is neurotoxic in vitro provides a hypothesis for the neuronal degeneration seen in the disease (Pike et al. 1991; Roher et al. 1991; Yankner et al. 1989, 1990). The mechanism of β-amyloid neurotoxicity has been proposed to involve production of reactive oxygen species followed by destabilization of Ca^{2+} homeostasis—two events that may ultimately lead to programmed cell death (reviewed in Iversen et al. 1995; Mattson 1995; Mattson et al. 1993a; see section, "Neuronal Degeneration," below). In addition, exposure of neurons to β-amyloid peptide can disrupt muscarinic cholinergic signal transduction and acetylcholine (ACh) synthesis, which implicates a role for β-amyloid in the impairment of cholinergic transmission that occurs in AD (Hoshi et al. 1997; Kelly et al. 1996; see section, "Cholinergic Deficits in Alzheimer's Disease," later in this chapter). The β-amyloid peptide can also promote the release of inflammatory cytokines and other mediators of inflammation from astrocytes and microglia that associate with senile plaques (reviewed in Mrak et al. 1995; see section, "Cerebral Inflammation in Alzheimer's Disease," later in this chapter). This β-amyloid-induced response may initiate the inflammation cascade that occurs in AD.

The hypothesis that β-amyloid has a central role in AD pathogenesis is supported by several lines of evidence. First, all of the known genetic perturbations associated with AD can be linked directly or indirectly to β-amyloid production. Second, transgenic mice programmed for increased β-APP expression (both wild type and "London" mutation) have many pathological features of AD. These transgenic animals have deposits of β-amyloid in their brains (Games et al. 1995; Higgins et al. 1994, 1995; Quon et al. 1991), deposit-associated inflammatory reactions (Games et al. 1995; Higgins et al. 1994), pre-NFT alterations (Higgins et al. 1994, 1995), and cognitive impairments (Moran et al. 1995). These pathological features become more severe with the age of the animal (Higgins et al. 1995; Moran et al. 1995). Hence, compelling evidence suggests that β-amyloid be used as a therapeutic target for the development of novel treatment strategies. Approaches to inhibit the enzymes that process β-APP to the β-amyloid peptide, to prevent β-amyloid aggregation, and to attenuate β-amyloid-induced neurotoxicity and inflammatory processes are under investigation.

Neurofibrillary Tangles

In AD, the neuronal cytoskeleton is progressively disrupted and replaced by NFTs composed of ultrastructural entities called paired helical filaments (PHFs). These NFTs are formed within the vast majority of neurons that degenerate during the course of the disease. NFTs are found in the neuronal cell body or extracellularly after neuronal death ("ghost" tangles). PHFs are also found in two structures related to NFTs—in dystrophic neurites associated with senile plaques and in diffusely distributed neuronal processes termed *neuropil threads*. NFTs develop selectively in specific sites within the cerebral cortex and spread in a predictable, nonrandom manner. This sequence of pathological progression provides a basis for distinguishing stages in the development of AD (Braak and Braak 1991). Neurofibrillary pathology and the associated synaptic loss correlate better with the degree of cognitive impairment than does the extent of β-amyloid deposition (Arriagada et al. 1992a; Brunelli et al. 1991; Terry et al. 1991; Tomlinson et al. 1970).

Protein chemistry and molecular cloning directly established that the microtubule-associated protein tau forms an integral component of all neurofibrillary structures (Goedert 1993; V. Y. M. Lee et al. 1991; Wischik et al. 1988). NFTs, dystrophic neurites, and neuropil threads are composed of the same cytoskeletal constituents; therefore, they probably originate by a common mechanism. This mechanism appears to involve phosphorylation of tau. NFT tau is abnormally hyperphosphorylated; unlike normal tau, which binds to microtubules to promote their assembly and cytoskeletal stability, hyperphosphorylated tau is functionally inactive (reviewed in Goedert 1993; Mandelkow and Mandelkow 1993; Trojanowski et al. 1993). Because hyperphosphorylated tau cannot bind to microtubules, the tau molecule tends to self-assemble into PHFs that form NFTs.

In a normal neuron, a regulated balance between phosphorylated and dephosphorylated tau exists. In the AD neuron, this dynamic equilibrium is disrupted in the direction of excessive phosphorylation. This imbalance does not appear to be caused by "runaway" kinase activity, as was previously believed (Biernat et al. 1993; Drewes et al. 1995); rather, it is more likely a result of inefficient phosphatase action (Matsuo et al. 1994). The basis for the apparent abnormal regulation of tau dephosphorylation in AD is not known.

Therapeutic strategies focused on neurofibrillary pathology have been largely confined to the application of microtubule-stabilizing agents and to methods of regulating tau phosphorylation. Agents that have been identified recently can inhibit aggregation of tau proteins in vitro (Wischik et al. 1996). These agents may represent a potential therapeutic avenue if they have in vivo activity against PHF formation.

Neuronal Degeneration

In AD, select neurons (e.g., large pyramidal cells of the neocortex) degenerate, whereas others (e.g., certain interneurons) are unaffected (Braak and Braak 1991; Hansen et al. 1988; Mountjoy et al. 1983; Whitehouse et al. 1982). Much of the cellular degeneration involves glutamatergic systems, which results in a disconnection between the hippocampus and neocortex (Braak and Braak 1991). The increased frequency of AD with age (Bachman et al. 1993) and the presence of AD pathological hallmarks in nondemented elderly individuals (Arriagada et al. 1992b; Katzman et al. 1988) suggest that the distinction between AD and normal aging may be merely quantitative. However, the pattern of loss of hippocampal neurons in AD is different from that in normal aging (West et al. 1994). This finding indicates that AD is not accelerated aging but a specific disease process.

Many factors have been proposed as the initiating cause of neuronal death in AD (reviewed in Yankner 1996). These factors include β-amyloid toxicity and abnormal phosphorylation of tau (discussed earlier in this chapter in "Neurofibrillary Tangles"), the effects of ApoE E4, and inflammatory and oxidative injury (discussed later in this chapter in "Cerebral Inflammation in Alzheimer's Disease"). Familial AD cases can be linked at present to one of four different genetic loci (see section, "Genetics of Alzheimer's Disease," below), yet all appear to share a common final pathway of neuropathological change and neuronal death, which is similar to that in AD cases with no apparent familial pattern (Lippa et al. 1996). Thus, although the initiating event may vary among AD cases, similar pathophysiological processes enter into the resulting neuronal degeneration.

Apoptosis, or programmed cell death, may be an important ultimate cause of neuronal degeneration in AD, regardless of the initiating event (reviewed in Cotman and Anderson 1995; Iversen et al. 1995). Apoptosis is an active intracellular process that occurs in a wide variety of cell types in response to different external stimuli. Molecular, biochemical, and morphological features that characterize apoptosis can be readily distinguished from events occurring in necrotic cell death.

To date, AD neurons have been shown to have only a limited set of the known apoptotic markers, including fragmentation of nuclear DNA (Su et al. 1994) and expression of immediate early genes *c-fos* and *c-jun* (Anderson et al. 1994). In contrast, in vitro studies, in which β-amyloid peptide was applied to cultured neurons, have reported many classical apoptotic events (reviewed in Cotman and Anderson 1995). Neuronal apoptosis mediated by excitotoxicity and neurotrophin withdrawal has been characterized in vitro and was found to have similar cell death responses (reviewed in Mattson 1995). These data imply that multiple diverse stimuli may induce a common neurodegenerative pathway in AD.

Much interest has focused on the potential role of neurotrophins in neuronal degeneration in AD as well as in treatment of AD. Nerve growth factor (NGF), the prototypical neurotrophin, can protect cholinergic neurons of the basal forebrain (which are lost in AD; see section, "Cholinergic Deficits in Alzheimer's Disease," below) from degeneration after experimental brain injury (Hefti 1986; Williams et al. 1986). Furthermore, withdrawal of neurotrophins can result in neuronal apoptosis (Jensen et al. 1992), and neurotrophins can prevent apoptosis of cholinergic neurons (Wilcox et al. 1995). However, despite considerable effort, it has been difficult to assign a definite role to NGF or other neurotrophins in the pathophysiology of AD (A. S. Scott and Crutcher 1994).

Attempts to use neurotrophins in the treatment of AD have been hindered by the impermeability of the blood-brain barrier to most of these agents, necessitating intracerebral delivery (Hefti 1994). However, because of the considerable potential of neurotrophins in treating AD and other CNS disorders, research interest in these agents remains strong.

CHOLINERGIC DEFICITS IN ALZHEIMER'S DISEASE

It has been known for many years that AD is characterized by deficits in CNS cholinergic function (Bartus et al. 1982; Coyle et al. 1983). Choline acetyltransferase, the enzyme responsible for the synthesis of ACh, is decreased in brains of patients with AD (Bowen et al. 1976), and this decrease is correlated with the degree of cognitive decline (Bierer et al. 1995; Perry et al. 1978). In AD, there is a loss of cholinergic neurons in the nucleus basalis of Meynert and related cholinergic nuclei of the basal forebrain (Whitehouse et al. 1982). Because these neurons provide most of the cholinergic input to the cerebral cortex and hippocampus in primates (Kitt et al. 1987; Struble et al. 1986), their loss results in a profound decrease in cholinergic innervation of these structures. This decreased cholinergic stimulation has been hypothesized to be a

cause of the deficits in memory and higher cortical functions in AD. In fact, experimental drug-induced cholinergic deficits in healthy humans and animals result in impaired learning and memory (Bartus and Johnson 1976; Drachman and Leavitt 1974; Sunderland et al. 1987). Furthermore, in AD, the number of NFTs in the nucleus basalis, which is an indicator of neuronal loss in this region, is a good predictor of degree of cognitive impairment (Samuel et al. 1994). In animals, lesions of basal forebrain and septal cholinergic nuclei result in deficits in attention, memory, and learning (Dekker et al. 1991; Dunnett et al. 1991; Muir et al. 1994; Voytko et al. 1994).

Various drug therapies for AD have been developed based on the cholinergic hypothesis. Currently, the acetylcholinesterase inhibitors tacrine and donepezil are marketed in the United States for the treatment of AD. These agents act to increase the availability of ACh at surviving cholinergic synapses by inhibiting the action of acetylcholinesterase, which degrades ACh to acetate and choline. However, clinical efficacy is limited, and pharmacological and toxic side effects are common, particularly with tacrine (Davis and Powchik 1995). An important source of side effects with nonspecific cholinesterase inhibitors such as these is an increase in activity at peripheral cholinergic synapses, which results in complaints such as gastrointestinal distress. Alternative strategies that are under development involve either selective inhibition of central acetylcholinesterases or specific activation of muscarinic cholinergic receptor subtypes (Fisher et al. 1996). Researchers hypothesize that these agents could have greater specificity for cholinergic systems related to memory and could generate fewer side effects than nonspecific cholinesterase inhibitors. Another potential approach would be to develop agonists that are specific for nicotinic cholinergic receptors, because these receptors are decreased in brains of patients with AD, and nicotinic agonists may enhance cognition (Whitehouse and Kalaria 1995; Whitehouse et al. 1986).

A criticism of cholinergic approaches to the treatment of AD is that many neurotransmitter systems, not only cholinergic, are profoundly affected by AD. Deficits in serotonergic, noradrenergic, and various peptidergic systems have been detected in brains of patients with AD (Auchus et al. 1994; Bondareff et al. 1987; D'Amato et al. 1987; Yamamoto and Hirano 1985), which suggests that the loss of cholinergic neurons is simply part of widespread neuronal death in AD. Furthermore, cholinergic neuronal death in AD is probably secondary to another more fundamental process responsible for other neuropathological changes such as the formation of senile plaques and NFTs.

Nevertheless, specific links may exist between cho-

finity for β-amyloid (Strittmatter et al. 1993), which suggests a pathophysiological role for ApoE in AD. Subsequent association studies detected the *APOE* ε4 allele with increased frequency in both late-onset familial and sporadic AD compared with control populations (Corder et al. 1993; Saunders et al. 1993; Strittmatter et al. 1993). Additional studies showed that the ε4 allele is also increased in early-onset sporadic AD and, perhaps, early-onset familial AD (Dai et al. 1994; Lehtovirta et al. 1995; St. Clair et al. 1995). However, some studies have not found an association between the ε4 allele and early-onset familial AD (Locke et al. 1995; Sorbi et al. 1994). At present, the ε4 allele is most strongly associated with late-onset familial AD and sporadic AD; these findings have been replicated in many studies. Although most studies of sporadic AD have been based on clinic patients with dementia or other samples of convenience, numerous population-based studies that have been conducted confirm the association of the ε4 allele in AD (Evans et al. 1997; A. S. Henderson et al. 1995; Myers et al. 1996).

The actual increase in the frequency of the ε4 allele varies from study to study. Depending on the sample, between 34% and 65% of subjects with AD carry the ε4 allele, whereas only 24%–31% of control subjects are ε4 allele carriers (Farrer et al. 1995). Although the ε4 allele clearly increases the risk for AD, the exact increase in risk over that for noncarriers is unclear (Farrer et al. 1995; Relkin et al. 1996), and the risk may be lower in the general population than in clinic samples or in affected families (Evans et al. 1997). Furthermore, although persons with two ε4 alleles appear to be at greater risk than heterozygous individuals, the exact amount of increased risk varies from study to study. Finally, some persons live until the tenth decade of life and carry the ε4 allele but do not develop AD (Rebeck et al. 1994). Likewise, many persons without ε4 alleles develop neuropathologically confirmed AD (Saunders et al. 1996). Thus, having an ε4 allele is not deterministic for AD, and AD can develop without an ε4 allele.

The current general consensus is that *APOE* ε4 carrier status should not be used to predict the risk of developing AD in noncognitively impaired individuals (Breitner 1996; Farrer et al. 1995; Relkin et al. 1996). Nonetheless, controversy surrounds the use of *APOE* genotyping as an adjunctive test in the diagnosis of AD; some researchers urge caution until additional data are obtained, whereas others see testing as a valuable clinical tool (Bird 1995; Post et al. 1997; Roses 1995). Prospective studies of patients with AD confirmed by autopsy will be of value in determining the utility of *APOE* genotyping in the diagnosis of AD (Saunders et al. 1996).

In addition to an increased frequency of the ε4 allele in AD, several other associations of potential clinical importance have emerged. First, the ε2 allele is found with decreased frequency in AD subjects and may be a protective factor in late-onset familial and sporadic AD (Corder et al. 1994). Some studies have reported that the ε2 allele has a protective role in early-onset AD (Locke et al. 1995), whereas others have not (van Duijn et al. 1995). Another interesting but controversial association of ApoE concerns age at onset in AD. Corder et al. (1993) originally proposed that in late-onset familial AD, ε4 predisposes to an earlier age at onset, ε2 predisposes to a later age at onset, and ε3 predisposes to an intermediate age at onset. However, other groups could not replicate this finding with different samples (St. Clair et al. 1995; van Duijn et al. 1994; Zubenko et al. 1994). In a recent study, Corder et al. (1995) reported that the ε4 allele was associated with earlier age at onset in late-onset familial AD but not in sporadic AD. A likely source of confusion is that the precise age at onset in AD is difficult to determine retrospectively.

Other than a possible association of the ε4 allele with earlier age at onset, clinical associations for the ε4 allele in AD have been difficult to detect. The number of NFTs and β-amyloid deposits in brains of patients with AD may be related to *APOE* genotype (see below). Several studies have found that rate of cognitive decline in AD is not affected by *APOE* genotype (Dal Forno et al. 1996; Gomez-Isla et al. 1996; Murphy et al. 1997b). Survival time of AD patients—the interval from disease onset to death—also does not appear to be affected by the ε4 allele (Corder et al. 1995). Two preliminary studies reported that psychiatric signs and symptoms in AD are more severe among ε4 carriers, even when degree of cognitive impairment is taken into account (Murphy et al. 1997c; Ramachandran et al. 1996). Longitudinal studies of clinical phenotypes in AD and their correlation with *APOE* genotype will clarify these issues.

The *APOE* ε4 allele may affect cognition in persons without dementia. One study found that cognitive decline in the elderly after cardiothoracic surgery was more likely in ε4 allele carriers (Newman et al. 1995) than in those without the allele. Survival in very elderly patients who do not have dementia may also be decreased by the presence of the ε4 allele (Corder et al. 1996). In a study of elderly nondemented fraternal twins discordant for the ε4 allele, the ε4 carrier had subtle deficits in cognitive performance (Reed et al. 1994). These intriguing results should be verified in larger longitudinal studies.

The neurobiological basis for the association of *APOE* ε4 with AD is unclear. Outside of the nervous system,

ApoE is involved in the transport and metabolism of lipids (Davignon et al. 1988). In the nervous system, ApoE is probably involved in the repair and maintenance of myelin and neuronal membranes, especially after injury (Ignatius et al. 1986), and in metabolism of cholesterol and phospholipids associated with the formation of new synapses (Poirier 1994). ApoE mRNA is found in astrocytes but not in neurons or microglia (Poirier et al. 1991). The lack of ApoE expression by microglia is somewhat unexpected, because macrophages, which have many similarities to microglia, express ApoE (Basu et al. 1981). However, ApoE immunoreactivity may be detected in neurons and macrophages after ischemic brain injury (Kida et al. 1995). In brains of persons with and without AD, ApoE immunoreactivity is found in neurons and microglia, as well as astrocytes (Han et al. 1994; Metzger et al. 1996; Uchichara et al. 1995). Presumably, ApoE synthesized by astrocytes is taken up by neurons and microglia. Neurons express the low-density lipoprotein receptor and the low-density lipoprotein receptor–related protein (Rebeck et al. 1993), both of which bind ApoE and may be involved in internalization.

In vitro assays showing ApoE binding to tau suggest a role for ApoE in NFT development in AD (Strittmatter et al. 1994). This hypothesis is based on the observation that ApoE E3 binds unphosphorylated tau, whereas ApoE E4 does not, and the speculation that ApoE E3 protects tau from hyperphosphorylation. This hypothesis is supported by studies of ApoE-deficient mice, in which levels of tau phosphorylation are increased (Genis et al. 1995), and by the observation that ApoE is present in NFTs (Namba et al. 1991). Furthermore, the ε4 allele may be associated with increased numbers of NFTs in AD (Nagy et al. 1995; Ohm et al. 1995). Because neurons do not express ApoE, receptor-mediated uptake is presumed to precede incorporation of ApoE into NFT.

ApoE and β-amyloid are also related. First, ApoE is associated with β-amyloid in senile plaques and in the cerebral vasculature (Namba et al. 1991; T. Wisniewski and Frangione 1992). Second, the levels of β-amyloid deposited in the brains of individuals with AD vary according to *APOE* genotype; *APOE* ε4 carriers have the largest amyloid burden (Premkumar et al. 1996; reviewed in Strittmatter and Roses 1995). Third, ApoE binds to β-amyloid and influences aggregation of the peptide in a genotype-specific manner in vitro (Ma et al. 1994; Strittmatter et al. 1993). Investigators speculate that the normal interaction between ApoE and β-amyloid is related to the clearance of β-amyloid and that in AD the *APOE* genotypes confer differences in the kinetics of this process. Whether the key pathogenic interaction is between ApoE and tau or ApoE

and β-amyloid is debatable, but both interactions may be important.

Three other genetic polymorphisms were recently associated with AD. Kamboh et al. (1995) reported an association between a polymorphism in the signal peptide of α_1-antichymotrypsin (ACT) and AD. However, two subsequent studies did not confirm the ACT A allele association with AD (Haines et al. 1996; Murphy et al. 1997a). Okuizumi et al. (1995) found that a trinucleotide repeat allelic variant at the very-low-density lipoprotein receptor locus was associated with AD. However, a subsequent study was unable to replicate this association (Chung et al. 1996). Finally, Wragg et al. (1996) found that a polymorphism in intron 8 of the presenilin 1 gene was associated with late-onset AD. Although this finding has been replicated by some groups (Higuchi et al. 1996; Kehoe et al. 1996), others have been unable to detect this association (W. K. Scott et al. 1996). These conflicting results among studies may be due to statistical error, differences in sampling methods, or differences in allele frequencies among populations sampled. Clearly, candidate genes for AD risk factors should be examined in multiple samples from diverse populations to assess generalizability.

CEREBRAL INFLAMMATION IN ALZHEIMER'S DISEASE

Although AD usually is not thought of as an inflammatory disease, considerable evidence indicates a low-level inflammatory state in brains of patients with AD, which may have adverse effects on brain function. For example, researchers have known for many years that neuritic plaques in AD are surrounded by large numbers of activated microglia and astrocytes (Haga et al. 1989; H. Wisniewski and Terry 1973). Proliferation of astrocytes and microglia may form a physical barrier to neuronal function; however, the more important effect is that in vitro these cells can secrete a variety of substances potentially toxic to neurons such as cytokines, eicosanoids, and reactive oxygen and nitrogen intermediates (Eddleston and Mucke 1993; Nakajima and Kohsaka 1993). Furthermore, neuropathological studies have identified markers for inflammation in brains of patients with AD, including increased expression of major histocompatibility class II antigens (Rogers et al. 1988), which are necessary for antigen presentation; inflammatory cytokines interleukin 1 (IL-1) (Griffin et al. 1989) and interleukin-6 (IL-6) (Bauer et al. 1991); and components of the classical complement pathway, which when activated can injure neurons (Eikelenboom et al. 1989; McGeer et al. 1989).

Evidence of oxidative injury and injury secondary to reactive nitrogen species can also be detected in brains of patients with AD (Good et al. 1996; Smith et al. 1996). The inflammatory reaction in AD is far less dramatic than that in, for example, a bacterial infection of the nervous system but nevertheless could injure neurons if active for many years.

According to the inflammatory hypothesis of AD, neurons are injured as a result of microglial and astrocyte activation and increased production of potentially cytotoxic cytokines, complement proteins, nitric oxide and its derivatives, oxidative agents, and other neuroactive substances (McGeer and Rogers 1992; Mrak et al. 1995). Little evidence, at present, supports infiltration of circulating leukocytes, tissue macrophages, or other peripheral immune effector cells in brains of patients with AD. Studies of peripheral inflammatory markers in AD have been largely negative. For example, although IL-1 is increased in brains of patients with AD (Griffin et al. 1989), production of IL-1 by lymphocytes and monocytes is unremarkable in AD (Bessler et al. 1989; Huberman et al. 1994). The inflammatory reaction in AD appears to be primarily associated with the endogenous immune effector cells of the CNS, microglia and astrocytes, and their secretory products.

Experimental evidence is increasing to support the hypothesis that inflammation is important in the pathophysiology of AD. Recent studies have reported that microglia secrete β-amyloid and that this secretion is augmented by immunologic stimuli and by β-amyloid itself (Bitting et al. 1996). This finding demonstrates that immune activation could lead to increased microglial β-amyloid secretion in the brain in AD and that once β-amyloid deposition begins, it could be perpetuated through an autocrine or paracrine mechanism.

β-Amyloid also stimulates astrocytes and microglia to produce cytokines such as IL-1 (Araujo and Cotman 1992; Walker et al. 1995). IL-1, in turn, can cause proliferation of glial cells (Giulian and Lachman 1985), cause secretion of other cytokines (Benveniste 1993), and alter expression of β-APP (Goldgaber et al. 1989), although whether these effects are accompanied by increased secretion of β-amyloid has not yet been determined (Vasilakos et al. 1994).

β-Amyloid can also induce cultured microglia and endothelial cells to secrete reactive nitrogen and oxygen intermediates, which may result in oxidative injury to nerve cells (Ii et al. 1996; Meda et al. 1995; Thomas et al. 1996). Evidence even indicates that in a cell-free aqueous solution, β-amyloid can generate reactive oxygen species (Hensley et al. 1994).

Finally, in vitro β-amyloid can activate the classical complement pathway (Rogers et al. 1992), which results in formation of the cytotoxic C5b-9 membrane attack complex, which is found on dystrophic neurites and NFTs in brains of patients with AD (McGeer et al. 1989). Although the actual initiating immune stimulus in AD remains uncertain, substantial evidence shows that β-amyloid alone may play an important role, even if only to sustain the reaction once it is initiated. Furthermore, mediators of the inflammatory reaction such as IL-1 may alter β-APP metabolism, resulting in a self-perpetuating pathogenic cycle.

As in most inflammatory processes, endogenous antiinflammatory or protective factors appear to be involved in AD. For example, β-amyloid induces microglia secretion of tumor necrosis factor (TNF)-α (Meda et al. 1995), and TNF-α may protect neurons from β-amyloid-mediated neurotoxicity (Barger et al. 1995). Transforming growth factor (TGF)-β, an antiinflammatory cytokine found in plaques in AD (van der Wal et al. 1993), may also protect neurons from β-amyloid toxicity (Chao et al. 1994). It may be possible to exploit these natural protective responses through pharmacological means in the treatment of AD. However, effects of cytokines in vivo are unpredictable; a recent report indicated that transgenic overexpression of TGF-β1 may enhance perivascular β-amyloid deposition (Wyss-Coray et al. 1997).

Clinical evidence supports the role of inflammation in the etiology of AD. Retrospective studies indicate that prior treatment with corticosteroids or nonsteroidal antiinflammatory drugs may delay the onset of AD or may result in milder cognitive deficits once the disease is manifest (Breitner et al. 1994; Corrada et al. 1996; Rich et al. 1995; Stewart et al. 1997). A small prospective, placebo-controlled study of the nonsteroidal agent indomethacin in AD reported that the rate of cognitive decline decreased in subjects treated for 6 months (Rogers et al. 1993). These results require replication.

CONCLUSION

Important advances in understanding the pathophysiology and genetics of AD have been made in recent years. Novel targets for therapeutic intervention have been identified, and many new therapeutic agents are being developed. Drugs that impede the formation of β-amyloid or inhibit its aggregation are under development. β-Amyloid secretase inhibitors should be available for clinical testing within several years; if these inhibitors have efficacy in AD, the hypothesis that β-amyloid is fundamental to the pathophysiology of AD will have substantial support.

Agents designed to decrease the risk of ApoE E4 by mimicking the effects of ApoE E2 in the brain are also under development, although the problem of delivering these agents across the blood-brain barrier may be limiting. Recent data indicate that existing antiinflammatory drugs may have efficacy in treating AD. In addition, a host of newer agents, including selective cyclooxygenase inhibitors, cytokine receptor antagonists, and cytokine convertase inhibitors, have potential use in preventing cerebral inflammation in AD (B. Henderson and Bodmer 1996; Vane and Botting 1996). Drug development aimed at cholinergic deficits in AD also continues at a brisk pace—newer acetylcholinesterase inhibitors with fewer side effects have been released, and release of selective cholinergic agonists is pending. Although prospective trials are lacking, retrospective studies suggest that estrogens can attenuate risk for AD (Paganini-Hill and Henderson 1996; Schneider et al. 1996), possibly by interfering with β-amyloid toxicity (Goodman et al. 1996), and hence may represent another therapeutic avenue.

It is not surprising that multiple therapeutic approaches to AD are under development. Genetic studies have shown that AD is etiologically heterogeneous, and additional predisposing or exacerbating factors—both biological and environmental—will undoubtedly be found. Future pharmacological therapy for AD may involve interrupting the cascade of pathological changes at multiple points to decrease incrementally the risk or progression of the disease.

REFERENCES

Anderson AJ, Cummins BJ, Cotman CW: Increased immunoreactivity for Jun- and Fos-related proteins in Alzheimer's disease: association with pathology. Exp Neurol 125: 286–295, 1994

Anwar R, Moynihan TP, Ardley H, et al: Molecular analysis of the presenilin 1 (S182) gene in "sporadic" cases of Alzheimer's disease: identification and characterisation of unusual splice variants. J Neurochem 66:1774–1777, 1996

Araujo DM, Cotman CW: β-amyloid stimulates glial cells in vitro to produce growth factors that accumulate in senile plaques in Alzheimer's disease. Brain Res 569:141–145, 1992

Arriagada PA, Growdon JH, Hedley-White ET, et al: Neurofibrillary tangles but not senile plaques parallel duration and severity of Alzheimer's disease. Neurology 42:631–639, 1992a

Arriagada PA, Marzloff K, Hyman BT: Distribution of Alzheimer-type pathologic changes in non-demented elderly individuals matches the pattern of Alzheimer's disease. Neurology 42:1681–1688, 1992b

Auchus AP, Green RC, Nemeroff CB: Cortical and subcortical neuropeptides in Alzheimer's disease. Neurobiol Aging 15:589–595, 1994

Bachman DL, Wolf PA, Linn RT, et al: Incidence of dementia and probable Alzheimer's disease in a general population: the Framingham study. Neurology 43:515–519, 1993

Barger SW, Horster D, Furukawa K, et al: Tumor necrosis factors α and β protect neurons against amyloid β-peptide toxicity: evidence for involvement of a κB-binding factor and attenuation of peroxide and Ca^{2+} accumulation. Proc Natl Acad Sci U S A 92:9328–9332, 1995

Bartus RT, Johnson HR: Short-term memory in the rhesus monkey: disruption from the anti-cholinergic scopolamine. Pharmacol Biochem Behav 5:39–46, 1976

Bartus RT, Dean RL, Beer B, et al: The cholinergic hypothesis of geriatric memory dysfunction. Science 217:408–417, 1982

Basu SK, Brown MS, Ho YK, et al: Mouse macrophages synthesize and secrete a protein resembling apolipoprotein E. Proc Natl Acad Sci U S A 78:7545–7549, 1981

Bauer J, Strauss S, Schreiter-Gasser U, et al: Interleukin-6 and alpha-2-macroglobulin indicate an acute-phase state in Alzheimer's disease cortices. FEBS Lett 285:111–114, 1991

Benveniste EN: Astrocyte-microglia interactions, in Astrocytes: Pharmacology and Function. Edited by Murphy J. New York, Academic Press, 1993, pp 355–382

Bessler H, Sirota P, Hart J, et al: Lymphokine production in patients with Alzheimer's disease. Age Ageing 18:21–25, 1989

Bierer LM, Haroutunian V, Gabriel S, et al: Neurochemical correlates of dementia severity in Alzheimer's disease: relative importance of the cholinergic deficits. J Neurochem 64:749–760, 1995

Biernat J, Gustke N, Drewes G, et al: Phosphorylation of Ser 262 strongly reduces binding of tau to microtubules: distinction between PHF-like immunoreactivity and microtubule binding. Neuron 11:153–163, 1993

Bird TD: Apolipoprotein E genotyping in the diagnosis of Alzheimer's disease: a cautionary view. Ann Neurol 38:2–3, 1995

Bird TD, Lampe TH, Nemens EJ, et al: Familial Alzheimer's disease in American descendants of the Volga Germans: probable genetic founder effect. Ann Neurol 23:25–31, 1988

Bitting L, Naidu A, Cordell B, et al: β-amyloid peptide secretion by a microglial cell line is induced by β-amyloid-(25–35) and lipopolysaccharide. J Biol Chem 271:16084–16088, 1996

Bondareff W, Mountjoy CQ, Roth M, et al: Neuronal degeneration in locus ceruleus and cortical correlates of Alzheimer's disease. Alzheimer Dis Assoc Disord 1:256–262, 1987

Borchelt DR, Thinakaran G, Eckman CB, et al: Familial Alzheimer's disease-linked presenilin I variants elevate Aβ1–42/1–40 ratios in vitro and in vivo. Neuron 17: 1005–1013, 1996

Bowen DM, Smith CB, White P, et al: Neurotransmitter-related enzymes and indices of hypoxia in senile dementia and other abiotrophies. Brain 99:459–496, 1976

Braak H, Braak E: Neuropathological staging of Alzheimer-related changes. Acta Neuropathol 82:239–259, 1991

Breen KC, Bruce M, Anderson BH: β-amyloid precursor protein mediates neuronal cell-cell and cell-surface adhesion. J Neurosci Res 26:90–100, 1991

Breitner JCS: APOE genotyping and Alzheimer's disease. Lancet 347:1184–1185, 1996

Breitner JCS, Gau BA, Welsh KA, et al: Inverse association of anti-inflammatory treatments and Alzheimer's disease. Neurology 44:227–232, 1994

Breitner JCS, Welsh KA, Gau BA, et al: Alzheimer's disease in the National Academy of Sciences—National Research Council registry of aging twin veterans, III: detection of cases, longitudinal results, and observations on twin concordance. Arch Neurol 52:763–771, 1995

Brunelli MP, Kowall NW, Lee JM, et al: Synaptophysin immunoreactivity is depleted in cortical laminae with dense dystrophic neurites and neurofibrillary tangles. J Neuropathol Exp Neurol 50:315–327, 1991

Busciglio J, Gabuzda D, Matsudeira P, et al: Generation of β-amyloid in the secretory pathway in neuronal and nonneuronal cells. Proc Natl Acad Sci U S A 90:2092–2096, 1993

Bush AI, Pettingell WH, Mulhaup G, et al: Rapid induction of Alzheimer Aβ amyloid formation by zinc. Science 265:1464–1467, 1994

Cai X, Golde TE, Younkin SG: Release of excess amyloid β protein from a mutant amyloid β protein precursor. Science 259:514–516, 1993

Chao C, Hu S, Kravitz FH, et al: Transforming growth factor-β protects human neurons against β-amyloid induced injury. Mol Chem Neuropathol 23:159–179, 1994

Chen M, Yankner BA: An antibody to β-amyloid and the amyloid precursor protein inhibits cell-substratum adhesion in many mammalian cell types. Neurosci Lett 125:223–226, 1991

Chung H, Roberts CT, Greenberg S, et al: Lack of association of trinucleotide repeat polymorphisms in the very-low-density lipoprotein receptor gene with Alzheimer's disease. Ann Neurol 6:800–803, 1996

Citron M, Oltersdorf T, Haass C, et al: Mutation of the β-amyloid precursor protein in familial Alzheimer's disease increases β-protein production. Nature 360:672–674, 1992

Citron M, Vigo-Pelfrey C, Teplow DB, et al: Excessive production of amyloid β-protein by peripheral cells of symptomatic and presymptomatic patients carrying the Swedish familial Alzheimer's disease mutation. Proc Natl Acad Sci U S A 91:11993–11997, 1994

Citron M, Westaway D, Xia W, et al: Mutant presenilins of Alzheimer's disease increase production of 42-residue amyloid β-protein in both transfected cells and transgenic mice. Nature Medicine 3:67–72, 1997

Clark RF, Hutton M, Fuldner RA, et al: The structure of the presenilin 1 (S182) gene and identification of six novel mutations in early onset AD families. Nat Genet 11:219–222, 1995

Corder EH, Saunders AM, Strittmatter WJ, et al: Gene dose of apolipoprotein E type 4 allele and the risk of Alzheimer's disease in late onset families. Science 261:921–923, 1993

Corder EH, Saunders AM, Risch NJ, et al: Protective effect of apolipoprotein E type 2 allele for late onset Alzheimer disease. Nat Genet 7:180–184, 1994

Corder EH, Saunders AM, Strittmatter WJ, et al: Apolipoprotein E, survival in Alzheimer's disease patients, and the competing risks of death and Alzheimer's disease. Neurology 45:1323–1328, 1995

Corder EH, Lannfelt L, Vittanen M, et al: Apolipoprotein E genotype determines survival in the oldest old (85 years or older) who have good cognition. Arch Neurol 53:418–422, 1996

Corrada M, Brookmeyer R, Kawas C: Sources of variability in prevalence rates of Alzheimer's disease. Int J Epidemiol 24:1000–1005, 1995

Corrada M, Stewart W, Kawas C: Non-steroidal anti-inflammatory drugs and the risk of Alzheimer's disease (abstract). Neurology 46:A433, 1996

Correy-Bloom J, Thal LJ, Galasko D, et al: Diagnosis and evaluation of dementia. Neurology 45:211–218, 1995

Cotman CW, Anderson AJ: A potential role for apoptosis in neurodegeneration and Alzheimer's disease. Mol Neurobiol 10:19–45, 1995

Coyle JT, Price DL, DeLong MR: Alzheimer's disease: a disorder of cortical cholinergic innervation. Science 219:1184–1190, 1983

Cribbs DH, Chen L-S, Bende SM, et al: Widespread neuronal expression of the presenilin-1 early onset Alzheimer's disease gene in the murine brain. Am J Pathol 148:1797–1806, 1996

Dai XY, Nanko S, Hattori M, et al: Association of apolipoprotein E4 with sporadic Alzheimer's disease is more pronounced in early onset type. Neurosci Lett 175:74–76, 1994

Dal Forno G, Rasmusson X, Brandt J, et al: Apolipoprotein E genotype and rate of decline in probable Alzheimer's disease. Arch Neurol 53:345–350, 1996

D'Amato RJ, Zweig RM, Whitehouse PJ, et al: Aminergic systems in Alzheimer's disease and Parkinson's disease. Ann Neurol 22:229–236, 1987

Davidson EA, Robertson EE: Alzheimer's disease with acne rosacea in one of identical twins. J Neurol Neurosurg Psychiatry 18:72–77, 1955

Davies P: The genetics of Alzheimer's disease: a review and a discussion of the implications. Neurobiol Aging 7: 459–466, 1986

Davignon J, Gregg RE, Sing CF: Apolipoprotein E polymorphism and atherosclerosis. Arteriosclerosis 8:1–21, 1988

Davis KL, Powchik P: Tacrine. Lancet 345:625–630, 1995

Dekker AJ, Connor DJ, Thal LJ: The role of cholinergic projections from the nucleus basalis in memory. Neurosci Biobehav Rev 15:299–317, 1991

Drachman DA, Leavitt J: Human memory and the cholinergic system. Arch Neurol 30:113–121, 1974

Drewes G, Trinczek B, Illenberger S, et al: Microtubule-associated protein/microtubule affinity-regulating kinase (p110^{mark}). J Biol Chem 270:7679–7688, 1995

Duff K, Eckman C, Zehr C, et al: Increased amyloid-β42(43) in brains of mice expressing mutant presenilin 1. Nature 383:710–713, 1996

Dunnett SB, Everitt BJ, Robbins TW: The basal forebrain-cortical cholinergic system: interpreting the functional consequences of excitotoxic lesions. Trends Neurosci 14:494–501, 1991

Eddleston M, Mucke L: Molecular profile of reactive astrocytes—implications for their role in neurologic disease. Neuroscience 54:15–36, 1993

Eikelenboom P, Hack CE, Rozemuller JM, et al: Complement activation in amyloid plaques in Alzheimer's dementia. Virchows Archiv B Cell Pathol 56:259–262, 1989

Ellis WG, McCulloch JR, Corley CL: Presenile dementia in Down's syndrome: ultrastructural identity with Alzheimer's disease. Neurology 24:101–106, 1974

Esch FS, Keim PS, Beattie EC, et al: Cleavage of amyloid β peptide during constitutive processing of its precursor. Science 248:1122–1124, 1990

Evans DA, Beckett LA, Field TS, et al: Apolipoprotein E ε4 and incidence of Alzheimer disease in a community population of older persons. JAMA 277:822–824, 1997

Evin G, Beyreuther K, Masters CL: Alzheimer's disease amyloid precursor protein (AβPP): proteolytic processing, secretases and βA4 amyloid production. International Journal of Experimental Clinical Investigation 1:263–280, 1994

Farrer L, Brin MF, Elsas L, et al: Statement on the use of apolipoprotein E testing for Alzheimer's disease. JAMA 274:1627–1629, 1995

Fisher A, Heldman E, Gurwitz D, et al: M1 agonists for the treatment of Alzheimer's disease: novel properties and clinical update. Ann N Y Acad Sci 777:189–196, 1996

Games D, Adams D, Alessandrini R, et al: Alzheimer-type neuropathology in transgenic mice over-expressing V717F β-amyloid precursor protein. Nature 373:523–527, 1995

Genis I, Gordon I, Sehayek E, et al: Phosphorylation of tau in apolipoprotein E-deficient mice. Neurosci Lett 199:5–8, 1995

Giovannelli L, Casamenti F, Scali C, et al: Differential effects of amyloid peptides β-(1–40) and β-(25–35) injections into the rat nucleus basalis. Neuroscience 66:781–792, 1995

Giulian D, Lachman LB: Interleukin-1 stimulation of astroglial proliferation after brain injury. Science 228:497–498, 1985

Glenner GG, Wong CW: Alzheimer's disease: initial report of the purification and characterization of a novel cerebrovascular amyloid protein. Biochem Biophys Res Commun 122:885–890, 1984

Goate A, Chartier-Harlin M-C, Mullan M, et al: Segregation of a missense mutation in the amyloid precursor protein gene with familial Alzheimer's disease. Nature 349:704–706, 1991

Goedert M: Tau protein and the neurofibrillary pathology of Alzheimer's disease. Trends Neurosci 16:460–465, 1993

Goldgaber D, Harris HW, Hla T, et al: Interleukin 1 regulates synthesis of amyloid beta-protein precursor mRNA in human endothelial cells. Proc Natl Acad Sci U S A 86:7606–7610, 1989

Gomez-Isla T, West HL, Rebeck GW, et al: Clinical and pathological correlates of apolipoprotein E ε4 in Alzheimer's disease. Ann Neurol 39:62–70, 1996

Good PF, Werner P, Hsu A, et al: Evidence of neuronal oxidative damage in Alzheimer's disease. Am J Pathol 149:21–28, 1996

Goodman Y, Bruce AJ, Cheng B, et al: Estrogens attenuate and corticosterone exacerbates excitotoxicity, oxidative injury, and amyloid β-peptide toxicity in hippocampal neurons. J Neurochem 66:1836–1844, 1996

Griffin WST, Stanley LC, Ling C, et al: Brain interleukin 1 and S-100 immunoreactivity are elevated in Down syndrome and Alzheimer disease. Proc Natl Acad Sci U S A 86: 7611–7615, 1989

Haass C, Schlossmacher MG, Hung MG, et al: Amyloid β-peptide is produced by cultured cells during normal metabolism. Nature 359:322–325, 1992

Haass C, Hung AY, Selkoe DJ, et al: Mutations associated with a locus from familial Alzheimer's disease result in alternative processing of amyloid β-protein precursor. J Biol Chem 269:17741–17748, 1994

Haga S, Akai K, Ishii T: Demonstration of microglial cells in and around senile (neuritic) plaques in Alzheimer brain. Acta Neuropathol 77:569–575, 1989

Haines JL, Pritchard ML, Saunders AM, et al: No genetic effect of α1-antichymotrypsin in Alzheimer disease. Genomics 33:53–56, 1996

Han S-H, Hulette C, Saunders AM, et al: Apolipoprotein E is present in hippocampal neurons without neurofibrillary tangles in Alzheimer's disease and in age-matched controls. Exp Neurol 128:13–26, 1994

Hansen LA, DeTeresa R, Davies P, et al: Neocortical morphometry, lesions counts, and choline acetyltransferase levels in the age spectrum of Alzheimer's disease. Neurology 38:48–54, 1988

Harkany T, De Jong GI, Soos K, et al: Beta-amyloid (1–42) affects cholinergic but not parvalbumin-containing neurons in the septal complex of the rat. Brain Res 698:270–274, 1995

Hefti F: Nerve growth factor promotes survival of septal cholinergic neurons after fimbrial transections. J Neurosci 6:2155–2162, 1986

Hefti F: Development of effective therapy for Alzheimer's disease based on neurotrophic factors. Neurobiol Aging 15:S193–S194, 1994

Henderson AS, Easteal S, Jorm AF, et al: Apolipoprotein E allele ε4, dementia, and cognitive decline in a population sample. Lancet 356:1387–1390, 1995

Henderson B, Bodmer MW (eds): Therapeutic Modulation of Cytokines. Boca Raton, FL, CRC Press, 1996

Hendriks L, van Duijn CM, Cras P, et al: Presenile dementia and cerebral haemorrhage linked to a mutation at codon 692 of the beta-amyloid precursor protein gene. Nat Genet 1:218–221, 1992

Hensley K, Carney JM, Mattson MP, et al: A model of β-amyloid aggregation and neurotoxicity based on free radical generation by the peptide: relevance to Alzheimer's disease. Proc Natl Acad Sci U S A 91:3270–3274, 1994

Heston LL, Mastri AR, Anderson E, et al: Dementia of the Alzheimer type: clinical genetics, natural history, and associated conditions. Arch Gen Psychiatry 38:1085–1090, 1981

Higaki J, Quon D, Zhong Z, et al: Inhibition of β-amyloid formation identifies proteolytic precursors and cellular site of processing. Neuron 14:651–659, 1995

Higgins LS, Holtzman DM, Rabin J, et al: Transgenic mouse brain histopathology resembles early Alzheimer's disease. Ann Neurol 35:8–13, 1994

Higgins LS, Rodems JM, Catalano R, et al: Early Alzheimer's disease-like histopathology increases in frequency with age in mice transgenic for β-APP 751. Proc Natl Acad Sci U S A 92:4402–4406, 1995

Higuchi S, Muramatsu T, Matsushita S, et al: Presenilin-1 polymorphism and Alzheimer's disease. Lancet 347:1186, 1996

Hoshi M, Takashima A, Murayama M, et al: Nontoxic amyloid β-peptide 1–42 suppresses acetylcholine synthesis. J Biol Chem 272:2038–2041, 1997

Huberman M, Shalit F, Roth-Deri I, et al: Correlation of cytokine secretion by mononuclear cells of Alzheimer patients and their disease stage. J Neuroimmunol 52:147–152, 1994

Ignatius MJ, Gebicke-Harter PJ, Skene JH, et al: Expression of apolipoprotein E during nerve degeneration and regeneration. Proc Natl Acad Sci U S A 83:1125–1129, 1986

Ii M, Sunamoto M, Ohnishi K, et al: β-amyloid protein-dependent nitric oxide production from microglial cells and neurotoxicity. Brain Res 720:93–100, 1996

Iversen LL, Mortshire-Smith RJ, Pollack SJ, et al: The toxicity in vitro of β-amyloid protein. Biochem J 311:1–16, 1995

Iwatsubo T, Odaka A, Suzuki N, et al: Visualization of Aβ42(43) and Aβ40 in senile plaques with end specific Aβ monoclonals: evidence that an initially deposited species is Aβ42(43). Neuron 13:45–53, 1994

Jarrett JT, Lansbury Jr PT: Seeding "one-dimensional crystallization" of amyloid: a pathogenic mechanism in Alzheimer's disease and scrapie? Cell 73:1055–1058, 1993

Jarrett JT, Berger EP, Lansbury Jr PT: The carboxy-terminus of β-amyloid protein is critical for the pathogenesis of Alzheimer's disease. Biochemistry 32:4693–4697, 1993

Jensen LM, Zhang Y, Shooter EM: Steady-state polypeptide modulations associated with nerve growth factor (NGF)-induced terminal differentiation and NGF deprivation-induced apoptosis in human neuroblastoma cells. J Biol Chem 267:19325–19333, 1992

Joachim CL, Morris JH, Kosik KS, et al: Tau antisera recognize neurofibrillary tangles in a range of neurodegenerative disorders. Ann Neurol 22:514–520, 1987

Johnson SA, McNeill T, Cordell B, et al: Neuronal β-APP 751/695 mRNA ratio correlates with neuritic plaque density in Alzheimer's disease. Science 248:854–857, 1990

Johnston JA, Cowburn RF, Norgren S, et al: Increased β-amyloid release and levels of amyloid precursor protein (APP) in fibroblast cell lines from family members with the Swedish Alzheimer's disease mutation. FEBS Lett 354:274–278, 1994

Kamboh MI, Sanghera DK, Ferrell RE, et al: APOE*4-associated Alzheimer's disease risk is modified by α1-antichymotrypsin polymorphism. Nat Genet 10:486–488, 1995

Kang J, Lemaire H, Unterbeck A, et al: The precursor of Alzheimer's disease amyloid A4 protein resembles a cell-surface receptor. Nature 325:733–736, 1987

Katzman R: The prevalence and malignancy of Alzheimer disease. Arch Neurol 33:217–218, 1976

Katzman R, Terry R, DeTeresa R, et al: Clinical, pathological, and neurochemical changes in dementia: a subgroup with preserved mental status and numerous neocortical plaques. Ann Neurol 23:138–144, 1988

Kehoe P, Williams J, Lovestone S, et al: Presenilin-1 polymorphism and Alzheimer's disease. Lancet 347:1185, 1996

Kelly JF, Furukawa K, Barger SW, et al: Amyloid β-peptide disrupts carbachol-induced muscarinic cholinergic signal transduction in cortical neurons. Proc Natl Acad Sci U S A 93:6753–6758, 1996

Khachaturian ZS: Diagnosis of Alzheimer's disease. Arch Neurol 42:1097–1105, 1985

Kida E, Pluta R, Lossinsky AS, et al: Complete cerebral ischemia with short-term survival in rat induced by cardiac arrest, II: extracellular and intracellular accumulation of apolipoproteins E and J in the brain. Brain Res 674: 341–346, 1995

Kirschner DA, Inouye H, Duffy LK, et al: Synthetic peptide homologous to β-protein from Alzheimer's disease forms amyloid-like fibrils. Proc Natl Acad Sci U S A 84: 6953–6969, 1987

Kitaguchi N, Takahashi Y, Tokushima Y, et al: Novel precursor of Alzheimer's disease amyloid protein shows protease inhibitory activity. Nature 331:530–532, 1988

Kitt CA, Mitchell SJ, DeLong MR, et al: Fiber pathways of basal forebrain cholinergic neurons in monkeys. Brain Res 406:192–206, 1987

Kokmen E, Beard CM, O'Brien PC, et al: Epidemiology of dementia in Rochester, Minnesota. Mayo Clin Proc 71:275–282, 1996

Kovacs DM, Fausett HJ, Page KJ, et al: Alzheimer-associated presenilins 1 and 2: neuronal expression in brain and localization to intracellular membranes in mammalian cells. Nature Medicine 2:224–229, 1996

Lee MK, Slunt HH, Martin LJ, et al: Expression of presenilin 1 and 2 (PS1 and PS2) in human and murine tissues. J Neurosci 16:7513–7525, 1996

Lee VYM, Balin BJ, Otvos L Jr, et al: A68: a major subunit of paired helical filaments and derivatized forms of normal tau. Science 251:675–678, 1991

Lehtovirta M, Helisalmi S, Mannermaa A, et al: Apolipoprotein E polymorphism and Alzheimer's disease in Eastern Finland. Neurosci Lett 185:13–15, 1995

Lendon CL, Ashall F, Goate AM: Exploring the etiology of Alzheimer disease using molecular genetics. JAMA 277:825–831, 1997

Levitan D, Greenwald I: Facilitation of *lin-12*-mediated signaling by *sel-12*, a *Caenorhabditis elegans* S182 Alzheimer's disease gene. Nature 377:351–354, 1995

Levy E, Carman MD, Fernandez-Madrid IJ, et al: Mutation of the Alzheimer's disease amyloid gene in hereditary cerebral hemorrhage, Dutch type. Science 248:1124–1126, 1990

Levy-Lahad E, Wasco W, Poorkaj P, et al: Candidate gene for the chromosome 1 familial Alzheimer's disease locus. Science 269:973–977, 1995a

Levy-Lahad E, Wijsman EM, Nemens E, et al: A familial Alzheimer's disease locus on chromosome 1. Science 269: 970–973, 1995b

L'Hernault SW, Arduengo PM: Mutation of a putative sperm membrane protein in *Caenorhabditis elegans* prevents sperm differentiation but not its associated meiotic divisions. J Cell Biol 119:55–68, 1992

Lippa CF, Saunders AM, Smith TW, et al: Familial and sporadic Alzheimer's disease: neuropathology cannot exclude a final common pathway. Neurology 46:406–412, 1996

Lobo A, Saz P, Marcos G, et al: The prevalence of dementia and depression in the elderly community in a southern European population. Arch Gen Psychiatry 52:497–506, 1995

Locke PA, Conneally PM, Tanzi RE, et al: Apolipoprotein E4 allele and Alzheimer disease: examination of allelic association and effect on age at onset in both early- and late-onset cases. Genetic Epidemiology 12:83–92, 1995

Ma J, Yee A, Brewer Jr AYH, et al: Amyloid associated proteins α1 antichymotrypsin and apolipoprotein E promote assembly of Alzheimer β-protein into filaments. Nature 372:92–94, 1994

Malamud N: Neuropathology of organic brain syndromes associated with aging, in Advances in Behavioral Biology, Vol 3: Aging and the Brain. Edited by Gaitz CM. New York, Plenum, 1972, pp 63–87

Mandelkow EM, Mandelkow E: Tau as a marker for Alzheimer's disease. Trends Biochem Sci 18:480–483, 1993

Masters CL, Simms G, Weinman NA, et al: Amyloid plaque core protein in Alzheimer's disease and Down syndrome. Proc Natl Acad Sci U S A 82:4245–4249, 1985

Matsuo ES, Shin RW, Billingsley ML, et al: Biopsy-derived adult human brain tau is phosphorylated at many of the same sites as Alzheimer's disease paired helical filament tau. Neuron 13:989–1002, 1994

Mattson MP: Untangling the pathophysiochemistry of β-amyloid. Nature Structural Biology 2:926–928, 1995

Mattson MP, Barger SW, Cheng B, et al: β-Amyloid precursor protein metabolites and loss of neuronal Ca^{2+} homeostasis in Alzheimer's disease. Trends Neurosci 16:409–414, 1993a

Mattson MP, Cheng B, Culerll AR, et al: Evidence for excitoprotective and intraneuronal calcium-regulating roles for secreted forms of the β-amyloid precursor protein. Neuron 10:243–254, 1993b

McGeer PL, Rogers J: Anti-inflammatory agents as a therapeutic approach to Alzheimer's disease. Neurology 42: 447–449, 1992

McGeer PL, Akiyama H, Itagaki S, et al: Activation of the classical complement pathway in brain tissue of Alzheimer patients. Neurosci Lett 107:341–356, 1989

McKhann G, Drachman D, Folstein M, et al: Clinical diagnosis of Alzheimer's disease: report of the NINCDS-ADRDA work group under the auspices of Department of Health and Human Services Task Force on Alzheimer's Disease. Neurology 34:939–944, 1984

Meda L, Cassatella MA, Szendrel GI, et al: Activation of microglial cells by β-amyloid protein and interferon-γ. Nature 374:647–650, 1995

Mercken M, Takahashi H, Honda T, et al: Characterization of human presenilin 1 using N-terminal specific monoclonal antibodies: evidence that Alzheimer mutations affect proteolytic processing. FEBS Lett 389:297–303, 1996

Metzger RE, LaDu MJ, Pan JB, et al: Neurons of the human frontal cortex display apolipoprotein E immunoreactivity: implications for Alzheimer's disease. J Neuropathol Exp Neurol 55:373–380, 1996

Milward EA, Papadopoulos R, Fuller SJ, et al: The amyloid protein precursor of Alzheimer's disease is a mediator of the effects of nerve growth factor on neurite outgrowth. Neuron 9:129–137, 1992

Moran P, Higgins LS, Cordell B, et al: Age-related learning deficits in transgenic mice expressing the 751-amino acid isoform of human β-amyloid precursor protein. Proc Natl Acad Sci U S A 92:5341–5345, 1995

Mountjoy CQ, Roth M, Evans NJR, et al: Cortical neuronal counts in normal elderly controls and demented patients. Neurobiol Aging 4:1–11, 1983

Moussaoui S, Czech C, Pradier L, et al: Immunohistochemical analysis of presenilin-1 expression in the mouse brain. FEBS Lett 383:219–222, 1996

Mrak RE, Shen JG, Griffin WST: Glial cytokines in Alzheimer's disease: review and pathogenic implications. Hum Pathol 26:816–823, 1995

Muir JL, Everitt BJ, Robbins TW: AMPA-induced excitotoxic lesions of the basal forebrain: a significant role for the cortical cholinergic system in attentional function. J Neurosci 14:2313–2326, 1994

Mullan M, Crawford F, Axelman K, et al: A pathogenic mutation for probable Alzheimer's disease in the APP gene at the N-terminus of beta-amyloid. Nat Genet 1:345–347, 1992a

Mullan M, Houlden H, Windelspecht M, et al: A locus for familial early onset Alzheimer's disease on the long arm of chromosome 14, proximal to the alpha 1-antichymotrypsin gene. Nat Genet 2:340–342, 1992b

Murphy GM, Forno LS, Ellis WG, et al: Antibodies to presenilin proteins detect neurofibrillary tangles in Alzheimer's disease. Am J Pathol 149:1839–1846, 1996

Murphy GM, Sullivan EV, Gallagher-Thompson D, et al: No association between the alpha 1-antichymotrypsin A allele and Alzheimer's Disease. Neurology 48:1313–1316, 1997a

Murphy GM, Taylor J, Kraemer HC, et al: No association between apolipoprotein E ε4 allele and rate of decline in Alzheimer's disease. Am J Psychiatry 154:603–608, 1997b

Murphy GM, Taylor J, Tinklenberg JR, et al: The apolipoprotein ε4 allele is associated with increased behavioral disturbance in Alzheimer's disease. American Journal of Geriatric Psychiatry 5:88–89, 1997c

Myers RH, Schaefer EJ, Wilson PWF, et al: Apolipoprotein E ε4 association with dementia in a population-based study: the Framingham study. Neurology 46:673–677, 1996

Nagy Z, Esiri MM, Jobst KA, et al: Influence of the apolipoprotein E genotype on amyloid deposition and neurofibrillary tangle formation in Alzheimer's disease. Neuroscience 69:757–761, 1995

Nakajima K, Kohsaka S: Functional roles of microglia in the brain. Neurosci Res 17:187–203, 1993

Namba Y, Tomonaga M, Kawasaki H, et al: Apolipoprotein E immunoreactivity in cerebral amyloid deposits and neurofibrillary tangles in Alzheimer's disease and kuru plaque amyloid in Creutzfeldt-Jakob disease. Brain Res 541:163–166, 1991

Newman MF, Croughwell ND, Blumenthal JA, et al: Predictors of cognitive decline after cardiac operation. Ann Thorac Surg 59:1326–1330, 1995

Nitsch RM, Growdon JH: Role of neurotransmission in the regulation of amyloid β-protein precursor processing. Biochem Pharmacol 47:1275–1284, 1994

Nitsch RM, Slack BE, Wurtman RJ, et al: Release of Alzheimer amyloid precursor protein derivatives stimulated by activation of muscarinic acetylcholine receptors. Science 258:304–307, 1992

Ohm TG, Kirca M, Bohl J, et al: Apolipoprotein E polymorphism influences not only cerebral senile plaque load but also Alzheimer-type neurofibrillary tangle formation. Neuroscience 66:583–587, 1995

Okuizumi K, Onodera O, Namba Y, et al: Genetic association of the very low density lipoprotein (VLDL) receptor gene with sporadic Alzheimer's disease. Nat Genet 11:207–209, 1995

Paganini-Hill A, Henderson VW: Estrogen replacement therapy and the risk of Alzheimer's disease. Arch Intern Med 156:2213–2217, 1996

Pericak-Vance MA, Bebout JL, Gaskell PC, et al: Linkage studies in familial Alzheimer's disease: evidence on chromosome 19 linkage. Am J Hum Genet 48:1034–1050, 1991

Perry EK, Tomlinson BE, Blessed G, et al: Correlation of cholinergic abnormalities with senile plaques and mental test scores in senile dementia. BMJ 2:1457–1459, 1978

Pike CJ, Walencewicz AJ, Glabe CG, et al: In vitro aging of β-amyloid protein causes peptide aggregation and neurotoxicity. Brain Res 563:311–314, 1991

Poirier J: Apolipoprotein E in animal models of CNS injury and in Alzheimer's disease. Trends Neurosci 17:525–530, 1994

Poirier J, Hess M, May PC, et al: Astrocytic apolipoprotein E mRNA and GFAP mRNA in hippocampus after entorhinal cortex lesioning. Molecular Brain Research 11:97–106, 1991

Poirier J, Delisle M-C, Quiron R, et al: Apolipoprotein E4 allele as a predictor of cholinergic deficits and treatment outcome in Alzheimer's disease. Proc Natl Acad Sci U S A 92:12260–12264, 1995

Ponte P, Gonzalez-De Whitt P, Shilling J, et al: A new A4 amyloid mRNA contains a domain homologous to serine proteinase inhibitors. Nature 331:525–527, 1988

Post SG, Whitehouse PJ, Binstock RH, et al: The clinical introduction of genetic testing for Alzheimer's disease: an ethical perspective. JAMA 277:832–836, 1997

Premkumar DRD, Cohen DL, Hedera P, et al: Apolipoprotein E-e4 alleles in cerebral amyloid angiopathy and cerebrovascular pathology associated with Alzheimer's disease. Am J Pathol 148:2083–2095, 1996

Quon D, Wang Y, Catalano R, et al: Formation of β-amyloid protein deposits in brains of transgenic mice. Nature 352:239–241, 1991

Ramachandran G, Marder K, Tang M, et al: A preliminary study of apolipoprotein E genotype and psychiatric manifestations of Alzheimer's disease. Neurology 47:256–259, 1996

Rebeck GW, Reitner JS, Strickland DK, et al: Apolipoprotein E in sporadic Alzheimer's disease: allelic variation and receptor interactions. Neuron 11:575–580, 1993

Rebeck GW, Perls TT, West HL, et al: Reduce apolipoprotein ε4 allele frequency in the oldest old Alzheimer's patients and cognitively normal individuals. Neurology 44:1513–1516, 1994

Reed T, Carmelli D, Swan GE, et al: Lower cognitive performance in normal older adult male twins carrying the apolipoprotein E ε4 allele. Arch Neurol 51:1189–1192, 1994

Relkin NR, Tanzi R, Breitner J, et al: Consensus statement: apolipoprotein E genotyping in Alzheimer's disease. Lancet 347:1091–1095, 1996

Rich JB, Rasmusson DX, Folstein MF, et al: Nonsteroidal anti-inflammatory drugs in Alzheimer's disease. Neurology 45:51–55, 1995

Rocca WA, Hofman A, Brayne C, et al: Frequency and distribution of Alzheimer's disease in Europe: a collaborative study of 1980–1990 prevalence findings. Ann Neurol 30:381–390, 1991

Rockwood K, Stadnyk K: The prevalence of dementia in the elderly: a review. Can J Psychiatry 39:253–257, 1994

Rogers J, Luber-Narod J, Styren SD, et al: Expression of immune system-associated antigens by cells of the human central nervous system: relationship to the pathology of Alzheimer's disease. Neurobiol Aging 9:339–349, 1988

Rogers J, Cooper NR, Webster S, et al: Complement activation by β-amyloid in Alzheimer disease. Proc Natl Acad Sci U S A 89:10016–10020, 1992

Rogers J, Kirby LC, Hempelman SR, et al: Clinical trial of indomethacin in Alzheimer's disease. Neurology 43:1609–1611, 1993

Roher AE, Ball MJ, Bhave SV, et al: β-Amyloid from Alzheimer's disease brain inhibits sprouting and survival of sympathetic neurons. Biochem Biophys Res Commun 174:572–579, 1991

Roses A: Apolipoprotein E genotyping in the differential diagnosis, not prediction, of Alzheimer's disease. Ann Neurol 38:6–14, 1995

Sahara N, Yahagi Y, Takagi H, et al: Identification and characterization of presenilin I-467, I-463 and I-373. FEBS Lett 381:7–11, 1996

Saitoh T, Sundsmo M, Roch JM, et al: Secreted form of amyloid β-protein precursor is involved in the growth regulation of fibroblasts. Cell 58:615–622, 1989

Samuel W, Terry RD, DeTeresa R, et al: Clinical correlates of cortical and nucleus basalis pathology in Alzheimer dementia. Arch Neurol 51:772–778, 1994

Saunders AM, Strittmatter WJ, Schmechel D, et al: Association of apolipoprotein E allele ε4 with late-onset familial and sporadic Alzheimer's disease. Neurology 43:1467–1472, 1993

Saunders AM, Hulette C, Welsh-Bohmer KA, et al: Specificity, sensitivity, and predictive value of apolipoprotein-E genotyping for sporadic Alzheimer's disease. Lancet 348:90–93, 1996

Schellenberg GD, Bird TD, Wijsman EM, et al: Absence of linkage of chromosome 21q21 markers to familial Alzheimer's disease. Science 241:1507–1510, 1988

Schellenberg GD, Bird TD, Wijsman EM, et al: Genetic linkage evidence for a familial Alzheimer's disease locus on chromosome 14. Science 258:668–671, 1992

Scheuner D, Eckman C, Jensen M, et al: Secreted amyloid β-protein similar to that in the senile plaques of Alzheimer's disease is increased *in vivo* by the presenilin 1 and 2 and APP mutations linked to familial Alzheimer's disease. Nature Medicine 2:864–870, 1996

Schneider LS, Farlow MR, Henderson VW, et al: Effects of estrogen replacement therapy on response to tacrine in patients with Alzheimer's disease. Neurology 46:1580–1584, 1996

Schubert D, Jin LW, Saitoh T, et al: The regulation of amyloid β-protein precursor secretion and its modulatory role in cell adhesion. Neuron 3:689–694, 1989

Scott AS, Crutcher KA: Nerve growth factor and Alzheimer's disease. Rev Neurosci 5:179–211, 1994

Scott WK, Growdon JH, Roses AD, et al: Presenilin-1 polymorphism and Alzheimer's disease. Lancet 347:1186–1187, 1996

Seubert P, Vigo-Pelfrey C, Esch F, et al: Isolation and quantification of soluble Alzheimer's beta-peptide from biological fluids. Nature 359:325–327, 1992

Sherrington R, Rogaev EI, Liang Y, et al: Cloning of a gene bearing missense mutations in early onset familial Alzheimer's disease. Nature 375:754–760, 1995

Shoji M, Golde TE, Ghiso J, et al: Production of the Alzheimer's amyloid β protein by normal proteolytic processing. Science 258:126–129, 1992

Sisodia SS: β-amyloid precursor protein cleavage by a membrane-bound protease. Proc Natl Acad Sci U S A 89:6075–6079, 1992

Sjogren T, Sjogren H, Lindgren GH: Morbus Alzheimer and morbus pick. Acta Psychiatr Neurol Scand Suppl 82:9–152, 1952

Slunt HH, Thinakaran G, Van Koch G, et al: Expression of a ubiquitous, cross-reactive homologue of the mouse β-amyloid precursor protein (APP). J Biol Chem 269:2637–2644, 1994

Smith MA, Perry G, Richey PL, et al: Oxidative damage in Alzheimer's. Nature 382:120–121, 1996

Snow AD, Willmer JP, Kisilevsky R: Sulphated glycosaminogly-cans in Alzheimer's disease. Hum Pathol 18:506–510, 1987

Sorbi A, Nacmias B, Forleo P, et al: ApoE allele frequencies in Italian sporadic and familial Alzheimer's disease. Neurosci Lett 177:100–102, 1994

Soto C, Brañes M, Alvarez J, et al: Structural determinants of the Alzheimer's amyloid β-peptide. J Neurochem 63:1191–1198, 1994

St.Clair D, Rennie M, Slrach E, et al: Apolipoprotein E ε4 allele is a risk factor for familial and sporadic presenile Alzheimer's disease in both homozygote and heterozygote carriers. J Med Genet 32:642–644, 1995

Stewart WF, Kawas C, Corrada M, et al: Risk of Alzheimer's disease and duration of NSAID use. Neurology 48:626–632, 1997

St George-Hyslop PH, Tanzi RH, Polinsky RJ, et al: The genetic defect causing familial Alzheimer's disease maps on chromosome 21. Science 235:885–889, 1987

Strittmatter WJ, Roses AD: Apolipoprotein E and Alzheimer's disease. Proc Natl Acad Sci U S A 92:4725–4727, 1995

Strittmatter WJ, Saunders AM, Schmechel D, et al: Apolipoprotein E: high-avidity binding to β-amyloid and increased frequency of type 4 allele in late-onset familial Alzheimer disease. Proc Natl Acad Sci U S A 90:1977–1981, 1993

Strittmatter WJ, Saunders AM, Goedert M, et al: Isoform-specific interactions of apolipoprotein E with microtubule associated protein tau: implications for Alzheimer's disease. Proc Natl Acad Sci U S A 91:11183–11186, 1994

Struble RG, Lehmann J, Mitchell SJ, et al: Basal forebrain neurons provide major cholinergic innervation of primate neocortex. Neurosci Lett 66:215–220, 1986

Su JH, Anderson AJ, Cummings BJ, et al: Immunohistochemistry evidence for apoptosis in Alzheimer's disease. Neuroreport 5:2529–2533, 1994

Sunderland T, Tariot PN, Cohen RM, et al: Anticholinergic sensitivity in patients with dementia of the Alzheimer type and age-matched controls. Arch Gen Psychiatry 44:418–426, 1987

Suzuki N, Cheung TT, Cai X, et al: An increased percentage of long amyloid β protein secreted by familial amyloid β protein precursor (βAPP_{717}) mutants. Science 264:1336–1340, 1994

Suzuki T, Nishiyama K, Murayama S, et al: Regional and cellular presenilin 1 gene expression in human and rat tissues. Biochem Biophys Res Commun 219:708–713, 1996

Tabaton M, Nunzi MG, Xue R, et al: Soluble amyloid β-protein is a marker of Alzheimer's amyloid in brain but not CSF. Biochem Biophys Res Commun 200:1598–1603, 1994

Tamaoka A, Kondo T, Odaka A, et al: Biochemical evidence for the long-tail form Aβ1–42/43 of amyloid β protein as a seed molecule in cerebral deposits of Alzheimer's disease. Biochem Biophys Res Commun 205:834–842, 1994

Tanzi RE, McClatchery AI, Lamperti ED, et al: Protease inhibitor domain encoded by an amyloid protein precursor mRNA associated with Alzheimer's disease. Nature 331:528–530, 1988

Teller JK, Russo C, DeBusk LM, et al: Presence of soluble amyloid β-peptide precedes amyloid plaque formation in Down's syndrome. Nature Medicine 2:93–95, 1996

Terry RD, Masliah E, Salmon DP, et al: Physical basis of cognitive alterations in Alzheimer's disease: synapse loss is the major correlate of cognitive impairment. Ann Neurol 30:572–580, 1991

Thinakaran G, Borchelt DR, Lee MK, et al: Endoproteolysis of presenilin 1 and accumulation of processed derivatives in vivo. Neuron 17:181–190, 1996

Thomas T, Thomas G, McLendon C, et al: β-Amyloid- mediated vasoactivity and vascular endothelial damage. Nature 380:168–171, 1996

Tomlinson BE, Blessed G, Roth M: Observations on the brains of demented old people. J Neurol 11:205–242, 1970

Trojanowski JQ, Schmidt ML, Shin RW, et al: Tau(A68): from pathological marker to potential mediator of neuronal dysfunction and degeneration in Alzheimer's disease. Clinical Neuroscience 1:184–191, 1993

Uchichara T, Duyckaerts C, He Y, et al: ApoE immunoreactivity and microglial cells in Alzheimer's disease brain. Neurosci Lett 195:5–8, 1995

van Broeckhoven C: Presenilins and Alzheimer disease. Nat Genet 11:230–232, 1995

van Broeckhoven C, Backhovens H, Cruts M, et al: Mapping of a gene predisposing to early onset Alzheimer's disease to chromosome 14q24.3. Nat Genet 2:335–339, 1992

van der Wal EA, Gomez-Pinilla F, Cotman CW: Transforming growth factor-beta 1 is in plaques in Alzheimer and Down pathologies. Neuroreport 4:69–72, 1993

van Duijn CM, de Knijff P, Cruts M, et al: Apolipoprotein E4 allele in a population-based study of early onset Alzheimer's disease. Nat Genet 7:74–78, 1994

van Duijn CM, de Knijff P, Wehnert A, et al: The apolipoprotein E ε2 allele is associated with an increased risk of early onset Alzheimer's disease and a reduced survival. Neurology 37:605–610, 1995

Vane JR, Botting RM: Mechanism of action of anti-inflammatory drugs. Scand J Rheumatol 25 (suppl 102):9–21, 1996

Van Hoesen GW, Solodkin A, Hyman BT: Neuroanatomy of Alzheimer's disease: hierarchical vulnerability and neural system compromise. Neurobiol Aging 16:278–280, 1995

Vasilakos P, Carroll RT, Emmerling MR, et al: Interleukin-1β dissociates β-amyloid precursor protein and β-amyloid peptide secretion. FEBS Lett 354:289–292, 1994

Vigo-Pelfrey C, Lee D, Keim P, et al: Characterization of β-amyloid peptide from human cerebrospinal fluid. J Neurochem 61:1965–1968, 1993

Vito P, Lacana W, D'Adamio L: Interfering with apoptosis: Ca^{2+}-binding protein ALG-2 and Alzheimer's disease gene ALG-3. Science 271:521–525, 1996

Voytko ML, Olton DS, Richardson RT, et al: Basal forebrain lesions in monkeys disrupt attention but not learning and memory. J Neurosci 14:167–186, 1994

Walker DG, Kim SU, McGeer PL: Complement and cytokine gene expression in cultured microglia derived from post-mortem human brains. J Neurosci Res 40:478–493, 1995

Wallace WC, Lieberburg I, Schenk D, et al: Chronic elevation of secreted amyloid precursor protein in subcortically lesioned rats, and its exacerbation in aged rats. J Neurosci 15:4896–4905, 1995

Ward RV, Davis JB, Gray CW, et al: Presenilin-1 is processed into two major cleavage products in neuronal cell lines. Neurodegeneration 5:293–298, 1996

Wasco W, Bupp K, Magendantz M, et al: Identification of a mouse brain cDNA that encodes a protein related to the Alzheimer's disease-associated amyloid β-protein precursor. Proc Natl Acad Sci U S A 89:10758–10762, 1992

Wasco W, Gurubhagavatula S, Paradis MD, et al: Isolation and characterization of APLP2 encoding a homologue of the Alzheimer's associated amyloid β-protein precursor. Nat Genet 5:95–100, 1993

West MJ, Coleman PD, Flood DG, et al: Differences in the pattern of hippocampal neuronal loss in normal aging and Alzheimer's disease. Lancet 344:769–772, 1994

Whitehouse PJ, Kalaria RN: Nicotinic receptors and neurodegenerative dementing diseases: basic research and clinical implications. Alzheimer Dis Assoc Disord 9 (suppl 2):3–5, 1995

Whitehouse PJ, Price DL, Struble RG, et al: Alzheimer's disease and senile dementia: loss of neurons in the basal forebrain. Science 215:1237–1239, 1982

Whitehouse PJ, Martino AM, Antuono PG, et al: Nicotinic acetylcholine binding sites in Alzheimer's disease. Brain Res 371:146–151, 1986

Wilcox BJ, Applegate MD, Portera-Cailliau C, et al: Nerve growth factor prevents apoptotic cell death in injured central cholinergic neurons. J Comp Neurol 59:573–585, 1995

Williams LR, Varon S, Peterson GM, et al: Continuous infusion of nerve growth factor prevents basal forebrain neuronal death after fimbria fornix transection. Proc Natl Acad Sci U S A 83:9231–9235, 1986

Wischik CM, Novak M, Thogersen HC, et al: Isolation of a fragment of tau derived from the core of the paired helical filament of Alzheimer disease. Proc Natl Acad Sci U S A 85:4506–4510, 1988

Wischik CM, Edwards PC, Lai RYK, et al: Selective inhibition of Alzheimer disease-like tau aggregation by phenothiazines. Proc Natl Acad Sci U S A 93:11213–11218, 1996

Wisniewski H, Terry R: Reexamination of the pathogenesis of the senile plaques, in Progress in Neuropathology, Vol II. Edited by Zimmerman H. New York, Grune & Stratton, 1973, pp 1–27

Wisniewski T, Frangione B: Apolipoprotein E: a pathological chaperone in patients with cerebral and systemic amyloid. Neurosci Lett 135:235–238, 1992

Wisniewski T, Ghiso J, Frangione B: Peptides homologous to the amyloid protein of Alzheimer's disease containing a glutamine for glutamic acid substitution have accelerated amyloid fibril formation. Biochem Biophys Res Commun 3:1247–1254, 1991

Wolf BA, Wertkin AM, Jolly YC, et al: Muscarinic regulation of Alzheimer's disease amyloid precursor protein and amyloid β-protein production in human neuronal NT2N cells. J Biol Chem 270:4916–4922, 1995

Wolozin B, Iwasaki K, Vito P, et al: Participation of presenilin 2 in apoptosis: enhanced basal activity conferred by an Alzheimer mutation. Science 274:1710–1713, 1996

Wong CW, Quaranta V, Glenner GG: Neuritic plaques and cerebrovascular amyloid in Alzheimer's disease are antigenically related. Proc Natl Acad Sci U S A 82:8729–8732, 1985

Wragg M, Hutton M, Talbot C, et al: Genetic association between intronic polymorphism in presenilin-1 gene and late-onset Alzheimer's disease. Lancet 347:509–512, 1996

Wyss-Coray T, Masliah E, Mallory M, et al: Amyloidogenic role of cytokine TGF-β1 in transgenic mice and in Alzheimer's disease. Nature 389:603–606, 1997

Yamamoto T, Hirano A: Nucleus raphe dorsalis in Alzheimer's disease: neurofibrillary tangles and loss of large neurons. Ann Neurol 17:573–577, 1985

Yankner B: Mechanisms of neuronal degeneration in Alzheimer's disease. Neuron 16:921–932, 1996

Yankner BA, Dawes RL, Fisher S, et al: Neurotoxicity of a fragment of the amyloid precursor protein associated with Alzheimer's disease. Science 245:417–429, 1989

Yankner BA, Duffy LK, Kirschner DA: Neurotrophic and neurotoxic effects of amyloid β-protein: reversal by tachykinin neuropeptides. Science 260:279–282, 1990

Zheng H, Jiang M, Trumbauer ME, et al: β-Amyloid precursor protein-deficient mice show reactive gliosis and decreased locomotor activity. Cell 81:525–531, 1995

Zhong Z, Quon D, Higgins LS, et al: Increased amyloid production from aberrant β-amyloid precursor molecules. J Biol Chem 269:12179–12184, 1994

Zubenko GS, Stiffler S, Stabler S, et al: Association of the apolipoprotein E ε4 allele with clinical subtypes of autopsy-confirmed Alzheimer's disease. Am J Med Genet 54:199–205, 1994

Biology of Psychoactive Substance Dependence Disorders: Cocaine, Opiates, and Ethanol

Roger E. Meyer, M.D., and S. Paul Berger, M.D.

Physicians have been intrigued with the causes of addictive disorders for more than 200 years (Rush 1791). There has been a surprising continuity of major themes of interest, even as science and clinical observation have brought greater sophistication to theory, methods, and practice. The current diagnostic nomenclature in DSM-IV (American Psychiatric Association 1994) and ICD-10 (World Health Organization 1992) emphasizes, as Benjamin Rush did in 1791, impaired control of substance use as the defining criterion for substance use disorders. Earlier constructs of addiction in this century (e.g., American Psychiatric Association 1980; World Health Organization 1964) emphasized physical dependence as part of the definition; however, the absence of a withdrawal syndrome associated with some substance dependence disorders and the presence of withdrawal symptoms associated with the termination of chronic treatment with non-dependence-producing psychotropic drugs helped to remove this criterion from its central place in the addiction puzzle. At the same time, the presence of physical dependence in relation to opiate, alcohol, or sedative-hypnotic drug dependence still merits consideration in the diagnosis according to DSM-IV.

Central to a consideration of etiology is the question of factors in the host, the agent, and the environment, which might explain risk and pathophysiology of the disorder. It is generally understood that most people who use addictive drugs do not progress to drug dependence, and certain characteristics of temperament, psychiatric comorbidity, and/or heritability appear to contribute to risk, but only informed speculation persists on the ways that (for example) family history, antisocial personality disorder, and differential alcohol sensitivity may contribute to heightened individual risk of alcohol dependence. Culture and age cohort can magnify or reduce individual risk because of differences in cultural (and subcultural) attitudes toward substance use over the same and different periods.

In contrast to human studies that focus on host- or environmentally based risk factors, the development of homologous animal models of drug-seeking and drug-consuming behavior during the past 25 years has emphasized the reinforcing properties of the agent (drugs of abuse, including ethanol). These animal models represent the best available biomedical approximation of a human behavioral disorder, and they offer powerful tools to study the relationship between behavioral, cellular (neuronal), and molecular biology.

Over the past decade, new methods such as in vivo microdialysis and in vivo voltammetry have enabled investigators to link the reinforcing properties of abused drugs to their effects on the mesolimbic dopamine system. More

---

Supported in part by a grant from the National Institute on Alcohol Abuse and Alcoholism (P50 AA 03 510-16) (R. E. M.) and a National Institute on Drug Abuse/Department of Veteran's Affairs Interagency Agreement (YOIDA50038-00) (S. P. B.).

recently, investigators have turned from studies of reinforcement to studies of the neurobiology of "anticipatory states," in efforts to understand the physiological basis for craving and relapse behaviors in human beings. Older models of craving and relapse phenomena were based on classical conditioning and theoretical models of "neuroadaptation."

In this decade, molecular neurobiologists have begun to examine changes in gene expression in mesolimbic dopamine neurons (and other behaviorally relevant systems), which might clarify the neuroadaptive processes consequent to chronic drug administration. "Knockout" methods of molecular genetics are being studied in rodent behavioral paradigms to clarify the relationship between specific serotonergic, γ-aminobutyric acid (GABA)ergic, and dopaminergic receptors and drug and alcohol self-administration. The addictions field is ready for the insights of molecular biology and genetics because of the availability of homologous animal behavioral models of well-described human disorders.

More than 30 years of behavioral research have shown the importance of the drug *self*-administration models, because results can differ depending on schedules of self-administration and on whether the drug was administered on a schedule determined by the investigator or by the animal subject. If molecular biologists can link their powerful new methodologies to drug self-administration behavioral paradigms, their insights would be of great significance to the addictions field. If they ignore behavior in their acute or chronic drug studies, their findings may not be relevant to an understanding of addictive behavior.

In this chapter, we highlight the range of issues relevant to a biological understanding of cocaine, opiate, and alcohol dependence: nosological considerations, putative individual risk factors, homologous animal behavioral models, and the cellular and molecular mechanisms associated with drug and alcohol reinforcement (as well as the putative mechanisms of neuroadaptation and other factors that may be associated with craving and risk of relapse).

NOSOLOGICAL CONSIDERATIONS

Psychoactive substance dependence has been defined as a "cluster of cognitive, behavioral, and physiological symp-

toms that indicate that the person has impaired control of psychoactive substance use and continues use of the substance despite adverse consequences" (DSM-III-R [American Psychiatric Association 1987], p. 166). The symptoms of the dependence syndrome are principally behavioral, as they have been described in DSM-III-R, DSM-IV, and ICD-10, with a focus on drug-seeking and drug-consuming behaviors.

The major changes in DSM-IV relative to DSM-III-R include 1) some modification in the language of the defining criteria;[1] 2) a change in the order that criteria are listed to give greater prominence to the presence of tolerance and withdrawal symptoms; 3) the addition of new modifying criteria;[2] 4) a reference to the possibility that the patient may experience subjective craving for the substance, without listing this as a defining criterion for the disorder; and 5) an attempt to stage the course of recovery from the disorder (i.e., early full remission, early partial remission, sustained full remission, sustained partial remission, on agonist therapy, in a controlled environment) (American Psychiatric Association 1994, pp. 175–182).

As with ICD-10 and DSM-III-R, the authors of DSM-IV recognized the persistent risk of relapse following withdrawal. In DSM-IV, the four remission specifiers can be applied only after none of the criteria for substance dependence or substance abuse has been met for at least 1 month. Twelve months of continuous (total) remission are required to denote "sustained full remission" in DSM-IV, and the term *partial remission* is used to denote the presence of symptoms of abuse or dependence that do not meet criteria. The remission stage specifiers in DSM-IV are compatible with "evidence that return to substance use after a period of abstinence leads to a more rapid reappearance of other features of the (dependence) syndrome than occurs with non-dependent individuals" (World Health Organization 1992, p. 75). In summary, DSM-IV continues to define the core dependence syndrome on the basis of drug-seeking behavior that persists despite adverse consequences and that includes a persistent risk of relapse following withdrawal.

The term *substance abuse* is applied to individuals who experience the harmful consequence of substance use but do not experience a pattern of compulsive use, tolerance, or withdrawal symptoms.

---

[1] Reducing the number of possible criteria from nine to seven without altering the requirement that at least three of the criteria must be present to diagnose substance dependence disorder

[2] Substance dependence with or without physiological dependence

ISSUES OF INDIVIDUAL VULNERABILITY AND RISK

For most of this century (in the case of illegal drugs) and during Prohibition (in the case of alcohol), public policy derived from the perspective that the problem of addiction and its consequences was largely a function of the "power" of the substance to overwhelm an individual. Efforts to understand addiction focused on the problem of physical dependence and the use of drugs to self-medicate the distressing symptoms of withdrawal (Wikler 1965). In contrast, until recently, many psychiatrists focused on addictive disorders as self-medication to treat underlying psychopathology (Meyer 1986b). These models linked individual risk to psychopathology. However, Meyer (1986b) described the association between drug use/abuse/dependence and psychopathology as more complex than a simple linear cause-and-effect relationship. Psychiatric symptoms may antedate drug use, will appear (or be exacerbated) in the context of chronic intoxication or withdrawal states, can modify the course of addictive disorders, and may affect response to treatment.

As a general rule, psychopathology is not a significant risk factor for substance use (or heavy use) in those cultures or environments where substance use (or heavy use) is normative. In countries where per capita alcohol consumption is high (e.g., France), significant comorbid psychopathology is less common among treated alcoholic patients than in countries where per capita alcohol consumption is low (e.g., Taiwan) (Babor et al. 1992; Helzer et al. 1990). Although, by definition, substance use is necessary for the development of substance dependence disorders, the latter develops in the context of individual risk factors (e.g., some types of psychopathology, family history), the environment, and the reinforcing potency (and mode of self-administration) of the drug. In clinical populations of alcoholic individuals, those with antisocial personality disorder report an earlier onset of drinking and a more rapid progression to alcohol dependence than do individuals without antisocial personality disorder (Hesselbrock et al. 1986).

Family history of alcoholism appears to be a risk factor for the development of alcohol dependence based on some still unspecified heritable risk factors (Cotton 1979). Several characteristics identified in sons of alcoholic individuals (e.g., electrophysiological markers and sensitivity to alcohol) have been studied to determine their relationship to the risk of alcohol dependence in these individuals (Begleiter et al. 1984; Schuckit 1984, 1994). Behavioral characteristics (e.g., shy aggressiveness) of children in first- and third-grade classrooms suggest an early sign of vulnerability to the later development of alcoholism (Kellam et al. 1983). This may or may not be related to the risk associated with childhood conduct disorder, a risk factor connected to the development of antisocial personality disorder (as well as alcoholism) in adults (Robins 1966) and/or to the heritable type II subtype of alcoholism associated with a family history of criminality (Cloninger et al. 1981).

In general, research on individual biological and behavioral risk factors associated with alcohol dependence has proceeded much further than efforts to identify individual risk factors related to other types of substance dependence. In contrast, alcohol is a less potent reinforcer in animal models than are opiates or stimulants. Moreover, the route of alcohol self-administration reduces reinforcing potency, whereas intravenous use or smoking of heroin or cocaine enhances reinforcing potency. The mode of administration of heroin and cocaine is probably a major risk factor for the development of dependence and may be a very significant factor in the rate of progression from use to dependence. At the same time, individual risk factors appear to play some role; "most people who use addictive drugs never come for treatment" because use does not progress to dependence (Jones 1992, p. 109).

Further research is clearly needed to identify the biological, psychological, and social characteristics of individuals who progress from drug experimentation to drug dependence. In this regard, longitudinal studies of individuals believed to be at risk are critically important. Schuckit's (1994) recent report that low levels of response to alcohol in young men with and without a family history of alcoholism predicted the development of alcohol dependence a decade later serves as a landmark study in this regard. At this juncture, it is unclear how (or if) differential alcohol sensitivity affects the differential reinforcing properties of alcohol or the progression from use to "liking" to dependence. The addictions field benefits from the availability of animal models that can help to clarify these issues.

BEHAVIORAL NEUROBIOLOGY OF DRUG-SEEKING BEHAVIOR

Of all the diagnostic categories within ICD-10 and DSM-IV, animal models are most similar to specific human disorders in the "drug-seeking behavior" identified as the core element in substance dependence disorders. In this section, we focus on homologous animal models of cocaine, opiate, and ethanol self-administration and the biological correlates of this behavior. In general, over the past

35 years, we have gained substantial understanding of drugs as reinforcers. However, questions persist regarding the specific "neuroadaptive" changes consequent to chronic drug self-administration that may account for human drug dependence and the persistent risk of relapse following drug withdrawal.

Drug Self-Administration Behavior

Weeks (1963) initially developed an animal model of intravenous drug self-administration 35 years ago. Restrained and freely moving rats and monkeys have been chronically catheterized (via intravenous catheter) for study in operant paradigms in which the animals are rewarded with a drug injection consequent to the performance of a task (usually some type of lever-pressing activity). Researchers who tested this self-administration procedure in monkeys reported that intravenous opiates (Weeks 1963), intravenous cocaine (Woods and Schuster 1968), and intragastric ethanol (Yanagita et al. 1969) all reinforced operant behavior. With the exception of ethanol (see following section), the intravenous self-administration of these drugs will also serve as reinforcers in rats.

Over time, the operant behavior associated with opiate or stimulant self-administration comes under stimulus control; that is, the behavior occurs at those times that the animal has learned that the drug will be "available." Moreover, if the dose per injection is lowered, the animal will increase operant work output to receive more injections (Koob and Bloom 1988). If the dose per injection is increased, operant work output will decrease. When access to opiates or stimulants is limited to several hours per day, animals will maintain a stable level of drug intake within a limited range of doses (Schuster and Thompson 1969). In contrast, under conditions of continuous access, animals will self-administer cocaine to the point of death (Deneau et al. 1969) or will develop substantial tolerance to and physical dependence on opiates (W. R. Martin et al. 1963). The behavior of monkeys and rats in intravenous cocaine, opiate, and stimulant self-administration paradigms is strikingly homologous to behavioral patterns of human drug dependence (Wise and Bozarth 1987). Knockout methods from molecular genetics are now being applied to studies of drug self-administration in order to better understand individual host differences in drug reinforcing potency (Uhl 1996).

Animal Models of Alcohol Self-Administration

Although many animal models of alcohol consumption have been developed over the past 25 years, the general consensus is that no animal model fully satisfies all the criteria for an animal model of alcohol dependence. The critical first step in the development of an animal model of alcoholism involves the initiation and maintenance of oral self-administration of alcohol; alcohol-related reinforcement must be associated with its pharmacological effects, not its nutritional value. Two conclusions can be derived from a review of the literature on animal models of alcohol consumption: 1) alcohol consumption can be significantly affected by schedules of reinforcement and by association with other reinforcers, and 2) alcohol consumption is influenced significantly by pharmacogenetic factors.

Selective breeding of rats that differ in their ethanol-drinking behavior has resulted in at least three groups of rats that differ strongly in their spontaneous drinking or avoidance of alcohol (Eriksson 1971; Li et al. 1987, 1991). The development of these stable traits of preferential alcohol drinking or avoidance has further enabled researchers to examine neurobiological differences in alcohol-preferring (P) rats and nonpreferring (NP) rats. The P rats will drink a 10% ethanol solution in a free-choice paradigm (Li et al. 1987). They will press a bar for an ethanol reward in a traditional operant paradigm, they will self-administer ethanol via an intragastric catheter, and they will consume enough alcohol to be physically dependent (Waller et al. 1984). Current evidence indicates that the P rats consume ethanol for its pharmacological effects, apart from its caloric value (Waller et al. 1984).

P rats have lower levels of serotonin in several regions of the central nervous system (CNS) and lower levels of both dopamine and serotonin in the nucleus accumbens (NA) when compared with NP rats (Li et al. 1988). The potential significance of these neurochemical data is described in subsequent sections on the neurobiology of drug reinforcement.

Newer techniques of molecular biology have been applied recently to ethanol drinking preference paradigms. The application of quantitative trait loci (QTL) gene mapping studies in mice with different responses to ethanol (including ethanol reinforcement) has suggested the importance of 5-HT_{1B} receptors in the regulation of ethanol drinking. Crabbe and Phillips (1996) compared ethanol drinking in knockout mice lacking the 5-HT_{1B} receptor with wild-type mice. They reported that compared with the wild-type mice, the mutant mice drank twice as much ethanol, were less sensitive to the effects of ethanol, and developed tolerance more slowly.

Three behavioral paradigms have been developed to initiate alcohol consumption in animals not specifically bred for alcohol preference. Falk and colleagues (1972) induced high levels of alcohol consumption in rats by using schedule-induced polydipsia. Unfortunately, alcohol drinking in this paradigm does not appear to be related to the pharmacological effects of ethanol. The sucrose- or saccharine-fading technique pairs sweet taste with alcohol consumption to facilitate initiation of drinking in rats not bred for ethanol preference (Samson 1986). When a stable pattern of consumption has been attained with a 10% ethanol solution, the sweet taste is gradually withdrawn, but the high levels of alcohol consumption continue. In general, the sucrose- or saccharine-fading technique produces stable alcohol-drinking behavior and moderate blood alcohol levels. The persistent alcohol consumption appears to be related to the pharmacological effects of ethanol. Another technique that was designed to produce moderate blood alcohol levels is the limited access paradigm in which rats are exposed to alcohol for a limited time (20 minutes) in a novel environment during their light cycle. Blood alcohol levels of 80 mg% have been obtained with this procedure (Gill et al. 1986).

In general, the stability of alcohol-drinking behavior in some of these models permits the analysis of biological correlates of alcohol reinforcement in freely moving animals, as described in the next section. The biological correlates of alcohol reinforcement in these paradigms can now be compared with the mechanisms of stimulant and opiate reinforcement in intravenous drug self-administration paradigms. In addition, intracerebral drug and alcohol self-administration procedures have provided additional insights on brain mechanisms involved in drug and alcohol reinforcement, as is described later in this chapter.

CONDITIONED PLACE PREFERENCE PARADIGMS

Clinicians have long noted that abstinent patients are more likely to experience drug craving leading to relapse in settings or circumstances previously associated with drug use. Although this observation has been explained by several different models of conditioning (see next section), it is curious that these patients purposely reexpose themselves to these high-risk settings despite the contrary advice of their clinicians. It is almost as though the setting previously associated with drug use has been paired with the reinforcing properties of the drug through classical conditioning. In this context, the "place preference" demonstrated by the abstinent patient is a measure of the reinforcing potency of past drug experiences. Conditioned place preference paradigms in animals involve an initial determination of spontaneous place preference within a maze or open field. Drug injection is then paired with non-preferred locations in the maze or open field. By a process

of classical conditioning, the animal eventually prefers the setting in which drugs have been administered. Chronic administration of most abused drugs (alcohol, nicotine, cocaine, and phencyclidine) is associated with the development of conditioned place preference behavior. This paradigm is routinely used to screen medications under clinical development for possible abuse potential (for review, see Schecter et al. 1993). Place preference paradigms have also been useful in examining the effects of pharmacological treatments in blocking or enhancing the reinforcing properties of addictive drugs (e.g., Brown et al. 1991).

BRAIN STIMULATION REWARD PARADIGMS

Brain stimulation reward (BSR) paradigms build on the observation that animals will press a lever to obtain electrical stimulation in certain brain regions (Olds and Milner 1954). In 1957, Killam and colleagues reported that some substances of abuse increased the response rate for brain stimulation in an operant paradigm. They also suspected that amphetamine lowered the threshold of electrical current sufficient to reinforce BSR behavior. In general, the effects of drugs on BSR may vary as a function of whether the investigator is reporting changes in the rate of responding for BSR or changes in the threshold of electrical current that reinforces behavior in this paradigm. Moreover, different results may be accounted for by differences in site selection for electrode implantation. The median forebrain bundle (MFB) and the ventral tegmental area (VTA) are the most common sites for electrode placement, although self-stimulation behavior can be elicited from other regions of the brain.

Just as opiates and cocaine are more potent reinforcers than alcohol in drug self-administration paradigms, these drugs also more reliably increase the sensitivity of animals to rewarding electrical brain stimulation. This is manifest most clearly by a decrease in threshold of the electrical impulse required for reinforcement (Kornetsky and Porrino 1992). The effects of ethanol on BSR have been somewhat more problematic (e.g., Schaefer and Michael 1987 compared with DeWitte and Bada 1983). Bain and Kornetsky (1989) found that response rate increased and BSR threshold declined only when animals orally self-administered ethanol. Moolten and Kornetsky (1990) replicated this finding in comparing BSR results in animals who self-administered ethanol via intragastric catheter with yoked animals receiving ethanol via intragastric catheter in the same dose and time. Only self-administered ethanol reliably lowered BSR thresholds. Lewis (1991) found that low doses (but not higher doses) of ethanol given intraperitoneally reduced BSR thresholds in the ventral noradrenergic bundle (VNB) but not at electrodes placed in the lateral hypothalamus (LH). Kornetsky and colleagues placed electrodes in the MFB at the level of the LH. The low doses of ethanol administered by Lewis were comparable to doses self-administered by Kornetsky's group and produced motoric stimulation rather than the suppression of motor activity found at higher doses. Lewis's data are also compatible with the psychomotor stimulant theory of addiction proposed by Wise and Bozarth (1987; see next section).

BSR has been used in studies of combined opiate-stimulant administration to demonstrate more profound effects from the drug combination (regarding reinforcing potency) than from the individual drug alone (Kornetsky and Porrino 1992). BSR has also been used to study the persistent (anhedonic) state following cocaine and other stimulant withdrawal (see next section). Although cocaine or other stimulant administration produces a decrease in BSR threshold, the withdrawal state following stimulant administration is characterized by a substantial elevation in BSR threshold (Koob 1992a).

Finally, the BSR paradigm has been used to investigate the neurochemical basis for drug reinforcement. Kornetsky and Porrino (1992) reported that naloxone (a narcotic-blocking drug) appeared to block or attenuate the threshold-lowering effects of a variety of stimulants when naloxone was administered prior to the stimulant. A dose of 2–4 mg/kg of naloxone was required to achieve this effect, but doses as low as 0.25 mg/kg would block the threshold-lowering effects of morphine. They also reported that pimozide (0.15 mg/kg) blocked the threshold-lowering effects of 2.0 mg/kg of morphine. They concluded that "although the abused psychomotor stimulants and opioids have independent actions that contribute to their reinforcing effects, there are common neuronal substrates for some of the rewarding effects" (Kornetsky and Porrino 1992, p. 74).

Substantial evidence now links BSR mechanisms to dopamine systems. Moreover, most investigators would agree that mesolimbic dopamine neurons mediate the reinforcement characteristics of different classes of drugs of abuse but that other neurotransmitters and receptors play a significant role in the reinforcement properties of drugs such as opiates and alcohol.

CELLULAR AND MOLECULAR MECHANISMS OF DRUG- AND ALCOHOL-SEEKING BEHAVIOR

Given the identical behavioral criteria for substance dependence disorders across drug classes and the evidence of reinforcement associated with most cocaine, opiate, and ethanol self-administration in animals, researchers are interested in identifying the common cellular and molecular mechanisms that might account for drug-seeking and drug-consuming behaviors across drug classes. As expected, just as animal models of cocaine and opiate self-administration are clearer than the models of alcohol consumption discussed earlier in this chapter, the picture is a bit clearer for biological mechanisms of cocaine and opiate reinforcement than for mechanisms of alcohol reinforcement.

Neurobiology of Stimulant Reinforcement

In 1987, Wise and Bozarth proposed a theory of addiction based on the neurobiology of psychomotor stimulant reinforcement. They argued that

> all addictive drugs have psychomotor stimulant actions, that the stimulant actions of these different drugs have a shared biological mechanism, and that the biological mechanism of these stimulant actions is homologous with the biological mechanisms of positive reinforcement. (p. 469)

Wise and Bozarth built their model on the theory of reinforcement of Glickman and Schiff (1967), who observed that electrical stimulation of the MFB elicited approach behaviors and positive reinforcement. Wise and Bozarth argued that the increased locomotor activity results from activation of the dopaminergic cells of the VTA and substantia nigra and that reinforcement is mediated by effects on dopamine neurons in the VTA and NA.

The evidence for a primary role for dopamine neurons in the reinforcing properties of drugs is strongest in the case of cocaine and other stimulants. Cocaine binds to the dopamine transporter and effectively blocks dopamine reuptake (Ritz et al. 1987). "Knockout" mice, in which the gene for the dopamine transporter has been eliminated, lack sensitivity to the pharmacological effects of cocaine and other stimulants (Balter 1996). After lesioning of dopamine neurons in the NA or the VTA with 6-hydroxydopamine, drug-naive rats will not learn to self-administer stimulants, and stimulant drug self-administration will be extinguished (Roberts et al. 1980). Lesions of the caudate nucleus are relatively ineffective unless accompanied by damage to the NA.

Parenteral administration of dopamine receptor antagonists results in increased stimulant self-administration (Yokel and Wise 1975), much as lowering the dose or injection of amphetamine or cocaine results in increased lever pressing for the drug (see section, "Drug Self-Administration Behavior," earlier in this chapter). The model has been supported by data derived from in vivo microdialysis in the NA. Extracellular dopamine concentrations in this region are increased by intraperitoneally or intravenously self-administered cocaine and amphetamine (DiChiara and Imperato 1988; Weiss et al. 1992). All of these data, together with studies of BSR, strongly argue that dopamine neurons have a primary role in the biology of stimulant drug reinforcement.

Both D_1 and D_2 receptor subtypes have been implicated in cocaine reinforcement (Koob 1992b). Self and colleagues (1996) recently demonstrated an important dissociation between D_1- and D_2-like receptor processes in cocaine-seeking behavior. These investigators noted that activation of the mesolimbic dopamine system will trigger relapse in animal models of cocaine-seeking behavior. This priming effect, which can be elicited by low doses of a stimulant, was selectively induced in rats by D_2 receptor agonists but not by a D_1 receptor agonist. Moreover, the D_1 receptor agonist prevented cocaine-seeking behavior induced by cocaine itself, whereas D_2 receptor agonists enhanced this behavior. From a neuroanatomical perspective, Koob (1992a) noted the relative paucity of data regarding the efferent mechanisms through which dopamine neurons in NA may mediate positive reinforcement. Koob suggested that the connection between the NA and the substantia innominata–ventral pallidum may be important in this regard. He also suggested a role for the amygdala system as a mediator of drug reinforcement and reward. Dopaminergic mechanisms in the amygdala have been related to reinforcement (Caine et al. 1995; LeDoux 1987), and Bechara and colleagues (1995) recently confirmed the importance of this region to the acquisition of emotional conditioning in human beings. As described later in this chapter (see subsection, "Conditioning Models of Relapse"), conditioning mechanisms play a critical role in the transition from drug use to dependence.

In addition to a specific role for dopamine in the pharmacology of cocaine and other stimulants, studies suggest that the excitatory amino acid glutamate has a role in drug-related reinforcement and conditioning. Glutamatergic projections to both dopaminergic cell bodies and nerve terminals arise from the hippocampus, amygdala, and cortex (Almaric and Koob 1993; Brog et al. 1993; Fuller et al. 1987). Application of glutamatergic agonists to either dopaminergic cell bodies or nerve terminals has been shown to increase dopamine release (Imperato et al. 1990; Lonart and Zigmond 1991; Westerink et al. 1992; Youngren et al. 1993). Increases in the excitation of striatal neurons following stimulant administration have been attributed to activation of the descending corticostriatal glutamatergic pathway. Glutamate antagonists have been reported to alter the behavioral effects of acutely administered psychomotor stimulants, which suggests that stimulants may induce increases in extracellular excitatory amino acid levels (Freed and Cannon 1990; Kelley and Throne 1992; Pulvirenti et al. 1991; Supko et al. 1992; Tschanz et al. 1991; Witkin 1992). Because learning is an important component to the conditioning of drug effects and sensitization and because excitatory amino acids have been implicated in long-term potentiation (which is an important component in learning and memory), excitatory amino acids likely play some role in the conditioning process.

Karler and colleagues (1989) reported that systemic injections of MK-801 (a noncompetitive antagonist of *N*-methyl-D-aspartate [NMDA] receptors) blocked the development of sensitization to cocaine and amphetamine. Stewart and Druhan (1991) followed up on this work and found that MK-801 blocked the development of all conditioned amphetamine effects as well as morphine-induced tolerance. More study is needed to determine the role, if any, of drug-induced glutamate release in reinforcement, conditioned drug effects, tolerance, and sensitization.

Neurobiology of Opiate Reinforcement

It has been known for decades that opiates have primary reinforcing properties that are not dependent on the presence of physical dependence (Schuster and Villareal 1968). Bozarth and Wise (1984) demonstrated the neurobiology of this phenomenon in an apparently unequivocal manner. Drug-naive rats rapidly learned to press a lever for microinjections of morphine directly into the VTA. Naloxone challenges failed to elicit the signs of physical dependence in these rats after the morphine injections. Moreover, signs of withdrawal were not seen after long-term morphine infusion in the VTA but were observed after chronic infusion into the periventricular gray region. The data strongly indicate that the pathways mediating opiate reinforcement (e.g., the VTA) were independent of pathways mediating the signs of opiate withdrawal. Opiates act as reinforcers in not only the VTA but also the NA (Almaric and Koob 1985).

More recently, Koob (1992b) showed that chronic morphine administration results in sensitization of specific brain regions to the effects of direct injections of opiate antagonists. These regions include the NA and the locus coeruleus (LC). Direct placement of a narcotic antagonist in the NA in morphine-dependent rats results in the disruption of food-motivated behaviors and conditioned place aversion. The LC is sensitive to the acute effects of opiates (resulting in a suppression of LC activity), as well as to the effects of opiate withdrawal (characterized by a large increase in LC activity; clonidine suppresses LC activity and is used to treat opiate withdrawal). Thus, it is clear that some neurons are affected by the acute effects of opiates as well as by opiate withdrawal. The data are consistent with the view that although opiates will serve as reinforcers in the absence of physical dependence, the "motivation" for opiate self-administration is enhanced during opiate withdrawal.

Evidence indicates that opiate reinforcement involves activation of dopamine neurons but through a different mechanism than reinforcement associated with stimulant administration. As with stimulants, the parenteral administration of opiates results in an increase in extracellular dopamine concentrations in the NA, as measured by in vivo microdialysis (DiChiara and Imperato 1988; Weiss et al. 1992). However, although lesioning of dopamine neurons in the NA with 6-hydroxydopamine eliminates stimulant self-administration (as discussed earlier in this chapter in the section, "Neurobiology of Stimulant Reinforcement"), it does not eliminate opiate self-administration in rats (Koob and Bloom 1988). Opiates may increase the firing rate of dopamine neurons by activating μ-receptors in the VTA and NA producing local disinhibitory effects on the dopamine neurons. Naloxone blocks the effects of opiates on the VTA (Britt and Wise 1983). Koob (1992a) theorized that the downstream circuitry from the NA to the substantia innominata–ventral pallidum is important in opiate and stimulant reinforcement.

As was described earlier in this chapter, Wise and Bozarth (1987) postulated that the reinforcing properties of opiates are mediated by the same mechanisms mediating forward movement and reward for stimulants. For opiates and other depressant drugs, these motoric properties are manifest most clearly at low doses and subsequent to the development of tolerance to the depressant effects. In contrast to the development of tolerance to the depressant effects of opiates, chronic administration of these drugs results in increased sensitization to their reinforcing properties. Chronic cocaine administration is also characterized by the development of sensitization (reverse tolerance) to the reinforcing properties of the drug. Recent work suggests that chronic opiate and stimulant administration affects gene expression of guanine nucleotide binding proteins (G proteins) and the cyclic adenosine monophosphate (cAMP) system (see below). These changes in the molecular biology of second messenger function may be related to the development of sensitization to the reinforcing properties of opiates (and stimulants).

Neurobiology of Alcohol Reinforcement

Several lines of evidence suggest that opioid peptides, serotonin, dopamine, and GABA are all involved in alcohol reinforcement (Koob and Bloom 1988). Pharmacological probes in the context of animal models of ethanol self-administration represent one line of research. Alcohol self-administration increases in association with morphine, whereas narcotic antagonists decrease ethanol drinking (Reid and Hunter 1984). It is unclear whether the effects of narcotic antagonists on alcohol consumption are more or less specific to alcohol, because narcotic antagonists have a general inhibitory effect on consummatory behavior. Nevertheless, one immediate implication of this experimental work has been the testing of the narcotic antagonist naltrexone in alcohol-dependent human subjects; this drug was found to be a promising adjunct to behavioral relapse prevention treatment (O'Malley et al. 1992; Volpicelli et al. 1992).

P rats have a relative deficit of serotonin compared with NP rats (Murphy et al. 1982), and patients with alcoholism have a relative deficit of 5-hydroxyindoleacetic acid (5-HIAA, the principal metabolite of serotonin) in cerebrospinal fluid (CSF) (Ballenger et al. 1979). Low levels of CSF 5-HIAA have also been reported in one group of impulsive individuals who were at high risk for alcoholism (Linnoila et al. 1989). Alcohol increases 5-HIAA levels in the NA and other brain regions (suggesting a role for serotonin in alcohol reinforcement; Murphy et al. 1988). Serotonin uptake inhibitors reduce alcohol consumption in animal models and, to a modest degree, in heavy-drinking human subjects (see Naranjo et al. 1987). Paradoxically, the results of several serotonin depletion studies in animal models have not established a consistent finding (summarized by Weiss and Koob 1991). The serotonin story is obviously complex and may become clearer as a result of greater understanding of receptor subtypes and their function. Alcohol may differentially affect one or more receptor subtypes, as demonstrated by the work of Crabbe and Phillips (1996; described earlier in this chapter in the section, "Animal Models of Alcohol Self-Administration") in relation to the 5-HT$_{1B}$ receptor in the mouse.

A possible role for dopamine in the reinforcing properties of ethanol is suggested by studies of P rats compared with NP rats, by studies of the effects of dopamine receptor antagonists on alcohol consumption in one of the animal behavioral models (see section, "Animal Models of Alcohol Self-Administration," earlier in this chapter), and by in vivo microdialysis measures of dopamine and dopamine metabolites in the NA following alcohol administration. Murphy and colleagues (1982) reported lower levels of dopamine in the NA of P rats than in the NA of NP rats. Pfeffer and Samson (1988) reported that dopamine receptor antagonists reduce operant behavior for alcohol, as well as alcohol consumption, in rats studied in the sucrose-fading procedure. DiChiara and Imperato (1988) reported that intraperitoneal injections of alcohol produced an increase in extraneuronal concentrations of dopamine in the NA, which is similar to effects of injections of other drugs of abuse studied by these investigators.

Not all investigators have observed this effect of alcohol (Vavrousek-Jakuba et al. 1990). However, two groups of investigators found that alcohol *self*-administration results in increased extraneuronal dopamine levels in the NA (Vavrousek-Jakuba et al. 1990; Weiss et al. 1992). These results are remarkably similar to the findings of Kornetsky and Porrino (1992) on the effects of *self*-administered ethanol on BSR thresholds (described earlier in this chapter in the section, "Brain Stimulation Reward Paradigms"). Weiss and colleagues (1992) also found strain differences in dopamine release by self-administered ethanol. Although average ethanol intake and blood alcohol levels were equivalent in P rats compared with genetically heterogeneous Wistar rats, self-administered ethanol produced a significantly greater increase in dopamine release in the P rats than in the Wistar rats.

Finally, some clinical evidence indicates that alcohol is reinforcing in some individuals because of its anxiolytic and intoxicating effects (summarized by Meyer 1986a). A large amount of evidence suggests that the anxiolytic effects of alcohol are mediated through its effects on the benzodiazepine/GABA receptor. As is described later in this chapter (see section, "Evidence of Protracted Abstinence to Ethanol"), in vitro studies of synaptoneurosomes show that alcohol increases chloride flux through the ion channel that is the second messenger of this receptor. Although the mechanism of alcohol's effects is different from that for benzodiazepines, the net effect—increased chloride flux—is the same. P. D. Suzdak and colleagues (1986) reported that this effect of alcohol was blocked by the benzodiazepine partial inverse agonist Ro 15-4513. Of interest to studies on the neurobiology of alcohol reinforcement is the report of Samson and colleagues (1987) that Ro 15-4513 also produced a dose-dependent reduction in alcohol consumption in rats involved in the sucrose-fading procedure.

Summary of Neurobiology of Stimulant, Opiate, and Ethanol Reinforcement

The last decade has been marked by substantial progress in understanding the neurobiology of drug reinforcement.

Beginning with robust animal models of intravenous (and later with region-specific intracerebral) stimulant and opiate self-administration (plus several different pharmacogenetic and behavioral models of voluntary oral alcohol consumption), neurobiologists have used a range of techniques to describe the CNS events associated with drug-seeking and drug-consuming behavior. These techniques range from lesion studies to pharmacological challenge strategies, electrophysiological studies, and in vivo microdialysis methods. The data strongly support a major role for dopamine neurons in the NA in the neurobiology of drug and alcohol reinforcement. The types of changes that occur in the NA and its circuits that may account for the high risk of relapse after drug or alcohol withdrawal remain unclear. The high risk of relapse appears to be a problem that is composed of two distinct elements: a tendency to use again after a period of abstinence and (as described in ICD-10) the rapid reinstatement of the elements of the dependence syndrome following the reinitiation of use.

BIOBEHAVIORAL THEORIES OF RELAPSE AND RAPID REINSTATEMENT OF DEPENDENCE

Biobehavioral theories that have been invoked to explain relapse and rapid reinstatement of dependence can be grouped into two general categories: conditioning models and homeostatic (or neuroadaptive) models. Although conditioning models date back to Pavlov's (1926) work, they were developed most clearly by an American psychiatrist Abraham Wikler. Conditioning models posit that relapse into drug or alcohol use occurs in those environments or circumstances that have been associated with past drug or alcohol use as a function of Pavlovian conditioning (discussed later in this chapter in the section, "Conditioning Models of Relapse"). Homeostatic (neuroadaptive) models postulate that chronic substance use results in a perturbation of homeostatic mechanisms, such that the addicted individual requires continued use of the substance to maintain homeostasis. The latter model is most clearly valid in the context of acute opiate and alcohol withdrawal syndromes (in which the preferred drug reverses the symptoms and signs of withdrawal). However, the high rate of relapse to cocaine, opiate, and alcohol use in the first 3–6 months after withdrawal has suggested that deficient homeostasis is persistent. This has been called "protracted abstinence" (W. A. Martin and Jasinski 1969, p. 7). To some extent, both models postulate an antecedent subjective state (craving or desire) that serves as a trigger to drug-seeking behavior, in the same way that hunger serves as a trigger for eating. The models are not mutually exclusive; both may be important in conceptualizing new approaches to treatment (including pharmacotherapy).

Koob (1996) recently highlighted the important distinction between within-system and between-system neuroadaptation. The former relates to the effects of repeated drug administration (compared with acute drug administration) on the primary reinforcing neurochemical system, whereas between-system adaptations involve the recruitment of different neurochemical system(s) with repeated drug administration. Although much of the work on neuroadaptation has focused recently on molecular changes in the primary system(s) affected by repeated drug administration (see below), these within-system changes represent only a portion of the process of neuroadaptation associated with the development of substance dependence.

Robinson and Berridge (1993) hypothesized that one special type of neuroadaptation—sensitization—could account for the development of craving following repeated administration of cocaine and other drugs of abuse. These authors differentiated the "liking" (reinforcing) effects of drugs from the "wanting" effects. They postulated that with repeated administration, sensitization to the "wanting" effects occurs. The model also appears to link neuroadaptation with conditioning phenomena in that "wanting" effects are thought to result from associative learning mechanisms that link the environmental cues proximal to drug reinforcing events with drug reinforcement. In this context, the environmental cues become conditioned reinforcers and acquire incentive motivational properties (see next subsection). Paradoxically, as tolerance develops to the acute pharmacological effects of opiates, stimulants, or alcohol, subjective awareness of "wanting" increases as a consequence of sensitization (Robinson and Berridge 1993). As proposed, the model developed by Robinson and Berridge would appear to agree with the between-system adaptation cited by Koob; however, as described later in this section, the "wanting" effects are probably mediated by dopamine release.

Conditioning Models of Relapse

Wikler first proposed a conditioning model to explain heroin addiction in 1948. He tested the model in studies of addicted persons incarcerated at the Addiction Research Center in Lexington, Kentucky, and in experiments in animal models of addicted behavior (Wikler and Pescor 1967; Wikler et al. 1963, 1971). Because Wikler viewed the development of physical dependence as the defining stage of opiate addiction, he believed that, by a process of Pavlovian conditioning, the symptoms and signs of withdrawal (the unconditioned stimulus) are paired with environmental stimuli in the addicted person's home community. Over time, these stimuli elicit withdrawal symptoms that result in relapse to heroin use, when a drug-free individual returns home after incarceration. Subsequently, Wikler postulated that environmental stimuli could elicit "counteradaptive interoceptive responses" (p. 18)—mirror opposites of the effects of opiates—as individuals anticipated the administration of heroin (Wikler 1974). O'Brien and colleagues (1977) confirmed the conditioning of opiate withdrawal symptoms in human subjects, whereas Siegel demonstrated a role for opponent process conditioning in the development of tolerance (summarized by Siegel et al. 1987). Ludwig and Wikler (1974) extended Wikler's theoretical approach to explain relapse to alcohol addiction by linking craving for alcohol by alcoholic patients to conditioned withdrawal symptoms.

In addition to evidence of conditioning of the signs and symptoms of abstinence and of opponent process conditioning, there has long been evidence of conditioning of drug effects. Pavlov first noted conditioning of morphine's effects in dogs in 1926. Conditioned place preference represents a behavioral example of the conditioning of the rewarding properties of stimulants, opiates, and alcohol. Meyer and Mirin (1979) reported evidence of conditioned heroin-like effects in individuals who continued to self-administer heroin (despite pharmacologically effective narcotic blockade) as long as the subjects experienced conditioned opiate-like effects. These investigators also observed that craving for heroin was highest while subjects anticipated and experienced the conditioned or unconditioned effects of heroin (a priming effect). Priming effects have also been observed in alcoholic individuals (Hodgson et al. 1979; Kaplan et al. 1983; Laberg 1986), and conditioned drug–like effects have been observed in cocaine-dependent subjects and in cocaine-dependent rats (O'Brien et al. 1992).

Stewart and colleagues (1984) postulated that conditioned drug–like effects are responsible for relapse. Their model is consistent with the priming effects of low doses of a preferred drug, as well as with data on sensitization that suggest enhanced reinforcing effects only when repeated drug use occurs in the same environmental setting (Stewart 1992; Stewart and Vezina 1988). Post and colleagues (1992) termed this *context-dependent sensitization*. Their research group used in vivo microdialysis and observed significantly increased dopamine release in the NA in animals given cocaine who had previously received this drug in the same environment compared with control animals exposed to the same amount of cocaine in a different setting.

Shippenberg and colleagues (1992) also presented evidence from lesioning studies that the mesolimbic dopamine system is important for the conditioned reinforcing effects of opiates (conditioned place preference). Increased locomotor activity associated with reinforcement has also been linked to the dopaminergic system. When cocaine or morphine injections are repeatedly paired with specific environmental stimuli, increased locomotor activity occurs when these stimuli are present (i.e., in the absence of drug injections; Stewart 1992)—another example of conditioned drug–like effects.

Two studies using different methods to assess dopamine release in the NA reported increased dopamine levels in association with *anticipated* voluntary alcohol consumption in rats (Vavrousek-Jakuba et al. 1990; Weiss et al. 1992). Parsons et al. (1996) found that stimuli associated with cocaine administration resulted in increased dopamine release in the NA and central amygdala, as measured by in vivo microdialysis. Indeed, after a period of 24 days during which animals were not exposed to the cocaine injections or associated stimuli, reexposure to the cocaine-associated stimuli for 1 hour resulted in continued responding to saline injections. The behavior continued for a period of 14 days (1 hour/day) despite the absence of the primary reinforcer (cocaine).

As may be clear from the preceding sections, the literature on the behavioral neurobiology of drug-related reinforcement was framed by Skinnerian models of learning, which posited that behavior is shaped by its consequences. The emerging literature is shifting the focus from reward to anticipation. By using techniques of in vivo voltammetry, Phillips and colleagues (1993; Blackburn et al. 1992; Fibiger and Phillips 1986) showed that dopamine release in the VTA and NA may occur prior to the delivery of a novel reward associated with "hardwired" appetites. For example, sexually naive male rats manifest increased dopamine levels in the NA, as measured by in vivo voltammetry, when they are exposed to the odor of female rats in estrus.

According to Montague et al. (1996), the totality of related functions of mesencephalic dopamine neurons (including their influence on synaptic plasticity) accounts for their critical role in the development of addictive behaviors. These neurons participate in motivational processes, reward processing, working memory, and conditioned behavior (Montague et al. 1996). Montague et al. (1996) postulated that a drug such as cocaine, which profoundly increases dopamine levels following acute administration,

will dramatically affect the power of sensory cues (associated with drug administration) to elicit dopamine release. "The model suggests that rather than reflecting direct pharmacological effects, the physiological and behavioral effects that attend drug taking or drug removal may relate in a complicated manner to learning effects that are slow to reverse or to accrue" (p. 1944).

Physiological recordings from alert monkeys indicate that midbrain dopamine neurons respond to food and fluid rewards, novel stimuli, conditioned stimuli, and stimuli eliciting a behavioral reaction (Schultz 1993). Once a task has been learned, the response pattern of these cells shifts from the delivery of the reward to the onset of the stimulus that had signaled the reward.

Gratton (1996) recently noted that "the increases in NA dopamine transmission" in the presence of cocaine- or opiate-related stimuli in monkeys trained to self-administer these drugs "would not have been predicted by simple opponent process conditioning models, nor do they conform to the notion that the motivation to self-administer more drug increases as a function of declining DA levels in NA" (p. 275). Indeed, Gratton (1996) reported that in all but the first few self-administered drug injections, phasic increases in dopamine release were observed during the anticipatory state and not in response to the receipt of the drug injection. In essence, once a pattern of drug self-administration has been learned, it is incorrect to state that the reinforcing properties of the drug are related to dopamine release in the VTA or NA (Gratton 1996).

The newly emerging literature on the neurobiology of anticipatory states appears to challenge the traditional Skinnerian view of drug dependence, because the anticipatory state has greater salience than the actual reward. The data are consistent with the concept that repeated drug administration is associated with "sensitization to the wanting effects of the drugs" (Robinson and Berridge 1993, p. 288). Indeed, the finding of Cador and colleagues (1992) that stress shows cross-sensitization with amphetamine raises interesting questions on differential vulnerability to drug dependence and/or risk of relapse as a consequence of exposure to antecedent stress. The exposure to stress may amplify the initial effects of stimulants by a process of cross-sensitization, just as environmental stimuli associated with previous episodes of drug use may contribute to sensitization and the risk of relapse.

Finally, the animal literature prompts new questions on the relevance of "cue reactivity" studies in human subjects, which have been based on conditioning models of addictive behavior. Until recently, conditioning models of addiction have been most useful in conceptualizing clinical approaches to relapse prevention. Clinicians have used cue exposure techniques in an attempt to extinguish drug-related responses (e.g., Childress et al. 1988). Some investigators have utilized the cue responsivity of cocaine-dependent individuals to screen for new anticraving medications. The results have been inconsistent (Dackis et al. 1987; Kranzler and Bauer 1992; Margolin et al. 1991; Robbins et al. 1992).

Meyer (1988) reported that in the absence of the opportunity to consume an alcoholic beverage, only 50% of alcohol-dependent patients reliably manifested autonomic arousal and increased craving in response to the olfactory, visual, and tactile stimuli of their favorite beverage. Results from cue reactivity studies in humans, coupled with the recent animal literature on the dopamine system response associated with anticipatory states, raise questions about the validity of cue exposure studies in relatively unfamiliar laboratory environments in which the subject is aware that drugs will not be administered. On the other hand, one of us (S. P. B.) found that exposure of cocaine-dependent subjects to cocaine cues (paraphernalia and a videotape depicting "crack" cocaine use) significantly increased plasma levels of homovanillic acid (HVA, a dopamine metabolite believed to reflect CNS dopamine release). Furthermore, haloperidol pretreatment (4 mg orally) in a single-dose, double-blind, crossover design significantly decreased cue-induced cocaine craving and anxiety (Berger et al. 1996). Whether better tolerated medications that interfere with the dopamine release associated with a cocaine anticipatory state would have any value in promoting abstinence remains to be determined.

Persistent Alterations in Homeostasis and Risk of Relapse

Relapse into heroin, cocaine, and alcohol addiction is most likely to occur in the first 3–6 months of abstinence (e.g., see Meyer 1989), a period that may be characterized by physiological abnormalities, mood dysregulation, and a variety of somatic symptoms theoretically linked to the relapse. Meyer (1989) and Kreek (1992b) suggested that the signs and symptoms of protracted abstinence represent potential targets for pharmacotherapy in the treatment of addiction. The construct should also be useful in applying the tools of molecular neurobiology to relevant animal models of drug or alcohol dependence.

Evidence of protracted abstinence to opiates.
W. A. Martin and Jasinski (1969) described persistent abnormalities in vital signs and neuroendocrine function in heroin-addicted subjects who had been detoxified and had been hospitalized at the Addiction Research Center in Lexington, Kentucky, for 6 months or longer. Prior to the discovery of opiate receptors and endogenous opioid peptides, Dole and Nyswander (1965) postulated that patients addicted to heroin required steady doses of an exogenous opioid to feel "normal." In formulating the rationale for methadone maintenance treatment of heroin addiction, these investigators postulated that, by analogy, methadone was the insulin of those addicted to heroin.

Kreek and colleagues (summarized in Kreek 1992b) assessed hypothalamic-pituitary reserve by administering a metyrapone challenge test in patients receiving methadone maintenance therapy, in drug-free heroin-addicted individuals during protracted withdrawal, and in control subjects. Metyrapone blocks the final step in the biosynthesis of cortisol in the adrenal cortex and results in increased plasma levels of adrenocorticotropic hormone (ACTH) and β-endorphin. Patients undergoing long-term methadone maintenance were indistinguishable from healthy volunteer subjects. Hyperresponsivity to the metyrapone injection was observed in formerly addicted individuals who were undergoing protracted abstinence (greater than normal increase in ACTH and β-endorphin levels). Opiate administration produced hyporesponsiveness to metyrapone. Subjects taking chronic high doses of methadone were tolerant to this effect.

With the discovery of opiate receptors and endogenous opioid peptides, it was anticipated that the development of tolerance and/or physical dependence would be reflected in changes in receptor binding or measurable changes in peptide levels. Although it is now clear that β-endorphin is the most potent ligand for the μ-receptor (which is associated with the reinforcing properties of opiate drugs), tolerance and physical dependence are not clearly associated with changes in receptor binding or total β-endorphin levels. Tolerance and physical dependence may be mediated by more than one neurotransmitter, and chronic opiate administration may affect gene expression of receptor-related structure and/or function.

Bronstein and colleagues (1990) reported that pro-opiomelanocortin (POMC) messenger ribonucleic acid (mRNA) levels decline with chronic morphine treatment. Because POMC yields several biologically active peptides, including β-endorphin, ACTH, melanocyte-stimulating hormone (MSH), and β-lipotropin, morphine may affect the biosynthesis of β-endorphin. The authors also reported that chronic morphine treatment appears to result in preferential production of β-endorphin 1-27 (which functions as an antagonist at the μ-receptor) relative to β-endorphin 1-31 (which functions as an agonist at the μ-receptor). Acute stress also favors the production of β-endorphin

1-27 relative to β-endorphin 1-31. Chronic treatment with naltrexone increases the mRNA for POMC and results in an increase in β-endorphin 1-31 relative to β-endorphin 1-27. The work suggests that the POMC system is quite sensitive to the effects of exogenous opiates as well as to acute stress. It would be useful to examine not only this system in the context of protracted withdrawal but also protracted withdrawal in the context of acute stress.

Chronic opiate treatment produces regionally specific changes in gene expression of several second messenger functions in the brain that are associated with the reinforcing effects of opiates (Beitner-Johnson et al. 1992). Taken together, these changes should result in decreased dopamine synthesis in NA (a prediction that is confirmed by in vivo microdialysis) (Acqua et al. 1992; Brock et al. 1990) and altered D_1 receptor function. Chronic morphine treatment results in a decrease in the phosphorylation state of tyrosine hydroxylase (the rate-limiting enzyme in the synthesis of dopamine) in the NA (Beitner-Johnson et al. 1992); thus, functional activity of the enzyme is decreased in the NA, whereas upregulation (and increased phosphorylation) of the enzyme occurs in the VTA. Chronic morphine treatment also results in a decrease in neurofilament (NF) proteins in dopamine neurons in the VTA (Beitner-Johnson et al. 1992). These effects are regionally specific. The NF proteins are a major component of the cytoskeleton. Chronic morphine treatment may alter the structural features of mesolimbic dopamine neurons, which reduces their ability to transmit dopamine signals to postsynaptic cells in the NA. The D_1 receptor, which uses cAMP as a second messenger, is also affected by chronic morphine treatment (Beitner-Johnson et al. 1992). Levels of G_i protein (the protein that inhibits adenylate cyclase) decrease, and levels of adenylate cyclase and cAMP-dependent protein kinase increase. Identical regionally specific changes in dopamine function occur with chronic cocaine administration (see section, "Evidence of Protracted Abstinence to Cocaine," below). Beitner-Johnson et al. (1992) postulated that these changes could result in impairment of the brain's endogenous reward system, with implications for motivation and affect in humans.

The LC is an important mediator of physical dependence on opiates. Nestler and associates (1989; Duman et al. 1988) reported that chronic morphine treatment results in upregulation of the intracellular cAMP system at multiple levels in the LC. Levels of G_i and G_o proteins (alpha subunits), adenylate cyclase, and cAMP-dependent protein kinase increase, and several phosphoprotein substrates for the protein kinase in this region also increase. Given the location of these changes, the upregulation of the adenylate cyclase system may play a role in the development of tolerance and physical dependence, as reflected in the activity of the LC neurons. Whether the specific changes in second messenger function in the LC and the mesolimbic dopamine system persist beyond the period of chronic opiate administration to account for some of the signs and symptoms of protracted abstinence remains to be determined.

Evidence of protracted abstinence to cocaine. In 1986, Gawin and Kleber described the stages and elements of a cocaine abstinence syndrome in a cohort of outpatients in treatment at Yale University. Phase 1 (9 hours to 4 days after the last dose of cocaine) was marked by progression from agitation, depression, anorexia, and high levels of cocaine craving to a later stage of fatigue, exhaustion, hypersomnia, hyperphagia, and the absence of cocaine craving. Phase 2 (1–10 weeks after the last dose of cocaine) was characterized in the first weeks by normal sleep, euthymic mood, low levels of cocaine craving, and low levels of anxiety, with anhedonia, anergia, anxiety, high levels of cocaine craving, and high levels of conditioned craving occurring episodically over the next 2 months. Following this period of protracted abstinence, subjects still had episodic craving and craving in response to specific environmental cues associated with past drug use. The specificity of the stages of cocaine withdrawal has not been confirmed by others (e.g., Weddington et al. 1990).

At present, apart from the acute symptom complex of exhaustion and hyperphagia immediately following binge use of cocaine, there is a relative paucity of data that point clearly to a period of persistent homeostatic dysregulation characteristic of protracted opiate and alcohol withdrawal. Indeed, acute intravenous injections of cocaine produced dose-dependent increases in plasma cortisol concentrations (Wilkins et al. 1992), whereas plasma cortisol levels remained normal across 4 weeks of inpatient care in cocaine-dependent male patients (Mendelson et al. 1988). Kreek (1992a) reported preliminary findings suggesting some abnormalities in hypothalamic-pituitary-adrenal (HPA) function in recently abstinent cocaine-abusing patients. However, systematic studies of HPA function using newer challenge strategies (metyrapone or corticotropin-releasing factor [CRF]) have not been done in recently detoxified cocaine-dependent patients. Reports of persistent hyperprolactinemia following cocaine withdrawal (Teoh et al. 1990) have not been confirmed by some investigators (Swartz et al. 1990).

Positron-emission tomography (PET) studies of cerebral metabolism suggest that acute cocaine administration results in a decrease in glucose metabolism, especially in

when the organism is drug- or alcohol-free. Evidence of residual dysfunction is most apparent in association with acute opiate and alcohol withdrawal syndromes. In this situation, homeostasis is restored by drug substitution and controlled detoxification. At another level, abnormalities of GABA and NMDA receptor sensitivity are most evident during chronic administration and acute withdrawal of ethanol. At present, the strongest evidence of persistent deficits in homeostasis in alcoholic patients comes from clinical studies. Further work is needed to identify persistent residual abnormalities in receptor function that may suggest appropriate pharmacotherapies. In this context, the collection of symptoms and signs of protracted abstinence in alcoholic patients offers an inviting target for clinical trials.

SUMMARY AND POSTSCRIPT

Current diagnostic criteria for opiate, stimulant, and alcohol dependence disorders have a high degree of reliability. The development of homologous animal models of opiate and stimulant drug dependence, plus some promising animal behavioral and pharmacogenetic models of alcohol consumption, add the potential dimension of validity to the criteria for these human disorders. The greatest progress on the biology of opiate, stimulant, and alcohol dependence has been made recently. Building on highly reliable behavioral models, new techniques in neurobiology have enabled investigators to clarify the CNS correlates of drug reinforcement. Much evidence points to the dopamine neurons of the NA and VTA. Although these neurons may form a "final common pathway" for drug reinforcement, the effects of different drug classes on these neurons clearly result from different mechanisms. The significance of the findings on the neurobiology of the acute reinforcing properties of abusable drugs cannot be overstated.

More recently, neurobiologists have begun to take on the challenge of defining the neurobiological correlates of some of the most important clinical phenomena associated with the dependence syndromes: the tendency to use again after a period of abstinence and the rapid reinstatement of the symptoms of the dependence syndrome once drug use has resumed. Two constructs are highlighted in the clinical literature: the role of conditioned cue responsiveness in relapse and the importance of persistent homeostatic dysregulation after drug and alcohol withdrawal (protracted abstinence).

Since the publication of the previous edition of this volume, neurobiologists have begun to unravel the basis of anticipatory states with specific relevance to craving for dependence-producing drugs. This literature is beginning to form a bridge between conditioning and neuroadaptation—particularly in models related to sensitization. The mesolimbic dopamine system plays a critical role in the development of dependence through its effects on working memory, motivational processes, mechanisms of reinforcement, and conditioned behavior. At some point in the dependence process, the reward salience of the environmental stimuli supersedes the importance of the reward stimulus. This probably represents both within- and between-system neurochemical adaptations within the CNS. In the near term, the findings are changing our models of addiction from behavioral (operant) psychology to cellular and molecular models that will become more syntonic with evolving biological models of emotional learning. At the same time, the growing literature on neuroadaptation has become more molecular based. If chronic exposure to opiates, cocaine, and alcohol results in changes in gene expression affecting receptor function in behaviorally relevant brain regions, then the clinical reports of patients in treatment (who argue that they "feel normal" when taking their drug of choice) seem more compelling. Neurobiologists would make a major contribution to clinicians if they defined the duration of these changes in gene expression affecting receptor function. Are these changes permanent? Do they respond to acute or chronic treatment with receptor antagonists or other drugs that may modify neurotransmitter, receptor, or second messenger function? Clinical investigators must describe the symptoms and signs of persistent homeostatic dysregulation more precisely to identify potential targets for pharmacotherapy. This need is particularly great for cocaine and stimulant dependence, in which the case for protracted abstinence has been less well developed than that for alcohol or opiates.

Finally, neurobiologists have begun to examine the question of individual and strain differences in vulnerability to drug and alcohol dependence in animal models in order to identify potential risk and/or protective factors that might generalize to human populations (in which individual differences are quite significant). Because pharmacogenetic differences in ethanol preference have been significant in developing animal models of alcohol consumption, much more progress has been made in comparing specific neurobiological characteristics of P and NP rats. The issue of individual or strain differences in the reinforcing potency of opiates and cocaine was not explored until relatively recently. Of special interest is the report by Beitner-Johnson et al. (1992) comparing the characteristics of mesolimbic dopamine neurons in Lewis and Fischer rats. Lewis rats develop greater degrees of conditioned place preference to parenteral morphine and cocaine compared with Fischer rats. The differences in the molecular neurobiology of mesolimbic dopamine neurons in drug-naive Lewis rats compared with Fischer rats resembled the differences between chronic morphine-treated and chronic cocaine-treated outbred Sprague-Dawley rats (compared with control animals). This study suggests that some aspects of vulnerability may be genetically determined.

Other investigators have observed that stress sensitizes rats to the reinforcing properties of stimulants (and vice versa) in a process that appears to involve CRF and the HPA axis (Cador et al. 1992). Monkeys reared in isolation spontaneously drink much greater quantities of ethanol than monkeys reared in a normal environment in proximity to their biological mothers (Higley et al. 1991). Environmental factors can seemingly affect gene expression related to CNS function. Over the next few years, neuroscientists will apply tools of increasing sophistication to tease apart the genetic and environmental factors that may contribute to the development of drug and alcohol dependence in homologous animal models of these well-characterized human disorders. As a result of this research, it is highly likely that clinicians will eventually have the tools to offer more effective programs of treatment and prevention.

REFERENCES

Acqua E, Carboni E, DiChiara G: Profound depression of mesolimbic dopamine release after morphine withdrawal in dependent rats. Eur J Pharmacol 193:133–134, 1992

Almaric M, Koob GF: Low doses of methylnaloxonium in the nucleus accumbens antagonize hyperactivity induced by heroin in the rat. Pharmacol Biochem Behav 23:411–415, 1985

Almaric M, Koob GF: Functionally selective neurochemical afferents and efferents of the mesocorticolimbic and nigrostriatal dopamine system. Prog Brain Res 99:209–226, 1993

American Psychiatric Association: Diagnostic and Statistical Manual of Mental Disorders, 3rd Edition. Washington, DC, American Psychiatric Association, 1980

American Psychiatric Association: Diagnostic and Statistical Manual of Mental Disorders, 3rd Edition, Revised. Washington, DC, American Psychiatric Association, 1987

American Psychiatric Association: Diagnostic and Statistical Manual of Mental Disorders, 4th Edition. Washington, DC, American Psychiatric Association, 1994

Babor TF, Wolfson A, Boivin D, et al: Alcoholism, culture and psychopathology: a comparative study of French, French Canadian, and American alcoholics, in Alcoholism in North America, Europe, and Asia. Edited by Helzer JE, Canino GH. New York, Oxford University Press, 1992, pp 182–195

Bain GT, Kornetsky C: Ethanol oral self-administration and rewarding brain stimulation. Alcohol 6:499–503, 1989

Ballenger J, Goodwin F, Major L, et al: Alcohol and central serotonin metabolism in man. Arch Gen Psychiatry 36:224–227, 1979

Balter M: New clues to brain dopamine control, cocaine addiction. Science 271:909–911, 1996

Bauer LO: Psychomotor and EEG sequelae of cocaine dependence, in Neurotoxicity and Neuropathology Associated With Cocaine Abuse (NIDA Research Monograph 163). Edited by Majewska MD. Washington, DC, U.S. Government Printing Office, 1996, pp 66–93

Bechara A, Tranel D, Damasio H, et al: Double dissociation of conditioning and declarative knowledge relative to the amygdala and hippocampus in humans. Science 269:1115–1118, 1995

Becker HT, Kaplan RF: Neurophysiological and neuropsychological concomitance of brain dysfunction in alcoholics, in Psychopathology and Addictive Disorders. Edited by Meyer RE. New York, Guilford, 1986, pp 262–292

Begleiter H, Porjesz B: Persistence of brain hyperexcitability following chronic alcoholic exposure in rats. Adv Exp Med Biol 85:209–222, 1977

Begleiter H, DeNoble V, Porjesz B: Protracted brain dysfunction after alcohol withdrawal in monkeys, in Biological Effects of Alcohol. Edited by Begleiter H. New York, Plenum, 1980, pp 231–239

Begleiter H, Porjesz B, Bihari B, et al: Event-related brain potentials in sons of alcoholic fathers. Alcohol Clin Exp Res 7:1493–1496, 1984

Beitner-Johnson D, Guitart X, Nestler EJ: Common intracellular actions of chronic morphine and cocaine in dopaminergic brain reward regions, in The Neurobiology of Drug and Alcohol Addiction. Edited by Kalivas PW, Sampson HH. New York, New York Academy of Sciences, 1992, pp 70–87

Berger SP, Hall S, Mickalian JD, et al: Haloperidol antagonism of cue-elicited cocaine craving. Lancet 347:504–508, 1996

Blackburn JR, Pfaus JC, Phillips AG: Dopamine function in appetitive and defensive behaviors. Prog Neurobiol 39:247–279, 1992

Bozarth MA, Wise RA: Anatomically distinct opiate receptor fields mediate reward and physical dependence. Science 224:516–517, 1984

Britt MD, Wise RA: Ventral tegmental site of opiate reward: antagonism by a hydrophilic opiate receptor blocker. Brain Res 258:105–108, 1983

Brock JW, Ng JP, Justice JB Jr: Effect of chronic cocaine on dopamine synthesis in the nucleus accumbens as determined by microdialysis with NSD-1015. Neurosci Lett 117:234–239, 1990

Brog JS, Salyapongse A, Deutch AY, et al: The patterns of afferent innervation of the core and shell in the "accumbens" part of the rat ventral striatum: immunohistochemical detection of retrogradely transported fluoro-gold. J Comp Neurol 338:255–278, 1993

Bronstein DM, Prezewlocki R, Akil H: Effects of morphine treatment on pro-opiomelanocortin systems in rat brain. Brain Res 519:102–111, 1990

Brown EE, Finlay JM, Wong JP, et al: Behavioral and neurochemical interactions between cocaine and buprenorphine: implications for the pharmacotherapy of cocaine abuse. J Pharmacol Exp Ther 256:119–126, 1991

Buck KJ, Harris RA: Benzodiazepine agonist and inverse agonist actions on GABAa receptor-operated chloride channels, I: acute effects of ethanol. J Pharmacol Exp Ther 253:706–712, 1990a

Buck KJ, Harris RA: Benzodiazepine agonist and inverse agonist actions on GABAa receptor-operated chloride channels, II: chronic effects of ethanol. J Pharmacol Exp Ther 253:713–719, 1990b

Cador M, Dumas S, Cole BJ, et al: Behavioral sensitization induced by psychostimulants or stress: search for a molecular basis and evidence for a CRF dependent phenomenon, in The Neurobiology of Drug and Alcohol Addiction. Edited by Kalivas PW, Samson HH. New York, New York Academy of Sciences, 1992, pp 416–420

Caine SB, Heinrichs SC, Coffin VL, et al: Effects of the dopamine D-1 antagonist SCH 23390 microinjected into the accumbens, amygdala or striatum on cocaine self-administration in the rat. Brain Res 692:47–56, 1995

Carlin PL, Wortzman G, Holgate RC, et al: Reversible cerebral atrophy in recently abstinent chronic alcoholics measured by computerized tomography scans. Science 200:1076–1078, 1978

Childress AR, McLellan AT, Ehrman R, et al: Classically conditioned responses in opioid and cocaine dependence: a role in relapse, in Learning Factors in Substance Abuse (DHHS Publ No ADM-88-1576). Edited by Ray BA. Rockville, MD, Alcohol, Drug Abuse and Mental Health Administration, 1988, pp 25–43

Cloninger CR, Bohman M, Sigvardsson S: Inheritance of alcohol abuse: cross-fostering analysis of adopted men. Arch Gen Psychiatry 38:861–868, 1981

Cotton NS: The familial incidence of alcoholism: a review. J Stud Alcohol 40:89–116, 1979

Crabbe JC, Phillips TJ: The serotonin 5-HT 1B receptor: a QTL for alcohol preference drinking. Paper presented at the annual meeting of the American College of Neuropsychopharmacology, San Juan, Puerto Rico, December 1996

Dackis CA, Gold MS, Sweeney DR, et al: Single-dose bromocriptine reverses cocaine craving. Psychiatry Res 20:261–264, 1987

Deneau G, Yanagita T, Seavers MH: Self administration of psychoactive substances by the monkey: a measure of psychological dependence. Psychopharmacologia 16:30–48, 1969

DeWitte P, Bada MF: Self-stimulation and alcohol administered orally or intraperitoneally. Exp Neurol 8:675–682, 1983

DiChiara G, Imperato A: Drugs abused by humans preferentially increase synaptic dopamine concentrations in the mesolimbic system of freely moving rats. Proc Natl Acad Sci U S A 85:5274–5278, 1988

Dole VP, Nyswander ME: A medical treatment for diacetylmorphine (heroin) addiction. JAMA 193:646–650, 1965

Dolin S, Little H, Hudspith M: Increased dihydropyridine-sensitive calcium channels in rat brain may underlie ethanol physical dependence. Neuropharmacology 26:275–279, 1987

Duman RS, Tallman JF, Nestler EJ: Acute and chronic opiate-regulation of adenylate cyclase in brain: specific effects in locus ceruleus. J Pharmacol Exp Ther 246:1033–1039, 1988

Eriksson K: Rat strains specially selected for their voluntary alcohol consumption. Annals of Medicine and Experimental Biology Finland 49:67–72, 1971

Erwin CW, Linnoila M, Hartwell J: Effects of buspirone and diazepam, alone and in combination with alcohol, on skill performance and evoked potentials. J Clin Psychopharmacol 6:199–209, 1986

Falk JL, Samson HH, Winger G: Behavioral maintenance of high concentrations of blood-ethanol and physical dependence in the rat. Science 177:811–813, 1972

Fibiger HC, Phillips AG: Reward, motivation, cognition: psychobiology of mesotelencephalic dopamine systems, in Handbook of Physiology: The Nervous System, Vol 4. Edited by Plum F. Bethesda, MD, American Physiological Society, 1986, pp 647–675

Fitzgerald LW, Nestler EJ: Molecular and cellular adaptations in signal transduction pathways following ethanol exposure. Clinical Neuroscience 3:165–174, 1995

Freed WJ, Cannon SH: A possible role for AA2 excitatory amino acid receptors in the expression of stimulant drug effects. Psychopharmacology (Berl) 101:456–464, 1990

Fuller TA, Russchen FT, Price JL: Sources of presumptive glutamatergic/aspartergic afferents to the rat ventral striatopallidal region. J Comp Neurol 258:317–338, 1987

Gawin FH, Kleber HD: Abstinence symptomatology and psychiatric diagnosis in cocaine abusers. Arch Gen Psychiatry 43:107–113, 1986

Gill K, France C, Amit Z: Voluntary ethanol consumption in rats: an examination of blood/brain ethanol levels and behavior. Alcohol Clin Exp Res 10:457–462, 1986

Gillin JC, Smith TL, Irwin M: EEG sleep studies in "pure" primary alcoholism during sub acute withdrawal: relationships to normal controls, age, and other clinical variables. Biol Psychiatry 27:477–488, 1990

Glickman SE, Schiff BB: A biological theory of reinforcement. Psychol Rev 74:81–109, 1967

Grant KA, Lovinger DM: Cellular and behavioral neurobiology of alcohol: receptor mediated neuronal processes. Clinical Neuroscience 3:155–164, 1995

Grant KA, Valverius P, Hudspith M: Ethanol withdrawal seizures and NMDA receptor complex. Eur J Pharmacol 176:289–296, 1990

Gratton A: In vivo analysis of the role of dopamine in stimulant and opiate self administration. J Psychiatry Neurosci 21:264–279, 1996

Helzer JE, Canino GJ, Yeh E, et al: Alcoholism—North America and Asia: a comparison of population surveys with the Diagnostic Interview Schedule. Arch Gen Psychiatry 47:313–319, 1990

Herning RI, Glover BJ, Guo X, et al: Excessive EEG fast activity in cocaine abusers: pharmacological interventions. Paper presented at the annual meeting of the American College of Psychopharmacology, San Juan, Puerto Rico, December 1992

Hesselbrock V, Hesselbrock MN, Workman-Daniels KL: The effect of major depression and antisocial personality disorder on alcoholism: course and motivational patterns. J Stud Alcohol 47:207–212, 1986

Higley JD, Hasert MF, Suomi SJ, et al: Nonhuman primate model of alcohol abuse: effects of early experience, personality, and stress on alcohol consumption. Proc Natl Acad Sci U S A 88:7261–7265, 1991

Hodgson R, Rankin H, Stockwell T: Alcohol dependence and the priming effect. Journal of Behavioral Research and Therapy 17:379–387, 1979

Imperato A, Honore T, Jensen LH: Dopamine release in the nucleus caudatus and in the nucleus accumbens is under glutamatergic control through non-NMDA receptors: a study in freely moving rats [published erratum appears in Brain Res 539:179, 1991]. Brain Res 530:223–228, 1990

Jones RT: What have we learned from nicotine, cocaine, and marijuana about addiction? in Addictive States. Edited by O'Brien CP, Chaffe JH. New York, Raven, 1992, pp 109–122

Kaplan RF, Meyer RE, Stroebel CF: Alcohol dependence and responsivity to an ethanol stimulus as predictors of alcohol consumption. British Journal of Addiction 78:259–267, 1983

Karler R, Calder LD, Chauhry IA: Blockade of "reverse tolerance" to cocaine and amphetamine by MK801. Life Sci 45:599–606, 1989

Kellam SG, Brown CH, Rubin BR, et al: Paths leading to teenage psychiatric symptoms and substance use: developmental epidemiological studies in Woodlawn, in Childhood Psychopathology and Development. Edited by Guze SB, Earls FJ, Barrett JE. New York, Raven, 1983, pp 17–51

Kelley AE, Throne LC: NMDA receptors mediate the behavioral effects of amphetamine infused into the nucleus accumbens. Brain Res Bull 29:247–254, 1992

Khan A, Ciraulo DA, Nelson WH, et al: Dexamethasone suppression tests in recently detoxified alcoholics: clinical implications. J Clin Psychopharmacol 4:94–97, 1984

Killam KF, Olds J, Sinclair J: Further studies on the effects of centrally acting drugs on the results of self-stimulation. J Pharmacol Exp Ther 119:157–163, 1957

Kissin B: The use of psychoactive drugs in the long term treatment of chronic alcoholics. Ann N Y Acad Sci 252:385–395, 1975

Koob GF: Neurobiological mechanism in cocaine and opiate dependence, in Addictive States. Edited by O'Brien CP, Jaffe JH. New York, Raven, 1992a, pp 79–92

Koob GF: Neural mechanisms of drug reinforcement, in The Neurobiology of Drug and Alcohol Addiction. Edited by Kalivas PW, Samson HH. New York, New York Academy of Sciences, 1992b, pp 171–191

Koob GF: Drug addiction: the yin and yang of hedonic homeostasis. Neuron 16:893–896, 1996

Koob GF, Bloom FE: Cellular and molecular mechanisms of drug dependence. Science 242:715–723, 1988

Kornetsky C, Porrino L: Brain mechanisms of drug-induced reinforcement, in Addictive States. Edited by O'Brien CP, Jaffe JH. New York, Raven, 1992, pp 59–77

Kranzler HR, Bauer LO: Bromocriptine and cocaine cue reactivity in cocaine-dependent patients. British Journal of Addiction 87:1537–1548, 1992

Kranzler H, Liebowitz N: Anxiety and depression in substance abuse: clinical implications. Med Clin North Am 72:867–885, 1985

Kreek MJ: Neuroendocrinology of cocaine abuse. Paper presented at the annual meeting of the American College of Neuropsychopharmacology, San Juan, Puerto Rico, December 1992a

Kreek MJ: Rational for maintenance pharmacotherapy of opiate dependents, in Addictive States. Edited by O'Brien CP, Jaffe JH. New York, Raven, 1992b, pp 205–230

Laberg JC: Alcohol and expectancies: subjective, psychophysiological, and behavioral responses to alcohol stimuli in severely, moderately, and non-dependent drinkers. British Journal of Addiction 81:797–808, 1986

LeDoux J: The amygdala, in Handbook of Physiology: The Nervous System, Vol 5. Edited by Plum F. Bethesda, MD, American Physiological Society, 1987, pp 419–459

Lewis MJ: Alcohol effects on brain stimulation reward: blood alcohol concentration and site specificity, in Neuropharmacology of Ethanol: New Approaches. Edited by Meyer RE, Koob GF, Lewis MJ, et al. Boston, MA, Birkhauser, 1991, pp 163–178

Li TK, Lumeng L, McBride WJ, et al: Rodent lines selected for factors effecting alcohol consumption. Alcohol Alcohol Suppl 1:91–96, 1987

Li TK, Lumeng L, McBride WJ: Pharmacology of alcohol preference in rodents. Advances in Alcoholism and Substance Abuse 7:73–86, 1988

Li TK, Crabb DW, Lumeng L: Molecular and genetic approaches to understanding alcohol seeking behavior, in Neuropharmacology of Ethanol: New Approaches. Edited by Meyer RE, Koob GF, Lewis MJ, et al. Boston, MA, Birkhauser, 1991, pp 107–124

Linnoila M, DeJong J, Virkkunen M: Family history of alcoholism in violent offenders and impulsive fire setters. Arch Gen Psychiatry 46:613–616, 1989

Little HJ, Dolin SJ, Halsey MJ: Calcium channel antagonists decrease the ethanol withdrawal syndrome. Life Sci 39:2059–2065, 1986

Little HJ, Gale R, Sellars N, et al: Chronic benzodiazepine treatment increases the effects of the inverse agonist FG 7142. Neuropharmacology 27:383–389, 1988

Lonart G, Zigmond MJ: High glutamate concentrations evoke Ca(++)-independent dopamine release from striatal slices: a possible role of reverse dopamine transport. J Pharmacol Exp Ther 256:1132–1138, 1991

London EK, Cascella NG, Wong DF, et al: Cocaine-induced reduction of glucose utilization in human brain: a study using positron emission tomography and (fluorine-18)-fluorodeoxyglucose. Arch Gen Psychiatry 47:567–574, 1990

Loosen PT, Prange AJ, Wilson IC: TRH (protireline) in depressed alcoholic men: behavioral changes and endocrine responses. Arch Gen Psychiatry 36:540–547, 1979

Lovinger DM, White G, Weight FF: Ethanol inhibits NMDA-activated ion current in hippocampal neurons. Science 243:1721–1724, 1989

Ludwig AM, Wikler A: Craving and relapse to drink. Quarterly Journal of Studies on Alcohol 35:108–130, 1974

Margolin AT, Kosten I, Petrakis SK, et al: Bupropion reduces cocaine abuse in methadone-maintained patients (letter). Arch Gen Psychiatry 48:87, 1991

Martin WA, Jasinski DR: Physiological parameters of morphine dependence in man—tolerance, early abstinence and protracted abstinence. J Psychiatr Res 7:7–9, 1969

Martin WR, Winkler A, Eades CG, et al: Tolerance to and physical dependence on morphine in rats. Psychopharmacologia 4:247–260, 1963

Mehta AK, Ticku MK: Ethanol potentiation of gamma amino butyric acid gated chloride channels. J Pharmacol Exp Ther 246:558–564, 1988

Mendelson JH, Teoh SK, Lange U, et al: Anterior pituitary, adrenal, and gonadal hormones during cocaine withdrawal. Am J Psychiatry 145:1094–1098, 1988

Meyer RE: Anxiolytics and the alcoholic patient. J Stud Alcohol 47:269–273, 1986a

Meyer RE: How to understand the relationship between psychopathology and addictive disorders: another example of the chicken and the egg, in Psychopathology and Addictive Disorders. Edited by Meyer RE. New York, Guilford, 1986b, pp 3–16

Meyer RE: Conditioning phenomena and the problem of relapse in opioid addicts and alcoholics, in Learning Factors in Substance Abuse (NIDA Research Monograph Series 84). Edited by Ray B. Rockville, MD, U.S. Government Printing Office, 1988, pp 61–79

Meyer RE: Prospects for a rational pharmacotherapy of alcoholism. J Clin Psychiatry 50:403–412, 1989

Meyer RE: New pharmacotherapies for cocaine dependence . . . revisited. Arch Gen Psychiatry 49:900–904, 1992

Meyer RE, Mirin SM: The Heroin Stimulus: Implications for a Theory of Addiction. New York, Plenum, 1979

Montague PR, Dayan P, Sejnowski TJ: A framework for mesencephalic dopamine systems based on predictive hebbian learning. J Neurosci 16:1936–1947, 1996

Moolten M, Kornetsky C: Oral self-administration of ethanol and not experimenter administered ethanol facilitates rewarding electrical brain stimulation. Alcohol Clin Exp Res 7:3–9, 1990

Morrow AL, Montpied P, Paul SM: Ethanol and the GABA receptor gated chloride ion channel, in Neuropharmacology of Ethanol: New Approaches. Edited by Meyer RE, Koob GF, Lewis MJ, et al. Boston, MA, Birkhauser, 1991, pp 49–76

Murphy JM, McBride WJ, Luming L, et al: Regional brain levels of monoamines in alcohol-preferring and non-preferring lines of rats. Pharmacol Biochem Behav 16:145–149, 1982

Murphy JM, McBride WJ, Gatto GJ, et al: Effects of acute ethanol administration on monoamine and metabolite content in four brain regions of ethanol-tolerant and nontolerant alcohol preferring rats. Pharmacol Biochem Behav 29:169–174, 1988

Naranjo C, Sellers EM, Sullivan JT, et al: The serotonin uptake inhibitor citalopram attenuates ethanol intake. Clin Pharmacol Ther 41:266–274, 1987

Nestler EJ, Urdos JJ, Derwilliger R, et al: Regulation of G-proteins by chronic morphine in the rat locus ceruleus. Brain Res 476:230–239, 1989

O'Brien CP, Testa T, O'Brien TJ, et al: Conditioned narcotic withdrawal in human. Science 195:1000–1002, 1977

O'Brien C, Childress AR, McLellan AT, et al: Classical conditioning in drug dependent humans, in The Neurobiology of Drug and Alcohol Addiction. Edited by Kalivas PW, Samson HH. New York, New York Academy of Sciences, 1992, pp 400–415

Olds J, Milner P: Positive reinforcement produced by electrical stimulation of septal area and other regions of the rat brain. Journal of Comparative Physiological Psychology 47:419–427, 1954

O'Malley SS, Jaffe AJ, Chang G, et al: Naltrexone and coping skills therapy for alcohol dependence: a controlled study. Arch Gen Psychiatry 49:881–887, 1992

Parsons LH, Markou A, Smith D, et al: Involvement of mesolimbic dopamine transmission in cocaine seeking behavior elicited by drug-related environmental cues in rats. Poster presented at the annual meeting of the American College of Neuropsychopharmacology, San Juan, Puerto Rico, December 1996

Pavlov IP: Conditioned Reflexes. New York, Dover Press, 1926

Pfeffer AO, Samson HH: Haloperidol and apomorphine effects on ethanol reinforcement in free-feeding rats. Pharmacol Biochem Behav 29:343–350, 1988

Phillips AG, Atkinson IJ, Blackburn JR, et al: Increased extra cellular dopamine in the nucleus accumbens of the rat elicited by a conditioned stimulus for food: an electrochemical study. Can J Physiol Pharmacol 71:387–393, 1993

Porjesz B, Begleiter H: Human brain electrophysiology and alcoholism, in Alcohol and the Brain: Chronic Effects. Edited by Tartar RE, Van Thiel DH. New York, Plenum, 1985, pp 139–182

Post RM, Weiss SRB, Fontana D, et al: Conditioned sensitization to the psychomotor stimulant cocaine, in The Neurobiology of Drug and Alcohol Addiction. Edited by Kalivas PW, Samson HH. New York, New York Academy of Sciences, 1992, pp 386–399

Pulvirenti L, Swerdlow NR, Koob GF: Nucleus accumbens NMDA antagonist decreases locomotor activity produced by cocaine, heroin or accumbens dopamine, but not caffeine. Pharmacol Biochem Behav 40:841–845, 1991

Reid LD, Hunter GA: Morphine and naloxone modulate intake of ethanol. Alcohol 1:33–37, 1984

Ritz RT, Lamb MC, Oldburg SR, et al: Effects of cocaine on the dopamine transporter. Science 237:1219–1223, 1987

Robbins SJ, Ehrman RN, Childress AR, et al: Using cue reactivity to screen medications for cocaine abuse: a test of amantadine hydrochloride. Addict Behav 17:491–499, 1992

Roberts DCS, Koob GF, Klonoff P, et al: Extinction and recovery of cocaine self-administration following 6-hydroxy-dopamine lesions of the nucleus accumbens. Pharmacol Biochem Behav 12:781–787, 1980

Robins LN: Deviant Children Grown Up. Baltimore, MD, Williams & Wilkins, 1966

Robinson TE, Berridge KC: The neural basis of drug craving: an incentive-sensitization theory of addiction. Brain Res Brain Res Rev 18:247–291, 1993

Rush B: An Inquiry Into the Effects of Spirituous Liquors Upon the Human Body and Their Influences Upon the Happiness of Society. Boston, MA, Thomas and Andrews, 1791

Samson HH: Initiation of ethanol reinforcement using a sucrose-substitution procedure in food-and-water-sated rats. Alcohol Clin Exp Res 10:436–442, 1986

Samson HH, Tolliver GA, Pfeffer AU, et al: Oral ethanol reinforcement in the rat: effects of the partial inverse benzodiazepine agonist Ro 15-4513. Pharmacol Biochem Behav 27:517–519, 1987

Schaefer GJ, Michael RP: Ethanol and current thresholds for brain self-stimulation in the lateral hypothalamus of the rat. Alcohol 4:209–213, 1987

Schecter MD, Calcagnetti DJ: Trends in place preference conditioning with a cross-indexed bibliography, 1957–1991. Neurosci Biobehav Rev 17:1957–1991, 1993

Schuckit MA: Subjective responses to alcohol in sons of alcoholics and control subjects. Arch Gen Psychiatry 41:879–884, 1984

Schuckit MA: Low level of response to alcohol as a predictor of future alcoholism. Am J Psychiatry 151:184–189, 1994

Schultz W: Responses of monkey dopamine neurons to reward and conditioned stimuli during successive steps of learning a delayed response task. J Neurosci 13:900–913, 1993

Schuster CR, Thompson T: Self-administration of and behavioral dependence on drugs. Annual Review of Pharmacology 9:483–502, 1969

Schuster CR, Villareal JE: The Experimental Analysis of Opioid Dependence—Psychopharmacology: A Review of Progress (PHS Publ No 1836). Edited by Efron EH. Washington, DC, U.S. Government Printing Office, 1968, pp 811–828

Self DW, Barnhart WJ, Lehman DA, et al: Opposite modulation of cocaine-seeking behavior by D1- and D2-like dopamine receptor agonists. Science 271:1586–1589, 1996

Shippenberg TS, Herz A, Spanagel R: Conditioning of opioid reinforcement: neuroanatomical and neurochemical substrates, in The Neurobiology of Drug and Alcohol Addiction. Edited by Kalivas PW, Sampson HH. New York, New York Academy of Sciences, 1992, pp 347–356

Siegel S, Hinson RE, Krank MD: Anticipation of pharmacological and non-pharmacological events: classical conditioning and addictive behavior. Journal of Drug Issues 17:83–110, 1987

Stewart J: Neurobiology of conditioning to drugs of abuse, in The Neurobiology of Drug and Alcohol Addiction. Edited by Kalivas PW, Samson HH. New York, New York Academy of Sciences, 1992, pp 335–344

Stewart J, Druhan JP: The non-competitive MDA antagonist, MK-801 blocks the development of conditioned activity to amphetamine. Society for Neuroscience Abstracts 557:12, 1991

Stewart J, Vezina P: Conditioning and behavioral sensitization, in Sensitization in the Nervous System. Edited by Kalivas PW, Barnes C. Caldwell, NJ, Telford Press, 1988, pp 207–224

Stewart J, deWitt H, Eikelboom R: Role of unconditioned and conditioned drug effects in the self-administration of opiates and stimulants. Psychol Rev 91:251–268, 1984

Supko DE, Uretsky NJ, Wallace LJ: AMPA/kainic acid glutamate receptor antagonism in the zona incerta dorsal to the subthalamic nucleus inhibits amphetamine-induced stereotypy but not locomotor activity. Brain Res 576:89–96, 1992

Suzdak PD, Schwartz RD, Scolnick O, et al: Ethanol stimulates gamma amino butyric acid receptor mediated chloride transport in rat brain synaptoneurosomes. Proc Natl Acad Sci U S A 83:4071–4075, 1986

Suzdak PT, Glowa JR, Crawley JN, et al: A selective imidazobenzodiazepine antagonist of ethanol in the rat. Science 234:1243–1247, 1986

Swartz CM, Breen MD, Leone F: Serum prolactin levels during extended cocaine abstinence. Am J Psychiatry 147:777–779, 1990

Tabakoff B, Rabie CS, Grant KA: Ethanol and NMDA receptor: insights into ethanol pharmacology, in Neuropharmacology of Ethanol: New Approaches. Edited by Meyer RE, Koob GF, Lewis MJ, et al. Boston, MA, Birkhauser, 1991, pp 42–56

Tennant FS, Sagherian AA: Double blind comparison of amantadine and bromocriptine for ambulatory withdrawal from cocaine dependence. Arch Intern Med 147:109–112, 1987

Teoh SK, Mendelson JH, Mello NK, et al: Hyperprolactinemia and risk for relapse of cocaine abuse. Biol Psychiatry 28:824–828, 1990

Tschanz JT, Haracz JL, Griffith KE, et al: Bilateral cortical ablations attenuate amphetamine-induced excitations of neostriatal motor-related neurons in freely moving rats. Neurosci Lett 134:127–130, 1991

Uhl GR: Dopamine transporter and cocaine therapeutic strategies. Paper presented at the annual meeting of the American College of Neuropsychopharmacology, San Juan, Puerto Rico, December 1996

Vavrousek-Jakuba E, Cohen CA, Shoemaker WJ: Ethanol effects of CNS dopamine receptors: in vivo binding following voluntary ethanol intake in rats, in Novel Pharmacological Interventions for Alcoholism. Edited by Naranjo CA, Sellers EM. New York, Springer-Verlag, 1990, pp 372–374

Volkow ND, Fowler JS, Wolf AP, et al: Changes in brain glucose metabolism in cocaine dependence and withdrawal. Am J Psychiatry 148:621–626, 1991

Volkow ND, Hitzemann R, Wang GJ, et al: Long term frontal brain metabolic changes in cocaine abusers. Synapse 11:184–190, 1992

Volpicelli JR, Alterman AI, Hayashadi M, et al: Naltrexone in the treatment of alcohol dependence. Arch Gen Psychiatry 49:876–880, 1992

Waller MB, McBride MC, Gatto GJ, et al: Intragastric self infusion of ethanol of the p and np (alcohol preferring and alcohol non-preferring) lines of rats. Science 225:78–80, 1984

Weddington WW, Brown BS, Haertzen CA, et al: Changes in mood, craving, and sleep during short term abstinence reported by male cocaine addicts: a controlled residential study. Arch Gen Psychiatry 47:861–868, 1990

Weeks JR: Experimental morphine addiction: methods for automatic intravenous injections in unrestrained rats. Science 138:143–144, 1963

Weiss F, Koob GF: The neuropharmacology of ethanol self-administration, in Neuropharmacology of Ethanol: New Approaches. Edited by Meyer RE, Koob GF, Lewis MJ, et al. Boston, MA, Birkhauser, 1991, pp 125–162

Weiss F, Herd YL, Ungerstedt U, et al: Neurochemical correlates of cocaine and ethanol self-administration, in The Neurobiology of Drug and Alcohol Addiction. Edited by Kalivas PW, Samson HH. New York, New York Academy of Sciences, 1992, pp 220–241

Westerink BH, Santiago M, De VJ: The release of dopamine from nerve terminals and dendrites of nigrostriatal neurons induced by excitatory amino acids in the conscious rat. Naunyn Schmiedebergs Arch Pharmacol 345:523–529, 1992

Wikler A: Recent progress in research on the neurophysiological basis of morphine addiction. Am J Psychiatry 105:329–338, 1948

Wikler A: Conditioning factors in opiate addiction and relapse, in Narcotics. Edited by Wilmer DM, Kassebaum GG. New York, McGraw-Hill, 1965, pp 85–100

Wikler A: Dynamics of drug dependent: implications of a conditioning theory for research and treatment, in Opiate Addiction: Origins and Treatment. Edited by Fisher S, Freedman AM. Washington, DC, Winston Press, 1974, pp 7–22

Wikler A, Pescor FT: Classical conditioning of morphine abstinence, reinforcement of opioid-drinking behavior and relapse in morphine-addicted rats. Psychopharmacologia 10:255–284, 1967

Wikler A, Martin WR, Pescor FT, et al: Factors regulating oral consumption or an opioid (etonitazine) by morphine-addicted rats. Psychopharmacologia 5:55–76, 1963

Wikler A, Pescor FT, Miller T, et al: Persistent potency of a secondary (conditioned) reinforcer following withdrawal of morphine from physically dependent rats. Psychopharmacologia 20:103–117, 1971

Wilkins J, Gorelick DA, Nademanee K, et al: Hypothalamic-pituitary function during alcohol exposure and withdrawal and cocaine exposure, in Recent Developments in Alcoholism, Vol 10: Alcohol and Cocaine Similarities and Differences. Edited by Galanter M. New York, Plenum, 1992, pp 57–71

Wise RA, Bozarth MA: A psychomotor stimulant theory of addiction. Psychol Rev 94:469–492, 1987

Witkin JM: Blockade of the locomotor stimulant effects of cocaine and methamphetamine by glutamate antagonists. J Pharmacol Exp Ther 261:476–483, 1992

Woods JH, Schuster CR: Reinforcement properties of morphine, cocaine, and SPA as a function of unit dose. Int J Addict 3:231–237, 1968

World Health Organization: International Statistical Classification of Diseases and Related Health Problems, 10th Revision. Geneva, Switzerland, World Health Organization, 1992

World Health Organization Expert Committee on Addiction Producing Drugs. World Health Organ Tech Rep Ser 273:3–20, 1964

Yanagita T, Kiyoshi A, Takahashi S, et al: Self-administration of barbiturates, alcohol (intragastric) and CNS stimulants (intravenous) in monkeys, in National Academy of Sciences–National Research Council Committee on Problems of Drug Dependence. Palo Alto, CA, Stanford University Press, 1969, pp 6039–6051

Yokel RA, Wise RA: Increased lever pressing for amphetamine after pimozide in rats: implications for a dopamine theory of reward. Science 187:547–549, 1975

Youngren KD, Daly DA, Moghaddam B: Distinct actions of endogenous excitatory amino acids on the outflow of dopamine in the nucleus accumbens. J Pharmacol Exp Ther 264:289–293, 1993

THIRTY-TWO

Biology of Eating Disorders

Regina C. Casper, M.D.

Anorexia nervosa and bulimia nervosa form a heterogeneous group of psychiatric disorders. There is a widespread belief that eating disorders are a product of American society and culture, as indeed they are; however, neither disorder is new, and similar disorders have existed throughout history (Bell 1985; Ziolko 1976). The incidence of anorexia nervosa has risen since 1980 (Szmukler et al. 1986; Wakeling 1996), whereas bulimia nervosa has only recently been described as a nosological syndrome (Casper 1983; Russell 1979).

The biological changes present in both disorders reflect mainly the body's adjustment to prolonged undernutrition and to changes in eating pattern; whether the changes are intrinsic to either disorder is uncertain. Nonetheless, the starvation-induced biological changes might well play a permissive role in reinforcing some psychopathological mechanisms. Based on wide-ranging constitutional differences, individual patients tolerate undernutrition and malnutrition in different ways. By and large, differences in the amount and speed of weight loss, use of laxatives or diuretics, variations in eating pattern and in the frequency of self-induced vomiting override all other factors in determining the medical condition. If treatment normalizes the eating pattern and body weight, virtually all physical, metabolic, and endocrine abnormalities normalize as well. Prolonged emesis and laxative or diuretic abuse, however, can lead to permanent gastrointestinal, renal, or dental damage.

In this chapter, I consider the physical changes associated with anorexia nervosa separately from those occurring in bulimia nervosa. It is now well known that the adaptation to prolonged starvation and the resulting pathological weight loss in the restricting subtype of anorexia nervosa (Casper et al. 1980a) differ in several ways from the body's adaptation to the emesis and/or cathartic or diuretic abuse commonly practiced in the binge-eating/purging subtype and in bulimia nervosa.

ANOREXIA NERVOSA

Anorexia nervosa typically develops in adolescent girls, whose profound weight loss is the direct consequence of reduced food intake, which is related to loss of appetite only in rare cases. The classic attitudinal and behavioral changes—denial of illness, an overriding and irrational fear of becoming overweight, distorted perception of body image, and often hypermotility—establish the diagnosis (American Psychiatric Association 1994; Bruch 1973). The starvation process in anorexia nervosa is personally sustained, even though the initial weight loss may not be self-imposed but may be initiated through appetite loss in depression, in physical illness, or through religious fasting (Casper and Davis 1977). To interpret the biological changes, clinicians must distinguish patients with the restricting subtype who consistently fast from those who also vomit and from those who fall prey to periodic bouts of overeating and subsequent emesis (Casper et al. 1980a).

Physical Changes

The human body is well equipped to deal with the consequences of temporary starvation and to recover functionally in times of plenty (Keys et al. 1950). Chronic weight loss is better tolerated than acute severe weight loss, and adults seem to adjust more easily to weight loss than do children or young adolescents. In adolescents, changes in body weight can be calculated as height and weight deviations from the norms published in the Iowa Growth Charts (Jackson and Kelby 1945). Ideal weights derived from the Metropolitan Life Insurance Company generally form the basis for calculating weight loss in adults. The Body Mass Index (BMI; weight in kilograms divided by height in meters, squared) (Keys et al. 1972) has become popular for standardizing weight loss, because the BMI has a high correlation with skinfold thickness and therefore with body fat mass. The most commonly observed physical changes in anorexia nervosa are listed in Table 32–1.

The starved skeleton-like appearance of the anorexic patient is the result of reduction in subcutaneous fat tissue. The skin acquires a dark, yellowish color with a rough texture. With advanced emaciation, a lanuginous coat of fine, silky hair can cover the back, extremities, and cheeks. Not infrequently, petechiae and ecchymoses develop, not nec-

essarily as a result of thrombocytopenia but secondary to increased capillary permeability. A decreased core temperature and an inability to adjust to environmental temperature changes have also been reported (Luck and Wakeling 1980; Mecklenburg et al. 1974; Vigersky et al. 1976), which are similar to the temperature changes reported by Vigersky and colleagues (1977) in underweight young women. Core body temperatures can decline to as low as 93°F, especially in children. Hypothermia and abnormal temperature regulation during starvation and anorexia nervosa seem to be caused by a dysregulation in hypothalamic areas.

Heart morphology and function can be profoundly affected in anorexia nervosa and starvation (Schocken et al. 1989). The heart rate can decrease to below 60 beats/minute, leading to sinus bradycardia, and can decrease to as low as 30 beats/minute in the sleeping state. Hypotension with systolic blood pressures below 70 mm Hg is common and can be associated with a reduction in heart size (Gottdiener et al. 1978). Mitral valve prolapse (despite structurally normal mitral valves), leading to systolic and diastolic ventricular dysfunction, is not infrequently detected on echocardiogram (Myers et al. 1987). In a study of 31 female and male adolescents with anorexia nervosa who on average had lost 26% of body weight, Fohlin (1977) reported reduced heart and blood volumes and decreased maximal heart rates during exercise compared with adolescents of normal weight. Loss of body weight alone could not explain the reduced maximal oxygen uptake; hence, hypothermia was thought to have contributed to the lower maximal heart rates. Some patients develop transitory systolic heart murmurs and peripheral edema (Halmi and Falk 1981). Peripheral edema most often occurs as a result of decreased renal perfusion and is not necessarily associated with a reduced plasma protein content or impaired renal function. In patients with anorexia nervosa of the restricting subtype, renal function is preserved despite a reduction in renal concentrating capacity.

Electrocardiographic abnormalities, such as sinus bradycardia associated with increased Q-T and Q-T$_c$ intervals, reflect an increased risk for cardiac arrest and ectopic atrial rhythm. Atrioventricular junctional blocks and other forms of arrhythmias have been reported (Powers 1982; Thurston and Marks 1974). For these reasons, the cardiac status of cachectic patients requires careful monitoring, especially during refeeding, because congestive heart failure may occur (Powers 1982).

Sensory perceptual changes, such as changes in taste perception with reduced acuity for sour, salty, and bitter tastes (sweet taste is preserved the longest), have been documented (Casper et al. 1980b). Such impaired taste

Table 32–1. Physical manifestations in restricting anorexia nervosa

Body weight loss (from 15% to 60%)	
Subcutaneous fat tissue loss	
Growth retardation (children)	
Metabolic	Hypothermia
	Hypometabolism
	Cold intolerance
	Carbohydrate intolerance
Central nervous system	Abnormal electroencephalogram findings
	Cerebral pseudoatrophy
Gastrointestinal	Delayed gastric emptying
	Superior mesenteric artery syndrome
	Constipation
Cardiovascular	Hypotension
	Bradycardia
	Arrhythmias
	Acrocyanosis
Renal	Dehydration
	Edema
	Polyuria
	Nocturia
Hematological	Anemia (rare)
	Leukopenia with relative lymphocytosis
	Thrombocytopenia
	Bone marrow hypoplasia

perception would be expected to facilitate food avoidance by making meals less palatable. Reduced gastric motility and delayed gastric emptying (Dubois et al. 1979; Saleh and Lebwohl 1980), leading to unpleasant sensations of feeling bloated after eating, are common. Constipation is always present, but patients rarely mention it or complain about it, except during refeeding.

Metabolic Changes

The metabolic rate in anorexia nervosa declines as a result of reduced body mass and decreased serum levels of triiodothyronine (T_3) (Casper et al. 1991). Depending on the nature and the severity of the starvation, the metabolic rate can decline to as low as 40% of the normal basal metabolic rate (Vaisman et al. 1988), at which point low T_3 plasma levels and reduced thyroxine (T_4) plasma levels are the rule.

Fasting hypoglycemia (Mecklenburg et al. 1974) and increased lipid mobilization, reflected in elevated free fatty acid levels (Casper et al. 1988a) and β-hydroxybutyric acid levels (Pirke et al. 1985), have been documented in patients with anorexia nervosa. Other functional metabolic changes include glucose intolerance similar to that reported in cases of total starvation (Unger et al. 1963), with an abnormal rise in postabsorptive plasma glucose levels and a slow decline (Casper et al. 1977). Fixed glucose plasma levels following glucose ingestion are most likely due to malabsorption. Impaired glucose tolerance is rarely the result of low circulating insulin levels. Instead, increased insulin receptor binding capacity has been reported in the cachectic state of anorexia nervosa (Wachslicht-Rodbard et al. 1979). Glucose tolerance (Casper et al. 1988a) and insulin receptor binding capacity normalize with weight restoration and a normal food intake. No correlation between circulating insulin levels and insulin binding has been found.

Table 32–2 shows the metabolic and hormonal factors that may affect the outcome of the glucose tolerance test in anorexia nervosa of either the restricting or the binge-eating/purging subtype.

Hypercarotenemia is not only the result of excessive ingestion of foods containing carotene but also, similar to the frequently observed hypercholesterolemia, which is characterized by low-density lipoproteins, caused by reduced enzymatic degradation and reduced metabolic clearance. Therefore, treatment to lower plasma cholesterol levels would, instead of reducing the intake of dietary fat, encourage high-calorie meals to achieve the positive metabolic balance necessary to metabolize plasma cholesterol more efficiently.

Table 32–2. Factors influencing glucose metabolism in anorexia nervosa

Low insulin plasma levels

Increased insulin binding to receptors on erythrocytes and monocytes

Increased glucocorticoids and human growth hormone

Malabsorption—oral versus intravenous route

Glucose tolerance and intolerance

Dietary carbohydrate deficiency

Excessive exercising

Hypokalemia

Increased free fatty acids and ketoacids

Increased gastric inhibitory peptides

Increased pancreatic polypeptides

Hematological changes, such as mild anemia and moderate to severe leukopenia, often associated with relative lymphocytosis, seem to be the result of reversible bone marrow hypoplasia with increased mucopolysaccharide content in bone marrow (Mant and Faragher 1972). Clinical observations do not support an increased susceptibility to infection in anorexia nervosa, even in patients with lymphopenia, except in advanced chronic cases (Bowers and Eckert 1978). Indeed, Silver and Chan (1996) reported no differences in the percentages or absolute counts of lymphocyte subsets CD3, CD4, CD8, and CD19 in partially renourished adolescents with anorexia nervosa compared with control subjects. Similarly, Fink et al. (1996) found normal CD4 counts in older patients with anorexia nervosa, both on admission and after weight gain, but surprisingly found diminished CD8 counts on both occasions; these observations are inconsistent with those in the previous literature.

Levels of serum proteins remain generally within the low-normal range, and hypoalbuminemia points to protracted and severe undernutrition (Casper et al. 1980b). Serum transferrin levels—measured directly or calculated from measurements of total iron-binding capacity (TIBC)—reflect protein deficiency much earlier than total serum albumin levels because of their shorter half-life. Transferrin levels are almost always reduced in patients with anorexia nervosa and are a sensitive measure of malnutrition.

Liver enzymes are occasionally elevated in anorexia nervosa. In a study by Mickley et al. (1996), a mere 4.1% of outpatients with eating disorders had increased liver enzymes, typically serum glutamic-pyruvic transaminase (SGPT), which were related to current and past levels of being underweight.

Sleep Changes

Insomnia and a reduction in sleep time with early-morning awakening are common in underweight and malnourished patients with anorexia nervosa, but few patients ever mention sleep disturbances. In fact, anorexic patients who awaken early feel animated and vigorous and might exercise or clean the house.

Polysomnographic studies have reported significant reductions in sleep efficiency, total sleep time, and amount of slow-wave sleep (SWS) (Kupfer and Bulik 1984; Lauer et al. 1988; Levy et al. 1987, 1988; Neil et al. 1980). Several studies noted reduced rapid eye movement (REM) latency (Katz et al. 1984; Lauer et al. 1990; Neil et al. 1980), an abnormality that has been considered specific for depression. Indeed, Katz and colleagues (1984) found a significant negative correlation between scores on the Hamilton Rating Scale for Depression (Hamilton 1960) and REM latency. However, Walsh and colleagues (1985) did not find an association between depressive symptoms and REM latency but did report shorter REM latency in anorexic patients with concurrent depressive disorders. Lauer et al. (1988) distinguished patients with depression and patients with eating disorders by showing that the REM sleep–inducing effects of the cholinergic agent RS-86 were more pronounced in depressed patients than in either control subjects or patients with eating disorders.

Several factors that influence sleep (e.g., age, chronicity, nutrition) must be considered when interpreting sleep changes in anorexia nervosa. Sleep studies have rarely included the typical adolescent with anorexia nervosa. Treatment-refractory patients in their 20s were most often monitored, but, even in these patients, their fairly young age might have prevented the full spectrum of sleep abnormalities characteristic of depression from coming into play. Treatment-refractory patients are also more likely to have comorbid disorders that could account for some of the associated sleep disturbances (Benca and Casper 1994). Food deprivation alone affects sleep in animals (McFayden et al. 1973) and in humans (Karacan et al. 1973). Consistent with this nutritional deficiency theory, once patients with anorexia nervosa gain weight, their total sleep time, SWS, and REM sleep increase significantly (Crisp et al. 1971; Evans 1983; Levy et al. 1987). However, some studies have not found a correlation between the amount of body weight and sleep variables (Lauer et al. 1990). Without comparisons to underweight or undernourished age-matched control groups, the abnormal sleep findings in anorexia nervosa are difficult to interpret.

Morphological Brain Changes

Atrophic brain changes are well documented from postmortem examinations of cachectic anorexia nervosa patients (Martin 1958).

Morphological brain changes are not uncommon. Brain imaging studies, such as computed tomography (CT) or magnetic resonance imaging (MRI), reveal enlarged inner and outer cerebrospinal fluid spaces in cases of advanced starvation, which suggest cerebral cortical and interhemispheric atrophy and, less so, cerebellar atrophy (Datlof et al. 1986; Enzmann and Lane 1977; Heinz et al. 1977; Katzman et al. 1996; Nussbaum et al. 1980; Sein et al. 1981). The enlargement of cortical sulcal width, expansion of the interhemispheric fissure, and widening of the ventricles are associated with the rapidity and amount of weight loss (Golden et al. 1996; Lankenau et al. 1985). Regional blood flow as assessed by single photon emission computed tomography (SPECT) does not seem significantly affected (Krieg et al. 1989).

Because the morphological brain changes can no longer be observed after patients with anorexia gain weight (Golden et al. 1996; Kohlmeyer et al. 1983; Krieg et al. 1989; Swayze et al. 1996), these changes would be more accurately described as pseudoatrophy or dystrophy. Herholz et al. (1987) used positron-emission tomography (PET) and found bilateral caudate hypermetabolism in 5 underweight females with anorexia nervosa who were compared with 15 male control subjects; caudate metabolism returned to normal after weight gain. In a PET study by Hoffman et al. (1989), the mean ventricular enlargement was significant only for patients with anorexia nervosa who were or had been vomiting. In contrast, Krieg et al. (1988) showed small, yet significant, correlations between ventricular enlargement, age, weight, and serum T_3 levels. Because the restricting subtype was not differentiated from the binge-eating/purging subtype in most studies of patients with anorexia nervosa, contributing factors are difficult to isolate.

Lowered plasma albumin levels and hypercortisolemia (Okuno et al. 1980) caused by undernutrition have been mentioned as possible causes of the movement of intravascular fluid to extracellular spaces, although serum albumin is rarely abnormally low in anorexia nervosa. Enhanced vasopressin release, which increases the permeability of the blood-brain barrier and which has been described in vomiting and anorexic behavior (Gold et al. 1983; Rowe et al. 1979), may contribute to the brain changes found in imaging studies.

The implications of these morphological brain changes for cognitive function and other clinical correlates are far from established (Maxwell et al. 1984). Kohlmeyer et al. (1983) reported that improved cognitive test performance paralleled a reduction in sulcal width in patients with anorexia nervosa who had gained weight. However, Laessle et al. (1989) found no relation between ventricular size and performance on a vigilance test. Kingston et al. (1996) tested attention, visual-spatial ability, and memory in underweight patients with anorexia nervosa and retested patients after a weight gain of at least 10% and also did not find a relation between MRI brain appearance and cognitive performance.

Electroencephalogram Changes

The most commonly found, yet by no means common, electroencephalogram (EEG) changes are generalized abnormalities of the EEG background activity that are related to duration of illness, low fasting blood glucose level, electrolyte abnormalities, vomiting, and diuretic and laxative abuse (Crisp et al. 1968; Kupfer and Bulik 1984; Neil et al. 1980). The functional significance of the EEG changes is not known. The EEG changes normalize once weight is regained (Lacey et al. 1976).

Adaptation of the Neuroendocrine System in Anorexia Nervosa

The conceptualization of anorexia nervosa as an endocrine disorder by Simmonds (1914) led to a wealth of studies describing hormonal deficiencies, all of which were presumably the result of pituitary insufficiency. The current consensus is that pituitary function overall is not impaired in anorexia nervosa (Dreyfus and Mamou 1947; Garfinkel et al. 1975; Scheithauer et al. 1988), even though imaging studies show that the size of the pituitary gland is reduced in underweight patients with anorexia nervosa (Doraiswamy et al. 1994). Current evidence suggests that the adaptive regulatory changes originate from functional changes in and/or above the hypothalamus. Factors associated with anorexia nervosa that alone or in combination have been shown to produce changes in hormone levels include the following:

- Pathological body weight loss
- Reduced caloric intake insufficient to maintain weight
- Selective food intake, leading to different kinds of malnutrition or undernutrition; for example, a vegetarian diet or an exclusive diet of cereals and bread may result in amino acid, trace element, or vitamin deficiencies, depending on individual habits and preferences

- Abnormal patterns of eating with gorging and emesis (anorexia nervosa, binge-eating/purging type)
- As yet unknown factors that could turn out to be specific to anorexia nervosa

The first three of the above factors far outweigh the others in their contribution to the dysregulation of endocrine systems.

The Hypothalamic-Pituitary-Adrenal Axis

Early reports of reduced urinary excretion of 17-ketosteroids were taken as a sign of pituitary-adrenal insufficiency in anorexia nervosa (Perloff et al. 1954). However, ketosteroids are poor indicators of adrenal function, because both gonadal and adrenal steroid hormones contribute to urinary ketosteroid excretion. In fact, the daily cortisol production rate in absolute terms and expressed as a function of body mass and body surface area has been found to be significantly increased in anorexia nervosa (Boyar et al. 1977; Walsh et al. 1978). Higher than normal resting plasma cortisol levels (but normal levels of cortisol-binding globulin with reduced affinity), increased number of secretory episodes and time spent in secretory activity, and flattened diurnal secretory rhythm are all common (Casper et al. 1979; Doerr et al. 1980; Fichter et al. 1986; Walsh et al. 1978). Thus, urinary free cortisol is elevated in anorexic patients relative to nonanorexic control subjects (Boyar et al. 1977). A reduced metabolic clearance rate, which prolongs the half-life of plasma cortisol, and altered steroid metabolic pathways contribute to the increase in circulating cortisol plasma levels. Aside from weight loss, motor hyperactivity (Casper et al. 1991) and emotional distress may be involved in the activation of the hypothalamic-pituitary-adrenal (HPA) axis. Whether a coexisting depression contributes to the HPA changes is difficult to establish, unless the patient is in metabolic balance and has regained at least 10%–15% of body weight (Doerr et al. 1980).

A study by Gold et al. (1986) suggested that the hyperactivity of the adrenal cortex in anorexia nervosa might be related to increased secretion of corticotropin-releasing hormone (CRH); indeed, elevated CRH levels have been reported (Glowa and Gold 1991; Hotta et al. 1991). The anorexiant effects of CRH could well facilitate food abstention in anorexia nervosa, although tolerance seems to develop after repeated CRH exposure (Krahn et al. 1990). Interestingly, Gold et al. (1986) reported a significantly reduced net adrenocorticotropic hormone (ACTH) response to CRH but normal baseline ACTH plasma levels in anorexic patients with the highest cortisol levels. The ACTH response to CRH continued to be markedly attenuated even after some weight gain, but when weight was fully restored to normal, patients with anorexia nervosa had a normal ACTH response and a normal ACTH-to-cortisol ratio on stimulation with CRH. The data suggest that the basal hypercortisolism in anorexia nervosa is related to a regulatory defect at or above the hypothalamic level and that with full weight recovery, eucortisolism is reestablished in most patients.

The dexamethasone suppression test (DST) lacks specificity for anorexia nervosa because most of the changes can be attributed to starvation. When dexamethasone, a highly potent synthetic corticosteroid, is given at 11:00 P.M. to block production of CRH and release of ACTH and cortisol, severely underweight and malnourished patients with anorexia nervosa invariably fail to show the dexamethasone-induced suppression of cortisol secretion the next morning or the next afternoon (Gerner and Gwirtsman 1981). In most patients who gain weight and are in positive caloric balance, morning and afternoon plasma cortisol levels are suppressed to less than 5 mg/dL after dexamethasone administration. Although patients with depression or other psychiatric disorders may also avert dexamethasone suppression, no consistent relationship in acute anorexia nervosa has been found between depressive symptoms or a diagnosis of depressive disorder and dexamethasone suppression. Herpertz-Dahlman and Remschmidt (1990) suggested that the DST might be of prognostic value to predict relapse in anorexia nervosa. From a clinical point of view, regular body weight measurements would seem more convenient for predicting relapse than would repeated DSTs.

Reduced caloric intake and weight loss clearly play a major role in this lack of dexamethasone suppression. Fasting, weight loss, and protein-calorie malnutrition can each cause alterations in the HPA axis in animals (Scapagnini et al. 1971) and in humans. Fichter et al. (1986) subjected healthy subjects to 3 weeks of total food abstinence and reported an increase in 24-hour plasma cortisol levels, with an attenuated circadian pattern of cortisol release but a greater number of secretory episodes and a prolonged half-life of plasma cortisol. Half of the DSTs done during the fasting state showed insufficient suppression after administration of 1.5 mg of dexamethasone, but dexamethasone suppression normalized with weight regain.

Because cortisol stimulates gluconeogenesis, increased cortisol levels would be expected to play a role in maintaining adequate blood glucose concentrations. Elevated cortisol levels also inhibit thyroid-stimulating hormone (TSH) release and thus decrease T_4 and consequently T_3 production. The decreased T_3 production has been shown to lead to changes in metabolic pathways of cortisol, with an increase in the ratio of tetrahydrocortisol to tetrahydrocortisone (Boyar and Bradlow 1977; Zumoff et al. 1983).

The Hypothalamic-Pituitary-Gonadal Axis

Primary or secondary amenorrhea in females (American Psychiatric Association 1994) and impotence in males are considered diagnostic for anorexia nervosa. Secondary amenorrhea is associated with markedly reduced estradiol and absent progesterone plasma levels. Depending on the degree of weight loss, a regression from the adult diurnal and nocturnal plasma luteinizing hormone (LH) pattern occurs, with reactivation of the typical mid- and prepubertal LH pattern and ultimately the continuous low LH plasma levels of early puberty (Boyar et al. 1974; Katz et al. 1978; Pirke et al. 1979). Thus, patients whose weight loss exceeds 45% of body weight invariably show the low sleep-dependent LH secretion pattern reminiscent of prepuberty.

Pituitary responsiveness can be tested through administration of synthetic gonadotropin-releasing hormones (GnRHs) at different levels of body weight loss. The blunted LH and less consistently blunted follicle-stimulating hormone (FSH) responses (Sherman and Halmi 1977) to GnRH typical of prepuberty suggest a hypothalamic or suprahypothalamic defect. Pulsatile GnRH administration can restore ovarian activity even in patients with anorexia nervosa who are markedly underweight (Guisti et al. 1988). After a substantial weight gain to about 70% of ideal body weight, anorexic patients may have not only normal but also occasionally excessive LH release following GnRH bolus injections (Beumont et al. 1976). The same transitory supersensitivity of the pituitary gonadotrophs occurs during normal puberty.

At about 80%–90% of ideal body weight, normal pituitary-gonadal responsiveness may be restored (Ferrari et al. 1989), but the timing of normalization varies substantially among individuals. As weight is regained, the diurnal and nocturnal LH plasma levels repeat the pubertal release pattern, with sequential changes in ovarian activity. Thus, the restitutive changes observed in anorexia nervosa mimic the normal sequential changes during puberty. Normal cyclical LH release and menstrual function may resume months after weight recovery, but more often several years pass before menstrual function is restored. The mechanism for the impaired GnRH secretion is unclear. Because naloxone infusion can restore LH pulses, endogenous opioid overactivity may be involved (Brambilla et al. 1991), although secretory changes in melatonin may well contribute (Ferrari et al. 1989).

The processes leading up to normal pubertal maturation are insufficiently understood. A theory proposed by Frisch and Revelle (1970) is relevant to anorexia nervosa. Frisch (1985) suggested that a certain amount of accumulated body fat is necessary to initiate puberty and that reproductive function depended on an optimal amount of body fat. Although this theory is still being debated, it would explain changes in reproductive function in patients with anorexia nervosa and in athletes whose excessive exercise might have led to increased muscle mass at the expense of body fat. However, this theory does not easily explain the frequently observed menstrual function changes in patients with bulimia nervosa whose body fat mass changes little. Serum leptin concentrations have been found to be correlated with percent body fat in anorexia nervosa in a similar way as in nonanorexic populations. A minimum leptin level, however, seems to be critical for maintaining menstruation (Brown et al. 1996; Grinspoon et al. 1996; Hebebrand et al. 1997).

Numerous studies have reported a decline in birth rate during famine or times of food scarcity, which underlines the importance of an adequate food supply for reproductive function (Wade and Schneider 1992; Wilmsen 1982). In view of the menstrual changes reported with undernutrition, the hypothesis that the secondary amenorrhea in anorexia nervosa reflects a primary hypothalamic deficit remains unconfirmed. The phenomenon of psychogenic amenorrhea, for example, suggests that stress may play a role in early-onset amenorrhea (Nillius 1978) as may alterations in the diet (e.g., a vegetarian diet; Goldin et al. 1982) and excessive exercise (Brooks et al. 1984; Dale et al. 1979; Frisch et al. 1980). Furthermore, large individual variations exist in the stability of the hypothalamic-pituitary-gonadal (HPG) axis.

Prolonged amenorrhea with low plasma estradiol levels has been associated with low bone density (Rigotti et al. 1984; Szmukler et al. 1985). A longer duration of anorexia nervosa with amenorrhea as well as greater body weight loss have all been related to reduced spinal bone mineral density, with exercise somewhat counteracting demineralization (Andersen et al. 1995; Siemers et al. 1996). These findings raise two as yet unanswered questions: 1) Is estrogen replacement necessary in young, normally active underweight adolescents or women? and 2) What are the long-term consequences of low plasma estradiol levels and the risks associated with reduced bone density? (Ettinger et al. 1985). First, no controlled studies have reported an increase in bone density with estradiol administration. In contrast, the risks of estradiol administration in the presence of protein-calorie malnutrition to the not fully grown adolescent patient may well exceed its benefits. Second,

the commonly observed physical activity (Casper et al. 1991) may well counteract the reduction in bone density.

In patients with anorexia nervosa, estradiol metabolism is shifted toward an increased production of 2-hydroxyestrone (2-OH estrone) at the expense of estriol (Fishman et al. 1975). Remarkably, this increase in the catechol estrogens and the decrease in estriol formation have been reported in hyperthyroidism rather than hypothyroidism (Fishman et al. 1976). This increased production of 2-OH estrone has two effects: 1) 2-OH estrone has a high binding capacity for estrogen receptors but little biological activity, and 2) 2-OH estrone inhibits tyrosine hydroxylase and catechol-O-methyltransferase (COMT), two enzymes that are important for the synthesis and disposition of catecholamines. These two mechanisms can reduce the biological activity of estradiol even further.

Plasma testosterone levels have been reported in the normal range (Casper et al. 1979). Boyar and Bradlow (1977) reported a decrease in 5-α-reductase activity (as in clinical hypothyroidism), which leads to diminished androsterone production at the expense of the β-route leading to etiocholanolone. Etiocholanolone has little androgen-like activity but tends to be pyrogenic. This enzymatic shift can be reversed by acute T_3 administration (Boyar and Bradlow 1977).

The Hypothalamic-Pituitary-Thyroid Axis

The hypometabolic adaptation to starvation is achieved not so much by changes in thyroid glandular function as by reduced peripheral conversion of T_4 to T_3. About 80%–90% of T_3 derives from extrathyroidal conversion of T_4. Moreover, within days of severe undernutrition with carbohydrate deprivation, the peripheral deiodination of T_4 to T_3 is shunted into the inactive form—reverse T_3—which further reduces T_3 levels (Vagenakis et al. 1975). This change may represent another protective mechanism during the catabolic state.

In patients with anorexia nervosa, T_3 serum levels can decline to as low as half of those of nonanorexic control subjects (Moshang and Utiger 1977; Moshang et al. 1975). Dialyzable free T_4 levels usually remain in the normal range. The low T_3 state contributes to symptoms such as constipation, dry skin and hair, bradycardia, cold intolerance, hypercarotenemia, and hypercholesterolemia, as well as to the decreased resting metabolic rate.

Hypothyroidism is ruled out by normal TSH serum levels in the presence of low serum T_3 levels; instead, the pituitary set point of TSH release seems to readjust. Similar changes in the hypothalamic-pituitary-thyroid (HPT) axis, termed the *euthyroid-sick syndrome*, have occurred in other forms of malnutrition and in patients with severe nonthyroidal illnesses (Bermuder et al. 1975). Low T_3 plasma levels help conserve muscular tissue during sickness and starvation. Exogenous administration of T_3 leads to an increase in nitrogen excretion in starvation and in anorexia nervosa (Gardner et al. 1979; Leslie et al. 1978).

Thus, it is not surprising that the administration of thyrotropin-releasing hormone (TRH) results in quantitatively normal and occasionally slightly delayed TSH release (Casper and Frohman 1982; Kiriike et al. 1986; Leslie et al. 1978; Miyai et al. 1975). In fact, Lesem et al. (1994) reported reduced cerebrospinal fluid TRH immunoreactivity not only in underweight patients but also in patients who had regained weight. During weight gain, temporary increases of T_3 into the hyperthyroid range and exaggerated TSH responses can be observed (Casper and Frohman 1982; Moore and Mills 1979).

Human Growth Hormone

Slightly or markedly elevated basal human growth hormone (HGH) levels have been found in acutely starving patients with anorexia nervosa (Casper et al. 1977). Growth hormone release is stimulated by other forms of undernutrition (Alvarez et al. 1972; Pimstone et al. 1967) and even by short-term fasting and will normalize promptly with refeeding, especially with ingestion of carbohydrates. The presence of normal or elevated plasma growth hormone and cortisol levels distinguishes anorexia nervosa from hypopituitarism. Paradoxical growth hormone release has been reported by Macaron and colleagues (1978) in response to TRH administration and by Casper and colleagues (1977) in response to glucose administration. Under normal conditions, growth hormone secretion is augmented during SWS onset early in the night. This association may be disrupted in patients with anorexia nervosa in whom nocturnal growth hormone surges have been found to be prolonged or decreased in amplitude (Kalucy et al. 1976). HGH and cortisol hormones are protective counterregulatory hormones that stimulate gluconeogenesis in response to the threat of hypoglycemia with undernutrition. Growth hormone also stimulates the mobilization of fatty acids from fat tissue and seems to play a synergistic role with sex steroids during the adolescent growth spurt in conjunction with somatomedin (Phillips and Vassilopoulou-Sellin 1980).

Arginine Vasopressin

In response to osmotic challenge tests, patients with anorexia nervosa have been shown to have erratically high or reduced vasopressin responses consistent with partial diabetes insipidus, which results in mild polyuria (Gold et al. 1983). In response to water deprivation, patients often do not sufficiently concentrate urine but respond normally when given vasopressin. Thus, most patients do have a relative, but not an absolute, deficiency of vasopressin secretion, which can also be observed after fasting (Drenick 1977). Even intermittent decreases in vasopressin may cause polyuria despite episodic high levels. The instability of the vasopressin response can persist in some patients even after they gain weight. However, in a study by Gold and colleagues (1983), most weight-improved patients were found to have normal vasopressin responses to sodium loading.

Prolactin

Prolactin is one of the few hormones that shows little, if any, alteration during the course of anorexia nervosa or in malnutrition (Beumont et al. 1974; Casper and Frohman 1982; Ferrari et al. 1990; Isaacs et al. 1980; Kiriike et al. 1986; Mecklenburg et al. 1974; Wakeling et al. 1979). Given that pituitary lactotrophs reflect central nervous system (CNS) dopaminergic tone, the normal prolactin plasma levels would argue against a dopamine deficiency theory of anorexia nervosa. Most investigators have found normal plasma prolactin secretion patterns in response to TRH administration, although some have observed elevated levels (Travaglini et al. 1976) or a temporary delay in peak prolactin responses (Vigersky et al. 1976).

Melatonin

Melatonin, produced by the pineal gland, is an important neuromodulator of reproductive function. In various mammalian species, melatonin has been shown to inhibit gonadal development and function (Rivest 1987). Changes in the circadian pattern of melatonin may modulate pubertal development and ovarian cyclicity.

The reports on the circadian rhythm of melatonin in anorexia nervosa are somewhat conflicting. Ferrari et al. (1989, 1990) reported that the circadian profile of plasma melatonin in patients with anorexia nervosa was similar to, albeit levels were significantly higher than concentrations in control subjects, with an increased ratio of day and night melatonin levels to abnormal daytime secretory peaks of melatonin. In contrast, Kennedy et al. (1991) reported similar melatonin plasma levels in underweight or weight-improved patients and healthy control subjects; however, the patients with the lowest weight tended to have the highest nocturnal melatonin levels. Thus, increases in melatonin levels and the persistence of melatonin secretion during the day might contribute to the inhibition of pituitary-gonadal function in patients with anorexia nervosa.

ANOREXIA NERVOSA, BINGE-EATING/PURGING SUBTYPE, AND BULIMIA NERVOSA

The starvation-induced changes in anorexia nervosa, binge-eating/purging subtype, and in bulimia nervosa resemble in many ways those seen in anorexia nervosa of the restricting subtype. The additional binge-eating, self-induced vomiting, and/or diuretic and laxative abuse produce a new set of medical complications (Table 32–3).

Physical Changes

Despite generally normal body weight in bulimia nervosa, large body weight fluctuations as a result of episodic fasting followed by periods of overeating are nevertheless possible. Binge eating can cause acute gastric dilatation and, in rare cases, gastric rupture (Backett 1985; Saul et al. 1981). Repeated vomiting has been found to lead to erosion of dental enamel, esophagitis, Mallory-Weiss syn-

Table 32–3. Physical manifestations in bulimia nervosa (and in anorexia nervosa, binge-eating/purging subtype)

Body weight fluctuations (2–50 lbs.)	
Metabolic	Hypothermia
	Hypometabolism
	Hypokalemia
	Hypochloremic alkalosis
Central nervous system	Abnormal electroencephalogram findings
Orogastrointestinal	Dental enamel erosion
	Swelling of salivary glands
	Parotid enlargement
	Esophagitis
	Mallory-Weiss tears
	Gastric dilation
	Gastric rupture
	Diarrhea
Cardiovascular	Electrocardiogram changes
	Arrhythmias
	Cardiac arrest
Renal	Dehydration
	Alkalosis
	Renal calculi
	Renal insufficiency
Pulmonary	Aspiration pneumonia

drome, and (rarely) esophageal rupture. Salivary gland enlargement is common, with the parotid glands most frequently affected, resulting in a "chipmunk" appearance, but its mechanism is unclear. It could be related to excess saliva production, rapid overeating, repeated vomiting, excess use of chewing gum, or alkalosis. Parotid biopsies have revealed normal hyperplastic tissue (Levin et al. 1980; Walsh et al. 1982). Salivary gland enlargement may be associated with elevated serum amylase levels, which need to be distinguished through isoenzyme assay from elevated serum amylase levels in pancreatitis. Cox and colleagues (1983) reported pancreatic abnormalities and pancreatitis (Marano and Sangree 1984; Zerbe 1992) in patients with bulimia nervosa. In patients who abuse alcohol or drugs, vomiting during semiconscious states can lead to aspiration and aspiration pneumonia and cause death.

Metabolic Changes

The intermittent caloric deficiency in patients with bulimia nervosa has been shown to elevate levels of free fatty acids and β-hydroxybutyric acid in plasma, which suggests excess lipid mobilization (Pirke et al. 1985). A serious and potentially life-threatening metabolic complication is hypokalemia. Potassium depletion is most often a result of emesis and/or laxative or diuretic abuse (Elkinton and Huth 1958; Wallace et al. 1968; Warren and Steinberg 1979). Because the potassium concentration of gastric fluid is fairly low, probably only a small portion of the potassium depletion is caused by potassium loss from gastric fluid or saliva. Most of the potassium is lost as a result of increased renal potassium excretion secondary to metabolic alkalosis, partly because of loss of hydrochloric acid from gastric fluid through vomiting.

On the other hand, hypokalemia can result from significant intestinal potassium loss through chronic diarrhea following laxative abuse. Moderate to severe hypokalemia leads to weakness in skeletal and smooth muscle; more dangerous effects are cardiac conduction abnormalities, arrhythmia, and (ultimately) cardiac arrest. Chronic metabolic alkalosis can be associated with hypokalemic nephropathy and occasionally simulates Bartter's syndrome, which is characterized by hypokalemic alkalosis, hyperaldosteronism, and hyperplasia of the renal juxtaglomerular apparatus. Urinary chloride levels distinguish chronic metabolic alkalosis from Bartter's syndrome. Clinicians often must prescribe potassium supplements for patients with bulimia nervosa; dosage adjustments depend on the frequency of vomiting. The orthostatic hypotension can be worsened by a reduction in plasma volume caused by significant electrolyte imbalances and intermittent dehydration as a result of vomiting. A serious renal complication, aside from renal calculi, is renal failure.

Sleep Changes

Patients with bulimia nervosa have less significant disruptions in sleep continuity than do patients with anorexia nervosa (Levy et al. 1987; Waller et al. 1989; Walsh et al. 1985). Most studies found that REM latency in patients with bulimia nervosa was indistinguishable from that of control subjects (Levy et al. 1988; Walsh et al. 1985). The increased incidence of drug abuse, alcoholism, and affective disorder can affect sleep parameters and must be monitored when evaluating sleep parameters in patients with bulimia nervosa. The phenomena of sleepwalking and sleep-related eating in bulimia nervosa doubtlessly deserve more systematic investigation (Guirguis 1986; Gupta 1991).

Morphological Brain Changes

In a brain PET study of a small group of bulimic patients, Lankenau et al. (1985) found no differences in comparison with nonbulimic control subjects, although all bulimic patients reported vomiting and some reported laxative abuse. A subsequent study by Krieg and colleagues (1987), which used brain CT scans, reported that nearly one-half of a group of normal-weight bulimic patients had sulcal widening, and one-fifth had enlarged ventricles. No relation was found between the brain changes and measures of starvation such as plasma cortisol, T_3, and β-hydroxybutyric acid levels; however, in later study, Krieg and Pirke (1989) found that ventricular size was inversely correlated with plasma levels of T_3. Hoffman et al. (1989) reported sulcal widening by MRI, but no ventricular expansion in bulimic patients. In a further assessment, Hoffman et al. (1990) measured proton longitudinal relaxation time (T1) through MRI and found a significant T1 decrease for inferior frontal gray matter in the bulimic group compared with control subjects. The T1 decrease was not associated with vomiting, but the study did not measure potassium levels, which have been implicated in T1 decreases.

Differences in the activation of various brain regions based on PET scanning between patients with bulimia nervosa and control subjects were documented by Hagman and colleagues (1990). These authors found reduced right-hemispheric metabolic rates, including the basal ganglia, which document a reversal of the right greater than left metabolic pattern in nonbulimic women. Depressed women in this study retained the right-hemisphere activa-

tion. Because the bulimic women were rated as equally depressed as the depressed women control subjects based on clinical rating scales, the findings point to specific changes associated with bulimia nervosa (Hagman et al. 1990; Wu et al. 1990). It cannot be ruled out that the specific changes are produced by an altered physiology, because the studies provided evidence supporting a correlation between binge-eating and vomiting frequency and abnormal eating attitudes and the abnormal metabolic pattern in several brain regions. Further support for the notion of a metabolic component is the finding by Hagman et al. (1990) of a positive correlation between the severity of the dynamic PET changes and the severity of the bulimia. As in anorexia nervosa, the functional consequences of the brain changes remain to be elucidated.

Electroencephalogram Changes

Green and Rau (1974) first noted abnormal EEG findings in bulimia nervosa; the most common abnormality is a paroxysmal 14- and 6-per-second spike pattern. This pattern, however, can also be observed in nonbulimic adolescents (Maulsby 1979). Indeed, Mitchell et al. (1983) confirmed the age dependence of these findings when they reported normal EEG recordings in more than 80% of adult patients with bulimia nervosa.

Neuroendocrine Changes

Far fewer endocrine investigations have been done in bulimia nervosa than in anorexia nervosa. Some patients with bulimia nervosa show endocrine changes; others do not (Mitchell et al. 1983; Wetzin et al. 1991). Dietary restriction and abnormal eating very likely play a role because few hormonal abnormalities are observed when food intake becomes normal (Casper et al. 1988b). For instance, Kiyohara et al. (1987) documented abnormal eating patterns in all bulimia nervosa patients who had abnormal TSH responses to TRH. Similarly, in normal-weight bulimic women, normal peak glucose and insulin levels after oral glucose administration have been reported (Blouin et al. 1991; Casper et al. 1988b; Mitchell and Bantle 1983; Weingarten et al. 1988), and insulin responses after intravenous glucose administration were in the normal range (Coiro et al. 1992); it is interesting that cortisol levels remained unchanged and HGH levels increased rather than declined, which suggests subtle metabolic alterations. Somatostatin levels are generally normal (Kaye et al. 1988). Oligomenorrhea or menstrual irregularities in bulimic women seem to exceed the rates in nonbulimic women (Pirke et al. 1987a; Stewart et al. 1987), and abnormalities in LH release have been reported (Pirke et al. 1987b).

Patients with bulimia nervosa show dexamethasone nonsuppression more often than would be expected based on their apparently normal body weight (Gwirtsman et al. 1983; Hudson et al. 1982, 1983; Levy and Dixon 1987; Walsh et al. 1987), but comorbid disorders were not ruled out in most studies. Walsh et al. (1987) measured 24-hour cortisol secretion patterns and cortisol release on ACTH stimulation in symptomatic patients with bulimia nervosa and found a normal cortisol secretion pattern and normal cortisol increase following ACTH administration. Similarly, Gold et al. (1986) reported normal ACTH levels following CRH administration in patients of normal weight with bulimia nervosa.

CONCLUSION

The prolonged and severe caloric restriction and the resultant catabolic state that characterize anorexia nervosa lead to innumerable biological changes. In fact, the restricting subtype of anorexia nervosa, with its profound and pathological weight loss, can be considered a model of long-term starvation without attendant organic illness. Anorexia nervosa provides a wealth of information about the physiological, metabolic, and endocrine consequences of various degrees of undernutrition and malnutrition.

Follow-up studies suggest that full biological recovery with normalization of all metabolic and endocrine parameters is likely in the fasting patient with anorexia nervosa if weight is restored to that appropriate for age and height and if nutritious, well-balanced meals are eaten. Whether undernutrition in early adolescence affects long-term skeletal growth and, from an orthopedic viewpoint, whether patients with anorexia nervosa are at greater risk for nontraumatic fractures in the long run deserve further study.

In the case of bulimia nervosa, in which episodic caloric deficiency (mostly as a result of emesis) can result in a puzzling array of generally moderate but sometimes life-threatening physiological, metabolic, and neuroendocrine disturbances, permanent physical damage has been reported. Such injury is invariably the result of vomiting behavior and abuse of laxatives or diuretics and other noxious substances (e.g., ipecac use can lead to cardiomyopathy).

Various efforts have been made to sort out the biological differences between eating disorders and depressive disorders. The remarkable similarities between the HPA axis abnormalities in anorexia nervosa and in depressive disorder require more careful examination against the background of either malnutrition and weight loss in depressive disorders or a comorbid affective disorder in an-

orexia nervosa before a common underlying mechanism can be postulated (Casper et al. 1987). The overlap in the HPA axis disturbances between the two disorders should not detract from obvious differences in the clinical picture. For instance, marked differences in mood and energy level at early-morning awakening (typically observed in both conditions) can easily differentiate the two disorders. Patients with anorexia nervosa usually awaken refreshed and full of energy, whereas depressed patients typically dwell on morbid worries and feel lethargic in the morning. Lethargy in the presence of abnormally low plasma cortisol levels would be highly suggestive of Addison's disease.

The thyroid axis is another system that can be used to distinguish the two disorders. The recently developed supersensitive TSH assays show normally low TSH plasma levels in anorexia nervosa, indicating a euthyroid sick syndrome, whereas elevated TSH levels would be suggestive of hypothyroidism with weight loss.

In the eating disorders, then, nutritional deficits and changes in body composition, eating pattern, dietary composition, comorbidity, age, and treatment status account for most of the variance in the biological findings. Unless more homogeneous populations can be investigated with superb experimental control of all the confounding variables, it would seem premature to assign etiological significance to any of the recorded biological changes.

REFERENCES

Alvarez LC, Dimas CO, Catro A, et al: Growth hormone in malnutrition. J Clin Endocrinol Metab 34:400–409, 1972

American Psychiatric Association: Diagnostic and Statistical Manual of Mental Disorders, 4th Edition, Washington, DC, American Psychiatric Association, 1994

Andersen AE, Woodward PJ, LaFrance N: Bone mineral density of eating disorder subgroups. Int J Eat Disord 18:335–342, 1995

Backett SA: Acute pancreatitis and gastric dilation in a patient with anorexia nervosa. Postgrad Med J 61:39–40, 1985

Bell RM: Holy Anorexia. Chicago, IL, University of Chicago Press, 1985

Benca RM, Casper RC: Sleep in eating disorders, in Principles and Practice of Sleep Medicine, 2nd Edition. Edited by Kryger MH, Roth T, Dement WC. Philadelphia, PA, WB Saunders, 1994, pp 927–933

Bermuder F, Surks MI, Oppenheimer JH: High incidence of decreased serum triiodothyronine concentration in patients with nonthyroidal disease. J Clin Endocrinol Metab 41:27–31, 1975

Beumont PJV, Freisen HG, Gelder MG, et al: Plasma prolactin and luteinizing hormone levels in anorexia nervosa. Psychol Med 4:219–221, 1974

Beumont PJV, George GCW, Pimstone BL, et al: Body weight and the pituitary response to hypothalamic-releasing hormones in patients with anorexia nervosa. J Clin Endocrinol Metab 40:221–227, 1976

Blouin AG, Blouin JH, Braaten JT, et al: Physiological and psychological responses to a glucose challenge in bulimia. Int J Eat Disord 10:285–296, 1991

Bowers TK, Eckert E: Leukopenia in anorexia nervosa: lack of increased risk of infection. Arch Intern Med 138:1520–1523, 1978

Boyar RM, Bradlow HL: Studies of testosterone metabolism in anorexia nervosa, in Anorexia Nervosa. Edited by Vigersky RA. New York, Raven, 1977, pp 271–276

Boyar RM, Katz J, Finkelstein JW, et al: Anorexia nervosa: immaturity of the 24-hour luteinizing hormone secretory pattern. N Engl J Med 291:861–865, 1974

Boyar RM, Hellman LD, Roffwarg HP, et al: Cortisol secretion and metabolism in anorexia nervosa. N Engl J Med 296:190–193, 1977

Brambilla F, Ferrari E, Petraglia F, et al: Peripheral opioid secretory pattern in anorexia nervosa. Psychiatry Res 39:115–127, 1991

Brooks SM, Sanborn CF, Albrecht BH, et al: Diet in athletic amenorrhoea (letter). Lancet 1:559–560, 1984

Brown N, Ward A, Treasure J, et al: Leptin levels in anorexia nervosa (acute and long term recovered) (abstract). Int J Obes 20:37, 1996

Bruch H: Eating Disorders. New York, Basic Books, 1973

Casper RC: On the emergence of bulimia nervosa as a syndrome: a historical view. Int J Eat Disord 2:3–16, 1983

Casper RC, Davis JM: On the course of anorexia nervosa. Am J Psychiatry 134:974–978, 1977

Casper RC, Frohman LA: Delayed TSH release in anorexia nervosa following injection of thyrotropin releasing hormone (TRH). Psychoneuroendocrinology 7:59–68, 1982

Casper RC, Davis JM, Pandey GN: The effect of nutritional status and weight changes on hypothalamic function tests in anorexia nervosa, in Anorexia Nervosa. Edited by Vigersky RA. New York, Raven, 1977, pp 137–147

Casper RC, Chatterton RT Jr, Davis M: Alterations in serum cortisol and its binding characteristics in anorexia nervosa. J Clin Endocrinol Metab 49:406–411, 1979

Casper RC, Eckert ED, Halmi KA, et al: Bulimia: its incidence and clinical importance in patients with anorexia nervosa. Arch Gen Psychiatry 37:1030–1035, 1980a

Casper RC, Kirschner B, Sandstead HH, et al: An evaluation of trace metals, vitamins, and taste function in anorexia nervosa. Am J Clin Nutr 33:1801–1808, 1980b

Casper RC, Swann AC, Stokes PE, et al: Weight loss, cortisol levels, and dexamethasone suppression in patients with major depressive disorder. Acta Psychiatr Scand 75:243–250, 1987

Casper RC, Pandey GN, Jaspan JB, et al: Eating attitudes and glucose tolerance in anorexia nervosa patients at 8-year followup compared to control subjects. Psychiatry Res 25:283–299, 1988a

Casper RC, Pandey GN, Jaspan JB, et al: Hormone and metabolite plasma levels after oral glucose in bulimia and healthy controls. Biol Psychiatry 24:663–674, 1988b

Casper RC, Schoeller DA, Kushner R, et al: Total daily energy expenditure and activity level in anorexia nervosa. Am J Clin Nutr 53:1143–1150, 1991

Coiro V, Volpi R, Marchesi C, et al: Abnormal growth hormone and cortisol, but not thyroid-stimulating hormone, responses to an intravenous glucose tolerance test in normal-weight, bulimic women. Psychoneuroendocrinology 17:639–645, 1992

Cox KL, Cannon RA, Ament ME, et al: Biochemical and ultrasound abnormalities of the pancreas in anorexia nervosa. Dig Dis Sci 28:225–229, 1983

Crisp AH, Fenton GW, Scotton L: A controlled study of the EEG in anorexia nervosa. Br J Psychiatry 114:1149–1160, 1968

Crisp AH, Stonehill E, Fenton GW: The relationship between sleep, nutrition and mood: a study of patients with anorexia nervosa. Postgrad Med J 47:207–213, 1971

Dale D, Gerlach DH, Wilhite AL: Menstrual dysfunction in distance runners. Obstet Gynecol 54:47–53, 1979

Datlof S, Coleman PD, Frobes GB, et al: Ventricular dilation on CAT scans of patients with anorexia nervosa. Am J Psychiatry 143:96–98, 1986

Doerr P, Fichter M, Pirke KM, et al: Relationship between weight gain and hypothalamic pituitary adrenal function in patients with anorexia nervosa. J Steroid Biochem Mol Biol 13:529–537, 1980

Doraiswamy PM, Massey EW, Enright K, et al: Wernicke-Korsakoff syndrome caused by psychogenic food refusal: MR findings. American Journal of Neuroradiology 15:594–596, 1994

Drenick H: Role of vasopressin and prolactin in abnormal salt and water metabolism of obese patients before and after fasting and during refeeding. Metabolism 26:309–317, 1977

Dreyfus G, Mamou H: Cachéxie cérébro-hypophysaire d'origine fonctionnelle et à évolution mortelle sans altérations histologiques à l'autopsie [Cachexia of central hypophyseal origin leading to death without histological changes at autopsy]. Ann Endocrinol (Paris) 8:540–544, 1947

Dubois A, Gross HA, Ebert MH, et al: Altered gastric emptying and secretion in primary anorexia nervosa. Gastroenterology 77:319–323, 1979

Elkinton JR, Huth EJ: Body fluid abnormalities in anorexia nervosa and undernutrition. Metabolism 5:376–403, 1958

Enzmann DR, Lane B: Cranial computer tomography findings in anorexia nervosa. J Comput Assist Tomogr 1:410–414, 1977

Ettinger B, Genant HK, Cann CE: Long-term estrogen replacement therapy prevents bone loss and fractures. Ann Intern Med 102:319–324, 1985

Evans FJ: Sleep, eating, and weight disorders, in Eating and Weight Disorders. Edited by Richard K. New York, Springer, 1983, pp 147–178

Ferrari E, Foppa S, Bossolo PA, et al: Melatonin and pituitary-gonadal function in disorders of eating behavior. J Pineal Res 7:115–124, 1989

Ferrari E, Fraschini F, Brambilla F: Hormonal circadian rhythms in eating disorders. Biol Psychiatry 27:1007–1020, 1990

Fichter M, Pirke KM, Holsboer F: Weight loss causes neuroendocrine disturbances: experimental study in healthy starving subjects. Psychiatry Res 17:61–72, 1986

Fink S, Eckert E, Mitchell J, et al: T-lymphocyte subsets in patients with abnormal body weight: longitudinal studies in anorexia nervosa and obesity. Int J Eat Disord 20:295–305, 1996

Fishman J, Boyar RM, Hellman L: Influence of body weight on estradiol metabolism in young women. J Clin Endocrinol Metab 41:989–991, 1975

Fishman J, Hellman L, Zumoff B, et al: Effect of thyroid on hydroxylation of estrogen in man. J Clin Endocrinol Metab 25:365–376, 1976

Fohlin L: Body composition, cardiovascular and renal function in adolescent patients with anorexia nervosa. Acta Paediatr Suppl 268:1–20, 1977

Frisch RL: Fatness, menarche, and female fertility. Perspect Biol Med 28:611–633, 1985

Frisch RL, Revelle R: Height and weight at menarche and a hypothesis of critical body weights and adolescent events. Science 169:397–398, 1970

Frisch RL, Wyshak G, Vincent L: Delayed menarche and amenorrhea in ballet dancers. N Engl J Med 303:17–19, 1980

Gardner DF, Kaplan MM, Stanley CA, et al: Effect of triiodothyronine replacement on the metabolic and pituitary responses to starvation. N Engl J Med 300:579–584, 1979

Garfinkel PE, Brown GH, Stancer HC, et al: Hypothalamic-pituitary function in anorexia nervosa. Arch Gen Psychiatry 32:739–744, 1975

Gerner RH, Gwirtsman HE: Abnormalities of dexamethasone suppression test and urinary MHPG in anorexia nervosa. Am J Psychiatry 138:650–653, 1981

Glowa JR, Gold PW: Corticotropin releasing hormone produced profound anorexigenic effects in the rhesus monkey. Neuropeptides 18:55–61, 1991

Gold PW, Kaye W, Robertson GL, et al: Abnormalities in plasma and cerebrospinal fluid arginine vasopressin in patients with anorexia nervosa. N Engl J Med 308:1117–1123, 1983

Gold PW, Gwirtsman H, Avgerinos PC, et al: Abnormal hypothalamic-pituitary-adrenal function in anorexia nervosa: pathophysiologic mechanisms in underweight and weight-corrected patients. N Engl J Med 314:1335–1342, 1986

Golden NH, Ashtari M, Kohn MR, et al: Reversibility of cerebral ventricular enlargement in anorexia nervosa, demonstrated by quantitative magnetic resonance imaging. J Pediatr 128:296–301, 1996

Goldin BR, Adlercrentz H, Gorbach SL: Estrogen excretion patterns and plasma levels in vegetarian and omnivorous women. N Engl J Med 307:1542–1547, 1982

Gottdiener JS, Gross HA, Henry WL, et al: Effects of self-induced starvation on cardiac size and function in anorexia nervosa. Circulation 58:426–433, 1978

Green RS, Rau JH: Treatment of compulsive eating disturbances with anticonvulsant medication. Am J Psychiatry 131:428–432, 1974

Grinspoon S, Gulick T, Askari H, et al: Serum leptin levels in women with anorexia nervosa. J Clin Endocrinol Metab 81:3361–3863, 1996

Guirguis WR: Sleepwalking as a symptom of bulimia. BMJ 293:587–588, 1986

Guisti M, Torre R, Traverso L: Endogenous opioid blockade and gonadotropin secretion: role of pulsatile luteinizing hormone-releasing hormone administration in anorexia nervosa and weight loss amenorrhea. Fertil Steril 49:797–801, 1988

Gupta MA: Sleep-related eating in bulimia nervosa—an underreported parasomnia disorder. Sleep Research 20:182–185, 1991

Gwirtsman HE, Roy-Byrne P, Yager J, et al: Neuroendocrine abnormalities in bulimia. Am J Psychiatry 140:559–563, 1983

Hagman JO, Buchsbaum MS, Wer JG, et al: Comparison of regional brain metabolism in bulimia nervosa and affective disorder assessed with positron emission tomography. J Affect Disord 19:153–162, 1990

Halmi KA, Falk JR: Common physiological changes in anorexia nervosa. Int J Eat Disord 1:16–27, 1981

Hamilton M: A rating scale for depression. J Neurol Neurosurg Psychiatry 23:56–62, 1960

Hebebrand J, Blum W, Barth N, et al: Leptin levels in patients with anorexia nervosa are reduced in the acute stage and elevated upon short-term weight restoration. Molecular Psychiatry 2:330–334, 1997

Heinz ER, Martinez J, Haenggeli A: Reversibility of cerebral atrophy in anorexia nervosa and Cushing's syndrome. J Comput Assist Tomogr 1:415–418, 1977

Herholz K, Krieg JC, Emrich HM, et al: Regional cerebral glucose metabolism in anorexia nervosa measured by positron emission tomography. Biol Psychiatry 22:43–51, 1987

Herpertz-Dahlman B, Remschmidt H: The prognostic value of the dexamethasone suppression test for the course of anorexia nervosa—comparison with depressive diseases. Z Kinder Jugenpsychiatr 18:5–11, 1990

Hoffman GW, Ellinwood EH, Rockwell WJK, et al: Cerebral atrophy in anorexia nervosa. Biol Psychiatry 26:321–324, 1989

Hoffman GW, Ellinwood EH, Rockwell WJK, et al: Cerebral atrophy and T1 measured by magnetic resonance imaging in bulimia. Biol Psychiatry 27:116–119, 1990

Hotta M, Shibasaki T, Yamauchi N, et al: The effects of chronic central administration of corticotropin-releasing factor on food intake, body weight, and hypothalamic-pituitary-adrenocortical hormones. Life Sci 48:1483–1491, 1991

Hudson JI, Laffer PS, Pope HG: Bulimia related to affective disorder by family history and response to the DST. Am J Psychiatry 139:685–687, 1982

Hudson JI, Pope HG, Jonas JM, et al: HPA axis hyperactivity in bulimia. Psychiatry Res 8:111–117, 1983

Isaacs AJ, Leslie D, Gomez J, et al: The effect of weight gain on gonadotrophins and prolactin in anorexia nervosa. Acta Endocrinologia (Copenh) 94:145–150, 1980

Jackson RL, Kelby AG: Growth charts for use in pediatric practice. J Pediatr 27:215–229, 1945

Kalucy RC, Crisp AH, Chard T, et al: Nocturnal hormonal profiles in massive obesity, anorexia nervosa and normal females. J Psychosom Res 20:595–604, 1976

Karacan I, Rosenbloom AL, Londono JH, et al: The effect of acute fasting on sleep and the sleep-growth hormone response. Psychosomatics 14:33–37, 1973

Katz JL, Boyar R, Roffwarg H, et al: Weight and circadian luteinizing hormone secretory pattern in anorexia nervosa. Psychosom Med 40:549–567, 1978

Katz JL, Kuperberg A, Pollack CP, et al: Is there a relationship between eating disorder and affective disorder? New evidence from sleep recordings. Am J Psychiatry 141:753–759, 1984

Katzman DK, Lambe EK, Mikulis DJ, et al: Cerebral gray matter and white matter volume deficits in adolescent girls with anorexia nervosa. J Pediatr 129:794–803, 1996

Kaye WH, Rubinow D, Gwirtsman HE, et al: CSF somatostatin in anorexia nervosa and bulimia: relationship to the hypothalamic-pituitary-adrenal cortical axis. Psychoneuroendocrinology 13:265–272, 1988

Kennedy SH, Brown GM, McVey G, et al: Pineal and adrenal function before and after refeeding in anorexia nervosa. Biol Psychiatry 30:216–224, 1991

Keys A, Brozek J, Henschel A, et al: The Biology of Human Starvation. Minneapolis, MN, University of Minnesota Press, 1950

Keys A, Fidanza F, Karvonan MJ, et al: Indices of relative weight and obesity. Journal of Chronic Disease 25:329–343, 1972

Kingston K, Szmukler G, Andrewes D, et al: Neuropsychological and structural brain changes in anorexia nervosa before and after refeeding. Psychol Med 26:15–28, 1996

Kiriike N, Nishiwaki S, Izumiya Y, et al: Thyrotropin, prolactin and growth hormone responses to thyrotropin-releasing hormone in anorexia nervosa and bulimia. Biol Psychiatry 21:167–176, 1986

Kiyohara K, Tamai H, Karibe C, et al: Serum thyrotropin (TSH) responses to thyrotropin-releasing hormone (TRH) in patients with anorexia nervosa and bulimia: influence of changes in body weight and eating disorders. Psychoneuroendocrinology 12:21–28, 1987

Kohlmeyer K, Lehmkul G, Poutska F: Computed tomography of anorexia nervosa. AJNR Am J Neuroradiol 4:437–438, 1983

Krahn DD, Gosnell BA, Majchrzak MG: The anorectic effects of CRH and restraint stress decrease with repeated exposures. Biol Psychiatry 27:1094–1102, 1990

Krieg JC, Pirke KM: Structural brain abnormalities in patients with bulimia nervosa. Psychiatry Res 27:39–48, 1989

Krieg JC, Backmund H, Pirke KM: Cranial computed tomography findings in bulimia. Acta Psychiatr Scand 75:144–149, 1987

Krieg JC, Pirke KM, Lauer C, et al: Endocrine, metabolic and cranial computed tomographic findings in anorexia nervosa. Biol Psychiatry 23:377–387, 1988

Krieg JC, Lauer C, Leinsinger G, et al: Brain morphology and regional cerebral blood flow in anorexia nervosa. Biol Psychiatry 25:1041–1048, 1989

Kupfer DJ, Bulik CM: Sleeping and waking EEG in anorexia nervosa, in The Psychobiology of Anorexia Nervosa. Edited by Pirke KM, Ploog D. Berlin, Springer-Verlag, 1984, pp 73–86

Lacey JH, Crisp AH, Kalucy RS, et al: Study of EEG sleep characteristics in patients with anorexia nervosa before and after restoration of matched population mean weight consequent on ingestion of a 'normal' diet. Postgrad Med J 52:45–49, 1976

Laessle RG, Krieg JC, Pirke KM: Cerebral atrophy and vigilance performance in patients with anorexia nervosa and bulimia nervosa. Neuropsychobiology 21:187–191, 1989

Lankenau H, Swigar ME, Bhimani S, et al: Cranial CT scans in eating disorder patients and controls. Compr Psychiatry 26:136–147, 1985

Lauer CJ, Zulley J, Krieg JC, et al: EEG sleep and the cholinergic REM induction test in anorexic and bulimic patients. Psychiatry Res 26:171–181, 1988

Lauer CJ, Krieg JC, Riemann D, et al: A polysomnographic study in young psychiatric inpatients: major depression, anorexia nervosa, bulimia nervosa. J Affect Disord 18:235–245, 1990

Lesem MD, Kaye WH, Bissette G, et al: Cerebrospinal fluid TRH immunoreactivity in anorexia nervosa. Biol Psychiatry 35:48–53, 1994

Leslie RD, Isaacs AJ, Gomez J, et al: Hypothalamo-pituitary-thyroid function in anorexia nervosa: influence of weight gain. BMJ 2:526–528, 1978

Levin PA, Falko JM, Dixon K, et al: Benign parotid enlargement in bulimia. Ann Intern Med 93:827–829, 1980

Levy AB, Dixon KN: DST in bulimia without endogenous depression. Biol Psychiatry 22:783–786, 1987

Levy AB, Dixon KN, Schmidt H: REM and delta sleep in anorexia nervosa and bulimia. Psychiatry Res 20:189–197, 1987

Levy AB, Dixon KN, Schmidt H: Sleep architecture in anorexia nervosa and bulimia. Biol Psychiatry 23:99–101, 1988

Luck P, Wakeling A: Altered thresholds for thermoregulatory sweating and vasodilation in anorexia nervosa. BMJ 281:906–908, 1980

Macaron C, Wilber JF, Green O, et al: Studies of growth hormone (GH), thyrotrophin (TSH) and prolactin (PRL) secretion in anorexia nervosa. Psychoneuroendocrinology 3:181–185, 1978

Mant MJ, Faragher BS: The haematology of anorexia nervosa. Br J Haematol 23:737–749, 1972

Marano AR, Sangree MH: Acute pancreatitis associated with bulimia. J Clin Gastroenterol 6:245–248, 1984

Martin F: Pathologie des aspects neurologiques et psychiatriques de quelques manifestitations carentielles avec troubles digestifs et neuro-endocriniens [The pathology of neurological and psychiatric aspects of certain manifestations with digestive and neuroendocrine problems as a result of fasting]. Acta Neurol Belg 58:816–830, 1958

Maulsby RL: EEG patterns of uncertain diagnostic significance, in Current Practice of Clinical Electroencephalography. Edited by Klass DW, Daly DD. New York, Raven, 1979, pp 251–267

Maxwell JK, Tuycker DM, Townes BD: Asymmetric cognitive function in anorexia nervosa. Int J Neurosci 24:37–44, 1984

McFayden UM, Oswald I, Lewis SA: Starvation and human slow-wave sleep. J Appl Physiol 35:391–394, 1973

Mecklenburg RS, Loriaux DL, Thompson RH, et al: Hypothalamic dysfunction in patients with anorexia nervosa. Medicine (Baltimore) 53:147–159, 1974

Mickley D, Greenfeld D, Quinlan DM, et al: Abnormal liver enzymes in outpatients with eating disorders. Int J Eat Disord 20:325–329, 1996

Mitchell JE, Bantle JP: Metabolic and endocrine investigations in women of normal weight with the bulimia syndrome. Biol Psychiatry 18:355–364, 1983

Mitchell JE, Hosfield W, Pyle RL: EEG findings in patients with the bulimia syndrome. Int J Eat Disord 2:17–23, 1983

Miyai K, Yamamoto T, Axukizawa M, et al: Serum thyroid hormones and thyrotropin in anorexia nervosa. J Clin Endocrinol Metab 40:334–338, 1975

Moore R, Mills H: Serum T_3 and T_4 levels in patients with anorexia nervosa showing transient hyperthyroidism during weight gain. Clin Endocrinol (Oxf) 10:433–439, 1979

Moshang T, Utiger RD: Low triiodothyronine euthyroidism in anorexia nervosa, in Anorexia Nervosa. Edited by Vigersky RA. New York, Raven, 1977, pp 263–270

Moshang T Jr, Parks JS, Balsor L, et al: Low serum triiodothyronine in patients with anorexia nervosa. J Clin Endocrinol Metab 40:470–473, 1975

Myers DG, Starke H, Pearson PH, et al: Leaflet to left ventricular size disproportion and prolapse of a structurally normal mitral valve in anorexia nervosa. Am J Cardiol 60:911–914, 1987

Neil JF, Merikangas JR, Foster FG, et al: Waking and all-night sleep EEG's in anorexia nervosa. Clin Electroencephalogr 11:9–15, 1980

Nillius SJ: Psycho-pathology of weight-related amenorrhea, in Advances in Gynaecological Endocrinology. Edited by Jacobs HS. London, Royal College of Obstetrics and Gynaecologists, 1978, pp 118–130

Nussbaum M, Shenker IR, Marc J, et al: Cerebral atrophy in anorexia nervosa. J Pediatr 96:867–869, 1980

Okuno T, Ito M, Konishi Y, et al: Cerebral atrophy following ACTH therapy. J Comput Assist Tomogr 4:20–23, 1980

Perloff WH, Lasche EM, Nodine JH, et al: The starvation state and functional hypopituitarism. JAMA 155:1307–1313, 1954

Phillips LS, Vassilopoulou-Sellin R: Somatomedins. N Engl J Med 312:438–446, 1980

Pimstone BL, Barbezat G, Hansen JPL, et al: Growth hormone and protein-calorie malnutrition. Lancet 2:1333–1334, 1967

Pirke KM, Fichter MM, Lund R, et al: Twenty-four hour sleep wake pattern of plasma LH in patients with anorexia nervosa. Acta Endocrinologia 92:193–204, 1979

Pirke KM, Pahl J, Schweiger U, et al: Metabolic and endocrine indices of starvation in bulimia: a comparison with anorexia nervosa. Psychiatry Res 15:33–39, 1985

Pirke KM, Fichter MM, Chlond C, et al: Disturbances of the menstrual cycle in bulimia nervosa. Clin Endocrinol (Oxf) 27:245–251, 1987a

Pirke KM, Fichter MM, Schweiger V, et al: Gonadotropin secretion pattern in bulimia nervosa. Int J Eat Disord 6:655–661, 1987b

Powers PS: Heart failure during treatment of anorexia nervosa. Am J Psychiatry 139:1167–1170, 1982

Rigotti NA, Nussbaum SR, Herzog DB, et al: Osteoporosis in women with anorexia nervosa. N Engl J Med 311:1601–1606, 1984

Rivest RW: The female rat as a model describing patterns of pulsatile LH secretion during puberty and their control by melatonin. Gynecol Endocrinol 1:279–293, 1987

Rowe JW, Shelton RL, Helderman JH, et al: Influence of the emetic response on vasopressin release in man. Kidney Int 16:729–735, 1979

Russell GFM: Bulimia nervosa: an ominous variant of anorexia nervosa. Psychol Med 9:429–448, 1979

Saleh JW, Lebwohl P: Metoclopramide-induced gastric emptying in patients with anorexia nervosa. Am J Gastroenterol 74:127–132, 1980

Saul SH, Dekker A, Watson CG: Acute gastric dilation with infarction and perforation. Gut 22:978–983, 1981

Scapagnini U, Moberg GP, Van Loon GR, et al: Relation of the brain 5-hydroxytryptamine content to the diurnal variation in plasma corticosterone in the rat. Neuroendocrinology 7:90–96, 1971

Scheithauer BW, Kovacs KT, Jariwala LK, et al: Anorexia nervosa: an immunohistochemical study of the pituitary gland. Mayo Clin Proc 63:23–28, 1988

Schocken DD, Holloway JD, Powers PS: Weight loss and the heart: effects of anorexia nervosa and starvation. Arch Intern Med 149:877–881, 1989

Sein P, Searson S, Nicol AR: Anorexia nervosa and pseudo-atrophy of the brain. Br J Psychiatry 139:257–258, 1981

Sherman BM, Halmi KA: Effect of nutritional rehabilitation on hypothalamic-pituitary function in anorexia nervosa, in Anorexia Nervosa. Edited by Vigersky RA. New York, Raven, 1977, pp 211–223

Siemers B, Chakmakjian Z, Gench B: Bone density patterns in women with anorexia nervosa. Int J Eat Disord 19:179–186, 1996

Silver TJ, Chan M: Immunologic cytofluorometric studies in adolescents with anorexia nervosa. Int J Eat Disord 19:415–418, 1996

Simmonds M: Ueber Hypophysisschwund mit toedlichem Ausgang [About atrophy of the pituitary gland leading to death]. Dtsch Med Wochenschr 40:322–323, 1914

Stewart DE, Raskin J, Garfinkel PE, et al: Anorexia nervosa, bulimia and pregnancy. Am J Obstet Gynecol 157:1194–1198, 1987

Swayze VW II, Andersen A, Arndt S, et al: Reversibility of brain tissue loss in anorexia nervosa assessed with a computerized Talairach 3-D proportional grid. Psychol Med 26:381–390, 1996

Szmukler GI, Brown SW, Parsons V, et al: Premature loss of bone in chronic anorexia nervosa. BMJ 290:26–27, 1985

Szmukler G, McCance C, McCrone L, et al: Anorexia nervosa: a psychiatric case register study from Aberdeen. Psychol Med 16:49–58, 1986

Thurston J, Marks P: Electrocardiographic abnormalities in patients with anorexia nervosa. Br Heart J 36:719–723, 1974

Travaglini P, Beck-Peccoz P, Ferrari C, et al: Some aspects of hypothalamic-pituitary function in patients with anorexia nervosa. Acta Endocrinologia (Copenh) 81:252–262, 1976

Unger RH, Eisentraut AM, Madison LL: The effects of total starvation upon the levels of circulating glucagon and insulin in man. J Clin Invest 42:1031–1039, 1963

Vagenakis AG, Portnay GI, Burger A, et al: Diversion of peripheral thyroxine metabolism from activating to inactivating pathways during complete fasting. J Clin Endocrinol Metab 41:191–194, 1975

Vaisman N, Rossi MF, Goldberg E, et al: Energy expenditure and body composition in patients with anorexia nervosa. J Pediatr 113:919–924, 1988

Vigersky RA, Loriaux DL, Andersen AE, et al: Delayed pituitary hormone response to LRF TRF in patients with anorexia nervosa and with secondary amenorrhea associated with simple weight loss. J Clin Endocrinol Metab 43:898–900, 1976

Vigersky RA, Andersen AE, Thompson RH, et al: Hypothalamic dysfunction in secondary amenorrhea associated with simple weight loss. N Engl J Med 296:1141–1145, 1977

Wachslicht-Rodbard H, Gross HA, Rodbard D, et al: Increased insulin binding to erythrocytes in anorexia nervosa. N Engl J Med 300:882–887, 1979

Wade GN, Schneider JE: Metabolic fuels and reproduction in female mammals. Neurosci Biobehav Rev 16:235–272, 1992

Wakeling A: Epidemiology of anorexia nervosa. Psychiatry Res 62:3–9, 1996

Wakeling A, DeSouza VA, Gore MBR, et al: Amenorrhea, body weight and serum hormone concentration, with particular reference to prolactin and thyroid hormones in anorexia nervosa. Psychol Med 9:265–272, 1979

Wallace M, Richards P, Chesser E, et al: Persistent alkalosis and hypokalaemia caused by surreptitious vomiting. QJM 37:577–588, 1968

Waller DA, Hardy BW, Pole R, et al: Sleep EEG in bulimic, depressed, and normal subjects. Biol Psychiatry 25:661–664, 1989

Walsh BT, Katz JK, Levin J, et al: Adrenal activity in anorexia nervosa. Psychosom Med 40:499–506, 1978

Walsh BT, Croft CB, Katz JA: Anorexia nervosa and salivary gland enlargement. Int J Psychiatry Med 11:255–261, 1982

Walsh BT, Goetz R, Roose SP, et al: EEG-monitored sleep in anorexia nervosa and bulimia. Biol Psychiatry 20:947–956, 1985

Walsh BT, Roose SP, Katz JL, et al: Hypothalamic-pituitary-adrenal-cortical activity in anorexia nervosa and bulimia. Psychoneuroendocrinology 12:131–140, 1987

Warren SE, Steinberg SM: Acid-base and electrolyte disturbances in anorexia nervosa. Am J Psychiatry 136:415–418, 1979

Weingarten HP, Hendler P, Rodin J: Metabolism and endocrine secretion in response to a test meal in normal weight bulimic women. Psychosom Med 50:273–285, 1988

Wetzin TE, McConaha C, McKee M, et al: Circadian patterns of cortisol, prolactin, and growth hormonal secretion during bingeing and vomiting in normal weight bulimic patients. Biol Psychiatry 30:37–40, 1991

Wilmsen EN: Studies in diet, nutrition, and fertility among a group of Kalahari Bushmen in Botswana. Social Science Information 21:95–125, 1982

Wu JC, Hagman J, Buchsbaum MS, et al: Greater left cerebral hemispheric metabolism in bulimia assessed by positron emission tomography. Am J Psychiatry 147:3, 1990

Zerbe KJ: Recurrent pancreatitis presenting as fever of unknown origin in a recovering bulimic. Int J Eat Disord 12:337–340, 1992

Ziolko HU: Hyperorexia nervosa. Psychother Psychosom Med Psychol 26:10–12, 1976

Zumoff B, Walsh BT, Katz JL, et al: Subnormal plasma dehydroisoandrosterone to cortisol ratio in anorexia nervosa: a second hormonal parameter of ontogenic regression. J Clin Endocrinol Metab 56:668–672, 1983

THIRTY-THREE

Biology of Personality Disorders

Richelle Kirrane, M.D., and Larry J. Siever, M.D.

Disorders of personality may be defined as constellations of character traits and patterns of behavior that are persistently maladaptive and lead to difficulties in functioning in interpersonal and occupational arenas. Personality types were first described in ancient Greece, where a system of four temperaments was elaborated, giving rise to familiar terms such as melancholic and sanguine. Despite this lengthy history, the biology of personality disorders as we know them today has been, until recently, quite ill-defined. Only in the past two decades has a clearer understanding of the mechanisms underlying their clinical manifestations come about, and this is reflected in the fact that a chapter on the biology of personality disorders appears for the first time in this volume.

Personality disorders are coded on Axis II in DSM-IV (American Psychiatric Association 1994); in contrast to Axis I disorders, which occur for the most part in discrete episodes, personality disorders are notably stable and unchanging over time. Recent studies that identify biological bases for these persisting traits of personality render the differentiation between DSM Axes I and II less clear and challenge this traditional separation of psychiatric disorders.

DSM-III-R (American Psychiatric Association 1987) included 11 personality disorders. In DSM-IV, criteria for some of these disorders were modified, and passive-aggressive personality disorder was placed in Appendix B. The 10 DSM-IV personality disorders are divided into three clusters: the "odd" cluster of paranoid, schizoid, and schizotypal (Cluster A); the "dramatic" cluster of antisocial, borderline, histrionic, and narcissistic (Cluster B); and the "anxious" cluster of avoidant, dependent, and obsessive-compulsive personality disorders (Cluster C).

The biological abnormalities that have been described may be elaborated on according to these clusters, affording a dimensional approach to their categorization and further study (Siever et al. 1994b). Along these lines, the domain of cognitive disorganization is prominent in Cluster A, impulsivity and affective lability are core features of Cluster B, and anxiety is the defining feature in Cluster C. Dimensions such as these cut across the boundaries of the specific personality disorders and may even blur the boundaries of the clusters; for example, the dimension of social anxiety overlaps both schizotypal personality disorder and avoidant personality disorder.

Cognitive organization is defined as the ability to organize relevant information and use it appropriately to interact with the environment. Difficulties in this realm are manifested in the psychotic-like symptoms of schizotypal personality disorder and in the less dramatic impairment in interpersonal interactions characteristic of this disorder. Cognitive organization is most profoundly impaired in chronic schizophrenia, in which reality testing is severely distorted. *Impulsivity* may be defined as a tendency to respond to environmental stimuli in an aggressive fashion and is a core characteristic in borderline, histrionic, and antisocial personality disorders. The dramatic cluster is also notable for the trait of *affective instability*, which may be defined as intense and rapid mood shifts, particularly in response to stressors in the environment. *Anxiety* is the most prominent characteristic of the anxious cluster; the fearfulness evident in these disorders is associated with simultaneous autonomic arousal, and assertive behaviors are inhibited.

In this chapter, we review the evidence supporting a biological basis for these four dimensions. The personality disorders about which most is known are schizotypal and borderline, and most attention will be devoted to the biological abnormalities present in these two disorders, along the above dimensions.

BIOLOGY OF PSYCHOTIC-LIKE SYMPTOMS

The odd cluster personality disorders are also known as the schizophrenia-related personality disorders. They are characterized by a pervasive interpersonal isolation; patients are perceived by others as eccentric and "loners." Little is known about the pathophysiology of paranoid or schizoid personality disorder, and these disorders overlap greatly with the third disorder in this category, schizotypal personality disorder; that is, most patients with symptoms that meet criteria for either paranoid or schizoid personality disorder also meet criteria for schizotypal personality disorder. The latter is the most severe personality disorder in this cluster and may be defined as the prototype. It has been well studied, and biological abnormalities have been defined (see Table 33–1). In many areas of study, including those of phenomenology, genetics, and biology, it has been

Table 33–1. Biological correlates of odd cluster personality disorders

Personality disorder	Biological correlates
Schizotypal	Elevated CSF HVA, correlated with positive symptoms
	Amphetamine reduces negative symptoms
	Psychophysiological abnormalities
	Eye movements
	Continuous performance
	Event-related potentials
	Orienting response
	Structural abnormalities
	Increased and decreased ventricle size
	Cognitive deficits
	Abnormal WCST results, correlated with deficit symptoms, decreased HVA
	Amphetamine improves performance
Schizoid	None
Paranoid	None

Note. CSF HVA = cerebrospinal fluid homovanillic acid; WCST = Wisconsin Card Sorting Test.

shown that schizotypal personality disorder is related to schizophrenia (Siever et al. 1993b). Patients have positive or psychotic-like symptoms, such as ideas of reference and magical thinking, and negative or deficit-type symptoms, including restricted emotion and social isolation. These two domains have been shown to be independently heritable (Kendler et al. 1991), and a recent approach to the investigation of schizotypal personality disorder examined the different correlates of the two symptom clusters. Studies of schizotypal personality disorder may help to elucidate the biology of schizophrenia, which may best be understood as part of a spectrum of disorders and not as an isolated entity. Patients with schizotypal personality disorder are less affected by confounding factors such as neuroleptics, institutionalization, and severe unremitting psychosis than are schizophrenic patients and therefore may provide an ideal population in which to study the biological basis of the schizophrenia spectrum.

Studies of schizotypal personality disorder reported that both plasma and cerebrospinal fluid (CSF) homovanillic acid (HVA) levels are elevated, and these elevations have been correlated with the sum of psychotic-like symptoms (Siever et al. 1991, 1993a). This finding lends credence to the hypothesis that these symptoms are associated with hyperdopaminergia, as are the psychotic symptoms of schizophrenia. No correlation was found between plasma or CSF HVA levels and negative symptoms in the studies of schizotypal personality disorder, but in relatives of schizophrenic patients with schizotypal traits, decreased plasma HVA levels were correlated with the deficit-like symptoms of schizotypal personality disorder (Amin et al. 1997). These results not only point toward some dopaminergic abnormality in schizotypal personality disorder but also suggest that in this disorder the two symptom domains may be disentangled.

In 1938, amphetamine, which was being used to treat narcolepsy, was noted to be responsible for the development of psychosis in some patients (Angrist and van Kammen 1984). A subsequent debate ensued about whether the patients had latent schizophrenia to begin with. Amphetamine was later used as a research tool in schizophrenia with varied results: some patients' conditions improved after taking amphetamine, but others worsened. Amphetamine was also used as a probe to determine whether patients would relapse rapidly after neuroleptics were discontinued (Angrist et al. 1985) and as a challenge paradigm in the investigation of borderline personality disorder (Schulz et al. 1987). Some studies examined the differential effects of amphetamine on positive and negative symptoms in schizophrenia; results were mixed and confounded by the fact that patients were taking neuroleptics

(Cesarec and Nyman 1985). More recently, investigators have hypothesized that the psychotic symptoms of schizophrenia are caused by hyperdopaminergia in subcortex, and negative symptoms are the result of hypodopaminergia in the frontal cortex (Davis et al. 1991). Amphetamine is a dopamine agonist. If psychotic-like symptoms in schizotypal personality disorder and in schizophrenia are a result of hyperdopaminergia, then neuroleptics should reduce these symptoms, and amphetamine should worsen them. In schizotypal personality disorder, neuroleptics have indeed diminished psychotic-like symptoms (Goldberg et al. 1986), and amphetamine has worsened psychotic-like symptoms (Schulz et al. 1988). Of note, however, is more recent work showing that patients with schizotypal personality disorder selected solely on the basis of meeting schizotypal personality disorder criteria did not have an increase in psychotic-like symptoms with amphetamine, lending support to the hypothesis that patients with schizotypal personality disorder may be less vulnerable to psychosis based on hyperdopaminergia (Siegel et al. 1996).

BIOLOGY OF NEGATIVE SYMPTOMS

Several psychophysiological tests have yielded abnormal results in schizotypal personality disorder and in schizophrenia, and these abnormalities are associated particularly with negative or deficit-type symptoms. More than one-half of schizophrenic patients have abnormal eye movements while tracking a smoothly moving target, as evidenced by a larger than expected number of saccadic intrusions and by decreased smooth pursuit velocity. Fewer than 10% of the nonschizophrenic population have this abnormality. Relatives of schizophrenic patients also have abnormal eye movements (Holzman et al. 1984). If schizotypal personality disorder is indeed part of the schizophrenia spectrum, patients with schizotypal personality disorder would be expected to have this abnormality, which is, in fact, the case. Studies of volunteers selected for their schizotypal traits had abnormal smooth pursuit eye movements, and volunteers selected for poor eye tracking showed schizotypal traits (Siever et al. 1984). Abnormal eye movements in schizotypal patients (Lencz et al. 1993; Siever et al. 1990) and volunteers are associated with deficit symptoms in these patients (Siever et al. 1994a).

The Continuous Performance Test (Cornblatt and Keilp 1994), a test of attention, produces abnormal results in patients with schizotypal personality disorder, volunteers with schizotypal traits, and patients with schizophrenia. In children of schizophrenic patients, abnormalities on this test are correlated with social isolation (Cornblatt et al. 1992). The Backward Masking Test (Braff 1993), a test of information processing, produces abnormal results in schizotypal and schizophrenic patients, although in one recent study, schizotypal patients performed within the normal range on this test, which raises the question of the relevance of this deficit to the schizophrenia spectrum (Harvey et al. 1996).

Event-related potentials provide a measure of selective attention. Patients with schizotypal personality disorder have abnormal event-related potentials. This abnormality, in which a positive wave at p300 is reduced in amplitude and increased in latency, has also been found in schizophrenic patients and has been linked with negative symptoms. In a recent study, patients with schizotypal personality disorder had significant abnormalities in p300 topography over the left posterior temporal area (Salisbury et al. 1996). However, the abnormality in schizotypal personality disorder is not as prominent as that in schizophrenia, giving rise to the possibility that patients with schizotypal personality disorder share some, but not all, abnormalities with patients with schizophrenia (Trestman et al. 1996). Furthermore, abnormal event-related potentials are not specific to schizotypal personality disorder because they are also found in borderline personality disorder (Kutcher et al. 1989).

The galvanic skin orienting response test measures autonomic responses to environmental stimuli. The findings are abnormal in patients with schizotypal personality disorder and those with schizophrenia, particularly those characterized by anhedonia, because they show hypoarousal to stimuli. Visual reaction time, another test of information processing, has abnormal results in patients with schizotypal personality disorder and schizophrenia; both groups manifested crossover, which represents attentional impairment (Siever 1985).

Structural abnormalities have been found in the brains of patients with schizotypal personality disorder and those with schizophrenia. In schizophrenia, increased ventricle size indexed by increased ventricular-to-brain ratios and cortical atrophy have been described. Ventricular enlargement has also been shown in teenagers with schizophrenia spectrum diagnoses (Schulz et al. 1983), but decreased ventricle size has been associated with schizotypal personality disorder in the children of schizophrenic patients (Schulsinger et al. 1984). This latter finding suggests that children with a genetic predisposition to schizophrenia but without the structural abnormalities may be protected from the disease. Increased ventricle size has also been reported in patients with schizotypal personality disorder and was associated with deficit symptoms in one study (Siever et al. 1993b) but not in a larger series of patients from the same study (Siever et al. 1995). It has been correlated with reduced plasma HVA levels and impaired performance on neuropsychological tasks (Siever et al. 1993b). Finally, in a magnetic resonance imaging study, reduced frontal size was correlated with schizotypal traits in nonschizophrenic volunteers (Raine et al. 1992).

Cognitive deficits have been reported in patients with schizotypal personality disorder and in those with schizophrenia and have been associated with deficit symptoms. In schizophrenia, performance is impaired on tests of frontal-lobe function, such as the Wisconsin Card Sorting Test (WCST), a test of ability to categorize objects in shifting sets, and the Trail Making Test Part B. This impairment has also been noted in volunteers with schizotypal traits (Lyons et al. 1991), in nonpsychotic relatives of schizophrenic patients (Keefe et al. 1994), and in patients with schizotypal personality disorder (Trestman et al. 1995). However, performance on Wechsler Intelligence Scale vocabulary and block design components does not differ from that of nonpsychotic control subjects; thus, a global impairment in functioning is unlikely.

Abnormal results on the WCST in schizotypal personality disorder have been correlated with both deficit symptoms and reduced concentrations of plasma HVA. In relatives of schizophrenic patients with schizotypal traits, deficit symptoms have been significantly correlated with hypodopaminergia (Amin et al. 1997). Therefore, dopamine agonism might reasonably be expected to reduce cognitive impairment in patients with schizotypal personality disorder. Further evidence supporting the involvement of dopamine receptors in cognition, specifically in the mnemonic processes of the prefrontal cortex, arises from the observation that dopamine antagonists administered in the frontal cortex in primates have resulted in a working memory deficit related to a delayed-response task (Sawaguchi and Goldman-Rakic 1991). Improved results on the WCST after administration of amphetamine in schizophrenic patients further suggest that hypodopaminergia is associated with impaired executive function and hypofrontality (Daniel et al. 1991). As noted earlier in this chapter, in preliminary studies, amphetamine improves cognitive performance in patients with schizotypal personality disorder. Of nine patients with schizotypal personality disorder who were given 30 mg of amphetamine or placebo, seven had a decreased WCST rate of perseverative errors with amphetamine, and no patient had worsening of positive symptoms (Siegel et al. 1996). When more selective D_1 agonists become available, they may also be effective.

To integrate the two different symptom domains of schizotypal personality disorder, it is helpful to view them in terms of both developmental and dopaminergic abnormalities. Positive symptoms are correlated with increased dopamine, and negative symptoms are correlated with decreased dopamine. Negative symptoms are also correlated with structural abnormalities and cognitive impairment. One hypothesis linking these two processes is a multidimensional one. Patients with milder cortical neurodevelopmental impairment develop the negative symptoms of schizotypal personality disorder. Because the primary neurodevelopmental lesion is less severe and/or subcortical dopamine circuits are less susceptible to upregulation, patients with schizotypal personality disorder are protected from developing a full-blown psychosis. However, schizophrenic patients are, for some as yet unclarified reason, possibly a genetic abnormality, especially vulnerable to upregulation of subcortical dopaminergic systems by cortical deafferentation, which leads to chronic psychosis. Patients with schizotypal personality disorder, therefore, may represent the most common expression of a genetic vulnerability to the schizophrenia spectrum and provide a unique window through which to study schizophrenia.

BIOLOGY OF IMPULSIVITY AND AGGRESSION

Antisocial, borderline, histrionic, and narcissistic personality disorders—the dramatic cluster (see Table 33–2)—are characterized by a tendency to react to the environment, often without thinking and in an aggressive manner, and by rapid mood shifts. The two dimensions relevant to the biology of these disorders are impulsivity-aggression and affective lability.

Impulsivity-aggression in the Cluster B personality disorders is treated as a single entity because the biological correlates that have been described relate only to impulsive acts with aggressive behaviors and not to nonaggressive-impulsive acts or to premeditated violence. Impulsive-aggressive behaviors are heritable to some degree; in healthy nonpsychiatric persons, indices relevant to aggressiveness and irritable impulsiveness are heritable, with environmental influences playing a small role (Coccaro et al. 1993). Most work on impulsivity-aggression in personality disorder focuses on the borderline and antisocial types. Borderline personality disorder itself does not seem to be inherited (Torgersen 1984), but evidence suggests that certain features of the syndrome, including impulsivity, may be inherited (Torgersen 1992). Relatives of borderline probands have been shown to be at greater risk

Table 33–2. Biological correlates of dramatic cluster personality disorders

Personality disorder	Biological correlates
Borderline	Impulsivity heritable
	Impulsivity associated with decreased serotonin
	Low CSF 5-HIAA associated with suicidal behavior
	Low 5-HT indices in impulsivity-aggression
	Prolactin response to fenfluramine
	Blunted in mood disorders and personality disorders
	Inversely correlated with impulsivity-aggression only in personality disorders
	Blunted in association with self-injurious behavior in personality disorders
	Prolactin response to m-CPP
	Inversely correlated with irritability in personality disorders
	Prolactin response to buspirone
	Inversely correlated with irritability in personality disorders
	Impulsivity-aggression correlated with TPH genotype
	GH response to clonidine correlated with irritability
	Increased endorphins associated with self-injurious behavior
	Response to amphetamine correlated with affective instability
	Dysphoric response to physostigmine correlated with affective instability
	Decreased REM latency, increased REM density
	Abnormal EEG findings
	Abnormal evoked potentials
	Neuropsychological deficits
	Neurological soft signs
Antisocial	Genetic basis of aggressivity shown in adoptees
	Seasonality in density of 5-HT$_{2A}$ in at-risk boys
	Prolactin response to fenfluramine blunted
	Abnormal EEG findings
	Abnormal electrodermal responses
Narcissistic	None
Histrionic	None

Note. CSF 5-HIAA = cerebrospinal fluid 5-hydroxyindoleacetic acid; 5-HT = 5-hydroxytryptamine; m-CPP = m-chlorophenylpiperazine; TPH = tryptophan hydroxylase; GH = growth hormone; REM = rapid eye movement; EEG = electroencephalogram; 5-HT$_{2A}$ = 5-hydroxytryptamine type 2A receptor.

for borderline personality disorder than relatives of control subjects without borderline personality disorder (Baron et al. 1985). More specifically, personality dimensions of impaired affective regulation and poor impulse control found in borderline personality disorder appear to aggregate independently in the relatives of patients with borderline personality disorder (Silverman et al. 1991).

Interaction between genetics and the environment in antisocial personality disorder has been the subject of recent work. In an adoptive study of antisocial behavior and aggressivity, a biological background of antisocial personality disorder interacted with adverse adoptive home environment to result in significantly increased aggressivity in adoptees (Cadoret et al. 1995). Another study reported

that genetic factors were more prominent in adult than in juvenile antisocial traits (Lyons et al. 1995). A genetic basis for antisocial personality traits is supported by these studies.

The serotonergic system is a behavioral inhibitory system that appears to play a defining role in the biology of impulsivity and aggression (Coccaro and Siever 1995). Rodents given an inhibitor of serotonin synthesis become more aggressive (Di Chiara et al. 1971). In primates, differences in serotonin metabolite concentrations and receptor sensitivity have been associated with aggressive behaviors (Higley et al. 1992; Raleigh et al. 1986). Consistent with animal data, decreased indices of serotonin are associated with impulsivity-aggression in humans, directed both toward the self in the form of suicide attempts and toward others (Brown et al. 1982). This association appears consistent across diagnoses. Thus, in patients with depression (Asberg et al. 1975), patients with personality disorders, and nondepressed patients with schizophrenia, low CSF 5-hydroxyindoleacetic acid (5-HIAA) levels are associated with suicidal behavior, which suggests that indices of low serotonin are related to suicidal behavior regardless of the primary psychiatric diagnosis (Ninan et al. 1984; van Praag 1983). Postmortem studies have reported reduced concentrations of serotonin metabolites in the brains of suicide victims and decreased tritiated imipramine binding sites, which are a measure of presynaptic 5-hydroxytryptamine (5-HT) receptors. However, postsynaptic 5-HT$_2$ receptor binding has been increased in the frontal cortex of suicide victims. This compensatory increase has been interpreted as reflecting decreased function presynaptically. In the CSF of patients with histories of suicide attempts, 5-HIAA concentrations are reduced.

With regard to aggression directed toward others, reduced 5-HT indices have been reported in patients who are physically aggressive, violent criminals, arsonists, and murderers of a sexual partner (Lidberg et al. 1985; Linnoila et al. 1983; Virkkunen et al. 1987). In a slightly different vein, the relation between serotonin, childhood antisocial behavior, and harsh parenting has been studied recently; no association was found between 5-HT receptor profile and aggressive behavior, but significant seasonal variation was found in the density of platelet 5-HT$_{2A}$ receptors in boys at risk for antisocial behavior, and the density of 5-HT$_2$ receptors was inversely related to parental factors known to place youth at risk for antisocial behavior (Pine et al. 1996).

Challenge studies have been helpful in studying the serotonergic system in the limbic-hypothalamic region of the brain. Fenfluramine releases endogenous 5-HT and inhibits its reuptake, which results in increased intrasynaptic 5-HT and leads to a prolactin response. The prolactin response to fenfluramine thus provides a measure of net function at the 5-HT synapses, reflecting information about both presynaptic and postsynaptic 5-HT indices (Coccaro et al. 1989b). Prolactin responses to fenfluramine are blunted in patients with personality disorders and patients with affective disorders, but only in patients with personality disorders is the prolactin response to fenfluramine specifically correlated inversely with externally directed impulsivity-aggression (Coccaro et al. 1989b). In a study of families of these probands, a blunted prolactin response to fenfluramine was associated with an increased risk of impulsivity-aggression in the probands' first-degree

relatives to a greater extent than impulsivity itself in the proband. This finding suggests that this assessment of central serotonin function may serve as a sensitive parameter for identification of this familial trait and is more likely to reflect genetic factors than the impulsive behavior that may be variably expressed (Coccaro et al. 1994).

A decreased prolactin response has been observed in self-injurious behavior in patients with personality disorders, which suggests that the serotonergic abnormality may be associated with self-directed aggression and not specifically with suicidal intent (New et al. 1995a). The prolactin response to fenfluramine is also blunted in patients with antisocial personality disorder (O'Keane et al. 1992). Other serotonergic agonists that have been studied in personality disorders include buspirone and m-chlorophenylpiperazine (m-CPP). The former is a 5-HT$_{1A}$ receptor agonist; the prolactin response to buspirone correlated negatively with irritability in patients with personality disorders (Coccaro et al. 1990). The latter is an active metabolite of trazodone and a direct 5-HT agonist; the prolactin response to m-CPP also correlated negatively with irritability and aggressiveness in these patients (Coccaro et al. 1989a). These data provide a strong basis for a serotonergic abnormality in the genesis of impulsivity-aggression, and further evidence comes from treatment studies: a 5-HT uptake inhibitor has been reported to decrease anger, irritability, and impulsivity in patients with borderline personality disorder (Norden 1989).

Tryptophan hydroxylase (TPH), one of a number of genes that may be important in controlling serotonergic activity, regulates the rate-limiting step in the synthesis of serotonin. In a group of impulsive patients, a significant association was found between TPH genotype and CSF 5-HIAA, but no association between TPH and impulsive behavior was detected (Nielsen et al. 1994). In a more recent, more heterogeneous sample, a TPH genotype was correlated with higher irritability scores, suggesting that in male patients, impulsivity-aggression may be linked to the TPH genotype (New et al. 1996). Monoamine oxidase A (MAO$_A$) metabolizes serotonin; thus, the gene for MAO$_A$ is also potentially important in regulating serotonergic activity. In a family of males with mental retardation and impulsivity-aggression, a complete deficiency of MAO$_A$, which resulted in a marked disturbance in monoamine metabolism, was identified (Brunner et al. 1993). In animal studies, mice with a deletion of the gene encoding MAO$_A$ had increased brain serotonin concentrations and increased aggression (Cases et al. 1995). Furthermore, when mutant mice lacking the 5-HT$_{1B}$ receptor were confronted with an intruder, they attacked faster and more intensely than did wild-type mice, suggesting that serotonin receptors play an important role in aggressive behavior (Saudou et al. 1994).

Involvement of noradrenergic pathways and neurotransmitters in the genesis of irritable aggression is suggested by early basic studies showing that threatening stimuli increase activity in the locus coeruleus of rodents (Aston-Jones and Bloom 1981) and that increased noradrenergic activity may be correlated with irritable aggression in rodents (Stolk et al. 1974). In humans, studies using indices of noradrenergic function imply that an increase in this neurotransmitter is associated with impulsivity-aggression; in pathological gamblers, the noradrenergic system is hyperactive, as evidenced by CSF and plasma levels of 3-methoxy-4-hydroxyphenylglycol (MHPG) and urinary metabolites of noradrenaline (Roy et al. 1989). Another measure of noradrenergic activity, the growth hormone response to clonidine, an α_2 agonist, has been shown to be correlated with irritability but not physical aggression measures in patients with personality disorders (Coccaro et al. 1991). These findings are supported by the observation that adrenergic antagonists, such as propranolol, have been helpful in the clinical management of aggression. Thus, noradrenergic indices may serve as biological correlates of irritability and aggression in patients with personality disorders.

Other biological abnormalities have been reported in patients with personality disorders who have impulsive or aggressive traits and support the theory of some cerebral dysfunction in these patients. In borderline personality disorder, dysrhythmias on electroencephalogram (EEG) monitoring have been noted (Cowdry et al. 1985–1986), and evidence indicates that anticonvulsant medication may be helpful in the treatment of the behavioral dyscontrol so common in this syndrome (Cowdry and Gardner 1987). Both of these facts support a possible limbic epileptic focus in the pathophysiology of this behavioral dyscontrol. However, in another study no association was found between abnormal EEG findings and impulsivity (Cornelius et al. 1986). Abnormal EEG findings have also been described in antisocial personality disorder, but in this case, the changes are reflective of decreased cortical arousal rather than an epileptogenic focus. Evoked potentials are abnormal in borderline personality disorder but are not specific to this disorder (Kutcher et al. 1989).

On neuropsychological testing, patients with borderline personality disorder perform poorly on the process of visual discrimination and filtering and have difficulty recalling complex material; these tests may be sensitive to abnormalities in the dominant temporal lobe (O'Leary et al. 1991). Neurological soft signs have been noted in borderline and antisocial personality disorder—specifically, increased left-sided signs, which correlate with neuropsychological deficits, and increased right-sided signs, which correlate with a history of aggression (Stein et al. 1993). A history of head injury has been associated with borderline personality disorder, but findings have been contradictory and not specific to this personality disorder (New et al. 1995b).

Some evidence suggests that endogenous opioids may play a role in impulsivity-aggression, specifically in the genesis of self-injurious behavior; plasma levels of β-endorphin are increased in patients with these traits (Konicki and Schulz 1989). Evidence also indicates that a high free testosterone level in CSF is associated with increased aggressiveness (Virkkunen et al. 1994).

Psychophysiological studies of antisocial patients have reported abnormal electrodermal responses in anticipation of an aversive stimulus, which has been interpreted as deficiency in fear conditioning. In a recent study of antisocial adolescents, measures of electrodermal and cardiovascular arousal were higher in those who did not progress to become adult criminals than in those who did. Thus, higher arousal may protect against development of criminal behavior (Raine et al. 1995).

BIOLOGY OF AFFECTIVE SYMPTOMS

Depressive symptoms are extremely common in patients with personality disorders, and affective-related traits constitute the second defining dimension common to the dramatic cluster. Patients who have borderline personality disorder and histrionic personality disorder manifest these traits at their most obvious, and most biological findings in this realm relate to borderline personality disorder. Patients with borderline personality disorder are affectively labile, and their mood changes dramatically, sometimes in the space of a few minutes. Patients with histrionic personality disorder show exaggerated displays of emotions, which seem shallow and superficial and shift rapidly. In the past, a familial relationship between borderline personality disorder and affective disorders was suspected, but more recent work indicates that this relationship may be the result of comorbid mood disorder in the patients with borderline personality disorder (Silverman et al. 1991; Zanarini et al. 1988). Affective and impulsive traits did, however, show familial transmission, which suggests a familial relationship between borderline personality disorder and these core traits.

Neuroendocrine abnormalities have been described in borderline personality disorder, but findings have not been reliable. Dexamethasone suppression in borderline personality disorder appears to be related to the presence of a comorbid mood disorder (Lahmeyer et al. 1989), and the thyrotropin-stimulating hormone (TSH) test has not been helpful in attempts to link abnormalities of the hypothalamic-pituitary-thyroid axis with affective symptoms in patients with personality disorders (Kavoussi et al. 1993). Abnormal test results were noted in prior studies of patients with personality disorders, but major depression and alcoholism were comorbid in many patients. The growth hormone response to clonidine is not consistently abnormal in patients with personality disorders, nor does the prolactin response to fenfluramine correlate with depressive symptoms in these patients.

More than one neurotransmitter may be involved in the production of affective instability. Amphetamine, which releases and prevents reuptake of catecholamines, improved mood in some patients with borderline personality disorder, and, furthermore, response to amphetamine has been shown to correlate with affective instability. In a group of nonborderline subjects, a dysphoric response to amphetamine was associated with increased scores on a scale measuring affective lability. Thus, mood response to amphetamine may serve as a marker for this trait (Kavoussi and Coccaro 1993). A heightened noradrenergic response to clonidine occurs in patients with irritability (Coccaro et al. 1991) compared with depressed patients, in whom the response is blunted.

Much evidence suggests that the cholinergic system is abnormal in major depressive illness. Cholinergic substances, including acetylcholinesterase inhibitors and muscarinic agonists, cause a syndrome resembling depression in animals and in humans (Risch et al. 1981) and also have some efficacy in the suppression of manic symptoms (Davis et al. 1978). Dysphoric response to physostigmine in healthy males is correlated with irritability and emotional lability. Therefore, the cholinergic system also may be abnormal in patients with personality disorders, specifically borderline, who have these traits. In one study, a dysphoric response to physostigmine compared with placebo was noted in patients with borderline personality disorder in contrast to patients with other personality disorders, and the extent of this response correlated with baseline affective instability (Steinberg et al. 1993). This suggests that increased cholinergic receptor responsiveness may play a role in affective instability in these patients.

Sleep studies in patients with borderline personality disorder report the same abnormalities seen in those with depressive disorders, including decreased rapid eye movement (REM) latency and increased REM density (Akiskal et al. 1985; McNamara et al. 1984). Because REM sleep is partially modulated by cholinergic activity, a role for cho-

linergic abnormalities in this disorder is further suggested.

Whether anticholinergic medication has efficacy in treating affective instability has not been examined; indeed, the treatment of affective instability with any medication rarely has been investigated. Trials of mood-stabilizing agents, such as carbamazepine and valproate, thus far show inconsistent results in borderline personality disorder but have not been extensively studied.

BIOLOGY OF ANXIETY-RELATED DISORDERS

Avoidant, dependent, and obsessive-compulsive personality disorders—the anxious cluster—are characterized by a propensity to excessive anxiety and patterns of behavior consistent with attempts to restrain this anxiety. Patients with avoidant personality disorder are anxious about being rejected and thus avoid social situations, and patients with dependent personality disorder are anxious lest they find themselves without a caregiver and thus submit to the wishes of others. The pathophysiology of this cluster of personality disorders has seldom been investigated and is poorly understood. Few solid biological findings are available apart from those relating to social anxiety, but these findings have been reported for the most part in social phobia and less so in the anxious cluster of personality disorders (Table 33–3). Nevertheless, the question of overlap between these disorders persists, and the biology of social phobia may help to elucidate that of these personality disorders.

The extensive comorbidity between avoidant personality disorder and social phobia has raised the question as to whether they are two distinct disorders (Noyes et al. 1995; Schneier et al. 1991). Obsessive-compulsive personality disorder is also common in patients with social phobia. Thus, the clarification of biological abnormalities in social phobia may provide some understanding of the biological basis of avoidant and other personality disorders in this cluster.

In family studies, traits of anxiety were increased in

Table 33–3. Biological correlates of anxious cluster personality disorders

Personality disorder	Biological correlates
Avoidant	Overlap with social phobia
	Genetic basis for social anxiety
Dependent	Anxiety traits increased in relatives
Obsessive-compulsive	None

the relatives of patients with dependent personality disorder and panic disorder, which suggests familial transmission of these traits (Reich 1991). Heritability of social anxiety is also evident in twin studies, and longitudinal studies of childhood traits of inhibition have shown that these traits are stable over years (Kagan et al. 1988). Thus, some evidence exists for a genetic basis for social anxiety.

Little evidence of other biological abnormalities in social phobia/avoidant personality disorder exists. The hypothalamic-pituitary-thyroid axis and the hypothalamic-pituitary-adrenal axis are not abnormal in social phobia (Tancer et al. 1990; Uhde 1994). Response to lactate, which stimulates panic attacks in patients with panic disorder, is inconsistent in social phobia (Liebowitz et al. 1985). Some evidence of serotonin receptor supersensitivity exists because patients with social phobia have a greater fenfluramine-induced rise in cortisol than do nonpsychiatric control subjects, but responses to adrenergic challenge tests have been inconsistent (Uhde 1994). Reduced dopamine metabolism has been suggested in one study of patients with social phobia, but evidence is limited (Potts and Davidson 1992). Dependent personality disorder is increased in phobic patients with panic disorder (Reich et al. 1987). However, pharmacological agents that induce panic in patients with panic disorder do not induce symptoms of social phobia in patients with a history of social phobia, and responses to these agents are not clear markers for anxiety-related personality disorders (Tancer 1993).

Treatment studies of social phobia reported that monoamine oxidase inhibitors were efficacious and also decreased symptoms of avoidant personality disorder (Deltito and Stam 1989). Therefore, the assumption that monoamines play some role in the pathogenesis of avoidant personality disorder seems reasonable. Similarly, serotonin reuptake inhibitors reduced symptoms in avoidant personality disorder, which implicates the serotonergic system. The efficacy of benzodiazepines in treating social phobia in some studies (Davidson et al. 1991) raises the possibility of an abnormality of γ-aminobutyric acid (GABA) in this disorder and perhaps in avoidant personality disorder as well.

CONCLUSION

Although insights have been gained into the pathophysiology of personality disorders, further investigations are required. The most solid biological findings are found in studies of schizotypal and borderline personality disorders. However, a dimensional approach is also useful. The dimensions of cognitive disorganization, impulsivity-aggression, affective lability, and anxiety appear to have neurochemical foundations, including those of the dopaminergic, serotonergic, and noradrenergic systems. Neurodevelopmental and neurophysiological defects also appear to play a role. Investigating these disorders in terms of such defining concepts allows an increased appreciation of their biology and proposes that dimensions such as these may be useful in formulating treatment or even prevention.

REFERENCES

Akiskal HS, Yerevanian BI, Davis GC, et al: The nosologic status of borderline personality: clinical and polysomnographic study. Am J Psychiatry 142:192–198, 1985

American Psychiatric Association: Diagnostic and Statistical Manual of Mental Disorders, 3rd Edition, Revised. Washington, DC, American Psychiatric Association, 1987

American Psychiatric Association: Diagnostic and Statistical Manual of Mental Disorders, 4th Edition. Washington, DC, American Psychiatric Association, 1994

Amin F, Siever LJ, Silverman J, et al: Plasma HVA in schizotypal personality disorder, in Plasma Homovanillic Acid in Schizophrenia: Implications for Presynaptic Dopamine Dysfunction. Edited by Friedhoff AJ, Amin F. Washington, DC, American Psychiatric Press, 1997, pp 133–149

Angrist B, van Kammen DP: Central nervous system stimulants as tools in the study of schizophrenia. Trends Neurosci 7:338–340, 1984

Angrist B, Peselow E, Rubinstein M, et al: Amphetamine response and relapse risk after neuroleptic discontinuation. Psychopharmacology 85:277–283, 1985

Asberg M, Thoren P, Traskman L: "Serotonin depression"—a biochemical subgroup within the affective disorders? Science 191:478–480, 1975

Aston-Jones G, Bloom FE: Norepinephrine-containing locus coeruleus neurons in behaving rats exhibit pronounced responses to non-noxious environmental stimuli. J Neurosci 1:887–900, 1981

Baron M, Gruen R, Asnis L, et al: Familial transmission of schizotypal and borderline personality disorders. Am J Psychiatry 142:927–934, 1985

Braff DL: Information processing and attention dysfunctions in schizophrenia. Schizophr Bull 19:233–259, 1993

Brown GL, Ebert MH, Goyer PF, et al: Aggression, suicide, and serotonin: relationships to CSF amine metabolites. Am J Psychiatry 139:741–746, 1982

Brunner HG, Nelen M, Breakefield XO, et al: Abnormal behavior associated with a point mutation in the structural gene for monoamine oxidase A. Science 262:578–580, 1993

Cadoret RJ, Yates WR, Troughton E, et al: Genetic-environmental interaction in the genesis of aggressivity and conduct disorders. Arch Gen Psychiatry 52:916–924, 1995

Cases O, Seif I, Grimsby J, et al: Aggressive behavior and altered amounts of brain serotonin and norepinephrine in mice lacking MAOA. Science 268:1763–1766, 1995

Cesarec Z, Nyman AK: Differential response to amphetamine in schizophrenia. Acta Psychiatr Scand 71:523–538, 1985

Coccaro EF, Siever LJ: The neuropsychopharmacology of personality disorders, in Psychopharmacology: The Fourth Generation of Progress. Edited by Bloom FE, Kupfer DJ. New York, Raven, 1995, pp 1567–1579

Coccaro EF, Siever LJ, Kavoussi R, et al: Impulsive aggression in personality disorder: evidence for involvement of 5-HT$_1$ receptors (abstract). Biol Psychiatry 25:86A, 1989a

Coccaro EF, Siever LJ, Klar HM, et al: Serotonergic studies in patients with affective and personality disorders. Arch Gen Psychiatry 46:587–599, 1989b

Coccaro EF, Gabriel S, Siever LJ: Buspirone challenge: preliminary evidence for a role for central 5-HT$_{1A}$ receptor function in impulsive aggressive behavior in humans. Psychopharmacol Bull 26:393–405, 1990

Coccaro EF, Lawrence T, Trestman RL, et al: Growth hormone responses to intravenous clonidine challenge correlate with behavioral irritability in psychiatric patients and healthy volunteers. Psychiatry Res 39:129–139, 1991

Coccaro EF, Bergeman CS, McClearn GE: Heritability of irritable impulsiveness: a study of twins reared together and apart. Psychiatry Res 48:229–242, 1993

Coccaro EF, Silverman JM, Klar HM, et al: Familial correlates of reduced central serotonergic system function in patients with personality disorders. Arch Gen Psychiatry 51:318–324, 1994

Cornblatt BA, Keilp JG: Impaired attention, genetics, and the pathophysiology of schizophrenia. Schizophr Bull 20:31–46, 1994

Cornblatt BA, Lenzenweger MF, Dworkin RH, et al: Childhood attentional dysfunctions predict social deficits in unaffected adults at risk for schizophrenia. Br J Psychiatry 161 (suppl 18):59–64, 1992

Cornelius JR, Brenner RP, Soloff PH, et al: EEG abnormalities in borderline personality disorder: specific or non-specific. Biol Psychiatry 21:974–977, 1986

Cowdry RW, Gardner DL: Pharmacotherapy of borderline personality disorder. Arch Gen Psychiatry 45:111–119, 1987

Cowdry R, Pickar D, Davies R: Symptoms and EEG findings in the borderline syndrome. Int J Psychiatry Med 15:201–211, 1985–1986

Daniel DG, Weinberger DR, Jones DW, et al: The effect of amphetamine on regional cerebral blood flow during cognitive activation in schizophrenia. J Neurosci 11:1907–1917, 1991

Davidson JR, Ford SM, Smith RD, et al: Long-term treatment of social phobia with clonazepam. J Clin Psychiatry 52 (suppl 11):16–20, 1991

Davis KL, Berger PA, Hollister LE, et al: Physostigmine in mania. Arch Gen Psychiatry 35:119–122, 1978

Davis KL, Kahn RS, Ko G, et al: Dopamine in schizophrenia: a review and reconceptualization. Am J Psychiatry 148:1474–1486, 1991

Deltito JA, Stam M: Psychopharmacological treatment of avoidant personality disorder. Compr Psychiatry 30:498–504, 1989

Di Chiara G, Camba R, Spano PF: Evidence for inhibition by brain serotonin of mouse killing behaviour in rats. Nature 233:272–273, 1971

Goldberg SC, Schulz SC, Schulz PM, et al: Borderline and schizotypal personality disorders treated with low-dose thiothixene versus placebo. Arch Gen Psychiatry 43:680–686, 1986

Harvey PD, Keefe RS, Mitroupoulou V, et al: Information-processing markers of vulnerability to schizophrenia: performance of patients with schizotypal and nonschizotypal personality disorders. Psychiatry Res 60:49–56, 1996

Higley JD, Mehlman PT, Taub DM, et al: Cerebrospinal fluid monoamine and adrenal correlates of aggression in free-ranging rhesus monkeys. Arch Gen Psychiatry 49:436–441, 1992

Holzman PS, Solomon CM, Levin S, et al: Pursuit eye movement dysfunctions in schizophrenia. Arch Gen Psychiatry 41:136–139, 1984

Kagan J, Reznick S, Snidman N, et al: Childhood derivatives of inhibition and lack of inhibition to the unfamiliar. Child Dev 59:1580–1589, 1988

Kavoussi RJ, Coccaro EF: The amphetamine challenge test correlates with affective lability in healthy volunteers. Psychiatry Res 48:219–228, 1993

Kavoussi RJ, Coccaro EF, Klar H, et al: The TRH stimulation test in DSM-III personality disorder. Biol Psychiatry 34:234–239, 1993

Keefe RS, Silverman JM, Lees Roitman SE, et al: Performance of nonpsychotic relatives of schizophrenic patients on cognitive tests. Psychiatry Res 53:1–12, 1994

Kendler KS, Ochs AL, Gorman AM, et al: The structure of schizotypy: a pilot multitrait twin study. Psychiatry Res 36:19–36, 1991

Konicki PE, Schulz SC: Rationale for clinical trials of opiate antagonists in treating patients with personality disorders and self-injurious behavior. Psychopharmacol Bull 25:556–563, 1989

Kutcher SP, Blackwood DH, Gaskell DF, et al: Auditory p300 does not differentiate borderline personality disorder from schizotypal personality disorder. Biol Psychiatry 26:766–774, 1989

Lahmeyer HW, Reynolds CF, Kupfer DJ, et al: Biologic markers in borderline personality disorder: a review. J Clin Psychiatry 50:217–225, 1989

Lencz T, Raine A, Scerbo A, et al: Impaired eye tracking in undergraduates with schizotypal personality disorder. Am J Psychiatry 150:152–154, 1993

Lidberg L, Tuck JR, Asberg M, et al: Homicide, suicide and CSF 5-HIAA. Acta Psychiatr Scand 71:230–236, 1985

Liebowitz MR, Fyer AJ, Gorman JM, et al: Specificity of lactate infusions in social phobia versus panic disorders. Am J Psychiatry 142:947–950, 1985

Linnoila M, Virkkunen M, Scheinin M, et al: Low 5-hydroxyindoleacetic acid concentration differentiates impulsive from nonimpulsive violent behavior. Life Sci 33:2609–2614, 1983

Lyons MJ, Merla ME, Young L, et al: Impaired neuropsychological functioning in symptomatic volunteers with schizotypy; preliminary findings. Biol Psychiatry 30:424–426, 1991

Lyons MJ, True WR, Eisen SA, et al: Differential heritability of adult and juvenile antisocial traits. Arch Gen Psychiatry 52:906–915, 1995

McNamara E, Reynolds CF, Soloff PH, et al: EEG sleep evaluation of depression in borderline patients. Am J Psychiatry 141:182–186, 1984

New AS, Trestman RL, Benishay DS, et al: Self-injurious behavior in personality disorders (abstract). Proceedings of the 148th Annual Meeting of the American Psychiatric Association, NR360, 1995a, p 152

New AS, Trestman RL, Siever LJ: Borderline personality disorder, in Impulsivity and Aggression. Edited by Hollander E, Stein DJ. Essex, England, Wiley, 1995b, pp 153–173

New AS, Gelernter J, Trestman RL, et al: A polymorphism in tryptophan hydroxylase and irritable aggression in personality disorders (abstract). Proceedings of the 149th Annual Meeting of the American Psychiatric Association, NR284, 1996, p 144

Nielsen DA, Goldman D, Virkkunen M, et al: Suicidality and 5-hydroxyindoleacetic acid concentration associated with a tryptophan hydroxylase polymorphism. Arch Gen Psychiatry 51:34–38, 1994

Ninan PT, van Kammen DP, Scheinin M, et al: CSF 5-hydroxyindoleacatic acid levels in suicidal schizophrenic patients. Am J Psychiatry 141:566–569, 1984

Norden MJ: Fluoxetine in borderline personality disorder. Prog Neuropsychopharmacol Biol Psychiatry 13:885–893, 1989

Noyes R, Woodman CL, Holt C, et al: Avoidant personality traits distinguish social phobic and panic disorder subjects. J Nerv Ment Dis 183:145–153, 1995

O'Keane V, Moloney E, O'Neill H, et al: Blunted prolactin responses to d-fenfluramine in sociopathy. Br J Psychiatry 160:643–646, 1992

O'Leary KM, Brouwers P, Gardner DL, et al: Neuropsychological testing of patients with borderline personality disorder. Am J Psychiatry 148:106–111, 1991

Pine DS, Wasserman GA, Coplan J, et al: Platelet serotonin 2A (5-HT$_{2A}$) receptor characteristics and parenting factors for boys at risk for delinquency: a preliminary report. Am J Psychiatry 153:538–544, 1996

Potts NL, Davidson JR: Social phobia: biological aspects and pharmacotherapy. Prog Neuropsychopharmacol Biol Psychiatry 16:635–646, 1992

Raine A, Sheard C, Reynolds GP, et al: Pre-frontal structural and functional deficits associated with individual differences in schizotypal personality. Schizophr Res 7:237–247, 1992

Raine A, Venables PH, Williams M: High autonomic arousal and electrodermal orienting at age 15 years as protective factors against criminal behavior at age 29 years. Am J Psychiatry 152:1595–1600, 1995

Raleigh MJ, Brammer GL, Ritvo ER, et al: Effects of chronic fenfluramine on blood serotonin, cerebrospinal fluid metabolites, and behavior in monkeys. Psychopharmacology 90:503–508, 1986

Reich J: Avoidant and dependent personality traits in relatives of patients with panic disorder, patients with dependent personality disorder and normal controls. Psychiatry Res 39:89–98, 1991

Reich J, Noyes R, Troughton E: Dependent personality disorder associated with phobic avoidance in patients with panic disorder. Am J Psychiatry 144:323–326, 1987

Risch SC, Cohen RM, Janowsky DS, et al: Physostigmine induction of depressive symptomatology in normal human subjects. Psychiatry Res 4:89–94, 1981

Roy A, De Jong J, Linnoila M: Extraversion in pathological gamblers correlates with indices of noradrenergic function. Arch Gen Psychiatry 46:679–681, 1989

Salisbury DF, Voglmaier MM, Seidman LJ, et al: Topographic abnormalities of P3 in schizotypal personality disorder. Biol Psychiatry 40:165–172, 1996

Saudou F, Arnara D, Dierich A, et al: Enhanced aggressive behavior in mice lacking 5-HT$_{1B}$ receptor. Science 265:1875–1878, 1994

Sawaguchi T, Goldman-Rakic P: D1 dopamine receptors in pre-frontal cortex: involvement in working memory. Science 251:947–950, 1991

Schneier FR, Spitzer RL, Gibbon M, et al: The relationship of social phobia subtypes and avoidant personality disorder. Compr Psychiatry 32:496–502, 1991

Schulsinger F, Parnas J, Petersen ET, et al: Cerebral ventricular size in the offspring of schizophrenic mothers. Arch Gen Psychiatry 41:602–606, 1984

Schulz SC, Koller MM, Kishore PR, et al: Ventricular enlargement in teenage patients with schizophrenia spectrum disorder. Am J Psychiatry 140:1592–1595, 1983

Schulz SC, Cornelius J, Jarret DB, et al: Pharmacodynamic probes in personality disorders. Psychopharmacol Bull 23:337–341, 1987

Schulz SC, Cornelius J, Schulz PM, et al: The amphetamine challenge test in patients with borderline personality disorder. Am J Psychiatry 145:809–814, 1988

Siegel BV, Trestman RL, O'Flaithbheartaigh SO, et al: D-Amphetamine challenge effects on Wisconsin Card Sort Test: performance in schizotypal personality disorder. Schizophr Res 20:29–32, 1996

Siever LJ: Biological markers in schizotypal personality disorder. Schizophr Bull 11:564–575, 1985

Siever LJ, Coursey RD, Alterman IS, et al: Impaired smooth pursuit eye movement: vulnerability marker for schizotypal personality disorder in a normal volunteer population. Am J Psychiatry 141:1560–1566, 1984

Siever LJ, Keefe R, Bernstein DP, et al: Eye tracking impairment in clinically identified patients with schizotypal personality disorder. Am J Psychiatry 147: 740–745, 1990

Siever LJ, Amin F, Coccaro EF, et al: Plasma homovanillic acid in schizotypal personality disorder. Am J Psychiatry 148:1246–1248, 1991

Siever LJ, Amin F, Coccaro EF, et al: Cerebrospinal fluid homovanillic acid in schizotypal personality disorder. Am J Psychiatry 150:149–151, 1993a

Siever LJ, Kalus OF, Keefe RS: The boundaries of schizophrenia. Psychiatr Clin North Am 16:217–244, 1993b

Siever LJ, Friedman L, Moskowitz J, et al: Eye movement impairment and schizotypal pathology. Am J Psychiatry 151:1209–1215, 1994a

Siever LJ, Steinberg BJ, Trestman RL, et al: Personality disorders, in American Psychiatric Press Review of Psychiatry, Vol 13. Edited by Oldham JM, Riba MB. Washington, DC, American Psychiatric Press, 1994b, pp 253–290

Siever LJ, Rotter M, Losonczy M, et al: Lateral ventricular enlargement in schizotypal personality disorder. Psychiatry Res 57:109–118, 1995

Silverman JM, Pinkham L, Horvath TB, et al: Affective and impulsive personality disorder traits in the relatives of patients with borderline personality disorder. Am J Psychiatry 148:1378–1385, 1991

Stein DJ, Hollander E, Cohen L, et al: Neuropsychiatric impairment in impulsive personality disorders. Psychiatry Res 48:257–266, 1993

Steinberg BJ, Weston S, Trestman RL, et al: Affective instability in personality disordered patients correlates with mood response to physostigmine challenge (abstract). Biol Psychiatry 33:86A, 1993

Stolk JM, Conner RL, Levine S, et al: Brain norepinephrine metabolism and shock-induced fighting behavior in rats: differential effects of shock and fighting on the neurochemical response to a common footshock stimulus. J Pharmacol Exp Ther 190:193–209, 1974

Tancer ME: Neurobiology of social phobia. J Clin Psychiatry 54 (suppl 12):26–30, 1993

Tancer ME, Stein MB, Gelernter CS, et al: The hypothalamic-pituitary-thyroid axis in social phobia. Am J Psychiatry 147:929–933, 1990

Torgersen S: Genetic and nosological aspects of schizotypal and borderline personality disorders. Arch Gen Psychiatry 41:546–554, 1984

Torgersen S: The genetic transmission of borderline personality features displays multidimensionality (abstract). Paper presented at the annual meeting of the American College of Neuropsychopharmacology, December 1992

Trestman RL, Keefe RS, Mitropoulou V, et al: Cognitive function and biological correlates of cognitive performance in schizotypal personality disorder. Psychiatry Res 59: 127–136, 1995

Trestman RL, Horvath T, Kalus O, et al: Event-related potentials in schizotypal personality disorder. J Neuropsychiatry Clin Neurosci 8:33–40, 1996

Uhde TW: Anxiety and growth disturbance: is there a connection? A review of biological studies in social phobia. J Clin Psychiatry 55 (suppl 6):17–27, 1994

van Praag H: CSF 5-HIAA and suicide in non-depressed schizophrenics. Lancet 2:977–978, 1983

Virkkunen M, Nuutila A, Goodwin F, et al: Cerebrospinal fluid monoamine metabolite levels in male arsonists. Arch Gen Psychiatry 44:241–247, 1987

Virkkunen M, Kallio E, Rawlings R, et al: Personality profiles and state aggressiveness in Finnish alcoholic, violent offenders, fire setters and healthy volunteers. Arch Gen Psychiatry 51:28–33, 1994

Zanarini MC, Gunderson JG, Marino MF, et al: DSM-III disorders in the families of borderline outpatients. Journal of Personality Disorders 2:292–302, 1988

SECTION IV

Psychopharmacological Treatment

Donald F. Klein, M.D., Section Editor

THIRTY-FOUR

Treatment of Depression

Dennis S. Charney, M.D.,
Robert M. Berman, M.D., and
Helen L. Miller, M.D.

The effectiveness of the pharmacological treatment of depression compares very favorably with the pharmacological treatment of chronic medical disorders, such as hypertension and diabetes. The spectrum of available antidepressant medications permits the clinician to select a specific antidepressant drug based on depressive subtype and coexisting medical conditions. For patients who do not respond to the initial antidepressant drug prescribed, a range of options exists for subsequent drug treatment approaches. In this chapter, we review the clinical strategies involved in the drug treatment of depressed patients, including initial medical and psychiatric evaluation, acute and maintenance antidepressant treatment, and therapeutic approaches to the treatment-refractory depressed patient.

HISTORICAL BACKGROUND

The most dramatic and fundamental discoveries in the pharmacotherapy of psychiatric disorders took place in the two decades after World War II. After witnessing the great progress made in the pharmacology of medical disorders, with the advent of chemotherapy for tuberculosis, syphilis, and other major medical disorders, research psychiatrists were committed to discovery of drugs that would cure (or at least ameliorate) psychiatric disorders. Major breakthroughs occurred with the observation that lithium was useful for manic states (Cade 1949) and that chlorpromazine was highly effective for psychotic symptoms (Delay and Deniker 1952). Nevertheless, it took years before these medications were commonly used in clinical practice.

In the early 1950s, several investigators noted that iproniazid, initially used to treat tuberculosis, caused an elevation of mood in some patients (Crane 1956). In the United States, Kline and colleagues started to use iproniazid in depressed patients. According to Kline, his original impetus to try iproniazid for treatment of depression was further supported not only by these clinical data but also by the effects (e.g., hyperalertness and hyperactivity) of that drug on laboratory animals. The clinical efficacy of iproniazid in the treatment of depression was quickly established (Kline 1970; Loomer et al. 1957, 1958). Consequently, additional irreversible monoamine oxidase inhibitors (MAOIs) were synthesized, found to be effective for depression, and approved for general use. After about 5 years of widespread use, the highly effective MAOIs became increasingly less popular in the treatment of depression because of their side-effect profile, particularly the cardiovascular responses following tyramine ingestion. Over the past decade, reversible selective MAOIs were introduced in Europe and South America, and these medications have a favorable side-effect profile with reduced tyramine sensitivity. The future availability of those compounds in the United States may enhance psychiatrists' interest in this class of antidepressant drugs.

At approximately the same time that iproniazid was reported to be an antidepressant, Roland Kuhn (1958) was testing the tricyclic compound G 2022355 (imipramine) in the treatment of psychiatric patients in Switzerland. Kuhn observed that imipramine, although lacking antipsychotic properties, improved depressed mood in some schizophrenic patients. Subsequently, imipramine was tested in depressed patients and was documented as an effective antidepressant (Kuhn 1970a, 1970b, 1989). The mechanism of action underlying imipramine's antidepressant properties was not initially known. Subsequently, it was determined that the ability of imipramine to inhibit the reuptake of norepinephrine and serotonin (5-HT) was related to its antidepressant activity (Carlsson et al. 1968; Glowinski and Axelrod 1964). This discovery facilitated the development of other tricyclic antidepressants (TCAs) that inhibited monoamine reuptake, with variable potency.

Based on the therapeutic properties of the MAOIs and TCAs and the monoamine hypothesis of depression, a search began in the 1970s for drugs that would selectively enhance the function of one of the monoamine systems rather than all three. A specific and potent dopamine reuptake inhibitor, nomifensine, was synthesized and used with success in the treatment of depression; however, hematological side effects (i.e., hemolytic anemia) have precluded its wide use. Note that nomifensine was effective in some depressed patients for whom other antidepressants were not helpful.

The search for drugs acting specifically at the level of one monoamine system also led to the development of compounds with primary actions on the serotonin system. Fluoxetine was the first available selective serotonin reuptake inhibitor (SSRI) to be marketed for the treatment of depression (Beasley et al. 1991, 1992). Subsequently, other SSRIs—sertraline (Amin et al. 1989), paroxetine (Rickels et al. 1992), fluvoxamine (Wilde et al. 1993), and citalopram (Montgomery and Djarv 1996)—have been developed and are useful for treating major depression. Further preclinical understanding of the role of monoamines in antidepressant action has led to the strategy of developing agents that specifically target multiple monoamine receptors or reuptake sites. Examples of this generation of antidepressant agents include venlafaxine (an SSRI and noradrenergic reuptake inhibitor), nefazodone (a specific 5-HT$_2$ antagonist and weak SSRI), and mirtazapine (a 5-HT$_2$, 5-HT$_3$, and α_2-adrenergic antagonist). Large-scale clinical experience with these agents is needed before their specific role in the treatment of depression can be delineated.

PHARMACOTHERAPY FOR THE ACUTE DEPRESSIVE EPISODE

Early recognition and treatment of depressive illness may have important implications for treatment responsiveness. Studies of the instantaneous probabilities of recovery indicate that the longer the patient is ill, the lower the chances are of recovering. The shorter the episode of depression prior to initiating treatment, the higher the chances of recovery are and the lower the impairment in social and vocational adjustment will be (Keller et al. 1982a, 1982b; Lavori et al. 1984).

Medical Evaluation

The initial evaluation of patients presenting with depressive symptoms should include a careful medical history, a physical examination, and appropriate laboratory testing. Clinicians must consider the possible existence of physical illnesses that may present as depression or have depression as an associated symptom. Medical conditions that should be considered when evaluating depressed patients are listed in Table 34–1. In some cases, treatment of the underlying medical condition is sufficient to eliminate depressive symptoms. However, in many cases, depressive symptoms will persist, necessitating the use of antidepressant drugs. Drug-induced depression will occasionally be encountered. The drug classes listed in Table 34–2 have been associated with depressive symptoms. The patient's medication should be reviewed and drugs that are less centrally active substituted when possible.

Another rationale for a comprehensive medical assessment is that the identification of specific medical disorders will influence the choice of antidepressant drugs. The blockade of neurotransmitter receptors by antidepressant drugs is related to numerous side effects of antidepressant drugs and drug-drug interactions. Knowledge of these pharmacological features of antidepressant drugs is therefore important in the selection of antidepressant drugs for the patient with depression and a coexisting major medical disorder. Table 34–3 summarizes the relationship between specific receptors and antidepressant-induced side effects. The antidepressants with the highest and lowest affinity for these receptors are listed (Richelson 1991; Richelson and Nelson 1984). Antidepressant drug recommendations based on coexisting specific medical disorders are reviewed later in this chapter (Table 34–4 [Richelson 1989]).

In addition, stimulants may be considered a treatment alternative in some medically ill populations. Although placebo-controlled trials offer little support for the antide-

Table 34–1. Medical conditions associated with depressive symptoms

Cardiovascular disease
Cardiomyopathy
Cerebral ischemia
Congestive heart failure
Myocardial infarction

Neurological disorders
Alzheimer's disease
Multiple sclerosis
Parkinson's disease
Head trauma
Narcolepsy
Brain tumors
Wilson's disease

Cancer
Pancreatic cancer
Lung cancer

Endocrine disorders
Hypothyroidism
Hyperthyroidism
Cushing's disease
Addison's disease
Hyperparathyroidism
Hypoparathyroidism
Hypoglycemia
Pheochromocytoma
Carcinoid
Ovarian failure
Testicular failure

Infectious diseases
Syphilis
Mononucleosis
Hepatitis
Acquired immunodeficiency syndrome
Tuberculosis
Influenza
Encephalitis
Lyme disease

Nutritional deficiencies
Folate
Vitamin B_{12}
Pyridoxine (B_6)
Riboflavin (B_2)
Thiamine (B_1)
Iron

Table 34–2. Classes of drugs associated with depressive symptoms

Drugs of abuse
Phencyclidine
Marijuana
Amphetamines
Cocaine
Opiates
Sedative-hypnotics
Alcohol

Antihypertensive drugs
Reserpine
Propranolol
Methyldopa
Guanethidine
Clonidine

Gastrointestinal drugs
Cimetidine

Cytotoxic agents

Corticosteroids

Oral contraceptives

pressant efficacy of stimulants in major depression, multiple studies support their usefulness in medically ill geriatric populations with depressive symptoms characterized by apathy (Satel and Nelson 1989).

Cardiovascular disease. The SSRIs (fluoxetine, sertraline, paroxetine) and bupropion are preferred in pa-

tients with heart conduction disease, orthostatic hypotension, ventricular arrhythmias, and/or ischemic heart disease. These drugs have little or no effect on heart rate, heart rhythm, or blood pressure. Although the SSRIs have not been systematically evaluated in patients with cardiovascular disease, they do not prolong either the P-R or the QRS intervals or cause orthostatic hypotension as TCAs do. No serious cardiovascular side effects have been reported with SSRIs, except for several cases of severe sinus node slowing (Buff et al. 1991; Ellison et al. 1990; Feder 1991; Glassman et al. 1993).

One investigation of bupropion in depressed patients with severe heart disease has been done (Roose et al. 1991). Bupropion was found to be free of effects on heart conduction or contractility. Neither SSRIs nor bupropion has yet been carefully investigated in patients with arrhythmias and heart failure (Glassman and Preud'homme 1993).

TCAs have been used safely in patients with preexisting cardiac disease for many years, but these drugs generally should be avoided as first-choice antidepressants in these patients. The effects of TCAs to slow intraventricular conduction, as reflected in the increased QRS, P-R, and $Q-T_c$ intervals on the electrocardiogram, may pose a risk to patients with prolonged conduction times or heart block and patients taking quinidine or other type 1 antiarrhythmics. The orthostatic hypotension and rebound tachycardia produced by TCAs are risks in patients with congestive heart failure, particularly those with left ventricular im-

Table 34–3.   Relationship between blockade of neurotransmitter receptors and antidepressant-induced side effects

Receptor subtype	Side effects	Receptor affinity[a]			
		High		Low	
Histamine-1 receptor	Sedation	Doxepin	+ + + +	Venlafaxine	0
	Weight gain	Trimipramine	+ + + +	Nefazodone	±
	Hypotension	Amitriptyline	+ + +	Bupropion	±
	Potentiation of CNS depressants	Maprotiline	+ + +	Trazodone	+
		Mirtazapine	+ + +	Desipramine	+
				Nortriptyline	+
Muscarinic receptors	Dry mouth	Amitriptyline	+ + +	Bupropion	0
	Blurred vision	Clomipramine	+ + +	Trazodone	0
	Urinary retention	Protriptyline	+ + +	Nefazodone	0
	Constipation			Venlafaxine	0
	Memory dysfunction			Mirtazapine	0
	Tachycardia			SSRIs	±
				Nortriptyline	+
				Desipramine	+
				SSRIs	+
α_1 Receptors	Postural hypotension	Doxepin	+ + + +	Venlafaxine	0
	Reflex tachycardia	Trimipramine	+ + + +	Bupropion	0
	Potentiation of antihypertensive effects of prazosin	Trazodone	+ + + +	Mirtazapine	+
		Nefazodone	+ + +	SSRIs	+
		Amoxapine	+ + +		
α_2 Receptors	Blockade of antihypertensive effects of clonidine, α-methyldopa, guanfacine	Mirtazapine	+ + +	Bupropion	0
		Trimipramine	+ +	Venlafaxine	0
		Amitriptyline	+ +	SSRIs	+
		Trazodone	+ +	Nefazodone	+
Serotonin-2 receptors	Ejaculatory dysfunction	Amoxapine	+ + + +	Bupropion	0
	Hypotension	Nefazodone	+ + +	Venlafaxine	0
	Alleviation of migraine headaches	Trazodone	+ + +	SSRIs	±
		Doxepin	+ +	Desipramine	±
		Amitriptyline	+ +		

Note.   0 = no affinity; ± = negligible affinity; + = weak affinity; + + = moderate affinity; + + + = high affinity; + + + + = very high affinity; CNS = central nervous system; SSRIs = selective serotonin reuptake inhibitors.
[a]Drugs with higher receptor affinity are associated with a greater frequency of receptor-mediated side effects.
Source.   Adapted from Cusack et al. 1994; Richelson 1991.

pairment, and in patients taking drugs such as diuretics or vasodilators (Glassman and Preud'homme 1993).

Until recently, it had been suggested that certain pre-existing arrhythmias would benefit from TCA treatment because, at therapeutic plasma concentrations, TCAs suppress arrhythmias, and their cardiac effects are similar to those of class I antiarrhythmic drugs (Glassman and Bigger 1981; Glassman et al. 1987; Rawling and Fozzard 1979; Weld and Bigger 1980). However, several multicenter studies reported that class I antiarrhythmic drugs are asso-

ciated with increased mortality when administered to patients with ventricular arrhythmias postmyocardial infarction (Cardiac Arrhythmia Suppression Trial Investigators 1989; Cardiac Arrhythmia Suppression Trial II Investigators 1992; Horowitz et al. 1987; Morganroth and Goin 1991; Pratt et al. 1990). Studies have also documented that these antiarrhythmic drugs may have a mortality risk when used in patients with atrial fibrillation (Coplen et al. 1990; Falk 1989; Selzer and Wray 1964). Class I antiarrhythmic drugs are sodium channel blockers. TCAs have

Table 34–4. Antidepressant drugs of choice for depressed patients with comorbid medical disorders

Comorbid disorder	Drugs of choice
Cardiovascular	
Congestive heart failure or ischemic heart disease	For each of these conditions, SSRIs (fluoxetine, sertraline, or paroxetine) or bupropion is preferred. Of the tricyclic antidepressants, nortriptyline or desipramine is best.
Conduction disturbance	
Tachycardia	
Orthostatic hypotension	
Neurological	
Seizure disorder	Desipramine, MAOIs, venlafaxine, SSRIs, mirtazapine (avoid bupropion, clomipramine, maprotiline)
Organic brain syndrome	SSRIs, bupropion, trazodone
Migraine headaches	Amitriptyline, trazodone, amoxapine, doxepin
Parkinson's disease	Amitriptyline, doxepin, SSRIs (avoid amoxapine)
Chronic pain	SSRIs, amitriptyline, doxepin
Stroke	SSRIs
Gastrointestinal	
Peptic ulcer disease	Doxepin, trimipramine
Chronic diarrhea	Doxepin, trimipramine, amitriptyline
Chronic constipation	SSRIs, bupropion, trazodone, nefazodone
Sexual	
Erectile failure	Bupropion, nefazodone, trazodone
Anorgasmia	Bupropion, desipramine, nefazodone, trazodone
Opthalmological	
Angle-closure glaucoma	SSRIs, bupropion, trazodone, nefazodone

Note. SSRIs = selective serotonin reuptake inhibitors; MAOIs = monoamine oxidase inhibitors.
Source. Adapted from Richelson 1989.

class I antiarrhythmic properties. Thus, Glassman and colleagues (1993) suggested that TCAs may have mortality risks similar to those of antiarrhythmics when used in depressed patients with a recent myocardial infarction and, perhaps, in a wider range of cardiac disease. Investigators have hypothesized that the risk of using class I antiarrhythmics increases proportionately with the severity of ischemic heart disease (Bigger 1990; Echt et al. 1991).

Venlafaxine has been associated with sustained elevated blood pressure in a dose-dependent manner, with approximately 13% of patients taking doses greater than 300 mg/day experiencing clinically significant elevations (Feighner 1995). In approximately one-third of patients, blood pressure will eventually diminish, as evidenced during 1-year follow-up studies (Feighner 1995). The risks of clinically relevant blood pressure increases (i.e., increases greater than 15 mm Hg or diastolic blood pressures greater than 90 mm Hg) must be weighed against the clinical benefits of continued venlafaxine dosing. Concurrent administration of antihypertensive medications may be warranted in some cases (Feighner 1995). Both trazodone and nefazodone have been associated with hypotension (Robinson et al. 1996). Further studies are needed to assess the

safety of these medications in patients with underlying conduction abnormalities and ischemic heart disease.

Neurological disease. Desipramine, MAOIs, SSRIs, and trazodone are preferred for depressed patients with seizure disorders or for patients at risk for seizures based on predisposing factors such as head trauma, multiple central nervous system (CNS) medications, and substance abuse. These drugs lower the seizure threshold less than other antidepressant drugs do, with a 1.0%–1.5% incidence of seizures during the first 2 years of treatment (see Rosenstein et al. 1993). Mirtazapine has also been associated with a low incidence of seizures (R. Davis and Wilde 1995). Three antidepressant drugs—maprotiline, clomipramine, and bupropion—should be particularly avoided in these patients at risk for seizures (Jick et al. 1983; Settle 1992; Trimble 1978). Maprotiline causes an increased incidence of seizures with rapid dose escalation and higher doses (Dessain et al. 1987). Clomipramine has been reported to have a high seizure risk (Peck et al. 1983; Trimble 1978). Bupropion should be avoided in patients at risk for seizure disorders because in doses higher than 300 mg/day, it has an observed seizure rate approximately twice that observed with most other antidepressants (Davidson 1989; Johnston et al. 1991).

Depression is a common sequela of stroke, occurring in an estimated 30% of patients. SSRIs may be safer than TCAs in treatment of these patients because of their lower incidence of cardiovascular side effects and lack of anticholinergic properties.

Confusion in patients with organic brain syndromes can be exacerbated by anticholinergic effects of antidepressant drugs. Therefore, drugs such as SSRIs, trazodone, maprotiline, amoxapine, bupropion, venlafaxine, and desipramine are indicated in those patients. These agents should also be used in patients with other conditions, such as neurogenic bladder and prostate disease, that may worsen as a result of cholinergic receptor blockade.

Evidence indicates that migraine headaches may be effectively treated with serotonin receptor antagonists, particularly the 5-HT$_{1D}$ receptor antagonist sumatriptan (Humphrey 1992). Therefore, antidepressant drugs such as amoxapine and trazodone, with high affinity for serotonin receptors, may be useful for depressed patients with migraines.

Depression occurs in approximately 50% of patients with Parkinson's disease. Reduced serotonin function is evident in parkinsonian patients with depression (Mayeux et al. 1984). SSRIs may be particularly helpful in these patients. The anticholinergic effects of antidepressants such as amitriptyline and doxepin reduce the motor deficits of Parkinson's disease. Amoxapine should be avoided because of its dopamine receptor blocking actions.

Cancer. About 25% of patients with cancer report clinically significant depressive symptoms. Selection of antidepressant drugs should be based on cancer-related somatic problems. Patients experiencing significant weight loss and reduced appetite may benefit from TCAs that increase appetite and produce weight gain. On the other hand, the anticholinergic effects of TCAs may be contraindicated in cancer patients recovering from abdominal surgery or stomatitis. SSRIs, bupropion, nefazodone, or trazodone should be used in these patients.

Allergic disease. Antidepressant drugs such as doxepin, trimipramine, amitriptyline, and maprotiline, which have strong antihistamine properties, are indicated for depressed patients with severe allergic disorders such as dermatological allergies and idiopathic pruritus.

Gastrointestinal disease. Depressed patients with peptic ulcer disease may particularly benefit from trimipramine and doxepin because of their strong anticholinergic and histamine-2 (H$_2$) antagonist properties. Drugs with potent anticholinergic effects should be avoided in treatment of depressed patients with chronic constipation. Conversely, these drugs may be useful for depressed patients with chronic diarrhea.

Sexual dysfunction. Erectile impotence may be caused by a variety of medical conditions generally related to endocrine, drug, local, neurological, and vascular problems (McConnell and Wilson 1991). TCAs, SSRIs, and MAOIs have been reported to reduce erectile function and, therefore, should be avoided in patients with erectile impotence (Segraves 1992). In contrast, bupropion does not produce erectile dysfunction and when used in patients with a history of TCA-induced erectile failure, normal function is restored (Gardner and Johnston 1985). Trazodone, nefazodone, and mirtazapine may also prove useful in this depressed population.

Inability to ejaculate, greatly delayed ejaculation, and anorgasmia have been reported with use of TCAs, MAOIs, and SSRIs (Segraves 1992). Bupropion is not associated with these side effects and is the drug of choice for patients prone to the development of these symptoms (Gardner and Johnston 1985).

Ophthalmic disease. Antidepressant drugs with little or no anticholinergic effects should be used in depressed patients with angle-closure glaucoma.

Psychiatric Evaluation

The initial psychiatric evaluation of the depressed patient should focus on determining whether other psychiatric disorders coexist with the depression and identifying depressive disorder subtype. The existence of comorbid psychiatric disorders will influence the choice of antidepressant. For example, SSRIs are the drug of choice for patients with comorbid depression and obsessive-compulsive disorder (OCD) (Goodman et al. 1990). Furthermore, preliminary evidence suggests that the SSRIs may be indicated for patients with posttraumatic stress disorder (PTSD) (Nagy et al. 1993) and for obese patients (Marcus et al. 1990). MAOIs may be the most effective agent for depressed patients with panic disorder (Sheehan et al. 1983a); however, SSRIs may be a preferable first-line agent in this population. Evidence (discussed in greater detail later in this chapter; see section, "Depressive Subtypes and Antidepressant Response") indicates that specific depressive subtypes (i.e., atypical depression, delusional depression, bipolar depression) respond preferentially to specific antidepressant agents.

FACTORS INFLUENCING THE ANTIDEPRESSANT DRUG OF CHOICE

Symptomatic Predictors of Antidepressant Response

Most studies indicate that depressed patients with melancholia characterized by key symptoms—pervasive anhedonia, nonreactivity of mood, diurnal variation, early-morning awakening, guilt, and psychomotor change—respond better to TCAs than do patients with nonmelancholic depression (Paykel 1972; Raskin and Crook 1976; Simpson et al. 1976). Of the individual symptoms, psychomotor retardation, loss of interest, and anhedonia are the best prognostic indicators of antidepressant response (Downing and Rickels 1973; Hollister and Overall 1965; Overall et al. 1966; Paykel 1972; Raskin and Crook 1976; Simpson et al. 1976). In contrast, sleep and appetite disturbances are not predictive of antidepressant response (for review, see Joyce and Paykel 1989).

Regarding specific antidepressant choice, multiple studies suggest that SSRIs and TCAs are equivalently effective in various depressed populations, including severely depressed inpatient and outpatient melancholic samples (e.g., Feighner et al. 1993; Moller et al. 1993; Stuppaeck et al. 1994). Furthermore, many melancholic patients who are refractory to TCAs have subsequently responded to SSRIs (e.g., Amsterdam et al. 1994). Nevertheless, in the subgroup of melancholic depressed inpatients, treatment efficacy has been best established for the TCAs, which may prove more efficacious than the SSRIs (Danish University Antidepressant Study Group 1990; Roose et al. 1994). Further studies are needed to confirm this latter conclusion.

In patients with nonmelancholic depression, TCAs are superior to placebo (Quitkin et al. 1989). Consistent evidence maintains that depressed patients with an associated personality disorder or narcissistic, hypochondriacal, or histrionic personality traits respond less well to TCAs than do subjects without personality disorders (Bielski and Friedel 1976; Hirschfeld et al. 1986; Paykel 1979; Pfohl et al. 1984; Shawcross and Tyrer 1985). MAOIs or SSRIs may be helpful for these patients.

Depressions of longer duration appear to be less likely to respond to antidepressants than are depressions of shorter duration (Keller et al. 1984). The chance of responding to antidepressants is reduced with each recurrence (Cassano et al. 1983; Keller et al. 1986). Both dysthymia (Keller et al. 1982a, 1982b, 1983) and depression secondary to medical disorders or other psychiatric conditions has been associated with less favorable outcomes (Keller et al. 1983, 1984).

Neurobiological Predictors of Antidepressant Response

Numerous research studies have attempted to identify neurobiological predictors of antidepressant response (Joyce and Paykel 1989). The results of these investigations have generally been disappointing. The hypothesis suggesting the existence of norepinephrine- and serotonin-deficient depressive subtypes has not been confirmed (Berman et al. 1996). Furthermore, characterization of the depression by levels of the norepinephrine metabolite 3-methoxy-4-hydroxyphenylglycol (MHPG) or the serotonin metabolite 5-hydroxyindoleacetic acid (5-HIAA) has not been of practical use in the selection of antidepressant drugs. Most studies have found that a low urinary MHPG level is associated with therapeutic responses to imipramine (Beckmann and Goodwin 1975; Fawcett et al. 1972; Janicak et al. 1986; Maas et al. 1972, 1982; A. H. Rosenbaum et al. 1980; Schatzberg et al. 1980). A similar relationship has been identified between low urinary MHPG level and therapeutic responses to nortriptyline (Hollister et al. 1980) and maprotiline (Schatzberg et al. 1980, 1981). However, the variability in these studies is too high for the findings to be clinically useful. No correlation has been found between urinary MHPG levels and therapeutic responses to amitriptyline (Beckmann and Goodwin 1975; Coppen et al. 1979; Gaertner et al. 1982; Maas et al. 1982; Spiker et al. 1980). Preliminary data suggest that low cerebrospinal fluid (CSF) 5-HIAA relates to therapeutic responses to zimeldine (Aberg-Wistedt et al. 1981), clomipramine (VanPraag 1977), imipramine (Goodwin et al. 1973), and nortriptyline (Asberg et al. 1973).

The ratio of serum tryptophan (the amino acid precursor of serotonin) to large neutral amino acids has been found to have modest value (25% of the variance) in predicting clinical response to amitriptyline, clomipramine, and paroxetine (Møller et al. 1983, 1990). The ratio of tyrosine (the amino acid precursor of norepinephrine and dopamine) to large neutral amino acids may relate to nortriptyline (Møller et al. 1985) and maprotiline (Møller et al. 1986) responses.

A series of investigations have examined whether the effect of single doses of a stimulant drug (e.g., amphetamine, methylphenidate) on mood is predictive of antidepressant response. Mood elevation after stimulant administration has been found to be associated with a therapeutic response to imipramine (P. Brown and Brawley 1983; Sabelli et al. 1983; van Kammen and Murphy 1978) and desipramine (Ettigi et al. 1983; Sabelli et al. 1983; Spar and La Rue 1985). An absent or dysphoric mood response after stimulant administration has been proposed to predict therapeutic responses to amitriptyline (P. Brown and Brawley 1983; Sabelli et al. 1983; Spar and La Rue 1985) and nortriptyline (Sabelli et al. 1983). Similar to the studies involving urinary MHPG and amino acid ratios, the high variability in the findings limits therapeutic application.

One of the most consistently documented neuroendocrine abnormalities in depressive illness is the blunted suppression of cortisol after dexamethasone administration (Carroll 1982). This abnormality usually normalizes during successful antidepressant treatment (Greden et al. 1983; Holsboer et al. 1982), and failure to normalize is associated with poor outcome and early relapse (Greden et al. 1983; Targum 1984). However, the lack of cortisol suppression by dexamethasone is not associated with a greater likelihood of responding to antidepressant treatment in general (W. A. Brown and Shuey 1980; Gitlin and Gerner 1986; Gitlin et al. 1984; Greden et al. 1983; McLeod et al. 1970; Peselow and Fieve 1982) or to specific antidepressant drugs (W. A. Brown and Qualls 1981; Fraser 1983; Gitlin and Gerner 1986; Greden et al. 1981). It has been suggested, however, that this neuroendocrine dysfunction is associated with lack of response to placebo or psychotherapy and the need for antidepressant drugs or electroconvulsive therapy (ECT) (Peselow et al. 1986; Rush 1983).

Shortened rapid eye movement (REM) latency is a well-documented sleep abnormality in patients with depression. Preliminary data indicate that a reduced REM latency is associated with a poor placebo response (Coble et al. 1979) and a positive response to TCAs (Coble et al. 1979; Hochli et al. 1986; Kupfer et al. 1976, 1980; Svendsen and Christensen 1981).

DEPRESSIVE SUBTYPES AND ANTIDEPRESSANT RESPONSE

The treatments of choice for depressive subtypes are considered in the following sections (Table 34–5).

Unipolar Major Depression

An extensive review of overall efficacy of antidepressant drug treatment in uncomplicated unipolar major depression indicates that approximately 65% of patients treated with antidepressants improve compared with 30% given placebos (J. M. Davis 1985). To date, one antidepressant drug does not stand out as having better efficacy than others. Therefore, the initial choice of an antidepressant drug for a patient with unipolar major depression, with or with-

out melancholia, depends on the associated medical conditions and the drug-induced side effects. Purchase price may be a factor to consider when selecting an antidepressant, because the generic TCAs are much less expensive than the SSRIs and bupropion.

The discovery of the TCAs represented a major breakthrough in clinical psychiatry. The efficacy of this class of

Table 34–5. Treatments of choice for depressive subtypes

Major depression

All antidepressants have equal efficacy.

Choice of antidepressant is based on side effects, comorbid medical conditions, family history of drug treatment response, and previous response to antidepressants.

Atypical depression

Monoamine oxidase inhibitors (MAOIs) have superior efficacy to tricyclic antidepressants (TCAs).

Selective serotonin reuptake inhibitors (SSRIs) need further study.

Delusional depression

Antidepressant alone usually is ineffective.

Antidepressant and antipsychotic combination is effective in many patients.

Electroconvulsive therapy is probably the most effective treatment.

Bipolar depression

All antidepressants may produce mania or hypomania (bupropion may be least likely).

MAOIs may be more effective than TCAs.

Lithium may be more effective than in unipolar depression.

Lithium-MAOI and lithium-carbamazepine combinations may be effective for refractory patients.

Dysthymic disorder

Antidepressant efficacy may be reduced compared with major depression.

MAOIs may be more effective than TCAs.

SSRIs need further study.

Geriatric depression

Drug of choice is based largely on side-effect profile.

Low or absent anticholinergic properties—desipramine, nortriptyline, SSRIs, bupropion.

Reduced cardiovascular adverse effects—desipramine, nortriptyline, SSRIs, bupropion.

Generally use lower doses.

Comorbid psychiatric disorders

Panic disorder—bupropion and trazodone are not effective.

Obsessive-compulsive disorder—SSRIs are the drugs of choice.

Eating disorders—SSRIs may be the drugs of choice.

antidepressants for moderate and severe depression is unquestioned. Although the use of these medications as a first-choice agent is appropriate in many cases, these compounds are being used less often because of the availability of newer antidepressant drugs with less adverse side-effect profiles and less lethality with overdose. As noted earlier in this chapter, in depressed patients with certain comorbid medical conditions, TCAs may be particularly indicated.

The availability of the SSRIs has provided another therapeutic option for the clinician. In fact, fluoxetine is the most widely used antidepressant in the United States. SSRIs are appropriate first-choice antidepressant drugs because of their broad spectrum of efficacy, favorable side-effect profile, and lack of lethality with overdose. The SSRIs are effective in psychiatric disorders that frequently occur in combination with depression. For example, the SSRIs have therapeutic efficacy in the treatment of OCD and PTSD, conditions for which TCAs (except clomipramine) are generally ineffective. Note that the SSRIs have adverse side effects, such as headache, tremor, nausea, diarrhea, insomnia, agitation, and nervousness, that may need to be attended to. Sexual dysfunction (particularly anorgasmia in men and women) and ejaculatory disturbances are more common with these drugs than with TCAs. In addition, paroxetine, sertraline, and fluoxetine inhibit cytochrome P450 (CYP) enzymes, thereby reducing the metabolism of drugs such as warfarin, phenytoin, and digoxin, which are metabolized by this system (Bergstrom et al. 1992; Crewe et al. 1992). Nefazodone, SSRIs, and TCAs may significantly inhibit metabolism of terfenadine and astemizole. Because the parent compounds of these antihistamines may cause fatal arrhythmias, these agents should not be prescribed with the aforementioned antidepressants (Nemeroff et al. 1996; Riesenman 1995).

Bupropion is an antidepressant with different neurochemical properties from those of other available antidepressant drugs. It has weak effects on noradrenergic and serotonin reuptake; its dopamine-enhancing actions are sufficiently weak to make this an unlikely mechanism of action. Bupropion is comparable in efficacy to the TCAs (Feighner et al. 1986; Ferguson et al. 1994) and the SSRIs (Feighner et al. 1991) for major depression. Anecdotal evidence indicates that bupropion may be useful in patients with bipolar disorder, particularly for maintenance prophylaxis (Haykal and Akiskal 1990; Shopsin 1983; Wright et al. 1985). Bupropion is generally well tolerated and has fewer side effects than do the TCAs. It does not cause sedation, weight gain, sexual dysfunction, or anticholinergic effects and has minimal cardiovascular toxicity and low lethality with overdose. A therapeutic disadvantage is that bupropion is not effective for treatment of panic disorder and OCD (Sheehan et al. 1983b).

MAOIs (e.g., tranylcypromine, phenelzine, isocarboxazid) are extremely effective antidepressant agents. As described later in this chapter, they may be superior to other antidepressants in the treatment of atypical depression (Liebowitz et al. 1988). In addition, they are effective for treatment of panic disorder (Sheehan et al. 1983b), PTSD (Kosten et al. 1991), social phobia (Liebowitz et al. 1986), and bulimia (Walsh et al. 1984). The factor limiting the use of MAOIs is their side-effect profile. The available MAOIs are irreversible inhibitors of the enzyme monoamine oxidase. Patients must avoid foods containing tyramine because the inability of peripheral monoamine oxidase to metabolize tyramine may lead to hypertension and (rarely) cerebral hemorrhage or death (Cooper 1989). Other MAOI side effects include weight gain, orthostatic hypotension, delayed ejaculation, insomnia, and the spectrum of anticholinergic signs and symptoms.

A relatively new development are short-acting reversible inhibitors such as moclobemide, which is currently not available in the United States. These drugs are less vulnerable to the tyramine reaction and often have fewer side effects compared with the MAOIs. Several preliminary treatment trials indicate that these drugs may have a therapeutic spectrum of action similar to that of reversible MAOIs (Lecrubier and Guelfi 1990).

Nefazodone and trazodone are antidepressants that are distinguished biochemically from the TCAs, SSRIs, and MAOIs. They have moderate serotonin reuptake inhibition properties but are also postsynaptic serotonin receptor antagonists. Their principal metabolite—m-chlorophenylpiperazine (m-CPP)—is a nonselective serotonin receptor agonist. Controlled trials indicate that nefazodone and trazodone are similar in efficacy to other antidepressants. However, they may not be particularly useful for treating panic disorder (Charney et al. 1986), and there is no evidence that they are effective for treating OCD. Their side-effect profiles are notable for a lack of anticholinergic effects and low lethality with overdose. Their principal adverse effects are sedation, lightheadedness, confusion, orthostatic hypotension, nausea, and (in rare cases with trazodone) priapism.

Mirtazapine is the newest addition to the pharmaceutical armamentarium for the treatment of depression in the United States. This medication has a novel pharmacological profile and is distinguished by its potent antagonist activity at the α_2-adrenergic, 5-HT$_2$, and 5-HT$_3$ receptors. Additionally, significant histaminergic antagonism may contribute to mirtazapine's potential side effects of drowsiness, dry mouth, and constipation. In multiple efficacy studies, mirtazapine was shown to be effective in treating moderate to severe major depression, with responsiveness similar to that of TCAs (R. Davis and Wilde 1995). Notably, preliminary experience with this drug worldwide suggests that it has a high therapeutic index, and no known deaths due to overdose have been cited to date. Further studies are needed to investigate the role of mirtazapine in patients with medical complications and those refractory to treatment.

Atypical Depression

The current general consensus is that a nonmelancholic atypical depressive syndrome exists that responds preferentially to MAOIs (Liebowitz et al. 1988; Quitkin et al. 1990, 1991). This syndrome generally meets criteria for unipolar depression, bipolar depression, or dysthymic disorder, but excessive mood reactivity (i.e., complete, transient remission from depressed mood in response to positive environmental factors) and two or more of the associated features of overeating, oversleeping, extreme fatigue, and chronic oversensitivity to rejection are also present (Liebowitz et al. 1988; F. Quitkin, personal communication, June 1993). In comparison to TCAs, MAOIs have superior efficacy for the symptoms associated with atypical depression, as well as for borderline and labile personality and self-rated interpersonal sensitivity (Liebowitz et al. 1988).

In considering the initial antidepressant drug trial in atypical depression, the clinician must balance the greater response to MAOIs (i.e., phenelzine) against their greater side-effect risk. MAOIs are appropriate as first-line treatment in this disorder. Alternatively, because some patients with atypical depression will respond to SSRIs (F. Quitkin, personal communication, June 1993), these drugs may be tested first.

Delusional Depression

Considerable data from descriptive, neurobiological, and treatment response investigations suggest that delusional depression is a distinct subtype of depressive illness (for review, see Joyce and Paykel 1989). The evidence is convincing that patients with delusional depression have a poorer response to TCAs than do patients with nondelusional depression. The recommended pharmacological treatment for delusional depression is a combination of antidepressant and antipsychotic drugs (Charney and Nelson 1981; Nelson and Bowers 1978; Spiker et al. 1985). The antipsychotic dose is generally less than that required to treat the psychotic symptoms associated with schizophrenia. The antipsychotic drug will elevate antidepressant blood levels, necessitating lower antidepressant drug doses and, when appropriate, monitoring blood levels. No evidence suggests that specific antidepressant or antipsychotic drugs are more effective in delusional depression. In patients with a medication-refractory delusional depression, ECT is a treatment alternative.

Bipolar Depression

The concept that bipolar and unipolar affective disorders are distinct entities is based on family studies, a variety of biological studies, clinical characteristics, course of illness, and treatment response (for review, see Joyce and Paykel 1989). During treatment of a patient's depressed phase of bipolar disorder, the clinician must avoid eliciting a manic episode. Most studies indicate that essentially all antidepressant drugs can induce mania in bipolar patients (Bunney 1977; Prien et al. 1973). Preliminary evidence suggests that bupropion and the SSRIs may potentially confer a reduced likelihood of a manic switch (Peet 1994; Stoll et al. 1994).

Some evidence indicates that bipolar depressed patients are more likely to have an antidepressant response to lithium than are unipolar depressed patients (Baron et al. 1975; Goodwin et al. 1972; Mendels et al. 1979; Noyes et al. 1974). Anecdotal reports propose that bipolar depression (especially when characterized by anergia, psychomotor retardation, and hypersomnia) may be more responsive to phenelzine, lithium, and tranylcypromine (Himmelhoch et al. 1972) than to TCAs. Of concern, a growing literature has suggested that antidepressant medications in bipolar depressed subjects may lead to cycle acceleration, with such acceleration potentially associated with greater treatment resistance (see Post and Weiss 1995). In some bipolar depressed patients refractory to standard treatment, carbamazepine alone or carbamazepine plus lithium is effective (Post 1991).

Dysthymic Disorder

Dysthymia was first recognized as a disorder in 1980, with the publication of DSM-III (American Psychiatric Association 1980). The inclusion of dysthymic disorder with the affective disorders represented a significant theoretical shift and led to new ways of thinking about the etiology and treatment of the illness (Kocsis and Frances 1987). Dysthymic disorder is generally conceptualized as an illness with an insidious onset that begins at an early age. Dysthymic disorder and major depression may be diagnosed simultaneously in some subjects. The coexistence of dysthymic disorder with a major depressive episode is referred to as *double depression* (Keller et al. 1983). This background is important when reviewing the dysthymia literature, because it has not been as well characterized as other affective disorders, and the biology and treatment of dysthymic disorder are not well understood.

Dysthymic disorder appears to respond to a variety of antidepressant agents, including TCAs, MAOIs, and SSRIs (Bakish et al. 1994; Howland 1991; Marin et al. 1994; Rosenthal et al. 1992; Thase et al. 1996). Data suggest that MAOIs may be superior to TCAs in the treatment of this disorder, but this issue is unresolved. Interpretation of treatment studies is complicated by the variability of diagnostic criteria used, by the high incidence of comorbidity of dysthymia with other illness (especially major depression), and by the lumping together of both patients with dysthymia and those with major depression in investigations of other depressive subtypes, such as atypical depression. Dysthymia and atypical depression also overlap in that both illnesses tend to be chronic. Moreover, there is a paucity of double-blind, placebo-controlled treatment trials.

Some theoretical issues cloud research into treatment of dysthymic disorder, particularly the degree to which it is distinct from major depression as opposed to a varying expression of the same illness. For example, although the concept of a double depression is a useful one, it is not clear that a person with both dysthymic disorder and major depression in fact has two illnesses as opposed to a single illness varying in severity over time (Garvey et al. 1989). Further research is needed to clarify the diagnostic classification of dysthymic disorder and to compare comparative efficacy of antidepressant agents in the treatment of this illness. However, despite the paucity of double-blind, placebo-controlled treatment trials, it has been well demonstrated that dysthymic disorder responds to antidepressant medication. The risks of nontreatment should be emphasized. Studies have found that most subjects with dysthymic disorder go on to develop major depression. Patients with double depression who recover from an episode of major depression but continue to have dysthymic symptoms are at greater risk for relapse into major depression. The risk of relapse increases the longer the episode of dysthymia continues (Keller et al. 1992).

Geriatric Depression

Depression in the geriatric population (older than 65 years) constitutes a major public health problem and is often underdiagnosed and undertreated (National Institutes of Health Consensus Development Panel 1992). These problems are partially a result of the insidious nature of depression in elderly people. In contrast to a young adult's presentation, depressed mood in an elderly person may be less prominent than other depressive symptoms such as changes in appetite and sleep, loss of interest, anergia, and social withdrawal; these changes may appear to be caused by aging and attendant medical problems.

Although relatively few controlled studies of antidepressant efficacy have been conducted in depressed patients older than 60, most antidepressants are believed to be equally efficacious for geriatric depression as for nongeriatric depression (for review, see Salzman 1993). Very little is known about antidepressant efficacy in very old depressed patients (those older than 85).

The risk of adverse drug side effects is increased in elderly people for several reasons. Elderly patients are more likely than younger patients to have concomitant medical disorders, to be more sensitive to drug side effects, and to take other medications, which increases drug-drug interactions. In addition, drugs are excreted more slowly and metabolized less efficiently in elderly people compared with younger people. Therefore, lower antidepressant doses may be warranted in the elderly, and treatment nonresponse or unexpected side effects should prompt therapeutic drug level monitoring. Antidepressant medications should be initiated at low doses and increased very gradually (Neshkes and Jarvik 1987).

The efficacy studies of TCAs favor nortriptyline and desipramine because they are less likely than other TCAs to produce orthostatic hypotension (which can lead to falls and fractures) and because they have fewer adverse anticholinergic, cardiovascular, and sedative effects. Monitoring plasma levels of nortriptyline and desipramine and electrocardiograms will facilitate effective and safe use (Reynolds et al. 1992; Salzman 1993).

SSRIs may be particularly useful for elderly patients. The low incidence of cardiovascular side effects and lack of anticholinergic properties offer advantages over most other antidepressant classes (Altamura et al. 1989; Cohn et al. 1990; Dunner et al. 1992). As with the TCAs, the SSRIs should be initiated at low doses (fluoxetine, 5 mg; sertraline, 12.5 mg; paroxetine, 10 mg) and increased slowly as needed. The shorter half-life of sertraline and reduced inhibition of cytochrome P450 compared with fluoxetine and paroxetine suggest that its use is favored over other SSRIs in treating elderly patients, especially those receiving a complex medication regimen.

Bupropion has been shown to be as efficacious for elderly patients as are other antidepressant drugs (Branconnier et al. 1983; Kane et al. 1983). Like the SSRIs, it does not produce anticholinergic side effects or orthostatic hypotension. The activating effects of bupropion may be a disadvantage for some individuals. As more experience is gained with bupropion in treating elderly patients, it may emerge as one of the drugs of choice for this population.

The sedative properties and lack of anticholinergic effects of nefazodone and trazodone may offer advantages to elderly depressed patients who are agitated. However, these agents may cause orthostatic hypotension and cardiac arrhythmias, which limit their usefulness in treating elderly patients.

Although the MAOIs (especially phenelzine) are not widely prescribed for elderly patients, these drugs are effective and safe for the treatment of geriatric depression. In low doses, psychomotor stimulants may diminish depressed mood, loss of interest, and anergia in some elderly individuals.

ECT is extremely effective in the treatment of depression in elderly patients. When the depression is very severe or is accompanied by delusions, ECT is the treatment of choice. A limitation of the use of ECT is that relapse after effective ECT is common, and usually alternative maintenance treatment is needed (Sackeim et al. 1990). Another disadvantage of ECT for elderly patients is that the probability of transient post-ECT confusion is elevated. Use of unilateral treatments with a brief-pulse current to reduce confusion after the procedure may be helpful (Kramer 1987).

DURATION OF TREATMENT

Many patients with depressive illness are prone to relapse if antidepressant treatment is not continued. Data indicate that 50% or more of patients experiencing an episode of depression will eventually have a recurrence (Angst 1990; Lee and Murray 1988). The continuation of TCAs for 6 months after resolution of depressive symptoms reduces the relapse rate by more than 50% compared with placebo (Prien and Kupfer 1986). These data have led to the recommendation that pharmacological treatment for a first episode of depression should continue for 6 months after a patient's symptoms have responded to an antidepressant medication.

Patients with recurrent major depression require longer-term antidepressant drug maintenance. The advice concerning the duration of antidepressant treatment provided by the 1985 National Institute of Mental Health (NIMH) Consensus Development Conference on the pharmacological prevention of depressive recurrences remains useful: "Duration of treatment must be determined on an individual basis depending upon the previous pattern of episodes, degree of impairment produced, the adverse consequences of a new recurrence, and the patient's ability to tolerate the drug" (p. 473).

This recommendation is helpful on a generic basis, but it needs to be more specific to be of practical use for the clinician. Unfortunately, long-term clinical trials designed to develop guidelines for chronic antidepressant drug use are limited. Most of the available data are based on studies of 1-year antidepressant drug maintenance. TCAs, MAOIs, and SSRIs have all been shown to reduce relapse rates by more than 50% during this period compared with placebo (Doogan and Caillard 1992; Eric 1991; Georgotas et al. 1989; Montgomery et al. 1988, 1991). In addition, patients maintained on a full dosage of imipramine for 3 years had a 20% relapse rate compared with an 80% relapse rate on placebo (Frank et al. 1990). Only one controlled study has evaluated the efficacy of an antidepressant beyond 3 years. An extension of the original 3-year maintenance study of imipramine to 5 years found that imipramine continued to have a clinically significant prophylactic effect (Kupfer et al. 1992).

These studies strongly support the continued efficacy of full-dose antidepressant therapy in preventing relapse over a period of several years. The clinical implications of this work are that patients who have recovered from an initial depressive episode or prior depressive episodes spaced far apart (i.e., greater than 5 years) should receive maintenance antidepressant therapy for 6 months to 1 year. However, patients with prior depressive episodes that occurred less than 3 years apart should probably be given full-dose maintenance antidepressant therapy for at least 3, and probably up to 5, years. Patients with frequent recurrent depressive episodes may require lifetime treatment with antidepressants.

Maintenance antidepressant therapy should be discontinued with a slow taper. Involvement of a significant other, friend, or close family member to help the patient monitor for the return of symptoms and, if necessary, alert the treating clinician is also helpful.

THERAPEUTIC MONITORING OF ANTIDEPRESSANT BLOOD LEVELS

Therapeutic plasma levels have been established only for imipramine, desipramine, and nortriptyline (American Psychiatric Association Task Force Report 1985). However, information is available on other antidepressants for which blood levels may be useful in the treatment of refractory patients or elderly depressed patients to determine whether drug dosage is adequate (for review, see Preskorn 1989; Preskorn and Fast 1991).

Pharmacokinetic studies indicate that the absorption, distribution, and excretion of antidepressants vary greatly among individuals; thus, some patients will require monitoring of plasma levels to determine optimal drug dosage. Therapeutic antidepressant drug monitoring may therefore enhance the safe and efficacious use of antidepressants and may help to determine compliance. It is well known that a substantial number of patients do not take their medications as prescribed. Noncompliance or partial compliance may reduce response to treatment because of wide fluctuations in plasma levels.

For some antidepressants, therapeutic drug monitoring enables the clinician to maximize therapeutic dosage. Most studies have reported an association between plasma levels of nortriptyline, imipramine, and desipramine and clinical efficacy (Glassman et al. 1977; Nelson et al. 1982; Risch et al. 1979). The available evidence suggests that a curvilinear relationship may exist between nortriptyline plasma levels and antidepressant efficacy, with maximal therapeutic efficacy achieved with levels of 50–175 ng/mL. Thus, if the nortriptyline plasma level is less than 50 ng/mL or greater than 175 ng/mL, a dose change may be warranted. Evidence supports a linear relationship between plasma levels of imipramine plus desipramine (to which imipramine is metabolized) and clinical response. A similar relationship has been identified between desipramine plasma levels and therapeutic efficacy. Therefore, increasing drug doses to raise serum levels of imipramine and desipramine above a threshold value may convert nonresponders to responders. For example, in one study, 10 desipramine-resistant depressed patients' conditions improved when dosage was adjusted to raise desipramine plasma concentrations to 125 ng/mL or higher (Nelson et al. 1982).

Most investigations support a more limited role for the plasma levels of antidepressants other than nortriptyline, imipramine, or desipramine. In these cases, a plasma level determination might be useful when abnormal metabolism or poor compliance is suspected. Less established documentation is available for antidepressant drugs such as amitriptyline, doxepin, trimipramine, protriptyline, amoxapine, maprotiline, trazodone, bupropion, and fluoxetine (Preskorn and Fast 1991).

Monitoring of antidepressant drug levels may also help the clinician avoid drug toxicity. For some antidepressant drugs, a relationship exists between plasma concentration and toxicity. Data indicate that the effects of TCAs on cardiac function (i.e., delayed intraventricular conduction and rhythm disturbances) and on brain neuronal activity (i.e., seizures, delirium) are concentration dependent (Preskorn 1989). The same may be true for other antidepressants such as bupropion that show a dose-dependent increase in drug-induced seizures (Preskorn 1991). The

SSRIs may not require therapeutic drug monitoring, because relationships to clinical response or adverse effects have not been identified.

Therapeutic antidepressant drug monitoring may assist in the evaluation of drug-drug interactions. Many pharmacological agents, which are commonly coadministered with antidepressants, may alter steady-state antidepressant drug levels. For example, drugs that stimulate the hepatic microsomal enzyme system (e.g., anticonvulsants, barbiturates, chronic alcohol use, glutethimide, chloral hydrate, nicotine, oral contraceptives) will lower drug levels of most antidepressant drugs. On the other hand, TCA levels are increased by neuroleptics and stimulants that inhibit hepatic metabolism. Coadministration of fluoxetine and TCAs increases TCA blood levels as a result of hepatic metabolism inhibition via CYP2D6 (Bergstrom et al. 1992). Sertraline may have less inhibitory effects on CYP2D6 than do other SSRIs (Crewe et al. 1992; Preskorn et al. 1994), but clinical experience with this drug in combination with TCAs is limited. Inhibition of CYP2D6 will also increase levels of anticonvulsants, neuroleptics, certain antiarrhythmic drugs, and β-adrenergic blocking drugs. Dosages of these drugs may need to be adjusted in patients receiving SSRIs.

ANTIDEPRESSANT DRUGS AND SUICIDE

As noted, there is excellent evidence that antidepressant drugs are extremely effective in both acute treatment of depression and prevention of recurrence. However, whether antidepressant drugs can reduce the incidence of suicide in depressed patients has not been established. Some data suggest that SSRIs may be more effective than standard antidepressants in decreasing suicidal ideation, but these data are preliminary and inconsistent. This issue has been a great concern for clinicians and patients because of the suggestion that the SSRI fluoxetine may precipitate or exacerbate suicidal ideation or behavior (Beasley et al. 1991; Mann and Kapur 1991; Power and Cowen 1992; Teicher et al. 1990).

Several reviews have examined the data relevant to the question of whether antidepressant pharmacotherapy is associated with the emergence of suicidal ideation and behavior. These studies indicate that although suicidal ideation may emerge rarely during antidepressant treatment of depressed patients, these responses occur with essentially all types of antidepressant drugs, and a causal relationship to antidepressant drugs has not been established. Furthermore, the emergence or intensification of suicidal ideation and behavior with antidepressant drugs is not limited to patients with primary depression. Patients with a history of impulsive-aggressive behavior appear to be particularly prone to these effects (Mann and Kapur 1991; Power and Cowen 1992).

The conclusions of Mann and Kapur (1991) are appropriate in this context:

> Clinicians should be aware that emergence or intensification of suicidal ideation or behavior in patients receiving antidepressant treatment has been reported in patients with various psychiatric diagnoses and has not been proven to be associated with any specific type of antidepressant. Whether certain antidepressants precipitate or aggravate suicidal ideation in a small, vulnerable subpopulation of psychiatric patients who require antidepressants is uncertain. In practice, whatever the antidepressant medication, the clinician should always monitor the patient to assess the severity of depression and suicidal ideation, aggressive ideational behavior, agitation, and akathisia. (p. 1032)

Suicidal ideation or behavior may be more frequent in patients who are nonresponsive, have unrecognized akathisia, and have attempted suicide previously. Patients should be informed of this rare adverse reaction and must be instructed to immediately contact their clinician should these symptoms occur (Mann and Kapur 1991).

APPROACHES TO TREATMENT OF REFRACTORY DEPRESSION

Despite the well-documented effectiveness of antidepressant drugs, a significant proportion—approximately 10%–30%—of the depressed patient population does not respond adequately to treatment. Based on the relatively high prevalence of depression, a substantial number of patients are not adequately responding to treatment (Nierenberg et al. 1991).

For the purposes of this discussion, we have used a definition that has a lower threshold than that generally used in clinical practice. *Refractory depression* is defined as an episode of major depression, not secondary to a medical or drug-induced condition, that fails to respond (or to maintain a response) to an adequate trial of an antidepressant drug of established efficacy. An *adequate trial* is defined as 6 weeks of treatment with the antidepressant at a dosage considered therapeutic.

Once it has been established that a patient is resistant to an antidepressant, several options are available to the treating clinician: maximizing the trial of that same antidepressant, changing to a different antidepressant, or select-

ing a drug combination or nonpharmacological treatment, such as ECT (Table 34–6).

Maximizing the Antidepressant Drug Trial

When a patient does not respond to an antidepressant, a clinician may maximize the response to that same antidepressant by increasing its dose and/or the duration of the trial. Measuring the plasma levels of certain antidepressants may help determine whether a dosage adjustment is needed. There is evidence that a substantial percentage (85%) of the monoamine oxidase enzyme must be inhibited to produce therapeutic responses. Some patients fail to respond to conventional doses of MAOIs because of inadequate inhibition of monoamine oxidase. Non-placebo-controlled studies have reported that higher than conventional doses of tranylcypromine (90–200 mg/day) may be a safe and effective treatment for refractory depression (Amsterdam 1991).

Use of higher than conventional doses of other antide-

Table 34–6. Therapeutic options for treatment-refractory depressed patients

Treatment	Efficacy	Replicability
Lithium augmentation of antidepressants	+++	+++
Electroconvulsive therapy	+++	+++
Thyroid (T$_3$) augmentation of antidepressants	++–+++	++
Stimulant augmentation of antidepressants	+–++	++
TCA and MAOI combination	+	++
Estrogen	0–+	++
Desipramine and fluoxetine combination	++–+++	+
High-dose MAOI	++	+
Repetitive transcranial magnetic stimulation	++	+
Antiglucocorticoid therapy	+–++	+
Pindolol augmentation of SSRIs	0–+++	+

Note. Efficacy was rated as follows: 0 = ineffective; + = slightly effective; ++ = moderately effective; +++ very effective. Replication refers to the extent to which the efficacy of the treatment has been investigated; it was rated as follows: + = open studies and/or only one controlled study conducted; ++ = several controlled studies conducted but further investigation indicated for complete evaluation; +++ = highly replicated and consistent degree of efficacy reported.
T$_3$ = triiodothyronine; TCA = tricyclic antidepressant; MAOI = monoamine oxidase inhibitor; SSRIs = selective serotonin reuptake inhibitor.

pressant medications may be considered in cases of highly refractory depression; however, dosages should be increased very slowly, with frequent monitoring for side effects, including serial electrocardiogram monitoring if indicated.

Changing Treatment Strategies

Medication substitution.   When a patient does not respond to an adequate antidepressant trial, the clinician often decides to change to a different antidepressant. The choice of the next antidepressant should involve those considerations ordinarily included in the initial selection of an antidepressant, such as side-effect profile, past antidepressant trial responses, family history of antidepressant responses, course of illness, premorbid personality, and depressive subtype.

Another method that has been advocated in selecting another antidepressant is consideration of its neuropharmacological properties. For example, if the patient's depression did not respond to an adequate trial with fluoxetine (a potent blocker of serotonin reuptake), then a trial with desipramine (a potent blocker of norepinephrine reuptake) is indicated. This rationale has become a basis for a common clinical practice, but its validity has not been confirmed in systematic clinical trials (Nolen et al. 1988). Some evidence suggests that two SSRIs—fluoxetine (Beasley et al. 1990) and fluvoxamine (Delgado et al. 1988)—may be effective in some patients in whom treatment with TCAs was unsuccessful.

Treatment with MAOIs may be useful for depressed patients whose condition has not responded to TCAs such as imipramine. In a double-blind crossover trial, phenelzine was reported to be effective in approximately two-thirds of patients whose symptoms had not responded to imipramine (McGrath et al. 1993). These chronically depressed, nonmelancholic, mood-reactive patients had many symptoms characteristic of atypical depression. In another double-blind crossover study, 75% of a group of anergic bipolar depressed patients had been refractory to treatment with imipramine, but many patients had therapeutic responses to tranylcypromine (Thase et al. 1992). This work was consistent with previous open-label trials in a similar patient population (Himmelhoch et al. 1991). Thus, these results suggest that many depressed patients characterized by anergia, psychomotor retardation, and symptoms of atypical depression will have therapeutic responses to MAOIs despite previous treatment resistance to TCAs.

Electroconvulsive therapy.   As discussed earlier in this chapter, most investigations suggest that ECT has ef-ficacy equal or superior to that of TCAs or MAOIs in the treatment of severe depression. A possible exception is that ECT is not effective for treating atypical depression. The results from several centers indicate that ECT is often effective in cases of depression unresponsive to TCAs (Avery and Winokur 1977; Devanand et al. 1991). For example, in the British Cooperative Study, ECT resulted in a 50% response rate in those patients whose conditions did not improve with imipramine (Clinical Psychiatry Committee of the British Medical Research Council 1965). Similarly, in another study, 6 of 9 patients' symptoms that did not respond to amitriptyline diminished with ECT (Browne and Kreeger 1963). In a study of 153 endogenously depressed patients who were imipramine nonresponders, 120 (78%) responded to ECT (Avery and Lubrano 1979). When Paul and colleagues (1981) reviewed their experience with ECT in intractably and seriously depressed patients over an 8-year period at NIMH, they found that only 1 of 9 patients did not respond favorably.

ECT is particularly indicated in patients with psychotic depression. Major depression with psychotic features appears to be relatively resistant to single-agent antidepressant treatment compared with major depression without psychotic features. Efficacy is substantially improved when an antipsychotic is combined with a conventional antidepressant in the treatment of delusional depression. In one study, coadministration of an antipsychotic and a TCA in a delusionally depressed sample resulted in a total drug response rate of 70% compared with 22% for a single agent (Charney and Nelson 1981). Nevertheless, seven of the eight who had inadequate responses to the antipsychotic-TCA treatment responded to ECT. For most patients with psychotic depression, ECT or the antipsychotic-TCA combination is the treatment of choice.

Selecting an Antidepressant Drug Combination

TCAs and MAOIs.   The rationale for combining a TCA with an MAOI was based on the monoamine deficiency hypothesis of depression. The combined ability of TCAs to inhibit presynaptic reuptake of biogenic amines and MAOIs to reduce metabolic breakdown of biogenic amines theoretically results in increased neurotransmitters in the synapse.

Most initial reports of combined TCA-MAOI therapy in the treatment of refractory depression were encouraging. However, most of these studies used open designs with no placebo control or comparison treatment groups (Pande et al. 1991; Razani et al. 1983; Schmauss et al.

1988; White and Simpson 1981). To date, no controlled study has confirmed an advantage in efficacy when a TCA is combined with an MAOI compared with either agent given alone. Most of the research supporting this combination approach in refractory depression comes from open clinical trials and anecdotal reports. On the other hand, despite early alarm about adverse side effects associated with this combination, the relative safety of this approach has been substantiated, provided low to moderate doses of an MAOI are added to an ongoing trial of a moderate dose of a TCA (Pande et al. 1991). An occasional patient may benefit from this treatment approach (Tyrer and Murphy 1990).

Desipramine and fluoxetine. Several uncontrolled studies have found that when desipramine and fluoxetine are used in combination, they have a synergistic effect. In several cases when desipramine was added to fluoxetine, patients rapidly improved. These patients had been unresponsive to desipramine or fluoxetine alone (Eisen 1989). A case series of 30 treatment-refractory depressed patients reported an 87% response rate to a combination of fluoxetine and non-MAOIs (Weilburg et al. 1989). Furthermore, preliminary data suggested a more rapid antidepressant response in depressed patients treated with combined desipramine and fluoxetine than in patients treated with desipramine alone (Nelson et al. 1991). Many anecdotal reports of the efficacy of this combination in treatment-refractory patients are available, and the combination is widely used in clinical practice. However, double-blind, placebo-controlled studies are needed to document the efficacy of this treatment combination.

Augmentation Strategies

Antidepressants and stimulants. The combination of a TCA and methylphenidate is usually mentioned as a treatment approach to refractory depression. However, to our knowledge, no studies of its efficacy have used a comparison treatment group. In the most frequently cited report, seven treatment-refractory patients with psychotic depression were given 20-mg doses of methylphenidate in addition to an imipramine regimen. Five of the seven patients had rapid and robust improvements (Wharton et al. 1971). However, the clinical improvement may have been the result of methylphenidate-induced increases in imipramine plasma levels. In a single case report, robust and rapid resolution of a patient's intractable depression occurred when methylphenidate was added to ongoing desipramine treatment. No concomitant change in plasma desipramine level occurred (Drimmer et al. 1983). In

more recent case series of SSRI-refractory depressed patients, methylphenidate (10–40 mg/day) (Stoll et al. 1996) and pemoline (9.875–37.5 mg/day) (Metz and Shader 1991) augmentation resulted in marked reduction in depressive symptoms.

A report on clinical experience with a combination of either pemoline or dextroamphetamine and an MAOI in 32 depressed patients who were severely refractory to treatment indicated that the combination was safe and effective (Fawcett et al. 1991). Six patients became manic ($n = 1$) or hypomanic ($n = 5$). This treatment approach may be a viable option for severely ill patients.

Lithium augmentation of antidepressant action. Unlike many pharmacological approaches to the treatment of refractory depressed patients, the investigations of the efficacy of lithium when added to a chronic antidepressant regimen were initiated because of a specific hypothesis that was based on preclinical neurobiological research (DeMontigny et al. 1981, 1983; Heninger et al. 1983). DeMontigny hypothesized that lithium's ability to increase presynaptic transmission of serotonin would potentiate TCA-induced postsynaptic serotonergic supersensitivity, resulting in enhanced efficacy of transmission in the brain serotonergic system. Although other mechanisms for lithium's effectiveness are possible, the discovery of this treatment approach represents the potential effect that a hypothesis generated from basic neuroscience research may have on the development and implementation of new treatment strategies.

Very strong data from more than 20 investigations support the effectiveness of adding lithium carbonate to ongoing antidepressant treatment in treatment-refractory depressed patients (Austin et al. 1991; Charney et al. 1991; Kramlinger and Post 1989). Whether starting an antidepressant and lithium concomitantly is equally efficacious in treating refractory depression has not been determined. Similarly, it is not known whether the lithium-antidepressant combination is necessary for preventing relapse and, if not, which agent should be used alone for prophylaxis. Preliminary observations indicate that the effectiveness of lithium augmentation is sustained and reduces the relapse rate—particularly in patients who had an acute, marked response to lithium augmentation (Nierenberg et al. 1990).

The earliest reports of lithium augmentation found that in patients whose symptoms did not respond to standard treatment with antidepressants, depressive symptomatology decreased dramatically within 48–72 hours after lithium was added (DeMontigny et al. 1981). Subsequent controlled investigations reported a more variable response to lithium. Only a fraction of patients whose condition responds to lithium augmentation will have dramatic responses within a week of adding lithium. More commonly, the response is gradual, with a response latency of up to 3 weeks.

The overall response rate of patients with treatment-refractory depression is approximately 50%, with patients with nonpsychotic melancholic depression or bipolar depression most likely to respond. However, many patients with nonmelancholic depression or delusional depression also respond to lithium augmentation. Lithium appears to be effective when added to all classes of antidepressant drugs, including carbamazepine. No evidence supports any superiority of one antidepressant type when lithium is added.

A controlled fixed-dose lithium investigation was conducted to determine proper lithium dose. This study and clinical experience suggest that lithium should be used in the typical fashion, titrating doses to a lithium level of 0.5–0.8 mEq/L (Stein and Bernadt 1993).

Lithium and monoamine oxidase inhibitors. Shortly after lithium carbonate was introduced in the United States for the treatment of bipolar disorders, two reports (Himmelhoch et al. 1972; Zall 1971) on using lithium and an MAOI together were published. The rationale seemed related less to biological theory and more to a growing awareness that lithium alone was not always effective in the acute treatment of bipolar depression. In these open, uncontrolled trials, an MAOI was added to ongoing lithium administration in 24 lithium-resistant subjects. Most had already failed to respond to TCAs alone. Nineteen of 24 had substantial improvement after the MAOI was added. In a more recent investigation, 11 of 12 well-defined refractory unipolar depressed patients who had not responded to other lithium-antidepressant combinations were successfully treated when tranylcypromine was added to lithium (Price et al. 1985).

The robustness of the responses reported suggests that the lithium-MAOI combination may be a potent antidepressant treatment appropriate for use in treatment-refractory patients. In addition, further investigation should help clarify whether the sequence in which an MAOI and lithium are combined affects efficacy (Nelson and Byck 1982).

Thyroid hormones and antidepressant drugs. In 1963, Prange reported a case of hyperthyroidism in which imipramine seemed to induce a toxic reaction. Based on this clinical observation and the preclinical evidence that thyroid hormone enhances adrenergic receptor sensitiv-

ity, Prange reasoned that modest amounts of triiodothyronine (T_3) might accelerate imipramine's antidepressant activity without producing toxicity. In a placebo-controlled study of 20 depressed (but not treatment-refractory) patients, a more rapid onset of antidepressant action was observed in the imipramine-T_3 group compared with the imipramine-placebo group (Prange et al. 1969). Several other studies also found that a T_3-TCA combination provided a more rapid relief of symptoms than a TCA alone. The general trend in these studies was for women to respond better than men.

These favorable reports of T_3's effect on the rate of TCA response stimulated investigation into the efficacy of the T_3-TCA combination in refractory depression. Open studies (Banki 1975; Earle 1969; Ogura et al. 1974; Schwartz et al. 1984; Tsutsui et al. 1979) showed that when T_3 was added to TCAs in treatment-refractory depressed patients, about two-thirds of the cases had a favorable outcome. The significance of any conclusion drawn from these studies is weakened by several methodological flaws, including the absence of standardized diagnostic and treatment response rating criteria and a nonblind design. The results of controlled studies are less consistent. Two studies reported antidepressant effects of T_3 augmentation (Goodwin et al. 1982; Joffe and Singer 1991), whereas two other investigations did not (Gitlin et al. 1987; Thase et al. 1989). However, a placebo-controlled comparison of lithium and T_3 augmentation of TCAs in treatment-refractory patients with unipolar depression found that both of these agents were equal in efficacy and superior to placebo (Joffe et al. 1993). The effectiveness of thyroid hormone augmentation is not related to varying degrees of subclinical hypothyroidism in depressed patients.

Estrogen. In the 1930s, several reports were published on the use of estrogen for depression occurring around the time of menopause. The rationale for the use of estrogen for treatment was that symptoms (including depression) occurring during menopause were the result of declining hormone levels. The findings of these studies were inconsistent, ranging from conclusions that estrogen had no proven value to assertions that it was a specific treatment for involutional melancholia. A more recent investigation failed to demonstrate an antidepressant effect of estrogen in perimenopausal patients (Coope 1981). However, a double-blind, placebo-controlled study used much higher doses of conjugated estrogen (Premarin at doses of up to 25 mg/day) in pre- and postmenopausal treatment-refractory depressed patients. Depression ratings significantly improved, but no complete remission occurred in the estrogen-treated patients (Klaiber et al. 1979). No significant association of estrogen response with menopausal status was found. Citing the catecholamine deficiency hypothesis of depression, the authors speculated that estrogen might exert an antidepressant action by augmenting central noradrenergic activity. However, preclinical studies indicated that the effect of estrogen on brain serotonin function may mediate some of its actions on depressed mood (Fischette et al. 1984).

Few reports of combined antidepressant-estrogen treatment have been published. In studies comparing imipramine plus estrogen with imipramine alone, the combination showed no clear advantage (Oppenheim 1984; Prange 1972; Shapira et al. 1985). Several case reports suggested possible beneficial effects of adding contraceptives to antidepressants for treatment of refractory depression (Sherwin 1991).

At present, insufficient data exist to support an estrogen trial early in the course of treatment for patients with treatment-refractory depression. An advantage to an antidepressant-estrogen combination has not yet been demonstrated. In addition, the side effects of long-term estrogen administration to pre- and postmenopausal depressed women have not been definitively determined.

PROMISING APPROACHES

The depression treatment literature is rich with a variety of other pharmacological and nonpharmacological approaches. However, their efficacy in refractory depression has not been studied sufficiently to warrant detailed inclusion in this chapter. Pharmacological approaches of interest include the use of S-adenosylmethionine (J. F. Rosenbaum et al. 1990). Examples of innovative nonpharmacological approaches for depressed patients with hypothesized biological rhythm disturbances include sleep deprivation and bright-light treatment (Levitt et al. 1991).

Another developing antidepressant strategy directly targets the hypothalamic-pituitary-adrenal (HPA) axis. Abnormalities of the HPA axis were among the first and most consistently identified findings in depressed subjects. Such findings include elevated CSF corticotropin-releasing hormone (CRH) levels, elevated cortisol levels, and diminished sensitivity to dexamethasone suppression. In preclinical and clinical studies, chronic antidepressant treatment normalized these findings. Therefore, agents that directly reduce the hypercortisolemia in depressed subjects were tested for antidepressant activity (Murphy and Wolkowitz 1993).

In two open-trial studies (Murphy et al. 1991;

Wolkowitz et al. 1993), refractory depressed patients consistently showed clinical improvement during administration of a regimen of steroid suppressant therapy, including aminoglutethimide, metyrapone, and ketoconazole. In the first study (Murphy et al. 1991), 6 of 10 initial study subjects who completed the trial had either a full ($n = 4$) or a partial ($n = 2$) remission. In the second study (Wolkowitz et al. 1993), 7 of 10 initial study subjects who completed the trial had an average 30% decrease in Hamilton Rating Scale for Depression scores. A preliminary placebo-controlled study of 20 medication-free depressed subjects reported no differences between ketoconazole- and placebo-treated patients; however, the subgroup of patients with high baseline cortisol levels did respond significantly better to ketoconazole than to placebo (Wolkowitz et al. 1996). Because of potential serious side effects, such as hepatotoxicity and hypoadrenalism, an antiglucocorticoid strategy should not be used in the general population until further placebo-controlled studies validate its effectiveness.

A novel strategy in the treatment of major depression is the concomitant use of a serotonin autoreceptor antagonist with an SSRI to enhance serotonergic function. In preliminary, open-label studies, pindolol, a serotonin antagonist and β-adrenergic blocker, has strongly augmented SSRIs in resistant depression and rapidly accelerated treatment response (Artigas et al. 1994; Blier and Bergeron 1995). To date, placebo-controlled studies of this strategy have reported mixed results. Results from our group with fluoxetine have not been favorable (Berman et al. 1996); however, other researchers have found that a fluoxetine-pindolol combination hastens response in a subgroup of patients who are predominantly treatment-naive with nonchronic depressions (Isaac et al. 1996). Further evaluation of this pharmacological approach is necessary.

A novel nonpharmacological approach to the treatment of depression involves the application of repetitive transcranial trains of magnetic stimulation (rTMS) over the left prefrontal cortex, an area consistently implicated in the pathophysiology of major depression in positron-emission tomography (PET) and single photon emission computed tomography (SPECT) studies. rTMS likely depolarizes cortical neurons in a generalized region; therefore, it bears some similarity to ECT. However, rTMS confers only a modest risk of seizure. rTMS was first applied to nondepressed subjects and had effects on mood (Bickford et al. 1987). In more recent studies, rTMS has been examined for efficacy in the treatment of major depression. In one study of five highly refractory depressed subjects, two patients had robust improvement after rTMS treatment, with 17-item Hamilton Rating Scale for Depression scores decreasing from 23 to 3 and 20 to 12 (George et al. 1995). Both patients had failed to respond to 10 or more previous antidepressant trials. Further work is under way to elaborate these findings. Controlled, blinded trials are needed to establish further the effectiveness of this potential treatment.

THE FUTURE OF PHARMACOLOGICAL TREATMENT OF DEPRESSIVE ILLNESS

Clinicians now have an impressive drug armamentarium from which to treat depressive illness. Severe depressive illness in most patients will have good therapeutic responses to antidepressant drugs, with an acceptable degree of adverse side effects. Furthermore, various effective drug treatment approaches have been developed for most patients whose symptoms do not respond to the initial antidepressant drug used.

However, important deficits persist in knowledge relevant to the pharmacological treatment of depression. Descriptive and biological markers capable of identifying subtypes of depressive illness characterized by therapeutic responses to specific antidepressants are lacking. The mechanisms of action of antidepressant drugs have not been established. This limits the discovery of new, more effective, rapid-acting antidepressant drugs.

The future development of antidepressant drugs likely will move beyond drugs with therapeutic properties related to monoamine reuptake or metabolism inhibition. Drugs with specific actions on monoamine receptor subtypes are being synthesized and tested in treatment of depressed patients. Psychopharmaceutical research will focus less on the monoamine systems because of recent data suggesting that these systems may not be primary in the pathophysiology of depression (Berman et al. 1996). Further understanding of the effects of antidepressant drug action at sites distal to receptor recognition sites may provide new approaches for developing new classes of antidepressant drugs.

REFERENCES

Aberg-Wistedt A, Jostell KG, Ross SB, et al: Effects of zimeldine and desipramine on serotonin and noradrenaline uptake mechanisms in relation to plasma concentrations and to therapeutic effects during treatment of depression. Psychopharmacology (Berl) 74:297–305, 1981

Altamura AC, DeNovelis F, Guercetti G, et al: Fluoxetine compared with amitriptyline in elderly depression: a controlled clinical trial. Int J Clin Pharmacol Res 9:391–396, 1989

American Psychiatric Association: Diagnostic and Statistical Manual of Mental Disorders, 3rd Edition. Washington, DC, American Psychiatric Association, 1980

American Psychiatric Association Task Force Report: Tricyclic antidepressants: blood level measurements and clinical outcome. Am J Psychiatry 142:155–182, 1985

Amin M, Lehmann H, Mirmiran J: A double-blind, placebo-controlled dose-finding study with sertraline. Psychopharmacol Bull 25:164–167, 1989

Amsterdam JD: Use of high dose tranylcypromine in resistant depression, in Advances in Neuropsychiatry and Psychopharmacology, Vol 2: Refractory Depression. Edited by Amsterdam JD. New York, Raven, 1991, pp 123–130

Amsterdam J, Maislin G, Potter L: Fluoxetine efficacy in treatment resistant depression. Prog Neuropsychopharmacol Biol Psychiatry 18:243–261, 1994

Angst J: Natural history and epidemiology of depression, in Results of Community Studies in Prediction and Treatment of Recurrent Depression. Edited by Cobb J, Goeting N. Southampton, England, Duphar Medical Relations, 1990, pp 121–154

Artigas F, Perez V, Alvarez E: Pindolol induces a rapid improvement of depressed patients treated with serotonin reuptake inhibitors. Arch Gen Psychiatry 51:248–251, 1994

Asberg M, Bertilsson L, Tuck D, et al: Indoleamine metabolites in cerebrospinal fluid of depressed patients before and during treatment with nortriptyline. Clin Pharmacol Ther 14:277–286, 1973

Austin MP, Souza FG, Goodwin GM: Lithium augmentation in antidepressant-resistant patients: a quantitative analysis. Br J Psychiatry 159:510–514, 1991

Avery D, Lubrano A: Depression treated with imipramine and ECT: the DeCardis study reconsidered. Am J Psychiatry 136:559–562, 1979

Avery D, Winokur G: The efficacy of electroconvulsive therapy and antidepressants in depression. Biol Psychiatry 12:507–524, 1977

Bakish D, Ravindran A, Hooper C, et al: Psychopharmacological treatment response of patients with a DSM-III diagnosis of dysthymic disorder. Psychopharmacol Bull 30:53–59, 1994

Banki CM: Triiodothyronine in the treatment of depression. Orv Hetil 116:2543–2546, 1975

Baron M, Gershon ES, Rudy V, et al: Lithium carbonate response in depression: prediction by unipolar/bipolar illness, average-evoked response, catechol-O-methyltransferase, and family history. Arch Gen Psychiatry 32:1107–1111, 1975

Beasley CM Jr, Sayler ME, Cunningham GE, et al: Fluoxetine in tricyclic refractory major depressive disorder. J Affect Disord 20:193–200, 1990

Beasley CM Jr, Dornseif BE, Bosomworth JC, et al: Fluoxetine and suicide: a meta-analysis of controlled trials of treatment for depression. BMJ 303:685–692, 1991

Beasley CM, Masica DN, Potvin JH: Fluoxetine: a review of receptor and functional effects and their clinical implications. Psychopharmacology (Berl) 107:1–10, 1992

Beckmann H, Goodwin FK: Antidepressant response to tricyclics and urinary MHPG in unipolar patients. Arch Gen Psychiatry 32:17–21, 1975

Bergstrom RF, Peyton AL, Lemberger L: Quantification and mechanism of the fluoxetine and tricyclic antidepressant interaction. Clin Pharmacol Ther 51:239–248, 1992

Berman RM, Krystal JH, Charney DS: Mechanism of action of antidepressants: monoamine hypotheses and beyond, in Biology of Schizophrenia and Affective Disease. Edited by Watson SJ. Washington, DC, American Psychiatric Press, 1996, pp 295–368

Bickford RG, Guidie N, Fortesque P, et al: Magnetic stimulation of human peripheral nerve and brain: response enhancement by magnetoelectrical technique. Neurosurgery 20:110–116, 1987

Bielski RJ, Friedel RO: Prediction of tricyclic antidepressant response: a critical review. Arch Gen Psychiatry 33:1479–1489, 1976

Bigger JT Jr: Implications of the Cardiac Arrhythmia Suppression Trial for antiarrhythmic drug treatment. Am J Cardiol 65:3D–10D, 1990

Blier P, Bergeron R: Effectiveness of pindolol with selected antidepressant drugs in the treatment of major depression. J Clin Psychopharmacol 15:217–222, 1995

Branconnier RJ, Cole JO, Ghazvinian S, et al: Clinical pharmacology of bupropion and imipramine in elderly depressives. J Clin Psychiatry 44 (5, sec 2):130–133, 1983

Brown P, Brawley P: Dexamethasone suppression test and mood response to methylphenidate in primary depression. Am J Psychiatry 140:990–993, 1983

Brown WA, Qualls CB: Pituitary-adrenal disinhibition in depression: marker of a subtype with characteristic clinical features and response to treatment. Psychiatry Res 4:115–128, 1981

Brown WA, Shuey I: Response to dexamethasone and subtype of depression. Arch Gen Psychiatry 37:747–751, 1980

Browne MW, Kreeger LC: A clinical trial of amitriptyline in depressive patients. Br J Psychiatry 109:692–694, 1963

Buff DD, Brenner R, Kirtane SS, et al: Dysrhythmia associated with fluoxetine treatment in an elderly patient with cardiac disease. J Clin Psychiatry 52:174–176, 1991

Bunney WE: The switch process in manic-depressive psychosis. Ann Intern Med 87:319–335, 1977

Cade JFJ: Lithium salts in the treatment of psychotic excitement. Med J Aust 36:349–352, 1949

Cardiac Arrhythmia Suppression Trial (CAST) Investigators: Preliminary report: effect of encainide and flecainide on mortality in a randomized trial of arrhythmia suppression after myocardial infarction. N Engl J Med 321:406–412, 1989

Cardiac Arrhythmia Suppression Trial II Investigators: Effect of the antiarrhythmic agent moricizine on survival after myocardial infarction. N Engl J Med 327:227–233, 1992

Carlsson A, Fuxe K, Ungerstedt U: The effect of imipramine on central 5-hydroxytryptamine neurons. J Pharm Pharmacol 20:150–151, 1968

Carroll BJ: The dexamethasone suppression test for melancholia. Br J Psychiatry 140:292–304, 1982

Cassano GB, Maggini C, Akiskal HS: Short-term, subchronic, and chronic sequelae of affective disorders. Psychiatr Clin North Am 6:55–67, 1983

Charney DS, Nelson JC: Delusional and nondelusional unipolar depression: further evidence for distinct subtypes. Am J Psychiatry 138:328–333, 1981

Charney DS, Woods SW, Goodman WK, et al: Drug treatment of panic disorder: the comparative efficacy of imipramine, alprazolam and trazodone. J Clin Psychiatry 47:580–585, 1986

Charney DS, Delgado PL, Southwick SM, et al: Current hypotheses of the mechanism of antidepressant treatments: implications for the treatment of refractory depression, in Advances in Neuropsychiatry and Psychopharmacology, Vol 2: Refractory Depression. Edited by Amsterdam JD. New York, Raven, 1991, pp 23–40

Clinical Psychiatry Committee of the British Medical Research Council: Clinical trial of the treatment of depressive illness. BMJ 1:881–886, 1965

Coble PA, Kupfer DJ, Spiker DG, et al: EEG sleep in primary depression: a longitudinal placebo study. J Affect Disord 1:131–138, 1979

Cohn CK, Shrivastava R, Mendels J, et al: Double-blind, multicenter comparison of sertraline and amitriptyline in elderly depressed patients. J Clin Psychiatry 51 (12, suppl B):28–33, 1990

Coope J: Is estrogen therapy effective in the treatment of menopausal depression? J R Coll Gen Pract 31:134–140, 1981

Cooper AJ: Tyramine and irreversible monoamine oxidase inhibitors in clinical practice. Br J Psychiatry 155 (suppl 6):38–45, 1989

Coplen SE, Antman EM, Berlin JA, et al: Efficacy and safety of quinidine therapy for maintenance of sinus rhythm after cardioversion: a metaanalysis of randomized control trials. Circulation 82:1106–1116, 1990

Coppen A, Rama Rao VA, Ruthven CRJ, et al: Urinary 4-hydroxy-3-methoxyphenylglycol is not a predictor for clinical response to amitriptyline in depressive illness. Psychopharmacology (Berl) 64:95–97, 1979

Crane GE: The psychiatric side-effects of iproniazid. Am J Psychiatry 112:494–501, 1956

Crewe HK, Lennard MS, Tucker GT, et al: The effect of selective serotonin re-uptake inhibitors on cytochrome P4502D6 (CYP2D6) activity in human liver microsomes. Br J Pharmacol 34:262–265, 1992

Cusack B, Nelson A, Richelson E: Binding of antidepressants to human brain receptors: focus on newer generation of compounds. Psychopharmacology 114:559–565, 1994

Danish University Antidepressant Study Group: Paroxetine: a selective serotonin reuptake inhibitor showing better tolerance, but weaker antidepressant effect than clomipramine in a controlled multicenter study. J Affect Disord 18:289–299, 1990

Davidson J: Seizures and bupropion: a review. J Clin Psychiatry 50:256–261, 1989

Davis JM: Antidepressant drugs, in Comprehensive Textbook of Psychiatry, Vol 4, 4th Edition. Edited by Kaplan HI, Saddock BJ. Baltimore, MD, Williams & Wilkins, 1985, pp 765–794

Davis R, Wilde MI: Mirtazapine: a review of its pharmacology and therapeutic potential in the management of major depression. CNS Drugs 5:389–402, 1995

Delay J, Deniker P: Trente-huit cas de psychoses traitées par la cure prolongée et continue de 4560 RP. Le Congrès des Medicins Alienistes et Neurologistes de France, Vol 50. In Compte redu du Congrès. Paris, Masson et Cie, 1952

Delgado PL, Price LH, Charney DS, et al: Efficacy of fluvoxamine in treatment-refractory depression. J Affect Disord 15:55–60, 1988

DeMontigny CF, Grunberg AF, Deschenes JP: Lithium induces rapid relief of depression in tricyclic antidepressant drug non-responders. Br J Psychiatry 138:252–256, 1981

DeMontigny CF, Ceurnoyer G, Morissette R, et al: Lithium carbonate addition in tricyclic antidepressant-resistant unipolar depression. Arch Gen Psychiatry 40:1327–1334, 1983

Dessain EC, Schatzberg AF, Woods BT, et al: Maprotiline treatment in depression. Arch Gen Psychiatry 43:86–90, 1987

Devanand DP, Sacheim HA, Prudic J: Electroconvulsive therapy in the treatment-resistant patient. Psychiatr Clin North Am 14:905–923, 1991

Doogan DP, Caillard V: Sertraline in the prevention of depression. Br J Psychiatry 160:217–222, 1992

Downing RW, Rickels K: Predictors of response to amitriptyline and placebo in three outpatient treatment settings. J Nerv Ment Dis 156:109–129, 1973

Drimmer EJ, Gitlin MJ, Gwirtouran HE: Desipramine and methylphenidate combination treatment of depression: case report. Am J Psychiatry 140:241–242, 1983

Dunner DL, Cohn JB, Walshe TI, et al: Two combined, multicenter double-blind studies of paroxetine and doxepin in geriatric patients with major depression. J Clin Psychiatry 53 (2 suppl):57–60, 1992

Earle BV: Thyroid hormone and tricyclic antidepressants in resistant depressions. Am J Psychiatry 126:1667–1669, 1969

Echt DS, Liebson PR, Mitchell LB, et al: Mortality and morbidity in patients receiving encainide, flecainide, or placebo: the Cardiac Arrhythmia Suppression Trial. N Engl J Med 324:781–788, 1991

Eisen A: Fluoxetine and desipramine: a strategy for augmenting antidepressant response. Pharmacopsychiatry 22:272–273, 1989

Ellison JM, Milofsky JE, Ely E: Fluoxetine-induced bradycardia and syncope in two patients. J Clin Psychiatry 51:385–386, 1990

Eric L: A prospective, double-blind, comparative, multicentre study of paroxetine and placebo in preventing recurrent major depressive episodes. Biol Psychiatry 29 (suppl 11):254S–255S, 1991

Ettigi PG, Hayes PE, Narasimhacharr N, et al: *d*-Amphetamine response and dexamethasone suppression test as predictors of treatment outcome in unipolar depression. Biol Psychiatry 18:499–504, 1983

Falk RH: Flecainide-induced ventricular tachycardia and fibrillation in patients treated for atrial fibrillation. Ann Intern Med 111:107–111, 1989

Fawcett J, Maas JW, Dekirmenjian H: Depression and MHPG excretion: response to dextroamphetamine and tricyclic antidepressants. Arch Gen Psychiatry 26:246–251, 1972

Fawcett J, Kravitz HM, Sajecka JM, et al: CNS stimulant potentiation of monoamine oxidase inhibitors in treatment-refractory depression. J Clin Psychopharmacol 11:127–132, 1991

Feder R: Bradycardia and syncope induced by fluoxetine (letter). J Clin Psychiatry 52:139, 1991

Feighner J: Cardiovascular safety in depressed patients: focus on venlafaxine. J Clin Psychiatry 56(12):574–579, 1995

Feighner J, Hendrickson G, Miller L, et al: Double-blind comparison of doxepin vs bupropion in outpatients with major depressive disorder. J Clin Psychopharmacol 6:27–32, 1986

Feighner J, Gardner E, Johnson J, et al: Double-blind comparison of bupropion and fluoxetine in depressed outpatients. J Clin Psychiatry 52:329–355, 1991

Feighner J, Cohn J, Fabre L, et al: A study comparing paroxetine, placebo and imipramine in depressed patients. J Affect Disord 28:71–79, 1993

Ferguson J, Cunningham L, Merideth C, et al: Bupropion in tricyclic antidepressant nonresponders with unipolar major depressive disorder. Ann Clin Psychiatry 6:153–160, 1994

Fischette CT, Biegon A, McEwen B: Sex steroid modulation of the serotonin behavioral syndrome. Life Sci 35:1197–1206, 1984

Frank E, Kupfer DJ, Perel JM, et al: Three-year outcomes for maintenance therapies in recurrent depression. Arch Gen Psychiatry 47:1093–1099, 1990

Fraser AR: Choice of anti-depressant based on test. Am J Psychiatry 140:786–787, 1983

Gaertner HJ, Kreuter F, Scharek G: Do urinary MHPG and plasma drug levels correlate with response to amitriptyline therapy? Psychopharmacology (Berl) 76:236–239, 1982

Gardner EA, Johnston JA: Bupropion: an antidepressant without sexual pathophysiological action. J Clin Psychopharmacol 5:24–29, 1985

Garvey MJ, Cook BL, Tollefson GD, et al: Antidepressant response in chronic major depression. Compr Psychiatry 30:214–217, 1989

George MS, Wassermann EM, Williams WA, et al: Daily repetitive transcranial magnetic stimulation (rTMS) improves mood in depression. NeuroReport 6:1853–1856, 1995

Georgotas A, McCue RE, Cooper TB: A placebo controlled comparison of nortriptyline and phenelzine in maintenance therapy of elderly depressed patients. Arch Gen Psychiatry 46:783–786, 1989

Gitlin MJ, Gerner RH: The dexamethasone suppression test and response to somatic treatment: a review. J Clin Psychiatry 47:16–21, 1986

Gitlin MJ, Gwirtsman H, Fairbanks L, et al: Dexamethasone suppression test and treatment response. J Clin Psychiatry 45:387–389, 1984

Gitlin MJ, Weiner H, Fairbanks L: Failure of T_3 to potentiate tricyclic antidepressant response. J Affect Disord 13:267–272, 1987

Glassman AH, Bigger JT Jr: Cardiovascular effects of therapeutic doses of tricyclic antidepressants: a review. Arch Gen Psychiatry 38:815–820, 1981

Glassman AH, Preud'homme XA: Review of the cardiovascular effects of heterocyclic antidepressants. J Clin Psychiatry 54 (2, suppl):16–22, 1993

Glassman AH, Perel JM, Shostak M, et al: Clinical implications of imipramine plasma levels for depressive illness. Arch Gen Psychiatry 34:197–204, 1977

Glassman AH, Roose SP, Giardina EGV, et al: Cardiovascular effects of tricyclic antidepressants, in Psychopharmacology: The Third Generation of Progress. Edited by Meltzer HY. New York, Raven, 1987, pp 1437–1442

Glassman AH, Roose SP, Bigger JT Jr: The safety of tricyclic antidepressants in cardiac patients: risk-benefit reconsidered. JAMA 269:2673–2675, 1993

Glowinski J, Axelrod J: Inhibition of uptake of tritiated-noradrenaline in the intact rat brain by imipramine and structurally related compounds. Nature 204:1318–1319, 1964

Goodman WK, Price LH, Delgado PL, et al: Specificity of serotonin reuptake inhibitors in the treatment of obsessive-compulsive disorder: comparison of fluvoxamine and desipramine. Arch Gen Psychiatry 47:577–585, 1990

Goodwin FK, Murphy DL, Dunner DL, et al: Lithium response in unipolar versus bipolar depression. Am J Psychiatry 129:44–47, 1972

Goodwin FK, Post RM, Murphy DL: CSF amine metabolites and therapies of depression. Scientific Proceedings in Summary Form: The One Hundred Twenty-Sixth Annual Meeting of the American Psychiatric Association, Honolulu, HI, May 7–11, 1973, pp 24–25

Goodwin FK, Prange AJ, Post RM, et al: Potentiation of antidepressant effects by L-tri-iodothyronine in tricyclic nonresponders. Am J Psychiatry 139:34–38, 1982

Greden JF, Kronfol Z, Gardner R, et al: Dexamethasone suppression test and selection of antidepressant medications. J Affect Disord 3:389–396, 1981

Greden JF, Gardner R, King D: Dexamethasone suppression tests in anti-depressant treatment of melancholia: the process of normalization and test-retest reproducibility. Arch Gen Psychiatry 40:493–500, 1983

Haykal RF, Akiskal HS: Bupropion as a promising approach to rapidly cycling bipolar II patients. J Clin Psychiatry 51:450–455, 1990

Heninger GR, Charney DS, Sternberg DE: Lithium carbonate augmentation of antidepressant treatment: an effective prescription for treatment-refractory depression. Arch Gen Psychiatry 40:1335–1342, 1983

Himmelhoch JM, Detre T, Kupfer DJ, et al: Treatment of previously intractable depressions with tranylcypromine and lithium. J Nerv Ment Dis 155:216–220, 1972

Himmelhoch JM, Thase ME, Mallinger AG, et al: Tranylcypromine versus imipramine in anergic bipolar depression. Am J Psychiatry 148:910–916, 1991

Hirschfeld RMA, Klerman GL, Andreasen NC, et al: Psychosocial predictors of chronicity in depressed patients. Br J Psychiatry 148:648–654, 1986

Hochli D, Riemann D, Zulley J, et al: Initial REM sleep suppression by clomipramine: a prognostic tool for treatment response in patients with a major depressive disorder. Biol Psychiatry 21:1217–1220, 1986

Hollister LE, Overall JE: Reflections on the specificity of action of antidepressants. Psychosomatics 6:361–365, 1965

Hollister LE, Davis KL, Berger PA: Subtypes of depression based on excretion of MHPG and response to nortriptyline. Arch Gen Psychiatry 37:1107–1110, 1980

Holsboer F, Liebl R, Hofschuster E: Repeated dexamethasone suppression test during depressive illness: normalization of test result compared with clinical improvement. J Affect Disord 4:93–101, 1982

Horowitz LN, Zipes DP, Bigger JT Jr, et al: Proarrhythmia, arrhythmogenesis or aggravation of arrhythmia—a status report. Am J Cardiol 59:54E–56E, 1987

Howland RH: Pharmacotherapy of dysthymia: a review. J Clin Psychopharmacol 11(2):83–92, 1991

Humphrey P: 5-Hydroxytryptamine receptors and drug discovery, in Serotonin Receptor Subtypes: Pharmacological Significance and Clinical Implications (International Academic and Biomedical Drug Research, Vol 1). Edited by Langer SZ, Brunello N, Racagni G, et al. Basel, Switzerland, Karger, 1992, pp 129–139

Isaac MT, Tome MB, Hart R: Serotonergic autoreceptor blockade in the reduction of antidepressant latency: a controlled trial. Program and Abstracts on New Research in Summary Form: the 149th Annual Meeting of the American Psychiatric Association, New York City, May 4–9, 1996, p 154

Janicak PG, Davis JM, Chan C, et al: Failure of urinary MHPG levels to predict treatment response in patients with unipolar depression. Am J Psychiatry 143:1398–1402, 1986

Jick H, Dinan BJ, Hunter JR, et al: Tricyclic antidepressants and convulsions. J Clin Psychopharmacol 3:182–185, 1983

Joffe RT, Singer W: Thyroid hormone potentiation of antidepressants, in Advances in Neuropsychiatry and Psychopharmacology, Vol 2: Refractory Depression. Edited by Amsterdam JD. New York, Raven, 1991, pp 185–190

Joffe RT, Singer W, Levitt AJ, et al: A placebo-controlled comparison of lithium and triiodothyronine augmentation of tricyclic antidepressants in unipolar refractory depression. Arch Gen Psychiatry 50:387–393, 1993

Johnston JA, Lineberry CG, Ascher JA, et al: A 102-center prospective study of seizure in association with bupropion. J Clin Psychiatry 52:450–456, 1991

Joyce PR, Paykel ES: Predictors of drug response in depression. Arch Gen Psychiatry 46:89–99, 1989

Kane JM, Cole K, Sarantakos S, et al: Safety and efficacy of bupropion in elderly patients: preliminary observations. J Clin Psychiatry 44 (5, sec 2):134–136, 1983

Keller MB, Shapiro RW, Lavori PW, et al: Recovery in major depressive disorder: analysis with the life table and regression models. Arch Gen Psychiatry 39:905–910, 1982a

Keller MB, Shapiro RW, Lavori PW, et al: Relapse in major depressive disorder: analysis with the life table. Arch Gen Psychiatry 39:911–915, 1982b

Keller MB, Lavori W, Endicott J, et al: "Double depression": two year follow-up. Am J Psychiatry 140:289–294, 1983

Keller MB, Klerman GL, Lavori PW, et al: Long-term outcome of episodes of major depression: clinical and public health significance. JAMA 252:788–792, 1984

Keller MB, Lavori PW, Rice J, et al: The persistent risk of chronicity in recurrent episodes of nonbipolar major depressive disorder: a prospective follow-up. Am J Psychiatry 143:24–28, 1986

Keller MB, Lavori PW, Mueller TI, et al: Time to recovery, chronicity, and levels of psychopathology in major depression: a 5-year prospective follow-up of 431 subjects. Arch Gen Psychiatry 49:809–816, 1992

Klaiber EL, Bouerman DM, Vogel W, et al: Estrogen therapy for severe persistent depression in women. Arch Gen Psychiatry 36:550–554, 1979

Kline NS: Monoamine oxidase inhibitors: an unfinished picaresque tale, in Discoveries in Biological Psychiatry. Edited by Ayd FJ, Blackwell B. Philadelphia, PA, JB Lippincott, 1970, pp 194–204

Kocsis JH, Frances AJ: A critical discussion of DSM-III dysthymic disorder. Am J Psychiatry 144:1534–1542, 1987

Kosten TR, Frank JB, Dan E, et al: Pharmacotherapy for posttraumatic stress disorder using phenelzine or imipramine. J Nerv Ment Dis 179:366–370, 1991

Kramer BA: Electroconvulsive therapy use in geriatric depression. J Nerv Ment Dis 175:233–235, 1987

Kramlinger KG, Post RM: The addition of lithium to carbamazepine: antidepressant efficacy in treatment-resistant depression. Arch Gen Psychiatry 46:794–800, 1989

Kuhn R: The treatment of depressive states with G22355 (imipramine) hydrochloride. Am J Psychiatry 115:459–464, 1958

Kuhn R: The imipramine story, in Discoveries in Biological Psychiatry. Edited by Ayd FJ, Blackwell B. Philadelphia, PA, JB Lippincott, 1970a, pp 205–217

Kuhn R: Foreword, in Tofranil® (Imipramine). Berne, Switzerland, Verlag Stamplfi, 1970b, pp vi–vii

Kuhn R: The discovery of modern antidepressants. Psychiatr J Univ Ottawa 14:249–252, 1989

Kupfer DJ, Foster FG, Reich L, et al: EEG sleep changes as predictors in depression. Am J Psychiatry 133:622–626, 1976

Kupfer DJ, Spiker DG, Coble PA, et al: Depression, EEG sleep, and clinical response. Compr Psychiatry 21:212–220, 1980

Kupfer DJ, Frank E, Perel JM, et al: Five-year outcome for maintenance therapies in recurrent depression. Arch Gen Psychiatry 49:769–773, 1992

Lavori PW, Keller MB, Klerman GL: Relapse in affective disorders: a reanalysis of the literature using life table methods. J Psychiatr Res 18:13–21, 1984

Lecrubier Y, Guelfi JD: Efficacy of reversible inhibitors of monoamine oxidase-A in various forms of depression. Acta Psychiatr Scand 360:18–23, 1990

Lee AS, Murray AM: The long term outcome of Maudsley depressives. Br J Psychiatry 153:741–751, 1988

Levitt AJ, Joffe RT, Kennedy SH: Bright light augmentation in antidepressant nonresponders. J Clin Psychiatry 52:336–337, 1991

Liebowitz MR, Fyer AJ, Gorman JM, et al: Phenelzine in social phobia. J Clin Psychopharmacol 6:93–98, 1986

Liebowitz MR, Quitkin FM, Stewart JW, et al: Antidepressant specificity in atypical depression. Arch Gen Psychiatry 45:129–137, 1988

Loomer HP, Saunders JC, Kline NS: Iproniazid, an amine oxidase inhibitor, as an example of a psychic energizer. Congressional Record, 1957, pp 1382–1390

Loomer HP, Saunders JC, Kline NS: A clinical and pharmacodynamic evaluation of iproniazid as a psychic energizer (Psychiatric Research Report No 8). Washington, DC, American Psychiatric Association, 1958, pp 129–141

Maas JW, Fawcett JA, Dekirmenjian H: Catecholamine metabolism, depressive illness, and drug response. Arch Gen Psychiatry 26:252–262, 1972

Maas JW, Kocsis JH, Bowden CL, et al: Pretreatment neurotransmitter metabolites and response to imipramine or amitriptyline treatment. Psychol Med 12:37–43, 1982

Mann JJ, Kapur S: The emergence of suicidal ideation and behavior during antidepressant pharmacotherapy. Arch Gen Psychiatry 48:1027–1033, 1991

Marcus MD, Wing RR, Ewing L, et al: A double blind, placebo-controlled trial of fluoxetine plus behavior modification in the treatment of obese binge-eaters and non-binge eaters. Am J Psychiatry 147:876–881, 1990

Marin D, Kocsis J, Frances A, et al: Desipramine for the treatment of "pure" dysthymia versus double depression. Am J Psychiatry 151:1079–1080, 1994

Mayeux R, Stern Y, Cote L, et al: Altered serotonin metabolism in depressed patients with Parkinson's disease. Neurology 34:642–646, 1984

McConnell JD, Wilson JDD: Impotence, in Harrison's Principles of Internal Medicine. Edited by Wilson JD, Braunwald E, Isselbagher KJ, et al. New York, McGraw-Hill, 1991, pp 296–299

McGrath PJ, Stewart JW, Nunes EV, et al: A double-blind crossover trial of imipramine and phenelzine for outpatients with treatment-refractory depression. Am J Psychiatry 150:118–123, 1993

McLeod WR, Carroll B, Davies B: Hypothalamic dysfunction and antidepressant drugs. BMJ 2:480–481, 1970

Mendels J, Ramsey TA, Dyson WL, et al: Lithium as an antidepressant. Arch Gen Psychiatry 36:845–846, 1979

Metz A, Shader RI: Combination of fluoxetine and pemoline in the treatment of major depressive disorder. Int Clin Psychopharmacol 6:93–96, 1991

Moller H, Berzewski H, Eckmann F, et al: Double-blind multicenter study of paroxetine and amitriptyline in depressed inpatients. Pharmacopsychiatry 26:75–78, 1993

Møller SE, Honore P, Larsen OB: Tryptophan and tyrosine ratios to neutral amino acids in endogenous depression: relation to antidepressant response to amitriptyline and lithium/L-tryptophan. J Affect Disord 5:67–79, 1983

Møller SE, Odum K, Kirk L, et al: Plasma tyrosine/neutral amino acid ratio correlated with clinical response to nortriptyline in endogenously depressed patients. J Affect Disord 9:223–229, 1985

Møller SE, de Beurs P, Timmerman L, et al: Plasma tryptophan and tyrosine ratios to competing amino acids in relation to antidepressant response to citalopram and maprotiline. Psychopharmacology (Berl) 88:96–110, 1986

Møller SE, Bech P, Bjerrum H, et al: Plasma ratio tryptophan/neutral amino acids in relation to clinical response to paroxetine and clomipramine in patients with major depression. J Affect Disord 18:59–66, 1990

Montgomery S, Djarv L: The antidepressant efficacy of citalopram. Int Clin Psychopharmacol 11S:29–33, 1996

Montgomery SA, Dufour H, Brion S, et al: The prophylactic efficacy of fluoxetine in unipolar depression. Br J Psychiatry 153 (suppl 3):69–76, 1988

Montgomery SA, Doogan DP, Burnside R: The influence of different relapse criteria on the assessment of long-term efficacy of sertraline. Int Clin Psychopharmacol 6 (suppl 2):37–46, 1991

Morganroth J, Goin JE: Quinidine-related mortality in the short-to-medium-term treatment of ventricular arrhythmias: a meta-analysis. Circulation 84:1977–1983, 1991

Murphy BEP, Wolkowitz OM: The pathophysiologic significance of hyperadrenocorticism: antiglucocorticoid strategies. Psychiatric Annals 23:682–690, 1993

Murphy BE, Dhar V, Ghadirian AM, et al: Response to steroid suppression in major depression resistant to antidepressant therapy. J Clin Psychopharmacol 11:121–126, 1991

Nagy LM, Morgan CA III, Southwick SM, et al: Open prospective trial of fluoxetine for posttraumatic stress disorder. J Clin Psychopharmacol 13:107–113, 1993

National Institutes of Health Consensus Development Panel on Depression in Late Life: Diagnosis and treatment of depression in late life (NIH consensus conference). JAMA 268:1018–1024, 1992

Nelson JC, Bowers MB: Delusional unipolar depression: description and drug response. Arch Gen Psychiatry 35:1321–1328, 1978

Nelson JC, Byck R: Rapid response to lithium in phenelzine non-responders. Br J Psychiatry 141:85–86, 1982

Nelson JC, Jatlow P, Quinlan DM, et al: Desipramine plasma concentration and antidepressant response. Arch Gen Psychiatry 39:1419–1422, 1982

Nelson JC, Mazure CM, Bowers MB, et al: A preliminary open study of the combination of fluoxetine and desipramine for rapid treatment of major depression. Arch Gen Psychiatry 48:303–307, 1991

Nemeroff CB, DeVane CL, Pollock BG: Newer antidepressants and the cytochrome P450 system. Am J Psychiatry 153:311–320, 1996

Neshkes RE, Jarvik LF: Affective disorders in the elderly. Annu Rev Med 38:445–456, 1987

Nierenberg AA, Price LH, Charney DS: After lithium augmentation: a retrospective follow-up of patients with antidepressant-refractory depression. J Affect Disord 18:167–175, 1990

Nierenberg AA, Keck PE Jr, Samson J, et al: Methodological considerations for the study of treatment-resistant depression, in Advances in Neuropsychiatry and Psychopharmacology, Vol 2: Refractory Depression. Edited by Amsterdam JD. New York, Raven, 1991, pp 1–12

Nolen WA, van de Putte JJ, Dijken WA, et al: Treatment strategy in depression, I: non-tricyclic and selective reuptake inhibitors in resistant depression: a double-blind partial crossover study on the effects of oxaprotiline and fluvoxamine. Acta Psychiatr Scand 78:668–675, 1988

Noyes R, Dempsey GM, Blum A, et al: Lithium treatment of depression. Compr Psychiatry 15:187–193, 1974

Ogura C, Okuma T, Uchida Y, et al: Combined thyroid (triiodothyronine)-tricyclic antidepressant treatment in depressive states. Folia Psychiatrica et Neurologica Japonica 28:179–186, 1974

Oppenheim G: Rapid mood cycling with estrogen: implications for therapy. J Clin Psychiatry 45:34–35, 1984

Overall JE, Hollister LE, Johnson M, et al: Nosology of depression and differential response to drugs. JAMA 195:946–948, 1966

Pande AC, Calarco MM, Grunhaus LJ: Combined MAOI-TCA treatment in refractory depression, in Advances in Neuropsychiatry and Psychopharmacology, Vol 2: Refractory Depression. Edited by Amsterdam JD. New York, Raven, 1991, pp 115–122

Paul SM, Extein I, Call HM, et al: Use of ECT with treatment-resistant depressed patients at the NIMH. Am J Psychiatry 134:486–489, 1981

Paykel ES: Depressive typologies and response to amitriptyline. Br J Psychiatry 120:147–156, 1972

Paykel ES: Predictors of treatment response, in Psychopharmacology of Affective Disorders. Edited by Paykel ES, Coppen A. Oxford, England, Oxford University Press, 1979, pp 193–220

Peck AW, Stern WC, Watkinson C: Incidence of seizures during treatment with tricyclic antidepressant drugs and bupropion. J Clin Psychiatry 44 (5, sec 2):197–201, 1983

Peet M: Induction of mania with selective serotonin re-uptake inhibitors and tricyclic antidepressants. Br J Psychiatry 164:549–550, 1994

Peselow ED, Fieve RR: Dexamethasone suppression test and response to antidepressants in depressed outpatients. N Engl J Med 307:1216–1217, 1982

Peselow ED, Loutin A, Wolkin A, et al: The dexamethasone suppression test and response to placebo. J Clin Psychopharmacol 6:286–291, 1986

Pfohl B, Stangl D, Zimmerman M: The implications of DSM-III personality disorders for patients with major depression. J Affect Disord 7:309–318, 1984

Post RM: Anticonvulsants as adjuncts or alternatives to lithium in refractory bipolar illness, in Advances in Neuropsychiatry and Psychopharmacology, Vol 2: Refractory Depression. Edited by Amsterdam JD. New York, Raven, 1991, pp 155–165

Post R, Weiss S: The neurobiology of treatment-resistant mood disorders, in Psychopharmacology: The Fourth Generation of Progress. Edited by Bloom F, Kupfer D. New York, Raven, 1995, pp 1605–1611

Power AC, Cowen PJ: Fluoxetine and suicidal behaviour: some clinical and theoretical aspects of a controversy. Br J Psychiatry 161:735–741, 1992

Prange AJ: Paroxysmal auricular tachycardia apparently resulting from combined thyroid-imipramine treatment. Am J Psychiatry 119:994–995, 1963

Prange AJ: Estrogen may well affect response to antidepressant. JAMA 219:143–144, 1972

Prange AJ, Wilson IC, Rabon AM, et al: Enhancement of imipramine antidepressant activity by thyroid hormone. Am J Psychiatry 126:457–469, 1969

Pratt GM, Brater DC, Harrell FE Jr, et al: Clinical and regulatory implications of the Cardiac Arrhythmia Suppression Trial. Am J Cardiol 65:103–105, 1990

Preskorn SH: Tricyclic antidepressants: the whys and hows of therapeutic drug monitoring. J Clin Psychiatry 50 (7, suppl):34–42, 1989

Preskorn SH: Should bupropion dosage be adjusted based upon therapeutic drug monitoring? Psychopharmacol Bull 27:637–643, 1991

Preskorn SH, Fast GA: Therapeutic drug monitoring for antidepressants: efficacy, safety, and cost effectiveness. J Clin Psychiatry 52 (6, suppl):23–33, 1991

Preskorn SH, Alderman J, Chung M, et al: Pharmacokinetics of desipramine coadministered with sertraline or fluoxetine. J Clin Psychopharmacol 14:90–98, 1994

Price LH, Gharney DS, Heninger GR: Efficacy of lithium-tranylcypromine treatment in refractory depression. Am J Psychiatry 142:619–623, 1985

Prien RF, Kupfer DJ: Continuation drug therapy for major depressive episodes: how long should it be maintained? Am J Psychiatry 143:18–23, 1986

Prien RF, Klett J, Caffey EM: Lithium carbonate and imipramine in prevention of affective episodes. Arch Gen Psychiatry 29:420–425, 1973

Quitkin FM, McGrath P, Liebowitz MR, et al: Monoamine oxidase inhibitors in bipolar endogenous depressives. J Clin Psychopharmacol 1:70–74, 1989

Quitkin FM, McGrath PJ, Stewart JW, et al: Atypical depression, panic attacks, and response to imipramine and phenelzine. Arch Gen Psychiatry 47:935–941, 1990

Quitkin FM, Harrison W, Stewart JW, et al: Response to phenelzine and imipramine in placebo nonresponders with atypical depression. Arch Gen Psychiatry 48:319–323, 1991

Raskin A, Crook TA: The endogenous-neurotic distinction as a predictor of response to antidepressant drugs. Psychol Med 6:59–70, 1976

Rawling DA, Fozzard HA: Effects of imipramine on cellular electrophysiological properties of cardiac Purkinje fibers. J Pharmacol Exp Ther 209:371–375, 1979

Razani J, White KL, White J, et al: The safety and efficacy of combined amitriptyline and tranylcypromine antidepressant treatment: a controlled trial. Arch Gen Psychiatry 40:657–661, 1983

Reynolds CF III, Frank E, Perel JM, et al: Combined pharmacotherapy and psychotherapy in the acute and continuation treatment of elderly patients with recurrent major depression: a preliminary report. Am J Psychiatry 149:1687–1692, 1992

Richelson E: Antidepressants: pharmacology and clinical use, in Treatments of Psychiatric Disorders: A Task Force Report of the American Psychiatric Association. Washington, DC, American Psychiatric Association, 1989, pp 1773–1786

Richelson E: Side effects of old and new generation antidepressants: a pharmacologic framework. J Clin Psychiatry 9:13–19, 1991

Richelson E, Nelson A: Antagonism by antidepressants of neurotransmitter receptors of normal human brain in vitro. J Pharmacol Exp Ther 230:94–102, 1984

Rickels K, Amsterdam J, Clary C, et al: The efficacy and safety of paroxetine compared with placebo in outpatients with major depression. J Clin Psychiatry 53 (suppl):30–32, 1992

Riesenman C: Antidepressant drug interactions and the cytochrome P450 system: a critical appraisal. Pharmacotherapy 15 (6, pt 2):84S–99S, 1995

Risch SC, Huey LY, Janowsky DS: Plasma levels of tricyclic antidepressants and clinical efficacy: review of the literature—parts I and II. J Clin Psychiatry 40:4–16, 58–69, 1979

Robinson DS, Roberts DL, Smith JM, et al: The safety profile of nefazodone. J Clin Psychiatry 57 (suppl 2):31–38, 1996

Roose SP, Palack GW, Glassman AH, et al: Cardiovascular effects of bupropion in depressed patients with heart disease. Am J Psychiatry 148:512–516, 1991

Roose S, Glassman A, Attia E, et al: Comparative efficacy of selective serotonin reuptake inhibitors and tricyclics in the treatment of melancholia. Am J Psychiatry 151: 1735–1739, 1994

Rosenbaum AH, Schatzberg AF, Maruta T, et al: MHPG as a predictor of antidepressant response to imipramine and maprotiline. Am J Psychiatry 137:1090–1092, 1980

Rosenbaum JF, Fava M, Falk WE, et al: The antidepressant potential of oral S-adenosyl-L-methionine. Acta Psychiatr Scand 81:432–436, 1990

Rosenstein D, Nelson J, Jacobs S: Seizures associated with antidepressants: a review. J Clin Psychiatry 54:289–299, 1993

Rosenthal J, Hemlock C, Hellerstein DJ, et al: A preliminary study of serotonergic antidepressants in treatment of dysthymia. Prog Neuropsychopharmacol Biol Psychiatry 16:933–941, 1992

Rush AJ: Cognitive therapy of depression: rationale, techniques and efficacy. Psychiatr Clin North Am 6:105–127, 1983

Sabelli HC, Fawcett J, Javaid JJ, et al: The methylphenidate test for differentiating desipramine responsive from nortriptyline responsive depression. Am J Psychiatry 140:212–214, 1983

Sackeim HA, Prudic J, Devanand DP, et al: The impact of medication resistance and continuation pharmacotherapy on relapse following response to electroconvulsive therapy in major depression. J Clin Psychopharmacol 10:96–104, 1990

Salzman C: Pharmacologic treatment of depression in the elderly. J Clin Psychiatry 54 (2, suppl):23–28, 1993

Satel S, Nelson J: Stimulants in the treatment of depression: a critical overview. J Clin Psychiatry 50:241–249, 1989

Schatzberg AF, Orsulak PJ, Rosenbaum AH, et al: Toward a biochemical classification of depressive disorders, IV: pretreatment urinary MHPG levels as predictors of antidepressant response to imipramine. Communications in Psychopharmacology 4:441–445, 1980

Schatzberg AF, Rosenbaum AH, Orsulak PJ: Toward a biochemical classification of depressive disorders, III: pretreatment urinary MHPG levels as predictors of response to treatment with maprotiline. Psychopharmacology (Berl) 75:34–38, 1981

Schmauss M, Kapfhammer HP, Meyer P, et al: Combined MAO-inhibitor and tri-(tetra) cyclic antidepressant treatment in therapy resistant depression. Prog Neuropsychopharmacol Biol Psychiatry 12:523–532, 1988

Schwartz G, Halaris A, Baxter L: Normal thyroid function in desipramine nonresponders compared to responders by the addition of L-tri-iodothyronine. Am J Psychiatry 141:1614–1616, 1984

Segraves RT: Sexual dysfunction complicating the treatment of depression. J Clin Psychiatry 10:75–83, 1992

Selzer A, Wray HW: Quinidine syncope: paroxysmal ventricular fibrillations occurring during treatment of chronic atrial arrhythmias. Circulation 30:17–26, 1964

Settle EC Jr: Antidepressant side effects: issues and options. J Clin Psychiatry 10:48–61, 1992

Shapira B, Oppenheim G, Zohar J, et al: Lack of efficacy of estrogen supplementation to imipramine in resistant female depressives. Biol Psychiatry 20:576–579, 1985

Shawcross CR, Tyrer P: Influence of personality on response to monoamine oxidase inhibitors and tricyclic antidepressants. J Psychiatr Res 19:557–562, 1985

Sheehan DV, Ballenger J, Jacobsen G: Treatment of endogenous anxiety with phobic, hysterical and hypochondriacal symptoms. Arch Gen Psychiatry 40:125–138, 1983a

Sheehan DV, Davidson J, Manschreck T, et al: Lack of efficacy of a new antidepressant (bupropion) in the treatment of panic disorder with phobias. J Clin Pharmacol 3:28–31, 1983b

Sherwin BB: Estrogen and refractory depression, in Advances in Neuropsychiatry and Psychopharmacology, Vol 2: Refractory Depression. Edited by Amsterdam JD. New York, Raven, 1991, pp 209–218

Shopsin B: Bupropion's prophylactic efficacy in bipolar affective illness. J Clin Psychiatry 44 (5, sec 2):163–169, 1983

Simpson GM, Lee HL, Cuche Z, et al: Two doses of imipramine in hospitalized endogenous and neurotic depressions. Arch Gen Psychiatry 33:1093–1102, 1976

Spar JA, La Rue A: Acute response to methylphenidate as a predictor of outcome of treatment with TCAs in the elderly. J Clin Psychiatry 46:466–469, 1985

Spiker DG, Edwards D, Hanin I, et al: Urinary MHPG and clinical response to amitriptyline in depressed patients. Am J Psychiatry 137:1183–1187, 1980

Spiker DG, Weiss JC, Dealy RS, et al: The pharmacological treatment of delusional depression. Am J Psychiatry 142:430–436, 1985

Stein G, Bernadt M: Lithium augmentation therapy in tricyclic-resistant depression: a controlled trial using lithium in low and normal doses. Br J Psychiatry 162:634–640, 1993

Stoll AL, Mayer PV, Kolbrener M, et al: Antidepressant-associated mania: a controlled comparison with spontaneous mania. Am J Psychiatry 151:1642–1645, 1994

Stoll AL, Srinavasan SP, Diamond L, et al: Methylphenidate augmentation of serotonin selective reuptake inhibitors: a case series. J Clin Psychiatry 75:73–76, 1996

Stuppaeck C, Geretsegger C, Whitworth A, et al: A multicenter double-blind trial of paroxetine versus amitriptyline in depressed inpatients. J Clin Psychopharmacol 14:241–246, 1994

Svendsen K, Christensen PDG: Duration of REM sleep latency as predictor of effect of antidepressant therapy. Acta Psychiatr Scand 64:238–243, 1981

Targum SD: Persistent neuroendocrine dysregulation in major depressive disorder: a marker for early relapse. Biol Psychiatry 19:305–318, 1984

Teicher MH, Glod C, Cole JO: Emergence of intense suicidal preoccupation during fluoxetine treatment. Am J Psychiatry 147:207–210, 1990

Thase ME, Kupfer DJ, Jarret DB: Treatment of imipramine-resistant recurrent depression, I: an open clinical trial of adjunctive L-triiodothyronine. J Clin Psychiatry 50:385–388, 1989

Thase ME, Mallinger AD, McKnight D, et al: Treatment of imipramine-resistant recurrent depression, IV: a double-blind crossover study of tranylcypromine for anergic bipolar depression. Am J Psychiatry 149:195–198, 1992

Thase M, Fava M, Halbreich U, et al: A placebo-controlled, randomized clinical trial comparing sertraline and imipramine for the treatment of dysthymia. Arch Gen Psychiatry 53:777–784, 1996

Trimble MR: Nonmonoamine oxidase inhibitor antidepressants and epilepsy: a review. Epilepsia 19:241–250, 1978

Tsutsui S, Yamazaki Y, Namba T, et al: Combined therapy of T_3 and antidepressants in depression. J Int Med Res 7:138–146, 1979

Tyrer P, Murphy S: Efficacy of combined antidepressant therapy in resistant neurotic disorder. Br J Psychiatry 156:115–118, 1990

van Kammen DP, Murphy DL: Prediction of imipramine antidepressant response by a one day d-amphetamine trial. Am J Psychiatry 135:1179–1184, 1978

VanPraag HM: New evidence of serotonin deficient depressions. Neuropsychobiology 3:56–63, 1977

Walsh BT, Stewart JW, Roose SP, et al: Treatment of bulimia with phenelzine: a double-blind, placebo-controlled study. Arch Gen Psychiatry 41:1105–1109, 1984

Weilburg JB, Rosenbaum JF, Biederman J, et al: Fluoxetine added to non-MAOI antidepressants converts nonresponders to responders: a preliminary report. J Clin Psychiatry 50:447–449, 1989

Weld FM, Bigger JT Jr: Electrophysiological effects of imipramine on ovine cardiac Purkinje and ventricular muscle fibers. Circ Res 46:167–175, 1980

Wharton RN, Perel JM, Dayton PG, et al: A potential clinical use for methylphenidate (Ritalin) with tricyclic antidepressants. Am J Psychiatry 127:1619–1625, 1971

White K, Simpson G: Combined MAOI-tricyclic antidepressant treatment: a reevaluation. J Clin Psychopharmacol 1:264–282, 1981

Wilde M, Plosker G, Benfield P: Fluvoxamine: an updated review of its pharmacology, and therapeutic use in depressive illness. Drugs 46:895–924, 1993

Wolkowitz OM, Reus VI, Manfredi F, et al: Ketoconazole administration in hypercortisolemic depression. Am J Psychiatry 150:810–812, 1993

Wolkowitz OM, Reus VI, Vinogradov S, et al: Antiglucocorticoids in depression and schizophrenia. Program and Abstracts on New Research in Summary Form: the 149th Annual Meeting of the American Psychiatric Association, New York City, May 4–9, 1996, p 152

Wright D, Galloway L, Kim J, et al: Bupropion in the long-term treatment of cyclic mood disorders: mood stabilizing effects. J Clin Psychiatry 46:22–25, 1985

Zall H: Lithium carbonate and isocarboxazid: an effective drug approach in severe depressions. Am J Psychiatry 127:136–139, 1971

THIRTY-FIVE

Treatment of Bipolar Disorder

Charles L. Bowden, M.D.

RATIONALE FOR TREATMENT

Bipolar disorder is unique among psychiatric diseases in the multiple factors associated with it that influence treatment strategies. It is chronic, recurrent, severely impairing, and usually present from adolescence or early adulthood, thus spanning the most vocationally productive years and childbearing years. Many of the treatments for bipolar disorder have established efficacy and provide not only symptomatic control but also excellent social and vocational function. These benefits are not achieved in most cases simply because of complexities of the disease and its treatments. The small number of comparative treatment studies further complicates selection of an optimal treatment plan at a particular point in the illness course. The subsyndromal variations of bipolar disorder—based on both symptom constellation and illness course—have major differences in prognosis and require different treatment strategies.

Bipolar disorder has been difficult to study because of the wide fluctuations in mood state intrinsic to the disease, the numerous factors that can confound treatment effects, and the impaired insight and psychotic function of patients during severe points of illness. I address these factors in this chapter, with the intent of providing guidelines both for overall treatment strategy and for handling details and special problems that arise on an individual basis.

SYMPTOMATIC AND ILLNESS COURSE FEATURES AFFECTING PHARMACOTHERAPY

Acute Mania and Hypomania

Although certain epidemiological differences appear to distinguish mania from hypomania, efficacy of treatments has not appeared to differ (Davis 1976). Also, many of the undesirable sequelae or concomitants of the illness (e.g., suicide risk, substance abuse) appear to be equivalent in the two groups (Cooke et al. 1995). Thus, although most studies of treatments have been with bipolar I patients, the recommendations here are intended for both bipolar I and II groups, with the caveat that experimental data from bipolar II patients are limited. A major difference between mania and hypomania affecting treatment is that hypomania is much more likely to escape detection by the psychiatrist and to be rationalized as healthy function by the patient. Both factors thus increase the possibility of incorrect diagnosis and of poor compliance with treatment.

A small percentage of patients have only manic or hypomanic episodes. Although treatment has been studied infrequently in these patients, standard antimanic regimens (for both acute and maintenance treatment) are generally instituted, without use of antidepressant medication.

Acute Depression

The current criteria for diagnosis of depression in bipolar disorder require the presence of a major depressive episode. This is in part based on evidence that the symptom profile and severity of the depression in bipolar disorder are relatively similar to those of major depression (Katz et al. 1982). This similarity poses problems that may result in incorrect diagnosis and, therefore, inappropriate treatment. Depressive episodes in bipolar patients are generally shorter than those in patients with major depression. This is most evident in rapid-cycling patients. The brevity of a hypomanic or depressive episode may result in failure to recognize that a patient has bipolar disorder or is experiencing a depressive episode.

The frequency of certain symptoms differs in bipolar patients compared with unipolar patients. Hypersomnia and psychomotor retardation are more common in bipolar depression, and anxiety and agitation are less common (Beigel and Murphy 1971; Katz et al. 1982). As many as 25% of bipolar patients may have three or four depressive episodes before their first manic episode (Angst et al. 1978). If the clinician does not recognize a bipolar pattern, then prolonged treatment of the patient with antidepressants, with the attendant risks of precipitating manic episodes and increasing cycle frequency, may result. Attention to several factors during assessment may reduce such erroneous diagnostic classification. The younger the patient at the first episode of depression, the greater the likelihood of an underlying bipolar disorder (Geller et al. 1994; Lewinsohn et al. 1995). The more frequent and the greater the number of depressive episodes, the greater the likelihood of bipolar disorder (Goodwin and Jamison 1990). A high frequency of either bipolar depression or major depression in a patient's relatives is positively associated with the likelihood that the patient's mood disorder is bipolar.

Severity of Illness

Severity of bipolar episodes varies both qualitatively and quantitatively. Cyclothymia is thought by most authorities to be linked to (or a mild form of) bipolar disorder, although the question has been little studied (Akiskal 1995). A decision to try medications indicated for bipolar disorder is thus largely made on the plausible basis that the patient senses that he or she has substantial dysfunction from the mood instability.

Approximately one-half of all manic patients will have psychotic symptoms. Patients with psychotic features have responded less well to lithium than patients without psychosis in some, but not all, studies (Goodwin and Jami-

son 1990). Psychotic symptomatology was reduced more in divalproex-treated than in lithium-treated patients in a large, well-designed study (Bowden et al. 1994). Schizoaffective patients refractory to standard antimanic therapies have been reported to respond well to clozapine (Suppes et al. 1992).

Patients who move from a depressive episode directly to a manic episode respond less well to standard lithium therapy than do those who characteristically move from depression to euthymia (Grof et al. 1987).

Comorbid Symptomatology

Bipolar disorder is strongly associated with several other disorders: migraine, obsessive-compulsive disorder (OCD), panic disorder, and attention-deficit/hyperactivity disorder (ADHD). Although some of this association may be a function of overlapping criteria (e.g., ADHD), much appears to indicate some shared etiopathology. The presence of these comorbid conditions does have treatment implications. Valproate is beneficial for migraine (for which it is approved by the U.S. Food and Drug Administration [FDA] for prophylaxis) and possibly for panic attacks and OCD (Deltito 1994; Herridge and Pope 1985; Lum et al. 1990; Primeau et al. 1990). Valproate also appears to be effective in mania comorbid with substance abuse, but this finding is only based on an open study (Brady et al. 1995). Therefore, the presence of such additional problems in a patient with bipolar disorder would predispose to initiation of treatment with valproate.

Open studies suggest that ADHD is responsive to bupropion (Sachs et al. 1994). Concurrent evidence of ADHD would therefore predispose to selection of bupropion for treatment of a depressive episode. Because of the lack of conclusive studies on many of these points, these recommendations are tentative, but the principle of assessing for additional factors linked to likelihood of response is a sound one.

Subsyndromal Variations

Mixed mania. Since 1980, strong evidence has been published for syndromal variations that have important treatment implications. Mixed or depressive manic patients respond less well to both acute and chronic treatment with lithium than do patients with pure or elated mania (Bowden 1995; Keller et al. 1986; Swann et al. 1997). Suggestive evidence of relatively favorable response to carbamazepine needs to be followed by randomized, blinded studies (Post et al. 1987). Additional features that may aid in identifying patients with mixed mania include older age at first onset of illness, fewer episodes per unit of time, a positive dexamethasone suppression test, and no family history of mood disorder.

Elated or pure mania. Patients whose symptoms are principally along the behavioral dimensions of elevated mood, elation, grandiosity, increased activity, and reduced need for sleep constitute the group that responds best to acute treatment with lithium (Bowden et al. 1994; Keller et al. 1986; Swann et al. 1986). Whether this advantage holds for maintenance-phase outcome is not well established. Additional features that may help to identify these patients include early first onset of illness and positive family history for mood disorders.

Rapid cycling. Patients with a greater frequency of episodes have quite low response rates to lithium during both acute and prophylactic treatment (Dunner and Fieve 1974; Kukopulos et al. 1983). *Rapid cycling* is defined as four or more episodes of any combination of depression and mania during a 12-month period. A smaller group of patients has much more frequent cycles, even within a day (Frye et al. 1996; Kramlinger and Post 1995). Drug-induced precipitation of mania in these patients appears to presage more frequent cycling (Altshuler et al. 1995; Keller et al. 1992). Much remains to be clarified about this group of patients. For example, whether most rapid cycling occurs over the full course of illness or, conversely, only for limited periods, perhaps principally secondary to exposure to mood-destabilizing agents, is unclear.

Comorbid Substance Abuse

Patients with concurrent substance abuse (including alcoholism) respond less well to lithium than do patients without substance abuse but may respond well to valproate (Brady et al. 1995). The substance abuse must be eliminated through direct intervention. Concurrent attention to the bipolar illness is warranted. Some substance abuse appears to be an effort either to extend manic symptoms or to alleviate dysphoric symptoms of the disorder, and it may resolve with alleviation of the manic or depressive episode. Because approximately one-half of both bipolar I and II patients have concurrent substance abuse, close attention to this problem during evaluation or at times of breakthrough episodes is important (Regier et al. 1988).

Secondary Bipolar Disorders

A wide range of medical disorders results in disturbance of mood, either concurrently or as sequelae of the medical disorder. Most late-onset bipolar disorders are in this category. When possible, treatment should concurrently be aimed at the primary disorder. Patients with secondary bipolar disorders tend to have mixed symptomatology and more manic than depressed episodes. Lithium is relatively ineffective in treatment of these conditions. Uncontrolled studies suggest more favorable responses with carbamazepine or valproate (D. Kahn et al. 1988; Tohen et al. 1990).

PHARMACOTHERAPIES

General Principles of Drug Treatment

Mood charting. Charting of mood, also known as *life charting*, has a special role in bipolar disorder management. Because of the fluctuating mood states and varying symptom presentations requiring changing medication regimens, as well as the nearly uniform long-term treatment required, it can be difficult to glean drug treatment–clinical response relationships from the traditional medical record with progress notes. Charting offers a graphically succinct means of capturing several domains of treatment and response on one sheet.

Many of the benefits of charting directly affect drug therapy. Evidence of partial response patterns, antidepressant-induced rapid cycling, gradual loss of efficacy, and the effectiveness of nondrug therapies such as bright lights are among the potential benefits of this approach. Charting is relatively labor intensive and requires regular updating. Patients' active participation in developing a life chart is desirable (Post et al. 1988). An example of a clinician-rated chart is shown in Figure 35–1. The ability of the form to capture in a temporally meaningful way stressors, illness episodes, and treatment interventions is evident.

Optimizing sleep. Benzodiazepines often relieve insomnia and related agitation and restlessness. Their adjunctive use is particularly important early in treatment, before the mood stabilizer becomes effective, and as needed to normalize sleep during maintenance treatment. Although standard doses of any benzodiazepine may be helpful, two drugs warrant special consideration. Lorazepam has the advantage of parenteral administration to the patient unable or unwilling to take oral medication. Clonazepam has a long duration of action, thus reducing the need for frequent dosing and producing consistent sedation both at night and (if needed) during the day. Additionally, clonazepam (one of a small number of drugs that is metabolized by nitrogen reduction) is not pharmacoki-

poor judgment) that are elevated in mania but not specific thereto were less responsive to either drug.

The quality and scope of double-blind, placebo-controlled studies of valproate effectiveness in acute mania are better than those for lithium. Two placebo-controlled studies have reported highly clinically significant clinical superiority of divalproex over placebo (Bowden et al. 1994; Pope et al. 1991). The divalproex form has better gastrointestinal tolerability than valproic acid (Wilder et al. 1983). Divalproex is as effective in acute treatment of patients with mixed mania as in those with pure mania and those with rapid cycling (Bowden et al. 1994; Calabrese and Delucchi 1990).

Divalproex can be administered in a loading dose of 20–30 mg/kg, which results in a partial response within 1–3 days (Keck et al. 1993). The adverse effects of divalproex most likely to occur during acute treatment include gastrointestinal irritation, tremor, sedation, and cognitive dulling. A serum level between 45 and 110 μg/mL provides a relatively wide range for therapeutically effective yet well tolerated treatment (Bowden et al. 1996).

Carbamazepine.   As was the case with divalproex, the effectiveness of carbamazepine in mania was initially observed serendipitously by practicing psychiatrists. This fact has contributed to the unusual way in which both drugs have been studied. In particular, no industry-sponsored placebo-controlled studies have been completed with carbamazepine. The one placebo-controlled study was a crossover design with 19 patients that did not allow comparison of relative efficacy. Nevertheless, more than a dozen controlled studies indicate that carbamazepine is effective in acute mania (Post et al. 1988). Comparisons with lithium indicate lesser efficacy for carbamazepine. Of the two parallel-group comparisons with lithium, one found a lower response rate with carbamazepine than with lithium (Lerer et al. 1987). The other, composed of a relatively treatment-refractory sample, reported only a 33% response rate for both drugs (Small et al. 1991). Comparisons with neuroleptics have shown equivalent response rates, whereas lithium was generally superior to neuroleptics in controlled trials (Goodwin and Jamison 1990). Carbamazepine was more effective in treatment of patients with mixed mania than in those with pure mania. It is less effective in rapid-cycling than in non-rapid-cycling patients (Denicoff et al. 1994; Okuma et al. 1990).

Carbamazepine requires cautious initial administration. A starting dose of 200 mg twice a day with a gradual increase to levels greater than 4 μg/mL will often prevent or reduce sedation, cognitive dulling, diplopia, gastrointes-

tinal irritability, and psychomotor slowing, which otherwise are relatively common early adverse effects. Carbamazepine causes induction of the 3A4 isoform of the P450 family of oxidative enzymes. This induction is generally clinically identifiable at about the fourth to eighth week of treatment. This complicates management, requiring relatively frequent plasma level measurement and dosage increases to return to the range at which initial response occurred. Similarly, other medications metabolized through 3A4 will likely require an increased dosage. In the case of several of these drugs (oral contraceptives, bupropion, alprazolam, nefazodone), concurrent use is inadvisable because of the marked lowering of plasma levels (Ketter et al. 1995). Rashes, which lead to discontinuation in 10%–15% of patients, can include severe hemorrhagic responses (e.g., Stevens-Johnson syndrome). Regular monitoring of white blood cell and platelet count is important, although the relatively common 20%–30% reduction in granulocyte count and platelet count warrants more frequent monitoring rather than discontinuation of the medication.

No fixed-dose-type studies that would be needed to determine whether plasma level–response relationships exist have been conducted with carbamazepine. The available data suggest only approximate relationships of plasma concentration to response. Therefore, dosage should be increased as tolerated until a response occurs or a carbamazepine concentration of 12 μg/mL is achieved. Despite the lack of strong plasma level–response guidelines, plasma concentration monitoring every 2–3 months is still warranted. This ensures that the concentration is not moving upward or downward despite a stable dosage, serves as a check on compliance, and establishes that the patient is within the concentration range at which a positive initial response occurred.

Verapamil.   In a few patients, mania has been reported to respond to verapamil (Dubovsky et al. 1986). These mixed results are sufficiently encouraging to warrant further study of calcium channel blockers. A recent single-blind, randomized study of acute mania reported that lithium was superior to verapamil, with response rates generally low in the latter group (Walton et al. 1995). Verapamil would seem to be an unlikely candidate because of its relatively low lipophilicity. Several newer calcium channel blockers (nimodipine and nifedipine) have higher lipid solubility (Brunet et al. 1990). Some authorities believe verapamil may be useful in patients who benefited from lithium but tolerated it poorly.

Clonidine has been found to be no better than placebo in a small, well-designed, double-blind, parallel-group study (Janicak et al. 1989).

Acute Depression

Direct experimental data about drug efficacy in bipolar depression are inadequate. Only one double-blind, randomized, parallel-group, placebo-controlled study of bipolar patients has been published (Cohn et al. 1989). Consequently, recommendations for treatment of bipolar depression are based largely on data that are either outdated, derived from research on a different disease (i.e., major depression), or both. The response rate of bipolar and unipolar depression to TCAs appears to be similar (Koslow et al. 1983). Bipolar depression specifically characterized by anergia is more responsive to monoamine oxidase inhibitors (MAOIs) than to TCAs (Himmelhoch et al. 1991). More than half of bipolar depressed patients who do not respond to imipramine subsequently respond to tranylcypromine. Initial dosages and patterns of dosage escalation and dosage ranges do not differ from those for major depression. With the exception of the risks of mood destabilization (expressed as either hypomania, rapid cycling, or both), the side-effect profile does not differ.

Because selective serotonin reuptake inhibitors (SSRIs) have a favorable side-effect profile, they are promising agents for bipolar depression. Positive results have been reported with fluoxetine and paroxetine. Fluoxetine was superior to placebo and nonsignificantly better than imipramine in one placebo-controlled study (Cohn et al. 1989). The patients treated with fluoxetine had fewer side effects than those treated with imipramine. Bupropion has also been reported to be more effective than a TCA with a lower rate of induction of mania in a randomized, blinded small open study (Shopsin 1983).

Results of a recent consensus survey of experts favored bupropion and SSRIs as initial treatment for bipolar depressive episodes (Frances et al. 1996). Given the greater likelihood of cognitive impairment, autonomic overstimulation, hypotension, sedation, and weight gain, as well as the potential lethality in suicide attempts, associated with all TCAs, their use should generally be limited to secondary choices or to patients who have benefited from and tolerated them well in previous depressive episodes. Among the SSRIs, the long half-life of fluoxetine is a potential disadvantage, because plasma levels would not decline by 50% for approximately 1 month after discontinuing the drug if the patient developed hypomania.

If the patient is unresponsive, is intolerant, or has a medical contraindication to these agents, electroconvulsive therapy (ECT) may be implemented. ECT has been reported to be superior to TCAs in bipolar depression, although the studies have substantial methodological limitations (Goodwin and Jamison 1990). A recent open trial suggested that lamotrigine, an approved antiepileptic drug, may be effective in bipolar depressive episodes.

Several studies—only one of which was prospective and controlled—indicated that all of the above classes of antidepressants can either precipitate manic or (more often) hypomanic episodes or destabilize the course of illness, which results in a rapid-cycling course (Frye et al. 1996; Prien et al. 1984; Wehr and Goodwin 1987). The frequency of development of drug-induced mania is not established, although studies suggest that it may occur in approximately 30% of patients with bipolar disorder (Frye et al. 1996). The few studies that have not reported this adverse effect have tended to exclude the very subjects who would be at risk for mood destabilization (Kupfer et al. 1988; Lewis and Winokur 1982). Furthermore, concurrent lithium does not consistently prevent the development of manic episodes (Quitkin et al. 1981). Based on this increasingly strong evidence for mood disturbance from antidepressants, the recommendation for use of antidepressants in bipolar disorder has changed to that of limiting them to administration during depressive episodes. Thus, once the patient is free of the symptoms of depression, the dose should be tapered over a period of several weeks and then discontinued. A small percentage of patients with bipolar disorder (mostly women) will have a preponderance of depressive rather than manic episodes. These episodes may necessitate maintenance use of an antidepressant.

Mood-stabilizing agents also have been tried for treatment of acute bipolar depression. Although most studies of lithium have shown that it is superior to placebo or equivalent to TCAs, methodological problems limit generalizability. Most of these studies included unipolar patients, lacked placebo control subjects, or both (Worrall et al. 1979). The one study that compared lithium, imipramine, and placebo in patients with bipolar depression found that both lithium and imipramine were superior to placebo, and imipramine was somewhat more effective than lithium (Fieve et al. 1968). In addition, reduction in depressive symptoms in patients treated with lithium often was not evident for 3–4 weeks.

Prophylactic studies uniformly indicate that lithium is much more effective in reducing the frequency of manic relapses than in reducing the frequency of depressive relapses. Thus, the use of lithium to treat acute depressive episodes has little current support. Uncontrolled studies with carbamazepine and valproate suggest that each is less effective in relieving depression than mania (Calabrese and Delucchi 1990; Post et al. 1989).

Maintenance Treatment

Although authorities debate the relative merits of mandatory maintenance treatment of newly diagnosed bipolar disorder, this is warranted in the large majority of cases. Bipolar disorder is in nearly all instances recurrent and chronic, with no tendency for the patient to mature out of the disease. Single episodes of mania are rare. Furthermore, the risks of not treating prophylactically include the disease's suicide rate of approximately 15%, the strong likelihood of recurrent episodes, and the serious social and vocational morbidity associated with the illness.

Post et al. (1992) presented suggestive evidence that discontinuation of lithium may lead to drug-induced treatment refractoriness, in which previously effective treatments become ineffective on readministration.

Exceptions to this recommendation for maintenance treatment include the patient in whom toxic precipitants of a manic episode have confounded the diagnostic picture (i.e., what appears as mania may represent a toxic psychosis rather than a first bipolar episode). A person whose mania spontaneously remits after a first, brief, apparent manic episode would not warrant initiation of maintenance treatment.

A recent, large, prospective study of maintenance treatment of bipolar disorder found that divalproex and lithium were associated with only modest advantage over placebo among patients with relatively mild illness severity. The result suggests that educational support and structured psychosocial support may be beneficial, at least for periods up to 1 year, among relatively mildly ill patients. Conversely, the urgency of prophylactic pharmacological treatment for patients with more active illness is underscored by the results (C. L. Bowden, J. R. Calabrese, S. L. McElroy, L. Gyulai, A. Wassef, F. Petty, H. G. Pope Jr, J. C.-Y. Chou, P. E. Keck Jr, L. J. Rhodes, A. C. Swann, R. M. A. Hirschfeld, P. J. Wozniak: "Randomized, Placebo-Controlled Trial of Divalproex Versus Lithium in Maintenance Therapy of Bipolar Disorder," manuscript in preparation, 1998). Further analyses of this and similar studies may warrant some revision in the recommendation for maintenance treatment, with the urgency of such treatment increased for patients with more active illness but assessed more on a case-by-case basis for patients with few and mild episodes.

Lithium.   Early maintenance-phase studies of lithium's superiority over placebo were substantially more conclusive for maintenance treatment than for acute treatment, with early studies showing an approximate 2:1 superiority of lithium over placebo (Baastrup et al. 1970; Davis

1976). Lithium discontinuation is followed by a high rate of relapse, with most new episodes being of manic rather than depressed type (Suppes et al. 1992).

Recent studies indicate that a substantial number of patients have inadequate long-term responses to lithium therapy. A naturalistic follow-up of outpatients with bipolar disorder found that the outcome was no better for patients given lithium maintenance therapy than for those taking no medication (Goldberg et al. 1995; Harrow et al. 1990). Even among patients with an initial successful response to lithium for 2 years, only about half continued to have an unequivocally good response in subsequent years (Maj et al. 1989).

Part of the poor response over time may be related to inadequate dosing. Gelenberg and colleagues (1989) found that relapse rates were higher among patients with plasma levels maintained at 0.4–0.6 mEq/L than among patients with plasma levels maintained at 0.8–1.0 mEq/L. The difference in relapse rates was only for manic episodes—suggesting, as do most studies, that lithium's prophylactic benefits are largely for new manic or hypomanic episodes. Additionally, the differences held only for patients with one or two prior episodes and thus cannot be generalized to patients with frequent episodes (Gelenberg et al. 1989).

The dosage of lithium needed to maintain a desired serum level is generally somewhat lower during maintenance treatment than during an acute manic episode (Vahip et al. 1995). Lithium's side effects are much more problematic during maintenance therapy than during acute therapy. Additional problems unlikely to occur during acute treatment include weight gain, acne, hypothyroidism, polydipsia, and polyuria. The group of side effects most likely to cause poor compliance or discontinuation of lithium are those that affect the central nervous system. These include impaired cognition, impaired short-term memory, poor coordination, muscular weakness, and lethargy (Jamison et al. 1979). Thyroid function should be assessed approximately every 6 months because of the high frequency of hypothyroidism during lithium treatment and the potential for hypothyroidism to then compromise the patient's clinical response (Citrome 1995).

The combination of a relatively low percentage of patients with good long-term outcomes, the frequency and functional severity of side effects, and lithium's very narrow therapeutic index has stimulated studies of alternative mood stabilizers.

Valproate.   A recent randomized, open comparison of valproate and lithium for an 18-month period reported good efficacy for both drugs, with somewhat more favorable results among valproate-treated patients (Lambert and Venaud 1995). An additional randomized, double-blind study of bipolar I patients treated for 1 year with divalproex, lithium, or placebo recently has been completed. Divalproex was somewhat more effective than lithium in time to relapse in duration in maintenance treatment. In fewer divalproex-treated than placebo-treated patients, treatment was prematurely terminated for mania or depression. Patients whose acute mania was treated with divalproex and who received divalproex during the maintenance phase also had better outcomes than those who received lithium or placebo. Divalproex was better tolerated than lithium (C. L. Bowden, J. R. Calabrese, S. L. McElroy, L. Gyulai, A. Wassef, F. Petty, H. G. Pope Jr, J. C.-Y. Chou, P. E. Keck Jr, L. J. Rhodes, A. C. Swann, R. M. A. Hirschfeld, P. J. Wozniak, "Randomized, Placebo-Controlled Trial of Divalproex Versus Lithium in Maintenance Therapy of Bipolar Disorder," manuscript in preparation, 1998). In both of these recent studies, valproate was better tolerated than lithium. Among numerous open trials of valproate, the best conceived and executed of these found that prophylactic effectiveness was high for patients who entered the study during a pure or mixed manic episode and was good for patients with rapid cycling. Patients who entered the study during a depressive episode fared much less well (Calabrese and Delucchi 1990).

Valproate's dosage and plasma levels appear to be the same for maintenance treatment as those used for acute treatment. As with lithium, additional side effects must be considered. Transient hair loss may occur after several weeks of therapy. Many authorities believe that selenium and zinc may provide some protection against hair loss. Increased appetite and weight gain may occur, in what is probably a dose-dependent response. Although cognitive dulling may occur, it appears to be dose related and generally manageable by adjustment of timing of valproate dosage or reduction of dosage. Single daily dosing of divalproex has been well tolerated and as effective as divided-dose regimens in a recent study (C. A. Masi, L. J. Rhodes, C. L. Bowden, "Changing Divalproex Dosing to Once Daily—Can Patients Tolerate It and Is It Still Effective?," unpublished data, December 1996). Although increased hepatic enzymes have been reported, the double-blind study of divalproex sodium in the treatment of acute mania did not indicate any trends for increased hepatic enzymes (Bowden et al. 1994).

Carbamazepine. Carbamazepine also has been inadequately studied in maintenance-phase treatment. Lusznat and colleagues (1988) found no significant differences between lithium and carbamazepine among patients treated for up to a year, although a larger percentage of carbamazepine-treated patients relapsed during treatment. Small and colleagues (1991) reported a trend favoring lithium over carbamazepine in the long-term maintenance-phase treatment of initially hospitalized, treatment-refractory manic patients. Carbamazepine was inferior to lithium in a random assignment study without concomitant medication (Lerer et al. 1987). Another small study found that carbamazepine was superior to placebo; however, nearly all patients received supplemental neuroleptics (Goncalves and Stoll 1985). This and the Lerer study suggest (albeit without much data) that antipsychotic medication may be needed when carbamazepine is used.

Retrospective analyses suggest that at least half of bipolar patients who initially respond to carbamazepine will relapse over a 3- to 4-year period (Frankenburg et al. 1988; Post et al. 1990). Although these results are not encouraging, they should not be viewed pessimistically in the light of similar long-term results reported from the analogous studies of lithium summarized earlier in this chapter. Definitive studies require an experimental design and prospective, randomized, double-blind, and generally placebo-controlled procedures, the sum of which is difficult to execute in patients with bipolar disorder.

Dosing approaches for carbamazepine require some modification during months 2–6 of treatment. Sometime during this period, most patients undergo hepatic enzyme induction, thus requiring a consequent increase in carbamazepine dose to restore the plasma level that was initially effective. In addition to the acute-phase side effects, several additional side effects require monitoring during maintenance-phase treatment. Hematological and hepatic function should be monitored. Hyponatremia may be clinically significant, particularly in older patients. Carbamazepine lowers not only its own levels but also those of all oxidatively metabolized drugs (Jann et al. 1985; E. M. Kahn et al. 1990). Careful inquiry as to continued efficacy of such other drugs and use of drug-level monitoring (when available) will ward off most problems of this type.

Selection of a Mood Stabilizer

As a result of recent randomized studies comparing divalproex and lithium, the rationale for selection of a primary mood-stabilizing agent has changed. Lithium appears to be most useful for patients with elated manic episodes and for patients who have shown good responses and tolerability during previous episodes (Bowden et al. 1994). Divalproex appears to be more effective than lithium for patients with mixed mania, rapid cycling, concurrent substance abuse, and secondary mania (Bowden and Rhodes 1997). Divalproex is generally better tolerated than lithium, especially regarding cognition, and poses fewer serious risks. These advantages are particularly clinically important in adolescents and elderly persons with bipolar disorder (Papatheodorou et al. 1995; Tohen et al. 1990). Overall, these studies suggest a broader spectrum of efficacy for divalproex than for lithium. However, lithium may be highly effective in the subset of patients for whom it provides benefit. Lithium is less expensive than the better tolerated divalproex form of valproate; however, studies suggest that the overall costs of divalproex-based treatment of mania are similar to and perhaps somewhat lower than those for lithium, as a function of earlier improvement and lower laboratory costs (Altshuler et al. 1995; Keck et al. 1995).

Less relevant data are available for carbamazepine. Based on the evidence, carbamazepine may be considered particularly in patients with secondary mania and mixed mania. Rapid-cycling patients have responded poorly to carbamazepine (Denicoff et al. 1994; Okuma et al. 1990).

The duration of a trial to determine efficacy does not need to be longer than 3 weeks. The duration of a maintenance trial is more a function of the characteristic cycle frequency and episode severity for the particular patient. When practical, continuation of a regimen through two episode cycles is advisable.

Adjunctive Treatment

Thyroid supplementation of lithium therapy has been reported in a small, open trial to be effective in alleviating rapid-cycling symptomatology (Bauer and Whybrow 1990). Although hypermetabolic doses were used, authorities differ on the merits of such a high-dose strategy because of the potential for adverse effects, such as tachycardia and bone demineralization, with elevated thyroid function (Lehmke et al. 1992).

The indications for benzodiazepines and neuroleptics are the same in maintenance treatment as in acute treatment. The principal difference is that the risk of tardive dyskinesia from neuroleptic therapy is, for practical purposes, limited to chronic treatment. Unless gradual withdrawal of the neuroleptic results in an exacerbation of delusional, hallucinatory, or severely aggressive behavior not otherwise controlled without neuroleptics, the medication should be discontinued. As with other psychotic conditions, even when long-term neuroleptic medication is required, the dosage can often be gradually reduced, thereby reducing side-effect burden and risk.

Open trials have suggested that clozapine treatment may improve otherwise treatment-refractory bipolar disorder and maintain this improvement (McElroy et al. 1991). The dosage range used has been 25–90 mg/day. Initially, only low dosages are characteristically well tolerated, and the dosage often must be increased slowly (McElroy et al. 1991). Because of the potential for agranulocytosis from both carbamazepine and clozapine, the two drugs should not be used together. The recognition of differing illness course and treatment responsiveness of subtypes of bipolar disorder and the approval of divalproex as a second effective treatment for mania have stimulated interest in other drugs for bipolar disorder.

CONCLUSION

Early studies are assessing the effectiveness of lamotrigine and gabapentin for various aspects of bipolar disorder. Both drugs were initially developed to treat epilepsy. Recent recognition of the complex presentations of bipolar disorder, the spectrum of conditions with elements of bipolar symptomatology, and its episodic course and the excitement engendered by evidence of the effectiveness of a new treatment—divalproex—have stimulated interest in the disorder. Important studies of symptomatology, illness course, and potential new treatments are in progress and are likely to affect patient care even beyond the information summarized in this chapter. Close attention to this developing information will substantially improve the quality of care psychiatrists can provide for patients with this disease.

REFERENCES

Akiskal HS: Depressive onset in pre-pubertal, pubertal, and possibly teenage and early adult years (age 21 and earlier) has been shown to presage eventual bipolarity. J Am Acad Child Adolesc Psychiatry 34:754–763, 1995

Altshuler LL, Post RM, Leverich GS, et al: Antidepressant-induced mania and cycle acceleration: a controversy revisited. Am J Psychiatry 152:1130–1138, 1995

Angst J, Felder W, Stassen HH: The course of affective disorders, I: change of diagnosis of monopolar, unipolar, and bipolar illness. Archiv für Psychiatrie Nervenkrankheiten 226:57–64, 1978

Baastrup PC, Poulsen JC, Schou M, et al: Prophylactic lithium: double-blind discontinuation in manic-depressive and recurrent-depressive disorders. Lancet 2:326–330, 1970

Bauer MS, Whybrow PC: Rapid cycling bipolar disorder, II: treatment of refractory rapid cycling with high-dose levothyroxine: a preliminary study. Arch Gen Psychiatry 47:435–440, 1990

Beigel A, Murphy DL: Assessing clinical characteristics of the manic state. Am J Psychiatry 128:688–694, 1971

Bowden CL: Predictors of response to divalproex and lithium. J Clin Psychiatry 56:25–30, 1995

Bowden CL, Rhodes LJ: Treatment of acute mania, in Current Psychiatric Therapy, 2nd Edition. Edited by Dunner DL. Philadelphia, PA, WB Saunders, 1997, pp 253–261

Bowden CL, Brugger AM, Swann AC, et al: Efficacy of divalproex vs lithium and placebo in the treatment of mania. JAMA 271:918–924, 1994

Bowden CL, Janicak PG, Orsulak P, et al: Relation of serum valproate concentration to response in mania. Am J Psychiatry 153:765–770, 1996

Brady KT, Sonne S, Anton R, et al: Valproate in the treatment of acute bipolar affective episodes complicated by substance abuse: a pilot study. J Clin Psychiatry 56:118–121, 1995

Brunet G, Cerlich B, Robert P, et al: Open trial of a calcium antagonist, nimodipine, in acute mania. Clin Neuropharmacol 13:224–228, 1990

Calabrese JR, Delucchi GA: Spectrum of efficacy of valproate in 55 patients with rapid-cycling bipolar disorder. Am J Psychiatry 147:431–434, 1990

Citrome L: The use of lithium, carbamazepine, and valproic acid in a state operated psychiatric hospital. Journal of Pharmacy Technology 11:55–59, 1995

Cohn JB, Collins G, Ashbrook E, et al: A comparison of fluoxetine, imipramine, and placebo in patients with bipolar depressive disorder. Int Clin Psychopharmacol 4:313–322, 1989

Cooke RG, Young T, Levitt AJ, et al: Bipolar II: not so different when co-morbidity excluded. Depression 3:154–156, 1995

Davis JM: Overview: maintenance therapy in psychiatry, II: affective disorders. Am J Psychiatry 133:1–13, 1976

Deltito JA: Valproate treatment for the difficult-to-treat patient with OCD (letter). J Clin Psychiatry 55:500, 1994

Denicoff KD, Blake KD, Smith-Jackson EE, et al: Morbidity in treated bipolar disorder: a one-year prospective study using daily life chart ratings. Depression 2:95–104, 1994

Dubovsky SI, Franks RD, Allen S, et al: Calcium antagonists in mania: a double blind study of verapamil. Psychiatry Res 18:309–320, 1986

Dunner DL, Fieve RR: Clinical factors in lithium carbonate prophylaxis failure. Arch Gen Psychiatry 30:229–233, 1974

Fieve RR, Platman SR, Plutchik RR: The use of lithium in affective disorders, I: acute endogenous depression. Am J Psychiatry 125:487–491, 1968

Frances A, Docherty JP, Kahn DA: The expert consensus guideline series: treatment of bipolar disorder. J Clin Psychiatry 57:3–88, 1996

Frankenburg FR, Tohen M, Cohen BM, et al: Long-term response to carbamazepine: a retrospective study. J Clin Psychopharmacol 8:130–132, 1988

Frye MA, Altshuler LL, Szuba MP, et al: The relationship between antimanic agent for treatment of classic or dysphoric mania and length of hospital stay. J Clin Psychiatry 57:17–21, 1996

Gelenberg AJ, Kane JM, Keller MB, et al: Comparison of standard and low serum levels of lithium for maintenance treatment of bipolar disorder. N Engl J Med 321:1489–1493, 1989

Geller B, Fox LW, Clark KA: Rate and predictors of prepubertal bipolarity during follow-up of 6 to 12 year-old depressed children. J Am Acad Child Adolesc Psychiatry 33:461–468, 1994

Goldberg JF, Harrow M, Grossman LS: Course and outcome in bipolar affective disorder. Am J Psychiatry 152:379–384, 1995

Goncalves N, Stoll KD: Carbam pin bei manischen syndromen. EINE kontrollierte doppel blind studie [Carbamazepine in manic syndromes: a controlled double-blind study]. Nervenerzt 56:43–47, 1985

Goodwin FK, Jamison KR: Manic-Depressive Illness. New York, Oxford University Press, 1990

Goodwin FK, Zis AP: Lithium in the treatment of mania: comparisons with neuroleptics. Arch Gen Psychiatry 36:840–844, 1979

Grof E, Haag M, Grof P, et al: Lithium response and the sequence of episode polarities: preliminary report on a Hamilton sample. Prog Neuropsychopharmacol Biol Psychiatry 11:199–203, 1987

Harrow M, Goldberg JF, Grossman LS, et al: Outcome in manic disorders: a naturalistic follow-up study. Arch Gen Psychiatry 47:665–671, 1990

Herridge PL, Pope HG Jr: Treatment of bulimia and rapid-cycling bipolar disorder with sodium valproate: a case report. J Clin Psychopharmacol 5:229–230, 1985

Himmelhoch JM, Thase MF, Mallinger AG, et al: Tranylcypromine versus imipramine in anergic bipolar depression. Am J Psychiatry 148:910–916, 1991

Jamison KR, Gerner RH, Goodwin FK: Patient and physician attitudes toward lithium: relationship to compliance. Arch Gen Psychiatry 36:866–869, 1979

Janicak PG, Sharma RP, Easton M, et al: A double-blind, placebo-controlled trial of clonidine in the treatment of acute mania. Psychopharmacol Bull 25:243–245, 1989

Jann MW, Ereshefsky L, Saklad SR, et al: Effects of carbamazepine on plasma haloperidol levels. J Clin Psychopharmacol 5:106–109, 1985

Kahn D, Stevenson E, Douglas CJ: Effect of sodium valproate in three patients with organic brain syndromes. Am J Psychiatry 145:101–111, 1988

Kahn EM, Schulz SC, Perel JM, et al: Change in haloperidol level due to carbamazepine—a complicating factor in combined medication for schizophrenia. J Clin Psychopharmacol 10:54–57, 1990

Katz MM, Robins E, Croughan J, et al: Behavioral measurement and drug response characteristics of unipolar and bipolar depression. Psychol Med 12:25–36, 1982

Keck PE Jr, McElroy SL, Tugrul KC, et al: Valproate oral loading in the treatment of acute mania. J Clin Psychiatry 54:305–308, 1993

Keck PE, Bennett JA, Stanton SP: Health economic aspects of the treatment of manic-depressive illness with divalproex. Reviews in Contemporary Pharmacotherapy 6:597–604, 1995

Keller MB, Lavori PW, Coryell W, et al: Differential outcome of pure manic, mixed/cycling, and pure depressive episodes in patients with bipolar illness. JAMA 255:3138–3142, 1986

Keller MB, Lavori PW, Kane JM, et al: Subsyndromal symptoms in bipolar disorder: a comparison of standard and low serum levels of lithium. Arch Gen Psychiatry 49:371–376, 1992

Ketter TA, Pazzaglia P, Post RM: Synergy of carbamazepine and valproic acid in affective illness: case report and review of literature. J Clin Psychopharmacol 12:276–282, 1992

Ketter TA, Jenkins JB, Schroeder DH, et al: Carbamazepine but not valproate induces bupropion metabolism. J Clin Psychopharmacol 15:327–330, 1995

Koslow SH, Maas JW, Bowden CL, et al: CSF and urinary biogenic amines and metabolites in depression and mania: a controlled, univariate analysis. Arch Gen Psychiatry 40:999–1010, 1983

Kramlinger KG, Post RM: The addition of lithium carbonate to carbamazepine: antidepressant efficacy in treatment-resistant depression. Arch Gen Psychiatry 46:794–800, 1989

Kramlinger KG, Post RM: Ultra-rapid and ultradian cycling in bipolar affective illness. Br J Psychiatry 167:95/31.1–95/31.10, 1995

Kukopulos A, Caliari B, Tundo A, et al: Rapid cyclers, temperament, and antidepressants. Compr Psychiatry 24:249–258, 1983

Kupfer DJ, Carpenter LL, Frank E: Possible role of antidepressants in precipitating mania and hypomania in recurrent depression. Am J Psychiatry 145:804–808, 1988

Lambert PA, Venaud G: Comparative study of valpromide versus lithium as prophylactic treatment in affective disorders. Nervure Journal de Psychiatrie 7:1–9, 1995

Lehmke J, Bogner U, Felsenberg D, et al: Determination of bone mineral density by quantitative-computed tomography and single photon absorptiometry in subclinical hyperthyroidism: a risk of early osteopaenia in post-menopausal women. Clin Endocrinol (Oxf) 36:511–517, 1992

Lerer B, Moore N, Meyendorff E, et al: Carbamazepine versus lithium in mania: a double-blind study. J Clin Psychiatry 48:89–93, 1987

Lewinsohn PM, Klein DN, Seeley JR: Bipolar disorders in a community sample of older adolescents: prevalence, phenomenology, comorbidity, and course. J Am Acad Child Adolesc Psychiatry 34:454–463, 1995

Lewis JL, Winokur G: The induction of mania: a natural history study with controls. Arch Gen Psychiatry 39:303–306, 1982

Lum M, Fontaine R, Elie R, et al: Divalproex sodium's antipanic effect in panic disorder: a placebo-controlled study. Biol Psychiatry 27:164A–165A, 1990

Lusznat R, Murphy DP, Nunn CMH: Carbamazepine vs lithium in the treatment and prophylaxis of mania. Br J Psychiatry 153:198–204, 1988

Maj M, Priozzi R, Kemali D: Long-term outcome of lithium prophylaxis in patients initially classified as complete responders. Psychopharmacology 98:535–538, 1989

McElroy SL, Dessain EC, Pope HG Jr, et al: Clozapine in the treatment of psychotic mood disorders, schizoaffective disorder, and schizophrenia. J Clin Psychiatry 52:411–414, 1991

Okuma T, Yamashita I, Takahashi R, et al: Comparison of the antimanic efficacy of carbamazepine and lithium carbonate by double-blind controlled study. Pharmacopsychiatry 23:143–150, 1990

Papatheodorou G, Kutcher SP, Katic M, et al: The efficacy and safety of divalproex sodium in the treatment of acute mania in adolescents and young adults. J Clin Psychopharmacol 15:110–116, 1995

Pope HG Jr, McElroy SL, Keck PE Jr, et al: Valproate in the treatment of acute mania: a placebo-controlled study. Arch Gen Psychiatry 48:62–68, 1991

Post RM, Uhde TW, Roy-Byrne PP, et al: Correlates of antimanic response to carbamazepine. Psychiatry Res 21:71–83, 1987

Post RM, Roy-Byrne PP, Uhde TW: Graphic representation of the life course of illness in patients with affective disorder. Am J Psychiatry 145:844–848, 1988

Post RM, Rubinow DR, Uhde TW, et al: Dysphoric mania: clinical and biological correlates. Arch Gen Psychiatry 46:353–358, 1989

Post RM, Leverich GS, Rosoff AS, et al: Carbamazepine prophylaxis in refractory affective disorders: a focus on long-term follow-up. J Clin Psychopharmacol 10:318–327, 1990

Post RM, Leverich GS, Altshuler L, et al: Lithium-discontinuation-induced refractoriness: preliminary observations. Am J Psychiatry 149:1727–1729, 1992

Prien RF, Kupfer DJ, Mansky PA, et al: Drug therapy in the prevention of recurrences in unipolar and bipolar affective disorders: report of the NIMH Collaborative Study Group comparing lithium carbonate, imipramine, and a lithium carbonate-imipramine combination. Arch Gen Psychiatry 41:1096–1104, 1984

Prien RF, Himmelhoch JM, Kupfer DJ: Treatment of mixed mania. J Affect Disord 15:9–15, 1988

Primeau F, Fontaine R, Beauclair L: Valproic acid and panic disorder. Can J Psychiatry 35:248–250, 1990

Quitkin FM, Kane J, Rifkin A, et al: Prophylactic lithium carbonate with and without imipramine for bipolar I patients: a double-blind study. Arch Gen Psychiatry 38:902–907, 1981

Regier DA, Boyd JH, Burke JDJ, et al: One-month prevalence of mental disorders in the United States: based on five Epidemiological Catchment Area sites. Arch Gen Psychiatry 45:977–986, 1988

Sachs GS, Lafer B, Stoll AL, et al: A double-blind trial of bupropion versus desipramine for bipolar depression. J Clin Psychiatry 55:391–393, 1994

Secunda S, Katz MM, Swann A, et al: Mania: diagnosis, state measurement and prediction of treatment response. J Affect Disord 8:113–121, 1985

Shopsin B: Bupropion's prophylactic efficacy in bipolar affective illness. J Clin Psychiatry 44:163–169, 1983

Shulman KI, Mackenzie S, Hardy B: The clinical use of lithium carbonate in old age: a review. Prog Neuropsychopharmacol Biol Psychiatry 11:159–164, 1987

Small JG, Klapper MH, Milstein V, et al: Carbamazepine compared with lithium in the treatment of mania. Arch Gen Psychiatry 48:915–921, 1991

Suppes T, McElroy SL, Gilbert J, et al: Clozapine in the treatment of dysphoric mania. Biol Psychiatry 32:270–280, 1992

Swann AC, Secunda SK, Katz MM, et al: Lithium treatment of mania: clinical characteristics, specificity of symptom change, and outcome. Psychiatry Res 18:127–141, 1986

Swann AC, Bowden CL, Morris D, et al: Depression during mania: treatment response to lithium or divalproex. Arch Gen Psychiatry 54:37–42, 1997

Tohen M, Watemaux CM, Tsuang MT, et al: Four-year follow-up of twenty-four first-episode manic patients. J Affect Disord 19:76–86, 1990

Vahip S, Ozkan B, Ayan A, et al: Elevation of plasma lithium at the end of mania and some biochemical correlates. Abstract presented at the Second International Conference on New Directions in Affective Disorders, Jerusalem, Israel, 1995, p 31

Walton SA, Berk M, Brook S: Superiority of lithium over verapamil in mania: a randomized, controlled, single-blind trial. J Clin Psychiatry 57:543–546, 1995

Wehr TA, Goodwin FK: Can antidepressants cause mania and worsen the course of affective illness? Am J Psychiatry 144:1403–1411, 1987

Wilder BJ, Karas BJ, Penry JK, et al: Gastrointestinal tolerance of divalproex sodium. Neurology 33:808–811, 1983

Worrall EP, Moody JP, Peet M, et al: Controlled studies of the acute antidepressant effects of lithium. Br J Psychiatry 135:255–262, 1979

THIRTY-SIX

Treatment of Schizophrenia

Herbert Y. Meltzer, M.D., and S. Hossein Fatemi, M.D., Ph.D.

The treatment of schizophrenia is based on the skillful integration of pharmaco-therapy and psychosocial interventions. Never before has there been as broad an array of drugs to treat the full range of deficits that are variably present in this illness, including positive, negative, and disorganization symptoms, depressive symptoms, and cognitive disturbances. These developments in pharmacological treatments are taking place in the context of significant changes in how treatment is provided to persons with schizophrenia; these changes are, in large part, the result of deinstitutionalization of even the most seriously and persistently ill schizophrenic patients and the increasingly prominent role of managed care in deciding who will provide treatment, what treatments will be available, and for how long. The pharmacoeconomic dimension of the assessment of treatment strategies has also become very prominent because of the introduction of new, patented drugs after a period of nearly 20 years during which mainly generic medications, which are relatively inexpensive, were available. The purpose of this chapter is to provide an integrative approach to the treatment of schizophrenia. Extensive discussion of specific antipsychotic drugs is found elsewhere in this volume (see Marder, Chapter 17; Owens and Risch, Chapter 18; and Stanilla and Simpson, Chapter 19, in this volume).

HISTORICAL BACKGROUND

Dementia praecox and schizophrenia were recognized by Emil Kraepelin and Eugen Bleuler approximately 100 and 90 years ago, respectively. The disorder that these concepts represent has, to the best of our knowledge, been present throughout human history. Before the introduction of pharmacotherapy in the 1950s, in the great majority of cases, schizophrenia led to lifelong psychosis with very poor outcome.

Opiates and sedatives, as well as insulin coma therapy, were used in the first half of the twentieth century without producing specific improvement in psychopathology or changing the course of illness. Psychosurgery, mainly frontal lobotomy, was introduced in the 1930s and was used until the late 1940s, with no noteworthy benefits except for, in some cases, reduction in agitated and violent behavior. The first effective somatic treatment was electroconvulsive therapy (ECT), which remains in limited use. Reserpine, which depletes the stores of biogenic amines such as serotonin, norepinephrine, and dopamine, was found, as early as 1950, to have some antipsychotic efficacy but was never widely used.

The discovery and testing of chlorpromazine, a tricyclic phenothiazine compound, in 1954 by Laborit, Delay, and Deniker in France was the beginning of the modern era

Preparation of this manuscript was supported by a Center Grant from the National Institute of Mental Health (MH-48481) and grants from the Esel, Lattner, and Lauerate Foundations, and Ms. Debra Schuller.

The excellent secretarial support of Ms. Diantha McLeod and Ms. Dina Kauffman is greatly appreciated.

of the pharmacotherapy of schizophrenia. Their careful, pioneering studies were the first reliable demonstration of pharmacological treatment of psychosis, which ranks as among the most important discoveries in all of medicine.

Elucidation of the role of receptor blockade in the action of chlorpromazine led to the discovery of many other phenothiazines with antipsychotic efficacy (e.g., fluphenazine, perphenazine, and thioridazine), as well as other classes of agents that included effective antipsychotic drugs (e.g., haloperidol, sulpiride, molindone, pimozide, and thiothixene). It was noted that all these agents produce extrapyramidal side effects (EPS)—that is, dystonic reactions, muscle rigidity, tremor, loss of associated movements, and akathisia (an intense restlessness that leads to repetitive limb movements and pacing [Adler et al. 1989]). After months to years of neuroleptic treatment, abnormal involuntary movement of the tongue, lips, face, and limbs, known as *tardive dyskinesia*, or permanent dystonias, referred to as *tardive dystonia*, developed in some, but not all, patients.

Antipsychotic drugs that are potent dopamine receptor antagonists are referred to as the *typical* or *conventional* neuroleptics because at usual clinical doses they produce the neurological side effects noted above. It is now established that the antipsychotic efficacy of these agents is the result of blockade of D_2 dopamine receptors in the mesolimbic system of the brain, whereas their EPS are the result of blockade of the same group of receptors in the basal ganglia (K. L. Davis et al. 1991). These two processes appear to be inextricably linked. However, as noted later in this chapter, there is controversy as to whether lower doses of these agents, which do not produce EPS, might be clinically effective by producing sufficient blockade of dopaminergic transmission in the mesolimbic system and sparing that in the basal ganglia (McEvoy et al. 1991). The introduction of these agents constitutes one of the great advances in the history of medicine, having led to enormous beneficial changes in the lives of most people with schizophrenia and their families. These agents also became essential tools in the study of dopaminergic neurotransmission and the identification of multiple types of dopamine receptors in the brain (K. L. Davis et al. 1991).

The search for medications that have antipsychotic properties but that do not produce as many or as severe EPS as the conventional neuroleptic drugs led to the discovery, in 1959, of clozapine, a dibenzodiazepine, which produces virtually no EPS in humans, even though other members of the same chemical class, loxapine and amoxapine, produce significant EPS at clinically effective doses (Meltzer 1996, 1997). Clozapine was introduced into clinical practice in 1969 but was withdrawn because of its ability to produce agranulocytosis (Meltzer 1997). (The side effects of clozapine, including agranulocytosis, are discussed in more detail later in this chapter.) It was reintroduced in 1989 after it was found to be more effective than the first generation of antipsychotic drugs in many patients with treatment-resistant schizophrenia (Kane et al. 1988). It had also been observed that clozapine did not produce tardive dyskinesia or tardive dystonia but, in fact, actively suppressed the symptoms of both conditions in many, but not all, patients; this finding disproved the strongly held belief that any antipsychotic drug that could alleviate the symptoms of tardive movement disorders would also produce them (Kane and Marder 1993).

Unlike the typical neuroleptic drugs mentioned earlier, clozapine is not a potent antagonist of the D_2 receptor in vivo or in vitro (Fatemi et al. 1996). As is discussed below, clozapine has a complex pharmacology (Fatemi et al. 1996).

The hypothesis that clozapine's novel effects derive from potent antagonism of the serotonin (5-HT) 5-HT_{2A} receptor (Meltzer et al. 1989), coupled with the earlier finding of weak blockade of the D_2 receptor, led to the development of a group of drugs with similar properties (e.g., risperidone, olanzapine, sertindole, quetiapine, and ziprasidone). However, as noted below, these drugs differ from clozapine in many other pharmacological properties (Schotte et al. 1996). It is still uncertain as to whether the potent 5-HT_{2A}/weak D_2 antagonism hypothesis is correct. These drugs, which are sometimes referred to as *serotonin-dopamine antagonists*, are currently being assessed for their superiority to the typical neuroleptic drugs and their advantages and disadvantages relative to clozapine. They are frequently referred to as *atypical* antipsychotic drugs because of the dissociation between antipsychotic activity and EPS (Meltzer 1995b). Other agents that are not serotonin-dopamine antagonists (e.g., remoxipride) may also have atypical properties.

TREATMENT OBJECTIVES

Psychopathology

Schizophrenia is usually first recognized during late adolescence or early adulthood with the appearance of positive symptoms (i.e., delusions, hallucinations, thought disturbance, and bizarre behavior) (Carpenter 1987). The onset of these symptoms may be gradual or abrupt. It is now recognized that there are antecedents to psychosis in childhood and early adolescence (e.g., disturbances in motor behavior, attention, interpersonal relationships in some patients with schizophrenia) (Baum and Walker 1995; Murray et al. 1992). So-called negative symptoms (i.e., lack of spontaneity, decreased motivation, flat affect, anhedonia, and anergia) may precede or follow the development of psychosis (Kibel et al. 1993; Liddle 1987; Murray et al. 1992). A third syndrome, disorganization (i.e., incoherence, inappropriate affect, loose associations, and poverty of thought content), has also been recognized as an independent domain of psychopathology (Liddle 1987; Liddle and Barnes 1990; Meltzer and Zureick 1989).

Patients will show varying levels of each of these three syndromes. DSM-IV (American Psychiatric Association 1994) criteria for schizophrenia require that delusions, hallucinations, disorganized speech, or disorganized behavior be present at least 1 month before the diagnosis can be made. Negative symptoms, along with at least one of the four positive or disorganization symptoms described above, can satisfy Criterion A in the DSM-IV diagnostic criteria.

When patients first present for treatment, they usually manifest one or more of the positive or disorganization symptoms mentioned above. These symptoms may be severe and of acute onset, in which case they are usually quite disturbing to the patient or family. However, they may be of gradual onset and may not be disturbing to the patient or family for a variety of reasons. In this case, the symptoms may have been present for some time and may not have received medical attention because they were not manifested in such a way as to be noticeable or because those in close contact with the individual did not recognize the need for medical attention. There is some evidence that prolonged psychosis prior to antipsychotic drug treatment may be associated with worse long-term outcome (Wyatt 1991; Wyatt et al. 1997).

The treatment of schizophrenia traditionally has focused—and, unfortunately, in many places still focuses—mainly on the treatment of positive symptoms. The primary reasons for this emphasis are that positive symptoms are relatively easy to detect and that the typical neuroleptic drugs have the ability to ameliorate these symptoms in the large majority of patients. Early studies (Meltzer et al. 1986) showed some, albeit small, effects of the conventional neuroleptic drugs on negative symptoms. Since the seminal paper of Crow (1980), the treatment of negative symptoms has been appreciated as an important, if elusive, target of antipsychotic drug treatment.

Carpenter (1987, 1994) has promoted the desirability of distinguishing between *primary negative symptoms*—negative symptoms that are enduring and unrelated to positive symptoms, EPS resulting from treatment with antipsychotic drugs, depression, or other types of psychopathology—and *secondary negative symptoms*—symptoms that result from one or more of the factors above and presumably would remit if that factor(s) was effectively treated. Although having obvious face validity, this distinction is not easy to make in clinical practice and from the patient's perspective is of little significance. However, to the extent that making such a distinction can lead to increased awareness of those components of the illness that are supposedly causing the secondary negative symptoms (i.e., positive symptoms, EPS, and depression), it is of some importance. Primary negative symptoms should be the target of therapeutic intervention in their own right.

Cognitive Impairment

Patients with schizophrenia have widespread, multifaceted impairments in neurocognitive measures such as executive function, attention, and working memory. Cognitive impairment in schizophrenia is an early feature of the illness (Saykin et al. 1991). Indeed, some aspects of this deficit may precede the development of psychotic symptoms. For most patients, once the deficit is established at the end of the first episode, the extent of impairment changes only marginally over time, although clearly there are significant numbers of patients in whom the impairment is progressive and reaches the proportions characteristic of severe dementia (Goldberg et al. 1993). It is important to treat the cognitive disturbance as well as the symptoms of schizophrenia and to assess the role of such disturbance on work and social function (Cassens et al. 1990; Green 1996).

The range of cognitive tests applied to patients with schizophrenia is enormous. The frequency and extent of abnormalities vary with the test. It has been estimated that about 40% of patients with schizophrenia have impaired neurocognition (Braff et al. 1991; Goldberg et al. 1988). The major deficits are in executive function (abstraction/flexibility), attention, verbal learning and memory, spatial and verbal working memory, semantic memory, and psychomotor performance (Braff et al. 1991; Saykin et al. 1991). These abnormalities in cognition are believed to be the result of abnormalities in the frontal and temporal lobes and in the connectivity between these regions (Weinberger 1987).

There is strong evidence for the functional significance of these cognitive impairments. In a recent review of the functional consequences of neurocognitive deficits in schizophrenia, Green (1996) concluded that the most consistent finding was that verbal memory was associated with three types of outcome measures: 1) community survival and function, 2) social problem solving, and 3) skill acquisition. Vigilance was related to social problem solving and skill acquisition. Executive function/abstraction was related to community functioning but not social problem solving. Cognitive impairment is also highly correlated with quality-of-life measures (Sevy and Davidson 1995).

Mood Disturbance

In addition to positive, negative, and disorganization symptoms and cognitive dysfunction, patients with schizophrenia have affective disturbances. Flat affect and inappropriate affect are components of negative symptoms and disorganization, respectively, but patients with schizophrenia may have varying degrees of depressive and hypomanic or manic symptoms as well. When these mood symptoms are a prominent part of the clinical picture and precede the core schizophrenic symptoms, patients are appropriately diagnosed as having *schizoaffective disorder, depressed or bipolar type.* The mood symptoms accompanying schizophrenia or schizoaffective disorder must be the target of therapy as well.

The importance of detecting and treating depressive symptoms in schizophrenia has been discussed by Siris et al. (1981). Approximately half of patients with schizophrenia will experience a significant depressive episode during the course of their illness. When this episode follows an acute exacerbation of positive symptoms, it is called a *postpsychotic depression.* Between 9% and 13% of patients with schizophrenia commit suicide, and as many as 50% make suicide attempts with varying severity of intent (Roy 1982). These attempts may reflect the despair patients with schizophrenia experience because of the disabling effects of their illness and the lack of efficacy of treatments offered to them.

Social and Work Function and Quality of Life

The positive, negative, disorganization, and affective symptoms experienced by patients with schizophrenia, together with the cognitive disturbance, lead to great *disability in social and work function.* This is particularly true in developed countries, where a high level of cognitive function may be needed for most jobs. Only about 20% of patients with schizophrenia are employed. It is less of a problem in undeveloped countries, where the skills required for participating in many work activities may be less cognitively demanding.

Another concept of importance in evaluating the adequacy of treatment in schizophrenia is *quality of life* (Awad 1992). Quality of life, which refers to the individual's subjective sense of well-being, has been surprisingly neglected in discussions of schizophrenia, in part because of the impairment in insight in many patients with schizophrenia and the limited goals that clinicians have established for themselves with regard to patients with this illness. There is no generally accepted definition of quality of life. The concept can entail the subjective assessment of both medical and nonmedical aspects of life. Nonmedical aspects include social status, economic well-being, and fulfillment of personal aspirations.

An individual's assessment of the quality of his or her life is affected by many factors. Premorbid level of functioning and, in many cases, the degree to which the individual compares his or her level of functioning with that of other members of the family and circle of friends or acquaintances are important factors. Patients with schizophrenia are sometimes aware of the severity of their impairment in cognition; they may complain greatly of impairments in attention, concentration, ability to remember, and so forth. Such awareness, in turn, produces demoralization and depression, which have been reported to be a factor in the decision of some patients who attempted or committed suicide. It is well known from research on expressed emotion in schizophrenia that familial critical comments and intrusiveness on autonomy can have a major impact on the function of patients with schizophrenia. This reflects the impact of the family members or caregivers who may be unrelated to the patient on quality of life. Somatic problems that may accompany schizophrenia can have a major impact on quality of life. Inadequate diagnosis and treatment of medical problems that may be secondary to or independent of schizophrenia (e.g., poor nutrition, infections due to institutionalization) is very common in schizophrenia and may contribute to poor quality of life.

The side effects of medication (e.g., EPS, weight gain, impaired sexual function not due to loss of libido) and the disfiguring aspects of tardive dyskinesia can lead to poor quality of life.

Substance Abuse

A large and growing proportion of patients with schizophrenia have substance abuse and dependence problems involving alcohol, stimulants (including cocaine), and even psychotomimetic agents such as phencyclidine (Buckley et al. 1994; Mueser et al. 1990). Although estimates vary widely, it can be safely concluded that between 25% and 50% of schizophrenia patients abuse alcohol or illicit drugs at some point in their illness. These agents may produce in some patients a transient sense of well-being that results from the temporary relief of depression or anhedonia. However, in the long run, use of these substances greatly diminishes quality of life because of the role of these substances in increasing psychotic symptomatology, impairing cognitive function, or producing medical problems such as liver failure. Substance abuse in schizophrenia is closely associated with, and often causally related to, medication noncompliance (Mueser et al. 1990; Weiden et al. 1991).

Summary

It is of essential importance in the treatment of schizophrenia to recognize that the major psychopathological dimensions of the schizophrenia syndrome (e.g., positive, negative disorganization and depressive symptoms) may be independent of one another and of cognitive dysfunction (Meltzer 1992). The severity of impairment in these domains is often very disparate. The Type I, Type II model of schizophrenia proposed by Crow (1980) suggested that positive symptoms and negative symptoms were independent and that the former, but not the latter, respond to typical neuroleptic drugs. We have found that negative symptoms and cognition are more relevant to quality of life than are positive symptoms. As mentioned previously, there is evidence that cognition is more relevant to work function in schizophrenia than are positive and negative symptoms. Because of this independence, clinicians must be willing to go beyond the usual attention to positive symptoms in developing disease management strategies for schizophrenia.

TREATMENT OF THE ACUTE PHASE OF PSYCHOSIS

Stages of the Illness

Acute Psychosis

The acute phase of schizophrenia is currently organized, for purposes of treatment, into three phases, although, as we shall argue, it may be important to consider a fourth phase.

1. *Period of markedly increased positive symptoms* (referred to as *acute exacerbations*). Control of positive symptoms and preparing the patient for long-term treatment are the essential components of treatment during this phase of the illness.
2. *Phase of symptom remission following an acute exacerbation*. There is evidence that during this period patients will relapse within days to months if neuro-

leptic treatment is stopped (Gilbert et al. 1995). The goals of treatment during this phase are suppression of symptoms, prevention of relapse, and rehabilitation of the work and social function of the patient.
3. *Residual phase*. In this period, which only some patients enter, the propensity for an acute exacerbation to recur when neuroleptic drugs are stopped is greatly diminished. During this period, patients may not require neuroleptics to remain nonpsychotic. They may still have negative symptoms and cognitive dysfunction, however. In rare cases, individuals show no major symptoms. The major goal of this period of treatment is to focus on reintegration and socialization.

Prodromal Phase

A fourth phase of schizophrenia emerging as a target for treatment, the *prodromal* phase, is actually the first phase of the illness, occurring before the onset of psychosis (McGorry et al. 1995). There is now evidence that incipient features of schizophrenia are present during this period, which may even begin at birth but for clinical purposes is usually considered to be the period several months to several years before the psychosis emerges (Baum and Walker 1995; Murray et al. 1992). During this period, patients exhibit some of the symptoms of schizotypal patients—for example, magical thinking, mildly bizarre behavior, increased problems with attention and concentration, decreased school or work performance, increased irritability or withdrawal, ritualistic or socially unacceptable behaviors, loss of or failure to develop appropriate interest in sexual activity. These symptoms are not very specific to schizophrenia, but it is possible that they can be discerned as prodromes of schizophrenia, particularly if there is a family history of the illness.

It is of great importance to determine 1) whether pharmacological and psychosocial interventions at this stage of the illness might be effective and 2) whether the benefits of treatment at this phase would outweigh the risks of the interventions, considering that a proportion of those individuals who would receive treatment would not be destined to develop schizophrenia even though they are manifesting schizotypal symptoms and have decreased social and intellectual function. Clearly, as biological tests to identify individuals with vulnerability to develop schizophrenia are developed, treatments for this phase of the evolution of schizophrenia will be of the greatest importance. It is conceivable that effective interventions in the prodromal phase will prevent the development of acute episodes and thus obviate treatment in that period as well as maintenance treatment.

Acute Phase of Psychosis

Periods of acute psychosis may occur during the first episode or any time thereafter, even when patients are compliant with previously effective dosages of medication. Acute psychosis may occur during periods of increased stress from the environment but can also occur without apparent exogenous events contributing. It is not uncommon for patients to experience as many as 20 to 30 acute episodes of psychosis; such recurrence may be the result of noncompliance, failure to prescribe clozapine, if needed, for patients with neuroleptic-, risperidone-, or olanzapine-resistant schizophrenia, or the poor organization of mental health services for patients who would otherwise be compliant. There is concern that each episode of psychosis or prolonged periods of psychosis without treatment may have long-term adverse consequences (Wyatt 1991). Clearly, frequent psychotic episodes have serious short-term consequences, and, therefore, it is critically important for mental health services to be organized in a way that helps prevent frequent relapses. Treatment of patients during the first episode of schizophrenia requires separate consideration from that of patients with recurrent psychotic episodes.

First-Episode Schizophrenia

The patient with first-episode schizophrenia may present with florid psychotic symptoms that have been present for as long as several years or as brief as a few days. The duration of psychosis prior to presentation depends on the severity and type of symptoms, the extent to which the patient can hide them from detection, the sensitivity of the observers in the environment, and the availability of treatments, among other factors. The first challenge with such patients is to establish the diagnosis and to rule out any other psychiatric or medical, especially neurological, conditions that may be present. Schizophrenia may be difficult to differentiate from mania during the first episode. Characteristic manic symptoms may be absent or less prominent than delusions and hallucinations, which may be paranoid rather than grandiose in some manic patients. It is, therefore, sometimes prudent to defer the diagnosis of schizophrenia until definitive information about the character and course of the illness is available. Of course, if the duration of illness at the time of presentation is less than 6 months, the diagnosis of schizophrenia is not yet applicable, and the diagnoses of brief reactive psychosis or schizophreniform disorder should be considered.

The initial decision to be made in the treatment of a patient with first-episode schizophrenia is whether hospitalization is required. Assuming that managed care does not preclude hospitalization because of failure to meet narrow criteria (e.g., danger to self or others), it is necessary to evaluate a number of factors to decide whether to hospitalize the patient. An intensive evaluation is necessary to rule out organic factors that may be producing the psychosis. It may not be possible to do this evaluation conveniently or safely on an outpatient basis. However, if symptoms are relatively mild and an evaluation of the family and environment suggests the availability of considerable support and the absence of stressors, it may be possible to conduct such an evaluation on an outpatient basis. However, first-episode patients who are initially treated as outpatients often fail to continue treatment because the clinician, in the limited time available, cannot establish a relationship with the patient in the initial interview. The nature of the hospital that is available to the clinician must also be considered in deciding whether to hospitalize the patient. The clinician may be reluctant to hospitalize a first-episode patient, or the patient, if judged competent, or family may be reluctant to consent, if the only hospital unit that is available is one that is physically unattractive, is poorly staffed, has mainly very chronic and older patients, and so forth. Hospitalization is strongly recommended for patients who are in severely stressful situations, whether these occur at home, school, or work. Removing the patient from these stressful situations, sometimes even without administering antipsychotic medication, can lead to a rapid remission (Young and Meltzer 1980).

It may be necessary to seek civil commitment for some patients. The clinician should avoid taking this step, if possible, by attempting to obtain a voluntary admission. This process may take additional time and, thus, can be difficult to carry out in a managed care environment in which time of contact with new patients is restricted—to as little as 45 minutes in some instances. In some jurisdictions, civil commitment requires prolonged hospitalization even if there is no clinical need for it after a relatively brief period of time.

The duration of hospitalization for first-episode patients should be kept relatively short, since there is no evidence that prolonged hospitalization achieves any greater benefit than brief hospitalizations. In a managed care environment, the duration of the first hospitalization may be only a few days. If this is the case, it is of great importance that the clinician establish a relationship with the patient that will lead to continuing contact after discharge and a good chance of compliance with treatment. Contact with the family during the hospitalization by the clinician is critical to ensuring continuing contact with the patient and compliance. In many settings, only a social worker has such contact—a situation that may preclude the possibility of an alliance between the clinician and the family, which may be essential if further treatment after discharge is to take place.

During the first episode, whether evaluation is on an outpatient or inpatient basis, it is essential to establish the history of the illness, the family history of mental illness, the use of illicit drugs or alcohol, the presence of other medical conditions that may be directly associated with psychosis (e.g., Huntington's disease, Cushing's disease), or the use of medications that may produce psychosis (e.g., corticosteroids for collagen vascular diseases or asthma). Generally, it is useful to obtain a brain imaging study to examine for structural abnormalities. A computed tomography (CT) or magnetic resonance imaging (MRI) examination will reveal any organic abnormalities that may be contributing to the clinical picture. It is essential to test for substance abuse.

Psychopharmacological Treatment of the Acute Phase

The initial treatment of an acute psychosis requires consideration of drug, dosage, and route of administration. Oral medication may be acceptable and sufficient for many patients. One of the atypical agents may be preferred because of their low risk of EPS. Patients who present in the emergency room with severe agitation or threatening harm to themselves or others require being isolated in a safe room. They may also require restraining of their limbs. The latter should be done with great care for the psychological well-being of the patient, but physical safety for patient and staff is the preeminent consideration. Patients who are this severely ill will ordinarily require parenteral medication. The most commonly used medication for this purpose at present is haloperidol, with chlorpromazine as a second choice. Haloperidol, 5 mg intramuscularly, is effective in calming many patients within 30 minutes. If the response is insufficient, the injection may be repeated at intervals of 1 hour after vital signs are checked. There is no clear evidence of a safe upper limit in such a situation. Parenteral administration of a benzodiazepine such as lorazepam may also be a useful augmentation of the neuroleptic. Monitoring vital signs is crucial during this period. In the most severe cases, emergency ECT may be needed. Short-acting parenteral forms of olanzapine and risperidone are under development. Ziprasidone is a novel antipsychotic that should be commercially available in the first half of 1998 in the United States and elsewhere in the world. It has been approved in Brazil. A parenteral form of ziprasidone is also being developed.

Conventional neuroleptics and the atypical antipsychotics are effective in treating an acute exacerbation of schizophrenia (Arvanitis et al. 1997; Beasley et al. 1996; Chouinard et al. 1993; J. M. Davis et al. 1989). As reviewed in detail in this volume in the chapters on the individual drugs, the conventional drugs effect remission of psychosis in about 75% of patients within days to months. The response rate is greater and more rapid in patients with first-episode schizophrenia than in patients with more chronic schizophrenia, but there is considerable variability in both groups (Loebel et al. 1992). Patients with first-episode schizophrenia usually require lower doses of antipsychotic drugs than do patients with more chronic schizophrenia and are more sensitive to EPS. About 10% of first-episode patients fail to respond to typical neuroleptics and may have to be treated with an atypical antipsychotic or clozapine. We discuss principles for choosing among the new antipsychotic drugs later in this section.

Time Course of Response in an Acute Episode

It may be expected that some decrease in agitation, anxiety, and sleeplessness will occur shortly after the initiation of antipsychotic treatment. Some patients show a rapid decrease in positive symptoms, but more often it is several days before any appreciable decrease is noted. Most patients show a near maximal response by 6 weeks of treatment. Loebel et al. (1992) demonstrated that treatment beyond 6 weeks with the same dose of a typical neuroleptic drug, with twice the dose, or after switching to another conventional neuroleptic drug of a different chemical class did not achieve significantly greater benefits. Therefore, if a satisfactory remission of positive symptoms is not achieved with a typical neuroleptic by 6 weeks, assuming that the dose is adequate, a switch to an atypical antipsychotic drug is indicated.

Choice of Antipsychotic for Acute Treatment

The choice of which oral medication to use during acute exacerbations depends on a number of factors. Until the introduction of clozapine and risperidone, only a few, simple principles were relevant to the choice of an antipsychotic medication. There is no convincing evidence for any advantages in efficacy among the conventional antipsychotic drugs (Baldessarini et al. 1988; Kane and Marder 1993). This has been attributed to the fact that the efficacy of these agents is based solely on their ability to block D_2 receptors in mesolimbic areas of the brain, including the nucleus accumbens, the stria terminalis, and the olfactory tubercle (K. L. Davis et al. 1991). These agents differ in affinities for other receptors, including α_1-

and α_2-adrenergic receptors, muscarinic receptors, and H_1 histamine receptors (Richelson and Nelson 1984). This suggests that the antipsychotic efficacy of these agents has little to do with actions at these receptors.

The differences in pharmacology among the conventional antipsychotic drugs are relevant to their side-effect profiles, which provide some basis for choosing among them. It is likely that the potent anticholinergic effects of thioridazine are the basis for its low EPS profile. However, there is no evidence that thioridazine is any *less* likely to produce tardive dyskinesia than any of the other conventional neuroleptic drugs. The antimuscarinic property of the conventional antipsychotic drugs may also contribute to memory impairment and urinary retention. H_1 receptors in brain have an important role in arousal and the regulation of appetite. Loxapine, *cis*-thiothixene, and chlorpromazine are conventional neuroleptics that have higher affinities for the H_1 receptor than does the classic antihistamine diphenhydramine. Haloperidol and molindone have low affinities for these receptors and thus might be chosen when it is of particular importance to minimize sedation and appetite stimulation. Neuroleptic drugs, with the exception of molindone, cause significant blockade of the α_1 receptor at clinically effective doses, which leads to varying degrees of postural hypotension, nasal congestion, dizziness, and tachycardia. The most potent of these neuroleptics in this regard are chlorpromazine, thioridazine, and haloperidol. The least potent α_1 antagonists are loxapine and molindone. The blockade of α_2 receptors by conventional neuroleptics is relatively weak and is not related to any particular side effect.

In recent years, haloperidol has been the most widely used antipsychotic in the United States, mainly because of its relatively low sedation. In England, chlorpromazine remains the most widely used conventional antipsychotic drug. In Italy and France, sulpiride and amisulpride, two substituted benzamide drugs, are the most frequently prescribed antipsychotic agents. Neither of these two drugs, or any other substituted benzamide with antipsychotic properties is available in the United States. The pharmacology of these compounds is of interest because they are highly selective for the D_2, D_3, and D_4 dopamine receptors.

Some patients develop preferences for or aversions to specific conventional antipsychotic drugs. These attitudes will limit the choice of antipsychotic drugs that clinicians can make without jeopardizing the chances for compliance.

Extrapyramidal Side Effects

The side effects associated with D_2 receptor blockade are more or less unavoidable with the conventional neurolep-

tic drugs. Low-potency agents such as chlorpromazine and thioridazine have the least EPS, whereas high-potency agents such as fluphenazine and haloperidol have the most. Parkinsonian side effects (e.g., dystonic reactions, including opisthotonos) may be manifest from the first dose. These side effects are usually treated by intravenous administration of diphenhydramine or intramuscular administration of trihexyphenidyl. More frequent are symptoms that occur after several days to weeks of treatment, such as muscle rigidity, loss of associated movement, masked facies, and drooling. These parkinsonian side effects are usually treated by lowering the dose and/or administering an oral antiparkinsonian agent (e.g., trihexyphenidyl or benztropine mesylate, which are potent anticholinergic agents, or amantadine, a dopaminomimetic agent). Increases in serum prolactin levels are present with all the conventional neuroleptic drugs (Meltzer and Fang 1976). The increases are greater in females than in males and sometimes produce galactorrhea, a condition that may be treated with pergolide mesylate or bromocriptine, both of which are direct-acting dopamine agonists.

Dosage of Neuroleptics

The dosages of conventional antipsychotic agents and galenic forms are given in Table 36–1. In general, the lowest dosages of the dosage ranges listed in Table 36–1 should be used. Recent fixed-dose studies reviewed by Marder (see Chapter 17 in this volume) suggest that low doses of haloperidol, and presumably the other conventional drugs as well, are as effective as higher dosages in the treatment of acute psychosis. (Groups of acutely psychotic patients were randomly assigned to groups receiving low, medium, or high doses of haloperidol.) Increasing the dose of these agents when patients fail to respond rapidly is not recommended. The addition of a benzodiazepine may produce a further calming effect prior to the onset of efficacy of lower doses of neuroleptic drugs. Some patients may require higher doses of neuroleptic drugs to respond adequately, but it is likely that such patients may actually be neuroleptic resistant, as described below, and should be treated with clozapine or perhaps another atypical antipsychotic drug.

Atypical Antipsychotic Drugs

Although clozapine was the first atypical antipsychotic drug discovered, it is not recommended at this time as a first-line treatment for patients with schizophrenia because of the increased risk of agranulocytosis. On the other hand, the side-effect burden of the newer atypical agents such as risperidone, olanzapine, quetiapine, sertin-

Table 36–1. Antipsychotic drugs available in the United States, dosage ranges, and dosage forms

Drug	Dosage range (mg)	Parenteral dosage (mg)	Galenic form(s)
Conventional			
Butyrophenone			
Haloperidol (Haldol)	5–30	5–10	Oral, liquid, injection
Haloperidol decanoate (Haldol-D)		25–100 q 1–4 weeks	
Dibenzoxazepine			
Loxapine succinate (Loxitane)	40–100	25	Oral, liquid, injection
Diphenylbutylpiperidine			
Pimozide (Orap)	2–6		Oral
Indole			
Molindone hydrochloride (Moban)	50–225		Oral, liquid
Phenothiazines			
Acetophenazine maleate (Tindal)	40–120	—	Oral
Chlorpromazine hydrochloride (Thorazine)	200–800	25–50	Oral, liquid, injection, suppository
Fluphenazine hydrochloride (Prolixin)	2–60	1.25–2.5	Oral, liquid, injection
Fluphenazine decanoate (Prolixin-D)		12.5–50 q 1–4 weeks	
Fluphenazine enanthate (Prolixin-E)		12.5–50 q 1–4 weeks	
Mesoridazine besylate (Serentil)	75–300	25	Oral, liquid, injection
Perphenazine (Trilafon)	8–32	5–10	Oral, liquid, injection
Thioridazine hydrochloride (Mellaril)	150–800		Oral, liquid
Trifluoperazine hydrochloride (Stelazine)	5–20	1–2	Oral, liquid, injection
Thioxanthenes			
Thiothixene hydrochloride (Navane)	5–30	2–4	Oral, liquid, injection
Atypical			
Benzisothiazolyl			
Ziprasidone (Zeldox)	40–160	10	Oral, liquid, injection
Benzisoxazole			
Risperidone (Risperdal)	4–8		Oral, liquid
Dibenzothiazepine			
Quetiapine fumarate (Seroquel)	150–600	—	Oral
Dibenzodiazepine			
Clozapine (Clozaril)	100–900	—	Oral
Imidazolidine			
Sertindole (SerLect)	20–24	—	Oral
Thienobenzodiazepine			
Olanzapine (Zyprexa)	10–20	—	Oral

dole, and ziprasidone is such that they may be considered as first-line agents. As will be discussed, sertindole has been found to prolong the Q-T$_c$ interval, a feature that may increase the risk of serious arrhythmias in some predisposed individuals (Van Kammen et al. 1996). It remains to be determined what precautions will be necessary in routine clinical practice because of this feature and whether the problem is serious enough to relegate this compound to use only in patients who do not respond adequately to other antipsychotic drugs. The clinical pharmacology of these drugs is discussed elsewhere in this volume (see Chapters 17–19). Remarks here will be confined to an overview of their role in the treatment of schizophrenia based on current knowledge.

The atypical drugs share an ability to produce fewer EPS than the conventional neuroleptics, although dose considerations are critical. As previously mentioned, many patients with schizophrenia will respond to low doses of typical neuroleptic drugs that produce few or no EPS. The problem is that many clinicians prescribe higher doses than are needed. It should be noted that there is no evidence that any of the newer atypical antipsychotic drugs produce agranulocytosis at the same level that clozapine does, so weekly monitoring of white blood cell (WBC) counts is not needed.

Risperidone.   Risperidone, a benzisoxazole compound, was the first novel atypical antipsychotic drug introduced after clozapine. It has been very rapidly adopted because of its low EPS and because its efficacy is at least as good as—and possibly superior to, especially for negative symptoms—that of conventional antipsychotics (Chouinard et al. 1993; Marder and Meibach 1994; Peuskens 1995). Like clozapine, risperidone is more potent as a 5-HT$_{2A}$ antagonist than as a D$_2$ antagonist.

The studies mentioned above, and reviewed by Owens and Risch in this volume (see Chapter 18), clearly indicate that risperidone is at least as effective as haloperidol for treating acute exacerbations and may be more effective for treating negative symptoms. A path analysis that considered the influence of positive symptoms, EPS, and depression on the improvement in negative symptoms associated with risperidone in a United States–Canada double-blind clinical trial of risperidone concluded that risperidone had an effect on primary negative symptoms (Möller et al. 1995). These advantages of risperidone over haloperidol in terms of EPS and negative symptoms have proven to be important for fostering compliance and preventing relapse. Risperidone has been found to produce improvement in working memory compared with haloperidol in a recent clinical trial (Green et al. 1997). These benefits are important for justifying the additional expense of this medication.

Clinical experience indicates that risperidone is sometimes effective in patients who fail to respond adequately to typical neuroleptic drugs, but the rate of positive response with this drug is not as high as that for clozapine. Indeed, in patients who are stable on clozapine, the attempt to switch to risperidone leads to a high rate of relapse. This should not be taken as an indication that risperidone is always ineffective in patients who do not respond adequately to typical neuroleptic drugs. There are no published reports of the efficacy of risperidone in patients who are clearly neuroleptic resistant. Comparisons with clozapine in this regard are of particular importance.

Risperidone, at the lower end of its dosage range (1–4 mg), has been shown to be comparable to olanzapine,

sertindole, ziprasidone, and quetiapine in EPS liability. If higher doses are used, however, risperidone may produce more EPS than do these agents. Risperidone at a mean dose of 6.1 mg/day produced more EPS and required benztropine more frequently than did clozapine (Daniel et al. 1996). Trials of 4–6 weeks at the lower doses (1–6 mg/day) are indicated to optimize the response to risperidone in relation to EPS. Doses as high as 16 mg/day are needed in some patients. There is no evidence at present to conclude that the risk of tardive dyskinesia is less with risperidone than with conventional neuroleptic drugs.

Risperidone produces less weight gain than clozapine (Daniel et al. 1996). Risperidone is associated with increases in serum prolactin levels that are comparable to those with typical neuroleptic drugs (Umbricht and Kane 1995). Risperidone has been found to induce activation (e.g., hypomanic symptoms) in some patients. Depot and skin patch formulations of risperidone are in development and should prove useful for patients who are unwilling or unable to take oral medication consistently.

Olanzapine.   Olanzapine, at doses of 10–15 mg/day, has been shown to be effective for the treatment of acute psychotic episodes in both first-episode and chronic schizophrenia patients (Beasley et al. 1996; Tollefson et al. 1997b). Once-a-day administration makes olanzapine convenient to use and appears not to produce significant EPS at recommended (10–15 mg/day) or even slightly higher doses (Beasley et al. 1996; Tollefson et al. 1997b). Thus, olanzapine may be better tolerated than risperidone in some patients who are very prone to develop EPS when higher doses are needed. Both drugs will prove useful in many patients with schizophrenia for whom compliance due to EPS is an issue at recommended doses.

A significant number of patients appear to require as much as 20 mg/day of olanzapine. As with risperidone, there is evidence that olanzapine is superior to haloperidol in the treatment of both negative and positive symptoms. A path analysis found evidence that olanzapine has a beneficial effect on primary negative symptoms (Tollefson and Sanger 1997).

Findings from a recent study suggest that olanzapine, compared with haloperidol, may be associated with lower risk for producing tardive dyskinesia. Treatment-emergent tardive dyskinesia in 707 olanzapine-treated patients over a median period of exposure of 237 days (range 42–964) was 7.0% compared with a rate of 16.2% in 197 patients treated with haloperidol for a median of 203 days (range 42–540 days; Fisher's two-tailed exact test; $P < 0.001$). Analysis of Abnormal Involuntary Movement Scale (AIMS) data showed the same results (Tollefson et al.

1997a). Much further work is needed in this regard.

The major side effects of olanzapine appear to be significant weight gain and sedation. Olanzapine does not produce increases in serum prolactin levels at clinically effective doses. Thus, some female patients may find olanzapine more acceptable than risperidone if they are sensitive to elevated prolactin levels. There is some evidence that compliance with olanzapine is superior to that with typical neuroleptic drugs. There is no evidence from controlled studies that olanzapine is effective in neuroleptic-resistant patients. Comparisons with clozapine are needed on this important issue. Preliminary data suggest that olanzapine has beneficial effects on some cognitive functions (H. Y. Meltzer and S. M. McGurk, unpublished observations). Like risperidone, olanzapine has been found to produce in some patients activation that may be hypomanic in nature. Skin patch formulations of olanzapine are in development.

Quetiapine. Quetiapine, another serotonin-dopamine antagonist, has preclinical effects in animal models of EPS that are very similar to those of clozapine. Quetiapine was shown to be superior to placebo and equivalent to chlorpromazine in early clinical trials in hospitalized schizophrenic patients (Goldstein and Arvanitis 1995; Small et al. 1997). There was no evidence that quetiapine was more effective than haloperidol in the treatment of positive or negative symptoms during a 6-week trial (Arvanitis et al. 1997). Data for more prolonged treatment periods are needed.

Twice-a-day administration is necessary for quetiapine (Casey 1996). The effective dosage range appears to be between 200 and 750 mg/day, with an optimal dosage of perhaps 300 mg/day (Arvanitis et al. 1997). There are no published data concerning its efficacy in patients with neuroleptic-resistant schizophrenia.

Quetiapine produces no increase in serum prolactin levels and has significant advantages in terms of EPS, appearing to be no more likely than placebo to produce EPS (Arvanitis et al. 1997; Casey 1996). As with olanzapine, the major side effects of quetiapine are weight gain, postural hypotension, and sedation. Quetiapine produces some increases in liver enzymes, but these do not appear to be clinically significant.

Sertindole. Sertindole, another serotonin-dopamine antagonist, is an imidazolidinone compound that appears to have particular selectivity for the limbic system. It has comparable potency in vitro for D_2 and 5-HT_{2A} and 5-HT_{2C} receptors. The application for its approval by the Food and Drug Administration (FDA) in the United States was withdrawn in January 1998. Clinical trials have demonstrated that sertindole is superior to placebo for the treatment of positive and negative symptoms (Van Kammen et al. 1996). Sertindole produces EPS that are comparable to those produced by placebo and does not elevate serum prolactin levels. Sertindole is associated with weight gain and sedation. It has minimal effect on extrapyramidal function throughout its effective dose range. Sertindole may be less likely than typical neuroleptics to produce tardive dyskinesia because of its very low liability to produce EPS.

As mentioned earlier in this section, sertindole prolongs the Q-T_c interval. There is little published evidence to date that this feature is associated with untoward clinical consequences (Casey 1996). However, additional evaluation of patients for the risk of an arrhythmia may be required before this compound can be marketed in the United States. Sertindole is also associated with decreased ejaculatory volume and nasal congestion. Twice-a-day administration is indicated.

Ziprasidone. Ziprasidone, the last of the serotonin-dopamine antagonists to be discussed here, should be available in the United States by 1998 (Seeger et al. 1995). In addition to its antagonism of 5-HT_{2A} and D_2 receptors, ziprasidone is a potent 5-HT_{1A} agonist—a feature that may have advantages for treating anxiety and depression in schizophrenia (Seeger et al. 1995). Early clinical trials indicate that ziprasidone is effective in treating positive and negative symptoms in patients with acute exacerbations. It is also effective in delaying relapse in patients with chronic schizophrenia.

Ziprasidone has a favorable profile with regard to elevations of serum prolactin and EPS. It appears to produce less weight gain than the other atypical antipsychotic drugs, although studies involving direct comparisons are needed to firmly establish this. It is not yet known whether ziprasidone is effective in treating patients with neuroleptic-resistant schizophrenia or in diminishing the risk of developing tardive dyskinesia.

Clozapine. Because of its ability to produce agranulocytosis, clozapine is not considered to be a first-line treatment (Marder and Van Putten 1988). However, it is highly effective in neuroleptic-responsive patients as well. Clozapine will be discussed in detail later in this chapter in the context of neuroleptic resistance.

There is some evidence that clozapine is superior to typical neuroleptic drugs in patients with non-treatment-resistant schizophrenia (see Meltzer and Ranjan 1996 for review), particularly in terms of cognitive measures (Lee et al. 1994). There is no evidence to date as to its superiority to other atypical neuroleptic drugs in non-treatment-resistant schizophrenia patients. However, until there is evidence to the contrary, it is reasonable to assume that clozapine has the least risk of producing EPS or tardive movement disorders of any of the atypical antipsychotic drugs.

It is not recommended at this point that clozapine be used for first-episode schizophrenia. However, clinicians should be alert to the possibility that if adequate trials of typical or other atypical antipsychotic drugs produce only control of positive symptoms, unsatisfactory outcome in other important dimensions (e.g., negative symptoms, cognition, mood, and suicidality) provides the basis for a clozapine trial.

Choice of an Atypical Antipsychotic Drug

For the clinician, choosing between the new, atypical antipsychotic drugs and the conventional neuroleptic agents represents a challenge. The benefits of the newer agents that have been demonstrated in controlled clinical trials are impressive. However, it is still necessary to show that these benefits can be achieved in routine clinical practice, where patients cannot be carefully selected and where polypharmacy may interfere with the actions of these agents.

The apparent advantages of risperidone and olanzapine over haloperidol in treating negative symptoms would appear to favor these two agents over quetiapine, sertindole, and ziprasidone. It must be emphasized, however, that the studies on which this suggestion is based did not directly compare these agents. The advantages these two drugs showed over haloperidol in their Phase 3 studies may not translate into real advantages over the last-mentioned three drugs in studies in which direct comparisons are made. In addition, effectiveness data from clinical practice would be invaluable for the identification of reliable and clinically significant differences between these agents.

It is also necessary to understand the magnitude of the advantages of atypical agents over conventional neuroleptic drugs in making the decision as to which drug to choose. Large-scale clinical trials can show statistically significant differences that are not very significant clinically.

Finally, the importance of significant advantages with regard to effects on cognitive function must be emphasized. As previously mentioned, risperidone, olanzapine, and clozapine have been shown in most, but not all, studies to have positive effects on certain aspects of cognitive function. Data for the effects of quetiapine, sertindole, and ziprasidone on cognition are needed. More data on the cognitive effects of all the atypical antipsychotic drugs,

along with follow-up data to indicate whether these effects translate into clinically significant differences (e.g., in the ability to work), are needed.

MAINTENANCE TREATMENT

Conventional neuroleptic drugs are still the most widely used treatment following the end of an acute episode, despite the evidence that the atypical antipsychotic drugs have considerable advantages for many patients. The choice between these classes of drugs is discussed later in this section. There is strong evidence that without continuous treatment with an effective antipsychotic agent, nearly all schizophrenic patients will relapse within a 12- to 24-month period. The rate of relapse is approximately 3.5% per month, so within 2 years of the acute episode nearly all schizophrenic patients will have relapsed. However, the rate of development of tardive dyskinesia is 4%–5% per year (Glazer et al. 1993; Kane et al. 1984), so those patients who continue to take conventional neuroleptic drugs indefinitely do so at some significant risk. For many patients, however, only mild forms of tardive dyskinesia develop, and these symptoms may be suppressed by the antipsychotic agent.

A number of studies have sought to define the most appropriate minimum dosage for effective maintenance treatment in schizophrenia (Hogarty et al. 1988; Kane et al. 1985; Marder et al. 1984, 1987). Markedly lower doses than those used to treat acute episodes may be effective. For most patients, doses in the moderate range are indicated for maintenance treatment (e.g., 5–15 mg/day of haloperidol or 12.5–25 mg of fluphenazine decanoate every 2 weeks) (Levinson et al. 1990; Rifkin et al. 1990; Van Putten et al. 1990). Hogarty et al. (1988) found that social adjustment was superior in patients receiving lower doses of neuroleptics for maintenance treatment. Higher doses provide little added protection and increase the risk or severity of EPS. Should moderate doses not prove satisfactory, the choice of the clinician is to raise the dose, with probable worsening of EPS, or to switch to an atypical antipsychotic drug. The latter may be the more satisfactory choice in most patients.

Depot neuroleptic drugs are used in many clinics to ensure adequate delivery of medication. Visiting nurses or case managers help ensure that patients receive injections at scheduled times. Either fluphenazine decanoate at doses of 12.5–25 mg every 2 weeks or haloperidol decanoate at doses of 50–100 mg every 2–4 weeks is of great value in ensuring compliance. Unfortunately, there are as yet no long-acting preparations of the novel antipsychotic drugs. However, as noted above, efforts are under way to develop long-activity formulations of risperidone and olanzapine.

Plasma-level determinations of neuroleptic drugs to guide dosage have not proven very helpful (Van Putten et al. 1991). Findings from some early studies suggested that there was a curvilinear relationship between plasma levels of some neuroleptics and therapeutic response—a "therapeutic window"—with both low and high plasma levels resulting in less successful treatment. Van Putten et al. (1991) found that the optimal range for plasma levels of haloperidol is 5–12 ng/mL. At present, plasma levels of neuroleptics, with the exception of clozapine, are rarely monitored (Hasegawa et al. 1993).

The importance of striving for compliance with treatment in schizophrenic patients cannot be overstated. Relapse rates due to noncompliance of as high as 50% within a year after discharge from hospital for an acute episode have been reported (Weiden et al. 1991). Factors associated with poor compliance include persistent psychotic symptoms, poor insight with denial of illness, dissatisfaction with care providers, persistent EPS, and poor social support. Case management and family education may decrease noncompliance. However, use of depot neuroleptics or more effective oral medications with low EPS potential is probably the most important element in a compliance program.

Management of Side Effects of Neuroleptics

Side effects of treatment with conventional neuroleptics are common (Ayd 1961; Casey 1991; Chakos et al. 1992) and are the chief reason for poor compliance with treatment (Van Putten 1974; Weiden et al. 1991). For sake of convenience, they may be divided into neurological (Table 36–2) and nonneurological adverse effects (Table 36–3).

Neurological Side Effects

The main neurological side effects of neuroleptics are EPS (acute dystonic reactions, parkinsonism, akathisia), tardive dyskinesia and other tardive movement disorders, neuroleptic malignant syndrome (NMS), and seizures (Table 36–2). Ayd (1961) reported on the incidence of side effects in more than 3,000 patients evaluated for as many as 6 years and noted that 38% of patients showed EPS: 2% had dystonia, 15% parkinsonism, and 21% akathisia. In a prospective study of 70 "first-episode" schizophrenic patients (Chakos et al. 1992), 38% of patients showed no EPS, whereas 38% had one form of EPS, 21% two forms, and 3% all three forms. Parkinsonism was

observed in 34% of patients, acute dystonia in 36%, and akathisia in 18%. Acute EPS were associated with both higher baseline psychopathology and better treatment outcome.

Acute dystonic reactions. Acute dystonic reactions typically occur within the first 4 days of neuroleptic treatment and are more common in young male patients who are receiving high-potency neuroleptics (Casey 1991). These reactions are characterized by sustained, involuntary muscular spasms, most often involving the facial, head, or neck muscles; examples include spasm of masticatory muscles (trismus), spasm of the orbicularis oculi (blepharospasm), oculogyric crises (fixed upward gazing of the eyes), torticollis, dysarthria, and dysphagia. Such spasms are painful and very distressing and may go undetected or be misinterpreted by staff.

The exact pathophysiological mechanism underlying acute dystonia is unclear. Acute dystonia is thought to be caused by an acute hypodopaminergic state in the basal ganglia due to neuroleptic blockade of dopamine receptors or, alternatively, a relative imbalance between neuroleptic-induced elevation in presynaptic dopamine turnover and postsynaptic receptor blockade.

Treatment of acute dystonia includes one or more parenteral injections of an anticholinergic (e.g., benztropine mesylate 2 mg intramuscularly) or antihistamine (e.g., diphenhydramine 50 mg intravenously) drug. Oral anticholinergic drugs are generally administered thereafter. If there is a recurrence, then the neuroleptic dosage should be reduced or a switch should be made to an atypical agent. Prophylactic use of anticholinergics to avoid the development of EPS is not indicated because of the risk of anticholinergic toxicity and the possible increase in the risk for tardive dyskinesia (Boodhood and Sadler 1991).

Parkinsonism. Parkinsonism, which is similar to idiopathic Parkinson's disease, consists of tremor, rigidity, and bradykinesia and appears to be a direct (i.e., dose-related) consequence of dopamine receptor blockade in the nigrostriatal pathway (Casey 1991). These symptoms generally emerge after a few days of neuroleptic treatment and are more common in older patients. More than 60% of patients may show one or more of the features of parkinsonism.

Early detection of parkinsonism is important because it is readily treated with the addition of an anticholinergic drug or a dopaminomimetic drug (e.g., amantadine 100 mg twice a day). With patients who manifest parkinsonism at low doses of neuroleptics, a switch should be made to an atypical agent, because these patients may be at increased risk for tardive dyskinesia (Barnes 1990).

Table 36–2.   Neurological side effects of conventional neuroleptic drugs

Side effect	Characteristics	Prevalence	Risk factors	Management
Acute dystonia	Oculogyric crises; dysarthria; acute neck and truncal spasms	2%–90%	Young males; high-potency neuroleptics	Reduce dosage or switch to a different drug class; administer anticholinergic (benztropine mesylate 2 mg im/po or diphenhydramine 50 mg im or po)
Parkinsonism	Tremor; cogwheel rigidity; bradykinesia	2%–90%	Dose related	Reduce dosage; administer anticholinergic
Akathisia	Subjective and objective motor restlessness	35%	Dose related; low serum iron status?	Reduce dosage or switch to another drug class; administer benzodiazepine (diazepam 2 mg three times a day), β-blocker (propranolol 10–40 mg twice a day)
Tardive dyskinesia	Involuntary choreic or athetoid movements, orofacial and peripheral	5%–50%	Female gender; age; brain disease; concomitant anti-parkinsonian treatments?; history of EPS; affective symptoms	Reduce or discontinue neuroleptic; administer vitamin E 400–1,200 mg, benzodiazepine, β-blocker (valproate 400–1,000 mg), clozapine
Neuroleptic malignant syndrome	Pyrexia; muscle rigidity; autonomic instability; clouding of consciousness; elevated CK	0.1%–1%	High, rapid neuroleptic dosing; agitation	Rule out other medical conditions; discontinue neuroleptic; use supportive measures; administer dopamine agonist (bromocriptine 15–30 mg); administer muscle relaxant (dantrolene 100–400 mg)
Seizures	Grand mal; myoclonic	0.1%	Dosage; epileptogenic tendency	Reduce dosage; administer concomitant anticonvulsant drug (valproate 400–1,000 mg)

Note.   im = intramuscular; po = oral; EPS = extrapyramidal side effects; CK = creatine kinase.

Table 36–3.   Nonneurological side effects of conventional neuroleptic drugs

Side effect	Characteristics	Prevalence	Management
Sedation	Tolerance developing over time	~70%	Reduce dosage; switch to nonsedating drug; add L-dopa or methylphenidate
Weight gain		15%–20%	Use practical measures
Hypotension	Antiadrenergic effect	10%–30%	Reduce dosage; switch to a different drug class
Anticholinergic effects	Cognitive impairment; blurred vision; dry mouth; constipation; sexual dysfunction	~60%	Reduce dosage; switch to a low anticholinergic drug
Hormonal	Elevated prolactin; reduced testosterone	Variable	Treat breast abscess if one develops; reduce dosage; add bromocriptine; switch to olanzapine
Marrow toxicity	Agranulocytosis	<0.1%	Obtain hematologist consult; discontinue neuroleptic
Jaundice	Cholestatic	<0.1%	Investigate for other causes; switch to another drug
Retinitis pigmentosa		Low	Avoid high doses of thioridazine

Akathisia.   Akathisia is a syndrome of subjective and objective motor restlessness associated with neuroleptic treatment. Patients experience anxiety, inner restlessness, inability to stand still, and constant pacing (Adler et al. 1989). It may be very distressing for the patient and is a chief cause of neuroleptic noncompliance (Van Putten 1974; Weiden et al. 1991). Akathisia is often overlooked or misinterpreted as anxiety or worsening of psychosis.

The pathophysiology of akathisia is the least understood of the acute EPS and does not appear solely to reflect nigrostriatal dopamine receptor blockade. Alterations in iron metabolism may be a predisposing factor for akathisia (Barnes et al. 1992).

Anticholinergic drugs are of limited use in the treatment of akathisia, but the addition of a β-blocker (e.g., propranolol 20 mg twice a day) or a benzodiazepine (e.g., diazepam 2 mg three times a day) may be more effective (Adler et al. 1989). Reducing neuroleptic dosage and switching to an atypical antipsychotic are the other alternatives for the management of akathisia.

Tardive dyskinesia and other tardive movement disorders.   Tardive dyskinesia and tardive dystonia are serious, potentially irreversible side effects of long-term neuroleptic treatment that are characterized by the late appearance of choreiform or athetoid movements of body regions, particularly in the orofacial and truncal regions (Barnes 1990; Casey 1991). Although neuroleptic dosage and duration of treatment have been implicated as risk factors, their association with tardive dyskinesia is inconsistent (Barnes 1990). Old age, female gender, affective disorders, and evidence of organic brain impairment are risk factors for tardive dyskinesia. Diabetes has also been established as a risk factor (Woerner et al. 1993). Acute EPS have been associated specifically with vulnerability to tardive dyskinesia (Barnes 1990).

Supersensitivity of nigrostriatal dopamine receptors due to chronic exposure to neuroleptics continues to have heuristic value in elucidating the pathophysiology of tardive dyskinesia (Casey 1991, 1993). However, modulatory effects of other neurotransmitter systems, such as the γ-aminobutyric acid (GABA)ergic and noradrenergic systems, are also considered to be of importance, with partial support for their involvement derived from animal studies and clinical studies (Casey 1991; J. Gerlach and Casey 1988).

Current management strategies for tardive dyskinesia reflect its proposed pathophysiology. First, the risk of tardive dyskinesia may be minimized through use of the lowest effective dose of neuroleptic for the shortest duration of time, clinical circumstances permitting. Discontinua-

tion of neuroleptics alone results in a 50% improvement in tardive dyskinesia by 3 months in more than a third of patients, with further improvement over time (Glazer et al. 1990). Second, reduction in neuroleptic dose may alleviate symptoms of tardive dyskinesia, although often these symptoms initially worsen as part of a withdrawal dyskinesia. Third, several classes of agents have been tried for the treatment of tardive dyskinesia. Both dopaminergic and dopamine-depleting agents have been tried in the treatment of tardive dyskinesia, but the results are at best inconsistent (Feltner and Hertzman 1993). GABAergic drugs (e.g., γ-vinyl GABA), adrenergic drugs (e.g., pindolol, γ-linoleic acid), calcium channel blockers (e.g., nifedipine, verapamil), and clonazepam have all been used, with limited success, in the treatment of tardive dyskinesia (Feltner and Hertzman 1993).

More recently, vitamin E has been advocated as an effective treatment on the basis of theories of oxidation and free-radical processes in the development of tardive dyskinesia. Although early findings led to initial optimism, more recent studies have not confirmed any significant benefit of vitamin E for tardive dyskinesia.

At present, clozapine is the best treatment option for moderate to severe, persistent tardive dyskinesia (Lieberman et al. 1991; Meltzer and Luchins 1984). Clozapine has, as of yet, not been directly implicated in the induction of tardive dyskinesia and may even actively ameliorate it. In a prospective study of tardive dyskinesia in 30 clozapine-treated schizophrenic patients, 16 patients showed a 50% or greater reduction in tardive dyskinesia; this effect was most marked in patients with severe tardive dyskinesia and dystonia (Lieberman et al. 1991). For patients with severe tardive dyskinesia or dystonia, switching to clozapine is usually desirable.

Neuroleptic malignant syndrome.   NMS is an uncommon (incidence < 0.9%), potentially fatal complication of neuroleptic treatment. It is characterized by the development of fever, rigidity, autonomic instability, altered consciousness, and elevated creatine kinase (CK) activity (the last-mentioned having poor diagnostic specificity) (Meltzer 1973) and raised WBC count in the absence of any other medical condition that might explain these symptoms (Kellam 1990; Rosebush and Stewart 1989). Rapid increases in dosage of neuroleptic drugs, parenteral administration, agitation, and diagnosis of affective disorder are all risk factors for the development of NMS (Kellam 1990). NMS may develop after removal of antiparkinsonian agents. The pathophysiology of NMS is suggested to involve acute dopaminergic blockade in the hypothalamus and/or basal ganglia.

When NMS is suspected, the patient must have a thorough physical examination and organic and septic workup to rule out other causes. If no other causes are evident, then immediate cessation of neuroleptics (and lithium, if present) and provision of full supportive measures are recommended. A dopamine agonist (e.g., bromocriptine 30 mg/day) and a muscle relaxant (e.g., dantrolene 400 mg/day) should be given as adjunctive therapy. ECT may also be given to manage acute psychotic symptoms during NMS (Hermesh et al. 1987). The risk of recurrence on reexposure to neuroleptics—approximately 30% of patients have a recurrence of NMS—may be minimized by delaying rechallenge by 2 weeks post NMS and by using an antipsychotic of an alternative class (Rosebush and Stewart 1989). Switching to a low-EPS atypical antipsychotic is recommended.

Seizures.   Standard neuroleptic drugs lower the seizure threshold. A history of epilepsy or organic brain impairment is a risk factor for the development of seizures in persons taking neuroleptics. However, seizures occur uncommonly during treatment and are more likely to arise during neuroleptic withdrawal, particularly when complicated by withdrawal from benzodiazepines or other agents.

Nonneurological Side Effects

Nonneurological adverse effects of standard antipsychotic medication (Table 36–3) are, in general, of lesser morbidity but may be distressing for patients and may limit the choice and ultimate dosage of neuroleptic.

Most patients experience some sedative effects while taking neuroleptics. Sedation is more commonly associated with low-potency agents that possess prominent antiadrenergic and antimuscarinic effects (e.g., mesoridazine) than with other, higher-potency agents. Tolerance usually develops, although if sedation persists, then divided doses and adjustment of time when doses are taken, neuroleptic dose reduction, *or* substitution is a worthwhile management strategy.

Weight gain is a particular problem with clozapine and olanzapine. Increases of 5%–10% of base weight are often noted. Dietary counseling and exercise programs are desirable. Weight gain with other atypical and typical antipsychotics is less frequent and less extensive.

Hypotension is a frequent cardiovascular side effect attributable to an α_1 antiadrenergic effect and more commonly seen with low-potency agents. Tachycardia may also be observed, as may nonspecific T-wave changes on the electrocardiogram (ECG), which result from atropine-like effects on the myocardium.

Common anticholinergic adverse effects include blurred vision, precipitation of glaucoma, dry mouth, reduced gastrointestinal tract motility, urinary hesitancy, and impotence. Anticholinergic toxicity, ranging from subtle memory impairment to delirium, may result from concomitant use of anticholinergic drugs; the elderly are particularly prone to this problem. These adverse effects may be avoided by careful clinical observation and judicious management of neuroleptic dosage and any concomitant medications.

Hyperprolactinemia, the chief endocrine side effect of standard neuroleptics, is a direct consequence of blockade of pituitary dopamine receptors (Meltzer and Fang 1976). Hyperprolactinemia accounts for amenorrhea in female patients and for galactorrhea, which may occasionally result in a breast abscess. Also, standard neuroleptics may reduce urinary concentrations of estrogen and progesterone.

Leukocytosis, eosinophilia, or leukopenia may occur with treatment with standard neuroleptics, especially phenothiazines. Agranulocytosis, however, occurs in only 1 of 2,000 patients receiving standard neuroleptics. Because WBC counts are typically not monitored with these drugs, a proportion of these cases are fatal, so the mortality rate may be comparable to that with clozapine. Leukopenia (WBC $\leq 3,000/mm^3$) may forewarn the clinician of impending agranulocytosis, and neuroleptic medication should be withdrawn.

Neuroleptics uncommonly induce hepatitis with a cholestatic pattern that generally is self-limiting and resolves with brief cessation of treatment.

Dermatological reactions, hypersensitivity urticaria, photosensitivity, or slate-gray hyperpigmentation occurs in fewer than 5% of patients receiving standard neuroleptics. These effects are managed conservatively, with dermatological consultation as necessary. Pigmentation retinopathy has been described in patients receiving doses of thioridazine above 1,000 mg/day, so low doses of thioridazine are advocated in long-term maintenance therapy.

It is also important to recognize that adverse effects can also occur from interactions with other drugs (Goff and Baldessarini 1993). Such effects may result from alterations in the metabolism of neuroleptics (e.g., carbamazepine induces the hepatic microsomal system that metabolizes haloperidol, with the result that plasma levels are lowered) or additive toxic effects (e.g., combined anticholinergic effects with concomitant use of tricyclic antidepressant medications). Almost all antidepressants will raise antipsychotic blood levels as a result of metabolic interactions. Although such an effect amounts to increasing the dose of neuroleptics, antidepressants increase vulnerability to psychosis. Lithium may induce neurotoxic reactions when combined with neuroleptics. Patients need to be alerted in advance to these potential adverse effects. Commonly prescribed drugs that interact with antipsychotics include alcohol, anticonvulsants, anxiolytics, antidepressants, antihypertensives, cimetidine, disulfiram, and lithium.

Discontinuation of Neuroleptic Treatment

Because of the high probability of relapse, indefinite maintenance treatment with an antipsychotic is prudent. A targeted, or intermittent, maintenance strategy has been used to reduce relapse in stable patients. This strategy relies heavily on the patient's and relatives' ability to recognize prodromal symptoms of relapse: anxiety, irritability, sleep disturbance, perceptual aberrations, oddity of behavior, and paranoid ideas of reference. Intensive psychosocial and educative support are also necessary.

Unfortunately, the optimism engendered by earlier studies (Carpenter et al. 1987; Herz et al. 1982) has not been maintained after further study (Carpenter et al. 1990; Herz et al. 1991; Jolley et al. 1989, 1990). More recent studies have indicated that patients on targeted strategies not only fare significantly worse in terms of relapse (both higher rates and greater severity) but also show only modest reductions in overall side effects when compared with patients who are continued on conventional maintenance treatment.

Augmentation of Neuroleptic Drugs

Various augmenting agents have been used to enhance conventional or atypical antipsychotic drug response and to treat other, specific associated symptoms (Table 36–4). In general, these drugs, when added to neuroleptics or atypical antipsychotics, have at best only marginal effects on both positive and negative symptoms (Christison et al. 1991; Meltzer 1992). Anticonvulsants and lithium may produce clinically significant improvement in aggression.

The initial optimism for the efficacy of lithium augmentation in schizophrenia (Schulz et al. 1990) does not appear to be justified. Moreover, lithium therapy needs to be closely monitored to avoid neurotoxicity associated with concomitant neuroleptic treatment and increased risk of NMS.

Recent interest has focused on the use of selective serotonin reuptake inhibitors (SSRIs), with some preliminary findings showing encouraging benefits in treating persistent positive and negative symptoms (Goff et al. 1991; Silver and Nassar 1992).

Benzodiazepines have also been shown to be helpful in ameliorating persistent psychotic symptoms in some patients (Meltzer 1992; Wolkowitz and Pickar 1991). However, these effects are, at best, modest and must be weighed against the adverse effects of these agents and also the potential for rebound psychotic and anxiety symptoms, which are particularly associated with the withdrawal of high-potency triazolobenzodiazepines such as alprazolam.

When negative symptoms predominate, the use of L-dopa or methylphenidate to accentuate dopaminergic activity may be of benefit, although this strategy may be associated with a risk of precipitating a relapse of positive symptoms.

Anticonvulsant drugs, such as valproate and carbamazepine, appear to be ineffective as a primary treatment for schizophrenia (Carpenter and Strauss 1991), but they may be of use in persistently psychotic patients who manifest impulsive or violent behavior (Meltzer 1992). Patients who have electroencephalogram (EEG) abnormalities or episodic dyscontrol behaviors may also derive benefit from adjunctive anticonvulsant therapy. There is a very extensive literature, previously well reviewed (Christison et al. 1991; Meltzer 1992), on the use of opioid drugs, β-blockers, calcium channel blockers, and neuropeptide analogues in treatment-refractory schizophrenia. With the possible exception of propranolol, there is as yet little evidence to support the use of these agents.

Finally, the role of ECT in the treatment of the persistently psychotic patient has recently come under renewed scrutiny (Sajatovic and Meltzer 1993). Maintenance ECT may be of value in the management of treatment-refractory schizophrenia and can result in reduction in positive symptoms and rates of rehospitalization (Sajatovic and Meltzer 1993). However, ECT needs to be given at least monthly.

Table 36–4.	Neuroleptic augmentation strategies in treatment-refractory schizophrenia
Symptom(s)	**Adjunctive treatment**
Persistent positive symptoms	Lithium, anticonvulsants, electroconvulsive therapy
Persistent negative symptoms	L-Dopa, bromocriptine, benzodiazepine
Depressive symptoms	Antidepressants, lithium
Hypomania	Lithium
Anxiety	Benzodiazepine
Aggression	Anticonvulsants

PHARMACOTHERAPY OF ANTIPSYCHOTIC DRUG–RESISTANT SCHIZOPHRENIA

Clozapine

Clozapine, a dibenzodiazepine chemically related to loxapine, was first identified as a promising antipsychotic that produces few or no EPS (for review, see Baldessarini and Frankenburg 1991). At least six controlled studies demonstrated that clozapine had superior efficacy compared with typical antipsychotic drugs for the treatment of neuroleptic-responsive schizophrenia (e.g., Ekblöm and Haggström 1974; Fischer-Cornelssen and Ferner 1976; I. Gerlach et al. 1974). However, in 1975, eight patients treated with clozapine died from agranulocytosis in southwestern Finland (Amsler et al. 1977). All of these cases of agranulocytosis occurred within the first 4 months of treatment. The overall incidence of agranulocytosis is thought to be 1%.

Clozapine was withdrawn from general use in Europe and from further clinical trials in the United States. However, because many of the schizophrenic patients who were withdrawn from clozapine had a marked relapse and did not respond well to reinstitution of typical neuroleptics, use of clozapine was permitted on a restricted basis in several western European countries. Clinical experience with clozapine over the next decade suggested that clozapine not only caused lower EPS but also was devoid of risk for tardive dyskinesia (Casey 1989). Moreover, additional clinical evidence for its superiority in efficacy was obtained, although not from controlled studies (Juul Povlsen et al. 1985; Kuha and Miettinen 1986; Lindström 1988).

These studies led to the first controlled trial of clozapine in treatment-resistant schizophrenia, which was conducted by one of the present authors (H. Y. M.) and colleagues (Kane et al. 1988). In a double-blind trial of 6 weeks' duration, clozapine and chlorpromazine were compared in nearly 300 hospitalized patients with treatment-resistant schizophrenia. Treatment resistance was defined as the failure to respond to at least three separate trials of neuroleptics, from at least two different chemical classes, over a 5-year period at dosages equivalent to 1,000 mg/day of chlorpromazine or greater for a period of 6 weeks.

During the initial, open-label phase of the study, patients were treated with haloperidol (up to 60 mg/day or more) for 6 weeks. Responders to haloperidol were excluded from the double-blind phase of the study. Nonresponders were randomly assigned to a 6-week, double-blind trial with either clozapine (up to 900 mg/day) or chlorpromazine (up to 1,800 mg/day) and benztropine (up to 6 mg/day). Improvement in this study was defined as 1) reduction of more than 20% from baseline in the Brief Psychiatric Rating Scale (BPRS) total score and 2) either a posttreatment CGI Scale score of 3 or less or a posttreatment BPRS total score of 35 or lower. Of all patients who completed at least 1 week of double-blind treatment, only 4% of patients treated with chlorpromazine and benztropine were responders, compared with 30% of clozapine-treated patients. Response onset was as brief as 1 week for some patients.

As a result of this study, clozapine was approved for use in neuroleptic-responsive and -resistant schizophrenic patients by the FDA in 1989. By the end of 1996, it had been administered to approximately 175,000 patients in the United States, with about 90,000 having remained in treatment for at least 6 months. Numerous other countries also approved clozapine as a result of this study.

The results of the Kane et al. study were confirmed in a crossover, placebo-controlled, double-blind comparison of long-term fluphenazine and clozapine treatment in 21 patients with either neuroleptic-resistant or -intolerant schizophrenia (Pickar et al. 1992). Clozapine, in comparison with both fluphenazine and placebo, was significantly superior in reducing psychopathology. Also, Breier et al. (1994) reported that in a 10-week, double-blind, parallel-groups comparison of clozapine and haloperidol, clozapine was superior to haloperidol in reducing symptoms among schizophrenic outpatients who had only a partial response to typical neuroleptics.

Subsequent experience has indicated that the response to clozapine may either be very rapid (≤ 6 weeks) in about 30% of patients (Stern et al. 1994) or delayed (6 weeks to 6 months) in another 30% (Lieberman et al. 1994; Meltzer 1995a). Thus, Meltzer et al. (1989) reported an open study of 51 schizophrenic patients in which 31 (60.8%) of the patients showed at least a 20% decrease in BPRS total score. The mean duration of treatment at the time of the report was 10.3 ± 8.1 months. In half of those who responded, the response occurred only after 3 months of treatment or longer. In a follow-up report on 85 patients with treatment-resistant schizophrenia, 51 of whom had been in the preliminary study, 81.5% of the patients who were still being administered clozapine at the end of 12 months showed a decrease of 20% or more in the BPRS total score (Meltzer 1992). Lieberman et al. (1994) reported that the probability of response to clozapine in 66 patients with treatment-resistant schizophrenia or schizoaffective disorder was about 0.35 through 6 weeks of treatment. It declined to 0.22 between 12 and 26 weeks and to 0.19 between 26 and 39 weeks. There were additional responders between weeks 26 and 39. Thirty-three (50%) of the patients in this study were responders by 52 weeks.

Efficacy

Effect on psychopathology. Clozapine has been found to be significantly superior to typical neuroleptics in reducing the total score on the BPRS Positive Symptoms subscale as well as the scores on individual items that constitute this subscale (i.e., Conceptual Disorganization, Hallucinatory Behavior, Suspiciousness, and Unusual Thought Content) (Claghorn et al. 1987; Kane et al. 1988; Pickar et al. 1992).

Effect on negative symptoms. Kane et al. (1988), in their controlled trial of clozapine in treatment-resistant schizophrenia, found clozapine to be clearly more effective than chlorpromazine in reducing scores on the BPRS Negative Symptoms subscale (i.e., Emotional Withdrawal, Blunted Affect, Psychomotor-Retardation, and Disorientation). Clozapine has been reported to decrease significantly scores on the BPRS Withdrawal/Retardation subscale (Meltzer 1989a). This subscale differs from the Negative Symptoms subscale in that it does not include Disorientation, which is more appropriately part of the Disorganization cluster. Furthermore, improvement in Withdrawal/Retardation subscale scores was independent of improvement in the Paranoid Disturbance subscale scores—an indication that the improvement in negative symptoms was independent of the improvement in positive symptoms.

Clozapine is also effective in ameliorating the negative symptoms in patients who do not have notable positive symptoms (Meltzer and Zureick 1989). Pickar et al. (1992) found significantly more improvement in scores on the BPRS Negative Symptoms subscale, but not in those on the Scale for the Assessment of Negative Symptoms (SANS), in clozapine-treated patients compared with fluphenazine-treated patients. Breier et al. (1994), in their comparison of clozapine and haloperidol treatment in outpatients with a partial neuroleptic response, did find significantly greater improvement, as measured by the SANS total score, with clozapine treatment. However, they found no differences between the effects of clozapine and those of haloperidol on negative symptoms among patients designated as having "deficit" schizophrenia, based on the Schedule for the Deficit Syndrome (Kirkpatrick et al. 1989). These findings raise the issue of whether clozapine's effect on negative symptoms may result from changes in associated features such as depression and EPS.

Clozapine has been reported to produce a significant decrease in ratings on the Schedule for Affective Disorders and Schizophrenia–C (SADS-C) Disorganization factor, which includes loose association, poverty of thought content, incoherence, and inappropriate affect (Meltzer 1992). The effect of clozapine on the Disorganization cluster of the SADS-C was superior to its effect on both the Positive and Negative subscales of that same schedule.

Clozapine is effective in improving some of these deficits in patients with treatment-resistant schizophrenia. Hagger et al. (1993) studied cognitive function and psychopathology in 36 patients with treatment-resistant schizophrenia before initiation of clozapine and at 6 weeks and 6 months of clozapine treatment. Compared with 26 healthy control subjects, the schizophrenic patients were noted to have deficits in measures of memory, executive function, and attention. With clozapine treatment, significant improvement occurred in retrieval from reference memory at 6 weeks and 6 months and in some measures of executive function (Wechsler Intelligence Scale for Children—Revised Maze Test), attention (Wechsler Adult Intelligence Scale—Revised [WAIS-R] Digit Symbol subtest), and recall memory (Verbal List Learning Test) at 6 months. Classen and Laux (1988) reported that 7 days of treatment with clozapine tended to produce better performance on the Stroop Color and Color Word Tests than with haloperidol or flupentixol. Goldberg et al. (1993) reported that after 3–24 months of clozapine treatment, clozapine had no beneficial effect on attention, memory, and higher-level problem solving in 15 psychotic, primarily schizophrenic, patients. Some of these patients also received a variety of other psychotropic drugs. In a recent study, two groups of 19 patients were treated with clozapine or haloperidol for 10 weeks. Clozapine produced significantly greater improvement than haloperidol in two tests: Category Fluency and WAIS-R Block Design. Thirty-three of these patients were treated with clozapine for a year; performance on both Category Fluency and WAIS-R Block Design, as well as on the Mooney Faces Closure Test, was found at 1 year to have improved (Buchanan et al. 1994).

Effect on mood symptoms. Clozapine has been reported to be effective in decreasing both manic and depressive symptoms in patients with treatment-resistant schizoaffective disorder (McElroy et al. 1991; Naber and Hippius 1990; Naber et al. 1989, 1992; Owen et al. 1993; Wood and Rubinstein 1990). Overall, clozapine was found to be more effective in schizoaffective patients than in schizophrenic patients. Naber et al. (1989) found that 45% of 229 patients with schizophrenia and 65% of 55 patients with schizoaffective disorder had marked improvement in symptoms with clozapine treatment. Owen et al.

(1993) reported that 112 schizoaffective patients, as compared with 37 schizophrenic patients, had significantly greater decreases in the BPRS total score. In a retrospective study of 39 patients with schizophrenia, 25 patients with schizoaffective disorder, and 14 patients with bipolar disorder with psychotic feelings, the patients with affective disorders and bipolar disorder showed significantly higher response rates to clozapine compared with the schizophrenic patients (McElroy et al. 1991).

In a recent prospective study, clozapine markedly reduced suicidality, especially low- and high-probability suicide attempts, in patients with treatment-resistant schizophrenia and schizoaffective disorder (Meltzer and Okayli 1995). This decrease in suicidality was associated with improvement in depression and hopelessness, as measured by the Hamilton Rating Scale for Depression (Hamilton 1960). These findings could be the basis for reevaluation of the risk-benefit assessment of clozapine. Thus, the overall morbidity and mortality for treatment-resistant schizophrenia could be less with clozapine than with typical neuroleptic drugs because of decreased suicidality. Suicide has been reported to occur in 9%–13% of schizophrenic patients, whereas the risk of agranulocytosis from clozapine is less than 1%, and the mortality is approximately 0.01% (Alvir et al. 1993).

Dosage and Administration

The recommended starting dosage of clozapine is 12.5–25 mg/day to test for possible hypotension. The dosage of clozapine may be increased by 25 mg every other day until it reaches 100 mg/day. This can be done on an outpatient basis if the patient is able to adhere to the prescribed schedule or if there are family members or case managers who can assist the patient. The total dose can then be increased by 50 mg every other day until a dosage of 300–450 mg/day is reached. Twice-a-day dosage is recommended, because the half-life of clozapine is 16 hours (Choc et al. 1987; Jann et al. 1993). The dosage need not exceed 450–600 mg/day in most adults age 60 years or younger in the initial phase of treatment. However, if response at 600 mg/day is unsatisfactory, the dosage should be further increased up to a maximum of 900 mg/day. The dosage of clozapine required in the elderly is usually 200–300 mg/day but may be as low as 5–100 mg/day (Kronig et al. 1995). No data are available as to whether lower dosages of clozapine are needed for maintenance treatment. Clozapine is effective in adolescent patients with schizophrenia (Birmaher et al. 1992). The dosage may have to be reduced because of sedation and hypersalivation.

To date, no fixed-dose studies have been done to determine the optimal dosage in treatment-resistant schizophrenia. In the United States, dosages of 400–600 mg/day (mean dosage 444 mg/day) are most common, whereas in Europe, dosages in the range of 200–500 mg/day or lower (mean dosage 284 mg/day) are most often used (Fleischhacker et al. 1994; Naber et al. 1989). The reasons for this discrepancy are unknown at this time but could be related to more common use of concomitant neuroleptic drugs in Europe.

In general, clozapine is best given as monotherapy from the start. If this is not clinically feasible, then the medication regimen should be simplified as much as possible so that the patient is receiving a single neuroleptic such as haloperidol (in oral form only). Patients should be withdrawn from typical neuroleptic drugs as the dosage of clozapine is increased to 450 mg/day. Benzodiazepines should be avoided because of the risk (based mainly on case reports) of respiratory depression with concomitant use of clozapine and benzodiazepines during the initial phases of treatment. The duration of a trial with clozapine before it is considered to be ineffective may be as long as 6 months (Lieberman et al. 1994; Meltzer 1989b, 1995a; Safferman et al. 1991).

Clozapine and Extrapyramidal Symptoms

Clozapine produces remarkably few EPS (Lieberman et al. 1991, 1994) and can suppress tardive dyskinesia or dystonia (Chengappa et al. 1994; Lieberman et al. 1994). The rate of suppression may be slow, with some patients showing no change until after 6 months of treatment. The rate of akathisia in clozapine-treated patients is also low (Chengappa et al. 1994; Claghorn et al. 1987). These features give clozapine very significant advantages over typical neuroleptics and possibly other atypical antipsychotic agents as well.

Side Effects

The side effects of clozapine have been reviewed by Safferman et al. (1991). Important side effects of clozapine and their management are highlighted in Table 36–5. The most serious of these is agranulocytosis, which is reported to occur in slightly fewer than 1% of patients receiving clozapine (Alvir et al. 1993). It is possible that after 1998, weekly monitoring of WBC counts will be required in the United States for only the first 6 months, after which time biweekly monitoring will be required. Currently, weekly monitoring on an indefinite basis is required. The peak risk period for developing agranulocytosis is in the first 18 weeks of treatment; as yet, there are no useful predictors

Table 36–5. Side effects of clozapine

Side effect	Incidence	Action
Agranulocytosis	0.8%	Monitor WBC weekly; if WBC < 2,000/mm^3: stop clozapine; hospitalize; treat infection aggressively; never give clozapine again
Seizures	3%, dose related	Decrease dose of clozapine; add phenytoin or valproate
Tachycardia	>25%	Treat if heart rate is >140 bpm or patient is symptomatic; add low dose of β-blocker
Hypertension	9%	Monitor; add β-blocker if BP high or persistent
Hypotension	9%	Monitor; encourage fluid intake; alter dosage regimen
Dizziness	20%	Tolerance often develops; monitor; alter dosage regimen
Sedation	40%, dose related	Give maximum dosage at night; reduce total daily dose; add methylphenidate 20–40 mg/day
Weight gain	Variable, >3%	Reduce diet; prescribe exercise
Hypersalivation	31%	Benztropine mesylate or clonidine may help
Constipation	14%	Prescribe laxative, if required
Nausea	5%	Use supportive measures

Note. WBC = white blood cell; bpm = beats per minute; BP = blood pressure.

as to which patients are likely to develop this side effect. Age and female gender may be risk factors for the development of clozapine-related agranulocytosis (Alvir et al. 1993). For patients who show an abrupt or marked fall in WBC count or whose WBC count falls to between 3,500/mm^3 and 3,000/mm^3 inclusive, the WBC count should be checked twice a week. If the WBC count falls below 3,000/mm^3 but is not less than 2,000/mm^3, clozapine should be stopped and the WBC count monitored daily. A WBC count of less than 2,000/mm^3 or an absolute neutrophil count of less than 1,000/mm^3 is an indication for immediate cessation of clozapine. When the WBC count falls below 1,500/mm^3 or the absolute neutrophil count reaches 500/mm^3, clozapine therapy should *never* be resumed.

Agranulocytosis is an indication for hospitalization and the institution of reverse isolation. A full infectious disease workup is mandatory, and often the prophylactic use of antibiotics is advisable. The use of one of the known granulocyte-stimulating factors will help to restore normal bone marrow production (Gerson and Meltzer 1992; Lieberman and Alvir 1992).

Major motor seizures occur at a rate of approximately 3% at 300 mg/day and 6% at 600 mg/day of clozapine (Sajatovic and Meltzer 1993). Myoclonus occurs less frequently. Neither major motor seizures nor myoclonus is a cause for discontinuation of clozapine; rather, they should be treated either by reduction in the dosage of clozapine or by addition of an anticonvulsant agent. Valproic acid is usually effective but may increase clozapine levels. Carbamazepine should be avoided be-

cause of the risk of agranulocytosis, but when necessary for seizure control, carbamazepine and clozapine can be given.

The other main side effects of clozapine are cardiovascular effects, sedation, weight gain, and hypersalivation. The chief cardiovascular effects are orthostatic hypotension, tachycardia, and ECG changes. Other than tachycardia, which is persistent, these effects are seen early in treatment, are short lived, and seldom result in discontinuation of clozapine. Sedation is a less serious but common and distressing side effect. It is generally observed early in treatment, and tolerance develops over time. Alterations in the dosage regimen are usually effective, although in severe cases the addition of methylphenidate or L-dopa may be warranted (H. Y. Meltzer et al., unpublished observations, 1990–1995). Another common side effect of clozapine is weight gain, with reported rates varying from 1% to 85% (average 38%); the weight gain associated with clozapine is greater than that associated with haloperidol (Hummer et al. 1995). Simple strategies, including dietary advice, exercise, and weight monitoring, are usually effective. Most of the gain occurs in the first 4 months. Hypersalivation, another common side effect of clozapine, generally occurs at night, again often in the initial phases of treatment (Ben-Aryeh et al. 1996). If the hypersalivation becomes troublesome or persistent, the addition of benztropine mesylate or clonidine (an α$_1$ receptor agonist) will usually relieve this side effect. Constipation and nausea are also side effects of clozapine. Some patients cannot tolerate clozapine or refuse to try it.

Availability

Numerous fiscal and political constraints influence the availability of clozapine for patients with treatment-refractory schizophrenia. When these constraints preclude a trial of clozapine, the use of the more traditional neuroleptic augmentation strategies is advisable. Some of the most commonly used augmenting agents, and their relative indications, are listed in Table 36–4.

Relationship Between Clinical Efficacy and Plasma Concentrations

The half-life of clozapine after twice-a-day dosing at the steady state is about 16 hours (range 6–33). Thus, a steady state is achieved after about 1 week of twice-a-day administration at a constant dosage (Choc et al. 1987). Current evidence suggests that of the major metabolites of clozapine, norclozapine may be partially active, and clozapine-N-oxide may be pharmacologically inactive, but this issue needs further elucidation.

There is some evidence that plasma levels of clozapine may be a useful guide to optimally efficacious dosage. It appears that dosages that achieve plasma levels higher than 350–370 ng/mL are maximally effective in treatment-resistant schizophrenia (Hasegawa et al. 1993; Lieberman et al. 1994; Perry et al. 1991). There is no evidence of a therapeutic window. Some patients do respond at lower plasma levels. Clozapine plasma levels are most commonly measured by high-pressure liquid chromatography (Lovdahl et al. 1991).

Plasma levels of clozapine should be obtained in patients who have inadequate response. Also, it may be useful to check clozapine levels once the dosage exceeds 600 mg/day, since the incidence of seizures increases significantly at dosages higher than 600 mg/day, and since high plasma concentrations of clozapine are associated with seizures (Simpson and Cooper 1978). Finally, it may be possible, in selected cases, to exceed the recommended limit of 900 mg/day if there is poor response, if plasma levels are lower than 370 ng/mL, and there are no serious or troublesome side effects.

Factors that have been found to affect plasma levels of clozapine include gender, smoking, and certain drugs. One study found that smoking decreased clozapine concentrations in men (Haring et al. 1990), whereas another study found no difference in clozapine concentrations among male smokers and nonsmokers (Hasegawa et al. 1993). Phenytoin has been reported to lower the clozapine concentration (Miller 1991). Valproate and fluvoxamine increase plasma levels of clozapine by decreasing its metabolism.

Partial Response to Clozapine

Partial response to clozapine may be approached in a variety of ways. Clinical experience indicates that addition of a low dose of a high-potency neuroleptic drug to clozapine has been found to be helpful in ameliorating positive symptoms in some partial responders. Concomitant ECT may also be useful in some of these patients, but maintenance ECT may be needed to sustain the benefits (Sajatovic and Meltzer 1993).

Antidepressants and mood stabilizers have also been used as adjuncts in treating depressive or manic symptoms among schizoaffective patients. SSRIs, including fluoxetine, sertraline, fluvoxamine, and paroxetine, are the antidepressants of choice (Cassady and Thacker 1992). It may be prudent not to initiate clozapine and lithium simultaneously given a few reports of increased neurotoxicity (Blake et al. 1992; Pope et al. 1991); but once a stable dosage of clozapine has been attained, lithium can safely be added in most cases. Valproic acid may also be used. Carbamazepine should be avoided because of increased risk of agranulocytosis.

For persistent anxiety symptoms, benzodiazepines or buspirone may be added. A few earlier reports of cardiorespiratory collapse with concomitant use of benzodiazepines caused great concern; however, subsequent clinical experience has shown that this combination is safe in most medically healthy patients. Again, benzodiazepines should be added preferably only after a stable dose of clozapine has been achieved.

Systematic studies assessing the usefulness and safety of various psychotropics as an adjunct to clozapine therapy in patients with persistent symptomatology are clearly lacking and are needed at this time.

Recommendations for Pharmacological Treatment of Resistant Schizophrenia

After determining that a patient has not had a satisfactory response to typical neuroleptic drugs, despite adequate dosage and duration of treatment, and that compliance has been adequate, the choice of pharmacotherapy is between initiating treatment with clozapine immediately or trying one or more of the novel antipsychotic drugs first. Controlled trials regarding this medical decision are urgently needed.

At present, clinical experience with risperidone and olanzapine indicates that some proportion of patients with neuroleptic-resistant schizophrenia will respond to adequate doses of these agents, but the appropriate dosage range and duration of a trial are not known. Higher dosages of risperidone (e.g., 6–12 mg/day) result in a higher incidence of EPS. Olanzapine was recently found, in a small study, not to be more effective than chlorpromazine in patients with neuroleptic-resistant schizophrenia (Conley et al., unpublished data, 1997). However, much more research is needed before the issue of how many patients with treatment-resistant schizophrenia will respond to risperidone or olanzapine, at what doses, and after how long is clarified.

What is known is that clozapine will be more effective than standard neuroleptics in a high proportion of such patients (i.e., at least 60%) (Lieberman et al. 1994; Meltzer and Ranjan 1996) but that there is somewhat increased risk and more difficult administration attached. At the current price of these agents, clozapine may be more expensive than olanzapine and risperidone, depending on the dosage of the latter agents. However, the true cost from the perspective of the third-party payer includes other factors such as the cost of treatment failures and hospitalization, so it is not possible to conclude on a cost-minimization basis that clozapine is not also favored over other atypical agents for patients with treatment-resistant schizophrenia.

Patients and their families should be given, when possible, sufficient information about the potential benefits and risks of all pharmacological treatment options and encouraged to make an informed choice. Because clozapine is the drug for which there is the best evidence for efficacy and tolerability in treatment-resistant schizophrenia patients, a decision to go directly to clozapine should be supported. However, some patients or mental health providers will wish to try olanzapine or risperidone before clozapine in order to avoid the need for weekly blood drawing and the risk of agranulocytosis. This, too, is a reasonable approach. Should there be an unsatisfactory response to either of these agents, it would appear prudent to proceed directly to clozapine without the need for a trial of the other agent—or of quetiapine, ziprasidone, or sertindole once they have been approved for use, in the absence of any empirical evidence that they are effective in cases of neuroleptic-resistant schizophrenia.

CONCLUSION

Significant advances have been made in defining appropriate treatment strategies for patients with schizophrenia (Meltzer and Ranjan 1995). A broad view of treatment objectives that includes much more than positive symptom control is essential. Neuroleptic drugs are still widely used for acute and maintenance treatment of schizophrenia, but atypical antipsychotic drugs are rapidly displacing them. Olanzapine and risperidone, which are expected to be joined by quetiapine and ziprasidone, qualify as first-line drugs because of fewer side effects and superior efficacy compared with standard neuroleptics. As a group, the atypical antipsychotic agents have advantages in terms of EPS, negative symptoms, and compliance. Clozapine is the treatment of choice in schizophrenic patients who fail to respond to other antipsychotic drugs and has demonstrated efficacy in a wide range of outcome measures. The efficacy of alternative treatments for patients with neuroleptic-resistant schizophrenia, including neuroleptic augmentation strategies or adjunctive ECT, is now less clear, and these treatments are probably best reserved for patients who either refuse or cannot tolerate clozapine treatment. The advent of clozapine and other new antipsychotics offers encouragement and optimism for the treatment of persons with schizophrenia and provides a neurobiological framework on which to explore the pathophysiology of schizophrenia.

REFERENCES

Adler LA, Angrist B, Reiter S, et al: Neuroleptic-induced akathisia: a review. Psychopharmacology (Berl) 97:1–11, 1989

Alvir JMJ, Lieberman JA, Safferman AZ, et al: Clozapine-induced agranulocytosis: incidence and risk factors in the United States. N Engl J Med 329:162–167, 1993

American Psychiatric Association: Diagnostic and Statistical Manual of Mental Disorders, 4th Edition. Washington, DC, American Psychiatric Association, 1994

Amsler HA, Teerenhovi L, Barth E, et al: Agranulocytosis in patients treated with clozapine: a study of the Finnish epidemic. Acta Psychiatr Scand 56:241–248, 1977

Arvanitis LA, Miller BG, Seroquel Trial 13 Study Group: Multiple fixed doses of "Seroquel" (quetiapine) in patients with acute exacerbation of schizophrenia: a comparison with haloperidol and placebo. Biol Psychiatry 42:233–246, 1997

Awad G: Quality of life of schizophrenic patients on medications and implications for new drug trials. Hospital and Community Psychiatry 43:262–265, 1992

Ayd FJ: A summary of drug-induced extrapyramidal reactions. JAMA 175:1054–1060, 1961

Baldessarini RJ, Frankenburg FF: Clozapine: a novel antipsychotic agent. N Engl J Med 324:746–754, 1991

Baldessarini RJ, Cohen BM, Teicher MH: Significance of neuroleptic dose and plasma level in the pharmacological treatment of psychoses. Arch Gen Psychiatry 45:79–91, 1988

Barnes TRE: Movement disorder associated with antipsychotic drugs: the tardive syndromes. International Review of Psychiatry 2:355–366, 1990

Barnes TRE, Halstead SM, Liddle PF: Relationship between iron status and chronic akathisia in an inpatient population with chronic schizophrenia. Br J Psychiatry 161:791–796, 1992

Baum KM, Walker EF: Childhood behavioral precursors of adult symptom dimensions in schizophrenia. Schizophr Res 16:111–120, 1995

Beasley CM, Tollefson G, Tran P, et al: Olanzapine versus placebo and haloperidol: acute phase results of the North American double-blind olanzapine trial. Neuropsychopharmacology 14:111–123, 1996

Ben-Aryeh H, Jungerman T, Szargel R, et al: Salivary flow-rate and composition in schizophrenic patients on clozapine: subjective reports and laboratory data. Biol Psychiatry 39:946–949, 1996

Birmaher B, Baker R, Kapur S, et al: Clozapine for the treatment of adolescents with schizophrenia. J Am Acad Child Adolesc Psychiatry 31:160–164, 1992

Blake LM, Marks RC, Luchins DJ: Reversible neuroleptic symptoms with clozapine. J Clin Psychopharmacol 12:297–299, 1992

Boodhood JA, Sadler WM: Anticholinergic antiparkinsonian drugs in psychiatry. Br J Hosp Med 46:167–169, 1991

Braff DL, Heaton R, Kuck J, et al: The generalized pattern of neuropsychological deficits in outpatients with chronic schizophrenia with heterogeneous Wisconsin Card Sorting Test results. Arch Gen Psychiatry 48:891–898, 1991

Breier A, Buchanan RW, Kirkpatrick B, et al: Effects of clozapine on positive and negative symptoms in outpatients with schizophrenia. Am J Psychiatry 151:20–26, 1994

Buchanan RW, Holstein C, Breier A: The comparative efficacy and long-term effect of clozapine treatment of neuropsychological test performance. Biol Psychiatry 36:717–725, 1994

Buckley P, Way L, Meltzer HY: Substance abuse among patients with treatment-resistant schizophrenia: characteristics and implications for clozapine therapy. Am J Psychiatry 151:154–159, 1994

Carpenter WT Jr: The phenomenology and course of schizophrenia: treatment implications, in Psychopharmacology: A Third Generation of Progress. Edited by Meltzer HY. New York, Raven, 1987, pp 1121–1128

Carpenter WT Jr: The deficit syndrome. Am J Psychiatry 151:327–329, 1994

Carpenter WT Jr, Strauss JS: The prediction of outcome in schizophrenia, IV: eleven-year follow up of the Washington IPSS Cohort. J Nerv Ment Dis 179:517–525, 1991

Carpenter WT Jr, Heinrichs DW, Hanlon TE: A comparative trial of pharmacologic strategies in schizophrenia. Am J Psychiatry 144:1466–1470, 1987

Carpenter WT, Hanlon TE, Heinrichs DW, et al: Continuous versus targeted medication in schizophrenic outpatients: outcome results. Am J Psychiatry 147:1138–1148, 1990

Casey DE: Clozapine: neuroleptic-induced EPS and tardive dyskinesia. Psychopharmacology (Berl) 99 (suppl): S47–S53, 1989

Casey DE: Neuroleptic drug-induced extrapyramidal syndromes and tardive dyskinesia. Schizophr Res 4:109–120, 1991

Casey DE: Neuroleptic-induced acute extrapyramidal syndromes and tardive dyskinesia. Psychiatr Clin North Am 16:589–610, 1993

Casey DE: 'Seroquel' (quetiapine): preclinical and clinical findings of a new atypical antipsychotic. Expert Opinion on Investigational Drugs 5:939–957, 1996

Cassady SL, Thacker GK: Addition of fluoxetine to clozapine (letter). Am J Psychiatry 149:1274, 1992

Cassens G, Inglis ALK, Appelbaum PS, et al: Neuroleptics: effects on neuropsychological function in chronic schizophrenic patients. Schizophr Bull 16:477–499, 1990

Chakos MH, Mayerhoff DI, Loebel AD, et al: Incidence and correlates of acute extrapyramidal symptoms in first episode of schizophrenia. Psychopharmacol Bull 28:81–86, 1992

Chengappa KN, Shelton M, Baker R, et al: The prevalence of akathisia in patients receiving stable doses of clozapine. J Clin Psychiatry 55:142–145, 1994

Choc MG, Lehr RG, Hsuan F, et al: Multiple-dose pharmacokinetics of clozapine in patients. Pharm Res 4:402–405, 1987

Chouinard G, Jones B, Remington G, et al: A Canadian multicenter placebo-controlled study of fixed doses of risperidone and haloperidol in the treatment of chronic schizophrenic patients. J Clin Psychopharmacol 13:25–40, 1993

Christison GW, Kirch DJ, Wyatt RJ: When symptoms persist: choosing among alternative somatic treatments for schizophrenia. Schizophr Bull 17: 217–245, 1991

Claghorn J, Honigfeld G, Abuzzahab FS, et al: The risks and benefits of clozapine versus chlorpromazine. J Clin Psychopharmacol 7:377–384, 1987

Classen W, Laux G: Sensorimotor and cognitive performance of schizophrenic inpatients treated with haloperidol, fluphenthixol or clozapine. Pharmacopsychiatry 21: 197–295, 1988

Crow TJ: Schizophrenia: more than one molecular process. BMJ 280:66–68, 1980

Daniel DG, Goldberg TE, Weinberger DR, et al: Different side-effect profiles of risperidone and clozapine in 20 outpatients with schizophrenia or schizoaffective disorder: a pilot study. Am J Psychiatry 153:417–419, 1996

Davis JM, Barter JT, Kane JM: Antipsychotic drugs, in Comprehensive Textbook of Psychiatry/V, 5th Edition. Edited by Kaplan HI, Sadock BJ. Baltimore, MD, Williams & Wilkins, 1989, pp 1591–1626

Davis KL, Kahn RS, Ko G, et al: Dopamine in schizophrenia: a review and reconceptualization. Am J Psychiatry 148: 1474–1486, 1991

Ekblöm B, Haggström JE: Clozapine (Leponex) compared with chlorpromazine: a double-blind evaluation of pharmacological and clinical properties. Current Therapeutic Research 16:945–957, 1974

Fatemi SH, Meltzer HY, Roth BL: Atypical antipsychotic drugs: clinical and preclinical studies, in Handbook of Experimental Pharmacology, Vol 120: Antipsychotics. Edited by Csernansky JG. Heidelberg, Springer-Verlag, 1996, pp 77–116

Feltner DE, Hertzman M: Progress in the treatment of tardive dyskinesia: theory and practice. Hospital and Community Psychiatry 44:25–34, 1993

Fischer-Cornelssen KA, Ferner VJ: An example of European multicenter trials: multispectral analysis of clozapine. Psychopharmacol Bull 2:34–39, 1976

Fleischhacker WW, Hummer M, Kurz M, et al: Clozapine dose in the United States and Europe: implications for therapeutic and adverse effects. J Clin Psychiatry 55 (no 9, suppl B):78–81, 1994

Gerlach I, Koppelhus P, Helweg E, et al: Clozapine and haloperidol in a single-blind cross-over trial: therapeutic and biochemical aspects in the treatment of schizophrenia. Acta Psychiatr Scand 50:410–424, 1974

Gerlach J, Casey DE: Tardive dyskinesia. Acta Psychiatr Scand 77:369–378, 1988

Gerson SL, Meltzer HY: Mechanisms of clozapine-induced agranulocytosis. Drug Saf 7:17–25, 1992

Gilbert PL, Harris MJ, McAdams LA, et al: Neuroleptic withdrawal in schizophrenic patients: a review of the literature. Arch Gen Psychiatry 52:173–188, 1995

Glazer WM, Morgenstein H, Schooler N, et al: Predictors of improvement in tardive dyskinesia following discontinuation of neuroleptic medication. Br J Psychiatry 157:585–592, 1990

Glazer WM, Morgenstein H, Doucette JT: Predicting the long-term risk of tardive dyskinesia in outpatients maintained on neuroleptic medication. J Clin Psychiatry 54:133–139, 1993

Goff DC, Baldessarini RJ: Drug interactions with antipsychotic agents. J Clin Psychopharmacol 13:57–65, 1993

Goff DC, Midha KK, Brotman AW, et al: An open trial of buspirone added to neuroleptics in schizophrenic patients. J Clin Psychopharmacol 11:193–197, 1991

Goldberg TE, Calls JR, Weinberger DR, et al: Performance of schizophrenic patients on putative neuropsychological tests of frontal lobe function. Int J Neurosci 42:51–58, 1988

Goldberg TE, Greenberg RD, Griffin SJ, et al: The effect of clozapine on cognition and psychiatric symptoms in patients with schizophrenia. Br J Psychiatry 162:43–48, 1993

Goldstein JF, Arvanitis LA: ICI204,636 (Seroquel); a dibenzthiazepine atypical antipsychotic: review of preclinical pharmacology and highlights of phase II clinical trial. CNS Drug Review 1:50–73, 1995

Green MF: What are the functional consequences of neurocognitive deficits in schizophrenia? Am J Psychiatry 153:321–330, 1996

Green MF, Marshall BD Jr, Wirshing WC, et al: Does risperidone improve verbal working memory in treatment-resistant schizophrenia? Am J Psychiatry 154:799–804, 1997

Hagger C, Buckley P, Kenny JT, et al: Improvement in cognitive functions and psychiatric symptoms in treatment-refractory schizophrenic patients receiving clozapine. Biol Psychiatry 34:702–712, 1993

Hamilton M: A rating scale for depression. J Neurol Neurosurg Psychiatry 23:56–62, 1960

Haring C, Fleishhacker W, Schett P, et al: Influence of patient-related variables on clozapine plasma levels. Am J Psychiatry 147:1471–1475, 1990

Hasegawa M, Gutierrez-Esteinou R, Way L, et al: Relationship between clinical efficacy and clozapine plasma concentrations in schizophrenia: effect of smoking. J Clin Psychopharmacol 13:383–390, 1993

Hermesh H, Aizenburg D, Weizman A: A successful electroconvulsive treatment of neuroleptic malignant syndrome. Acta Psychiatr Scand 75:237–239, 1987

Herz MI, Szymanski HV, Simon JC: Intermittent medication for stable schizophrenic outpatients: an alternative to maintenance medication. Am J Psychiatry 139:918–922, 1982

Herz MI, Glazer WM, Mostert MA, et al: Intermittent vs maintenance medication in schizophrenia: two-year results. Arch Gen Psychiatry 48:333–339, 1991

Hogarty GE, Anderson CM, Reiss DJ, et al: Family psychoeducation, social skills training, and maintenance chemotherapy in the aftercare treatment of schizophrenia, II: two-year effects of a controlled study on relapse and adjustment. Arch Gen Psychiatry 48:340–347, 1988

Hummer M, Kemmler G, Kurz M, et al: Weight gain induced by clozapine. Eur Neuropsychopharmacol 5:437–440, 1995

Jann MW, Grimstey SR, Gray EC, et al: Pharmacokinetics and pharmaco-dynamics of clozapine. Clin Pharmacokinet 24:161–176, 1993

Jolley AG, Hirsch SR, McRink A, et al: Trial of brief intermittent neuroleptic prophylaxis for selected schizophrenic outpatients: clinical outcome at one year. BMJ 298:985–990, 1989

Jolley AG, Hirsch SR, Morrison E, et al: Trial of brief intermittent neuroleptic prophylaxis for selected schizophrenic outpatients: clinical outcome at two years. BMJ 301:837–847, 1990

Juul Povlsen U, Noring V, Fog R, et al: Tolerability and therapeutic effect of clozapine: a retrospective investigation of 216 patients treated with clozapine for up to 12 years. Acta Psychiatr Scand 71:176–185, 1985

Kane J, Marder SR: Psychopharmacologic treatment of schizophrenia. Schizophr Bull 19:287–302, 1993

Kane JM, Woener M, Weinhold P, et al: Incidence of tardive dyskinesia: five-year data from a prospective study. Psychopharmacol Bull 20:39–40, 1984

Kane JM, Rifkin A, Woerner M, et al: High-dose versus low-dose strategies in the treatment of schizophrenia. Psychopharmacol Bull 21:533–537, 1985

Kane J, Honigfeld G, Singer J, et al [Clozaril Collaborative Study Group]: Clozapine for the treatment-resistant schizophrenic: a double-blind comparison with chlorpromazine. Arch Gen Psychiatry 45:789–796, 1988

Kellam AMP: The (frequently) neuroleptic malignant syndrome. Br J Psychiatry 157:169–173, 1990

Kibel DA, Laffont I, Liddle PF: The composition of the negative syndrome of chronic schizophrenia. Br J Psychiatry 162:744–750, 1993

Kirkpatrick B, Buchanan RW, McKenney PD, et al: The Schedule for the Deficit Syndrome: an instrument for research in schizophrenia. Psychiatry Res 30:119–123, 1989

Kronig M, Munne R, Szymanski S, et al: Plasma clozapine levels and clinical response for treatment refractory schizophrenic patients. Am J Psychiatry 152:179–182, 1995

Kuha S, Miettinen E: Long-term effect of clozapine in schizophrenia: a retrospective study of 108 chronic schizophrenics treated with clozapine for up to 7 years. Nordisk Psykiatrisk Tidsskrift 40:225–230, 1986

Lee MA, Thompson P, Meltzer HY: Effects of clozapine on cognitive function in schizophrenia. J Clin Psychiatry 55 (no 9, suppl B):82–87, 1994

Levinson DF, Simpson GM, Single H, et al: Fluphenazine dose, clinical response and extrapyramidal symptoms during acute treatment. Arch Gen Psychiatry 47:761–768, 1990

Liddle PF: The symptoms of chronic schizophrenia: a reexamination of the positive-negative dichotomy. Br J Psychiatry 151:145–15l, 1987

Liddle PF, Barnes TR: Syndromes of chronic schizophrenia. Br J Psychiatry 157:558–561, 1990

Lieberman JA, Alvir JMJ: A report of clozapine induced agranulocytosis in the United States: incidence and risk factors. Drug Saf 7 (suppl):1–2, 1992

Lieberman JA, Saltz BL, Johns CA, et al: The effects of clozapine on tardive dyskinesia. Br J Psychiatry 158:503–510, 1991

Lieberman J, Safferman A, Pollack S, et al: Clinical effects of clozapine in chronic schizophrenia: response to treatment and predictors of outcome. Am J Psychiatry 151:1744–1752, 1994

Lindström LH: The effect of long-term treatment with clozapine in schizophrenia: a retrospective study in 96 patients treated with clozapine for up to 13 years. Acta Psychiatr Scand 77:524–529, 1988

Loebel AD, Lieberman JA, Alvir J, et al: Duration of psychosis and outcome in first-episode schizophrenia. Am J Psychiatry 149:1183–1188, 1992

Lovdahl MJ, Perry PJ, Miller DD: The assay of clozapine and N-desmethylclozapine in human plasma by high-performance liquid chromatography. Ther Drug Monit 13:69–72, 1991

Marder SR, Meibach RC: Risperidone in the treatment of schizophrenia. Am J Psychiatry 151:825–835, 1994

Marder SR, Van Putten T: Who should receive clozapine? Arch Gen Psychiatry 45:865–867, 1988

Marder SR, Van Putten T, Mentz J, et al: Costs and benefits of two doses of fluphenazine. Arch Gen Psychiatry 41:1025–1029, 1984

Marder SR, Van Putten T, Mintz J, et al: Low- and conventional-dose maintenance therapy with fluphenazine decanoate: two-year outcome. Arch Gen Psychiatry 44:518–521, 1987

McElroy SL, Dessain EC, Pope HG Jr, et al: Clozapine in the treatment of psychotic mood disorders, schizoaffective disorder, and schizophrenia. J Clin Psychiatry 52:411–414, 1991

McEvoy JP, Hogarty GE, Steingard S: Optimal dose of neuroleptic in acute schizophrenia: a controlled study of neuroleptic threshold and higher haloperidol dose. Arch Gen Psychiatry 48:739–745, 1991

McGorry PD, McFarlane C, Patton GC, et al: The prevalence of prodromal features of schizophrenia in adolescence: a preliminary survey. Acta Psychiatr Scand 92:241–249, 1995

Meltzer HY: Rigidity, hyperpyrexia and coma following fluphenazine enthanate. Psychopharmacologia 29:337–346, 1973

Meltzer HY: Clinical studies on the mechanism of action of clozapine: the dopamine-serotonin hypothesis of schizophrenia. Psychopharmacology (Berl) 99 (suppl):S18–S27, 1989a

Meltzer HY: Duration of a clozapine trial in neuroleptic-resistant schizophrenia (letter). Arch Gen Psychiatry 46:672, 1989b

Meltzer HY: Dimensions of outcome with clozapine. Br J Psychiatry 160:46–53, 1992

Meltzer HY: Clozapine: is another view valid? Am J Psychiatry 152:821–825, 1995a

Meltzer HY: The concept of atypical antipsychotics, in Advances in the Neurobiology of Schizophrenia, Vol 1. Edited by den Boer JA, Westenberg HGM, van Praag HM. London, Wiley, 1995b, pp 265–273

Meltzer HY: A career in biological psychiatry, in The Psychopharmacologists: Interviews by David Healy. London, Chapman & Hall, 1996, pp 509–538

Meltzer HY: The clozapine story, in The Handbook of Psychopharmacology Trials. Edited by Hertzman M, Feltner DE. New York, New York University Press, 1997, pp 137–156

Meltzer HY, Fang VS: Effect of neuroleptics on serum prolactin in schizophrenic patients. Arch Gen Psychiatry 33:279–286, 1976

Meltzer HY, Luchins DJ: Effect of clozapine in severe tardive dyskinesia: a case report. J Clin Psychopharmacol 4:286–287, 1984

Meltzer HY, Okayli G: The reduction of suicidality during clozapine treatment in neuroleptic-resistant schizophrenia: impact on risk-benefit assessment. Am J Psychiatry 152:183–190, 1995

Meltzer HY, Ranjan R: Recent advances in the pharmacotherapy of schizophrenia. Acta Psychiatr Scand Suppl 384:95–101, 1995

Meltzer HY, Ranjan R: Efficacy of novel antipsychotic drugs in treatment-refractory schizophrenia, in Handbook of Experimental Pharmacology, Vol 120: Antipsychotics. Edited by Csernansky JG. Heidelberg, Springer-Verlag, 1996, pp 333–358

Meltzer HY, Zureick JL: Negative symptoms in schizophrenia. A target for new drug development, in Clinical Pharmacology in Psychiatry, Vol 1. Edited by Dahl SG, Gram LF. Berlin, Springer, 1989, pp 68–77

Meltzer HY, Sommers AA, Luchins DJ: The effect of neuroleptics and other psychotropic drugs on negative symptoms in schizophrenia. J Clin Psychopharmacol 6:329–338, 1986

Meltzer HY, Matsubara S, Lee JC: Classification of typical and atypical antipsychotic drugs on the basis of dopamine D-1, D-2 and serotonin$_2$ pKi values. J Pharmacol Exp Ther 251:238–246, 1989

Miller DD: Effect of phenytoin on plasma clozapine concentrations in two patients. J Clin Psychiatry 52:23–25, 1991

Möller J-J, Müller H, Borison RL, et al: A path-analytical approach to differentiate between direct and indirect drug effects on negative symptoms in schizophrenic patients: evaluation of the North American Risperidone Study. Eur Arch Psychiatry Clin Neurosci 245:45–49, 1995

Mueser KT, Yarnold PR, Levinson DF, et al: Prevalence of substance abuse in schizophrenia: demographic and clinical correlates. Schizophr Bull 16:31–53, 1990

Murray RM, O'Callaghan E, Castle DJ, et al: A neurodevelopmental approach to the classification of schizophrenia. Schizophr Bull 18:319–331, 1992

Naber D, Hippius H: The European experience with use of clozapine. Hospital and Community Psychiatry 41:886–890, 1990

Naber D, Leppig M, Grohman R, et al: Efficacy and adverse effects of clozapine in the treatment of schizophrenia and tardive dyskinesia—a retrospective study of 387 patients. Psychopharmacology (Berl) 99 (suppl):S73–S76, 1989

Naber D, Holzbach R, Perro C, et al: Clinical management of clozapine patients in relation to efficacy and side-effects. Br J Psychiatry 160:54–59, 1992

Owen RR, Gutierrez-Esteinou R, Hsiao J, et al: Effects of clozapine and fluphenazine treatment on responses to m-chlorophenylpiperazine infusions in schizophrenia. Arch Gen Psychiatry 50:636–644, 1993

Perry PJ, Miller DD, Arndt SV, et al: Clozapine and norclozapine plasma concentrations and clinical response of treatment-refractory schizophrenic patients. Am J Psychiatry 148:231–235, 1991

Peuskens J: Risperidone in the treatment of patients with chronic schizophrenia: a multi-national multi-centre, double-blind parallel-group study versus haloperidol. Br J Psychiatry 166:712–726, 1995

Pickar D, Owen RR, Litman RE, et al: Clinical and biological response to clozapine in patients with schizophrenia. Arch Gen Psychiatry 49:345–353, 1992

Pollack S, Lieberman J, Kleiner D, et al: High plasma clozapine levels in tardive dyskinesia. Psychopharmacol Bull 29:257–262, 1993

Pope HG Jr, McElroy SL, Keck PE, et al: Valproate in the treatment of acute mania. Arch Gen Psychiatry 44:113–118, 1991

Richelson E, Nelson A: Antagonism by neuroleptics of neurotransmitter receptors of normal human brain in vitro. Eur J Pharmacol 103:197–204, 1984

Rifkin A, Karajgi B, Doddi S, et al: Dose and blood levels of haloperidol in treatment of mania. Psychopharmacol Bull 76:144–146, 1990

Rosebush PI, Stewart TD: A prospective analysis of 24 episodes of neuroleptic malignant syndrome. Am J Psychiatry 146:717–725, 1989

Roy A: Suicide in chronic schizophrenia. Br J Psychiatry 141:171–177, 1982

Safferman A, Lieberman J, Kane J, et al: Update on the clinical efficacy and side effects of clozapine. Schizophr Bull 17:247–261, 1991

Sajatovic M, Meltzer HY: The effect of short-term electroconvulsive treatment plus neuroleptic in treatment-resistant schizophrenia and schizoaffective disorder. Convuls Ther 9:167–175, 1993

Saykin AJ, Gur RC, Gur RJ, et al: Neuropsychological function in schizophrenia: selective impairment in learning and memory. Arch Gen Psychiatry 48:618–624, 1991

Schotte A, Janssen PFM, Gommeren W, et al: Risperidone compared with new and reference antipsychotic drugs: in vitro and in vivo receptor binding. Psychopharmacology (Berl) 124:57–73, 1996

Schulz SC, Kahn EM, Baker RW, et al: Lithium and carbamazepine augmentation in treatment-refractory schizophrenia, in The Neuroleptic Nonresponsive Patient: Characterization and Treatment. Edited by Angrist B, Schulz SC. Washington, DC, American Psychiatric Press, 1990, pp 109–136

Seeger TF, Seymour PA, Schmidt AW, et al: Ziprasidone (CP-88,059): a new antipsychotic with combined dopamine and serotonin receptor antagonist activity. J Pharmacol Exp Ther 275:101–113, 1995

Sevy S, Davidson M: The cost of cognitive impairment in schizophrenia. Schizophr Res 17:1–3, 1995

Silver H, Nassar A: Fluvoxamine improves negative symptoms in treated chronic schizophrenia: an add-on double-blind, placebo-controlled study. Biol Psychiatry 31:698–704, 1992

Simpson GM, Cooper TA: Clozapine plasma levels and convulsions. Am J Psychiatry 135:99–100, 1978

Siris SG, Harmon GK, Endicott J: Postpsychotic depressive symptoms in hospitalized schizophrenic patients. Arch Gen Psychiatry 38:1122–1123, 1981

Small JG, Hirsch SR, Arvanitis LA, et al [Seroquel Study Group]: Quetiapine in patients with schizophrenia: a high- and low-dose double-blind comparison with placebo. Arch Gen Psychiatry 54:549–557, 1997

Stern R, Kahn R, Davidson M, et al: Early response to clozapine in schizophrenia. Am J Psychiatry 151:1817–1818, 1994

Tollefson GD, Sanger TM: Negative symptoms: a path analytic approach to a double-blind, placebo- and haloperidol-controlled clinical trial with olanzapine. Am J Psychiatry 154:466–474, 1997

Tollefson GD, Beasley CM, Tamura RN, et al: Blind, controlled long-term study of the comparative incidence of treatment-emergent tardive dyskinesia with olanzapine or haloperidol. Am J Psychiatry 154:1248–1259, 1997a

Tollefson GD, Beasley CM, Tran PV, et al: Olanzapine versus haloperidol in the treatment of schizophrenia and schizoaffective and schizophreniform disorders: results of an international collaborative trial. Am J Psychiatry 154:457–465, 1997b

Umbricht D, Kane JM: Risperidone: efficacy and safety. Schizophr Bull 21:593–604, 1995

Van Kammen DP, McEvoy JP, Targum S, et al: A randomized controlled, dose-ranging trial of sertindole in patients with schizophrenia. Psychopharmacology (Berl) 124:168–175, 1996

Van Putten T: Why do schizophrenic patients refuse to take their drugs? Arch Gen Psychiatry 31:67–72, 1974

Van Putten T, Marder SR, Mintz J: A controlled dose comparison of haloperidol in newly admitted schizophrenic patients. Arch Gen Psychiatry 47:754–758, 1990

Van Putten T, Marder SR, Wirshing WC, et al: Neuroleptic plasma levels. Schizophr Bull 17:197–216, 1991

Weiden PJ, Dixon L, Frances A, et al: Neuroleptic noncompliance in schizophrenia, in Schizophrenia Research. Edited by Tamminga CA, Schulz SC. New York, Raven, 1991, pp 285–296

Weinberger DR: Implications of normal brain development for the pathogenesis of schizophrenia. Arch Gen Psychiatry 44:660–669, 1987

Woerner MG, Saltz BL, Kane JM, et al: Diabetes and the development of tardive dyskinesia. Am J Psychiatry 150:966–968, 1993

Wolkowitz OM, Pickar D: Benzodiazepines in the treatment of schizophrenia: a review and reappraisal. Am J Psychiatry 148:714–726, 1991

Wood MJ, Rubinstein M: An atypical responder to clozapine. Am J Psychiatry 147:369, 1990

Wyatt RJ: Neuroleptics and the natural course of schizophrenia. Schizophr Bull 17:325–351, 1991

Wyatt RJ, Green MF, Tuma AH: Long-term morbidity associated with delayed treatment of first admission schizophrenic patients: a re-analysis of the Camarillo State Hospital data. Psychol Med 27:261–268, 1997

Young MA, Meltzer HY: The relationship of demographic, clinical, and outcome variables to neuroleptic treatment requirements. Schizophr Bull 6:88–101, 1980

THIRTY-SEVEN

Treatment of Anxiety Disorders

C. Barr Taylor, M.D.

The psychopharmacological treatment of panic and other anxiety disorders has changed dramatically in the past 10 years. The changes in treatment were enhanced by the publication of DSM-III (American Psychiatric Association 1980), which allowed for uniform diagnoses, by the epidemiological evidence of the high prevalence of these disorders, by the development of new pharmacological and cognitive therapies, and by a general increase in research in this area. Even 10 years ago, benzodiazepines were the customary psychopharmacological treatment in the United States for most anxiety disorders. Now a variety of agents has been shown to be effective. The psychological treatment of anxiety disorders also has expanded and has been better integrated into the pharmacological treatment (Taylor and Arnow 1988).

PANIC DISORDER

Panic disorder (with and without agoraphobia) is the most common anxiety disorder, occurring in 2%–6% of the population (Myers et al. 1984). The target symptoms of panic disorder include panic attacks, anticipatory and generalized anxiety, avoidance (agoraphobia), and, to varying degrees, worry, somatic symptoms, and even obsessions. Panic disorder is a long-term disorder, with frequent relapses, changes in symptomatology, and comorbidity. Of the latter, depression and alcohol use and abuse are particularly relevant in considering which psychopharmacological agents to use. The psychopharmacological treatment of panic disorder can be conceptualized as occurring in two phases—short- and long-term—with much more being known about the former than the latter.

Short-Term, Acute Treatment

The short-term goals of psychopharmacological treatment are symptom relief and initiation of psychoeducational or psychological therapies. In many patients, the target symptoms are alleviated and work, family, and social functioning improve within 8 weeks of treatment with combinations of psychological and pharmacological therapies.

Antidepressants

Antidepressants should be considered the first line of treatment for patients with panic disorder, especially if depression is present. Of all the antidepressants, imipramine has been used the longest and has been most extensively investigated. However, recent studies have substantiated the benefit of serotonin reuptake inhibitors (SRIs). Based on their effectiveness and favorable side-effect profile, they should now be considered the first drug of choice (Coplan et al. 1996). Advantages and disadvantages of SRIs for anxiety disorders are listed in Table 37–1.

Serotonin reuptake inhibitors. The SRIs, including fluoxetine, paroxetine, fluvoxamine, and clomipramine, have proven to be effective antipanic agents at least in the short term (Den Boer and Westenberg 1990; Modigh et al. 1992; Oehrberg et al. 1995; Pecknold et al. 1995). Boyer (1995) reviewed 27 placebo-controlled, double-blind studies in which an SRI was used to treat panic disorder.

Table 37–1. Advantages and disadvantages of serotonin reuptake inhibitors for anxiety disorders

Advantages	Disadvantages
Single daily dose	Delayed onset of action
Antidepressant	Few well-controlled studies
No dependence/withdrawal	Side effects
	Insomnia
	Irritability
	Sexual dysfunction

The SRIs were at least as effective as imipramine or alprazolam. There are few data comparing efficacy among the SRIs. Paroxetine has been approved by the U.S. Food and Drug Administration (FDA) for treating panic disorder. Although clomipramine is not approved as an antipanic medication, it is widely used for that purpose in Europe.

Patients with panic disorder sometimes have a reaction, characterized by feelings of restlessness, sweating, flushing, or even increased anxiety, to SRIs at the usual starting dose. This reaction is similar to that with other antidepressants and may even be more common with SRIs, especially clomipramine, than with other psychopharmacological treatments. To avoid or minimize this "jitteriness reaction," many clinicians begin with one-quarter to one-half the usual SRI dose, increasing the medication as tolerated and needed. Low doses of benzodiazepines can also be used on an as-needed basis to counteract this syndrome temporarily.

Sexual dysfunction is a common side effect of SRIs. Sexual dysfunction can involve loss of interest in sex and/or alteration in physiological arousal, including difficulty with orgasm and ejaculation (Gitlin 1994). The etiology of these changes is not known. Some patients can be switched to another SRI to avoid this side effect. Cyproheptadine, an antihistaminic and antiserotonergic agent, has been used to reverse the effects of the SRI temporarily. Case studies report some improvement in orgasm when cyproheptadine, 2–16 mg, is administered 1–2 hours before sex (Aizenberg et al. 1995; Gitlin 1994). However, cyproheptadine also appears to block the antipanic effects of the SRIs. Patients with loss of sexual interest who were given yohimbine, an α_2 blocking agent, had some improvement in sexual functioning. Yohimbine has been given at doses of 5.4–16.2 mg 2–4 hours before sex (Keller Ashton et al. 1997). Amantadine and bethanechol, two cholinergic agents, have also been used with some anecdotal success. If the patient is very troubled by this side effect and switching to another SRI does not work, then another drug class should be considered. Because SRIs (and other antidepressants) can precipitate manic episodes, a careful history of

hypomanic episodes should be obtained and/or a positive family history of bipolarity should be documented and other medications considered as appropriate. Some patients report dizziness, paresthesias, tremor, anxiety, nausea, and other symptoms when SRIs are abruptly discontinued. This so-called serotonin withdrawal syndrome usually occurs after 2 days and resolves within 3 weeks (Price et al. 1996; Zajecka et al. 1997). The syndrome appears to be minimized if SRIs are discontinued over a few weeks.

Tricyclics. The benefits of imipramine for reducing the frequency of panic attacks were first noted more than 30 years ago by D. F. Klein and Fink (1962). Since then, several studies have substantiated its benefits. The largest study involved 1,168 patients in 14 countries and compared imipramine, alprazolam, and placebo (Cross-National Collaborative Panic Study 1992). At 4 weeks, 52% of patients taking imipramine, 63% of patients taking alprazolam, and 45% of patients taking placebo had no panic attacks. At the end of the study, the effects of the two active drugs were similar to each other, and both drugs were superior to placebo for most outcome measures. It was surprising that no differences were found between the active treatments and placebo in the number of panic attacks per week at 8 weeks. However, the dropout rate was high for the placebo group: only 56% of the placebo patients completed the study compared with 70% of the imipramine and 83% of the alprazolam patients; therefore, the 8-week data for completers are difficult to interpret. The mean daily dose of imipramine was 155 mg. Some patients may need a higher dose. Of interest, in a reanalysis of the data set, Briggs et al. (1993) found that for those patients with dyspnea as a major feature of their panic attacks, imipramine was superior to alprazolam, and for those who did not have dyspnea, the reverse was true.

Imipramine should be started at doses of 25–50 mg and increased gradually. Most patients achieve a therapeutic benefit at 150–250 mg, although the dose can be increased to 300 mg. Mavissakalian and Perel (1995) found a positive dose-response relationship between imipramine and clinical improvement. Different dose ranges had different clinical effects. For phobias, the best total drug plasma level was in the range of 110–140 ng/mL; higher levels had a detrimental effect. For panic, the probability of response increased quickly with greater plasma levels and then tapered off, with no improvement at levels beyond 140 ng/mL. About 25% of patients with panic disorder who begin taking imipramine experience the "jitteriness syndrome" mentioned above. In patients who find these symptoms intolerable, imipramine can be reduced to very low doses (10 mg) and increased gradually. Advantages and disadvantages of tricyclic antidepressants for anxiety disorders are listed in Table 37–2.

Desipramine would theoretically work as well as imipramine because it is the main metabolite of imipramine. However, imipramine may be more serotonergic than desipramine, which may give imipramine greater efficacy, assuming that the serotonin system is important in panic disorder. Clomipramine has been shown to be effective for panic in European studies (Amin et al. 1977). Amitriptyline and nortriptyline may also be effective, but fewer and less-well-designed studies are available (Ballenger 1986).

Monoamine oxidase inhibitors. Monoamine oxidase inhibitors (MAOIs) are also effective antipanic and antiphobic agents. Of the three available MAOIs, phenelzine has been studied most extensively and has been shown to be as efficacious as imipramine. Isocarboxazid and tranylcypromine are probably also effective. Recently, so-called reversible and selective MAOIs have been developed. In theory, they should be effective for panic disorder, and at least one study has found this to be the case (Bakish et al. 1993). They appear to be as effective as traditional MAOIs. In comparison with irreversible and nonselective MAOIs, such drugs have reduced tyramine-potentiating effects. Advantages and disadvantages of MAOIs for anxiety disorders are listed in Table 37–3.

Other antidepressants. Trazodone has been shown to be less effective than imipramine or alprazolam (Charney et al. 1986). Nefazodone, which is chemically related to trazodone, has been shown to reduce anxiety in depressed patients, but little information is available on its effect in patients with panic disorder (Fawcett et al. 1995). Bupropion, an atypical antidepressant, and maprotiline, a noradrenaline uptake inhibitor, do not appear to be effective (Den Boer and Westenberg 1988; Sheehan et

al. 1983). Some of the newer antidepressants may prove to be of benefit. Case reports suggest, for instance, that venlafaxine, a drug that inhibits the neuronal reuptake of both serotonin and norepinephrine and has been shown to be an effective antidepressant, may help to reduce panic attacks (Geracioti 1995).

Benzodiazepines

The benzodiazepines are effective for reducing panic attacks, phobic behavior, and anticipatory anxiety. Of the many benzodiazepines, alprazolam has been studied most extensively. The results of two large cross-national trials have been reported (Ballenger et al. 1988; Cross-National Collaborative Panic Study 1992). In the first large multicenter trial, 526 patients were randomized to receive either alprazolam or placebo. Of these, 86% of the alprazolam subjects completed the trial compared with only 50% of the placebo subjects. At the primary comparison point (week 4 of the study), 82% of the subjects receiving alprazolam were considered moderately improved or better compared with 42% of the placebo group. At that point, 50% of the alprazolam group compared with 28% of the placebo group had no panic attacks. For those subjects who completed the trial, no significant difference in total number of panic attacks or in disability ratings was found between subjects taking alprazolam and those taking placebo, although the former were much less fearful and avoidant than the latter.

As noted earlier in this chapter, in the Cross-National Collaborative Panic Study, Phase 2, which compared imipramine and alprazolam with placebo, a significant placebo effect occurred, particularly for frequency of panic attacks. However, the placebo group dropout rate was high, which caused difficulty in detecting differences between the active medications and placebo. The subjects taking

Table 37–2. Advantages and disadvantages of tricyclic antidepressants for anxiety disorders

Advantages	Disadvantages
Single daily dose	Delayed onset of action
Antidepressant	Activation syndrome
Generics available	Side effects
Well studied	Anticholinergic
	Orthostatic hypotension
	Weight gain
	? Blood pressure increase
	Overdosage

Table 37–3. Advantages and disadvantages of classic monoamine oxidase inhibitors for anxiety disorders

Advantages	Disadvantages
Single daily dose	Delayed onset of action
Antidepressant	Diet/hypertensive crises
Generics available	Hyperpyrexic reactions
	Side effects
	Insomnia
	Anticholinergic
	Orthostatic hypotension
	Weight gain
	Overdosage

Several studies have found that imipramine combined with cognitive-behavior therapy works better than either alone (Telch et al. 1985). However, Marks and Swinson (1990) found no advantage for alprazolam combined with exposure therapy, and Klosko et al. (1990) argued that benzodiazepines may impede the effects of behavior therapy.

In our experience, thoughtful integration of cognitive-behavior therapy and pharmacotherapy produces an optimal outcome (Taylor and Arnow 1988). For instance, many patients require some medication before they are able to undergo intensive exposure therapy. Psychological interventions can facilitate withdrawal of medication and prepare patients for long-term treatment.

Long-Term Treatment

Panic disorder is a chronic, long-term condition, and the length of pharmacological treatment remains controversial. Most of the studies reported in the previous section have focused on only short-term outcomes. Current clinical practice generally involves a trial of 3–6 months of an effective medication. More controversial is continued therapy for an additional 6–12 months or longer. We do know that relapse rates are very high after medication is discontinued. Depending on the medication, concomitant psychological treatment, the length of follow-up, and the criteria, relapse rates of between 20% and 80% have been reported (Ballenger 1992). With medication alone, probably fewer than half of patients remain well after medication has been discontinued for 6 months or longer. Ballenger (1992) asserted that the medications shown to be effective have few adverse physical effects; therefore, the length of treatment should only be based on questions of effectiveness.

In several series of patients with panic disorder, no evidence indicated that patients developed an abusive pattern during long-term use of benzodiazepines to treat panic disorder symptoms (Rifkin et al. 1989). The evidence that patients with depression, another long-term condition, have better outcomes with maintenance medication should also be considered (Kupfer et al. 1992). In light of the controversies surrounding long-term medication use, and because the medication may no longer be necessary, it is good practice to routinely discontinue the medication after 6 months to a year, especially if patients are taking benzodiazepines. Patients should remain off of the medication for at least a month before being restarted on it to give adequate time for adjustment after discontinuation.

Clinicians usually reinstate the medication previously used if it was successful or prescribe a new medication if it might have an advantage over the medication previously used.

Refractory Cases

Most panic disorders can be treated successfully with one medication, often the first one tried. However, some patients may require combinations of medications. The combinations that have been reported to be successful tend to be similar to those reported for depression, such as the use of a tricyclic and an SRI (Coplan et al. 1996; Tiffon et al. 1994). If such combined therapy fails, then addition of a benzodiazepine or some of the other agents mentioned earlier in this chapter can be considered.

GENERALIZED ANXIETY DISORDER

Generalized anxiety disorder (GAD), like panic disorder, is common, occurring in at least 2%–3% of the population (Weissman et al. 1978). The main features of GAD are chronic cognitive, behavioral, and physiological symptoms of hyperarousal and anxiety. GAD commonly occurs with other anxiety disorders and depression, and the latter should always be considered when symptoms of GAD are present. When depression or panic disorder is present, it should be treated first.

Benzodiazepines have been the mainstay of treatment for patients with GAD (Thompson 1996). Benzodiazepines are effective in the short run for reducing symptoms of GAD. Different types of benzodiazepines at equivalent doses are equally effective for generalized anxiety, and the agent used should be chosen on the basis of potency, half-life, and side effects.

The issues discussed earlier in this chapter regarding the use of benzodiazepines for panic disorder apply to GAD. In 1980, after reviewing studies on benzodiazepine effects, the British Medical Association concluded that the effects of such drugs do not persist beyond 3–4 months. However, other experts have argued that benzodiazepines are effective for much longer. For instance, Haskell et al. (1986) studied 194 patients with a history of diazepam use. The patients taking long-term diazepam were as symptomatic as patients presenting for anxiety treatment. Yet, 158 of the 194 had tried to discontinue diazepam at some time, and, of these, 142 reported the reemergence of anxiety symptoms. However, the patients believed that they were deriving benefit from treatment.

Rickels et al. (1991) followed up 123 patients who had participated in a benzodiazepine discontinuation program. At follow-up, a mean of 2.9 years later, 55 (45%) of the patients were not taking benzodiazepines. Discontinuing chronic benzodiazepine use did not result in significant worsening of anxious or depressive symptoms. Of these patients, 25% still had substantial levels of anxiety. The study provided more evidence that GAD is chronic or recurrent and may benefit from long-term treatment. However, the use of benzodiazepines for long-term treatment remains controversial. Discontinuance of benzodiazepines allows for adequate reassessment and institution of new treatments (Rickels et al. 1991).

The problems with benzodiazepines have prompted an intensive search for alternative agents effective in reducing symptoms of GAD. Buspirone, an azapirone derivative and a 5-HT$_{1A}$ partial agonist, has been shown to be as effective as benzodiazepines and significantly better than placebo in controlled clinical trials (Goldberg and Finnerty 1979; Napoliello 1986; Rickels et al. 1982; Wheatley 1982) at doses of 20–40 mg. In these trials, improvement continued from pretreatment through the fourth week of treatment and paralleled but was somewhat slower than that of the benzodiazepines (Rickels et al. 1990).

In a 40-month follow-up of 34 patients participating in a comparison of buspirone and clorazepate, 30% of patients treated with clorazepate were still taking a benzodiazepine regularly, and 25% were taking benzodiazepines on an as-needed basis, whereas none of those treated with buspirone was still receiving medication. This study suggests that buspirone can be discontinued more easily than benzodiazepines. Buspirone produces less drowsiness, psychomotor impairment, and alcohol potentiation and has less potential for addiction or abuse compared with the benzodiazepines. Buspirone has a slow onset (its major drawback) and does not have anticonvulsive effects. A comparison of alprazolam and buspirone found both to be equally effective for GAD and superior to placebo (Enkelmann 1991). The buspirone group had a higher dropout rate than the alprazolam group (36% vs. 13%). Buspirone seems to be most helpful in anxious patients who do not demand immediate relief of symptoms, including patients who have taken benzodiazepines (Rickels 1990). A meta-analysis of GAD treatment studies found that diazepam had a somewhat greater effect than buspirone (Cox et al. 1992). Some investigators add buspirone to reduce rebound symptoms during discontinuation from benzodiazepines (Udelman and Udelman 1990). Buspirone will not block the potential serious withdrawal effects of benzodiazepines and should not be used instead of a gradual benzodiazepine withdrawal.

An important and perhaps overlooked finding is that imipramine may have anxiolytic effects (Hoehn-Saric et al. 1988; Kahn et al. 1986; McLeod et al. 1990). Imipramine had a significant effect on reducing anticipatory anxiety in the cross-national alprazolam and imipramine trial, but the effect was only significantly different by the eighth week of treatment. Doses lower than those used for panic disorder are often effective in GAD. Treatment may not be effective until patients have been taking medication for a month or longer.

Serotonin reuptake blockers may prove to have significant antianxiety effects. Clomipramine has been shown to be effective in at least one uncontrolled study (Wingerson et al. 1992).

Several new antianxiety agents are being developed. The partial benzodiazepine receptor agonists bretazenil and abecarnil have some antianxiety effects (Ballenger et al. 1992; Haefely et al. 1992). These newer agents may have the advantages of benzodiazepines such as less risk of physical dependence. However, it is still too early to know how useful they will be for treating anxiety disorders.

The cognitive-behavioral treatment of GAD has been less well evaluated than that of panic disorder. A combination of relaxation and related techniques aimed at decreasing hyperarousal—cognitive-behavior therapy, skills training and coping, and alteration in lifestyle factors as appropriate—is often beneficial (Borkovec and Costello 1993; Miller et al. 1995; Taylor 1978; Taylor and Arnow 1988), but long-term controlled studies are lacking. Traditional psychodynamic therapies are often effective in alleviating symptoms of chronic anxiety.

SOCIAL PHOBIA

Social phobia is a common, disabling, and often unrecognized anxiety disorder, occurring in about 1%–2% of the population (Myers et al. 1984). Although social phobia shares many features of panic disorder and often occurs with it, it has separate phenomenological features. For instance, the five most common fears of people with social phobia are 1) public speaking, 2) eating in public, 3) writing in public, 4) using public lavatories, and 5) being stared at or being the center of attention, whereas the most common fears of people with panic disorder are 1) driving or traveling, 2) going to stores, 3) being in crowds, 4) eating in restaurants, and 5) using elevators (Uhde et al. 1991). People with social phobia do not have spontaneous panic attacks and do not panic when they are alone or asleep. They also have low rates of dyspnea. Fear of negative evaluation is the critical cognitive feature of social phobia. Many people with social phobia also have avoidant personality disorder, characterized by chronic patterns of shyness and avoidance. Patients with avoidant personality disorder appear very similar to patients with generalized social phobia (Hofmann et al. 1995). Social phobia is often quite disabling and results in extreme anxiety, avoidance, work and social impairment, depression, and substance abuse (Liebowitz et al. 1985).

The pharmacological treatment of social phobia has lagged behind that of other anxiety disorders. However, recent studies found that fluoxetine, sertraline, fluvoxamine, and paroxetine can be effective treatments of social phobia (Marshall and Schneier 1996). Although these have all been small-scale studies, the safety and favorable side-effect profile of the SRIs, combined with their apparent efficacy, suggest that they should be considered the drugs of choice over the MAOIs, which have more established efficacy. Because MAOIs should not be used for at least 5 weeks after fluoxetine has been discontinued, SRIs with shorter half-lives might be preferred in cases in which MAOIs need to be started (e.g., patients whose severe symptoms have not responded to an SRI).

High-potency benzodiazepines, particularly alprazolam and clonazepam, have been reported to reduce symptoms of social phobia (Lydiard et al. 1988; Reiter et al. 1990). For instance, in an uncontrolled study of 26 patients (most of whom had other diagnoses and had received various previous treatments), 85% of patients had moderate to significant improvement with doses of clonazepam ranging from 0.5 to 5.0 mg/day (mean dose 2.1) (Davidson et al. 1991).

Liebowitz et al. (1988) decided to use MAOIs to treat social phobia after observing that MAOIs are useful in a variety of phobias and reduce excessive interpersonal sensitivity in patients with atypical depression. Because such sensitivity to criticism is typical of patients with social phobia, it made sense to determine whether an MAOI would be effective in this condition. In a sample of 74 patients, phenelzine was superior to both atenolol and placebo, with no significant differences between the latter two agents (Liebowitz et al. 1992).

In a controlled trial with 45 patients randomized to receive phenelzine, alprazolam, or placebo for 23 weeks, all three groups showed improvement, and no differences in self-reported data were noted. However, subjects who were given alprazolam or phenelzine had better scores on the clinician-rated Work and Social Disability Scale (Uhde et al. 1991). After a 4-week drug-free period, the phenelzine-treated group remained significantly improved compared with the placebo group on this measure, whereas the alprazolam-treated group did not differ from the placebo group.

Reversible MAOIs, a class of medications that is selective for isoenyzme A of monoamine oxidase and that binds reversibly so that it has less risk for hypertensive crises than the standard MAOIs, may also be effective for social phobia. For instance, Versiani et al. (1992) found that moclobemide, an experimental reversible MAOI, was nearly as effective as phenelzine and superior to placebo. However, these medications have not been submitted for approval by the FDA.

β-Blockers also have been used to treat social phobia, with mixed results. For performance anxiety, β-blockers have been shown to benefit activities such as pistol shooting, bowling, stringed instrument playing, and public speaking (Liebowitz et al. 1991). Doses of 10–40 mg of propranolol taken about 1 hour before such performances can reduce symptoms of sympathetic activity, such as sweating and tremor, that may serve as cues for anxiety and fear. The early β-blocker studies focused on performance anxiety, and this subgroup of persons with social phobia may respond differently from individuals with generalized social fears. As noted earlier in this chapter, Liebowitz et al. (1992) found that atenolol had no significant effects on social phobia. A small controlled trial found that propranolol and placebo had no effect in patients receiving behavioral treatment (Falloon et al. 1981).

Uncontrolled trials also found that buspirone, in doses up to 60 mg/day, had some benefits in patients with social phobia (Liebowitz et al. 1991). Buspirone had no effect on exposure therapy in a controlled clinical trial (Clark and Agras 1991).

As with panic disorder, cognitive-behavior therapy is an appropriate adjunctive treatment to psychopharmacology in social phobia. A major line of basic research in behavior therapy has been devoted to one type of social phobia—that of speech phobia. This research has led to a number of treatment approaches, including systematic desensitization, social skills training, imaginal flooding, applied relaxation training, graduated exposure, anxiety management, and a variety of cognitive-restructuring procedures (i.e., self-instructional training, rational-emotive therapy, and cognitive-behavior group therapy) (Liebowitz et al. 1985). These approaches are often effective, at least for the more circumscribed phobias (Heimberg and Barlow 1991).

Several studies have found that pharmacological treatments did not improve outcome over cognitive-behavior therapy alone. For example, concomitant use of buspirone did not improve outcome of exposure therapy with performance phobia, and propranolol did not improve outcome with social skills treatment (Clark and Agras 1991; Stravynski et al. 1982). This finding is not surprising because buspirone has not been shown to be an effective medication for social phobia. In another study, cognitive-behavior treatment programs were compared with phenelzine, alprazolam, or placebo administered to patients with social phobia (Gelernter et al. 1991). All patients improved in all groups. Patients treated with phenelzine plus self-exposure had greater improvement than other groups did on a measure of trait anxiety. On one fear measure, patients treated with cognitive-behavior group therapy showed additional improvement from the posttest to follow-up assessment, whereas patients treated with alprazolam plus exposure therapy showed deterioration on this measure. Comparative studies are needed before the relative benefits of psychopharmacological and psychological treatments alone and in combination are known.

OBSESSIVE-COMPULSIVE DISORDER

Obsessive-compulsive disorder (OCD) is much more common than formerly thought, with a 6-month point prevalence of 1%–2% and a lifetime prevalence of 2%–3% (Myers et al. 1984; Robins et al. 1984). Until recently, therapists treating patients with OCD were often frustrated. Now, five medications—clomipramine, fluoxetine, fluvoxamine, paroxetine, and sertraline—have proven effective in reducing OCD symptoms (Jefferson and Greist 1996). Nevertheless, many patients continue to experience symptoms.

Given apparent comparable efficacy, either clomipramine or an SRI should be considered the drug of first choice for OCD, after taking into account the relatively different side effects of clomipramine (a tricyclic) compared with the SRIs. Case reports of the value of clomipramine appeared more than 20 years ago. Since then, its effectiveness has been confirmed in a number of double-blind trials of patients with OCD (Goodman et al. 1992). At the end of one large trial, obsessive and compulsive symptoms in patients given clomipramine had decreased by 35%–42% on the Yale-Brown Obsessive-Compulsive Scale, the standard instrument for measuring improvement, compared with 2%–5% in placebo groups (Clomipramine Collaborative Study Group 1991). Significant improvement was generally not seen until after about 6 weeks of clomipramine treatment with doses up to 300 mg. Fewer than 20% of patients discontinued clomipramine prematurely because of side effects. Although few studies have compared clomipramine with other antidepressants, a consistent pattern seems to emerge. Drugs that are less potent blockers of serotonin reuptake than clomipramine are generally ineffective in OCD. For instance, clomipramine was more effective than nortrip-tyline (Thoren et al. 1980) and desipramine (Leonard et al. 1988).

Recent studies have provided more information on the effectiveness and use of SRIs for OCD. Many patients' symptoms decline in 2–3 weeks, but clinical response may be delayed considerably (4 weeks in the fluoxetine and 6 weeks in the fluvoxamine multicenter trials); thus, a trial of 10–12 weeks is recommended before concluding lack of efficacy (Jefferson and Greist 1996). In the early studies, relatively high doses of SRIs were used. However, it is not clear if patients would have responded to lower doses if given more time. A preliminary fixed-dose study comparing 10 weeks of single daily doses of 20, 40, or 60 mg of fluoxetine with placebo did not find a clear-cut advantage of the 40- or 60-mg doses over the 20-mg dose (Wheadon 1991). With paroxetine, doses of 40 and 60 mg/day were more effective than placebo but 20-mg doses were not (Jefferson and Greist 1996). Jefferson and Greist (1996) recommended that an OCD drug trial should not be considered complete until a patient has been treated with a minimum daily dose of the following (assuming tolerability): clomipramine 250 mg, fluoxetine 60 mg, fluvoxamine 300 mg, paroxetine 60 mg, and sertraline 200 mg.

If patients' symptoms do not respond to clomipramine or an SRI at adequate doses and time, then another SRI (or clomipramine) should be tried. If a partial response occurs, initiation of combined treatment may be appropriate. At this point in the history of OCD, combined treatments are largely based on case reports and single-case design rather than rigorous studies. Currently recommended strategies are to add agents such as buspirone, lithium, or fenfluramine, which may modify serotonergic function, to ongoing SRI or clomipramine therapy. In an open-label study, Hollander et al. (1990) reported that the addition of the serotonin releaser and reuptake blocker fenfluramine to ongoing treatment with various SRIs led to reduction in OCD symptoms in 6 of 7 patients. The use of lithium to treat OCD has been more equivocal. One study reported reduced OCD symptoms in 3 of 4 patients treated with fluoxetine and lithium, but no treatment was effective in 16 patients who had had a partial response to clomipramine (Pigott et al. 1991). When lithium was added to fluvoxamine in patients refractory to treatment, only 3 of 30 patients' conditions improved (McDougle et al. 1991).

Buspirone has also been studied in treatment-resistant OCD patients. The results have been mixed; some studies show a benefit and others do not (Goodman et al. 1992). Interestingly, one small study found that buspirone alone was equal in efficacy to clomipramine (Pato et al. 1991). One author suggested that buspirone might be added to the regimen in anxious patients who are taking SRIs.

de Beurs E, van Balkom AJ, Lange A, et al: Treatment of panic disorder with agoraphobia: comparison of fluvoxamine, placebo, and psychological panic management combined with exposure and of exposure in vivo alone. Am J Psychiatry 152:683–691, 1995

Den Boer JA, Westenberg HG: Effect of a serotonin and noradrenaline uptake inhibitor in panic disorder: a double-blind comparative study with fluvoxamine and maprotiline. Int Clin Psychopharmacol 3:59–74, 1988

Den Boer JA, Westenberg HG: Serotonin function in panic disorder: a double blind placebo controlled study with fluvoxamine and ritanserin. Psychopharmacology 102:85–94, 1990

Dunner DL, Ishiki D, Avery DH, et al: Effect of alprazolam and diazepam on anxiety and panic attacks in panic disorder: a controlled study. J Clin Psychiatry 47:458–460, 1986

Enkelmann R: Alprazolam versus buspirone in the treatment of outpatients with generalized anxiety disorder. Psychopharmacology 105:428–432, 1991

Falcon S, Ryan C, Chamberlain K, et al: Tricyclics: possible treatment for posttraumatic stress disorder. J Clin Psychiatry 46:385–388, 1985

Falloon IR, Lloyd GG, Harpin RE: The treatment of social phobia: real-life rehearsal with non-professional therapists. J Nerv Ment Dis 169:180–184, 1981

Fawcett J, Marcus RN, Anton SF, et al: Response of anxiety and agitation symptoms during nefazodone treatment of major depression. J Clin Psychiatry 56 (suppl 6):37–42, 1995

Feldman TB: Alprazolam in the treatment of posttraumatic stress disorder (letter). J Clin Psychiatry 48:216–217, 1987

Fesler FA: Valproate in combat-related posttraumatic stress disorder. J Clin Psychiatry 52:361–364, 1991

Foa EB, Kozak MJ, Steketee GS, et al: Treatment of depressive and obsessive-compulsive symptoms in OCD by imipramine and behavioral therapy. Br J Clin Psychol 31:279–292, 1992

Frank JB, Kosten TR, Giller EL Jr, et al: A randomized clinical trial of phenelzine and imipramine for posttraumatic stress disorder. Am J Psychiatry 145:1289–1291, 1988

Gelernter CS, Uhde TW, Cimbolic P, et al: Cognitive-behavioral and pharmacological treatments for social phobia: a controlled study. Arch Gen Psychiatry 48:938–945, 1991

Geracioti TD Jr: Venlafaxine treatment of panic disorder: a case series. J Clin Psychiatry 56:408–410, 1995

Gitlin MJ: Psychotropic medications and their effects on sexual function: diagnosis, biology, and treatment approaches. J Clin Psychiatry 55:406–413, 1994

Goldberg HL, Finnerty RJ: The comparative efficacy of buspirone and diazepam in the treatment of anxiety. Am J Psychiatry 136:1184–1187, 1979

Goodman WK, McDougle CJ, Price LH: Pharmacotherapy of obsessive compulsive disorder. J Clin Psychiatry 53 (suppl 4):29–37, 1992

Haefely W, Facklam M, Schoch P, et al: Partial agonists of benzodiazepine receptors for the treatment of epilepsy, sleep, and anxiety disorders, in GABAergic Synaptic Transmission. Edited by Biggio G, Concas A, Costa E. New York, Raven, 1992, pp 379–394

Haskell D, Cole JO, Schniebolk S, et al: A survey of diazepam patients. Psychopharmacol Bull 22:434–438, 1986

Heimberg RG, Barlow DH: New developments in cognitive-behavioral therapy for social phobia. J Clin Psychiatry 52 (suppl 11):21–30, 1991

Helzer JE, Robins LN, McEvoy L: Post-traumatic stress disorder in the general population: findings of the Epidemiological Catchment Area Survey. N Engl J Med 317:1630–1634, 1987

Hewlett WA, Vinogradov S, Agras WS: Clonazepam treatment of obsessions and compulsions. J Clin Psychiatry 51:158–161, 1990

Hoehn-Saric R, McLeod DR, Zimmerli WD: Differential effects of alprazolam and imipramine in generalized anxiety disorder: somatic versus psychiatric symptoms. J Clin Psychiatry 49:293–301, 1988

Hofmann SG, Newman ME, Becker E, et al: Social phobia with and without avoidant personality disorder: preliminary behavior therapy outcome findings. Journal of Anxiety Disorders 9:1–13, 1995

Hogben GL, Cornfield RB: Treatment of traumatic war neurosis with phenelzine. Arch Gen Psychiatry 38:440–445, 1981

Hollander E, DeCaria CM, Schneier FR, et al: Fenfluramine augmentation of serotonin reuptake blockade antiobsessional treatment. J Clin Psychiatry 51:119–123, 1990

Jefferson JW, Greist JH: The pharmacotherapy of obsessive-compulsive disorder. Psychiatric Annals 26:202–209, 1996

Kahn RJ, McNair DM, Lipman RS, et al: Imipramine and chlordiazepoxide in depression and anxiety disorders, II: efficacy in anxious outpatients. Arch Gen Psychiatry 43:79–95 , 1986

Kauffman CD, Reist C, Djenderedijan A, et al: Biological markers of affective disorders and posttraumatic stress disorder: a pilot study with desipramine. J Clin Psychiatry 48:366–367, 1987

Keck PE Jr, McElroy SL, Tugrul KC, et al: Antiepileptic drugs for the treatment of panic disorder. Neuropsychobiology 27:150–153, 1993

Keller Ashton A, Hamer R, Rosen RC: Serotonin reuptake inhibitor-induced sexual dysfunction and its treatment: a large-scale retrospective study of 596 psychiatric outpatients. J Sex Marital Ther 23:165–175, 1997

Kinzie JD, Leung P: Clonidine in Cambodian patients with posttraumatic stress disorder. J Nerv Ment Dis 177:546–550, 1989

Kitchner I, Greenstein R: Low dose lithium carbonate in the treatment of posttraumatic stress disorder: brief communication. Mil Med 150:378–381, 1985

Klein DF, Fink M: Psychiatric reaction patterns to imipramine. Am J Psychiatry 119:4324–4338, 1962

Klein E, Colin V, Stolk J, et al: Alprazolam withdrawal in patients with panic disorder and generalized anxiety disorder: vulnerability and effect of carbamazepine. Am J Psychiatry 151:1760–1766, 1994

Klosko J, Barlow D, Tassinari R, et al: A comparison of alprazolam and behavior therapy in treatment of panic disorder. J Consult Clin Psychol 58:77–84, 1990

Kupfer DJ, Frank E, Perel JM, et al: Five-year outcome for maintenance therapies in recurrent depression. Arch Gen Psychiatry 49:769–773, 1992

Lennane KJ: Treatment of benzodiazepine dependence. Med J Aust 144:594–597, 1986

Leonard H, Swedo S, Coffey M, et al: Clomipramine vs. desipramine in childhood obsessive-compulsive disorder. Psychopharmacol Bull 24:43–45, 1988

Lidren DM, Watkins PL, Gould RA, et al: A comparison of bibliotherapy and group therapy in the treatment of panic disorder. J Consult Clin Psychol 62:865–869, 1994

Liebowitz MR, Gorman JM, Fyer AJ, et al: Social phobia: review of a neglected anxiety disorder. Arch Gen Psychiatry 42:729–736, 1985

Liebowitz MR, Gorman JM, Fyer AJ, et al: Pharmacotherapy of social phobia: an interim report of a placebo-controlled comparisons of phenelzine and atenolol. J Clin Psychiatry 49:252–257, 1988

Liebowitz MR, Schneier FR, Hollander E, et al: Treatment of social phobia with drugs other than benzodiazepines. J Clin Psychiatry 52 (suppl 11):10–15, 1991

Liebowitz MR, Schneier F, Campeas R, et al: Phenelzine vs. atenolol in social phobia: a placebo-controlled comparison. Arch Gen Psychiatry 49:290–300, 1992

Lipper S, Davidson JR, Grady TA, et al: Preliminary study of carbamazepine in post-traumatic stress disorder. Psychosomatics 27:849–854, 1986

Lydiard RB, Laraia MT, Howell EF, et al: Alprazolam in the treatment of social phobia. J Clin Psychiatry 49:17–19, 1988

Lydiard RB, Lesser IM, Ballenger JC, et al: A fixed-dose study of alprazolam 2 mg, alprazolam 6 mg, and placebo in panic disorder. J Clin Psychopharmacol 12:96–103, 1992

Marks IM, Swinson RP: Alprazolam and exposure for panic disorder with agoraphobia: summary of London/Toronto results. J Psychiatr Res 24:100–101, 1990

Marshall RD, Schneier FR: An algorithm for the pharmacotherapy for social phobia. Psychiatric Annals 26:210–216, 1996

Marshall RD, Stein DJ, Liebowitz MR, et al: A pharmacotherapy algorithm in the treatment of posttraumatic stress disorder. Psychiatric Annals 26:217–226, 1996

Mavissakalian MR, Perel JM: Imipramine treatment of panic disorder with agoraphobia: dose ranging and plasma level-response relationships. Am J Psychiatry 152:673–682, 1995

McDougle CJ, Price LH, Goodman WK, et al: A controlled trial of lithium augmentation in fluvoxamine-refractory obsessive-compulsive disorder: lack of efficacy. J Clin Psychopharmacol 11:175–184, 1991

McLeod DR, Hoehn-Saric R, Zimmerli WD, et al: Treatment effects of alprazolam and imipramine: physiological versus subjective changes in patients with generalized anxiety disorder. Biol Psychiatry 28:849–861, 1990

Miller JJ, Fletcher K, Kabat-Zinn J: Three-year follow-up and clinical implications of a mindfulness meditation-based stress reduction intervention in the treatment of anxiety disorders. Gen Hosp Psychiatry 17:192–200, 1995

Modigh K, Westberg P, Erickson E: Superiority of clomipramine over imipramine in the treatment of panic disorder: a placebo-controlled trial. J Clin Psychopharmacol 12:251–261, 1992

Myers JK, Weissman MM, Tischler GL, et al: Six-month prevalence of psychiatric disorders in three communities: 1980–1982. Arch Gen Psychiatry 41:959–967, 1984

Napoliello MJ: An interim multicentre report on 7,677 anxious geriatric out-patients treated with buspirone. Br J Clin Pract 40:71–73, 1986

Newman MG, Kenardy J, Herman S, et al: Comparison of palmtop-computer-assisted brief cognitive-behavioral treatment to cognitive-behavioral treatment for panic disorder. J Consult Clin Psychol 65:178–183, 1997

Nierenberg AA, Cole JO, Glass L: Possible trazodone potentiation of fluoxetine: a case series. J Clin Psychiatry 53:83–85, 1992

Noyes R Jr, Perry PJ, Crowe R, et al: Seizures following the withdrawal of alprazolam. J Nerv Ment Dis 174:50–52, 1986

Oehrberg S, Christiansen PE, Behnke K, et al: Paroxetine in the treatment of panic disorder: a randomised, double-blind, placebo-controlled study. Br J Psychiatry 167:374–379, 1995

Ost LG: Applied relaxation vs progressive relaxation in the treatment of panic disorder. Behav Res Ther 26:13–22, 1988

O'Sullivan G, Noshirvani H, Marks I, et al: Six-year follow-up after exposure and clomipramine therapy for obsessive compulsive disorder. J Clin Psychiatry 52:150–155, 1991

Owen RT, Tyrer P: Benzodiazepine dependence: a review of the evidence. Drugs 25:385–398, 1983

Pato MT, Zohar-Kadouch R, Zohar J, et al: Return of symptoms after discontinuation of clomipramine in patients with obsessive-compulsive disorder. Am J Psychiatry 145:1521–1525, 1988

Pato MT, Pigott TA, Hill JL, et al: Controlled comparison of buspirone and clomipramine in obsessive-compulsive disorder. Am J Psychiatry 148:127–129, 1991

Patterson JF: Withdrawal from alprazolam dependency using clonazepam: clinical observations. J Clin Psychiatry 51 (suppl):47–49, 1990

Pecknold JC, Swinson RP, Krich K, et al: Alprazolam in panic disorder and agoraphobia: results from a multicenter trial, III: discontinuation effects. Arch Gen Psychiatry 45:429–436, 1988

Pecknold JC, Luthe L, Iny L, et al: Fluoxetine in panic disorder: pharmacologic and tritiated platelet imipramine and paroxetine binding study. J Psychiatry Neurosci 20:193–198, 1995

Pigott TA, Pato MT, L'Heureux F, et al: A controlled comparison of adjuvant lithium carbonate or thyroid hormone in clomipramine-treated patients with obsessive-compulsive disorder. J Clin Psychopharmacol 11:242–248, 1991

Pigott TA, L'Heureux F, Rubenstein CS, et al: A double-blind, placebo controlled study of trazodone in patients with obsessive-compulsive disorder. J Clin Psychopharmacol 12:156–162, 1992

Price JS, Waller PC, Wood SM, et al: A comparison of the post-marketing safety of four selective serotonin re-uptake inhibitors including the investigation of symptoms occurring on withdrawal. Br J Clin Pharmacol 42:757–763, 1996

Reist C, Kauffmann CD, Haier RJ, et al: A controlled trial of desipramine in 18 men with posttraumatic stress disorder. Am J Psychiatry 146:513–516, 1989

Reiter SR, Pollack MH, Rosenbaum JF, et al: Clonazepam for the treatment of social phobia. J Clin Psychiatry 51:470–472, 1990

Rickels K: Buspirone in clinical practice. J Clin Psychiatry 51 (suppl):51–54, 1990

Rickels K, Weisman K, Norstad N, et al: Buspirone and diazepam in anxiety: a controlled study. J Clin Psychiatry 43:81–86, 1982

Rickels K, Schweizer E, Case WG, et al: Long-term therapeutic use of benzodiazepines, I: effects of abrupt discontinuation. Arch Gen Psychiatry 47:899–907, 1990

Rickels K, Case WG, Schweizer E, et al: Long-term benzodiazepine users 3 years after participation in a discontinuation program. Am J Psychiatry 148:757–761, 1991

Rickels K, Schweizer E, Weiss S, et al: Maintenance drug treatment for panic disorder, II: short- and long-term outcome after drug taper. Arch Gen Psychiatry 50:61–68, 1993

Rifkin A, Doddi S, Karajgi B, et al: Benzodiazepine use and abuse by patients at outpatient clinics. Am J Psychiatry 146:1331–1332, 1989

Robins LN, Helzer JE, Weissman MM, et al: Lifetime prevalence of specific psychiatric disorders in three sites. Arch Gen Psychiatry 412:958–967, 1984

Salzman C: Anxiety in the elderly: treatment strategies. J Clin Psychiatry 51 (suppl):18–21, 1990

Schweizer E, Pohl R, Balon R, et al: Lorazepam vs. alprazolam in the treatment of panic disorder. Pharmacopsychiatry 23:90–93, 1990

Schweizer E, Rickels K, Weiss S, et al: Maintenance drug treatment of panic disorder, I: results of a prospective, placebo-controlled comparison of alprazolam and imipramine. Arch Gen Psychiatry 50:51–60, 1993

Sharp DM, Power KG, Simpson RJ, et al: Fluvoxamine, placebo, and cognitive behaviour therapy used alone and in combination in the treatment of panic disorder and agoraphobia. Journal of Anxiety Disorders 10:219–242, 1996

Shear MK, Pilkonis PA, Cloitre M, et al: Cognitive behavioral treatment compared with nonprescriptive treatment of panic disorder. Arch Gen Psychiatry 51:395–401, 1994

Sheehan DV, Davidson J, Manschreck TC, et al: Lack of efficacy of a new antidepressant (bupropion) in the treatment of panic disorder with phobias. J Clin Psychopharmacol 3:23–31, 1983

Sheehan DV, Raj AB, Sheehan KH, et al: Is buspirone effective for panic disorder? J Clin Psychopharmacol 10:3–11, 1990

Shen WW, Park S: The use of monoamine oxidase inhibitors in the treatment of traumatic war neurosis: case report. Mil Med 148:430–431, 1983

Silver JM, Sandberg DP, Hales RE: New approaches in the pharmacotherapy of post-traumatic stress disorder. J Clin Psychiatry 51 (suppl 10):33–38, 1990

Spealman RD: Disruption of schedule-controlled behavior by Ro 15-1788 one day after acute treatment with benzodiazepines. Psychopharmacology 88:398–400, 1986

Stravynski A, Marks I, Yule W: Social skills problems in neurotic outpatients: social skills training with and without cognitive modification. Arch Gen Psychiatry 39:1378–1385, 1982

Swinson RP, Fergus KD, Cox BJ, et al: Efficacy of telephone-administered behavioral therapy for panic disorder with agoraphobia. Behav Res Ther 33:465–469, 1995

Taylor CB: Relaxation training and related techniques, in Behavior Modification: Principles and Clinical Applications. Edited by Agras WS. Boston, MA, Little, Brown, 1978, pp 134–162

Taylor CB, Arnow B: The Nature and Treatment of Anxiety Disorders. New York, Free Press, 1988

Telch MJ, Agras WS, Taylor CB, et al: Combined pharmacological and behavioral treatment for agoraphobia. Behav Res Ther 23:325–335, 1985

Tesar GE, Rosenbaum JF, Pollack MH, et al: Double-blind, placebo-controlled comparison of clonazepam and alprazolam for panic disorder. J Clin Psychiatry 52:69–76, 1991

Thompson PM: Generalized anxiety disorder treatment algorithm. Psychiatric Annals 26:227–232, 1996

Thoren P, Asberg M, Cronholm B, et al: Clomipramine treatment of obsessive-compulsive disorder, I: a controlled clinical trial. Arch Gen Psychiatry 37:1281–1285, 1980

Tiffon L, Coplan JD, Papp LA, et al: Augmentation strategies with tricyclic or fluoxetine treatment in seven partially responsive panic disorder patients. J Clin Psychiatry 55:66–69, 1994

Udelman HD, Udelman DL: Concurrent use of buspirone in anxious patients during withdrawal from alprazolam therapy. J Clin Psychiatry 51 (suppl):46–50, 1990

Uhde TW, Tancer ME, Black B, et al: Phenomenology and neurobiology of social phobia: comparison with panic disorder. J Clin Psychiatry 52 (suppl 11):31–40, 1991

van der Kolk BA, Dreyfuss D, Michaels M, et al: Fluoxetine in posttraumatic stress disorder. J Clin Psychiatry 55:517–522, 1994

Versiani M, Nardi AE, Mundim FD, et al: Pharmacotherapy of social phobia: a controlled study with moclobemide and phenelzine. Br J Psychiatry 161:353–360, 1992

Weissman MM, Myers JK, Harding PS: Psychiatric disorders in a U.S. urban community. Am J Psychiatry 135:459–462, 1978

Welkowitz LA, Papp LA, Cloitre M, et al: Cognitive-behavior therapy for panic disorder delivered by psychopharmacologically oriented clinicians. J Nerv Ment Dis 179:473–477, 1991

Wheadon DE: Placebo controlled multi-center trial of fluoxetine in OCD. Paper presented at the 5th World Congress of Biological Psychiatry, Florence, Italy, June 12, 1991

Wheatley D: Buspirone: multicenter efficacy study. J Clin Psychiatry 43:92–94, 1982

Wincor MZ, Munjack DJ, Palmer R: Alprazolam levels and response in panic disorder: preliminary results. J Clin Psychopharmacol 11:48–51, 1991

Wingerson D, Nguyen C, Roy-Byrne PP: Clomipramine treatment for generalized anxiety disorder (letter). J Clin Psychopharmacol 12:214–215, 1992

Wolf ME, Alavi A, Mosnaim AD: Posttraumatic stress disorder in Vietnam veterans: clinical and EEG findings; possible therapeutic effects of carbamazepine. Biol Psychiatry 23:642–644, 1988

Zajecka J, Tracy KA, Mitchell S: Discontinuation symptoms after treatment with serotonin reuptake inhibitors: a literature review. J Clin Psychiatry 58:291–297, 1997

Zinbarg RT, Barlow DH, Brown JA, et al: Cognitive-behavioral approaches to the nature and treatment of anxiety disorders. Annu Rev Psychol 43:235–267, 1992

THIRTY-EIGHT

Treatment of Noncognitive Symptoms in Alzheimer's Disease and Other Dementias

Murray A. Raskind, M.D., and Elaine R. Peskind, M.D.

Alzheimer's disease (AD) is the most common disorder causing dementia in later life, afflicting at least 4 million people in the United States (Katzman 1976). As in all disorders causing dementia, the primary symptoms of AD are acquired impairment of memory and other intellectual functions. AD is specifically characterized by insidious onset, gradual but inexorable progression, and development of fluent aphasia and apraxia as the disease progresses into its later stages. In addition to these primary cognitive and neurological deficits, AD is characterized by noncognitive behavioral problems (Ballard et al. 1995; Wragg and Jeste 1989). These noncognitive problems are highly prevalent in AD and in other late-life disorders causing dementia and are the most common precipitants of institutional placement (O'Donnell et al. 1992). The most troublesome of these noncognitive behavioral problems are disruptive agitated behaviors, such as physical and verbal aggression, uncooperativeness with activities necessary for personal hygiene and safety, wandering, delusions and hallucinations, and motoric hyperactivity.

In this chapter, we review the evidence for efficacy of psychopharmacological approaches to the management of these disruptive agitated behaviors in AD and other disorders causing dementia. We also review the management of depression (or depressive signs and symptoms) complicating dementia. The chapter's focus is on the results of placebo-controlled studies evaluating psychopharmacological therapies. However, because well-designed pla-

cebo-controlled studies are scarce (despite the extensive use of a wide variety of psychotropic medications to control agitated disruptive behaviors in AD), data from studies that are not placebo controlled but are nevertheless informative are also presented.

PREVALENCE OF PSYCHOTROPIC DRUG USE IN DISORDERS CAUSING DEMENTIA

Disruptive behaviors occur in at least 40% of patients with AD during the course of their illness (Reisberg et al. 1987), and the true prevalence is probably even higher. Most of these patients with AD (as well as patients with other disorders causing dementia who manifest disruptive behaviors) are given some type of psychotropic medication as a part of their treatment regimens (Salzman 1987). The epidemiology of disruptive behaviors and psychotropic drug prescribing patterns in nursing home settings has been well studied. Rovner and colleagues (1986) documented noncognitive behavioral problems in the majority of patients ($n = 38$) from a random sample of 50 residents of a proprietary nursing home. Among the 40% ($n = 20$) of patients with five or more behavioral problems, the most frequently reported were disruptiveness, restlessness, noisiness, and aggressive behaviors.

With this high prevalence of noncognitive behaviors complicating the management of AD and other disorders causing dementia, it is not surprising that the use of psychotropic medications in long-term-care facilities is common. Beers et al. (1988) reviewed psychotropic medication use in intermediate-care-facility residents in the state of Massachusetts. To ensure that the homes represented typical geriatric facilities rather than those caring for deinstitutionalized mental hospital patients, homes were not studied if they had admitted more than 20% of their residents from inpatient psychiatric hospitals. Beers and colleagues found that more than 50% of all elderly residents were receiving a psychotropic medication, 26% were receiving antipsychotic medication, and 28% were receiving sedative-hypnotics (primarily benzodiazepines and sedating antihistamines).

Buck (1988) examined the administration of psychotropic medications to Medicaid recipients residing continuously in nursing homes in Illinois. Of these residents, 60% received at least one psychotropic medication during the year. The antipsychotic drugs haloperidol and thioridazine and the benzodiazepine flurazepam were the most frequently prescribed medications. Avorn and colleagues (1989) surveyed a random sample of 55 nursing homes in Massachusetts and found that more than 50% of the residents were taking at least one psychoactive medication. Antipsychotic medications were being administered to 39% of patients. In a follow-up investigation, they studied 837 residents in 44 nursing homes with particularly high levels of antipsychotic drug use.

PSYCHOPHARMACOLOGICAL MANAGEMENT OF DISRUPTIVE AGITATED BEHAVIORS

Antipsychotic Drugs

General clinical issues. The antipsychotic drugs are widely prescribed to patients with AD and other disorders causing dementia that are complicated by disruptive behaviors (Harrington et al. 1992). The rationale for the use of these drugs is partially based on phenomenological similarities of at least some disruptive agitated behaviors in elderly patients with dementia to signs and symptoms of psychotic disorders such as schizophrenia in nonelderly patients. For example, delusions and hallucinations are common in AD (Wragg and Jeste 1989). Cummings and colleagues (1987) reported that persecutory delusions occurred in 30% of patients with AD and in 40% of patients with multi-infarct dementia. Hallucinations were frequent but somewhat less common in this study. However, it should be emphasized that psychotic behaviors in AD are often qualitatively different from those that complicate schizophrenia.

In AD and in other disorders causing dementia, the most common delusions are relatively unelaborated paranoid beliefs, such as that money or property has been stolen. Systematized complex delusions with bizarre content and grandiose delusions are uncommon. Often, the delusions accompanying AD appear to be related to underlying memory deficits. For example, the patient with AD forgets where he or she has placed an item and then believes that it has been stolen; or, when an article of clothing discarded many years earlier cannot be located, the patient believes that it has been taken. Patients with AD often stubbornly insist in a delusion-like manner that long-deceased people are alive, that their current residence is not their home, or that their spouse is an impostor. Although these beliefs meet formal criteria for delusions, they are in some ways unlike the delusions of schizophrenia for which the antipsychotic drugs have proved so effective. The phenomenological differences between psychotic features of AD and psychotic features of schizophrenia may explain why treatment outcome studies suggest that the antipsychotic drugs are less effective in patients with AD than they are in patients with schizophrenia (Schneider et al. 1990).

Nonpsychotic disruptive behaviors, such as motor restlessness, aggressive verbal and physical outbursts, persistent pacing, and uncooperativeness, also may occur in the absence of delusions and/or hallucinations. Patients with AD who have disruptive agitated behaviors but no discernible psychosis often have been included in antipsychotic drug outcome trials. Inclusion of such agitated but not psychotic patients with AD in treatment trials of antipsychotic drugs may have contributed to the relatively small magnitude of reported antipsychotic efficacy in patients with AD (see the next subsection).

Because the adverse effects of antipsychotic drugs, particularly extrapyramidal effects, can be very troubling for elderly patients with dementia (Devanand et al. 1989), the clinician should carefully weigh risks and benefits before prescribing antipsychotic drugs for delusions and hallucinations that are not bothersome either to the patient or to caregivers. In these instances, the potential adverse effects of antipsychotic medications, such as extrapyramidal rigidity and excessive sedation, may complicate management more than they improve the patient's quality of life. On the other hand, several studies have reported that psychotic symptoms in AD are associated with more rapid cognitive deterioration (Drevets and Rubin 1989; Jeste et al. 1992; Lopez et al. 1991; Y. Stern et al. 1987). Long-term studies are needed to clarify whether pharmacological control of psychotic symptoms would modify disease progression.

Outcome trials.   More clinical outcome trials of antipsychotic drug therapy in dementia patients with disruptive behaviors have been done than for any other class of psychotropic medication. Even so, relatively few placebo-controlled studies have provided interpretable data. Furthermore, many of the studies completed before publication of DSM-III (American Psychiatric Association 1980) used somewhat confusing diagnostic nomenclature and occasionally used the term *psychotic* to connote severe dementia rather than the presence of delusions and/or hallucinations. Also, these earlier studies frequently used state hospital populations of chronically ill inpatients and included both patients with degenerative neurological disorders such as AD and patients with chronic schizophrenia who had grown old.

In one of these early studies, chlorpromazine was compared with placebo in a double-blind crossover design that included 29 patients with the diagnosis of dementia (Seager 1955). Global ratings of disturbed behaviors favored chlorpromazine over placebo, but sedation and falls were more common in the chlorpromazine group. Acetophenazine was compared with placebo in 14 patients with the diagnosis of dementia and associated hyperactive behaviors, such as assaultiveness, nocturnal wandering, irritability, hyperexcitability, and abnormal fear (L. D. Hamilton and Bennett 1962a). Attenuation of these hyperactive behaviors was greater in the acetophenazine group than in the placebo group, but excessive sedation was a major adverse effect of acetophenazine.

Haloperidol was compared with placebo in 18 patients with dementia (mean age 72) for the control of agitation, overactivity, and hostility (Sugerman et al. 1964). Significant differences favoring haloperidol compared with placebo were noted in ratings of hallucinations, restlessness, and uncooperativeness. In the haloperidol group, a substantial number of subjects developed unsteady gait and/or pseudoparkinsonian signs. In this study, the patients who were most severely agitated prior to randomization had the best response to haloperidol.

In contrast to these three studies (L. D. Hamilton and Bennett 1962a; Seager 1955; Sugerman et al. 1964), other studies completed before DSM-III was published did not report an advantage for antipsychotic medications compared with placebo in patients with dementia. A common feature of these studies was the absence of target signs and symptoms (e.g., hallucinations, delusions, severe agitation, and severe hyperactivity) that responded better to antipsychotic medication than to placebo in the three studies described above. Trifluoperazine was compared with placebo in 27 patients with severe dementia (mean age 71) (L. D. Hamilton and Bennett 1962b). In this study,

target symptoms were apathy, withdrawal, and cognitive and behavioral deterioration (e.g., incontinence, loss of ambulation, and severe disorientation). Trifluoperazine was no more effective than placebo in this study, and the antipsychotic drug induced troublesome sedation and parkinsonian signs and symptoms in most of the patients taking active medication.

Thiothixene was compared with placebo in a study of patients with dementia in whom the target symptoms were primarily cognitive deficits (Rada and Kellner 1976). Global improvement was noted equally in the thiothixene and placebo groups. Thirteen of 22 patients receiving thiothixene were rated as at least minimally globally improved, and 11 of 20 patients in the placebo group were rated as at least minimally globally improved. The apparent placebo response in this study is of interest and has also been found in some of the more recent placebo-controlled trials of antipsychotic medications in well-characterized dementia patients (see later in this section).

Several studies have been done since the publication of DSM-III and DSM-III-R (American Psychiatric Association 1987). In these studies, the use of explicit diagnostic criteria for primary degenerative dementia of the Alzheimer type and multi-infarct dementia increased confidence that elderly patients with chronic schizophrenia and other chronic psychotic psychiatric disorders beginning in early life were excluded from the study populations. In addition, these studies required that either psychotic symptoms (i.e., delusions and hallucinations) or disruptive nonpsychotic behaviors be present as target symptoms.

Two studies have been carried out in very elderly typical community nursing home patients (mean age > 80 years). In the first study, Barnes et al. (1982) randomized 60 patients (mean age 83 years) whose symptoms met criteria for either AD or multi-infarct dementia and who had psychotic or nonpsychotic disruptive behaviors to receive either thioridazine, loxapine, or placebo. Ratings of excitement and uncooperativeness on the Brief Psychiatric Rating Scale (BPRS; Overall and Gorham 1962) had significantly greater improvement with either active drug than with placebo. However, suspiciousness and hostility decreased both with active drug and with placebo, and the differences between active drug and placebo responses were not statistically significant for these latter symptoms. Global improvement was greater for active drug than for placebo, but only one-third of the patients taking active medication were rated as either moderately or markedly improved on a clinical global impression of change scale. In the second study, Finkel et al. (1995) randomized 33 nursing home residents (mean age 85 years) with agitated behavior to receive either thiothixene or placebo. Behavioral improvement as quantified by the Cohen-Mansfield Agitation Inventory (Cohen-Mansfield 1986) significantly favored thiothixene, but the magnitude of difference between active drug and placebo was modest. The lack of persistent differences in extrapyramidal symptoms between groups was attributed to a flexible dosage schedule and the use of short-term benztropine (1–3 weeks) when extrapyramidal signs and symptoms emerged. Psychotic signs and symptoms per se were not identified or quantified in this study. These two studies suggest real but limited efficacy for antipsychotic drugs in typical nursing home populations of behaviorally disturbed and very old patients with dementia. Note that these studies included dementia patients with disruptive behaviors regardless of whether they had psychotic symptoms.

In a study conducted in a younger (mean age 73 years) state psychiatric hospital sample of behaviorally disturbed patients with AD and multi-infarct dementia, haloperidol or loxapine was compared with placebo (Petrie et al. 1982). Both antipsychotic medications were significantly more effective than placebo, particularly for treating suspiciousness, hallucinatory behavior, excitement, hostility, and uncooperativeness. Global ratings of improvement, however, were similar to those found by Barnes et al. (1982) and Finkel et al. (1995). Thirty-two percent of loxapine patients and 35% of haloperidol patients were rated as moderately or markedly improved compared with 9% of patients who had been randomized to the placebo condition.

In a pilot study that used a single-blind ABA (A = 4 weeks of placebo, B = 8 weeks of haloperidol) design, haloperidol in doses of 1–5 mg/day was efficacious in the treatment of nine outpatients with AD and behavioral complications (Devanand et al. 1989). However, some patients could not tolerate the higher doses (>4 mg/day) primarily because of extrapyramidal symptoms. Haloperidol treatment was associated with a small but significant decline in cognitive function, assessed by the modified Mini-Mental State Exam (Folstein et al. 1975). These findings suggested that even lower doses may be necessary; that is, very low doses might retain the efficacy seen at higher doses, while avoiding side effects. To address this issue, Devanand and colleagues (personal communication, December 1997) are in the process of completing a random assignment, parallel-group, double-blind, placebo-controlled study in which "standard"-dose haloperidol (2–3 mg/day), low-dose haloperidol (0.5–0.75 mg/day), and placebo are being compared in a 6-week trial with a subsequent crossover phase. In preliminary analyses, haloperidol at 2–3 mg/day showed moderate efficacy and

was significantly superior to low-dose haloperidol and placebo, which did not differ from each other in measures of both efficacy and side effects (Devanand, personal communication, December 1997). These findings, if confirmed, suggest that doses of haloperidol below 1 mg/day are often subtherapeutic.

The Lewy body variant of AD presents clinically with extrapyramidal rigidity, fluctuating cognitive impairment, and an increased incidence of psychotic symptoms as compared with typical AD (Byrne et al. 1991). In addition to the diffuse neuritic plaques characteristic of AD, this variant shows subcortical, limbic, and neocortical Lewy bodies (Perry et al. 1990) at postmortem examination. Patients with the Lewy body variant of AD appear particularly susceptible to extrapyramidal adverse effects of typical antipsychotic drugs (McKeith et al. 1992); thus, a treatment dilemma presents when psychotic symptoms emerge. Anecdotal reports suggest that the antipsychotic drug risperidone potentially may reduce psychotic symptoms with fewer parkinsonian adverse effects than those of typical antipsychotics (e.g., haloperidol) in Lewy body variant AD (Allen et al. 1995; Lee et al. 1994).

The important question of long-term antipsychotic drug maintenance was addressed by an antipsychotic drug discontinuation study in patients with dementia whose disturbed behaviors appeared to decline with antipsychotic medication and who had then been given chronic antipsychotic maintenance therapy. Risse et al. (1987) substituted placebo for maintenance antipsychotic medication in nine male patients with dementia (mean age 65 years) who had symptomatically improved after standard clinical treatment with antipsychotic medication to control agitated behaviors and who had been given maintenance antipsychotic medication for at least 90 days. At the end of the 6-week substitution period, only one patient had developed disruptive behavior severe enough to warrant reinstitution of antipsychotic medication. Of the remaining eight patients, one was rated as more agitated, two were unchanged, and five actually were rated as less agitated. These results suggest the need for further study of antipsychotic medication discontinuation trials in behaviorally stable patients with dementia who appear to have benefited from past antipsychotic treatment. Such discontinuation trials also are consistent with federal policies as stipulated in the Omnibus Budget Reconciliation Act (OBRA) of 1987 (Kelly 1989).

Drugs With Pharmacological Effects on Serotonin Systems

The loss of serotonergic neurons in the brain stem raphe nuclei and decreased concentrations of the serotonin metabolite 5-hydroxyindoleacetic acid (5-HIAA) in post-mortem brain tissue and in cerebrospinal fluid (Blenow et al. 1991; Zweig et al. 1988) indicate a serotonergic deficiency in AD. The efficacy of serotonergic drugs, such as trazodone, buspirone, and selective serotonin uptake inhibitors (SSRIs), for treatment of disruptive agitated behaviors in AD is suggested by anecdotal reports and a few placebo-controlled studies.

Simpson and Foster (1986) treated two patients with AD and two patients with alcoholic dementia with trazodone. At doses of 200–500 mg/day, trazodone appeared to decrease agitation, combative behavior, and violent outbursts. In a similar open trial, Pinner and Rich (1988) treated seven patients with dementia with trazodone for symptomatic aggressive behavior. Patients had various dementia diagnoses, including AD, dementia due to head trauma, alcoholic dementia, and schizophrenia with dementia. Three of the seven patients (all of whom had not shown a therapeutic response to prior treatment with antipsychotic drugs) had a marked decrease in aggressive behavior following 4–6 weeks of trazodone treatment at 200–300 mg/day. Three other patients had no response, and one patient was unable to take the drug for more than 11 days because of unspecified adverse effects.

An advantage of trazodone compared with antipsychotics that supports further evaluation of this compound in the treatment of AD patients with disruptive behaviors is its lack of extrapyramidal adverse effects. Although trazodone is sedating and can produce orthostatic hypotension (as well as rarely producing priapism), it appears to be well tolerated in older patients with dementia.

Buspirone has an even more benign adverse-effect profile than does trazodone. Colenda (1988) studied a 74-year-old woman with AD who manifested agitated behaviors, including constant rocking, angry outbursts, and oppositional behavior, and who had failed to respond therapeutically to haloperidol. After a 2-month course of buspirone at 45 mg/day, the patient's agitated behaviors were markedly reduced. Tiller and colleagues (1988) reported a similarly positive response to buspirone (15 mg/day) in a patient with multi-infarct dementia complicated by agitated behaviors. Sakauye and colleagues (1993) reported an open-label study of buspirone in 10 patients with AD complicated by agitated behaviors. At doses of 30–40 mg/day of buspirone, a modest but significant overall reduction (22%) on the Cohen-Mansfield Agitated Behavior Scale (Cohen-Mansfield et al. 1989) occurred. A substantial variability in response was seen: 4 patients apparently had marked declines in disruptive behaviors, 4 patients had minimal or no change, and 2 had slight elevations in ratings of agitated behaviors.

In a double-blind, placebo-controlled crossover study, Lawlor et al. (1994) treated 10 patients with AD and behavioral complications (troublesome agitation, depression, psychosis, or anxiety) with trazodone (up to 150 mg/day), buspirone (30 mg/day), and placebo. Trazodone produced a small but significant behavioral improvement compared with placebo, whereas buspirone had no apparent effect. Levy (1994) used buspirone to treat 20 patients with AD and behavioral disturbances rated as at least moderately troublesome on the Behavioral Pathology in Alzheimer's Disease Rating Scale (BEHAVE-AD) (Reisberg et al. 1987) in a single-blind dose-escalation study. After a 2- to 4-week psychotropic drug washout period, subjects were given placebo for 1 week and then progressively increasing weekly doses (15, 30, 45, and 60 mg) of buspirone. At least one dose of buspirone was significantly more effective than placebo for global behavioral score, aggression, and anxiety. A dose-response improvement in anxiety rating occurred. As with the Barnes et al. (1982) study of antipsychotic drugs, placebo had a significant effect on delusions.

Because trazodone and buspirone have relatively low toxicity, both drugs merit further investigation in parallel-group studies that encourage titration to relatively high dosage levels. There have been surprisingly few reports of the use of SSRIs in the treatment of disruptive agitated behaviors complicating AD. Lebert et al. (1994) conducted an open 8-week pilot study of fluoxetine (20 mg/day) in 10 patients with AD. Ratings of emotional lability, irritability, anxiety, and fear-panic were significantly improved following fluoxetine treatment. Surprisingly, the rating of "reduced mood" was unaffected by fluoxetine. Positive effects of the SSRI citalopram as compared with placebo on both anxiety and affective symptoms in patients with dementia also have been reported (Nyth and Gottfries 1990). The efficacy of citalopram in depression complicating AD is discussed later in this chapter (see section, "Depression Complicating AD and Other Disorders Causing Dementia").

Antimanic Drugs

The effectiveness of antimanic drugs for the hyperactivity, aggressive behaviors, and temper outbursts seen in patients in the manic phase of bipolar disorder has prompted trials of these drugs for treatment of disruptive agitated behaviors in patients with AD or other disorders causing dementia. As with information on the drugs acting on serotonergic systems, information on the antimanic drugs in dementia patients with disruptive behaviors is largely anecdotal. In an open study of carbamazepine (Marin and Greenwald 1989), two patients with AD and one patient with multi-infarct dementia who did not respond to haloperidol for treatment of combative agitated behaviors appeared to improve markedly within 2 weeks of starting carbamazepine treatment at doses ranging from 100 to 300 mg/day.

In a more extensive open study of carbamazepine in patients with AD who had no response to antipsychotic drugs (Gleason and Schneider 1990), disruptive agitation clinically improved in five of nine patients. Particular symptomatic reduction of hostility, agitation, and uncooperativeness in responders was noted. Ataxia and confusion occurred in two of the patients whose agitated behaviors had declined with carbamazepine therapy. These adverse effects resolved with dose reduction. The mean dose of carbamazepine in this study was 480 mg/day, and the mean plasma level achieved was 6.5 µg/mL. Tempering these enthusiastic but uncontrolled open studies is an earlier study in which 19 elderly patients with dementia were prescribed carbamazepine (100–300 mg/day) or placebo in a crossover design (Chambers et al. 1982). No overall benefit from carbamazepine was detected for the target symptoms of wandering, overactivity, and restlessness, but the low doses of carbamazepine prescribed may have limited the possibility of detecting efficacy. The most convincing data supporting carbamazepine efficacy were reported by Tariot et al. (1994). In a nonrandomized, placebo-controlled pilot study, they reported decreased agitation with minimal adverse effects in 25 nursing home patients with dementia.

The anticonvulsant and antimanic drug sodium valproate was evaluated in an open-label study of 4 patients who had AD complicated by disruptive agitated behaviors but who did not have clear psychotic signs or symptoms (Mellow et al. 1993). Sodium valproate was prescribed for periods of 1–3 months at doses ranging from 500 mg twice a day to 500 mg three times a day. Substantial behavioral improvement was observed in 2 of the 4 patients, and no adverse effects were noted. Lithium, the classic antimanic drug, has also been evaluated in open studies in patients with dementia and disruptive behaviors. Holton and George (1985) prescribed a low dose of lithium (250 mg/day) for 4 weeks to 10 such patients who ranged in age from 72 to 85. Disruptive behaviors were not ameliorated during the 4-week open lithium trial, but the low dose of lithium prescribed may have been outside a potential therapeutic range.

Benzodiazepines

The use of benzodiazepines in patients with dementia and disturbed behaviors was reviewed by R. G. Stern and colleagues (1991). Several placebo-controlled studies of benzodiazepines were completed in the 1960s and 1970s. Although specific subject diagnoses are difficult to determine, these studies probably included mostly patients with AD and other disorders causing dementia.

Sanders (1965) compared oxazepam with placebo in elderly (mean age 81) "emotionally disturbed" patients. Although oxazepam was superior to placebo after 6 weeks of treatment, no difference was found between the placebo-treated and oxazepam-treated patients at the end of the 8-week treatment period. Agitation and anxiety had the most favorable response to active treatment. These data suggest that tolerance to the benzodiazepine may have developed by the end of the treatment protocol.

Thioridazine and diazepam were compared in a non-placebo-controlled study of the control of behavioral symptoms associated with "senility" (Kirven and Montero 1973). Although both drugs were associated with symptomatic reduction, the trend was in favor of thioridazine. As with the Sanders (1965) study, the data suggested that tolerance may have developed to the benzodiazepine by the end of the treatment protocol. In both of these studies, psychotic symptoms, such as delusions and/or hallucinations, were not specifically rated.

In another study (Coccaro et al. 1990), the efficacy of an antipsychotic drug (haloperidol), a benzodiazepine (oxazepam), and a sedating antihistamine (diphenhydramine) were compared for the treatment of agitated behaviors in a group of elderly institutionalized patients, most of whom met criteria for AD. The patients' mean age was 75, and target signs and symptoms included tension, excitement, verbal aggressiveness, physical aggressiveness, pacing, fidgeting, and increased motor activity. These behaviors decreased in all treatment groups over the 8-week period, but there was no differential response to the three psychotropic drugs. The trend was for modestly greater improvement with diphenhydramine and haloperidol than with oxazepam. Because this study lacked a placebo group, the investigators acknowledged that the modest improvements in objective ratings of behavioral problems may have been a result of factors other than drug treatment. This study is of interest because it suggests that sedation (a common effect of these otherwise markedly different drugs) may have been the factor producing improvement. This study also does not provide evidence favoring benzodiazepines for the treatment of behaviorally disturbed patients with dementia, given that oxazepam appeared to be even less effective than the other two drugs.

Cholinesterase Inhibitors

Cholinesterase inhibitor therapy was conceptualized as a specific therapy for the cognitive deficits presumably secondary to the presynaptic cholinergic lesion of AD (Whitehouse et al. 1982). Recent uncontrolled studies suggest possible efficacy of cholinesterase inhibitors for noncognitive symptoms, such as apathy, agitation, and delusions (Cummings and Kaufer 1996). In the 30-week pivotal study establishing the efficacy of tacrine for memory and other cognitive deficits of AD (Knapp et al. 1994), effects of tacrine on noncognitive symptoms as quantified by the noncognitive subscale of the Alzheimer's Disease Assessment Scale (Rosen et al. 1984) were evaluated in an exploratory analysis (Raskind et al. 1997). Subjects with AD randomized to receive tacrine (160 mg/day—the recommended target dose) more frequently showed improvement or stabilization of pacing, delusions, and poor cooperation than did subjects with AD randomized to receive placebo. These data suggest that the cholinergic deficiency of AD may contribute to at least some noncognitive behavioral disturbances in this disorder.

PRACTICAL MANAGEMENT OF DISRUPTIVE BEHAVIORS IN AD AND OTHER DISORDERS CAUSING DEMENTIA

The available data suggest that antipsychotic drugs should still be the first agents tried for the management of disruptive behaviors in dementia. Before antipsychotic medications are instituted, the clinician must evaluate the general medical condition of the patient to rule out a medical etiology for disruptive behaviors (e.g., pain, thyrotoxicosis) or an adverse effect of a nonpsychotropic medication (e.g., theophylline, L-dopa). Environmental and behavioral approaches also should be instituted when possible. For example, the pacing behavior of patients in the middle stages of AD is best treated by providing a secure environment in which patients can get up and walk around at any time of the day or night. Pacing not clearly attributable to delusions or hallucinations appears unresponsive to psychotropic medication, and akathisia from antipsychotic medications may exacerbate pacing. Although research evaluating the efficacy of behavioral approaches to disruptive behaviors is limited (Teri et al. 1992), collaboration with a clinical psychologist or other mental health professional knowledgeable in behavioral techniques can prove rewarding.

It appears that the closer the disruptive behaviors of the patient with AD resemble the psychotic signs and symptoms seen in schizophrenia, the more effective antipsychotic drugs will be. Clinical experience suggests that the choice of a particular antipsychotic drug should be based on the tolerability of the adverse effects of a given agent by the patient to whom it will be prescribed. Haloperidol and other high-potency drugs are more likely to produce parkinsonian signs and symptoms than are low-potency antipsychotic drugs such as thioridazine. However, thioridazine and other low-potency drugs are more likely to produce anticholinergic adverse effects (e.g., urinary retention, constipation, dry mouth, blurred vision, central anticholinergic delirium), orthostatic hypotension, and excess sedation than are high-potency antipsychotic drugs such as haloperidol. The newer antipsychotic drug risperidone has a relatively low propensity to produce either extrapyramidal or anticholinergic adverse effects at doses that are antipsychotic (Owens 1994). This drug offers a potentially attractive alternative to typical antipsychotics for behaviorally disturbed patients with dementia. A large multicenter trial comparing risperidone with haloperidol in behaviorally disturbed patients with dementia is in progress. Given these considerations, haloperidol would be a reasonable choice of medication for an elderly male patient with prostatic hypertrophy and no parkinsonian-like motor signs (e.g., bradykinesia or rigidity). Because rigidity is common in the later stages of AD, a patient with such rigidity might better tolerate a lower-potency drug such as thioridazine.

All drugs should be started at a low but constantly prescribed dose, such as 1 mg of haloperidol, 25 mg of thioridazine, or 0.5 mg of risperidone every day. Because the therapeutic action of these drugs may not be immediately apparent, the dose should be increased gradually, perhaps every week, if the desired therapeutic effect has not been achieved and adverse effects are either not present or well tolerated. As the dose increases, clinical experience suggests that in the more frail elderly patient, dividing the total dose into a three-times-a-day regimen may avoid excessive peak plasma drug concentrations that could increase acute adverse effects such as orthostatic hypotension. Divided dosing does, however, increase demands on caregivers and nursing personnel. In the elderly patient with AD or another disorder causing dementia, a dose of haloperidol higher than 3 mg/day or thioridazine greater than 75 mg/day often is poorly tolerated. On the other hand, the less common patient with early-onset AD who is in his or her 50s or 60s and whose general medical condition is sound may both tolerate and need higher doses of antipsychotic medication for adequate management of disruptive agitated behaviors.

As should be apparent from this review of clinical outcome trials of psychotropic drugs other than antipsychotics for disruptive behaviors in AD and other disorders causing dementia, no well-established guidelines are available for selecting a psychotropic medication for patients in whom antipsychotic drugs are either ineffective or poorly tolerated. Buspirone at a starting dose of 5 mg three times a day but with gradual increases up to 15 mg three times a day has the advantage of a relatively benign adverse-effect profile. Trazodone starting at 50 mg/day with gradual increases to 50 or 100 mg three times a day may also be effective, but orthostatic hypotension or excessive sedation may complicate the use of trazodone in some patients. Violent behavior may respond to carbamazepine or valproate. These drugs are reasonably well tolerated, although sedation and ataxia may occur. Short-half-life benzodiazepines may be useful if subjective anxiety is prominent or can be reasonably inferred from the patient's behavioral problems. However, benzodiazepines have a high incidence of ataxia and excessive sedation and can impair cognitive function in elderly patients (Sunderland et al. 1989). Furthermore, tolerance to the therapeutic antianxiety or anti-agitation effects of the benzodiazepines is common. It also appears likely that cholinesterase inhibitors prescribed as cognitive enhancers will have positive effects on noncognitive behavioral problems in some patients with AD.

DEPRESSION COMPLICATING AD AND OTHER DISORDERS CAUSING DEMENTIA

Because depression per se can impair cognitive function (Cohen et al. 1982), the recognition and effective treatment of depression complicating a disorder causing dementia offer the potential for both improving mood and maximizing the patient's cognitive abilities. However, the recognition of a true depressive disorder in the patient with AD or another illness causing dementia can be difficult. The overlap of signs and symptoms between depression and dementia can make diagnosis of depression in the patient with dementia confusing. Common to both disorders are apathy, sleep disturbances, loss of interest in previously interesting activities, and changes in psychomotor activity. Even with these diagnostic difficulties, a number of studies have found a high prevalence of depressive signs and symptoms in AD (Reifler et al. 1986; Rovner et al. 1986). Depressive signs and symptoms in patients with AD have also been shown to be associated with added functional impairment (Pearson et al. 1989).

Although anecdotal reports suggest that antidepressant drugs are effective in the treatment of depression complicating AD and other disorders causing dementia (Jenike 1985), only a few placebo-controlled studies have actually addressed the question of efficacy in these patients. Reifler and colleagues (1989) compared imipramine with placebo in a double-blind outcome study of the treatment of major depressive episode complicating AD. Subjects in this study had symptoms that met DSM-III-R criteria for both primary degenerative dementia of the Alzheimer type and major depressive episode. Patients were still living in the community but were in the middle stages of AD (Mini-Mental State Exam mean score = 17) and had depression of mild to moderate severity (Hamilton Rating Scale for Depression [M. Hamilton 1960] mean score = 19). Patients were given imipramine (mean dose 83 mg/day; mean plasma level of imipramine plus desmethylimipramine 116 ng/mL) or placebo and were evaluated with their caregivers at weekly visits for 8 weeks. Substantial and highly significant reduction in depressive signs and symptoms was documented in both the imipramine and the placebo groups, but the amount of improvement was indistinguishable between groups. This study suggests that AD outpatients with depressive symptoms (and probably their caregivers) respond positively to participation in an antidepressant treatment outcome trial. Whether a tricyclic antidepressant specifically ameliorates depressive symptomatology in doses well tolerated in patients with AD has yet to be confirmed.

Because Reifler et al. (1989) did not include patients with severe depression in their study, their results are applicable only to patients with mild to moderate dementia and a modest amount of depressive symptomatology. However, the latter type of patient accounts for the bulk of depressive signs and symptoms complicating AD. Interpretation of this study is also complicated because the emergence of adverse effects limited the amount of imipramine prescribed. A higher dose of imipramine might have been even more effective than the substantial placebo group response.

Tricyclic antidepressants also have been evaluated in a placebo-controlled study of depression (both major depressive episode and dysthymia) complicating stroke (Lipsey et al. 1984). A substantial proportion of the subjects in this study likely had at least mild multi-infarct dementia. In this study (Lipsey et al. 1984), nortriptyline was more effective than placebo for depressive signs and symptoms. The SSRI citalopram, which is available in Europe and Canada but not in the United States, was compared with placebo in a small group of patients with dementia (unspecified type) with depressive symptomatology (Nyth et al. 1992). Citalopram was modestly but significantly more effective than placebo and was well tolerated. Sertraline also has been reported to improve depressed affect in advanced AD (Volicer et al. 1994). Placebo-controlled studies of SSRIs for the treatment of depression complicating AD and other neurodegenerative disorders causing dementia are needed.

CONCLUSION

Further studies are necessary to provide rational guidelines for the psychopharmacological management of noncognitive behavioral problems complicating AD and other disorders causing dementia. Extrapolations from the large body of psychotherapeutic drug outcome studies in younger patients with diseases such as schizophrenia and depression starting in adolescence or middle age often are not relevant to elderly patients with dementia who are behaviorally disturbed. Careful evaluations of newer antipsychotic agents with reduced extrapyramidal toxicity, such as risperidone and olanzapine, may improve the applicability of the general class of antipsychotic drugs for behaviorally disturbed patients with dementia. Placebo-controlled outcome studies of drugs such as buspirone and trazodone can establish or refute the hints of efficacy derived from anecdotal reports. The antimanic drugs, particularly carbamazepine and sodium valproate, also deserve evaluations in well-designed clinical trials. The potential positive effects of "cognitive-acting" drugs such as the cholinesterase inhibitors tacrine and donepezil should not be discounted in future outcome trials. Careful attention to accurate phenomenological descriptions of specific types of behavioral problems may help to establish therapeutic specificity of a drug for a given behavioral problem.

REFERENCES

Allen RL, Walker Z, D'Ath PJ, et al: Risperidone for psychotic and behavioural symptoms in Lewy body dementia (letter). Lancet 346:185, 1995

American Psychiatric Association: Diagnostic and Statistical Manual of Mental Disorders, 3rd Edition. Washington, DC, American Psychiatric Association, 1980

American Psychiatric Association: Diagnostic and Statistical Manual of Mental Disorders, 3rd Edition, Revised. Washington, DC, American Psychiatric Association, 1987

Avorn J, Dreyer P, Connelly MA, et al: Use of psychoactive medication and the quality of care in rest homes. N Engl J Med 320:227–232, 1989

Ballard CG, Saad K, Patel A, et al: The prevalence and phenomenology of psychotic symptoms in dementia sufferers. International Journal of Geriatric Psychiatry 10:477–485, 1995

Barnes R, Veith R, Okimoto J, et al: Efficacy of antipsychotic medications in behaviorally disturbed dementia patients. Am J Psychiatry 139:1170–1174, 1982

Beers M, Avorn J, Soumerai SB, et al: Psychoactive medication use in intermediate-care facility residents. JAMA 260:3016–3020, 1988

Blenow KAJ, Wallin A, Gottfries CG, et al: Significance of decreased lumbar CSF levels of HVA and 5-HIAA in Alzheimer's disease. Neurobiol Aging 13:107–113, 1991

Buck JA: Psychotropic drug practice in nursing homes. J Am Geriatr Soc 36:409–418, 1988

Byrne EJ, Lennox GG, Godwin-Austen RB, et al: Dementia associated with cortical Lewy bodies: proposed clinical diagnostic criteria. Dementia 2:283–284, 1991

Chambers CA, Bain J, Rosbottom R, et al: Carbamazepine in senile dementia and overactivity—a placebo controlled double blind trial. IRCS Journal of Medical Science 10:505–506, 1982

Coccaro EF, Kramer E, Zemishlany Z, et al: Pharmacologic treatment of noncognitive behavioral disturbances in elderly demented patients. Am J Psychiatry 147:1640–1656, 1990

Cohen RM, Weingartner HW, Smallberg A, et al: Effort and cognition in depression. Arch Gen Psychiatry 39:593–597, 1982

Cohen-Mansfield J: Agitated behaviors in the elderly, II: preliminary results in the cognitively deteriorated. J Am Geriatr Soc 34:722–727, 1986

Cohen-Mansfield J, Marx MS, Rosenthal AS: A description of agitation in a nursing home. J Gerontol 44:77–84, 1989

Colenda CC: Buspirone in treatment of agitated demented patient (letter). Lancet 1:1169, 1988

Cummings JL, Kaufer D: Neuropsychiatric aspects of Alzheimer's disease: the cholinergic hypothesis revisited. Neurology 47:876–883, 1996

Cummings JL, Miller B, Hill MA, et al: Neuropsychiatric aspects of multi-infarct dementia and dementia of the Alzheimer type. Arch Neurol 44:389–393, 1987

Devanand DP, Sackheim HA, Brown RP, et al: A pilot study of haloperidol treatment of psychosis and behavioral disturbance in Alzheimer's disease. Arch Neurol 46:854–857, 1989

Drevets WC, Rubin E: Psychotic symptoms and the longitudinal course of senile dementia of the Alzheimer type. Biol Psychiatry 25:39–48, 1989

Finkel SI, Lyons JS, Anderson RL, et al: A randomized, placebo-controlled trial of thiothixene in agitated, demented nursing home patients. International Journal of Geriatric Psychiatry 10:129–136, 1995

Folstein MF, Folstein SE, McHugh PR: Mini-Mental State: a practical method for grading the cognitive state of patients for the clinician. J Psychiatr Res 12:189–198, 1975

Gleason RP, Schneider LS: Carbamazepine treatment of agitation in Alzheimer's outpatients refractory to neuroleptics. J Clin Psychiatry 51:115–118, 1990

Hamilton LD, Bennett JL: Acetophenazine for hyperactive geriatric patients. Geriatrics 17:596–601, 1962a

Hamilton LD, Bennett JL: The use of trifluoperazine in geriatric patients with chronic brain syndrome. J Am Geriatr Soc 10:140–147, 1962b

Hamilton M: A rating scale for depression. J Neurol Neurosurg Psychiatry 23:56–62, 1960

Harrington C, Tompkins C, Curtis M, et al: Psychotropic drug use in long-term care facilities: a review of the literature. Gerontologist 32:822–833, 1992

Holton A, George K: The use of lithium in severely demented patients with behavioral disturbance. Br J Psychiatry 146:99–100, 1985

Jenike MA: MAO inhibitors as treatment for depressed patients with primary degenerative dementia (Alzheimer's disease). Am J Psychiatry 142:763–764, 1985

Jeste DV, Wragg RE, Salmon DP, et al: Cognitive deficits with Alzheimer's disease with and without delusions. Am J Psychiatry 149:184–189, 1992

Katzman R: The prevalence and malignancy of Alzheimer's disease: a major killer. Arch Neurol 33:217–218, 1976

Kelly M: The Omnibus Budget Reconciliation Act of 1987: a policy analysis. Nurs Clin North Am 24:791–794, 1989

Kirven LE, Montero EF: Comparison of thioridazine and diazepam in the control of nonpsychotic symptoms associated with senility: double-blind study. J Am Geriatr Soc 21:546–551, 1973

Knapp MJ, Knopman DS, Solomon PR, et al: A 30 week randomized controlled trial of high dose tacrine in patients with Alzheimer's disease. JAMA 271:985–991, 1994

Lawlor BA, Radcliffe J, Molchan SE, et al: A pilot placebo-controlled study of trazodone and buspirone in Alzheimer's disease. International Journal of Geriatric Psychiatry 9:55–59, 1994

Lebert F, Pasquier F, Petit H: Behavioural effects of fluoxetine in dementia of Alzheimer type (letter). International Journal of Geriatric Society 9:590–591, 1994

Lee H, Cooney JM, Lawlor BA: The use of risperidone, an atypical neuroleptic, in Lewy body disease. International Journal of Geriatric Psychiatry 9:415–417, 1994

Levy MA: A trial of buspirone for the control of disruptive behaviors in community-dwelling patients with dementia. International Journal of Geriatric Psychiatry 9:841–848, 1994

Lipsey JR, Pearlson GD, Robinson RG, et al: Nortriptyline treatment of post-stroke depression: a double blind study. Lancet 1:297–300, 1984

Lopez OL, Becker JT, Brenner RP, et al: Alzheimer's disease with delusions and hallucinations: neuropsychological and electroencephalographs correlates. Neurology 41:906–912, 1991

Marin DB, Greenwald BS: Carbamazepine for aggressive agitation in demented patients (letter). Am J Psychiatry 146:805, 1989

McKeith I, Fairbairn A, Perry R, et al: Neuroleptic sensitivity in patients with senile dementia of Lewy body type. BMJ 305:673–678, 1992

Mellow AM, Solano-Lopez C, Davis S: Sodium valproate in the treatment of behavioral disturbance in dementia. J Geriatr Psychiatry Neurol 6:28–32, 1993

Nyth AL, Gottfries CG: The clinical efficacy of citalopram in treatment of emotional disturbances in dementia disorders (a Nordic multicenter study). Br J Psychiatry 157:894–901, 1990

Nyth AL, Gottfries CG, Lyby K, et al: A controlled multicenter clinical study of citalopram and placebo in elderly depressed patients with and without concomitant dementia. Acta Psychiatr Scand 86:138–145, 1992

O'Donnell BF, Drachman DA, Barnes HJ, et al: Incontinence and troublesome behaviors predict institutionalization in dementia. J Geriatr Psychiatry Neurol 5:45–52, 1992

Overall JE, Gorham DR: The Brief Psychiatric Rating Scale. Psychol Rep 10:799–812, 1962

Owens DGS: Extrapyramidal side effects and tolerability of risperidone: a review. J Clin Psychiatry 55 (suppl):29–35, 1994

Pearson JL, Teri L, Reifler BV, et al: Functional status and cognitive impairment in Alzheimer's disease patients with and without depression. J Am Geriatr Soc 37:1117–1121, 1989

Perry RH, Irving D, Blessed G, et al: Senile dementia of Lewy body type: a clinically and neuropathologically distinct form of Lewy body dementia in the elderly. J Neurol Sci 95:119–139, 1990

Petrie WM, Ban TA, Berney S, et al: Loxapine in psychogeriatrics: a placebo- and standard-controlled clinical investigation. J Clin Psychopharmacol 2:122–126, 1982

Pinner E, Rich CL: Effects of trazodone on aggressive behavior in seven patients with organic mental disorders. Am J Psychiatry 145:1295–1296, 1988

Rada RT, Kellner R: Thiothixene in the treatment of geriatric patients with chronic organic brain syndrome. J Am Geriatr Soc 24:105–107, 1976

Raskind MA, Sadowsky CH, Sigmund WR, et al: Effect of tacrine on language, praxis and noncognitive behavioral problems in Alzheimer's disease. Arch Neurol 54:836–840, 1997

Reifler BV, Larson E, Teri L, et al: Dementia of Alzheimer's type and depression. J Am Geriatr Soc 34:855–859, 1986

Reifler BV, Teri L, Raskind M, et al: Double-blind trial of imipramine in Alzheimer's disease patients with and without depression. Am J Psychiatry 146:45–49, 1989

Reisberg B, Borenstein J, Salob SP, et al: Behavioural symptoms in Alzheimer's disease: phenomenology and treatment. J Clin Psychiatry 48 (5, suppl):9–15, 1987

Reisberg B, Auer SR, Monteiro IM: Behavioral Pathology in Alzheimer's Disease (BEHAVE-AD) rating scale. Int Psychogeriatr 8 (suppl 3):301–308, 1996

Risse SC, Cubberly L, Lampe TH, et al: Acute effects of neuroleptic withdrawal in elderly dementia patients. Journal of Geriatric Drug Therapy 2:65–67, 1987

Rosen WG, Mohs RC, Davis KL: A new rating scale for Alzheimer's disease. Am J Psychiatry 141:1356–1364, 1984

Rovner BW, Kafonek S, Filipp L, et al: Prevalence of mental illness in a community nursing home. Am J Psychiatry 143:1446–1449, 1986

Sakauye KM, Camp CJ, Ford PA: Effects of buspirone on agitation associated with dementia. Am J Geriatr Psychiatry 1:82–84, 1993

Salzman C: Treatment of the elderly agitated patient. J Clin Psychiatry 48 (5, suppl):19–22, 1987

Sanders JF: Evaluation of oxazepam and placebo in emotionally disturbed aged patients. Geriatrics 20:739–746, 1965

Schneider LS, Pollock VE, Lyness SA: A metaanalysis of controlled trials of neuroleptic treatment in dementia. J Am Geriatr Soc 38:553–563, 1990

Seager CP: Chlorpromazine in treatment of elderly psychotic women. BMJ 1:882–885, 1955

Simpson DM, Foster D: Improvement in organically disturbed behavior with trazodone treatment. J Clin Psychiatry 47:191–193, 1986

Stern RG, Duffelmeyer ME, Zemishlani Z, et al: The use of benzodiazepines in the management of behavioral symptoms in dementia patients. Psychiatr Clin North Am 14:375–384, 1991

Stern Y, Mayeux R, Sano M, et al: Predictions of disease course in patients with probable Alzheimer's disease. Neurology 37:1649–1653, 1987

Sugerman AA, Williams BH, Adlerstein AM: Haloperidol in the psychiatric disorders of old age. Am J Psychiatry 120:1190–1192, 1964

Sunderland T, Weingartner T, Cohen RM, et al: Low-dose oral lorazepam administration in Alzheimer subjects and age-matched controls. Psychopharmacology (Berl) 99:129–133, 1989

Tariot PN, Erb R, Leibovici A, et al: Carbamazepine treatment of agitation in nursing home patients with dementia: a preliminary study. J Am Geriatr Soc 42:1160–1166, 1994

Teri L, Rabins P, Whitehouse P, et al: Management of behavior disturbance in Alzheimer disease: current knowledge and future directions. Alzheimer Dis Assoc Disord 6:77–88, 1992

Tiller JW, Dakis JA, Shaw JM: Short-term buspirone treatment in disinhibition with dementia (letter). Lancet 2:510, 1988

Volicer L, Rheaume Y, Cyr D: Treatment of depression in advanced Alzheimer's disease using sertraline. J Geriatr Psychiatry Neurol 7:227–229, 1994

Whitehouse PJ, Price DL, Struble RG, et al: Alzheimer's disease and senile dementia: loss of neurons in the basal forebrain. Science 215:1237–1239, 1982

Wragg RE, Jeste DV: Overview of depression and psychosis in Alzheimer's disease. Am J Psychiatry 146:577–587, 1989

Zweig RM, Ross CA, Hedreen J, et al: The neuropathology of aminergic nuclei in Alzheimer's disease. Ann Neurol 24:233–242, 1988

THIRTY-NINE

Treatment of Childhood and Adolescent Disorders

Mina K. Dulcan, M.D., Joel Bregman, M.D.,
Elizabeth B. Weller, M.D., and Ronald Weller, M.D.

SPECIAL ISSUES IN THE PSYCHOPHARMACOLOGICAL TREATMENT OF CHILDREN AND ADOLESCENTS

In this chapter, we emphasize the ways in which the practice of psychopharmacology with children and adolescents differs from that with adults. Unless otherwise specified, *children* refers to individuals age 4 years through adolescence. Detailed discussions of specific drugs can be found in Section II of this textbook. For those disorders and their respective treatments that are similar in youths and adults, the reader should also refer to other chapters in this section. This chapter details the treatment of disorders that occur in both adults and children that are not covered in other chapters of this text, such as attention-deficit/hyperactivity disorder (ADHD), Tourette's disorder, mental retardation, and autistic disorder. A number of texts provide more extensive information on the use of medications in pediatric psychiatry (e.g., Green 1995; Greenhill and Osman 1991; Riddle 1995a, 1995b; Rosenberg et al. 1994; Werry and Aman 1993; Wiener 1996). In-depth discussions of the clinical aspects of the diagnosis and treatment of developmental psychopathology may be found in M. Lewis (1996) and Wiener (1996).

Whenever possible, DSM-IV (American Psychiatric Association 1994) terminology is used. Unfortunately, most drug studies conducted with children have used other diagnostic systems, and it is difficult to know how well the results generalize to contemporary diagnoses.

The clinical practice of pediatric psychopharmacology is impeded by the relative lack of controlled empirical trials. There are numerous examples of medications that appeared to be effective in anecdotal reports, case series, and open trials that were not shown to be more effective than placebo in double-blind studies. Caution is therefore advised in the interpretation of publications based on only clinical experience.

Evaluation

The evaluation of a young person is complicated by the interaction of psychopathology with the child's environment and with developmental processes. An interview with at least one parent or adult caregiver is essential. Information from teachers is desirable in all cases, and indispensable in ADHD. Standardized symptom rating scales supplement the clinical interview regarding the primary diagnosis, possible comorbidity, and baseline levels of target symptoms (Achenbach 1991). A recent medical history and physical examination are necessary, with laboratory follow-up as indicated. A drug screen or pregnancy test may be required. Whenever a student's functioning in school is impaired, psychoeducational testing (including, at a minimum, intelligence quotient [IQ] and academic achievement tests) should be obtained. Additional testing for learning disabilities may be needed.

Treatment Planning

Psychiatric diagnosis, specific target symptoms, and the strengths and weaknesses of the patient, the family, the school, and the community all enter into the choice of intervention strategies. Parents and their child (as clinically and developmentally appropriate) are included in a discussion about the disorder and a review of treatment options, parent and child motivation, available resources, potential risks and benefits of each intervention, and the risks of no treatment. In clinical psychopharmacology, therapeutic contact to form and maintain a treatment alliance is essential. Other interventions may be primary or used together with medications as determined by target symptoms and data on efficacy for the specific diagnosis. These may include parent guidance or training in behavior modification; special assistance at school; and individual, family, and group psychotherapy. For the most seriously impaired children, hospitalization or day treatment may be needed.

Ethical Issues

The careful physician attempts to balance the risks of medication, the risks of the untreated disorder, and the expected benefits of medication relative to other treatments. It is usually prudent to delay the use of a new psychotropic drug in children and young adolescents until substantial clinical experience has been accumulated for their use in adults.

Children are under the supervision of adults. These adults may misinterpret a youngster's response to the environment either as evidence for a need for medication or as improvement because of a medication. Adults may seek to use drugs to control or eliminate a child's troublesome behavior instead of investigating the family or institutional dynamics that may be provoking and maintaining such behavior and/or implementing more time-consuming, difficult, and expensive therapeutic or behavioral management strategies. Perceived levels of a child's symptoms may be more closely related to the adult's tolerance of the behaviors than to objective data. Often the most appropriate response to a child's behavioral problem is to develop a behavior modification program or change the classroom placement or teaching strategy rather than to start administering medication to the child or to increase the dosage of a medication. This method is particularly useful when evidence indicates that the disturbance is localized to a single classroom or teacher or when the child has a learning disability.

Consent for drug treatment of children is a complex issue (Popper 1987) that can be made even more difficult in clinical situations, such as when divorced parents are feuding over the child's treatment. Informed consent is best considered an ongoing process rather than a single event. The legal minimum age for giving informed consent varies from state to state, but "assent" to medication use is considered possible to obtain from a patient older than 7 years (Popper 1987). Formal consent forms (although often required by law or by institutional guidelines) are less useful than a discussion documented in the medical record that includes the topic, parties present, understanding of the disorder and prognosis, therapeutic options with risks and benefits, questions asked, subsequent consent, and the opportunity to ask further questions (Schouten and Duckworth 1993). Published information sheets for parents, youths, and teachers are now available to supplement discussion with the physician regarding specific medications (Dulcan, in press).

The Food and Drug Administration

Once a drug is approved for any indication, the U.S. Food and Drug Administration (FDA) regulates only the company's advertising of the drug, not the prescribing behavior of physicians. In addition, the "administration of an approved drug in a way that is not approved by the FDA is not research and does not call for special consent or review if it is given solely in the patient's interest" (American Academy of Pediatrics 1996, p. 144). Because pharmaceutical companies have had little incentive to undertake the time, expense, and perceived excessive potential liability associated with testing drugs in children, nearly all psychopharmacological agents and indications (and three-fourths of the drugs used in pediatrics as well; American Academy of Pediatrics 1996) lack pediatric labeling and are "unapproved" or "off-label" for children. As a result, the FDA guidelines as published in the *Physicians' Desk Reference* (PDR) cannot be relied on for appropriate indications, age ranges, or doses for children. Although lack of approval for an age group or a disorder does not imply improper or illegal use, it is prudent to inform the family of these labeling issues, as well as of evidence in the literature for safe and effective use (Appler and McMann 1989). Recent FDA regulations recognizing additional methods (including data from existing nonindustry sponsored trials) to support pediatric labeling claims and the FDA's encouragement of drug manufacturers to establish safety and efficacy and to determine pharmacokinetics and appropriate doses in children may lead to more complete labeling information and to commercial sponsorship of more drug trials in children (Coté et al. 1996).

The Meaning of Medication

Emanative effects are the indirect and inadvertent cognitive and social (i.e., nonpharmacological) consequences of prescribing a drug. These can be positive or negative and may influence the child's self-esteem or attributions of the source of problems and their solution (Henker and Whalen 1980) or the parent's or teacher's view of the child (Amirkhan 1982).

A placebo response may occur, especially in ADHD, Tourette's disorder, depression, overanxious disorder, and autistic disorder. This result is not surprising, given children's suggestibility, the power of adult influence, the "magical thinking" that is normal in young children, and the natural waxing and waning of symptoms. In the clinical situation, the parent, teacher, or child may have such significant positive or negative expectancies about the drug that a single-blind, placebo-drug crossover trial is indicated. Examples of situations that may require such a trial include initiating stimulant medication for ADHD or determining whether a chronically administered drug is still required and effective, is no longer needed, is ineffective, or is even exacerbating the condition (Doherty et al. 1987; Fine and Jewesson 1989; McBride 1988; Ullmann and Sleator 1986; Varley and Trupin 1983).

Measurement of Outcome

The physician should specify target symptoms and obtain affective, behavioral, and physical baseline and posttreatment data. Side effects that are tolerable in adults may be unacceptable in the long-term treatment of children. Children's cognitive limitations in identifying and reporting physical symptoms or changes in mood require a skilled clinician to detect drug-induced changes. Therapeutic and side effects can be assessed by interviews and rating scales for patients, parents, and other relevant adults such as teachers and nurses (in an inpatient setting) (Garvey et al. 1991). (See Aman 1993; Klein et al. 1994; and Zametkin and Yamada 1993 for compendia of scales.) Other means of assessment include direct observation by the clinician, physical examination, and where appropriate, laboratory or psychometric tests to evaluate attention or learning (Barkley 1990; Conners 1985; Gadow and Swanson 1985).

Compliance

Faithful adherence to a prescribed regimen requires the cooperation of one or both parents, the child, and often additional caregivers and school personnel. Pediatric medications may be incorrectly used because of parental factors such as lack of perceived need for drug, carelessness, inability to afford medication, misunderstanding of instructions, complex schedules of administration (Briant 1978), and family dynamics. Both developmental and psychopathological factors may impede the patient's cooperation. Even in intensively monitored protocols, missed doses and unilateral discontinuation by a parent (even when the child has responded positively) are common (R. T. Brown et al. 1987; Firestone 1982). Recent media attention to alleged inappropriate use of medications (especially Ritalin and Prozac) has made some families and teachers highly resistant to pharmacotherapy. Small group teaching (Knight et al. 1990) or a medication manual (Bastiaens 1992; Bastiaens and Bastiaens 1993) may be useful in educating young patients about their medications and may improve adherence.

Some children cannot or will not swallow pills. Some drugs are available in elixir form or can be dissolved in juice. Problems with this method of administration may include unpleasant taste, incompatibility resulting in precipitation of the medication, and inaccurate dosing (J. L. Geller et al. 1992). If necessary, a behavior modification program may be implemented to shape pill-swallowing behavior (Pelco et al. 1987).

Developmental Toxicology

Developmental toxicology refers to the unique or especially severe side effects resulting from interaction between a drug and a patient's stage or process of physical, cognitive, or emotional development. Interference with a child's learning in school or development of social relationships within the family or with peers can have lasting effects. Behavioral toxicity (negative effects on mood, behavior, or learning) often develops before physical side effects are observed, especially in young children (Campbell et al. 1985).

Metabolism and Kinetics

Dosage may be determined empirically or by extrapolation from adult doses according to weight or age. Unfortunately, dosage studies in children are rare. Few data exist on the parameters that determine pharmacokinetics in children (Briant 1978). Young children absorb some drugs more rapidly than adults, leading to higher peak levels (Jatlow 1987). Young children may require divided doses to minimize fluctuations in blood level (particularly for tricyclic antidepressants [TCAs]), although more frequent doses may reduce medication compliance. Age-related factors that may influence distribution include uptake by actively growing tissue and proportional size of organs and tissue masses. In children, drugs such as lithium (which are primarily distributed in body water) have a proportionally larger volume of distribution and, therefore, lower concentration (Jatlow 1987). By age 1 year,

some children who have attention deficits without hyperactivity (Famularo and Fenton 1987).

Bupropion

Bupropion may decrease hyperactivity and aggression and perhaps improve cognitive performance of children with ADHD and conduct disorder (Conners et al. 1996). One blind, controlled crossover study found that efficacy of bupropion was statistically equal to that of methylphenidate in decreasing behavioral and cognitive symptoms of ADHD (Barrickman et al. 1995).

α-Adrenergic Agonists

Despite limited empirical data, the antihypertensive agents clonidine and guanfacine are used as adjuncts to stimulant medication or as third-line alternative drugs. Clonidine is useful in modulating mood and activity level and improving cooperation and frustration tolerance in a subgroup of children with ADHD, especially those who are very highly aroused, hyperactive, impulsive, defiant, irritable, explosive, and labile (Hunt et al. 1990). Clonidine often improves ability to fall asleep, whether insomnia is a result of ADHD overarousal, oppositional refusal to go to bed, or stimulant effect or rebound (T. E. Brown and Gammon 1992). Although clonidine has no direct effect on attention, it may be used alone in children with a family or personal history of tics or those who are nonresponders or negative responders to stimulants. It is most useful in combination with a stimulant when stimulant response is only partial or when stimulant dose is limited by side effects (Hunt et al. 1991). The addition of clonidine may allow a lower dose of stimulant medication (Hunt et al. 1991). Questions have been raised about the safety of the combination of clonidine and methylphenidate, however (see later subsection on clonidine and Fenichel 1995).

Guanfacine hydrochloride has a longer half-life and a more favorable side-effect profile than does clonidine. Preliminary animal and human data suggest positive cognitive effects. Guanfacine hydrochloride recently has been used for similar indications as those for clonidine—that is, for children who cannot tolerate clonidine's sedative effect or in whom clonidine has too short a duration of action, leading to rebound effects on tics, sleep, or behavior. Only data from open trials are available (Chappell et al. 1995; Horrigan and Barnhill 1995; Hunt et al. 1995).

Tricyclic Antidepressants

A TCA may be used to treat ADHD if stimulants exacerbate tics or Tourette's disorder (Riddle et al. 1988) or if the patient or a parent is at high risk for abusing or selling a stimulant. In addition, a TCA may be indicated if stimulants are ineffective or if side effects (especially dysphoria, weight loss, or severe rebound) are unacceptable. Although it has been suggested that TCAs be considered first if the family history and patient symptoms strongly suggest comorbid anxiety or depression (Kutcher et al. 1992), their narrower margin of safety typically makes them a second or third choice, especially in prepubertal children. Although depressive symptoms in children with ADHD have not been found to differentially predict positive outcome of TCA treatment, a TCA may decrease depressive symptoms in youngsters with ADHD, and it avoids the risk of stimulant-induced dysphoria (Biederman et al. 1989a). The longer duration of action does not require a dose at school and minimizes rebound effects. Drawbacks include the inconvenience and expense of electrocardiogram (ECG) monitoring, serious potential cardiac side effects (especially in prepubertal children), the danger of accidental or intentional overdose, and troublesome anticholinergic and sedating side effects. There have been case reports of sudden death in children taking desipramine (Riddle et al. 1993). (See section, "Mood Disorders," later in this chapter for a discussion.)

TCAs reduce symptoms of ADHD better than placebo does but not as well as stimulants do (Pliszka 1987). TCAs do not cause impairment on cognitive tests, but they yield minimal improvement on these measures, in comparison to stimulant effects (Biederman et al. 1989a; Donnelly et al. 1986; Rapport et al. 1993). At present, the TCAs used most often for ADHD are nortriptyline and imipramine, although desipramine is occasionally used (especially in older adolescents). Amitriptyline has an unacceptable level of anticholinergic and sedative side effects. (The use of TCAs in young patients is discussed later in this chapter in "Depressive Disorders.")

Selective Serotonin Reuptake Inhibitors (SSRIs)

Although there has been considerable clinical interest in the use of SSRIs in the treatment of ADHD, only anecdotal data are available. SSRIs do not appear to be efficacious for the core symptoms of ADHD but may be useful as adjuncts for secondary or comorbid mood and behavior symptoms (Gammon and Brown 1993).

Assessment of Response

Multiple outcome measures are essential. The direction and magnitude of effects in various domains (i.e., cognitive, behavioral, social) are typically inconsistent among children and even for a specific child. A particular dose of medication often produces improvement in some areas of functioning, but no change or worsening in others, and stimulant dose-response curves vary in shape (Rapport et al. 1987). Data from parents and teachers on behavior and academic performance are essential prior to initiating stimulant medication and at regular intervals during treatment (Barkley et al. 1988). The Child Attention Problems (CAP; Barkley 1990) is a brief teacher rating scale derived from the Teacher Report Form of the Child Behavior Checklist (Achenbach 1991) that is convenient to use weekly to assess treatment outcome (see Table 39–1 and Table 39–2). It covers both overactivity/impulsivity and inattention symptoms. In the absence of any intervention, rating scale scores tend to decline from the first administration to the second and then rise with frequent repeated administration (Diamond and Deane 1988). The Conners Abbreviated Teacher Rating Scale (Goyette et al. 1978) can be used to measure drug response. It is not ideal as a diagnostic screen, however, because it overlooks children with attention deficits without hyperactivity (Ullmann et al. 1985) and is overinclusive of oppositional and aggressive children, even without ADHD. The IOWA Conners is a short form that was developed to separate inattention and overactivity ratings from oppositional defiance (Loney and Milich 1982; Pelham et al. 1989). It is useful in following treatment progress in children with comorbid ADHD and oppositional defiant disorder. Use of the Academic Performance Rating Scale (DuPaul et al. 1991) ensures that learning as well as behavior receives attention in the school setting. Systematic observations of behavior (Barkley et al. 1988) and measures of academic productivity and accuracy (Gadow and Swanson 1985; Pelham 1985) may also be useful in assessing a drug's effect.

Use of Stimulants

Stimulants include methylphenidate, dextroamphetamine, and magnesium pemoline.

Table 39–1. Child Attention Problems (CAP) Rating Scale

Child's name: _____   Child's age: _____

Today's date: _____   Child's sex: Male   [ ]

Filled out by: _____   Female   [ ]

Below is a list of items that describes pupils. For each item that describes the pupil **now or within the past week,** check whether the item is **Not true, Somewhat** or **Sometimes true,** or **Very** or **Often true.** Please check all items as well as you can, even if some do not seem to apply to this pupil.

	Not true	Somewhat or Sometimes true	Very or Often true
1. Fails to finish things he/she starts	[ ]	[ ]	[ ]
2. Can't concentrate, can't pay attention for long	[ ]	[ ]	[ ]
3. Can't sit still, restless, or hyperactive	[ ]	[ ]	[ ]
4. Fidgets	[ ]	[ ]	[ ]
5. Daydreams or gets lost in his/her thoughts	[ ]	[ ]	[ ]
6. Impulsive or acts without thinking	[ ]	[ ]	[ ]
7. Difficulty following directions	[ ]	[ ]	[ ]
8. Talks out of turn	[ ]	[ ]	[ ]
9. Messy work	[ ]	[ ]	[ ]
10. Inattentive, easily distracted	[ ]	[ ]	[ ]
11. Talks too much	[ ]	[ ]	[ ]
12. Fails to carry out assigned tasks	[ ]	[ ]	[ ]

Please feel free to write any comments about the pupil's work or behavior in the last week.

Source.   Reprinted with permission of Craig Edelbrock, Ph.D.

Table 39–2. Child Attention Problems (CAP) Rating Scale scoring

Each of the 12 items is scored 0, 1, or 2.

Total score = sum of the scores on all items

Subscores:

    Inattention: Sum of scores on items 1, 2, 5, 7, 9, 10, and 12

    Overactivity: Sum of scores on items 3, 4, 6, 8, and 11

Scores recommended as the upper limit of the normal range (93rd percentile):

	Boys	Girls
Inattention	9	7
Overactivity	6	5
Total score	15	11

Source. Reprinted with permission of Craig Edelbrock, Ph.D.

Initiation of Treatment

The physician should explicitly debunk common myths about stimulant treatment. Stimulants do not have a paradoxical sedative action, do not lead to drug abuse, and often continue to be indicated and effective after puberty.

No predictors are available to help specify which stimulant will be best for a particular child. A substantial number of children respond to one stimulant but not to another (Elia et al. 1991). Therefore, if one stimulant is insufficiently effective, another should be tried before using another drug class. Methylphenidate is the most commonly used and best studied stimulant. It may be more effective in reducing motor activity than is dextroamphetamine (Borcherding et al. 1989). Dextroamphetamine is less expensive and has a longer duration of action than methylphenidate. Disadvantages include negative attitudes of pharmacists toward dextroamphetamine (some are unwilling to stock it), its exclusion from many formularies, and higher potential for abuse. Dextroamphetamine may have a mildly increased incidence of side effects such as growth retardation (Greenhill 1981), appetite suppression, and compulsive behaviors.

Once-a-day dosing may be sufficient for magnesium pemoline, which has the least potential for abuse compared with other stimulants, although absorption and metabolism vary widely, and some children need twice-daily doses. Although it was previously believed that pemoline action was delayed, later research has shown effects within the first 1–2 hours after a dose, lasting for 7–8 hours after ingestion (Pelham et al. 1990, 1995; Sallee et al. 1992). The half-life increases with chronic administration (Sallee et al. 1985). At currently recommended doses, pemoline

may be as effective as the other stimulants. The risk of pemoline-induced chemical hepatitis (Nehra et al. 1990), although rare, and the higher incidence of involuntary movements limit the usefulness of pemoline.

Longer-acting stimulant preparations are appealing when the duration of action of the standard formulations is very short (2.5–3 hours), severe rebound occurs, or the administration of medication every 4 hours (or at school) is inconvenient, stigmatizing, or impossible. The most commonly used long-acting forms are Ritalin Sustained Release [SR] and Dexedrine Spansule. Cylert (pemoline), Adderall (a mixture of amphetamine salts), and Desoxyn Gradumets (methamphetamine) are also available. For some children, Ritalin SR is less reliable and less effective than two doses of the standard preparation, although SR works better for a few children. Onset of action may be delayed up to 2 hours and may be more variable from day to day (Pelham et al. 1990). On the other hand, Dexedrine Spansule appears to have more consistent results than standard methylphenidate and to be more effective for some children (Pelham et al. 1990). It also has a greater range of available doses (see Table 39–3). Excessively high doses may result if a child chews a SR tablet or a spansule instead of swallowing it.

Stimulant medication should be initiated with a low dose and titrated every week or two, using half or whole pills, within the usual recommended range, according to response and side effects, using body weight as a rough guide (see Table 39–3). An alternative strategy is a systematic trial using a range of doses (Greenhill et al. 1996). Preschool children or patients with ADHD, predominantly inattentive type, may be more sensitive to both therapeutic and side effects of stimulants; therefore, lower doses may be indicated. Starting with only a morning dose may be useful in assessing drug effect through comparing morning and afternoon school performance. The need for an after-school dose or medication on weekends is individually determined by considering target symptoms. A third dose after school improves behavior without increasing sleep problems (Kent et al. 1995).

Continuation, Maintenance, and Monitoring

The physician should work closely with parents on dose adjustments and obtain regular reports from teachers and annual academic testing. Children should not be responsible for their own medications because these youngsters are impulsive and forgetful at best, and most dislike the idea of taking medication, even when they can verbalize its positive effects and cannot identify any side effects. They will often avoid, "forget," or simply refuse to take a dose of

Table 39–3.   Clinical use of most commonly prescribed stimulant medications

	Methylphenidate	Dextroamphetamine	Pemoline
How supplied (mg)	5, 10, 20	5, 10	18.75, 37.5, 75
	Sustained release: 20	Elixir (5 mg/5 mL)	
		Spansule: 5, 10, 15	
Usual starting dose (mg)	5–10 once or twice per day	2.5 or 5.0 once or twice per day	37.5 or 56.25 per day
Usual single dose range (mg/kg/dose)	0.3–0.7	0.15–0.5	0.5–2.5
Usual daily dose range (mg/day)	10–60	5–40	37.5–112.5
Maintenance number of doses per day	2–4	2–3	1–2
Behaviorally equivalent doses (Pelham et al. 1995)	10 mg twice a day	5 mg twice a day	56.25 mg every morning
	Sustained release: 20 mg every morning	Spansule: 10 mg every morning	
Monitor	Pulse	Pulse	Pulse
	Blood pressure	Blood pressure	Blood pressure
	Weight	Weight	Weight
	Height	Height	Height
	Dysphoria	Dysphoria	Dysphoria
	Tics	Tics	Tics
			Liver functions

medication. Pemoline requires obtaining baseline liver enzyme measures and clinical monitoring (routine liver function studies are not useful in detecting idiosyncratic liver failure). Parents should be instructed to notify the clinician promptly if the child develops vomiting or persistent abdominal distress, nausea, lethargy, or malaise.

Management of Side Effects

Most side effects are similar for all stimulants (see Table 39–4). Giving medication after meals minimizes anorexia. Insomnia may be caused by ADHD symptoms, oppositional refusal to go to bed, separation anxiety, or stimulant rebound or effect. Preexisting sleep problems are common in patients with ADHD. Stimulants may either worsen or improve irritable mood (Gadow 1992). Children with comorbid anxiety and African American male adolescents may be at risk for mildly elevated blood pressure while taking stimulants (R. T. Brown and Sexson 1989; Urman et al. 1995), but other cardiovascular side effects are exceedingly rare (Safer 1992).

The use of stimulants in patients with a personal or family history of tics has been controversial because of concern that new, persistent tics might be precipitated. Existing data suggest that tics may appear or worsen in some children who are at genetic risk. The physician must balance the impairment resulting from tics compared with

that from ADHD symptoms, considering the efficacy and side-effect profile of alternative medications. With appropriate informed consent and careful clinical monitoring, stimulants may still be the medication of first choice.

Although stimulant-induced growth retardation has been a concern, any decrease in expected weight gain is small, despite statistical significance in studies. The effect on height is rarely clinically significant. The magnitude is dose related and appears to be greater with dextroamphetamine than with methylphenidate or pemoline (Greenhill 1981). Growth retardation can be minimized by using drug holidays. The mechanism is not through effects on growth hormone (Greenhill 1981). Tolerance to this effect has been reported. Medication-free summers (if clinically appropriate) may facilitate height or weight normalization (Klein et al. 1988). A study of young adults treated in childhood with methylphenidate showed no decrement in final height (Klein and Mannuzza 1988).

Rebound effects, increased excitability, activity, talkativeness, irritability, and insomnia, beginning 3–15 hours after a dose, may be seen daily or for up to several days after sudden withdrawal of high daily doses of stimulants. These effects may resemble a worsening of the original symptoms (Zahn et al. 1980). Management strategies include increased structure after school, a dose of medication in the afternoon that is smaller than the midday dose, the use of a long-acting formulation,

Table 39–4.   Side effects of stimulant medications

Common initial side effects (try dose reduction)

Anorexia

Weight loss

Irritability

Abdominal pain

Headaches

Emotional oversensitivity, crying easily

Less common side effects

Insomnia

Dysphoria (especially at higher doses)

Decreased social interest

Impaired cognitive test performance (especially at very high doses)

Less than expected weight gain

Rebound overactivity and irritability (as dose wears off)

Anxiety

Nervous habits (e.g., picking at skin, pulling hair)

Hypersensitivity, rash, conjunctivitis, or hives

Withdrawal effects

Insomnia

Rebound attention-deficit/hyperactivity disorder symptoms

Depression (rare)

Rare but potentially serious side effects

Motor tics

Exacerbation or precipitation of Tourette's disorder

Depression

Growth retardation (reversible when drug stopped)

Tachycardia

Hypertension

Psychosis with hallucinations

Stereotyped activities or compulsions

Side effects reported with pemoline only

Choreiform movements

Dyskinesias

Night terrors

Lip licking or biting

Chemical hepatitis (elevated serum glutamic-oxaloacetic transaminase and serum glutamic-pyruvic transaminase, jaundice, epigastric pain) (very rare) (Patterson 1984)

Source.   Adapted from Dulcan MK, Popper CW: *Concise Guide to Child and Adolescent Psychiatry.* Washington, DC, American Psychiatric Press, 1991. Copyright 1991, American Psychiatric Press. Used with permission.

and the addition of either clonidine or guanfacine.

There is no evidence that stimulants produce a decrease in the seizure threshold. In contrast to popular lay belief, taking stimulants prescribed for ADHD does not result in addiction.

Discontinuation

If symptoms are not severe outside of the school setting, the young person should have an annual drug-free trial in the summer of at least 2 weeks but longer if possible. If school behavior and academic performance are stable, a carefully monitored trial off medication during the school year (but *not* at the beginning) will provide data on whether medication is still needed. The duration of medication treatment is individually determined by whether drug-responsive target symptoms are still present. Treatment may be required through adolescence and into adulthood.

Treatment Resistance

Stimulant tolerance is reported anecdotally, but noncompliance should be the first possibility considered when medication appears to have become ineffective. Decreased drug effect may also be due to a reaction to stress at home or school, attenuation of an initial positive placebo effect, or lower efficacy of a generic preparation. True tolerance may be more likely with the long-acting formulations (Birmaher et al. 1989). If tolerance occurs, another stimulant may be substituted.

If several stimulants in appropriate doses have been found to be ineffective for an individual child, several strategies are possible. More intensive psychosocial treatment may be indicated. An innovative strategy for difficult-to-manage cases is the combination of short-acting and longer-acting stimulant medications (Fitzpatrick et al. 1992). Bupropion is an alternative possibility. If a stimulant is partially effective, clonidine or guanfacine may be added. A TCA trial may be successful in stimulant nonresponders. Anecdotal data suggest the use of fluoxetine in combination with methylphenidate (Gammon and Brown 1993), but there is little evidence of efficacy for the core symptoms of ADHD.

Use of Bupropion

The clinical history should include a search for seizures and factors that predispose to seizures (e.g., head trauma, other central nervous system pathology, other drugs that lower the seizure threshold, or eating disorders). An EEG may be indicated prior to starting bupropion if an eating disorder or a seizure diathesis is possible. Bupropion is administered in two or three daily doses, beginning with a dose of 37.5 or 50 mg twice a day, with gradual titration over 2 weeks to a usual maximum of 250 mg/day

(300–400 mg/day in adolescents). A single dose should not exceed 150 mg. Blood levels do not appear to be useful. Allergic reactions are relatively common, including rash, urticaria, and rare serum sickness. Other side effects include drowsiness, fatigue, nausea, anorexia, dizziness, and "spaciness" (Barrickman et al. 1995; Conners et al. 1996). Bupropion may exacerbate tics (T. Spencer et al. 1993). Side effects seen in adults may be expected, and seizures are possible at daily doses greater than 450 mg.

Use of Clonidine

Initiation of Treatment

The clinician should take reasonable precautions before starting clonidine, including a thorough cardiovascular history, a recent clinical cardiac examination, measurement of baseline blood pressure and pulse, and an ECG. History of syncope and finding of bradycardia or heart block on baseline ECG are relative contraindications. Laboratory blood studies may include a complete blood count (CBC) with differential and fasting glucose (if personal or family history suggests diabetes). Clonidine is initiated at a low dose of 0.05 mg (one-half of the smallest manufactured tablet) at bedtime. This converts the side effect of initial sedation into a benefit. An alternative strategy is to begin with 0.025 mg four times a day.

Continuation, Maintenance, and Monitoring

The dose of clonidine is titrated gradually over several weeks to 0.15–0.30 mg/day (0.003–0.01 mg/kg/day) in three or four divided doses. Very young children (age 5–7 years) may require lower initial and maintenance doses. The transdermal form (skin patch) may improve compliance and reduce variability in blood levels. It lasts only 5 days in children (compared with 7 days in adults) (Hunt et al. 1990). Once the daily dose is determined using pills, an equivalent size patch may be substituted (0.1, 0.2, or 0.3 mg/day). The patch may be cut to adjust the dose. Note that patches do not adhere well in hot, humid climates.

Clonidine has a slow onset of therapeutic action, in part because of the gradual dose increase needed to minimize side effects, and perhaps due to the time required for receptor downregulation (Hunt et al. 1991). Significant clinical response is not seen for as long as a month, and maximal effect may be delayed for another several months.

Management of Side Effects

Clonidine's most troublesome side effect is sedation, but this effect tends to decrease after several weeks. Dry mouth, nausea, and photophobia have been reported, with hypotension and dizziness possible at high doses. The skin patch often causes local pruritic dermatitis and may cause a toxic reaction if chewed or swallowed. Depression may occur, most often in patients with a history of depressive symptoms in themselves or their families (Hunt et al. 1991). Glucose tolerance may decrease, especially in those at risk for diabetes.

Four deaths have been reported to the FDA of children who at one time had been taking both methylphenidate and clonidine, but the evidence linking the drugs to the deaths is tenuous, at best (Fenichel 1995). Pending further clarification, extra caution is advised when treating children with cardiac or cardiovascular disease or when combining clonidine with other medications. Erratic compliance with medication increases the risk of adverse cardiovascular events. Families should be cautioned repeatedly about this problem, and clonidine should not be prescribed if it cannot be administered reliably. The acute onset of dizziness, fatigue, light-headedness, sedation, syncope, or near-syncope, especially if they occur during or after exercise, should prompt closer clinical monitoring and cardiology consultation (Cantwell et al. 1997).

Discontinuation

When clonidine is discontinued, it should be tapered rather than stopped suddenly to avoid a withdrawal syndrome consisting of increased motor restlessness, headache, agitation, and elevated blood pressure and pulse rate (Leckman et al. 1986).

Use of Guanfacine

The use of guanfacine is similar to that of clonidine. Compared with clonidine, guanfacine has fewer and less significant side effects (particularly sedation and hypotension) and a longer half-life. It is typically given in divided doses two or three times a day, starting with 0.5 mg (one-half of a 1-mg tablet) in the morning or at bedtime. The daily dose is increased by 0.5-mg increments every 3–4 days. The usual maximum dose is 3 mg/day. One mg of guanfacine is equivalent to 0.1 mg of clonidine. When switching between the two agents, one can be tapered down as the other is increased.

Use of Tricyclic Antidepressants

When treating ADHD, the clinician may start nortriptyline at 10 or 25 mg/day and may increase the dosage as tolerated until a clinical effect or a maximum of 4.5 mg/kg/day (usual dose 2 mg/kg/day), given in two divided doses, is reached. The serum level (50–150 ng/mL) may relate to therapeutic response (Wilens et al. 1993). Imipramine (or desipramine) is begun at 10 or 25 mg/day and increased weekly to a maximum dose of 5 mg/kg/day (divided into three doses per day in prepubertal children). Plasma levels do not predict efficacy. Some patients respond to a daily dose as low as 2 mg/kg. The use of TCAs in children and adolescents is discussed in the next section.

A note of caution is necessary: The combination of imipramine and methylphenidate has been associated with a syndrome of confusion, affective lability, marked aggression, and severe agitation that disappeared when the medications were stopped (Grob and Coyle 1986). The mechanism may be methylphenidate's interference with hepatic metabolism of imipramine, resulting in a longer half-life and elevated blood levels.

MOOD DISORDERS

Bipolar Disorders

Assessment for Treatment

In the past, mania was underdiagnosed in children and adolescents (Weller et al. 1986c). Many clinicians still are not aware of the existence of mania in children and adolescents or do not encounter it often enough to fully master its assessment and treatment. The clinician may consider referring such patients to centers that specialize in childhood mood disorders. Clinical assessment should be done by interviewing the child and the parents together and then each individually. When assessing the child, it is important to ask age-specific questions that cover the DSM-IV criteria. Useful but lengthy standardized instruments include the Diagnostic Interview for Children and Adolescents—Revised (DICA-R; Reich and Welner 1988; DSM-IV version in preparation) and the Schedule for Affective Disorders and Schizophrenia for School-Age Children (K-SADS; Chambers et al. 1985; DSM-IV version—Kaufman et al. 1997). The DICA-R can be used by a well-trained psychometrician; however, the K-SADS requires both clinical training in child and adolescent psychopathology and additional training on the interview. The DICA-R yields a high rate of false-positive diagnoses of mania in children who have conduct disorders or ADHD. Children with mania can be distinguished from children with ADHD by their higher total score and distinctive pattern of item endorsement on the clinician-completed Mania Rating Scale (MRS; Fristad et al. 1995). The widely used Conners Parent and Conners Teacher Rating Scales (Goyette et al. 1978) do not discriminate between ADHD and mania. A careful history can often

differentiate the child with mania from a child with hyperactivity or conduct disorder. In mania, a cyclic history is more common; in conduct disorder and ADHD, symptoms are more chronic. Obtaining a family psychiatric history may also be useful.

Medical conditions that may cause secondary mania, such as multiple sclerosis, seizure disorders, brain tumors, treatment with steroids, and drug abuse, must be ruled out. Similar to the workup for any child with a first episode of psychosis, the baseline workup for a youth with mania might include magnetic resonance imaging (MRI) or computed tomography (CT) scan. The medical evaluation should include routine blood studies, including CBC with differential, electrolytes, thyroid function tests, blood urea nitrogen (BUN), creatinine, and creatinine clearance. A baseline ECG is advisable because children with mania often become depressed and may need TCAs in addition to mood-stabilizing medications.

Selection of Treatment

Despite the lack of published double-blind, placebo-controlled studies of medications for children and adolescents with bipolar disorder, many clinicians use mood-stabilizing drugs in an effort to help their patients with this potentially devastating illness. The physician must extrapolate from data on the successful psychopharmacological treatment of adults with bipolar disorder.

Lithium carbonate is the drug most commonly used to stabilize mood in children (Weller et al. 1986a). Although mania in children and adolescents that is treated with lithium may become easier to manage, the dramatic positive response to lithium observed in adults with mania is uncommon. Youngsters with mania who have preadolescent onset of psychopathology have a poorer response to lithium than those with adolescent-onset mania without prepubertal psychopathology (Strober et al. 1988). In a study in which researchers used lithium to treat aggressive behavior in children and adolescents, positive responders had mood symptoms, a family history of mood disorders, and/or lithium-responsive relatives (Youngerman and Canino 1978).

Because the degree of symptom abatement with lithium is often disappointing, other medications such as carbamazepine and valproic acid have been tried, although no double-blind, placebo-controlled studies have been done in children and adolescents with bipolar disorder. Some clinicians advocate using valproate even before a trial of lithium and/or carbamazepine. Practice is based on anecdotal clinical experience (West et al. 1994) and extrapolation from the treatment of adults. The clinician should obtain consent from parents or guardians and assent from the patient before starting mood-stabilizing medication in a child or adolescent. The clinician should make clear to the responsible adult that data substantiating the efficacy of treating children and adolescents with mania or hypomania with these agents are limited. (The use of carbamazepine is discussed in the section, "Aggression," later in this chapter.)

Assessment of Response

Treatment of bipolar disorder in youths is best done by experienced clinicians who can assess response. The MRS can be used to assess response because total scores decrease with successful treatment. The Beigel-Murphy (Beigel et al. 1971) scale can also be used with adolescents.

Use of Lithium

Initiation of treatment. In children, traditional practice is to start lithium at 300 mg/day for several weeks and slowly increase the dose to 900 mg/day. If the clinician uses a weight-based dosage guide for prepubertal children, therapeutic levels can be safely attained in a much shorter time (Weller et al. 1986a). The higher glomerular filtration rate in children, compared with adults, usually requires a higher mg/kg dose before puberty. Published nomograms can be used to calculate dosages based on blood levels after single test doses (Alessi et al. 1994; B. Geller and Fetner 1989; Malone et al. 1995b). Lithium's half-life could permit once-a-day dosing in adolescents, although children have more rapid lithium clearance than do adults, and multiple divided doses may be necessary to maintain therapeutic levels. In addition, some patients have gastrointestinal distress when they take the entire day's dose at bedtime. Lithium is therefore usually given two or three times a day with meals. Divided doses have the disadvantage of potentially decreasing adherence to the prescribed regimen, however. Some clinicians use slow-release lithium to sustain the therapeutic effect throughout the day while avoiding multiple doses. No systematic studies in children have compared the efficacy and side effects of different dosing schedules.

In general, the blood level should not exceed 1.4 mEq/L. Peak serum levels will occur within 1–2 hours after ingestion. Steady-state serum levels are achieved after 5 days. Blood should be drawn for a serum level 8–12 hours after the patient ingested the last evening dose and before the first morning dose. For children, an 8:00 A.M. sampling time is most commonly used. Some clinicians suggest that lithium may be maintained at higher blood levels in preschool-aged children. There are, however, no published data supporting the safety and efficacy of this practice.

Although lithium comes in different forms, in our practice (E. B. W. and R. W.), we have found little advantage to using compounds other than lithium carbonate, which has reliable serum levels and reasonable cost.

Continuation, maintenance, and monitoring. A child or adolescent being treated with lithium carbonate should have a psychiatric evaluation at least once a month to ensure that the lithium is tolerated well and to monitor compliance. Although in the acute manic phase, serum levels up to 1.4 mEq/L are tolerated well, clinical experience suggests that maintenance levels can be lower (i.e., 0.6–1.2 mEq/L). Although it is theoretically possible to substitute saliva levels of lithium for serum levels (Weller et al. 1987), this approach has not yet become common in clinical practice. BUN, creatinine, and creatinine clearance should be periodically measured because lithium may cause alterations in kidney function. Lithium may produce goiter and/or hypothyroidism; therefore, a thyroid-stimulating hormone (TSH) test should be obtained every 4–6 months.

Management of side effects. Lithium is well tolerated by most children and adolescents, although children younger than 7 years are more prone to side effects, especially with higher lithium doses and serum levels (Hagino et al. 1995). The most common side effects in children (i.e., tremor, weight gain, development or exacerbation of enuresis, polyuria, polydypsia, and polyphagia; Weller et al. 1986a) rarely require discontinuation of lithium. Acne may be induced or aggravated, especially in adolescents. Lithium carbonate is deposited in bones, but it is not known whether this has any significant effect on a growing child whose epiphyseal plate is not closed. Lithium has not been reported to interfere with the growth of children. The effect of lithium on cognitive functioning in children has not been studied in detail. Hypokalemia is a very rare side effect that can be managed by dietary supplementation (e.g., two bananas, two large carrots, two cups of skim milk, half of a honeydew melon, or an avocado daily). Such supplementation may be preferable to giving potassium tablets, which can further irritate the gastrointestinal tract and which have a taste that most children dislike.

When a child is taking lithium carbonate, the patient and the family should be taught to be especially cautious when the patient develops an illness with fever, vomiting, or diarrhea; uses rigorous dieting to lose weight; or takes diuretics or nonsteroidal antiinflammatory agents. Any of these situations should immediately be brought to the psychiatrist's attention. Lithium should be discontinued while a patient has fever, vomiting, or diarrhea. Vigorous exercise in hot weather can also lead to lithium toxicity, and parents should be cautioned to be sure the patient drinks enough water. Nonsteroidal antiinflammatory agents (other than aspirin), which are often taken by adolescent girls to relieve menstrual distress, can increase lithium levels and even lead to lithium intoxication. Wide swings in salt intake can produce erratic lithium levels, between ineffective and toxic.

Discontinuation. Gradual tapering off of medication is recommended. The patient should be followed up closely after discontinuing medication and should be checked for signs of relapse to mania or for symptoms of depression so that episodes can be treated early and hospitalization avoided. The kindling hypothesis and data on adult treatment resistance following intermittent treatment suggest special caution regarding discontinuation of mood stabilizers.

No studies address the issue of how long lithium should be continued. A naturalistic study (Strober et al. 1990) found that adolescents who discontinued their lithium were three times more likely to relapse compared with those who continued the medication. Most relapses occurred within the first year after cessation of treatment. Once lithium is started, it seems advisable to continue for at least 6 months and preferably for a year. If studies of lithium termination in adults are applicable, an even longer duration of treatment might be considered.

Use of Valproate

Initiation of treatment. Baseline liver function tests are necessary before starting treatment with valproate because it can cause hepatotoxicity, although this effect is extremely rare in patients older than 10 years; the greatest risk is for patients younger than 3 years (Trimble 1990). Other initial laboratory studies include CBC with differential, creatinine, BUN, and TSH.

Valproic acid is available in tablets, capsules (Depakene), and an elixir of 250 mg/5 mL (16-ounce bottles). Depakote, an enteric-coated tablet combining sodium valproate and valproic acid (available in 125, 250, and 500 mg), is recommended to avoid gastrointestinal side effects. Valproic acid should be started at a dose of 250 mg/day (500 mg in adolescents) and increased by 250 mg every 4 days, not to exceed 60 mg/kg/day. The usual range for adolescent acute mania is 1,000–1,750 mg/day. Although valproic acid can be given in a single bedtime dose, it is usu-

ally administered in two divided daily doses. Plasma levels are minimally useful.

Continuation, maintenance, and monitoring. Liver function tests should be done periodically, although routine liver function studies may not detect idiosyncratic liver failure. Parents should be instructed to notify the clinician promptly if the child develops vomiting, easy bruising, or persistent abdominal distress, nausea, lethargy, or malaise.

Management of side effects. Side effects of valproate include nausea, vomiting, anorexia, lethargy, and abdominal pain, although these may be minimized by starting with a low dose and titrating up slowly. Hepatotoxicity is possible, but when valproate is discontinued, recovery of liver enzymes occurs within several weeks. A very rare complication of valproate treatment of children and adolescents is (potentially fatal) pancreatitis, which usually occurs within the first 12 months of treatment (Trimble 1990). However, most patients who experience this complication are taking multiple anticonvulsants. Neutropenia and thrombocytopenia as well as macrocytic anemia have been reported in valproate-treated patients. Little is known about the longer-term effects of the use of valproate during development, although data from its use to treat children with seizure disorders do not suggest unique problems, with the exception of mildly decreased bone mineral density (Sheth et al. 1995) and, in girls, polycystic ovaries and/or hyperandrogenism following chronic valproate use (Geller 1998).

Treatment resistance. If mania is resistant to treatment, several options can be considered. However, it should always be remembered that although such strategies have been used in adults, few, if any, studies of their efficacy or safety have been done in children and adolescents.

A possible strategy is the addition of an antipsychotic agent, most commonly haloperidol, although the newer atypical antipsychotics may have fewer side effects. Despite an isolated report of complications from the simultaneous use of haloperidol and lithium in adult patients, most patients tolerate this combination fairly well. Clinical experience (E. B. W.) suggests that the use of haloperidol should be considered in treating mania in patients with psychosis who have obsessive or compulsive traits and frequent rumination or who have comorbid diagnoses (e.g., Tourette's disorder) that might respond to haloperidol.

Other medications that have occasionally been used in treatment-resistant mania include clonazepam, lorazepam, clonidine, verapamil, propranolol, and physostigmine. Electroconvulsive therapy has rarely been used in treatment-resistant manic teenagers. Because of the paucity of even clinical anecdotal data with most of these treatments in children, the reader is referred to the chapter on treatment of bipolar disorder in adults (see Bowden, Chapter 35, in this volume).

Depressive Disorders

In the past 20 years, recognition that mood disorders can present in children and adolescents has resulted in increased interest in diagnosing and treating depression in young patients (Weller and Weller 1990). The successful pharmacological treatment of mood disorders in this age group awaits well-designed multicenter double-blind, placebo-controlled studies.

Assessment for Treatment

The clinician should conduct an assessment using DSM-IV criteria, including interviewing both the parents and the child and obtaining information from the child's school. It is important to remember that most children with mood disorders have a family history of such disorders. Parental depression may color the reporting of the child's psychopathology. However, the child and a parent may be simultaneously depressed. Reports from the teacher, who can observe the child objectively in comparison with other students, can be a very important part of the evaluation. Although teacher evaluations may be more difficult to obtain and may be less accurate for high school students, information from the school is still valuable. The most disturbed youths often come to the attention of the school counselor, the school nurse, or the principal because of poor attendance or declining academic performance.

Interview-based assessment measures include the diagnostic interviews discussed in the section above on mania as well as the Child Depression Rating Scale—Revised (CDRS-R; Poznanski et al. 1985), which is similar to the Hamilton Rating Scale for Depression (Hamilton 1967) and combines information from the clinician, child, parent, and teacher. Self-report is also important. In children, the Children's Depression Inventory (CDI; Kovacs 1985) is frequently used, although it performs better as a screen than as a diagnostic instrument. It may underestimate the degree of depression because children can determine the "normal" response and answer accordingly. In one study, the CDI did not differentiate children with depression from those with conduct disorder (Fristad et al. 1988). In adolescents, the Beck Depression Inventory (BDI; Beck et al. 1961) can be used.

The proper role of the laboratory assessment of depression is controversial. This is particularly true of the dexamethasone suppression test (DST; Weller and Weller 1988). The DST is positive in approximately 50% of prepubertal depressed children and 40% of depressed adolescents. In a study of hospitalized children, the DST was positive in 70% of the depressed subjects (Weller et al. 1984). Normalization of the DST with treatment has been reported in a small group of depressed children (Weller et al. 1986b). To perform the DST, 0.5 mg of dexamethasone is given to prepubertal children and 1 mg is given to adolescents at 11:00 P.M. Plasma cortisol levels are measured at 4:00 P.M. and 11:00 P.M. the next day. If the cortisol level is greater than or equal to 5 ng/mL, cortisol is nonsuppressed and the DST is considered positive. A positive DST is most frequently observed in hospitalized, suicidal, or "endogenously depressed" children and adolescents.

Selection of Treatment

The clinician should not underestimate the importance of working with school personnel and parents by educating them about the illness. Also, individual and/or group therapies may address social deficits that cannot be remedied with medication alone.

Published algorithms exist based on clinical experience and extrapolation from data on adults (e.g., see Alessi 1991; Ambrosini et al. 1995; Johnston and Fruehling 1994), but experts disagree. Selection of the first drug may be influenced by the patient's target symptoms, comorbidity, risk of impulsive behavior, family history of disorder and drug response, and side-effect profile of the drugs. Remarkably few empirical data on children and adolescents are available to guide therapeutic choices.

The TCAs have been the most studied medications in the treatment of depression in children and adolescents. In open studies, 75% of patients whose depression was treated with antidepressants responded positively. However, only one of the (relatively few) double-blind, placebo-controlled studies found an advantage of imipramine over placebo (Preskorn et al. 1987). In this small sample of hospitalized prepubertal children, dexamethasone nonsuppression and comorbid anxiety symptoms were associated with a positive response to imipramine. In adolescents, no double-blind study shows the efficacy of TCAs over placebo. Existing studies, however, have small sample sizes, lack of data on how subtypes and predictors of response differ with development, and problems with limited duration of treatment and insufficiently sensitive measures of response (Conners 1992; Strober et al. 1992).

SSRIs, including fluoxetine, sertraline, paroxetine,

and venlafaxine, may be effective in the treatment of depression in children and adolescents. Long-term effects of these medications on growing children are not known. Their advantages over TCAs include the absence of cardiac side effects and relative safety in overdose. As with other antidepressants, hypomania or mania can be precipitated.

Several open-label studies report improvement in depressed children and adolescents (some of whom did not respond to TCAs) treated with fluoxetine. One rigorous double-blind, placebo-controlled trial in children and adolescents with depression found that fluoxetine yielded significantly greater improvement in depressive symptoms than did placebo (Emslie et al. 1997). Fluoxetine is started at 20 mg/day or less. Most patients do not need more than 40 mg/day. Fluoxetine is sometimes prescribed on an every-other-day basis because of the long half-life of the drug and its active metabolites. (The use of fluoxetine is discussed in the subsection, "Obsessive-Compulsive Disorder," later in this chapter.)

An open trial of sertraline (dose range 25–200 mg/day, mean daily dose 110 mg) in adolescents with a major depressive episode was promising in reducing symptoms of depression and anxiety. The most troublesome side effects were insomnia, feelings of tension and restlessness, drowsiness, anorexia, weight change, headaches, and nightmares (McConville et al. 1996). An open trial of bupropion in adolescents with major depressive disorder was promising (Arredondo et al. 1993). Additional agents (including monoamine oxidase inhibitors [MAOIs]) are discussed in the subsection on treatment resistance.

Assessment of Response

To fully assess response to medication, the clinician should obtain input from the child, parent, and school personnel. Depending on the patient's age, the CDI, the BDI, or the abbreviated CDRS-R can be used to assess changes in symptomatology (Overholser et al. 1995).

Use of Tricyclic Antidepressants

Initiation of treatment.   Pharmacokinetics for TCAs are different in children than in adolescents or adults. The smaller fat-to-muscle ratio in children leads to a decreased volume of distribution, and most children do not have the buffer of a relatively large volume of fat in which the drug can be stored. Children have larger livers relative to body size, leading to faster metabolism (Sallee et al. 1986), more rapid absorption, and lower protein binding than in adults (Winsberg et al. 1974); these factors all contribute to a shorter half-life in younger children. As a result, children probably need a higher weight-corrected dose of

TCAs than do adults. Prepubertal children are prone to rapid dramatic swings in blood levels from toxic to ineffective and should be given divided doses to produce more stable levels (Ryan 1992). Plasma levels vary widely at a given fixed dose.

TCAs' quinidine-like effect slows cardiac conduction time and repolarization. Children and adolescents may develop mildly increased pulse and blood pressure and small, statistically significant, but usually clinically benign, ECG changes (intraventricular conduction defects; e.g., lengthened P-R interval that may progress to a first-degree atrioventricular heart block and occasional widening of the QRS complex), especially at doses equivalent to greater than 3 mg/kg/day of imipramine or desipramine (Bartels et al. 1991; Biederman et al. 1989b, 1993; Fletcher et al. 1993; Leonard et al. 1995; Schroeder et al. 1989; Winsberg et al. 1975). In one carefully monitored sample of nearly 200 children and adolescents, desipramine in doses up to 5 mg/kg/day produced increases in diastolic blood pressure, heart rate, and ECG conduction parameters that were statistically significant but not clinically meaningful or symptomatic (Biederman 1991). Prolongation of the Q-T$_c$ interval may be a sensitive indicator of cardiac effect (Wilens et al. 1996). The tendency of prepubertal children to have wider swings in blood levels may place them at higher risk for serious cardiac conduction changes. Approximately 5% of the population has a genetic defect in TCA metabolism, which causes these individuals to be "slow hydroxylators," increasing risk for toxicity.

Five cases (three prepubertal children, one 12-year-old girl, and one 14-year-old boy) have been reported of unexplained sudden death during desipramine treatment, and in three of these cases, death occurred following exercise (Popper and Zimnitzky 1995; Riddle et al. 1990/1991, 1993). A causal relationship between the medication and the deaths has not been established. The evidence appears to suggest that treatment with desipramine in usual doses is associated with only a slight added risk of sudden death beyond that occurring naturally (Biederman et al. 1995). Desipramine may represent a greater risk than other TCAs, however. Because of these concerns, clinical practice now favors nortriptyline or imipramine as the first choice among the tricyclics in the treatment of prepubertal children.

Before initiating treatment with a TCA, the clinician should perform a complete physical examination, including baseline vital signs. He or she should obtain a careful history for cardiac symptoms such as chest pain, dyspnea, actual or near syncope, palpitation, or tachycardia. Congenital hearing impairment may signal Jervell-DeLange syndrome, which is associated with cardiac abnormalities and increased risk of sudden death (Ambrosini et al. 1995). The clinician should examine the family history for possible contraindications to TCA use, such as arrhythmias (especially long–Q-T syndrome), unexplained fainting, conduction defects, cardiomyopathy, early cardiac disease, or sudden death (Liberthson 1996).

An ECG should be performed prior to initiating treatment. If abnormalities are seen in a routine ECG, an ECG with a rhythm strip should be obtained and interpreted by a pediatric cardiologist. A CBC with differential, BUN, creatinine, creatinine clearance, and thyroid function tests are recommended as part of a baseline laboratory evaluation; approximately 20%–30% of depressed children and adolescents subsequently develop bipolar disorder and may require mood-stabilizing medications. If the history suggests head trauma or seizures, an EEG is indicated prior to starting treatment because TCAs lower the seizure threshold. Parents must be reminded to supervise closely the administration of medication and to keep pills in a safe place.

Treatment should be initiated with a small dose of the TCA and gradually increased. Some experts believe that plasma level monitoring may be helpful in determining optimum dose (if a laboratory that measures TCA levels reliably is available) (Preskorn et al. 1988), although this is controversial. TCAs have long half-lives; hence, once-a-day dosing is adequate for antidepressant effect. The short half-life of TCAs in prepubertal children can produce daily withdrawal symptoms if medication is given only once a day. If this occurs, or if comorbid ADHD is present, a thrice-daily regimen may be preferred. For imipramine, the daily dose should not exceed 5 mg/kg or 200 mg, whichever is smaller. Equivalent doses for other TCAs should be used. Most studies of TCAs in childhood depression have used imipramine and nortriptyline. Serial ECGs after each dose increase of 50–100 mg/day are recommended when the daily dose is above 2.5 mg/kg of imipramine or 1.0 mg/kg/day of nortriptyline (Wilens et al. 1996). Table 39–5 lists titration parameters for monitoring vital signs and ECG.

Continuation, maintenance, and monitoring.

Once the symptoms respond to the antidepressant (after approximately 3–8 weeks), the medication should be continued for at least 4–6 months. Throughout this period, the clinician should continue to monitor side effects and response. Monitoring the medication with plasma levels is recommended by some to ensure compliance and avoid toxicity (Preskorn et al. 1988). Periodic ECGs should be obtained if the dose exceeds 3 mg/kg/day. Unexplained withdrawal symptoms may indicate that poor compliance is resulting in missed doses. Because of the predictability

Table 39–5. Guidelines for the use of tricyclic antidepressants in children and adolescents

	Children	Adolescents
P-R interval (seconds)	0.2	0.2
QRS interval (seconds)	0.12	0.12
	130% of baseline	
Q-T$_c$ interval (seconds)	0.48	0.48
Resting heart rate (beats/minute)	110–130	110–120
Chronic blood pressure (mm Hg)	120/80	140/90

Note. **Electrocardiogram and vital sign limits to titration:** reduce dose or discontinue drug if reached.
Source. Wilens et al. 1996.

of TCA-induced ECG changes, a rhythm strip is useful in monitoring compliance.

Management of side effects. If ECG changes appear, alternatives include decreasing the dose or switching to another antidepressant. The most common side effects of TCAs are dry mouth, tremor, constipation, and tachycardia. Drowsiness and dizziness sometimes occur at initiation of treatment. However, with proper instruction in how to manage transient postural hypotension, most children tolerate this side effect and adjust to it. Dry mouth can usually be managed by instructing the patient to chew sugarless gum or wax or to sip water or diet drinks. These techniques will help keep the mouth moist while minimizing the risk of dental cavities and weight gain. In extreme cases that do not respond to these measures, xerulobe mouth wash can be used. If a TCA-induced tremor becomes intolerable, decreasing the dosage should be considered. Constipation is a common problem, for which a regular toileting schedule, a high-fiber diet, and increased liquids are helpful. Bedtime snacks of popcorn are fun for children and provide good roughage. In the occasional situation in which a stool softener is needed, Colace (200 mg at bedtime) can be used. Behavioral toxicity may be manifested by irritability, mania, agitation, anger, aggression, forgetfulness, or confusion. A drug blood level is often required to differentiate central nervous system toxicity from exacerbation of the primary condition. The physician should be alert to the risk of intentional overdose or accidental poisoning, not only by the patient but also by other family members, especially young children. Switching to mania may occur, which would demand discontinuation of the TCA and addition of a mood stabilizer (B. Geller et al. 1993).

Discontinuation.   After a child or adolescent has been asymptomatic for 4–6 months, stopping the medication should be considered. It is not advisable to stop the medication when the patient is confronting stressful life events. Some clinicians now maintain their young patients on TCAs chronically, especially when a patient has had multiple episodes of unipolar depression.

Sudden cessation of moderate or higher doses results in a flulike anticholinergic withdrawal syndrome with malaise, nausea, cramps, vomiting, headaches, and muscle pains. Other manifestations may include social withdrawal, hyperactivity, depression, agitation, and insomnia (Petti and Law 1981; Ryan 1990). TCAs should therefore be tapered off over a 2- to 3-week period, especially if the patient has been taking medication for a long time.

Treatment resistance.   Open-label studies have suggested that lithium augmentation of a TCA may be useful in adolescents who have not responded or had only a partial response (Ryan et al. 1988a; Strober et al. 1992). There are anecdotal reports (E. B. W. and R. W.) of some success in using lithium augmentation in prepubertal children with residual symptoms of depression after antidepressant treatment. Lithium augmentation may be especially helpful in children with a family history of bipolar illness or those with comorbid aggressive conduct disorder. Although there are no empirical guidelines as to the optimum blood level in lithium augmentation, lithium serum levels should not exceed 1 mEq/L. There are anecdotal reports of the usefulness of triiodothyronine (T_3) augmentation.

MAOIs have rarely been used to treat children and adolescents because of the concern that the required dietary restrictions present problems for this age group. The most common dietary risks for children and adolescents are pepperoni and sausage pizza and chocolate. Chianti, aged cheese, and anchovies, which may cause problems for adults taking MAOIs, are rarely part of children's or even adolescents' diets. Ryan and colleagues (1988b) have successfully used MAOIs in teenagers to treat symptoms that did not respond to TCAs. We (E. B. W. and R. W.) have used MAOIs in prepubertal children whose conditions are unresponsive to TCAs and lithium in cases in which both the child and the family were reliable and responsible.

SCHIZOPHRENIA

Assessment for Treatment

Schizophrenia is often difficult to diagnose prior to adulthood, especially in prepubertal children. In addition to thorough medical, neurological, psychiatric, and developmental assessment, target symptoms for treatment should be identified. Before beginning medication, the clinician should ensure that a complete physical examination and baseline laboratory workup (including CBC with differential, liver profile, and urinalysis) have been done.

Selection of Treatment

The cornerstone of treatment is an intensive and comprehensive program that may include a highly structured environment, remediation of specific developmental deficits, social skills training, family psychoeducational treatment, and supportive reality-based individual psychotherapy. Special education placement or the assistance of a full-time aide in a mainstream classroom is commonly required. Day treatment, hospitalization, or long-term residential treatment may be needed. Medication is indicated if positive psychotic symptoms (e.g., delusions or hallucinations) cause significant impairment or interfere with other interventions. Disabling negative symptoms (e.g., apathy and social withdrawal) may also be indications for drug treatment, given the potential therapeutic effects of the newer neuroleptics.

A variety of neuroleptics appear to have modest efficacy in children and adolescents (Teicher and Glod 1990; Whitaker and Rao 1992). In general, however, schizophrenia in young patients is less responsive to pharmacotherapy than is that in adults, and substantial impairment continues, even if the more florid symptoms such as hallucinations, anxiety, and agitation abate (Campbell et al. 1985). Although no evidence suggests superior efficacy of one traditional neuroleptic over another, the lower-potency compounds (e.g., chlorpromazine and thioridazine) are best avoided because of sedation, cognitive dulling, and memory deficits that can interfere with learning in school and in treatment programs. Concerns regarding the development of tardive dyskinesia (TD) in long-term use of the typical neuroleptics and the prominence of negative symptoms in young schizophrenic patients suggest that clozapine may prove to be useful (Teicher and Glod 1990), although it is likely to be replaced by the even newer antipsychotic medications being developed. A double-blind trial found clozapine to be superior to haloperidol for both positive and negative symptoms in children and adolescents with early-onset schizophrenia (Kumra et al. 1996). Risperidone is rapidly becoming a preferred drug in adults and may be indicated for young schizophrenic patients as well, but only small case series reports have been published (Armenteros et al. 1997; Quintana and Keshavan 1995; Simeon et al. 1995). Negative as well as positive symptoms may improve. Although risperidone's side-effect profile is more benign than that of other neuroleptics, children appear to be more sensitive than adults to developing extrapyramidal symptoms on this drug (Mandoki 1995).

Assessment of Response

Full efficacy may require several months to appear (as long as 6–9 months for clozapine and risperidone). Parent and teacher reports are essential, in addition to self-report from adolescents. Standardized clinician ratings such as the Positive and Negative Syndrome Scales derived from the Children's Psychiatric Rating Scale are sensitive to neuroleptic-induced improvement in children (E. K. Spencer et al. 1994).

Initiation of Treatment

TD has been documented in children and adolescents after as brief a period of treatment as 5 months (Herskowitz 1987), and it may appear even during periods of constant medication dose (see Wolf and Wagner 1993 for a review). Initiation of chronic neuroleptic treatment during the developmental period may yield a greater risk of TD than exposure that begins in adulthood. Before the clinician prescribes a neuroleptic and periodically thereafter, he or she should carefully examine each patient for abnormal movements by using a scale such as the Abnormal Involuntary Movement Scale (AIMS; Munetz and Benjamin 1988). Parents and patients (as they are able) should receive regular explanations of the risk of movement disorders.

Prior to clozapine treatment, an EEG is needed because of the increased frequency of seizures and EEG abnormalities in adolescents while taking this drug.

Antipsychotic drugs are highly lipophilic. Chlorpromazine has been reported to have a lower plasma concentration in children than in adults after the same weight-adjusted dose (Rivera-Calimlim et al. 1979). However, the magnitude of the difference exceeds that expected from the small proportional excess of adipose tissue in children compared with adults, probably because of children's increased efficiency of hepatic biotransformation (Jatlow 1987). Developmental changes in protein binding may be influential as well.

Doses must be titrated with careful attention to positive and negative effects. Age, weight, and severity of symptoms do not provide clear dose guidelines. The initial dose should be very low, with gradual increments, no more than once or twice a week. Loading doses or rapid titration does not accelerate clinical improvement but does increase side effects and decrease compliance. Children metabolize these drugs more rapidly than do adults but also re-

quire lower plasma levels for efficacy (Teicher and Glod 1990). Common doses for children are 0.25–6.0 mg of haloperidol or 10–200 mg of chlorpromazine, or the equivalent, per day. Older adolescents with schizophrenia may require doses of neuroleptics in the adult range. Young adolescents fall in between, and doses must be empirically determined. Even less is known about optimal doses of the atypical neuroleptics. Although a single daily dose (usually at bedtime) is generally preferred for maintenance, divided doses may be used during titration (especially in hospitalized patients) to minimize side effects and permit finer dose adjustments.

Continuation, Maintenance, and Monitoring

Efficacy and side effects must be monitored regularly. A standard protocol should be followed for clozapine (see Towbin et al. 1994 for recommendations). Neuroleptics should be maintained at the lowest effective dose. Although current practice with adults with schizophrenia is to maintain neuroleptic treatment indefinitely, for children the lack of clarity in diagnosis and the possibility of developmental toxicity make firm recommendations about the advisability of periodic withdrawal of medication difficult. If medication is to be stopped, it should be withdrawn gradually to prevent rebound psychiatric symptoms. Withdrawal dyskinesias are relatively common.

Management of Side Effects

Sedation, weight gain, and hypersalivation are the most common side effects. Weight gain may be especially problematic in the long-term use of the low-potency neuroleptics and risperidone. Neutropenia and seizures at rates significantly higher than seen in adults may limit the usefulness of clozapine (Kumra et al. 1996).

Acute extrapyramidal side effects (EPS), including dystonic reactions, parkinsonian tremor and rigidity, drooling, and akathisia, occur as in adults. Laryngeal dystonia is potentially fatal. Acute dystonia may be treated with oral or intramuscular diphenhydramine, 25 or 50 mg, or benztropine, 0.5–2.0 mg. When medication is initiated for an outpatient, the clinician should instruct a responsible adult to watch for a dystonic reaction and should provide a supply of medication for dystonia to be given to the patient if needed. Adolescent boys seem to be more vulnerable to acute dystonic reactions than are adult patients, so the physician may be more inclined to use prophylactic anti-parkinsonian medication. Clinical experience suggests that children do not respond well to anticholinergics, and reduction of neuroleptic dose is therefore preferable

(Campbell et al. 1985). For treatment or prevention of parkinsonian symptoms, adolescents may be given benztropine, 1–2 mg/day, in divided doses. Chronic parkinsonian symptoms are often drastically underrecognized by clinicians (Richardson et al. 1991). The neuromuscular consequences may impair performance of age-appropriate activities, and the subjective effects may lead to noncompliance with medication. Akathisia may be especially difficult to identify in very young patients or those with limited verbal ability. It may be misinterpreted as anxiety or agitation and mistakenly exacerbated with an increase in neuroleptic dose. Clonazepam (0.5 mg/day) may reduce neuroleptic-induced akathisia (Kutcher et al. 1987) in adolescents.

Potentially fatal neuroleptic malignant syndrome (NMS) has been reported in children and adolescents (Latz and McCracken 1992; Steingard et al. 1992). Adolescents may present with serious medical complications (S. E. Peterson et al. 1995) or may have NMS without fever (Hynes and Vickar 1996). NMS is treated by discontinuation of the neuroleptic and aggressive supportive measures. The use of specific medications to treat NMS has not been studied in adolescents.

Abnormal laboratory findings are less often reported in studies of children than in studies of adults, but the clinician should be alert to their possibility, especially agranulocytosis or hepatic dysfunction. If an acute febrile illness or easy bruising occurs, medication should be withheld, and a CBC with differential and liver enzymes should be obtained (Campbell et al. 1985). Children may be at greater risk for neuroleptic-induced seizures than are adults, because of their immature nervous systems and the very high prevalence of abnormal EEG findings in seriously disturbed children (Teicher and Glod 1990).

Of particular concern is behavioral toxicity, which is manifested as worsening of preexisting symptoms or development of new symptoms such as hyper- or hypoactivity, irritability, apathy, withdrawal, stereotypies, tics, or hallucinations (Campbell et al. 1985). Children and adolescents are more sensitive than adults are to cognitive dulling and sedation resulting from low-potency antipsychotic drugs (e.g., chlorpromazine and thioridazine) that interfere with ability to benefit from school (Campbell et al. 1985; Realmuto et al. 1984).

Anticholinergic side effects are unusual. Miscellaneous side effects include abdominal pain, enuresis (Realmuto et al. 1984), photosensitivity, and various neuroendocrine effects that may be especially distressing to adolescents. For a more detailed discussion of neuroleptic side effects and their management, see Whitaker and Rao (1992).

Discontinuation

Withdrawal dyskinesias, which are usually transient but potentially irreversible, are seen in 8%–51% of neuroleptic-treated children and adolescents (Campbell et al. 1985). Other withdrawal-emergent symptoms include nausea, vomiting, loss of appetite, diaphoresis, and hyperactivity (Gualtieri and Hawk 1980). A variety of behavioral symptoms may appear up to several weeks after neuroleptic withdrawal and persist for as long as 8 weeks (Gualtieri et al. 1984). These must be distinguished from a return of manifestations of the original disorder. A prolonged drug-free trial may be indicated, if possible, to determine whether neuroleptics are truly needed.

Treatment Resistance

Neuroleptic resistance is common in young schizophrenic patients, although a child whose symptoms have not responded to one neuroleptic may respond to another. If the response is insufficient after a 6-week trial at adequate doses (and assured compliance), another neuroleptic (usually in a different class) should be tried (McClellan and Werry 1994). In open trials and case studies, clozapine has been reported to be effective in a substantial proportion of neuroleptic-resistant adolescents and several children with schizophrenia (Blanz and Schmidt 1993; Frazier et al. 1994; Kowatch et al. 1995; Mozes et al. 1994; Remschmidt et al. 1994). (See Towbin et al. 1994 for suggestions regarding informed consent.)

Common therapeutic errors leading to the perception of neuroleptic resistance include incorrect diagnosis, subtherapeutic or excessive medication doses, premature changes in medication before efficacy can appear, failure to monitor target symptoms or ensure patient compliance, hasty or irrational polypharmacy, and failure to provide psychosocial therapies (McClellan and Werry 1992).

AGGRESSION

Assessment for Treatment

Many aggressive patients have a primary or secondary diagnosis of conduct disorder. When aggression is secondary to another psychiatric diagnosis, such as ADHD (impulsivity, low frustration tolerance), depression (increased irritability), mania (psychosis, irritability), schizophrenia (paranoid delusions or hallucinations), pervasive developmental disorder (decreased ability to communicate verbally), or substance abuse (intoxication or withdrawal), the primary disorder is the appropriate focus of treatment. Adults such as parents, teachers, juvenile justice authorities, and child care and nursing staff are quick to report verbal or physical aggression and demand its elimination. The physician's first duty is to perform a careful evaluation to identify any primary medical or psychiatric disorders. The frequency of brain damage is high in patients with violent conduct disorders, and a focused history may disclose symptoms suggestive of temporal lobe, psychomotor, or complex partial seizures (D. W. Lewis et al. 1982).

The youth's environment must be considered in detail, because aggression is often a response to the dynamics or reinforcement structure of a family, school, neighborhood, group home, or inpatient unit. Psychodynamic, systems, and behavioral theories may all be useful in understanding the conditions that precipitate and maintain aggressive behavior and in reducing its frequency and severity. Parents and school personnel are likely to be unsophisticated regarding behavior modification, and they may require strong encouragement to institute appropriate contingency management programs. The physician should guard against being persuaded to use medication alone when other interventions instead of or in addition to medication would be more appropriate (e.g., aggression secondary to frustration at overly high academic demands or in response to peer bullying). No evidence indicates that premeditated, predatory aggression (Vitiello et al. 1990) will respond to any drug, unless the patient is so sedated that virtually all activities are limited. On the other hand, at times, a chemical restraint is preferable to a physical restraint and may facilitate other forms of treatment or permit the child to be placed in a less restrictive environment. A wide variety of medications are used on an as-needed basis in hospital settings to control aggressive behavior. Empirical data on the efficacy of this practice are essentially lacking.

Selection of Treatment

Various classes of medication may be prescribed in an attempt to reduce aggression. If the aggression is impulsive and the youth also has a diagnosis of ADHD, the first choice is a stimulant. In children with ADHD that responds positively to stimulants, oppositional and defiant behavior and aggression are reduced, and activity level and attention improve (Amery et al. 1984; Hinshaw 1991; Hinshaw et al. 1989; Klorman et al. 1989; Murphy et al. 1992; Whalen et al. 1987). Case reports suggest that pemoline may be more efficacious than methylphenidate (Shah et al. 1994). Although stimulants have been suggested for the treatment of conduct disorder without ADHD, no data are yet available to support this strategy.

Lithium may be considered in the treatment of children with severe aggression, especially when such aggression is impulsive and accompanied by explosive affect and poor self-control. Although studies have not had consistent results (see Campbell et al. 1995b for a discussion), efficacy has been reported for some hospitalized prepubertal explosively aggressive children with conduct disorder in a double-blind, placebo-controlled trial (Campbell et al. 1995a). Lithium may be the first pharmacological choice for an aggressive child with a family history of bipolar mood disorder (especially if a family member has responded to lithium). (The use of lithium in children is described in the section, "Mood Disorders," earlier in this chapter.)

In patients with severe impulsive aggression with emotional lability and irritability who have abnormal EEG findings or a strong clinical suggestion of episodic phenomena, a trial of carbamazepine may be warranted, although deliberate aggression is rarely part of a frank seizure (R. W. Evans et al. 1987). Preliminary data suggest efficacy in children younger than 12 years with severe explosive aggression, even in the absence of neurological findings (Kafantaris et al. 1992). Efficacy was not shown, however, in a placebo-controlled trial of 22 hospitalized children with a DSM-III-R (American Psychiatric Association 1987) diagnosis of conduct disorder, solitary aggressive type (Cueva et al. 1996). Valproic acid has been used, although there are no systematic data on its efficacy.

β-Adrenergic blockers may be useful in patients with otherwise uncontrollable rage reactions and impulsive aggression, especially those with evidence of organicity (Kuperman and Stewart 1987; Williams et al. 1982). Evidence of organicity does not appear to be a prerequisite for efficacy, however (Grizenko and Vida 1988).

Historically, neuroleptics have been used to control aggression. In view of the risk of cognitive dulling and TD, neuroleptics should be low on the list of medication options. Studies of hospitalized severely aggressive children ages 6–12 years have reported the short-term efficacy of haloperidol (1–6 mg/day or 0.04–0.21 mg/kg/day), thioridazine (mean 170 mg/day), and molindone (mean 26.8 mg/day) compared with placebo in reducing, although not eliminating, aggression, hostility, negativism, and explosiveness (Campbell et al. 1985; Greenhill et al. 1985). (The use of neuroleptics in children is discussed in the section, "Schizophrenia," earlier in this chapter.)

Use of many other drugs is speculative at present. One pilot study found that bupropion reduced symptoms of conduct disorder regardless of whether ADHD was also present (Simeon et al. 1986). (The use of bupropion is discussed in the section, "Attention-Deficit/Hyperactivity Disorder," earlier in this chapter.) Trazodone may be useful in decreasing aggression in children with disruptive behavior disorders (Ghaziuddin and Alessi 1992). Clonidine may reduce aggression even in the absence of ADHD (Kemph et al. 1993). (See the earlier section on ADHD regarding the use of clonidine.) A small open-case series suggested that venlafaxine might be useful in conduct disorder, with or without ADHD (Derivan et al. 1995). Reports of several clinical cases noted reduction in aggression in nonpsychotic youngsters after initiation of risperidone (Fras and Major 1995). Based on data from adults and from animal studies, buspirone has been suggested as an option when aggression is presumed to result from anxiety.

Assessment of Response

Careful documentation of precipitants, severity, frequency, type (predatory vs. affective; verbal vs. physical), and targets (property, self, animals, children, adults) of aggression is necessary for evaluating efficacy of treatment. An instrument such as the Overt Aggression Scale (Kafantaris et al. 1996) or the Modified Overt Aggression Scale (Kay et al. 1988) can facilitate this process. Baseline measures are important. Even in samples of children with severe aggression resistant to outpatient treatment, 20%–45% respond (at least temporarily) to hospitalization alone or hospitalization plus a placebo with an immediate and significant decrease in aggressive behavior (Campbell et al. 1995b; Cueva et al. 1996; Malone et al. 1995a).

Use of Carbamazepine

Initiation of Treatment

Baseline hemoglobin, hematocrit, CBC with differential, and liver functions should be measured before starting carbamazepine in a child. The initial dose is 100 mg/day, with food. Use of the brand Tegretol is advised because of reports of both reduced serum levels and toxicity when generic formulations are substituted (Gilman et al. 1993). Children eliminate carbamazepine more rapidly than do adults (Jatlow 1987). Plasma levels (drawn approximately 12 hours after the last dose) are crucial because dosage calculated by weight correlates poorly with plasma concentration. The half-life is approximately 9 hours. Titration is gradual (increased weekly by 100 mg/day), guided by plasma levels, to a usual plateau of 8–12 mEq/mL. Therapeutic levels have not been empirically determined for psychiatric symptoms, but those established for epilepsy help define guides to compliance and toxicity. The usual daily dose range is 10–50 mg/kg, divided into three doses for children and two for older adolescents. Slow-release carbamazepine may be given twice a day for more consistent blood levels. Autoinduction of hepatic enzymes may lead to declining plasma concentration (especially in the first 6 weeks) requiring periodic increases in dose. Carbamazepine lowers the plasma levels of neuroleptics, imipramine, and valproic acid and may reduce the effectiveness of oral contraceptives. Erythromycin causes a clinically significant increase in carbamazepine levels and may result in toxicity.

Continuation, Maintenance, and Monitoring

The degree of ongoing laboratory monitoring necessary is controversial. A conservative recommendation includes CBC and liver function studies weekly for the first 4 weeks, monthly for 4 months, and every 3 months thereafter (Silverstein et al. 1983). A more modest regimen is CBC (with differential and platelet count), serum iron, BUN, and creatinine measurements after the first month and every 3–6 months thereafter (Trimble 1990). Routine monitoring is likely to be ineffective in detecting life-threatening idiosyncratic toxicity. Parents should be instructed to notify the physician, and tests should be ordered if a rash, sore throat, skin infection, facial or periorbital edema, fever, malaise, lethargy, weakness, vomiting, increased urinary frequency, anorexia, jaundice, easy bruising, bleeding, or mouth ulcers develop. If the neutrophil count drops below 1,000 or hepatitis occurs, the drug should be stopped (Silverstein et al. 1983).

Management of Side Effects

The most common adverse effects are drowsiness, headache, incoordination, vertigo, rash, and reversible dose-related leukopenia (especially when carbamazepine is started). Less common side effects include abdominal pain, nausea, vomiting, diplopia, nystagmus, ataxia, tics, muscle cramps, and exacerbation of seizures. Very rare but serious effects are blood dyscrasias (such as thrombocytopenia, agranulocytosis, or aplastic anemia), hepatotoxicity, severe skin reactions (e.g., Stevens-Johnson or systemic lupuslike syndromes), hypersensitivity syndrome (Bellman et al. 1995), and inappropriate secretion of antidiuretic hormone (in rare cases leading to acute renal failure) (Pellock 1987; Trimble 1990). Teratogenic effects have been reported. Adverse behavioral reactions (e.g., extreme irritability, agitation, insomnia, obsessive thinking, hyperactivity, aggression, mania, and psychosis or delirium with hallucinations and/or paranoia) may be seen during the first 1–4 weeks of treatment (R. W. Evans et al. 1987; Herskowitz 1987; Pleak et al. 1988).

Use of β-Adrenergic Blockers

In the drug class of β-adrenergic blockers (see Connor 1993 for a review), the most clinical experience has been accumulated with propranolol. Pindolol and nadolol have been suggested as alternatives with fewer side effects and longer half-lives. Pindolol was modestly effective in a double-blind, placebo-controlled study of children with comorbid ADHD and conduct problems but resulted in frequent paresthesias and distressing nightmares and hallucinations (Buitelaar et al. 1996). Nadolol has not been tested in children.

Initiation of Treatment

The premedication workup should include a recent history and physical examination, with particular attention to medical contraindications: asthma, diabetes, bradycardia, heart block, cardiac failure, and hypothyroidism. Fasting blood sugar and a glucose tolerance test may be indicated if the patient is at risk for diabetes. An ECG may be considered.

In children and adolescents, the initial dose of propranolol is 10 mg three times a day, increasing by 10–20 mg every 3–4 days, monitoring pulse and blood pressure (minimum pulse 50 beats/minute, blood pressure 80/50 mm Hg). The standard daily dose range is 10–120 mg for children and 20–300 mg for adolescents, divided into three doses (2–8 mg/kg/day) (Coffey 1990). The short elimination half-life in children (2–4 hours) may necessitate four daily doses. Dose is titrated to clinical effect or side effects. Maximum improvement at a given dose may not be seen for up to 12 weeks. When propranolol or pindolol are used together with chlorpromazine or thioridazine (but not haloperidol), blood levels of both drugs are elevated.

Side Effects

Side effects are generally the same as those in adults. Tiredness, mild hypotension, and bradycardia are the most common side effects.

Discontinuation

β-Blockers should be tapered gradually to avoid rebound hypertension and tachycardia.

Use of Trazodone

The dose of trazodone used in the few reported cases has been 75 mg/day (mean 0.35 mg/kg/day) (Ghaziuddin and Alessi 1992). Reported side effects in youths include mild sedation and increased penile erections. Priapism is possible, with the potential for severe irreversible consequences.

Treatment Resistance

If aggression is not reduced at the highest appropriate drug dose, a different class of drug should be considered. A closer look at the family and school environment is indicated, with initiation of more intensive psychosocial treatment, perhaps including hospitalization.

ANXIETY DISORDERS

Anxiety disorders are one of the most prevalent categories of psychiatric disorders in children and adolescents. Prevalence in community samples is as high as 10% by self-report. Although symptoms of anxiety are widespread in children and often resolve spontaneously or with supportive treatment, when severity and chronicity are sufficient to lead to impairment of functioning and a brief trial of psychosocial intervention is ineffective, pharmacotherapy may be considered. Unfortunately, few controlled trials exist (except in patients with obsessive-compulsive disorder), and establishment of efficacy is confounded by extensive comorbidity and high placebo response rates.

Symptoms of the anxiety disorders overlap, and several trials have included subjects with heterogeneous disorders. A case series review of open clinical trials of fluoxetine (mean dose 25.7 mg/day) for children and adolescents with overanxious disorder, social phobia, or separation disorder (*N* = 21) found moderate to marked improvement in a substantial majority of patients (Birmaher et al. 1994). Interestingly, improvement typically did not begin until after 6–8 weeks of treatment. All patients had been unresponsive to psychotherapy before the drug trial.

A small open trial of buspirone in children and adolescents with various anxiety disorders, some of which were comorbid with other anxiety disorders or with ADHD, was promising in the reduction of anxiety, mood, and behavioral symptoms (Simeon et al. 1994).

Separation Anxiety Disorder

Assessment for Treatment

In separation anxiety disorder, cognitive, affective, somatic, or behavioral symptoms appear in response to genuine or fantasied separation from attachment figures. Common presenting problems are school refusal and insomnia. The differential diagnosis of school avoidance (formerly called *school phobia*) includes medical illness, realistic fear of something at school (e.g., bullies or a punitive teacher), simple phobia, social phobia, agoraphobia, mood disorder, schizophrenia, truancy (secondary to conduct or oppositional defiant disorder), or substance abuse. Certain medications, such as propranolol (prescribed for headache) or haloperidol (prescribed for Tourette's disorder), may produce symptoms of separation anxiety and school refusal.

Selection of Treatment

Psychological interventions such as family therapy, collaboration with school personnel, and behavior modification using contingencies and systematic desensitization are primary (American Academy of Child and Adolescent Psychiatry 1993). If the child's separation anxiety is being exacerbated by a parent's anxiety or mood disorder, then the parent should also receive direct psychiatric treatment (possibly including medication) as well as guidance in child management. Medication for the child or adolescent may be useful as an adjunct if psychosocial treatment is ineffective after 3–4 weeks.

The efficacy of imipramine in separation anxiety disorder is controversial (Bernstein et al. 1990; Klein et al. 1992), and clear guidelines for its use do not exist. Typical starting doses are low: for example, for children ages 6–8 years, 10 mg at bedtime; for older children, 25 mg at bedtime (McDaniel 1986). The dose may be increased by 10–50 mg/week, depending on the age of the child. Clinical experience suggests that some children respond at a low dose, whereas others may require the antidepressant dose range. As long as 6–8 weeks may be required for response. Medication is continued for at least another 8 weeks and then gradually withdrawn. (See section, "Mood Disorders," earlier in this chapter for more detail on the use of imipramine.)

Benzodiazepines may be used in the short-term treatment of children with severe anticipatory anxiety. Alprazolam (0.03 mg/kg or 0.5–6.0 mg/day) may be useful in the treatment of separation anxiety disorder or school avoidance (Bernstein et al. 1990; Kutcher et al. 1992). In a recent small ($N = 15$) double-blind, placebo-controlled study of clonazepam (up to 2 mg/day) in children with separation anxiety disorder (and a variety of comorbid anxiety and behavior disorders), some patients appeared to improve, but the results were not statistically significant (Graae et al. 1994). Two subjects experienced serious disinhibition with irritability, tantrums, aggression, and attempted self-injury.

Assessment of Response

Response is measured behaviorally (e.g., return to school, ability to sleep alone) and by questions about subjective distress.

Overanxious Disorder and Generalized Anxiety Disorder

Assessment for Treatment

Overanxious disorder has been eliminated from DSM-IV, and the adult category—generalized anxiety disorder—is now used. Existing studies have used a variety of DSM and non-DSM criteria to select anxious children who experience a variety of worries, almost always including unrealistic worry about future events. These children often appear shy, self-doubting, and self-deprecating and have multiple somatic complaints. They may show habit disturbances, such as nail-biting, hair-pulling, or thumb-sucking.

Selection of Treatment

Several treatment modalities are typically used, although systematic data exist only for behavioral interventions. Behavioral methods include relaxation, desensitization by progressive exposure or in imagination, and contingent reinforcement of approach to feared objects or situations. Psychotherapy is often oriented toward promoting psychological individuation and autonomy in the child and family. Cognitive therapy is directed at changing self-defeating and pessimistic attitudes. Assertiveness training can be helpful, especially in a group setting. Treatment of any parental anxiety disorder is important.

Controlled drug studies of children who have only anxiety disorders are lacking. Benzodiazepines may be used in the short-term treatment of severe anticipatory anxiety in children. Although an open trial of alprazolam (0.5–1.5 mg/day) for children with avoidant and overanxious disorders was promising (Simeon and Ferguson 1987), a double-blind study did not find that alprazolam was superior to placebo in the context of an intensive treatment program (Simeon et al. 1992). Efficacy may have been limited by low doses and the short duration of treatment. Antihistamines are commonly prescribed, but no empirical data exist regarding their use. Anecdotal reports suggest the efficacy of buspirone (15–30 mg/day divided into three doses) in the treatment of overanxious disorder in adolescents (Kranzler 1988; Kutcher et al. 1992).

Assessment of Response

Both behavioral reports from parents and patient ratings of anxiety in target domains are useful.

Use of Benzodiazepines

Initiation of Treatment

Children absorb diazepam faster and metabolize it more quickly than adults do (Simeon and Ferguson 1985). The usual daily dose ranges for children and adolescents are lorazepam, 0.25–6.0 mg; diazepam, 1–20 mg; and alprazolam, 0.25–4.0 mg. The dosage schedule depends on age (i.e., more frequent dosing in young children) and the specific drug (Coffey 1990; Kutcher et al. 1992).

Continuation, Maintenance, and Monitoring

Generally, benzodiazepines should be used for relatively brief periods.

Management of Side Effects

In addition to the risks of substance abuse and physical or psychological dependence, side effects include sedation, cognitive dulling, ataxia, confusion, and emotional lability. Paradoxical or disinhibition reactions may occur, manifested by acute excitation, irritability, increased anxiety, hallucinations, increased aggression and hostility, rage reactions, insomnia, euphoria, and/or incoordination (Coffey 1990; Reiter and Kutcher 1991; Simeon and Ferguson 1985).

Discontinuation

When treatment with benzodiazepines is being discontinued, the dose should be tapered gradually to avoid withdrawal seizures or rebound anxiety.

Use of Antihistamines

Initiation of Treatment

The initial dose of diphenhydramine or hydroxyzine in children and adolescents is 10 or 25 mg/day. Either drug is titrated gradually up to a maximum of 200–300 mg/day (5 mg/kg/day) (Coffey 1990).

Side Effects

The most common side effects are dizziness and oversedation. Some children become paradoxically agitated. Occasionally, incoordination, blurred vision, dry mouth, nausea, or abdominal pain may occur. At high doses, the seizure threshold is lowered. Leukopenia and agranulocytosis are extremely rare. Antihistamines have been reported to cause acute dystonic reactions, tics, and possibly (with chronic administration) TD. They should not be prescribed for children with asthma because anticholinergic effects dry the mucous membranes.

Use of Buspirone

Initiation of Treatment

Tentative guidelines for use of buspirone in children and adolescents suggest a starting dose of 2.5–5.0 mg/day, increasing to three times a day over 2–3 days (Kutcher et al. 1992). The therapeutic effects may be delayed for 1–2 weeks after reaching the proper dose, with maximal effects not seen for an additional 2 weeks (Coffey 1990). After a 10-day interval to assess efficacy, the dose may be increased gradually to a maximum of 10 mg twice a day in children and 10 mg three times a day in adolescents.

Management of Side Effects and Discontinuation

Reported adverse effects of buspirone in adults include insomnia, dizziness, anxiety, nausea, headache, restlessness, agitation, depression, and confusion (Coffey 1990). Clinical experience with children and adolescents is limited, but side effects appear to be minimal. It is important to distinguish preexisting somatic complaints related to the generalized anxiety disorder from medication side effects. Buspirone can be discontinued relatively rapidly (i.e., over 4 days; Kutcher et al. 1992).

Selective Mutism

Selective mutism, a rare disorder characterized by the child's refusal to speak to certain people and in certain situations, despite the ability to do so, is considered by some to be related to social phobia in adolescents and adults. Psychosocial interventions typically include behavior modification and family therapy. Following several anecdotal reports and open trials, a 12-week double-blind, placebo-controlled study ($N = 15$) of fluoxetine (0.6 mg/kg/day) reported modest efficacy over placebo according to parent ratings but not clinician or teacher ratings (Black and Uhde 1994). Subjects in both the placebo and the fluoxetine groups showed improvement over baseline ratings, but most subjects remained very symptomatic.

Obsessive-Compulsive Disorder

Assessment for Treatment

Obsessive-compulsive disorder is a chronic and often disabling disorder in childhood and adolescence. In community samples, the point prevalence is 3%–4% (Valleni-Basile et al. 1994; Zohar et al. 1992). Subclinical obsessive-compulsive symptomatology has been reported to occur in approximately 8% of adolescents (Apter et al.

1996; Valleni-Basile et al. 1996). Between one-third and one-half of adult patients with obsessive-compulsive disorder report an onset of the disorder early in life. The clinical manifestations of obsessive-compulsive disorder are similar at all ages, although in children rituals are more common than obsessions (Rapoport et al. 1992).

Selection of Treatment

Pharmacotherapy plays a central role in the treatment of obsessive-compulsive disorder, although patients with childhood onset have a lower response rate to medications (Ackerman et al. 1994). *Within* the child and adolescent population, however, age does not appear to predict treatment response (D. A. Geller et al. 1995). Clinical experience suggests that individual children respond to one medication but not to others. No factors predicting differential response have yet been identified.

Successful treatment often requires the implementation of combined modalities. Recently developed cognitive-behavioral techniques have been reported to be efficacious for children with obsessive-compulsive disorder (March et al. 1994), often in combination with medication. Family and individual psychotherapy may be useful for residual symptoms that do not respond to pharmacotherapy.

Double-blind, placebo-controlled studies of clomipramine in youths have reported a 35%–75% reduction in obsessive-compulsive disorder symptoms in 60% of subjects, independent of depression (DeVeaugh-Geiss et al. 1992; Flament et al. 1985; Leonard et al. 1989). Plasma levels of clomipramine and its metabolites correlated with the presence of side effects but not with clinical response. Efficacy appears to be specific for serotonin reuptake blockade because desipramine failed to reduce obsessive-compulsive symptomatology.

Both open and double-blind, placebo-controlled studies of fluoxetine (20–80 mg/day) alone or in combination with low doses of clomipramine have found moderate to marked improvement in obsessive-compulsive symptomatology, including reductions of more than 50% in the level of functional impairment (Riddle et al. 1990, 1992; Simeon et al. 1990). Approximately half of subjects are responders, regardless of the presence of comorbid Tourette's disorder. Preliminary findings from a retrospective study suggest that higher doses of fluoxetine (i.e., 1 mg/kg/day) may result in response rates as high as 74% among both children and adolescents with obsessive-compulsive disorder (D. A. Geller et al. 1995). Other serotonin reuptake inhibitors (SRIs) also may be effective in the treatment of obsessive-compulsive disorder in children and

adolescents. Apter et al. (1994) reported that fluvoxamine in doses of 100–300 mg/day resulted in a significant reduction in obsessive-compulsive severity, based on scores on the Yale-Brown Obsessive-Compulsive Scale (Y-BOCS; Goodman et al. 1989) in 14 adolescents with obsessive-compulsive disorder who were treated for 8 weeks. Efficacy did not become apparent until week 6. Neither comorbid disorders (present in 11 subjects) nor the use of other psychotropic medications influenced treatment response to fluvoxamine. A multicenter controlled trial supported both safety and efficacy of fluvoxamine in the treatment of obsessive-compulsive disorder in children and adolescents (Riddle and Pediatric OCD Research Group 1996).

In a substantial minority of children with obsessive-compulsive disorder, response to medication is delayed for 8 or even 12 weeks after reaching the expected therapeutic dose. Therefore, the physician should wait at least 10–12 weeks before changing drugs, adding an augmenting drug, or using a high-dose strategy. Early in treatment, some patients experience an exacerbation of obsessive-compulsive symptoms or complain of feeling agitated or "jittery." This phenomenon usually subsides after a few weeks.

Strategies developed for the treatment of treatment-resistant obsessive-compulsive disorder in adults are largely untested in children and adolescents. In general, trials of sufficient dose and duration of two or three different drugs used alone should precede the use of drug combinations to augment response. The addition of low-dose neuroleptics (e.g., haloperidol, pimozide, or risperidone) to SRIs has been reported to improve efficacy in the treatment of SRI-refractory adult patients, especially those with comorbid tic disorders (McDougle et al. 1994, 1995). Augmenting strategies suggested for children include adding clonazepam to an SRI (Leonard et al. 1994) or combining clomipramine and fluoxetine (Simeon et al. 1990).

Clomipramine. A starting dose of clomipramine, 25 mg/day, has been recommended with increases of 25–50 mg/day every 4–7 days. The maximum recommended dose is 3 mg/kg/day, up to 200 mg/day, although 50 mg/day (1 mg/kg/day) may be sufficient. Response is delayed for 10 days to 2 weeks (as in the treatment of depression), unlike the immediate response seen in the treatment of ADHD or enuresis (Rapoport 1986).

Children's experience of side effects is similar to that of adults, including tremor, fatigue, anticholinergic effects, dizziness, and sweating. Dose-dependent paranoia and aggression have been reported in two case studies. Cardiovascular monitoring (see Table 39–5) is necessary, given the potential for tachycardia, hypertension (and rarely, hypotension), and arrhythmias related to the use of TCAs in children. (See section, "Mood Disorders," for more detail on the use of TCAs.)

Fluoxetine. Fluoxetine is begun at a dose of 5–20 mg/day, usually in the morning. Although early reports cited higher doses, clinical experience suggests that relatively few youths require a dose greater than 20 mg/day for the treatment of obsessive-compulsive disorder, and some may respond to as low as 5 mg/day. Dose adjustments may require alternate-day regimens, use of the liquid formulation, or dissolving medication in juice and dispensing aliquots.

Although children have relatively few somatic side effects (anorexia, weight loss, headaches, nausea, vomiting, tremor), behavioral toxicity is common, perhaps related in part to akathisia. Symptoms include restlessness, insomnia, social disinhibition, agitation (Riddle et al. 1990/1991), and mania (Venkataraman et al. 1992). Suicidal ideation, self-destructive behavior, aggression, and psychotic symptoms have also been reported, although many children with these symptoms had preexisting risk factors for the development of these clinical features (King et al. 1991). Fluoxetine may interfere with sleep architecture, resulting in daytime tiredness.

Treatment typically is required for years. Relapse is common when fluoxetine is discontinued (Leonard et al. 1991).

Fluvoxamine. A typical starting dose of fluvoxamine is 25 mg/day, with a usual treatment range of 100–175 mg/day. Side effects most commonly seen in children are insomnia, agitation, somnolence, and upset stomach.

Assessment of Response

The Leyton Obsessional Inventory—Child Version (Berg et al. 1988) or the Children's Version of the Y-BOCS (Goodman et al. 1989) may be used to quantify symptom severity.

Panic Disorder

Assessment for Treatment

Both panic disorder and agoraphobia occur in children and adolescents (Ballenger et al. 1989). The diagnostic criteria and physical symptom profile are the same as those in adults. Cognitive immaturity may preclude anticipatory anxiety or the characteristic cognitions during an attack (i.e., fear of dying, going crazy, or doing something uncontrolled) (Nelles and Barlow 1988).

Selection of Treatment

There are virtually no systematic data on the treatment of panic disorder in youths. Treatment strategies that have proven successful in adults may be cautiously tried in children and adolescents. Medication doses used are typically conservative to avoid sedation that would impede the patient's academic learning. Supportive and educational individual and family psychotherapy may be useful. Case reports suggest that alprazolam (0.25–2.5 mg/day divided into three or four doses) or imipramine may be effective (Ballenger et al. 1989; Biederman 1987; Kutcher et al. 1992). Clonazepam efficacy (at 1–4 mg/day divided into two or three doses) is supported by preliminary controlled data (Reiter et al. 1992). The benzodiazepines can cause disinhibition and angry outbursts, however (Reiter and Kutcher 1991). Initial titration should be slow. If the patient responds, a maintenance period of 4–6 months should be followed by a drug-free trial to assess continuing need for medication. When discontinuing benzodiazepines, the dose should be tapered gradually (e.g., decreasing by 25% of the initial amount every 3–5 days) to avoid withdrawal symptoms. Other medications that have been used in adults (e.g., SSRIs) may be considered.

Posttraumatic Stress Disorder

Assessment for Treatment

Although the diagnostic criteria for posttraumatic stress disorder (PTSD) are essentially the same at all ages, the symptoms in children differ in some ways from those seen in adults (Terr 1987). Immediate effects include fear of separation from parent(s), of death, and of further fear, leading to withdrawal from new experiences. Perceptual distortions occur, most commonly in time sense and in vision, but auditory, touch, and olfactory misperceptions have been described. Children are likely to reexperience the event in the form of nightmares, daydreams, and/or repetitive, potentially dangerous reenactment in symbolic play or in actual behavior, rather than in intrusive flashbacks. Children may later develop a variety of fears, such as fear of repetition of the experience and fear of other situations that may involve separation or danger or may remind the child of the event. Children may experience somatic symptoms, such as headaches and stomachaches. Increased arousal in children is most often manifested as sleep disturbances, which may add to functional impairment in other areas (Pynoos et al. 1987). Regression and guilt are common. Key items in the assessment include preexisting stressors; previous loss, anxiety, or depression; the nature and degree of exposure to the threat; and life changes secondary to the stressor itself.

Selection of Treatment

Controlled trials of any treatments are lacking. Individual or group insight-oriented play or verbal psychotherapy have been used most often. Systematic desensitization of specific trauma-related fears may be useful in conjunction with other interventions. Supportive therapy for parents and siblings to help them deal with the trauma can reduce contagion. Parents may require therapeutic attention for their own posttraumatic symptoms and/or to help them deal appropriately with their child's symptoms and re-enactment.

The use of psychotropic medication to treat PTSD in children has not been systematically evaluated. Anecdotal reports suggest that propranolol may be effective in the treatment of agitated, hyperaroused children and adolescents with PTSD (Famularo et al. 1988). Propranolol was started at 0.8 mg/kg/day, divided into three doses, with titration to 2.5 mg/kg/day, unless limited by hypotension, bradycardia, or sedation. Case reports suggested the use of carbamazepine (Looff et al. 1995) or guanfacine (Horrigan 1996).

TOURETTE'S DISORDER

Assessment for Treatment

Tourette's disorder (or Tourette's syndrome) is a chronic motor and vocal tic disorder with a duration of more than 1 year, an onset during childhood or adolescence, and a prevalence of 0.03%–1.6%. The tics wax and wane over time and vary in complexity from simple movements or vocalizations (e.g., eye blinks, coughs) to complex, seemingly purposeful behaviors or verbalizations (e.g., facial expressions, coprolalia) (D. Cohen et al. 1992). Genetic studies suggest that Tourette's disorder is an autosomal dominant condition with incomplete, gender-specific penetrance and variable expression (Pauls and Leckman 1986). Linkage studies point to a clinical spectrum that includes Tourette's disorder proper, chronic tic disorder (CTD), obsessive-compulsive disorder, and probably transient tic disorder (TTD). Tourette's disorder is complicated by obsessive-compulsive disorder in 40% of cases. Although about half of the children with Tourette's disorder referred for treatment have ADHD, a genetic association with Tourette's disorder appears unlikely (Pauls and Leckman 1986).

Selection of Treatment

The treatment of Tourette's disorder and associated conditions should be comprehensive and directed toward fostering adaptive development and improving overall functioning rather than simply reducing tic symptoms. Psychopharmacological treatment can be quite effective. Careful monitoring for several months before starting medication is possible because Tourette's disorder is chronic and not usually an emergency. Monitoring permits establishing a baseline of symptoms and assessing the need for psychological and educational interventions.

Neuroleptics

Studies have focused primarily on blockade of dopamine D_2 and α-adrenergic receptors, because hypersensitivity of these neurochemical systems has been hypothesized to underlie Tourette's disorder. Dopamine antagonists have been the mainstay of treatment and are effective in 60%–70% of cases, reducing tic symptoms by approximately 60%–70% (Regeur et al. 1986; A. K. Shapiro and Shapiro 1984; E. Shapiro et al. 1989). Double-blind, placebo-controlled crossover studies using standardized assessments have found that both haloperidol and pimozide (which also acts as a calcium channel blocker) are effective in reducing tics (A. K. Shapiro and Shapiro 1984; E. Shapiro et al. 1989). In a double-blind, placebo-controlled head-to-head comparison, at equivalent doses, pimozide was more effective and had fewer side effects than haloperidol in children and adolescents with Tourette's disorder (Sallee et al. 1997). Other dopamine antagonists, including fluphenazine and piquindone, have been reported to be effective in open clinical trials.

Risperidone, which has both serotonin-2 (5-HT_2) and D_2 receptor antagonism, has undergone preliminary study in the treatment of Tourette's disorder. In open trials of adults with Tourette's disorder, risperidone was effective in decreasing the frequency and severity of both motor and phonic tics in more than half of the patients, including some for whom neuroleptics and/or clonidine were ineffective or poorly tolerated (Bruun and Budman 1996; Van der Linden et al. 1994). Side effects leading patients to discontinue medication were relatively common, however. Clinically and statistically significant reductions in tic frequency and intensity were reported in an open-label study of seven children and adolescents (age 11–16 years) with Tourette's disorder whose symptoms had not responded to treatment with haloperidol or clonidine (Lambroso et al. 1995). Five patients were receiving concurrent clonidine or an SSRI.

Unfortunately, the neuroleptics have a troublesome

side-effect profile. In one clinical sample, 81% of consecutive patients treated with haloperidol for Tourette's disorder discontinued treatment because of side effects (Silva et al. 1996).

α-*Adrenergic Agonists*

Clonidine is effective in ameliorating Tourette's disorder symptoms in a subgroup of patients. Some studies report a 35%–50% reduction in both tic and behavioral symptoms in a substantial minority of patients (Leckman et al. 1991), although other studies report no benefit (Goetz et al. 1987). Vocal tics and associated behavioral manifestations such as impulsivity and restlessness are the most responsive symptoms. Obsessive-compulsive symptoms do not improve. Because of side effects often associated with clonidine (particularly sedation and hypotension), guanfacine, a selective α_{2a}-receptor agonist, has been considered as a possible alternative (Chappell et al. 1995). Guanfacine differs from clonidine in having a longer half-life (17 vs. 12.7 hours) and in producing less sedation and hypotension at clinically comparable doses. In a recent study, 10 subjects with Tourette's disorder and comorbid ADHD experienced a significant reduction in the severity of motor and phonic tics when treated with approximately 1.5 mg/day of guanfacine (in two to three divided doses) (Chappell et al. 1995). The authors noted that guanfacine produced less fatigue and sedation than did clonidine.

Alternative Drugs

Preliminary reports regarding the use of calcium channel blockers and opioid antagonists have been promising, although findings have been inconsistent (Micheli et al. 1990). In one study, clonazepam (when added to clonidine) further reduced tic frequency and severity among seven children with Tourette's disorder, without affecting comorbid ADHD symptomatology (Steingard et al. 1994). In addition, anticholinergic stimulation through the use of nicotine gum has been reported to augment the efficacy of neuroleptics (McConville et al. 1991). Novel treatments are being considered, particularly for refractory cases. Nonsteroidal androgen receptor blocking agents (e.g., flutamide) have yielded modest benefits for some patients with Tourette's disorder (B. S. Peterson et al. 1994).

Treatment of Tourette's Disorder With Comorbidity

Several studies have focused on the treatment of comorbid neuropsychiatric conditions that frequently complicate Tourette's disorder. More than one-half of patients with Tourette's disorder also have obsessive-compulsive disorder. In an open trial, fluoxetine significantly reduced obsessive-compulsive symptomatology (Riddle et al. 1990). Tic frequency and severity were unaffected. These findings were not replicated, however, in a very small controlled trial with less symptomatic patients (Kurlan et al. 1993). Clomipramine, with or without a neuroleptic, has also been advocated for the treatment of Tourette's disorder and obsessive-compulsive disorder (D. Cohen et al. 1992). Patients with Tourette's disorder and obsessive-compulsive symptoms that are refractory to SRIs (e.g., fluvoxamine) may derive substantial benefit from the addition of neuroleptics (e.g., haloperidol) (McDougle et al. 1996). Depression is common among children and adults with Tourette's disorder. If pharmacological treatment is elected, an antidepressant may be used in conjunction with clonidine or a neuroleptic.

For children and adolescents with Tourette's disorder, symptoms of hyperactivity, impulsivity, and distractibility may be more impairing than the tics themselves. Accordingly, treatment is often focused on reducing ADHD symptomatology. The treatment of comorbid ADHD is complicated and controversial. Stimulant medications have been reported to exacerbate or precipitate tics in as many as half of children with Tourette's disorder (Riddle et al. 1995; see Robertson and Eapen 1992 for a review). Other studies report no change in tics or actual reduction in tic frequency and/or severity among children with Tourette's disorder. In a recent double-blind study, Gadow et al. (1995a, 1995b) found that 34 prepubertal children with Tourette's disorder and ADHD had a marked reduction in hyperactivity, disruptive behavior, and aggression during methylphenidate treatment phases, without an exacerbation of tics. Although all three dosages (0.1 mg/kg, 0.3 mg/kg, 0.5 mg/kg) were beneficial, 0.3 mg/kg was the optimum minimum effective dose. The severity of either motor or phonic tics across all three observational settings (classroom, lunchroom, and playground) did not increase. Although a small but statistically significant increase in motor tic frequency occurred during classroom observations, vocal tics decreased during lunchroom observations. Current practice suggests that clinicians can give stimulants to children with comorbid ADHD and Tourette's disorder with informed consent and careful observation when behavioral symptoms cause more impairment than the tics and when other drugs are insufficiently effective or have problematic side effects.

Clonidine and desipramine (alone or in combination with neuroleptics) have been suggested as useful treatments for children with Tourette's disorder and comorbid ADHD (D. Cohen et al. 1992). In a double-blind, placebo-controlled, crossover study of 37 children with Tourette's disorder and ADHD (age 7–13 years), 25 mg four times a day of desipramine was superior to 0.05 mg four times a day of clonidine as shown by reductions in parent and teacher ratings of ADHD symptomatology (Singer et al. 1995). Clinical response was not correlated with blood levels of desipramine. Neither medication affected tics. Clinical observation suggests efficacy of nortriptyline in reducing both tics and ADHD symptoms (T. Spencer et al. 1993). Guanfacine recently has been reported to significantly reduce errors of commission and omission on vigilance tasks and to decrease ADHD symptoms in some patients with Tourette's disorder (Chappell et al. 1995).

Pimozide appears to have less risk than other neuroleptics of cognitive dulling (except at high doses) and may even enhance attention and memory in Tourette's disorder with comorbid ADHD (Sallee et al. 1994). Some clinicians advocate the combination of a neuroleptic and a stimulant (with careful monitoring).

Assessment of Response

The natural waxing and waning course of Tourette's disorder makes evaluation of medication efficacy difficult. A variety of symptom rating scales may be used to quantify the number and severity of tics as well as the patient's school and social impairment (Walkup et al. 1992).

Use of Neuroleptics

Initiation of Treatment

The initial dose of haloperidol is 0.5 mg/day. It may be slowly increased up to 1–3 mg/day, divided in twice-daily doses (D. Cohen et al. 1992). Pimozide, which may be given in a single daily dose, is started at 1 mg/day and may be gradually increased to a maximum of 6–8 mg/day (0.2 mg/kg). Risperidone doses are typically 0.5–9.0 mg/day.

Management of Side Effects

Neuroleptic side effects in children include akathisia, sedation, lethargy, feelings of being like a "zombie," intellectual dulling, weight gain, anxiety, irritability, dysphoria, parkinsonian symptoms, and TD (D. Cohen et al. 1992). In patients with Tourette's disorder, it may be especially difficult to distinguish medication-induced movements from those characteristic of the disorder. Dysphoria and school avoidance have also been reported (Mikkelsen et al. 1981). The side-effect profiles of haloperidol and pimozide are generally similar, although pimozide may cause less sedation and EPS. Pimozide can affect cardiac electrophysiological functioning, including lengthening of the

Q-T$_c$ interval. ECGs should, therefore, be monitored before and during pimozide treatment. Risperidone side effects in children include increased appetite, fatigue, dystonia, muscle stiffness, and almost universal weight gain (8–14 pounds) (Lambroso et al. 1995).

Discontinuation

When haloperidol (and sometimes pimozide) is withdrawn, severe exacerbation of symptoms lasting for up to several months may occur.

Use of α-Adrenergic Agonists

Initiation of Treatment

For clonidine, a gradual increase in dosage to a maximum of approximately 5 µg/kg/day (or 0.25 mg/day) is recommended. A typical guanfacine regimen is 0.5 mg three times per day, titrated up from a starting dose of 0.5 mg/day. (See section, "Attention-Deficit/Hyperactivity Disorder," earlier in this chapter for more information on the use of clonidine and guanfacine.)

Management of Side Effects

Among youths with Tourette's disorder treated with clonidine, 90% experienced transient sedation, and one-third to one-half reported dry mouth, dizziness, and irritability (Goetz et al. 1987; Leckman et al. 1991). Guanfacine has a similar side-effect profile, although it is generally better tolerated than clonidine. In a recent open-label study, side effects included fatigue, headache, insomnia, sedation, and dizziness/light-headedness (Chappell et al. 1995).

Discontinuation

If the α-adrenergic agonists are to be discontinued, gradual tapering off is recommended to avoid rebound tic symptoms and elevations in blood pressure and pulse.

AUTISTIC DISORDERS

Assessment for Treatment

Autism is a relatively rare developmental disorder of early onset that involves significant deficits in social reciprocity, pragmatic (social) communication, and the range and nature of preferred interests and activities. Autism differs from mental retardation in that there are qualitative deviations of development, not simply delays. Behavioral exacerbations in patients with autism may be a result of changes in routine, environmental stressors, an occult medical problem, or a comorbid psychiatric disorder.

Evaluation is made more difficult by the limited communication abilities of many children with autism. Before starting medication, target symptoms should be selected and their baseline level measured. The core symptoms of autism are not generally drug responsive.

Selection of Treatment

Clinicians have used virtually all of the psychotropic medications in attempts to ameliorate the developmental deficits and behavioral difficulties associated with autism. Unfortunately, no medication has yet been identified that fundamentally changes the core social and linguistic deficits. However, medications can often reduce the frequency and intensity of associated behavioral disturbances, which include hyperactivity, agitation, mood instability, aggression, self-injury, and stereotypy, as well as comorbid Axis I disorders. Several neurochemical systems have been implicated in the etiology of the social and behavioral manifestations of the disorder, including the dopaminergic, serotonergic, and endogenous opioid systems. Treatment selection is complicated by the tendency of persons with autism to experience idiosyncratic reactions to psychotropic medications.

Neuroleptics

Drugs such as haloperidol, trifluoperazine, or pimozide result in behavioral improvement in most cases. For example, haloperidol has been evaluated in a series of elegant placebo-controlled studies involving more than 100 autistic children (Anderson et al. 1984, 1989; Campbell et al. 1978). In doses of 0.5–4.0 mg/day, haloperidol significantly reduced hyperactivity, stereotypy, and withdrawal, without adversely affecting cognitive performance. In addition, haloperidol improved discrimination learning and language acquisition when used in combination with positive reinforcement and behavioral interventions (Campbell et al. 1982). The more sedating neuroleptics such as chlorpromazine often cause excessive sedation without significant clinical improvement, however. In a recent case report, risperidone reduced aggression and other behavioral symptoms manifested by three prepubertal children with autistic disorder and mental retardation (Demb 1996).

The use of neuroleptics is discussed in the section, "Schizophrenia," earlier in this chapter. The trial must be of sufficient length to determine whether the drug is efficacious, barring serious side effects requiring immediate discontinuation. If the drug appears to be helpful, it should be continued for at least several months. Although few short-term side effects occur, prospective studies have indicated that withdrawal dyskinesias develop in 25%–30%

of children, leading to concern about the potential for development of TD. Birth complications (during delivery) are associated with increased risk of withdrawal dyskinesias and TD in children with autism (Armenteros et al. 1995). Dyskinesias may be difficult to distinguish from the stereotyped movements characteristic of autism. Baseline and periodic follow-up AIMS ratings (and perhaps even videotaping) are indicated (Shay et al. 1993). At 3- to 6-month intervals, the drug should be discontinued so that the child may be observed for withdrawal dyskinesias and to determine whether the drug is still necessary. Some children may have physical withdrawal symptoms or a rebound phenomenon consisting of worsening of behavior for up to 8 weeks after the medication is stopped (Campbell et al. 1985).

Stimulants

Methylphenidate may reduce target symptoms of inattention, impulsivity, and overactivity in some higher-functioning children and adolescents with autistic disorder (Birmaher et al. 1988; Strayhorn et al. 1988). Although preoccupation, withdrawal, and stereotypy may increase, this is not always the case. In a double-blind, crossover study of 10 children ages 7–11 years with autistic disorder and mild cognitive impairment, methylphenidate resulted in modest but statistically significant reductions in hyperactivity without worsening behavior or increasing stereotypy (Quintana et al. 1995). On the basis of behavioral checklist data, hyperactivity decreased in the classroom but not at home. Other behavioral problems (e.g., aggression and self-injury) did not respond. No differences were found between dosages of 10 and 20 mg twice daily. (See section, "Attention-Deficit/Hyperactivity Disorder," earlier in this chapter for information on the use of stimulants.)

Results of controlled studies of fenfluramine (involving about 200 subjects) are mixed (see Aman and Kern 1989). Clinical benefit was reported in about half of the studies for a third of the subjects. Responsive symptoms included hyperactivity, stereotypy, and withdrawal. There were no consistent improvements in learning, IQ, or language. Side effects were common and included weight loss, irritability, and sedation. Neurotoxicity has been reported in animals but not in humans. Methylphenidate appears to be a better choice than fenfluramine if a stimulant medication is indicated.

Opioid Antagonists

Opioid antagonists have been studied in autism because of their possible involvement in attachment behavior and suggestions that endogenous opioid levels may be abnormal in some autistic individuals. Several controlled, acute-dose trials of naltrexone found modest improvements in activity level, attention, and irritability but no significant changes in social behavior (Willemsen-Swinkels et al. 1995b). A longer-term controlled study reported improvements in activity level, social withdrawal, and communication on global assessments but not on more systematic measures (Campbell et al. 1990). In two double-blind, placebo-controlled crossover studies of naltrexone (mean daily dose 1 mg/kg) administration in children (ages 3–8 years) with autism, results were mixed. One study found statistically significant improvements in parent and teacher global impressions and hyperactivity-impulsivity ratings. Eight of the 13 subjects improved in at least two of the three observational settings (home, school, and clinical laboratory). Hyperactivity and restlessness improved most consistently (Kolmen et al. 1995). The other study found positive effects of naltrexone on teacher reports of hyperactivity and irritability but no effect on parent ratings or playroom observations. Social behaviors and stereotypies did not change (Willemsen-Swinkels et al. 1995b). Negative findings were reported in a double-blind, crossover study of naltrexone with 24 young to middle-aged adults with autism (17 of whom engaged in self-injurious behavior) (Willemsen-Swinkels et al. 1995a). Plasma naltrexone levels do not correlate with clinical response (Gonzalez et al. 1994). Some children experience mild sedation, but no significant side effects have been reported. Reversible hepatic inflammation may occur at higher doses.

Other Drugs

Several other medications have received preliminary study. Two small controlled trials of clonidine reported modest reductions in hyperactivity, overstimulation, and irritability (Frankhauser et al. 1992). Clinical experience suggests that tolerance often develops to the positive effects of clonidine. Lithium has been reported to reduce symptomatology among autistic individuals with cyclic mood disturbances.

The SRIs have attracted attention because of the frequent occurrence of compulsive, ritualistic behavior among autistic individuals. Two small controlled studies of clomipramine (Gordon et al. 1992, 1993) and several case reports of clomipramine, fluoxetine, and fluvoxamine suggested improvement in compulsive behavior, withdrawal, and irritability. However, in an open-label study of eight autistic children (ages 3–8 years), clomipramine was not effective in ameliorating symptoms associated with autism (based on evaluation with several standard instruments)

despite optimal doses (50–175 mg/day or 2.5–4.64 mg/kg/day). In fact, six children were rated as worse on the CGI Consensus Ratings (Sanchez et al. 1996). In a double-blind, placebo-controlled study of adults with autistic disorder, half of the subjects who received fluvoxamine were positive responders (compared with none who received placebo), with reductions in repetitive thoughts and behavior, maladaptive behavior, and aggression and improvement in language use. Several of the fluvoxamine responders had significant improvements in overall adaptive functioning (e.g., moving from a group home to a supervised apartment or obtaining and maintaining full-time employment). Side effects were limited to mild sedation and nausea (McDougle et al. 1996). Sedation may become problematic if it limits energy available for communication or learning.

The combination of vitamin B_6 and magnesium has been reported to improve various symptoms associated with autism. Pfeiffer et al. (1995) reviewed 12 published studies, most of which reported favorable results. They noted, however, that the studies have serious methodological problems, including small sample sizes, imprecise outcome measures, no adjustments for regression effects, and no long-term follow-up. Finally, several case reports suggest that β-blockers, buspirone, and trazodone may reduce agitation and explosive outbursts in some autistic individuals (Ratey et al. 1987).

ENURESIS

Assessment for Treatment

Functional enuresis is diagnosed when the frequency of medically unexplained urinary incontinence exceeds developmental (age-specific) expected norms. Enuresis is strongly familial, especially in males. Neurodevelopmental delays are common in enuretic boys, whereas frequent physiological causes of diurnal enuresis in girls include vaginal reflux of urine, "giggle incontinence," and urgency incontinence. Enuresis is occasionally caused by psychiatric disorders. Anxious children may experience urinary frequency, resulting in daytime incontinence if toilet facilities are not readily available or if the child is fearful of certain bathrooms. In oppositional defiant disorder, refusal to use the toilet may be part of the child's battle for control. Many children with ADHD wait until the last minute to urinate and then lose continence on the way to the bathroom. Secondary enuresis may be related to stress, trauma, or a psychosocial or developmental crisis.

Before starting any treatment, the clinician should obtain baseline measures of frequency of wetting.

Selection of Treatment

For younger children with nocturnal enuresis, the most useful strategy is to minimize secondary symptoms by discouraging the parents from punishing or ridiculing the child while awaiting the child's maturation. For older children who are motivated to stop bed-wetting, a monitoring and reward procedure may be effective. "Bladder training" exercises may be helpful. If these simple interventions are unsuccessful, a urine alarm combined with behavior modification may be useful. Children may need treatment of comorbid psychiatric disorders and management of psychosocial stressors before they are motivated to participate in or respond to behavioral techniques.

Low doses of a TCA or desmopressin (DDAVP) can be helpful if behavioral interventions are ineffective, an associated mood or anxiety disorder is present, special occasions (such as overnight camp) arise. Behavioral treatments are the first choice, however, because they avoid medication side effects and last longer. The combination of DDAVP with the urine alarm has been shown to increase the rate of dryness in children with severe wetting and those with family and behavioral problems (Bradbury and Meadow 1995).

All of the TCAs are equally effective in the treatment of nocturnal enuresis. The mechanism is unclear, but it does not seem to work by altering sleep architecture, by treating depression, or via peripheral anticholinergic activity. In 80% of patients, TCAs reduce the frequency of bed-wetting within the first week. Total remission, however, occurs in relatively few. Wetting returns when the drug is discontinued.

DDAVP is an analogue of antidiuretic hormone administered as a nasal spray to treat nocturnal enuresis (see Thompson and Rey 1995 for a review). A major drawback is its expense: $32 to $240 per month. A minority of patients become completely dry but usually relapse when medication is stopped (Klauber 1989).

Assessment of Response

Daily charts are used to monitor progress.

Use of Tricyclic Antidepressants

Initiation of Treatment

The treatment of enuresis requires much lower doses of TCAs than does the treatment of depression. As a result, ECG monitoring is not necessary. Imipramine is started at 10–25 mg at bedtime and increased by 10- to 25-mg increments weekly to 50 mg (75 mg in preadolescents), if necessary. Maximum dose is 2.5 mg/kg/day (Ryan 1990). At these doses, side effects are rare.

Treatment Resistance

Tolerance to TCAs may develop, requiring a dose increase. For some children, TCAs lose their effect entirely.

Use of Desmopressin

Onset of action of DDAVP is rapid (several days), and side effects are negligible (rare headache or nasal mucosa dryness or irritation) in patients with normal electrolyte regulation. It acts by increasing water absorption in the kidneys, thereby reducing the volume of urine. Evening fluid restriction is advised, to avoid hyponatremia (possibly resulting in seizures; Beach et al. 1992). The usual dose is 5–40 μg intranasally at bedtime. The likelihood of relapse may be decreased by tapering the drug slowly.

Discontinuation

Because enuresis has a high spontaneous remission rate, children and adolescents taking chronic medication should have a drug-free trial at least every 6 months.

SLEEP DISORDERS

Insomnia

Assessment for Treatment

Chronic insomnia is much more frequent in children with psychiatric disorders than in children without psychiatric disorders. What parents report as the child's insomnia is often related to behavioral or habit problems in settling down for the night, especially in the child with ADHD, oppositional defiant disorder, or separation anxiety disorder. Difficulty falling asleep, sleep continuity disturbance, and/or early-morning awakening can be secondary to depression, psychosis, or separation anxiety. A decreased need for sleep can be a symptom of mania. Insomnia may also be secondary to prescribed or over-the-counter medication (e.g., phenobarbital, theophylline, decongestants, or stimulants) or to substance abuse. A detailed sleep diary is needed before initiating any treatment. Sleep laboratory studies may be useful in complex cases.

Selection of Treatment

The first step is treatment of any primary psychiatric disorder. To address true insomnia, parents or adolescents are taught to remove environmental factors interfering with sleep and to develop a bedtime routine, which may include the use of a transitional object or a night-light. Behavioral treatment removes the secondary gain of parental attention for night wakening and provides positive reinforcement for appropriate sleep behavior, or at least for staying quietly in the child's own room. Older children and adolescents may benefit from hypnosis or systematic instruction in relaxation techniques. Short-term medication may facilitate faster results of a behavioral program with less distress to parent and child or may provide parents with a respite to regain enough energy to pursue other solutions.

Many children respond with paradoxical agitation to sedatives. Hypnotic medications are not recommended for chronic use. Chloral hydrate (25–50 mg/kg 30 minutes before bedtime with a maximum dose of 1,000 mg) or diazepam (0.2 mg/kg in preschool-aged children or 1–2 mg in school-aged children) may be indicated for short-term (3–5 days) use in a crisis or for severe insomnia that has not responded to psychological interventions (Dahl 1995).

Sleep Terror Disorder (Pavor Nocturnus) and Sleepwalking Disorder (Somnambulism)

Assessment for Treatment

Episodes of sleep terror typically occur during the first third of the night, in non–rapid eye movement (REM) sleep Stages 3 and 4, lasting 1–10 minutes. The child appears terrified, screams, stares, has dilated pupils, sweats, and has rapid pulse and hyperventilation. He or she is agitated and confused and cannot be comforted. When alert, the child most commonly has no memory of the episode. Return to sleep is rapid when the episode is over, with complete amnesia in the morning. Stress, anxiety, change in sleep schedule, exhaustion, or a febrile illness may increase the frequency of episodes. In children, no associated psychopathology is usually found. Various sedative, neuroleptic, and antidepressant medications, alone or in combination, have been reported to cause night terrors and/or somnambulism (Nino-Murcia and Dement 1987).

Sleepwalking is characterized by repeated episodes of arising from bed and engaging in motor activities while still asleep. Episodes (which last a few minutes to a half-hour) typically occur 1–3 hours after falling asleep, during Stage 3 and 4 delta (non-REM) sleep. The child or adolescent engages in perseverative, stereotyped movements (e.g., picking at blankets) that may progress to walking and other complex behaviors. The child is difficult to awaken, and his or her coordination is poor. Speech, when present, is usually incomprehensible. The youngster may awaken and be confused, may return to bed, or may lie down somewhere else and continue sleeping. The risk of injury is high.

Morning amnesia is typical. Sleepwalking is often seen in children who had night terrors when younger. Likelihood of sleepwalking is increased when the child is overtired or under stress.

Selection of Treatment

For both sleep terror disorder and sleepwalking, restricting fluids prior to bedtime may avoid episodes that are triggered by a full bladder (Nino-Murcia and Dement 1987). Most cases of both disorders respond to support and education while waiting for the child to outgrow the problem. An adequate sleep schedule should be arranged and any specific anxieties or fears addressed. Parents of sleepwalkers should be guided to remove hazards in the environment, and they may need to lock the child's door. Medication (i.e., low doses of imipramine, diazepam, or clonazepam at bedtime) is used only if the episodes are frequent, are dangerous, severely disrupt the family, or interfere with the child's daytime functioning (Nino-Murcia and Dement 1987; Pesikoff and Davis 1971). Imipramine may be given at a dose of 10–50 mg (depending on weight) at bedtime.

EMOTIONAL AND BEHAVIORAL SYMPTOMS IN MENTALLY RETARDED CHILDREN AND ADOLESCENTS

Assessment for Treatment

Mental retardation is a developmental condition that includes subaverage intellectual functioning, impairments in adaptive behavior, and an onset during the developmental period. As such, mental retardation is not amenable to pharmacological treatment. Most people with mental retardation do not have emotional and behavioral difficulties. If such difficulties do occur, the clinician should conduct a thorough assessment to identify a psychiatric disorder and/or psychosocial stressors responsible for the symptoms and then should develop a comprehensive treatment plan. Community-based epidemiological studies indicate that the prevalence of psychiatric disorders among people with mental retardation is higher than in the general population (Gillberg et al. 1986). The full range of psychopathology is present. To improve the validity and reliability of psychiatric diagnosis, standardized assessment instruments can be used, such as the BDI, the CDI, the Aberrant Behavior Checklist (Aman et al. 1985), the Psychopathology Instrument for Mentally Retarded Adults (Aman et al. 1986), and others (Sturmey et al. 1991).

Selection of Treatment

Psychotropic medications can play an important role in the treatment of psychiatric disorders affecting individuals with mental retardation (Aman and Singh 1988; Bregman 1991). Drug selection is made according to the specific disorder that is comorbid with mental retardation.

ADHD

About 10%–20% of children with mental retardation manifest symptoms of ADHD. Well-controlled studies involving more than 100 subjects indicated that methylphenidate significantly reduces hyperactivity, impulsivity, and inattention and improves performance on laboratory measures of attention and memory (Handen et al. 1990, 1992). Responders (60%–75% of those studied) tend to have milder cognitive deficits and to be free from comorbid disorders such as autism and schizophrenia. Other predictors of a positive response to methylphenidate include higher baseline parent and teacher ratings of impulsivity and activity level, higher baseline teacher ratings of inattention and conduct problems, male gender, higher socioeconomic status, and Caucasian heritage (Handen et al. 1994). Children with mental retardation may be particularly prone to side effects such as irritability, social withdrawal, stereotypy, and overinclusive attention.

Schizophrenia

Schizophrenia affects 1%–2% of the mentally retarded population. Neuroleptic medications appear to be as efficacious among patients with mental retardation as they are among those in the general population (Menolascino et al. 1986). Treatment-resistant schizophrenia with cognitive impairments may respond to atypical neuroleptics. Sajatovic et al. (1994) reported that four of five treatment-resistant patients with borderline IQ or mental retardation and either schizophrenia or schizophreniform disorder had a favorable response to clozapine. Progressive improvements were reported in psychopathology, social functioning, and adaptive behavior.

Mood Disorders

Major and minor depression are common among mentally retarded individuals, and case reports documented the efficacy of antidepressants. However, double-blind studies are greatly needed. Mood-stabilizing agents (e.g., lithium carbonate, anticonvulsants) have received preliminary study for the treatment of bipolar disorder and aggressive behavior among individuals with mental retardation. For example, clinical reports and two placebo-controlled trials found that lithium was useful in reducing the frequency and severity of affective cycles and of aggressive and self-injurious behavior in as many as two-thirds to three-quarters of patients (Craft et al. 1987).

Obsessive-Compulsive Disorder

Obsessive-compulsive disorder has been reported among persons with mental retardation. An open-label trial of sustained-release clomipramine was reported recently for the treatment of disabling cleaning and collecting compulsions affecting 11 young adults with mild mental retardation (Barak et al. 1995). An 8-week trial of sustained-release clomipramine, 75 mg/day, resulted in a statistically significant decrease in the severity of compulsive rituals as assessed by several standardized obsessive-compulsive disorder instruments.

Behavioral Symptoms

Most medication studies that have targeted the treatment of stereotypy and destructive behavior in patients with mental retardation have not considered psychiatric diagnosis. Researchers have tried psychotropic medications of various classes, with inconsistent results. The neuroleptics have been studied most extensively. Some reports have been very favorable; however, several well-controlled studies have been discouraging. Recent data suggest that dopamine D_1 receptor supersensitivity may underlie some forms of self-injurious behavior. Preliminary studies of mixed D_1/D_2 receptor antagonists have been encouraging. Definitive results must await controlled studies. The use of neuroleptics for these behavioral difficulties must be weighed against their potential side effects, which include impairment in cognitive performance and the development of akathisia or TD (affecting 15%–35% of mentally retarded patients receiving chronic neuroleptic treatment). The rate of dyskinesia among women with mental retardation has been reported to be negatively correlated with IQ (Farren and Dinan 1994). Low-potency neuroleptics may actually increase aggression. When discontinuing neuroleptics, gradual tapering off is recommended because withdrawal-induced symptomatic deterioration (e.g., anxiety, insomnia) may occur. Clonidine has been reported to reduce these symptoms, suggesting that withdrawal symptoms are caused by adrenergic hyperactivity (Sovner 1995).

Medications that enhance serotonergic activity, including lithium, buspirone, trazodone, and fluoxetine, have been reported to decrease aggressive behavior toward self and others. However, only lithium has been evaluated in controlled studies. The endogenous opioid system has been implicated in at least some forms of self-injury and stereotypy. Preliminary studies (some well controlled) of the opioid antagonists naloxone and naltrexone have reported favorable results; however, others have not. In a recent double-blind, placebo-controlled study of mentally retarded adults with self-injurious behavior, dosages of 50 mg/day for 4 weeks (six subjects) and 150 mg/day for 4 weeks (three subjects) did not have any clinical benefit (Willemsen-Swinkels et al. 1995a). Self-injurious behavior tended to increase with the higher dose. In another double-blind study, 0.5 mg/kg/day of naltrexone administered for 1 month was marginally superior to placebo in decreasing self-injurious behavior (Bouvard et al. 1995).

Some investigators have suggested that heightened noradrenergic activity may result in hyperarousal and may lead to explosive, destructive behavior. Several open clinical trials have reported that β-blockers such as propranolol are effective in some cases (Ratey et al. 1987). Propranolol increases levels of thorazine and imipramine (Gillette and Tannery 1994). Although benzodiazepines and other sedative-hypnotics are often prescribed for the treatment of destructive behavior among people with mental retardation, exacerbation of aggression and self-injurious behavior and paradoxical excitement may occur. Buspirone has been suggested for reducing anxiety (Ratey et al. 1991) and self-injurious behavior (Ricketts et al. 1994) among patients with mental retardation.

CONCLUSION

Psychopharmacological agents that are used carefully can be powerful additions to the therapeutic armamentarium for children and adolescents. Far more empirical work is required, however, to identify and document optimal treatments.

REFERENCES

Abikoff H, Gittelman R: Does behavior therapy normalize the classroom behavior of hyperactive children? Arch Gen Psychiatry 41:449–454, 1984

Achenbach TM: Integrative Guide for the 1991 CBCL/4–18, YSR, and TRF profiles. Burlington, VT, University of Vermont Department of Psychiatry, 1991

Ackerman DL, Greenland S, Bystritsky A, et al: Predictors of treatment response in obsessive-compulsive disorder: multivariate analyses from a multicenter trial of clomipramine. J Clin Psychopharmacol 14:247–254, 1994

Alessi NE: Refractory childhood depressive disorders from a pharmacotherapeutic perspective, in Advances in Neuropsychiatry and Psychopharmacology, Vol 2: Refractory Depression. Edited by Amsterdam JD. New York, Raven, 1991, pp 53–63

Alessi N, Naylor MW, Ghaziuddin M, et al: Update on lithium carbonate therapy in children and adolescents. J Am Acad Child Adolesc Psychiatry 33:291–304, 1994

Aman MG: Monitoring and measuring drug effects, II: behavioral, emotional, and cognitive effects, in Practitioner's Guide to Psychoactive Drugs for Children and Adolescents. Edited by Werry JS, Aman MG. New York, Plenum Medical Book, 1993, pp 99–159

Aman M, Kern R: Review of fenfluramine in the treatment of the developmental disabilities. J Am Acad Child Adolesc Psychiatry 28:549–565, 1989

Aman MG, Singh NN (eds): Psychopharmacology of the Developmental Disabilities. New York, Springer-Verlag, 1988

Aman MG, Singh NN, Stewart AW, et al: The Aberrant Behavior Checklist: a behavior rating scale for the assessment of treatment effects. American Journal of Mental Deficiency 89:485–491, 1985

Aman MG, Watson JE, Singh NN, et al: Psychometric and demographic characteristics of the Psychopathology Instrument for Mentally Retarded Adults. Psychopharmacol Bull 22:1072–1076, 1986

Ambrosini PJ, Emslie GJ, Greenhill LL, et al: Selecting a sequence of antidepressants for treating depression in youth. Journal of Child and Adolescent Psychopharmacology 5:233–240, 1995

American Academy of Child and Adolescent Psychiatry: Practice parameters for the assessment and treatment of anxiety disorders. J Am Acad Child Adolesc Psychiatry 32:1089–1098, 1993

American Academy of Pediatrics: Unapproved uses of approved drugs: the physician, the package insert, and the Food and Drug Administration: subject review. Pediatrics 98:143–145, 1996

American Psychiatric Association: Diagnostic and Statistical Manual of Mental Disorders, 3rd Edition, Revised. Washington, DC, American Psychiatric Association, 1987

American Psychiatric Association: Diagnostic and Statistical Manual of Mental Disorders, 4th Edition. Washington, DC, American Psychiatric Association, 1994

Amery B, Minichiello MD, Brown GL: Aggression in hyperactive boys: response to *d*-amphetamine. J Am Acad Child Adolesc Psychiatry 23:291–294, 1984

Amirkhan J: Expectancies and attributions for hyperactive and medicated hyperactive students. J Abnorm Child Psychol 10:265–276, 1982

Anderson LT, Campbell M, Grega DM, et al: Haloperidol in the treatment of infantile autism: effects on learning and behavioral symptoms. Am J Psychiatry 141:1195–1202, 1984

Anderson LT, Campbell M, Adams P, et al: The effects of haloperidol on discrimination learning and behavioral symptoms in autistic children. J Autism Dev Disord 19:227–239, 1989

Appler WD, McMann GL: Off-label uses of approved drugs: limits on physicians' prescribing behavior. J Clin Psychopharmacol 9:368–370, 1989

Apter A, Ratzoni G, King RA, et al: Fluvoxamine open-label treatment of adolescent inpatients with obsessive-compulsive disorder or depression. J Am Acad Child Adolesc Psychiatry 33:342–348, 1994

Apter A, Fallon, TJ, King RA, et al: Obsessive-compulsive characteristics: from symptoms to syndrome. J Am Acad Child Adolesc Psychiatry 35:907–912, 1996

Armenteros JL, Adams PB, Campbell M, et al.: Haloperidol-related dyskinesias and pre- and perinatal complications in autistic children. Psychopharmacol Bull 31:363–369, 1995

Armenteros JL, Whitaker AH, Welikson M, et al: Risperidone in adolescents with schizophrenia: an open pilot study. J Am Acad Child Adolesc Psychiatry 36:694–700, 1997

Arredondo DE, Docherty JP, Streeter BA: Bupropion treatment of adolescent depression. Paper presented at the 146th annual meeting of the American Psychiatric Association, San Francisco, CA, May 22–27, 1993

Ayllon T, Rosenbaum MS: The behavioral treatment of disruption and hyperactivity in school settings, in Advances in Clinical Child Psychology, Vol 2. Edited by Lahey BB, Kazdin AE. New York, Plenum, 1977, pp 83–118

Ballenger JC, Carek DJ, Steele JJ, et al: Three cases of panic disorder with agoraphobia in children. Am J Psychiatry 146:922–924, 1989

Barak Y, Ring A, Levy D, et al: Disabling compulsions in 11 mentally retarded adults: an open trial of clomipramine SR. J Clin Psychiatry 56:526–528, 1995

Barkley RA: The effects of methylphenidate on the interactions of preschool ADHD children with their mothers. J Am Acad Child Adolesc Psychiatry 27:336–341, 1988

Barkley RA: Attention Deficit Hyperactivity Disorder: A Handbook for Diagnosis and Treatment. New York, Guilford, 1990

Barkley RA, Fischer M, Newby RF, et al: Development of a multimethod clinical protocol for assessing stimulant drug response in children with attention deficit disorder. Journal of Clinical Child Psychology 17:14–24, 1988

Barrickman LL, Perry PJ, Allen AJ, et al: Bupropion versus methylphenidate in the treatment of attention-deficit hyperactivity disorder. J Am Acad Child Adolesc Psychiatry 34:649–657, 1995

Bartels MG, Varley CK, Mitchell J, et al: Pediatric cardiovascular effects of imipramine and desipramine. J Am Acad Child Adolesc Psychiatry 30:100–103, 1991

Bastiaens L: The impact of an intensive educational program on knowledge, attitudes, and side effects of psychotropic medications among adolescent inpatients. Journal of Child and Adolescent Psychopharmacology 2:249–258, 1992

Bastiaens L, Bastiaens DK: A manual of psychiatric medications for teenagers. Journal of Child and Adolescent Psychopharmacology 3:M1–M59, 1993

Beach PS, Beach RE, Smith LR: Hyponatremic seizures in a child treated with desmopressin to control enuresis: a rational approach to fluid intake. Clin Pediatr (Phila) 31:566–569, 1992

Beck AT, Ward CH, Mendelson M, et al: An inventory for measuring depression. Arch Gen Psychiatry 4:561–571, 1961

Beigel A, Murphy DL, Bunney WE Jr: The Manic-State Rating Scale. Arch Gen Psychiatry 25:256–262, 1971

Bellman B, Schachner LA, Pravder L, et al: Carbamazepine hypersensitivity. J Am Acad Child Adolesc Psychiatry 34:1405–1406, 1995

Berg CZ, Whitaker A, Davies M, et al: The survey form of the Leyton Obsessional Inventory—Child Version: norms from an epidemiological study. J Am Acad Child Adolesc Psychiatry 27:759–763, 1988

Bernstein GA, Garfinkel BD, Borchardt CM: Comparative studies of pharmacotherapy for school refusal. J Am Acad Child Adolesc Psychiatry 29:773–781, 1990

Biederman J: Clonazepam in the treatment of prepubertal children with panic-like symptoms. J Clin Psychiatry 48 (suppl):38–41, 1987

Biederman J: Sudden death in children treated with a tricyclic antidepressant. J Am Acad Child Adolesc Psychiatry 30:495–498, 1991

Biederman J, Baldessarini RJ, Wright V, et al: A double-blind placebo controlled study of desipramine in the treatment of ADD, I: efficacy. J Am Acad Child Adolesc Psychiatry 28:777–784, 1989a

Biederman J, Baldessarini RJ, Wright V, et al: A double-blind placebo controlled study of desipramine in the treatment of ADD, II: serum drug levels and cardiovascular findings. J Am Acad Child Adolesc Psychiatry 28:903–911, 1989b

Biederman J, Baldessarini RJ, Goldblatt A: A naturalistic study of 24-hour electrocardiographic recordings and echocardiographic findings in children and adolescents treated with desipramine. J Am Acad Child Adolesc Psychiatry 32:805–813, 1993

Biederman J, Thisted RA, Greenhill LL, et al: Estimation of the association between desipramine and the risk for sudden death in 5- to 14-year-old children. J Clin Psychiatry 56:87–93, 1995

Birmaher B, Quintana H, Greenhill LL: Methylphenidate treatment of hyperactive autistic children. J Am Acad Child Adolesc Psychiatry 27:248–251, 1988

Birmaher B, Greenhill L, Cooper T, et al: Sustained release methylphenidate: pharmacokinetic studies in ADHD males. J Am Acad Child Adolesc Psychiatry 28:768–772, 1989

Birmaher B, Waterman GS, Ryan N, et al: Fluoxetine for childhood anxiety disorders. J Am Acad Child Adolesc Psychiatry 33:993–999, 1994

Black B, Uhde TW: Treatment of elective mutism with fluoxetine: a double-blind, placebo-controlled study. J Am Acad Child Adolesc Psychiatry 33:1000–1006, 1994

Blanz B, Schmidt MH: Clozapine for schizophrenia (letter). J Am Acad Child Adolesc Psychiatry 32:223, 1993

Borcherding GB, Keysor CS, Cooper TB, et al: Differential effects of methylphenidate and dextroamphetamine on the motor activity level of hyperactive children. Neuropsychopharmacology 2:255–263, 1989

Bouvard MP, Leboyer M, Launay JM, et al: Low dose naltrexone effects on plasma chemistries and clinical symptoms in autism: a double-blind, placebo-controlled study. Psychiatry Res 58:191–201, 1995

Bradbury MG, Meadow SR: Combined treatment with enuresis alarm and desmopressin for nocturnal enuresis. Acta Paediatr 84:1014–1018, 1995

Bregman JD: Current developments in the understanding of mental retardation, part II: psychopathology. J Am Acad Child Adolesc Psychiatry 30:861–872, 1991

Briant RH: An introduction to clinical pharmacology, in Pediatric Psychopharmacology: The Use of Behavior Modifying Drugs in Children. Edited by Werry JS. New York, Brunner/Mazel, 1978, pp 3–28

Brown RT, Sexson SB: Effects of methylphenidate on cardiovascular responses in attention deficit hyperactivity disordered adolescents. J Adolesc Health 10:179–183, 1989

Brown RT, Borden KA, Wynne ME, et al: Compliance with pharmacological and cognitive treatments for attention deficit disorder. J Am Acad Child Adolesc Psychiatry 26:521–526, 1987

Brown TE, Gammon GD: ADHD-associated difficulties falling asleep and awakening: clonidine and methylphenidate treatments. Paper presented at the annual meeting of the American Academy of Child and Adolescent Psychiatry, Washington, DC, October 1992

Bruun RD, Budman CL: Risperidone as a treatment for Tourette's syndrome. J Clin Psychiatry 57:29–31, 1996

Buitelaar JK, van der Gaag RJ, Swaab-Barneveld H, et al: Pindolol and methylphenidate in children with attention-deficit hyperactivity disorder: clinical efficacy and side-effects. J Child Psychol Psychiatry 37:587–595, 1996

Campbell M, Anderson LT, Meier M, et al: A comparison of haloperidol, behavior therapy, and their interaction in autistic children. Journal of the American Academy of Child Psychiatry 17:640–655, 1978

Campbell M, Anderson LT, Small AM, et al: The effects of haloperidol on learning and behavior in autistic children. J Autism Dev Disord 12:167–175, 1982

Campbell M, Green WH, Deutsch SI (eds): Child and Adolescent Psychopharmacology. Beverly Hills, CA, Sage, 1985

Campbell M, Anderson LT, Small AM, et al: Naltrexone in autistic children: a double-blind and placebo-controlled study. Psychopharmacol Bull 26:130–135, 1990

Campbell M, Adams PB, Small AM, et al: Lithium in hospitalized aggressive children with conduct disorder: a double-blind and placebo-controlled study. J Am Acad Child Adolesc Psychiatry 34:445–453, 1995a

Campbell M, Kafantaris V, Cueva JE: An update on the use of lithium carbonate in aggressive children and adolescents with conduct disorder. Psychopharmacol Bull 31:93–102, 1995b

Cantwell DP, Swanson J, Connor DF: Case study: adverse response to clonidine. J Am Acad Child Adolesc Psychiatry 36:539–544, 1997

Carlson CL, Pelham WE, Milich R, et al: Single and combined effects of methylphenidate and behavior therapy on the classroom performance of children with attention-deficit hyperactivity disorder. J Abnorm Child Psychol 20:213–232, 1992

Chambers WJ, Puig-Antioch J, Hirsch MT, et al: The assessment of affective disorders in children and adolescents by structured interview. Arch Gen Psychiatry 42:696–702, 1985

Chappell PB, Riddle MA, Scahill L, et al: Guanfacine treatment of comorbid attention-deficit hyperactivity disorder and Tourette's syndrome: preliminary clinical experience. J Am Acad Child Adolesc Psychiatry 34:1140–1146, 1995

Coffey BJ: Anxiolytics for children and adolescents: traditional and new drugs. Journal of Child and Adolescent Psychopharmacology 1:57–83, 1990

Cohen D, Riddle M, Leckman J: Pharmacotherapy of Tourette's syndrome and associated disorders. Psychiatr Clin North Am 15:109–129, 1992

Cohen NJ, Sullivan J, Minde K, et al: Evaluation of the relative effectiveness of methylphenidate and cognitive behavior modification in the treatment of kindergarten-aged hyperactive children. J Abnorm Child Psychol 9:43–54, 1981

Conners CK: A teacher rating scale for use in drug studies with children. Am J Psychiatry 126:884–888, 1969

Conners CK: Controlled trial of methylphenidate in preschool children with minimal brain dysfunction. International Journal of Mental Health 4:61–74, 1975

Conners CK: The computerized continuous performance test. Psychopharmacol Bull 21:891–892, 1985

Conners CK: Methodology of antidepressant drug trials for treating depression in adolescents. Journal of Child and Adolescent Psychopharmacology 2:11–22, 1992

Conners CK, Casat CD, Gualtieri CT, et al: Bupropion hydrochloride in attention deficit disorder with hyperactivity. J Am Acad Child Adolesc Psychiatry 35:1314–1321, 1996

Connor DF: Beta blockers for aggression: a review of the pediatric experience. Journal of Child and Adolescent Psychopharmacology 3:99–114, 1993

Coté CJ, Kauffman RE, Troendle GJ, et al: Is the "therapeutic orphan" about to be adopted? Pediatrics 98:118–123, 1996

Craft M, Ismail IA, Krishnamurti D, et al: Lithium in the treatment of aggression in mentally handicapped patients: a double-blind trial. Br J Psychiatry 150:685–689, 1987

Cueva JE, Overall JE, Small AM, et al: Carbamazepine in aggressive children with conduct disorder: a double-blind and placebo-controlled study. J Am Acad Child Adolesc Psychiatry 35:480–490, 1996

Dahl RE: Child and adolescent sleep disorders. Child and Adolescent Psychiatric Clinics of North America 4:323–341, 1995

Demb HB: Risperidone in young children with pervasive developmental disorders and other developmental disabilities. Journal of Child and Adolescent Psychopharmacology 6:79–80, 1996

Derivan A, Agular L, Upton GV, et al: A study of venlafaxine in children and adolescents with conduct disorder. Paper presented at the 42nd annual meeting of the American Academy of Child and Adolescent Psychiatry, New Orleans, LA, October 1995

DeVeaugh-Geiss J, Moroz G, Biederman J, et al: Clomipramine hydrochloride in childhood and adolescent obsessive compulsive disorder: multicenter trial. J Am Acad Child Adolesc Psychiatry 31:45–49, 1992

Diamond JM, Deane FP: Conners Teacher's Questionnaire: is frequent administration clinically useful? Paper presented at annual meeting of the American Academy of Child and Adolescent Psychiatry, Seattle, WA, October 1988

Doherty M, Gordon A, Brown J, et al: Placebo substitution during medication reductions: controlling for expectancies. Paper presented at the annual meeting of the American Academy of Child and Adolescent Psychiatry, October 1987

Donnelly M, Zametkin AJ, Rapoport JL, et al: Treatment of childhood hyperactivity with desipramine: plasma drug concentration, cardiovascular effects, plasma and urinary catecholamine levels, and clinical response. Clin Pharmacol Ther 39:72–81, 1986

Dubey DR, O'Leary SG, Kaufman KF: Training parents of hyperactive children in child management: a comparative outcome study. J Abnorm Child Psychol 11:229–246, 1983

Dulcan MK (ed): Information for Parents, Youth, and Teachers on Medications for Feelings and Behavior. Washington, DC, American Psychiatric Press (in press)

Dulcan MK, Popper CW: Concise Guide to Child and Adolescent Psychiatry. Washington, DC, American Psychiatric Press, 1991

DuPaul GJ, Rapport MD: Does methylphenidate normalize the classroom performance of children with attention deficit disorder? J Am Acad Child Adolesc Psychiatry 32:190–198, 1993

DuPaul GJ, Rapport MD, Perriello LM: Teacher ratings of academic skills: the development of the Academic Performance Rating Scale. School Psychology Review 20:284–300, 1991

DuPaul GJ, Barkley RA, McMurray MB: Response of children with ADHD to methylphenidate: interaction with internalizing symptoms. J Am Acad Child Adolesc Psychiatry 33: 894–903, 1994

Edelbrock C, Costello AJ, Kessler MK: Empirical corroboration of attention deficit disorder. J Am Acad Child Psychiatry 23:285–290, 1984

Elia J, Borcherding BG, Rapoport JL, et al: Methylphenidate and dextroamphetamine treatments of hyperactivity: are there true nonresponders? Psychiatry Res 36:141–155, 1991

Emslie GJ, Rush AJ, Weinberg WA: A double-blind, randomized placebo-controlled trial of fluoxetine in depressed children and adolescents. Arch Gen Psychiatry 54:1031–1037, 1997

Evans RW, Clay TH, Gualtieri CT: Carbamazepine in pediatric psychiatry. J Am Acad Child Psychiatry 26:2–8, 1987

Evans SW, Pelham WE: Psychostimulant effects on academic and behavioral measures for ADHD junior high school students in a lecture format classroom. J Abnorm Child Psychol 19:537–552, 1991

Famularo R, Fenton T: The effect of methylphenidate on school grades in children with attention deficit disorder without hyperactivity. J Clin Psychiatry 48:112–114, 1987

Famularo R, Kinscherff R, Fenton T: Propranolol treatment for childhood posttraumatic stress disorder, acute type. Am J Dis Child 142:1244–1247, 1988

Farren CK, Dinan TG: Dyskinesia in mentally handicapped women: relationship to level of handicap, age and neuroleptic exposure. Acta Psychiatr Scand 90:210–213, 1994

Fenichel RR: Combining methylphenidate and clonidine: the role of post-marketing surveillance. Journal of Child and Adolescent Psychopharmacology 5:155–156, 1995

Fine S, Jewesson B: Active drug placebo trial of methylphenidate: a clinical service for children with an attention deficit disorder. Can J Psychiatry 34:447–449, 1989

Firestone P: Factors associated with children's adherence to stimulant medication. Am J Orthopsychiatry 52:447–457, 1982

Firestone P, Kelly MJ, Goodman JT, et al: Differential effects of parent training and stimulant medication with hyperactives: a progress report. J Am Acad Child Adolesc Psychiatry 20:135–147, 1981

Fitzpatrick PA, Klorman F, Brumaghim JT, et al: Effects of sustained-release and standard preparations of methylphenidate on attention deficit disorder. J Am Acad Child Adolesc Psychiatry 31:226–234, 1992

Flament MF, Rapoport JL, Berg CZ, et al: Clomipramine treatment of childhood obsessive-compulsive disorder. Arch Gen Psychiatry 42:977–983, 1985

Fletcher SE, Case CL, Sallee FR, et al: Prospective study of the electrocardiographic effects of imipramine in children. J Pediatr 122:652–654, 1993

Frankhauser M, Karumanchi V, German M, et al: A double-blind, placebo-controlled study of the efficacy of transdermal clonidine in autism. J Clin Psychiatry 53:77–82, 1992

Fras I, Major LF: Clinical experience with risperidone (letter). J Am Acad Child Adolesc Psychiatry 34:833, 1995

Frazier JA, Gordon CT, McKenna K, et al: An open trial of clozapine in 11 adolescents with childhood-onset schizophrenia. J Am Acad Child Adolesc Psychiatry 33:658–663, 1994

Fristad MA, Weller EB, Weller RA, et al: Self-report vs. biological markers in assessment of childhood depression. J Affect Disord 15:339–345, 1988

Fristad MA, Weller RA, Weller EB: The Mania Rating Scale (MRS): further reliability and validity studies with children. Ann Clin Psychiatry 7:127–132, 1995

Gadow KD: Pediatric psychopharmacology: a review of recent research. J Child Psychol Psychiatry 33:153–195, 1992

Gadow KD, Swanson HL: Assessing drug effects on academic performance. Psychopharmacol Bull 21:877–886, 1985

Gadow KD, Nolan EE, Sprafkin J, et al: School observations of children with attention-deficit hyperactivity disorder and comorbid tic disorder: effects of methylphenidate treatment. J Dev Behav Pediatr 16:167–176, 1995a

Gadow KD, Sverd J, Sprafkin J, et al: Efficacy of methylphenidate for attention-deficit hyperactivity disorder in children with tic disorder. Arch Gen Psychiatry 52:444–455, 1995b

Gammon GD, Brown TE: Fluoxetine and methylphenidate in combination for treatment of attention deficit disorder and comorbid depressive disorder. Journal of Child and Adolescent Psychopharmacology 3:1–10, 1993

Garvey CA, Gross D, Freeman L: Assessing psychotropic medication side effects among children: a reliability study. Journal of Clinical Psychiatric Nursing 4:127–131, 1991

Geller B: Valproate and polycystic ovaries: reply. J Am Acad Child Adolesc Psychiatry 37:9–10, 1998

Geller B, Fetner HH: Children's 24-hour serum lithium level after a single dose predicts initial dose and steady state plasma levels (letter). J Clin Psychopharmacol 9:155, 1989

Geller B, Fox LW, Fletcher M: Effect of tricyclic antidepressants on switching to mania and on the onset of bipolarity in depressed 6- to 12-year-olds. J Am Acad Child Adolesc Psychiatry 32:43–50, 1993

Geller DA, Biederman J, Reed ED, et al: Similarities in response to fluoxetine in the treatment of children and adolescents with obsessive-compulsive disorder. J Am Acad Child Adolesc Psychiatry 34:36–44, 1995

Geller JL, Gaulin BD, Barreira PJ: A practitioner's guide to use of psychotropic medication in liquid form. Hosp Community Psychiatry 43:969–971, 1992

Ghaziuddin N, Alessi NE: An open clinical trial of trazodone in aggressive children. Journal of Child and Adolescent Psychopharmacology 2:291–297, 1992

Gillberg C, Persson E, Grufman M, et al: Psychiatric disorders in mildly and severely mentally retarded urban children and adolescents: epidemiological aspects. Br J Psychiatry 149:68–74, 1986

Gillette DW, Tannery LP: Beta blocker inhibits tricyclic metabolism. J Am Acad Child Adolesc Psychiatry 33:223–224, 1994

Gilman JT, Alvarez LA, Duchowny M: Carbamazepine toxicity resulting from generic substitution. Neurology 43:2696–2697, 1993

Gittelman R, Abikoff H, Pollack E, et al: A controlled trial of behavior modification and methylphenidate in hyperactive children, in Hyperactive Children: The Social Ecology of Identification and Treatment. Edited by Whalen CK, Henker B. New York, Academic Press, 1980, pp 221–243

Goetz CG, Tanner CM, Wilson RS, et al: Clonidine and Gilles de la Tourette's syndrome: double-blind study using objective rating methods. Ann Neurol 21:307–310, 1987

Gonzalez NM, Campbell M, Small AM, et al: Naltrexone plasma levels, clinical response and effect on weight in autistic children. Psychopharmacol Bull 30:203–208, 1994

Goodman WK, Price LH, Rasmussen SA, et al: The Yale-Brown Obsessive Compulsive Scale, I: development, use, and reliability. Arch Gen Psychiatry 46:1006–1011, 1989

Gordon C, Rapoport J, Hamburger S, et al: Differential response of seven subjects with autistic disorder to clomipramine and desipramine. Am J Psychiatry 149:363–366, 1992

Gordon CT, State RC, Nelson JE, et al: A double-blind comparison of clomipramine, desipramine, and placebo in the treatment of autistic disorder. Arch Gen Psychiatry 50:441–447, 1993

Goyette CH, Conners CK, Ulrich RF: Normative data on revised Conners Parent and Teacher Rating Scales. J Abnorm Child Psychol 6:221–236, 1978

Graae F, Milner J, Rizzotto L, et al: Clonazepam in childhood anxiety disorders. J Am Acad Child Adolesc Psychiatry 33:372–376, 1994

Green WH: Child and Adolescent Clinical Psychopharmacology, 2nd Edition. Baltimore, MD, Williams & Wilkins, 1995

Greenhill LL: Stimulant-related growth inhibition in children: a review, in Strategic Interventions for Hyperactive Children. Edited by Gittleman M. New York, ME Sharpe, 1981, pp 39–63

Greenhill LL, Osman BB (eds): Ritalin: Theory and Patient Management. New York, Mary Ann Liebert, 1991

Greenhill LL, Solomon M, Pleak R, et al: Molindone hydrochloride treatment of hospitalized children with conduct disorder. J Clin Psychiatry 46:20–25, 1985

Greenhill LL, Abikoff HB, Arnold LE, et al: Medication treatment strategies in the MTA study: relevance to clinicians and researchers. J Am Acad Child Adolesc Psychiatry 35:1304–1313, 1996

Grizenko N, Vida S: Propranolol treatment of episodic dyscontrol and aggressive behavior in children. Can J Psychiatry 33:776–778, 1988

Grob CS, Coyle JT: Suspected adverse methylphenidate-imipramine interactions in children. Dev Behav Pediatr 7:265–267, 1986

Gualtieri CT, Hawk B: Tardive dyskinesia and other drug-induced movement disorders among handicapped children and youth. Applied Research in Mental Retardation 1:55–69, 1980

Gualtieri CT, Quade D, Hicks RE, et al: Tardive dyskinesia and other clinical consequences of neuroleptic treatment in children and adolescents. Am J Psychiatry 141:20–23, 1984

Hagino OR, Weller EB, Weller RA, et al: Untoward effects of lithium treatment in children aged four through six years. J Am Acad Child Adolesc Psychiatry 34:1584–1590, 1995

Halperin JM, Gittelman R, Katz S, et al: Relationship between stimulant effect, electroencephalogram, and clinical neurological findings in hyperactive children. J Am Acad Child Adolesc Psychiatry 25:820–825, 1986

Hamilton M: Development of a rating scale for primary depressive illness. British Journal of Social and Clinical Psychology 6:278–296, 1967

Handen BL, Breaux AM, Gosling A, et al: Efficacy of Ritalin among mentally retarded children with ADHD. Pediatrics 86:922–930, 1990

Handen B, Breaux A, Janosky J, et al: Effects and noneffects of methylphenidate in children with mental retardation and ADHD. J Am Acad Child Adolesc Psychiatry 31:455–461, 1992

Handen BL, Janosky J, McAuliffe S, et al: Prediction of response to methylphenidate among children with ADHD and mental retardation. J Am Acad Child Adolesc Psychiatry 33:1185–1193, 1994

Henker B, Whalen CK: The many messages of medication: hyperactive children's perceptions and attributions, in The Ecosystem of the "Sick" Child. Edited by Salzinger S, Antrobus J, Glick J. New York, Academic Press, 1980, pp 141–166

Herskowitz J: Developmental toxicology, in Psychiatric Pharmacosciences of Children and Adolescents. Edited by Popper C. Washington, DC, American Psychiatric Press, 1987, pp 81–123

Hinshaw SP: Stimulant medication and the treatment of aggression in children with attentional deficits. Journal of Clinical Child Psychology 20:301–312, 1991

Hinshaw SP, Henker B, Whalen CK, et al: Aggressive, prosocial, and nonsocial behavior in hyperactive boys: dose effects of methylphenidate in naturalistic settings. J Consult Clin Psychol 57:636–643, 1989

Horrigan JP: Guanfacine for PTSD nightmares (letter). J Am Acad Child Adolesc Psychiatry 35:975, 1996

Horrigan JP, Barnhill LJ: Guanfacine for treatment of attention-deficit hyperactivity disorder in boys. Journal of Child and Adolescent Psychopharmacology 5:215–223, 1995

Hunt RD, Capper S, O'Connell P: Clonidine in child and adolescent psychiatry. Journal of Child and Adolescent Psychopharmacology 1:87–102, 1990

Hunt RD, Lau S, Ryu J: Alternative therapies for ADHD, in Ritalin: Theory and Patient Management. Edited by Greenhill LL, Osman BB. New York, Mary Ann Liebert, 1991, pp 75–95

Hunt RD, Arnsten AFT, Asbell MD: An open trial of guanfacine in the treatment of attention-deficit hyperactivity disorder. J Am Acad Child Adolesc Psychiatry 34:50–54, 1995

Hynes AFM, Vickar EL: Case study: neuroleptic malignant syndrome without pyrexia. J Am. Acad Child Adolesc Psychiatry 35:959–962, 1996

Jatlow PI: Psychotropic drug disposition during development, in Psychiatric Pharmacosciences of Children and Adolescents. Edited by Popper C. Washington, DC, American Psychiatric Press, 1987, pp 27–44

Johnston HF, Fruehling JJ: Using antidepressant medication in depressed children: an algorithm. Psychiatric Annals 24:348–356, 1994

Kafantaris V, Campbell M, Padron-Gayol MV, et al: Carbamazepine in hospitalized aggressive conduct disorder children: an open pilot study. Psychopharmacol Bull 28:193–199, 1992

Kafantaris V, Lee DO, Magee H, et al: Assessment of children with the Overt Aggression Scale. J Neuropsychiatry Clin Neurosci 8:186–193, 1996

Kaufman J, Birmaher B, Brent D, et al: Schedule for Affective Disorders and Schizophrenia for School-Age Children—Present and Lifetime Version (K-SADS-PL): initial reliability and validity data. J Am Acad Child Adolesc Psychiatry 36:980–988, 1997

Kay SR, Wolkenfeld F, Murrill LM: Profiles of aggression among psychiatric patients. J Nerv Ment Dis 176:539–546, 1988

Kemph JP, DeVane CL, Levin GM, et al: Treatment of aggressive children with clonidine: results of an open pilot study. J Am Acad Child Adolesc Psychiatry 32:577–581, 1993

Kent JD, Bladfer JC, Koplewicz HS, et al: Effects of late-afternoon methylphenidate administration on behavior and sleep in attention-deficit hyperactivity disorder. Pediatrics 96:320–325, 1995

King RA, Riddle MA, Chappell PB, et al: Emergence of self-destructive phenomena in children and adolescents during fluoxetine treatment. J Am Acad Child Adolesc Psychiatry 30:179–186, 1991

Klauber GT: Clinical efficacy and safety of desmopressin in the treatment of nocturnal enuresis. J Pediatr 114:719–722, 1989

Klein RG, Mannuzza S: Hyperactive boys almost grown up, III: methylphenidate effects on ultimate height. Arch Gen Psychiatry 45:1131–1134, 1988

Klein RG, Landa B, Mattes JA, et al: Methylphenidate and growth in hyperactive children. Arch Gen Psychiatry 45:1127–1130, 1988

Klein RG, Koplewicz HS, Kanner A: Imipramine treatment of children with separation anxiety disorder. J Am Acad Child Adolesc Psychiatry 31:21–28, 1992

Klein RG, Abikoff H, Barkley RA, et al: Clinical trials in children and adolescents, in Clinical Evaluation of Psychotropic Drugs: Principles and Guidelines. Edited by Prien RF, Robinson DS. New York, Raven, 1994, pp 501–546

Klorman R, Brumaghim JT, Salzman LF, et al: Comparative effects of methylphenidate on attention-deficit hyperactivity disorder with and without aggressive/noncompliant features. Psychopharmacol Bull 25:109–113, 1989

Klorman R, Brumaghim JT, Fitzpatrick P, et al: Clinical effects of a controlled trial of methylphenidate on adolescents with attention deficit disorder. J Am Acad Child Adolesc Psychiatry 29:702–709, 1990

Knight MM, Wigder KS, Fortsch MM, et al: Medication education for children: is it worthwhile? Journal of Child Psychiatric Nursing 3:25–28, 1990

Kolmen BK, Feldman HM, Handen BL, et al: Naltrexone in young autistic children: a double-blind, placebo-controlled cross-over study. J Am Acad Child Adolesc Psychiatry 34:223–231, 1995

Kovacs M: The Children's Depression Inventory (CDI). Psychopharmacol Bull 21:995–998, 1985

Kowatch RA, Suppes T, Gilfillan SK, et al: Clozapine treatment of children and adolescents with bipolar disorder and schizophrenia: a clinical case series. Journal of Child and Adolescent Psychopharmacology 5:241–253, 1995

Kranzler HR: Use of buspirone in an adolescent with overanxious disorder. J Am Acad Child Adolesc Psychiatry 27:789–790, 1988

Kumra S, Frazier JA, Jacobsen LK, et al: Childhood-onset schizophrenia: A double-blind clozapine-haloperidol comparison. Arch Gen Psychiatry 53:1090–1097, 1996

Kuperman S, Stewart MA: Use of propranolol to decrease aggressive outbursts in younger patients. Psychosomatics 28:315–319, 1987

Kurlan R, Como PG, Deeley C, et al: A pilot controlled study of fluoxetine for obsessive-compulsive symptoms in children with Tourette's syndrome. Clin Neuropharmacol 16:167–172, 1993

Kutcher SP, MacKenzie S, Galarraga W, et al: Clonazepam treatment of adolescents with neuroleptic-induced akathisia. Am J Psychiatry 144:823–824, 1987

Kutcher SP, Reiter S, Gardner DM, et al: The pharmacotherapy of anxiety disorders in children and adolescents. Psychiatr Clin North Am 15:41–67, 1992

Lambroso PJ, Scahill L, King RA, et al: Risperidone treatment of children and adolescents with chronic tic disorders: a preliminary report. J Am Acad Child Adolesc Psychiatry 34:1147–1152, 1995

Latz SR, McCracken JT: Neuroleptic malignant syndrome in children and adolescents: two case reports and a warning. Journal of Child and Adolescent Psychopharmacology 2:123–129, 1992

Leckman JF, Ort S, Caruso KA, et al: Rebound phenomena in Tourette's syndrome after abrupt withdrawal of clonidine. Arch Gen Psychiatry 43:1168–1176, 1986

Leckman J, Hardin M, Riddle M, et al: Clonidine treatment of Gilles de la Tourette's syndrome. Arch Gen Psychiatry 48:324–328, 1991

Leonard HL, Swedo SE, Rapoport JL, et al: Treatment of obsessive compulsive disorder with clomipramine and desipramine in children and adolescents. Arch Gen Psychiatry 46:1088–1092, 1989

Leonard HL, Swedo SE, Lenane MC, et al: A double-blind desipramine substitution during long-term clomipramine treatment in children and adolescents with obsessive-compulsive disorder. Arch Gen Psychiatry 48:922–927, 1991

Leonard HL, Topol D, Bukstein O, et al: Clonazepam as an augmenting agent in the treatment of childhood-onset obsessive-compulsive disorder. J Am Acad Child Adolesc Psychiatry 33:792–794, 1994

Leonard HL, Meyer MC, Swedo SE, et al: Electrocardiographic changes during desipramine and clomipramine treatment in children and adolescents. J Am Acad Child Adolesc Psychiatry 34:1460–1468, 1995

Lewis DW, Pincus JH, Shanok SS, et al: Psychomotor epilepsy and violence in a group of incarcerated adolescent boys. Am J Psychiatry 139:882–887, 1982

Lewis M (ed): Child and Adolescent Psychiatry: A Comprehensive Textbook, 2nd Edition. Baltimore, MD, Williams & Wilkins, 1996

Liberthson RR: Sudden death from cardiac causes in children and young adults. N Engl J Med 334:1039–1044, 1996

Livingston RL, Dykman RA, Ackerman PT: Psychiatric comorbidity and response to two doses of methylphenidate in children with attention deficit disorder. Journal of Child and Adolescent Psychopharmacology 2:115–122, 1992

Loney J, Milich R: Hyperactivity, inattention, and aggression in clinical practice. Advances in Developmental and Behavioral Pediatrics 3:113–147, 1982

Looff D, Grimley P, Kuller F, et al: Carbamazepine for PTSD. J Am Acad Child Adolesc Psychiatry 34:703–704, 1995

Malone RP, Biesecker KA, Luebbert JF, et al: Importance of placebo baseline in clinical drug trials involving aggressive children (abstract). Psychopharmacol Bull 31:593, 1995a

Malone RP, Delaney MA, Luebbert JF, et al: The lithium test dose prediction method in aggressive children. Psychopharmacol Bull 31:379–381, 1995b

Mandoki MW: Risperidone treatment of children and adolescents: increased risk of extrapyramidal side effects? Journal of Child and Adolescent Psychopharmacology 5:49–67, 1995

March JS, Mulle K, Herbel B: Behavioral psychotherapy for children and adolescents with obsessive-compulsive disorder: an open trial of a new protocol-driven treatment package. J Am Acad Child Adolesc Psychiatry 33:333–341, 1994

Mash EJ, Dalby JT: Behavioral interventions in hyperactivity, in Hyperactivity in Children: Etiology, Measurement and Treatment Implications. Edited by Trites RL. Baltimore, MD, University Park Press, 1979, pp 161–216

McBride MC: An individual double-blind cross-over trial for assessing methylphenidate response in children with attention deficit disorder. J Pediatr 113:137–145, 1988

McClellan JM, Werry JS: Schizophrenia. Psychiatr Clin North Am 15:131–148, 1992

McClellan J, Werry J: Practice parameters for the assessment and treatment of children and adolescents with schizophrenia. J Am Acad Child Adolesc Psychiatry 33:616–635, 1994

McConville BJ, Fogelson MH, Norman AB, et al: Nicotine potentiation of haloperidol in reducing tic frequency in Tourette's disorder. Am J Psychiatry 148:793–794, 1991

McConville BJ, Minnery KL, Sorter MT, et al: An open study of the effects of sertraline on adolescent major depression. Journal of Child and Adolescent Psychopharmacology 6:41–51, 1996

McDaniel KD: Pharmacologic treatment of psychiatric and neurodevelopmental disorders in children and adolescents (part 1). Clin Pediatr (Phila) 25:65–71, 1986

McDougle CJ, Goodman WK, Leckman JF, et al: Haloperidol addition in fluvoxamine-refractory obsessive-compulsive disorder: a double-blind, placebo-controlled study in patients with and without tics. Arch Gen Psychiatry 51:302–308, 1994

McDougle CJ, Fleischmann RL, Epperson CN, et al: Risperidone addition in fluvoxamine-refractory obsessive-compulsive disorder: three cases. J Clin Psychiatry 56:526–528, 1995

McDougle CJ, Naylor ST, Cohen DJ, et al: A double-blind, placebo-controlled study of fluvoxamine in adults with autistic disorder. Arch Gen Psychiatry 53:1001–1008, 1996

Menolascino F, Wilson J, Golden C, et al: Medication and treatment of schizophrenia in persons with mental retardation. Ment Retard 24:277–283, 1986

Micheli F, Gatto M, Lekhuniec E, et al: Treatment of Tourette's syndrome with calcium antagonists. Clin Neuropharmacol 13:77–83, 1990

Mikkelsen EJ, Detlor J, Cohen DJ: School avoidance and social phobia triggered by haloperidol in patients with Tourette's disorder. Am J Psychiatry 138:1572–1576, 1981

Mozes T, Toren P, Chernauzan N, et al: Clozapine treatment in very early onset schizophrenia. J Am Acad Child Adolesc Psychiatry 33:65–70, 1994

Munetz MR, Benjamin S: How to examine patients using the Abnormal Involuntary Movement Scale. Hosp Community Psychiatry 39:1172–1177, 1988

Murphy DA, Pelham WE, Lang AR: Aggression in boys with attention deficit-hyperactivity disorder: methylphenidate effects on naturalistically observed aggression, response to provocation, and social information processing. J Abnorm Child Psychol 20:451–466, 1992

Nehra A, Mullick F, Ishak KG, et al: Pemoline-associated hepatic injury. Gastroenterology 99:1517–1519, 1990

Nelles WB, Barlow DH: Do children panic? Clinical Psychology Review 8:359–372, 1988

Nino-Murcia G, Dement WC: Psychophysiological and pharmacological aspects of somnambulism and night terrors in children, in Psychopharmacology: The Third Generation of Progress. Edited by Meltzer HY. New York, Raven, 1987, pp 873–879

Overholser JC, Brinkman DC, Lehnert KL, et al: Children's Depression Rating Scale—Revised: development of a short form. Journal of Clinical Child Psychology 24:443–452, 1995

Patterson JF: Hepatitis associated with pemoline (letter). South Med J 77:938, 1984

Pauls DL, Leckman JF: The inheritance of Gilles de la Tourette syndrome and associated behaviors: evidence for an autosomal dominant transmission. N Engl J Med 315:993–997, 1986

Pelco LE, Kissel RC, Parrish JM, et al: Behavioral management of oral medication administration difficulties among children: a review of literature with case illustrations. Dev Behav Pediatr 8:90–96, 1987

Pelham WE: The effects of stimulant drugs on learning and achievement in hyperactive and learning disabled children, in Psychological and Educational Perspectives on Learning Disabilities. Edited by Torgesen JK, Wong B. New York, Academic Press, 1985, pp 259–295

Pelham WE, Bender ME: Peer relationships in hyperactive children: description and treatment. Advances in Learning and Behavioral Disabilities 1:365–436, 1982

Pelham WE, Murphy HA: Attention deficit and conduct disorders, in Pharmacological and Behavioral Treatment: An Integrative Approach. Edited by Hersen M. New York, Wiley, 1986, pp 108–148

Pelham WE, Schnedler RW, Bologna NC, et al: Behavioral and stimulant treatment of hyperactive children: a therapy study with methylphenidate probes in a within-subject design. J Appl Behav Anal 13:221–236, 1980

Pelham WE, Milich R, Walker JL: Effects of continuous and partial reinforcement and methylphenidate on learning in children with attention deficit disorder. J Abnorm Psychol 95:319–325, 1986

Pelham WE, Milich R, Murphy DA, et al: Normative data on the IOWA Conners Teacher Rating Scale. Journal of Clinical Child Psychology 18:259–262, 1989

Pelham WE, Greenslade KE, Vodde-Hamilton M, et al: Relative efficacy of long-acting stimulants on children with attention deficit-hyperactivity disorder: a comparison of standard methylphenidate, sustained-release methylphenidate, sustained-release dextroamphetamine, and pemoline. Pediatrics 86:226–237, 1990

Pelham WE, Swanson JM, Furman MB, et al: Pemoline effects on children with ADHD: a time-response by dose-response analysis on classroom measures. J Am Acad Child Adolesc Psychiatry 34:1504–1513, 1995

Pellock JM: Carbamazepine side effects in children and adults. Epilepsia 28 (suppl 3):564–570, 1987

Pesikoff RB, Davis PC: Treatment of pavor nocturnus and somnambulism in children. Am J Psychiatry 128:778–781, 1971

Peterson BS, Leckman JF, Scahill L, et al: Steroid hormones and Tourette's syndrome: early experience with antiandrogen therapy. J Clin Psychopharmacol 14:131–135, 1994

Peterson SE, Myers KM, McClellan J, et al: Neuroleptic malignant syndrome: three adolescents with complicated courses. Journal of Child and Adolescent Psychopharmacology 5:139–149, 1995

Petti TA, Law W: Abrupt cessation of high-dose imipramine treatment in children. JAMA 246:768–769, 1981

Pfeiffer SI, Norton J, Nelson L, et al: Efficacy of Vitamin B6 and magnesium in the treatment of autism: a methodological review and summary of outcomes. J Autism Dev Disord 25:481–493, 1995

Pleak RR, Birmaher B, Gavrilescu A, et al: Mania and neuropsychiatric excitation following carbamazepine. J Am Acad Child Adolesc Psychiatry 27:500–503, 1988

Pliszka SR: Tricyclic antidepressants in the treatment of children with attention deficit disorder. J Am Acad Child Adolesc Psychiatry 26:127–132, 1987

Pliszka SR: Effect of anxiety on cognition, behavior, and stimulant response in ADHD. J Am Acad Child Adolesc Psychiatry 28:882–887, 1989

Popper C: Medical unknowns and ethical consent, in Psychiatric Pharmacosciences of Children and Adolescents. Edited by Popper C. Washington, DC, American Psychiatric Press, 1987, pp 127–161

Popper CW, Zimnitzky B: Sudden death putatively related to desipramine treatment in youth: a fifth case and a review of speculative mechanisms. Journal of Child and Adolescent Psychopharmacology 5:283–300, 1995

Poznanski EO, Freeman LN, Mokros HB: Children's Depression Rating Scale—Revised. Psychopharmacol Bull 21:979–989, 1985

Preskorn SH, Weller E, Hughes CW, et al: Depression in prepubertal children: dexamethasone nonsuppression predicts differential response to imipramine vs. placebo. Psychopharmacol Bull 23:128–133, 1987

Preskorn SH, Weller E, Jerkovich G, et al: Depression in children: concentration-dependent CNS toxicity of tricyclic antidepressants. Psychopharmacol Bull 24:140–142, 1988

Pynoos RS, Frederick C, Nader K, et al: Life threat and posttraumatic stress in school-age children. Arch Gen Psychiatry 44:1057–1063, 1987

Quintana H, Keshavan M: Case study: risperidone in children and adolescents with schizophrenia. J Am Acad Child Adolesc Psychiatry 34:1292–1296, 1995

Quintana H, Birmaher B, Stedge D, et al: Use of methylphenidate in the treatment of children with autistic disorder. J Autism Dev Disord 25:283–294, 1995

Rapoport JL: Antidepressants in childhood attention deficit disorder and obsessive-compulsive disorder. Psychosomatics 27:30–36, 1986

Rapoport JL, Swedo SE, Leonard HL: Childhood obsessive compulsive disorder. J Clin Psychiatry 53 (suppl):11–16, 1992

Rapport MD, Jones JT, DuPaul GJ, et al: Attention deficit disorder and methylphenidate: group and single-subject analyses of dose effects on attention in clinic and classroom settings. Journal of Clinicial Child Psychology 16:329–338, 1987

Rapport MD, Carlson GA, Kelly KL, et al: Methylphenidate and desipramine in hospitalized children, I: separate and combined effects on cognitive function. J Am Acad Child Adolesc Psychiatry 32:333–342, 1993

Ratey J, Bemporad J, Sorgi P, et al: Brief report: open trial effects of beta-blockers on speech and social behaviors in 8 autistic adults. J Autism Dev Disord 17:439–446, 1987

Ratey J, Sovner R, Parks A, et al: Buspirone treatment of aggression and anxiety in mentally retarded patients: a multiple-baseline, placebo lead-in study. J Clin Psychiatry 52:159–162, 1991

Realmuto GM, Erickson WD, Yellin AM, et al: Clinical comparison of thiothixene and thioridazine in schizophrenic adolescents. Am J Psychiatry 141:440–442, 1984

Regeur L, Pakkenberg B, Fog R, et al: Clinical features and long-term treatment with pimozide in 65 patients with Gilles de la Tourette's syndrome. J Neurol Neurosurg Psychiatry 49:791–795, 1986

Reich W, Welner Z: The Diagnostic Interview for Children and Adolescents—Revised. St. Louis, MO, Washington University, 1988

Reiter S, Kutcher SP: Disinhibition and anger outbursts in adolescents treated with clonazepam (letter). J Clin Psychopharmacol 11:268, 1991

Reiter S, Kutcher S, Gardner D: Anxiety disorders in children and adolescents: clinical and related issues in pharmacological treatment. Can J Psychiatry 37:432–438, 1992

Remschmidt H, Schulz E, Martin PDM: An open trial of clozapine in thirty-six adolescents with schizophrenia. Journal of Child and Adolescent Psychopharmacology 4:31–41, 1994

Richardson MA, Haugland G, Craig TJ: Neuroleptic use, parkinsonian symptoms, tardive dyskinesia, and associated factors in child and adolescent psychiatric patients. Am J Psychiatry 148:1322–1328, 1991

Ricketts RW, Goza AB, Ellis CR, et al: Clinical effects of buspirone on intractable self-injury in adults with mental retardation. J Am Acad Child Adolesc Psychiatry 33:270–276, 1994

Riddle MA (guest ed): Pediatric psychopharmacology I. Child and Adolescent Psychiatric Clinics of North America 4(1), 1995a

Riddle MA (guest ed): Pediatric psychopharmacology II. Child and Adolescent Psychiatric Clinics of North America 4(2), 1995b

Riddle MA, Pediatric OCD Research Group: Fluvoxamine in the treatment of OCD in children and adolescents: a multicenter, double-blind, placebo-controlled trial. American Psychiatric Association 1996 Annual Meeting New Research Program and Abstracts (NR 197). Washington, DC, American Psychiatric Association, 1996, p 121

Riddle MA, Hardin MT, Cho SC, et al: Desipramine treatment of boys with attention-deficit hyperactivity disorder and tics: preliminary clinical experience. J Am Acad Child Adolesc Psychiatry 27:811–814, 1988

Riddle MA, Hardin MT, King RA, et al: Fluoxetine treatment of children and adolescents with Tourette's and obsessive compulsive disorders: preliminary clinical experience. J Am Acad Child Adolesc Psychiatry 29:45–48, 1990

Riddle MA, King RA, Hardin MT, et al: Behavioral side effects of fluoxetine in children and adolescents. Journal of Child and Adolescent Psychopharmacology 1:193–198, 1990/1991

Riddle MA, Scahill L, King RA, et al: Double-blind, cross-over trial of fluoxetine and placebo in children and adolescents with obsessive compulsive disorder. J Am Acad Child Adolesc Psychiatry 31:1062–1069, 1992

Riddle MA, Geller B, Ryan N: Another sudden death in a child treated with desipramine. J Am Acad Child Adolesc Psychiatry 32:792–797, 1993

Riddle MA, Lynch KA, Scahill L, et al: Methylphenidate discontinuation and reinitiation during long-term treatment of children with Tourette's disorder and attention-deficit hyperactivity disorder: a pilot study. Journal of Child and Adolescent Psychopharmacology 5:205–214, 1995

Rivera-Calimlim L, Griesbach PH, Perlmutter R: Plasma chlorpromazine concentrations in children with behavioral disorders and mental illness. Clin Pharmacol Ther 26:114–121, 1979

Robertson MM, Eapen V: Pharmacologic controversy of CNS stimulants in Gilles de la Tourette's syndrome. Clin Neuropharmacol 15:408–425, 1992

Rosenberg DR, Holttum J, Gershon S: Textbook of Pharmacotherapy for Child and Adolescent Psychiatric Disorders. New York, Brunner/Mazel, 1994

Ryan ND: Heterocyclic antidepressants in children and adolescents. Journal of Child and Adolescent Psychopharmacology 1:21–31, 1990

Ryan ND: The pharmacologic treatment of child and adolescent depression. Psychiatr Clin North Am 15:29–40, 1992

Ryan ND, Puig-Antioch J, Cooper T, et al: Imipramine in adolescent major depression: plasma level and clinical response. Acta Psychiatr Scand 73:275–288, 1986

Ryan N, Meyer VA, Dachille S, et al: Lithium antidepressant augmentation in TCA-refractory depression in adolescents. J Am Acad Child Adolesc Psychiatry 27:371–376, 1988a

Ryan ND, Puig-Antioch J, Rabinovich H, et al: MAOIs in adolescent major depression unresponsive to tricyclic antidepressants. J Am Acad Child Adolesc Psychiatry 27:755–758, 1988b

Safer DJ: Relative cardiovascular safety of psychostimulants used to treat attention-deficit hyperactivity disorder. Journal of Child and Adolescent Psychopharmacology 2:279–290, 1992

Sajatovic M, Ramirez LF, Kenny JT, et al: The use of clozapine in borderline-intellectual-functioning and mentally retarded schizophrenic patients. Compr Psychiatry 35:29–33, 1994

Sallee F, Stiller R, Perel J, et al: Oral pemoline kinetics in hyperactive children. Clin Pharmacol Ther 37:606–609, 1985

Sallee F, Stiller R, Perel J, et al: Targeting imipramine dose in children with depression. Clin Pharmacol Ther 40:8–13, 1986

Sallee FR, Stiller RL, Perel JM: Pharmacodynamics of pemoline in attention deficit disorder with hyperactivity. J Am Acad Child Adolesc Psychiatry 31:244–251, 1992

Sallee FR, Sethuraman G, Rock CM: Effects of pimozide on cognition in children with Tourette syndrome: interaction with comorbid attention deficit disorder. Acta Psychiatr Scand 90:4–9, 1994

Sallee FR, Nesbitt L, Jackson C, et al: Relative efficacy of haloperidol and pimozide in children and adolescents with Tourette's disorder. Am J Psychiatry 154:1057–1062, 1997

Sanchez LE, Campbell M, Small AM, et al: A pilot study of clomipramine in young autistic children. J Am Acad Child Adolesc Psychiatry 35:537–544, 1996

Satterfield JH, Satterfield BT, Schell AM: Therapeutic interventions to prevent delinquency in hyperactive boys. J Am Acad Child Adolesc Psychiatry 26:56–64, 1987

Schleifer M, Weiss G, Cohen N, et al: Hyperactivity in preschoolers and the effect of methylphenidate. Am J Orthopsychiatry 45:38–50, 1975

Schouten R, Duckworth KS: Medicolegal and ethical issues in the pharmacologic treatment of children, in Practitioner's Guide to Psychoactive Drugs for Children and Adolescents. Edited by Werry JS, Aman MG. New York, Plenum Medical Book, 1993, pp 161–178

Schroeder JS, Mullin AV, Elliott GR, et al: Cardiovascular effects of desipramine in children. J Am Acad Child Adolesc Psychiatry 28:376–379, 1989

Shah MR, Seese LM, Abikoff H, et al: Pemoline for children and adolescents with conduct disorder: a pilot investigation. Journal of Child and Adolescent Psychopharmacology 4:255–261, 1994

Shapiro AK, Shapiro E: Controlled study of pimozide vs. placebo in Tourette's syndrome. J Am Acad Child Adolesc Psychiatry 23:161–173, 1984

Shapiro E, Shapiro A, Fulop G, et al: Controlled study of haloperidol, pimozide, and placebo for the treatment of Gilles de la Tourette's syndrome. Arch Gen Psychiatry 46:722–730, 1989

Shay J, Sanchez LE, Cueva JE, et al: Neuroleptic-related dyskinesias and stereotypies in autistic children: videotaped ratings. Psychopharmacol Bull 29:359–363, 1993

Sheth RD, Wesolowski CA, Jacob JC, et al: Effect of carbamazepine and valproate on bone mineral density. J Pediatr 127:256–262, 1995

Silva RR, Munoz DM, Daniel W, et al: Causes of haloperidol discontinuation in patients with Tourette's syndrome. J Clin Psychiatry 57:129–135, 1996

Silverstein FS, Boxer L, Johnston MV: Hematological monitoring during therapy with carbamazepine in children. Ann Neurol 13:685–686, 1983

Simeon JG, Ferguson HB: Recent developments in the use of antidepressant and anxiolytic medications. Psychiatr Clin North Am 8:893–907, 1985

Simeon JG, Ferguson HB: Alprazolam effects in children with anxiety disorders. Can J Psychiatry 32:570–574, 1987

Simeon JG, Ferguson HB, Fleet JVW: Bupropion exacerbates tics in children with attention-deficit hyperactivity disorder and Tourette's syndrome. J Am Acad Child Adolesc Psychiatry 32:211–214, 1986

Simeon JG, Thatte S, Wiggins D: Treatment of adolescent obsessive-compulsive disorder with a clomipramine-fluoxetine combination. Psychopharmacol Bull 26:285–290, 1990

Simeon JG, Ferguson HB, Knott V, et al: Clinical, cognitive, and neurophysiological effects of alprazolam in children and adolescents with overanxious and avoidant disorders. J Am Acad Child Adolesc Psychiatry 31:29–33, 1992

Simeon JG, Knott VJ, Dubois C, et al: Buspirone therapy of mixed anxiety disorders in childhood and adolescence: a pilot study. Journal of Child and Adolescent Psychopharmacology 4:159–170, 1994

Simeon JG, Carrey NJ, Wiggins DM, et al: Risperidone effects in treatment-resistant adolescents: preliminary case reports. Journal of Child and Adolescent Psychopharmacology 5:69–79, 1995

Singer HS, Brown J, Quaskey S, et al: The treatment of attention deficit hyperactivity disorder in Tourette's syndrome: a double-blind placebo-controlled study with clonidine and desipramine. Pediatrics 95:74–81, 1995

Sovner R: Thioridazine withdrawal-induced behavioral deterioration treated with clonidine: two case reports. Ment Retard 33:221–225, 1995

Speltz ML, Varley CK, Peterson K, et al: Effects of dextroamphetamine and contingency management on a preschooler with ADHD and oppositional defiant disorder. J Am Acad Child Adolesc Psychiatry 27:175–178, 1987

Spencer EK, Alpert M, Pouget ER: Scales for the assessment of neuroleptic response in schizophrenic children: specific measures derived from the CPRS. Psychopharmacol Bull 30:199–202, 1994

Spencer T, Biederman J, Steingard R, et al: Bupropion exacerbates tics in children with attention-deficit hyperactivity disorder and Tourette's syndrome. J Am Acad Child Adolesc Psychiatry 32:211–214, 1993

Steingard R, Khan A, Gonzalez A, et al: Neuroleptic malignant syndrome: review of experience with children and adolescents. Journal of Child and Adolescent Psychopharmacology 2:183–198, 1992

Steingard RJ, Goldberg M, Lee D, et al: Adjunctive clonazepam treatment of tic symptoms in children with comorbid tic disorders and ADHD. J Am Acad Child Adolesc Psychiatry 33:394–399, 1994

Strayhorn JM, Rapp N, Donina W, et al: Randomized trial of methylphenidate for an autistic child. J Am Acad Child Adolesc Psychiatry 27:244–247, 1988

Strober M, Morrell W, Lampert C, et al: A family study of bipolar I illness in adolescence: early onset of symptoms linked to increased familial loading and lithium resistance. J Affect Disord 15:255–268, 1988

Strober M, Morrell W, Lampert C, et al: Relapse following discontinuation of lithium maintenance therapy in adolescents with bipolar I illness: a naturalistic study. Am J Psychiatry 147:457–461, 1990

Strober M, Freeman R, Rigali J, et al: The pharmacotherapy of depressive illness in adolescence, II: effects of lithium augmentation in nonresponders to imipramine. J Am Acad Child Adolesc Psychiatry 31:16–20, 1992

Sturmey P, Reed J, Corbett J: Psychometric assessment of psychiatric disorders in people with learning difficulties (mental handicap): a review of measures. Psychol Med 21:143–155, 1991

Tannock R, Ickowicz A, Schachar R: Differential effects of methylphenidate on working memory in ADHD children with and without comorbid anxiety. J Am Acad Child Adolesc Psychiatry 7:886–896, 1995

Teicher MH, Glod CA: Neuroleptic drugs: indications and guidelines for their rational use in children and adolescents. Journal of Child and Adolescent Psychopharmacology 1:33–56, 1990

Terr LC: Childhood psychic trauma, in Basic Handbook of Child Psychiatry, Vol V. Edited by Call JD, Cohen RL, Harrison SI, et al. New York, Basic Books, 1987, pp 262–272

Thompson S, Rey JM: Functional enuresis: is desmopressin the answer? J Am Acad Child Adolesc Psychiatry 34:266–271, 1995

Thurston LP: Comparison of the effects of parent training and of Ritalin in treating hyperactive children, in Strategic Interventions for Hyperactive Children. Edited by Gittelman M. New York, ME Sharpe, 1981, pp 178–185

Towbin KE, Dykens EM, Pugliese RG: Clozapine for early developmental delays with childhood-onset schizophrenia: protocol and 15-month outcome. J Am Acad Child Adolesc Psychiatry 33:651–657, 1994

Trimble MR: Anticonvulsants in children and adolescents. Journal of Child and Adolescent Psychopharmacology 1:107–124, 1990

Ullmann RK, Sleator EK: Attention deficit disorder children with or without hyperactivity: which behaviors are helped by stimulants? Clin Pediatr (Phila) 24:547–551, 1985

Ullmann RK, Sleator EK: Responders, nonresponders, and placebo responders among children with attention deficit disorder. Clin Pediatr (Phila) 25:594–599, 1986

Ullmann RK, Sleator EK, Sprague RL: A change of mind: the Conners abbreviated rating scales reconsidered. J Abnorm Child Psychol 13:553–565, 1985

Urman R, Ickowicz A, Fulford P, et al: An exaggerated cardiovascular response to methylphenidate in ADHD children with anxiety. Journal of Child and Adolescent Psychopharmacology 2:29–37, 1995

Valleni-Basile LA, Garrison CZ, Jackson KL, et al: Frequency of obsessive-compulsive disorder in a community sample of young adolescents. J Am Acad Child Adolesc Psychiatry 33:782–791, 1994

Valleni-Basile LA, Garrison CZ, Waller JL, et al: Incidence of obsessive-compulsive disorder in a community sample of young adolescents. J Am Acad Child Adolesc Psychiatry 35:898–906, 1996

Van der Linden C, Bruggeman R, Van Woerkom T: Serotonin-dopamine antagonist and Gilles de La Tourette's syndrome: an open pilot dose-titration study with risperidone. Mov Disord 9:687–688, 1994

Varley CK, Trupin EW: Double-blind assessment of stimulant medication for attention deficit disorder: a model for clinical application. Am J Orthopsychiatry 53:542–547, 1983

Venkataraman S, Naylor MW, King CA: Mania associated with fluoxetine treatment in adolescents. J Am Acad Child Adolesc Psychiatry 31:276–281, 1992

Vitiello B, Behar D, Hunt J, et al: Subtyping aggression in children and adolescents. J Neuropsychiatry Clin Neurosci 2:189–192, 1990

Walkup JT, Rosenberg LA, Brown J, et al: The validity of instruments measuring tic severity in Tourette's syndrome. J Am Acad Child Adolesc Psychiatry 31:472–477, 1992

Weller E, Weller R: Neuroendocrine changes in affectively ill children and adolescents. Neurol Clin 6:41–54, 1988

Weller E, Weller R: Depressive disorders in children and adolescents, in Psychiatric Disorders in Children and Adolescents. Edited by Garfinkle BD, Carlson G, Weller EB. Philadelphia, PA, WB Saunders, 1990, pp 3–20

Weller E, Weller R, Fristad M, et al: The dexamethasone suppression test in hospitalized prepubertal depressed children. Am J Psychiatry 141:290–291, 1984

Weller E, Weller R, Fristad M: Lithium dosage guide for prepubertal children: a preliminary report. J Am Acad Child Psychiatry 25:92–95, 1986a

Weller E, Weller R, Fristad M, et al: Dexamethasone suppression test and clinical outcome in prepubertal depressed children. Am J Psychiatry 143:1469–1470, 1986b

Weller R, Weller E, Tucker S, et al: Mania in prepubertal children: has it been underdiagnosed? J Affect Disord 11:151–154, 1986c

Weller E, Weller R, Fristad M, et al: Saliva monitoring in prepubertal children. J Am Acad Child Adolesc Psychiatry 26:173–175, 1987

Wender PH: Attention-Deficit Hyperactivity Disorder in Adults. New York, Oxford University Press, 1995

Werry JS, Aman MG: Practitioner's Guide to Psychoactive Drugs for Children and Adolescents. New York, Plenum Medical Book, 1993

West SA, Keck PE, McElroy SL, et al: Open trial of valproate in the treatment of adolescent mania. Journal of Child and Adolescent Psychopharmacology 4:263–267, 1994

Whalen CK, Henker B: Therapies for hyperactive children: comparisons, combinations, and compromises. J Consult Clin Psychol 59:126–137, 1991

Whalen CK, Henker B, Castro J, et al: Peer perceptions of hyperactivity and medication effects. Child Dev 58:816–828, 1987

Whalen CK, Henker B, Buhrmester D, et al: Does stimulant medication improve the peer status of hyperactive children? J Consult Clin Psychol 57:545–549, 1989

Whitaker A, Rao U: Neuroleptics in pediatric psychiatry. Psychiatr Clin North Am 15:243–276, 1992

Wiener JM (ed): Diagnosis and Psychopharmacology of Childhood and Adolescent Disorders, 2nd Edition. New York, Wiley, 1996

Wilens TE, Biederman J, Geist DE, et al: Nortriptyline in the treatment of ADHD: a chart review of 58 cases. J Am Acad Child Adolesc Psychiatry 32:343–349, 1993

Wilens TE, Biederman J, Baldessarini RJ, et al: Cardiovascular effects of therapeutic doses of tricyclic antidepressants in children and adolescents. J Am Acad Child Adolesc Psychiatry 35:1491–1501, 1996

Willemsen-Swinkels SH, Buitelaar JK, Nijhof GJ, et al: Failure of naltrexone hydrochloride to reduce self-injurious and autistic behavior in mentally retarded adults. Arch Gen Psychiatry 52:766–773, 1995a

Willemsen-Swinkels SH, Buitelaar JK, Weijnen FG, et al: Placebo-controlled acute dosage naltrexone study in young autistic children. Psychiatry Res 16:203–215, 1995b

Williams DT, Mehl R, Yudofsky S, et al: The effect of propranolol on uncontrolled rage outbursts in children and adolescents with organic brain dysfunction. J Am Acad Child Psychiatry 21:129–135, 1982

Winsberg BG, Perel JM, Hurwic MJ, et al: Imipramine protein binding and pharmacokinetics in children, in The Phenothiazines and Structurally Related Drugs. Edited by Forrest IS, Carr CJ, Usdin E. New York, Raven, 1974, pp 425–431

Winsberg BG, Goldstein S, Yepes LE, et al: Imipramine and electrocardiographic abnormalities in hyperactive children. Am J Psychiatry 132:542–545, 1975

Wolf DV, Wagner KD: Tardive dyskinesia, tardive dystonia, and tardive Tourette's syndrome in children and adolescents. Journal of Child and Adolescent Psychopharmacology 3:175–198, 1993

Youngerman J, Canino IA: Lithium carbonate use in children and adolescents. Arch Gen Psychiatry 35:216–224, 1978

Zahn TP, Rapoport, JL, Thompson CL: Autonomic and behavioral effects of dextroamphetamine and placebo in normal and hyperactive prepubertal boys. J Abnorm Child Psychol 8:145–160, 1980

Zametkin A, Yamada EM: Monitoring and measuring drug effects, I: physical effects, in Practitioner's Guide to Psychoactive Drugs for Children and Adolescents. Edited by Werry JS, Aman MG. New York, Plenum Medical Book, 1993, pp 75–97

Zametkin AJ, Linnoila M, Karoum F, et al: Pemoline and urinary excretion of catecholamines and indoleamines in children with attention deficit disorder. Am J Psychiatry 143:359–362, 1986

Zohar AH, Ratzoni G, Paul DL, et al: An epidemiological study of obsessive compulsive disorder and related disorders in Israeli adolescents. J Am Acad Child Adolesc Psychiatry 31:1057–1061, 1992

FORTY

Treatment of Substance-Related Disorders

James W. Cornish, M.D.,
Laura F. McNicholas, M.D., Ph.D., and
Charles P. O'Brien, M.D., Ph.D.

ALCOHOL

Alcoholism is the most prevalent substance use disorder in the United States, affecting approximately 14% of the population at some point in their lifetime (Robins et al. 1984). The magnitude of this problem is huge, involving the loss of 65,000 lives and costs of $136 billion per year (National Institute of Alcoholism and Alcohol Abuse 1990). The natural history of excessive alcohol consumption is known. The amount and pattern of alcohol consumption and the harmful effects of drinking are associated in a predictable manner (Kranzler et al. 1990).

The principal forms of treatment for alcoholism have been self-help/support groups, such as Alcoholics Anonymous (see section, "Self-Help Groups," later in this chapter), or psychosocial treatments in inpatient or outpatient rehabilitation programs or sheltered living situations. Many 28-day treatment programs provide group and individual therapy for alcoholic rehabilitation. Unfortunately, psychosocial treatments for alcohol-dependent persons have had only limited success in reducing alcohol use (Holder et al. 1991). Although there is ample room for improvement over psychosocial treatment alone, only a few controlled clinical studies have been conducted to test the efficacy of pharmacotherapies in the rehabilitation of alcohol-dependent patients (Meyer 1989). Pharmacotherapy has been directed at specific indications that often occur during the course of treatment for alcoholism. Studies have been conducted involving alcohol detoxification treatments, alcohol sensitization agents, anticraving agents, and agents to diminish drinking by treating associated psychiatric disorders.

Alcohol Detoxification

Detoxification refers to the clearing of alcohol from the body and the readjustment of all systems to functioning in the absence of alcohol. The alcohol withdrawal syndrome at the mild end may include only headache and irritability, but about 5% of alcoholic patients have severe withdrawal symptoms (Schuckit 1991) manifested by tremulousness, tachycardia, perspiration, and even seizures (rum fits). The presence of malnutrition, electrolyte imbalance, or infection increases the possibility of cardiovascular collapse.

Significant progress has been made in establishing safe and effective medications for alcohol withdrawal. Pharmacotherapy with a benzodiazepine is the treatment of choice for the prevention and treatment of the signs and symptoms of alcohol withdrawal (Nutt et al. 1989). Many patients detoxify from alcohol without specific treatment or medications. However, it is difficult to determine accurately which patients require medication for alcohol withdrawal. Patients in good physical condition with uncomplicated, mild to moderate alcohol withdrawal symptoms can usually be treated as outpatients (Hayashida et al. 1989).

A typical regimen requires the patient to attend the clinic daily for 5–10 days to receive clinical evaluations, multiple vitamins, and benzodiazepine pharmacotherapy.

A typical medication dosing regimen involves giving enough benzodiazepine on the first day of treatment to relieve withdrawal symptoms; the dose should be adjusted if withdrawal symptoms increase or if the patient complains of excessive sedation. Over the next 5–7 days, the dose of benzodiazepine is tapered to zero. Most clinicians use longer-acting benzodiazepines such as clonazepam, chlordiazepoxide, or diazepam. The usual starting dose of medication on the first day is 25–50 mg of chlordiazepoxide or 10 mg of diazepam given every 6 hours (Schuckit 1991). The diagnosis of delirium tremens is given to patients who have marked confusion and severe agitation in addition to the usual alcohol withdrawal symptoms (Goodwin 1992).

It is important to remember that the risk of mortality is 5% in patients with severe alcohol withdrawal symptoms (Schuckit 1987). Patients who have medically complicated or severe alcoholic withdrawal must be treated in a hospital. Benzodiazepines will usually be sufficient to calm agitated patients; however, some patients may require intravenous barbiturates to control extreme agitation (Goodwin 1992).

Alcohol Sensitizing Agents

In 1951, disulfiram was the first medication approved by the U.S. Food and Drug Administration (FDA) for the treatment of alcohol dependence other than detoxification. Disulfiram inhibits a key enzyme, aldehyde dehydrogenase, involved in breakdown of ethyl alcohol. After drinking, the alcohol-disulfiram reaction produces excess blood levels of acetaldehyde, which is toxic in that it produces facial flushing, tachycardia, hypotension, nausea and vomiting, and physical discomfort. The usual maintenance dose of disulfiram is 250 mg/day.

There have been only a few randomized controlled trials, and these trials have had mixed results for drug efficacy (Peachy and Naranjo 1984). The most comprehensive trial was the Veterans Administration (VA) Cooperative Study of disulfiram treatment of alcoholism. This study was conducted with male veterans and found no differences between disulfiram, 250 mg/day and 1 mg/day (an ineffective dose), and placebo groups in total abstinence, time to first drink, employment, or social stability. Among patients who drank, those in the 250-mg disulfiram group reported significantly fewer drinking days (Fuller et al. 1986).

The main problem with disulfiram is that frequently patients stop taking it and relapse to drinking (Goodwin 1992). Disulfiram is most effective when it is used in a clinical setting that emphasizes abstinence and offers a mechanism to ensure that the medication is taken. Drug compliance may be successfully ensured by giving the medication at 3- to 4-day intervals in the physician's office, or at the treatment center, or by having a spouse or family member administer it.

Alcohol Anticraving Agents

According to Volpicelli et al. (1992), an ideal pharmacotherapy has few, if any, side effects; decreases patients' craving for alcohol so that they have less motivation to drink; and blocks the reinforcing effects of alcohol so that if they resume drinking, they experience neither pleasant nor unpleasant effects.

Several animal models have implicated the involvement of neurotransmitter systems, including endogenous opioid peptides, catecholamine, serotonin, dopamine, and γ-aminobutyric acid (GABA), in alcohol craving and consumption. The only pharmacological intervention that has thus far shown substantial promise involves blocking opioid receptors. Evidence from animal studies and some human research shows that alcohol increases endogenous opioid activity. Activation of opioid receptors, therefore, may be involved in the reinforcing properties of alcohol. Opioid antagonists, such as naloxone and naltrexone, that block opioid receptors have been found to decrease alcohol consumption in animal models (Altshuler et al. 1980; Myers et al. 1986; Volpicelli et al. 1986). Conversely, rats pretreated with small doses of an opioid agonist, such as morphine, show increased alcohol drinking (Hubbell et al. 1986), whereas higher doses reduce alcohol drinking. Rats bred for alcohol preference have not only high alcohol consumption but also high endogenous opioid activity, and naltrexone blocks alcohol drinking in these rodents in a dose-related fashion (Froehlich et al. 1990). Collectively, these findings suggest that alcohol consumption is reinforced by an interaction with the endogenous opioid system and that blocking opioid receptors with specific antagonists lessens behavioral reinforcement, which decreases drinking. This hypothesis also explains why higher doses of opioids, which are an external supply of opioid activity, can reduce drinking.

The first human study of the efficacy and safety of naltrexone in the treatment of alcoholism was a 12-week double-blind trial conducted by Volpicelli et al. (1992), in which 72 subjects were randomly assigned to receive either naltrexone 50 mg/day or placebo in addition to standard psychosocial treatment. The naltrexone group had lower rates of relapse, fewer drinking days, and reduced alcohol craving compared with the placebo group. The results indicated that half as many naltrexone-treated patients (23%) relapsed as those receiving placebo (54.3%).

The most striking effects were seen in those who sampled alcohol. Of the 20 placebo patients, 19 (95%) relapsed after they sampled alcohol, compared with only 8 of 16 (50%) of the naltrexone patients. In the other double-blind, placebo-controlled study, 97 alcohol-dependent subjects were randomized to receive either naltrexone or placebo and either coping skills/relapse prevention therapy or a supportive therapy (O'Malley et al. 1992). Compared with the placebo group, the naltrexone-treated patients drank on half as many days, drank one-third as much alcohol during occasions of drinking, and had less severe alcohol-related problems. As in the prior study, those randomly assigned to naltrexone had significantly fewer relapses during the 3-month treatment period, and this difference was still present at follow-up 6 months later. In a series of laboratory studies involving social drinkers, Swift and associates (1994) found that naltrexone altered human alcohol intoxication. They reported that following a standard dose of alcohol, subjects who were treated with naltrexone had less euphoria than did placebo-treated subjects. These studies supplement prior clinical studies and indicate that naltrexone may reduce the pleasurable aspects of drinking to some degree. In addition to studies on naltrexone, research has been done with the opiate antagonist nalmefene as a treatment for alcohol dependence. In a preliminary 12-week study, Mason and associates (1994) reported that nalmefene-treated subjects had a significantly better outcome than that of the placebo-treated subjects.

In 1995, some 44 years after disulfiram was approved, the FDA approved naltrexone, under the trade name ReVia, for the treatment of alcohol dependence. Other studies of naltrexone in alcoholism are under way and should help to clarify the role of naltrexone in this disorder. It will be important to determine which patients are most likely to be helped by this opioid antagonist and what is the optimal amount of psychosocial treatment. The evidence so far suggests that naltrexone is most likely to improve relapse rates when combined with a strong psychosocial rehabilitation program.

Another promising pharmacotherapy for alcohol dependence is acamprosate, whose chemical name is calcium acetyl homotaurinate. Structurally, acamprosate is similar to the amino acid taurine and is believed to act as a GABA receptor agonist. Acamprosate has been reported as a safe and effective treatment for alcoholism in several controlled studies. In 1985, Lhuintre et al. (1985) published the results of a double-blind study in which 85 subjects, described as severely alcoholic, were randomized to 3 months of treatment with either acamprosate or placebo. Seventy subjects completed the trial, and of these, 20 of

33 (60%) acamprosate-treated subjects and 12 of 37 (32%) placebo-treated subjects were abstinent during the study. Positive results were reported for two subsequent placebo-controlled trials (Lhuintre et al. 1990; Paille et al. 1995) in which the total number of abstinent days was lower for acamprosate-treated subjects compared with placebo-treated subjects. In 1996, the reports of two German double-blind, placebo-controlled studies were published. In the first trial, Sass et al. (1996) studied 272 subjects randomly assigned to a year of treatment with either acamprosate or placebo and evaluated for an additional 12 months following the discontinuation of study medication. Compared with placebo-treated subjects, the subjects who received acamprosate had a significantly lower dropout rate, a greater number of days before their first drink, and a greater number of days of total abstinence during the study.

The second study, which had a similar design, involved 455 subjects and was conducted by Whitworth and colleagues (1996). The results of this trial were that acamprosate was superior to placebo with respect to the number of dropouts, relapse rate, and total days of abstinence. Interestingly, 18% of the acamprosate-treated subjects compared with 7% of the placebo-treated subjects remained continuously abstinent a year after discontinuation of study medication. These impressive clinical results for acamprosate warrant further study of this potentially beneficial medication.

Less encouraging results have recently been reported for two drugs that target the serotonin system. Kranzler and colleagues (1995b) studied fluoxetine, a serotonin reuptake inhibitor, as a treatment for alcoholism. There were no differences in outcomes measures between the fluoxetine-treated and placebo-treated subjects. B. A. Johnson et al. (1996) studied ritanserin, a serotonin type 2 receptor antagonist, in a large multicenter trial. In this study, ritanserin showed no advantage over placebo as a pharmacotherapy for alcohol dependence.

Agents Used to Diminish Drinking by Treating Associated Psychiatric Disorders

Depressed alcoholic patients treated with lithium showed no difference compared with those treated with placebo in a multiple center VA study (Dorus et al. 1989). In a study in which desipramine was the pharmacotherapy for alcoholism, the results indicate a trend toward decreased drinking in both depressed and nondepressed subjects (Mason and Kocsis 1991).

McGrath et al. (1993) studied alcoholic patients (93% met DSM-III-R [American Psychiatric Association 1987]

al. 1995) and found to have no advantage over placebo treatment. Kampman et al. (1996) completed a trial for amantadine but were unable to replicate the positive findings of a prior study (Alterman et al. 1992).

Another approach has been based on animal studies that indicate that cocaine can produce kindling of seizure activity. *Kindling* is an electrical phenomenon that refers to the increase in seizure activity when a standard subthreshold stimulus is applied repeatedly to certain brain structures, especially the amygdaloid nucleus. Small doses of cocaine applied to the amygdala have also been shown to produce kindling, and thus the drug carbamazepine, which blocks kindling (Post 1988), might have a role in the treatment of cocaine dependence. Unfortunately, double-blind studies thus far have not shown any benefit from carbamazepine in preventing relapse to cocaine use (Cornish et al. 1995; Halikas et al. 1992; Kranzler et al. 1995a; Montoya et al. 1995).

The lack of success in identifying an effective medication for treating cocaine dependence has not dampened scientific enthusiasm or impeded further research. On the contrary, there is renewed interest in studying various methods of altering the physiological effects of cocaine. Some of the most exciting work involves schemes for either blocking the effects of cocaine or hastening the destruction of cocaine.

The first area of research is based on the fact that cocaine must attach to its binding site on the dopamine transporter in order to produce pharmacological effects. New work (Bagasra et al. 1992; Fox et al. 1996) focuses on making anticocaine antibodies for this specific cocaine-binding site with the hope of developing a cocaine vaccine.

The second area involves the catabolism of cocaine. The strategy is to accelerate the inactivation of cocaine by augmenting the natural cholinesterase activity (Hoffman et al. 1996; Schwartz and Johnson 1996). If successful, the resultant medication regimen would be crucial to the treatment of cocaine overdose (Gorelick 1997; Mattes et al. 1996) and would be a possible pharmacological adjunct to the psychosocial treatment for cocaine dependence.

Summary

No medication is clearly identified as an effective pharmacotherapeutic agent for cocaine-dependent persons. Desipramine, which has been studied in several double-blind studies, appears to be moderately effective at inducing abstinence. New research to develop a cocaine vaccine as well as to find methods of accelerating the catabolism of cocaine offer innovative approaches in the search for a medication treatment for cocaine dependence.

OPIOIDS

Pharmacotherapy of opioid dependence has a long history, in part, because "heroinism" was one of the first recognized drug problems in the United States and because therapeutically used congeners of the drug of abuse, heroin, were readily available. Later studies have shown only limited success with nonpharmacological treatment.

Detoxification From Opioid Dependence

The classical method of opioid detoxification was, and remains, short-term substitution therapy. The medication traditionally used has been methadone, at a sufficient dose to suppress signs and symptoms of heroin withdrawal abstinence; the methadone is then tapered over a period ranging from 1 week to 6 months. The idea behind a rapid (i.e., 1- to 2-week) detoxification regimen is to achieve total opioid abstinence quickly so that treatment can be continued in a drug-free setting. Detoxification can usually be accomplished in 4–7 days in an inpatient setting, whereas more time is often required in the outpatient setting to minimize patient discomfort. Most practitioners consider 21 days sufficient for short-term outpatient detoxification. However, many patients have very chaotic lives when presenting for treatment and require a period of stabilization before they can hope to maintain a drug-free lifestyle. As discussed below, the regulations for opioid treatment facilities require that patients be dependent on opioids for the majority of a year before they may be admitted to methadone maintenance. The 6-month stabilization/detoxification regimen allows these patients to work on the most acute personal and employment problems while they are stabilized on a relatively low dose (30–40 mg/day) of methadone and then are detoxified from methadone to continue treatment in a drug-free setting.

More recently, a partial agonist, buprenorphine, has been studied for efficacy in suppressing withdrawal abstinence signs and symptoms. In outpatient trials, Bickel et al. (1988) showed that buprenorphine is as effective as methadone in a 10-week double-blind trial (4 weeks on medication taper followed by 6 weeks of placebo). In an open trial, Kosten and Kleber (1988) compared three doses of buprenorphine and found that 4 mg, administered sublingually, was superior to 2 or 8 mg of buprenorphine in suppressing signs and symptoms of withdrawal abstinence, although illicit opiates were present in the urine of approximately equal numbers of patients in both 2- and 4-mg dose groups.

There has always been concern about substitution detoxification on the basis that the physician is prolonging the problem by prescribing an addictive medication, even with a tapering regimen. Many of the symptoms of opioid withdrawal abstinence (e.g., diaphoresis, hyperactivity, and irritability) appear to be mediated by overactivity in the sympathetic nervous system. This led Gold and his associates (1978, 1980) to attempt to depress this overactivity and thereby ameliorate the withdrawal abstinence syndrome by using adrenergic agents that have no abuse potential. Clonidine, an α-adrenergic agonist with inhibitory action primarily at the locus coeruleus, was effective in inpatient populations in decreasing the signs and symptoms of opioid withdrawal abstinence. Outpatient detoxification with clonidine has not been as successful as inpatient treatment. Inpatient studies reported an 80%–90% success rate, whereas outpatient studies have reported success rates as low as 31% in detoxifying patients from methadone and 36% in detoxifying patients from heroin. The problems identified in outpatient clonidine detoxification include 1) access to heroin and other opioids, 2) lethargy, 3) insomnia, 4) dizziness, and 5) oversedation. The last four adverse effects were noted in inpatient populations during detoxification with clonidine but were easily managed in the hospital setting.

Because the side effects of clonidine were unacceptable to many patients, other α-agonists have been investigated for use in detoxifying opioid-dependent patients. Lofexidine, guanabenz, and guanfacine have all been investigated, to varying degrees, as detoxification agents. The data thus far would indicate that all of these agents have fewer cardiovascular side effects than clonidine. In a double-blind, randomized trial comparing methadone, clonidine, and guanfacine in a rapid (12-day) inpatient detoxification program, methadone was significantly better in suppressing signs and symptoms of withdrawal abstinence than either of the α-agonists. The authors further concluded that guanfacine was more effective than clonidine in suppressing abstinence and had fewer cardiovascular side effects (San et al. 1990).

Because clonidine was much less successful in the outpatient setting than in the inpatient setting, various approaches, including the previously mentioned alternative α-agonists, were studied in efforts to improve the efficacy of clonidine. One of the major reasons clonidine was less successful in the outpatient setting was that heroin and other opioids were available to the patient. Naltrexone, a competitive opioid antagonist, was added to the clonidine regimen in efforts both to speed up the time course of withdrawal and to block the effect of any opioid used illicitly by the patient. As reported by Stine and Kosten (1992), Kosten showed that 82% of patients were successfully detoxified, as outpatients, in 4–5 days using a single daily dose regimen of clonidine and 12.5 mg of naltrexone. This significantly decreased the time necessary for detoxification. Furthermore, the patients reported few signs or symptoms of withdrawal except restlessness, insomnia, and muscle aches. This protocol not only allowed the patients to detoxify from opioids but also simultaneously began naltrexone maintenance in patients (see section, "Relapse Prevention," later in this chapter).

Loimer and colleagues have studied very rapid opioid detoxification. These methods have involved anesthetizing patients with either methohexital (Loimer et al. 1990) or midazolam (Loimer et al. 1991) and then using naltrexone to precipitate abstinence. These protocols successfully detoxified patients in 48 hours but required major medical intervention (intubation, mechanical ventilation, and intravenous fluids) and exposed the patient to the risks of general anesthesia. This very rapid detoxification procedure has gained acceptance in some areas in treating opioid-dependent patients. However, no follow-up studies of patients undergoing rapid detoxification, to determine the patients' drug use or adherence to outpatient therapy, have been done.

Two major problems with detoxification (either rapid or slow) have been identified over the years by clinicians and researchers working in this area. The first is that all regimens, regardless of the detoxification agent involved, must be individualized; this eliminates the possibility of standard protocols for opioid detoxification. The second problem is more serious in terms of patient management: opioid-abusing and -dependent patients in drug-free treatment have an extremely high relapse rate. Maddux and Desmond (1992) reported on six long-term (3 years or longer) follow-up studies of drug-free treatment of opiate abuse and dependence. Methadone was used for initial withdrawal, and one study used naltrexone to increase the chances of compliance with a drug-free program. Abstinence rates at follow-up in these studies ranged from 10% to 19%; the percentage of patients with unknown status at follow-up ranged from 10% to 32%. Because drug-free treatment of opioid users has such high relapse rates, other modalities of treatment have been developed.

Maintenance Treatment of Opioid Dependence

Methadone maintenance has been the mainstay of the pharmacotherapy of opioid dependence since its introduction by Dole and Nyswander (1965). Since the 1970s, levomethadyl acetate (LAAM), a long-acting congener of methadone, has been used experimentally for maintenance treatment. It was approved by the FDA for this purpose in 1993 and is now available for general use in opioid-dependence treatment programs. More recently, buprenorphine has been studied in clinical trials as a maintenance therapy in opioid-dependent patients; it has not yet received FDA approval but does show a great deal of promise as an alternative to methadone maintenance.

Methadone. As discussed earlier in this chapter, methadone has been used for both short- and long-term detoxification from opioids. Methadone maintenance, however, is designed to support patients with opioid dependence for months or years while the patient engages in counseling and other therapy to change his or her lifestyle. Since methadone was introduced, experience has accumulated in approximately 1.5 million person-years (Gerstein 1992), strongly showing methadone to be safe and effective. Further, this experience has shown that although patients on methadone maintenance show physiological signs of opioid tolerance, there are minimal side effects, and patients' general health and nutritional status improve.

This approach to the treatment of opioid dependence has been controversial since its beginning. Physicians and other treatment professionals who regard opioid dependence using a disease model have little or no problem treating patients with an active drug for long periods of time, especially in light of repeated treatment failures in the absence of active medication therapy. However, many people view methadone maintenance as simply substituting a legal drug for an illegal one and refuse to accept any outcome other than total abstinence from all drugs. These people point to long-term follow-up studies of methadone maintenance patients (see Maddux and Desmond 1992) that show that 5 years after discharge from the maintenance program, only 10%–20% of the patients are completely abstinent, which is defined as not being enrolled in methadone maintenance and not using illicit opioids. However, long-term follow-up studies of patients discharged from drug-free treatment programs show that only 10%–19% of opioid-dependent patients are abstinent at 3- or 5-year time points (see Maddux and Desmond 1992) using the same definition.

Despite these results of patients discharged from programs, studies of outcome measures other than total abstinence done on patients in maintenance treatment consistently show that these patients have marked improvement in various measures. Investigators have shown up to an 85% decrease in criminal behavior, measured by self-report or arrest records, in patients in treatment, whereas employment among maintenance patients ranges from 40% to 80%. Gerstein (1992) quoted a Swedish study published in 1984 showing the results over 5 years in 34 patients who applied for treatment to the only methadone clinic in Sweden at the time. The 34 patients were randomly assigned to either methadone maintenance or outpatient drug-free therapy; those patients in drug-free treatment could not apply for methadone for a minimum of 24 months after being accepted into the study. After 2 years, 71% of methadone patients were doing well, compared with 6% of patients admitted to drug-free treatment. After 5 years, 13 of 17 patients remained on methadone and were free of illicit drugs, whereas 4 of 17 patients had been discharged from treatment for continued drug use. Of the 17 drug-free treatment patients, 9 had subsequently been switched to methadone treatment, were free of illicit drug use, and were "socially productive." Of the remaining 8 patients, 5 were dead (allegedly from overdose), 2 were in prison, and 1 was drug-free.

Furthermore, although previous generations of drug abusers had hepatitis B, endocarditis, and other infections, in this age when intravenous drug use and concomitant sharing of needles and syringes place a patient at risk for human immunodeficiency virus (HIV) infection, the medical consequences of heroin dependence must be taken into account when determining appropriate therapy for a patient. These issues are currently being studied by a variety of methods, but the overall clinical impression of increased general health in methadone maintenance patients is very strong. Additionally, Metzger et al. (1993) have undertaken a study of HIV seroconversion rates in opioid-dependent subjects. In this study, 152 subjects were in methadone maintenance treatment, and 103 subjects were out of treatment. At baseline, 12% of the subjects were HIV positive (10% of in-treatment and 16% of out-of-treatment subjects); follow-up of HIV-negative subjects over 18 months showed conversion rates of 3.5% for in-treatment subjects and 22% for those remaining out of treatment. These data suggest that although transmission of HIV still occurs, opioid-abusing intravenous drug users in methadone maintenance programs have a significantly lower likelihood of becoming infected than do patients who are not in treatment.

Methadone maintenance programs are licensed and regulated by the FDA and the Drug Enforcement Agency (DEA). A program and its physician must be licensed for a methadone maintenance program in order to prescribe or dispense more than a 2-week supply of any opioid to a patient known or suspected to be dependent on opioids. Most clinics are ambulatory and open 6–7 days per week, requiring patients to come into the clinic daily to receive medication unless and until a patient has "earned" privileges (take-home medication) by compliance with the clinic rules and abstinence from illicit substances. For a person to be eligible for methadone maintenance, she or he must be at least 18 years old (or have consent of the legal guardian) and must be physiologically dependent on heroin or other opioids for at least 1 year. The treatment regulations define a 1-year history of addiction to mean that the patient was addicted to an opioid narcotic at some time at least 1 year before admission and was addicted, either continuously or episodically, for most of the year immediately before admission to the methadone maintenance program. A physician must document evidence of current physiological dependence on opioids before a patient can be admitted to the program; such evidence may be a precipitated abstinence syndrome in response to a naloxone challenge or, more commonly, signs and symptoms of opioid withdrawal, evidence of intravenous injections, or evidence of medical complications of intravenous injections. Exceptions to these requirements are patients who have recently been in penal or chronic care, previously treated patients, or pregnant patients; in these cases, patients need not show evidence of current physiological dependence, but the physician must justify their enrollment in methadone maintenance. A person younger than 18 years must have documented evidence of at least two attempts at short-term detoxification or drug-free treatment (the episodes must be separated by at least 1 week) and have the consent of his or her parent or legal guardian.

Each clinic sets its own rules within the guidelines set by state and federal agencies. Many clinics are open only 6 days a week, thus giving all patients at least one dose of take-home medication weekly; others are open 7 days a week. All clinics must obtain urine toxicologies on patients, but the frequency varies from two to three times per week to one time per month. Some clinics have set upper limits on the dose of methadone, such that no patient receives higher than a dose specified by clinic rules; some clinics have dose limits of 30 or 40 mg, others go as high as 80 mg, whereas still others have no predetermined dosage limit (although the FDA must give approval for any patient to receive more than 100 mg/day). All methadone maintenance clinics must provide counseling for patients, but the amount required is up to the clinic's discretion.

The variability in clinic practice is widespread and, as with the issue of limiting doses, sometimes mandated by state regulators who take a stand with the people advocating total abstinence. These practices continue despite studies showing that doses of at least 60 mg/day were associated with longer retention in treatment, decreased use of illicit drugs, and a lower incidence of HIV infection (Hartel et al. 1988, 1989). Among patients receiving at least 71 mg/day of methadone, no heroin use was detected,

whereas patients receiving doses of 46 mg/day of methadone or lower were five times more likely to use heroin than those receiving higher doses (Ball and Ross 1991). Further, McLellan et al. (1993) showed, in a comparison of three levels of treatment services in which all patients received at least 60 mg/day of methadone, "enhanced methadone services" patients (methadone plus counseling and on-site medical/psychiatric, employment, and family therapy) had fewer positive urine tests for illicit substances than did patients in the "standard services" (methadone plus counseling) group, or the "minimum services" (methadone alone). The standard services group did significantly better in treatment than did the minimum services group, and in fact, 69% of the minimum services group required transfer to a standard program 12 weeks into the study because of unremitting use of opioids or other illicit drugs.

Yet another issue that has engendered a great deal of controversy is the treatment of opioid-dependent pregnant women. Those who are philosophically opposed to methadone treatment would advocate that any woman using illicit opioids (heroin) or enrolled in methadone maintenance who became pregnant should be detoxified. It is currently estimated that up to 2%–3% of babies born each year have had intrauterine exposure to opioids. Because many women with substance abuse problems fear all organizations, including medical ones, they frequently have little or no prenatal care, exposing themselves and their children to the complications of unsupervised pregnancy in addition to the severe stressor of maternal addiction. The complications and treatment of maternal opioid addiction and the effects on the fetus and neonate have been discussed by Finnegan (1991) and Finnegan and Kandall (1992). For the purposes of this chapter, it should be noted that current evidence shows that pregnant women who wish to be detoxified from opioids (either heroin or methadone) should *not* be detoxified before the 14th week of gestation because of the potential risk of inducing abortion or after the 32nd week of gestation because of possible withdrawal-induced fetal stress (see Finnegan 1991). Most clinicians dealing with pregnant opioid-dependent patients advocate methadone maintenance at a dose of methadone that maintains homeostasis and eliminates opioid craving; this dose must be individualized for each patient and managed in concert with the obstetrician.

LAAM. LAAM is a long-acting opioid agonist recently approved for marketing as a treatment for opioid dependence. Clinical trials conducted in the 1970s showed LAAM to be as effective as methadone in keeping heroin users from using illicit opioids (Jaffe et al. 1970, 1972; Ling et al. 1976). There is currently extensive literature on the safety and efficacy of LAAM in the treatment of opioid dependence. The major difference between methadone and LAAM is the duration of action, which is based on the metabolism of the two drugs. Methadone is slowly metabolized to inactive metabolites; LAAM, on the other hand, is metabolized to two congeners, nor-LAAM and dinor-LAAM, both of which are more potent opioid agonists than LAAM itself. Further, the plasma half-life of methadone is about 35 hours (Gilman et al. 1990), whereas the half-lives for LAAM, nor-LAAM, and dinor-LAAM are estimated to be 47, 62, and 162 hours, respectively (Finkle et al. 1982). These prolonged half-lives of LAAM and its active metabolites allow for every-other-day dosing or three times a week dosing, without the problem of diverted take-home medication that is inherent in methadone maintenance programs that allow take-home medication. It is also crucial to remember that LAAM will not reach steady-state plasma levels for 2–3 weeks after the medication is started or the dose changed and that too rapid an escalation in LAAM dose may result in an unintentional overdose because of drug accumulation, whereas too slow an escalation may result in the patient having withdrawal symptoms and using illicit opioids.

LAAM has now been approved by the FDA and is available in clinics, regulated by the FDA and DEA, for the treatment of opioid dependence. In general, a patient who is eligible for methadone maintenance would also be eligible for LAAM maintenance; however, LAAM has not been studied in pregnant women. LAAM would obviously have advantages for the patient who does not wish to come to a clinic on a daily basis and who does not require the structure of daily clinic attendance.

Buprenorphine.   Buprenorphine is a partial agonist of μ-opioid type and is a clinically effective analgesic agent with an estimated potency of 25–40 times that of morphine (Cowan et al. 1977). Buprenorphine is currently approved only for use as an analgesic agent and not yet for treatment of opioid dependence. Human pharmacology studies have shown buprenorphine to be 25–30 times as potent as morphine in producing pupillary constriction, but buprenorphine was less effective in producing morphinelike subjective effects (Jasinski et al. 1978). Further, these studies showed that the physiological and subjective effects of morphine (15–120 mg) were significantly attenuated when morphine was administered 3 hours after buprenorphine in patients maintained on 8 mg/day of buprenorphine; the physiological and subjective effects of 30 mg of morphine were also tested at 29.5 hours after the last dose of chronically administered buprenorphine and

were again significantly attenuated. Studies in opiate-abusing patients have shown that buprenorphine can be administered sublingually (SL) rather than subcutaneously (SC), the route most commonly used for analgesic effect, with only a moderate difference in potency, 1.0 mg SC being equal to 1.5 mg SL (Jasinski et al. 1989). In early clinical trials with opioid-dependent patients, it was found that patients would tolerate the SL route and that the dose of buprenorphine could be rapidly escalated to effective doses without significant side effects or toxicity (R. E. Johnson et al. 1989) and that detoxification from heroin dependence using buprenorphine was as effective as methadone (Bickel et al. 1988) or clonidine (Kosten and Kleber 1988). R. E. Johnson et al. (1992) compared buprenorphine, 8 mg/day SL, and methadone, 20 mg/day or 60 mg/day, in a 25-week maintenance study and found that buprenorphine was as effective as 60 mg/day of methadone in reducing illicit opioid use and keeping patients in treatment. Both buprenorphine and methadone, 60 mg/day, were superior to methadone, 20 mg/day, in this study. Recently, a multicenter study comparing sublingual doses of 1 mg of buprenorphine with 8 mg of buprenorphine was completed; more than 700 patients were studied. Preliminary results show that the 8-mg dose was significantly better than the 1-mg dose on outcome measures of opiate-free urine tests and retention in treatment (W. Ling, personal communication, June 1997). Both detoxification and maintenance studies have shown that the abrupt discontinuation of buprenorphine in a blind fashion causes only very minor elevations in withdrawal scores on any withdrawal scale (Bickel et al. 1988; Fudala et al. 1990; Jasinski et al. 1978; R. E. Johnson et al. 1989; Kosten and Kleber 1988).

Because the issue of take-home medication is likely to arise in any opiate maintenance program and because methadone take-home medication is likely to be diverted, the option of every-other-day buprenorphine dosing was explored. After 19 heroin-dependent patients were stabilized on buprenorphine, 8 mg/day, for 2 weeks, 9 patients continued to receive buprenorphine daily while the other 10 patients, in a blind fashion, received alternate-day buprenorphine doses, 8 mg/dose, for 4 weeks. Patients reported some dysphoria on days on which they received placebos, and it was also noted that pupils were less constricted on placebo days in the patients on alternate-day therapy, but patients tolerated the 48-hour dosing interval without significant signs or symptoms of opiate withdrawal abstinence (Fudala et al. 1990). This leaves open the possibility of alternate-day medication in the treatment setting, much like dosing regimens utilizing LAAM, eliminating the need for take-home medication, but, unlike LAAM, buprenorphine can be administered on a daily basis until the patient "earns" days away from the clinic. Another alternative is currently being explored in clinical trials. The main concern with buprenorphine take-home medication would be diversion of the sublingual tablets, and particularly, diversion to the injection route. At the time of this writing, clinical trials of a buprenorphine/naloxone combination sublingual tablet are nearing completion in an effort to address the potential diversion issues.

Relapse Prevention

As has been noted earlier in this chapter, various methods of detoxifying patients from opioids have been developed, from substitution and rapidly tapering the dose of opioid to long-term methadone maintenance and a very gradual methadone taper. These methodologies were, by and large, unsuccessful in achieving permanent opioid abstinence in patients. It has long been thought that both conditioned reactivity to drug-associated cues (Wikler 1973) and protracted withdrawal symptoms (Martin and Jasinski 1969) contribute to the high rate of opioid relapse. The use of a blocking dose of a pure opioid antagonist would allow the patient to extinguish the conditioned responses to opioids by blocking the positive reinforcing effects of the illicit drugs. Naltrexone was shown to be orally effective in blocking the subjective effects of morphine for up to 24 hours (Martin et al. 1973). Patients using naltrexone maintenance for relapse prevention need to be carefully screened as they *must* be opioid-free at the start of naltrexone administration. Many practitioners administer a naloxone challenge, which must be negative, before starting naltrexone. Naltrexone is usually administered either daily (50 mg) or three times weekly (100 mg, 100 mg, and 150 mg). Although naltrexone is pharmacologically able to block the reinforcing effects of opioids, the patient must take the medication in order for it to be effective. Many opioid-addicted patients have very little motivation to remain abstinent. Fram et al. (1989) reported that of 300 inner-city patients offered naltrexone, only 15 (5%) agreed to take the medication, and 2 months later, only 3 patients were still taking naltrexone. However, patients with better identified motivation, among them groups of recovering professionals (e.g., physicians, attorneys) and federal probationers, who face loss of license to practice a profession or legal consequences, have significantly better success with naltrexone.

Summary

Thus, there are a variety of well-developed and well-studied treatments for opiate-dependent patients, including detoxification from opioids, maintenance therapy, and effective, if not well accepted, relapse prevention pharmacotherapies. However, even though the area of opioid dependence is probably the most widely studied of the areas of drug abuse, we can "cure" only a small percentage of patients seeking help. We must be content with assisting the rest of this patient population to improve their lives and the lives of their families while they continue to deal with the effects of ongoing opioid dependence.

SELF-HELP GROUPS

Self-help groups, such as Alcoholics Anonymous, Narcotics Anonymous, and Cocaine Anonymous among others, which are based on a 12-step method of recovery, can be a valuable source of support for the recovering patient. These groups are a fellowship of recovering people interested in helping themselves and others lead drug-free lives. The groups are very good for reminding people of the adverse consequences of relapse and of the benefits of maintaining abstinence. Many recovering people feel that it is easier and more relevant to hear about some aspects of recovery from another recovering person. Patients can attend meetings as frequently as necessary and can learn more effective management of leisure time. A sponsor, a person in the group with a prolonged time in a drug-free lifestyle, can provide a good role model for a person in recovery, in addition to providing support and encouragement. Self-help groups are also available to non-drug-abusing family members to help them understand the addictive process and how family member dynamics can affect the drug-abusing or recovering family member.

HALLUCINOGENS

The use and abuse of hallucinogens wax and wane much more than the use of some other drugs, such as alcohol and opioids. The major drugs of abuse that fall into this classification are cannabis and related compounds, lysergic acid diethylamide (LSD) and other indolealkylamines (psilocybin), and phencyclidine (PCP) and its congeners. Cannabis has a relatively constant rate of use, but its use alone almost never causes the user to seek medical attention. LSD (and related compounds) use has changed from the pattern set in the 1960s, when users lived together communally, and the lifestyle of the group frequently revolved around the psychedelic experience. Today LSD use occurs in isolated groups, polysubstance abusers, and adolescents and young adults who frequent "rave" clubs. Most users of

It is unclear what role smoking plays in psychopathology of these disorders. There is some information supporting smoking in these populations as a maladaptive coping strategy (Revell et al. 1985). Future research on smoking in these targeted populations may indicate the most efficient treatment approaches for patients who have both nicotine dependence and a psychiatric disorder.

Summary

Nicotine replacement combined with behavior modification therapy is very effective in relieving nicotine withdrawal symptoms and in initiating smoking cessation. The antidepressant bupropion was recently approved by the FDA as a treatment for smoking cessation. We must await the results of future research in order to establish methods of improving long-term nicotine abstinence.

REFERENCES

Alterman AI, Droba M, Antelo RE, et al: Amantadine may facilitate detoxification of cocaine addicts. Drug Alcohol Depend 31:19–29, 1992

Altshuler HL, Phillips PE, Feinhandler DA: Alteration of ethanol self-administration by naltrexone. Life Sci 26:679–688, 1980

American Psychiatric Association: Diagnostic and Statistical Manual of Mental Disorders, 3rd Edition, Revised. Washington, DC, American Psychiatric Association, 1987

American Psychiatric Association: Diagnostic and Statistical Manual of Mental Disorders, 4th Edition. Washington, DC, American Psychiatric Association, 1994

Arndt IO, Dorozynsky L, Woody GE, et al: Desipramine treatment of cocaine dependence in methadone-maintained patients. Arch Gen Psychiatry 49:888–893, 1992

Bagasra O, Forman LJ, Howeedy A, et al: A potential vaccine for cocaine abuse prophylaxis [see comments]. Immunopharmacology 23(3):173–179, 1992

Ball JC, Ross A: The Effectiveness of Methadone Maintenance Treatment. New York, Springer-Verlag, 1991

Beary MD, Christofides J, Fry D, et al: The benzodiazepines as substances of abuse. Practitioner 231:19–20, 1987

Benowitz NL: Nicotine replacement therapy: what has been accomplished—can we do better? Drugs 45:157–170, 1993

Benwell ME, Balfour DJ: The effects of nicotine administration on 5-HT uptake and biosynthesis in rat brain. Eur J Pharmacol 84:71–77, 1982

Bickel WE, Stitzer ML, Bigelow GE, et al: A clinical trial of buprenorphine: comparison with methadone in the detoxification of heroin addicts. Clin Pharmacol Ther 43:72–78, 1988

Burling TA, Ziff DC: Tobacco smoking: a comparison between alcohol and drug abuse in patients. Addict Behav 13:185–190, 1988

Cornish JW, Maany I, Fudala PJ, et al: Carbamazepine treatment for cocaine dependence. Drug Alcohol Depend 38:221–227, 1995

Covey LS, Glassman AH, Ststner F: Depression and depressive symptoms in smoking cessation. Compr Psychiatry 31:350–354, 1990

Cowan A, Lewis JW, Macfarlane IR: Agonist and antagonist properties of buprenorphine, a new antinociceptive agent. Br J Pharmacol 60:537–545, 1977

Crane M, Sereny G, Gordis E: Drug use among alcoholism detoxification patients: prevalence and impact on alcoholism treatment. Drug Alcohol Depend 22:33–36, 1988

Daughton DM, Heatley SA, Pendergast JJ, et al: Effect of transdermal nicotine delivery as an adjunct to low-intervention smoking cessation therapy. Arch Intern Med 151:749–752, 1991

Dole VP, Nyswander M: A medical treatment for diacetylmorphine (heroin) addiction: a clinical trial with methadone hydrochloride. JAMA 193:646–650, 1965

Dorus W, Ostrow DG, Anton R, et al: Lithium treatment of depressed and nondepressed alcoholics. JAMA 262:1646–1652, 1989

Edwards NB, Simmons RC, Rosenthal TL, et al: Doxepin in the treatment of nicotine withdrawal. Psychosomatics 29:203–206, 1988

Edwards NB, Murphy JK, Downs AD, et al: Doxepin as an adjunct to smoking cessation. Am J Psychiatry 146:373–376, 1989

Farebrother MJB, Pearce SJ, Turner P, et al: Propranolol and giving up smoking. British Journal of Diseases of the Chest 74:95–96, 1980

Ferry LH, Robbins AS, Scariati PD, et al: Enhancement of smoking cessation using the antidepressant bupropion hydrochloride. Abstract from the 65th Scientific Sessions of the American Heart Association, New Orleans, LA. Circulation 86 (suppl 1):671, 1992

Finkle BS, Jennison TA, Chinn DM, et al: Plasma and urine disposition of 1-alpha-acetylmethado and its principal metabolites in man. J Anal Toxicol 6:100–105, 1982

Finnegan LP: Treatment issues for opioid-dependent women during the perinatal period. J Psychoactive Drugs 23:191–201, 1991

Finnegan LP, Kandall SR: Maternal and neonatal effects of alcohol and drugs, in Substance Abuse: A Comprehensive Textbook. Edited by Lowinson JH, Ruiz P, Millman RB, et al. Baltimore, MD, Williams & Wilkins, 1992, pp 628–656

Fox BS, Kantak KM, Edwards MA, et al: Efficacy of a therapeutic cocaine vaccine in rodent models [see comments]. Nat Med 2(10):1129–1132, 1996

Fram DH, Marmo J, Holden R: Naltrexone treatment—the problem of patient acceptance. J Subst Abuse Treat 6:119–122, 1989

Franks P, Harp J, Bell B: Randomized controlled trial of clonidine for smoking cessation in a primary care setting. JAMA 262:3011–3013, 1989

Froehlich JC, Harts J, Lumeng L, et al: Naloxone attenuates voluntary ethanol intake in rats selectively bred for high ethanol preference. Pharmacol Biochem Behav 35: 385–390, 1990

Fudala PJ, Jaffe JH, Dax EM, et al: Use of buprenorphine in the treatment of opiate addiction, II: physiologic and behavioral effects of daily and alternate-day administration and abrupt withdrawal. Clin Pharmacol Ther 47:525–534, 1990

Fuller RK, Branchey L, Brightwell DR, et al: Disulfiram treatment of alcoholism: a Veterans Administration cooperative study. JAMA 256:1449–1455, 1986

Gawin FH, Kleber HD: Abstinence symptomatology and psychiatric diagnosis in cocaine abusers. Arch Gen Psychiatry 43:107–113, 1986

Gawin FH, Kleber HD, Byck R, et al: Desipramine facilitation of initial cocaine abstinence. Arch Gen Psychiatry 46:117–121, 1989

Gerstein DR: The effectiveness of drug treatment, in Addictive States, Vol 70. Edited by O'Brien CP, Jaffe JH. New York, Raven, 1992, pp 253–282

Gilman AG, Rall TW, Nies AS, et al (eds): Goodman and Gilman's The Pharmacological Basis of Therapeutics, 8th Edition. New York, Pergamon, 1990

Glassman AH: Cigarette smoking: implications for psychiatric illness. Am J Psychiatry 150:546–553, 1993

Glassman AH, Jackson WK, Walsh BT, et al: Cigarette craving, smoking withdrawal, and clonidine. Science 226:864–866, 1984

Glassman AH, Stetner F, Walsh Raizman PS, et al: Heavy smokers, smoking cessation, and clonidine: results of a double-blind, randomized trial. JAMA 259:2863–2866, 1988

Glassman AH, Helzer JE, Covey LS, et al: Smoking, smoking cessation, and major depression. JAMA 264:1546–1549, 1990

Goff DC, Henderson DC, Amico E: Cigarette smoking in schizophrenia: relationship to psychopathology and medication side effects. Am J Psychiatry 149:1189–1194, 1992

Gold MS, Redmond DE, Kleber HD: Clonidine blocks acute opiate withdrawal symptoms. Lancet 2:599–602, 1978

Gold MS, Pottach AC, Sweeney DR, et al: Opiate withdrawal using clonidine. JAMA 243:343–346, 1980

Goodwin DW: Alcohol: clinical aspects, in Substance Abuse—A Comprehensive Textbook. Edited by Lowinson JH, Ruiz P, Millman RB. Baltimore, MD, Williams & Wilkins, 1992, pp 144–151

Gorelick DA: Enhancing cocaine metabolism with butyrylcholinesterase as a treatment strategy. Drug Alcohol Depend 48:159–165, 1997

Grabowski J, Rhoades H, Elk R, et al: Fluoxetine is ineffective for treatment of cocaine dependence or concurrent opiate and cocaine dependence: two placebo controlled double-blind trials. J Clin Psychopharmacol 15:163–173, 1995

Gross J, Stitzer ML: Nicotine replacement: ten-week effects on tobacco withdrawal symptoms. Psychopharmacology 93:334–341, 1989

Halikas J, Crosby RD, Graves N: Double-blind carbamazepine enhancement in the treatment of cocaine abuse, in Abstracts: Annual Meeting of the American College of Neuropsychopharmacology, San Juan, Puerto Rico, 1992, p 231

Hall SM, Killen JD: Psychological and pharmacological approaches to smoking relapse prevention. NIDA Res Monogr 53:131–143, 1985

Hall SM, Tunstall C, Rugg D, et al: Nicotine gum and behavioral treatment in smoking cessation. J Consult Clin Psychol 53:256–258, 1985

Hartel D, Selwyn PA, Schoenbaum EE: Methadone maintenance and reduced risk of AIDS and AIDS-specific mortality in intravenous drug users, in Fourth International Conference on AIDS. Stockholm, Sweden, Abstract 8526, 1988

Hartel D, Schoenbaum EE, Selwyn PA: Temporal patterns of cocaine use and AIDS in intravenous drug users in methadone maintenance, in Fifth International Conference on AIDS. Montreal, Canada, Abstract, 1989

Hayashida M, Alterman AI, McLellan AT, et al: Comparative effectiveness and costs of inpatient and outpatient detoxification of patients with mild-to-moderate alcohol withdrawal syndrome. N Engl J Med 320:358–365, 1989

Hoffman RS, Morasco R, Goldfrank LR: Administration of purified human plasma cholinesterase protects against cocaine toxicity in mice. J Toxicol Clin Toxicol 34:259–266, 1996

Holder H, Longabaugh R, Miller W, et al: The cost effectiveness of treatment for alcoholism: a first approximation. J Stud Alcohol 52:517–540, 1991

Hubbell CL, Czirr SA, Hunter GA, et al: Consumption of ethanol solution is potentiated by morphine and attenuated by naloxone persistently across repeated daily administrations. Alcohol 3:39–54, 1986

Hughes JR, Hatsukami D: Signs and symptoms of tobacco withdrawal. Arch Gen Psychiatry 43:289–294, 1986

Jacobs MA, Spilken AA, Norman MM, et al: Interaction of personality and treatment conditions associated with success in a smoking control program. Psychosom Med 33:545–546, 1971

Jaffe JH, Kranzler M: Smoking as an addictive disorder. NIDA Res Monogr 23:4–23, 1979

Jaffe JH, Schuster CR, Smith BB, et al: Comparison of acetylmethadol and methadone in the treatment of long-term heroin users. JAMA 211:1834–1836, 1970

Jaffe JH, Senay EC, Schuster CR, et al: Methadyl acetate vs methadone: a double-blind study in heroin users. JAMA 222:437–442, 1972

Jasinski DR, Pevnick JS, Griffith JD: Human pharmacology and abuse potential of the analgesic buprenorphine. Arch Gen Psychiatry 35:501–516, 1978

Jasinski DR, Fudala PJ, Johnson RE: Sublingual versus subcutaneous buprenorphine in opiate abusers. Clin Pharmacol Ther 45:513–519, 1989

Johnson BA, Jasinski DR, Galloway GP, et al: Ritanserin in the treatment of alcohol dependence—a multi-center clinical trial. Ritanserin Study Group. Psychopharmacology (Berl) 128:206–215, 1996

Johnson RE, Cone EJ, Henningfield JE, et al: Use of buprenorphine in the treatment of opiate addiction, I: physiologic and behavioral effects during a rapid dose induction. Clin Pharmacol Ther 46:335–343, 1989

Johnson RE, Jaffe JH, Fudala PJ: A controlled trial of buprenorphine treatment for opioid dependence. JAMA 267:2750–2755, 1992

Kampman K, Volpicelli JR, Alterman A, et al: Amantadine in the early treatment of cocaine dependence: a double-blind, placebo-controlled trial. Drug Alcohol Depend 41:25–33, 1996

Killen JD, Maccoby N, Taylor CB: Nicotine gum and self-regulation training in smoking relapse prevention. Behav Res Ther 15:234–248, 1984

Kornetsky C, Porrino LJ: Brain mechanisms of drug-induced reinforcement, in Addictive States, Vol 70. Edited by O'Brien CP, Jaffe JH. New York, Raven, 1992, pp 59–78

Kosten TR, Kleber HD: Buprenorphine detoxification from opioid dependence: a pilot study. Life Sci 42:635–641, 1988

Kosten TR, Morgan CM, Falcione J, et al: Pharmacotherapy for cocaine-abusing methadone-maintained patients using amantadine or desipramine. Arch Gen Psychiatry 49:894–898, 1992

Kranzler HR, Babor TF, Laureman RJ: Problems associated with average alcohol consumption and frequency of intoxication in a medical population. Alcoholism Clin Exp Res 14:119–126, 1990

Kranzler HR, Bauer LO, Hersh D, et al: Carbamazepine treatment of cocaine dependence: a placebo-controlled trial. Drug Alcohol Depend 38:203–211, 1995a

Kranzler HR, Burleson JA, Korner P, et al: Placebo-controlled trial of fluoxetine as an adjunct to relapse prevention in alcoholics. Am J Psychiatry 152:391–397, 1995b

Leventhal H, Cleary P: The smoking problem: a review of the research and theory in behavioral risk modification. Psychol Bull 88:370–405, 1980

Lhuintre JP, Daoust M, Moore ND, et al: Ability of calcium bis acetyl homotaurine, a GABA agonist, to prevent relapse in weaned alcoholics. Lancet 1(8436):1014–1016, 1985

Lhuintre JP, Moore N, Tran G, et al: Acamprosate appears to decrease alcohol intake in weaned alcoholics. Alcohol Alcohol 25:613–622, 1990

Ling W, Charuvastra C, Kiam SC, et al: Methadyl acetate and methadone as maintenance treatments for heroin addicts. Arch Gen Psychiatry 33:709–720, 1976

Lipsedge MS, Cook CCH: Prescribing for drug addicts. Lancet 2:451–452, 1987

Loimer N, Schmid R, Lenz K, et al: Acute blocking of naloxone-precipitated opiate withdrawal symptoms by methohexitone. Br J Psychiatry 157:748–752, 1990

Loimer N, Lenz K, Schmid R, et al: Technique for greatly shortening the transition from methadone to naltrexone maintenance of patients addicted to opiates. Am J Psychiatry 148:933–935, 1991

Maddux JF, Desmond DP: Methadone maintenance and recovery from opioid dependence. Am J Drug Alcohol Abuse 18:63–74, 1992

Magura S, Goldsmith D, Casriel C, et al: The validity of methadone clients' self-reported drug use. Int J Addict 22:727–750, 1987

Margolin A, Kosten TR, Avants SK, et al: A multicenter trial of bupropion for cocaine dependence in methadone-maintained patients. Drug Alcohol Depend 40:125–131, 1995

Martin WR, Jasinski DR: Physical parameters of morphine dependence in man: tolerance, early abstinence, protracted abstinence. J Psychiatr Res 7:9–17, 1969

Martin WR, Jasinski D, Mansky P: Naltrexone, an antagonist for the treatment of heroin dependence. Arch Gen Psychiatry 28:784–791, 1973

Mason BJ, Kocsis JH: Desipramine treatment of alcoholism. Psychopharmacol Bull 27:155–161, 1991

Mason BJ, Ritvo EC, Morgan RO, et al: A double-blind, placebo-controlled pilot study to evaluate the efficacy and safety of oral nalmefene HCl for alcohol dependence. Alcohol Clin Exp Res 18:1162–1167, 1994

Matherson E, O'Shea B: Smoking and malignancy in schizophrenia. Br J Psychiatry 145:429–432, 1984

Mattes C, Bradley R, Slaughter E, et al: Cocaine and butyryl-cholinesterase (BChE): determination of enzymatic parameters. Life Sci 58:L257–L261, 1996

McGrath PJ, Nunes EV, Delivannides D, et al: Imipramine treatment of depressed alcoholics. Paper presented at the 33rd annual meeting of the New Clinical Drug Evaluation Unit Program (NCDEU), Boca Raton, FL, June 1993

McLellan AT, Arndt IO, Metzger DS, et al: The effects of psychosocial services on substance abuse treatment. JAMA 269:1953–1959, 1993

Metzger DS, Woody GE, McLellan AT, et al: Human immunodeficiency virus seroconversion among in- and out-of-treatment intravenous drug users: an 18-month prospective follow-up. J Acquir Immune Defic Syndr Hum Retrovirol 6:1049–1056, 1993

Meyer RE: Prospects for a rational pharmacotherapy of alcoholism. J Clin Psychiatry 50:403–412, 1989

Montoya ID, Levin FR, Fudala PJ, et al: Double-blind comparison of carbamazepine and placebo for treatment of cocaine dependence. Drug Alcohol Depend 38:213–219, 1995

Myers RD, Borg S, Mossberg R: Antagonism by naltrexone of voluntary alcohol selection in the chronically drinking macaque monkey. Alcohol 3:383–388, 1986

National Institute of Alcoholism and Alcohol Abuse: Seventh Special Report to the US Congress on Alcohol and Health. Rockville, MD, U.S. Department of Health and Human Services, 1990

Nutt D, Adinoff B, Linnoila M: Benzodiazepines in the treatment of alcoholism, in Recent Developments in Alcoholism, Treatment Research, Vol 7. Edited by Galanter M. New York, Plenum, 1989, pp 283–313

Ogborne AC, Kapur BM: Drug use among a sample of males admitted to an alcohol detoxification center. Alcohol Clin Exp Res 11:183–185, 1987

O'Malley SS, Jaffe AJ, Chang G, et al: Naltrexone and coping skills therapy for alcohol dependence. Arch Gen Psychiatry 49:881–887, 1992

Paille FM, Guelfi JD, Perkins AC, et al: Double-blind randomized multicentre trial of acamprosate in maintaining abstinence from alcohol. Alcohol Alcohol 30:239–247, 1995

Palmer KJ, Buckley MM, Faulds D: Transdermal nicotine: a review of its pharmacodynamic and pharmacokinetic properties and therapeutic efficacy as an aid to smoking cessation. Drugs 44:498–529, 1992

Peachy JE, Naranjo CA: The role of drugs in the treatment of alcoholism. Drugs 27:171–182, 1984

Post R: Time course of clinical effects of carbamazepine: implications for mechanisms of action. J Clin Psychiatry 49 (suppl 1):35–46, 1988

Regier DA, Myers JK, Kramer M, et al: The NIMH Epidemiologic Catchment Area Program: historical context, major objectives, and study population characteristics. Arch Gen Psychiatry 41:934–941, 1984

Revell AD, Warburton DM, Wesnes K: Smoking as a coping strategy. Addict Behav 10:209–224, 1985

Robins LN, Helzer JE, Weissman MM, et al: Lifetime prevalence of specific psychiatric disorders in three sites. Arch Gen Psychiatry 41:949–958, 1984

San L, Cami J, Peri JM, et al: Efficacy of clonidine, guanfacine and methadone in the rapid detoxification of heroin addicts: a controlled clinical trial. British Journal of Addictions 85:141–147, 1990

Sass H, Soyka M, Mann K, et al: Relapse prevention by acamprosate: results from a placebo-controlled study on alcohol dependence. Arch Gen Psychiatry 53:673–680, 1996

Schneider NG, Jarvik ME, Forsythe AB, et al: Nicotine gum in smoking cessation: a placebo controlled, double-blind trial. Addict Behav 8:253–261, 1983

Schuckit MA: Alcohol and alcoholism, in Harrison's Principles of Internal Medicine. Edited by Braunwald E, Isselbacher KJ, Petersdorf RG, et al. New York, McGraw-Hill, 1987, pp 2106–2111

Schuckit MA: Alcohol and alcoholism, in Harrison's Principles of Internal Medicine, Vol 2. Edited by Wilson JD, Braunwald E, Isselbacher KJ, et al. New York, McGraw-Hill, 1991, pp 2149–2151

Schwartz HJ, Johnson D: In vitro competitive inhibition of plasma cholinesterase by cocaine: normal and variant genotypes. J Toxicol Clin Toxicol 34:77–81, 1996

Soyka M, Lutz W, Kauert G, et al: Epileptic seizures and alcohol withdrawal: significance of additional use (and misuse) of drugs and electroencephalographic findings. Epilepsy 2:109–113, 1989

Stine SM, Kosten TR: Use of drug combinations in treatment of opioid withdrawal. J Clin Psychopharmacol 12:203–209, 1992

Stitzer ML: Nicotine-delivery products: demonstrated and desirable effects, in New Developments in Nicotine-Delivery Systems. Edited by Henningfield JE, Stitzer ML. Ossining, NY, Cortland Communications, 1991, pp 35–45

Substance Abuse and Mental Health Services Administration: Preliminary Estimates From the Drug Abuse Warning Network—Third Quarter 1992 Estimates of Drug-Related Emergency Room Episodes (Advance Report No 2). Washington, DC, U.S. Government Printing Office, 1993

Substance Abuse and Mental Health Services Administration: Preliminary Estimates From the 1994 National Household Survey on Drug Abuse (Advance Report No 3). Washington, DC, U.S. Government Printing Office, 1995

Sutherland G, Stapleton JA, Russell MAH, et al: Randomised controlled trial of nasal nicotine spray in smoking cessation. Lancet 340:324–329, 1992

Swift RM, Whelihan W, Kuznetsov O, et al: Naltrexone-induced alterations in human ethanol intoxication. Am J Psychiatry 151:1463–1467, 1994

Tonnesen P, Norrezaard J, Simonsen K, et al: A double-blind trial of a 16-hour transdermal nicotine patch in smoking cessation. N Engl J Med 325:311–315, 1991

Tonnesen P, Norregaard J, Mikkelson K, et al: A double-blind trial of a nicotine inhaler for smoking cessation. JAMA 269:1268–1271, 1993

U.S. Department of Health and Human Services: Reducing the health consequences of smoking: 25 years of progress: a report of the Surgeon General. Washington, DC, U.S. Government Printing Office, 1989

U.S. Department of Health and Human Services: The health benefits of smoking cessation: a report of the Surgeon General. Washington, DC, U.S. Government Printing Office, 1990

Volpicelli JR, Davis MA, Olgin JE: Naltrexone blocks the postshock increase of ethanol consumption. Life Sci 38:841–847, 1986

Volpicelli JR, Alterman AI, Hayashida MD, et al: Naltrexone in the treatment of alcohol dependence. Arch Gen Psychiatry 49:886–880, 1992

Whitworth AB, Fischer F, Lesch OM, et al: Comparison of acamprosate and placebo in long-term treatment of alcohol dependence [see comments]. Lancet 347(9013):1438–1442, 1996

Wikler A: Dynamics of drug dependence. Arch Gen Psychiatry 28:611–616, 1973

FORTY-ONE

Treatment of Eating Disorders

W. Stewart Agras, M.D.

In this chapter, the pharmacological treatment of two classic eating disorders—anorexia nervosa (AN) and bulimia nervosa (BN)—is considered, together with that of binge-eating disorder, which is included as a new entity in DSM-IV (American Psychiatric Association 1994). Of the three disorders, most is known about the pharmacological treatment of BN, because it is a relatively common problem that has been studied extensively during the past 15–20 years. Less is known about the pharmacological treatment of AN. Because it is a relatively uncommon disorder, thus militating against controlled research, it is difficult to attain an adequate sample size to evaluate treatment effects.

The treatment of binge-eating disorder has been formally studied only in the past several years. Hence, few studies are available, although it can be argued that much of what we know about the treatment of BN is applicable to binge-eating disorder. Because we know most about the treatment of BN, this disorder is considered first, followed by the closely related binge-eating disorder, and finally AN.

BULIMIA NERVOSA

BN is a relatively common disorder affecting some 1%–2% of young women (Fairburn and Beglin 1990). The disorder usually has an onset in late adolescence or early adult life, with a prodromal period characterized by dissatisfaction with body shape and a fear of becoming overweight, followed by marked dietary restriction. Sooner or later periods of dietary restriction are followed by episodes of binge eating experienced as a loss of control over dietary intake, often accompanied by the consumption of large amounts of food. This, in turn, further aggravates both the dissatisfaction with body shape and the fears of weight gain. Ultimately, the bulimic person discovers purging, usually in the form of self-induced vomiting, with or without laxative use, or (in rare cases) by chewing food and spitting it out.

The DSM-IV diagnosis of BN requires that at least an average of two episodes of binge eating per week for at least 3 months with compensatory behaviors occur. Purging, which should be directed toward the prevention of weight gain, includes self-induced vomiting, laxative misuse, diuretic misuse, enemas, fasting, and excessive exercise. The diagnosis also requires that the disorder does not occur exclusively during episodes of AN. DSM-IV distinguishes two forms of BN—namely, purging and nonpurging types, the latter characterized by the use of exercise or fasting rather than other types of compensatory behavior (American Psychiatric Association 1994). The implications of this classification for treatment are unknown. Medical complications of BN are relatively rare; the most frequent are potassium depletion and dental caries. Comorbid psychopathology includes major depression; various anxiety disorders, including generalized anxiety disorder, social phobia, and panic disorder; alcoholism; and personality disorders, particularly those in the Cluster B spectrum. It is now recognized that the natural history of the disorder is frequently one of chronicity (Keller et al. 1992), which emphasizes the importance of adequate and early treatment.

Binge Eating

The form and content of binge-eating episodes have been studied in two ways: 1) in the natural environment by self-monitoring and 2) in the laboratory. Despite reports by bulimic patients that their binges are typically very large, often greater than 5,000 kcal (Johnson et al. 1982), self-monitoring studies of patients with BN reported a different picture. In the first of these studies, binge-eating episodes averaged 1,459 calories (range 45–5,138 kcal) compared with 321 calories (range 10–1,652 kcal) in non-binge-eating episodes (Rosen et al. 1986). Sixty-five percent of binge episodes were within the range of non-binge episodes. This finding suggests that when loss of control is made an additional criterion for a binge, the quantity of food eaten during a binge varies greatly among and even within individuals. In addition, bulimic patients ate more desserts and snacks and fewer fruits and vegetables in their binge-eating episodes than in their non-binge-eating episodes. Subsequent self-monitoring studies essentially confirmed the findings of Rosen and colleagues (1986).

Laboratory studies have reported a somewhat different picture from that of self-monitoring studies. The average binge is larger than that found in the self-monitoring studies; caloric consumption varies from a mean of 3,031 kcal to 7,774 kcal across studies, with a range of 83–25,755 kcal for binge episodes (Hadigan et al. 1989; Mitchell and Laine 1985). These differences between laboratory and field studies may be partly a result of differences in sample selection, because many of the participants in laboratory studies were inpatients with more severe BN. Self-monitoring is also likely to underestimate the caloric content of binges because of deficiencies in recording. One interpretation of the differences between laboratory and field studies is that laboratory studies may overestimate caloric consumption during binge episodes, whereas field studies may underestimate such consumption.

Overall, both laboratory and field studies of the form and content of binge eating in patients with BN suggest the following:

- The average binge is larger than the average nonbinge episode.
- Caloric consumption during a binge varies considerably within and between individuals.
- Content (particularly when assessed as food types) may differ between binges and nonbinges.
- Less certainly, eating rate may be more rapid during binges than during nonbinge episodes.

Factors maintaining binge eating. Differentiating between factors that cause and those that maintain binge eating is important, because the latter may be more critical in the treatment of BN. Two factors—dietary restraint and transient negative moods—appear to be important in maintaining binge eating and subsequent purging. Chronic dietary restraint is often accompanied by long periods between meals (e.g., skipping breakfast and lunch), after which the bulimic person loses control over eating and begins to binge eat. This pattern of restraint is fueled by cognitive distortions regarding food intake and an exaggerated sense of the importance of body shape and weight. Laboratory studies report that a preload such as a milkshake may potentiate overeating in nonbulimic women with high dietary restraint as compared with women with low restraint (Polivy 1976). However, this phenomenon has been difficult to replicate in bulimic patients, even though some patients report that a snack will trigger a binge.

The effects of negative mood on binge eating have been suggested by the fact that bulimic patients report negative mood to be the most frequent trigger of binge eating (Bruce and Agras 1992). Laboratory studies have confirmed this observation: negative mood leads to loss of control over eating, provokes binge eating, and leads bulimic patients to classify their eating episodes as binges (Telch and Agras 1996). From a clinical perspective, patients with atypical depression often develop hyperphagia, which disappears with the resolution of the depressive episode. No systematic studies of the eating behavior of such patients have been published.

Etiology of Bulimia Nervosa

Relatively little is known about the etiology of BN. Studies suggest that the disorder is heritable and that familial aggregation is most likely explained in part by heritability and in part by familial psychological influences specific to the affected individual (Kendler et al. 1991). Various neurochemical hypotheses have been proposed; the most frequent is reduction in brain serotonin (5-hydroxytryptamine [5-HT]) synthesis. Recently, dietary restriction has been shown to lead to decreased plasma tryptophan levels, which would likely reduce 5-HT synthesis. It is possible that bulimic patients may be particularly sensitive to such changes and become locked in a vicious circle of neurochemical changes once they begin dieting, resulting in an effect on satiety. On the other hand, it must be remembered that food intake is controlled by several neurochemical systems, including norepinephrine and peptide YY, both of which potentiate eating; hence, it may be too early to implicate one particular system. In addition, nutritional state markedly affects these neurochemical systems, making the task of detailing the abnormalities in BN even more complicated.

Social factors are also implicated in BN. During the 1980s, the number of cases of BN seen in clinics around the world increased dramatically (Garner et al. 1985). This increase occurred concurrently with the portrayal of a thin body shape as the ideal for women, despite the fact that few women can meet this social demand (Brownell 1991). Such social pressure may have led more young women to diet, increasing the risk of binge eating and purging in the biologically susceptible individual. Patton et al. (1990), in a 1-year follow-up study of schoolgirls in London, found that dieting was associated with a relative risk eight times higher than that of nondieters for the development of an eating disorder. Moreover, dieters had a higher maximum weight at initial interview and reported a greater discrepancy between ideal and actual body weight than nondieters. This study confirmed that dieting after weight gain is a risk factor for the development of BN. However, even though the vast majority of female adolescents diet, only 2%–3% develop an eating disorder. This finding poses an interesting dilemma for public health policy. On the one hand, the prevalence of obesity is increasing, which suggests that dietary interventions are important, but on the other hand, a small proportion of women may respond to dieting by developing an eating disorder. Education about healthy eating habits would seem important, particularly in adolescents, in an effort to stop the development of highly restrictive dieting. Also, certain personality types (e.g., those in the Cluster B spectrum) may be more affected by societal pressures to maintain a thin body shape, perhaps explaining the comorbidity between BN and Cluster B personality disorder.

Psychopharmacological Treatment of Bulimia Nervosa

The first controlled pharmacological study of binge eaters (a group of patients with BN and binge-eating disorder because purging was not required for entry into the study) compared phenytoin with placebo based on an earlier observation that bulimic patients may have abnormal electroencephalogram (EEG) findings (Wermuth et al. 1977). In this relatively brief crossover study, no evidence was found that phenytoin was effective in reducing binge eating, and no relation was found between EEG abnormalities and reduction in binge eating. Subsequent studies have focused on the use of antidepressants.

Antidepressant treatment. The use of antidepressants in the treatment of BN was sparked by the observation that depression is often a comorbid feature of the disorder (Pope and Hudson 1982). Disturbances of eating frequently accompany depression, suggesting a link between the two disorders. In 1982, two groups of researchers conducted small-scale uncontrolled studies indicating that both monoamine oxidase inhibitors and tricyclic antidepressants reduced binge eating and purging (Pope and Hudson 1982; Walsh et al. 1982). These observations were followed by a series of double-blind, placebo-controlled studies confirming the utility of antidepressants in treating BN, at least in the short term. A wide range of antidepressant drugs have been found effective, including imipramine (Agras et al. 1987; Mitchell et al. 1990; Pope et al. 1983), desipramine (Agras et al. 1991; Barlow et al. 1988; Blouin et al. 1989; Hughes et al. 1986), phenelzine (Walsh et al. 1984, 1988), bromofarin (Kennedy et al. 1993), trazodone (Pope et al. 1989), bupropion (Horne et al. 1988), and fluoxetine (Fluoxetine Bulimia Nervosa Collaborative Study Group 1992). In these studies, the rate of decrease in binge eating and purging ranged from 30% to 91% (median 69%). Complete recovery from binge eating and purging ranged from 10% to 60% (median 32%), and the dropout rate from the medication groups ranged from 0% to 48% (median 23%). In other words, of 100 patients with BN, about 77 will continue taking medication, and 25 will be in remission at the end of treatment with a single antidepressant.

Antidepressants are prescribed for BN in the same dosage used for treating depression, with the exception of fluoxetine, because a dosage of 60 mg/day was found to be more effective than 20 mg/day in reducing binge eating and purging in a placebo-controlled trial involving 387 bulimic women (Fluoxetine Bulimia Nervosa Collaborative Study Group 1992). One problem with medication given at times other than bedtime is that a significant amount of medication may be purged through subsequent vomiting. Side effects and reasons for dropout from the various medications were similar to those observed in the treatment of depression, with the exception of bupropion, for which a higher than expected proportion of patients with BN had a grand mal seizure (Horne et al. 1988). The authors concluded that bupropion should not be used in patients with BN until the reason for the high proportion of seizures in these patients was established.

In light of the widespread publicity regarding suicidality and fluoxetine, it is reassuring that a large-scale study of the use of fluoxetine in BN found no differences in suicidal thoughts or actions between the subjects taking active drug and those taking placebo (Wheadon et al. 1992).

Only two antidepressants have been found to be no more effective than placebo: mianserin (Sabine et al. 1983) and amitriptyline (Mitchell and Groat 1984). In the first of these studies, the dosage may have been too low for maximal efficacy. In the second study, a simple form of behavior therapy that was used in both groups may have masked the differences between placebo and medication because both groups had good and equivalent improvement.

Overall, most antidepressants appear to be effective in the short-term treatment of BN, but the effects are limited, with about one-quarter to one-third of patients achieving remission on average. Less is known about the long-term effectiveness of antidepressants. In one uncontrolled study (Pope et al. 1985) in which a variety of antidepressants were used over the course of a 2-year follow-up, 50% of patients achieved and maintained remission from binge eating and purging. The only controlled longer-term follow-up studies have been plagued by sample size problems, with relatively few participants' symptoms meeting criteria for entry into the follow-up phase of treatment (Pyle et al. 1990; Walsh et al. 1991). Even with continued medication treatment, about one-third of patients in these studies relapsed. Little evidence indicated that continued treatment with a single antidepressant was more effective than the placebo condition. This outcome raises the question of whether treatment with a different antidepressant for patients who do not respond initially (or who relapse) would be more effective. One open-label study suggested that about half of such patients will respond to a different antidepressant, with complete remission of symptoms (Mitchell et al. 1989). This would raise the remission rate for the hypothetical cohort of 100 patients to 50. Hence, sequential trials of different antidepressants would seem useful in the treatment of BN.

To date, only one study has compared different lengths of antidepressant treatment, in this case with desipramine. Patients with BN treated for 16 weeks relapsed to pretreatment levels of binge eating when medication was withdrawn. On the other hand, those treated for 24 weeks maintained remission after withdrawal and at 1-year follow-up (Agras et al. 1991, 1994a). This study suggests that patients responding to antidepressant treatment should be given a minimum trial of 6 months on medication.

Finally, two studies bear on subpopulations of bulimic patients. In a placebo-controlled study of 30 women with BN treated with 60 mg of fluoxetine or placebo, no relation was found between a history of sexual abuse and response of binge eating to medication (McCarthy et al. 1994). In the second study of 24 bulimic patients with comorbid atypical depression, Rothschild et al. (1994) found that phenelzine was superior to both imipramine and placebo in reducing both binge eating and depressive symptoms.

Combined treatment. Cognitive-behavior therapy for BN was developed in parallel with the use of antidepressants, and numerous controlled studies suggest that such treatment is effective (Fairburn et al. 1992). Cognitive-behavior therapy has four distinct phases. First, the extent of the problem is examined by careful history taking and the use of self-monitoring of food intake, binge eating, and purging. Second, dietary intake is slowly normalized by shaping at least three adequate meals each day. This diet shortens the long intervals between eating episodes that are typical of patients with bulimia and lessens dietary restraint; thus, the probability of binge eating is reduced. Third, distorted cognitions regarding caloric intake and body shape and weight are corrected. Finally, relapse prevention procedures (e.g., coping with high-risk situations) are practiced. Treatment usually extends over a 6-month period, averaging about 20 sessions.

Cognitive-behavior therapy in either individual or group format has been shown to be more effective in reducing binge eating and/or purging than placebo (Mitchell et al. 1990), supportive psychotherapy plus self-monitoring of eating behavior (Agras et al. 1989), stress management (Laessle et al. 1991), behavior therapy (Fairburn et al. 1993), and psychodynamic forms of psychotherapy (Garner et al. 1993; Walsh et al. 1997). For the most part, cognitive-behavior therapy reduces both measures of general psychopathology and measures of eating-specific psychopathology (e.g., dietary restraint, concerns about shape and weight) more effectively than the comparison conditions noted above. Hence, cognitive-behavior therapy that has been documented in treatment manuals appears to be more effective than credible and active control conditions. Note, however, that there has been some variability in the components of treatment used under the rubric of cognitive-behavior therapy. Moreover, it appears that some forms of psychotherapy may be as effective as cognitive-behavior therapy. For example, Fairburn et al. (1993) found that interpersonal therapy adapted to the treatment of BN was as effective as cognitive-behavior therapy. This study is particularly convincing because elements of overlap between the two treatment conditions were carefully controlled for. Further research comparing interpersonal therapy and cognitive-behavior therapy is under way.

The existence of two different and effective treatments—antidepressant medications and cognitive-behavior therapy—naturally leads to the question of whether the combination of such treatments would be more effective than either treatment alone.

The first study of this question used a randomized 2 × 2 design with four experimental groups: 1) imipramine combined with group psychosocial treatment, 2) imipramine with no psychosocial treatment, 3) placebo combined with group psychosocial treatment, and 4) placebo with no psychosocial treatment (Mitchell et al. 1990). The treatment phase was preceded by a single-blind placebo washout phase. One hundred and seventy-one women with BN entered the treatment phase, which lasted for 10 weeks. The psychosocial treatment was an intensive group variant of cognitive-behavior therapy, with 5 daily sessions in the first week and 22 treatment sessions overall. The mean daily dose of imipramine was 217 mg for the psychosocial treatment group and 266 mg for the group receiving medication alone. As might be expected, the dropout rate was significantly higher for those in the medication groups (34%) compared with those taking placebo (15%). The results for reductions in binge eating and purging were quite straightforward. Imipramine was found to be superior to placebo, which confirmed previous study results. However, cognitive-behavioral treatment, with a remission rate of 51%, was superior to imipramine, with a remission rate of 16%, and combining the two treatments did not result in any additional advantage in reducing binge eating and purging. The combined treatment was, however, significantly superior to cognitive-behavioral treatment in reducing depression.

In the second study (Agras et al. 1991, 1994b), 71 participants were randomly allocated to one of three groups: 1) desipramine (mean dose 168 mg), 2) cognitive-behavioral treatment, and 3) combined treatment. In half of the desipramine participants, medication was withdrawn at 16 weeks, and in the remaining half, desipramine was discontinued at 24 weeks. Cognitive-behavioral treatment lasted for 24 weeks. This study examined longer-lasting treatments than did the 1990 study by Mitchell and colleagues. However, the results were comparable. Eighteen percent of participants stopped taking desipramine before medication was withdrawn compared with 4.3% of subjects receiving cognitive-behavior therapy. Cognitive-behavioral treatment, with a 48% remission rate, was significantly superior to desipramine, with a 33% remission rate, in reducing the frequency of binge eating and purging, and the combined treatment was no more effective than cognitive-behavioral treatment alone. At 1-year follow-up of 61 of the original 71 patients, 77% of the combined 24-week medication and cognitive-behavior therapy group were abstinent compared with 54% of those receiving cognitive-behavior therapy alone (Agras et al. 1994b); this difference was not statistically significant. The combina-

tion of medication and cognitive-behavior therapy was superior to cognitive-behavior therapy alone in reducing dietary preoccupation, hunger, and disinhibited eating, pointing to some degree of added effectiveness for the combined treatment group. However, the group receiving desipramine alone for 24 weeks was the most cost-effective in terms of the cost of treatment per recovered patient at 1-year follow-up (Koran et al. 1995).

A more recent study involved 120 women with BN and used a more sophisticated medication regimen consisting of desipramine followed by fluoxetine if the first medication was either ineffective or poorly tolerated (Walsh et al. 1997). It is important to note that the two-medication combination was used by two-thirds of the patients assigned to active medication, which suggests that a two-medication combination is an experimental design closer to clinical reality than a single medication is. This study used a five-cell design: cognitive-behavior therapy combined with placebo or active medication, psychodynamically oriented therapy combined with placebo or active medication, and medication alone. Cognitive-behavior therapy (plus placebo) was more effective than psychodynamic therapy (plus placebo) in reducing both binge eating and purging. The average dose of desipramine was 188 mg/day and of fluoxetine was 55 mg/day. Of patients receiving medication, 43% dropped out of the study compared with 32% of those receiving psychotherapy, which is a nonsignificant difference. Patients receiving active medication (in combination with psychological treatments) reduced binge eating significantly more than those receiving placebo. Finally, antidepressant medication combined with cognitive-behavior therapy was superior to medication alone in reducing purging frequency. Of those receiving cognitive-behavior therapy plus medication, 50% were in remission compared with 25% of those receiving medication alone.

Predictors of treatment response. Because the use of antidepressants to treat BN was based on the hypothesis that BN is a variant of depression, researchers thought that pretreatment level of depression would predict the outcome of antidepressant treatment. In fact, studies that have examined this proposition have found no evidence that level of depression predicts outcome. Both depressed and nondepressed patients respond equally well to antidepressant treatment (Mitchell and Groat 1984). In addition, different factors predicted the antibulimic and antidepressant responses to desipramine in 24 patients with BN enrolled in a placebo-controlled crossover study (Blouin et al. 1989). Thus, degree of depression was not a predictor of antibulimic response, although a higher frequency of purging and a lower bulimia scale score on the Eating Disorders Inventory (Garner et al. 1983) did predict a good antibulimic response. On the other hand, those whose depression diminished had abnormal dexamethasone suppression test scores and were more likely to have a family history of depression. The only other factor to predict outcome is the patient's lowest weight since early adolescence; those with lower weights (i.e., those who were more anorexic) had worse outcomes (Agras et al. 1987). Note, however, that all studies that examined predictors of response had sample sizes too small to determine accurately the characteristics of treatment responders.

Mechanism of action.   If antidepressants do not exert their effect in BN by decreasing depression, then what is the mechanism of action? Two alternative hypotheses have been proposed (Agras and McCann 1987). The first hypothesis suggests that although the state of depression does not predict outcome, fluctuant negative moods arising during the day may promote binge eating. The second hypothesis, based on the finding that desipramine is an anorexic agent in rats, suggests that antidepressants may work by reducing hunger. These hypotheses were tested directly in a study by Rossiter and colleagues (1991). No evidence was found that desipramine reduced fluctuant negative moods. However, desipramine did reduce hunger levels significantly. This effect was confirmed in a study of binge-eating disorder in which participants taking desipramine had significantly greater reductions in hunger than those receiving placebo (McCann and Agras 1990). Reductions in levels of hunger would likely reduce the urge of bulimic patients to binge eat.

Other medications.   Although considerable evidence from controlled trials indicates that most antidepressants are useful in the treatment of BN, few studies of other pharmacological agents have been done. Based on the possibility that antidepressants work by reducing hunger in patients with BN, studies of appetite suppressants are of interest. In one controlled study of 42 patients, 30 mg of *d*-fenfluramine was significantly more effective in reducing the frequency of binge eating and purging than was placebo (Russell et al. 1988). However, 40% of patients dropped out of this study. This dropout rate is high but did not appear to be due to medication side effects. The high, unexplained dropout rate led the authors to conclude that *d*-fenfluramine may be useful as an adjunctive treatment of BN but that further study is needed before making definitive conclusions about its efficacy. In a second study of 43 patients, 45 mg of *d*-fenfluramine or placebo was added to cognitive-behavior therapy in an 8-week trial (Fahy et al. 1993). Only 4 subjects dropped out of this study. Both groups had significant reductions in binge eating and purging, but no evidence indicated that the active medication added to the effectiveness of cognitive-behavior therapy. It is likely, however, that the effects of cognitive-behavior therapy were too large, and the sample size too small, to allow an additive effect of *d*-fenfluramine to be detected. Further studies of appetite suppressants appear warranted.

Because opioids are involved in the control of eating, there has been some interest in using opiate antagonists to treat eating disorders. One study of 16 women with BN compared low (50–100 mg/day) and high (200–300 mg/day) doses of naltrexone and found that high doses in patients with BN reduced binge eating and purging more than low doses (Jonas and Gold 1988). However, this was a short-term study, and no data on full recovery were provided. In addition, one patient in the high-dose group had elevations on liver function tests that normalized after the dose was reduced. The authors suggested that liver function should be monitored at frequent intervals in patients who are taking high-dose naltrexone. Another study found no effect of naltrexone (100 mg/day) over placebo on the frequency of binge eating and purging in patients with BN, although the duration of binges was reduced significantly (Alger et al. 1991). Finally, one placebo-controlled study of lithium in the treatment of BN in 91 women found no evidence for effectiveness (Hsu et al. 1991). However, the mean serum lithium level was 0.62 mEq/L, which is lower than the usual therapeutic range. Nonetheless, little evidence indicates that medications other than antidepressants are of use in the treatment of BN.

Comprehensive Treatment of Bulimia Nervosa

For the most part, patients with BN are best treated as outpatients, unless there are either medical or psychiatric reasons for hospitalization (e.g., an intercurrent physical illness or comorbid psychiatric disorder requiring hospitalization, such as major depression with suicidality). One reason that outpatient treatment is useful is that gains made in the hospital may not carry over to the patient's home, where more complex food stimuli and greater stress are present than in the hospital.

At present, no clear guidelines exist for the sequence of pharmacological and psychological therapies. It can be argued that because cognitive-behavior therapy is superior to medication, psychological treatment might be the best initial approach in uncomplicated cases of BN, and medication could be added if the response to cognitive-behavior therapy were unsatisfactory. On the other hand, antidepressant medication appears to be more cost-effective than cognitive-behavior therapy. Patients should be advised of these facts so that they can make an informed choice. When marked depression accompanies the bulimic symptoms, antidepressant therapy should be used either alone or in combination with cognitive-behavior therapy, because depressive symptoms have a superior response to antidepressants used in the treatment of BN. Similarly, when the patient has marked preoccupation with food and/or hunger, the clinician should consider the use of antidepressants. If the first antidepressant does not lead to therapeutic gains in a reasonable time, the use of alternative antidepressants should be considered, followed by the addition of cognitive-behavior therapy if the response is not satisfactory.

BINGE-EATING DISORDER

Although the association between binge eating and obesity has been noted from time to time in case reports in the literature, it was not until the upsurge of research into the psychopathology and treatment of BN that systematic attention was paid to binge-eating disorder. The principal features of binge-eating disorder include episodes of binge eating at a frequency of at least twice a week for 6 months, marked distress caused by binge eating, and binge eating that does not occur during the course of BN or AN.

A self-monitoring study found that patients with binge-eating disorder consumed about 600 calories during each binge, with high variability among and within subjects (Rossiter et al. 1992). This finding suggests that binges in patients with binge-eating disorder are smaller than those of patients with BN, which has been confirmed in laboratory studies (Telch and Agras 1996). Also, patients with binge-eating disorder consumed about 900 kcal less on nonbinge days than on binge days, which suggests that binge eating alternates with dietary restriction.

About 2% of women in the general population have symptoms that meet criteria for binge-eating disorder (Bruce and Agras 1992). In clinical populations, the ratio of women to men with binge-eating disorder is approximately 3:2, the highest rate for men for any eating disorder. Although obesity is not a requirement for the diagnosis of binge-eating disorder, a substantial overlap exists between binge-eating disorder and obesity. Studies have shown that more than one-quarter of obese subjects have symptoms that meet criteria for binge-eating disorder and that the prevalence of binge eating increases as body mass index increases (Marcus et al. 1985; Telch et al. 1988). Because binge eating often precedes the onset of becoming overweight, binge eating may be a risk factor for obesity and the multiple health problems associated with being overweight. Moreover, the syndrome is associated with comorbid psychopathology similar to that of BN and causes much distress; hence, it is an entity deserving of treatment in its own right. One study that compared individuals with binge-eating disorder with weight-matched non-binge-eating obese individuals found that subjects with binge-eating disorder were significantly more likely to receive diagnoses of major depression (51%), panic disorder (9%), and borderline personality disorder (9%) than those without binge-eating disorder (Yanovski et al. 1992).

Antidepressant Treatment

As noted earlier in this chapter, research into the treatment of binge-eating disorder is in its infancy. Nonetheless, because of the similarity between BN and binge-eating disorder, investigators have suggested that treatments effective for BN should also be effective for binge-eating disorder. To date, two double-blind, placebo-controlled studies of the use of antidepressants in binge-eating disorder have been done (Alger et al. 1991; McCann and Agras 1990). One of these studies involved 23 women with binge-eating disorder; patients who received desipramine reduced their binge eating significantly more than those who received placebo, and 60% of the desipramine group was abstinent at the end of 12 weeks' treatment (McCann and Agras 1990). In addition, hunger was significantly reduced and dietary restraint was increased in those assigned to the active drug condition. When medication was withdrawn, rapid relapse across all parameters occurred. The second study had a large placebo effect with no differences between imipramine and placebo in reducing binge eating (Alger et al. 1991).

Although the McCann and Agras (1990) study suggested that antidepressants are useful in the treatment of binge-eating disorder, patients who stopped binge eating did not lose weight in this short-term study. This finding is in accord with the two controlled psychological treatment studies of this disorder (Telch et al. 1990; Wilfley et al. 1993), neither of which reported significant weight loss in the treated group. Hence, a comprehensive treatment approach would of necessity require combining antidepressants with weight loss therapy. In one controlled study of 108 overweight women with binge-eating disorder treated for 3 months with cognitive-behavior therapy, followed by 6 months of weight loss treatment combined with desipramine. No additive effect of desipramine on binge eating

Hadigan C, Kissileff HR, Walsh BT: Patterns of food selection during meals in women with bulimia. Am J Clin Nutr 50:759–766, 1989

Halmi CA, Eckert E, LaDu TJ, et al: Treatment efficacy of cyproheptadine and amitriptyline. Arch Gen Psychiatry 43:177–181, 1986

Horne RL, Ferguson JM, Pope HG, et al: Treatment of bulimia with bupropion: a multicenter controlled trial. J Clin Psychiatry 49:262–266, 1988

Hsu LKG, Clement L, Santhouse R, et al: Treatment of bulimia nervosa with lithium carbonate: a controlled study. J Nerv Ment Dis 179:351–355, 1991

Hughes PL, Wells LA, Cunningham CJ, et al: Treating bulimia with desipramine. Arch Gen Psychiatry 43:182–187, 1986

Johnson WG, Stuckey MK, Lewis LD, et al: Bulimia: a descriptive survey of 316 cases. Int J Eat Disord 2:3–16, 1982

Jonas JM, Gold MS: The use of opiate antagonists in treating bulimia: a study of low-dose versus high-dose naltrexone. Psychiatry Res 24:195–199, 1988

Kaye WH, Weltzin TE, Hsu G, et al: An open trial of fluoxetine in patients with anorexia nervosa. J Clin Psychiatry 52:464–471, 1991

Keller MB, Herzog DB, Lavori PW, et al: The naturalistic history of bulimia nervosa: extraordinarily high rates of chronicity, relapse, recurrence, and psychosocial morbidity. Int J Eat Disord 12:1–10, 1992

Kendler KS, MacLean C, Neale M, et al: The genetic epidemiology of bulimia nervosa. Am J Psychiatry 148:1627–1637, 1991

Kennedy SH, Goldbloom DS, Ralevski E, et al: Is there a role for selective monoamine oxidase inhibitor therapy in bulimia nervosa? A placebo-controlled trial. J Clin Psychopharmacol 13:415–422, 1993

Koran LM, Agras WS, Rossiter E, et al: Comparing the cost-effectiveness of psychiatric treatments: bulimia nervosa. Psychiatry Res 58:13–21, 1995

Laessle PJ, Beumont PJV, Butow P, et al: A comparison of nutritional management with stress management in the treatment of bulimia nervosa. Br J Psychiatry 159:250–261, 1991

Marcus MD, Wing RR, Lamparski DM: Binge-eating and dietary restraint in obese patients. Addict Behav 10:163–168, 1985

Marrazzi MA, Luby ED: An auto-addiction opioid model of chronic anorexia nervosa. Int J Eat Disord 5:1191–1208, 1986

Marrazzi MA, Bacon JP, Kinzie J, et al: Naltrexone use in the treatment of anorexia nervosa and bulimia nervosa. International Journal of Clinical Psychopharmacology 10:163–172, 1995

McCann UD, Agras WS: Successful treatment of compulsive binge-eating with desipramine: a double-blind placebo-controlled study. Am J Psychiatry 147:1509–1513, 1990

McCarthy MK, Goff DC, Baer L, et al: Dissociation, childhood trauma, and the response to fluoxetine in bulimic patients. Int J Eating Disord 15:219–226, 1994

Mitchell JE, Groat R: A placebo-controlled, double-blind trial of amitryptiline in bulimia. J Clin Psychopharmacol 4:186–193, 1984

Mitchell JE, Laine DC: Monitored binge-eating behavior in patients with bulimia. Int J Eat Disord 4:177–183, 1985

Mitchell JE, Pyle RL, Eckert ED, et al: Response to alternative antidepressants in imipramine nonresponders with bulimia nervosa. J Clin Psychopharmacol 9:291–293, 1989

Mitchell JE, Pyle RL, Eckert ED, et al: A comparison study of antidepressants and structured intensive group psychotherapy in the treatment of bulimia nervosa. Arch Gen Psychiatry 47:149–160, 1990

Patton E, Johnson-Sabine E, Wood A, et al: Abnormal eating attitudes in London schoolgirls—a prospective epidemiological study: outcome at twelve-month follow-up. Psychol Med 20:383–394, 1990

Polivy J: Perception of calories and regulation of intake in restrained and unrestrained subjects. Addict Behav 1:237–243, 1976

Pope HG, Hudson JI: Treatment of bulimia with antidepressants. Psychopharmacology (Berl) 78:176–179, 1982

Pope HG, Hudson JI, Jonas JM, et al: Bulimia treated with imipramine: a placebo-controlled double-blind study. Am J Psychiatry 140:554–558, 1983

Pope HG, Hudson JI, Jonas JM, et al: Antidepressant treatment of bulimia: a two-year follow-up study. J Clin Psychopharmacol 5:320–327, 1985

Pope HG, Keck PE, McElroy SL, et al: A placebo-controlled study of trazodone in bulimia nervosa. J Clin Psychopharmacol 9:254–259, 1989

Pyle RL, Mitchell JE, Eckert ED, et al: Maintenance treatment and 6-month outcome for bulimic patients who respond to initial treatment. Am J Psychiatry 147:871–875, 1990

Rosen JC, Leitenberg H, Fisher C, et al: Binge-eating episodes in bulimia nervosa: the amount and type of food consumed. Int J Eat Disord 5:255–267, 1986

Rossiter EM, Agras WS, McCann U: Are antidepressants appetite suppressants in bulimia nervosa? European Journal of Psychiatry 5:224–231, 1991

Rossiter EM, Agras WS, Telch CF, et al: The eating patterns of non-purging bulimic subjects. Int J Eat Disord 11:111–120, 1992

Rothschild R, Quitkin HM, Stewart JW, et al: A double-blind placebo comparison of phenelzine and imipramine in the treatment of atypical depressives. Int J Eat Disord 15:1–9, 1994

Russell GFM, Checkley SA, Feldman J, et al: A controlled trial of d-fenfluramine in bulimia nervosa. Clin Neuropharmacol 11 (suppl 1):146–159, 1988

Sabine EJ, Yonace A, Farrington AJ, et al: Bulimia nervosa: a placebo-controlled double blind therapeutic trial of mianserin. Br J Clin Pharmacol 15:195–202, 1983

Telch CF, Agras WS: Do emotional states influence binge eating in the obese? Int J Eat Disord 20:271–280, 1996

Telch CF, Agras WS, Rossiter EM: Binge-eating increases with increasing adiposity. Int J Eat Disord 7:115–119, 1988

Telch CF, Agras WS, Rossiter EM, et al: Group cognitive-behavioral treatment for the non-purging bulimic: an initial evaluation. J Consult Clin Psychol 58:629–635, 1990

Vandereycken W: Neuroleptics in the short-term treatment of anorexia nervosa: a double-blind placebo-controlled study with sulpiride. Br J Psychiatry 144:288–292, 1984

Vandereycken W, Pierloot R: Pimozide combined with behavior therapy in the short-term treatment of anorexia nervosa: a double-blind placebo-controlled cross over study. Acta Psychiatr Scand 66:445–450, 1982

Walsh BT, Stewart JW, Wright L, et al: Treatment of bulimia with monoamine oxidase inhibitors. Am J Psychiatry 139:1629–1630, 1982

Walsh BT, Stewart JW, Roose SP, et al: Treatment of bulimia with phenelzine: a double-blind, placebo-controlled study. Arch Gen Psychiatry 41:1105–1109, 1984

Walsh BT, Gladis M, Roose SP, et al: Phenelzine vs placebo in 50 patients with bulimia. Arch Gen Psychiatry 45:471–475, 1988

Walsh BT, Hadigan CM, Devlin MJ, et al: Long-term outcome of antidepressant treatment for bulimia nervosa. Am J Psychiatry 148:1206–1212, 1991

Walsh BT, Wilson GT, Loeb KL, et al: Medication and psychotherapy in the treatment of bulimia nervosa. Am J Psychiatry 154:523–531, 1997

Wermuth BM, Davis KL, Hollister LE, et al: Phenytoin treatment of the binge-eating syndrome. Am J Psychiatry 134:1249–1253, 1977

Wheadon DE, Rampey AH, Thompson VL, et al: Lack of association between fluoxetine and suicidality in bulimia nervosa. J Clin Psychiatry 53:235–241, 1992

Wilfley DE, Agras WS, Telch CF, et al: Group cognitive-behavioral therapy and group interpersonal psychotherapy for the non-purging bulimic: a controlled comparison. J Consult Clin Psychol 61:296–305, 1993

Yanovski SZ, Nelson JE, Dubbert BK, et al: Association of binge-eating disorder and psychiatric comorbidity in the obese. Am J Psychiatry 150:1472–1479, 1992

State Senate Select Committee on Mental and Physical Handicaps 1977; Tardiff 1987). In Veterans Administration hospitals, 12,000 assaultive incidents were reported over a 5-year period (Reid et al. 1985).

Aggression among psychiatric patients exacts an even greater toll on family members and other primary caregivers than it does on mental health professionals. Rabins and co-workers (1982) studied the families and primary caregivers of 55 patients whose symptoms met DSM-III (American Psychiatric Association 1980) criteria for dementia. Sixty percent of the patients had clinical diagnoses of Alzheimer's disease, 18% had multiinfarct dementia, and 22% had other etiologies for their dementia. In response to the first question posed by Rabins to the families, "What is the biggest problem you have in caring for the patient?," 22 different problems were isolated. The highest on the list of "the most serious" problems faced by the families was aggressive behavior, which 28 of 55 families studied reported to have occurred regularly. When aggression occurred, 75% of the families rated this behavior as the most serious problem with which they were confronted.

In our clinical experience, agitation, rageful affects, and aggressive behaviors are frequent precipitants of referral of elderly patients to psychiatrists for assessment and management. However, a significant percentage of elderly patients with agitation and aggression are *not* referred to psychiatrists but to nursing home facilities or other restrictive institutional environments such as state hospitals. We strongly believe that with appropriate diagnosis and treatment of the medical disorders underlying the agitation and aggression (such as delirium secondary to anticholinergic agents) as well as with the enlightened pharmacological management of their symptoms (such as the use of β-blockers to treat agitation and aggression associated with Alzheimer's disease), institutionalization could be avoided for a larger proportion of these elderly patients (Yudofsky et al. 1990). Psychiatrists are far better trained in and familiar with assessing and treating people who direct aggression toward themselves (i.e., suicidal individuals) than those who are aggressive toward others (violent and homicidal). With approximately 30,000 recorded suicides and 22,000–24,000 homicides occurring in the United States annually (Malmquist 1996; Reid et al. 1985), these categories of aggression offer great potential for improved preventive and interventive strategies.

In this chapter, we review nosological, diagnostic, and pathophysiological aspects of agitation and aggression and, thereafter, focus on the pharmacotherapy of agitation and aggression in the context of a comprehensive treatment plan.

DEFINITION AND CATEGORIZATION OF AGITATION AND AGGRESSION

Agitation and Aggression as Disorders

Agitation is almost universally conceptualized as a symptom that is the result of a primary medical disorder. On the other hand, largely on the basis of the various theoretical and clinical approaches of the numerous scientific and professional disciplines studying aggressive behaviors in animal models or in humans, aggression is conceptualized and diagnosed in an unusually broad and disparate fashion. In the same manner that anxiety and depression may be conceptualized as either symptoms or specific disorders, aggressive behavior may be categorized as a symptom or as a distinct disorder.

DSM-IV (American Psychiatric Association 1994) separates aggressive disorders into two diagnoses: 1) personality change due to a general medical condition, aggressive type (Table 42–1), and 2) intermittent explosive disorder (Table 42–2). We disagree with these diagnostic categorizations and have proposed an alternative diagnostic category—neuroaggressive disorder (Table 42–3)—to describe the specific condition of dyscontrol or rage and violence secondary to brain lesions (Ghosh and Victor 1994; Rabins et al. 1982; Yudofsky et al. 1990).

We view personality change due to a general medical condition as imprecise and nonspecific. We have seen many patients with brain lesions whose single symptom caused by the brain impairment is aggressive outbursts that are out of proportion to the precipitating stimulus. If, for example, a brain lesion results, on rare occasions, in an individual's vehemently pounding the seat of his car while being frustrated by a traffic jam, does this constitute a change in his "personality"? The concept of personality encompasses a multifaceted constellation of emotional, behavioral, and interactive patterns that are unique to an individual. If patients with aggressive episodes are categorized as having a "personality change," why would not those who develop anxiety, psychosis, or affective disorders also be characterized as having personality changes? Brain lesions that were made in specific brain regions of animal models caused increased aggression in response to irritating stimuli (Eichelman 1971; Leavitt et al. 1989), but otherwise the animals behaved quite normally.

We also have reservations about whether the diagnosis of intermittent explosive disorder actually exists. According to DSM-IV, this diagnosis does *not* apply if the episodes of aggression occur during the course of psychosis (i.e., general medical conditions, organic mental disorders, antisocial or borderline personality disorder, conduct disorder,

Table 42–1. DSM-IV diagnostic criteria for personality change due to a general medical condition

A. A persistent personality disturbance that represents a change from the individual's previous characteristic personality pattern. (In children, the disturbance involves a marked deviation from normal development or a significant change in the child's usual behavior patterns lasting at least 1 year).

B. There is evidence from the history, physical examination, or laboratory findings that the disturbance is the direct physiological consequence of a general medical condition.

C. The disturbance is not better accounted for by another mental disorder (including other mental disorders due to a general medical condition).

D. The disturbance does not occur exclusively during the course of a delirium and does not meet criteria for a dementia.

E. The disturbance causes clinically significant distress or impairment in social, occupational, or other important areas of functioning.

■ *Specify* type:

Labile type: if the predominant feature is affective lability
Disinhibited type: if the predominant feature is poor impulse control as evidenced by sexual indiscretions, etc.
Aggressive type: if the predominant feature is aggressive behavior
Apathetic type: if the predominant feature is marked apathy and indifference
Paranoid type: if the predominant feature is suspiciousness or paranoid ideation
Other type: if the predominant feature is not one of the above, e.g., personality change associated with a seizure disorder
Combined type: if more than one feature predominates in the clinical picture
Unspecified type

Table 42–2. DSM-IV diagnostic criteria for intermittent explosive disorder

A. Several discrete episodes of failure to resist aggressive impulses that result in serious assaultive acts or destruction of property.

B. The degree of aggressiveness expressed during the episodes is grossly out of proportion to any precipitating psychosocial stressors.

C. The aggressive episodes are not better accounted for by another mental disorder (e.g., antisocial personality disorder, borderline personality disorder, a psychotic disorder, a manic episode, conduct disorder, or attention-deficit/hyperactivity disorder) and are not due to the direct physiological effects of a substance (e.g., a drug of abuse, a medication) or a general medical condition (e.g., head trauma, Alzheimer's disease).

Table 42–3. Diagnostic criteria for proposed neuroaggressive disorder

Persistent or recurrent aggressive outbursts, whether of a verbal or physical nature.

The outbursts are out of proportion to the precipitating stress or provocation.

Evidence from history, physical examination, or laboratory tests of a specific organic factor that is judged to be etiologically related to the disturbance.

The outbursts are not primarily related to the following disorders: paranoia, mania, schizophrenia, narcissistic personality disorder, borderline personality disorder, antisocial personality disorder, or conduct disorder.

Source. Reprinted from Yudofsky SC, Silver J, Yudofsky B: "Organic Personality Disorder, Explosive Type," in *Treatments of Psychiatric Disorders: A Task Force Report of the American Psychiatric Association.* Washington, DC, American Psychiatric Association, 1989, pp. 839–852. Copyright 1989, American Psychiatric Association. Used with permission.

Agitation and Aggression as Symptoms

Agitation and aggression most often occur as consequences of experiential and biological predispositions in the context of current evocative situations or environments. Far more attention has been devoted to the neurobiology and neuropathology of aggression than to those of agitation. (A review of the brain pathways involved in aggression and the ways in which neuropathology and psychopathology combine to provoke aggression can be found in a chapter by Ovsiew and Yudofsky 1993.) Table 42–4 summarizes brain loci that are associated with aggressive behaviors, and Table 42–5 reviews the work of Valzelli (1981) on brain regions that trigger or suppress agitation and aggression. As we discuss later in this chapter, a broad range of conditions and disorders that affect the brain can

or as the result of physiological responses to substances of abuse or medications). These exclusions are so broad that our group, which specializes in the assessment and treatment of aggressive disorders, rarely, if ever, encounters a patient whose condition meets criteria for this diagnosis.

Our experience is consistent with the report of neurologist Frank Elliott (1976), who also found that 94% of 286 patients with histories of recurrent uncontrolled rage attacks that occurred with little or no provocation had objective evidence of developmental or acquired brain deficits. We believe that this nosological confusion and imprecision deriving from official diagnostic categorizations account, in part, for the pervasive failure of clinicians to diagnose and, consequently, to treat specifically and effectively aggressive symptomatology in all categories of patients.

Table 42–4.　Neuropathology of aggression

Locus	Activity
Hypothalamus	Orchestrates neuroendocrine response via sympathetic arousal
	Monitors and regulates somatic status
Limbic system	
Amygdala	Activates and/or suppresses hypothalamus
	Receives input from neocortex
Temporal cortex	Associated with aggression in both ictal and interictal states; associated with experiential memory for pain and danger
Frontal neocortex	Modulates limbic and hypothalamic states
	Associated with social and judgment aspects of aggression

Source.　Reprinted from Silver JM, Hales RE, Yudofsky SC: "Neuropsychiatric Aspects of Traumatic Brain Injury," in *The American Psychiatric Press Textbook of Neuropsychiatry*, 2nd Edition. Edited by Yudofsky SC, Hales RE. Washington, DC, American Psychiatric Press, 1992, pp. 363–395. Copyright 1992, American Psychiatric Press. Used with permission.

Table 42–5.　Areas of the brain that mediate aggressive behaviors

Triggers	Suppressors
Medial hypothalamus	Frontal lobes
Posteromedial hypothalamus	Septal nuclei
Thalamic center median	Cerebellar lobes
Thalamic lamella medialis	Cerebellar fastigium
Dorsomedial thalamus	
Anterior cingulum	
Anterior (ventral) hypothalamus	
Centromedial amygdala	

result in symptoms of agitation and aggression. Unfortunately, these aggressive symptoms are often not afforded diagnostic primacy and are, therefore, either not treated at all or "mistreated" with agents that do not have antiaggressive properties. In this regard, Yudofsky (1991) has written about the *monosymptomatic mischaracterization of neuropsychiatric disorders*, in which neuropsychiatric conditions with a broad range of symptoms are misconceptualized as being a uniform illness as defined by a singular predominant sign or symptom. An example is misconceptualizing Alzheimer's disease as a disorder of memory and cognition without recognizing the agitation, depres-

sion, and anxiety that are reported to be among the most common and disabling aspects of this disorder.

Similarly, Parkinson's disease is conventionally regarded as a movement disorder, but depression, delirium, and dementia are also well-documented common concomitant disorders. When schizophrenia is misconceptualized as a psychotic disorder, symptoms of depression, agitation, and aggression often are untreated or mistreated. For example, antipsychotic agents may be used to treat agitation in a patient with schizophrenia, but the agitation does not stem from psychotic ideation. This practice usually results in the patient being oversedated and unnecessarily placed at risk for many side effects associated with antipsychotic drugs, including irreversible tardive dyskinesia and potentially fatal neuroleptic malignant syndrome. We have evaluated and treated an overwhelming percentage of agitated or aggressive patients with schizophrenia who had been taking high doses of neuroleptics. Uniformly, neither their psychoses nor their disruptive behaviors diminished after the antipsychotic drug was discontinued. In most cases, the initiation of medications to treat specifically agitation or aggression reduced these behaviors without sedating the patients or placing them at risk for dangerous, irreversible side effects. In these cases, precise nosology would have aided the referring clinician in arriving at an accurate diagnosis, which would have led to specific and effective treatment.

Differentiating Aggression, Agitation, and Anxiety

We developed a rating scale, the OAS (Yudofsky et al. 1986; see Figure 42–1 and the next section of this chapter), which encompasses the definition, diagnosis, and operationalization of aggression. Although several rating scales are used to measure agitation, we believe that, for the purposes of documenting and monitoring the responses of agitation to pharmacological intervention, no existing rating scale is adequate. One major problem is that most currently used rating scales blur the boundaries between anxiety, agitation, and aggression; they also depend too heavily on the inferences or idiosyncratic theoretical approaches of the rater.

Figure 42–2 shows a newer rating scale we developed—the Overt Agitation Severity Scale (OASS)—that has undergone reliability and validity testing. The OASS currently is being peer reviewed by a scientific journal. The reader, by briefly reviewing this scale and comparing it with the OAS, can be helped to differentiate between agitation and aggression. Anxiety and neuropsychiatric syndromes or side effects such as akathisia also must be

Overt Aggression Scale (OAS)

Stuart Yudofsky, M.D., Jonathan Silver, M.D., Wynn Jackson M.D., and Jean Endicott, Ph.D.

Identifying Data

Name of patient	Name of rater
Sex of patient: 1 male 2 female	Date / / (mo/da/yr) Shift: 1 night 2 day 3 evening

☐ No aggressive incident(s) (verbal or physical) against self, others, or objects during the shift (check here).

Aggressive Behavior (check all that apply)

Verbal aggression	Physical aggression against self
☐ Makes loud noises, shouts angrily	☐ Picks or scratches skin, hits self, pulls hair (with no or minor injury only)
☐ Yells mild personal insults (e.g., "You're stupid!")	☐ Bangs head, hits fist into objects, throws self onto floor or into objects (hurts self without serious injury)
☐ Curses viciously, uses foul language in anger, makes moderate threats to others or self	☐ Small cuts or bruises, minor burns
☐ Makes clear threats of violence toward others or self (I'm going to kill you.) or requests to help to control self	☐ Mutilates self, makes deep cuts, bites that bleed, internal injury, fracture, loss of consciousness, loss of teeth

Physical aggression against objects	Physical aggression against other people
☐ Slams door, scatters clothing, makes a mess	☐ Makes threatening gesture, swings at people, grabs at clothes
☐ Throws objects down, kicks furniture without breaking it, marks the wall	☐ Strikes, kicks, pushes, pulls hair (without injury to them)
☐ Breaks objects, smashes windows	☐ Attacks others, causing mild to moderate physical injury (bruises, sprain, welts)
☐ Sets fires, throws objects dangerously	☐ Attacks others, causing severe physical injury (broken bones, deep lacerations, internal injury)

| Time incident began: ___ ___ : ___ ___ am/pm | Duration of incident: ___ ___ : ___ ___ (hours/minutes) |

Intervention (check all that apply)

☐ None	☐ Immediate medication given by mouth	☐ Use of restraints
☐ Talking to patient	☐ Immediate medication given by injection	☐ Injury requires immediate medical treatment for patient
☐ Closer observation	☐ Isolation without seclusion (time out)	☐ Injury requires immediate treatment for other person
☐ Holding patient	☐ Seclusion	

Comments

Figure 42–1. Overt Aggression Scale. *Source.* Reprinted from Yudofsky SC, Silver JM, Jackson W, et al: "The Overt Aggression Scale for the Objective Rating of Verbal and Physical Aggression." *American Journal of Psychiatry* 143:35–39, 1986. Copyright 1986, American Psychiatric Association. Used with permission.

Overt Agitation Severity Scale (OASS)

Intensity (I)	Behavior	Frequency (F)					Severity score (SS)
		Not present	Rarely	Some of the time	Most of the time	Always present	($I \times F = SS$)
A.	**Vocalizations and oral/facial movements**						
1	Whimpering, whining, moaning, grunting, crying	0	1	2	3	4	= _____
2	Smacking or licking of lips, chewing, clenching jaw, licking, grimacing, spitting	0	1	2	3	4	= _____
3	Rocking, twisting, banging of head	0	1	2	3	4	= _____
4	Vocal perseverating, screaming, cursing, threatening, wailing	0	1	2	3	4	= _____
B.	**Upper torso and upper extremity movements**						
1	Tapping fingers, fidgeting, wringing of hands, swinging or flailing arms	0	1	2	3	4	= _____
2	Task perseverating (e.g., opening and closing drawers, folding and unfolding clothes, picking at objects, clothes, or self)	0	1	2	3	4	= _____
3	Rocking (back and forth), bobbing (up and down), twisting or writhing of torso, rubbing or masturbating self	0	1	2	3	4	= _____
4	Slapping, swatting, hitting at objects or others	0	1	2	3	4	= _____
C.	**Lower extremity movements**						
1	Tapping toes, clenching toes, tapping heel, extending, flexing, or twisting foot	0	1	2	3	4	= _____
2	Shaking legs, tapping knees and/or thighs, thrusting pelvis, stomping	0	1	2	3	4	= _____
3	Pacing, wandering	0	1	2	3	4	= _____
4	Thrashing legs, kicking at objects or others	0	1	2	3	4	= _____

Total OASS = _____

Subtract baseline OASS = _____

Revised OASS = _____

Instructions for completing form

Step one: For each behavior, circle the corresponding frequency.

Step two: For every behavior *exhibited*, multiply the intensity score (I) by the frequency (F) and record as the severity score (SS).

Step three: For the Overt Agitation Severity Score (OASS), total all severity scores and record as total OASS.

Step four: Does this patient have a neuromuscular disorder (i.e., Parkinson's disease, tardive dyskinesia) affecting total OASS?   Yes   No

Step five: If yes, please establish a baseline OASS in nonagitated state and subtract from above total OASS for revised OASS.

Comments: _____

_____

Diagnosis: _____   Name of rater: _____

Sex of patient: Male   (1); Female   (2)   Time of observation: _____

Age: _____   Date: _____

Current medication:

Name: _____   Dose: _____   Frequency: _____

Name: _____   Dose: _____   Frequency: _____

Name: _____   Dose: _____   Frequency: _____

Name: _____   Dose: _____   Frequency: _____

Figure 42–2.   Overt Agitation Severity Scale. *Source.*   Reprinted from Yudofsky SC, Kopecky HJ, Kunik M, et al: "The Overt Agitation Severity Scale for the Objective Rating of Agitation." *Journal of Neuropsychiatry and Clinical Neurosciences* 9:541–548, 1997. Copyright 1997, American Psychiatric Press. Used with permission.

differentiated from agitation and aggression. When the clinician confuses akathisia with agitation or aggression, he or she may increase the patient's antipsychotic dose. Apart from the increased sedation from the antipsychotic, the misuse of a neuroleptic in this circumstance ultimately will aggravate the akathisia and result in a vicious cycle of ever-increasing doses of antipsychotic drug and consequent intensification of the akathisia. We advise clinicians to use standardized rating scales such as the OAS and the OASS to help diagnose, document, distinguish, and monitor aggression, agitation, and anxiety. Figure 42–3 depicts the overlap of agitation with other symptomatologies, and Figure 42–4 shows agitation on an objectivity-subjectivity continuum with aggression and anxiety.

DOCUMENTATION AND RATING OF AGITATION AND AGGRESSION

Aggression

Accurate documentation of episodes of agitation and aggression is critical to recording characteristics of such episodes when they occur, to assessing the effectiveness of interventions in the treatment of agitated and aggressive patients, and to conducting research related to disorders of agitation and aggression. The OAS and the OASS are 1-page rating scales that were developed to assess the effects of pharmacological agents in the treatment of agitation and aggression (Silver and Yudofsky 1991). In the OAS, aggressive behaviors are divided into four categories: verbal aggression, physical aggression against objects, physical aggression against self, and physical aggression against other people. Within each category, descriptive statements and numerical scores are used to define and rate four levels of severity. All behaviors shown by a patient during an aggressive episode are checked off by an observer (such as routine hospital staff or a family member). Therapeutic interventions used in response to these aggressive episodes are also listed, rated on the OAS, and checked off by the rater. These interventions are documented because they may indicate the observer's interpretation of the relative severity of the aggressive behaviors.

Our research, which evaluated more than 5,000 episodes of aggression in chronically hospitalized psychiatric inpatients, indicated that hospital records and other official communications and documentation did not include descriptions of most aggressive behaviors that occurred. Simultaneous use of the OAS ensured that a significantly greater percentage of aggressive episodes and behaviors was documented (Silver and Yudofsky 1987b).

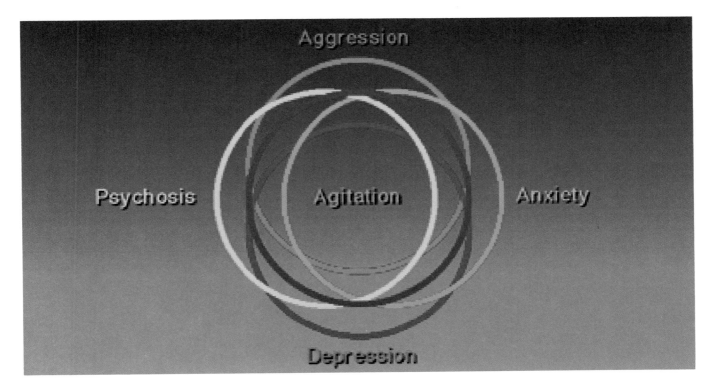

Figure 42–3. Present conceptualization of agitation.

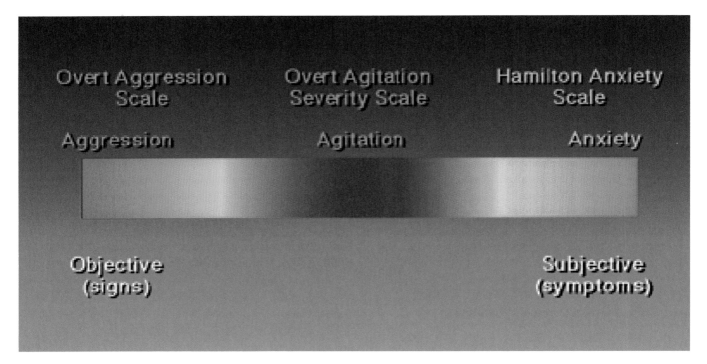

Figure 42–4. Continuum of the three *A's*.

Agitation

An article describing the validity and reliability testing of the OASS has recently been published (Yudofsky et al. 1997). The OASS includes 47 observable characteristics of agitation that are subcategorized into 12 behaviorally related units. The characteristics were identified as representative of the full content domain of agitation from the clinical and theoretical literature. Further subcategorization, for the purposes of enhancing its ease of use, are anatomically based: 1) vocalizations and oral/facial movements, 2) upper torso and upper extremity movements, and 3) lower extremity movements.

Each behavioral subgroup is rated with a likert-type frequency score from 1 (mild signs) to 4 (very severe signs). For each subgroup, a corresponding 5-point likert-type frequency score is selected by the rater from 0 (behavior is not present) to 4 (behavior is always present). The total OASS score is obtained by multiplying each item's frequency response by a weight that corresponds to the intensity of the symptom being measured. The total of the weighted responses indicates the severity of agitation. For patients with neuromuscular disorders (e.g., Parkinson's disease, akathisia, tardive dyskinesia), in which impaired motor activity can mimic agitation, a baseline nonagitated OASS score is obtained and subtracted from the score obtained during an agitated state to determine the revised OASS score.

We encourage practitioners to utilize the OAS and OASS to establish baseline scores for aggression before initiating psychopharmacological intervention and, thereafter, to document the efficacy (or lack thereof) of any therapeutic intervention. The documentation of aggression and agitation through the rating scales is often essential to *maintaining* a psychopharmacological treatment plan. We are often consulted by other physicians or by family members who contend that the psychopharmacological intervention "has stopped working." In these circumstances, professionals and family members are so alarmed by the patient's single episode of violence or agitation and its implications that they demand significant revisions in the treatment plan, which often entail the abrupt discontinuation of the current pharmacological agent and the initiation of another medication. In a significant percentage of these cases, the pharmacological agent has been highly, but not entirely, effective; however, for a variety of reasons (such as increased stress, poor compliance, concomitant use of alcohol or illicit substances), the agitation and aggression have "broken through" the pharmacological intervention. Documentation of agitation and aggression with rating scales is very useful in proving to patients, their families, and caregivers that a pharmacological intervention has been partially effective (e.g., the number of events may have been reduced by 80%, and the intensity of the events may have diminished by 94%). These data from rating scales may obviate a potentially deleterious "overreaction" by caregivers to a single extreme event and the discontinuation of an effective pharmacological regimen.

NEUROTRANSMITTER INVOLVEMENT IN AGITATION AND AGGRESSION

Multiple neurotransmitters and neurotransmitter systems are involved in the mediation of agitation and aggression; serotonin, norepinephrine, dopamine, acetylcholine, and γ-aminobutyric acid (GABA) play important roles. In neuropsychiatric disorders, it is the rule rather than the exception that multiple neurotransmitter systems are involved simultaneously in diffuse regions of the brain. In addition, different transmitters may affect one another in influencing agitation and aggression, which we have learned from the roles of neurotransmitters in depression. Most frequently, the critical factor relative to the role of neurotransmitters in agitation and aggression is the *relationship* among the neurotransmitters in both function and dysfunction.

Norepinephrine tracks originate in the locus coeruleus in the lateral tegmental system and course to the forebrain—an area frequently involved in traumatic brain injury and associated with dyscontrol of rage and violent behavior. The β_1-adrenergic receptors have been implicated through their localization in this region (limbic forebrain and cerebral cortex) and have been judged to be involved in the mediation of aggressive behavior (Alexander et al. 1979). Animal studies suggest that norepinephrine is involved in many aspects of aggressive behavior, including sham rage, affective aggression, and shock-induced fighting (Eichelman 1987). Higley et al. (1992) documented an association between aggression in free-ranging rhesus monkeys and cerebrospinal fluid (CSF) norepinephrine levels. Brown et al. (1979) reported that humans who have aggressive or impulsive behavior have increased levels of the norepinephrine metabolite 5-hydroxy-3-methoxyphenylglycol (5-MHPG).

Currently, dysfunction in serotonergic systems is receiving the most scientific attention with regard to the roles these systems play in agitation and aggression (Coccaro 1992; Wetzler et al. 1991). Serotonergic neurons originate in the raphe, are located in the pons and upper brain stem, and project to the frontal cortex. Clinical studies have implicated the role of lowered levels of serotonin in the central nervous system in the expression of aggression and impulsivity, particularly violent self-destructive acts, in humans (Coccaro et al. 1992; Kruesi et al. 1992; Linnoila and Virkkunen 1992). Dopamine systems are prominent in both mesolimbic and mesocortical regions of the brain. A variety of indirect evidence indicates that increased dopamine in the brain—particularly the release of dopamine after brain lesions—leads to increased agitation and aggression in animal models and in humans (Bareggi et al. 1975; Blackburn et al. 1992; Hamill et al. 1987; Kruesi et al. 1990). The profound increases in aggressive behavior after severe traumatic brain injury are thought to be closely associated with subsequent changes in dopaminergic systems (Eichelman et al. 1972).

DIFFERENTIAL DIAGNOSIS OF AGITATION AND AGGRESSION

In establishing a treatment plan for patients with agitation or aggression, the overarching principle is that diagnosis precedes treatment. The history of the development of the symptoms in a biopsychosocial context is usually the most critical part of the evaluation.

As stated earlier in this chapter, brain disorders are strongly associated with agitation and the dyscontrol of rage and violence. Table 42–6 includes common etiologies of neurologically induced agitation and aggression, and Table 42–7 lists categories of medications and drugs that are associated with engendering agitation and aggression (Yudofsky et al. 1990). Characteristic features that alert the clinician to the potential presence of neurologically induced aggression are summarized in Table 42–8.

In soliciting the patient's history of agitation and aggression, the clinician must interview family members, teachers, friends, work associates, and others because patients with these symptoms—as opposed to their families—tend to minimize the presence and importance of these behaviors (Silver and Yudofsky 1994a). In addition, in crafting a multifaceted treatment plan, the clinician must secure from the patient and observers the context in which agitation or aggression occurs. Determination of the mental status of the patient *before* the agitated or aggressive event, the nature of the precipitant, the physical and social environment in which the behavior occurs, the ways in which the event is mitigated, and the primary and secondary gains related to agitation and aggression is essential. If the agitation or aggression occurs in the context of a psychiatric disorder, a review of both the individual's and the family's psychiatric history should be emphasized. For *all* patients with agitation or aggression, the clinician must obtain a history of physical illness, review neurological signs and symptoms in detail, and conduct a thorough physical examination. Special focus should be placed on the neurological evaluation and on relevant laboratory testing as

Table 42–6. Common etiologies of neurologically induced agitation and aggression

Traumatic brain injury

Stroke and other cerebrovascular disease

Medications, alcohol and other abused substances, over-the-counter drugs

Delirium (e.g., hypoxia, electrolyte imbalance, anesthesia and surgery, uremia)

Alzheimer's disease

Chronic neurological disorders: Huntington's disease, Wilson's disease, Parkinson's disease, multiple sclerosis, systemic lupus erythematosus

Brain tumors

Infectious diseases: encephalitis, meningitis, acquired immunodeficiency syndrome (AIDS)

Epilepsy (ictal, postictal, and interictal)

Metabolic disorders: hyperthyroidism or hypothyroidism, hypoglycemia, vitamin deficiencies, porphyria

Source. Reprinted from Yudofsky SC, Silver JM, Hales RE: "Pharmacologic Management of Aggression in the Elderly. *Journal of Clinical Psychiatry* 51 (10 suppl):22–28, 1990. Copyright 1990, Physicians Postgraduate Press. Used with permission.

guided by information from the history and physical and neurological examinations. We find neuropsychological tests such as the Halstead-Reitan Battery and the Luria-Nebraska Neuropsychological Battery more useful than standard psychological tests such as the Minnesota Multiphasic Personality Inventory (MMPI) or projective psychological tests in evaluating patients with agitated and/or aggressive symptoms and disorders.

TREATMENT OF AGITATION AND AGGRESSION

Overview

Treatment of agitation and aggression is guided by the following four *D's:*

1. **D**etermining the etiologies of the psychological and/or organic disorder(s) that may contribute to the agitation or aggression
2. **D**elineating the biopsychosocial context in which the behaviors occur
3. **D**ocumenting and rating the agitation or aggression with the OAS and/or the OASS
4. **D**eveloping a multifaceted treatment plan

Almost without exception, treatment of agitation or aggression requires a multifaceted approach that often

Table 42–7. Categories of medications and drugs associated with agitation and aggression

Sedative, hypnotic, and antianxiety agents

  Alcohol

  Central nervous system depressants

  Barbiturates

  Benzodiazepines (intoxication and withdrawal states)

Analgesics

  Opiates and other narcotics (intoxication and withdrawal states)

Steroids

  Prednisone

  Cortisone

  Anabolic steroids (therapeutic doses and withdrawal states)

Antidepressants

  All categories (especially in initial phases of treatment)

Stimulants

  Amphetamines

  Cocaine (associated with manic excitement in early stages of abuse and secondary to paranoid ideation in later stages of use)

  Caffeine (in high doses)

Antipsychotics

  Phenothiazines

  Butyrophenones (high-potency dopamine antagonists that lead to akathisia)

Anticholinergics

  Over-the-counter sedatives (associated with delirium and central anticholinergic syndrome)

Hallucinogens

  Lysergic diethylamide (LSD)

  Phencyclidine

  Psilocybin (intoxication states)

Source. Reprinted from Yudofsky SC, Silver JM, Hales RE: "Pharmacologic Management of Aggression in the Elderly." *Journal of Clinical Psychiatry* 51 (10 suppl):22–28, 1990. Copyright 1990, Physicians Postgraduate Press. Used with permission.

combines pharmacological treatments, behavioral treatments, psychodynamically informed psychotherapy, family treatment, and (as indicated) other specific approaches such as spiritual counseling, occupational therapy, and couples treatment.

The review of the psychopharmacological management of agitation and aggression is the focus of this chapter; therefore, we do not expand on the other therapeutic approaches that also have been shown to have efficacy in the treatment of agitation and aggression. For a comprehensive review of behavioral treatments of aggression in

Table 42–8.   Characteristic features of neuroaggressive disorder

Reactive	Triggered by modest or trivial stimuli
Nonreflective	Usually does not involve premeditation or planning
Nonpurposeful	Aggression serves no obvious long-term goals
Explosive	Buildup is *not* gradual
Periodic	Brief outbursts of rage and aggression; punctuated by long periods of relative calm
Ego-dystonic	After outbursts, patients are upset, concerned, and embarrassed as opposed to blaming others or justifying behavior

Source.   Reprinted from Yudofsky SC, Silver JM, Hales RE: "Pharmacologic Management of Aggression in the Elderly." *Journal of Clinical Psychiatry* 51 (10 suppl):22–28, 1990. Copyright 1990, Physicians Postgraduate Press. Used with permission.

psychiatric patients, the reader is referred to a review article published in collaboration with us (Corrigan et al. 1993). A summary of the behavioral treatments of aggression that may be used in combination with pharmacological interventions is shown in Table 42–9 (Corrigan et al. 1993).

In conceptualizing an approach to the pharmacological treatment of agitation and aggression, we differentiate between the management of acute agitation and aggression (often constitutes a medical emergency) and the pharmacological treatment of chronic agitation and aggression (often constitutes a prophylactic and maintenance approach). Currently, no medication has U.S. Food and Drug Administration (FDA) approval for the treatment of these behaviors. Most frequently, when medications are used (and often misused), it is their sedating side effects that are sought. Although this may be appropriate in emergency or specific situations, such as using antipsychotics to treat both psychosis and agitation in a patient with delusional depression, prolonged use of sedation to "cover over" agitation or aggression has disadvantages. For example, when neuroleptics are used to manage agitation or aggression, side effects, including oversedation, hypotension, confusion, neuroleptic malignant syndrome, parkinsonism, akathisia, dystonia, and tardive dyskinesia, may emerge. When benzodiazepines are administered for prolonged periods to manage agitation or aggression, side effects, such as oversedation, motor disturbances including poor coordination, mood disturbances, memory impairment, confusion, dependency, overdoses, withdrawal syndromes, and paradoxical violence, often complicate treatment.

Pharmacological Management of Acute Agitation and Aggression

Antipsychotic medications.   Antipsychotics are the most commonly prescribed medications for the treatment of both acute and chronic agitation and aggression. These agents are appropriate and effective in the treatment of agitation or aggression that derives from psychosis. An example would be to use an antipsychotic drug in a manic patient who appeared at the gates of the White House in an angry and agitated state after she had sent hundreds of letters to the president detailing his scheme to redecorate the White House "in a more vivid color scheme." Another example would be to use an antipsychotic in a patient with paranoid schizophrenia who hears voices commanding him to use physical force to protect himself from a neighbor "who is monitoring my thoughts through a dental device that was surgically implanted during my sleep."

Unfortunately, however, in our experience, the most common use of antipsychotic medications is in the treatment of chronic agitation or aggression associated with brain disorders (including schizophrenia). Over time (i.e., days to months), tolerance to the sedative side effects of the neuroleptics develops, and the clinician must increase the dose to maintain the sedation. A vicious cycle often emerges—neuroleptics are increased to "treat" akathisias that are mistaken for increased irritability and agitation of the associated illness. Herrera et al. (1988) noted a marked increase in violent behavior when patients with schizophrenia were treated with haloperidol in doses ranging to 60 mg/day, when compared with violent behaviors that occurred during treatment with chlorpromazine in doses up to 1,800 mg/day or with clozapine in doses ranging to 900 mg/day. We interpret these findings to be the result of haloperidol's increased risk of causing akathisia as compared with chlorpromazine or clozapine. These complications and side effects can be avoided by establishing, before initiating neuroleptics to treat acute agitation or aggression, a treatment plan that includes 1) operationalized ratings of agitation and aggression with the OAS and OASS, 2) the reduction of neuroleptics when symptoms remit, and 3) prospectively specified dates when the antipsychotic agent will be tapered and discontinued.

Unless agitation or aggression is clearly related to psychotic ideation that is responding to treatment with antipsychotic agents, we limit the use of both antipsychotics and benzodiazepines for "sedating" agitation or aggression to a maximum period of 4 weeks. Beyond this time, clinicians must consider whether the agitation or aggression is chronic and alter the treatment plan accordingly to utilize medications that are recommended for

Table 42–9. Behavioral treatment of aggression

Strategy	Indications	Special considerations
Token economy	Provides both proactive and reactive strategies for aggressive behaviors	A strict format for implementing contingency management
Aggression replacement		
Differential reinforcement schedules	Replace punishing contingency for previolent behavior	Differential reinforcement of other behaviors is resource-intensive; differential reinforcement of incompatible behaviors requires identification of suitable interfering behaviors
Assertiveness training	Effective for patients who become angry when their needs are not met	Patients must work well in skills training groups
Activity programming	Diminishes opportunities for unstructured, frustrating interactions	Activities that patients find reinforcing should be identified
Decelerative techniques		
Social extinction	Effective with previolent patients who respond to social reinforcements	May not work with schizoid patients
Contingent observation	Effective with previolent patients who respond to social reinforcements	Patients must be sufficiently organized to perceive models accurately
Self-controlled timeout	Effective with violent patients immediately after incidents	May diminish risky attempts to seclude or restrain
Overcorrection	Effective with relatively docile patients	Stop if patient struggles with guided practice
Contingent restraint	Effective with violent patients who do not comply with self-controlled timeout and are resistant to guided practice	Decreases inadvertent reinforcement of behaviors that covary with seclusion and restraint

Source. Reprinted from Corrigan PW, Yudofsky SC, Silver JM: "Pharmacological and Behavioral Treatments for Aggressive Psychiatric Inpatients." *Hospital and Community Psychiatry* 44(2):125–133, 1993. Copyright 1993, American Psychiatric Association. Used with permission.

treatment of chronic behaviors (see next section).

The essence of managing acute episodes of agitation or aggression by using neuroleptics for sedation is to increase the dose of the neuroleptic, often every 1–2 hours, to achieve the lowest dose that will produce the sedation necessary to "control" the violent behaviors. Despite the aforementioned disadvantages of haloperidol in the management of chronic agitation or aggression, this medication—because it can be taken orally, intramuscularly, and intravenously, and because it has a low level of cardiovascular side effects compared with other classes of neuroleptics—is used most often. Summarized guidelines for the use of haloperidol in the management of acute agitation or aggression are provided in Table 42–10.

Clozapine has been used to treat agitation and aggression in patients with a broad variety of neuropsychiatric disorders, including traumatic brain injury (Michals et al. 1993) and mental retardation (Cohen and Underwood 1994). These and other similar studies used open trial methodologies to report that clozapine reduced agitated, aggressive, and self-injurious behaviors. The clinician must be cautioned, however, that clozapine significantly lowers

seizure thresholds, which is an especially dangerous side effect in patients with brain disorders. Seizures occurred in two of nine brain-injured patients who received clozapine to treat refractory aggression (Michals et al. 1993).

Benzodiazepines. Benzodiazepines may also be indicated for the management of acute agitation and aggression. Intramuscular lorazepam has advantages over other benzodiazepines as an effective medication for the emergency treatment of agitated or aggressive patients (Bick and Hannah 1986). In the management of acute agitation or aggression, lorazepam's advantages are similar to those of haloperidol, including flexible routes of administration (intravenous, intramuscular, or oral). In addition, lorazepam has a relatively brief half-life compared with other benzodiazepines such as diazepam or chlordiazepoxide, which can result in oversedation of the patient through the buildup of overly high plasma levels of the respective benzodiazepine. Table 42–11 contains guidelines for the use of lorazepam in the acute management of agitation or aggression.

Table 42–10. Use of haloperidol in the acute management of agitation or aggression

1. Initiate haloperidol—1 mg orally or 0.5 mg intravenously or intramuscularly every hour.
2. Increase dose by 1 mg every hour until agitation or aggression is controlled.
3. Administer haloperidol as 2 mg orally or 1 mg intravenously or intramuscularly every 8 hours.
4. When patient is not agitated or violent for at least 48 hours, taper at rate of 25% of highest daily dose.
5. If agitation or violent behavior reemerges while tapering drug, reevaluate etiology and consider switching to a more specific medication to manage chronic behavioral dysfunction.
6. Do not continue haloperidol administration for more than 6 weeks—unless agitation or aggression is secondary to psychosis.

Source. Adapted from Yudofsky SC, Silver JM, Hales RE: "Pharmacologic Management of Aggression in the Elderly." *Journal of Clinical Psychiatry* 51 (10 suppl):22–28, 1990. Copyright 1990, Physicians Postgraduate Press. Used with permission.

Table 42–11. Use of lorazepam in the acute management of agitation or aggression

1. Initiate lorazepam—1–2 mg orally or intramuscularly.
2. Repeat dose every hour until agitation or aggression is controlled.
3. If intravenous dose must be given, push slowly! Do not exceed 2 mg (1 mL) per minute to avoid respiratory depression and laryngospasm; may be repeated in 30 minutes if required.
4. When patient is no longer agitated or violent, maintain dose at maximum of 2 mg orally or intramuscularly every 4 hours.
5. When patient is not agitated or violent for 48 hours, taper at rate of 10% of highest total daily dose.
6. If agitation or violent behavior reemerges while tapering drug, reevaluate etiology and consider switching to a more specific medication to manage chronic aggression.
7. After 6 weeks, if lorazepam cannot be tapered without reemergence of agitation or aggression, reevaluate and revise treatment plan to include a more specific medication to manage chronic behavioral dysfunction.

Source. Adapted from Yudofsky SC, Silver JM, Hales RE: "Pharmacologic Management of Aggression in the Elderly." *Journal of Clinical Psychiatry* 51 (10 suppl):22–28, 1990. Copyright 1990, Physicians Postgraduate Press. Used with permission.

In a randomized, double-blind study, Lenox et al. (1992) compared lorazepam with haloperidol in the treatment of manic agitation in 20 hospitalized patients with bipolar disorder who were also taking lithium. The investigators found no significant difference in the treatment groups in the degree of or time to response.

Other categories of medication. Other medications such as paraldehyde, chloral hydrate, and diphenhydramine may also be prescribed to sedate patients with acute agitation or aggression. However, in general, benzodiazepines and neuroleptics are the preferred medications because they are safe and convenient and because their use, benefits, and risks are familiar to psychiatrists and hospital staff.

The scientific literature is replete with case reports of a broad range of medications that mitigate acute agitation or aggression in special clinical circumstances. For example, a study by Gualtieri et al. (1989) reported that amantadine, a dopamine agonist, reduced aggressive behavior in patients recovering from traumatic brain injury. Intensive care specialists who treat the medical sequelae of trauma may use succinylcholine with requisite ventilatory support to induce pharmacological paralysis in patients in intensive care units who have severe agitation following traumatic brain injury or surgical procedures. Clearly, the application of such interventions is best limited to those professionals who, by virtue of their subspecialty focus, have sufficient experience and resources necessary to use these novel approaches safely in the treatment of acute agitation and aggression.

Pharmacological Management of Chronic Agitation and Aggression

When patients' agitation and aggression persist beyond several weeks, *maintenance approaches* should be considered. We advocate that the decision about the choice of the specific psychopharmacological agent be guided by the determination of the underlying illness that causes the chronic behavior and by the co-occurrence of other psychiatric symptoms such as anxiety, mania, or depression. Table 42–12 outlines our approach to the pharmacological treatment of chronic agitation or aggression.

Antipsychotic medications. As we discussed earlier in this chapter, restricting the use of antipsychotic medications to the treatment of agitation or aggression that is directly related to psychotic ideation or perception, such as paranoid delusions or command hallucinations, is generally clinically indicated. The clinician should attempt to taper the antipsychotic agent at regular intervals to gauge its efficacy in treating both the psychosis and the atten-

Table 42–12.   Psychopharmacological treatment of chronic agitation or aggression

Medication class	Indications	Side effects and special clinical considerations
Antipsychotic	Agitation or aggression secondary to psychotic symptoms	Oversedation, akathisias, multiple extrapyramidal side effects
Antianxiety		
Benzodiazepines	Comorbid anxiety symptoms	Oversedation, confusion, paradoxical rage, dependency
Buspirone	Comorbid anxiety and/or depression	Delayed onset of action (3–5 weeks)
Anticonvulsant	Seizure disorder, organic brain syndrome, manic states	Bone marrow suppression, hepatoxicity
Carbamazepine		
Valproate		
Antimanic	Manic excitement, bipolar disorder, cyclothymia	Neurotoxicity and confusion
Lithium		
Valproate		
Cardiovascular	Organic brain syndromes	Delayed onset of action (4–6 weeks)
Propranolol (and other β-blockers)		
Antidepressant		
SSRIs	Depression; mood lability; irritability	Require standard doses for treatment of depression
Trazodone	Depression with insomnia	Oversedation, brief half-life

Note.   SSRIs = selective serotonin reuptake inhibitors.
Source.   Adapted from Yudofsky SC, Silver JM, Hales RE: "Pharmacologic Management of Aggression in the Elderly." *Journal of Clinical Psychiatry* 51 (10 suppl):22–28, 1990. Copyright 1990, Physicians Postgraduate Press. Used with permission.

dant agitation and aggression in such patients. If the agitated or aggressive behavior persists in the absence of psychosis, or if the psychosis is unaffected by the discontinuation of the antipsychotic medication, other approaches to the pharmacotherapy of agitation and aggression must be considered.

The Omnibus Budget Reconciliation Act (OBRA) of 1987 was designed to curtail the overuse and misuse of antipsychotics in elderly persons in intermediate-care and skilled nursing homes. This federal ruling specifically prohibited the use of neuroleptics to treat agitation. In a retrospective cohort study of residents in a large intermediate-care facility, Semla and colleagues (1994) found that agitation was the most common clinical condition for which antipsychotics were prescribed prior to OBRA regulations. It is important to emphasize that these OBRA regulations that now mandate how physicians prescribe antipsychotics and benzodiazepines in nursing home residents came about because of misuse of these agents in the treatment of agitation and aggression in the elderly. There are far-reaching public policy implications of this initiative and important messages for American medicine. Because most physicians failed to realize that, as with delirium, the underlying causes, as well as the target symptoms, of agitation and aggression must be diagnosed and treated and because they failed to use safe and ef-

fective medications in appropriate doses for responsible durations, governmental control was necessary.

Antianxiety medications.   Various case reports and prospective studies have reported that buspirone, a serotonin-1A (5-HT$_{1A}$) agonist, was effective in the management of aggression and agitation associated with brain disorders (Colenda 1988; Gualtieri 1991; Ratey et al. 1992a; Stanislav et al. 1994; Tiller et al. 1988) and developmental disabilities and autism (Ratey et al. 1989, 1991; Realmuto et al. 1989). Because we have observed that some patients become more agitated or aggressive in the initial phases of treatment with buspirone, we advocate beginning treatment at low doses (e.g., 5 mg twice a day) and increasing the dose by 5 mg every 3–5 days. Doses ranging from 45 to 60 mg/day and a latency of 3–6 weeks may be required before therapeutic effects are observed.

Although no double-blind, controlled studies of clonazepam in the management of chronic agitation or aggression have been done, several case reports indicate that it was beneficial in the treatment of agitation in elderly persons (Freinhar and Alvarez 1986) and in a patient with schizophrenia and seizures (Keats and Mukherjee 1988). We also prescribe clonazepam when agitation or aggression occurs in patients with pronounced anxiety or with neurologically induced tics and disinhibited motor behavior. Initial dosages are 0.5 mg twice a day and rarely exceed a total daily dose of 6 mg. Oversedation is the most common side effect, and daytime sedation may be mitigated by prescribing a single dose before bedtime.

Anticonvulsant medications. Overall, we prioritize the use of anticonvulsant medications, particularly carbamazepine and valproate, for the treatment of chronic agitation or aggression that is associated with seizure disorders or manic affects. Anticonvulsants are our second choice to β-blockers for disruptive behaviors related to diffuse neuronal destruction (e.g., those that occur subsequent to traumatic brain injury, middle cerebral artery stroke, and Alzheimer's disease).

One nonrandomized, placebo-controlled crossover study of 25 patients with dementia showed that low doses of carbamazepine (modal dose of 300 mg/day) reduced agitated behavior in some patients (Tariot et al. 1994). Several open studies indicated that carbamazepine may be effective in reducing aggressive behavior associated with organic brain disorders (Mattes 1988), schizophrenia (Hakoloa and Laulumaa 1982; Luchins 1983), developmental disabilities (Folks et al. 1982; Yatham and McHale 1988), and dementia (Gleason and Schneider 1990; Leibovici and Tariot 1988; Lemke 1995). Carbamazepine has also been used in combination with other medications to treat agitation and aggression. Lemke (1995) conducted an open, prospective study of 15 elderly patients with Alzheimer's disease whose severe agitation had not responded to neuroleptics. When carbamazepine was combined with haloperidol, a "significant improvement" was reported after 4 weeks of treatment. We use carbamazepine to treat agitation and aggression in the same doses and with the same blood levels that we use in the treatment of bipolar disorder.

Several studies have reported that valproate is efficacious in the treatment of agitation and aggression in patients with a wide variety of medical disorders. Most of these studies were published as case reports of valproate's usefulness in reducing agitation and aggression in patients with dementias and other organic brain syndromes (Giakas et al. 1990; Kahn et al. 1988; Lemke 1995; Mattes 1992; Mellow et al. 1993). Loft et al. (1995) conducted an open-label trial of 10 elderly nursing home patients with dementia and agitation. These patients were prospectively treated with valproate at doses ranging from 375 to 750 mg/day. Eight of the patients had a 50% or greater reduction in the frequency of agitation, and the intensity of the behavioral outbursts also diminished in many of these patients. Valproate was well tolerated by all patients in this study. Because of valproate's favorable side-effect profile (e.g., lower incidence of ataxia, rashes, behavioral changes), we prefer to use valproate rather than carbamazepine in the treatment of agitation and aggression.

Antimanic medications. Because aggressive behavior may be present in the manic state of bipolar disorder and because agitation is a frequent concomitant of both manic and depressed states, mood-stabilizing medications such as lithium and valproate (Wilcox 1994) treat these behaviors by treating the underlying illness. In addition, many reports suggest that lithium is of value in the treatment of agitation and aggression in patients without bipolar illness but with other specific underlying medical disorders. Included in this group are patients who have mental retardation with self-directed aggression (Luchins and Dojka 1989) or aggression toward others (Dale 1980) and patients who have traumatic brain injury (Haas and Cope 1985). Aggressive people from special segments of the population such as children and adolescents (Vetro et al. 1976) or prison inmates (Sheard et al. 1976) also have been reported to respond to lithium. Our clinical group limits the use of lithium to the treatment of agitation and aggression in patients with mania. The dosages and blood levels of lithium we use are the same as those recommended for nonagitated patients with bipolar disorder. One caveat, however, is that many patients with brain injury have increased sensitivity to the neurotoxic effects of lithium (Hornstein and Seliger 1989; Moskowitz and Altshuler 1991) and, therefore, must be followed up very closely with neuropsychiatric examinations and serum lithium level measurements.

Antidepressant medications. Although many antidepressants have been suggested for the treatment of agitation and aggression in patients with a wide range of neuropsychiatric disorders, most of these medications act either preferentially or specifically on the serotonergic system of the brain. Amitriptyline (Jackson et al. 1985; Szlabowicz and Stewart 1990) and trazodone (Lebert et al. 1994; Pinner and Rich 1988) have been reported to be useful in the treatment of agitation and aggression; however, most recent reports focus on the use of the selective serotonin reuptake inhibitors (SSRIs) (Albritton and Borison 1995; Bass and Beltis 1991; Coccaro et al. 1990; Fava et al. 1993). We have used SSRIs to treat agitation and aggression associated with brain lesions successfully and have found this category of antidepressant to be especially effective in patients with concomitant depression or dysthymia. We initiate treatment with relatively low doses (e.g., 10 mg of fluoxetine, 25 mg of sertraline, 50 mg of nefazodone). If effects are not achieved over a period of several weeks, we gradually increase the dose to relatively high ranges (e.g., 80–100 mg/day of fluoxetine, up to 200–300 mg/day of sertraline, 400 mg/day of nefazodone). For patients without comorbid depression, we prefer to prescribe β-blockers or anticonvulsants before initiating a trial of antidepressants.

Although we just reviewed the use of antidepressants to treat agitation that stems from disorders other than depression, clinicians should be aware that depression is underdiagnosed, occurs in all age groups, and presents in atypical ways that include symptoms of agitation and aggression. For these patients, the accurate diagnosis of and a multifaceted treatment approach to depression are more critical than the specific agent chosen. Friedman et al. (1992) identified 17 of 154 elderly patients in a Canadian chronic-care facility who had disruptive vocalizations. Eight had a previous diagnosis of depression but were not taking antidepressants. Five of these patients who were given the antidepressant doxepin had significant reductions in their noisiness and agitation. We interpret the results of this study to mean that the agitation and disruptive vocalizations of patients with untreated depression are best addressed by treating the underlying mood disorder with antidepressants.

β-Blockers.   More than 15 years have passed since β-blockers were first reported to be effective in treating chronic aggression in adults and children with organic brain syndromes (Yudofsky et al. 1981, 1984). Subsequently, more than 25 papers have been published in the neurological and psychiatric literature that report on the use of β-blockers to treat aggression (Silver and Yudofsky 1994b). The β-blockers that have been shown to have therapeutic effects in prospective, placebo-controlled studies include propranolol (a lipid-soluble, nonselective receptor antagonist) (Brooke et al. 1992b; Greendyke et al. 1986; Mattes 1988), nadolol (a water-soluble, nonselective receptor antagonist) (Brooke et al. 1992b; Greendyke et al. 1986; Mattes 1988; Ratey et al. 1992b), and pindolol (a lipid-soluble, nonselective antagonist with partial sympathomimetic activity) (Greendyke and Kanter 1986). Because much of this evidence from the scientific literature suggests that β-adrenergic receptor antagonists are specific and effective agents for the treatment of agitation and aggression in patients with organic brain syndromes, and because of our own extensive clinical experience with β-blockers to treat aggressive patients with neuropsychiatric disorders, this approach has become our "first line" of treatment of neurologically induced agitation and aggression.

Our guidelines for the clinical use of propranolol for treatment of agitation and aggression are summarized in Table 42–13 (Silver and Yudofsky 1987a). Several key clinical points are related to the use of propranolol:

■ Peripheral effects of β-blockade (e.g., lowered blood pressure, bradycardia) are frequently saturated when the patient achieves a dose of approximately 280 mg/day. If orthostatic hypotension occurs, one measure should be to ensure that the patient's salt

Table 42–13.   Clinical use of propranolol in the management of chronic agitation or aggression

1. Conduct a thorough medical examination.
2. Exclude patients with bronchial asthma, chronic obstructive pulmonary disease, insulin-dependent diabetes mellitus, congestive heart failure, persistent angina, significant peripheral vascular disease, and hyperthyroidism.
3. Avoid sudden discontinuation of propranolol (particularly in patients with hypertension).
4. Begin with a single test dose of 20 mg/day in patients in whom hypotension or bradycardia are clinical concerns. Increase the dose by 20 mg/day every 3 days.
5. Administer 20 mg of propranolol three times a day in patients without cardiovascular or cardiopulmonary disorder.
6. Increase the dose of propranolol by 60 mg/day every 3 days.
7. Increase medication unless the pulse rate declines to less than 50 beats per minute or systolic blood pressure is lower than 90 mm Hg.
8. Do not administer medication if severe dizziness, ataxia, or wheezing occurs. Reduce or discontinue propranolol if such symptoms persist.
9. Increase the dose of propranolol to 12 mg/kg or until agitated or aggressive behavior is controlled.
10. Doses of greater than 800 mg are not usually required to control aggressive behavior.
11. Continue administration of the highest dose of propranolol for at least 8 weeks before concluding that the patient is not responding to the medication. Some patients, however, may respond rapidly to propranolol.
12. Use caution when prescribing concurrent medications. Monitor plasma levels of all antipsychotic and anticonvulsant medications.

Source.   Reprinted from Silver JM, Hales RE, Yudofsky SC: "Neuropsychiatric Aspects of Traumatic Brain Injury," in *The American Psychiatric Press Textbook of Neuropsychiatry,* 3rd Edition. Edited by Yudofsky SC, Hales RE. Washington, DC, American Psychiatric Press, 1997, p. 546. Copyright 1997, American Psychiatric Press. Used with permission.

Table 42–14. Pharmacological characteristics of β-adrenergic receptor antagonists

Drug name (by receptor selectivity)	Trade name	Potency[a]	Local anesthetic activity	Intrinsic sympathomimetic activity	Lipid solubility	Plasma half-life (hours)
Nonselective (β₁ and β₂) antagonists						
Alprenolol	Aptine	0.3–1.0	+	+ +	+ +	2–3
Nadolol	Corgard	0.5	0	0	0	14–18
Pindolol	Visken	5.0–10.0	±	+ +	+	3–4
Propranolol	Inderal	1.0	+ +	0	+ +	3–5
Sotalol	Sotalex	0.3	0	0	0	5–12
Timolol	Blockadren	5.0–10.0	0	±	0	4
Selective (β₁) antagonists						
Acebutolol	Sectral	0.3	+	+	0	3
Atenolol	Tenormin	1.0	0	0	0	6–8
Metoprolol	Lopressor	0.5–2.0	±	0	+	3–4

Note. 0 = none; ± = questionable; + = intermediate; + + = significant.
[a]Propranolol = 1.
Source. Data from Hoffman and Lefkowitz 1990 and American Medical Association Division of Drugs 1986.

intake is adequate because many contemporary diets encourage the avoidance of salt. Thereafter, increasing the β-blocker dose is not usually associated with cardiovascular side effects.

■ Encouragement and support of the family and other members of the treatment team by the clinician are an essential component of care because of the long latency of 6–8 weeks before a therapeutic response occurs.

■ Controlled trials and our own extensive clinical experience indicate that depression is a rare side effect of use of β-blockers, despite reports that depression is commonly associated with their use (Yudofsky 1992).

■ The combination of propranolol and thioridazine should be avoided whenever possible because the use of propranolol is associated with a significant increase in plasma levels of thioridazine, which has an absolute dosage ceiling of 800 mg/day (Silver et al. 1986). The pharmacological characteristics of β-blockers are summarized in Table 42–14.

CONCLUSION

Agitation and aggression occur commonly and have serious and far-reaching consequences for patients with respect to their functioning at home, at work, and in other social settings. When assessing patients who have these behaviors, the clinician should focus on careful history

taking, thorough physical examination, and relevant laboratory testing to diagnose any medical condition that could underlie and/or aggravate the symptoms.

Although pharmacological treatment of agitation and aggression may be highly effective, medications for this purpose should be used in the context of a carefully crafted treatment plan involving the full range of biopsychosocial approaches. When medications are used to treat acute agitation or aggression, the sedative side effects of antipsychotics or benzodiazepines are commonly required. However, prolonged use of neuroleptics or benzodiazepines frequently leads to disabling side effects and, therefore, should be avoided for the treatment of chronic disruptive behaviors. A wide range of medications are helpful in the prophylaxis of chronic agitation and aggression. The underlying etiology of the symptomatologies guides the choice of the specific pharmacological agent for the treatment of chronic behavioral disturbances.

REFERENCES

Albritton J, Borison R: Paroxetine treatment of anger associated with depression. J Nerv Ment Dis 183:666–667, 1995

Alexander RW, Davis JN, Lefkowitz RJ: Direct identification and characterization of β-adrenergic receptors in rat brain. Nature 258:437–440, 1979

American Psychiatric Association: Diagnostic and Statistical Manual of Mental Disorders, 3rd Edition. Washington, DC, American Psychiatric Association, 1980

American Psychiatric Association: Diagnostic and Statistical Manual of Mental Disorders, 3rd Edition, Revised. Washington, DC, American Psychiatric Association, 1987

American Psychiatric Association: Diagnostic and Statistical Manual of Mental Disorders, 4th Edition. Washington, DC, American Psychiatric Association, 1994

Bareggi SR, Porta M, Selentati A, et al: Homovanillic acid and 5-hydroxyindole-acetic acid in the CSF of patients after a severe head injury, I: lumbar CSF concentration in chronic brain post-traumatic syndromes. Eur Neurol 13:528–544, 1975

Bass JN, Beltis J: Therapeutic effect of fluoxetine on naltrexone-resistant self-injurious behavior in an adolescent with mental retardation. Journal of Child and Adolescent Psychopharmacology 1:331–340, 1991

Bick PA, Hannah AL: Intramuscular lorazepam to restrain violent patients (letter). Lancet 1:206, 1986

Blackburn JR, Pfaus JG, Phillips AG: Dopamine functions in appetitive and defensive behaviors. Prog Neurobiol 39:247–279, 1992

Brooke MM, Questad KA, Patterson R, et al: Agitation and restlessness after closed head injury: a prospective study of 100 consecutive admissions. Arch Phys Med Rehabil 73:320–323, 1992a

Brooke MM, Patterson DR, Questad KA, et al: The treatment of agitation during initial hospitalization after traumatic brain injury. Arch Phys Med Rehabil 73:917–921, 1992b

Brown GL, Goodwin FK, Ballenger JC, et al: Aggression in human correlates with cerebrospinal fluid amine metabolites. Psychiatry Res 1:131–139, 1979

Chandler JD, Chandler JE: The prevalence of neuropsychiatric disorders in a nursing home population. J Geriatr Psychiatry Neurol 1:71–76, 1988

Coccaro EF: Impulsive aggression and central serotonergic system function in humans: an example of a dimensional brain-behavioral relationship. Int J Clin Psychopharmacol 7:3–12, 1992

Coccaro EF, Astill JL, Herbert JL, et al: Fluoxetine treatment of impulsive aggression in DSM-III-R personality disorder patients. J Clin Psychopharmacol 10:373–375, 1990

Coccaro EF, Kavoussi RJ, Lesser J: Self- and other-directed human aggression: the role of the central serotonergic system. Int J Clin Psychopharmacol 6 (suppl 6):70–83, 1992

Cohen SA, Underwood MT: The use of clozapine in a mentally retarded and aggressive population. J Clin Psychiatry 55:440–444, 1994

Colenda CC: Buspirone in treatment of agitated demented patients (letter). Lancet 1:1169, 1988

Corrigan PW, Yudofsky SC, Silver JM: Pharmacological and behavioral treatments for aggressive psychiatric inpatients. Hosp Community Psychiatry 44:125–133, 1993

Dale PG: Lithium therapy in aggressive mentally subnormal patients. Br J Psychiatry 137:469–474, 1980

Eichelman BS: Effect of subcortical lesions on shock-induced aggression in the rat following 7-hydroxydopamine administration. Journal of Comparative and Physiologic Psychology 74:331–339, 1971

Eichelman B: Neurochemical and psychopharmacologic aspects of aggressive behavior, in Psychopharmacology: The Third Generation of Progress. Edited by Meltzer HY. New York, Raven, 1987, pp 697–704

Eichelman B, Thoa NB, Ng KY: Facilitated aggression in the rat following 6-hydroxydopamine administration. Physiol Behav 8:1–3, 1972

Elliott FA: The neurology of explosive rage. Practitioner 217:51–59, 1976

Elliott FA: Violence: the neurologic contribution: an overview. Arch Neurol 49:595–603, 1992

Fava M, Rosenbaum JF, Pava JA, et al: Anger attacks in unipolar depression, part 1: clinical correlates and response to fluoxetine treatment. Am J Psychiatry 150:1158–1163, 1993

Folks DG, King LD, Dowdy SB, et al: Carbamazepine treatment of selective affectively disordered inpatients. Am J Psychiatry 139:115–117, 1982

Freinhar JP, Alvarez WA: Clonazepam treatment of organic brain syndromes in three elderly patients. J Clin Psychiatry 47:525–526, 1986

Friedman R, Gryfe CI, Tal DT, et al: The noisy elderly patient: prevalence, assessment, and response to the antidepressant doxepin. J Geriatr Psychiatry Neurol 5:187–191, 1992

Ghosh TB, Victor BS: Suicide, in American Psychiatric Press Textbook of Psychiatry, 2nd Edition. Edited by Hales RE, Yudofsky SC, Talbott JA. Washington, DC, American Psychiatric Press, 1994, pp 1251–1271

Giakas WJ, Seibyl JP, Mazure CM: Valproate in the treatment of temper outbursts (letter). J Clin Psychiatry 51:525, 1990

Gleason RP, Schneider LS: Carbamazepine treatment of agitation in Alzheimer's outpatients refractory to neuroleptics. J Clin Psychiatry 51:115–118, 1990

Greendyke RM, Kanter DR: Therapeutic effects of pindolol on behavioral disturbances associated with organic brain disease: a double-blind study. J Clin Psychiatry 47:423–426, 1986

Greendyke RM, Kanter DR, Schuster DB, et al: Propranolol treatment of assaultive patients with organic brain disease: a double-blind crossover, placebo-controlled study. J Nerv Ment Dis 174:290–294, 1986

Gualtieri CT: Buspirone for the behavior problems of patients with organic brain disorders. J Clin Psychopharmacol 11:280–281, 1991

Gualtieri CT, Chandler M, Coons TB, et al: Amantadine: a new clinical profile for traumatic brain injury. Clin Neuropharmacol 12:258–270, 1989

Haas JF, Cope N: Neuropharmacologic management of behavior sequelae in head injury: a case report. Arch Phys Med Rehabil 66:472–474, 1985

Hakoloa HP, Laulumaa VA: Carbamazepine in treatment of violent schizophrenics (letter). Lancet 1:1358, 1982

Hamill RW, Woolf PD, McDonald JV, et al: Catecholamines predict outcome in traumatic brain injury. Ann Neurol 21:438–443, 1987

Herrera JN, Sramek JJ, Costa JF, et al: High potency neuroleptics and violence in schizophrenics. J Nerv Ment Dis 176:558–561, 1988

Higley JD, Mehlman PT, Taum DM, et al: Cerebrospinal fluid monoamine and adrenal correlates of aggression in free-ranging rhesus monkeys. Arch Gen Psychiatry 49:436–441, 1992

Hoffman BB, Lefkowitz RJ: Adrenergic receptor antagonists, in Goodman and Gilman's The Pharmacological Basis of Therapeutics, 8th Edition. Edited by Gilman AG, Rall TW, Neiw AS, et al. New York, Pergamon, 1990, pp 221–243

Hornstein A, Seliger G: Cognitive side effects of lithium in closed head injury (letter). J Neuropsychiatry Clin Neurosci 1:446–447, 1989

Jackson RD, Corrigan JD, Arnett JA: Amitriptyline for agitation in head injury. Arch Phys Med Rehabil 66:180–181, 1985

Kahn D, Stevenson E, Douglas CJ: Effect of sodium valproate in three patients with organic brain syndromes. Am J Psychiatry 145:1010–1011, 1988

Keats MM, Mukherjee S: Antiaggressive effect of adjunctive clonazepam in schizophrenia associated with seizure disorder. J Clin Psychiatry 49:117–118, 1988

Kruesi MJ, Rapoport JL, Hamburger S, et al: Cerebrospinal fluid monoamine metabolites, aggression, and impulsivity in disruptive behavior disorders of children and adolescents. Arch Gen Psychiatry 47:419–426, 1990

Kruesi MJP, Hibbs ED, Zahn TP, et al: A 2-year prospective follow-up study of children and adolescents with disruptive behavior disorders: prediction by cerebrospinal fluid 5-hydroxyindoleacetic acid, homovanillic acid, and autonomic measures. Arch Gen Psychiatry 49:429–435, 1992

Leavitt ML, Yudofsky SC, Maroon JC, et al: Effect of intraventricular nadolol infusion on shock-induced aggression in 6-hydroxydopamine-treated rats. J Neuropsychiatry Clin Neurosci 1:167–172, 1989

Lebert F, Pasquier F, Petit H: Behavioral effects of trazodone in Alzheimer's disease. J Clin Psychiatry 55:536–538, 1994

Leibovici A, Tariot PN: Carbamazepine treatment of agitation associated with dementia. J Geriatr Psychiatry Neurol l:110–112, 1988

Lemke MR: Effect of carbamazepine on agitation in Alzheimer's inpatients refractory to neuroleptics. J Clin Psychiatry 56:354–357, 1995

Lenox RH, Newhouse PA, Creelman WL, et al: Adjunctive treatment of manic agitation with lorazepam versus haloperidol: a double-blind study. J Clin Psychiatry 53:47–52, 1992

Linnoila VMI, Virkkunen M: Aggression, suicidality, and serotonin. J Clin Psychiatry 53 (10 suppl):46–51, 1992

Lott AD, McElroy SL, Keys MA: Valproate in the treatment of behavioral agitation in elderly patients with dementia. J Neuropsychiatry Clin Neurosci 7:314–319, 1995

Luchins DJ: Carbamazepine for the violent psychiatric patient (letter). Lancet 2:755, 1983

Luchins DJ, Dojka D: Lithium and propranolol in aggression and self-injurious behavior in the mentally retarded. Psychopharmacol Bull 25:372–375, 1989

Malmquist CP: Homicide: A Psychiatric Perspective. Washington, DC, American Psychiatric Press, 1996

Mattes JA: Carbamazepine vs propranolol for rage outbursts. Psychopharmacol Bull 24:179–182, 1988

Mattes JA: Valproic acid for nonaffective aggression in the mentally retarded. J Nerv Ment Dis 180:601–602, 1992

Mellow AM, Solano-Lopez C, Davis S: Sodium valproate in the treatment of behavioral disturbance in dementia. J Geriatr Psychiatry Neurol 6:205–209, 1993

Michals ML, Crismon ML, Roberts S, et al: Clozapine response and adverse affects in nine brain-injured patients. J Clin Psychopharmacol 13:198–203, 1993

Monahan J: Mental disorder and violent behavior: perceptions and evidence. Am Psychol 47:511–521, 1992

Moskowitz AS, Altshuler L: Increased sensitivity to lithium-induced neurotoxicity after stroke: a case report. J Clin Psychopharmacol 11:272–273, 1991

Oddy M, Caughlan T, Tyerman A, et al: Social adjustment after closed head injury: a further follow-up seven years after injury. J Neurol Neurosurg Psychiatry 44:564–568, 1985

Ovsiew F, Yudofsky SC: Aggression: a neuropsychiatric perspective, in Rage, Power and Aggression. Edited by Glick RA, Roose SP. New Haven, CT, Yale University Press, 1993, pp 213–230

Pinner E, Rich CL: Effects of trazodone on aggressive behavior in seven patients with organic mental disorders. Am J Psychiatry 145:1295–1296, 1988

Rabins PV, Mace NL, Lucas MJ: The impact of dementia on the family. JAMA 248:333–335, 1982

Rao N, Jellinek HM, Woolson DC: Agitation in closed head injury: haloperidol effects on rehabilitation outcome. Arch Phys Med Rehabil 66:30–34, 1985

Ratey J, Sovner R, Mikkelsen E, et al: Buspirone therapy for maladaptive behavior and anxiety in developmentally disabled persons. J Clin Psychiatry 50:382–384, 1989

Ratey J, Sovner R, Parks A, et al: Buspirone treatment of aggression and anxiety in mentally retarded patients: a multiple-baseline, placebo lead-in study. J Clin Psychiatry 52:159–162, 1991

Ratey JJ, Leveroni CL, Miller AC, et al: Low-dose buspirone to treat agitation and maladaptive behavior in brain-injured patients: two case reports. J Clin Psychopharmacol 12:362–364, 1992a

Ratey JJ, Sorgi P, O'Driscoll GA, et al: Nadolol to treat aggression and psychiatric symptomatology in chronic psychiatric inpatients: a double-blind, placebo-controlled study. J Clin Psychiatry 53:41–46, 1992b

Realmuto FM, August GJ, Garfinkel BD: Clinical effect of buspirone in autistic children. J Clin Psychopharmacol 9:122–124, 1989

Reid HW, Bollinger MF, Edwards G: Assaults in hospital. Bull Am Acad Psychiatry Law 13:1–4, 1985

Reisberg B, Borenstein J, Salob SP, et al: Behavioral symptoms in Alzheimer's disease: phenomenology and treatment. J Clin Psychiatry 48 (5 suppl):9–15, 1987

Rovner BW, Kavonek S, Filipp L, et al: Prevalence of mental illness in a community nursing home. Am J Psychiatry 143:1446–1449, 1986

Semla TP, Palla K, Poddig B, et al: Effect of the Omnibus Reconciliation Act 1987 on antipsychotic prescribing in nursing home residents. J Am Geriatr Soc 42:648–652, 1994

Sheard MH, Marini JL, Bridges C, et al: The effects of lithium in impulsive aggressive behavior in man. Am J Psychiatry 133:1409–1413, 1976

Silver JM, Yudofsky SC: Aggressive behavior in patients with neuropsychiatric disorders: the scope of the problem. Psychiatric Annals 17:367–370, 1987a

Silver JM, Yudofsky SC: Documentation of aggression in the assessment of the violent patient. Psychiatric Annals 17:375–384, 1987b

Silver JM, Yudofsky SC: The Overt Aggression Scale: overview and guiding principles. J Neuropsychiatry Clin Neurosci 3 (suppl 1):S22–S29, 1991

Silver JM, Yudofsky SC: Aggressive disorders, in Neuropsychiatry of Traumatic Brain Injury. Edited by Silver JM, Yudofsky SC, Hales RE. Washington, DC, American Psychiatric Press, 1994a, pp 313–353

Silver JM, Yudofsky SC: Pharmacology, in Neuropsychiatry of Traumatic Brain Injury. Edited by Silver JM, Yudofsky SC, Hales RE. Washington, DC, American Psychiatric Press, 1994b, pp 631–670

Silver JM, Yudofsky S, Kogan M, et al: Elevation of thioridazine plasma levels by propranolol. Am J Psychiatry 143:1290–1292, 1986

Stanislav SW, Fabre T, Crismon ML, et al: Buspirone's efficacy in organic-induced aggression. J Clin Psychopharmacol 14:126–130, 1994

Szlabowicz JW, Stewart JT: Amitriptyline treatment of agitation associated with anoxic encephalopathy. Arch Phys Med Rehabil 71:612–613, 1990

Tardiff K: A survey of assault by chronic patients, in Assaults Within Psychiatric Facilities. Edited by Lion JR, Reid WH. New York, Grune & Stratton, 1983, pp 3–19

Tardiff K: Foreword to violence and the violent patient, in Psychiatric Update: American Psychiatric Association Annual Review, Vol 6. Edited by Hales RE, Frances AJ. Washington, DC, American Psychiatric Press, 1987, pp 447–450

Tardiff K, Sweillam A: The occurrence of assaultive behavior among chronic psychiatric inpatients. Am J Psychiatry 139:212–215, 1982

Tariot PN, Erb R, Leibovici A, et al: Carbamazepine treatment of agitation in nursing home patients with dementia: a preliminary study. J Am Geriatr Soc 42:1160–1166, 1994

Tiller JWG, Dakis JA, Shaw JM: Short-term buspirone treatment in disinhibition with dementia (letter). Lancet 2:510, 1988

Valzelli L: Psychobiology of Aggression and Violence. New York, Raven, 1981

Vetro A, Szentistvanyi L, Pallag M, et al: Therapeutic experience with lithium in childhood aggressivity. Pharmacopsychiatry 133:1409–1413, 1976

Wetzler S, Kahn RS, Asnis GM, et al: Serotonin receptor sensitivity and aggression. Psychiatry Res 37:271–279, 1991

Wilcox J: Divalproex sodium in the treatment of aggressive behavior. Ann Clin Psychiatry 6(1):17–20, 1994

Yatham LN, McHale PA: Carbamazepine in the treatment of aggression: a case report and a review of the literature. Acta Psychiatr Scand 78:188–190, 1988

Yudofsky SC: Psychoanalysis, psychopharmacology, and the influence of neuropsychiatry. J Neuropsychiatry Clin Neurosci 3:1–5, 1991

Yudofsky SC: β-Blockers and depression: the clinician's dilemma. JAMA 267:1826–1827, 1992

Yudofsky SC, Williams D, Gorman J: Propranolol in the treatment of rage and violent behavior in patients with organic brain syndromes. Am J Psychiatry 138:218–220, 1981

Yudofsky SC, Stevens L, Silver J, et al: Propranolol in the treatment of rage and violent behavior associated with 5 patients with Korsakoff's psychosis. Am J Psychiatry 141:114–115, 1984

Yudofsky SC, Silver JM, Jackson M, et al: The Overt Aggression Scale: an operationalized rating scale for verbal and physical aggression. Am J Psychiatry 143:35–39, 1986

Yudofsky SC, Silver J, Yudofsky B: Organic personality disorder, explosive type, in Treatments of Psychiatric Disorders: A Task Force Report of the American Psychiatric Association. Washington, DC, American Psychiatric Association, 1989, pp 839–852

Yudofsky SC, Silver JM, Hales RE: Pharmacologic management of aggression in the elderly. J Clin Psychiatry 51 (10 suppl):1–58, 1990

Yudofsky SC, Kopecky HJ, Kunik M, et al: The Overt Agitation Severity Scale for the objective rating of agitation. J Neuropsychiatry Clin Neurosci 9:541–548, 1997

FORTY-THREE

Treatment of Personality Disorders

Robert L. Trestman, Ph.D., M.D., Ann Marie Woo-Ming, M.D.,
Marie deVegvar, M.D., and Larry J. Siever, M.D.

Although pharmacotherapy has long been a therapeutic mainstay of the major Axis I syndromes, more recently, psychopharmacology has gained acceptance as a treatment option for severe personality disorders. This shift reflects the fact that personality disorders have historically been explained in terms of psychodynamic and developmental models that imply that psychotherapy, whether individual, group, or milieu, would be the major or even sole form of treatment. However, the important role of biological factors in the pathogenesis of personality disorders is increasingly appreciated. By definition, a *personality disorder* is constituted by enduring maladaptive symptoms or behaviors that have an early onset and persist without periods of remission. More recently, it has been viewed that this very pattern may actually represent chronic disorders in mood, impulsivity, aggression, cognition, or anxiety. This so-called dimensional approach to character disorders has been supported by research suggesting biological correlates of these various dimensions, as discussed later in this chapter (see also Kirrane and Siever, Chapter 33, in this volume). In turn, the use of psychopharmacology has more fully emerged as a treatment of personality disorders, for example, by targeting affective instability as one would in a chronic affective disorder.

Furthermore, the specific etiology of the disorder may not necessarily determine its treatment: whether symptoms of anxiety or depression evolved from environmental circumstances or from underlying genetic susceptibilities, they may nonetheless be amenable to psychopharmacological treatment. Thus, the clinician working with individuals with personality disorders must be aware of the important role pharmacological treatment may play in these disorders.

Pioneering studies of patients with personality disorders showed that pharmacological interventions used in affective and schizophrenic disorders might be of benefit (Klein 1968; Klein and Greenberg 1967; Liebowitz and Klein 1981; Rifkin et al. 1972b). However, years passed before the field made use of these early findings; for example, disorders such as cyclothymia were still considered a personality disorder. More recent studies that categorized syndromes with DSM-III-R or DSM-IV (American Psychiatric Association 1987, 1994) criteria, in conjunction with work focused on clinical dimensions, suggested that pharmacological intervention may be beneficial in personality disorders for affective symptoms, including affective

The authors' research was supported in part by grants from the National Institutes of Health, National Center for Research Resources (RR00071) to the Mt. Sinai Medical Center, National Institutes of Mental Health (R01-MH41131), and Department of Veterans Affairs Merit Award (7609004).

instability or transient depression, impulsivity/aggression, psychotic-like symptoms or cognitive/perceptual distortions, and anxiety. These results are complemented by evidence implicating both genetic and biological factors in the pathogenesis of these disorders. A growing body of studies suggests that genetic factors play an important role in the development of normal personality (Goldsmith 1982; Tellegen et al. 1988). Although the heritability of the personality disorders has been less extensively studied, twin studies (Torgersen 1984), adoptive studies (Cloninger et al. 1978), and family studies (Siever et al. 1990; Silverman et al., in press) suggest that underlying dimensions of personality may be heritable. Developmental studies demonstrate a long-term continuity of behavioral traits such as fearfulness or shyness, which may have specific psychophysiological correlates (Kagan et al. 1988). Comparable studies in primates also suggest behavioral and biological continuity for behavioral dimensions such as aggression or affective sensitivity to separation (Suomi 1991).

In this chapter, we discuss issues of pharmacotherapy for patients with personality disorders. Appropriate selection and assessment of patients for pharmacotherapy are initially addressed, as are issues of initiating and maintaining psychopharmacological treatment in this population. Subsequent sections focus on specific syndromes and behavioral dimensions that have received adequate research interest to tentatively suggest appropriate psychopharmacological intervention. However, many Axis II syndromes do not lend themselves to pharmacological treatment and have not been the focus of controlled treatment studies (e.g., schizoid, narcissistic, histrionic, dependent, and obsessive-compulsive personality disorders); therefore, they are not discussed in this chapter.

Furthermore, it is important to note that, although we address in this chapter the pharmacological treatment of personality disorders, a wide array of psychotherapies exist and are in use. With the exception of the cognitive-behavior-based psychotherapy used by Linehan (1993) in patients with borderline personality disorder (BPD), there are no good controlled trials on the rational selection, use, and efficacy of psychotherapies in patients with personality disorders.

ASSESSMENT FOR TREATMENT

Before considering psychopharmacological treatment of signs and symptoms of a presumed personality disorder, the clinician should conduct a formal assessment to evaluate the differential diagnosis and possible complicating medical factors. A proposed sequence for this assessment is a detailed psychiatric history, substance abuse history, family history, medical history, and physical and laboratory examination. Specific issues of differential diagnosis are addressed in subsequent sections of this chapter.

Psychiatric History

Now that effective interventions and therapeutics exist for the treatment of many signs and symptoms of psychiatric illness, differential diagnosis becomes increasingly important. Assessments of psychiatric symptomatology, clinical contacts, medication history, and specific response to each of the psychotherapeutic and psychopharmacological interventions are basic to all psychiatric diagnosis and are critical to the evaluation of this patient population, many of whom will present with a bewildering array of problems and complaints.

Usually, Axis I and Axis II diagnoses must be differentiated initially. In general, Axis I disorders such as schizophrenia, major depression, and bipolar disorder take precedence in the differential diagnosis and treatment priority. For example, if bipolar disorder, type I, is diagnosed, it will usually be the initial target of treatment. When the bipolar disorder is optimally treated and residual mood disturbances ruled out, personality disorder disturbances may then appropriately be addressed.

In the process of obtaining a detailed past and present psychiatric history, the clinician must pay careful attention not only to the signs and symptoms of psychiatric illness per se but also to the pattern and timing of their presentation. One explicit example is the presence of impulsive-aggressive behavior, sexual promiscuity, and labile affect. If this symptom cluster is stable over time and has been present since adolescence, dramatic cluster personality disorders might head the differential diagnosis list. However, if the symptoms are episodic and associated with increased energy and decreased sleep, Axis I disorders such as bipolar disorder (mania) or organic mental disorder associated with substance intoxication or withdrawal become more probable as primary diagnoses.

Medication history is critical in this assessment. Optimally, for each psychotropic medication taken, the target symptoms, dose, duration, and efficacy should be determined. Given the frequent ambiguity of the behavioral, affective, and cognitive complaints, it is particularly important to operationally define each of the target symptoms assessed.

Substance Abuse and Dependence History

Drug and alcohol use must be carefully assessed and monitored. Before attempting to diagnose and treat personality disorders, the clinician should determine whether the patient has substance abuse and/or dependence and, when it is found, should treat it. Symptoms such as affective lability, impulsivity, and aggression that might otherwise be ascribed to personality disorders may remit with the resolution of substance abuse or dependence.

Interviewing of Family Members

Because of the nature of personality disorder diagnoses, it is frequently difficult for these patients to describe adequately the extent and severity of interpersonal difficulties. It is therefore important in this population to interview family members, with the knowledge and permission of the patient, to improve the database from which therapeutic interventions will be made. The information to be elicited from the family members is intended to elaborate the nature, extent, and severity of the intra- and interpersonal disturbances experienced by the patient. This is especially relevant regarding a history of substance abuse, which can have a profound effect on symptomatology and is frequently an area of patient denial. Families may provide information that would be otherwise inaccessible. Interviewing family members both separately and jointly often yields the most information, particularly when sharply differing viewpoints are endorsed. Patient refusal of family interviews should raise the question of the reliability of the patient's stated information.

Family History

A thorough family history is of the utmost importance because it may suggest the existence of biological vulnerabilities to mood disorders, drug or alcohol abuse, and perhaps personality disorders. Even if the patient is unaware of psychiatric illness in the family, it may prove valuable to speak with family members directly (again, with the permission of the patient) to evaluate more fully the potential presence of psychiatric illness in relatives of the proband.

Medical History

Many medical illnesses may present as psychiatric illness. Examples include endocrine, neurological, rheumatological, and metabolic disorders that have been reviewed elsewhere (Horvath et al. 1989). Further, medications prescribed for the treatment of other disorders may have cognitive, behavioral, or affective consequences. One common example is the use of steroids in the treatment of severe asthma, chronic obstructive pulmonary disease, or systemic lupus erythematosus. Some of the potential complications arising from the use of high-dose steroids

may include agitation, aggressive behavior, and affective lability. Therefore, a careful medical history and review of all medications taken (including nonpsychiatric medications) contribute to the overall accuracy of the diagnostic assessment.

Physical and Laboratory Examinations

A complete physical examination and routine laboratory studies, including blood counts and chemistries, thyroid function tests, serology (for syphilis and human immunodeficiency virus [HIV]), and computed tomography (CT)/magnetic resonance imaging (MRI) of the head, if indicated, should be obtained. Clinical indications should be used to guide the clinician in selecting further tests. If an individual presents with episodic impulsivity and aggression, electroencephalography might be considered in conjunction with structural imaging of the brain (CT or MRI); antibody testing might also be conducted if autoimmune diseases, such as systemic lupus erythematosus, are a possibility.

Treatment of underlying conditions may not completely correct the disorder but may at least ameliorate the symptoms. Only when the clinician is convinced that 1) no other treatable physical illness is present and 2) substance abuse and dependence diagnoses are controlled, he or she should make personality disorder diagnoses and initiate pharmacological interventions.

TREATMENT INITIATION AND MANAGEMENT OF TOXIC EFFECTS

When beginning any psychotropic medication in a patient with a personality disorder diagnosis, the clinician should discuss the treatment in detail with the patient and, when possible, the patient's family. Specific issues to be addressed include 1) clinician-patient agreement about the existence of a problem and the desirability of treating that problem; 2) discussion of the logic of the medication selection, its target symptoms, and potential toxic effects; and 3) an objective procedure for the assessment of treatment progress, or lack thereof.

All medications have predictable dose-dependent toxic effects and idiosyncratic toxic effects. To enhance the probability of a successful medication trial, the clinician should attempt to minimize or avoid toxic effects initially. Given the frequent sensitivity to medication side, or toxic, effects in patients with personality disorders and the chronic nature of the disturbances to be treated, a recommended treatment algorithm is to begin with a minimal dose of medication and incrementally and gradually increase to a therapeutic level. Operationally, it might be suggested to start with half the dose and half the rate of dosage increase that might be used in an Axis I condition. If toxic effects become manifest, they would then be managed as normal standards of care dictate, with discontinuation, dose reduction, or symptomatic treatment as indicated.

In this chapter, we address management of toxicity issues only as they relate specifically to patients with personality disorders; general management of toxic effects is beyond the scope of this chapter and is addressed elsewhere in this volume.

ASSESSMENT OF RESPONSE

With any patient, it is important to define desired target symptoms and to operationalize the outcome measures. Although this may sound more like a research paradigm than a clinical treatment plan, this approach to the treatment of behavioral, cognitive, anxiety, and/or affective symptoms in patients with personality disorders will reduce the risk of inappropriate expectations, ambiguous results, and power struggles between the patient and the clinician. For example, if the target symptom is reduction of affective instability, a simple 10-cm visual analogue scale might be used: one end might be behaviorally anchored with "most erratic, unstable emotions I have ever experienced," whereas the other might be anchored with "most stable I have ever experienced my emotions to be. " The patient would place a mark on this scale to describe his or her experience for the preceding week at baseline and at each subsequent office visit. This provides the clinician with an easy way to objectively chart target symptom change and provides the patient with objective criteria to justify either continuing medication if improvement is noted or altering the medication dose or selection if inadequate progress is noted. Another straightforward alternative is a calendar diary in which the patient marks whether it has been a good day or a bad day and why. This provides a focal point from which further exploration of the patient's response to the medications can be easily carried out. Informants may also be involved; for example, by monitoring patient compliance with medication.

MAINTENANCE AND MONITORING

Many of the symptoms in patients with personality disorders that are a target for pharmacotherapy (such as affective lability or impulsivity) are themselves inconstant. It may then be necessary for the clinician to be willing to work with the patient to modify the dosing of medications appropriately, increasing selected medications at times of stress and reducing others at times that toxic side effects outweigh benefits.

Blood levels of medications, if available, may be monitored to ensure appropriate adherence to the medication regimen and to confirm that therapeutic levels are being maintained. As with any medication, when indicated by normal standards of care, blood chemistry, electrocardiography, and hematological indices should be periodically monitored.

TREATMENT RESISTANCE

Given that, by definition, interpersonal relationships are disturbed in patients with personality disorders, these disturbances will likely intrude on the therapeutic relationship. It is important to realize that these intrusions are by no means limited to psychotherapy. Issues involving patients' adherence to a prescribed medication regimen, consistently and accurately reporting missed doses or side effects, and a willingness to discuss potential problems with medication all may evolve in the psychopharmacological management of any individual patient. It is essential, therefore, for the psychiatrist to be sensitive to these issues and to discuss them openly with the patient. Such discussions should be held at the outset of treatment and at appropriate intervals to ensure each other of concern on the clinician's part and cooperation and collaboration on the patient's part.

SPECIFIC SYNDROMAL TREATMENT

Not all personality disorder syndromes have received psychopharmacological research attention; indeed, even the most carefully studied of the syndromes is lacking in adequate numbers of well-defined, full-scale, placebo-controlled, double-blind studies. What follows are discussions of the psychobiology and psychopharmacological treatment of syndromes that, in our opinion, have received enough attention to support even tentative psychopharmacological treatment recommendations.

ECCENTRIC PERSONALITY DISORDERS: SCHIZOTYPAL PERSONALITY DISORDER

Regarded as part of the schizophrenia spectrum, the Cluster A ("odd cluster") personality disorders include schizotypal, schizoid, and paranoid types. Of the three, schizotypal personality disorder (SPD) has been the most clearly defined from clinical, psychobiological, and genetic perspectives. For example, in common with schizophrenic patients, SPD subjects have neuropsychological abnormalities, as well as impairment in attention and information processing, in auditory event-related potentials, and in smooth pursuit eye movements (Siever et al. 1990, 1993b). From the area of genetic studies, it has been shown that in comparison with relatives of healthy volunteers, the relatives of schizophrenic patients have significantly higher rates of SPD (Silverman et al. 1986, 1993). Similarly, assessments of the siblings of schizophrenic patients have found them to be at higher risk for both schizophrenia and SPD if either or both parents had SPD (Baron et al. 1985).

From a phenomenological viewpoint, psychotic-like and deficit-like symptoms are two defining dimensions of SPD, paralleling the positive and negative symptomatology of the schizophrenia. Magical thinking, ideas of reference, and perceptual disorders are included in the psychotic-like aspect of SPD, whereas poor interpersonal relatedness and social isolation are descriptive of the deficit-like syndrome. Plasma levels of the dopamine metabolite homovanillic acid (HVA) have been found to correlate with psychotic-like symptoms in patients with SPD (Amin et al. 1997; Siever et al. 1993a); similarly, this biological index is associated with psychosis in patients with schizophrenia (M. Davidson and Davis 1988; Davis et al. 1985). Furthermore, the dopaminergic agent amphetamine exacerbated these positive-like symptoms among a group of eight patients with SPD and BPD compared with eight patients with only BPD (Schulz et al. 1988). However, among schizophrenic patients receiving intravenous dextroamphetamine while on and off pimozide, negative symptoms improved, with little effect on positive symptoms (Van Kammen and Boronow 1988). On the other hand, decreased plasma HVA levels may be associated with deficit-like symptoms in relatives of schizophrenic patients (Amin et al. 1997), as well as diminished cognitive performance on neuropsychological testing of patients with SPD (Siever et al. 1993b). In turn, these cognitive test outcomes have been found to correlate with deficit-like symptoms (Trestman et al. 1995).

These psychobiological, genetic, and clinical perspectives support the concept of SPD as a schizophrenia-related disorder and suggest a role for psychopharmacological treatments for SPD as for schizophrenia. The agents most studied to date have been the antipsychotic drugs.

Differential Diagnoses

Other diagnoses to be considered include schizophrenia, residual schizophrenia, delusional disorder, and the interictal personality sometimes associated with temporal-lobe epilepsy. It is also important to consider the social context of the patient. The patient may come from a culture in which superstitiousness and forms of magical thinking are accepted; if so, it must be determined that the signs and symptoms go beyond that person's cultural norms. Interviews with family members may often be helpful in making this distinction.

Treatment Selection

Antipsychotics.   Low-dose antipsychotic medications have received the most attention in studies conducted over the past two decades in patients with personality disorders. In one early open-label study, patients ($N = 120$) with several DSM-II (American Psychiatric Association 1968) personality disorder diagnoses (borderline, schizoid, paranoid, obsessive-compulsive, hysterical) were treated with an average dose of 3 mg/day of pimozide (Reyntjens 1972). Results demonstrated global improvement in 69% of the group (Reyntjens 1972). Similar results were obtained in another early study that used mesoridazine (Barnes 1977). Both studies, therefore, concluded that antipsychotics were of benefit for the treatment of cognitive disorganization in these patients.

Seventeen patients with SPD were given haloperidol (maximum 12 mg/day) in a 6-week open-label study (Hymowitz et al. 1986). Mild to moderate improvement in target symptoms of social isolation, odd communication, and ideas of reference was observed in the 50% of patients who remained in the study. This high attrition rate speaks to the intolerance of, and sensitivity to, side effects in this patient population.

Low doses of thiothixene (mean dose 9 mg/day) or haloperidol (mean dose 3 mg/day) were used in a blinded comparison study of 52 patients with histories of recent transient psychotic episodes whose symptoms met DSM-III-R BPD or SPD criteria (Serban and Siegel 1984); 84% of the patients were moderately to markedly improved at 3-month follow up, with decreased derealization, paranoid ideation, anxiety, and depression.

In a 12-week double-blind, placebo-controlled study, 50 patients with BPD or SPD received thiothixene (mean dose 8.7 mg/day) (Goldberg et al. 1986). In the group receiving the drug, significant decreases were observed in measures of illusions, psychoticism, phobic anxiety, and ideas of reference; depressive symptoms were unaffected;

and no improvement was noted in measures of global functioning.

Although these results appear promising, note that all but one of these studies were uncontrolled, and the single double-blind, placebo-controlled study (Goldberg et al. 1986) used a heterogeneous sample. Furthermore, there is no evidence that any given agent or class of antipsychotic agent is more effective than another. At this time, medication selection must be based on expected side-effect profile at the minimum effective dose.

In summary, preliminary evidence indicates that low doses of antipsychotic medication (1–2 mg/day of haloperidol equivalent) are effective in at least temporarily reducing or relieving the symptoms of cognitive/perceptual dysfunction in patients with personality disorders. Because there are no studies of which we are aware that have examined long-term, chronic use of antipsychotic medications in SPD or related personality disorders, no guidelines grounded in research may be proposed. Clinical caution, coupled with concerns for the development of tardive dyskinesia or dystonia, argue that if antipsychotic medications are to be used in this population, they should be administered for short-term use (months) with subsequent medication withdrawal (if clinically tolerated) and reassessment. To date, no information is available on the efficacy of the atypical antipsychotic agents risperidone, clozapine, olanzapine, or sertindole in SPD.

Given the high rates of comorbidity—30%–50% in clinic settings—between SPD and major depression, antidepressants may be useful in the treatment of SPD. Clinical trials using antidepressants in subjects with personality disorders have also suggested a role for these drugs among patients with SPD. So far, however, mixed samples of subjects with only a limited number of actual patients with SPD have been described. Markovitz et al. (1991) found a decrease in obsessive symptoms, rejection sensitivity, depressive symptoms, anxiety, and psychoticism among a group of patients with BPD and SPD who were given 20–80 mg of open-label fluoxetine over 12 weeks. Notably, improvements were significant regardless of concurrent major depression or Axis II diagnosis. In contrast, amitriptyline, 100–175 mg given over 5 weeks (placebo-controlled), was less effective than haloperidol in mitigating either psychotic-like or depressive symptoms in a mixed BPD/SPD subject sample (Soloff et al. 1989).

Thus, controlled clinical trials in groups of patients with primarily SPD are needed to evaluate 1) antipsychotic and antidepressant efficacy, 2) optimal dosing regimens, 3) treatment duration, and 4) risk-benefit ratios. Furthermore, with the advent of new antipsychotic medications that are mixed serotonergic and dopamine D_2 antagonists with putatively minimal hematological risk (e.g., risperidone), improved treatment of the deficit-like symptoms and a reduced risk of tardive dyskinesia or dystonia may be possible.

Treatment Initiation

It is recommended that antipsychotic medication in this population be started at the level of 1 mg/day or less of haloperidol equivalent. After 1–2 weeks, if no untoward effects emerge, this treatment dose may be increased to 2 mg/day of haloperidol equivalent. Before initiating treatment, it is advisable to document any evidence of dyskinesias or dystonias at baseline to determine whether any subsequent changes occur. No definitive recommendations can be made about the use of antidepressants at this time; however, their judicious use following standard clinical guidelines would be appropriate in the depressed patient with SPD.

Management of Side Effects

At low antipsychotic doses, minimal side effects are expected. However, side effects such as akinesia, akathisia, and dystonia or dyskinesia are possible. These would be treated as usual. Periodic assessment should be made for occurrence of or change in medication-induced movement disorders.

Assessment of Response

Beyond global assessment of functioning, the clinician may operationalize target symptoms and follow them up at each visit to determine treatment efficacy. Although commonly conducted during an unstructured clinical interview, this may also be done with relevant sections of brief standardized instruments (e.g., the Brief Psychiatric Rating Scale [BPRS]) or with patient-specific visual analogue scales as described earlier in this chapter.

Treatment Resistance

Some patients with SPD are uncomfortable even taking low doses of antipsychotic medication, primarily because of behavioral toxicity: dysphoria or a worsening of some of the deficit-like symptoms. If such symptoms arise in the context of otherwise successful pharmacotherapy, the clinician should consider reducing the dose of antipsychotic to the lowest effective level and initiating supportive psychotherapy. If the symptoms persist and the benefit of the antipsychotic argues against discontinuation, a trial with an antidepressant may be considered.

IMPULSIVE AND AFFECTIVELY UNSTABLE PERSONALITY DISORDERS: BORDERLINE PERSONALITY DISORDER

Cluster B ("dramatic cluster") personality disorders, particularly BPD, can be conceptualized as including two dimensions: impulsive aggression and affective lability. The diagnosis of BPD, for example, is defined in DSM-IV (p. 650) as "a pervasive pattern of instability of interpersonal relationships, self-image, and affects" and characterized by criteria that include potentially self-damaging impulsivity, inappropriate or uncontrolled anger, recurrent suicidal threats or gestures, and physically self-damaging acts. Impulsive aggression is also characteristic of other personality disorders, although it is expressed somewhat differently in each. For example, in antisocial personality disorder, a disregard for social norms coupled with impulsive aggression may lead to behaviors such as lying, stealing, and destruction of property. Impulsivity/aggression may also play a part in the low frustration tolerance of the histrionic patient and in the rage of the narcissistic patient in response to criticism. This suggests that impulsivity/aggression may be a dimension of behavior that is not restricted to a single psychiatric diagnosis but may occur in both the Cluster B personality disorders and certain Axis I disorders (i.e., intermittent explosive disorder; bipolar disorder, manic type; and conduct disorder). A number of biological determinants can be associated with impulsive aggression, further supporting the notion of this dimension as a final common pathway to a variety of distinct categorical causes.

Family studies, for example, show significantly greater occurrences of impulsive-aggressive behaviors in first-degree relatives of patients with BPD than in relatives of other patients with personality disorders (Silverman et al. 1991); whereas preliminary results from a twin study point to genetic heritability for BPD criteria such as impulsivity and anger (Torgersen 1992).

Serotonin is thought to be a modulatory neurotransmitter with inhibitory effects on a variety of functions, including mood, arousal, cognition, and feeding behavior. There is evidence of an association between increased aggression toward self and/or others and reduced serotonergic function. Support for this relationship comes from a convergence of studies using serotonergic markers, including 5-hydroxyindoleacetic acid (5-HIAA) in cerebrospinal fluid (Brown et al. 1982; Linnoila et al. 1983), platelet imipramine binding and receptor sites (Marazziti et al. 1989; Meltzer and Arora 1986), human autopsy studies of metabolites and receptors (Arango et al. 1990; Mann and

Arango 1992), and neuroendocrine challenge studies (Coccaro et al. 1989). For example, "net" serotonergic functioning may be measured by the prolactin response to fenfluramine, a serotonin-releasing/uptake inhibiting agent. A decreased prolactin response to fenfluramine reflects diminished serotonergic function. One study examined 45 patients with personality disorder and/or affective disorder and found that reduced prolactin responses to fenfluramine correlated with measures of assault, irritability, and motoric impulsivity in the patients with personality disorders and with suicidal behavior in all patients (Coccaro et al. 1989).

Another key aspect of BPD is affective instability, which may be characterized as rapid, exaggerated shifts in affect in response to emotionally charged environmental stimuli such as criticism, separation from a significant person, or frustration (American Psychiatric Association 1987; Siever and Davis 1991). Affective instability may impair the ability to maintain a stable sense of self and thus disrupt interpersonal relationships. The inability to consistently modulate these mood shifts may also impair learning and the development of cognitive processes, as affective states may influence state-dependent learning (Bartlett and Santruck 1979), and selective memory may be the result of inadequate memory storage and recall. For example, the intense rage of a patient with BPD during an argument with a friend may distort the patient's memory of the event to the degree that he or she sees the friend as "all bad" (Kalus and Siever 1993).

To date, there is no definitive biological correlate of affective instability in personality disorders. However, because it is an enduring pattern of behavior, it is likely correlated with a trait abnormality (Siever and Davis 1991). There is evidence of an increased prevalence of affectively labile subjects in the first-degree relatives of patients with BPD, suggesting a heritable component to the dimensional characteristic (Silverman et al. 1991). Some of our preliminary studies demonstrate that patients with personality disorders who have affective instability have a heightened depressive response to the acetylcholinesterase inhibitor physostigmine, when compared with patients with personality disorders without this descriptive characteristic. These findings suggest that the cholinergic system may play a role in the modulation of affective instability in patients with personality disorders (Steinberg et al. 1994).

The noradrenergic system may also play a part in the regulation of affective instability. One study of compulsive gamblers, for example, observed an increase in noradrenergic function associated with extroversion (Roy et al. 1989). In a preliminary study, we examined 31 patients with DSM-III (American Psychiatric Association 1980) personality disorder and found positive correlations between increased measures of noradrenergic function and measures of irritability and verbal hostility (Trestman et al. 1993). Psychopharmacological interventions might therefore logically target serotonergic or catecholaminergic systems in an attempt to treat patients with BPD who are impulsive, aggressive, or affectively labile.

Differential Diagnoses of Impulsivity

Other diagnoses to consider in the differential include the Axis I impulse dyscontrol disorders; bipolar disorder, rapid-cycling or mixed subtypes; and organic syndromes secondary to epilepsy, trauma, or substance abuse. Although impulsive aggression associated with temporal-lobe epilepsy is often mentioned in the differential diagnosis, it is uncommonly the sole presenting symptom and is most often a postictal or interictal phenomenon (Fenwick 1989; Treiman 1991).

Differential Diagnoses of Affective Lability

Clinically, it is important to distinguish affective lability from a major mood disorder such as major depression or rapid-cycling bipolar disorder (Coccaro and Siever 1995). The diagnosis of major mood disorder is further complicated by the potential presence of comorbid atypical depression or of hysteroid dysphoria (Liebowitz and Klein 1981) in patients with personality disorders and affective lability.

Atypical depression is not uncommon in patients with personality disorder who have affective lability and is characterized by dysphoria with prominent mood reactivity, anxiety, rejection hypersensitivity and markedly decreased energy sometimes described as *leaden paralysis*. Other features of this disorder include hypersomnia and hyperphagia (especially carbohydrate craving or binge eating; Coccaro and Siever 1995). It is potentially valuable to probe for these symptoms during the initial evaluation given the benefits of monoamine oxidase inhibitors (MAOIs) for atypical depressive features (Coccaro 1993; Parsons et al. 1989).

Substance abuse, intoxication, and withdrawal syndromes may also present initially with affective lability, as may connective tissue disorders such as systemic lupus erythematosus, infectious diseases such as HIV-associated encephalopathy, or neurological disorders such as multiple sclerosis or the dementias.

Treatment Selection

Serotonin reuptake inhibitors.   The serotonin reuptake inhibitor fluoxetine has been used in several studies with dramatic cluster patients. In a double-blind, placebo-controlled study, 20–60 mg of fluoxetine given for 12 weeks reduced scores of overt aggression and irritability among a group of patients with personality disorders with histories of impulsive-aggressive behavior (Coccaro and Kavoussi 1995). In 22 volunteers with BPD symptoms without a history of suicidal behavior, significant reductions in impulsive-aggressive behavior, irritability, and anger occurred in a 12-week fluoxetine double-blind, placebo-controlled study (Salzman et al. 1992). An analysis of covariance demonstrated significant decreases in anger that did not correlate with depression scores, a finding consistent with other studies (Coccaro et al. 1990; Markovitz et al. 1991). Furthermore, a preliminary study of patients with BPD suggested that fluoxetine may decrease affective lability per se (Teicher et al. 1989).

Although many other studies are preliminary, have a small sample size, or are not double blind, the general results seem to also support the efficacy of fluoxetine in patients with BPD in a nonspecific manner or for symptoms of impulsive aggression or affective instability. Twelve patients with BPD were treated in an open-label trial with fluoxetine in doses ranging from 5 to 40 mg/day (Norden 1989). The patients had a variety of Axis I diagnoses, but none met criteria for a current major depressive episode. Results of the Clinical Global Rating Scale were as follows: 75% of the patients were very much improved or much improved, and the remaining 25% were moderately improved (Norden 1989). It is interesting that, in contrast to the treatment of major depression, with an expected response time of 3 weeks or more, patients in this treatment study of impulsive aggression improved within 1 week of treatment. Given the absence of a placebo washout period, the results may in part be due to placebo response. Two additional small, open-label studies have also suggested that fluoxetine may specifically reduce symptoms of impulsivity or aggression in patients with BPD (Coccaro et al. 1990; Cornelius et al. 1991).

Twenty-two patients whose symptoms met DSM-III criteria for BPD and/or SPD were treated in an open-label trial of fluoxetine (12 weeks duration, 80 mg/day) (Markovitz et al. 1991). Both affective and impulsive symptoms and the frequency of self-mutilation decreased significantly; self-injurious behavior did not decrease significantly until 9 weeks into the trial. Given the high dosing schedule of 80 mg/day, the delayed response is unlikely attributable to an "underdosing" effect and raises the possibility that the full effects of the drug, regardless of dose, may not be apparent until 9 weeks or longer. In addition, the presence or absence of depression did not appear to influence the outcome with regard to impulsive-aggressive behavior, suggesting the possibility of a differential effect of fluoxetine on depression and on impulsive-aggressive behavior.

Recently, the effect of open-label sertraline on impulsive aggression was examined among 11 patients meeting criteria for at least one personality disorder (Kavoussi et al. 1994). After 4 weeks, significant decreases in irritability and overt aggression were noted, suggesting a role for the serotonin uptake inhibitors as a group in this dimension of behavior.

Recently, two double-blind, placebo-controlled studies have indicated that fluoxetine is effective in the treatment of BPD symptoms. Fluoxetine treatment reduced anger in symptomatic volunteers (Salzman et al. 1995) and impulsive aggression in patients with personality disorder. In the second study, 40 patients with irritable aggression, meeting criteria for a personality disorder, who were not currently depressed were started on 20 mg of fluoxetine. Fluoxetine was superior to placebo in reducing irritability and aggression; treatment response was first apparent during the second month of treatment for irritability and third month for aggression. These results were not due to secondary measures such as anxiety or alcohol use (Coccaro and Kavoussi 1997).

Overall, fluoxetine is a reasonable first choice for the treatment of impulsive-aggressive behavior, because it is relatively safe in overdose and may also treat depression and affective lability. Controlled treatment trials have not as yet been conducted with the newer alternative selective serotonin reuptake inhibitors sertraline and paroxetine. Such trials may prove these agents to be useful alternatives to fluoxetine, given the differing pharmacokinetics and pharmacodynamics of these agents.

Tricyclic antidepressants. Studies conducted in patients with BPD using tricyclic antidepressants have generally shown a poor response to treatment (Cole et al. 1984; Soloff et al. 1986a, 1986b, 1989). Coupled with the lethal potential of overdose and the anticholinergic toxicity of these medications, tricyclic antidepressants are not generally recommended for the treatment of BPD.

Monoamine oxidase inhibitors. MAOIs are a class of antidepressants that alter the noradrenergic system (Cowdry and Gardner 1982; Liebowitz and Klein 1981). One relevant study targeted the treatment of hysteroid dysphoria, a disorder with characteristics of affective la-

bility and rejection sensitivity similar to those seen in patients with BPD (Liebowitz and Klein 1981). Three months of open-label treatment with phenelzine was followed with randomization to continued drug or placebo. The results of this preliminary study ($N = 11$) marginally supported the use of MAOIs in this condition; 40% taking active medication relapsed compared with 66% taking placebo who relapsed (Liebowitz and Klein 1981). Consistent with these early findings, a more recent treatment trial of BPD (Cowdry and Gardner 1988) demonstrated that patients taking tranylcypromine, even without current major depression, significantly improved with regard to the target symptoms of impulsivity and affective lability. Furthermore, one study has found that phenelzine may be more effective in the treatment of atypical depression even when patients have a comorbid diagnosis of BPD (Parsons et al. 1989). However, more recently, phenelzine was found to be less effective than haloperidol in decreasing impulsivity/hostile belligerence among a group of patients with BPD, although hostility scores were overall decreased with phenelzine (Soloff et al. 1993).

Given the available, if limited, evidence of MAOI efficacy, one of the practical concerns limiting their more widespread use is the risk of a hypertensive crisis. One common clinical practice is to give nifedipine to patients, with instructions to use it should symptoms of crisis such as sudden severe headache occur. However, patients who may also have difficulties with impulse regulation may still be liable to overdose on the MAOI. Reversible inhibitors of MAO-A, which are less likely to induce a hypertensive crisis, may therefore provide an excellent alternative if proven to be as effective as the present nonselective MAOIs for the treatment of affective instability (Liebowitz et al. 1990).

Lithium carbonate. Beyond its role in the treatment of bipolar disorder, lithium may treat affective lability (Van der Kolk 1986), regardless of the syndrome per se. Further, lithium may be effective in decreasing impulsivity in general (Shader et al. 1974), impulsivity associated with affective lability (Rifkin et al. 1972a), and episodic violence, especially in patients with antisocial personality disorder (Schiff et al. 1982). Sixty-six impulsive-aggressive prison inmates were treated with lithium carbonate for 3 months in a double-blind, placebo-controlled study; a significant reduction in the number of aggressive acts was observed (Sheard et al. 1976). A more recent controlled trial also found lithium to decrease therapist perceptions of irritability, anger, and suicidality among borderline patients (Links et al. 1990). The antiaggressive effects of lithium carbonate may be due to its enhancement of serotonergic postsynaptic receptors and/or its possible inhibition of catecholaminergic function (Coccaro et al. 1990) and a decrease in mood lability often associated with impulsivity. More double-blind, placebo-controlled studies of patients with a full range of impulsive-aggressive personality disorders would be useful at this time. It may also prove useful to compare the efficacy of fluoxetine and lithium and, in a controlled study, assess the efficacy of combination therapy in otherwise treatment-refractory patients.

Although clearly documented periods of hypomania or major depressive disorder may not be evident in a given patient, if periods of dysthymia or cyclothymia are noted, a trial of lithium may also be useful (Akiskal 1981; Rifkin et al. 1972b). Lithium carbonate has also been shown to have mood-stabilizing effects in patients with "emotionally unstable personality disorder," a diagnosis that is characterized by significant affective lability (Rifkin et al. 1972b). An additional indication for the use of lithium may be the presence of bipolar disorder in a first-degree relative of a proband with affective lability.

Anticonvulsants. The presence of mood lability, rage episodes, brief psychotic disturbances, and soft neurological signs in some patients with BPD suggested similarities with temporal-lobe epilepsy (despite a normal electroencephalogram result) and led to trials of anticonvulsants (Klein and Greenberg 1967; Gardner and Cowdry 1986a). One comprehensive double-blind, placebo-controlled 6-week study with a crossover design was conducted to examine the effects of four medications, including carbamazepine, in 16 female patients with DSM-III-R BPD (Cowdry and Gardner 1988). Target symptoms included impulsive self-injurious behavior and severe dysphoria. The average dose of carbamazepine was 820 mg/day, and those receiving the medication had a significant decrease in behavioral dyscontrol. Reduction of impulsive-aggressive behavior was associated with the capacity to delay action and "reflect." Although the mechanism of action is not yet understood, this study, along with other preliminary trials (Gardner and Cowdry 1986a; Luchins 1984), suggests that carbamazepine may be useful, either alone or as an adjunct to a serotonin reuptake inhibitor, for the control of impulsive aggression. Overall, carbamazepine's most significant effect has been demonstrated with behavioral dyscontrol (Cowdry and Gardner 1988).

Valproic acid has gained popularity in clinical practice as a mood stabilizer and has also been recently investigated in BPD. Modest reductions in irritability, anger, and impulsivity were noted for some among 8 outpatients with BPD who were given open-label valproate, up to 500 mg/day for 8 weeks (Stein et al. 1995). Similarly, 10 adolescents with mood lability/temper outbursts were all found to have clear improvement in frequency and severity of their symptoms with the use of divalproex sodium up to 1 g/day orally for 5 weeks, administered in an open-label fashion (Donovan et al. 1997). As with carbamazepine, case reports have similarly described the efficacy of valproate in dyscontrol syndromes such as dementia or episodic dyscontrol disorder (Giakas et al. 1990; Keck et al. 1992). Its established role in the treatment of BPD symptoms awaits further controlled investigation.

Adrenergic antagonists. Given evidence of increased noradrenergic responsivity in affective lability, the use of adrenergic antagonists such as propranolol may have merit. Propranolol has been shown to diminish explosive behaviors among a diverse group of patients including adolescents with rage outbursts or destructive behavior, among mentally retarded patients, or in Huntington's disease patients with aggressive behavior (Campbell et al. 1992; Stewart 1993). When used as an antiaggressive agent, divided doses of up to 200 mg/day or even higher have been reported, with careful cardiovascular and respiratory status monitoring. Formal investigations with patients who have personality disorders remain to be carried out.

Antipsychotics. A number of studies have suggested the general benefits of low-dose antipsychotics in individuals with impulsivity, depression, paranoid and schizotypal features, and rejection sensitivity. For example, haloperidol was found to be more effective than phenelzine in decreasing impulsivity/hostile belligerence among a group of 92 subjects with BPD (Soloff et al. 1993). The use of 4–16 mg/day of haloperidol for 5 weeks among a large sample of inpatients with BPD led to global improvements in hostile depression and impulsive ward behaviors (Soloff et al. 1989).

Support for the efficacy of these medications comes from other trials as well. Patients with BPD ($N = 80$) were treated with loxapine (mean dose 14 mg/day) compared with chlorpromazine (mean dose 110 mg/day) in a 6-week double-blind protocol. A decrease in suspiciousness, hostility, and anxiety, as well as improvement in depressed mood, was reported with both agents (Leone 1982). One double-blind, placebo-controlled study using a crossover design examined the effects of carbamazepine (mean dose 820 mg/day), tranylcypromine (mean dose 40 mg/day), trifluoperazine (mean dose 7.8 mg/day), and alprazolam (mean dose 4.7 mg/day) on 16 patients with DSM-III BPD (Cowdry and Gardner 1988). Although trifluoperazine was not well tolerated, the outcome was moderately favorable: objective ratings noted improvement in suicidality and anxiety.

A significant improvement in hostility, depression, and cognitive/perceptual disturbances was observed in a 12-week thioridazine (mean dose 92 mg/day) open-label study of 11 patients with DSM-III-R BPD (Teicher et al. 1989). Six of the 11 patients who completed the study showed decreased symptomatology on the impulse action patterns and psychosis subscales of the Diagnostic Interview for Borderline Personality Disorder. In addition, anxiety, interpersonal sensitivity, and paranoid ideation diminished. However, it is interesting that, contrary to expectations, the 3 individuals whose condition met many schizoid and schizotypal criteria became severely depressed and had to discontinue the study. This antipsychotic-induced dysphoria seems, on the basis of clinical experience, to occur more often in patients with SPD or related diagnoses, in contrast to an antidepressant-like effect in patients with BPD.

Low-dose antipsychotics, in summary, appear potentially useful in the treatment of patients with BPD who are more severely impaired, regardless of specific symptoms (Goldberg et al. 1986; Soloff et al. 1986a). It must be kept in mind, however, that these agents have been tested in patients with BPD only for relatively short periods (less than 4 months). Because of the potential for tardive dyskinesia, it may be most prudent to minimize both dose and duration of antipsychotic treatment in patients with BPD. Also, because of common antipsychotic side effects, compliance is often a problem. As with most medications, a careful risk-benefit assessment must be made for the specific indication and individual being treated.

Stimulants. One case report using methylphenidate has described improvement of mood lability and impulsivity in an adult with a diagnosis of BPD and comorbid attention-deficit disorder (Hooberman and Stern 1984). One finding associated with BPD improvement on tranylcypromine (an MAOI with psychostimulant actions) is a history of childhood attention-deficit/hyperactivity disorder (ADHD) (Cowdry and Gardner 1988). Furthermore, there is evidence that some patients with antisocial personality disorder have certain electrophysiological responses such as decreased galvanic skin response and diminished cortical electroencephalographic response to novel stimuli (Bloomingdale and Bloomingdale 1988). Because electrophysiological findings of a similar nature have been found in children with ADHD, this could be a biological correlate of adult residual ADHD, which may be characterized by impulsivity, irritability, mood lability,

difficulty in focusing, and subtle learning disabilities. Stimulants have proven effective in treating some of these symptoms (Wender 1995).

Although psychostimulants have received only minimal research attention, they may find a useful role in the treatment of impulsive aggression and affective lability. Psychostimulants such as methylphenidate may be considered for the treatment of carefully selected adult patients with BPD who had well-documented cases of childhood ADHD and no significant history of drug or alcohol dependence. Carefully controlled studies are needed to evaluate this possibility.

Benzodiazepines. Benzodiazepines have received little controlled attention in the treatment of BPD. One early report with alprazolam in three male patients with BPD (average dose 2.7 mg/day) suggested a general improvement in overall functioning (Faltus 1984). In a subsequent double-blind, placebo-controlled study, 7 of 12 patients (58%) developed serious behavioral dyscontrol (self-mutilation, drug overdoses, aggression) while taking alprazolam compared with 1 of 12 (8%) taking placebo (Gardner and Cowdry 1986b). Given the potential dyscontrol problem and the risk of drug dependency, therapy with alprazolam or other benzodiazepines is not currently indicated in this population.

Treatment Initiation

Because of the myriad symptoms that patients with BPD may present, it is important to directly state to the patient what symptoms are being targeted with medication. It may also help the patient cooperate fully with treatment if it is specified 1) that only limited success from psychopharmacological intervention is expected and 2) that a logical progression of medication interventions will be made, based on the responses of the individual to treatment.

Assessment of Response

Given that several symptoms may be targeted, it will benefit both patient and clinician to define objectively each of the target symptoms with either visual analogue scales or structured instruments (self-report or interview). The clinician should assess each symptom for severity at baseline and at each session and record a clinical global impression at these same visits to balance general progress with symptom-specific progress.

Treatment Resistance

Patients with BPD may often, intentionally or unintentionally, resist treatment. As many, if not all, of the targeted symptoms fluctuate, patients may benefit from specific psychoeducation as to the nature of the disturbances and the expected response to treatment. This may help them tolerate the occasional problems without discontinuing treatment.

ANXIOUS PERSONALITY DISORDERS: AVOIDANT PERSONALITY DISORDER

Anxiety is an alerting signal that warns of threats to safety, but it can also become maladaptive and interfere with productivity and well-being. It may be reflected in personality characteristics such as shyness, rejection sensitivity, and a diminished ability to perceive and take advantage of positive opportunities. Physiological manifestations include diaphoresis, palpitations, and gastrointestinal disturbances. Cognitively, it may impair concentration and lead to confusion and perceptual distortion. One study examined shyness, a trait that appears to be rather stable during childhood development. As youngsters, shy toddlers avoid strangers; as adults, they continue to be uncomfortable and anxious in new situations and social gatherings (Kagan et al. 1988).

It would seem that people who have a low threshold for physiological arousal in anticipation of threatening consequences might develop avoidant behavior (Kalus and Siever 1993). Although anxiety is a prominent feature of several Axis I disorders (i.e., social phobia, anxiety disorders, or obsessive-compulsive disorder [OCD]), hyperarousal as a concomitant of a low stimulation threshold may also contribute to the pathology of the anxious cluster diagnoses. Because anxiety may be a prominent feature of many of the personality disorder diagnoses, a target symptom approach may be particularly useful when examining the biological correlates and psychopharmacology of anxiety/inhibition (Siever et al. 1991).

Anxious individuals have increased tonic levels of sympathetic activity and cortical arousal, slower habituation to new stimuli, and lower sedation thresholds than do nonanxious individuals (Claridge 1967, 1985; Gray 1982). Studies suggest that the γ-aminobutyric acid (GABA)ergic, serotonergic, and noradrenergic systems each may be involved in the regulation of anxiety/inhibition. However, clear-cut biological markers are not established. Studies of the noradrenergic system in social phobia, for example, yield equivocal results in the growth hormone response to clonidine (Tancer 1993; Uhde 1994). Preliminary evidence of serotonergic involvement may be reflected in the increased cortisol response to fenfluramine among subjects with social phobia (Uhde 1994).

Stimulation of the locus coeruleus in primates is associated with responses that closely mimic anxiety in people (Redmond 1987). One hypothesis suggests a role for serotonergic function in harm avoidance, with a positive correlation between serotonin activity and increased avoidance behavior (Cloninger 1986). Consistent with this hypothesis, the postsynaptic serotonin agonist m-chlorophenylpiperazine (m-CPP) increases hormonal release as well as measures of anxiety in patients with panic disorder as compared with control subjects or patients with major depressive disorder (Kahn 1988). m-CPP has also been shown to increase obsessions in patients with OCD (Insel and Zohar 1987). Given high rates of comorbidity between social phobia and avoidant personality disorder (some authors suggest that the two are the same disorder), the biological findings in the Axis I diagnosis may best represent the psychobiological understanding of avoidant personality disorder at present.

Differential Diagnoses

Axis I anxiety disorders constitute most of the potentially confounding diagnoses. Most notably, generalized anxiety disorder, panic disorder, OCD, and phobic disorders should be carefully assessed. When identified, these Axis I disorders may take priority in treatment. Furthermore, avoidant and dependent personality disorders may coexist with, and be secondary to, a major depressive disorder or OCD; following treatment of the depression or OCD into remission, these apparent personality disorders may also resolve (Ricciardi et al. 1992). Further, when appropriately treated, symptoms of anxiety/excessive inhibition (otherwise attributed to an Axis II disorder) may remit. Thus, what is viewed as a personality disorder with associated affective symptoms may in actuality be an affective disorder with associated personality problems.

Treatment Selection

By extension to their use in related Axis I disorders, medications such as β-adrenergic receptor antagonists (Gorman et al. 1985), the benzodiazepine alprazolam, and the MAOI phenelzine (Liebowitz et al. 1986) may each be effective in the treatment of some patients with personality disorders with anxiety.

Cowdry and Gardner (1988) found the MAOI tranylcypromine helpful in alleviating anxiety in most patients who had avoidant personality disorder. Phenelzine led to a significant decrease in avoidant personality features among subjects with social phobia in two controlled situations (Liebowitz et al. 1992; Versiani et al. 1992). Alprazolam, used for the treatment of social phobia, also diminished specific symptoms of avoidant personality disorder (being fearful of saying something foolish or avoiding social and occupational situations requiring interpersonal contact) (Cowdry and Gardner 1988). Similar results were produced with the use of clonazepam (J. T. Davidson et al. 1993).

Case reports have described patients with avoidant personality disorder who were treated with tranylcypromine (30 mg/day), phenelzine (60 mg/day), or fluoxetine (20 mg/day) for a period of 2–3 months (Deltito and Stam 1989); marked improvement in each case was observed with regard to increased assertiveness, improved occupational and social functioning, and decreased social sensitivity. The improvement in target symptoms was independent of other Axis I diagnoses such as social phobia. Increased self-confidence, assertiveness, and socialization within several weeks were also described with the use of fluoxetine in case reports of patients with avoidant personality and social phobia (Goldman and Grinspoon 1990; Sternbach 1990).

Double-blind, placebo-controlled studies are needed to confirm these observations, but there is evidence that MAOIs, selective serotonin reuptake inhibitors, β-adrenergic receptor antagonists, and benzodiazepines may each be considered an adjunctive therapy to the overall treatment of patients with personality disorders characterized by anxiety or excessive inhibition.

CONCLUSION

Substantial evidence now suggests that biological components contribute to some of the more severe personality disorder syndromes such as SPD and BPD and to some of the troubling characteristics of personality disorders. These areas include, but may not be limited to, cognitive and perceptual dysfunction, impulsivity and aggression, affective instability, and anxiety/excessive inhibition. Furthermore, there is growing evidence from controlled treatment trials demonstrating the efficacy of psychopharmacological interventions in the treatment of these signs and symptoms.

It is important to emphasize, however, that it may be specific clusters of signs and symptoms that are being treated and not syndromal personality disorders per se. Although the advantages of categorical, syndromal nosologies are clear and include enhanced interrater reliability and operationalized criteria that encourage careful research, certain pathological disturbances cut across nosological boundaries. The observed personality disorders may therefore arise from the patterns of the underlying disturbances acting in concert. Given a growing armamentarium of research tools, the next decade may begin to yield many insights into the pathophysiology that underlies the cognitive, affective, and behavioral disturbances characteristic of the personality disorders.

REFERENCES

Akiskal HS: Subaffective disorders: dysthymic, cyclothymic and bipolar II disorders in the "borderline" realm. Psychiatr Clin North Am 4:26–46, 1981

American Psychiatric Association: Diagnostic and Statistical Manual of Mental Disorders, 2nd Edition. Washington, DC, American Psychiatric Association, 1968

American Psychiatric Association: Diagnostic and Statistical Manual of Mental Disorders, 3rd Edition. Washington, DC, American Psychiatric Association, 1980

American Psychiatric Association: Diagnostic and Statistical Manual of Mental Disorders, 3rd Edition, Revised. Washington, DC, American Psychiatric Association, 1987

American Psychiatric Association: Diagnostic and Statistical Manual of Mental Disorders, 4th Edition. Washington, DC, American Psychiatric Association, 1994

Amin F, Siever LJ, Silverman J, et al: Plasma HVA in schizotypal personality disorder, in Plasma Homovanillic Acid in Schizophrenia: Implications for Presynaptic Dopamine Dysfunction. Edited by Friedhoff AJ, Amin F. Washington, DC, American Psychiatric Press, 1997, pp 133–180

Arango V, Ernsberger P, Marzuk P, et al: Autoradiographic demonstration of increased serotonin 5-HT2 and beta-adrenergic receptor binding sites in the brain of suicide victims. Arch Gen Psychiatry 47:1038–1047, 1990

Barnes RJ: Mesoridazine in personality disorders: a controlled trial in adolescent patients. Diseases of the Nervous System 38:258–264, 1977

Baron M, Gruen R, Asnis L: Familial transmission of schizotypal and borderline personality disorders. Am J Psychiatry 142:927–933, 1985

Bartlett JC, Santruck JW: Affect-dependent episodic memory in young children. Child Dev 50:513–518, 1979

Bloomingdale LM, Bloomingdale EC: Childhood identification and prophylaxis of antisocial personality disorder. J Forensic Sci 33:187–199, 1988

Brown GL, Ebert M, Goyer P, et al: Aggression, suicide and serotonin: relationship to CSF amine metabolites. Am J Psychiatry 139:741–746, 1982

Campbell M, Gonzalez NM, Silva RR: The pharmacologic treatment of conduct disorders and rage outbursts. Psychiatr Clin North Am 15:69–85, 1992

Claridge G: Personality and Arousal. Oxford, England, Pergamon, 1967

Claridge G: Origins of Mental Illness. New York, Blackwell, 1985

Cloninger CR: A unified theory of personality and its role in the development of anxiety states. Psychiatric Developments 3:167–226, 1986

Cloninger CR, Christiansen KO, Reich T, et al: Implications of sex differences in the prevalence of antisocial personality, alcoholism, and criminality for familial transmission. Arch Gen Psychiatry 35:941–951, 1978

Coccaro EF: Psychopharmacologic studies in patients with personality disorders: review and perspective. Journal of Personality Disorders 7 (suppl):181–192, 1993

Coccaro EF, Kavoussi RJ: Fluoxetine in aggression in personality disorders. American Psychiatric Association 1995 Annual Meeting New Research Program and Abstracts. Washington, DC, American Psychiatric Association, 1995

Coccaro EF, Kavoussi RJ: Fluoxetine and impulsive aggressive behavior in personality disordered subjects. Arch Gen Psychiatry 54:1081–1088, 1997

Coccaro EF, Siever LJ: The neuropsychopharmacology of personality disorders, in Psychopharmacology: The Fourth Generation of Progress. Edited by Bloom F, Kupfer D. New York, Raven, 1995, pp 1567–1579

Coccaro EF, Siever LJ, Klar H: Serotonergic studies in patients with affective and personality disorders: correlates with suicidal and impulsive aggressive behavior. Arch Gen Psychiatry 45:177–185, 1989

Coccaro EF, Astill JL, Herbert JA, et al: Fluoxetine treatment of impulsive aggression in DSM-III-R personality disorder patients. J Clin Psychopharmacol 10:373–375, 1990

Cole JO, Salomon M, Gunderson J: Drug therapy in borderline patients. Compr Psychiatry 25:249–254, 1984

Cornelius JR, Soloff PH, Perel JM, et al: A preliminary trial of fluoxetine in refractory borderline patients. J Clin Psychopharmacol 11:116–120, 1991

Cowdry RW, Gardner DL: Pharmacology of borderline personality disorder. Arch Gen Psychiatry 139:741–746, 1982

Cowdry RW, Gardner DL: Pharmacotherapy of borderline personality disorder: alprazolam, carbamazepine, trifluoperazine, and tranylcypromine. Arch Gen Psychiatry 45:111–119, 1988

Davidson JT, Potts NS, Richichi EA, et al: Treatment of social phobia with clonazepam and placebo. J Clin Psychopharmacol 13:423–428, 1993

Davidson M, Davis KL: A comparison of plasma homovanillic acid concentrations in schizophrenic patients and normal controls. Arch Gen Psychiatry 45:561–563, 1988

Davis KL, Davidson M, Mohs RC, et al: Plasma homovanillic acid concentration and the severity of schizophrenic illness. Science 227:1601–1602, 1985

Deltito JA, Stam M: Psychopharmacological treatment of avoidant personality disorder. Compr Psychiatry 30:498–504, 1989

Donovan SJ, Susser ES, Nunes EV, et al: Divalproex treatment of disruptive adolescents: a report of ten cases. J Clin Psychiatry 58:1, 12–15, 1997

Faltus F: The positive effect of alprazolam in the treatment of three patients with borderline personality disorder. Am J Psychiatry 141:802–803, 1984

Fenwick P: The nature and management of aggression in epilepsy. Neuropsychiatric Practice and Opinion 1:418–425, 1989

Gardner DL, Cowdry RW: Positive effects of carbamazepine on behavioral dyscontrol in borderline personality disorder. Am J Psychiatry 143:519–522, 1986a

Gardner DL, Cowdry RW: Alprazolam induced discontrol in borderline personality disorder. Am J Psychiatry 142:98–100, 1986b

Giakas WJ, Seibyl JP, Mazure CM: Valproate in the treatment of temper outbursts (letter). J Clin Psychiatry 51:525, 1990

Goldberg SC, Schulz SC, Schulz PM, et al: Borderline and schizotypal personality disorders treated with low-dose thiothixene versus placebo. Arch Gen Psychiatry 43:680–686, 1986

Goldman MJ, Grinspoon L: Ritualistic use of fluoxetine by a former substance abuser (letter). Am J Psychiatry 147:1377, 1990

Goldsmith HH: Genetic influences on personality from infancy to adulthood. Child Dev 54:331–355, 1982

Gorman JM, Liebowitz MR, Fyer AJ, et al: Treatment of social phobia with atenolol. J Clin Psychopharmacol 5:298–301, 1985

Gray JA: The Neuropsychology of Anxiety. Oxford, England, Oxford University Press, 1982

Hooberman D, Stern TA: Treatment of attention deficit and borderline personality disorders with psychostimulants: case report. J Clin Psychiatry 45:441–442, 1984

Horvath TB, Siever LJ, Mohs RC, et al: Organic mental syndromes and disorders, in Comprehensive Textbook of Psychiatry/V. Edited by Kaplan HI, Sadock BJ. Baltimore, MD, Williams & Wilkins, 1989, pp 599–641

Hymowitz P, Frances A, Jacobsberg LB, et al: Neuroleptic treatment of schizotypal personality disorders. Compr Psychiatry 27:267–271, 1986

Insel TR, Zohar J: Psychopharmarcologic approaches to obsessive compulsive disorder, in Psychopharmacology: The Third Generation of Progress. Edited by Meltzer H. New York, Raven, 1987, pp 1205–1209

Kagan J, Reznick S, Snidman N, et al: Childhood derivatives of inhibition and lack of inhibition to the unfamiliar. Child Dev 59:1580–1589, 1988

Kahn RS, Wetzler S, Van Praag H, et al: Behavioral indications for serotonin receptor hypersensitivity in panic disorder. Psychiatry Res 25:101–104, 1988

Kalus O, Siever LJ: The biology of personality disorders, in An Examination of Illness Subtypes: State vs Trait and Comorbid Psychiatric Disorders. Edited by Mann JJ, Kupfer DJ. New York, Plenum, 1993, pp 89–107

Kavoussi RJ, Liu J, Coccaro EF: An open trial of sertraline in personality disordered patients with impulsive aggression. J Clin Psychiatry 55:137–141, 1994

Keck PE, McElroy SL, Friedman LM: Valproate and carbamazepine in the treatment of panic and posttraumatic stress disorder, withdrawal states, and behavioral dyscontrol syndromes. J Clin Psychopharmacol 12 (suppl 1): 36–41, 1992

Klein DF: Psychiatric diagnosis and a typology of clinical drug effects. Psychopharmacology 13:359–386, 1968

Klein DF, Greenberg IM: Behavioral effects of diphenylhydantoin in severe psychiatric disorders. Am J Psychiatry 124:847–849, 1967

Leone NF: Response of borderline patients to loxapine and chlorpromazine. J Clin Psychiatry 43:148–150, 1982

Liebowitz MR, Klein DF: Interrelationship of hysteroid dysphoria and borderline personality disorder. Psychiatr Clin North Am 4:67–87, 1981

Liebowitz MR, Fyer AJ, Gorman JM, et al: Phenelzine in social phobia. J Clin Psychopharmacol 6:93–98, 1986

Liebowitz MR, Hollander E, Schneier F, et al: Reversible and irreversible monoamine oxidase inhibitors in other psychiatric disorders. Acta Psychiatr Scand Suppl 360:29–34, 1990

Liebowitz MR, Schneier FR, Campeas R, et al: Phenelzine vs. atenolol in social phobia: a placebo-controlled comparison. Arch Gen Psychiatry 49:290–300, 1992

Linehan MM: Cognitive Behavioral Treatment of Borderline Personality Disorder. New York, Guilford, 1993

Links PS, Steiner M, Boiago I, et al: Lithium therapy for borderline patients: preliminary findings. Journal of Personality Disorders 4:173–181, 1990

Linnoila M, Virkunnen M, Scheinin M, et al: Low cerebrospinal fluid 5-hydroxyindoleacetic acid concentration differentiates impulsive from nonimpulsive violent behavior. Life Sci 33:2609–2614, 1983

Luchins DJ: Carbamazepine in violent non-epileptic schizophrenics. Psychopharmacol Bull 20:569–571, 1984

Mann JJ, Arango V: Integration of neurobiology and psychopathology in a unified model of suicidal behavior. J Clin Psychopharmacol 12 (suppl 2):2S–7S, 1992

Marazziti D, Leo D, Conti L: Further evidence supporting the role of the serotonin system in suicidal behavior: a preliminary study of suicide attempters. Acta Psychiatr Scand 80:322–324, 1989

Markovitz PJ, Calabrese JR, Schulz SC, et al: Fluoxetine in the treatment of borderline and schizotypal personality disorders. Am J Psychiatry 148:1064–1067, 1991

Meltzer HY, Arora RC: Platelet markers of suicidality. Ann N Y Acad Sci 487:271–280, 1986

Norden MJ: Fluoxetine in borderline personality disorder. Prog Neuropsychopharmacol Biol Psychiatry 13:885–893, 1989

Parsons B, Quitkin FM, McGrath PJ: Phenylzine, imipramine, and placebo in borderline patients meeting criteria for atypical depression. Psychopharmacol Bull 25:524–534, 1989

Redmond DE: Studies of the nucleus locus coeruleus in monkeys and hypotheses for neuropsychopharmacology, in Neuropsychopharmacology: The Third Generation of Progress. Edited by Meltzer H. New York, Raven, 1987, pp 967–975

Reyntjens AM: A series of multicentric pilot trials with pimozide in psychiatric practice, I: pimozide in the treatment of personality disorders. Acta Psychiatr Belg 72:653–661, 1972

Ricciardi JN, Baer L, Jenike MA, et al: Changes in DSM-III-R Axis II diagnoses following treatment of obsessive-compulsive disorder. Am J Psychiatry 149:829–831, 1992

Rifkin A, Levitan SJ, Galewski J, et al: Emotionally unstable personality disorder—a follow-up study. Biol Psychiatry 4:65–79, 1972a

Rifkin A, Quitkin F, Curillo C, et al: Lithium carbonate in emotionally unstable character disorders. Arch Gen Psychiatry 27:519–523, 1972b

Roy A, DeJong J, Linnoila M: Extraversion in pathological gamblers correlates with indices of noradrenergic function. Arch Gen Psychiatry 46:679–681, 1989

Salzman C, Wolfson AN, Miyawaki E, et al: Fluoxetine treatment of anger in borderline personality disorder (abstract). Proceedings of the American College of Neuropsychopharmacology, 1992, p 24

Salzman C, Wolfson AN, Schatzberg A, et al: Effect of fluoxetine on anger in symptomatic volunteers with borderline personality disorder. J Clin Psychopharmacol 15:23–29, 1995

Schiff HB, Sabin TD, Geller A, et al: Lithium in aggressive behavior. Am J Psychiatry 139:1346–1348, 1982

Schulz SC, Cornelius J, Schulz PM, et al: The amphetamine challenge test in patients with borderline personality disorder. Am J Psychiatry 145:809–814, 1988

Serban G, Siegel S: Response of borderline and schizotypal patients to small doses of thiothixene and haloperidol. Am J Psychiatry 141:1455–1458, 1984

Shader RI, Jackson AH, Dodes LM: The anti-aggressive effects of lithium in man. Psychopharmacologia 40:17–24, 1974

Sheard MH, Marini JL, Bridges DL, et al: The effect of lithium on impulsive aggressive behavior in man. Am J Psychiatry 133:1409–1413, 1976

Siever LJ, Davis KL: A psychobiological perspective on the personality disorders. Am J Psychiatry 148:1647–1658, 1991

Siever LJ, Silverman JM, Horvath T, et al: Increased morbid risk for schizophrenia-related disorders in relatives of schizotypal personality disordered patients. Arch Gen Psychiatry 47:634–640, 1990

Siever LJ, Amin F, Coccaro EF, et al: Plasma homovanillic acid in schizotypal personality disorder. Am J Psychiatry 148:1246–1248, 1991

Siever LJ, Amin F, Coccaro EF, et al: Cerebrospinal fluid homovanillic acid in schizotypal personality disorder. Am J Psychiatry 150:149–151, 1993a

Siever LJ, Kalus OF, Keefe RSE: The boundaries of schizophrenia. Psychiatr Clin North Am 16:217–244, 1993b

Silverman JM, Mohs RC, Siever LJ, et al: Heritability for schizophrenia-spectrum disorder in schizophrenic and schizophrenia related personality disorder patients. Clinical Neuropsychopharmacology 9:271–273, 1986

Silverman JM, Pinkham L, Horvath TB, et al: Affective and impulsive personality disorder traits in the relatives of borderline personality disorder patients. Am J Psychiatry 148:1378–1385, 1991

Silverman JM, Siever LJ, Horvath TB, et al: Schizophrenia-related and affective personality disorder traits in relatives of probands with schizophrenia and personality disorders. Am J Psychiatry 150:435–442, 1993

Silverman JM, Greenberg DA, Altsteil LD, et al: Evidence of a locus for schizophrenia and related disorders on the short arm of chromosome 5 in a large pedigree. Am J Med Genet (in press)

Soloff PH, George A, Nathan RS, et al: Progress in pharmacotherapy of borderline disorders. Arch Gen Psychiatry 43:691–697, 1986a

Soloff PH, George A, Nathan RS, et al: Paradoxical effects of amytriptyline in borderline patients. Am J Psychiatry 143:1603–1605, 1986b

Soloff PH, George A, Nathan RS, et al: Amytriptyline vs haloperidol in borderlines: final outcomes and predictors of response. J Clin Psychopharmacol 9:238–246, 1989

Soloff PH, Cornelius JR, George A, et al: Efficacy of phenelzine and haloperidol in borderline personality disorder. Arch Gen Psychiatry 50:377–385, 1993

Stein DJ, Simeon D, Frenkel M, et al: An open trial of valproate in borderline personality disorder. J Clin Psychiatry 56:506–510, 1995

Steinberg BJ, Trestman RL, Siever LJ: The cholinergic and noradrenergic neurotransmitter systems and affective instability in borderline personality disorder, in Biological and Neurobehavioral Studies in Borderline Personality Disorder. Edited by Silk KR. Washington, DC, American Psychiatric Press, 1994, pp 41–62

Sternbach HA: Fluoxetine treatment in social phobia (letter). J Clin Psychopharmacol 10:230, 1990

Stewart JT: Huntington's disease and propranolol. Am J Psychiatry 150:166–167, 1993

Suomi SJ: Primate separation models of affective disorders, in Neurobiology of Learning, Emotion and Affect. Edited by Madden J. New York, Raven, 1991, pp 321–334

Tancer ME: Neurobiology of social phobia. J Clin Psychiatry 54 (suppl 12):26–30, 1993

Teicher MH, Glod CA, Aaronson ST, et al: Open assessment of the safety and efficacy of thioridazine in the treatment of patients with borderline personality disorder. Psychopharmacol Bull 25:535–549, 1989

Tellegen A, Lykken DT, Bouchard TJ, et al: Personality similarity in twins reared apart and together. J Pers Soc Psychol 54:1031–1039, 1988

Torgersen S: Genetic and nosological aspects of schizotypal and borderline personality disorders. Arch Gen Psychiatry 41:546–554, 1984

Torgersen S: The genetic transmission of borderline personality features displays multidimensionality. Abstract presented at the annual meeting of the American College of Neuropsychopharmacology, San Juan, Puerto Rico, December 14–18, 1992

Treiman DM: Psychobiology of ictal aggression, in Advances in Neurology. Edited by Smith D, Treiman D, Trimble M. New York, Raven, 1991, pp 341–356

Trestman RL, deVegvar M-L, Coccaro EF, et al: The differential biology of impulsivity, suicide, and aggression in depression and in personality disorders. Biol Psychiatry 33:46A–47A, 1993

Trestman RL, Keefe RS, Mitropoulou V, et al: Cognitive function and biological correlates of cognitive performance in schizotypal personality disorder. Psychiatry Res 59:127–136, 1995

Uhde TW: A review of biological studies in social phobia. J Clin Psychiatry 55 (suppl 6):17–27, 1994

Van der Kolk BA: Uses of lithium in patients without major affective illness (letter). Hosp Community Psychiatry 37:675, 1986

Van Kammen DP, Boronow JJ: Dextroamphetamine diminishes negative symptoms in schizophrenia. Int Clin Psychopharmacol 3:111–121, 1988

Versiani M, Nardi AE, Mundim FD, et al: Pharmacotherapy of social phobia: a controlled study with moclobemide and phenelzine. Br J Psychiatry 161:353–360, 1992

Wender PH: Attention-Deficit Hyperactivity Disorder in Adults. New York, Oxford University Press, 1995

FORTY-FOUR

Treatment of Psychiatric Emergencies

Michael J. Tueth, M.D.,
C. Lindsay DeVane, Pharm.D., and
Dwight L. Evans, M.D.

Psychiatric emergencies are not found only in the emergency department. They can occur on a medical or surgical floor, in the intensive care unit, on a psychiatric unit, or in an outpatient facility. Regardless of the site of the emergency, the psychiatrist should assess the patient based on subjective complaints and objective findings and then develop a provisional diagnostic impression and a rational treatment plan.

Often the psychiatrist must make decisions based on very limited information. It is usually best to rely heavily on objective findings of the mental status examination. In addition, when only limited data are available, the clinician's treatment plan should be conservative. Although it is important to choose the least restrictive environment for the patient, the safety of the patient and others should be foremost in mind. Table 44–1 lists levels of the restrictive environments that may be used, ranging from no hospitalization to physical and chemical restraints.

In this chapter, we discuss the treatment of psychiatric emergencies from the standpoint of requirements for nonpharmacological, limited pharmacological, and primarily pharmacological intervention. Although most psychiatric emergencies require both pharmacological and psychotherapeutic intervention, many also require that legal action or procedures be followed.

PSYCHIATRIC EMERGENCIES REQUIRING NONPHARMACOLOGICAL INTERVENTION

Areas of nonpharmacological interventions include decisions regarding admission to the hospital versus discharge to the community, involuntary versus voluntary admission to a psychiatric facility, and legal action requiring involvement or notification of third parties. Although most physicians treat patients who present for treatment voluntarily, emergency physicians and psychiatrists sometimes confine patients to designated psychiatric facilities against the patients' will. All 50 states have statutes requiring physicians to detain a patient involuntarily in a designated psychiatric facility if the patient is judged to be dangerous to self or others. In most states, this concept extends to self-neglect and psychotic conditions. Similarly, all states have statutes that require reporting of suspected child abuse to state and/or county authorities. In addition, some states have included suspected abuse of elderly people as a mandatory reportable situation. Universal statutes also require physicians to contact an intended victim and/or the law enforcement agency in the intended victim's locality if a patient with a psychiatric disorder is judged likely to harm that person in the near future.

Table 44–2. Recommended psychopharmacological drug use in psychiatric emergencies

For healthy adult psychiatric patients

For agitation or substance withdrawal

Lorazepam 1–2 mg po, im, or iv every 1–2 hours as needed or

Diazepam 5–10 mg po, im, or iv every 1–2 hours as needed

For psychotic symptoms

Haloperidol 10–20 mg/day po or im as needed (higher dosages usually are not needed)

For medically ill, delirious, or elderly psychiatric patients

For agitation or substance withdrawal

Lorazepam 0.25–1.0 mg po, im, or iv every 1–2 hours as needed

For psychotic symptoms

Haloperidol 1–5 mg/day as needed (higher dosages usually are not needed)

Note.   po = orally; im = intramuscularly; iv = intravenously.

stressor and that has persisted for no longer than 6 months. Symptoms associated with adjustment disorder include anxiety, depression, disturbance of conduct, and mixed symptoms (American Psychiatric Association 1994). However, the usual presentation is an adjustment disorder with mixed emotional features. Crisis intervention psychotherapy has proven to be the best treatment for an adjustment disorder. Most crises are self-limited and resolve naturally, but they can definitely be helped by skilled psychotherapeutic intervention. The essential elements of this intervention include establishing rapport with the patient, demonstrating empathy, listening, obtaining a thorough history, and constructing a plan to deal with the reality of the situation. The therapist helps the patient reestablish his or her defenses, draws on the patient's own resources as well as social support resources, and attempts to increase the patient's confidence and self-esteem (Hyman 1988). Involvement of the patient's family or significant other in resolution of the crisis situation is equally important. It is important to note that hallucinations or delusions are not symptoms of an adjustment disorder but reflect a psychotic disorder. If the initial crisis intervention interview is successful and the patient establishes control of his or her emotions, hospitalization is not usually necessary, but a follow-up outpatient appointment is recommended.

Acute Bereavement

Although acute bereavement is an adjustment disorder, it is discussed separately here because of the magnitude of

the adjustment. It usually involves the loss of a significant family member or a reaction to an unusual event, such as a natural disaster. Allowing the patient to ventilate his or her feelings is essential. Also, it is imperative that the patient's family or friends be involved in ongoing support of the patient.

Rape and Assault

In addition to necessary medical and surgical evaluation and treatment, the rape or assault victim may need psychiatric intervention and follow-up care. As with the treatment of other acute adjustment disorders, the psychiatrist should follow the lead of the patient in discussing feelings about the assault. Although it is important for the patient to know that full psychological recovery from rape may take months or years, providing hope that the crisis can sometimes be addressed and successfully treated in a brief period is equally significant. In either case, the clinician should convey that psychotherapy can be extremely helpful in the recovery process (Hyman 1988).

Borderline Personality Disorder

Patients undergoing acute adjustment disorders who also have a borderline personality disorder usually have much difficulty with recovery. Sometimes they experience intermittent psychotic symptoms, suicidal urges, and loss of emotional control. These patients often need a brief psychiatric admission to prevent further deterioration. Borderline personalities often deteriorate along three lines: affective instability, transient psychotic phenomenon, and impulsive-aggressive behavior. Affective instability has responded to mood stabilizers such as carbamazepine and valproate or antidepressants. The role of monoamine oxidase inhibitors (MAOIs) or tricyclic antidepressants (TCAs) is not completely understood. Liebowitz and Klein (1981) suggested that core borderline features might respond to MAOIs. Within the context of atypical depression, such patients respond better to phenelzine than to imipramine (McGrath et al. 1993; Parsons et al. 1989). Transient psychotic symptoms often respond to low-dose neuroleptic medication, and impulsive-aggressive behavior has responded to serotonergic agents (Coccaro and Kavoussi 1991).

Conditions Requiring Organic Workup

Panic Attack

When for the first time a patient develops signs and symptoms consistent with the diagnosis of panic disorder, he or she should be evaluated medically (by an internist if necessary) to rule out physical causes. The symptoms of a panic attack (including shortness of breath, tachycardia, sweating, and chest pain) are consistent with many medical illnesses, including hypoglycemia, hyperthyroidism, and myocardial infarction or angina. Not until medical conditions have been excluded should a psychiatrist make a diagnosis of panic disorder. Following an initial panic attack, a patient may need a short course of a benzodiazepine to treat the accompanying anxiety and fear before obtaining a medical evaluation. Interestingly, clinical experience and physiological data suggest that patients with panic disorder sense impending suffocation, thus triggering a suffocation false-alarm and response, that accounts for symptoms (Klein 1993).

Dissociative Episodes

Dissociative amnesia is a relatively rare condition compared with physical causes for the amnestic syndrome. Amnesia is a frequent accompaniment of medical-surgical abnormalities such as head injury, brain tumor, cardiovascular incidents, and substance use. Not until organic amnestic disorder has been ruled out should the psychiatrist assume a psychogenic basis for memory loss. Any other dissociative episodes occurring for the first time, such as dissociative fugue or depersonalization experiences, need an organic evaluation to rule out physical causes.

Dissociative episodes may accompany posttraumatic stress disorder (PTSD). Patients who have experienced extreme traumatic stress can dissociate both at the time of the stressor and intermittently, for years. Vietnam veterans who had increased levels of combat exposure were reported to have an increased number of dissociative symptoms years after their combat experiences (Bremner et al. 1992). Although there is no specific emergency treatment for this condition, the patient should be evaluated for possible hospital admission if he or she is in an unstable emotional state. Patients who have experienced an unusual traumatic event such as a natural disaster could in some situations benefit from outpatient treatment to minimize the likelihood of developing PTSD.

Catatonia

Although major depression and schizophrenia (catatonic type) are the most common psychiatric disorders that are associated with catatonia, some medical and neurological conditions also cause this syndrome. Medical causes include hypercalcemia and hepatic encephalopathy. Catatonia may also appear as an adverse drug side effect from neuroleptic medication and phencyclidine (PCP). Neurological causes for catatonia include parkinsonism and en-

cephalitis. Unless the patient has had a previous episode of catatonia with an established causative psychiatric diagnosis, he or she should be fully evaluated by medical and/or neurological consultants. After eliminating physical causes, the clinician may find that catatonia improves temporarily through intravenous administration of amobarbital or lorazepam as in conversion states (Perry and Jacobs 1982; Rosebush et al. 1990).

Mania

In patients older than 50, the initial onset of mania is relatively uncommon. Any patient with an initial onset of mania (but especially a patient who is older than 50) should be evaluated for organic causes. Various drugs, medical illness, and neurological disease can cause this syndrome. For example, TCAs, MAOIs, and alprazolam have precipitated hypomania in susceptible patients. Medical illness and neurological disease that can cause the manic syndrome include a hyperthyroid state, multiple sclerosis, and various brain tumors.

Conversion Disorder

A patient with a rather sudden onset of unexplained neurological symptoms should have a full neurological workup before the diagnosis of "conversion hysteria" can be made. Traditionally, the amobarbital interview has been useful for assessment, initial management, and recovery of function in conversion disorders (Perry and Jacobs 1982). It has been reported that intravenous administration of lorazepam accompanied by repeated hypnotic suggestions resulted in full recovery in conversion disorder (Stevens 1990).

PSYCHIATRIC EMERGENCIES USUALLY REQUIRING PHARMACOLOGICAL INTERVENTION

Many psychiatric patients require pharmacological intervention as the primary treatment of their condition. These patients include most assaultive or aggressive patients, agitated psychotic patients, patients undergoing substance withdrawal, and substance-intoxicated patients with aggressivity.

Assaultive Behavior From Any Cause

On initial presentation, it is often impossible to accurately diagnose psychiatrically an assaultive or aggressive individual. Treatment usually precedes a definitive diagnosis. When a patient is assessed to be actively or potentially violent, then quick, decisive, and well-planned action is mandatory. The level of restriction that the psychiatrist chooses for each patient is based on good medical judgment, making use of the least restrictive environment (Table 44–1). However, when a patient is judged to be eminently violent, often a more restrictive environment is needed to minimize potential injury to the patient and others. Every emergency room and psychiatric unit in which potentially violent patients are treated should have a seclusion room with leather restraints available. In implementing the decision to restrain a violent patient, staff must act decisively with sufficient strength to fully control the situation. This usually requires at least five strong assistants. Often, when patients see a sufficient show of force, they will voluntarily allow themselves to be restrained.

Most patients who are physically restrained will also require psychopharmacological treatment. Intramuscular or intravenous medication can be used without a patient's consent to treat a life-threatening emergency. The three drugs most often used in this situation are lorazepam, diazepam, and haloperidol (Table 44–2). Any of these drugs can be given intravenously but are usually given intramuscularly. They are well absorbed if given in a deltoid muscle, but absorption of benzodiazepines may occasionally be erratic (Arana and Hyman 1991). For a healthy adult, the recommended dosage of lorazepam is 1–2 mg every hour as needed; of diazepam, 5–10 mg every hour as needed; and of haloperidol, 5–10 mg twice a day. Haloperidol is usually only required for patients who are clearly psychotic. However, haloperidol can worsen certain substance intoxications (e.g., PCP), and it frequently causes acute dystonia early in the course of treatment especially in younger adult patients. In these cases, chlorpromazine, 900 mg two or three times a day, might be substituted for haloperidol. An alternative is intramuscular chlorpromazine (30–150 mg/day), which is associated with fewer extrapyramidal side effects (EPS) than haloperidol but greater anticholinergic effects and orthostatic hypotension. Unless the patient is clearly delusional or hallucinating, lorazepam or diazepam is the recommended medication for emergency use.

Agitated Psychosis

Psychosis without accompanying behavioral or suicidal problems is not usually considered a psychiatric emergency and can be routinely treated with antipsychotic medication. However, psychosis with agitation, aggression, or violence is probably the most common psychiatric emergency encountered. Again, symptomatic treatment often precedes definitive diagnosis because of the urgency of the situation. Most agitated psychotic patients are given a diagnosis of bipolar disorder, schizophrenia, brief reactive psychosis, delirium, or dementia.

Bipolar Disorder

Agitated psychosis can occur in bipolar disorder in two forms: major depression and mania. Electroconvulsive therapy (ECT) is quite effective in the treatment of major depression, especially with catatonia, as well as in severe mania. Moreover, these disorders are more commonly managed psychopharmacologically. Although these disorders have traditionally been treated with neuroleptic medication, more recently, alternative therapies have been suggested. Studies have shown that lithium and valproate are both effective in reducing manic symptoms. However, valproate has a broader spectrum of response and has approximately equal benefit for patients with pure mania as for those with mixed mania, rapid cycling, comorbid substance abuse, and secondary bipolar disorder (Bowden 1995; Bowden et al. 1994; Freeman et al. 1992). Pope and colleagues (1991) concluded that valproate was an effective alternative for manic patients who did not tolerate or respond to lithium. Divalproex oral loading in the treatment of acute mania is often effective. It can be given at 20 mg/kg/day orally in divided doses for 5 days, resulting in therapeutic blood levels and rapid onset of antimanic response in some patients (Keck et al. 1993). Furthermore, it has been reported that oral loading with divalproex is as effective as haloperidol in treating acute psychotic mania (McElroy et al. 1996).

Investigations have demonstrated the therapeutic benefits of lorazepam and clonazepam in treating mania. However, one study showed lorazepam to be clearly superior to clonazepam in the treatment of manic symptoms. Of 13 acutely manic patients, 8 (62%) responded to treatment with lorazepam, and 5 (39%) achieved remission. This compared with an 18% ($n = 2$) response rate and 0% remission rate in 11 patients treated with clonazepam (Bradwejn et al. 1990). Lorazepam given orally or intravenously has also been shown to be effective in treating the catatonic syndrome. In one study, 12 of 15 (80%) patients responded completely and dramatically to lorazepam (Rosebush et al. 1990).

Schizophrenia

Treatment of schizophrenic exacerbation has changed markedly in the past 5 years. Rapid neuroleptization (tranquilization) with antipsychotics such as haloperidol in 5-mg doses administered every hour as needed has been replaced by 10–20 mg/day of haloperidol in combination with a benzodiazepine (usually lorazepam) as needed. Several studies have clearly shown that 10–20 mg/day of haloperidol, or the equivalent dose of another antipsychotic, is sufficient as an antipsychotic dose (McEvoy et al. 1991; Rifkin et al. 1991; Van Putten et al. 1990; Volavka et al. 1992). Likewise, benzodiazepine augmentation of neuroleptic medication has been shown to control agitation during exacerbations of schizophrenia (Barbee et al. 1992; Bodkin 1990; Salzman et al. 1991).

Brief Psychotic Disorder

A diagnosis of brief psychotic disorder is common in patients who have a comorbid personality disorder (often borderline personality disorder) and who decompensate under stress. However, it includes any brief psychotic episode not explained by another Axis I disorder. The treatment of agitated psychosis in this disorder is the same as in an exacerbation of schizophrenia, although the neuroleptic drug is usually needed for a shorter time. However, controlled studies addressing effectiveness of therapy for this disorder are lacking.

Delirium

Delirium is defined as a mental disorder with a physical cause that develops over a short period of time and fluctuates over the course of a day. Patients have disturbances of consciousness, poor attention, and a change in cognition or development of perceptual disturbances (American Psychiatric Association 1994). Delirium must always be considered as a cause of agitated psychotic behavior, especially in medically ill and elderly patients.

In addition to treating underlying organic causes of delirium and protecting the patient and others from harm while he or she is in a delirious state, medications can help to calm the patient's agitation. Low doses of haloperidol or lorazepam are usually employed. If the delirium is thought to be due to a substance withdrawal state, lorazepam is the drug of choice. It is important to remember that delirium can be accurately diagnosed by electroencephalogram (EEG). An abnormal EEG finding is virtually always present in delirium (Boutros 1992; Engel and Romano 1959).

Dementia

A patient with dementia can become agitatedly psychotic for various reasons, including delirium, catastrophic reaction, or a reaction to delusions and/or hallucinations. The best treatment for a patient with dementia is nonpharmacological—that is, behavior modification and supportive approaches. However, pharmacotherapy may be indicated, but very low doses of neuroleptics and/or benzodiazepines are recommended because of the high incidence of side effects including delirium, pseudoparkinsonism, and increased falls. Aggressive behavior in elderly patients with brain damage and dementia can respond to other medications, including serotonin reuptake inhibitors, propranolol, and carbamazepine (Deutsch et al. 1991; Maletta 1990). In addition, buspirone in daily doses of 15–45 mg has been reported to be effective in reducing aggressive behavior in brain-damaged patients (Ratey et al. 1991).

Substance Withdrawal

Withdrawal signs and symptoms from alcohol, sedatives and hypnotics, and benzodiazepines are similar. The major signs include tremulousness and autonomic instability (American Psychiatric Association 1994). Also, insomnia and weakness that are not commonly caused by anxiety often present as symptoms of alcohol or sedative withdrawal. The treatment of withdrawal and prevention of Wernicke-Korsakoff syndrome are important considerations. Alcohol withdrawal is probably best treated with benzodiazepines, although barbiturates might have advantages such as preferential renal excretion. Diazepam, because of its relatively long duration of action, has the advantage of providing a smoother tapering-off period. However, lorazepam is recommended for patients with significant liver disease because its metabolism is less impaired in these patients.

Alcohol withdrawal delirium is a life-threatening illness that usually should be treated in an intensive care unit. It is characterized by delirium developing within a week of the cessation of or reduction of alcohol consumption, usually accompanied by excessive autonomic activity, fever, perceptual disturbances, and agitation. The presence of a concomitant physical illness predisposes to the syndrome (American Psychiatric Association 1994). Administration of intramuscular thiamine before administration of an intravenous or oral carbohydrate load is necessary in an alcohol-dependent patient to prevent the development of Wernicke-Korsakoff syndrome (Hyman 1988). Although use of benzodiazepines to treat agitation is recommended, neuroleptic medication should not be used because of the frequency of adverse events.

Substance Intoxication With Violent Behavior

The major substances that lead to violent behavior are cocaine and PCP and, to a lesser extent, amphetamines, hallucinogens, and cannabis. The treatment of psychosis in substance intoxication is similar to the treatment of agitated psychosis (Tables 44–1 and 44–2).

Cocaine

Cocaine use is frequently associated with violence. One study showed transient paranoid states following the use of cocaine in 68% of subjects (Satel et al. 1991). Another study showed that 53% of users became psychotic, and of that group, 90% had paranoid delusions and 96% experienced hallucinations, mostly of the auditory type (Brady et al. 1991). Cocaine abuse is common among schizophrenic patients. Compared with those who were abstinent, schizophrenic individuals who used cocaine were hospitalized more frequently, were more likely to be of the paranoid subtype, and were more likely to be depressed during the course of their illness (Brady et al. 1990).

Phencyclidine

The presentation of PCP intoxication can include virtually any combination of psychiatric signs and symptoms. Agitation and violence are particularly common in these patients. Violence can be unprovoked, sudden, and even lethal. Any patient suspected of having PCP intoxication should be treated very cautiously. The person should usually be placed in an isolation room to decrease the amount of external stimuli. If the patient becomes combative, restraints will often be needed. Moderate doses of lorazepam or diazepam (sometimes in combination with haloperidol) are often needed to help calm the patient. Physical restraint may be necessary for a patient intoxicated with PCP if he or she shows aggressive behavior (Hyman 1988).

Other Substance Intoxications

Amphetamines, hallucinogens, and cannabis abuse can cause psychiatric behavioral emergencies but less often than with the substances already discussed. Any of these substances (including cannabis) can induce psychosis in susceptible individuals. One study found that schizophrenia was six times more likely to develop during a 15-year period in heavy cannabis users than in nonusers (Thornicroft 1990).

Psychoactive Drug Side Effects

Adverse drug effects necessitating prompt remedial action can occur at any time during pharmacotherapy with psychoactive drugs. One basis for selection of initial therapy is to avoid those drugs producing a high incidence of certain side effects. Informing patients and family of expected side effects can be comforting. Nevertheless, the clinician can expect patients who experience unanticipated and untoward drug reactions to be frightened and to often require immediate intervention.

The possible adverse effects from psychoactive drug therapy involve all organ systems. The most urgent side effects requiring attention involve the blood, eyes, and cardiovascular and neurological systems. The prominent drug side effects discussed in the following subsections may present as psychiatric emergencies. Many less common effects may be equally important and are discussed in standard references.

Antipsychotic Agents

Extrapyramidal side effects. Because all currently available antipsychotic drugs (with the relative exception of clozapine) block the dopamine, subtype 2 (D_2), receptor in the nigrostriatal tract, EPS may emerge during therapy (Goetz and Klawans 1981). Symptoms include acute dystonic reactions, akathisias, and parkinsonism (i.e., akinesia, tremor, rigidity). Antipsychotic drug-induced laryngeal and/or pharyngeal dystonia can precipitate cardiac arrhythmias, presumably through vagal reflexes. In addition, akathisia can be distressing and may result in maladaptive reactions, even contributing to suicidal behavior. These reactions require that antipsychotic dosage be kept as low as possible, but EPS are not consistently dose-related. When EPS appear, anticholinergic agents (e.g., benztropine, 0.5–4.0 mg/day; trihexyphenidyl, 2–10 mg/day; or diphenhydramine, 25–100 mg/day) may be used in treatment. Acute dystonias respond most rapidly to intravenous administration. Caution should be exercised to follow up adequately, because the duration of therapeutic effects following parenteral administration may be brief, and acute EPS can reoccur. There is no consistent evidence that one antiparkinsonian drug is consistently superior to another for treatment of EPS.

Neuroleptic malignant syndrome. An increasingly recognized adverse effect of antipsychotic drugs is the neuroleptic malignant syndrome (NMS). This is an acute and potentially lethal reaction manifested by fever, muscular rigidity, central nervous system (CNS) abnormalities, and autonomic dysfunction (Caroff 1980). It may occur at any time during antipsychotic drug treatment, even after the drug has been recently discontinued. The treatment consists of discontinuing the suspected drug and providing supportive treatment and pharmacotherapy. Appropriate cooling methods, such as hydration, sponge baths, and cooling blankets, are needed for high fever. Anticholinergic drugs may act to restore the central balance of dopamine and acetylcholine, one of the purported central mechanisms causing this reaction (Hashimoto et al. 1984). Benztropine (1–2 mg intramuscularly) or diphenhydramine (25–50 mg intramuscularly) is recommended. Anticholinergic drugs may also be useful to prevent a rebound of EPS or cholinergic withdrawal symptoms in patients previously taking an antipsychotic with a high degree of antimuscarinic activity. Early reintroduction of an antipsychotic drug runs the risk of a return to NMS symptoms. Dopamine agonists have been used orally, either amantadine (200 mg/day) or bromocriptine (15 mg/day) (McCarron et al. 1982; Mueller et al. 1983). Finally, dantrolene sodium (100–300 mg/day) has been successful in relieving skeletal muscle stiffness (May et al. 1983). Treatment may need to be continued for 1–3 weeks. Note that there is a relative lack of controlled and comparative treatment studies for NMS.

Cardiovascular side effects. Antipsychotics produce a variety of cardiovascular effects. In addition to orthostasis, hypotension, and tachycardia, electrocardiogram (ECG) changes are common. The risk of hypotension is increased in elderly patients, with parenteral administration, or with large changes in dosage. General recommendations to prevent hypotensive episodes would include making gradual dose increments, instructing patients to stand slowly when they rise from a reclining position, or recommending that elderly patients wear elastic stockings. Many of these patients are voluntarily salt deprived, and salt supplementation of their diet is often very useful. If systolic pressure falls below 90 mm Hg, the dosage should be held or reduced. It may be necessary to position the patient with legs elevated. In cases in which shock develops, drug treatment may be necessary. The unopposed β-agonist activity of epinephrine can lead to further decreases in blood pressure, and this drug is therefore not recommended. Preferred pressor treatment would be norepinephrine, phenylephrine, or metaraminol.

ECG changes can include prolongation of Q-T interval; S-T segment depression; blunted, notched, or inverted T waves; or appearance of U waves. The occurrence of serious arrhythmias is rare but can be life threatening. Factors that predispose to ECG changes include hypokalemia, recent food intake, heavy exercise, and alcohol abuse (Nasrallah 1978). Taking a baseline and follow-up ECGs on patients with increased risk factors is recommended. Avoiding the use of strongly anticholinergic phenothiazines, especially in elderly patients, may minimize the risk of causing cardiac effects of antipsychotics (Risch et al. 1982).

Anticholinergic side effects. Anticholinergic side effects may be prominent with the antipsychotics and can include dry mouth, blurred vision, urinary retention, and constipation. Many of these side effects can be distressing to patients. The avoidance of drugs with high degrees of muscarinic receptor-binding properties is a useful guide in drug selection. A patient with urinary retention may present with overdistension of the bladder, discomfort, or pain. Reducing drug dosage is usually helpful, or a trial of bethanechol (10–50 mg three or four times per day) can be considered. Constipation can be accompanied by pain, abdominal rigidity, and vomiting. Mild cases can be treated with diet, increased fluid intake, and exercise. Laxatives should be used in the lowest effective dose. Constipation may be a symptom of paralytic ileus, which (if left untreated) may be fatal. Treatment consists of lowering the drug dose when possible, correcting fluid and electrolyte balance, and (if necessary) restoring bowel continuity and function by intubation of the gut and relief of abdominal distension and pressure.

The anticholinergic effects of the antipsychotics and antidepressants may aggravate glaucoma, especially the narrow-angle type. Blurred vision from these drugs results from relaxation of the ciliary muscle and loss of accommodation for near vision. Complaints of eye pain, especially in patients older than 40, should prompt an ophthalmic examination. It may be necessary to decrease the dose of the offending drug or to change to another agent with lower anticholinergic properties. The short-term use of 1% pilocarpine eyedrops may be beneficial for treatment of mydriasis and cycloplegia (Malone et al. 1992).

Alteration of seizure threshold. Drug-induced EEG changes and alteration of the seizure threshold may occur with the antipsychotic drugs (Oliver et al. 1982). Most drug-induced seizures are of the generalized tonic-clonic type. The aliphatic phenothiazines and clozapine appear to be the worst offenders, although the occurrence of seizures is considered rare, with fewer than 1% of patients who receive these drugs being affected. At clozapine doses of 600 mg/day and higher, the risk of seizures appears to increase (Simpson and Cooper 1978). The butyrophenone and piperazine phenothiazines are reported to be associated with a lesser incidence of seizures. Factors that may contribute to the seizure incidence include large or sudden dosage changes; the presence of an organic brain syndrome or a preexisting seizure disorder; and a history of head trauma. EEG abnormalities may be present without the occurrence of seizures. In patients already receiving an anticonvulsant regimen to which an antipsychotic is added, plasma concentration of the anticonvulsant should be followed to ensure maintenance of a therapeutic level. The dosage must be adjusted if seizure activity increases.

For terminating status epilepticus, lorazepam has emerged as the agent of first choice at many centers (Treiman 1990). It is as effective as diazepam. Lorazepam can be given intramuscularly or by intravenous infusion (0.05–0.2 mg/kg at 2 mg/min; 8 mg maximal). If lorazepam fails to terminate status epilepticus, then phenytoin is the drug of choice. Attention should be paid to basic life-support measures (i.e., airway and cardiovascular control) and prevention of complications (e.g., rhabdomyolysis, hyperthermia, cerebral edema).

Clozapine-specific effects.   Patients taking clozapine may experience profound hypotension with or without syncope shortly following initiation of therapy, as early as the first or second dose. Although the documented incidence is less than 0.03%, respiratory and/or cardiac arrest has occurred. The most serious reaction to clozapine is agranulocytosis, which can be fatal. Most cases of bone marrow suppression occur between 6 weeks and 6 months after therapy begins, but weekly monitoring of the blood count is justified for the duration of treatment. Prodromal signs of bone marrow suppression include sore throat, low-grade fever, or flulike symptoms. If the white blood cell (WBC) count is below 3,500, then it should be rechecked biweekly. If the WBC count falls below 3,000 or the granulocyte count below 1,500, then the drug should be discontinued. Preventive measures against infection may be necessary, including isolation and antibiotic therapy. Most patients will need hospitalization for close monitoring while bone marrow function returns to normal.

Severe psychiatric side effects can appear when patients are switched abruptly from one antipsychotic, usually a phenothiazine or clozapine, to one of the newer atypical antipsychotics (Baldessarini et al. 1995). The newer drugs, currently represented by risperidone and olanzapine, generally lack the anticholinergic receptor effects of the traditional antipsychotics. Abruptly switching to a newer antipsychotic can result in appearance of cholinergic withdrawal symptoms, including somatic complaints, insomnia, and agitation lasting for several days. With clozapine, especially, abrupt discontinuation, which may be medically necessary with impending agranulocytosis or with NMS, may result in a return of flagrant psychotic symptoms. When switching drugs, a gradual reduction lasting from 1 to 3 weeks may be appropriate with an overlap of the newer drug. For clozapine, a slower withdrawal may be necessary. To prevent agitation or cholinergic rebound symptoms, coverage with benztro-

pine (1.0–2.0 mg/day) may be useful during the switch process.

Cyclic Antidepressants

Anticholinergic toxicity (i.e., a delirium or psychosis) can occur from use of any anticholinergic drug, including many of the cyclic antidepressants, antipsychotics, and the antiparkinsonian drugs used to treat EPS. The syndrome results from competitive inhibition of acetylcholine at central and peripheral cholinergic muscarinic receptors. Elderly patients are believed to be especially vulnerable, as well as patients in whom combinations or high doses of anticholinergic agents are used. Recommendations for treatment include discontinuing the offending drug or drugs, conducting a medical and mental status examination to confirm the diagnosis, and restricting the patient's environment (Table 44–1) as necessary to minimize accidental injury. If agitation is present, benzodiazepines may be used (Table 44–2). For severely ill patients, physostigmine (1 mg intramuscularly) has been useful. This reversible cholinesterase inhibitor results in enhanced central and peripheral cholinergic actions. Cardiac monitoring is recommended when using physostigmine.

Hypertensive crisis.   The most serious adverse effect of MAOIs is the precipitation of a hypertensive crisis, usually following ingestion of dietary products containing large amounts of tyramine or other substances coadministered with sympathomimetic properties. Management includes discontinuing the MAOI and treating the hypertension. The recommended treatment is intravenous administration of an α-adrenergic blocker. Phentolamine (up to 5 mg intravenously) has been used. An alternative would be chlorpromazine (25–50 mg intramuscularly or orally), which has the advantage of being routinely available in emergency rooms and psychiatric units. Oral nifedipine has been recommended for patients to carry with them to treat a hypertensive crisis, but it is important to be aware of the potential risk of hypotension following ingestion of nifedipine if the patient is not actually hypertensive (Hesselink 1991). An early indication of the need for oral nifedipine is the sudden onset of a severe bilateral pounding occipital headache.

Priapism.   Priapism may appear in male patients receiving trazodone (often after 1 or 2 weeks of therapy) and, to a much lesser extent, with antipsychotic drugs (Scher et al. 1983). This situation constitutes an emergency, because if left untreated, permanent erectile dysfunction may result. Immediate urological consultation should be sought, as surgical intervention may be necessary. Complaints of unusual erectile activity should be viewed with suspicion as a prodromal symptom of priapism and the drug immediately discontinued.

Alteration of seizure threshold. Epileptogenic effects may occur with the cyclic antidepressants in a similar fashion as with the antipsychotics (Jabbari et al. 1985). The incidence with bupropion at doses less than 450 mg/day is 0.4% but rises to nearly 3.0% above 600 mg/day. The incidence may be higher for patients receiving maprotiline. Patients without a history of a seizure disorder and with normal EEG results are considered to be at low risk. If an isolated seizure occurs, a thorough medical and neurological examination should be performed. Either the drug dosage should be lowered or (preferably) the regimen changed to another antidepressant. Prophylactic anticonvulsants are usually not necessary but may be considered for patients who are at high risk for seizure activity (e.g., presence of organicity). Benzodiazepines may be used to terminate seizure activity (as described previously for the antipsychotics) if seizures continue.

SPECIAL PSYCHIATRIC EMERGENCIES

Adolescence

Crisis intervention counseling is frequently indicated in the care of adolescent crises. When psychotherapeutic treatment approaches are unsuccessful, neuroleptics, lithium, anticonvulsants, antidepressants, and β-adrenergic blockers have all been recommended for treating violent adolescent behavior. Factors associated with adolescent violence include alcohol and substance use, depression and suicidality, overstimulation, and family issues. Often violence in the adolescent erupts from a strong wish for affectionate contact. Behavioral change through cognitive restructuring can provide adolescents with tools for self-improvement.

Geriatrics

Elderly patients are much more likely than younger patients to experience adverse effects of psychotropic medication. Therefore, treating behavioral emergencies in elderly people should be tempered by using a lower initial dosage of medication and slowly raising the total daily dosage (Table 44–2).

Another important statistic is the relatively high suicide rate in elderly people, especially white men older than 75. Whenever an elderly patient talks of suicide ideas or plans or demonstrates suicidal behavior, he or she should be fully evaluated (usually on an inpatient psychiatric unit) for psychopathology.

Psychiatric Drug Overdose

Although it is beyond the scope of this chapter to discuss the specific treatment for each psychotropic drug overdose, several points are of particular importance. It is very problematic to treat an acute overdose in a patient on a psychiatric unit, unless it is a medical-psychiatric unit equipped to handle medical emergencies. Often what appears to be a simple benzodiazepine overdose on admission, for example, turns out to be a multiple drug ingestion. Patients who have overdosed on a TCA, even those who appear stable, need 24–48 hours of cardiac monitoring, preferably in an intensive care unit, because of the risk of the development of potentially fatal arrhythmias. Sodium bicarbonate is usually considered the first line of treatment for serious tricyclic overdosage. Alkalinization of the serum acts to increase the protein binding of the tricyclic, thus decreasing the amount of free drug to block the conducting system in the heart (Jenkins and Loscalzo 1990; Kulig 1992). Although cyclic antidepressants and lithium can be fatal in overdosage, the newer antidepressants (i.e., fluoxetine and sertraline) and the benzodiazepines have few if any reported overdose fatalities when taken as the sole ingestant (Arana and Hyman 1991). The neuroleptics may produce electrocardiographic changes resembling conduction defects, but the occurrence of serious arrhythmias is rare (Wilson and Weilser 1984).

REFERENCES

American Psychiatric Association: Diagnostic and Statistical Manual of Mental Disorders, 4th Edition. Washington, DC, American Psychiatric Association, 1994

Apter A, Kotler M, Sevy S, et al: Correlates of risk of suicide in violent and nonviolent psychiatric patients. Am J Psychiatry 148:833–877, 1991

Arana GW, Hyman SE: Handbook of Psychiatric Drug Therapy, 2nd Edition. Boston, MA, Little, Brown, 1991

Bagby RM, Thompson JS, Dickens SE, et al: Decision making in psychiatric civil commitment: an experimental analysis. Am J Psychiatry 148:28–33, 1991

Baldessarini RJ, Gardner DM, Garver DL. Conversion from clozapine to other antipsychotic drugs. Arch Gen Psychiatry 52:1071–1072, 1995

Barbee JG, Mancuso DM, Freed CR, et al: Alprazolam as a neuroleptic adjunct in the emergency treatment of schizophrenia. Am J Psychiatry 149:506–510, 1992

Beck JC, White KA, Gage B: Emergency psychiatric assessment of violence. Am J Psychiatry 148:1562–1565, 1991

Bodkin JA: Emerging uses for high-potency benzodiazepines in psychotic disorders. J Clin Psychiatry 51 (suppl):41–46, 1990

Boutros NN: A review of indications for routine EEG in clinical psychiatry. Hosp Community Psychiatry 43:716–719, 1992

Bowden CL: Predictors of response to divalproex and lithium. J Clin Psychiatry 56 (suppl 3):25–30, 1995

Bowden CL, Brugger AM, Swann AC, et al: Efficacy of divalproex vs. Lithium and placebo in the treatment of mania. JAMA 271:918–924, 1994

Bradwejn J, Shriqui C, Koszycki D, et al: Double-blind comparison of the effects of clonazepam and lorazepam in acute mania. J Clin Psychopharmacol 10:403–408, 1990

Brady K, Anton R, Ballenger JC, et al: Cocaine abuse among schizophrenic patients. Am J Psychiatry 147:1164–1169, 1990

Brady KT, Lydiard RB, Malcolm R, et al: Cocaine-induced psychosis. J Clin Psychiatry 52:509–512, 1991

Bremner JD, Southwick S, Brett E, et al: Dissociation in post-traumatic stress disorder in Vietnam combat veterans. Am J Psychiatry 149:328–332, 1992

Caroff SN: The neuroleptic malignant syndrome. J Clin Psychiatry 41:79–82, 1980

Coccaro EF, Kavoussi RJ: Biological and pharmacological aspects of borderline personality disorder. Hosp Community Psychiatry 42:1029–1033, 1991

Coté TR, Biggar RJ, Dannenberg AL: Risk of suicide among persons with AIDS: a national assessment. JAMA 268:2066–2068, 1992

Deutsch LH, Bylsma FW, Rovner BW, et al: Psychosis and physical aggression in probable Alzheimer's disease. Am J Psychiatry 148:1159–1163, 1991

Engel GL, Romano J: Delirium: a syndrome of cerebral insufficiency. Journal of Chronic Disease 9:260–277, 1959

Freeman TW, Clothier JL, Pazzaglia P, et al: A double-blind comparison of valproate and lithium in the treatment of acute mania. Am J Psychiatry 149:108–111, 1992

Friedman S, Jones JC, Chernen L, et al: Suicidal ideation and suicide attempts among patients with panic disorder: a survey of two outpatient clinics. Am J Psychiatry 149:680–685, 1992

Goetz CG, Klawans HL: Drug-induced extrapyramidal disorders—a neuropsychiatric interface. J Clin Psychopharmacol 1:297–303, 1981

Goldstein RB, Black DW, Nasrallah A, et al: The prediction of suicide. Arch Gen Psychiatry 48:418–422, 1991

Hashimoto F, Sherman C, Jeffery W: Neuroleptic malignant syndrome and dopaminergic blockade. Arch Intern Med 144:629–630, 1984

Hesselink JMK: Safer use of MAOIs with nifedipine to counteract potential hypertensive crisis (letter). Am J Psychiatry 148:1616, 1991

Hoge SK, Appelbaum PS, Lawlor T, et al: A prospective, multicenter study of patients' refusal of antipsychotic medication. Arch Gen Psychiatry 47:949–956, 1990

Hyman SE: Manual of Psychiatric Emergencies, 2nd Edition. Boston, MA, Little, Brown, 1988

Jabbari B, Bryan GE, Marsh EE, et al: Incidence of seizures with tricyclic and tetracyclic antidepressants. Arch Neurol 42:480–481, 1985

Jenkins JL, Loscalzo J: Manual of Emergency Medicine, Diagnosis and Treatment, 2nd Edition. Boston, MA, Little, Brown, 1990

Keck PE, McElroy SL, Tugrul KC, et al: Valproate oral loading in the treatment of acute mania. J Clin Psychiatry 54:305–308, 1993

Klein DF: False suffocation alarms, spontaneous panics, and related conditions: an integrative hypothesis. Arch Gen Psychiatry 50:306–317, 1993.

Kulig K: Initial management of ingestion of toxic substances. N Engl J Med 326:1677–1681, 1992

Liebowitz MR, Klein DF: Interrelationship of hysteroid dysphoria and borderline personality disorder. Psychiatr Clin North Am 4:67–87, 1981.

Maletta GJ: Pharmacologic treatment and management of the aggressive demented patient. Psychiatric Annals 20:446–455, 1990

Malone DA Jr, Camara EG, Krug JH Jr: Ophthalmologic effects of psychotropic medications. Psychosomatics 33:271–277, 1992

Marttunen MJ, Aro HM, Henriksson MM, et al: Mental disorders in adolescent suicide. Arch Gen Psychiatry 48:834–839, 1991

May DC, Morris SW, Stewart RM, et al: Neuroleptic malignant syndrome: response to dantrolene sodium. Ann Intern Med 98:183–184, 1983

McCarron MM, Boettger ML, Peck JJ: A case of neuroleptic malignant syndrome successfully treated with amantadine. J Clin Psychiatry 43:381–382, 1982

McElroy SL, Keck PE, Stanton SP, et al: A randomized comparison of divalproex oral loading versus haloperidol in the initial treatment of acute psychotic mania. J Clin Psychiatry 57:142–146, 1996

McEvoy JP, Hogarty GE, Steingard S: Optimal dose of neuroleptic in acute schizophrenia: a controlled study of the neuroleptic threshold and higher haloperidol dose. Arch Gen Psychiatry 48:739–745, 1991

McGrath PJ, Stewart JW, Nunes EV, et al: A double-blind crossover trial of imipramine and phenelzine for outpatients with treatment-refractory depression. Am J Psychiatry 150:118–123, 1993

McKegney FP, O'Dowd MA: Suicidality and HIV status. Am J Psychiatry 149:396–398, 1992

McNiel DE, Myers RS, Zeiner HK, et al: The role of violence in decisions about hospitalization from the psychiatric emergency room. Am J Psychiatry 149:207–212, 1992

Merson S, Tyrer P, Onyett S, et al: Early intervention in psychiatric emergencies: a controlled clinical trial. Lancet 339:1311–1314, 1992

Mueller PS, Vester JW, Fermaglich J: Neuroleptic malignant syndrome—successful treatment with bromocriptine. JAMA 249:386–388, 1983

Murphy GE, Wetzel RD, Robins E, et al: Multiple risk factors predict suicide in alcoholism. Arch Gen Psychiatry 49:459–463, 1992

Nasrallah HA: Factors influencing phenothiazine-induced ECG changes. Am J Psychiatry 135:118–199, 1978

Oliver PA, Luchins DJ, Wyall RJ: Neuroleptic-induced seizures. Arch Gen Psychiatry 39:206–209, 1982

Parsons B, Quitkin FM, McGrath PJ, et al: Phenelzine, imipramine, and placebo in borderline patients meeting criteria for atypical depression. Psychopharmacol Bull 25:524–534, 1989

Perry JC, Jacobs D: Overview: clinical applications of the amytal interview in psychiatric emergency settings. Am J Psychiatry 139:552–559, 1982

Pope HG, McElroy SL, Keck PE, et al: Valproate in the treatment of acute mania: a placebo-controlled study. Arch Gen Psychiatry 48:62–68, 1991

Ratey J, Sovner R, Parks A, et al: Buspirone treatment of aggression and anxiety in mentally retarded patients: a multiple-baseline, placebo lead-in study. J Clin Psychiatry 52:159–162, 1991

Rifkin A, Doddi S, Karajgi B, et al: Dosage of haloperidol for schizophrenia. Arch Gen Psychiatry 48:166–170, 1991

Risch SC, Groom GP, Janowsky DS: The effects of psychotropic drugs on the cardiovascular system. J Clin Psychiatry 43 (5, sect 2):16–26, 1982

Rosebush PI, Hildebrand AM, Fulong BG, et al: Catatonic syndrome in a general psychiatric inpatient population: frequency, clinical presentation, and response to lorazepam. J Clin Psychiatry 51:357–362, 1990

Salzman C, Solomon D, Miyawaki E, et al: Parenteral lorazepam versus parenteral haloperidol for the control of psychotic disruptive behavior. J Clin Psychiatry 52:177–180, 1991

Satel SL, Southwick SM, Gawin FH: Clinical features of cocaine-induced paranoia. Am J Psychiatry 148:495–498, 1991

Scher M, Drieger JN, Juergens S: Trazodone and priapism. Am J Psychiatry 140:1362–1363, 1983

Simpson GM, Cooper TA: Clozapine plasma levels and convulsions. Am J Psychiatry 135:99–100, 1978

Spar JE, LaRue A: Geriatric Psychiatry. Washington, DC, American Psychiatric Press, 1990

Stanford EJ, Goetz RR, Bloom JD: The no harm contract in the emergency room assessment of suicidal risk. J Clin Psychiatry 55:344–348, 1994

Stevens CB: Lorazepam in the treatment of acute conversion disorder. Hosp Community Psychiatry 41:1255–1257, 1990

Thornicroft G: Cannabis and psychosis: is there epidemiological evidence for an association? Br J Psychiatry 157:25–33, 1990

Treiman DM: The role of benzodiazepines in the management of status epilepticus. Neurology 40 (suppl 2):32–42, 1990

Van Putten T, Marder SR, Mintz J: A controlled dose comparison of haloperidol in newly admitted schizophrenic patients. Arch Gen Psychiatry 47:754–758, 1990

Volavka J, Cooper T, Czobor P, et al: Haloperidol blood levels and clinical effects. Arch Gen Psychiatry 49:354–361, 1992

Wilson WH, Weilser SJ: Case report of phenothiazine induced torsades de pointes. Am J Psychiatry 141:1265–1266, 1984

Winchel RM, Stanley M: Self-injurious behavior: a review of the behavior in biology of self-mutilation. Am J Psychiatry 148:306–317, 1991

Zito JM, Craig TJ, Wanderling J: New York under the Rivers decision: an epidemiologic study of drug treatment refusal. Am J Psychiatry 48:904–909, 1991

FORTY-FIVE

Psychopharmacology in the Medically Ill Patient

Alan Stoudemire, M.D., and Michael G. Moran, M.D.

Prescribing psychotropic medications in medically ill patients requires careful risk-benefit assessment. In this chapter, the special psychopharmacological considerations that are required in making such risk-benefit assessments for the medical-psychiatric population are reviewed, including 1) potential interactions between psychotropic medications and drugs used for primary medical disorders; 2) effects of impaired renal, hepatic, or gastrointestinal functioning on psychotropic drug metabolism; and 3) side effects of psychotropic drugs that may complicate preexisting medical conditions.

Drug interactions of major clinical importance are listed in the tables (Rizos et al. 1988; Sargenti et al. 1988). More extensive critical reviews of the use of psychotropic agents may be found in our more expanded discussions of the area of psychopharmacology (Fogel and Stoudemire 1993; Stoudemire 1996; Stoudemire and Fogel 1987, 1995; Stoudemire et al. 1991, 1993). The use of psychotropic agents in pregnancy (Altshuler et al. 1996; Cohen et al. 1989, 1991), rapid tranquilization of the agitated medical-surgical patient (Goldstein and Haltzman 1993), and the use of psychotropic drugs to treat symptoms associated with primary medical disorders (e.g., chronic pain, peptic ulcer disease) are discussed elsewhere (Max et al. 1992).

A WORD ON NOMENCLATURE

The most consistent definition of *heterocyclic* compounds is that they are "cyclic compounds in which the rings in-clude at least one atom of an element different from the rest"—in contrast to *homocyclic* compounds, in which all the ring atoms are the same (Parker 1993, p. 472). Richelson (1993, p. 232) stated that heterocyclic "describes any ring compound that contains within one or more rings an atom different from carbon," which is consistent with other definitions of the term (Grant and Grant 1987). The breakdown of heterocyclic and homocyclic antidepressants according to these definitions is shown in Table 45–1 (Jefferson 1995). Following the recommendation of Jefferson, we use the general term *cyclic antidepressants* (CyADs) to refer to non–monoamine oxidase inhibitor (MAOI) antidepressants; specific antidepressant classes, such as tricyclic antidepressants (TCAs) or selective serotonin reuptake inhibitors (SSRIs), are designated more specifically.

CYCLIC ANTIDEPRESSANTS IN PATIENTS WITH CARDIAC DISEASE

At therapeutic doses, the cardiovascular risks involved in prescribing CyADs are relatively small in the vast majority of patients. TCAs (e.g., imipramine, amitriptyline) have quinidine-like properties that can increase the P-R interval, QRS duration, and Q-T interval and "flatten" the T wave on the electrocardiogram (ECG). These effects are almost never of major clinical significance unless patients have preexisting or latent cardiac conduction defects, congestive heart failure, or experienced a recent myocardial infarction (Jefferson 1975).

Table 45–1. Breakdown of heterocyclic and homocyclic antidepressants

Heterocyclic	Homocyclic
Amoxapine	Amitriptyline
Desipramine	Bupropion
Doxepin	Fluoxetine
Imipramine	Maprotiline
Paroxetine	Nortriptyline
Trazodone	Sertraline
	Venlafaxine

Source. Adapted from Jefferson 1995.

Because of their quinidine-like effects, TCAs have antiarrhythmic properties and may prolong the refractory period of the action potential of the cardiac conduction system. This quinidine-like effect may suppress ectopic pacemakers that cause atrial flutter, atrial fibrillation, ventricular tachycardia, and premature ventricular contractions (PVCs). Thus, if tricyclic agents are used in depressed patients with cardiovascular disease, they may actually suppress PVCs (Bigger et al. 1977).

TCAs may cause ECG changes at therapeutic serum levels in patients with preexisting conduction delays such as atrioventricular (AV) block. Patients with preexisting intraventricular conduction delays (defined as a QRS interval greater than 0.11 seconds), sick sinus syndrome, second-degree heart block, bifascicular heart block, and prolonged Q-T$_c$ intervals are at higher risk for arrhythmias (Roose et al. 1987). Patients with relatively benign types of heart block, such as uncomplicated left bundle branch block, isolated left anterior or left posterior fascicular block, or right bundle branch block, are at a relatively lower risk for aggravation of heart block by TCAs (Stoudemire and Atkinson 1988).

A prolonged Q-T interval presents a relative contraindication to TCA treatment because of the hazard of malignant ventricular arrhythmias (torsades de pointes; an approximate guideline for the relatively safe use of TCAs is a Q-T interval of no more than 0.440 seconds). Prolonged Q-T intervals may also occur on a congenital basis and present problems in using TCAs. Such patients may not be symptomatic and may only be detected with a routine ECG. In patients without cardiac disease, dangerous prolongations of the Q-T interval (i.e., beyond 0.440 seconds) occur most often in situations involving TCA overdose (Fricchione and Vlay 1986; Schwartz and Wolf 1978). The Q-T interval may also be prolonged iatrogenically from use of antiarrhythmic agents, often in combination, that prolong the Q-T interval over the 0.440-second limit. Note

that trazodone, fluoxetine, sertraline, paroxetine, nefazodone, venlafaxine, and bupropion have few, if any, quinidine-like side effects compared with TCAs (Fisch 1985; Preskorn and Othmer 1984; Sommi et al. 1987). These drugs are much safer than tricyclic agents in patients with cardiac conduction disease.

Although haloperidol is not an antidepressant, a series of reports have identified intravenous haloperidol as a rare potential cause of torsades de pointes (Hunt and Stern 1995). Oral haloperidol has not been reported to have clinically significant effects on the ECG, but the use of relatively high intravenous doses for severe agitation in intensive care settings can precipitate this arrhythmia. Potential risk factors include hypokalemia, hypomagnesemia, liver failure, and congestive heart failure (see also psychopharmacology review chapter by Stoudemire and Fogel 1995). Most patients in intensive care settings can, from the cardiovascular standpoint, be treated with intravenous haloperidol, although more attention should likely be given to monitoring the duration of the Q-T interval during aggressive haloperidol therapy (particularly in patients with the risk factors noted above).

Fluoxetine, sertraline, paroxetine, fluvoxamine, venlafaxine, and bupropion have a low affinity for α-adrenergic receptors. Thus, they have minimal effects on pulse and blood pressure and therefore may offer significant advantages in elderly medically ill patients.

In extremely rare reports, various arrhythmias, particularly bradycardia, are attributed to fluoxetine. Reports of arrhythmias associated with fluoxetine have been primarily in patients who have concomitant serious medical illness and who are taking multiple medications. In our experience, cardiac effects with fluoxetine, as with other SSRIs, are extremely rare; these drugs are preferred in patients with a history of cardiac conduction delays, orthostatic hypotension, and congestive heart failure. Bupropion should be considered for such patients as well.

Venlafaxine has been reported to raise diastolic blood pressure in about 5%–13% of patients when used in doses greater than 200–225 mg/day, but in patients with preexisting propensity for hypertension, pressor effects may occur at lower doses (Feighner 1995). Bupropion may also elevate blood pressure. Both of these drugs may be used safely in patients with preexisting hypertension, but monitoring of blood pressure should be more frequent (weekly) until stable maintenance doses are reached.

MAOIs, which do not have quinidine-like effects, may also be considered for patients with heart block, as can electroconvulsive therapy (ECT). The use of antidepressants in patients with cardiac conduction disease is reviewed in more detail elsewhere (Roose et al. 1987;

Stoudemire and Atkinson 1988; Stoudemire and Fogel 1987; Stoudemire et al. 1993).

Myocardial Infarction

Whether a recent myocardial infarction (MI) in itself is a risk factor for cardiotoxicity from CyADs is not known definitively. Secondary complications of MI, such as heart failure, arrhythmias, orthostatic hypotension, and cardiac conduction abnormalities—and the potential influence of CyADs on cardiac rhythm, conduction, and blood pressure and the potential interactions with other drugs—are all important in assessing the relative safety of CyADs in the post-MI period (Stoudemire and Fogel 1987). No information is available from prospective studies to show increased morbidity or mortality associated with the use of TCAs by post-MI patients. Recent reports from studies of post-MI antiarrhythmic prophylaxis protocols, however, suggest a possible increased risk of morbidity and mortality after MI when drugs with properties similar to those of the tricyclics on cardiac conduction are used. In the Cardiac Arrhythmia Suppression Trials (CAST), which were designed to assess the prophylactic benefit of antiarrhythmics post-MI, two of the type IC antiarrhythmics being studied—flecainide and encainide—were discontinued less than 2 years into the study (A. H. Glassman et al. 1993). These two drugs appeared to increase rather than decrease mortality rates compared with placebo-treated patients (A. H. Glassman et al. 1993).

Flecainide and encainide were the first two antiarrhythmics examined. It was hoped that the increased post-MI mortality would be confined to this class of antiarrhythmics and that the antiarrhythmic moricizine (a type IA antiarrhythmic) would have a beneficial effect. Moricizine eventually also was associated with increased mortality and was discontinued (Epstein et al. 1993). A meta-analysis of patients with ventricular arrhythmias treated with the type IA antiarrhythmic quinidine (Morganroth and Goin 1991; Teo et al. 1993) found an increased risk of mortality. Until more definitive data are available, a conservative approach would be to avoid tricyclics in the post-MI period, if possible, and to treat depression in such patients with SSRIs, venlafaxine, or bupropion.

Cardiac arrhythmias have been observed to emerge after TCAs are discontinued, particularly if the withdrawal is rapid (Regan et al. 1989; Van Sweden 1988). The decision to continue or discontinue TCAs after a cardiac event must be made on an individual basis and depends on multiple medical factors, such as the presence of heart block, orthostatic hypotension, and concurrent arrhythmias. Moreover, the complications caused by abrupt tricyclic withdrawal, or exacerbation or relapse of depression in the post-MI period, also should be considered. Hence, the use of antidepressants in the peri- and post-MI period must always be based on risk-benefit ratio assessment done in consultation with the patient's cardiologist.

The risk of depressive relapse in withdrawing a tricyclic after a cardiac event would have to be weighed against the extrapolated risk of their continued use based on their type IA quinidine-like (sodium channel blocking) effects. Most clinicians would likely opt to convert patients to an SSRI or bupropion post-MI or if significant cardiac conduction effects emerge. Venlafaxine might be a reasonable choice, because its effects at the presynaptic level are similar to those of the tricyclics.

Orthostatic Hypotension and Congestive Heart Failure

Orthostatic hypotension creates the most problems in medically ill patients treated with traditional tricyclics such as imipramine. Patients with preexisting hypotensive symptoms, impaired left ventricular functioning, or bundle branch block are at increased risk for orthostatic hypotension with tricyclic treatment (Rizos et al. 1988). Although in middle-aged and relatively healthy patients, the use of salt supplements and support hose can partially relieve orthostatic hypotension, these measures are of less benefit in elderly medical patients and, in the case of salt loading, may be contraindicated in patients with congestive heart failure or hypertension.

Imipramine has little or no effect on cardiac output in most patients, although it may produce orthostatic hypotension, a serious side effect that often prevents its use (A. H. Glassman et al. 1983). In patients with normal cardiac output and even in patients with stable or well-compensated congestive heart failure, nortriptyline usually has little or no effect on cardiac output and appears to have significantly fewer orthostatic hypotensive effects than does imipramine (Roose et al. 1981, 1986). At very low levels of cardiac output (20%–25% or less) or in decompensated heart failure, however, tricyclics may exacerbate congestive heart failure.

Bupropion appears to have minimal effects on the cardiovascular system, does not cause orthostatic hypotension, and, as noted earlier in this chapter, may actually cause an elevation in blood pressure, particularly in patients with preexisting hypertension. SSRIs appear to have little or no effect on blood pressure (Cooper 1988). Nefazodone has minimal effects on α-adrenergic receptors but can cause some degree of mild orthostatic hypotension (Taylor et al. 1995). Of the tricyclic agents, nortriptyline has been studied the most extensively in relation to blood pressure changes and has relatively less tendency to cause orthostatic hypotension than do tertiary tricyclic compounds such as imipramine and amitriptyline. In patients who have preexisting symptomatic orthostatic hypotension or who develop this condition, drugs such as fluoxetine, sertraline, paroxetine, venlafaxine, or bupropion should be used. For patients requiring more sedation (i.e., patients with persistent insomnia, anxiety, agitation), nefazodone or mirtazapine might be considered.

CYCLIC ANTIDEPRESSANTS IN PATIENTS WITH OTHER MEDICAL CONDITIONS

Glaucoma

Narrow-angle glaucoma can be exacerbated by antidepressants with high anticholinergic side effects, but patients with open-angle glaucoma generally can take TCAs with minimal risk. Patients with narrow-angle glaucoma may safely take TCAs if their glaucoma is being treated and monitored (E. Lieberman and Stoudemire 1987). In general, agents with low or no anticholinergic side effects would be preferred in treating this patient population.

Urogenital Tract Problems

Patients with known and untreated prostatic hypertrophy are at particular risk for urinary retention from traditional anticholinergic tricyclics. More typically, urinary retention that develops after use of a tricyclic often leads to the identification of latent prostatic disease. As with glaucoma, use of drugs with low or no anticholinergic effects would be the preferred choice in patients prone to urinary retention. Trazodone, which has low anticholinergic properties, can cause priapism, although the risk of this complication is low (about 1 in 7,000 men treated) (Falk 1987). Nefazodone, which has some similarities to trazodone, has not yet been reported to cause priapism.

Seizure Disorders

Human and animal reports vary in their conclusions as to the effects of CyADs on the seizure threshold (Edwards et al. 1986). Although antidepressants, particularly tricyclics, can cause seizures in overdose, their propensity to cause seizures in the general population and in patients with overt or latent epilepsy indicates some likelihood of lowering the seizure threshold. On the other hand, some antidepressants, such as doxepin, actually have been reported to have anticonvulsant effects on the electroencephalogram (EEG) when these drugs were given by injection to nonclinical volunteers (Simeon et al. 1969).

Some evidence suggests a higher rate of seizures for clomipramine than for the standard tricyclic imipramine (Burley 1977; Trimble 1978). It is relatively clear that maprotiline and bupropion should be avoided in patients prone to seizures. The data for bupropion indicate that—aside from certain groups at high risk for seizures—its effects on seizure threshold may not be significantly greater than those for other antidepressants. Nevertheless, bupropion should be avoided in patients with epilepsy and in other high-risk patients, such as those with a history of head trauma or patients with abnormal foci on the EEG, indicating potential enhanced central nervous system (CNS) irritability (Davidson 1989). Among the traditional tricyclic agents, amitriptyline appears most likely to aggravate seizures (Edwards et al. 1986).

When CyADs are given to treated epileptic patients, anticonvulsant levels should be periodically checked and dosages adjusted to maintain the level in the therapeutic range because of possible drug interactions between CyADs and anticonvulsants (Table 45–2). For example, carbamazepine will *lower* tricyclic levels, and sodium valproate may *elevate* tricyclic levels.

Pharmacokinetic Considerations

When treating frail, medically ill elderly patients, starting dosages of TCAs should be low (e.g., 10 mg/day of nortriptyline). Dosage should be raised gradually, depending on a patient's toleration of side effects and response to treatment. Cases have been reported of toxic serum tricyclic levels in elderly patients taking as little as 25 mg/day (J. N. Glassman et al. 1985).

Insufficient information exists regarding the effects of medical illness on TCA metabolism, but some general observations can be made from limited studies of the use of these drugs in elderly patients (Rockwell et al. 1988). Impaired hepatic protein synthesis (leading to decreased serum albumin levels) may decrease the availability of protein for drug binding, leaving more unbound drug active at receptor sites, and hence more bioactive drug availability at a given dose as compared with that in patients with normal serum albumin levels. Plasma levels of the tertiary tricyclics amitriptyline and imipramine also tend to be positively correlated with age (i.e., increased age equals increased serum level for a given dose; Nies et al. 1977). Metabolism of demethylated tricyclics such as nortriptyline and desipramine appears to be less affected by age than is metabolism of imipramine and amitriptyline (Abernethy et al. 1985; Antal et al. 1982; Cutler and Narang 1984; Cutler et al. 1981; Neshkes et al. 1985; Nies et al. 1977).

Table 45–2. Reported drug interactions with psychotropic agents: cyclic antidepressants (CyADs)

Medication	Interactive effect
Type IA antiarrhythmics (quinidine, procainamide)	May prolong cardiac conduction time
Phenothiazines	May prolong Q-T interval and raise CyAD levels
Reserpine Guanethidine Clonidine	May decrease antihypertensive effect
Prazosin and other α-adrenergic blocking agents	Potentiate hypotensive effect
Parenteral sympathomimetic pressor amines (e.g., epinephrine, norepinephrine, phenylephrine)	May cause slight increases in blood pressure
Disulfiram Methylphenidate Cimetidine	Raise CyAD levels
Warfarin	May increase prothrombin time (fluoxetine probably more likely to cause this effect)
Oral contraceptives Ethanol Barbiturates Phenytoin	May lower CyAD levels
Anticholinergic agents	TCA may potentiate side effects
Carbamazepine	Additive cardiotoxicity possible and lower tricyclic levels
Propafenone (type IC antiarrhythmic)	May elevate tricyclic levels
Digitoxin	Fluoxetine may displace digitoxin from protein-binding sites and increase bioactive levels of digitoxin; converse is also true
High-fiber diets Cholestyramine	May lower TCA serum levels

Note. TCA = tricyclic antidepressant.

Elderly and medically ill patients do not necessarily always need lower doses of TCAs, and elderly patients may show either great sensitivity or great tolerance to these drugs (J. N. Glassman et al. 1985; Rockwell et al. 1988; Stoudemire and Fogel 1987). Primary liver disease and hepatic dysfunction from diseases as well as congestive heart failure may result in slower metabolism of TCAs (and thus a longer half-life) compared with that in healthy patients.

A number of drugs may inhibit hepatic enzymes (e.g., SSRIs, antipsychotics, valproate, disulfiram, cimetidine, and methylphenidate) and may thereby increase plasma levels of TCAs (Table 45–2).

The various SSRIs differentially inhibit the cytochrome P450 (CYP) 2D6 enzyme to different degrees, and *all* of the SSRIs have the capacity to inhibit this isoenzyme (Harvey and Preskorn 1996). Paroxetine has the most potent in vitro inhibition of this isoenzyme, but fluoxetine (including its metabolite norfluoxetine) and sertraline also have inhibitory effects. A general trend in most studies evaluating the effects of SSRIs on the CYP2D6 system is that sertraline has relatively fewer inhibitory effects on CYP2D6 than does either fluoxetine or paroxetine (Brosen 1996). The effects of fluoxetine on desipramine levels are much more persistent, lasting as long as 3 weeks, which is consistent with norfluoxetine's long elimination half-life.

Paroxetine is almost exclusively metabolized by CYP2D6 and may saturate the enzyme at higher dose levels. Paroxetine thus has nonlinear pharmacokinetics, and its half-life increases with increasing doses and plasma concentrations as a result of this effect. The half-life of paroxetine is 10 hours after a single dose and 20 hours at steady state.

A second isoenzyme system of relevance is CYP3A3/4. This isoenzyme metabolizes the triazolobenzodiazepines triazolam, alprazolam, and midazolam; the antidepressant nefazodone; as well as erythromycin, cisapride, cyclosporine, lidocaine, nifedipine, quinidine, terfenadine, and astemizole (Table 45–3). CYP3A3/4 also participates in the *demethylation* of tricyclics such as imipramine and amitriptyline (Lemoine et al. 1993; Ohmori et al. 1993; von Moltke et al. 1994). Nefazodone increases the serum levels of alprazolam and triazolam, which are also metabolized by the CYP3A3/4 isoenzymes. This enzymatic system is *not* subject to genetic variability (polymorphism; i.e., all patients have this isoenzyme), and it is present in both liver and gastrointestinal tissue. CYP3A3/4 is also a major metabolic isoenzyme in the metabolism of sertraline (Ketter et al. 1995a).

Nefazodone appears to be metabolized primarily via the CYP3A3/4 system. The package insert recommends that nefazodone not be used with the antihistamines terfenadine and astemizole because ventricular arrhythmias may occur by blocking their metabolism of CYP3A3/4. Deleterious interactions, however, between nefazodone and the antihistamines terfenadine and astemizole are theoretical in nature and have not been reported.

Table 45–3. Substrates for and inhibitors of the cytochrome P450 (CYP) 3A3/4 isoenzyme

Drugs metabolized by CYP3A4 isoenzyme

Alprazolam

Astemizole

Cyclosporine

Imipramine, amitriptyline (demethylation)

Lidocaine

Midazolam

Nefazodone

Nifedipine

Quinidine

Sertraline

Terfenadine

Triazolam

Inhibitors of CYP3A4 activity

Cimetidine

Erythromycin (and other macrolide antibiotics)

Itraconazole

Ketoconazole

Selective serotonin reuptake inhibitors (weak effect)

Source. Reprinted from Stoudemire A, Fogel BS: "Psychopharmacology in Medical Patients: An Update," in *Medical-Psychiatric Practice*, Vol. 3. Washington, DC, American Psychiatric Press, 1995, pp. 79–149. Copyright 1995, American Psychiatric Press. Used with permission.

Among the nonsedating antihistamines, both terfenadine and astemizole (as well as the gastrointestinal medication cisapride, which promotes motility), even in recommended doses, can cause small increases in the Q-T$_c$ interval. This effect is of almost no clinical significance in normal dose ranges, but in overdose situations in patients with hepatic disease or when the medications are used with drugs that impair their metabolism via CYP3A3/4 (e.g., erythromycin, ketoconazole, clarithromycin, troleandomycin), ventricular arrhythmias such as torsades de pointes may develop.

This effect is of interest to psychiatrists because, as has been noted above, both nefazodone and sertraline and other SSRIs such as fluoxetine are metabolized via CYP3A3/4, but the extent that these antidepressants would inhibit terfenadine or astemizole (or cisapride) metabolism to cause an arrhythmia is not known. In patients being treated with nefazodone and sertraline, both fexofenadine and loratadine are good alternative antihistamines to consider. Fexofenadine is a nonsedating histamine (H$_1$) receptor antagonist with no anticholinergic or α-adrenergic blocking effects; the drug does not cross the blood-brain barrier. Unlike terfenadine, it does not block

cardiac cell potassium channels, which is the primary mechanism of terfenadine's proarrhythmic effects. Hence, if clinicians are concerned about the use of antihistamines with either nefazodone or sertraline, fexofenadine and loratadine would be the drugs to consider (Medical Letter 1996). Loratadine appears to be metabolized by CYP3A3/4, and its metabolism is inhibited by erythromycin, which results in elevation of loratadine serum levels and the levels of its principal metabolite (descarboethoxyloratadine). These relative elevations do *not* appear to have effects on the ECG such as Q-T$_c$ prolongation (Brannan et al. 1995).

It should also be noted that the parent compound nefazodone is metabolized predominantly by CYP3A3/4, whereas a major metabolite of nefazodone, m-CPP (meta-chloro-phenylpiperazine, a serotonin agonist), is metabolized predominantly by CYP2D6. If a patient is switched from an antidepressant (e.g., fluoxetine or paroxetine) that inhibits CYP2D6 to nefazodone, the metabolism of the m-CPP metabolite would be temporarily inhibited. This inhibition of m-CPP metabolism would increase the anxiogenic properties of this metabolite, possibly causing increased anxiety and agitation despite nefazodone's serotonin-2 (5-HT$_2$) receptor blockade effects. Hence, switching from a long-acting CYP2D6 inhibitor (such as fluoxetine) to nefazodone should allow sufficient time for fluoxetine to wash out (3–4 weeks), and starting doses of nefazodone should be conservative to prevent m-CPP toxicity.

Carbamazepine is metabolized by CYP3A3/4 and induces the enzyme's activity. Erythromycin and ketoconazole competitively inhibit CYP3A3/4 and therefore will inhibit the metabolism of carbamazepine.

The major metabolic pathway for sertraline is CYP3A3/4; CYP2D6 is a relatively minor pathway. Venlafaxine is metabolized (demethylated) by CYP2D6 and CYP3A3/4. Venlafaxine is weaker than any of the other SSRIs in inhibiting the 2D6 isoenzyme.

Space does not permit a detailed review of all of the reported drug interactions with the SSRIs. Table 45–4 summarizes drug interactions that have been reported over the past several years that appear to have the most clinical relevance. The mechanisms for these interactions vary: some may be related to direct metabolic effects on the cytochrome enzymatic systems, whereas others may be more related to pharmacodynamic interactions. Extensive details of side effects and drug interactions with fluoxetine may be found elsewhere (Ereshefsky et al. 1996; Messiha 1993; Nemeroff et al. 1996).

Because fluoxetine is tightly bound to plasma protein, the administration of fluoxetine to a patient taking another

Table 45–4. Reported drug interactions with selective serotonin reuptake inhibitors

Fluvoxamine

Drug	Effect	Reference
Propranolol	Five-time increase in propranolol levels	Benfield and Ward 1986; van Harten et al. 1992b
Warfarin	Increase in warfarin concentrations by 60%; increased prothrombin time	Benfield and Ward 1986
Theophylline	Increase in theophylline levels by factor of three	Sperber 1991
Carbamazepine	Conflicting reports: increase in carbamazepine levels as well as stable carbamazepine levels reported when fluvoxamine added	Fritze et al. 1991; Spina et al. 1993a
Amitriptyline	Increase in tricyclic antidepressant serum levels	Bertschy et al. 1991
Clomipramine	No increase in demethylated metabolites of clomipramine	
Atenolol	Some decrease in clinical effect of atenolol	Benfield and Ward 1986
Terfenadine	Possible elevation of terfenadine levels	von Moltke et al. 1996
Bromazepam	Increase in bromazepam levels	van Harten et al. 1992a
Imipramine	Increase in imipramine levels	Spina et al. 1993b, 1993c
Desipramine	Slight increase in desipramine levels when fluvoxamine added to patients with stable serum levels of desipramine	Spina et al. 1993b
Lorazepam	No effect	van Harten et al. 1992a

Fluoxetine

Drug	Effect	Reference
Imipramine	Increase in imipramine levels	Bergstrom et al. 1992
Desipramine	Increase in desipramine levels	Bergstrom et al. 1992
Nortriptyline	Increase in nortriptyline levels	Ciraulo and Shader 1990
Haloperidol	Increase in haloperidol levels	Goff et al. 1991; Tate 1989
Perphenazine	Increase in perphenazine levels	Lock et al. 1990
Diazepam	Increase in diazepam levels	Lemberger et al. 1988
Alprazolam	Increase in alprazolam levels	Ciraulo and Shader 1990; Lasher et al. 1991
Terfenadine	Increase in terfenadine levels	von Moltke et al. 1996
Carbamazepine	Increase in both carbamazepine and carbamazepine 10,11-epoxide levels	Gidal et al. 1993; Grimsley et al. 1991
Warfarin	No effect on half-life of warfarin or the prothrombin time	Rowe et al. 1978
Pimozide	Bradycardia when fluoxetine was added; delirium also reported, probably caused by increased pimozide levels	Ahmed et al. 1993; Hansen-Grant et al. 1993
Cyclosporine	No effect of fluoxetine on cyclosporine levels	Strouse et al. 1993
Valproic acid	Increase in valproate serum levels	Sovner and Davis 1991
Clozapine	Increase in clozapine levels	Centorrino et al. 1994
Clonazepam	No effect of fluoxetine on clonazepam levels	Greenblatt et al. 1992
Phenytoin	Possible increase in phenytoin levels	D. J. Woods et al. 1994
Metoprolol	Bradycardia when fluoxetine was added	Walley et al. 1993

Paroxetine

Drug	Effect	Reference
Cimetidine	Increase in paroxetine levels by 50%	Bannister et al. 1989
Phenobarbital	Decrease in paroxetine levels by 25%	Greb et al. 1989

(continued)

Table 45–4.   Reported drug interactions with selective serotonin reuptake inhibitors *(continued)*

	Paroxetine *(continued)*	
Drug	**Effect**	**Reference**
Carbamazepine, valproate, and phenytoin	No effect on carbamazepine serum levels when paroxetine coadministered with these anticonvulsants	Andersen et al. 1991
Phenytoin and carbamazepine	Possible decrease in paroxetine levels	Andersen et al. 1991
Molindone	Increase in extrapyramidal side effects	Malek-Ahmadi and Allen 1995
Drugs metabolized via CYP2D6 (includes tricyclics)	Increase in serum levels	See Table 45–3
Terfenadine	Possible elevation of terfenadine levels	von Moltke et al. 1996
	Sertraline	
Drug	**Effect**	**Reference**
Tolbutamide	Decrease in tolbutamide levels	Warrington 1991
Warfarin	Increased prothrombin time	Wilner et al. 1991
Atenolol	No effect on atenolol level	Warrington 1991
Terfenadine	Possible elevation of terfenadine levels	von Moltke et al. 1996
Drugs metabolized by CYP2D6	Increase in serum levels	See Table 45–3
Tricyclics (including desipramine)	Elevation of tricyclic antidepressant levels	Barros and Asnis 1993

Source.   Reprinted from Stoudemire A, Fogel BS: "Psychopharmacology in Medical Patients: An Update," in *Medical-Psychiatric Practice*, Vol. 3. Washington, DC, American Psychiatric Press, 1995, pp. 79–149. Copyright 1995, American Psychiatric Press. Used with permission.

drug that is tightly bound to protein (e.g., warfarin, digitoxin) could theoretically cause a shift in plasma concentrations that results in an adverse effect. Conversely, adverse effects may result from displacement of protein-bound fluoxetine by other tightly bound drugs. (These qualities also apply to sertraline and paroxetine, which are also highly protein bound.) Interactions between SSRIs and warfarin may increase coagulation time (prothrombin time [PT], or INR). The potential interaction is theoretically based on SSRIs possibly displacing warfarin from protein-binding sites, leaving more unbound (free) warfarin to be biologically active. The most extensive studies have been done with fluoxetine, but fluoxetine does not appear to alter the pharmacological effects of warfarin (Rowe et al. 1978). In contrast, both fluvoxamine and sertraline (Wilner et al. 1991) *have* been reported to increase *total* warfarin levels and increase PTs presumably by enzyme inhibition. For example, fluvoxamine has been noted to increase warfarin levels by 60% and subsequently increase PTs (Benfield and Ward 1986). Although paroxetine has been reported to have no effect on total warfarin levels, bleeding time nevertheless increased when the two drugs were coadministered (Bannister et al. 1989). Little

clinical evidence suggests these properties regarding protein binding are of major clinical significance; nevertheless, clinicians are advised to monitor clotting studies carefully when SSRIs are used with warfarin until steady-state levels are reached.

SSRIs and Hematological Effects

Fluoxetine may have hematological side effects. Fluoxetine diminishes granular storage of serotonin in platelets and has been reported to increase bleeding times. Petechiae, ecchymoses, and even melena have been reported rarely with fluoxetine treatment; evidence suggests that these hematological effects are dose related (Alderman et al. 1992). Impaired platelet aggregation has been described with fluoxetine in doses greater than 20 mg/day; platelet activity normalized several days after the drug was discontinued. This implies that the parent drug (fluoxetine) is responsible for hematological effects because the principal metabolite (norfluoxetine) would not be eliminated for at least several weeks. Whether other SSRIs clinically affect platelet functioning is not fully known. Based on the current state of knowledge, obtaining bleeding times in patients taking fluoxetine should be considered if these patients have planned elective surgery; however, screening of patients being treated with other SSRIs is not necessary.

A series of studies have investigated the use of sertraline with several drugs commonly used in general medicine. These studies have found the following results in healthy male volunteer subjects:

- Sertraline does not alter the β-blocking activity of atenolol (Ziegler and Wilner 1996).
- Sertraline does not appear to have a clinically significant effect on digoxin pharmacokinetics or ECG findings (Rapeport et al. 1996a).
- Sertraline does not change levels of carbamazepine or levels of its intermediate (more toxic) metabolite 10,11-epoxide when these drugs are used together (Rapeport et al. 1996c). Sertraline does not have any significant effect on phenytoin levels (Rapeport et al. 1996b).

These findings from controlled pharmacokinetic studies in healthy volunteers do not eliminate the possibility of drug interactions in older medically ill patients, and they do not define sertraline as the preferred SSRI in patients taking concomitant medications. They do lend support for a relatively low likelihood of sertraline affecting the serum levels of the above medications in most patients.

SSRIs and Extrapyramidal Side Effects

SSRIs can cause extrapyramidal side effects (EPS), including akathisia, dyskinesias, dystonias, and drug-induced parkinsonism (Arya and Szabadi 1993; Baldwin et al. 1991; Nicholson 1992; Wils 1992), via antidopaminergic effects. EPS are most likely to occur in older patients, particularly those whose histories or prior drug responses suggest preclinical Parkinson's disease (Dave 1994). Parkinsonian-like side effects may be caused by inhibition of neuronal production and release of dopamine caused by increases in synaptic serotonin. Inhibition of dopamine systems by serotonin and SSRIs has been demonstrated in animals (Baldessarini and Marsh 1990; Kapur and Remington 1996).

SSRIs have been reported to exacerbate symptoms of preexisting Parkinson's disease (Steur 1993), although some clinicians observe that such effects are rarely of clinical significance. Several of the reported cases of SSRIs causing EPS have occurred in patients treated with neuroleptics. Inhibition of neuroleptic metabolism by SSRIs may have played a role in the observed effect (Arya and

Szabadi 1993; Nicholson 1992; Wils 1992). Attempts to use medications with serotonin-dopamine interaction profiles suggest the possibility of reduced EPS and negative symptoms, but the benefits may appear in only a narrow dose range. Much work remains to be done to clarify this interaction and specify optimal therapeutic conditions (Kapur and Remington 1996).

Akathisia, however, is the most common neurological symptom caused by SSRIs. It may be seen in patients at any age. Akathisia can be managed by dose reduction of the SSRI or by treatment with low doses of propranolol (20–40 mg/day).

Renal Failure and Dialysis

The hydroxylated metabolites of TCAs have been found to be markedly elevated in patients with renal disease and on dialysis (Dawling et al. 1982; J. A. Lieberman et al. 1985) as compared with control subjects. Serum levels of the parent tricyclic compounds (amitriptyline and nortriptyline) after oral doses also tend to be somewhat higher in dialysis patients than in control subjects (J. A. Lieberman et al. 1985). However, no data indicate the need for routine measurement of the hydroxylated metabolites of TCAs in patients with chronic renal failure or in those on dialysis. Some toxicity may be accrued from these (unmeasured) hydroxylated tricyclic metabolites, but their effects are likely minimal unless patients have advanced end-stage organ failure. The fact that these hydroxylated metabolites contribute to side-effect hypersensitivity urges more conservative titration of doses in severely medically ill populations. In contrast, the serum levels of fluoxetine do not appear to be affected in the face of renal disease when patients are undergoing hemodialysis (Levy et al. 1996). Table 45–5 (Stoudemire et al. 1991) summarizes the side-effect profiles of the currently available non-MAOI CyADs.

MIRTAZAPINE

Mirtazapine, an antidepressant with a tetracyclic structure and a complex mechanism of action, was recently introduced into the United States. Mirtazapine blocks *presynaptic* noradrenergic α₂ autoreceptors that regulate biogenic amine release (deBoer 1996). This antagonism of central presynaptic α₂-adrenergic autoreceptors results in disinhibition of norepinephrine release and enhanced noradrenergic neurotransmission. Norepinephrine stimulation of α₁-adrenergic receptors increases serotonergic neurotransmission. Mirtazapine also blocks serotonin in-

Table 45–5.   Side-effect profiles of cyclic antidepressants (CyADs)

	Effect on serotonin reuptake	Effect on norepinephrine reuptake	Sedating effect	Anticholinergic effect	Orthostatic effect	Dose range[d] (mg)
Amitriptyline[a]	++++	++	++++	++++	++++	75–300
Imipramine[a]	++++	++	+++	+++	++++	75–300
Nortriptyline	+++	+++	++	++	+	40–150
Protriptyline	+++	++++	+	+++	+	10–60
Trazodone	+++	±	+++	±[b]	++	200–600
Desipramine	+++	++++	+	+	++	75–300
Amoxapine[c]	++	+++	++	++	++	75–600
Maprotiline	+	++	++	+	++	150–200
Doxepin	+++	++	+++	++	++	75–300
Trimipramine[c]	+	+	++	++	++	50–300
Fluoxetine	++++	–	–	–	–	20–60
Paroxetine	++++	–	–	++	–	20–40
Sertraline	++++	–	–	–	–	50–200
Bupropion	–	–	–	±	–	150–450

Note.   Relative potencies (some ratings are approximated) based partly on affinities of these agents for brain receptors in competitive binding studies. – = none, + = slight, ++ = moderate, +++ = marked, ++++ = pronounced, ± = indeterminant.
[a]Available in injectable form.
[b]Most in vivo and clinical studies report the absence of anticholinergic effects (or no difference from placebo). There have been case reports, however, of apparent anticholinergic effects.
[c]Amoxapine and trimipramine have dopamine receptor blocking activity.
[d]Dose ranges are for treatment of major depression. Lower doses may be appropriate for other therapeutic uses.
Source.   Reprinted from Stoudemire A, Fogel BS, Gulley L: "Psychopharmacology in the Medically Ill: An Update," in *Medical Psychiatric Practice*, Vol. 1. Edited by Stoudemire A, Fogel BS. Washington, DC, American Psychiatric Press, 1991, pp. 29–97. Copyright 1991, American Psychiatric Press. Used with permission.

hibiting α_2 adrenoreceptors located on serotonergic nerve terminals, which also causes an increase in serotonergic neurotransmission. Because 5-HT$_2$ and 5-HT$_3$ receptor subtypes are blocked by mirtazapine, the increased release of serotonin is exerted predominantly on 5-HT$_1$ receptors. Mirtazapine does not block 5-HT$_{1A}$ or 5-HT$_{1B}$ receptors. Mirtazapine is a potent antagonist of H$_1$ receptors, which accounts for its sedating properties.

Mirtazapine follows linear pharmacokinetics in the therapeutic dose range of 15–45 mg/day; its average half-life of 20–40 hours makes it suitable for once-a-day (nocturnal) dosing (Hoyberg et al. 1996). Major metabolic pathways for mirtazapine are demethylation and hydroxylation followed by glucuronide conjugation. In vitro data from human liver microsomes indicate that CYP2D6 and CYP1A2 are involved in the hydroxylated 8-OH metabolites, and CYP3A forms the *N*-desmethyl and *N*-oxide metabolites (Package Insert, Organow, Inc., West Orange, NJ).

The manufacturer reports that the half-life of the drug is more extended in women than in men (mean 37 hours for women and 26 hours for men). The oral clearance of

mirtazapine was decreased by 30% in patients with liver disease as compared with healthy control subjects. Compared with patients who have normal renal functioning, in patients with both moderate (glomerular filtration rate [GFR] 11–39 mL/min/1.73 m^2) and severe (GFR < 10 mL/min/1.73 m^2) renal impairment, the average oral clearance of mirtazapine was reduced by 30% and 50%, respectively (Package Insert data). Clearance of the drug is reduced in the elderly, with the most striking reductions in men (40% lower clearance in elderly men compared with younger men vs. only a 10% difference between older and younger women).

In premarketing trials, 2 of 2,796 patients taking mirtazapine developed agranulocytosis, and one-third developed neutropenia. All patients recovered after drug discontinuation. Whether bone marrow suppression will be a problem when the drug is used on a more widespread basis is unknown.

Mirtazapine has not been studied in patients post-MI or with cardiovascular disease, but in noncardiac patients, use of the drug is not associated with clinically significant ECG changes. It can be associated with orthostatic blood pressure to a mild degree and symptomatic complaints of dizziness.

Compared with placebo, mirtazapine use in elderly patients was significantly associated with dry mouth, sedation, and dizziness; rates of urinary retention and constipation were not significantly greater than those with placebo (Halikas 1995). Studies in younger adults, however, have shown that subjects reported frequency of dry mouth, constipation, blurred vision, fatigue, dizziness, and headache to be almost comparable to that of amitriptyline (Hoyberg et al. 1996).

The overall clinical picture of mirtazapine could be summarized as follows:

- It is a relatively sedating drug that can be given once daily at night, although its sedative properties may diminish over time.

- Its side-effect profile has been associated with dry mouth, constipation, dizziness, and blurred vision (more than placebo) in some studies, particularly in elderly patients.

- Its safety in patients with heart disease has not been studied, but ECG effects in persons without heart disease do not appear to be clinically significant.

- Its clearance is reduced in patients with liver and renal disease, and the drug rarely may cause agranulocytosis.

- Its mechanism of action is as a potent and highly selective presynaptic α_2-adrenoreceptor antagonist that increases noradrenergic neurotransmission by causing increased noradrenergic cell firing and norepinephrine release. Effects on serotonin are the result of norepinephrine-regulated stimulation of α_1 receptors that activate serotonin cells in the raphe nucleus (deBoer 1996). By blocking inhibitory α_2 adrenoreceptors that suppress serotonin activity, the overall effect is to enhance serotonin neurotransmission via this mechanism as well.

MAOIs IN MEDICALLY ILL PATIENTS

MAOIs may raise special problems in medically ill patients because of their effects on blood pressure and body weight as well as interactions with medications used in internal medicine. With respect to elderly medically ill patients, the most common effect of MAOIs is orthostatic hypotension. As compared with traditional tricyclics, there is relatively little difference between the orthostatic blood pressure effects of phenelzine compared with those of nortriptyline in patients age 55 and older (Georgotas et al. 1987). Effects on blood pressure may be ameliorated by slow, conservative dosing strategies. Divided-dose strategies also will help in minimizing blood pressure effects.

Hypertensive crises may be precipitated by drug interactions with MAOIs. The most consistent offenders are the *indirect* pressor amines (e.g., ephedrine, pseudoephedrine, and phenylpropanolamine; Table 45–6). *Direct* pressors (e.g., norepinephrine, epinephrine, and isoproterenol) are relatively safer, and in one well-designed animal study, they showed almost no pressor effects (Braverman et al. 1987). Nevertheless, close monitoring of blood pressure would be strongly advised if these drugs were administered to a patient taking MAOIs. Methylphenidate or an amphetamine is sometimes combined with an MAOI in treatment-resistant depression. Caution should be used in these situations because of possible hypertensive reactions (Feighner et al. 1985). Patients receiving bronchodilators are at a higher risk for side effects when taking MAOIs; however, at least theoretically, these patients should not have unusual problems as long as indirect sympathomimetics such as ephedrine are clearly avoided. Xanthines and cromolyn usually would be preferable to sympathomimetic drugs in asthmatic patients taking MAOIs.

Drug-induced hypertensive episodes would be particularly hazardous in patients with cardiovascular or cerebrovascular disease and in patients taking oral anticoagulants because of their greater risk for a cerebral hemorrhage. The first symptoms may include sudden fatigue or a pounding bilateral occipital headache. All patients treated with MAOIs (even those at relatively low risk) should carry 10-mg nifedipine tablets to be chewed or dissolved under the tongue at the first signs of a hypertensive reaction (Clary and Schweizer 1987). Nifedipine's hypotensive effect is relatively proportional to the degree of hypertension and has a direct antianginal effect that would be of benefit for patients with coronary insufficiency. Despite the U.S. Food and Drug Administration's (FDA) recent warning about nifedipine's capacity to produce hypotension, we believe that the risk is irrelevant to the danger of a sudden hypertensive episode during MAOI treatment. Verapamil, at a dose of 80 mg orally, has been used for treatment of hypertensive crises (Merikangas and Merikangas 1988). Drug interactions with MAOIs are summarized in Table 45–6.

All MAOIs—especially the hydrazines, such as phenelzine and isocarboxazid—are associated with carbohydrate craving and weight gain. Weight gain would be of particular importance in patients with diabetes mellitus and hyperlipidemia. For patients with these and other medical

Table 45–6.   Reported drug interactions with psychotropic agents: monoamine oxidase inhibitors (MAOIs)

Medication	Interactive effect
Meperidine	Fatal reaction
L-Dopa, methyldopa, dopamine, buspirone, guanethidine, cyclic antidepressants, carbamazepine, cyclobenzaprine	Elevation of blood pressure
Direct-acting sympathomimetics Epinephrine, norepinephrine, isoproterenol, methoxamine	Elevation of blood pressure
Indirect-acting sympathomimetics Cocaine, amphetamines, tyramine, methylphenidate, phenethylamine, metaraminol, ephedrine, phenylpropanolamine	Severe hypertension
Direct- and indirect-acting sympathomimetics Pseudoephedrine, metaraminol, phenylephrine	Severe hypertension
Serotonergic agents Fluoxetine, tryptophan	"Serotonin syndrome" (ataxia, nystagmus, confusion, fever, tremor)
Caffeine Theophylline Aminophylline	Mild elevation of blood pressure
Hypoglycemic agents	Lower blood glucose
Anticoagulants	Prolonged prothrombin time
Succinylcholine	Phenelzine prolongs action
Diuretics Propranolol Prazosin Calcium channel blockers	Increased hypotensive effect
Midrin	Midrin contains isometheptene, a sympathomimetic (Kraft and Dore 1996), and can cause hypertension in combination with an MAOI.

disorders that would be complicated by substantial weight gain, tranylcypromine typically would be the MAOI of choice. The "reversible" MAOI moclobemide is not manufactured in the United States but is often imported for use here. Moclobemide is not associated with weight gain and

would theoretically be the preferred MAOI in a diabetic patient based on potential for weight gain. The use of the MAOI diet is not required for this drug, up to a dose of 900 mg/day.

Clinical tradition has usually mandated that MAOIs should always be discontinued prior to anesthesia and surgery. However, more recent evidence suggests that surgery or ECT can be safely performed during concurrent use of MAOIs (El Ganzouri et al. 1985; Stack et al. 1988; Wells and Bjorksten 1989), providing that there is no chance the patient would receive meperidine in the postoperative period. Sedation may occur when MAOIs are used in conjunction with benzodiazepines and may be misinterpreted as a worsening of depression.

OTHER SPECIAL CONSIDERATIONS IN THE USE OF MAOIs

As has been noted earlier in this chapter, MAOIs do not significantly affect cardiac conduction, although few data are available on the use of these drugs in patients with advanced cardiovascular disease (McGrath et al. 1987). Phenelzine may slightly reduce heart rate and may actually shorten the Q-T interval (McGrath et al. 1987; Robinson et al. 1982). MAOIs may even have some antiarrhythmic effects; in one animal model of ventricular fibrillation, phenelzine had an antiarrhythmic effect (Verrier 1986).

MAOIs appear less likely than TCAs to aggravate seizures (Edwards 1985; Trinidad and Silver 1994), but their pharmacodynamic interactions with some anticonvulsants may create other problems, such as excessive sedation if barbiturate anticonvulsants are used. MAOIs, however, may be preferable in many situations to tricyclics in epileptic patients needing antidepressant therapy.

MAOIs may cause a pyridoxine (vitamin B_6) deficiency manifested as peripheral polyneuropathy or as susceptibility to nerve entrapment neuropathy conditions such as carpal tunnel syndrome (Robinson and Kurtz 1987). Pyridoxine deficiency can be treated with 50–100 mg/day of vitamin B_6. The MAOIs also influence thiamine metabolism (decreasing erythrocyte transketolase; Ali 1985). In malnourished or alcoholic patients, this effect could theoretically increase the likelihood of clinical symptoms of thiamine deficiency.

Recently, guidelines for more liberal dietary (tyramine) parameters for patients taking MAOIs have been published based on a critical literature review and a scientific assessment of the actual tyramine content of previously proscribed foods. These revised dietary recommendations are summarized in Table 45–7 (Gardner et al. 1996).

Table 45–7. Relative restrictions of foods and beverages with monoamine oxidase inhibitor (MAOI) use

Restriction	Foods
Absolute	Aged cheeses; aged and cured meats; banana peel; broad bean pods; improperly stored or spoiled meats, poultry, and fish; Marmite; sauerkraut; soy sauce and other soybean condiments; tap beer
Moderate	Red or white wine, bottled or canned beer (including nonalcoholic varieties)
Unnecessary	Avocados; bananas; beef/chicken bouillon; chocolate; fresh and mild cheeses (e.g., ricotta, cottage, cream cheese; processed slices); fresh meat, poultry, or fish; gravy (fresh); monosodium glutamate; peanuts; properly stored pickled or smoked fish (e.g., herring); raspberries; soy milk; yeast extracts (except Marmite)

Source. Reprinted from Gardner DM, Shulman KI, Walker SE, et al: "The Making of a User Friendly MAOI Diet." *The Journal of Clinical Psychiatry* 57:99–104, 1996. Copyright 1996, Physicians Postgraduate Press. Used with permission.

BENZODIAZEPINES

Complaints of anxiety and disturbed sleep are the most common indications for use of benzodiazepines among medically ill patients. However, when these complaints arise in medically ill patients who are taking several medications or who are in the hospital, care should be exercised in formulating the differential diagnosis. For example, anxiety in a pulmonary patient may be caused by toxic levels of methylxanthines, excessive use of β-adrenergic inhalers, or use of high-dose corticosteroids, none of which should be treated with benzodiazepines alone.

Benzodiazepines in Medically Ill Elderly Patients

As with most psychotropics, benzodiazepines present greater risks for elderly patients than for younger ones (Meyer 1982; Thompson et al. 1983). The high prevalence of anxiety disorders among elderly patients means that they are likely to be prescribed these drugs frequently (Markovitz 1993). Although no benzodiazepines are especially safe for medically ill elderly patients, ultrashort-acting agents such as triazolam are more likely than longer-acting agents to cause confusion, dissociation, and anterograde amnesia (Morris and Estes 1987; Rickels et al. 1988).

Long half-life drugs accumulate and reach steady state slowly, tend to be highly lipophilic, and are cleared slowly after the drug is stopped. These drugs are generally metabolized by oxidation, a hepatic mechanism that decays in efficacy with age and hepatic dysfunction and, for those additional reasons, should be used cautiously in medically ill elderly patients. For example, adjustments downward in dose, greater time intervals between doses, and close follow-up assessment of cognitive functioning and mood would be indicated. Prototypical benzodiazepines in this group include diazepam, flurazepam, and quazepam.

Shorter-acting drugs are less lipophilic, accumulate less, and clear more rapidly after cessation than long-acting drugs. Rather than being oxidized, they are primarily conjugated and renally excreted in a metabolic process that is minimally affected by aging or hepatic disease. Although the adjustments necessary for medically ill elderly patients may be proportionately *less* among this group of conjugated benzodiazepines than for the longer-acting agents, adjustments are usually needed, and close follow-up is indicated (Grad 1995; Greenblatt et al. 1983). Drugs with a medium to short half-life include temazepam, oxazepam, and lorazepam. In patients with hepatic dysfunction due to cirrhosis, active hepatitis, or metabolic damage, one of these three drugs should be selected.

Benzodiazepines can induce ventilatory suppression in the setting of certain pulmonary conditions. Those patients who chronically retain CO_2 are at greatest risk, because benzodiazepines reduce the hypoxic response to ventilation—their only remaining ventilatory stimulus (Lakshminarayan et al. 1976; Modeo and Berry 1974). Another high-risk category is that of patients with sleep apnea (the periodic cessation of ventilation during sleep) caused by either obstruction or failure of central drive.

When using benzodiazepines as hypnotics or anxiolytics, a thorough differential diagnosis and evaluation of etiology should precede reflexive prescription of a drug (Mendelson 1992). Patients with hepatic or pulmonary disease and elderly patients should probably avoid drugs metabolized by oxidation, and, in general, shorter-acting drugs that are conjugated are preferable. Special attention should be given to the patient's need to get up at night, because some drugs, such as triazolam, can cause ataxia and confusion. A key strategy for the psychiatrist treating these patients is frequent follow-up in a manner that allows assessment of cognitive functioning, mood, gait, and (when indicated) ventilatory status with blood gases.

Newer Benzodiazepines

Estazolam is a new drug for insomnia. Its elimination half-life increases moderately in elderly patients from the usual range of 8–24 hours to a range of 13–34 hours. It is effective in elderly patients at half the usual 2-mg dose for younger patients. Little rebound insomnia occurs after abrupt cessation (Pierce and Shu 1990). Risk to elderly patients (of cognitive impairment) and chronic pulmonary patients (of ventilatory suppression) should be considered moderate to high.

Quazepam is a long-acting benzodiazepine that appears to have preferential BZ1 receptor affinity (Wamsley and Hunt 1991). Because the drug is highly lipophilic and rapidly absorbed, its onset of action is rapid. The duration of action of single doses is brief because of movement to fat stores, but repeated doses will result in accumulation there. The fact that quazepam and flurazepam share a major active metabolite argues for caution in the use of quazepam in medically ill elderly patients, patients with pulmonary disease, and patients with hepatic dysfunction.

Zolpidem has largely supplanted the use of triazolam as a short-acting sedative-hypnotic. Zolpidem does not seem to be associated with many of the problems with triazolam (rebound insomnia, anterograde amnesia); nevertheless, zolpidem may affect memory, and adverse reactions have been reported with this agent (Rush and Griffiths 1996), including possible interactions with SSRIs causing drug-induced delirium (Katz 1995). Acute psychotic reactions have also been reported, particularly when zolpidem has been taken with SSRIs (Markowitz and Brewerton 1996). One of the authors (A. S.) observed rebound daytime anxiety following acute discontinuation of zolpidem after prolonged use.

BUSPIRONE

The use of buspirone, a nonbenzodiazepine anxiolytic, has not been studied extensively in medically ill patients. Buspirone may have advantages in patients with chronic lung disease, because in animal studies it appears to stimulate respiratory drive, as opposed to the general depressant effect on respiration observed with benzodiazepines (Garner et al. 1989; Mendelson et al. 1989). Diazepam may markedly depress ventilatory response to exogenous CO_2 administration, whereas buspirone has no such overall effect (Rapoport 1989; Rapoport et al. 1988). In addition, buspirone does not depress ventilatory response to increasing CO_2 levels. Therefore, buspirone appears to be a potentially safe long-term anxiolytic for treatment of patients with respiratory disease.

Pharmacokinetic studies with buspirone indicate no clinically significant differences between young and elderly patients in standard pharmacokinetic measures with either acute or chronic dosing (Gammans et al. 1989).

There appears to be no need to alter the initial doses of buspirone based solely on the patient's age.

NEUROLEPTICS

Apart from schizophrenia, delirium is perhaps the most common disorder treated with neuroleptics among elderly and medically ill patients. The therapeutic efficacy among the various available antipsychotics is essentially the same, and the choice of a particular agent is thus guided by the side-effect profile most likely to be tolerated or to cause the fewest problems in an individual patient. The antipsychotics can be arbitrarily divided into "high-potency" drugs (e.g., haloperidol and fluphenazine), which are relatively low in sedating and anticholinergic effects and high in EPS, and "low-potency" agents (e.g., chlorpromazine and thioridazine), which have opposite characteristics.

The same influences that merge to produce cerebral dysfunction in medically ill patients (i.e., electrolyte disturbances, hypoxemia, volume shifts, systemic infections, medications) make them vulnerable to side effects of any added medication, including neuroleptics. The neuroleptic alone may reduce symptoms in a delirium and thereby induce complacency about the underlying pathogenic cause. Thus, a careful differential diagnosis is necessary for the target syndrome (such as delirium) or symptom (such as agitation). Elderly and medically ill patients are generally more sensitive than younger patients to a given oral dose of low-potency agents, especially for chlorpromazine. As a result, most psychiatrists use high-potency agents, such as haloperidol, in the settings described.

Human data regarding the use of antipsychotic agents in the presence of epilepsy reveal few reliable guidelines for the clinician to follow. A review of the animal literature suggests that chlorpromazine may be the more proepileptic agent of traditional agents. Among newer agents, clozapine has a well-documented seizure-inducing potential (Trinidad and Silver 1994). Molindone may lower the seizure threshold less than other antipsychotics.

Clinicians should be aware that concurrent use of certain SSRIs will result in elevations of clozapine levels and its primary metabolite norclozapine. Such an effect can be expected to varying degrees with all of the available SSRIs and perhaps with fluvoxamine in particular (Centorrino et al. 1996; Dumortier et al. 1996).

Neuroleptics in Patients With Cardiac Disease

Patients with cardiac conduction disease may be susceptible to quinidine-like effects of neuroleptics. The effects on the ECG and on the clinical examination are usually negligible. However, if the patient concurrently takes a type I antiarrhythmic—including a tricyclic—or has a significant preexisting conduction delay, the effect may be less benign and may require close monitoring or even cardiological consultation. If the Q-T$_c$ interval before starting the neuroleptic is 0.440 seconds or longer, added quinidine-like effects may result in fatal ventricular arrhythmias. Among antipsychotics, thioridazine appears to be the most dangerous drug in this regard (Stoudemire et al. 1993). Drug interactions with neuroleptics are listed in Table 45–8.

The psychiatrist should avoid prescribing low-potency agents such as chlorpromazine to patients with symptomatic orthostatic hypotension. These drugs cause a notable degree of α-adrenergic blockade and can worsen blood pressure regulation. High-potency agents are preferred in this setting.

For the patient with an acute MI, the greatest risk again occurs among low-potency drugs, chiefly because of orthostatic hypotension but also because of tachycardia induced by vagolytic anticholinergic effects. High-potency neuroleptics present much lower risk for the cardiac patient.

Neuroleptics in Patients With Other Medical Disorders

The anticholinergic effects of the lower-potency agents (e.g., thioridazine) may cause or exacerbate cognitive dysfunction in elderly patients and may also lead to increased intraocular pressure in patients with narrow-angle glaucoma. The antimuscarinic effects of these drugs may exacerbate prostatism and contribute to male sexual dysfunction. Thioridazine may induce impotence and retrograde ejaculation (Mitchell and Popkin 1983). The higher-potency drugs are less likely to cause these types of anticholinergic problems; however, these drugs are more likely to cause EPS.

Other Side Effects of Neuroleptics

EPS occur with all neuroleptics except clozapine and occur at a much lower rate with risperidone, olanzapine, and sertindole. The high-potency agents produce EPS more commonly than do low-potency agents. Elderly patients are most susceptible to parkinsonian effects, and young male patients are most susceptible to dystonias. The hematological effects of clozapine will likely limit its general use, but the patient with Parkinson's disease and psychotic symptoms may be an ideal candidate for the drug.

Although all antipsychotics lower the seizure thresh-

Table 45–8. Reported drug interactions with neuroleptics

Medication	Interactive effect
Type IA antiarrhythmics	Chlorpromazine or thioridazine may prolong cardiac conduction
Alprazolam Tricyclics β-Blockers Chloramphenicol Disulfiram MAOIs Acetaminophen Buspirone Fluoxetine	May increase neuroleptic levels
Barbiturates Hypnotics Rifampin Griseofulvin Phenylbutazone Carbamazepine Phenytoin	Lower neuroleptic levels through induction of hepatic enzymes
Gel-type antacids with Al^{3+} and Mg^{2+}	May interfere with neuroleptic absorption
Narcotics Epinephrine Enflurane Isoflurane	Potentiate hypotensive effects of neuroleptics
α-Methyldopa Prazosin ACE-inhibitors (captopril, enalapril)	Increase hypotensive effect
Narcotics Tricyclics Barbiturates	May increase sedative effects of neuroleptics
Iproniazid	May cause encephalopathy and hepatotoxicity when used with neuroleptics
Guanethidine Clonidine	Neuroleptics may decrease blood pressure control
Sodium valproate	Chlorpromazine increases valproate levels
Carbamazepine	Carbamazepine treatment lowers clozapine levels

Note.   MAOI = monoamine oxidase inhibitor; ACE = angiotensin-converting enzyme.

old, molindone, fluphenazine (Luchins et al. 1984), thioridazine, and mesoridazine (Edwards et al. 1986) appear to be the least proconvulsant. Reports suggest that chlorpromazine and clozapine are the most problematic in this regard. Combinations of neuroleptics may synergistically lower the seizure threshold. Because neuroleptics may alter the serum levels of anticonvulsant medications, these levels should be monitored during concomitant treatment (Edwards et al. 1986).

Medically debilitated, dehydrated, and neurologically impaired patients appear to be at risk for two potentially catastrophic conditions: neuroleptic malignant syndrome and neuroleptic-induced catatonia. Patients with delirium who are taking antipsychotics thus require close monitoring of fluid status and vital signs (Harpe and Stoudemire 1987; Stoudemire and Luther 1984).

Increasing evidence indicates that antipsychotics have a therapeutic window of efficacy. Thus, in some patients, a dose increase may cause only more side effects and little therapeutic effect. However, in patients who have not yet responded, continued careful upward titration of the dose is indicated. Medically ill and elderly patients may respond to doses of haloperidol as low as 0.5–1.0 mg. Low doses of a benzodiazepine may act synergistically with neuroleptics, producing therapeutic effects without depressing the patient's level of consciousness (Levine 1994).

Clozapine

Clozapine is a novel antipsychotic with minimal EPS. Problems associated with its use include orthostatic hypotension, lowering of the seizure threshold, anticholinergic toxicity, and significant incidence of agranulocytosis (1%–2%). As a consequence, its FDA-approved indications are restricted to psychosis in Parkinson's disease and refractory schizophrenia. Clozapine may reduce the symptoms of Parkinson's disease (Roberts et al. 1989) and may be useful in the treatment of refractory bipolar disorder. The danger of seizure increases with increasing dose. The hematological risk is so grave as to require complete blood counts weekly.

In patients with medical and neurological illness, the major side effects of concern for clozapine are its high anticholinergic profile, its propensity to cause orthostatic hypertension, its potential to lower the seizure threshold, and the development of clozapine-induced fever and leukopenia. The reported problems with agranulocytosis require weekly blood monitoring. Of these patients, 1%–2% taking low doses (below 300 mg/day) are at risk for seizure; this risk increases to 3%–4% for those patients taking intermediate doses and to about 5% at higher doses (600–900 mg/day). Nevertheless, clozapine may have advantages in treatment of patients who are prone to EPS and tardive dyskinesia because it has minimal EPS and has not been reported to cause tardive dyskinesia. The drug may in fact have some beneficial effect in the treatment of tardive

dyskinesia caused by traditional neuroleptics.

Clozapine has been used to treat patients with psychosis in Parkinson's disease and has actually been found to reduce parkinsonian symptoms (Musser and Akil 1996; Roberts et al. 1989). Treatment of psychosis in Parkinson's disease should begin with low doses of clozapine (6.25–12.5 mg twice a day) and be titrated upward slowly if needed. Clozapine's prominent anticholinergic effects may actually decrease the EPS of Parkinson's disease.

Risperidone

Risperidone is a relatively new high-potency antipsychotic that researchers initially hoped would offer some advantages for patients with Parkinson's-related psychotic symptoms and elderly patients prone to EPS. This drug has been reported to cause EPS in elderly patients even at relatively low doses of 1–2 mg, and reliable reports indicate that it causes neuroleptic malignant syndrome (Tarsy 1996). No evidence suggests that this agent necessarily offers major advantages in the treatment of psychosis in patients with Parkinson's disease. Whether sertindole or olanzapine will be less likely to cause EPS in patients with Parkinson's disease remains to be determined.

Sertindole

The newer antipsychotic drug sertindole may have cardiotoxic effects. Sertindole appears to be as effective as haloperidol for the treatment of schizophrenia but with a low EPS profile. Sertindole prolongs the Q-T interval in healthy subjects by an average of 0.21 milliseconds (Schizophrenia Letter 1996). Therefore, if this drug becomes available, it should not yet be used in patients with preexisting cardiac conduction disease.

Olanzapine

Olanzapine is a recently introduced antipsychotic agent of the thienobenzodiazepine class. Its mechanism of antipsychotic activity is via combination of dopamine (D_{1-4}) and 5-HT_2 antagonism. The drug also has moderate antihistaminic, antimuscarinic, and anti-α_1-adrenergic effects. In vitro studies indicate that CYP1A2 and CYP2D6 are involved in olanzapine's oxidation, with 1A2 being the primary route of metabolism. The pharmacokinetics of the drug do not appear to be altered in the presence of advanced renal failure; its elimination half-life is increased by approximately 1.5 times in patients older than 65.

Mild elevations in the alanine aminotransferase (ALT; serum glutamic-pyruvic transaminase [SGPT]) levels were observed in about 2% of patients treated with olanzapine in placebo-controlled studies; none experienced jaundice or symptoms of hepatic impairment. These enzyme elevations tended to normalize as treatment continued. Seizures occurred in 0.9% (22/2,500) patients treated with olanzapine in a premarketing trial. (Information supplied by Bruce Kinon, Eli Lilly Laboratories, 1996.)

Because olanzapine is metabolized by multiple enzyme systems, inhibition of a single cytochrome P450 isoenzyme is unlikely to appreciably decrease olanzapine clearance. Drugs that have been studied as potentially interacting with olanzapine include imipramine, desipramine, and warfarin; pharmacokinetics of these drugs were not affected by a single dose of olanzapine. Multiple doses of olanzapine do not appear to affect the pharmacokinetics of theophylline or its metabolites (predominantly metabolized by CYP1A2). Carbamazepine causes about a 50% *increase* in the clearance of olanzapine, probably because carbamazepine is a potent inducer of CYP1A2 activity.

The most frequent treatment-emergent adverse side effects of olanzapine include postural hypotension, constipation, weight gain, dizziness, and akathisia. The drug may have some selectivity for D_4 receptor blockade and less affinity for nigrostriatal dopamine receptors. In dose ranges of 5–15 mg, akathisia, dystonic events, and parkinsonian events were substantially greater than with placebo. Hence, the drug is not free of EPS; whether it offers advantages for the treatment of psychosis in Parkinson's disease is not known.

The effects on the ECG appear to be benign, and no clinically significant effects on the ECG have been observed. The primary cardiovascular effects of the drug appear to be the propensity for mild degrees of orthostatic hypotension. There have been no reports of neutropenia with olanzapine. (Information supplied by Bruce Kinon, Eli Lilly Laboratories, 1996.)

LITHIUM IN PATIENTS WITH RENAL DISEASE

Because the kidney is the route for lithium excretion, renal competence and alterations in intravascular volume status are impediments to the prescription of the drug. Lithium occupies the "sodium space"; thus, any condition altering sodium movement will likely affect the body's handling of lithium. Volume depletion and traditional diuretic use are the most common clinical examples of conditions that raise serum lithium levels. Volume depletion occurs in conditions associated with vomiting, diarrhea, polyuria, and excessive sweating. Physical disability and diminished responsiveness to thirst could also hinder attempts at normal salt and water replacement. The result would be volume contraction and increased renal reabsorption of sodium and of lithium, with higher lithium levels on an unchanged oral dose. Among the diuretics, the thiazides have the most and furosemide the least effect on lithium concentration (Rizos et al. 1988). Indeed, the thiazides are used for the symptomatic treatment of lithium-induced diabetes insipidus. Potassium-sparing diuretics such as spironolactone may also reduce lithium clearance, but they have been less studied than other diuretics. Drug interactions with lithium are summarized in Table 45–9. Lithium levels may be elevated when angiotensin-converting enzyme inhibitors are added to a preexisting lithium regimen (Finley et al. 1996; Teitelbaum 1993).

Renal failure patients on dialysis do not eliminate lithium between dialyses, and they therefore require only one dose in this interim. Levels are checked 2–3 hours after the dose, which is given after the dialysis. The dosage range is 300–600 mg/day (Levy 1993).

Advancing age itself generally brings a 30%–40% reduction in glomerular filtration rate and necessitates a proportional reduction in oral dose (Hardy et al. 1987). Older

Table 45–9. Reported drug interactions with lithium (Li^+)

Medication	Interactive effect
Thiazide diuretics Spironolactone Triamterene Nonsteroidal antiinflammatants (e.g., indomethacin, ibuprofen, phenylbutazone, piroxicam)	Raise Li^+ levels
Acetazolamide Theophylline Aminophylline	Lower Li^+ levels
Calcium channel blockers	May either raise or lower Li^+ levels, effects not clear; verapamil may cause bradycardia when used with Li^+
Metronidazole	May raise Li^+ levels; may increase chances of nephrotoxicity
Tetracycline	Minor elevation of Li^+ levels
Enalapril and other angiotensin-converting enzyme (ACE) inhibitors	Anecdotally reported to raise Li^+ levels; systematic studies show little overall effect

patients and others with CNS disease may show confusion and sedation at levels therapeutic for younger patients (DePaulo 1984). The psychiatrist should closely monitor lithium levels in these patients and aim for the lower end of the therapeutic range.

Almost all patients taking lithium experience some polyuria because of its effect in reducing the kidney's ability to concentrate urine. This symptom may be ameliorated by giving the lithium once daily, preferably early in the day. In some cases, the concomitant use of thiazide diuretics may be needed to control polyuria. In elderly or debilitated patients, dehydration may become significant (Minden et al. 1993).

Other Side Effects of Lithium

Lithium induces hypothyroidism in 2%–15% of patients and goiter in 3%–4%. People with pretreatment elevated levels of thyroid-stimulating hormone (TSH) are probably at greatest risk for these effects. Diminished effectiveness of antidepressant medication may be the clinical result. Monitoring of TSH and free thyroxine (T_4) levels may detect hypothyroidism and prompt appropriate replacement treatment. Lithium cessation is rarely required.

Cardiac effects are generally quite benign and are restricted to nonspecific T-wave changes in the ECG and some increased susceptibility to digitalis toxicity (Mittal et al. 1985; Tilkian et al. 1976a, 1976b). Extreme sensitivity to side effects of lithium argues for consideration of alternative treatments, such as sodium valproate, for bipolar patients.

A significant risk in the use of lithium is its potential to exacerbate arrhythmias in patients with sinus node dysfunction (Steckler 1994). Although this condition is relatively rare, the propensity of lithium to unmask or aggravate sinus node dysfunction should prompt clinicians to be more judicious in the use of lithium in patients with this condition or who develop sinus arrhythmias in the context of lithium therapy. Pacemaker insertion would usually make the use of lithium safe in such patients, but if lithium actually precipitated sinus node dysfunction, use of valproic acid would be an alternative for an elderly bipolar patient requiring long-term prophylaxis. The use of carbamazepine, with its quinidine-like effect, has been suspected of contributing to the arrhythmogenic potential of lithium in patients prone to sinus node dysfunction (Steckler 1994).

PSYCHOSTIMULANTS

Psychostimulants such as methylphenidate, dextroamphetamine, and pemoline may be used for the treatment of depressed, medically debilitated patients (Kaufmann

et al. 1982; Kayton and Raskind 1980; S. W. Woods 1986) and cancer patients (Olin and Masand 1996; Weitzner et al. 1995). In addition, methylphenidate has been reported to be effective in the treatment of depression in patients with acquired immunodeficiency syndrome (AIDS) (Fernandez et al. 1988). The dose ranges suggested for methylphenidate vary from 10 to 40 mg/day and for dextroamphetamine from 10 to 20 mg/day given in divided doses early in the day. The half-life for methylphenidate is much shorter than that for dextroamphetamine (2 vs. 12 hours).

Psychostimulants, particularly dextroamphetamine, may cause rebound depression, agitation, psychotic reactions, and dependency (Chiarello and Cole 1987). A less controversial indication for their use is in the treatment of pain in cancer patients to counteract the sedation of narcotics (Goldberg and Tull 1984). In this setting, problems with dependency are moot because most of these patients will have limited life expectancies. Drug interactions are summarized in Table 45–10.

Pemoline is a mild CNS psychostimulant with minimal sympathomimetic activity and a very low abuse potential. Pemoline is used primarily in the treatment of atten-

Table 45–10. Reported drug interactions with benzodiazepines and psychostimulants

Medication	Interactive effect
Benzodiazepines	
Cimetidine	May elevate serum levels of benzodiazepines metabolized predominantly by oxidation
Disulfiram	
Ethanol	
Isoniazid	
Estrogens	Tend to lower benzodiazepine levels
Cigarettes	
Methylxanthine derivatives	
Rifampin	
Sodium valproate	Enhanced sedative effect of benzodiazepines (not applicable to lorazepam)
Psychostimulants	
Guanethidine	Decreased antihypertensive effect
Vasopressors	Increased pressor effect
Oral anticoagulants	Increased prothrombin time
Anticonvulsants	Increased phenobarbital, primidone, phenytoin levels
Tricyclics	Increased blood levels of cyclic antidepressants
MAOIs	Hypertension

Note. MAOI = monoamine oxidase inhibitor.

tion-deficit/hyperactivity disorder (ADHD) but also has been shown to have antidepressant (Conners and Taylor 1980) and cognitive-enhancing properties (Elizur et al. 1979; Small et al. 1968; Talland et al. 1967). Pemoline has been reported to be effective in depressed, debilitated cancer patients, with effects similar to those of methylphenidate and dextroamphetamine. The usual dose in adults with medical illness is initially 18.75 mg once or twice a day, which can be increased over several days to 37.5 mg twice a day. Reported side effects include agitation, anorexia, and manic behavior. Rare cases of the development or induction of motor tics have been reported in children. Pemoline may also cause a reversible elevation in liver enzymes as well as more severe hepatic injury. One death has been reported (Nehra et al. 1990).

A major advantage of pemoline is that it can be given as a chewable tablet and is reliably absorbed through the buccal mucosa—a route for patients with gastrointestinal motility or absorptive dysfunction (Breitbart and Mermelstein 1992). Masand and Tesar (1996) recently published a definitive review of the use of psychostimulants in medically ill patients.

CARBAMAZEPINE

Carbamazepine's dose-related toxicities include ataxia, diplopia, and sedation. Several additional toxicities that are particularly relevant when carbamazepine is used in patients with concurrent medical illness include hematological toxicity, hepatic toxicity, hyponatremia, quinidine-like cardiac effects, and effects on the pituitary-thyroid axis.

Carbamazepine may produce a transient reduction in white blood cell (WBC) count in approximately 10% of patients during the first 4 months of treatment (Rall and Schleifer 1985) and in extremely rare cases produces potentially fatal agranulocytosis and aplastic anemia. The incidence of aplastic anemia has been estimated at 0.5 cases per 100,000 treatment-years (Hart and Easton 1982), but neither the age of the patient nor the duration of treatment predicts the development of aplastic anemia (Pisciotta 1975).

Because of the risk of early neutropenia, weekly or biweekly monitoring of WBC count is usually advised during the first few months of therapy. Carbamazepine should usually be discontinued if the WBC count declines to below 3,500. However, exceptions may be necessary if the indications for carbamazepine are very strong or if a concurrent medical problem or drug treatment might be contributing to the decreased blood count. In such situations, hematological consultation will help to determine the appropriate frequency of monitoring and cutoff point for drug discontinuation. Administration of lithium and carbamazepine lowers the risk for neutropenia because lithium stimulates WBC production. Therefore, the lithium-carbamazepine combination might be an option for patients who have concurrent medical or hematological problems that suppress the WBC count and who have bipolar disorder unresponsive to lithium alone (Brewerton 1986; Vieweg et al. 1986).

Hepatic toxicity from carbamazepine, like hematological toxicity, comes in benign and relatively benign forms as well as in a rare and malignant form. Mild asymptomatic elevations in serum glutamic-oxaloacetic transaminase (SGOT), SGPT, and γ-glutamyl transpeptidase (GGTP) occur in 5%–10% of patients treated with carbamazepine (Jeavons 1983; Pellock 1987). Life-threatening acute hepatitis with liver failure occurs on an allergic basis in fewer than 1 in 10,000 treated patients (Jeavons 1983). This toxicity most often occurs during the first month of therapy. In patients with preexisting liver disease, carbamazepine would be relatively (but not absolutely) contraindicated. However, frequent monitoring of liver enzymes and PT would be a reasonable precaution. In patients without liver disease, elevations of SGOT and SGPT to twice normal levels would generally be acceptable. The upper bounds of transaminase elevation might need to be higher in patients with preexisting hepatic disease who required carbamazepine therapy. Consultation with a gastroenterologist would be indicated to determine both an appropriate schedule for monitoring and criteria for drug discontinuation.

Hyponatremia is a relatively frequent side effect of carbamazepine for which advanced age and higher serum levels are risk factors (Kalff et al. 1984; Lahr 1985; Perucca et al. 1978) and may be aggravated by other conditions predisposing to hyponatremia such as diuretic use, congestive heart failure, and occult malignancy. Patients with risk factors for hyponatremia should have weekly electrolyte measurements during the first month of carbamazepine therapy. If hyponatremia develops, the clinician's response should depend on the severity of the condition, and sodium levels of less than 125 mEq/L would usually be a reason to discontinue carbamazepine. Lesser degrees of hyponatremia should be considered in relation to the necessity of the drug for the patient. In some cases, drugs aggravating hyponatremia, such as diuretics, can be discontinued instead. Persistent hyponatremia after discontinuation of carbamazepine would warrant a full evaluation for inappropriate antidiuretic hormone (ADH) secretion.

Carbamazepine has a tricyclic structure similar to that

of TCAs and has quinidine-like cardiac effects. Clinically significant aggravation of heart block has been reported (Beerman and Edhag 1978; Benassi et al. 1987). Patients older than 40 years or with known cardiac risk factors should have a pretreatment ECG before receiving carbamazepine.

Carbamazepine has been implicated in numerous drug interactions that are summarized in Table 45–11. A major effect of carbamazepine is related to its potent effect on inducing drug metabolism by the hepatic microsomal system (Perucca and Richens 1989), which causes lower serum levels of other drugs metabolized by the liver, including (among many others) TCAs, neuroleptics, propranolol, quinidine, phenytoin, valproic acid, and warfarin. Levels of drugs metabolized by the hepatic microsomal system should probably be obtained more often in patients taking carbamazepine, and repeated levels of the other medications may be needed if carbamazepine doses are significantly changed.

Because carbamazepine is metabolized by the liver, drugs that inhibit the hepatic metabolic enzymes may raise carbamazepine levels and lead to acute carbamazepine toxicity after a new drug is added. These types of clinically significant interactions have been reported for fluoxetine, cimetidine, verapamil (Beattie et al. 1988; MacPhee et al. 1986), diltiazem (Brodie and MacPhee 1986), danazol (Kramer et al. 1986), propoxyphene (Dam et al. 1977), and the antibiotic erythromycin (Wong et al. 1983) and are listed in Table 45–11. More recently, carbamazepine levels were elevated to toxic proportions when nefazodone was added to a maintenance regimen of carbamazepine—an effect most likely the result of interactions at the CYP3A3/4 isoenzyme (Ashton and Wolin 1996).

Carbamazepine can decrease bupropion (and increase hydroxybupropion) levels; this effect is likely via enhancement of the hydroxylation and oxidative pathways of the parent drug's metabolism. In contrast, valproate does not affect bupropion levels but does increase hydroxybupropion serum concentrations (Ketter et al. 1995b) possibly by *inhibition* of hydroxybupropion metabolism. Because carbamazepine induces the CYP3A3/4 isoenzyme, this isoenzyme is likely responsible for bupropion's hydroxylation. Hence, both carbamazepine and valproate raise hydroxylated bupropion levels. The clinical implications of these findings for therapy are not clear because the psychotropic effects of increased OH-bupropion are not fully understood. It may well be that concurrent therapy with bupropion and carbamazepine could decrease the effectiveness of bupropion's antidepressant effect. On the other hand, carbamazepine appears to enhance the antidepressant effects of trazodone, perhaps by intensifying sero-

Table 45–11. Reported drug interactions with carbamazepine

Medication	Interactive effect
Erythromycin	May raise carbamazepine to toxic levels and precipitate heart block
Antiarrhythmics	May have additive effects on cardiac conduction time
Fluoxetine Cimetidine Diltiazem Verapamil Danazol Propoxyphene Nefazodone	May raise carbamazepine levels to toxic levels
Quinidine Phenytoin Warfarin Tricyclic antidepressants Neuroleptics Propranolol Valproate Clonazepam	Serum levels lowered by carbamazepine
Phenobarbital	Decreases serum levels of carbamazepine and increases concentrations of carbamazepine's epoxide metabolite
Phenytoin	Decreases levels of carbamazepine; phenytoin levels decrease when used with carbamazepine
Warfarin	Carbamazepine causes increased metabolism of anticoagulants due to hepatic enzyme induction
Oral contraceptives	Carbamazepine reduces efficacy; loss of contraceptive effect possible

tonin function (Otani et al. 1996). Plasma trazodone levels decrease when the two drugs are used together.

Phenytoin- and carbamazepine-treated patients may have decreased free T_4 and triiodothyronine (T_3) concentrations but appear clinically euthyroid and have normal TSH levels. This effect is explained primarily by the fact that therapeutic levels of phenytoin and carbamazepine displace T_4 and T_3 from serum binding proteins. When added to serum, these drugs effect an *increase* in free hormone fractions and free T_4 and T_3 concentrations. The most likely sequence is that in patients beginning anticonvulsant therapy:

1. A transient *increase* in serum free T_4 concentration
2. A transient decrease in TSH
3. A decrease in total T_4 concentration

4. Normal serum free T_4 concentration
5. Normal steady-state TSH levels

The concentrations of serum free T_4 and free T_3 are essentially unchanged and remain in the normal ranges with long-term therapy with phenytoin and carbamazepine. These findings are based on special techniques using an ultrafiltration assay of free T_4 fractions in undiluted serum, a technique that is not used in most laboratories. Hence, routine measurement of free T_4 will likely show decreased free T_4 concentrations in patients taking phenytoin or carbamazepine. Clinicians should rely on the TSH level to confirm the euthyroid state of these patients (Surks and DeFesi 1996).

VALPROATE

Valproic acid is increasingly being given to patients with bipolar spectrum disorders. The drug's gastrointestinal effects are well known. These problems are markedly reduced by the availability of enteric-coated preparations and by patients taking the medications after meals. Although hepatic failure was a major concern with valproate in the past, this problem is encountered almost exclusively in children younger than 2 years. The incidence of valproate-related hepatic necrosis in adults is less than 1 in 10,000 (Eadie et al. 1988). In adults, serum ammonia may be elevated as a result of inhibition of urea synthesis, but this effect is almost always benign and is of concern only in patients with preexisting liver disease. Significant liver disease is a relative contraindication to valproate treatment. A recent review found that between 1987 and 1993, fatal hepatotoxicity from anticonvulsant *monotherapy* with valproate occurred in only one patient older than 20; the chances of hepatotoxicity increase by a factor of 6 with anticonvulsant polytherapy. Risk factors for valproate hepatotoxicity include children younger than 10 years, polytherapy, developmental delays, and coincident metabolic disorders (such as cytochrome and oxidase deficiency) (Bryant and Dreifuss 1996). The drug appears to be safe and effective in the elderly (Puryear et al. 1995). Pancreatitis is a rare side effect but may be more common among mentally retarded adults (Buzan et al. 1995).

Valproate can increase the PT and decrease fibrinogen levels and platelet counts, but such effects very rarely lead to clinically significant bleeding (Stoudemire et al. 1991). Patients should have a coagulation panel (PT/partial thromboplastin time [PTT]) and a platelet count before undergoing surgery.

With respect to drug interactions, valproate tends to inhibit hepatic enzymes involved in drug metabolism. This effect is in contrast to that of carbamazepine, which is a hepatic enzyme inducer. Note that if carbamazepine and valproate are used together, valproate will raise the concentration of the 10-11-epoxide metabolite of carbamazepine. This epoxide metabolite has additional toxicity with carbamazepine and is usually not measured. Hence, the capacity for carbamazepine toxicity is increased when the two drugs are used together. In addition, valproate may displace carbamazepine from serum protein-binding sites, which increases the bioavailable fraction of carbamazepine but does not change the absolute blood level; thus, side effects may increase at a given carbamazepine level.

Valproate appears to interact with felbamate, a new anticonvulsant that recently has been withdrawn from the market. Seizures and psychotic symptoms have resulted with the combination of these two drugs. The psychotic symptoms accompanied a delirious state in the reported patients (McConnell et al. 1996). The mechanism of interaction may be potentiation of γ-aminobutyric acid (GABA)ergic systems.

Valproic acid's primary route of metabolism is via glucuronidation and β-oxidation, although the drug may be metabolized by the cytochrome P450 system when cytochrome P450 is induced by other drugs such as carbamazepine. This alternative pathway gives rise to the potentially more toxic 4-en-VPA metabolite, which may cause microvesicular steatosis, the characteristic histopathological lesion of valproic-induced hepatotoxicity (Bryant and Dreifuss 1996).

With valproate, protein-binding sites are readily saturated. Dose increases beyond the point of saturation may lead to enhanced side effects, even though dose increases are relatively small and absolute serum levels increase only slightly. Drug interactions with valproate are listed in Tables 45–12 and 45–13 (Abbott Laboratories data). More detailed discussions of the use of valproate in the medical patient may be found elsewhere (Fogel and Stoudemire 1993; Stoudemire et al. 1991, 1993).

Newer anticonvulsants include a product from Japan, zonisamide, which is structurally similar to serotonin. In small studies, zonisamide has proved effective in patients with mood disorders. Its pharmacological profile is similar to that of carbamazepine (Kanba et al. 1994). Zonisamide may produce leukocytosis and elevated liver function tests in a minority of patients.

ECT IN MEDICALLY ILL PATIENTS

ECT should be considered as a primary treatment for many severely depressed medically ill patients. In medi-

Table 45–12.   Reported drug interactions with valproate

Medication	Interactive effect
Benzodiazepines (except lorazepam)	Sedative effects and serum levels of benzodiazepine increased by valproate
Carbamazepine Phenytoin Phenobarbital	Lower levels of valproate
Phenobarbital	Phenobarbital levels increased by valproate
Phenytoin Carbamazepine	Bioavailable phenytoin and carbamazepine increased by valproate by displacing these drugs from serum protein-binding sites
10-11-epoxide metabolite of carbamazepine	This metabolite's levels increased by valproate
Tricyclic antidepressants (TCAs)	TCA levels increased by valproate
Chlorpromazine Cimetidine Salicylates	Increase levels of valproate
Anticoagulants (warfarin)	Increase prothrombin times; valproate also inhibits secondary phase of platelet aggregation

cally debilitated depressed patients and those with advanced cardiovascular disease, appropriate pharmacological management before and during anesthesia can usually attenuate the autonomic responses (i.e., hypertension and tachycardia) that pose the primary risks for elderly patients with cerebrovascular or cardiovascular disease. Advanced technical reviews of the use of ECT and special anesthetic considerations in medically ill patients may be found elsewhere (Knos and Sung 1991, 1993; Silver et al. 1986).

REFERENCES

Abernethy DR, Greenblatt DJ, Shader RI: Imipramine and desipramine disposition in the elderly. J Pharmacol Exp Ther 232:183–188, 1985

Ahmed I, Dagincourt PG, Miller LG, et al: Possible interaction between fluoxetine and pimozide causing sinus bradycardia. Can J Psychiatry 38:62–63, 1993

Alderman CP, Moritz CK, Ben-Tovim DI: Abnormal platelet aggregation associated with fluoxetine therapy. Ann Pharmacother 26:1517–1519, 1992

Ali BH: Effect of some monoamine oxidase inhibitors on the thiamine status of rabbits. Br J Pharmacol 86:869–875, 1985

Altshuler LL, Cohen L, Szuba MP, et al: Pharmacologic management of psychiatric illness during pregnancy: dilemmas and guidelines. Am J Psychiatry 153:592–606, 1996

Andersen BB, Mikkelsen M, Vesterager A, et al: No influence of the antidepressant paroxetine on carbamazepine, valproate and phenytoin. Epilepsy Res 10:201–204, 1991

Antal EJ, Lawson IR, Alderson LM, et al: Estimating steady-state desipramine levels in noninstitutionalized elderly patients using single dose disposition parameters. J Clin Psychopharmacol 2:193–198, 1982

Arya DK, Szabadi E: Dyskinesia associated with fluvoxamine (letter). J Clin Psychopharmacol 13:365–366, 1993

Ashton A, Wolin R: Nefazodone-induced carbamazepine toxicity (letter). Am J Psychiatry 153:733, 1996

Baldessarini R, Marsh E: Fluoxetine and side effects (letter). Arch Gen Psychiatry 47:191–192, 1990

Baldwin D, Fineberg N, Montgomery S: Fluoxetine, fluvoxamine and extrapyramidal tract disorders. Int Clin Psychopharmacol 6:51–58, 1991

Bannister SJ, Houser VP, Hulse JD, et al: Evaluation of the potential for interactions of paroxetine with diazepam, cimetidine, warfarin, and digoxin. Acta Psychiatr Scand 80 (suppl 350):102–106, 1989

Barros J, Asnis G: An interaction of sertraline and desipramine (letter). Am J Psychiatry 150:1751, 1993

Beattie B, Biller J, Mehlhaus B, et al: Verapamil-induced carbamazepine neurotoxicity: a report of two cases. Eur Neurol 28:104–105, 1988

Beerman B, Edhag O: Depressive effects of carbamazepine on idioventricular rhythm in man. BMJ 2:171–172, 1978

Benassi E, Bo GP, Cociot L, et al: Carbamazepine and cardiac conduction disturbances. Ann Neurol 22:280–281, 1987

Benfield P, Ward A: Fluvoxamine: a review of its pharmacodynamic and pharmacokinetic properties, and therapeutic efficacy in depressive illness. Drugs 32:313–334, 1986

Bergstrom RF, Peyton AL, Lemberger L: Quantification and mechanism of fluoxetine and tricyclic antidepressant interaction. Clin Pharmacol Ther 51:239–248, 1992

Bertschy G, Vandel S, Bandel B, et al: Fluvoxamine-tricyclic antidepressant interaction. Eur J Clin Pharmacol 40:119–120, 1991

Bigger JT, Giardina EGV, Perel JM, et al: Cardiac antiarrhythmic effect of imipramine hydrochloride. N Engl J Med 296:206–208, 1977

Brannan P, Reidenberg E, Radwanski L, et al: Loratadine (Claritin) and 3A4 inhibition: effects on cardiac (and hepatic) function. Clin Pharmacol Ther 58:269–278, 1995

Braverman B, McCarthy RJ, Ivankovich AD: Vasopressor challenges during chronic MAOI or TCA treatment in anesthetized dogs. Life Sci 40:2587–2595, 1987

Breitbart W, Mermelstein H: Pemoline: an alternative psychostimulant for the management of depressive disorders in cancer patients. Psychosomatics 33:352–356, 1992

Table 45–13.   Effects of valproate on other drugs: potentially important interactions

Drug administered with divalproex sodium	Interaction
Carbamazepine	Serum levels of carbamazepine decreased by 17%
10,11-Epoxide	Levels of carbamazepine-10,11-epoxide increased by 45% in patients with epilepsy taking valproate and carbamazepine.
Clonazepam	Concomitant use with valproic acid may induce absence status in patients with a history of absence-type seizures.
Diazepam	Valproate displaced diazepam from plasma albumin-binding sites and inhibited its metabolism. Coadministration of valproate 1,500 mg/day to healthy volunteers increased the free fraction of diazepam (10 mg) by 90%; diazepam plasma clearance decreased by 25% and volume of distribution by 20%. Elimination half-life of diazepam did not change.
Ethosuximide	Valproate inhibited ethosuximide metabolism. Administration of a single 500-mg dose of ethosuximide with valproate (800–1,600 mg/day) to healthy volunteers increased ethosuximide elimination half-life by 25% and decreased its total clearance by 15%. Serum levels of both drugs should be monitored in patients receiving valproate and ethosuximide, especially with other anticonvulsants.
Lamotrigine	Coadministration of valproate to healthy volunteers increased lamotrigine elimination half-life from 26 to 70 hours. The dose of lamotrigine should be reduced when coadministered with valproate.
Phenobarbital	Valproate inhibited phenobarbital metabolism, resulting in a 50% increase in phenobarbital half-life and a 30% decrease in plasma clearance. The fraction of phenobarbital dose excreted unchanged increased by 50%. There is evidence for severe central nervous system depression, with or without significant elevations of barbiturate or valproate serum concentrations. All patients receiving concomitant barbiturate therapy should be monitored closely for neurological toxicity.
Primidone	Primidone is metabolized to a barbiturate and may be involved in a similar interaction with valproate.
Phenytoin	Valproate displaced phenytoin from its plasma albumin-binding sites and inhibited its hepatic metabolism. Coadministration of valproate 400 mg twice a day with phenytoin 250 mg to healthy volunteers increased the free fraction of phenytoin by 60%; total plasma clearance and apparent volume of distribution increased by 30%. Both the clearance and the apparent volume of distribution of free phenytoin were reduced by 25%. In patients with epilepsy, breakthrough seizures have occurred with the combination of valproate and phenytoin.
Tolbutamide	In vitro, the unbound fraction of tolbutamide was increased from 20% to 50% when added to plasma samples from patients treated with valproate. The clinical relevance of this displacement is unknown.
Warfarin	The potential exists for valproate to displace warfarin from its plasma albumin-binding sites. The therapeutic relevance of this displacement is unknown; coagulation tests should be monitored if divalproex sodium is initiated in patients taking anticoagulants.
Zidovudine	In HIV-positive patients, the clearance of zidovudine 100 mg every 8 hours decreased by 38% after administration of valproate 250 or 500 mg every 8 hours; zidovudine half-life was unaffected.

Source.   Reprinted from "Advancing the Treatment of Mania Associated With Bipolar Disorder." North Chicago, IL, Abbott Laboratories, 1995.

Brewerton TD: Lithium counteracts carbamazepine-induced leukopenia while increasing its therapeutic effect. Biol Psychiatry 21:677–685, 1986

Brodie MM, MacPhee GJA: Carbamazepine neurotoxicity precipitated by diltiazem. BMJ 292:1170–1171, 1986

Brosen K: Are pharmacokinetic drug interactions with the SSRIs an issue? Int Clin Psychopharmacol 11:23–27, 1996

Bryant AE, Dreifuss FE: Valproic acid hepatic fatalities, III: U.S. experience since 1986. Neurology 46:465–469, 1996

Burley DM: A brief note on the problem of epilepsy in antidepressant treatment, in Depression—The Biochemical and Physiologic Role of Ludiomil. Edited by Jukes A. Newark, NJ, Ciba, 1977, pp 201–203

Buzan RD, Firestone D, Thomas M, et al: Valproate-associated pancreatitis and cholecystitis in six mentally retarded adults. J Clin Psychiatry 56:529–532, 1995

Centorrino F, Baldessarini RJ, Kando J, et al: Serum concentrations of clozapine and its major metabolites: effects of cotreatment with fluoxetine or valproate. Am J Psychiatry 151:123–125, 1994

Centorrino F, Baldessarini RJ, Frankenburg FR, et al: Serum levels of clozapine and norclozapine in patients treated with SSRIs. Am J Psychiatry 153:820–822, 1996

Chiarello RJ, Cole JO: The use of psychostimulants in general psychiatry: a reconsideration. Arch Gen Psychiatry 44:286–295, 1987

Ciraulo DA, Shader RI: Fluoxetine drug-drug interactions, I: antidepressants and antipsychotics. J Clin Psychopharmacol 10:48–50, 1990

Clary C, Schweizer E: Treatment of MAOI hypertensive crisis with sublingual nifedipine. J Clin Psychiatry 48:249–250, 1987

Cohen LS, Heller VL, Rosenbaum JF: Treatment guidelines for psychotropic drug use in pregnancy. Psychosomatics 30:25–33, 1989

Cohen LS, Heller VL, Rosenbaum JF: Psychotropic drug use in pregnancy: an update, in Medical Psychiatric Practice, Vol 1. Edited by Stoudemire A, Fogel BS. Washington, DC, American Psychiatric Press, 1991, pp 615–634

Conners K, Taylor E: Pemoline, methylphenidate and placebo in children with minimal brain dysfunction. Arch Gen Psychiatry 37:923–930, 1980

Cooper GL: The safety of fluoxetine—an update. Br J Psychiatry 153 (suppl 3):77–86, 1988

Cutler NR, Narang PK: Implications of dosing tricyclic antidepressants and benzodiazepines in geriatrics. Psychiatr Clin North Am 7:845–861, 1984

Cutler NR, Zavadil AP III, Eisdorfer C: Concentrations of desipramine in elderly women are not elevated. Am J Psychiatry 138:1235–1237, 1981

Dam M, Kristensen CB, Hensen BS, et al: Interaction between carbamazepine and propoxyphene in man. Acta Neurol Scand 56:603–607, 1977

Dave M: Fluoxetine-associated dystonia (letter). Am J Psychiatry 151:149, 1994

Davidson J: Seizures and bupropion: a review. J Clin Psychiatry 50:256–261, 1989

Dawling S, Lynn K, Rosser R, et al: Nortriptyline metabolism in chronic renal failure: metabolite elimination. Clin Pharmacol Ther 32:322–329, 1982

deBoer T: The pharmacologic profile of mirtazapine. J Clin Psychiatry 57 (suppl 4):19–25, 1996

DePaulo JR: Lithium. Psychiatr Clin North Am 7:587–599, 1984

Dumortier G, Lochu A, DeMelo PC, et al: Elevated clozapine plasma concentrations after fluvoxamine initiation. Am J Psychiatry 153:738–739, 1996

Eadie MJ, Hooper WD, Dickinson RG: Valproate-associated hepatotoxicity and its biochemical mechanisms. Medical Toxicology Adverse Drug Experience 3:85–106, 1988

Edwards JG: Antidepressants and seizures: epidemiological and clinical aspects, in The Psychopharmacology of Epilepsy. Edited by Trimble MR. Chichester, England, Wiley, 1985, pp 119–139

Edwards JG, Long SK, Sedgwick EM, et al: Antidepressants and convulsive seizures: clinical, electroencephalographic, and pharmacological aspects. Clin Neuropharmacol 9:329–360, 1986

El Ganzouri AR, Ivankovich AD, Braverman B, et al: Monoamine inhibitors: should they be discontinued preoperatively? Anesth Analg 64:592–596, 1985

Elizur A, Wintner I, Davidson S: The clinical and psychological effects of pemoline in depressed patients: a controlled study. International Pharmacopsychiatry 14:127–134, 1979

Epstein AE, Hallstrom AP, Rogers WJ, et al: Mortality following ventricular arrhythmia suppression by encainide, flecainide, and moricizine after myocardial infarction. JAMA 270:2451–2455, 1993

Ereshefsky L, Riesenman C, Lam YWF: Serotonin selective reuptake inhibitor drug interactions and the cytochrome P450 system. J Clin Psychiatry 57 (suppl 8):17–25, 1996

Falk WE: Trazodone and priapism. Biological Therapies in Psychiatry 10:9–10, 1987

Feighner JP: Cardiovascular safety in depressed patients: focus on venlafaxine. J Clin Psychiatry 56:574–579, 1995

Feighner JP, Herbstein J, Damlouji N: Combined MAOI, TCA, and direct stimulant therapy of treatment-resistant depression. J Clin Psychiatry 46:206–209, 1985

Fernandez F, Adams F, Levy JK, et al: Cognitive impairment due to AIDS-related complex and its response to psychostimulants. Psychosomatics 29:38–46, 1988

Finley PR, O'Brien JG, Coleman RW: Lithium and angiotensin-converting enzyme inhibitors: evaluation of a potential interaction. J Clin Psychopharmacol 16:68–71, 1996

Fisch C: Effect of fluoxetine on the electrocardiogram. J Clin Psychiatry 46:42–44, 1985

Fogel BS, Stoudemire A: New psychotropics in medically ill patients, in Medical-Psychiatric Practice, Vol 2. Edited by Stoudemire A, Fogel BS. Washington, DC, American Psychiatric Press, 1993, pp 69–111

Fricchione GL, Vlay SC: Psychiatric aspects of patients with malignant ventricular arrhythmias. Am J Psychiatry 143:1518–1526, 1986

Fritze J, Unsorg B, Lanczik M: Interaction between carbamazepine and fluvoxamine. Acta Psychiatr Scand 84:538–584, 1991

Gammans RE, Westrick ML, Shea JP, et al: Pharmacokinetics of buspirone in elderly subjects. J Clin Pharmacol 29:72–78, 1989

Gardner DM, Shulman KI, Walker SE, et al: The making of a user friendly MAOI diet. J Clin Psychiatry 57:99–104, 1996

Garner SJ, Eldridge FL, Wagner PG, et al: Buspirone, an anxiolytic drug that stimulates respiration. Am Rev Respir Dis 139:946–950, 1989

Georgotas A, McCue RE, Friedman E, et al: A placebo-controlled comparison of the effect of nortriptyline and phenelzine on orthostatic hypotension in elderly depressed patients. J Clin Psychopharmacol 7:413–416, 1987

Gidal BE, Aderson GD, Seaton TL, et al: Evaluation of the effect of fluoxetine on the formation of carbamazepine epoxide. Ther Drug Monit 15:405–409, 1993

Glassman AH, Johnson LL, Giardina EV, et al: The use of imipramine in depressed patients with congestive heart failure. JAMA 250:1977–2001, 1983

Glassman AH, Roose SP, Bigger JT: The safety of tricyclic antidepressants in cardiac patients: risk-benefit reconsidered. JAMA 269:2673–2675, 1993

Glassman JN, Dugas JE, Tsuang MT: Idiosyncratic pharmacokinetics complicating treatment of major depression in an elderly woman. J Nerv Ment Dis 173:573–576, 1985

Goff DC, Midha KK, Brotman AW, et al: Elevation of plasma concentrations of haloperidol after the addition of fluoxetine. Am J Psychiatry 148:790–792, 1991

Goldberg RG, Tull RM: Psychosocial Dimensions of Cancer: A Practical Guide for Health Care Providers. New York, Free Press, 1984, pp 111–169

Goldstein MG, Haltzman SD: Intensive care, in Psychiatric Care of the Medical Patient. Edited by Stoudemire A, Fogel BS. New York, Oxford University Press, 1993, pp 241–265

Grad RM: Benzodiazepines for insomnia in community-dwelling elderly: a review of benefit and risk. J Fam Pract 41:473–481, 1995

Grant R, Grant C (eds): Grant and Hackh's Chemical Dictionary, 5th Edition. New York, McGraw-Hill, 1987, p 282

Greb WH, Buscher G, Dierdorf H-D, et al: Effect of liver enzyme inhibition by cimetidine and enzyme induction by phenobarbitone on the pharmacokinetics of paroxetine. Acta Psychiatr Scand 80 (suppl 350):95–98, 1989

Greenblatt DJ, Divoll M, Abernethy DR, et al: Benzodiazepine kinetics: implications for therapeutics and pharmacogeriatrics. Drug Metab Rev 14:251–292, 1983

Greenblatt DJ, Preskorn SH, Cotreau MM, et al: Fluoxetine impairs clearance of alprazolam but not of clonazepam. Clin Pharmacol Ther 52:479–486, 1992

Grimsley SR, Jann MW, Carter JG, et al: Increased carbamazepine plasma concentrations after fluoxetine coadministration. Clin Pharmacol Ther 50:10–15, 1991

Halikas JA: Org 3770 (mirtazapine) versus trazodone: a placebo controlled trial in depressed elderly patients. Human Psychopharmacology 10:S125–S133, 1995

Hansen-Grant S, Silk KR, Guthrie S: Fluoxetine-pimozide interaction (letter). Am J Psychiatry 150:1751–1752, 1993

Hardy BG, Shulman KI, MacKenzie SE, et al: Pharmacokinetics of lithium in the elderly. J Clin Psychopharmacol 7:153–158, 1987

Harpe C, Stoudemire A: Aetiology and treatment of the neuroleptic malignant syndrome. Medical Toxicology Adverse Drug Experience 2:166–176, 1987

Hart RG, Easton JD: Carbamazepine and hematological monitoring. Ann Neurol 11:309–312, 1982

Harvey AT, Preskorn SH: Cytochrome P450 enzymes: interpretation of their interactions with selective serotonin reuptake inhibitors, part I. J Clin Psychopharmacol 16:273–285, 1996

Hoyberg OJ, Maragakis B, Mullin J, et al: A double-blind multicentre comparison of mirtazapine and amitriptyline in elderly depressed patients. Acta Psychiatr Scand 93:184–190, 1996

Hunt N, Stern TA: The association between intravenous haloperidol and torsades de pointes. Psychosomatics 36:541–549, 1995

Jeavons PM: Hepatoxicity in antiepileptic drugs, in Chronic Toxicity of Antiepileptic Drugs. Edited by Oxley J, Janz D, Meinardi H. New York, Raven, 1983, pp 1–46

Jefferson JW: A review of the cardiovascular effects and toxicity of tricyclic antidepressants. Psychosom Med 37:160–179, 1975

Jefferson JW: Just what is a heterocyclic antidepressant? (letter) J Clin Psychiatry 56:433, 1995

Kalff R, Houtkooper HA, Meyer JWA, et al: Carbamazepine and sodium levels. Epilepsia 25:390–397, 1984

Kanba S, Yagi G, Kamijima K, et al: The first open study of zonisamide, a novel anticonvulsant, shows efficacy in mania. Prog Neuropsychopharmacol Biol Psychiatry 18:707–715, 1994

Kapur S, Remington G: Serotonin-dopamine interaction and its relevance to schizophrenia. Am J Psychiatry 153:466–476, 1996

Katz SE: Possible paroxetine-zolpidem interaction (letter). Am J Psychiatry 152:1689, 1995

Kaufmann MW, Murray GB, Cassem NH: Use of psychostimulants in medically ill depressed patients. Psychosomatics 23:817–819, 1982

Kayton W, Raskind M: Treatment of depression in the medically ill elderly with methylphenidate. Am J Psychiatry 137:963–965, 1980

Ketter TA, Flockhart DA, Post RM, et al: The emerging role of cytochrome P450 3A in psychopharmacology. J Clin Psychopharmacol 15:387–398, 1995a

Ketter TA, Jenkins JB, Schroeder DH, et al: Carbamazepine but not valproate induces bupropion metabolism. J Clin Psychopharmacol 15:327–333, 1995b

Knos GB, Sung Y-F: Anesthetic management of the high-risk medical patient receiving electroconvulsive therapy, in Medical Psychiatric Practice, Vol 1. Edited by Stoudemire A, Fogel BS. Washington, DC, American Psychiatric Press, 1991, pp 99–144

Knos GB, Sung Y-F: ECT anesthesia strategies in the high risk medical patient, in Psychiatric Care of the Medical Patient. Edited by Stoudemire A, Fogel BS. New York, Oxford University Press, 1993, pp 225–240

Kraft K, Dore F: Computerized drug interaction programs: how reliable? (letter) JAMA 275:1087, 1996

Kramer G, Theisohn M, von Unruh GE, et al: Carbamazepine-danazol interaction: its mechanism examined by a stable isotope technique. Ther Drug Monit 8:387–392, 1986

Lahr MB: Hyponatremia during carbamazepine therapy. Clin Pharmacol Ther 37:693–696, 1985

Lakshminarayan S, Sahn SA, Hudson LD, et al: Effect of diazepam on ventilatory responses. Clin Pharmacol Ther 20:178–183, 1976

Lasher TA, Fleishaker JC, Steenwyk RC, et al: Pharmacokinetic pharmacodynamic evaluation of the combined administration of alprazolam and fluoxetine. Psychopharmacology 104:323–327, 1991

Lemberger L, Rowe H, Bosomworth JC, et al: The effect of fluoxetine on the pharmacokinetics and psychomotor responses of diazepam. Clin Pharmacol Ther 43:412–419, 1988

Lemoine A, Gautier JC, Azoulay D, et al: Major pathway of imipramine metabolism is catalyzed by cytochromes P-450 1A2 and P-450 3A4 in human liver. Mol Pharmacol 43:827–832, 1993

Levine RL: Pharmacology of intravenous sedatives and opioids in critically ill patients. Crit Care Clin 10:709–731, 1994

Levy NG: Chronic renal failure, in Psychiatric Care of the Medical Patient. Edited by Stoudemire A, Fogel BS. New York, Oxford University Press, 1993, pp 627–635

Levy NG, Blumenfield M, Beasley CM, et al: Fluoxetine in depressed patients with renal failure and in depressed patients with normal kidney function. Gen Hosp Psychiatry 18:8–13, 1996

Lieberman E, Stoudemire A: Use of tricyclic antidepressants in patients with glaucoma. Psychosomatics 28:145–148, 1987

Lieberman JA, Cooper TB, Suckow RF, et al: Tricyclic antidepressant and metabolite levels in chronic renal failure. Clin Pharmacol Ther 37:301–307, 1985

Lock JD, Gwirtsman HE, Targ EF: Possible adverse drug interactions between fluoxetine and other psychotropics. J Clin Psychopharmacol 10:383–384, 1990

Luchins DJ, Oliver AP, Wyatt RJ: Seizures with antidepressants: an in vitro technique to assess relative risk. Epilepsia 25:25–32, 1984

MacPhee GJ, McInnes GT, Thompson GG, et al: Verapamil potentiates carbamazepine neurotoxicity: a clinically important inhibitory interaction. Lancet 1(8483):700–703, 1986

Malek-Ahmadi P, Allen SA: Paroxetine-molindone interaction. J Clin Psychiatry 56:82–83, 1995

Markovitz PJ: Treatment of anxiety in the elderly. J Clin Psychiatry 54 (suppl):64–80, 1993

Markowitz J, Brewerton T: Zolpidem-induced psychosis. Ann Clin Psychiatry 8:89–91, 1996

Masand PS, Tesar GE: Use of stimulants in the medically ill. Psychiatr Clin North Am 19:515–547, 1996

Max MB, Lynch SA, Muir J, et al: Effects of desipramine, amitriptyline, and fluoxetine on pain in diabetic neuropathy. N Engl J Med 326:1250–1256, 1992

McConnell H, Snyder PJ, Duffy JD, et al: Neuropsychiatric side effects related to treatment with felbamate. J Neuropsychiatry Clin Neurosci 8:341–346, 1996

McGrath PJ, Blood DK, Stewart JW, et al: A comparative study of the electrocardiographic effects of phenelzine, tricyclic antidepressants, mianserin, and placebo. J Clin Psychopharmacol 7:335–339, 1987

Medical Letter: Fexofenadine. 38(986):95–96, October 25, 1996

Mendelson WB: Neuropharmacology of sleep induction by benzodiazepines. Crit Rev Neurobiol 6:221–232, 1992

Mendelson WB, Martin JV, Rapoport D, et al: Buspirone: stimulation of respiratory rate in freely moving rats (abstract). Sleep Research 18:62, 1989

Merikangas JR, Merikangas KR: Calcium channel blockers in MAOI-induced hypertensive crisis (abstract). Psychopharmacology 96 (suppl):229, 1988

Messiha FS: Fluoxetine: adverse effects and drug-drug interactions. Clinical Toxicology 31:603–630, 1993

Meyer BR: Benzodiazepines in the elderly. Med Clin North Am 66:1017–1035, 1982

Minden SL, Bassuk EL, Nadler SP: Lithium intoxication: a coordinated treatment approach. J Gen Intern Med 8:33–40, 1993

Mitchell J, Popkin M: The pathophysiology of sexual dysfunction associated with antipsychotic drug therapy in males: a review. Arch Sex Behav 12:173–183, 1983

Mittal SR, Mathur AK, Advani GB: Genesis of lithium-induced T wave flattening. Int J Cardiol 7:164–166, 1985

Modeo DG, Berry DJ: Effects of chlordiazepoxide in respiratory failure due to chronic bronchitis. Lancet 2:869–870, 1974

Morganroth J, Goin JE: Quinidine-related mortality in the short-to-medium-term treatment of ventricular arrhythmias: a meta-analysis. Circulation 84:1977–1983, 1991

Morris HH, Estes ML: Traveler's amnesia: transient global amnesia secondary to triazolam. JAMA 258:945–946, 1987

Musser WS, Akil M: Clozapine as a treatment for psychosis in Parkinson's disease: a review. J Neuropsychiatry Clin Neurosci 8:1–9, 1996

Nehra A, Mullick F, Ishak KG, et al: Pemoline-associated hepatic injury. Gastroenterology 99:1517–1519, 1990

Nemeroff CB, DeVane L, Pollock BG: Newer antidepressants and the cytochrome P450 system. Am J Psychiatry 153:311–320, 1996

Neshkes RE, Gerner R, Jarvik LF, et al: Orthostatic effect of imipramine and doxepin in depressed geriatric outpatients. J Clin Psychopharmacol 5:102–106, 1985

Nicholson SD: Extra pyramidal side effects associated with paroxetine. West of England Medical Journal 7(3):90–91, 1992

Nies A, Robinson DS, Friedman MJ, et al: Relationship between age and tricyclic antidepressant plasma levels. Am J Psychiatry 134:790–793, 1977

Ohmori S, Takeda S, Rikihisa T, et al: Studies on cytochrome P450 responsible for oxidative metabolism of imipramine in human liver microsomes. Biol Pharm Bull 16:571–575, 1993

Olin J, Masand P: Psychostimulants for depression in hospitalized cancer patients. Psychosomatics 37:57–62, 1996

Otani K, Yasui N, Kaneko S, et al: Carbamazepine augmentation therapy in three patients with trazodone-resistant unipolar depression. Int Clin Psychopharmacol 11:55–57, 1996

Parker SP (ed): McGraw-Hill Encyclopedia of Chemistry, 2nd Edition. New York, McGraw-Hill, 1993, p 472

Pellock JM: Carbamazepine side effects in children and adults. Epilepsia 28 (suppl 3):S64–S70, 1987

Perucca E, Richens A: General principles: biotransformation, in Antiepileptic Drugs, 3rd Edition. Edited by Levy R, Mattson R, Meldrum B, et al. New York, Raven, 1989, pp 23–48

Perucca E, Garratt A, Hebdige S, et al: Water intoxication in epileptic patients receiving carbamazepine. J Neurol Neurosurg Psychiatry 41:713–718, 1978

Pierce MW, Shu VS: Efficacy of estazolam: the United States clinical experience. Am J Med 88 (suppl 3A):6S–11S, 1990

Pisciotta AV: Hematological toxicity of carbamazepine. Adv Neurol 11:355–368, 1975

Preskorn SH, Othmer SC: Evaluation of bupropion hydrochloride: the first of a new class of atypical antidepressants. Pharmacotherapy 4:20–34, 1984

Puryear LJ, Kunik ME, Workman R Jr: Tolerability of divalproex sodium in elderly psychiatric patients with mixed diagnoses. J Geriatr Psychiatry Neurol 8:234–237, 1995

Rall TW, Schleifer LS: Drugs effective in the therapy of the epilepsies, in The Pharmacological Basis of Therapeutics, 7th Edition. Edited by Gilman AG, Goodman LS, Rall TW, et al. New York, Macmillan, 1985, pp 446–472

Rapeport WG, Coates PE, Dewland PM, et al: Absence of a sertraline-mediated effect on digoxin pharmacokinetics and electrocardiographic findings. J Clin Psychiatry 57 (suppl 1):16–19, 1996a

Rapeport WG, Muirhead DC, Williams SA, et al: Absence of effect of sertraline on the pharmacokinetics and pharmacodynamics of phenytoin. J Clin Psychiatry 57 (suppl 1):24–28, 1996b

Rapeport WG, Williams SA, Muirhead DC, et al: Absence of a sertraline-mediated effect on the pharmacokinetics and pharmacodynamics of carbamazepine. J Clin Psychiatry 57 (suppl 1):20–23, 1996c

Rapoport DM: Buspirone: anxiolytic therapy with respiratory implications. Family Practice Recertification 11 (suppl):33–41, 1989

Rapoport DM, Greenberg HE, Goldring RM: Comparison of the effects of buspirone and diazepam on control of breathing (abstract). Federation of American Societies for Experimental Biology 2:A1507, 1988

Regan WM, Margolin RA, Mathew RJ: Cardiac arrhythmia following rapid imipramine withdrawal. Biol Psychiatry 25:482–484, 1989

Richelson E: Review of antidepressants in the treatment of mood disorders, in Current Psychiatric Therapy. Edited by Dunner DL. Philadelphia, PA, WB Saunders, 1993, pp 232–238

Rickels K, Fox IL, Greenblatt DJ, et al: Clorazepate and lorazepam: clinical improvement and rebound anxiety. Am J Psychiatry 145:312–317, 1988

Rizos AL, Sargenti CJ, Jeste DV: Psychotropic drug interactions in the patient with late-onset depression or psychosis, part 2. Psychiatr Clin North Am 11:253–277, 1988

Roberts HE, Dean RC, Stoudemire A: Clozapine treatment of psychosis in Parkinson's disease. J Neuropsychiatry Clin Neurosci 1:190–192, 1989

Robinson DS, Kurtz NM: Question the experts: what is the degree of risk of hepatotoxicity for depressed patients receiving phenelzine therapy? J Clin Psychopharmacol 7:61–62, 1987

Robinson DS, Nies A, Corcella J, et al: Cardiovascular effects of phenelzine and amitriptyline in depressed outpatients. J Clin Psychiatry 43 (5, part 2):8–15, 1982

Rockwell E, Lam RW, Zisook S: Antidepressant drug studies in the elderly. Psychiatr Clin North Am 11:215–233, 1988

Roose SP, Glassman AH, Siris S, et al: Comparison of imipramine- and nortriptyline-induced orthostatic hypotension: a meaningful difference. J Clin Psychopharmacol 1:316–319, 1981

Roose SP, Glassman AH, Giardina EGV, et al: Nortriptyline in depressed patients with left ventricular impairment. JAMA 256:3253–3257, 1986

Roose SP, Glassman AH, Giardina EGV, et al: Tricyclic antidepressants in depressed patients with cardiac conduction disease. Arch Gen Psychiatry 44:273–275, 1987

Rowe H, Carmichael R, Lemberger L: The effect of fluoxetine on warfarin metabolism in the rat and man. Life Sci 23:807–812, 1978

Rush CR, Griffiths RR: Zolpidem, triazolam, and temazepam: behavioral and subject-rated effects in normal volunteers. J Clin Psychopharmacol 16:146–157, 1996

Sargenti CJ, Rizos AL, Jeste DV: Psychotropic drug interactions in the patient with late-onset psychosis and mood disorder, part 1. Psychiatr Clin North Am 11:235–252, 1988

Schizophrenia Letter: FDA panel recommends sertindole for approval. Psychiatric Times (suppl), September 1996, pp 1, 3

Schwartz P, Wolf S: QT interval prolongation as predictor of sudden death in patients with myocardial infarction. Circulation 57:1074–1077, 1978

Silver JM, Yudofsky SC, Kogan M, et al: Elevation of thiorida-zine plasma levels by propranolol. Am J Psychiatry 143:1290–1292, 1986

Simeon J, Spero M, Fink M: Clinical and EEG studies of doxepin. Psychosomatics 10:14–17, 1969

Small IF, Sharpley P, Small JG: Influence of Cylert upon memory changes with ECT. Am J Psychiatry 125:837–840, 1968

Sommi RW, Crismon ML, Bowden CL, et al: Fluoxetine: a serotonin-specific second-generation antidepressant. Pharmacotherapy 7:1–15, 1987

Sovner R, Davis JM: A potential drug interaction between fluoxetine and valproic acid (letter). J Clin Psychopharmacol 11:389, 1991

Sperber AD: Toxic interaction between fluvoxamine and sustained release theophylline in an 11-year-old boy. Drug Saf 6:460–462, 1991

Spina E, Avenoso A, Pollicino AM, et al: Carbamazepine coadministration with fluoxetine or fluvoxamine. Ther Drug Monit 15:247–250, 1993a

Spina E, Pollicino AM, Avenoso A, et al: Fluvoxamine-induced alterations in plasma concentrations of imipramine and desipramine in depressed patients. Int J Clin Pharmacol Res 13:167–171, 1993b

Spina E, Pollicino AM, Avenoso A, et al: Effect of fluvoxamine on the pharmacokinetics of imipramine and desipramine in healthy subjects. Ther Drug Monit 15:243–246, 1993c

Stack CG, Rogers P, Linter SPK: Monoamine oxidase inhibitors and anaesthesia. Br J Anaesth 60:222–227, 1988

Steckler TL: Lithium- and carbamazepine-associated sinus node dysfunction: nine-year experience in a psychiatric hospital. J Clin Psychopharmacol 14:336–339, 1994

Steur ENHJ: Increase of Parkinson disability after fluoxetine medication. Neurology 43:211–213, 1993

Stoudemire A: New antidepressant drugs and the treatment of depression in the medically ill patient. Psychiatr Clin North Am 19:495–514, 1996

Stoudemire A, Atkinson P: Use of cyclic antidepressants in patients with cardiac conduction disturbances. Gen Hosp Psychiatry 10:389–397, 1988

Stoudemire A, Fogel BS: Psychopharmacology in the medically ill, in Principles of Medical Psychiatry. Edited by Stoudemire A, Fogel BS. Orlando, FL, Grune & Stratton, 1987, pp 79–112

Stoudemire A, Fogel BS: Psychopharmacology in medical patients: an update, in Medical-Psychiatric Practice, Vol 3. Washington, DC, American Psychiatric Press, 1995, pp 79–149

Stoudemire A, Luther J: Neuroleptic malignant syndrome and neuroleptic-induced catatonia: differential diagnosis and treatment. Int J Psychiatry Med 14:57–63, 1984

Stoudemire A, Fogel BS, Gulley LR: Psychopharmacology in the medically ill: an update, in Medical Psychiatric Practice, Vol 1. Edited by Stoudemire A, Fogel BS. Washington, DC, American Psychiatric Press, 1991, pp 29–97

Stoudemire A, Fogel BS, Gulley LR, et al: Psychopharmacology in the medically ill, in Psychiatric Care of the Medical Patient. Edited by Stoudemire A, Fogel BS. New York, Oxford University Press, 1993, pp 155–206

Strouse TB, Skotzko CE, Fawzy FI: Absence of adverse drug interactions between fluoxetine and cyclosporine in organ transplant recipients (Abstract 46). Presented at the annual meeting of the Academy of Psychosomatic Medicine, New Orleans, LA, November 1993, p 19

Surks MI, DeFesi CR: Normal serum free thyroid hormone concentrations in patients treated with phenytoin or carbamazepine: a paradox resolved. JAMA 275:1495–1498, 1996

Talland GA, Hagen DQ, James M: Performance tests of amnestic patients with Cylert. J Nerv Ment Dis 144:421–429, 1967

Tarsy D: Risperidone and neuroleptic malignant syndrome (letter). JAMA 275:446, 1996

Tate JL: Extrapyramidal symptoms in a patient taking haloperidol and fluoxetine. Am J Psychiatry 146:399–400, 1989

Taylor DP, Carter RB, Eison AS, et al: Pharmacology and neurochemistry of nefazodone, a novel antidepressant drug. J Clin Psychiatry 56 (suppl 6):3–11, 1995

Teitelbaum M: A significant increase in lithium levels after concomitant ACE inhibitor administration. Psychosomatics 34:450–453, 1993

Teo KK, Yusuf S, Furberg CD: Effects of prophylactic antiarrhythmic drug therapy in acute myocardial infarction. JAMA 270:1589–1595, 1993

Thompson TL II, Moran MG, Nies AS: Psychotropic drug use in the elderly. N Engl J Med 308:134–138, 194–199, 1983

Tilkian JG, Schroeder JS, Kao JJ, et al: The cardiovascular effects of lithium in man. Am J Med 61:665–670, 1976a

Tilkian JG, Schroeder JS, Kao J, et al: Effect of lithium on cardiovascular performance: a report on extended ambulatory monitoring and exercise testing before and during lithium. Am J Cardiol 38:701–798, 1976b

Trimble M: Non-monoamine oxidase inhibitor antidepressants and epilepsy: a review. Epilepsia 19:241–250, 1978

Trinidad A, Silver PA: Use of psychotropic medication in the neurologically ill, in Psychotropic Drug Use in the Medically Ill. Edited by Silver PA. Adv Psychosom Med 21:61–89, 1994

van Harten J, Holland RL, Wesnes K: Influence of multiple-dose administration of fluvoxamine on the pharmacokinetics of the benzodiazepines bromazepam and lorazepam: a randomised, cross-over study (abstract). Eur Neuropsychopharmacol 2:381, 1992a

van Harten J, Holland RL, Wesnes K, et al: Kinetic and dynamic interaction study between fluvoxamine and benzodiazepines. Poster presented at the Second Jerusalem Conference on Pharmaceutical Sciences and Clinical Pharmacology, Jerusalem, Israel, May 24–29, 1992b

Van Sweden B: Rebound antidepressant cardiac arrhythmia. Biol Psychiatry 24:360–369, 1988

Verrier RL: Neurochemical approaches to the prevention of ventricular fibrillation. Federation Proceedings 445:2191–2196, 1986

Vieweg WVR, Yank GR, Row WT, et al: Increase in white blood cell count and serum sodium level following the addition of lithium to carbamazepine treatment among three chronically psychotic male patients with disturbed affective states. Psychiatr Q 58:213–217, 1986

von Moltke LL, Greenblatt DJ, Harmatz JS, et al: Cytochromes in psychopharmacology (editorial). J Clin Psychopharmacol 14:1–4, 1994

von Moltke LL, Greenblatt DJ, Duan SX, et al: Inhibition of terfenadine metabolism in vitro by azole antifungal agents and by selective serotonin reuptake inhibitor antidepressants: relation to pharmacokinetic interactions in vivo. J Clin Psychopharmacol 16:104–112, 1996

Walley T, Pirmohamed M, Proudlove C, et al: Interaction of metoprolol and fluoxetine (letter). Lancet 341:967–968, 1993

Wamsley JK, Hunt ME: Relative affinity of quazepam for type-1 benzodiazepine receptors. J Clin Psychiatry 52 (suppl):15–20, 1991

Warrington SJ: Clinical implications of the pharmacology of sertraline. Int Clin Psychopharmacol 6 (suppl 2):11–21, 1991

Weitzner MA, Meyers CA, Valentine AD: Methylphenidate in the treatment of neurobehavioral slowing associated with cancer and cancer treatment. J Neuropsychiatry Clin Neurosci 7:347–350, 1995

Wells DG, Bjorksten AR: Monoamine oxidase inhibitors revisited. Can J Anaesth 36:64–74, 1989

Wilner KD, Lazar JD, Apseloff G, et al: The effects of sertraline on the pharmacodynamics of warfarin in healthy volunteers (abstract). Biol Psychiatry 29:354S–355S, 1991

Wils V: Extrapyramidal symptoms in a patient treated with fluvoxamine (letter). J Neurol Neurosurg Psychiatry 55:330–331, 1992

Wong YY, Ludden TM, Bell RD: Effect of erythromycin on carbamazepine kinetics. Clin Pharmacol Ther 33:460–464, 1983

Woods DJ, Coulter DM, Pillans P: Interaction of phenytoin and fluoxetine (letter). N Z Med J 107(970):19, 1994

Woods SW: Psychostimulant treatment of depressive disorders secondary to medical illness. J Clin Psychiatry 47:12–15, 1986

Ziegler MG, Wilner KD: Sertraline does not alter the beta-adrenergic blocking activity of atenolol in healthy male volunteers. J Clin Psychiatry 57 (suppl 1):12–15, 1996

FORTY-SIX

Geriatric Psychopharmacology

Carl Salzman, M.D., Andrew Satlin, M.D., and
Adam B. Burrows, M.D.

Psychotropic drugs play an important (but not exclusive) role in the treatment of late-life psychopathology. In this chapter, we review specific uses of psychotropic drugs to treat disorders characterized by disruptive behavior, depression, mania, anxiety, sleep dysfunction, and impaired cognition.

OVERVIEW

There are important differences in the use of psychoactive medications for elderly and younger adult patients. An appreciation of these differences is essential for optimal prescribing of these drugs. Before prescribing, the clinician must consider several processes: 1) physiological changes associated with aging, 2) physiological changes caused by disease, 3) the potential influence of concurrent medications, and 4) the social context of illness and treatment.

PHYSIOLOGICAL CHANGES ASSOCIATED WITH AGING

The aging process varies considerably, and the effects of aging and disease may be difficult to distinguish. Despite the clinical heterogeneity of the aging population, certain physiological changes are observed consistently. These include changes in nervous system structure and function, such as enhancement of some brain enzymes with aging and increased receptor site sensitivity in several neurotransmitter systems (Morgan et al. 1987; Oreland and Gottfries 1986; Robinson et al. 1977). Age-related

changes are also evident in the sensory, respiratory, cardiovascular, gastrointestinal, genitourinary, endocrine, and neuromuscular systems.

A useful generalization often applied to age-related physiological changes is the concept of diminished physiological reserve. In this model, age-related changes in central nervous system (CNS) function may not become clinically apparent until an individual confronts a physiological challenge, such as an acute illness or medical intervention. Under the stress of these circumstances, clinical problems such as disruptive behavior, affective symptoms, and diminished sleep and cognition are revealed through symptoms in a vulnerable system. Thus, illness is typically expressed nonspecifically in elderly patients, and neuropsychiatric symptoms may represent the expression of diverse clinical problems.

DISEASE AND DISABILITY

Chronic disease and functional disability characterize the aging population. More than 80% of Americans older than 65 report at least one chronic medical condition, and most have multiple chronic problems (National Center for Health Statistics 1987). Chronic diseases impose functional limitations such that by age 85, half of all Americans have difficulty with at least one daily self-care activity (Dawson et al. 1987). Dementias impose growing challenges on individuals and the health care system. Community-based surveys suggest that 25%–50% of people age 85 and older have dementia, with 40%–70% of dementia cases attributed to Alzheimer's disease and the remainder primarily to vascular causes (Aronson et al. 1991; Evans et al. 1989; Skoog et al. 1993).

MEDICATIONS AND ELDERLY PATIENTS

It is not surprising that older individuals consume a disproportionate share of prescription drugs. Although elderly people constitute 12% of the American population, those older than 65 receive one-third of all prescriptions. Polypharmacy is common; community-dwelling Americans older than 65 fill, on average, 13 prescriptions each year and take twice as many medications as younger Americans (Institute of Medicine 1991; National Center for Health Statistics 1987; Office of Epidemiology and Biostatistics 1987; Stewart et al. 1989). After cardiovascular drugs and analgesics, psychotropic drugs are most frequently prescribed in the treatment of elderly patients.

The risks of medication use in elderly patients are well documented. Adverse drug reactions are more common among elderly people than among younger people and account for 10%–30% of their hospitalizations (Ancill et al. 1988; Antonijoan et al. 1990; Col et al. 1990; Grymonpre et al. 1988; Institute of Medicine 1991; Ives et al. 1987; Ray et al. 1992). It appears that the risk of adverse drug reactions is not simply a result of age-related vulnerability but rather is a function of complex interactions between medical frailty and the prescription of multiple medications (Avorn et al. 1989; Carbonin et al. 1991; Gurwitz and Avorn 1991). Medications that require monitoring of therapeutic levels, such as antidepressants, may be more likely than other drugs to cause adverse reactions in elderly outpatients (J. K. Schneider et al. 1992). Consultation-liaison by clinical pharmacists may reduce adverse drug effects (Kroenke and Pinholt 1990; J. K. Schneider et al. 1992).

THE SOCIAL CONTEXT OF AGING

Clinicians must consider the following questions: How and where will a drug be taken by an elderly patient? Will the cost of the drug be an issue? Will the drug be administered by a caregiver? Is the patient in a nursing home or other long-term care facility?

Approximately 5% of individuals older than 65 and more than 20% of those older than 85 live in nursing homes (National Center for Health Statistics 1987). Many other elderly persons receive formal and informal care and assistance with daily activities in community settings. As would be expected, nursing home residents have more disability, disease, and dependence than do community-dwelling elderly persons. Also, not surprisingly, polypharmacy is common in nursing homes; reports indicate an average of eight medications prescribed per resident (Beers et al. 1988). Psychotropic drugs are among the most frequently prescribed medications in nursing homes. Antipsychotic neuroleptics are prescribed for 20%–30% of residents (Avorn et al. 1992; Beardsley et al. 1989; Beers et al. 1988; Garrard et al. 1991).

Unfortunately, medications are commonly prescribed without clear documentation of an appropriate indication (Beardsley et al. 1989; Garrard et al. 1991; Ray et al. 1980; Saban et al. 1982; Zimmer et al. 1986). This problem has been a particular concern with regard to psychotropic medications and was the subject of federal regulation through the Nursing Home Reform Amendments of the Omnibus Budget Reconciliation Act (OBRA) of 1987.

THERAPEUTIC CONSIDERATIONS: PSYCHOTROPIC MEDICATIONS

Effect of Aging and Disease

Aging and disease contribute to physiological changes that alter the effect and availability of medications. Pharmacodynamic changes affect the physiological effect produced by a given concentration of drug. Pharmacokinetic changes affect the amount of drug that is made available for clinical effect after a given dose. Aging is associated with both pharmacodynamic and pharmacokinetic changes, and the coexistence of chronic diseases can further alter the body's response to drugs.

Pharmacodynamics.   Elderly patients are more sensitive than younger patients to the therapeutic and toxic effects of psychotropic agents. For a given concentration of drug, elderly patients usually experience more sedation, anticholinergic toxicity, extrapyramidal side effects (EPS), and orthostatic hypotension. In the setting of degenerative brain diseases, such as Alzheimer's disease and Parkinson's disease, drug sensitivities may increase as the amount of neuronal tissue in key brain areas declines. Patients with Alzheimer's disease and acetylcholine deficiency are more sensitive to anticholinergic side effects, whereas patients with Parkinson's disease are more sensitive to dopamine blockade.

Pharmacokinetics.   Four pharmacokinetic parameters determine the bioavailability of a drug after administration: absorption, distribution, metabolism, and clearance. Two significant changes occur with aging. First, distribution changes significantly. An almost universal decrease in lean body mass and a corresponding increase in body fat composition occur. Fat-soluble drugs such as benzodiazepine sedative-hypnotics, neuroleptics, and cyclic antidepressants distribute more widely in the body and will thus take longer to clear. Water-soluble drugs such as lithium distribute through a smaller volume and thus can reach higher tissue concentrations. Second, age-related changes in hepatic metabolism of psychotropic drugs occur. An age-related decrement in phase I oxidative biotransformation results. This process is generally controlled by the hepatic cytochrome P450 (CYP) drug-metabolizing system. The activity of several specific cytochromes, including CYP3A4, decreases in older as compared with younger patients. The extent of the impairment may be greater in elderly men than in women (von Moltke et al. 1998). The decrease in phase I oxidative biotransformation further delays hepatic metabolism and contributes to the prolonged half-lives of many psychotropic drugs and the delayed and prolonged appearance of active intermediate metabolites. The cumulative effect of large volumes of distribution for fat-soluble drugs and delayed hepatic metabolism results in a dramatic prolongation of clinical effect for many drugs, especially long-acting benzodiazepines.

Chronic diseases and the aging process alter the pharmacokinetic patterns of psychotropic drugs. Malnutrition or chronic inflammatory conditions can reduce the synthesis of plasma-binding proteins, resulting in higher free (or bioavailable) drug concentrations. Chronic liver disease or congestion will further delay clearance, leading to higher drug levels for even longer periods. Many older people have reduced glomerular filtration rates. For these individuals, renal clearance of drugs such as lithium will be impaired, and higher drug concentrations will result. Altogether, pharmacological changes associated with aging and disease mean that for a given dose of most psychoactive drugs, the bioavailable concentration at the target tissue will be higher, and for a given concentration at a CNS site of action, the physiological effect will be greater. These generalizations support the maxim to "start low and go slow" when prescribing drugs to geriatric patients.

Side effects. In elderly patients, side effects typically occur in vulnerable physiological systems. In the cardiovascular system, for example, decreased baroreceptor sensitivity predisposes to orthostatic hypotension, and diminished reserve in the cardiac conduction system predisposes to heart block. Changes in bowel motility predispose to constipation and impaction, whereas bladder weakness and prostatic enlargement predispose to urinary retention. In the CNS, changes in the extrapyramidal and vestibular systems predispose to problems with gait, balance, and posture. Dementia (even early in the course) predisposes to delirium.

POLYPHARMACY: ISSUES IN PRESCRIBING PSYCHOACTIVE DRUGS

The high prevalence of polypharmacy in elderly patients leads to three common prescribing problems:

1. A correlation exists between an increasing number of medications prescribed and an increasing risk of medication noncompliance.
2. One drug can impair the absorption, metabolism, or clearance of another drug or displace it from a protein-binding site.
3. A confluence of adverse effects may result. For example, additive effects of vasodilators and antidepressants on blood pressure are common, as are the additive toxic effects from multiple drugs with anticholinergic properties. Monoamine oxidase inhibitors (MAOIs) present special problems with regard to potentially catastrophic interactions with sympathomimetic agents and catecholamine precursors.

TREATMENT OF PSYCHOSIS, AGITATION, AND BEHAVIORAL DISRUPTION

Elderly patients who have psychosis, severe illness, or dementia often manifest behavioral symptoms that require treatment. Prevalence rates of agitation are particularly high in nursing homes (Billig et al. 1991; Cohen-Mansfield et al. 1989; Peabody et al. 1987; Rovner et al. 1986; Wragg and Jeste 1988; Zimmer et al. 1984). Severe agitation, screaming, and assaultiveness are seen frequently in the moderate to severe stages of dementia (particularly Alzheimer's disease) as well as in late-life schizophrenia.

Treatment Guidelines

Although medications are commonly used to treat severe agitation and psychosis in elderly patients, they are not the only form of treatment. Agitation and psychosis may be caused by drug toxicity, medical illness, pain, frustration, loneliness, reduced sensory input, new environment, diminished nutritional status, and environmental factors. Treatment approaches include using orienting stimuli, avoiding patient isolation, and using nonpharmacological treatments such as music, exercise, pets, and social contact.

Medications that are commonly used to treat disruptive behavior include neuroleptics, β-blockers, drugs with serotonergic effects, mood stabilizers, and hormones.

Neuroleptics

Neuroleptics are the most commonly used drugs to treat severe disruptive behavior in elderly patients (Devanand et al. 1988; Helms 1985; Maletta 1984; Phillipson et al. 1990; Risse and Barnes 1986; Salzman 1987; L. S. Schneider et al. 1990b; Small 1988; Wragg and Jeste 1988). Neuroleptics undergo a complicated stepwise hepatic metabolism. The effects of the aging process on this metabolism have not been extensively studied. However, limited data suggest that blood levels of parent compounds and active metabolites are 1.5–2 times higher in older patients compared with younger adult control subjects (Aoba et al. 1985; Cohen and Sommer 1988; Forsman and Ohman 1977) but not in all patients.

No current data suggest that any one neuroleptic is better at controlling agitated behavior or psychotic thinking than any other, given comparable therapeutic doses. Selection of a particular neuroleptic (or subclass of neuroleptics) is guided by the side-effect profile of each drug or drug class in relation to the patient's history of drug response (or lack of response) and the nature of concomitant chronic illness and medication.

Three categories of neuroleptic side effects occur regularly and may be particularly troublesome for older patients. These side effects are sedation, orthostatic hypotension, and EPS. Low-potency neuroleptics, such as chlorpromazine and thioridazine, commonly cause sedation or orthostatic hypotension. Although sedation may be helpful at bedtime for disruptive elderly patients, the sedative effect often continues through the next day because of the medications' prolonged elimination half-lives. During the day, a sedated elderly person may actually become more agitated and disruptive. For this reason and because of the risk of orthostatic hypotension, low-potency neuroleptics may present a risk in this population. In clinical practice, however, low doses of thioridazine are still used with considerable success for the treatment of agitation. High-potency neuroleptics, such as haloperidol and fluphenazine, are a commonly used alternative to low-potency neuroleptics because high-potency medications lack sedating and orthostatic hypotensive properties. Unfortunately, these high-potency compounds are more likely to produce EPS than are the low-potency medications. Among the latter, drug-induced parkinsonian-like

EPS may be associated with a lack of behavioral improvement (Ganzini et al. 1991).

Therefore, the clinician must evaluate the risks and benefits of different neuroleptics when selecting one to treat behavioral disruption. Current clinical practice tends to favor the use of high-potency medications, with an attempt to prevent or minimize EPS by using exceedingly low doses (Devanand et al. 1988, 1989, 1992; Petrie et al. 1982). Clinical experience suggests, for example, that doses of haloperidol in the range of 0.25–1.0 mg one to four times a day may help diminish disruptive behavior without producing undue EPS.

In elderly patients who have not previously taken neuroleptics, tardive dyskinesia develops rapidly and at lower doses than in younger patients (Karson et al. 1990; Lieberman et al. 1984; Saltz et al. 1989; Yassa et al. 1988). Tardive dyskinesia is more common in patients with evidence of cortical atrophy (Sweet et al. 1992). When neuroleptics are discontinued, tardive dyskinesia symptoms are less likely to disappear in older patients than in younger adults (De Veaugh-Geiss 1988; Smith and Baldessarini 1980; Yassa et al. 1984). However, for some elderly patients with tardive dyskinesia who are given maintenance neuroleptics, the symptoms do not increase (Huang 1986; Yassa 1991).

Neuroleptic malignant syndrome may also occur in older patients taking neuroleptics. This syndrome was more common in elderly patients who had either dementia or Parkinson's disease while taking neuroleptics (Addonizio 1992).

Nonneuroleptics

A growing body of clinical experience and anecdotal reports (summarized in Salzman 1990c) suggests that drugs such as β-blockers, trazodone, buspirone, serotonergic antidepressants, anticonvulsants, and lithium may help manage a variety of agitated behaviors refractory to more conventional treatment.

β-Blockers. β-Blockers, sometimes modestly helpful in reducing agitated and assaultive behavior in elderly patients, are given in low doses (10–100 mg/day). Not all studies, however, are positive (Risse and Barnes 1986; Weiler et al. 1988). These drugs can be given only to those elderly patients without cardiovascular disorder and chronic obstructive pulmonary disease (particularly asthma). Side effects include sedation, orthostatic hypotension, and decreased cardiac output.

Trazodone. The antidepressant drug trazodone has been reported to be an effective treatment for agitation and severely disruptive behavior (Greenwald et al. 1986; Pinner and Rich 1988; Simpson and Foster 1986; Tingle 1986). Although no double-blind studies to date compare this drug with placebo or with neuroleptics, clinical experience suggests that it is effective in doses of 50–200 mg/day, with few side effects other than sedation.

Buspirone. Buspirone, a nonbenzodiazepine antianxiety agent, has been reported to be effective in controlling disruptive behavior in older patients in one study (Colenda 1988) but not in another (Strauss 1988). However, oral dyskinesia was reported in an elderly patient with dementia who was given buspirone, and this symptom persisted for at least 4 months after symptom onset (Strauss 1988). Research studies have not yet compared its effect with that of placebo or other drugs for treating agitation. The average daily dose range is 20–80 mg in divided doses; side effects are reported to be relatively mild.

Selective serotonin reuptake inhibitors. Current clinical experience suggests that the antidepressant fluoxetine has some antiagitation properties in elderly patients. However, a study (Olafsson et al. 1992) failed to demonstrate effectiveness of fluvoxamine in the treatment of behavioral disruption in elderly patients with dementia. Careful research into the antiagitation properties of the selective serotonin reuptake inhibitors (SSRIs) is essential, because these drugs also tend to be activating and may actually increase agitation in some older patients. Although the SSRIs may also be helpful in states of dementia-associated agitation, they often cause severe worsening of agitation in the late stages of a dementing illness.

Anticonvulsants and lithium carbonate. In doses of 50–200 mg/day, carbamazepine has controlled chronic disruptive behavior and agitation in older patients, particularly those with dementia (Leibovici and Tariot 1988). Like carbamazepine, lithium carbonate is sometimes useful in managing disruptive behavior (Holton and George 1985). The therapeutic range is 150–900 mg in divided doses. Because both of these drugs may produce neurotoxicity characterized by increased agitation, confusion, and disorientation, the lowest possible therapeutic dosage should be given, and the drugs should be discontinued if behavior worsens.

Experience with valproate in managing disruptive behavior is limited but suggests that this drug, like carbamazepine, may be effective in controlling severe agitation.

Estrogen. A single case report (Kyomen et al. 1991) suggests that estrogen (e.g., diethylstilbestrol 1 mg/day or conjugated estrogen 0.625 mg/day) reduces the number of incidents of physical aggression but not of verbal aggression or physical or verbal repetitive behaviors in elderly male patients with dementia.

TREATMENT OF DEPRESSION

Depression is the most common psychiatric illness in the older population (Blazer and Williams 1980). Prevalence rates of depressive disorders in older people reach 20% for major depression and are even higher for milder forms. Suicide rates among depressed elderly people are particularly high (Alexopoulos et al. 1988). Research points to the high prevalence of diagnosed major depression in nursing home residents and the unusually high mortality (from causes other than suicide) of patients with depression (Parmelee et al. 1993; Rovner et al. 1991).

Although older people with depressive disorders can present with signs and symptoms similar to those in younger adults, late-life depression is characterized by diagnostic and symptomatic heterogeneity (Alexopoulos 1990). Ascribing diagnostic significance to individual depressive symptoms may be misleading. For example, early-morning awakening, appetite disturbance, and low energy level (which are characteristic vegetative signs of depression) may each result from the normal aging process, from drugs commonly taken by elderly patients, from medical conditions more common in elderly people, or from a combination of these factors (Salzman et al. 1992).

In addition to the heterogeneity of depressive symptom patterns, people older than 65 have remarkably diverse psychological functioning. Although precise age boundaries are lacking, elderly people are occasionally subdivided into the "young-old" (65 to 75 or 79) and the "old-old" (75 to 80+). Symptomatic presentation of depression may differ between these two groups, although considerable similarities and overlap of symptoms are also found. For example, the appearance of depression in very old (80+), frail nursing home residents may differ from that in younger, healthier nursing home residents and may confuse the diagnostician (Burrows et al. 1995). Factors of pharmacokinetic disposition and pharmacodynamic drug sensitivity may be quite different in old-old patients. Response to antidepressant treatment may also be different between these two general categories (Salzman et al. 1993), although, once again, similarities of response also exist, and overlap between the two groups is common. Virtually all studies of the pharmacological treatment of late-life depression have focused on the young-old group. One review (Salzman et al. 1993) noted that only one controlled study of depressed patients who were older than 75 has been done, and just 171 identifiable patients older than 75 have been studied in all antidepressant studies of elderly subjects. Consequently, treatment guidelines for very old patients are based on treatment of young-old or even of young and middle-aged adults and may be misleading.

As a general principle, elderly patients (especially those who are old-old) are more sensitive to the effects of antidepressants than are younger adults, although wide interindividual variability is seen. Elderly patients are more likely than younger adults to experience the side effects of sedation, orthostatic hypotension, and anticholinergic symptoms. Orthostatic hypotension (due to reduced central and peripheral controls of blood pressure) may lead to falls and serious fractures. For unclear reasons, pretreatment systolic orthostatic blood pressure may predict clinical response: patients who have large pretreatment systolic orthostatic blood pressure changes in the morning before treatment with antidepressants have a significantly greater response to antidepressant or electroconvulsive therapy (ECT) (Jarvik et al. 1983; L. S. Schneider et al. 1986; Stack et al. 1988). In some older patients, sensitivity to anticholinergic side effects of tricyclic antidepressants (TCAs) may limit dosing levels and may cause CNS symptoms of delirium even at therapeutic doses. A review of anticholinergic side effects in elderly patients found that cognitive impairment, which occurs in normal aging, is enhanced and also may be associated with behavioral disturbances (Meyers 1992). Activation and insomnia resulting from SSRIs may be greater in older patients than in younger patients, although these differences have not been carefully defined by controlled research studies.

Antidepressants, like neuroleptics, undergo complicated hepatic metabolism requiring both phase I (dealkylation, aromatic hydroxylation) and phase II (conjugation) reactions. The aging process may affect the first set of processes. As a general rule, dealkylation becomes less efficient, which leads to higher levels of tertiary tricyclic amines compared with the secondary amine metabolite and reduced clearance of these compounds, with accumulation and higher blood levels. For these reasons, older patients, on average, need lower doses of antidepressants to achieve therapeutic effect; old-old patients may need even lower doses than young-old patients. Pharmacokinetic data also suggest that for drugs with established therapeutic blood level ranges (e.g., nortriptyline and desipramine), older patients respond to the same levels as younger adult counterparts (Cutler et al. 1981; Dawling et al. 1980a, 1980b, 1981; Kanba et al. 1992; Katz et al. 1989; Kitanka et al. 1982; Nelson et al. 1985, 1988). However, the wide range of interindividual variability and limited research

data design suggest that the pharmacokinetics of antidepressants in elderly patients have not yet been consistently characterized in comparison with younger patients (von Moltke et al. 1993).

Phase I metabolism of TCAs also produces a water-soluble hydroxymetabolite whose clearance depends on renal function. This metabolite was previously thought to be inactive; however, in some patients, it may be associated with quinidine-like cardiotoxicity (McCue et al. 1989; Nelson et al. 1988; L. S. Schneider et al. 1990a; Young et al. 1984, 1985). Impaired renal function in older patients or in very elderly individuals may lead to higher levels of hydroxymetabolites and the potential for cardiotoxicity (Kutcher et al. 1986).

Treatment Guidelines

Traditionally, treatment of the depressed elderly patient with antidepressants has followed recommendations for younger and middle-aged adults. ECT or TCAs plus neuroleptics are usually prescribed for patients with delusional depression (Kroessler and Fogel 1993). TCAs have been the primary treatment for melancholic major depressive disorder, especially on an inpatient service, and MAOIs have been used for less severely depressed patients who do not require hospitalization. The new class of SSRIs has been studied primarily in depressed elderly outpatients and found to be useful for mild to moderately severe depression. These recommendations, however, are based on a small number of studies, with an age sample skewed toward young-old subjects.

Increased clinical experience and more recent studies have suggested that precise boundaries between these prescribing guidelines may not exist, and treatment recommendations for depressed elderly patients may be changing. For example, the combination of fluoxetine and perphenazine has been found effective in the treatment of psychotic depression in a study that included a few patients older than 60 (Rothschild et al. 1993). There are many reviews of antidepressant treatment in elderly patients (Alexopoulos 1992; Caine et al. 1993; Dewan et al. 1992; Kim 1988; Koenig and Breitner 1990; Magni et al. 1988; Peabody et al. 1986; Rockwell et al. 1988; Salzman 1990a, 1990c, 1993; Smith and Buckwalter 1992; Weissman et al. 1992).

Tricyclic Antidepressants

More than 400 studies of the treatment of serious major depression, nondelusional type, in elderly subjects have been done (Salzman 1994). In general, all TCAs are helpful for depressed elderly patients, although secondary amines are preferred. Regardless of the type of antidepressant used, however, one study suggested that elderly patients who have had major depression should continue taking their antidepressant to prevent relapse (Old Age Depression Interest Group 1993).

Although secondary amine TCAs are preferred to tertiary amines because side effects of secondary amines are usually less intense, the severity of tricyclic-related side effects in elderly patients may be correlated with dose. Because therapeutic blood levels of TCAs in elderly patients may be achieved with lower-than-usual doses, use of tertiary amines in elderly patients may be possible if doses remain low. A study of low-dose doxepin, for example, reported efficacy without serious side effects (Lakshmanan et al. 1986).

Before initiating treatment with TCAs in elderly patients, clinicians should do a physical examination and obtain an electrocardiogram (ECG). Starting doses should be extremely low (e.g., 10–25 mg/day), and dosage increments should be of a similar magnitude. The adage "start low and go slow" is applicable to the use of antidepressants in elderly patients. In addition, clinicians should try to prescribe the dose of antidepressant that produces the best therapeutic response with the fewest side effects, regardless of the final dose. Using the ECG to monitor potential cardiotoxicity will help determine the upper limit of doses.

Trazodone

The antidepressant effects of trazodone are unpredictable; thus, it is a less reliable first choice among the various available antidepressants. It is recommended, however, for older patients who have not responded to other compounds, and sometimes it has surprising therapeutic effects in the previously treatment-refractory older patient. Although trazodone causes sedation and orthostatic hypotension (Gerner et al. 1980), it has minimal anticholinergic properties and does not interfere with memory (Branconnier and Cole 1981).

Bupropion

Bupropion has been found to be effective for elderly subjects in research studies (Branconnier et al. 1983; Halaris 1986). A few elderly patients have reported an unusual side effect of falling backward that may be dose related (Szuba and Leuchter 1992).

Selective Serotonin Reuptake Inhibitors

SSRIs have been prescribed to elderly patients with major depression, less serious dysthymic disorders, and atypical depressions. The advantages of these drugs is the lack of anticholinergic side effects, cardiotoxicity, and orthostatic hypotension. In research studies, the efficacy of the SSRIs fluoxetine, paroxetine, sertraline, and fluvoxamine is equivalent to that of the TCAs (Dunner et al. 1992; Feighner and Cohn 1985; Feighner et al. 1988; Salzman 1994). For these reasons, the SSRIs have become the first choice among the various categories of antidepressants for elderly patients. However, in some elderly patients, these drugs cause unacceptable agitation and insomnia. Another report (Brymer and Winograd 1992) also noted that fluoxetine use may be associated with unacceptable weight loss in patients older than 75. Low starting doses and small dosage increments are recommended.

Monoamine Oxidase Inhibitors

MAOIs may be both safe and effective for some older patients with atypical depression characterized by withdrawal, lack of motivation, apathy, and lack of energy (Georgotas et al. 1981, 1983, 1986; Lazarus et al. 1986). Clinical overviews of the use of MAOIs include those of Jenike (1985), Zisook (1985), and Salzman (1992). These drugs are rarely the first-choice antidepressant for major depression. As with TCAs and SSRIs, older patients are likely to experience side effects. Lower doses (e.g., phenelzine 15–20 mg/day, tranylcypromine 10–40 mg/day) than those prescribed for younger adult patients are advised.

MAOIs can be given only to responsible, compliant elderly patients or to those whose medication is carefully supervised. The high risk of toxic drug interactions resulting from the large average number of drugs prescribed for the geriatric population may prevent these drugs from being recommended for many older outpatients.

TREATMENT OF MANIA

Elderly bipolar patients who have had many episodes tend to have rapid cycling and severe symptomatology, but bipolar disorder rarely appears for the first time in late life. Several studies suggest that first-onset mania in elderly patients is more likely to be associated with neurological impairment than is depression in this age group (Berrios and Bakshi 1991; Shulman et al. 1992; Snowdon 1991) and carries a greater risk for mortality than does depression (Dhingra and Rabins 1991; Shulman et al. 1992). Thus, late-onset mania may represent a different disorder from early-onset mania, or it may be secondary to other conditions.

Treatment Guidelines

Lithium is the primary treatment and prophylaxis for mania in elderly patients, as it is for younger adults. However, a review (Foster 1992) identified only five studies of antimanic efficacy of lithium in elderly subjects and concluded that the efficacy in elderly bipolar patients is not yet clearly established in the literature. Reviews of lithium effects in older patients include those of Foster (1992), Liptzin (1992), Stone (1989), Jefferson et al. (1987), and Glasser and Rabins (1984).

Age-associated reduction in renal clearance of lithium leads to accumulation and increased plasma levels in elderly patients more readily than in younger adults taking the same dosage. This effect is magnified by the reduction in the volume of distribution of lithium in elderly patients as a result of the relative loss of total body water. Therapeutic plasma levels for older patients with mania may need to be only 0.2–0.6 mEq/L. The daily dose necessary to achieve lower blood levels varies among older patients. As a general rule, starting lithium doses are low (e.g., 150–450 mg/day), with dosage increments of 150–300 mg at weekly intervals. However, it is important to recognize that some older patients with mania, particularly those with other psychiatric illnesses, may require doses and blood levels equivalent to those needed by younger patients. One prospective, double-blind, randomized lithium dose-reduction study found that dose reductions of 25%–50% to achieve serum levels of 0.45 mEq/L resulted in significantly increased affective symptoms in the elderly subjects (Abou-Saleh and Coppen 1989).

Older patients are more sensitive than younger patients to the therapeutic and toxic effects of lithium. The toxic profile of lithium in older patients differs in several important aspects from that of younger patients. Side effects of tremor and gastrointestinal upset occur in all age groups. In older patients, however, the first and often the most prominent side effects consist of a spectrum of neurotoxic symptoms, even at low therapeutic levels. In some patients, neurotoxicity may be associated with the presence of underlying neurological disease (Himmelhoch et al. 1980; Kemperman et al. 1989). Subtle but progressive impairment of recent recall (anterograde amnesia), disorientation, aphasia, restlessness, and irritability may appear as the first signs of excessive lithium dosage. This presents a double hazard: overdose and inaccurate interpretation of symptoms of cognitive impairment. Movement disorders also are early signs of toxicity—particularly EPS, dyskinesias, and cerebellar dysfunction, including irregular gait, decreased coordination, and dysarthria. Impaired consciousness also may develop at blood levels therapeutic for younger adults.

Other medical side effects may be common in elderly patients taking lithium. Cardiac effects include altered conduction due to sinus node dysfunction, sinoatrial block, bundle branch block, ventricular irritability, and possible myocardial injury. Lithium may impair urine concentration by the kidneys; this may be more severe in elderly patients with preexisting deficits in renal concentrating ability. Acute lithium toxicity may result in decreased glomerular filtration rate, and long-term use may be associated with tubular atrophy, glomerular sclerosis, and interstitial fibrosis. Hypothyroidism may be more common in elderly patients taking lithium and can present with more profound consequences such as myxedema coma.

Alternative medications for the treatment of mania in elderly patients have been less well studied than lithium. Neuroleptics are sometimes recommended for elderly patients as adjunctive treatment of severe agitation, insomnia, and potentially harmful behavior in patients with mania, particularly in the early stages of treatment before lithium exerts its effect. Among the alternatives to lithium, anticonvulsants have been used with increased frequency. Valproic acid is generally well tolerated in older patients (McFarland et al. 1990; Satlin and Liptzin, in press). Valproic acid pharmacokinetics are affected by the aging process; higher unbound fractions may be present in the cerebrospinal fluid. Thus, total concentrations as measured in blood may be misleading, and doses may need to be lower in elderly patients than in younger patients. The most common reported side effects are neurological symptoms (tremor, sedation, and ataxia), asymptomatic serum hepatic transaminase elevations, alopecia, increased appetite, and weight gain. The initial sedative effect, which generally lasts only about a week, may be helpful for elderly patients with mania who are agitated and have insomnia. Carbamazepine, like valproic acid, may be useful in the treatment and prevention of mania. In the elderly, however, fewer reports of use of carbamazepine are available than for valproic acid. Side effects of carbamazepine include bradycardia, confusion, ataxia, and impairment of water excretion. The most serious toxic effect of carbamazepine is depression of bone marrow function, which may result in leukopenia and potentially fatal infections, but this effect appears to be less common in the elderly. Other drugs that have been used to treat mania in younger adults include benzodiazepines and calcium channel blockers; these compounds have not been well studied in elderly patients. ECT is as useful for severe mania in elderly patients as in younger adults.

TREATMENT OF ANXIETY

In older patients, symptoms of anxiety are common, and the diagnosis of generalized anxiety disorder is not as clearly defined as in younger adults. Clinically significant anxiety symptoms commonly occur in states of depression and dementia as well as secondary to physical illness or as a result of drug treatment. Panic and phobic anxiety disorders may also occur in older people but are less prevalent than in younger adults and are often associated with physical illness and concomitant psychiatric disorder (Sheikh 1990). Various reviews of the pharmacological treatment of generalized anxiety in elderly patients have been conducted (Allen 1986; Hershey and Kim 1988; Salzman 1990b).

Treatment Guidelines

Benzodiazepines, the primary treatment of anxiety, are widely used in the treatment of anxious elderly patients (Beardsley et al. 1989; Beers et al. 1988; Buck 1988; Koepke et al. 1982; Pinsker and Suljaga-Petchel 1984). Elderly patients generally are more sensitive than younger patients to both the therapeutic and the toxic effects of benzodiazepines, or interindividual variability may be great. Low doses are generally recommended; side effects of sedation, impaired coordination, and cognitive impairment may result from higher doses that are commonly therapeutic for younger adults.

Like other psychotropic drugs, benzodiazepines undergo stepwise hepatic metabolism. The long-half-life benzodiazepines that are currently available in the United States undergo both phase I and phase II reactions. Phase I reactions tend to be prolonged in elderly patients and lead to drug accumulation and increased half-life. Phase II reactions are unaffected by age. Because short-half-life benzodiazepines undergo only phase II metabolism, they are preferred for older patients (Greenblatt and Shader 1990).

Benzodiazepines often cause four types of toxicity in older patients: 1) sedation, 2) ataxia and falls (Hale et al. 1988; Rashi and Logan 1986; Ray et al. 1987), 3) psychomotor slowing, and 4) cognitive impairment (Salzman 1990b). The last type—an increasing public health concern—is characterized by anterograde amnesia, diminished short-term recall, increased forgetfulness, and decreased attention. Discontinuing the drug is associated with improved memory and heightened concentration (Salzman et al. 1992).

Buspirone

Buspirone, a nonbenzodiazepine anxiolytic, has antianxiety properties in elderly patients. Although research data suggest that it is as effective as benzodiazepines (Napoliello 1986), clinical experience favors benzodiazepines as more rapid and reliable anxiolytics. Because research and clinical experience differ, recommendations for its use remain tentative: buspirone is recommended when benzodiazepines are ineffective or cannot be prescribed.

TREATMENT OF SLEEP DISORDERS

Disordered sleep is a common complaint among elderly people (Ancoli-Israel 1989; Pollack and Perlick 1991). Of people older than 65, 12% report persistent insomnia, and 1.6% report persistent daytime hypersomnia (Ford and Kamerow 1989). Although only about 12% of Americans are elderly, they receive 35%–40% of all prescriptions for sedative-hypnotics (Gottlieb 1990).

Treatment Guidelines

Sedative-hypnotic medications are indicated for the short-term treatment of insomnia associated with situational, psychological, psychiatric, or medical conditions that are expected to be time limited or to respond to appropriate therapy. For some elderly patients, long-term use can be justified by the morbidity of chronic sleep deprivation. Regular nightly use, however, may cause significant worsening of cognition, disorientation, confusion, and socially inappropriate behavior in some older people (Regestein 1992). Selection of a particular drug to alleviate sleep problems (like the selection of an antianxiety drug) is guided by the drug's pharmacokinetic properties, the drug's side-effect profile, the patient's medical and emotional health, and the patient's history of sedative-hypnotic use. Reviews of psychotropic drugs to treat sleep disorders in older patients include those of Regestein (1992), Reynolds (1991), and Prinz and colleagues (1990).

Benzodiazepines are the most commonly prescribed sedative-hypnotics. Five are currently marketed for this indication: flurazepam, quazepam, triazolam, temazepam, and estazolam. In general, the benzodiazepines with a long half-life (e.g., flurazepam and, to a lesser extent, quazepam) accumulate and are likely to produce daytime sedation in elderly patients. Long-term use can gradually produce a dementia syndrome of cognitive loss, psychomotor retardation, and apathy. Drugs with a shorter half-life cause less daytime sedation and hangover. For example, triazolam, when used in the recommended dose of 0.125 mg, is effective in older patients with sleep fragmentation, daytime sleepiness, and periodic limb movements of sleep (PLMS) (Bonnet and Arand 1991). Withdrawal symptoms and interdose rebound are common. Use of benzodiazepines with an intermediate half-life may be especially useful in elderly patients. Temazepam, which has a half-life of 10–20 hours, has been found to be effective in elderly patients and to cause little hangover, but it has a slow onset of action. The anxiolytic drugs lorazepam and oxazepam are pharmacokinetically similar and are as effective as temazepam for inducing sleep. Estazolam, another benzodiazepine with an intermediate half-life of 12–15 hours, is an effective hypnotic in elderly patients (Vogel and Morris 1992). With intermediate-half-life benzodiazepines, daytime performance and memory are not adversely affected, and rebound insomnia rarely extends beyond one night after discontinuation.

Other classes of psychotropic drugs are also given to older patients to induce sleep. Sedating neuroleptics such as thioridazine in low doses or antidepressants with sedating side effects such as trazodone and doxepin may be beneficial. Antihistaminic drugs such as diphenhydramine and hydroxyzine also may be helpful in some patients, although these drugs have the potential for anticholinergic, hypotensive, and cardiac side effects. Chloral hydrate is also effective and safe for short-term use. Barbiturates should not be given to elderly patients.

Two hypnotics that increase delta sleep are available. Because delta sleep typically decreases with aging, these medications may be of particular benefit to older people. Zolpidem, a clinically effective imidazopyridine hypnotic, does not appear to impair memory (Frattola et al. 1990). Zopiclone, a cyclopyrrolone derivative with a half-life of 5 hours, is as effective as triazolam (Mouret et al. 1990).

TREATMENT OF DEMENTIA

Some degree of memory loss and a slowing of other cognitive processes are common with advancing age. Dementia is diagnosed when other cognitive impairments and impaired social or occupational functioning accompany the memory loss. Dementia due to neurodegenerative disorders typically follows a slowly progressive course, with worsening attention, orientation, ability to concentrate, visual recognition, and language function in addition to declining short-term and long-term memory. Clinical overviews of the diagnosis and treatment of memory loss include those of Foster and Martin (1990), Crook (1989), and Rosebush and Salzman (1988).

Alzheimer's disease is the most common cause of degenerative dementia in elderly people. This idiopathic condition, characterized pathologically by senile plaques and neurofibrillary tangles in the brain, may affect as many as 10% of all people older than 65 and nearly 50% of those older than 85 (Evans et al. 1989). Alzheimer's disease also may cause various psychiatric syndromes, including depression, anxiety, psychosis, and behavioral disturbances such as agitation, sleep-wake cycle disorders, and aggression. At present, no known effective treatment is available to ameliorate or reverse the cognitive impairment caused by Alzheimer's disease. Numerous drugs have been studied, based on their presumed effects on those aspects of brain neurochemistry that appear abnormal in Alzheimer's disease. Comprehensive reviews of this research include those of Tariot (1992), Miller and colleagues (1992), and Crook and colleagues (1990).

Evidence has suggested that the degree of cognitive impairment in patients with Alzheimer's disease is correlated with CNS cholinergic deficits (Perry et al. 1978). Restitutive therapies using choline or lecithin as cholinergic precursors have not yielded clinically significant results. Other approaches have used acetylcholinesterase inhibitors to block the enzyme that metabolizes acetylcholine. Three examples are physostigmine, tetrahydroaminoacridine (tacrine, THA), and velnacrine maleate. Most studies of physostigmine showed small improvements in cognition, but the effect was brief (Jenike et al. 1990; Stern et al. 1988). The effects of THA have been both negative and positive. Two trials showed no benefit, but the effect may have been compromised by low doses of the drug (Chatellier and Lacomblez 1990; Gauthier et al. 1990). Three other trials found improvements that ranged from modest to clinically noticeable by physicians and caregivers (Davis et al. 1992; Eagger et al. 1991; Farlow et al. 1992).

In all of these studies, high rates of liver enzyme elevations—often more than three times normal—were found. Overall, however, the modest therapeutic effects of THA seemed to outweigh the possible toxic consequences so that this compound will be available for clinical use in the United States. Other restitutive cholinergic approaches involve the use of muscarinic or nicotinic agonists, or agents that purportedly enhance the potassium-evoked release of acetylcholine (Lavretsky and Jarvik 1992; Spagnoli et al. 1991). Acetylcarnitine may have some direct cholinergic activity, although its mechanism of action is uncertain.

Restitutive therapies based on known deficits of other neurotransmitters in Alzheimer's disease also have been tested. These include attempts to improve

- Noradrenergic transmission using clonidine or guanfacine
- Serotonergic function using alaproclate or minaprine

■ γ-Aminobutyric acid (GABA)ergic function using tetrahydroisoxazolopyridinol (THIP)

■ Peptide neurotransmission using somatostatin analogues, arginine vasopressin, adrenocorticotropic hormone (ACTH) agonists, thyrotropin-releasing hormone (TRH) analogues, and opiate receptor antagonists

No therapy improved cognition, although effects on mood were occasionally reported (Tariot 1992). Studies of selegiline, an MAOI that at low doses appears to be selective for MAO-B, have been encouraging.

Evidence indicates that neuronal death in neurodegenerative disorders such as Alzheimer's disease may be mediated by a sustained increase in cytosolic free calcium (Branconnier et al. 1992). Increased calcium influx into the cell may be a result of changes in the receptor for glutamate, which is part of the N-methyl-D-aspartate (NMDA) receptor complex. Newer therapeutic approaches to Alzheimer's disease involve attempts to block calcium channels with antagonists such as nimodipine. One study of nimodipine found significantly less deterioration on some cognitive measures than with placebo, but the short duration of the treatment period limited its clinical relevance (Tollefson 1990).

Another approach to the treatment of Alzheimer's disease involves attempts to enhance CNS cellular metabolism. Ergoloid mesylates is classified as a metabolic enhancer based on its ability to change levels of cyclic adenosine monophosphate. Although ergoloid mesylates has been studied for more than 20 years, evidence indicates that its efficacy is questionable (Thompson et al. 1990).

"Nootropics" are putative metabolic enhancers that were originally synthesized as GABA derivatives. The first of these was piracetam, and the class now includes oxiracetam, pramiracetam, aniracetam, and vinpocetine. Studies of these drugs indicate variable effects on mood and overall functional status but no clear cognitive effect (Tariot 1992).

Future research on treating the cognitive disorders of Alzheimer's disease may be directed at preventing the accumulation of β-amyloid protein fragments, which result from the abnormal processing of the amyloid precursor protein and constitute the core of the senile plaque. Additional research will be directed at targeted drug delivery systems to overcome the problems with drug delivery to the brain caused by peripheral metabolism, poor blood-brain barrier penetration, erratic drug absorption, serum protein binding, systemic adverse effects, and poor patient compliance (Miller et al. 1992).

SUMMARY AND CONCLUSION

Psychotropic drugs can benefit the older patient in acute emotional crisis or with chronic recurrent symptoms of severe mental distress that cannot be alleviated solely by other interventions. Regardless of the symptoms being treated or the class of drug being used, sound psychotropic treatment may be guided by the following principles:

■ The clinician must carefully review the elderly patient's current physical illness and medication regimen before beginning treatment.

■ The likelihood that concomitant medication for physical illness taken by an older patient may interact adversely with psychotropic drugs is increased.

■ An older patient is more likely to develop toxic effects from psychotropic drugs, even at doses and blood levels usually considered nontoxic in younger adults.

■ The average older patient's greater sensitivity to psychotropic drug effects (pharmacodynamics) and the tendency of psychotropic drugs to accumulate and exert greater effects for longer periods (pharmacokinetics) signify the need for low starting doses, low dosage increments, and low therapeutic and maintenance doses to avoid toxicity.

■ Drug response varies greatly among elderly people. An old-old patient may be even more sensitive to drugs than would a young-old patient.

■ As a corollary, fixed dosing guidelines are not useful when treating an elderly patient. Some older people require doses equal to those prescribed for younger adults.

■ The clinician should maintain close contact and have frequent meetings with the older patient being treated to ensure optimal compliance and to monitor effects and reactions.

REFERENCES

Abou-Saleh MT, Coppen A: The efficacy of low-dose lithium: clinical, psychological and biological correlates. J Psychiatr Res 23:157–162, 1989

Addonizio G: Neuroleptic malignant syndrome in the elderly, in Psychopharmacological Treatment Complications in the Elderly. Edited by Shamoian CA. Washington, DC, American Psychiatric Press, 1992, pp 63–70

Alexopoulos GS: Clinical and biological findings in late-onset depression, in American Psychiatric Press Review of Psychiatry, Vol 9. Edited by Tasman A, Goldfinger SM, Kaufmann CA. Washington, DC, American Psychiatric Press, 1990, pp 249–262

Alexopoulos GS: Treatment of depression, in Clinical Geriatric Psychopharmacology, 2nd Edition. Edited by Salzman C. Baltimore, MD, Williams & Wilkins, 1992, pp 137–174

Alexopoulos GS, Young RC, Meyers BS, et al: Late-onset depression. Psychiatr Clin North Am 11:101–115, 1988

Allen RM: Tranquilizers and sedative/hypnotics: appropriate use in the elderly. Geriatrics 41:75–88, 1986

Ancill RJ, Embury GD, MacEwan GW, et al: The use and misuse of psychotropic prescribing for elderly psychiatric patients. Can J Psychiatry 33:585–589, 1988

Ancoli-Israel S: Epidemiology of sleep disorders. Clin Geriatr Med 5:347–362, 1989

Antonijoan RM, Barbanoj MJ, Torrent J, et al: Evaluation of psychotropic drug consumption related to psychological distress in the elderly: hospitalized vs. nonhospitalized. Neuropsychobiology 23:25–30, 1990

Aoba A, Kakita Y, Yamaguchi N, et al: Absence of age effect on plasma haloperidol neuroleptic levels in psychiatric patients. J Gerontol 40:303–308, 1985

Aronson MK, Ooi WL, Geva DL, et al: Dementia: age-dependent incidence, prevalence, and mortality in the old-old. Arch Intern Med 151:989–992, 1991

Avorn J, Dreyer P, Connelly K, et al: Use of psychoactive medication and the quality of care in rest homes. N Engl J Med 320:227–232, 1989

Avorn J, Soumerai SB, Everett DE, et al: A randomized controlled trial of a program to reduce the use of psychoactive drugs in nursing homes. N Engl J Med 327:168–173, 1992

Beardsley RS, Larson DB, Burns BJ, et al: Prescribing of psychotropics in elderly nursing home residents. J Am Geriatr Soc 37:327–330, 1989

Beers M, Avorn J, Soumerai SB, et al: Psychoactive medication use in intermediate care facility residents. JAMA 260:3016–3020, 1988

Berrios GE, Bakshi N: Manic and depressive symptoms in the elderly: their relationships to treatment outcome, cognition and motor symptoms. Psychopathology 24:31–38, 1991

Billig N, Cohen-Mansfield J, Lipson S: Pharmacological treatment of agitation in a nursing home. J Am Geriatr Soc 39:1002–1005, 1991

Blazer D, Williams CD: Epidemiology of dysphoria and depression in an elderly population. Am J Psychiatry 137:439–444, 1980

Bonnet MH, Arand DL: Chronic use of triazolam in patients with periodic leg movements, fragmented sleep and daytime sleepiness. Aging 3:313–324, 1991

Branconnier RJ, Cole JO: Effects of acute administration of trazodone and amitriptyline on cognition, cardiovascular function, and salivation in the normal geriatric subject. J Clin Psychopharmacol 1:82S–88S, 1981

Branconnier RJ, Cole JO, Ghazvinian S, et al: Clinical pharmacology of bupropion and imipramine in elderly depressives. J Clin Psychiatry 44:130–133, 1983

Branconnier RJ, Branconnier ME, Walshe TM, et al: Blocking the Ca 2+-activated cytotoxic mechanisms of cholinergic neuronal death: a novel treatment strategy for Alzheimer's disease. Psychopharmacol Bull 28:175–181, 1992

Brymer C, Winograd CH: Fluoxetine in elderly patients: is there cause for concern? J Am Geriatr Soc 40:902–905, 1992

Buck JA: Psychotropic drug practice in nursing homes. J Am Geriatr Soc 36:409–418, 1988

Burrows AB, Satlin A, Salzman C, et al: Depression in a long-term care facility: clinical features and discordance between nursing assessment and patient interviews. J Am Geriatr Soc 43:1118–1122, 1995

Caine ED, Lyness JM, King DA: Reconsidering depression in the elderly. American Journal of Geriatric Psychiatry 1:4–20, 1993

Carbonin R, Pahor M, Bernabei R: Is age an independent risk factor for adverse drug reactions in hospitalized medical patients? J Am Geriatr Soc 39:1093–1099, 1991

Chatellier G, Lacomblez L: Tacrine (tetrahydroaminoacridine; THA) and lecithin in senile dementia of the Alzheimer type: a multicentre trial. BMJ 300:495–499, 1990

Cohen BM, Sommer BR: Metabolism of thioridazine in the elderly. J Clin Psychopharmacol 8:336–339, 1988

Cohen-Mansfield J, Marx MS, Rosenthal AS: A description of agitation in a nursing home. J Gerontol 44:77–84, 1989

Col N, Fanale JE, Kronholm P: The role of medication noncompliance and adverse drug reactions in hospitalizations of the elderly. Arch Intern Med 150:841–845, 1990

Colenda CC: Buspirone in treatment of agitated demented patient. Lancet 2:1169, 1988

Crook TH: Diagnosis and treatment of normal and pathologic memory impairment in later life. Semin Neurol 9:20–30, 1989

Crook TH, Johnson BA, Larrabee GJ: Evaluation of drugs in Alzheimer's disease and age-associated memory impairment. Psychopharmacology (Berl) 26:37–55, 1990

Cutler NR, Zavadil AP, Eisdorfer C, et al: Concentrations of desipramine in elderly women. Am J Psychiatry 138:1235–1237, 1981

Davis KL, Thal LJ, Gamzu ER, et al: A double-blind, placebo-controlled multicenter study of tacrine for Alzheimer's disease. N Engl J Med 327:1253–1259, 1992

Dawling S, Crome P, Braithwaite RA, et al: Nortriptyline therapy in elderly patients: dosage prediction after single dose pharmacokinetic study. Eur J Clin Pharmacol 18:147–150, 1980a

Dawling S, Crome P, Braithwaite RA: Pharmacokinetics of single oral doses of nortriptyline in depressed elderly hospital patients and young healthy volunteers. Clin Pharmacokinet 5:394–401, 1980b

Dawling S, Crome P, Heyer EJ, et al: Nortriptyline therapy in elderly patients: dosage prediction from plasma concentration at 24 hours after a single 50mg dose. Br J Psychiatry 139:413–416, 1981

Dawson D, Hundershot G, Fulton J: Aging in the eighties: functional limitations of individuals age 65 and over (Advance Data No. 133, June 1987), in Aging America: Trends and Projections, 1986–1987. Washington, DC, U.S. Department of Health and Human Services, 1987

Devanand DP, Sackeim HA, Mayeux R: Psychosis, behavioral disturbance, and the use of neuroleptics in dementia. Compr Psychiatry 29:387–401, 1988

Devanand DP, Sackeim HA, Brown RP, et al: A pilot study of haloperidol treatment of psychosis and behavioral disturbance in Alzheimer's disease. Arch Neurol 46:854–857, 1989

Devanand DP, Cooper T, Sackeim HA, et al: Low dose oral haloperidol and blood levels in Alzheimer's disease: a preliminary study. Psychopharmacol Bull 28:169–173, 1992

De Veaugh-Geiss J: Clinical changes in tardive dyskinesia during long-term follow-up, in Tardive Dyskinesia: Biological Mechanisms and Clinical Aspects. Edited by Wolf ME, Mosnaim AD. Washington, DC, American Psychiatric Press, 1988, pp 89–105

Dewan MJ, Huszonek J, Koss M, et al: The use of antidepressants in the elderly: 1986 and 1989. J Geriatr Psychiatry Neurol 5:40–44, 1992

Dhingra U, Rabins PV: Mania in the elderly: a 5–7 year follow-up. J Am Geriatr Soc 39:581–583, 1991

Dunner DL, Cohn JB, Walshe T III, et al: Two combined, multicenter double-blind studies of paroxetine and doxepin in geriatric patients with major depression. J Clin Psychiatry 53:57–60, 1992

Eagger SA, Levy R, Sahakian BJ: Tacrine in Alzheimer's disease. Lancet 337:989–992, 1991

Evans DA, Funkenstein H, Albert MS, et al: Prevalence of Alzheimer's disease in a community population of older persons. JAMA 262:2551–2556, 1989

Farlow M, Gracon SI, Hershey LA, et al: A controlled trial of tacrine in Alzheimer's disease. JAMA 268:2523–2529, 1992

Feighner JP, Cohn JB: Double-blind comparative trials of fluoxetine and doxepin in geriatric patients with major depressive disorder. J Clin Psychiatry 46:20–25, 1985

Feighner JP, Boyer WF, Meredith CH, et al: An overview of fluoxetine in geriatric depression. Br J Psychiatry 153 (suppl 3):105–108, 1988

Ford DE, Kamerow DB: Epidemiological studies of sleep disturbances and psychiatric disorders: an opportunity for prevention? JAMA 262:1479–1484, 1989

Forsman A, Ohman R: Applied pharmacokinetics of haloperidol in man. Current Therapeutic Research 21:396–411, 1977

Foster JR: Use of lithium in elderly psychiatric patients: a review of the literature. Lithium 3:77–93, 1992

Foster JR, Martin CE: Dementia, in Verwoerdt's Clinical Geropsychiatry, 3rd Edition. Edited by Bienenfeld D. Baltimore, MD, Williams & Wilkins, 1990, pp 66–84

Frattola L, Maggioni M, Cesana B, et al: Double blind comparison of zolpidem 20 mg versus flunitrazepam 2 mg in insomniac in-patients. Drugs Exp Clin Res 16:371–376, 1990

Ganzini L, Heintz R, Hoffman WF, et al: Acute extrapyramidal syndromes in neuroleptic-treated elders: a pilot study. J Geriatr Psychiatry Neurol 4:222–225, 1991

Garrard J, Makris L, Dunham T, et al: Evaluation of neuroleptic drug use under proposed Medicare and Medicaid regulations. JAMA 265:463–467, 1991

Gauthier S, Bouchard R, Lamontagne A, et al: Tetrahydroaminoacridine-lecithin combination treatment in patients with intermediate stage Alzheimer's disease. N Engl J Med 322:1272–1276, 1990

Georgotas A, Mann J, Friedman E: Platelet monoamine oxidase inhibitors as a potential indicator of favorable response to MAOIs in geriatric depression. Biol Psychiatry 16:997–1001, 1981

Georgotas A, Friedman E, McCarthy M, et al: Resistant geriatric depressions and therapeutic response to monoamine oxidase inhibitors. Biol Psychiatry 18:195–205, 1983

Georgotas A, McCue RE, Hapworth W, et al: Comparative efficacy and safety of MAOIs versus TCAs in treating depression in the elderly. Biol Psychiatry 21:1155–1166, 1986

Gerner R, Estabrook W, Steuer J, et al: Treatment of depression with trazodone, imipramine, and placebo: a double-blind study. J Clin Psychiatry 41:216–220, 1980

Glasser M, Rabins P: Mania in the elderly. Age Ageing 13:210–213, 1984

Gottlieb GL: Sleep disorders and their management: special considerations in the elderly. Am J Med 88 (3A):29S–33S, 1990

Greenblatt DJ, Shader RI: Benzodiazepines in the elderly: pharmacokinetics and drug sensitivity, in Anxiety in the Elderly. Edited by Salzman C, Lebowitz B. New York, Springer, 1990, pp 131–145

Greenwald BS, Marin DB, Silverman SM: Serotonergic treatment of screaming and banging in dementia (letter). Lancet 2:1464–1465, 1986

Grymonpre RE, Mitenko PA, Sitar DS, et al: Drug-associated hospital admissions in older medical patients. J Am Geriatr Soc 36:1092–1098, 1988

Gurwitz JH, Avorn J: The ambiguous relationship between aging and adverse drug reactions. Ann Intern Med 114:956–966, 1991

Halaris A: Antidepressant drug therapy in the elderly: enhancing safety and compliance. Int J Psychiatry Med 16:1986–1987, 1986

Hale WE, May FE, Moore MT, et al: Meprobamate use in the elderly. J Am Geriatr Soc 36:1003–1005, 1988

Helms PM: Efficacy of antipsychotics in the treatment of the behavioral complications of dementia: a review of the literature. J Am Geriatr Soc 33:206–209, 1985

Hershey LA, Kim KY: Diagnosis and treatment of anxiety in the elderly. Rational Drug Therapy 22:3–6, 1988

Himmelhoch JM, Neil JF, May F, et al: Age, dementia, dyskinesias, and lithium response. Am J Psychiatry 137:941–945, 1980

Holton A, George K: The use of lithium in severely demented patients with behavioral disturbance. Br J Psychiatry 146:99–104, 1985

Huang CC: Comparison of two groups of tardive dyskinesia patients. Psychiatry Res 19:335–336, 1986

Institute of Medicine: Extending Life, Enhancing Life: A National Research Agenda on Aging. Washington, DC, National Academy Press, 1991

Ives TJ, Bentz EJ, Gwyther RE: Drug-related admissions to a family medicine inpatient service. Arch Intern Med 147:1117–1120, 1987

Jarvik LF, Read SL, Mintz J, et al: Pretreatment orthostatic hypotension in geriatric depression: predictor of response to imipramine and doxepin. J Clin Psychopharmacol 3:368–372, 1983

Jefferson JW, Griest JH, Ackerman DL, et al: Lithium Encyclopedia for Clinical Practice. Washington, DC, American Psychiatric Press, 1987

Jenike MA: The use of monoamine oxidase inhibitors in the treatment of elderly depressed patients. J Am Geriatric Soc 32:571–575, 1985

Jenike MA, Albert M, Heller H, et al: Oral physostigmine treatment for patients with presenile and senile dementia of the Alzheimer's-type: a double-blind, placebo-controlled trial. J Clin Psychiatry 51:3–7, 1990

Kanba S, Matsumoto K, Nibuya M, et al: Nortriptyline response in elderly depressed patients. Prog Neuropsychopharmacol Biol Psychiatry 16:301–309, 1992

Karson CG, Bracha HS, Powell A, et al: Dyskinetic movements, cognitive impairment, and negative symptoms in elderly neuropsychiatric patients. Am J Psychiatry 147:1646–1649, 1990

Katz IR, Simpson GM, Jethanandani V, et al: Steady state pharmacokinetics of nortriptyline in the frail elderly. Neuropsychopharmacology 2:229–236, 1989

Kemperman CJF, Gerdes JH, De Rooij J, et al: Reversible lithium neurotoxicity at normal serum level may refer to intracranial pathology. J Neurol Neurosurg Psychiatry 52:679–680, 1989

Kim KY: Diagnosis and treatment of depression in the elderly. Int J Psychiatry Med 18:211–221, 1988

Kitanka I, Ross RJ, Cutler NR, et al: Altered hydroxydesipramine concentrations in elderly depressed patients. Clin Pharmacol Ther 31:51–55, 1982

Koenig HG, Breitner JCS: Use of antidepressants in medically ill older patients. Psychosomatics 31:22–32, 1990

Koepke HH, Gold RL, Linden ME, et al: Multicenter controlled study of oxazepam in anxious elderly outpatients. Pychosomatics 23:641–645, 1982

Kroenke K, Pinholt EM: Reducing polypharmacy in the elderly: a controlled trial of physician feedback. J Am Geriatr Soc 38:31–36, 1990

Kroessler D, Fogel BS: Electroconvulsive therapy for major depression in the oldest old: effects of medical comorbidity on post-treatment survival. American Journal of Geriatric Psychiatry 1:30–37, 1993

Kutcher SP, Reid K, Dubbin JD, et al: Electrocardiogram changes and therapeutic desipramine and 2-hydroxydesipramine concentrations in elderly depressives. Br J Psychiatry 148:676–679, 1986

Kyomen HH, Nobel KW, Wei JY: The use of estrogen to decrease aggressive physical behavior in elderly men with dementia. J Am Geriatr Soc 39:1110–1112, 1991

Lakshmanan EB, Mion CC, Frengley JD: Effective low dose tricyclic antidepressant treatment for depressed geriatric rehabilitation patients. J Am Geriatr Soc 34:421–426, 1986

Lavretsky EP, Jarvik LF: A group of potassium-channel blockers-acetylcholine releasers: new potentials for Alzheimer disease? a review. J Clin Psychopharmacol 12:110–118, 1992

Lazarus LW, Groves L, Gierl B, et al: Efficacy of phenelzine in geriatric depression. Biol Psychiatry 21:699–701, 1986

Leibovici A, Tariot N: Carbamazepine treatment of agitation associated with dementia. J Geriatr Psychiatry Neurol 1:110–112, 1988

Lieberman J, Kane JM, Woerner M, et al: Prevalence of tardive dyskinesia in elderly samples. Psychopharmacol Bull 20:22–26, 1984

Liptzin B: Treatment of mania, in Clinical Geriatric Psychopharmacology, 2nd Edition. Edited by Salzman C. Baltimore, MD, Williams & Wilkins, 1992, pp 175–188

Magni G, Palazzolo O, Bianchin G: The course of depression in elderly outpatients. Can J Psychiatry 33:21–24, 1988

Maletta GS: Use of antipsychotic medications, in Annual Review of Gerontology and Geriatrics, Vol 4. Edited by Eisdorfer C. New York, Springer, 1984, pp 175–220

McCue RE, Georgotas A, Nagachandran N, et al: Plasma levels of nortriptyline and 10-hydroxynortriptyline and treatment-related electrocardiographic changes in the elderly depressed. J Psychiatr Res 23:73–79, 1989

McFarland BH, Miller MR, Straumfjord AA: Valproate use in the older manic patient. J Clin Psychiatry 51:479–481, 1990

Meyers BS: Adverse cognitive effects of tricyclic antidepressants in the treatment of geriatric depression: fact or fiction?, in Psychopharmacological Treatment Complications in the Elderly. Edited by Shamoian CA. Washington, DC, American Psychiatric Press, 1992, pp 1–16

Miller SW, Mahoney JM, Jann MW: Therapeutic frontiers in Alzheimer's disease. Pharmacotherapy 12:217–231, 1992

Morgan DG, May PC, Finch LE: Dopamine and serotonin systems in human and rodent brain: effects of age and neurodegenerative disease. J Am Geriatr Soc 35:334–345, 1987

Mouret J, Ruel D, Maillard F, et al: Zopiclone versus triazolam in insomniac geriatric patients: a specific increase in delta sleep with zopiclone. Int Clin Psychopharmacol 5 (suppl 2):47–55, 1990

Napoliello MJ: An interim multicentre report on 677 anxious geriatric out-patients treated with buspirone. Br J Clin Pract 40:71–73, 1986

National Center for Health Statistics: Current estimates from the National Health Interview Survey: Vital and Health Statistics 1987, No. 10, in Aging America: Trends and Projections, 1986–1987. Washington, DC, U.S. Government Printing Office, 1987, p 164

Nelson JC, Atillasoy E, Mazure C: Desipramine plasma levels and response in elderly melancholic patients. J Clin Psychopharmacol 5:217–220, 1985

Nelson JC, Atillasoy E, Mazure C, et al: Hydroxydesipramine in the elderly. J Clin Psychopharmacol 8:428–433, 1988

Office of Epidemiology and Biostatistics, Center for Drug Evaluation and Research: Drug Utilization in the United States, 1986. Washington, DC, National Technical Information Service, 1987

Olafsson K, Jorgensen S, Jensen HV, et al: Fluvoxamine in the treatment of demented elderly patients: a double-blind, placebo-controlled study. Acta Psychiatr Scand 85:453–456, 1992

Old Age Depression Interest Group: How long should the elderly take antidepressants? A double-blind placebo-controlled study of continuation/prophylaxis therapy with dothiepin. Br J Psychiatry 162:175–182, 1993

Oreland L, Gottfries CG: Brain monoamine oxidase in aging and in dementia of the Alzheimer type. Prog Neuropsychopharmacol Biol Psychiatry 10:533–540, 1986

Parmelee PA, Katz IR, Lawton MP: Anxiety and association with depression among institutionalized elderly. American Journal of Geriatric Psychiatry 1:46–58, 1993

Peabody CA, Whiteford HA, Hollister LE: Antidepressants and the elderly. J Am Geriatr Soc 34:869–874, 1986

Peabody CA, Warner MD, Whiteford HA, et al: Neuroleptics and the elderly. J Am Geriatr Soc 35:233–238, 1987

Perry E, Tomlinson B, Blessed G, et al: Correlation of cholinergic abnormalities with senile plaques and mental test scores in senile dementia. BMJ 2:1457–1459, 1978

Petrie WM, Ban TA, Berney S, et al: Loxapine in psychogeriatrics: a placebo and standard controlled clinical investigation. J Clin Psychopharmacol 2:122–126, 1982

Phillipson M, Moranville JT, Jeste DV, et al: Antipsychotics. Clin Geriatr Med 6:411–422, 1990

Pinner E, Rich CL: Effects of trazodone on aggressive behavior in seven patients with organic mental disorders. Am J Psychiatry 145:1295–1296, 1988

Pinsker H, Suljaga-Petchel K: Use of benzodiazepines in primary-care geriatric patients. J Am Geriatr Soc 32:595–598, 1984

Pollack CP, Perlick D: Sleep problems and institutionalization of the elderly. J Geriatr Psychiatry Neurol 4:204–210, 1991

Prinz PN, Vitiello MV, Raskind MA, et al: Geriatrics: sleep disorders and aging. N Engl J Med 323:520–526, 1990

Rashi S, Logan RFA: Role of drugs in fractures of the femoral neck. BMJ 292:86, 1986

Ray WA, Federspiel CF, Schaffner W: A study of anti-psychotic drug use in nursing homes: epidemiologic evidence suggesting misuse. Am J Public Health 70:485–491, 1980

Ray WA, Griffin MR, Shaffner W, et al: Psychotropic drug use and the risk of hip fracture. N Engl J Med 316:363–369, 1987

Ray WA, Fought RL, Decker MD: Psychoactive drugs and the risk of injurious motor vehicle crashes in elderly drivers. Am J Epidemiol 136:873–883, 1992

Regestein QR: Treatment of insomnia in the elderly, in Clinical Geriatric Psychopharmacology, 2nd Edition. Edited by Salzman C. Baltimore, MD, Williams & Wilkins, 1992, pp 235–253

Reynolds CF: Sleep disorders, in Comprehensive Review of Geriatric Psychiatry. Edited by Sadavoy J, Lazarus LW, Jarvik LF. Washington, DC, American Psychiatric Press, 1991, pp 403–418

Risse SC, Barnes R: Pharmacologic treatment of agitation associated with dementia. J Am Geriatr Soc 34:368–376, 1986

Robinson DS, Sourkes TL, Nies A, et al: Monoamine metabolism in human brain. Arch Gen Psychiatry 34:89–92, 1977

Rockwell E, Lam RW, Zisook S: Antidepressant drug studies in the elderly. Psychiatr Clin North Am 11:215–233, 1988

Rosebush PI, Salzman C: Memory disturbance and cognitive impairment in the elderly, in Handbook of Clinical Psychopharmacology. Edited by Tupin JP, Shader RI, Harnett DS. New York, Jason Aronson, 1988, pp 159–210

Rothschild AJ, Samson AJ, Bessette MP, et al: Efficacy of the combination of fluoxetine and perphenazine in the treatment of psychotic depression. J Clin Psychiatry 54:338–342, 1993

Rovner B, Kafonek S, Filipp L, et al: Prevalence of mental illness in a nursing home. Am J Psychiatry 143:1146–1149, 1986

Rovner BW, German PS, Brant LJ, et al: Depression and mortality in nursing homes. JAMA 265:993–996, 1991

Saban RJ, Vitug AJ, Mark VH: Are nursing home diagnosis and treatment inadequate? JAMA 243:321–322, 1982

Saltz BL, Kane JM, Woerner MG, et al: Prospective study of tardive dyskinesia in the elderly. Psychopharmacol Bull 25:52–56, 1989

Salzman C: Treatment of agitation in the elderly, in Psychopharmacology: The Third Generation of Progress. Edited by Meltzer HY. New York, Raven, 1987, pp 1167–1176

Salzman C: The American Psychiatric Association Task Force Report on Benzodiazepine Dependency, Toxicity, and Abuse. J Psychiatr Res 24:35–37, 1990a

Salzman C: Practical considerations of the pharmacologic treatment of depression and anxiety in the elderly. J Clin Psychiatry 51 (1 suppl):40–43, 1990b

Salzman C: Recent advances in geriatric psychopharmacology, in American Psychiatric Press Review of Psychiatry, Vol 9. Edited by Tasman A, Goldfinger SM, Kaufmann C. Washington, DC, American Psychiatric Press, 1990c, pp 279–292

Salzman C: Monoamine oxidase inhibitors and atypical antidepressants. Clin Geriatr Med 8:335–348, 1992

Salzman C: Pharmacologic treatment of depression in the elderly. J Clin Psychiatry 54 (suppl):23–28, 1993

Salzman C: Pharmacological treatment of depression in elderly patients, in Diagnosis and Treatment of Depression in Late Life: Results of the NIH Consensus Development Conference. Edited by Schneider LS, Reynolds CF, Lebowitz BD, et al. Washington, DC, American Psychiatric Press, 1994, pp 181–244

Salzman C, Fisher J, Nobel K, et al: Cognitive improvement following benzodiazepine discontinuation in elderly nursing home residents. International Journal of Geriatric Psychiatry 7:89–93, 1992

Salzman C, Schneider LS, Lebowitz BD: Antidepressant treatment of very old patients. American Journal of Geriatric Psychiatry 1:21–29, 1993

Satlin A, Liptzin B: Treatment of mania, in Clinical Geriatric Psychopharmacology, 3rd Edition. Edited by Salzman C. Baltimore, MD, Williams & Wilkins, 1998, pp 310–332

Schneider LS, Sloane RB, Staples FR, et al: Pretreatment orthostatic hypotension as a predictor of response to nortriptyline in geriatric depression. J Clin Psychopharmacol 6:172–176, 1986

Schneider LS, Cooper TB, Suckow RF, et al: Relationship of hydroxynortriptyline to nortriptyline concentration and creatinine clearance in depressed elderly outpatients. J Clin Psychopharmacol 10:333–337, 1990a

Schneider LS, Pollock VE, Lyness SA: A metaanalysis of controlled trials of neuroleptic treatment in dementia. J Am Geriatr Soc 38:553–563, 1990b

Schneider JK, Mion LC, Frengley JD: Adverse drug reactions in an elderly outpatient population. Am J Hosp Pharm 49:90–96, 1992

Sheikh JI: Panic disorder, in Anxiety in the Elderly. Edited by Salzman C, Lebowitz B. New York, Springer, 1990, pp 251–266

Shulman KI, Tohen M, Satlin A, et al: Mania compared with unipolar depression in old age. Am J Psychiatry 149:341–345, 1992

Simpson DM, Foster D: Improvement in organically disturbed behavior with trazodone treatment. J Clin Psychiatry 47:191–193, 1986

Skoog I, Nilsson L, Palmertz B, et al: A population-based study of dementia in 85-year-olds. N Engl J Med 328:153–158, 1993

Small GW: Psychopharmacological treatment of elderly demented patients. J Clin Psychiatry 49 (suppl):8–13, 1988

Smith JM, Baldessarini RJ: Changes in prevalence, severity and recovery in tardive dyskinesia with age. Arch Gen Psychiatry 37:1368–1373, 1980

Smith M, Buckwalter KC: Medication management, antidepressant drugs, and the elderly: an overview. Journal of Psychosocial Nursing 30:30–36, 1992

Snowdon J: A retrospective case-note study of bipolar disorder in old age. Br J Psychiatry 158:485–490, 1991

Spagnoli A, Lucca U, Menasce G, et al: Long-term acetyl-L-carnitine treatment in Alzheimer's disease. Neurology 41:1726–1732, 1991

Stack JA, Reynolds CF III, Perel JM, et al: Pretreatment systolic orthostatic blood pressure (PSOP) and treatment response in elderly depressed inpatients. J Clin Psychopharmacol 8:116–120, 1988

Stern Y, Sano M, Mayeux R: Long-term administration of oral physostigmine in Alzheimer's disease. Neurology 38:1837–1841, 1988

Stewart RB, May FE, Moore MY, et al: Changing patterns of psychotropic drug use in the elderly: a five-year update. Ann Pharmacother 23:610–613, 1989

Stone K: Mania in the elderly. Br J Psychiatry 155:220–229, 1989

Strauss A: Oral dyskinesia associated with buspirone use in an elderly woman. J Clin Psychiatry 49:322–323, 1988

Sweet RA, Benoit H, Mulsant MD, et al: Dyskinesia and neuroleptic exposure in elderly psychiatric inpatients. J Geriatr Psychiatry Neurol 5:156–161, 1992

Szuba MP, Leuchter AF: Falling backward in two elderly patients taking bupropion. J Clin Psychiatry 53:157–159, 1992

Tariot PN: Neurobiology and treatment of dementia, in Clinical Geriatric Psychopharmacology, 2nd Edition. Edited by Salzman C. Baltimore, MD, Williams & Wilkins, 1992, pp 277–299

Thompson TL, Filley CM, Mitchell WD, et al: Lack of efficacy of hydergine in patients with Alzheimer's disease. N Engl J Med 323:445–448, 1990

Tingle D: Trazodone in dementia (letter). J Clin Psychiatry 47:482, 1986

Tollefson GD: Short-term effects of the calcium channel blocker nimodipine (Bay-e-9736) in the management of primary degenerative dementia. Biol Psychiatry 27:1133–1142, 1990

Vogel GW, Morris D: The effects of estazolam on sleep, performance, and memory: a long-term sleep laboratory study of elderly insomniacs. J Clin Pharmacol 32:647–651, 1992

von Moltke LL, Greenblatt DJ, Shader RI: Clinical pharmacokinetics of antidepressants in the elderly. Clin Pharmacokinet 24:141–160, 1993 von Moltke LL, Abernethy DR, Greenblatt DJ: Kinetics and dynamics of psychotropic drugs in the elderly, in Clinical Geriatric Psychopharmacology, 3rd Edition. Edited by Salzman C. Baltimore, MD, Williams & Wilkins, 1998, pp 70–96

Weiler PG, Mungo D, Bernick C: Propranolol for the control of disruptive behavior in senile dementia. J Geriatr Psychiatry Neurol 1:226–230, 1988

Weissman MM, Prusoff B, Sholomskas AJ, et al: A double-blind clinical trial of alprazolam, imipramine, or placebo in the depressed elderly. J Clin Psychopharmacol 12:175–182, 1992

Wragg RE, Jeste DV: Neuroleptics and alternative treatments: management of behavioral symptoms and psychosis in Alzheimer's disease and related conditions. Psychiatr Clin North Am 11:195–213, 1988

Yassa R: The course of tardive dyskinesia in newly treated psychogeriatric patients. Acta Psychiatr Scand 83:347–349, 1991

Yassa R, Nair V, Schwartz G: Tardive dyskinesia: a two-year follow-up study. Psychosomatics 25:852–855, 1984

Yassa R, Nastase C, Camille Y, et al: Tardive dyskinesia in a psychogeriatric population, in Tardive Dyskinesia: Biological Mechanisms and Clinical Aspects. Edited by Wolf ME, Mosnaim AD. Washington, DC, American Psychiatric Press, 1988, pp 125–133

Young RC, Alexopoulos GS, Shamoian CA, et al: Plasma 10-hydroxynortriptyline in elderly depressed patients. Clin Pharmacol Ther 35:540–544, 1984

Young RC, Alexopoulos GS, Shamoian CA, et al: Plasma 10-hydroxynortriptyline and ECG changes in elderly depressed patients. Am J Psychiatry 142:866–868, 1985

Zimmer JG, Watson N, Trent A: Behavior problems among patients in skilled nursing facilities. Am J Public Health 74:1118–1121, 1984

Zimmer JG, Bentley DW, Valente WM: Systemic antibiotic use in nursing homes: a quality assessment. J Am Geriatr Soc 34:703–710, 1986

Zisook S: A clinical overview of monoamine oxidase inhibitors. Psychosomatics 26:240–246, 1985

FORTY-SEVEN

Psychopharmacology During Pregnancy and Lactation

Zachary N. Stowe, M.D.,
James R. Strader, Jr., B.S., and
Charles B. Nemeroff, M.D., Ph.D.

The management of mental illness during pregnancy and lactation represents a unique and complex clinical situation. Given the high incidence of mental illness in women during the childbearing years and the rise in the number of women who plan to nurse, there is a high probability that the clinician will encounter such situations. The use of psychotropic medications during pregnancy and lactation has been comprehensively reviewed by several groups (Altshuler et al. 1996; Cohen 1989; Cohen et al. 1989; Kerns 1986; Miller 1991, 1994; Robinson et al. 1986; Stowe and Nemeroff 1995; Wisner and Perel 1988). The most common situations that the clinician will encounter in patients who are pregnant or lactating include the following:

- New-onset mental illness
- Exacerbation of psychiatric symptoms in the presence of preexisting mental illness
- Inadvertent conception during treatment with psychotropic medications
- Prepregnancy consultation for women who have a history of mental illness and/or are currently taking psychotropic medications
- Prophylactic treatment planning for women at high risk for a postpartum mental illness who plan to nurse

The literature, although expanding rapidly, provides little definitive data to develop scientifically derived guidelines in such situations. The clinician must have all available data on potential teratogenic, toxic, and neurobehavioral effects of psychotropic medications.

In this chapter, we provide a brief review of the normal physiological changes associated with pregnancy, lactation, and fetal and early infant life as a preamble to expanding previously suggested treatment guidelines (Cohen et al. 1989; Miller 1991). Knowledge of these basic physiological alterations has some empirical value in selecting medications based on their pharmacokinetic and pharmacodynamic properties in the event that prior pharmacological agents are not options and nonpharmacological interventions fail to provide adequate control of symptoms. This discussion is followed by the available data on the possible risks of individual agents from different classes. Such information is important for patient education, as well as for medical-legal issues. Finally, we review the individual classes of medications and discuss potential modifications of previously suggested treatment guidelines, emphasizing the need for an individualized risk-benefit assessment.

Review of the current literature on the use of psychotropic medications during pregnancy and lactation reveals a cadre of obstacles to the establishment of definitive guidelines. The most prominent confounding factors in these studies include 1) the failure of adequate sample size to establish a significant causal relationship for teratogenic or toxic effects of psychotropic medications, 2) the reliance on case reports, and 3) limited methodological consistency. In addition to these limitations, the clinician should be aware of factors related to obstetrical and neonatal outcome. Of all documented pregnancies, 84.5% result in the birth of a viable infant (Kiely 1991; McBride 1972). Of these infants, 2%–4% have malformations that impair function and/or require surgical correction, and up to 12% of these have minor malformations (Riccardi 1977).

The Collaborative Perinatal Project followed up a cohort of 50,282 mother-infant pairs from 12 medical centers and found an overall infant malformation rate of 6.5% (Heinonen et al. 1977). Studies on embryonic development have shown that most major malformations occur during the embryonic period (i.e., the third through the eighth week of gestation). After week 11 of gestation, most of the organ systems (except for the central nervous system, teeth, ears, eyes, and external genitalia) are developed (Sadler 1985). A second major issue, noted in previous reviews (Cohen et al. 1989), is that up to 80% of pregnant women are prescribed medications, and more than one-third of pregnant women may take psychotropic medications at some point in their pregnancy (Doering and Stewart 1978). Most previous case reports fail to control for maternal age, tobacco use, alcohol and drug abuse, potential exposure to environmental toxins, duration and timing of exposure, and the extent of prenatal care received.

There is also evidence that bias may exist in associating birth defects with psychotropic medications. For example, the association of in utero exposure to lithium with Ebstein's anomaly of the heart is still a widely held view, yet comprehensive reviews of the available data by Cohen et al. (1994) place the risk for this malformation at less than 0.1%. The potential adverse effect of untreated psychiatric illness on the rate of obstetrical complications, as well as the rate of spontaneous miscarriage, remains unknown. In contrast, considerable data suggest that untreated maternal illness during the early neonatal period poses considerable risk to the infant.

PHYSIOLOGY—PREGNANCY

Physiological alterations during pregnancy and data derived from studies of nonpsychotropic medications support several suggestions for the choice of a psychotropic medication from within a given class. One area of growing interest concerns the potential effects of gender differences and the effects of alterations in serum gonadal hormone concentrations on the pharmacokinetics of psychotropic medications (Yonkers et al. 1992). Most relevant data concerning the physiological changes associated with pregnancy are derived from monitoring therapeutic plasma levels of nonpsychotropic medications (Boobis and Lewis 1983).

Physiological changes during pregnancy that may alter maternal serum concentrations of psychotropic medications include the following:

- Delayed gastric emptying, which results in increased exposure to an acidic environment and degradative enzymes
- Decreased gastrointestinal motility, presumably related to increased progesterone, which potentially enhances complete absorption of medication
- Increased volume of distribution (increased body fat, plasma volume, total body water), which produces decreased serum concentrations for a given dose
- Decreased protein binding capacity, which increases serum free drug concentrations (Wood and Hytten 1981)
- Increased hepatic metabolism, which results in more rapid degradation of certain medications

With the exception of psychiatric inpatients treated with tricyclic antidepressants (TCAs), a clear relation between therapeutic response and serum concentrations has not been established. In fact, studies with all of the newly released antidepressants, including the four selective serotonin reuptake inhibitors (SSRIs), venlafaxine, nefazodone, and mirtazapine, report no relation between plasma drug concentrations and clinical response. Nevertheless, all of the factors listed above may alter the drug concentration to which the fetus is exposed.

Although no evidence of placental filtering of psychotropic medications exists, formal studies are lacking. All psychotropic medications are assumed to cross the blood-placental barrier. Our group (Stowe et al. 1997a) studied the placental passage of antidepressants in women treated during pregnancy and found significant differences among the SSRIs, a finding that warrants more formal study to minimize fetal exposure within a given class of medication. The mechanism of placental transport is thought to be simple diffusion that is dependent on several properties of the individual medication (molecular size, percentage of protein binding, polarity, lipid solubility) and, of course, duration of exposure (Rayburn and Andresen 1982). Although the fetus and mother are at equilibrium with respect to circulation, the fetus has several distinct physiological attributes that may result in its increased exposure to medications and potentially greater drug concentrations in the central nervous system. These attributes include increased cardiac output, increased blood-brain barrier permeability, decreased plasma protein and plasma protein binding affinity, and decreased hepatic enzyme activity.

PHYSIOLOGY—LACTATION

After childbirth, the neonate continues to exhibit unique physiological characteristics, including decreased activity of certain hepatic metabolic enzyme systems. Hepatic maturation in the infant appears to occur at a highly variable rate (Warner 1986) and is more delayed in premature infants. Both glucuronidation and oxidation systems are initially immature at birth (as low as 20% of adult levels). The latter system typically matures by age 3 months (Atkinson et al. 1988). In addition, rates of glomerular filtration and tubular secretion are relatively low in neonates—30%–40% and 20%–30% lower than adult levels, respectively (Welch and Findlay 1981). Hence, the potential for the infant to be exposed to higher serum concentrations of parent compounds and metabolites of any drug needs to be considered.

Neonates and infants are exposed to psychotropic medications when the mother breast-feeds during pharmacological treatment. The number of women who breast-feed is increasing; recent estimates indicate that more than 50% of new mothers leaving the hospital plan to nurse (Briggs et al. 1994). The excretion of psychotropic medications in breast milk has been reviewed elsewhere (Buist et al. 1990; Wisner et al. 1996). The literature is again difficult to interpret because of differences in the methodology of drug concentration assays as well as an identified gradient in breast milk with respect to lipophilic characteristics and protein content (Kauffman et al. 1994; Vorherr 1974). Most data have not controlled for which aliquot of the breast milk was used for assay nor the time after maternal dose when the aliquot was obtained.

Because medications enter breast milk predominantly by passive diffusion of the nonionized, unbound fraction (J. T. Wilson et al. 1980), the pH gradient between maternal serum and breast milk plays a significant role in the amount of medication that is excreted into breast milk. The physiochemical properties of an individual medication appear to be the best predictor of the amount of medication present in breast milk (see Kacew 1993 for review). These properties include the degree of ionization, molecular weight, protein binding, and lipid solubility. Maternal protein binding affects the quantity of free drug available for diffusion across the mammillary epithelium, and most medications have a higher affinity for maternal plasma proteins than for milk proteins (Kacew 1993).

The American Academy of Pediatrics (1994) recently published a committee report on the excretion of drugs and other chemicals into human breast milk. Although admittedly not complete, the report's list of psychotropic medications underscores the need to encourage further collaborative work with pediatricians. The academy's classification of individual psychotropic medications includes 1) drugs that are contraindicated during breast-feeding, 2) drugs whose effect on nursing infants is unknown but may be of concern (i.e., no adverse events have been reported, but the medications are present in human milk and thus conceivably alter development of the central nervous system), and 3) maternal medications usually compatible with breast-feeding. The information contained in the academy's report is included later in this chapter in our discussion of the individual classes of psychotropic medications.

ASSESSMENT OF RISK-BENEFIT RATIO

The morbidity and mortality of untreated mental illness during pregnancy and lactation have received limited attention. The sparse data that are available suggest some salient illness-specific features about the course of illness during pregnancy that should be considered in the risk-benefit assessment. Some psychiatric disorders, such as panic disorder, may improve or abate during pregnancy (Klein et al. 1994/1995). In contrast, obsessive-compulsive disorder appears to be more prevalent during pregnancy: in one study, more than 25% of women reported symptom onset during pregnancy (Neziroglu et al. 1992). Psychiatric disorders with a psychotic component (e.g., schizophrenia, schizoaffective disorder) were observed to generally worsen during pregnancy (McNeil et al. 1984a, 1984b). Finally, the rates and severity of depression during pregnancy span a wide range based on the diagnostic criteria employed (Buesching et al. 1986; Cutrona 1983; Kumar and Robson 1984; Manley et al. 1982; O'Hara et al. 1982, 1984; Raskin et al. 1990; Watson et al. 1984).

Furthermore, at least one group has assessed the rates of "normal depressive symptomatology" that accompany the somatic changes of pregnancy in women whose symptoms did not meet criteria for depression (Affonso et al. 1993). Their findings suggest that, to some extent, the epidemiology of depression during pregnancy may be confounded by the natural occurrence of symptoms inventoried on many depression screening tools and rating scales.

Together, these data depict a much more complex relationship between psychiatric illness and pregnancy, making general guidelines difficult to establish. The limited number of studies dictate a cautious prediction of the course of illness when treating pregnant women with psychiatric illness.

The risk to the fetus of untreated psychiatric illness during pregnancy is unclear. Although untreated schizophrenia is known to be associated with an increased incidence of perinatal death (Rieder et al. 1975), little is known of the effects, if any, of other psychiatric disorders on the fetus. One group that administered the General Health Questionnaire (Perkin et al. 1993) concluded that depressive and anxiety symptoms did not adversely affect obstetrical outcome. In contrast, Steer et al. (1992) found a risk of 3.97 for lower birth weight (<2,500 g), a risk of 3.39 for preterm delivery (<37 weeks' gestation), and a risk of 3.02 for small for gestational age (<10th percentile) in a group of adult women derived from an inner-city population with Beck Depression Inventory (Beck 1978) scores of 21 or higher. Similarly, preclinical studies have found an adverse effect of both maternal stress and increased maternal glucocorticoid concentrations on brain development (Meaney et al. 1996).

These preclinical data suggest that, if extreme stress during pregnancy results in increased maternal serum concentrations of cortisol, it may be detrimental to infant brain development. Untreated maternal mental illness clearly has an adverse effect on infant well-being. The vast majority of studies focus on untreated maternal depression. Taken together, these studies show deleterious effects on maternal-infant attachment and child development (Avant 1981; Brazelton 1975; Campbell et al. 1995; Cradon 1979; Cutrona 1983; Murray 1992; Teti et al. 1995; Zahn-Waxler et al. 1984).

The lack of large-scale epidemiological studies on the adverse effects of untreated major psychiatric illness on the fetus, as weighed against the potential adverse effects of psychopharmacological treatment, prevents the development of widely applicable treatment algorithms for managing existing and/or new-onset psychiatric illness in pregnant women. Because most pregnant women are not aware of their pregnancy until at least 6 weeks of gestation, psychotropic medications may be discontinued after the period of greatest potential risk to the fetus has passed. Abrupt discontinuation of medications may also carry an increased risk of relapse or development of withdrawal symptoms. Both situations may result in increased risk to the mother and/or greater fetal exposure to medication. Clinicians assessing the risks and benefits of treating pregnant women with concurrent psychiatric illness should take into account personal and family psychiatric histories; the possible course of illness; the effects of untreated illness on the fetus; and the teratogenic, perinatal, and neurobehavioral effects of individual psychotropic medications. A salient feature of most mental illness is impairment of function (DSM-IV [American Psychiatric Association 1994]), and intervention is clearly warranted if the impairment is sufficient to preclude a woman's participation in prenatal care or directly jeopardizes the pregnancy or the infant.

It is equally important for clinicians to obtain obstetrical histories, particularly of placental insufficiency, preeclampsia, and urinary or gastrointestinal difficulties. Potential drug interactions with analgesic and anesthetic medications also need to be considered. The clinician must be aware of such issues in the event that pharmacological intervention is warranted.

To date, the U.S. Food and Drug Administration (FDA) has not approved any psychotropic medication for use during pregnancy or lactation. The current classification system is presented in Table 47–1. One potential confounder of this system is that adverse case reports are more likely to have been filed for medications that have been available longer. The significance of these adverse case reports is difficult to evaluate.

The decision of whether to use psychotropic medica-

Table 47–1. U.S. Food and Drug Administration (FDA) use-in-pregnancy ratings

Category	Interpretation
A	**Controlled studies show no risk:** Adequate, well-controlled studies in pregnant women have failed to demonstrate risk to the fetus.
B	**No evidence of risk in humans:** Either animal findings show risk, but human findings do not; or, if no adequate human studies have been done, animal findings are negative.
C	**Risk cannot be ruled out:** Human studies are lacking, and animal studies are either positive for fetal risk or lacking as well. However, potential benefits may justify the potential risk.
D	**Positive evidence of risk:** Investigational or postmarketing data show risk to the fetus. Nevertheless, potential benefits may outweigh risks.
X	**Contraindicated in pregnancy:** Studies in animals or humans, or investigational or postmarketing reports, have shown fetal risk that clearly outweighs any possible benefit to the patient.

Source. Physicians' Desk Reference, 50th Edition. Montvale, NJ, Medical Economics, 1996.

tions during pregnancy and/or lactation not only is a difficult clinical judgment but also carries ethical and potentially legal ramifications regardless of what decision is made. It has been suggested that nonpharmacological interventions be used before psychotropic agents or electroconvulsive therapy (Cohen et al. 1989; Miller 1991). In the rapidly changing environment of health care reimbursement and managed health care, however, nonpharmacological options such as frequent psychotherapy sessions and inpatient hospitalizations may not be readily available.

Altshuler et al. (1996) determined the risk of psychotropic medication during pregnancy to fall into one of three categories: 1) somatic teratogenicity and organ malformation; 2) neonatal toxicity, including perinatal syndromes and withdrawal symptomatology; and 3) long-term neurobehavioral and developmental teratogenic effects. We address each of these issues in the discussions to follow as we describe the individual classes of psychotropic medications. It is important to note that little is known about how most psychotropic medications affect these three axes.

ANTIDEPRESSANTS

TCAs have been available in the United States since 1963, and their use has extended well beyond treating depression. The development of non-TCAs has further broadened the spectrum of the clinical utility of antidepressants as a class to include obsessive-compulsive disorder (clomipramine, fluvoxamine, paroxetine, sertraline, fluoxetine), panic disorder (imipramine, fluoxetine, paroxetine, sertraline), pain syndromes (amitriptyline, nortriptyline, doxepin, paroxetine, venlafaxine), bulimia (fluoxetine), and premenstrual syndromes (fluoxetine, nortriptyline, clomipramine). Whereas earlier studies (A. J. Rosenberg and Silver 1965; Sim 1963; Zajicek 1981) and clinical lore describe pregnancy as a time of psychiatric "well-being," investigations indicate that 9%–18% of women have symptoms that meet criteria for a mood disorder (both minor and major) during pregnancy (Kumar and Robson 1984; O'Hara et al. 1984, 1990; Watson et al. 1984).

Despite the widespread use of TCAs during pregnancy, no clear association with congenital malformations has been demonstrated (see Table 47–2 for information on individual medications). Earlier studies suggested an association between TCA exposure and various anomalies; the most commonly noted are those affecting the limbs (Barson 1972; Elia et al. 1987; McBride 1972). Altshuler et al. (1996) reviewed 14 studies, both prospective and retrospective in design, of in utero exposure to TCAs representing more than 300,000 total live births. Only 13 malformations were noted in 414 first-trimester exposures—an incidence of 3.14%. Similar rates were noted by McElhatton et al. (1996) in a review of data from the European Network of Teratology Information Services. This rate is within the normal baseline incidence of 2%–4%. A prospective study (Misri and Sivertz 1991) with a relatively small sample ($N = 18$) found no increased risk of fetal anomalies and no increase in complications during labor and delivery, although short-term withdrawal symptoms were noted in the neonates. In contrast, there have been reports of fetal tachycardia (Prentice and Brown 1989).

The issue of neonatal withdrawal is complicated by the lack of data about maternal dosing during labor. Symptoms reported include tachypnea, tachycardia, cyanosis, irritability, hypertonia, clonus, and spasm (Eggermont 1973; Miller 1991; Webster 1973). Wisner et al. (1993) reported that the TCA dosage for women with depression during pregnancy may need to be increased over the course of pregnancy to maintain adequate therapeutic serum concentrations and response. Unfortunately, although these researchers did not report any complications, they did not comment on the presence or absence of neonatal withdrawal phenomena.

Human data on the use of monoamine oxidase inhibitors (MAOIs) during pregnancy and lactation are limited. Although the MAOIs are all FDA category C medications, one prospective study in a small group of patients indicated that in utero tranylcypromine exposure is associated with fetal malformations. Studies in animals (Poulson and Robson 1964) have reported teratogenic effects associated with the MAOIs. The dietary constraints and potential for hypertensive crisis are relative contraindications to the use of MAOIs during pregnancy (Wisner and Perel 1988).

Data on the use of SSRIs during pregnancy are steadily accumulating. In one of the first investigations of first-trimester exposure to fluoxetine (mean dose 25.8 mg/day), no demonstrable increase in fetal anomalies was noted among 128 women (Pastuszak et al. 1993). The manufacturer's index currently lists more than 1,700 cases of first-trimester exposure to fluoxetine with no evidence of an increased incidence of congenital malformations or of a clustering of any particular anomaly (Eli Lilly, Inc., personal communication, January 1997). More recently, McElhatton et al. (1996) reported that of 92 women who received SSRI monotherapy during pregnancy, only two cases of infant major malformations were noted. The only study to date of known first-trimester exposure to paroxetine found no congenital malformations among 63 pregnancies (Inman et al. 1993). The postmarketing data

Table 47–2. Antidepressant medications

Generic name	Trade name	Daily dose (mg/day)[a]	Half-life (hours)[b]	Risk category[c]	American Academy of Pediatrics rating[d]
Tricyclic/heterocyclic antidepressants					
Amitriptyline	Elavil, Endep	150–300	10–22	D	Unknown, but of concern
Amoxapine	Asendin	150–400	8–20	C_m	Unknown, but of concern
Clomipramine	Anafranil	150–250	19–37	C_m	Unknown, but of concern[e]
Desipramine	Norpramin	150–300	12–76	C	Unknown, but of concern
Doxepin	Sinequan, Adapin	150–300	11–23	C	Unknown, but of concern
Imipramine	Tofranil	150–300	11–25	D	Unknown, but of concern
Nortriptyline	Pamelor, Aventyl	75–150	15–93	D	N/A
Maprotiline	Ludiomil	140–225	21–66	B_m	N/A
Protriptyline	Vivactil	15–60	54–198	C	N/A
Monoamine oxidase inhibitors					
Isocarboxazid	Marplan	30–60	N/A	C	N/A
Phenelzine	Nardil	45–90	N/A	C	N/A
Tranylcypromine	Parnate	30–60	N/A	C	N/A
Selective serotonin reuptake inhibitors					
Fluoxetine	Prozac	20–60	24–96	C	Unknown, but of concern
Fluvoxamine[f]	Luvox	50–300	17–22	C	Unknown, but of concern
Paroxetine[f]	Paxil	20–50	24	C	N/A
Sertraline	Zoloft	50–200	26	C	N/A
Other antidepressants					
Bupropion	Wellbutrin	150–450	8–24	B_m	N/A
Mirtazapine	Remeron	15–45	20–40	C	N/A
Nefazodone	Serzone	300–600	2–4	C	N/A
Trazodone	Desyrel	200–300	4–13	C_m	Unknown, but of concern
Venlafaxine[f]	Effexor	150–375	5–11	C_m	N/A

Note. N/A = not applicable.

[a]Dosing strategies adapted from Schatzberg and Cole 1991; Kaplan and Sadock 1993; and, for newer medications, the manufacturers' package inserts.

[b]Half-life of elimination is listed for parent compound.

[c]Risk category adapted from Briggs et al. 1994; "m" subscript is for data taken from the manufacturer's package insert.

[d]American Academy of Pediatrics 1994.

[e]Original committee report 1994 listed as "compatible," and a correction was later published.

[f]Not listed in Briggs et al. 1994. Risk category taken from Physicians' Desk Reference 1992, 1993, 1994, 1996.

on fluvoxamine from its use in Europe and the data from clinical trials with sertraline do not demonstrate teratogenic effects, but these data have not been published in peer-reviewed journals.

Obstetrical outcome is not confined to physical malformations. Pastuszak et al. (1993) noted that the rate of spontaneous abortion was higher among SSRI- and TCA-treated women than among control subjects (14.8%, 12.2%, and 7.8%, respectively). Two groups have found a slight increase in birth weight among neonates exposed to fluoxetine during pregnancy, but these differences did not achieve statistical significance (Chambers et al. 1993; Nulman et al. 1997). In one report, third-trimester fluoxetine exposure was associated with decreased birth weight and increased minor anomalies (Chambers et al. 1996). The numerous confounding factors present in this study, however, render definitive conclusions speculative at best.

In a landmark study, Nulman et al. (1997) conducted extensive neurodevelopmental assessment of children exposed in utero to antidepressant medications (TCA-treated subjects, $n = 80$; fluoxetine-treated subjects, $n = 55$; no exposure, $n = 84$). Children between ages 16 and 86 months were assessed with numerous study measures and diagnostic tools for factors such as global intelligence quotient (IQ), language development, temperament, mood, activity level, and behavior. The children whose mothers received antidepressants during pregnancy—either fluoxetine or a TCA—did not differ from the no-exposure control children on any measure of neurodevelopment. Furthermore, global IQ and language development scores were nearly identical among all groups. In conclusion, in utero exposure to fluoxetine or TCAs did not affect either neurodevelopment or behavior in preschool-aged children.

Perhaps the only criticism that can be leveled at the Nulman et al. (1997) study is that it did not assess neonatal exposure to breast milk as an important measure. To date, studies on drug excretion in breast milk have demonstrated that antidepressants are present in breast milk with a milk-to-serum ratio that is typically ≥1.0 (Buist et al. 1990). Wisner et al. (1996) reviewed the extant literature on the serum concentrations of antidepressants and their metabolites in nursing infants. They found that, although TCAs readily enter breast milk, most parent compounds and metabolites are undetectable in infant serum by 10 weeks, and there is no evidence of drug or metabolite accumulation in the neonate. The only exception to this was doxepin, which was present in concentrations of 3 ng/mL. Doxepin was also the only TCA to be associated with an adverse outcome (respiratory depression) during lactation in one study (Matheson et al. 1985). Those authors concluded that most TCAs (amitriptyline, nortriptyline, desipramine, clomipramine, and dothiepin) are safe for use during breast-feeding. The data on SSRIs were somewhat less benign. Analysis showed that some of the SSRIs may accumulate in nursing infants whose mothers are receiving these drugs. This seems to be particularly true of fluoxetine, which was found in one case to be disproportionately elevated in infant serum compared with the maternal dose (Lester et al. 1993). It is noteworthy that this may not have represented accumulation but rather a higher steady state because repeat infant serum measures have not been completed.

In contrast, two groups (C. S. Birnbaum, personal communication, August 1997; Kim et al. 1997) did not find evidence of accumulation of fluoxetine in breast-feeding infants. Only a single case report is available for fluvoxamine (Wright et al. 1991). Expanding experience with sertraline (Altshuler et al. 1995; DeVane 1992; Stowe et al. 1997b) has indicated predominantly undetectable concentrations in infant serum. The follow-up data on infants exposed during breast-feeding are sparse. Llewellyn et al. (1997) found no adverse effects on growth and milestone achievement in 12 infants exposed to sertraline. What is most remarkable about this literature is the small number of patients and infants that constitute the total number of studies.

The elapsed time between maternal dosing and infant feeding has been shown to affect the amount of antidepressant medication to which the nursling is exposed. Amitriptyline (Pittard and O'Neal 1986), desipramine (Stancer and Reed 1986), and trazodone (Verbeeck et al. 1986) appear to reach a peak in breast milk at 4–6 hours after an oral dose. A detailed study (Stowe et al. 1997b) of sertraline excretion into breast milk identified both a concentration gradient from "fore" milk to "hind" milk and a time course of excretion that paralleled the gastrointestinal absorptive phase. Peak concentrations occurred 7–10 hours after maternal dose, and by simply discarding one feeding (at 7–8 hours after the maternal dose), we determined that the total daily dose to which an infant would be exposed could be decreased by nearly 25%. The clinical utility of such calculations is obvious and substantial. The ability to estimate accurate levels of medication in breast milk would allow the development of individually tailored therapeutic regimens that maximize maternal care while minimizing infant exposure.

In summary, most earlier reviews recommend using the secondary amine TCAs (nortriptyline and desipramine) (Miller 1991; Wisner et al. 1996). In light of the increasing data on SSRIs and the lack of adverse reports, however, these recommendations are likely to be revised.

ANTIPSYCHOTICS

In contrast with other classes of psychotropic medications, antipsychotic agents have a considerably larger database that addresses concerns of neurobehavioral teratogenicity. Additionally, phenothiazines have been widely prescribed to treat pregnancy-associated emesis (typically at lower dose ranges), thereby aiding in separating the effects on pregnancy outcome of a concurrent neuropsychiatric diagnosis from the use of antipsychotic drugs. Chlorpromazine, haloperidol, and perphenazine have received the greatest scrutiny, and investigators have failed to find a significant association between the use of these drugs and major congenital malformations (Goldberg and DiMascio 1978; Hill and Stern 1979; Nurnberg and Prudic 1984). Commonly prescribed antipsychotic medications, as well as agents used to treat their side effects, are listed in Table 47–3.

In a study (Van Waes and Van de Velde 1969) of 100 women treated with haloperidol (mean dose 1.2 mg/day) for hyperemesis gravidarum, no differences in gestational duration, fetal viability, or birth weight were noted. In a large prospective study, Milkovich and Van den Berg (1976) followed up almost 20,000 women treated for emesis, mostly with phenothiazines. When maternal age, medication, and gestational age at exposure were controlled, the authors found no significant increase in severe anomalies or neonatal survival rates.

Similar results have been obtained in several retro-

Table 47–3. Antipsychotic medications

Generic name	Trade name	Daily dose (mg/day)[a]	Half-life (hours)[b]	Risk category[c]	American Academy of Pediatrics rating[d]
Chlorpromazine	Thorazine	200–800	8–35	C	Unknown, but of concern
Clozapine	Clozaril	100–800	4–66	B$_m$	N/A
Fluphenazine	Prolixin	5–10	14–24	C	N/A
Haloperidol	Haldol	5–10	12–36	C$_m$	Unknown, but of concern
Loxapine	Loxitane	20–80	4–12	C	N/A
Mesoridazine	Serentil	100–400	24–48	C	Unknown, but of concern
Molindone	Moban	20–80	24–36	C	N/A
Olanzapine	Zyprexa	5–20	21–54	C$_m$	N/A
Perphenazine	Trilafon	8–32	8–21	C	Unknown, but of concern
Pimozide[e]	Orap	1–10	50–70	C	N/A
Risperidone[e]	Risperdal	1–16	3–20	C	N/A
Thioridazine	Mellaril	200–600	9–30	C	N/A
Thiothixene	Navane	10–40	34	C	N/A
Trifluoperazine	Stelazine	10–40	18–30	C	N/A
Medications for antipsychotic side effects					
Amantadine	Symmetrel	100–400	15	C$_m$	N/A
Benztropine	Cogentin	0.5–6.0	10–12	C	N/A
Diphenhydramine	Benadryl	25–150	5–11	C	N/A
Propranolol	Inderal	20–120	3.5–4.5	C$_m$	Compatible
Trihexyphenidyl	Artane	2–15	10–12	C	N/A

Note. N/A = not applicable.
[a]Dosing strategies adapted from Schatzberg and Cole 1991; Kaplan and Sadock 1993; and, for newer medications, the manufacturers' package inserts.
[b]Half-life of elimination is listed for parent compounds.
[c]Risk category adapted from Briggs et al. 1994; "m" subscript is for data taken from the manufacturer's package insert.
[d]American Academy of Pediatrics 1994.
[e]Not listed in Briggs et al. 1994. Risk category taken from Physicians' Desk Reference 1992, 1993, 1994, 1996.

spective studies of women treated with trifluoperazine for repeated abortions and emesis (Moriarty and Nance 1963; Rawlings et al. 1963). In contrast, Rumeau-Rouquette et al. (1977) reported a significant association of major anomalies with prenatal exposure to phenothiazines with an aliphatic side chain but not with piperazine or piperidine class agents. Reanalysis of the data obtained by Milkovich and Van den Berg (1976) did find a significant risk of malformations associated with phenothiazine exposure in week 4 through 10 of gestation (Edlund and Craig 1976).

Beyond the potential teratogenic risks of these agents is the potential for other side effects of antipsychotic drugs, such as neuroleptic malignant syndrome (James 1988) and extrapyramidal side effects. The symptoms of extrapyramidal side effects in the neonate may include increased muscle tone and increased rooting and tendon reflexes that may persist for several months (Cleary 1977; Hill et al. 1966; O'Connor et al. 1981). In addition, in utero exposure to antipsychotics may produce neonatal jaundice (Scokel and Jones 1962) and intestinal obstruction (Falterman and Richardson 1980) postnatally.

Several studies in animals (Hoffeld et al. 1968; Ordy et al. 1966; Robertson et al. 1980) have shown that prenatal exposure to antipsychotic medications can cause persistent abnormalities in learning and memory; others (e.g., Dallemagne and Weiss 1982) have not observed such drug-induced alterations. Studies in humans have not detected significant differences in IQ scores at age 4 years among children exposed to antipsychotic drugs and control subjects (n = 52 [Kris 1965] and n = 151 [Slone et al. 1977]). However, these studies included women exposed to relatively low doses of phenothiazines (Kris 1965).

Antipsychotic drugs, like other psychotropics, are excreted into breast milk (see Buist et al. 1990 for a review). The most widely studied of these drugs is chlorpromazine: seven infants exposed to chlorpromazine did not have any developmental deficits at 16-month and 5-year follow-up evaluations (Kris and Carmichael 1957). The concentrations of several other antipsychotics in breast milk have been measured, including haloperidol (Stewart et al. 1980; Whalley et al. 1981), trifluoperazine and perphenazine (J. T. Wilson et al. 1980), and thioxanthenes (Matheson and Skjaeraasen 1988); the milk-to-serum ratio was consistently ≤1. J. T. Wilson et al. (1980) suggested that the physicochemical properties of perphenazine could cause it to become "trapped" in breast milk.

Various agents are available for the treatment of extrapyramidal side effects. In utero exposure to diphenhydramine has been the most widely reported. The Collaborative Perinatal Project found an association between first-trimester exposure to diphenhydramine and major and minor anomalies (see Miller 1991 and Wisner and Perel 1988 for reviews). One study in which 599 children with oral clefts were compared with 590 control subjects found a significantly higher rate of exposure to diphenhydramine in the children with oral clefts (Saxen 1974). Another group (Parkin 1974) described a possible neonatal withdrawal syndrome associated with diphenhydramine that included tremulousness and diarrhea. The cautious use of anticholinergic agents is warranted by case reports of intestinal obstruction after perinatal exposure to antipsychotic drugs and benztropine (Falterman and Richardson 1980), as well as the potential adverse effects on maternal gastrointestinal motility. Studies in animals have shown that amantadine is a known teratogen (Hirsch and Swartz 1980), but reports in humans are lacking.

In summary, antipsychotic medications have been widely used for more than three decades, and the paucity of data linking these agents to either congenital or neurobehavioral deficits suggests that the risk of these medications is minimal. However, as with all medications, their use should be avoided during the first trimester. Moreover, piperazine phenothiazines (e.g., trifluoperazine and perphenazine) may have less teratogenic potential (Rumeau-Rouquette et al. 1977).

ANXIOLYTICS

Benzodiazepines and antidepressants are the most commonly used drugs for the treatment of anxiety disorders, and benzodiazepines are the most widely prescribed psychotropic medications. A retrospective survey of Medicaid records (1980–1983) of 104,339 pregnant women found that at least 2% received one or more prescriptions for a benzodiazepine (Bergman et al. 1992). As a class, benzodiazepines readily traverse the placenta, and the presence of benzodiazepines in umbilical cord plasma demonstrates that these drugs accumulate in the fetus after prolonged administration (Mandelli et al. 1975; Shannon et al. 1972). We know that these medications are found in fetal brain, lungs, and heart (Mandelli et al. 1975). Mandelli et al. (1975) also found that the metabolism of diazepam in the fetus is slower than in the adult; the half-life of the parent compound is 31 hours in the fetus.

In contrast to concentrations of other benzodiazepines that have been studied, lorazepam concentrations were found to be lower in cord blood than in maternal serum but were excreted at a slower rate; detectable levels were excreted 8 days after delivery (Whitelaw et al. 1981).

Earlier studies reported an increased risk of oral clefts after in utero exposure to diazepam (Aarkog 1975; Saxen 1975; Saxen and Saxen 1974), but later studies failed to confirm this association (Entman and Vaughn 1984; L. Rosenberg et al. 1984; Shiono and Mills 1984). Altshuler et al. (1996) pooled data from several studies investigating the association of oral cleft with in utero exposure to benzodiazepines. They found that, although exposure does confer an increased risk of oral cleft, the absolute risk increased by only 0.01%, from 6 in 10,000 to 7 in 10,000.

Alprazolam, a triazolobenzodiazepine, is widely prescribed for a variety of anxiety states, including panic disorder. As of December 1991, the Upjohn voluntary reporting system database on exposure to alprazolam during pregnancy contained the following information: elective abortion, 15%; spontaneous abortion, 7%; and stillborn or neonatal death, 2%. These rates are comparable to those found in studies of non-medication-associated pregnancy outcome. Congenital anomalies occurred in fewer than 6% of infants who were exposed to alprazolam in utero. Table 47–4 lists benzodiazepine and nonbenzodiazepine anxiolytics and sedative-hypnotics used in the treatment of anxiety disorders and insomnia, respectively.

Long-term, longitudinal follow-up studies are urgently needed. One group described a "benzodiazepine exposure syndrome" that included growth retardation, dysmorphism, and both mental and psychomotor retardation in infants exposed in utero to benzodiazepines (Laegreid et al. 1987). The same group later reported predominantly neonatal sedation and withdrawal (Laegreid et al. 1989).

Table 47–4.   Anxiolytic medications

Generic name	Trade name	Daily dose (mg/day)[a]	Half-life (hours)[b]	Risk category[c]	American Academy of Pediatrics rating[d]
Benzodiazepines					
Alprazolam	Xanax	0.5–6.0	12	D$_m$	N/A
Chlordiazepoxide	Librium	15–100	>100	D	N/A
Clonazepam	Klonopin	0.5–10	34	C	N/A
Clorazepate	Tranxene	7.5–60	>100	D	N/A
Diazepam	Valium	2–60	>100	D	Unknown, but of concern
Halazepam[e]	Paxipam	60–160	>100	N/A	N/A
Lorazepam	Ativan	2–6	15	D$_m$	Unknown, but of concern
Oxazepam	Serax	30–120	8	D	N/A
Prazepam[e]	Centrax	20–60	>100	D	Unknown, but of concern
Benzodiazepines for insomnia					
Estazolam[e]	ProSom	1–2	1–2	X	N/A
Flurazepam	Dalmane	15–30	>100	X$_m$	N/A
Quazepam[e]	Doral	7.5–30	>100	X	Unknown, but of concern
Temazepam	Restoril	15–30	11	X$_m$	Unknown, but of concern
Triazolam	Halcion	0.125–0.25	2	X$_m$	N/A
Nonbenzodiazepine anxiolytics and hypnotics					
Buspirone[e]	BuSpar	20–30	2–3	B	N/A
Chloral hydrate	Noctec	500–1,500	4–8	C$_m$	Compatible
Zolpidem tartrate[e]	Ambien	5–10	2–3	C	N/A

Note.   N/A = not applicable.
[a]Dosing strategies adapted from Kaplan and Sadock 1993; and, for newer medications, the manufacturers' package inserts.
[b]Average half-life of elimination is listed for major metabolites.
[c]Risk category adapted from Briggs et al. 1994; "m" subscript is for data taken from the manufacturer's package insert.
[d]American Academy of Pediatrics 1994.
[e]Not listed in Briggs et al. 1994. Risk category taken from Physicians' Desk Reference 1992, 1993, 1994, 1996.

A second group failed to find an increased incidence of behavioral abnormalities at age 8 months, and no difference in IQ scores at age 4 years, for children exposed to chlordiazepoxide in utero (Hartz et al. 1975). Although the data on the teratogenetic effects of fetal exposure to benzodiazepines remain somewhat controversial, the presence of infant withdrawal syndromes has been described by several groups, and symptoms can persist for as long as 3 months (see Miller 1991 for a review).

Buist et al. (1990) concluded that benzodiazepines at relatively low doses present no contraindications to nursing. In contrast to other classes of psychotropic medications, benzodiazepines appear to have lower milk-to-maternal serum ratios. Wreitland (1987) found a ratio of 0.1:0.3 for oxazepam and estimated that the infant would be exposed to 1/1,000th of the maternal dose. The percentage of the maternal dose of lorazepam to which a nursing infant is exposed has been estimated to be 2.2% (Summerfield and Nielsen 1985).

In summary, benzodiazepines should not be abruptly withdrawn during pregnancy, and, if possible, these drugs should be tapered sufficiently before delivery to limit neonatal withdrawal. Evidence from umbilical cord sampling indicates that lorazepam may not cross the placenta to the same degree as other benzodiazepines. Lorazepam and oxazepam bypass hepatic metabolism and may therefore have less potential for accumulation in the neonate. Finally, as noted in the comprehensive review by Miller (1991), diazepam with sodium benzoate as a preservative may also present some potential difficulties. Clonazepam (FDA category C) appears to have minimal teratogenic risks (Sullivan and McElhatton 1977).

MOOD-STABILIZING MEDICATIONS

The management of bipolar disorder during pregnancy has received considerable attention. Unlike affective anxiety and formal thought disorders, the number of clinically efficacious medications for bipolar disorder is quite limited (Table 47–5).

Lithium carbonate remains the cornerstone of the available treatments for bipolar disorder. The Registry of Lithium Babies was established in 1969 for Danish women after case reports were made of congenital malformations after in utero exposure to lithium (Schou 1976; Schou and Amdisen 1973). Further registers were established in Canada and the United States, culminating in the International Register of Lithium Babies.

Initial studies suggested a marked increase in cardiovascular malformations, particularly Ebstein's anomaly (Nora et al. 1974; Weinstein and Goldfield 1975). However, as noted earlier in this chapter, Cohen et al. (1994) completed an extensive survey of the available information and found an increase in the relative risk ratio for cardiac malformations of 1.2–7.7 and an overall increase in the relative risk for congenital malformations of 1.5–3.0 for in utero lithium exposure. Altshuler et al. (1996) determined that the risk for Ebstein's anomaly after in utero lithium exposure rose from 1 in 20,000 to 1 in 1,000. In contrast to the results of studies in animals, a 5-year follow-up study failed to find any significant behavioral teratogenetic sequelae associated with lithium exposure antenatally (Schou 1976).

The outcome studies for lithium discontinuation and

Table 47–5. Mood-stabilizing medications

Generic name	Trade name	Daily dose (mg/day)[a]	Half-life (hours)[b]	Risk category[c]	American Academy of Pediatrics rating[d]
Carbamazepine	Tegretol	400–1,600	12–17	C_m	Compatible
Clonazepam	Klonopin	0.5–10	34	C	N/A
Gabapentin	Neurontin	900–1,800	5–7	C	N/A
Lamotrigine	Lamictal	300–500	25	C	N/A
Valproic acid	Depakote (divalproex sodium)	750–1,500	8–10	D	Compatible
Lithium carbonate	Eskalith, Lithobid, Lithonate	900–2,100	20	D	Contraindicated

Note. N/A = not applicable.
[a]Dosing strategies adapted from Kaplan and Sadock 1993; and, for newer medications, the manufacturers' package inserts.
[b]Average half-life of elimination is listed for parent compound.
[c]Risk category adapted from Briggs 1994; "m" subscript is for data taken from the manufacturer's package insert.
[d]American Academy of Pediatrics 1994.

relapse rates for patients with bipolar disorder (Suppes et al. 1991; Tohen et al. 1990) underscore the need to carefully assess the severity of illness, as outlined by Cohen et al. (1994). Briefly, it is recommended that women receive prepregnancy counseling and that those with a single episode should have medication tapered gradually and an attempt at lithium-free pregnancy or, if indicated, reinstitution of lithium after the first trimester. It is recommended that the clinician offer a fetal echocardiogram between week 16 and 18 of gestation for women who were treated with lithium during their first trimester of pregnancy.

The previously noted physiological alterations are of importance in the management of lithium therapy during pregnancy and parturition. The changes in glomerular filtration rate during parturition and the potential for dehydration at that time, along with the associated rapid changes in fluid status, warrant close monitoring of lithium levels at delivery. The neonate may be at risk for lithium toxicity at serum concentrations lower than maternal concentrations, and the clinician should avoid the use of nonsteroidal antiinflammatory drugs in both the mother and the infant during the early postpartum period. Symptoms of toxicity include flaccidity, lethargy, and poor suck reflexes that may persist for more than 7 days (Woody et al. 1971). Lithium can also produce reversible changes in thyroid function (Karlsson et al. 1975), cardiac arrhythmias (N. Wilson et al. 1983), hypoglycemia, and diabetes insipidus (Mizrahi et al. 1979).

Several anticonvulsants have also been shown to be effective in the treatment of bipolar disorder. These include carbamazepine, valproic acid, and perhaps clonazepam. The bulk of the literature on the teratogenic risk of these compounds is derived from studies on the treatment of epilepsy during pregnancy. As noted by Cohen et al. (1994), these agents have not yet been proven to provide comparable levels of prophylaxis for manic episodes.

In utero exposure to both carbamazepine and valproic acid increases the congenital malformation rate in infants of epileptic mothers (Jones et al. 1989; Lindhout and Schmidt 1986). Fetal serum concentrations of carbamazepine are approximately 50%–80% of the maternal concentrations (Nau et al. 1982). The risk for spina bifida associated with fetal exposure to carbamazepine is 1% (relative risk is about 13.7%) (Rosa 1991). Similarly, valproic acid is a known human teratogen and confers a 1%–2% risk of neural tube defects.

As noted by Janz (1982), almost all major and minor fetal malformations associated with mood-stabilizing medications have been reported for infants of epileptic mothers treated with anticonvulsants. Intrauterine growth retardation is one of the most commonly cited potential complications of in utero exposure to valproic acid (see Briggs et al. 1994 for a review). Gaily et al. (1988) compared the intelligence of 148 children of epileptic mothers (both treated and untreated) and 105 control subjects at age 5½ years; of the children of epileptic mothers, 4 were considered mentally deficient or of borderline intelligence, whereas none of the control children fulfilled those criteria. Such findings underscore the difficulty in assigning definitive neurobehavioral risk potential to psychotropic medications.

All of the commonly used mood-stabilizing medications except clonazepam appear to carry an increased risk of fetal malformations and a potentially deleterious effect on later cognitive development. Like other psychotropic medications, mood-stabilizing medications are present in breast milk. Nursing infants can achieve serum lithium concentrations that are 40%–50% of maternal levels (Kirksey and Groziak 1984; Schou and Amdisen 1973). Although no reports of toxic effects are associated with lithium and nursing, the potential for such toxicity warrants close observation of the infant's hydration status. In contrast, both carbamazepine and valproic acid appear in low concentrations in human milk, and both are considered compatible with breast-feeding (American Academy of Pediatrics 1994). The clinician may consider avoiding medications that increase the potential for liver toxicity, such as acetaminophen, in these infants.

In summary, the management of bipolar disorder during pregnancy requires careful assessment of the disorder and its severity. If possible, mood-stabilizing medications should be avoided during the first trimester. The guidelines suggested by Cohen et al. (1994) underscore the potentially favorable risk-benefit ratio of lithium use during pregnancy.

SUMMARY

There is a paucity of clinical data supporting the view that psychotropic medications are teratogenic; in contrast, preclinical studies in laboratory animals, in which high doses of these agents are typically used, reveal definite physical and neurobehavioral teratogenetic effects (Elia et al. 1987). Pregnant and nursing women are generally excluded in clinical studies of novel pharmacological agents, and routine postmarketing registries are not maintained by most pharmaceutical companies, thereby limiting the available data. It is doubtful that well-controlled studies will ever be conducted. Although some investigators have suggested that conducting such studies in pregnant and nursing women is unethical (Kerns 1986), it could be argued that failure to conduct such studies increases the overall risk to women and infants over time and may deprive some women of adequate treatment. Several characteristics (route of metabolism, protein binding affinity, lipid partitioning) warrant further study to determine whether these physicochemical features affect placental transfer and excretion into breast milk.

In the light of the higher prevalence of depressive and anxiety disorders in women than in men and the particularly high rates of these disorders during the childbearing years, it is likely that the clinician will be presented with complex issues of prescribing psychotropic medications during pregnancy and lactation. A thorough risk-benefit analysis should be completed for each woman presenting with concerns of psychiatric illness during pregnancy and lactation. This risk-benefit analysis should take into account factors such as maternal psychiatric history; potential deleterious effects of untreated illness on both the mother and the fetus; and what is known in regard to somatic, perinatal, and long-term neurobehavioral teratogenicity of the different classes of psychotropic medications. Tables 47–6 and 47–7 summarize the basic risk-benefit assessment that should be individualized based on the patient's history and treatment goals.

Included in the risk-benefit assessment is the need for infant monitoring. Although no guidelines have been established in this regard, the type and frequency of infant serum monitoring should be consistent with adult monitoring as a minimum and should be repeated with any adjustment in maternal daily dose.

In light of the lack of data demonstrating the superior clinical efficacy of a single medication within a given class, we offer the following general treatment recommendations. We assume that the clinician has already exhausted reasonable nonpharmacological interventions:

- *Informed consent*—It is not possible to provide a complete list of all the risks for any given psychotropic medication. It is important to discuss with the patient the risks of using or not using psychotropic medications and to document that other treatment options have been attempted or considered. It is equally important to document the risk of the untreated illness to both the mother and the infant.

- *Choice of medication*—The most important factor is treatment history. A novel agent should not be used during these periods if a history of positive response exists. Such a decision only increases the risk of exposure to a second medication and continued risk of the illness. In the absence of a treatment history, medications with the following characteristics should be sought:

Table 47–6. Risk-benefit assessment for pregnancy: summary of facts

Known

85% of all pregnancies result in live births.

7%–14% of deliveries are preterm.

2%–4% of live births result in infants with significant malformations, and up to 12% have minor anomalies.

>60% of all women take at least one prescription medication during pregnancy.

In the ideal pregnancy, as defined by the Centers for Disease Control and Prevention, maternal weight is ±15% of ideal body weight, and the mother was taking prenatal vitamins with folic acid for 6 weeks before conception.

Most women learn of pregnancy at 5–8 weeks' gestation and therefore may be past the window of risk for fetal anomalies associated with psychotropic medication.

Increasing data

Pregnancy is not protective against psychiatric illness.

Major depressive episodes occur with similar incidence during pregnancy as during nongravid periods.

Obsessive-compulsive disorder may have its onset or may worsen during pregnancy.

The incidence of psychotic disorders varies throughout pregnancy; there are limited data suggesting a need to decrease dosage of antipsychotic medications.

Panic disorder may improve during pregnancy for some women.

The teratogenic risk of psychotropic medications, if any, has been historically overestimated.

Increasing data on obstetrical outcome and follow-up of infants of mothers taking psychotropic medications are comparable in study sample sizes to data on most other prescription drugs.

Untreated maternal mental illness may adversely affect obstetrical outcome.

Unknown

The potential long-term effect of untreated maternal psychiatric illness during pregnancy on infant development is unknown.

The long-term neurobehavioral effects of in utero exposure to psychotropic medications are unknown, although initial studies have not reported adverse effects for several medications.

- *Greatest documentation of prior use*—Medications with some published data on relative safety. Being the first to use a particular medication in pregnancy or lactation is not recommended. Medications that have been available

Table 47–7. Risk-benefit assessment for lactation: summary of facts

Known: Postpartum

>60% of women plan to breast-feed during the puerperium.

5%–17% of all nursing women take a prescription medication during breast-feeding.

12%–20% of nursing women smoke cigarettes.

Breast-feeding is beneficial for the infant.

Breast-feeding is supported by all professional organizations as the ideal form of nutrition for the infant.

The postnatal period is a high-risk time for onset or relapse of psychiatric illness.

All psychotropic medications studied to date are excreted in breast milk.

Increasing data

Untreated maternal mental illness has an adverse effect on mother-infant attachment and later infant development.

The adverse effects of psychotropic agents on infants are limited to case reports.

The nursing infant's daily dose of psychotropic agents is less than the maternal daily dose.

Psychotropic medications are excreted into breast milk with a specific individual time course, allowing the minimization of infant exposure with continuation of breast-feeding.

Unknown

The long-term neurobehavioral effects of infant exposure to psychotropic medications through breast-feeding are unknown.

for a longer time have a larger database, although this usually consists predominantly of case reports, in pregnancy and lactation.

- ■ *Lower FDA risk category (B > C > D)*—The FDA is empirically conservative and has access to the most pre- and postmarketing data. Whereas this rating may be controversial for some medications, as evidenced by the recent reclassification of the SSRIs to category C in the absence of any new data, it is reasonable that medical-legal considerations would support this approach.

- ■ *Few or no metabolites*—Data from both pregnancy and lactation suggest that drug metabolites, which typically have longer elimination half-lives, may achieve higher steady states in both fetal circulation and infant serum. The issue of active versus inactive metabolites is unresolved with respect to teratogenic effects.

- ■ *Fewer side effects*—Medications with fewer hypotensive and anticholinergic side effects

are preferable. Additionally, the effect on seizure threshold and potential interaction with commonly used obstetrical anesthetic and analgesic agents should be minimized.

- ■ *Concordant data*—Medications with conflicting data should be avoided; a clinically comparable alternative should be used, if available. This recommendation should also reduce any potential legal liability.

- ■ *Dosage*—In contrast to previous recommendations (Cohen 1989; Stowe and Nemeroff 1995), the goal of treatment during pregnancy and lactation should be adequate treatment for syndrome resolution. Partial treatment only enhances the risk by exposing mother and infant to both illness and medications. The minimum effective dose should be maintained throughout treatment, and the clinician should remain mindful that often dosage requirements may be increased during pregnancy. Such increases do not increase fetal exposure beyond the initial treatment decision because the fetal circulation is exposed to maternal serum, not maternal dose. Adjustments may be indicated later in pregnancy as the volume of distribution changes. To minimize the potential for neonatal withdrawal and maternal toxicity after delivery, careful monitoring of side effects and serum concentrations may be indicated. Exposure of nursing infants can be minimized by adjusting the feeding and dose schedule and discarding the peak breast milk concentrations for several agents.

- ■ *Communication with the pediatrician*—It is highly recommended that the psychiatric clinician discuss the medication and potential interactions with the infant's pediatrician. The delay in hepatic maturity may affect the metabolism of psychotropic agents and potentially alter the serum levels of other medications prescribed for the infant.

REFERENCES

Aarkog D: Association between maternal intake of diazepam and oral clefts (letter). Lancet 2:921, 1975

Affonso DD, Mayberry LJ, Lovett S, et al: Pregnancy and postpartum depressive symptoms. Journal of Women's Health 2(2):157–164, 1993

Altshuler LL, Burt VK, McMullen M, et al: Breastfeeding and sertraline: a 24-hour analysis. J Clin Psychiatry 56:243–245, 1995

Altshuler LL, Cohen L, Szuba MP, et al: Pharmacologic management of psychiatric illness during pregnancy: dilemmas and guidelines. Am J Psychiatry 153:592–606, 1996

American Academy of Pediatrics, Committee on Drugs: The transfer of drugs and other chemicals into human breast milk. Pediatrics 93:137–150, 1994

American Psychiatric Association: Diagnostic and Statistical Manual of Mental Disorders, 4th Edition. Washington, DC, American Psychiatric Association, 1994

Atkinson HC, Begg EJ, Darlow BA: Drugs in human milk: clinical pharmacokinetic considerations. Clin Pharmacokinet 14:217–240, 1988

Avant K: Anxiety as a potential factor affecting maternal attachment. J Obstet Gynecol Neonatal Nurs 10:416–419, 1981

Barson AJ: Malformed infants. BMJ 2:45, 1972

Beck AT: Depression Inventory. Philadelphia, PA, Philadelphia Center for Cognitive Therapy, 1978

Bergman U, Rosa FW, Baum C, et al: Effects of exposure to benzodiazepine during fetal life. Lancet 340:694–696, 1992

Boobis AR, Lewis PJ: Pharmacokinetics in pregnancy, in Clinical Pharmacology in Obstetrics. Edited by Lewis P. Boston, MA, Wright-PSG, 1983, pp 6–54

Brazelton TB: Mother infant reciprocity, in Maternal Attachment and Mothering Disorders: A Roundtable. Edited by Klaus MH, Leger T, Trause MA. North Brunswick, NJ, Johnson and Johnson, 1975, pp 49–54

Briggs GG, Freeman RK, Yaffe SJ: Drugs in Pregnancy and Lactation, 4th Edition. Baltimore, MD, Williams & Wilkins, 1994

Buesching DP, Glasser ML, Frate DA: Progression of depression in the prenatal and postpartum periods. Women and Health 11:61–77, 1986

Buist A, Norman TR, Dennerstein L: Breastfeeding and the use of psychotropic medication: a review. J Affect Disord 19:197–206, 1990

Campbell SB, Cohn JF, Meyers T: Depression in first-time mothers: mother-infant interaction and depression chronicity. Dev Psychol 31:349–357, 1995

Chambers CD, Johnson KA, Jones KL: Pregnancy outcome in women exposed to fluoxetine. Reprod Toxicol 7:155–156, 1993

Chambers CD, Johnson KA, Dick LM, et al: Birth outcomes in pregnant women taking fluoxetine. N Engl J Med 335:1010–1015, 1996

Cleary MF: Fluphenazine decanoate during pregnancy. Am J Psychiatry 134:815–816, 1977

Cohen LS: Psychotropic drug use in pregnancy. Hosp Community Psychiatry 40:566–567, 1989

Cohen LS, Heller VL, Rosenbaum JF: Treatment guidelines for psychotropic drug use in pregnancy. Psychosomatics 30:25–33, 1989

Cohen LS, Friedman JM, Jefferson JW, et al: A reevaluation of risk of in utero exposures to lithium. JAMA 271:146–150, 1994

Cradon AJ: Maternal anxiety and neonatal wellbeing. J Psychosom Res 23:113–115, 1979

Cutrona CE: Causal attributions and perinatal depression. J Abnorm Psychol 92:161–172, 1983

Dallemagne G, Weiss B: Altered behavior of mice following postnatal treatment with haloperidol. Pharmacol Biochem Behav 16:761–767, 1982

DeVane CL: Pharmacokinetics of the selective serotonin reuptake inhibitors. J Clin Psychiatry 53 (suppl):13–20, 1992

Doering JC, Stewart RB: The extent and character of drug consumption during pregnancy. JAMA 239:843–846, 1978

Edlund MJ, Craig TJ: Antipsychotic drug use and birth defects: an epidemiologic reassessment. Compr Psychiatry 25:244–248, 1976

Eggermont E: Withdrawal symptoms in neonates associated with maternal imipramine therapy. Lancet 2:680, 1973

Elia J, Katz IR, Simpson GM: Teratogenicity of psychotherapeutic medications. Psychopharmacol Bull 23:531–586, 1987

Entman SS, Vaughn WK: Lack of relation of oral clefts to diazepam use in pregnancy. N Engl J Med 310:1121–1122, 1984

Falterman CG, Richardson CJ: Small left colon syndrome associated with maternal ingestion of psychotropic drugs. J Pediatr 97:308–310, 1980

Gaily E, Kantola-Sorsa E, Granstrom ML: Intelligence of children of epileptic mothers. J Pediatr 113:677–684, 1988

Goldberg HL, DiMascio A: Psychotropic drugs in pregnancy, in Psychopharmacology: A Generation of Progress. Edited by Lipton HL, DiMascio A, Killam KF. New York, Raven, 1978, pp 1047–1055

Hartz SC, Heinonen OP, Shapiro S, et al: Antenatal exposure to meprobamate and chlordiazepoxide in relation to malformations, mental development, and childhood mortality. N Engl J Med 292:726–728, 1975

Heinonen OP, Stone D, Shapiro S: Birth Defects and Drugs in Pregnancy. Littleton, MA, Publishing Sciences Group, 1977

Hill RM, Stern L: Drugs in pregnancy: effects on the fetus and newborn. Current Therapeutics 20:131–150, 1979

Hill RM, Desmond MM, Kay JL: Extrapyramidal dysfunction in an infant of a schizophrenic mother. J Pediatr 69:589–595, 1966

Hirsch MS, Swartz MN: Antiviral agents. N Engl J Med 302:903–907, 1980

Hoffeld DR, McNew J, Webster RL: Effect of tranquilizing drugs during pregnancy on activity of offspring. Nature 218:357–358, 1968

Inman W, Kubotu K, Pearce G: Prescription event monitoring of paroxetine. Prescription Event Monitoring Reports, 1–44, 1993

James ME: Neuroleptic malignant syndrome in pregnancy. Psychosomatics 29:112–119, 1988

Janz D: Antiepileptic drugs and pregnancy: altered utilization patterns and teratogenesis. Epilepsia 23 (suppl 1):S53–S63, 1982

Jones KL, Larco RV, Johnson KA, et al: Pattern of malformations in the children of women treated with carbamazepine during pregnancy. N Engl J Med 320:1661–1669, 1989

Kacew S: Adverse effects of drugs and chemicals in breast milk on the nursing infant. J Clin Pharmacol Ther 33:213–219, 1993

Kaplan HI, Sadock BJ: Pocket Handbook of Psychiatric Drug Treatment. Baltimore, MD, Williams & Wilkins, 1993

Karlsson K, Lindstedt G, Lundberg PA: Transplacental lithium poisoning: reversible inhibition of fetal thyroid (letter). Lancet 1:1295, 1975

Kauffman RE, Banner W Jr, Berline CM Jr: The transfer of drugs and other chemicals into human milk. Pediatrics 93:137–150, 1994

Kerns LL: Treatment of mental disorders in pregnancy: a review of psychotropic drug risks and benefits. J Nerv Ment Dis 174:652–659, 1986

Kiely M: Reproductive and Perinatal Epidemiology. Boca Raton, FL, CRC Press, 1991

Kim J, Misri S, Riggs KW, et al: Steroselective excretion of fluoxetine and norfluoxetine in breast milk and neonatal exposures. Paper presented at the 150th annual meeting of the American Psychiatric Association, San Diego, CA, May 17–22, 1997

Kirksey A, Groziak SM: Maternal drug use: evaluation of risks to breast-fed infants. World Rev Nutr Diet 43:60–79, 1984

Klein DF, Skrobala AM, Garfinkel RS: Preliminary look at the effects of pregnancy on panic disorder. Anxiety 1:227–232, 1994/1995

Kris EB: Children of mothers maintained on pharmacotherapy during pregnancy and postpartum. Current Therapeutic Research 7:785–789, 1965

Kris E, Carmichael D: Chlorpromazine maintenance therapy during pregnancy and confinement. Psychiatr Q 31:690–695, 1957

Kumar R, Robson KM: A prospective study of emotional disorders in childbearing women. Br J Psychiatry 144:35–47, 1984

Laegreid L, Olegard R, Wahlstrom J, et al: Abnormalities in children exposed to benzodiazepines in utero. Lancet 1:108–109, 1987

Laegreid L, Olegard R, Walstrom J, et al: Teratogenic effects of benzodiazepine use during pregnancy. J Pediatr 114:126–131, 1989

Lester BM, Cucca J, Andreozzi L, et al: Possible association between fluoxetine hydrochloride and colic in an infant. J Am Acad Child Adolesc Psychiatry 32:1253–1255, 1993

Lindhout D, Schmidt D: In utero exposure to valproate and neural tube defects. Lancet 1:329–333, 1986

Llewellyn AM, Stowe ZN, Nemeroff CB: Infant outcome after sertraline exposure. Paper presented at the 150th annual meeting of the American Psychiatric Association, San Diego, CA, May 17–22, 1997

Mandelli M, Morselli PL, Nordio S, et al: Placental transfer of diazepam and its disposition in the newborn. Clin Pharmacol Ther 17:564–572, 1975

Manley PC, McMahon RJ, Bradley CF, et al: Depressive attributional style and depression following childbirth. J Abnorm Psychol 91:245–254, 1982

Matheson I, Skjaeraasen J: Milk concentrations of flupenthixol, nortriptyline and zuclopenthixol and between breast differences in two patients. Eur J Clin Pharmacol 35:217–220, 1988

Matheson I, Pande H, Alertson AR: Respiratory depression caused by N-desmethyldoxepine in breast milk. Lancet 2(8464):1124, 1985

McBride WG: Limb deformities associated with iminodibenzyl hydrochloride, Med J Aust 1:175–178, 1972

McElhatton PR, Garbis HM, Elefant E, et al: The outcome of pregnancy in 689 women exposed to therapeutic doses of antidepressants: a collaborative study of the European Network of Teratology Information Services (ENTIS). Reprod Toxicol 10(4):285–294, 1996

McNeil TF, Kaij L, Malmquist-Larson A: Women with nonorganic psychosis: mental disturbance during pregnancy. Acta Psychiatr Scand 70:127–139, 1984a

McNeil TF, Kaij L, Malmquist-Larson A: Women with nonorganic psychosis: pregnancy's effect on mental health during pregnancy. Acta Psychiatr Scand 70:140–148, 1984b

Meaney MJ, Diorio L, Francis D, et al: Early environmental regulation of forebrain glucocorticoid receptor gene expression: implications for adrenocortical responses to stress. Dev Neurosci 18:49–72, 1996

Milkovich L, Van den Berg BJ: An evaluation of the teratogenicity of certain antinauseant drugs. Am J Obstet Gynecol 125:244–248, 1976

Miller LJ: Clinical strategies for the use of psychotropic drugs during pregnancy. Psychiatr Med 9:275–299, 1991

Miller LJ: Psychiatric medication during pregnancy: understanding and minimizing the risks. Psychiatr Ann 24(2):69–75, 1994

Misri S, Sivertz K: Tricyclic drugs in pregnancy and lactation: a preliminary report. Int J Psychiatry Med 21:157–171, 1991

Mizrahi EM, Hobbs JF, Goldsmith DI: Nephrogenic diabetes insipidus in transplacental lithium intoxication. J Pediatr 94:493–495, 1979

Moriarty AJ, Nance NR: Trifluoperazine and pregnancy. Can Med Assoc J 88:375–376, 1963

Murray L: The impact of postnatal depression on infant development. J Child Psychol Psychiatry 33:543–561, 1992

Nau H, Kuhnz W, Egger HJ, et al: Anticonvulsants during pregnancy and lactation: transplacental maternal and neonatal pharmacokinetics. Clin Pharmacokinet 7:508–543, 1982

Neziroglu FN, Anemone MA, Yaryura-Tobias JA: Onset of obsessive-compulsive disorder in pregnancy. Am J Psychiatry 149:947–950, 1992

Nora JJ, Nora AH, Toews WH: Lithium, Ebstein's anomaly, and other congenital heart defects. Lancet 2:594–595, 1974

Nulman I, Rovet J, Stewart DE, et al: Neurodevelopment of children exposed in utero to antidepressant drugs. N Engl J Med 336:258–262, 1997

Nurnberg HG, Prudic J: Guidelines for treatment of psychosis during pregnancy. Hosp Community Psychiatry 35:67–71, 1984

O'Connor MO, Johnson GH, James DI: Intrauterine effect of phenothiazines. Med J Aust 1:416–417, 1981

O'Hara MW, Rehm LP, Campbell SB: Predicting depressive symptomatology: cognitive-behavioral models and post-partum depression. J Abnorm Psychol 91:457–461, 1982

O'Hara MW, Neunaber DJ, Zekoski EM: Prospective study of postpartum depression: prevalence, course, and predictive factors. J Abnorm Psychol 93:158–171, 1984

O'Hara MW, Zekoski EM, Phillips LH, et al: Controlled prospective study of postpartum mood disorders: comparison of childbearing and non-childbearing women. J Abnorm Psychol 99:3–15, 1990

Ordy JM, Samorajski T, Collins RL: Prenatal chlorpromazine effects on liver survival and behavior of mice offspring. J Pharmacol Exp Ther 151:110–125, 1966

Parkin DE: Probable benadryl withdrawal manifestations in a newborn infant. J Pediatr 85:580, 1974

Pastuszak A, Schick-Boschetto B, Zuber C, et al: Pregnancy outcome following first trimester exposure to fluoxetine (Prozac). JAMA 269:2246–2248, 1993

Perkin R, Bland JM, Peacock JL, et al: The effect of anxiety and depression during pregnancy on obstetrical complications. J Obstet Gynecol 100:629–634, 1993

Pittard WB, O'Neal W: Amitriptyline excretion in human milk. J Clin Psychopharmacol 6:383–384, 1986

Poulson E, Robson JM: Effect of phenelzine and some related compounds in pregnancy. J Endocrinol 30:205–215, 1964

Prentice A, Brown R: Fetal tachyarrhythmia and maternal antidepressant treatment. BMJ 298:190, 1989

Raskin VD, Richman JA, Gaines C: Patterns of depressive symptoms in expectant and new parents. Am J Psychiatry 147:658–660, 1990

Rawlings WJ, Ferguson R, Maddison TG: Phenmetrazine and trifluoperazine. Med J Aust 1:370, 1963

Rayburn WF, Andresen BD: Principles of perinatal pharmacology, in Drug Therapy in Obstetrics and Gynecology. Edited by Rayburn WF, Zuspan F. Norwalk, CT, Appleton-Century-Crofts, 1982, pp 1–8

Riccardi VM: The Genetic Approach to Human Disease. New York, Oxford University Press, 1977

Rieder RO, Rosenthal D, Wender P, et al: The offspring of schizophrenics: fetal and neonatal deaths. Arch Gen Psychiatry 32:200–211, 1975

Robertson RT, Majka JA, Peter CP, et al: Effects of prenatal exposure to chlorpromazine on postnatal development and behavior of rats. Toxicol Appl Pharmacol 53:541–549, 1980

Robinson HE, Stewart DE, Flak E: The rational use of psychotropic drugs in pregnancy and postpartum. Can J Psychiatry 31:183–190, 1986

Rosa FW: Spina bifida in infants of women treated with carbamazepine during pregnancy. N Engl J Med 324:674–677, 1991

Rosenberg AJ, Silver E: Suicide, psychiatrists, and therapeutic abortion. California Medicine 102:407–411, 1965

Rosenberg L, Mitchell AA, Parsells JL, et al: Lack of relation of oral clefts to diazepam use during pregnancy. N Engl J Med 309:1281–1285, 1984

Rumeau-Rouquette C, Goujard J, Huel G: Possible teratogenic effect of phenothiazines in human beings. Teratology 15:57–64, 1977

Sadler TW (ed): Langman's Medical Embryology, 5th Edition. Baltimore, MD, Williams & Wilkins, 1985, pp 58–88

Saxen I: Cleft palate and maternal diphenhydramine intake. Lancet 1:407–408, 1974

Saxen I: Association between oral clefts and drugs taken during pregnancy. Int J Epidemiol 4:37–44, 1975

Saxen I, Saxen L: Association between maternal intake of diazepam and oral clefts (letter). Lancet 2:498, 1974

Schatzberg AF, Cole JO: Manual of Clinical Psychopharmacology. Washington, DC, American Psychiatric Press, 1991

Schou M: What happened later to the lithium babies?: follow-up study of children born without malformations. Acta Psychiatr Scand 54:193–197, 1976

Schou M, Amdisen A: Lithium and pregnancy, III: lithium ingestion by children breast-fed by women on lithium treatment. BMJ 2:138, 1973

Scokel PW, Jones WD: Infant jaundice after phenothiazine drugs for labor: an enigma. Obstet Gynecol 20:124–127, 1962

Shannon RW, Fraser GP, Aitken RG, et al: Diazepam in preeclamptic toxaemia with special reference to its effect on the newborn infant. Br J Clin Pract 26:271–275, 1972

Shiono PH, Mills JL: Oral clefts and diazepam use during pregnancy (letter). N Engl J Med 311:919–920, 1984

Sim M: Abortion and the psychiatrist. BMJ 5350:145–148, 1963

Slone D, Siskind V, Heinonen OP, et al: Antenatal exposure to the phenothiazines in relation to congenital malformations, perinatal mortality rate, birth weight, and intelligence quotient score. Am J Obstet Gynecol 128:468–486, 1977

Stancer HC, Reed KL: Desipramine and 2-hydroxydesipramine in human breast milk and the nursing infant's serum. Am J Psychiatry 143:12, 1597–1600, 1986

Steer RA, Scholl TO, Hediger ML, et al: Self-reported depression and negative pregnancy outcomes. Epidemiology 45:1093–1099, 1992

Stewart R, Karas B, Springer P: Haloperidol excretion in human milk. Am J Psychiatry 137:849–850, 1980

Stowe ZN, Nemeroff CB: Psychopharmacology during pregnancy and lactation, in The American Psychiatric Press Textbook of Psychopharmacology. Edited by Schatzberg AF, Nemeroff CB. Washington, DC, American Psychiatric Press, 1995, pp 823–837

Stowe ZN, Lllewellyn AM, Strader JR, et al: Placental passage of antidepressants. Paper presented at the 150th annual meeting of the American Psychiatric Association, San Diego, CA, May 17–22, 1997a

Stowe ZN, Owens M, Landry JC, et al: Sertraline and desmethylsertraline in human breast milk and nursing infants. Am J Psychiatry 154:1255–1260, 1997b

Sullivan FM, McElhatton PR: A comparison of the teratogenic activity of the antiepileptic drugs carbamazepine, clonazepam, ethosuximide, phenobarbital, phenytoin, and pyrimidone in mice. Toxicol Appl Pharmacol 40:365–378, 1977

Summerfield RJ, Nielsen MS: Excretion of lorazepam into breast milk. Br J Anaesth 57:1042–1043, 1985

Suppes T, Baldessarini RJ, Faedda GL, et al: Risk of recurrence following discontinuation of lithium treatment in bipolar disorder. Arch Gen Psychiatry 47:1082–1088, 1991

Teti DM, Messinger DS, Gelfand DM, et al: Maternal depression and the quality of early attachment: an examination of infants, preschoolers, and their mothers. Dev Psychol 31:364–376, 1995

Tohen M, Waternaux CM, Tsuang MT: Outcome in mania: a 4-year prospective follow-up of 75 patients utilizing survival analysis. Arch Gen Psychiatry 47:1106–1111, 1990

Van Waes A, Van de Velde EJ: Safety evaluation of haloperidol in the treatment of hyperemesis gravidarum. J Clin Pharmacol 9:224–227, 1969

Verbeeck RK, Ross SG, McKenna EA: Excretion of trazodone in breast milk. Br J Clin Pharmacol 22:367–370, 1986

Vorherr H: Drug excretion in breast milk. Postgrad Med 56:97–104, 1974

Warner A: Drug use in the neonate: inter-relationships of pharmacokinetics, toxicity and biochemical maturity. Clin Chem 32:721–727, 1986

Watson JP, Elliot SA, Rugg AJ, et al: Psychiatric disorder in pregnancy and the first postnatal year. Br J Psychiatry 147:453–462, 1984

Webster PAC: Withdrawal symptoms in neonates associated with maternal antidepressant therapy. Lancet 2:318–319, 1973

Weinstein MR, Goldfield MD: Cardiovascular malformations with lithium use during pregnancy. Am J Psychiatry 132:529–531, 1975

Welch R, Findlay J: Excretion of drugs in human breast milk. Drug Metab Rev 12:261–277, 1981

Whalley LJ, Blain PG, Prime JK: Haloperidol secreted in breast milk. BMJ 282:1746–1747, 1981

Whitelaw AGL, Cummings AJ, McFadyen IR: Effect of maternal lorazepam on the neonate. BMJ 282:1106–1108, 1981

Wilson JT, Brown RD, Cherek DR, et al: Drug excretion in human breast milk: principles, pharmacokinetics and projected consequences. Clin Pharmacokinet 5:1–66, 1980

Wilson N, Forfar JC, Godman MJ: Atrial flutter in the newborn resulting from maternal lithium ingestion. Arch Dis Child 58:538–549, 1983

Wisner KL, Perel JM: Psychopharmacologic agents and electroconvulsive therapy during pregnancy and the puerperium, in Psychiatric Consultation in Childbirth Settings: Parent- and Child-Oriented Approaches. Edited by Cohen RL. New York, Plenum, 1988, pp 165–206

Wisner KL, Perel JM, Wheeler SB: Tricyclic dosage requirements across pregnancy. Am J Psychiatry 150:1541–1542, 1993

Wisner KL, Perel JM, Findling RL: Antidepressant treatment during breast-feeding. Am J Psychiatry 153:1132–1137, 1996

Wood SM, Hytten FE: The fate of drugs in pregnancy. Clin Obstet Gynecol 8:255–259, 1981

Woody JN, London WL, Wilbanks GD: Lithium toxicity in a newborn. Pediatrics 47:94–96, 1971

Wreitland MA: Excretion of oxazepam in breastmilk. Eur J Clin Pharmacol 33:209–210, 1987

Wright S, Dawling S, Ashford JJ: Excretion of fluvoxamine in breast milk. Br J Clin Pharmacol 31:209, 1991

Yonkers KA, Kando JC, Cole JO: Gender differences in pharmacokinetics and pharmacodynamics of psychotropic medication. Am J Psychiatry 149:587–595, 1992

Zahn-Waxler C, Cummings EM, Ianoff RJ, et al: Young offspring of depressed patients: a population of risk for affective problems and childhood depression, in Childhood Depression. Edited by Cichetti D, Schneider-Rosen K. San Francisco, CA, Jossey-Bass, 1984, pp 81–105

Zajicek E: Psychiatric problems during pregnancy, in Pregnancy: A Psychological and Social Study. Edited by Wolkind S, Zajicek E. London, Academic Press, 1981, pp 57–73

FORTY-EIGHT

Treatment of Insomnia

Martin Reite, M.D.

Three things should be remembered when considering treatment of an insomnia complaint. First, insomnia is a symptom, not a disease. Second, it is important to perform a systematic differential diagnosis, keeping in mind the possibility that there will very likely be more than one cause of an insomnia complaint. And finally, most patients complaining of insomnia can be helped significantly.

The complaint of insomnia is essentially that sleep is difficult to initiate or maintain or is nonrestorative or not refreshing. There will usually be some associated daytime consequences as well, such as fatigue, sleepiness, or performance difficulties. Insomnia is among the most frequent of complaints. One recent Gallup poll found that nearly 40% of the general population complained of intermittent or chronic insomnia (Gallup Organization 1995). A telephone interview of 1,722 French-speaking Montrealers conducted in 1993 (Ohayon et al. 1997) also found that dissatisfaction with sleep was a common complaint, greater in women and in elderly and socially isolated persons. Although 17.8% of the population was dissatisfied with sleep, only 7% met DSM-IV (American Psychiatric Association 1994) criteria for insomnia disorder.

CONSEQUENCES OF SLEEP LOSS

Although insomnia usually is associated with a varying degree of sleep loss, the complaint is not identical to reduced sleep, and it is useful to consider as well the known effects of sleep loss or sleep restriction in normal sleepers as well as in those with insomnia.

Normal sleepers who undergo sleep loss, as well as po-

tentially normal sleepers who have medical or other conditions that lead to sleep loss and result in insomnia complaints, can experience significant consequences of that sleep loss. Sleep loss contributes to impairments in mood and in motor and cognitive performance (Pilcher and Huffcutt 1996; Singh et al. 1997), increases the likelihood of motor vehicle and other accidents (Leger 1994), and may contribute to impaired health.

Many individuals experience significant restriction of sleep as a consequence of job pressures and similar demands, and this restriction can have adverse consequences as well. Physician house staff members have been reported to fall asleep frequently while driving, seemingly as a direct result of sleep loss (Marcus and Loughlin 1996). A study of 80 long-distance truck drivers found that drivers obtained less sleep than required for alertness on the job; the greatest vulnerability to sleep or sleeplike states occurred in the late-night or early-morning hours (Mitler et al. 1997). A study of 102 European noncommercial vacation drivers compared with 50 control subjects found that 88% of drivers had experienced acute sleep deprivation within 1 day before their departure on vacation, and a two-nap Multiple Sleep Latency Test (MSLT; a test that quantifies the degree of sleepiness) found that the vacation drivers were significantly more sleepy than control subjects (Philip et al. 1997). A recent study demonstrated that healthy persons with no sleep complaints who remained awake for as long as 17 hours had performance impairment equivalent to that seen after ingestion of sufficient alcohol to raise blood alcohol concentration to 0.05%, which is the level for legal intoxication in many Western industrialized nations (Dawson and Reid 1997). This may help explain the increase in accidents and performance decrements associated with prolonged wakefulness. A recent study by Stoller (1994) estimated the direct and indirect costs of insomnia as between $92.5 billion and $107.5 billion per year.

Thus, insufficient sleep constitutes a significant public health problem, but clearly such a problem could be averted by preventing excessive sleep loss, and the sleepy individuals involved, because they are normal sleepers, would have no difficulty in making up lost sleep if given the opportunity. Patients with insomnia, on the other hand, would likely not recoup the lost sleep even given the opportunity.

Persistent sleep difficulties have been found to be predictive of future health problems as well. In a long-term follow-up study of 1,053 men questioned about insomnia while in medical school and evaluated for incidence of depression about 34 years later, self-reported insomnia and difficulty with sleeping were associated with a higher incidence of depression in later life (Chang et al. 1997). Epidemiological studies have suggested that a complaint of sleep problems might help predict as many as 47% of new cases of depression in the following year (Eaton et al. 1995).

Some sleep loss is voluntary. The National Commission on Sleep Disorders Research (1993) has suggested that many individuals in modern society voluntarily restrict sleep and as a consequence are more sleepy than were individuals in the past. In a study comparing answers about daytime fatigue from the Minnesota Multiphasic Personality Inventory (MMPI) scores of Midwestern adult populations in the 1930s and 1980s (Bliwise 1996), individuals in the 1980s were more likely to respond that they had greater daytime fatigue, a result that supports the notion of greater voluntary sleep restriction in recent times. Whether this voluntary restriction of sleep has any long-term adverse health consequences is unclear. But because mild voluntary sleep restriction in industrialized nations has been occurring in concert with an increase in life expectancy, such a relationship seems unlikely.

Although it is clear that normal sleepers (and potentially normal sleepers with insomnia complaints due to definable causes) deprived of sleep have performance decrements that are potentially dangerous, there appears to be a group of persons with chronic insomnia in whom the relationship between sleep loss and performance decrements is not as clear. Many individuals with chronic insomnia underestimate the amount of sleep they actually obtain (Edinger and Fins 1995), and in spite of obtaining less sleep on the whole than normal sleepers, those with chronic insomnia may not show similar objective evidence of excessive daytime sleepiness on the MSLT (Lichstein et al. 1994). It has been suggested that they may exhibit a state of general hyperarousal, which in some sense may serve to protect them from other consequences of reduced sleep (Bonnet and Arand 1995). Thus, researchers do not yet understand well the relationship between the effects of sleep restriction or sleep loss in otherwise normal or potentially normal sleepers and the effects of sleep restriction in individuals with certain chronic insomnia complaints.

THE INSOMNIA COMPLAINT

Insomnia can include difficulty in getting to sleep (sleep onset insomnia), difficulty staying asleep (sleep maintenance insomnia), or early-morning awakening (terminal insomnia). It does not appear that such subtypes are stable over time, however, and therefore, this method of subtyping may have little clinical utility (Hohagen et al. 1994a). As a rule, insomnia complaints are more frequent in women (Karacan and Williams 1983), elderly persons (Morin and Gramling 1989), and patients of lower socioeconomic status (Ford and Kamerow 1989).

Insomnia complaints are normally grouped into three types by duration of complaint. Transient insomnia lasts only a few days, short-term insomnia perhaps 2–3 weeks, and chronic insomnia from 3 weeks to many years.

Transient Insomnia

Transient insomnia is essentially ubiquitous and is caused by stressful events or experiences that are usually well defined and known to the subject. Anxiety about a forthcoming examination, job interview, or vacation departure, or even concern about having to get up early enough, are all common conditions that can result in a transient insomnia complaint. Physicians rarely see transient insomnias (although they experience them themselves), because these insomnias usually resolve with the event. Transient insomnia can be effectively managed with a short-half-life hypnotic agent, such as triazolam (0.125 mg) or zolpidem (5 mg) at bedtime for one or perhaps several nights. It is not unreasonable for individuals whose sleep is easily and predictably disrupted by stress to keep a hypnotic agent on hand for situations likely to disrupt sleep. The risk of using an occasional hypnotic agent appears to be outweighed by the performance decrements induced by one or more nights of poor sleep.

Several physiological causes of transient insomnia are sleep disruptions associated with high altitude, jet lag, and shift work. Travel from sea level to higher altitude, even that of several North American ski areas, can be associated with disruptions in sleep. Altitude-induced changes include frequent awakenings, periodic breathing with associated arousals (Reite et al. 1975), and, in more severe cases, related symptoms of acute mountain sickness. The periodic breathing per se can fragment sleep and produce an insomnia complaint; acute mountain sickness also includes insomnia as a component. The pathophysiology of acute mountain sickness is not well understood, but it may include disturbances of fluid balance associated with tissue hypoxia. Short-half-life hypnotics (e.g., zolpidem, 5 mg) can temporarily relieve high-altitude insomnia. Perhaps a better choice is acetazolamide (250 mg twice a day), which prevents or reduces symptoms of acute mountain sickness and improves sleep (Roberts 1994).

Two other transient insomnias, those associated with jet lag and work shift change, can be considered disturbances in circadian biology. Jet lag is a syndrome endured by travelers who traverse several time zones quickly, then try to sleep at a time when their circadian system would normally be in the wakeful state and try to remain awake when their circadian system is timed for sleep. The body temperature and serum cortisol rhythms are normally synchronized with sleep rhythm so that the low point (or *nadir*) of the body temperature rhythm occurs in the early morning hours, typically between 3:00 and 5:00 A.M., and the high point in the late afternoon or evening. We typically arise in the morning as body temperature is rising and fall asleep in the evening after body temperature has begun to fall. We normally fall asleep about 60 minutes after body temperature has begun its maximum rate of decline, and it has been suggested that a rapid decline in body temperature may serve as a signal to the brain that the individual is ready to sleep (Murphy and Campbell 1997).

Cortisol also reaches the low point in the midpoint of the night and begins to rise and reach its high point in the early morning about the time of arising. Body temperature and cortisol rhythms appear to have a common pacemaker, and when desynchronized from the sleep rhythm, as for example after an 8-hour time zone change, slowly return to synchronization, moving about 1 hour per day. The time when they are out of normal synchronization with the sleep rhythm is termed *internal desynchrony;* it can be associated with the typical symptoms of jet lag, including increased daytime sleepiness and insomnia during the new sleep time. How much of the jet lag syndrome is due to a state of circadian desynchrony and how much is due to sleep loss is still unclear. Preservation of sleep clearly diminishes the symptoms, however.

Shift work can also be associated with sleep complaints, for reasons similar to those encountered with jet lag. Individuals, for example, who move from day to night shifts are required to stay awake during the time they would previously have been sleeping and to try to sleep during the day when they would previously have been awake. A "shift workers' maladaptation syndrome" has been described; it includes impaired sleep, increases in gastrointestinal and cardiovascular complaints, excessive substance use, and social and family difficulties (Gordon et al. 1986). DSM-IV recognizes a circadian rhythm sleep disorder, shift work type (307.45).

Symptoms of both jet lag and work shift change can be effectively managed by appropriate use of bright light, as well as sedative-hypnotic agents, possibly including melatonin. Bright light is a potent synchronizer of the circadian system. Acting primarily at the retina, where it activates the pineal gland through a complex pathway, including the suprachiasmatic nucleus of the hypothalamus and the sympathetic nervous system, it modulates the synthesis and release of melatonin (Brzezinski 1997). Light exposure can either phase-advance or phase-delay the circadian system, depending on the time of exposure. It is most active near the nadir of the circadian temperature rhythm. Bright-light exposure prior to the temperature nadir can further phase-delay the system, whereas exposure shortly following the nadir can phase-advance the circadian system. An example of the human phase response curve to bright-light exposure is illustrated in Figure 48–1.

Appropriately timed bright-light exposure can also be useful for shift-work changes and for jet lag. Appropriate timing for light exposure to minimize jet lag should be based on knowledge of the phase response curve to light, considering the traveler's place of origin (Reite et al. 1997). Exposure should be timed to maximize phase shift in either an advanced or a delayed direction on the basis of the likely temperature nadir. An example of the use of light to minimize jet lag is provided in Figure 48–2.

The top panel of Figure 48–2 illustrates the use of light in travel from the eastern United States to Europe, for which a phase advance of the circadian system is desired. Typically, travelers depart the United States in the evening and arrive in Europe in the early morning (European time), which is the time when bright-light exposure will phase-delay the circadian system (not desired). Protection from light until about noon the first day will permit light exposure to phase-advance the circadian system in the desired direction. Subsequent days' light exposure can be advanced, further advancing the circadian system until it is entrained to the new time. The bottom panel of Figure 48–2 illustrates the use of natural light when it is desired to phase-delay the circadian system, as when traveling from the United States to Asia. On arrival in Asia, light exposure at midday will have little effect, but light exposure in the late afternoon will most likely be in the phase-advance portion of the temperature rhythm, promoting the desired phase advance (postnadir) of the circadian system. On

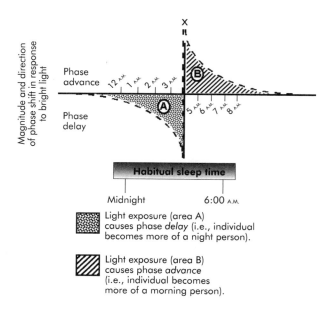

Figure 48–1. Type and magnitude of the response of the circadian rhythm to bright-light exposure.
Straight line represents time; period of habitual sleep is indicated at the bottom. Dashed line represents response of the circadian system to bright light, which is minimal during the midday hours. As the night progresses (and body temperature declines), light exposure progressively delays the circadian system. The effect is reversed at the time of the body temperature's lowest point (nadir); after this point, bright light causes an advancement of the circadian rhythm. The maximal response is found shortly before and shortly after the time of core body temperature minimum (x).

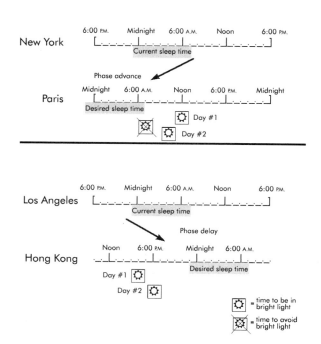

Figure 48–2. Examples of how to use bright light to reentrain the circadian system in west to east (phase advance) and east to west (phase delay) travel.

subsequent days, light exposure is encouraged later in the afternoon until entrainment is achieved.

Light exposure can also be manipulated to assist in adapting to shift work. Exposure to bright light (approximately 5,000 lux) during simulated night work for periods of 3–6 hours was experimentally shown to phase-shift the circadian temperature rhythm in the direction of circadian adaptation to the night work schedule (Eastman et al. 1995). Exposure to dim light (< 500 lux) had no such effect, and 6 hours of bright-light exposure were no better than 3 hours. Individuals with the greatest phase shifts also had more vigor, more sleep, and less mood disturbance, and overall they adapted better to night work. The timing of light exposure was thought to be important in inducing the reported phase shifts. Most subjects in the Eastman et al. study showed phase advance of temperature rhythms, possibly because the effective light exposure was maximum shortly after the time of the body temperature minimum, which is optimal sensitivity for phase advances. Manipulation of light exposure has been used successfully by

the National Aeronautics and Space Administration (NASA) on space shuttle missions (Eastman et al. 1995), but this process has yet to be widely adopted in other industries.

The use of temazepam (20 mg) to facilitate daytime sleep in individuals required to stay awake at night in a simulated shift work condition demonstrated that temazepam increased daytime sleep and improved both performance and ability to stay awake at night (Porcu et al. 1997). The chronic use of a benzodiazepine agent to preserve sleep in shift workers, however, probably cannot be generally recommended.

Melatonin has been found useful in the alleviation of jet lag (Arendt et al. 1986) and in improving accommodation to schedule changes in shift work (Dawson et al. 1995). Petrie et al. (1993) described melatonin administration as useful for reducing symptoms of jet lag in international cabin crews. Melatonin, or N-acetyl-5-methoxytryptamine, is synthesized from serotonin by two enzymes (arylalkylamine N-acetyltransferase and hydroxyindole-O-methyltransferase) that are largely confined to the pineal gland (Axelrod and Weissbach 1960; Coon et al. 1995). The hormone, secreted as light decreases, passively diffuses into the bloodstream, reaching maximum levels around 2:00–4:00 A.M. Normal young adults' average daytime and nighttime levels are about 10 and 60 pg/mL, respectively (Waldhauser and Dietzel 1985). Melatonin has not been approved for therapeutic use in humans by the U.S. Food and Drug Administration (FDA); thus, there is little control over type of manufacture, relative purity, or accuracy of dosage. There is relatively little information on optimal dosage, safety, and potential long-term side effects. Nonetheless, there is considerable interest in its putative hypnotic properties as well as in its ability to modulate the circadian system. It has been shown to have apparent time-dependent hypnotic properties (Tzischinsky and Lavie 1994), which are possibly due in part to its tendency to decrease body temperature (Hughes and Badia 1997). Melatonin may play a role in the treatment of certain insomnia disorders, especially those involving impaired regulation of the circadian system (Jan et al. 1994; Tomoda et al. 1994), although optimal dose and timing of administration are yet to be clarified.

Short-Term Insomnia

Short-term insomnia is usually caused by stressful events of greater severity or duration than those associated with transient insomnia. Significant job-related stress, job loss, major marital or family difficulties, bereavement, and major medical concerns or illnesses are all conditions prone to produce short-term insomnia complaints. Short-term insomnia can be effectively managed by hypnotic agents at bedtime for a week or two if necessary, or until the stress has subsided, although behavioral strategies such as attention to good sleep hygiene should also be invoked for these longer-lasting conditions. There is concern that if short-term insomnias do not resolve spontaneously, or are inadequately treated, they may lead, in susceptible individuals, to a more chronic insomnia complaint, such as a conditioned or psychophysiological insomnia.

Chronic Insomnias

Chronic insomnias last from many weeks to many years, and in these cases an accurate differential diagnosis is necessary for effective treatment. Although the stressful events leading to transient or short-term insomnias are usually apparent, this is most often not the case in the chronic insomnias, in which several diverse causations can lead to a similar symptom pattern. It is also the rule rather than the exception that a given chronic insomnia condition has more than one cause; thus, it is important to examine systematically all possible causes, recognizing that several may be present and require treatment. It is sometimes helpful to conceptualize a chronic insomnia complaint as

having two broad categories: 1) insomnia in potentially normal sleepers whose sleep is significantly disturbed by medical, psychiatric, circadian-rhythm, or other conditions that disrupt or limit sleep and therefore result in an insomnia complaint; and 2) psychophysiological or primary insomnia, representing a state of chronic physiological hyperarousal in susceptible individuals, thus leading to the insomnia complaints. These two broad categories may overlap, and they often cannot be clearly separated. The differentiation is further complicated by the fact that there are as of this time no objective physiological abnormalities specific to primary insomnia disorders.

There is increasing evidence, however, that there is in fact a true primary insomnia disorder. Patients with this putative disorder present with impaired sleep, as well as associated symptoms such as increased body temperature (Adam et al. 1986), heart rate (Monroe 1967), and possibly metabolic rate (Bonnet and Arand 1995). These symptoms all reflect a state of central nervous system (CNS) hyperarousal, in which case the insomnia complaint is likely one symptom of a more complex underlying disorder. Regestein et al. (1993) found 1) that patients with primary insomnia had increased amplitudes of auditory evoked potential components P_1N_1 that correlated with scores on a 26-item hyperarousal scale and 2) that they had greater electroencephalographic (EEG) activity across the frequency spectrum. Lamarche and Ogilvie (1997) found evidence that individuals with primary or psychophysiological insomnia evidenced high cortical arousal, based on EEG patterns during the sleep onset period, which may contribute to their difficulty in discriminating wakefulness from sleep. One would assume (although confirmatory data are not yet present) that a condition of chronic sleep deprivation, with associated symptoms of insufficient sleep, would be an additional complication of such a disorder.

In an effort to determine how experimentally induced hyperarousal compared with insomnia hyperarousal, Bonnet and Arand (1992) gave 400 mg of caffeine three times a day to a group of 12 normal volunteers, in whom a state of chronic hyperarousal was produced. The experimental subjects experienced increased anxiety, impaired sleep, and increased whole body metabolic rate, not dissimilar to that seen in chronic insomnia. These potentially normal sleepers had no trouble sleeping well after discontinuation of the medications, however, and experienced rapid resolution of symptoms.

These authors recently conducted another study (Bonnet and Arand 1996) to address the possibility that the disturbed sleep patterns of persons with insomnia were themselves responsible for other insomnia-related symptoms, as has often been speculated to be the case in chronic insomnia. In this study, a group of normal sleepers experimentally experienced for a 1-week period the same disturbed sleep patterns exhibited by a group of persons with chronic insomnia, and the effects of this exposure were quantified. The changes produced in the normally sleeping control subjects by the experience of yoked poor sleep for a period of a week were quite different from the symptoms and signs found in chronic insomnia. Many measures moved in directions opposite to those seen in subjects with chronic insomnia. Body temperature and metabolic rate were decreased, not increased, as were measures of tension and depression. Control subjects accurately estimated the time spent awake at night; persons with insomnia overestimated the time spent awake (which is characteristic of the patient with chronic insomnia; Edinger and Fins 1995). The symptoms produced in control subjects were more compatible with a state of mild sleep deprivation than were the symptoms in persons with chronic insomnia. And overall, the findings supported the thesis that the poor sleep experienced by patients with primary or psychophysiological insomnia is a symptom of another underlying disorder characterized by hyperarousal, perhaps not the primary disorder per se.

Evaluation of Insomnia Complaint

The first issue when presented with a patient complaining of insomnia is to ensure that a sleep problem is indeed present and that the patient is not simply a short sleeper. Sleep need is likely genetically determined to a significant degree, and it approximates a normal distribution; most individuals require about 7½–8 hours of sleep to feel rested the next day. There are, however, individuals on both ends of the distribution. Some short sleepers can seemingly get along fine on 4–5 hours of sleep, and some individuals habitually require 10 hours of sleep to feel rested the next day. Not infrequently, family members of a short sleeper think there must be something wrong with that individual because he or she is up and about while other family members are still sleeping, and they request that the person have a sleep evaluation.

In other situations, individuals who nap during the day may complain of not sleeping through the night. It is important to determine how many hours of sleep the person is getting. If, for example, he or she is napping 1½ hours in the afternoon, going to bed at 10:00 P.M., and awakening at 3:30 A.M., he or she is still getting a total of 7 hours of sleep, which might be all he or she requires. No physiological measure can predict a given individual's sleep need. We basically require sufficient sleep to feel rested and not excessively sleepy the next day.

Many patients do not inform their physicians of their sleep difficulty unless directly questioned. For this reason, it is worthwhile to include several brief questions about sleep during each new patient workup. In our experience, three routine questions will detect most significant sleep problems:

1. Are you content with your sleep? (This will identify most insomnia complaints.)
2. Are you excessively sleepy during the day? (This will identify most disorders of excessive sleepiness.)
3. Does your bed partner complain about your sleep? (This will identify most parasomnia disorders.)

A positive answer to any of these questions merits consideration of a more detailed sleep history to determine whether in fact a sleep disorder is likely present. Such a sleep history should include the following items:

- When did the symptoms begin?
- What has been their pattern since onset?
- Were there associated stress-related factors (e.g., job, school, family, health) at onset?
- What makes symptoms better or worse?
- What is a typical daily schedule (in detail—by the hour)?
- What treatments and medications have been tried to date, and how did they work?

Sources of diagnostic information should include the bed partner whenever possible, because many sleep-related symptoms are apparent only to the bed partner. A sleep diary can also be useful at this stage of the evaluation, because it can provide a detailed daily description of sleep/wake/activity patterns.

SLEEP LABORATORY STUDIES

Laboratory studies useful in diagnosing sleep disturbances include all-night sleep recordings (polysomnography, or PSG), which monitor multiple physiological variables during sleep, either in the sleep laboratory or at home, and the MSLT, which quantifies the degree of sleepiness.

The MSLT is usually performed the day after the PSG. The subject remains in the sleep laboratory and is asked to return to bed and try to go to sleep on four or five occasions (nap opportunities) at 2-hour intervals. Individuals with no sleep problems and who have obtained sufficient sleep the previous night will not go to sleep during these 20-

minute nap opportunities or will have mean sleep latencies (for all nap opportunities) of greater than 15 minutes. Individuals who are excessively sleepy will have much shorter mean sleep latencies, often ranging down to less than 5 minutes for persons with narcolepsy or severe sleep apnea.

PSG studies are used most often in the evaluation of complaints of excessive daytime sleepiness, especially when sleep apnea or narcolepsy is being considered. PSG studies are rarely needed in the evaluation of insomnia complaints. Two exceptions, periodic limb movements of sleep (PLMS) and central apnea, are described below.

DIFFERENTIAL DIAGNOSIS

Assuming that a true chronic insomnia condition is present, the next step is to conduct a thorough differential diagnostic evaluation, which includes systematically considering the conditions that are most likely to result in insomnia complaints. Common causes (not necessarily listed in order of frequency) that should be systematically considered in the evaluation of a chronic insomnia complaint include the following:

- Medical conditions or treatments of medical conditions
- Psychiatric disorders
- Circadian rhythm disorders presenting as insomnia
- PLMS
- Substance abuse disorders
- Central sleep apnea
- Primary or conditioned (psychophysiological) insomnia

I consider each cause in turn, but more than one cause may be present, and many if not most insomnia complaints will include a conditioned component that will likely require separate treatment. Most of these causes of insomnia (with the exception of PLMS and central apnea) do not require a PSG for diagnosis. A clinical assessment is usually adequate for establishing a diagnosis with a high degree of probability, at least to the extent that specific treatments can be tried.

Medical Conditions and Pharmacological Treatments of Medical Conditions

Medical conditions, or the pharmacological treatments of medical conditions, can result in insomnia complaints. The endocrinopathies are notorious for being associated with sleep-related complaints, as are conditions associated with chronic pain, breathing difficulties, cardiac ar-

rhythmias, arthritis, fibromyalgia, and chronic fatigue syndrome. Similarly, a number of medications frequently used for treatment of medical conditions can, in susceptible patients, result in insomnia as a side effect. A list of the more commonly used medications that can result in insomnia complaints is provided in Table 48–1.

No specific sleep abnormalities are associated with medical disorders, other than usually a decrease in total sleep, an increase in awakenings, and perhaps decreases in rapid eye movement (REM) sleep. On occasion, fibromyalgia is associated with an alpha-delta type of sleep abnormality, in which alpha frequency activity is accentuated in the slow-wave-sleep background, with a complaint of nonrestorative sleep. Chronic fatigue syndrome is frequently accompanied by sleep complaints, but such complaints can include insomnia, hypersomnia, nonrestorative sleep, and sleeping at the wrong time of the 24-hour period. No PSG-based sleep findings are specific to chronic fatigue syndrome as yet (Krupp et al. 1993).

The treatment of insomnia associated with medical conditions is first to isolate and appropriately treat the medical condition, and if the insomnia complaint persists, to evaluate the possibility of a separate additional sleep disorder. Conditioned insomnia can complicate insomnia complaints in this population, and it must be separately addressed (as outlined below). Similarly, it is quite possible for a patient with primary insomnia to also have a medical condition that further disrupts sleep.

Insomnia associated with acute medical conditions is appropriately treated with short-half-life hypnotic agents (e.g., zolpidem, 5–10 mg, or triazolam, 0.125–0.25 mg, at bedtime) if no other contraindication to their use exists.

Table 48–1. Common drugs with insomnia as a side effect

β-Blockers
Stimulating tricyclics
Corticosteroids
Stimulants
Adrenocorticotropic hormone
Thyroid hormones
Monoamine oxidase inhibitors
Oral contraceptives
Diphenylhydantoin
Antimetabolites
Calcium blockers
Some decongestants
α-Methyldopa
Thiazides
Bronchodilators

Zolpidem might be safer for patients with compromised pulmonary function because it does not appear to significantly depress the respiratory system (Murciano et al. 1993). Insomnia complaints associated with fibromyalgia and chronic fatigue syndrome are frequently resistant to treatment, although small doses of amitriptyline (10–50 mg at bedtime) or cyclobenzaprine (10 mg three times a day) have been reported to be helpful, and occasionally zolpidem (5–10 mg) will help with the associated insomnia complaints.

Psychiatric Disorders

Psychiatric disorders, especially disorders associated with anxiety or depression, frequently include insomnia as an associated symptom. Chronic anxiety is not infrequently associated with sleep onset insomnia or sleep maintenance insomnia, whereas depression is not infrequently associated with early-morning awakening. These associations are not specific enough to be diagnostic, however, and a

systematic psychiatric evaluation is necessary. Many depressive disorders appear to be accompanied by shortened REM latency, increased REM density during the first REM period of the night, and deficient slow-wave sleep. To date, however, such findings are not sufficiently specific to merit the cost of a PSG.

Antidepressant agents, although effective for the patient's depression, may have significantly different effects on sleep—a possibility that is useful to bear in mind. Table 48–2 shows sleep-related effects of the major antidepressant groups.

The choice of an antidepressant agent for a specific patient, all other things being equal, might well take into account the type of accompanying sleep complaint and the therapeutic effect on sleep desired. Typically, resolution of the depression will be accompanied by reduction in the sleep complaints. If, for a patient already complaining of insomnia, an antidepressant with a known high incidence of insomnia side effects is chosen, it may be useful to augment it with a hypnotic agent early in the course of treat-

Table 48–2. Overview of effects of antidepressant therapies on sleep

| Drug | EEG sleep effects | | | Sedation |
	Continuity	SWS	REM	
Tricyclics				
Amitriptyline	↑↑↑	↑	↓↓↓	++++
Doxepin	↑↑↑	↑↑	↓↓	++++
Imipramine	↔↑	↑	↓↓	++
Nortriptyline	↑	↑	↓↓	++
Desipramine	↔	↑	↓↓	+
Clomipramine	↑↔	↑	↓↓↓↓	±
MAOIs				
Phenelzine	↓	↔	↓↓↓↓	↔
Tranylcypromine	↓↓	↔	↓↓↓↓	↔
SSRIs				
Fluoxetine	↓	↔↓	↔↓	±
Paroxetine	↓↓	↔↓	↓↓	ND
Sertraline	↔	↔	↓↓	↔
Other antidepressants				
Bupropion	↓	↔	↑	↔
Venlafaxine	↓	↔	↓↓	++
SRMs				
Trazodone	↑↑↑	↔	↓	++++
Nefazodone	↑	↔	↑	↔

Note. ↑ = increased; ↓ = decreased; ↔ = no change; + = slight effect; ++ = small effect; +++ = moderate effect; ++++ = great effect; ± = no significant effect. EEG = electroencephalogram; SWS = slow-wave sleep; REM = rapid eye movement; MAOI = monoamine oxidase inhibitor; SSRI = selective serotonin reuptake inhibitor; ND = no data available; SRM = serotonin receptor modulator.
Source. Adapted from Winokur A, Reynolds C: "Overview of Effects of Antidepressant Therapies on Sleep," *Primary Psychiatry* 1:22–27, 1994. Used with permission of MBL Communications. Copyright 1994. All rights reserved.

ment. On the other hand, in a recent study (Satterlee and Faries 1995) of 89 outpatients with major depression treated with fluoxetine, an SSRI with insomnia as a relatively frequent side effect, fluoxetine did not exacerbate the sleep disturbance, and both depression and symptoms of the sleep disturbance improved compared with placebo.

For patients with seasonal affective disorder (SAD), a disturbance in circadian rhythm control may underlie their symptoms. A study of 20 patients with SAD demonstrated evidence of a significant phase delay and relatively poor entrainment of the circadian system (Teicher et al. 1997). Such findings may explain the utility of bright-light treatment to reentrain the system and provide symptom relief. As further evidence accumulates that disturbances in the regulation of circadian rhythms are implicated in the regulation of affective and mood states, additional therapeutic strategies emphasizing circadian regulation and entrainment in the treatment of mood disorders will likely emerge.

Treatment of insomnia associated with anxiety can incorporate a benzodiazepine with sedative-hypnotic properties with a sufficient bedtime dose to augment sleep. Many antianxiety agents, such as sedative tricyclics, have sedative-hypnotic properties as well, which facilitates the management of the insomnia component. Panic attacks can occasionally arise exclusively from sleep (Rosenfeld and Furman 1994); treatment in such cases should probably follow conventional panic attack treatment strategies.

Bipolar disorder may be accompanied by prominent sleep disruption. Manic and hypomanic episodes may be accompanied by marked decreases in sleep, although not necessarily insomnia complaints. Sedative antidepressants have been shown to increase the risk of a shift to mania in treating insomnia complaints in bipolar depressed patients (Saiz-Ruiz et al. 1994), and the use of other hypnotic agents would therefore be more advisable in these patients. Milder cyclic mood disorders may also have associated insomnia complaints, which can be mistaken for a psychophysiological insomnia or conditioned arousal insofar as the patients find it difficult to turn off their thinking at sleep onset or after awakening during the night. If these patients are questioned carefully, evidence of a cyclic mood component will suggest that treatment with a mood stabilizer might be appropriate for the chronic insomnia complaint in these patients.

Posttraumatic stress disorder (PTSD) is a psychiatric disorder in which sleep disturbances are a hallmark. Patients with PTSD have increased sleep latency, decreased sleep efficiency, recurrent traumatic dreams, and evidence of increased REM density (Mellman et al. 1997), as well as evidence of impaired skeletal muscle inhibition during REM sleep (Ross et al. 1994). The treatment of disordered sleep accompanying PTSD is usually not separated from the treatment of the entire PTSD syndrome, but many medications used for PTSD have been described as helpful for the sleep complaints that accompany PTSD. These medications include tricyclic and monoamine oxidase inhibitor (MAOI) antidepressants, the presynaptic α-adrenergic agonist clonidine and the β-receptor agonist propranolol, mood stabilizers lithium and carbamazepine, as well as benzodiazepines (Silver et al. 1990).

Circadian Rhythm Disorders

Circadian rhythm disorders usually present as sleep complaints. The most common is the *delayed sleep phase syndrome (DSPS)*, which presents as sleep onset insomnia. Typically, individuals with DSPS cannot get to sleep until 3:00–4:00 A.M. If they can then sleep until 10:00 A.M. or noon the next day, they can do fine, indicating that they have no trouble initiating or maintaining sleep, but if they are required to arise early to get to school or work, they complain of insomnia, and they are of course sleep deprived. They typically sleep in on weekends to recoup lost sleep. They often have already tried hypnotics, which are generally ineffective other than in inducing drowsiness, and their complaints are usually long standing. DSPS typically appears in adolescence or early adulthood, and it is frequently familial. Often first-degree relatives have a history of similar sleep patterns. In DSPS patients, evidence indicates that temperature rhythms and sleep rhythms are delayed and that possibly sleep persists for a longer time following the body temperature low point, suggesting that these patients may continue to sleep through the period when bright light would be most effective in phase-advancing their circadian system (Ozaki et al. 1988). The incidence of DSPS in the population is not known, but it may constitute as much as 10% of insomnia patients presenting to sleep disorders clinics (Weitzman et al. 1981). About 50% of these cases presenting to sleep disorders clinics (presumably the more severe cases) respond favorably to treatment (Regestein and Monk 1995).

Other forms of circadian rhythm disorders presenting as sleep complaints include advanced sleep phase syndrome and non-24-hour sleep-wake syndrome, also known as hypernychthemeral syndrome (Richardson and Malin 1996). Advanced sleep phase syndrome is accompanied by retiring very early in the evening and correspondingly arising very early in the morning, a schedule that sometimes mimics that of terminal insomnia. Patients with the hypernychthemeral syndrome experience a failure of the circadian clock to entrain normally to the 24-

hour day, and they sometimes experience a free-running 25-hour rhythm. This disorder is especially prevalent in blind persons, for whom light is unable to synchronize the circadian system. Some blind persons, however, are sensitive to light as an entrainer of the circadian system, so long as the retina and retinohypothalamic tract are normally functioning.

Treatment of circadian rhythm–based sleep disorders now most often includes both bright light and melatonin. Early-morning bright-light exposure, with restriction of light exposure in the evening, has been found to be effective for phase-advancing the circadian system in DSPS (Regestein and Pavlova 1995 [review]; Rosenthal et al. 1990). Evening bright-light treatment has been found to be effective in phase-delaying the circadian system and effectively treating advanced sleep phase syndrome. Bright light is usually ineffective in treating non-24-hour sleep-wake rhythms.

Melatonin has also been used successfully in the treatment of DSPS (Dahlitz et al. 1991; Lamberg 1996), and a case report indicated its successful use in entraining the circadian system in a blind retarded child who was unresponsive to bright light (Lapierre and Dumont 1995). Methylcobalamin (vitamin B_{12}) has also been reported to treat DSPS successfully, but well-controlled studies of its effectiveness have yet to be reported (Ohta et al. 1991; Yamadera et al. 1996).

Periodic Limb Movements of Sleep and Restless Legs Syndrome

PLMS and the related *restless legs syndrome (RLS)* are not infrequent causes of chronic insomnia complaints. PLMS can be transmitted as an autosomal dominant trait with onset in the second decade, and both PLMS and RLS can accompany a variety of medical illnesses, including peripheral neuropathies, anemia, uremia, and chronic pulmonary disease (Reite et al. 1997). The pathophysiology of the disorders remains unclear. PLMS, with dorsiflexion of the foot and toe, resembles a Babinski response, suggesting a lower motor neuron release phenomenon (Wechsler et al. 1986). RLS is not a true sleep disorder in that the uncomfortable sensations in the lower legs occur during wakefulness and that persons are aware of them. If RLS interferes with ability to sleep, however, it is perceived as an insomnia-like complaint. RLS is a common complaint, increasing in frequency with age and found in up to 23% of individuals older than 60 years (Montplaisir et al. 1997).

The involuntary limb movements, or leg (and occasionally arm) twitches or jerks, constituting PLMS are usu-

ally not recognized by the patient, because they occur during sleep. They may first be recognized as a problem by the bed partner, who complains of the patient's repeated bouts of kicking during the night. Patients who sleep alone may kick their bedcovers onto the floor during the night. PSG is required for accurate diagnosis of a PLMS disorder, quantifying both number of events and their association with awakenings or arousals. The isolated findings of PLMS (without associated arousals) during a sleep recording may have no clinical significance, but if occurrences of PLMS produce numerous short arousals during the night and so fragment sleep, they will likely be experienced as an insomnia complaint. Both RLS and PLMS have been associated with a variety of medical conditions, but they may occur in otherwise healthy individuals. They often but not always occur together, and, although most common in older individuals, they can have their onset in childhood.

Dopamine agonists such as carbidopa/levodopa and pergolide have been shown to be effective treatments in a large percentage of patients with RLS and PLMS. In general, patients with severe RLS have responded best to pergolide, whereas patients with PLMS but only mild to moderate RLS respond best to carbidopa/levodopa (Earley and Allen 1996). Alternative treatments have included opioid agents and benzodiazepines (Silber 1997; Trenkwalder et al. 1996). A recent study compared cognitive-behavior therapy (CBT) with clonazepam in the treatment of insomnia due to PLMS. Both treatments produced approximately equal subjective improvement. Patients treated with CBT showed decreased daytime napping; those treated with clonazepam showed increases in napping but greater decreases in polysomnographically determined PLMS arousals compared with those treated with CBT (Edinger et al. 1996).

Substance Use Sleep Disorders

Substance use sleep disorders are disorders of sleep that include insomnia as a prominent component and that are associated with use or abuse of psychoactive substances, including nicotine (Phillips and Danner 1995). Now relatively infrequent, abuse of barbiturate hypnotic agents was formerly a frequent cause of chronic insomnia complaints. Alcohol remains a significant problem, as do stimulants and other drugs of abuse. Alcohol-dependent sleep disorder occurs in those who habitually "self-medicate" with alcohol to induce sleep. Alcohol does tend to decrease sleep latency and wakefulness during the first 3–4 hours of sleep. It also suppresses REM sleep and leads to REM rebound (with the possibility of vivid dreams or nightmares) with fragmented sleep the latter part of the night. Treatment includes withdrawal of alcohol, with long-term abstinence as the goal. When necessary, sedation can be provided by judicious use of antihistamines (e.g., diphenhydramine, 25–50 mg, or cyproheptadine, 4–24 mg).

Chronic use of stimulants leads to prolonged sleeplessness, and their withdrawal is followed by a period of hypersomnolence. A chronic insomnia complaint is often seen in long-term stimulant abusers even when they are not actively abusing the agents. Treatment is similar to that of alcohol-induced sleep disorder. Antikindling agents such as carbamazepine (100–600 mg/day) or divalproex (250–1,500 mg/day) may help when CNS hyperarousal/kindling is evident, as is sometimes seen in postcocaine panic disorder in polysubstance abusers.

Habituation to benzodiazepine agents does not usually result in insomnia unless they are too rapidly withdrawn, in which case the withdrawal syndrome may include insomnia. Doses should be tapered by one therapeutic dose per week.

In all cases of substance abuse sleep disorders, the insomnia complaint should emphasize behavioral treatment strategies to the fullest extent possible, because psychoactive agents have already proved to be a problem. A more detailed account of the treatment of substance abuse sleep disorders can be found in Chapter 3 of Reite et al. (1997).

Central Sleep Apnea

Central sleep apnea is a relatively rare cause of chronic insomnia and requires PSG for accurate diagnosis. This disorder can be missed because the typical presentation of sleep apnea (excessive daytime sleepiness, sonorous snoring, recent weight gain, hypertension) is not present. The patient may not be aware of the pauses in breathing and the arousals associated with resumption of breathing, although the bed partner will often be aware of the frequent breathing pauses. The frequent apneas cause sleep fragmentation, which results in insomnia complaints and often complaints of increased daytime sleepiness (Bonnet and Arand 1996). Central sleep apnea is frequently associated with medical and neurological disorders (Thalhofer and Dorow 1997), but it may also occur in otherwise healthy individuals. It is more frequently encountered in older individuals (Ancoli-Israel 1997). Both oxygen and continuous positive airway pressure (CPAP) can be used in the treatment of central apnea in patients with medical disorders (Franklin et al. 1997; Granton et al. 1996). The pharmacological treatment of central sleep apnea is less than optimal. Therapeutic options might include protriptyline (5–20 mg at bedtime), fluoxetine (10–20 mg/day),

or theophylline (300–600 mg/day) (Ancoli-Israel 1997), although their efficacy has yet to be clearly established in well-controlled studies. Acetazolamide (250 mg twice a day) may be effective for high altitude–induced central apnea.

Primary Insomnia

Although there are several more rare causes of a chronic insomnia complaint, most often it is generally safe to assume that once the above specific causes have been systematically excluded, we are in all probability left with a possible primary insomnia diagnosis (DSM-IV 307.42). The nomenclature for this group is not clear, because specific pathophysiological mechanisms have yet to be identified. Whereas many individuals in these categories may experience a state of learned or conditioned arousal, there is likely another group of individuals with primary insomnia related to a state of chronic physiological hyperarousal of uncertain etiology, as outlined previously. The foregoing categories are often grouped under the term *psychophysiological insomnia*. These categories also include a group of individuals who complain of insomnia but who, when studied in the sleep laboratory, demonstrate normal sleep. This is termed the *sleep state misperception syndrome*.

Conditioned arousal (a term still sometimes used interchangeably with *psychophysiological insomnia*) characteristically begins when a susceptible individual experiences a stress-related transient insomnia and, after several nights of poor sleep, begins to fear going to bed because of concern that sleep will once again be difficult to initiate or maintain. This fear is associated with increased arousal, and soon a vicious circle is established in which merely going into the bedroom to prepare for sleep results in a conditioned arousal response sufficient to interfere with sleep. The conditioned arousal can persist long after the stress that caused the initial transient insomnia has resolved. Often, the conditioned arousal is limited to the individual's own bedroom and is not transferred to other sleeping locations. Such patients may be able to sleep on the living room couch, for example, and they may not necessarily have difficulty in napping during the day or sleeping well while on vacation in a new environment. They may also sleep normally if studied polysomnographically in the sleep laboratory, which is a new sleep environment in which they may not experience conditioned arousal. Thus, a normal PSG result does not mean that the patient does not experience insomnia in his or her usual sleep environment. Conditioned insomnia appears to occur most often in individuals who have a history of *fragile sleep*, in which stressful events have been prone to interfere with their sleep.

Normal sleep on PSG also raises the question of a possible sleep state misperception syndrome. Patients with conditioned arousal insomnia who sleep normally in the laboratory, however, often comment that the laboratory sleep was an unusually good night of sleep, and they are able to differentiate it from their usual nighttime insomnia. Patients with sleep state misperception syndrome, on the other hand, still complain that the night spent in the sleep laboratory was illustrative of their usual poor sleep, even though the laboratory sleep may have been objectively normal. Bonnet and Arand (1997) described evidence of increased metabolism in subjects with sleep state misperception syndrome and have raised the possibility that this syndrome may represent either a milder version of or a natural precursor to a primary insomnia disorder.

There is no clear, agreed-on demarcation between conditioned arousal insomnia and "primary" insomnia characterized by evidence of physiological hyperarousal. Both conditions are often subsumed under the term *psychophysiological insomnia*, a term suggesting more pathophysiological understanding than in fact exists. Indeed, there is probably overlap in that both appear to be characterized by a state of hyperarousal. Treatment should be addressed to the hyperarousal, whose etiology may not always be apparent.

COMBINED TREATMENT APPROACH FOR CHRONIC PSYCHOPHYSIOLOGICAL (PRIMARY) INSOMNIA

A treatment approach that combines both behavioral and pharmacological approaches is generally recommended for chronic psychophysiological or conditioned insomnia (Hajak et al. 1997; Mendelson and Jain 1995 [review]; Riemann 1996). Such approaches often work as well for sleep state misperception syndrome. Such a combined treatment approach offers the advantage of a pharmacological agent that can produce rapid relief of the sleep complaint, along with behavioral strategies, which take longer to become effective but provide long-term strategies that are under patients' control. Active and continued involvement of the patient is important for any chronic insomnia treatment. One facet of an insomnia complaint that fosters hyperarousal is the sense of helplessness in the face of sleeplessness that many patients describe, which further increases anxiety and concern, which in turn further delays sleep. It is important to avoid merely prescribing a hypnotic agent without also providing additional coping strategies for the patient. Morin and colleagues (1994), in a meta-analysis of treatment efficacy of non-

pharmacological interventions, found that such treatments required on the average only 5 hours of therapy time and were effective in producing reliable changes in two of the four variables measured (sleep latency and time awake after sleep onset). Furthermore, these beneficial changes persisted at a 6-month follow-up. Murtagh and Greenwood (1995) found that active behavioral treatments were all superior to placebo but that different behavioral treatment strategies did not differ significantly from one another in efficacy. Several studies have suggested that combinations of behavioral treatment strategies are better than single strategies (Jacobs and Benson 1993; Jacobs et al. 1993). I first consider the behavioral strategies most likely to be beneficial for chronic primary insomnia, then the pharmacological options.

BEHAVIORAL TREATMENTS

Behavioral treatment strategies are aimed at 1) breaking up bad sleep habits and replacing them with sleep-promoting habits, 2) directly decreasing physiological arousal levels, and 3) providing the patient with cognitive strategies to deal with sleep difficulties, thus promoting a sense of competence and diminishing anxiety about sleep.

First and foremost among the behavioral strategies is good *sleep hygiene*: the behaviors and habits that foster good sleep. Good sleep hygiene includes the following:

- Establish a regular sleep schedule, ideally including early-morning arising that does not vary more than an hour on different days of the week.
- Maintain a state of good aerobic fitness with regular exercise (but not within 3 hours of sleep onset).
- Do not use caffeine or alcohol to excess. Caffeine can have a long-lasting effect on some individuals, and they should restrict it to mornings.
- Ensure a quiet, dark, cool bedroom.
- Provide a time to wind down in the evening before sleeping. Stop working 30 minutes before bedtime, and engage in a low-stress activity, such as reading or listening to music.
- Consider a high-tryptophan snack (milk, cookies, banana) before bed.
- Use the bedroom for sleep and sex but not for reviewing or thinking about the affairs of the day. If not asleep in 30 minutes, get up and read, or complete a task, returning to bed after sleepiness returns.
- Minimize exposure to bright light to avoid phase-delaying the circadian system. Most reading lights and computer screens are not sufficiently bright to be troublesome in this regard.

Good sleep hygiene is appropriate for all, not just those with insomnia. Not infrequently, poor sleep hygiene contributes materially to an insomnia complaint. Careful questioning can identify such cases, and sometimes merely changing sleep habits in an appropriate manner is sufficient to significantly relieve the sleep complaint. As simple a procedure as improving regularity of sleep has been shown to improve sleep and diminish daytime sleepiness (Manber et al. 1996).

Several behavioral strategies discussed below are targeted directly at decreasing arousal level.

Biofeedback

Biofeedback involves monitoring physiological variables, such as electromyographic (EMG; muscle tension) responses, skin temperature, or EEG activity patterns (alpha, theta, or sensorimotor rhythms); providing the patient with an auditory or visual cue that levels are not meeting a target threshold; and allowing the patient to develop strategies to modify the physiological indicators and so decrease arousal level. Biofeedback can be an important adjunct to the treatment of chronic insomnia, and it is especially useful for patients with high arousal levels. Although EMG and skin temperature are perhaps the most widely available forms of biofeedback, EEG theta feedback has been shown to be useful in tense, anxious patients with chronic insomnia, and sensorimotor rhythm feedback may be useful in individuals who are not particularly tense or anxious but nonetheless have trouble sustaining sleep (Hauri 1981, 1983).

Progressive Relaxation

Progressive relaxation is designed to make the patient aware of increased muscle tension and thus high arousal level. Patients contract muscle groups, become aware of the tense state, and then systematically relax them. Attention is paid to the feeling accompanying the relaxation response. As a result, patients can learn to avoid the high muscle tension that interferes with sleep onset, to lower their arousal level, and thus to permit (rather than induce) sleep (Jacobson 1974).

Sleep Restriction

Sleep restriction is useful for individuals who spend a considerable amount of time in bed but much of that time awake. Older patients are especially prone to spending more and more time in bed and achieving less and less sleep—for example, they may be spending 10 hours in bed yet claim to be sleeping only 6 hours. The essence of sleep restriction is to restrict the time in bed, which tends to consolidate sleep. A typical sleep restriction protocol might include the following:

1. Have the patient keep a sleep diary for 5–7 days indicating when he or she went to bed, when sleep began, how often and how long he or she awoke during the night, and what time he or she awoke and arose in the morning. Compute from the diary the total sleep time (TST). Compute the percentage of sleep efficiency from the formula

$$\frac{\text{time asleep}}{\text{total time in bed}} \times 100$$

2. Restrict the patient's time in bed to the estimate of TST obtained from the sleep diary. Discuss with the patient the fact that he or she will experience daytime sleepiness for the first few days of this procedure.

3. Have the patient call in every morning to report sleep data from the preceding night, including time in bed, sleep latency, awakenings, time of final awakening, and time out of bed. Keep a running account of TST and sleep efficiency.

4. When mean sleep efficiency for 5 nights reaches 85%, increase time in bed by 15 minutes (allow the patient to go to bed 15 minutes earlier).

5. Repeat the steps above until sleep efficiency is maintained at 85% and the patient is obtaining what he or she considers an adequate amount of sleep.

An increase in daytime sleepiness will accompany the early stages of sleep restriction, and patients may need considerable encouragement to complete the procedure, but it can be successful in consolidation of sleep in a sizable percentage of patients (Spielman et al. 1987 [review]).

Several other forms of cognitive therapy have been described as useful in the treatment of chronic insomnia, including stimulus control and paradoxical intention (Baillargeon 1997; Bootzin and Perlis 1992). Referral to a psychologist experienced in the various forms of cognitive therapy can be useful for these patients.

PHARMACOLOGICAL TREATMENT

Mendelson and Jain (1995) have suggested that the ideal hypnotic would have a therapeutic profile characterized by rapid sleep induction and no residual effects (including memory effects). Its pharmacokinetic profile would include rapid absorption and optimal half-life, as well as specific receptor binding and lack of active metabolites. Its pharmacodynamic profile would include lack of tolerance or physical dependence and no CNS or respiratory depression.

Although the ideal hypnotic agent has yet to be developed, these agents are being systematically improved with respect to most of the foregoing issues. Benzodiazepine compounds and nonbenzodiazepine agents active at the level of the benzodiazepine receptor are the most commonly used hypnotic agents today. These agents are relatively safe and have a good therapeutic profile; patients with insomnia do not appear to demonstrate short-term dose escalation (Roehrs et al. 1996). Older hypnotic agents (chloral hydrate, paraldehyde, barbiturates) may have a limited utility for very short-term use in specific patients, but they cannot be recommended for the treatment of chronic insomnia.

The benzodiazepine compounds differ substantially in terms of half-life, and the clinician can choose the agent with a half-life most appropriate for the clinical situation. A long-half-life hypnotic such as flurazepam (15–30 mg) or quazepam (7.5–15.0 mg) might be appropriate for an anxious patient in whom daytime anxiolytic effects are helpful, if the interference with psychomotor performance is acceptable and tolerable and if both patient and physician realize that considerable buildup in blood level can be expected. Patients with difficulty sleeping through the night might benefit from intermediate-half-life agents such as temazepam (15–30 mg) or estazolam (1–2 mg). Patients who must be alert in the morning without residual daytime sedation would best be managed by a short-half-life agent such as triazolam (0.125–0.25 mg) or zolpidem (5–10 mg). Zolpidem is an imidazopyridine agent active at the ω_1 benzodiazepine receptor but without the same degree of potential for tolerance or rebound as seen with conventional benzodiazepines. Zolpidem has shown no evidence of rebound insomnia after being used at 10 mg/day for up to 35 days (Monti et al. 1994; Scharf et al. 1994; Ware et al. 1997).

Antidepressant agents, especially sedative tricyclics, are frequently used to manage chronic insomnia despite the relative lack of well-controlled double-blind studies demonstrating efficacy (Kupfer and Reynolds 1997). These agents are clearly indicated in insomnia that accompanies depressive disorders, where their effectiveness is clear. When used for other types of insomnia complaints, they are usually used at a dose lower than that of a typical antidepressant. A single-blind study of 19 patients with insomnia found that trimipramine is effective in relieving insomnia complaints (Hohagen et al. 1994b). Over-the-

counter sleep agents, or various herbal remedies found in health food stores, have generally not been evaluated for hypnotic efficacy in well-controlled double-blind studies. Although some have modest sedative effects, consumers should be cautious, especially as concerns regular or excessive use of such agents.

INSOMNIA IN ELDERLY PERSONS

Sleep complaints are greater in elderly persons than in other age groups (Ganguli et al. 1996). More than 50% of persons older than 65 years complain of poor sleep (Ancoli-Israel 1997). Whereas it was once thought that elderly persons required less sleep, it now appears that they in fact get less sleep, but primarily because the conditions known to disrupt sleep and produce insomnia complaints increase with age. Sleep-related breathing disturbances (Ancoli-Israel et al. 1991b), depression, PLMS (Ancoli-Israel et al. 1991a), and medical conditions all increase with age, as do associated insomnia complaints. As a result of obtaining less sleep than needed, elderly persons tend to be sleepier during the day, as indicated by shorter mean sleep latencies on the MSLT (Dement et al. 1982).

The diagnosis and treatment of insomnia complaints in the elderly should proceed in a fashion no different from that outlined in this chapter. A systematic differential diagnosis, appropriate treatment of the specific medical, psychiatric, or other conditions that might adversely influence sleep, and a combined approach for the chronic insomnia component are indicated. Behavioral treatment should be emphasized, because many patients will be taking medications for other medical illnesses, thus increasing the possibility of drug interactions. Additionally, the metabolic breakdown of sedative-hypnotic agents might be diminished in elderly patients; thus, doses should begin lower, and caution should be exercised in the use of long-half-life agents (e.g., flurazepam) whose period of activity may be further prolonged.

Melatonin levels in elderly persons with insomnia have been found to be lower, with later onset of peak blood levels (Haimov et al. 1994). Some studies have suggested that melatonin replacement therapy might be a helpful treatment strategy for certain elderly individuals with sleep complaints (Garfinkel et al. 1995; Haimov et al. 1995). Elderly persons are at special risk for bereavement, and sleep disturbance associated with bereavement-related depression has been found to respond favorably to nortriptyline treatment in elderly individuals (Pasternak et al. 1994).

Especially important are good sleep hygiene, and reinforcing optimal circadian sleep/activity patterns. Often, elderly individuals are less active than their younger counterparts and are in less than optimal aerobic condition. Regular weight-lifting exercise in a cohort of 32 subjects ages 60–84 years was found to improve subjective sleep quality, depression, strength, and overall quality of life (Singh et al. 1997).

SUMMARY

Insomnia can be a complex symptom with a multifaceted causation. Careful attention to a systematic differential diagnostic procedure, keeping in mind the likelihood of comorbidity, contributes to accurate diagnosis and effective treatment.

Effective treatment is dependent on accurate diagnosis and tailoring the several behavioral and pharmacological treatment options to the specific patient. When this process is done with care, there is a high probability of a favorable outcome.

REFERENCES

Adam K, Tomeny M, Oswald I: Physiological and psychological differences between good and poor sleepers. J Psychiatr Res 20:301–316, 1986

American Psychiatric Association: Diagnostic and Statistical Manual of Mental Disorders, 4th Edition. Washington, DC, American Psychiatric Association, 1994

Ancoli-Israel S: Sleep problems in older adults: putting myths to bed. Geriatrics 52:20–30, 1997

Ancoli-Israel S, Kripke DF, Klauber MR, et al: Periodic limb movements in sleep in community-dwelling elderly. Sleep 14:496–500, 1991a

Ancoli-Israel S, Kripke DF, Klauber MR, et al: Sleep-disordered breathing in community-dwelling elderly. Sleep 14:486–495, 1991b

Arendt J, Aldhous M, Marks V: Alleviation of "jet lag" by melatonin: preliminary results of controlled double blind trial. BMJ 292:1170, 1986

Axelrod J, Weissbach H: Enzymatic O-methylation of N-acetylserotonin to melatonin. Science 131:1312–1313, 1960

Baillargeon L: Traitements cognitifs et comportementaux de l'insomnie: une alternative a la pharmacotherapie [Behavior and cognitive treatments for insomnia: an alternative to pharmacotherapy]. Can Fam Physician 43:290–296, 1997

Bliwise DL: Historical change in the report of daytime fatigue. Sleep 19:462–464, 1996

Bonnet MH, Arand DL: Caffeine use as a model of acute and chronic insomnia. Sleep 15:526–536, 1992

Bonnet MH, Arand D: 24-hour metabolic rate in insomniacs and matched normal sleepers. Sleep 18:581–588, 1995

Bonnet MH, Arand DL: The consequences of a week of insomnia. Sleep 19:453–461, 1996

Bonnet MH, Arand DL: Physiological activation in patients with sleep state misperception. Psychosom Med 59:533–540, 1997

Bootzin RR, Perlis ML: Nonpharmacologic treatments of insomnia. J Clin Psychiatry 53 (suppl):37–41, 1992

Brzezinski A: Melatonin in humans. N Engl J Med 336:186–195, 1997

Chang PP, Ford DE, Mead LA, et al: Insomnia in young men and subsequent depression. Am J Epidemiol 146:105–114, 1997

Coon SL, Roseboom PH, Baler R: Pineal serotonin N-acetyltransferase: expression cloning and molecular analysis. Science 270:1681–1683, 1995

Dahlitz M, Alvarez B, Vignau J, et al: Delayed sleep phase syndrome response to melatonin. Lancet 337:1121–1124, 1991

Dawson D, Reid K: Fatigue, alcohol and performance impairment (scientific correspondence). Nature 388:235, 1997

Dawson D, Encel N, Lushington K: Improving adaptation to simulated night shift: timed exposure to bright light versus daytime melatonin administration. Sleep 18:11–21, 1995

Dement WC, Seidel W, Carskadon MA: Daytime alertness, insomnia and benzodiazepines. Sleep 5:S28–S45, 1982

Earley CJ, Allen RP: Pergolide and carbidopa/levodopa treatment of the restless legs syndrome and periodic leg movements in sleep in a consecutive series of patients. Sleep 19:801–810, 1996

Eastman CI, Boulos Z, Terman M, et al: Light treatment for sleep disorders: consensus report, VI: shift work. J Biol Rhythms 10:157–164, 1995

Eaton WW, Badawi M, Melton B: Prodromes and precursors: epidemiologic data for primary prevention of disorders with slow onset. Am J Psychiatry 152:967–972, 1995

Edinger JD, Fins AI: The distribution and clinical significance of sleep time misperceptions among insomniacs. Sleep 18:232–239, 1995

Edinger JD, Fins AI, Goeke JM, et al: The empirical identification of insomnia subtypes: a cluster analytic approach. Sleep 19:398–411, 1996

Ford DE, Kamerow DB: Epidemiologic study of sleep disturbances and psychiatric disorders: an opportunity for prevention? JAMA 262:1479–1484, 1989

Franklin KA, Eriksson P, Sahlin C, et al: Reversal of central sleep apnea with oxygen. Chest 111:163–169, 1997

Gallup Organization: Sleep in America. Princeton, NJ, The Gallup Organization, 1995, pp 1–10

Ganguli M, Reynolds CF, Gilby JE: Prevalence and persistence of sleep complaints in a rural older community sample: the movies project. J Am Geriatr Soc 44:778–784, 1996

Garfinkel D, Laudon M, Nof D, et al: Improvement of sleep quality in elderly people by controlled-release melatonin. Lancet 346:541–544, 1995

Gordon NP, Cleary PD, Parker CE: The prevalence and health impact of shiftwork. Am J Public Health 76:1225–1228, 1986

Granton JT, Naughton MT, Benard DC, et al: CPAP improves inspiratory muscle strength in patients with heart failure and central sleep apnea. Am J Respir Crit Care Med 153:277–282, 1996

Haimov I, Laudon M, Zisapel N, et al: Sleep disorders and melatonin rhythms in elderly people. BMJ 309:167, 1994

Haimov I, Lavie P, Laudon M, et al: Melatonin replacement therapy of elderly insomniacs. Sleep 18:598–603, 1995

Hajak G, Muller-Popkes K, Riemann D, et al: Psychological, psychotherapeutic and other non-pharmacologic forms of therapy in treatment of insomnia. Fortschr Neurol Psychiatr 65:133–144, 1997

Hauri P: Treating psychophysiologic insomnia with biofeedback. Arch Gen Psychiatry 38:752–758, 1981

Hauri P: A cluster analysis of insomnia. Sleep 6:326–338, 1983

Hohagen F, Kappler C, Schramm E, et al: Sleep onset insomnia, sleep maintaining insomnia and insomnia with early morning awakening—temporal stability of subtypes in a longitudinal study on general practice attenders. Sleep 17:551–554, 1994a

Hohagen F, Montero RF, Weiss E: Treatment of primary insomnia with trimipramine: an alternative to benzodiazepine hypnotics? Eur Arch Psychiatry Clin Neurosci 244:65–72, 1994b

Hughes RJ, Badia P: Sleep-promoting and hypothermic effects of daytime melatonin administration in humans. Sleep 20:124–131, 1997

Jacobs GD, Benson H: Home-based central nervous system assessment of a multifactor behavioral intervention for chronic sleep-onset insomnia. Behavior Therapy 24:159–174, 1993

Jacobs GD, Rosenberg PA, Friedman R, et al: Multifactor behavioral treatment of chronic sleep-onset insomnia using stimulus control and the relaxation response. Behav Modif 17:498–509, 1993

Jacobson E: Progressive Relaxation. Chicago, IL, University of Chicago Press, Midway Reprint, 1974

Jan JE, Espezel H, Appleton RE: The treatment of sleep disorders with melatonin. Dev Med Child Neurol 36:97–107, 1994

Karacan I, Williams RL: Sleep disorders in the elderly. Am Fam Physician 27:143–152, 1983

Krupp LB, Jandorf L, Coyle PK, et al: Sleep disturbance in chronic fatigue syndrome. J Psychosom Res 37:325–331, 1993

Kupfer DJ, Reynolds CF: Management of insomnia. N Engl J Med 336:341–346, 1997

Lamarche CH, Ogilvie RD: Electrophysiological changes during the sleep onset period of psychophysiological insomniacs, psychiatric insomniacs, and normal sleepers. Sleep 20:724–733, 1997

Lamberg L: Melatonin potentially useful but safety, efficacy remain uncertain. JAMA 276:1011–1014, 1996

Lapierre O, Dumont M: Melatonin treatment of a non-24-hour sleep-wake cycle in a blind retarded child. Biol Psychiatry 38:119–122, 1995

Leger D: The cost of sleep-related accidents: a report for the national commission on sleep disorders research. Sleep 17:84–93, 1994

Lichstein KL, Wilson NM, Noe SL, et al: Daytime sleepiness in insomnia: behavioral, biological and subjective indices. Sleep 17:693–702, 1994

Manber R, Bootzin RR, Acebo C, et al: The effects of regularizing sleep-wake schedules on daytime sleepiness. Sleep 19:432–441, 1996

Marcus CL, Loughlin GM: Effect of sleep deprivation on driving safety in housestaff. Sleep 19:763–766, 1996

Mellman TA, Nolan B, Hebding J, et al: A polysomnographic comparison of veterans with combat-related PTSD, depressed men, non-ill controls. Sleep 20:46–51, 1997

Mendelson WB, Jain B: An assessment of short-acting hypnotics. Drug Saf 13:257–270, 1995

Mitler MM, Miller JC, Lipsitz JJ, et al: The sleep of long-haul truck drivers. N Engl J Med 337:755–761, 1997

Monroe LJ: Psychological and physiological differences between good and poor sleepers. J Abnorm Psychol 72:255–264, 1967

Monti JM, Attali P, Monti D, et al: Zolpidem and rebound insomnia: a double-blind, controlled polysomnographic study in chronic insomniac patients. Pharmacopsychiatry 27:166–175, 1994

Montplaisir J, Boucher S, Poirer G, et al: Clinical, polysomnographic, and genetic characteristics of restless legs syndrome: a study of 133 patients diagnosed with new standards criteria. Mov Disord 12:61–65, 1997

Morin CM, Gramling SE: Sleep patterns and aging: comparison of older adults with and without insomnia complaints. Psychol Aging 4:290–294, 1989

Morin CM, Culbert JP, Schwartz SM: Nonpharmacological interventions for insomnia: a meta-analysis of treatment efficacy. Am J Psychiatry 151:1172–1180, 1994

Murciano D, Armengaud MH, Cramer PH, et al: Acute effects of zolpidem, triazolam, and flunitrazepam on arterial blood gases and control of breathing in severe COPD. Eur Respir J 6:625–629, 1993

Murphy PJ, Campbell SS: Nighttime drop in body temperature: a physiological trigger for sleep onset? Sleep 20:505–511, 1997

Murtagh DRR, Greenwood KM: Identifying effective psychological treatments for insomnia: a meta-analysis. J Consult Clin Psychol 63:79–89, 1995

National Commission on Sleep Disorders Research: Wake Up America: A National Sleep Alert: Report of the National Commission on Sleep Disorders Research, Vol 1. Washington, DC, National Commission on Sleep Disorders Research, 1993

Ohayon MM, Malijai C, Guilleminault C: How a general population perceives its sleep and how this relates to the complaint of insomnia. Sleep 20:715–723, 1997

Ohta T, Ando K, Iwata T, et al: Treatment of persistent sleep-wake schedule disorders in adolescents with methylcobalamin (vitamin B12). Sleep 14:414–418, 1991

Ozaki N, Iwata T, Itoh A, et al: Body temperature monitoring in subjects with delayed sleep phase syndrome. Neuropsychobiology 20:174–177, 1988

Pasternak RE, Reynolds CF, Houck PR, et al: Sleep in bereavement-related depression during and after pharmacotherapy with nortriptyline. J Geriatr Psychiatry Neurol 7:69–73, 1994

Petrie K, Dawson AG, Thompson L, et al: A double-blind trial of melatonin as a treatment for jet lag in international cabin crew. Biol Psychiatry 33:526–530, 1993

Philip P, Ghorayeb I, Leger D, et al: Objective measurement of sleepiness in summer vacation long-distance drivers. Electroencephalogr Clin Neurophysiol 102:383–389, 1997

Phillips BA, Danner FJ: Cigarette smoking and sleep disturbance. Arch Intern Med 155:734–737, 1995

Pilcher JJ, Huffcutt AI: Effects of sleep deprivation on performance: a meta-analysis. Sleep 19:318–326, 1996

Porcu S, Bellatreccia A, Ferrara M, et al: Acutely shifting the sleep-wake cycle: nighttime sleepiness after diurnal administration of temazepam or placebo. Aviat Space Environ Med 68:688–694, 1997

Regestein QR, Monk TH: Delayed sleep phase syndrome: a review of its clinical aspects. Am J Psychiatry 152:602–608, 1995

Regestein QR, Pavlova M: Treatment of delayed sleep phase syndrome. Gen Hosp Psychiatry 17:335–345, 1995

Regestein QR, Dambrosia J, Hallett M, et al: Daytime alertness in patients with primary insomnia. Am J Psychiatry 150:1529–1534, 1993

Reite M, Jackson D, Cahoon R, et al: Sleep physiology at high altitude. Electroencephalogr Clin Neurophysiol 38:463–471, 1975

Reite M, Ruddy J, Nagel K: Concise Guide to the Evaluation and Management of Sleep Disorders, 2nd Edition. Washington, DC, American Psychiatric Press, 1997

Richardson GS, Malin HV: Circadian rhythm sleep disorders: pathophysiology and treatment. J Clin Neurophysiol 13:17–31, 1996

Riemann D: Insomnia: diagnostic and therapeutic procedure, 2: non-medicamentous and medicamentous therapy in general practice. Fortschritte der Medizin 114(30):399–401, 1996

Roberts MJ: Acute mountain sickness—experience on the roof of Africa expedition and military implications. J R Army Med Corps 140:49–51, 1994

Roehrs T, Shore E, Papineau K, et al: A two-week sleep extension in sleepy normals. Sleep 19:576–582, 1996

Rosenfeld DS, Furman Y: Pure sleep panic: two case reports and a review of the literature. Sleep 17:462–465, 1994

Rosenthal NE, Joseph-Vanderpool JR, Levendosky AA, et al: Phase-shifting effects of bright morning light as treatment for delayed sleep phase syndrome. Sleep 13:354–361, 1990

Ross RJ, Ball WA, Dinges DF: Rapid eye movement sleep disturbance in posttraumatic stress disorder. Biol Psychiatry 35:195–202, 1994

Saiz-Ruiz J, Cebollada A, Ibanez A: Sleep disorders in bipolar depression: hypnotics vs. sedative antidepressants. J Psychosom Res 38 (suppl):55–60, 1994

Satterlee WG, Faries D: The effects of fluoxetine on symptoms of insomnia in depressed patients. Psychopharmacol Bull 31:227–237, 1995

Scharf MB, Roth T, Vogel GW, et al: A multicenter, placebo-controlled study evaluating zolpidem in the treatment of chronic insomnia. J Clin Psychiatry 55:192–199, 1994

Silber MH: Restless legs syndrome. Mayo Clin Proc 72:261–264, 1997

Silver JM, Sandberg DP, Hales RE: New approaches in the pharmacotherapy of posttraumatic stress disorder. J Clin Psychiatry 51 (10, suppl):33–38, 1990

Singh NA, Clements KM, Fiatarone MA: Sleep, sleep deprivation, and daytime activities: a randomized controlled trial of the effect of exercise on sleep. Sleep 20:95–101, 1997

Spielman AJ, Caruso LS, Glovinsky PB: A behavioral perspective on insomnia treatment. Psychiatr Clin North Am 10:541–553, 1987

Stoller MK: Economic effects of insomnia. Clin Ther 16:873–897, 1994

Teicher MH, Glod CA, Magnus E, et al: Circadian rest-activity disturbances in seasonal affective disorder. Arch Gen Psychiatry 54:124–130, 1997

Thalhofer S, Dorow P: Central sleep apnea. Respiration 64:2–9, 1997

Tomoda A, Miike T, Uezono K, et al: A school refusal case with biological rhythm disturbance and melatonin therapy. Brain Dev 16:71–76, 1994

Trenkwalder C, Walters AS, Hening W: Periodic limb movements and restless legs syndrome. Neurol Clin 14:629–650, 1996

Tzischinsky O, Lavie P: Melatonin possesses time-dependent hypnotic effects. Sleep 17:638–645, 1994

Waldhauser F, Dietzel M: Daily and annual rhythms in human melatonin secretion: role in puberty control. Ann N Y Acad Sci 453:205–214, 1985

Ware JC, Walsh JK, Scharf MB, et al: Minimal rebound insomnia after treatment with 10-mg zolpidem. Clin Neuropharmacol 20:116–125, 1997

Wechsler LR, Stakes JW, Shahani BT: Periodic leg movements of sleep (nocturnal myoclonus): an electrophysiological study. Ann Neurol 19:168–173, 1986

Weitzman ED, Czeisler CA, Coleman RM, et al: Delayed sleep phase syndrome. Arch Gen Psychiatry 38:737–746, 1981

Winokur A, Reynolds C: Overview of effects of antidepressant therapies on sleep. Primary Psychiatry 1:22–27, 1994

Yamadera H, Takahashi K, Okawa M: A multicenter study of sleep-wake rhythm disorders: therapeutic effects of vitamin B12, bright light therapy, chronotherapy and hypnotics. Psychiatry and Clinical Neurosciences 50:203–209, 1996

APPENDIX

New Psychotropic Drugs for Axis I Disorders: Recently Arrived, in Development, and Never Arrived

Joseph K. Belanoff, M.D., and Ira D. Glick, M.D.

The vitality of the field of psychopharmacology depends on the continued introduction of new medications for treatment. In this chapter, we identify the current status of medications for schizophrenia, mood disorders, and anxiety. We discuss the mechanisms of these new drugs and compare them with drugs currently approved by the U.S. Food and Drug Administration (FDA). Although this chapter is intended to be inclusive, a realistic caveat is that both medical and marketing decisions can dramatically influence the actual availability of any medication. We apologize in advance for any inadvertent omissions.

The reason for discussing these drugs in an American psychopharmacology text is that current FDA and customs policy, influenced by pressures from patients with acquired immunodeficiency syndrome (AIDS), allows 3-month supplies of drugs that are not available in the United States to be imported to treat treatment-resistant patients. It is not clear that any of these drugs is so different and so superior (as was clearly the case with clomipramine in the treatment of obsessive-compulsive disorder) as to impel many psychiatrists to arrange to bring one or more of these drugs to the United States to treat their patients, but in special situations this might be worth doing. In addition, our thought was that with the addition of the material in this text, it would be more useful for Canadian and European investigators.

METHODOLOGY AND RESULTS

We collected data from three sources: controlled trials from the literature (Ballenger et al. 1991; Borison et al. 1996; Patris et al. 1996), psychopharmacologists in eight countries, and representatives of the pharmaceutical industry (Glick et al. 1996). In our discussions, we identified a number of drugs that seem to promote equal or better efficacy than current medications with equivalent or less adverse side effects. The clinical use of medications not available in the United States, together with the toxicity of drugs, dosage, and comparison with other drugs, is listed in Table A–1.

SCHIZOPHRENIA

The key objectives in the treatment of schizophrenia are

1. To find medications that more effectively treat the symptoms of schizophrenia (particularly the negative symptoms)
2. To find medications for patients whose illness does not respond to conventional antipsychotic agents
3. To find medications that will cause less frequent, less severe, and potentially not permanent movement disorders

Table A–1. Clinical features of new and newest psychotropics

Drug (generic name)	Chemical classification	Presumed pharmacological effects	Comparison with standard drugs	Major side effects	Daily dose (mg)	Comment	Molecular structure
Antipsychotics							
Risperidone	Benzisoxazole derivative	5-HT$_2$, D$_2$ blocker	Better than placebo and equal to standard	Anxiety, dizziness, rhinitis	3–6	?↑ efficacy with negative symptoms; dose-related EPS	
Olanzapine	Thieno-benzodiazepine	Complicated	Better than placebo and equal to standard	Sedation, orthostatic hypotension, anticholinergic	5–20	Low EPS, no agranulocytosis	
Sertindole	Phenylindole	5-HT$_2$, D$_2$ blocker, α-blocker	Better than placebo and equal to standard	Nasal congestion, ↓ ejaculatory volume	20–24	Low EPS, ↑ Q-T interval?	
Quetiapine	Dibenzothiazepine	Complicated	Better than placebo and equal to standard	Mild somnolence, mild constipation, dry mouth	200–400	?↑ efficacy with negative symptoms, low EPS, no prolactinemia	
Ziprasidone	Substituted benzisothiazolyl-piperazine	5-HT$_2$, D$_2$ blocker	Better than placebo and equal to standard	Mild orthostatic hypotension	?50–150	Low EPS, ?↑ efficacy with negative symptoms and affective symptoms	
MDL 100,907	Novel piperidine-methanol	5-HT$_{2A}$ blocker	Better than placebo and equal to standard	Mild sedation	?40–60	No EPS or prolactinemia	

Drug	Chemical class	Mechanism	Efficacy	Side effects	Dose	Comments
Aripiprazole	Quinolinone derivative	Postsynaptic D_2 blocker, presynaptic dopamine agonist	Better than placebo and equal to standard	Insomnia, headache	20–30	Low EPS
Zotepine	Dibenzothiophene	5-HT_2, D_2 blocker	Better than placebo and equal to standard	Moderate EPS, akathisia	250–350	Improvement in negative & positive symptoms, ? ↓ anxiety and depression
Nemonapride	Benzamide derivative	Selective D_2 antagonist	Better than placebo and equal to standard	Akathisia, drowsiness	15–25	Low EPS, ? improvement in negative symptoms
Antidepressants						
Nefazodone	Phenylpiperazine	5-HT reuptake inhibitor, 5-HT_2 blocker	Better than placebo and equal to standard	Sedation	300–600	? Useful in PMS and chronic pain
Mirtazapine	Tetracyclic	α_2 autoreceptor blocker, 5-HT_2 blocker, 5-HT_3 blocker, ↑5-HT release	Better than placebo and equal to standard	Sedation, dry mouth, weight gain	30–45	? Anxiolytic, sleep enhancer
Tianeptine	Tricyclic	5-HT reuptake enhancer	Better than placebo and equal to standard	Insomnia, ↑ anxiety	25–50	Few somatic complaints
Citalopram	Tertiary amine	SSRI	Better than placebo and equal to standard	Mild nausea, sedation	30–60	No cardiotoxicity
Flesinoxan	Piperazine derivative	5-HT_{1A} agonist	Better than placebo and equal to standard	Headache, dizziness, nausea	4–8	More study needed
Reboxetine	Methane-sulfonate salt	SNRI	Better than placebo and equal to standard	Somnolence, tremor, hypotension, dry mouth	8–10	Available in the U.K.

(continued)

Table A–1. Clinical features of new and newest psychotropics *(continued)*

Drug (generic name)	Chemical classification	Presumed pharmacological effects	Comparison with standard drugs	Major side effects	Daily dose (mg)	Comment	Molecular structure
Moclobemide	Benzamide derivative	Reversible MAO$_A$-selective inhibitor	Better than placebo and equal to standard	Insomnia, headache, dry mouth, dizziness, fatigue, nausea, diarrhea	300–900	No dietary restrictions; not marketed in U.S.	
Brofaromine	Piperidine derivative	Reversible MAO$_A$-selective inhibitor; 5-HT reuptake inhibitor	Better than placebo and equal to standard	Insomnia, dizziness, headache, dry mouth, anorexia	25–150	No dietary restrictions; not marketed in U.S.	
Anxiolytics							
Abecarnil	β-Carboline	Benzodiazepine partial agonist	Better than placebo and equal to standard	Drowsiness, fatigue	3–9	Any interest?	
Mood stabilizers							
Lamotrigine	Phenyltriazine	Inhibits release of glutamate	None so far	Dizziness, headache, rash	150–250	? Efficacy in bipolar depression	
Gabapentin	GABA derivative	?	None so far	Somnolence, dizziness, ataxia	900–1,800	No interaction with CBZ or VPA	
Tiagabine	Nipecotic acid derivative	GABA uptake inhibitor	None so far	Dizziness	800 divided	Short half-life	
Topiramate	Sulfamate-substituted monosaccharide	Complicated	None so far	Headache, somnolence, dizziness	600 divided	Stops spread of seizures, as opposed to raising the seizure threshold, ? relevance to BAD	

| Vigabatrin | Gamma-vinyl GABA | Irreversible inhibitor of GABA-aminotransferase | None so far | Sedation, dizziness | 1,500–3,000 | ? of increase in depression and psychosis in patients with epilepsy |

Note. 5-HT = 5-hydroxytryptamine (serotonin); D_2 = dopamine type 2 [receptor]; EPS = extrapyramidal side effects; PMS = premenstrual syndrome; SSRI = selective serotonin reuptake inhibitor; SNRI = selective norepinephrine reuptake inhibitor; MAO = monoamine oxidase; GABA = γ-aminobutyric acid; CBZ = carbamazepine; VPA = valproic acid; BAD = bipolar affective disorder.

At present, a large number of new medications are being developed for the treatment of psychotic symptoms. One way to quickly grasp the overall picture is to characterize them on the basis of their (primary) receptor profile, as shown in Table A–2 (J. Lieberman, personal communication, August 1997).

Drugs That Recently Arrived

Although risperidone and olanzapine are discussed earlier in this textbook (see Marder, Chapter 17), we briefly describe them here to provide contrast and context to drugs currently in development.

Risperidone. Risperidone is a serotonin-dopamine antagonist. Like clozapine, it is a serotonin type 2 (5-HT$_2$) receptor blocker; unlike clozapine, it is a dopamine type 2 (D_2) receptor blocker, particularly in higher doses. Data indicate that risperidone is as effective as standard antipsychotics in treatment of positive symptoms, and perhaps more effective in the treatment of negative symptoms, of schizophrenia (Marder and Meibach 1994). At lower doses (≤6 mg), extrapyramidal side effects (EPS) of risperidone are often negligible, but their incidence rises with higher doses (Schotte et al. 1996). Early studies showed efficacy in 20 treatment-resistant schizophrenic patients. Adverse effects include anxiety, dizziness, and rhinitis. Dose-related adverse effects include sedation, fatigue, and accommodation disturbance (Borison et al. 1992).

Olanzapine. Olanzapine, a recently released antipsychotic agent, has a binding profile that is similar to that of clozapine (an antagonist to dopamine, serotonin, muscarinic cholinergic, α-adrenergic, and histamine receptors) but has a much higher dose potency. Olanzapine appears to have very little propensity to cause EPS (or prolactinemia) (Baldwin and Montgomery 1995). It may have efficacy in patients whose schizophrenia did not improve with clozapine or in those who could not tolerate clozapine's side effects (Tollefson et al. 1997b). In addition, olanzapine has been tried in patients with new-onset psychosis for whom standard antipsychotics have not been helpful. Because it does not appear to cause agranulocytosis (or reduce the seizure threshold), some propose that it even be used in "first-break" schizophrenia (Tollefson et al. 1997a), but data from controlled trials are needed to fully answer this question.

Drugs That Are in Development

Sertindole. Sertindole, another serotonin-dopamine antagonist, has now been shown to be effective in improv-

Table A–2.　Novel antipsychotic compounds

Compound	Pharmacological mechanism	Pharmaceutical company
Selective dopamine receptor agents		
SCH-39166	D_1 antagonist	Schering-Plough
NN22-0010	D_1 antagonist	Novo Nordisk
Remoxipride	D_2 antagonist	Astra
Raclopride	D_2 antagonist	Astra
NGD 94-1	D_4 antagonist	Neurogen
L-745,870	D_4 antagonist	Merck
SDZ-MAR-327	Partial D_2 agonist/antagonist	Sandoz
OPC-14597	D_2, D_3 antagonist, D_2 partial agonist 5-HT_{2A} antagonist	Otsuka
Mixed neuroreceptor antagonists		
Clozapine	D_2, D_1, 5-HT_{2A}, $NE\alpha_1$, α_2, H_1, ACH	Sandoz
Iloperidone (HP-873)	D_2, $NE\alpha_1$, α_2, 5-HT_{2A}	Roussel Uclaf SA
Mazapertine	D_2, D_3, $NE\alpha_1$, α_2, 5-HT_{1A}	Janssen
Olanzapine (LY 170053)	D_1, D_2, D_4, 5-HT_{2A}, $NE\alpha_1$, H_1	Lilly
Risperidone	D_2, 5-HT_{2A}, $NE\alpha_1$, α_2, H_1	Janssen
Quetiapine	D_2, D_1, 5-HT_{2A}, $NE\alpha_1$, α_2, ACH	Zeneca
Sertindole	D_2, D_1, 5-HT_{2A}, $NE\alpha_1$	Abbott/Lundbeck
Ziprasidone (CP-88059)	D_2, D_1, 5-HT_{2A}, $NE\alpha_1$	Pfizer
Serotonin antagonists		
Amperozide	$5\text{-HT}_{2A}/D_2$, D_1	Kabi-Pharmacia, Sandoz
MDL 100,907	5-HT_{2A} antagonist	Hoechst Merrell Dow

Note.　Affinities for (the common) neuroreceptors for which all drugs have been tested. D_1, D_2, D_3, and D_4 refer to dopamine receptors; 5-HT_{1A} and 5-HT_{2A} refer to serotonin receptors; $NE\alpha_2$, α_1 are norepinephrine alpha receptors; ACH refers to muscarinic receptors; H_1 refers to histamine receptor. This list of neuroreceptor effects is not comprehensive and does not reflect the proportional affinity that the drugs have for respective neuroreceptors.
Source.　Jeffrey Lieberman, M.D.

ing both the positive and the negative symptoms of schizophrenia. Like the other "atypicals," sertindole has a favorable EPS profile, although it is a more potent D_2 receptor blocker than clozapine and olanzapine. Sertindole appears to show greater selectivity for limbic as opposed to nigrostriatal D_2 receptors and has a relatively high affinity for 5-HT_2 receptors. Side effects include nasal congestion and decreased ejaculatory volume, which are probably related to α-adrenergic receptor blockade. Sertindole also appears to increase the Q-T interval on electrocardiogram. Data available as of this writing suggest that this side effect has little clinical significance (Borison 1995; Daniel et al. 1996), but the company has decided not to market the drug in the United States.

Quetiapine.　Quetiapine, a serotonin-dopamine antagonist, has shown efficacy in improving the positive and negative symptoms of schizophrenia (Casey 1996). It also appears to be comparable to haloperidol and chlorpromazine in acutely improving psychotic symptoms (Wetzel et

al. 1995). Quetiapine has a favorable EPS profile and does not produce sustained increased levels of prolactin (Hirsch et al. 1996). In fact, the drug is generally well tolerated, complaints of mild somnolence and mild anticholinergic effects appearing most commonly. The drug is now approved.

Ziprasidone.　Ziprasidone, also a serotonin-dopamine antagonist, has proven efficacy in blocking dopaminergic behaviors in animal models without producing severe motor side effects (Reeves and Harrigan 1996). However, it is also a potent 5-HT_{2A} receptor antagonist. Early studies report efficacy in positive and negative symptoms with few EPS in patients with schizophrenia. Clinical trials are now under way. Analysis of safety measures indicates that the agent is well tolerated and has a low incidence of EPS and orthostatic hypotension, only transient effects on prolactin levels, and no significant adverse effects on laboratory safety tests (Seeger et al. 1995).

MDL 100,907. MDL 100,907 is a potent and selective 5-HT_{2A} receptor antagonist with no dopamine effects (Sramek et al. 1996). In preclinical studies, it provided better ratings on central nervous system safety indices than did haloperidol, clozapine, risperidone, amperozide, and ritanserin. Early clinical trials have shown it to be well tolerated and to have no significant neurological side effects, no rise in serum prolactin levels, and very little orthostatic hypotension while significantly lowering scores on the Brief Psychiatric Rating Scale (Kehne et al. 1996; Overall and Gorham 1962). Phase 2 and 3 trials are in progress to determine efficacy.

Aripiprazole. Aripiprazole (ORL-N597) is an antagonist at postsynaptic D_2 receptors but an agonist at presynaptic dopamine autoreceptors. Animal models indicate that aripiprazole has less potential to cause EPS than do conventional antipsychotics. Early clinical studies show reduction in positive symptoms without significant neurological side effects (Otsuka Pharmaceuticals 1997).

Zotepine. Zotepine is currently being marketed in Japan, the United Kingdom, and Germany (Ott 1992). It appears to show some efficacy in reducing anxiety, depression, and negative as well as positive symptoms of schizophrenia (Fleischhacker et al. 1989). It also appears to produce fewer EPS than standard antipsychotic agents do (Barnas et al. 1992; Fleischhacker et al. 1989). Its adverse effects include fatigue, dry mouth, and constipation (Kondo et al. 1994). Like risperidone, zotepine is a more potent D_2 receptor blocker at higher doses and has a similar propensity to cause neurological side effects.

Nemonapride. Nemonapride has been released in Japan. It is a benzamide derivative and a potent and highly selective D_2 receptor antagonist (Yamamoto et al. 1982). It has shown efficacy in treating both the positive and the negative symptoms of schizophrenia while maintaining a surprisingly favorable EPS profile. Its adverse effects include akathisia and drowsiness (Satoh et al. 1997).

Drugs That Never Arrived

Remoxipride. Remoxipride was selected as a candidate atypical antipsychotic in 1978 (Lewander et al. 1990). It had a favorable EPS profile even though it was a potent D_2 receptor antagonist and had little effect on serotonin receptors. Remoxipride was not antihistaminergic and as a consequence was not sedating nor did it cause much weight gain. It had clear efficacy in treating the posi-

tive symptoms of schizophrenia, but in November 1993, it was dropped because of several cases of aplastic anemia (Lewander et al. 1992).

Raclopride. Raclopride had high affinity for D_2 and D_3 receptors compared with D_4 receptors. It had a favorable EPS profile compared with haloperidol. It was dropped because there was a suggestion that it increased tumor activity.

Amperozide. Amperozide had a significant effect on mesolimbic dopamine transmission as well as being a potent 5-HT_2 receptor antagonist (Svartengren and Celander 1994). It has been at least temporarily dropped from clinical trials.

Amisulpride. Amisulpride is available in Europe but was never marketed in the United States. It is a specific dopamine receptor antagonist with high affinity for D_2 and D_3 receptors. It seems to have selectivity for the limbic pathways. In clinical studies, patients showed improvement in negative symptoms of schizophrenia with amisulpride (Paillere-Martinot et al. 1995) while reporting fewer neurological side effects than with haloperidol (Perrault et al. 1997). It does produce galactorrhea. Clinicians report that it is particularly effective in helping patients with mild to moderate symptoms but not those with severe symptoms.

MAJOR DEPRESSION

The key objectives in treating major depression are to find antidepressants that

1. Consistently offer a higher response rate than the standard 65% rate
2. Work faster than the standard 3–6 weeks
3. Are better tolerated and safer than standard antidepressants

Drugs That Recently Arrived

The two most recently released antidepressants in the United States are nefazodone and mirtazapine.

Nefazodone. Nefazodone is a phenylpiperazine analogue of trazodone. Like trazodone, nefazodone blocks serotonin reuptake but with less potency than either the tricyclic antidepressants or the selective serotonin reuptake inhibitors (SSRIs). Nefazodone (and trazodone) are, however, significant blockers of 5-HT_2 receptors. This combination may result in stimulation of 5-HT_{1A} receptors in the dorsal raphe nucleus (which in turn may help depression) while avoiding stimulation of 5-HT_2 receptors in the forebrain (avoiding agitation or anxiety) or in the spinal cord (avoiding sexual dysfunction).

Nefazodone (and trazodone) are readily absorbed from the gastrointestinal tract, reach peak plasma levels in 1–2 hours, and have half-lives of 6–12 hours. Both are metabolized in the liver, and 75% of their metabolites are excreted in the urine.

Nefazodone has three main metabolites. Hydroxynefazodone has a pharmacodynamic profile similar to that of nefazodone, with SSRI and 5-HT_2 receptor antagonism. A second metabolite, a triazoledione, is a weaker 5-HT_2 antagonist than nefazodone and does not inhibit serotonin reuptake. *M*-Chlorphenylpiperazide is a metabolite of nefazodone (and trazodone) and has some serotonin antagonist activity at the 5-HT_2 receptor but agonist activity at serotonin receptor types 1A, 1B, 1C, and 1D (Cyr and Brown 1996).

Nefazodone has been shown to be effective in both first-episode and recurrent major depression. It may also be useful in premenstrual syndrome and pain management. Researchers are currently probing for a therapeutic window for nefazodone. It has a benign side-effect profile with much less sedation than trazodone.

Mirtazapine. Mirtazapine enhances both norepinephrine and serotonin release (de Boer 1995). It also blocks 5-HT_2 and 5-HT_3 receptors, an effect that directs the increase in serotonin function through the 5-HT_1 class of receptors (Davis and Wilde 1996). Mirtazapine has a low to moderate affinity for histamine H_1 receptors, which may explain its sedating properties (Stimmel et al. 1997).

Analysis of all United States controlled studies involving mirtazapine reveals an efficacy equal to that of tricyclic antidepressants and a lower dropout rate (Kasper 1997). The most common side effects of mirtazapine ($\geq 5\%$, and twice placebo) were increased appetite, weight gain, somnolence, dry mouth, and dizziness. Nausea, vomiting, insomnia, and sexual dysfunction were equally or less frequently noted in mirtazapine-treated patients compared with tricyclic-treated patients (Montgomery 1995).

Drugs That Are in Development

Tianeptine. Tianeptine is actually a serotonin uptake enhancer (Mitchell 1995). Although theoretically it might be presumed that tianeptine causes depression, it has actually been shown (in placebo-controlled studies) to

be an effective antidepressant (Dalery et al. 1997; Invernizzi et al. 1994). It has few anticholinergic (Wilde and Benfield 1995) or cardiovascular side effects but does occasionally cause insomnia and nausea. Interestingly, it appears to have some efficacy in the treatment of chronic alcoholism.

Citalopram. Citalopram is a potent SSRI (Lader 1996). Several studies have shown it to be better than placebo and equal in efficacy to standard antidepressant drugs (Montgomery and Djarv 1996). Citalopram is reported to have few side effects other than nausea, although one would presume that it also causes the type of sexual side effects that are seen with the other SSRIs (Muldoon 1996). It has few direct drug interactions but is an inhibitor of the cytochrome P450 (CYP) 2DC system (Brosen 1996).

Flesinoxan. Flesinoxan is a potent and selective 5-HT_{1A} agonist. No double-blind, placebo-controlled study of flesinoxan efficacy as an antidepressant has been published to date. In an open study of treatment-refractory depressed patients, flesinoxan was found to provide successful antidepressant effects (Grof et al. 1993). The most common side effects among patients in this study were headache, dizziness, and nausea.

Reboxetine. Reboxetine is a nontricyclic, selective norepinephrine reuptake inhibitor that is more potent than the older norepinephrine blocker desipramine. (However, it is not a cholinergic receptor blocker.) It does not significantly induce glucuronosyltransferase or the CYP3A4 system and has no interaction with the CYP2D6 system. As a consequence, reboxetine is unlikely to have any significant interaction with lorazepam, alprazolam, the tricyclic antidepressants, or the SSRIs. It has been released in the United Kingdom.

In early studies, reboxetine appeared to be significantly superior to placebo in treating major depression and dysthymia and may be as effective as imipramine in treating severe major depression (Berzewski et al. 1997). It tentatively appears that 8–10 mg/day is the optimum dosage. However, truly optimal doses have not yet been fully determined. Somnolence, tremor, hypotension, and dry mouth have been reported more frequently with reboxetine than with fluoxetine but not as frequently as with imipramine (Berzewski et al. 1997; Montgomery and Kasper 1995). Reboxetine does produce less gastrointestinal upset than does fluoxetine. Reboxetine is currently in early study in the United States.

Olanzapine. It has been suggested that olanzapine may be an effective monotherapy for psychotic major depression (DeBattista et al. 1997). The pharmacological properties of olanzapine include antagonism of dopamine (types 1–4) receptors, as well as 5-HT$_2$, muscarinic, α_1, and histamine receptors. It is conceivable that olanzapine, with its moderate 5-HT$_2$ antagonism and broad dopamine antagonism, has both primary antidepressant effects and antipsychotic effects. Interestingly, a number of case reports have suggested that clozapine, which has a similarly broad range of pharmacological activity, may also be useful in the monotherapy of psychotic depression (Ranjan and Meltzer 1996).

Drugs That Never Arrived

Reversible inhibitors of monoamine oxidase. The monoamine oxidase inhibitors currently available in the United States irreversibly bind their monoamine oxidase substrates. Reversible inhibitors of monoamine oxidase (RIMAs) are being developed. These drugs bind reversibly to monoamine oxidase, resulting in the full restoration of enzyme activity within 2–5 days after their discontinuation. Moreover, because RIMAs are competitive inhibitors, large amounts of ingested tyramine will displace the drug from the enzyme, limiting the potential for an extreme tyramine-induced reaction.

Moclobemide, an RIMA, has been shown to be better than placebo and equal to standard medication in treating major depression (Angst and Stabl 1992). Its adverse effects include nausea and agitation, and, like irreversible monoamine oxidase inhibitors, it has a significant interaction with SSRIs, particularly in overdose (Rihmer et al. 1994). Unfortunately, moclobemide is not likely to be introduced in the United States any time soon. Similarly, **brofaromine,** another RIMA, has also been found to be an effective agent in depression (Chouinard et al. 1993) and even treatment-resistant depression (Volz et al. 1994). Its adverse effects include insomnia, dizziness, dry mouth, and anorexia. The manufacturer of brofaromine does not appear to have plans to market it in the United States in the near future.

Nomifensine. Nomifensine was available in the mid-1980s, but its manufacturer elected to stop its distribution. It had a reputation for being an effective stimulating antidepressant with good efficacy in treatment-resistant cases. Unfortunately, a few patients in England who were using nomifensine died from hemolytic anemia, and the company (perhaps fearful of the product liability litigation) withdrew the drug from the market (Cole 1988).

BIPOLAR DISORDER

Bipolar disorder is chronic, recurrent, often severely impairing, and usually present from adolescence or early adulthood (Bowden 1995). The established pharmacological treatments for bipolar disorder (lithium, carbamazepine, and valproic acid) have clear efficacy. Unfortunately, they also have multiple adverse effects ranging from the annoying to the potentially lethal, so the search for new agents is in full swing.

Drugs That Recently Arrived

Lamotrigine. Lamotrigine was approved by the FDA in December 1997 for use as adjunctive therapy in the treatment of partial seizures in adults with epilepsy (Gilman 1995). It is believed to inhibit the stimulated presynaptic release of glutamate and may have significant mood-stabilizing properties (Walden et al. 1996). Moreover, it may be effective in the treatment of bipolar depression (which is often difficult to treat with standard mood stabilizers). In order of decreasing frequency, the side effects associated with lamotrigine include dizziness, headaches, diplopia, ataxia, gastrointestinal upset, somnolence, and rash (Calabrese et al. 1996). (Slow titration may significantly reduce the chances of a rash.)

Gabapentin. Gabapentin is a new antiseizure medication used as adjunctive therapy in patients with refractory partial seizures. The mechanism of action is unknown, and although it is structurally related to the neurotransmitter γ-aminobutyric acid (GABA), it does not interact with the GABA receptor (Singh et al. 1996). Gabapentin has a unique pharmacological profile for an anticonvulsant, including lack of binding to plasma proteins, primary elimination by the kidney, and no induction of hepatic enzymes (Andrews and Fischer 1994). Moreover, in clinical trials, no interactions have been observed between gabapentin and carbamazepine or valproic acid (Ramsay 1994). In a small inpatient study of patients with bipolar disorder that was refractory to standard treatment, gabapentin was used as adjunctive medicine with impressive results (Bennett et al. 1997). No serious side effects were seen, although somnolence, dizziness, and ataxia (usually resolving in 1–2 weeks) have been noted in earlier studies with epileptic patients (Andrews and Fischer 1994; Ramsay 1994).

Drugs That Are in Development

Tiagabine. Tiagabine, a GABA uptake inhibitor (Gram 1994), has shown efficacy in a wide range of seizure models (Mengel 1994). Because it does not inhibit or induce drug metabolism, it does not alter the concentration of other antiseizure medications. Potential problems that have emerged in clinical studies include dizziness (which has been transient) and a short (5- to 8-hour) half-life (which could be offset by a controlled-release formulation) (Brodie 1995).

Topiramate.   Topiramate is a new antiseizure medication that appears to have several possible mechanisms of action, including a modulation effect on voltage-dependent sodium conductance (Coulter et al. 1993) and enhancement of $GABA_A$ submediated C_1-flu (Brown et al. 1993). It appears to stop the spread of seizures as opposed to raising the seizure threshold. In both open trials (Rangel et al. 1988; Wilder et al. 1988) and controlled trials (Ben-Menachem et al. 1996; Tassinari et al. 1996) in patients with refractory partial seizures, it was quite effective. Side effects included dizziness, sedation, weight loss, and increased incidence of renal calculi.

Vigabatrin.   Vigabatrin is a specific, irreversible inhibitor of GABA-aminotransferase, the principal catabolic enzyme of GABA (Lippert et al. 1977). It has been shown to be effective in multiple double-blind, placebo-controlled studies of patients with refractory seizures (Gram et al. 1985; Loiseau et al. 1986; Tassinari et al. 1987). (Interestingly, by preventing the transmission of GABA to succinic semialdehyde, it is used to treat 4-hydroxybutyric aciduria, a rare inborn error of metabolism caused by the deficiency of succinic semialdehyde dehydrogenase [Rahbeeni et al. 1994].) It has few drug interactions but does cause sedation and dizziness in some patients (Tartara et al. 1986). There have been occasional reports of both psychosis and an increase in depressive symptoms in patients with epilepsy, so further clinical research is obviously needed.

ANXIETY DISORDERS

Anxiety disorders are almost always chronic and relapsing. It is probably necessary to find anxiolytics that may be used for long-term treatment. Effective anxiolytic medication that lacks the potential for abuse or dependence would be a major advance. The main choice today is between benzodiazepines, which are fast in onset but are associated with dependence, and antidepressants, which are effective and do not cause dependence but are slower in onset.

Drugs That Never Arrived

Abecarnil.   Abecarnil is a β-carboline and a benzodiazepine partial agonist. Phase 1 studies in healthy volunteers have yielded findings typical of anxiolytic compounds while producing relatively few side effects. An extensive double-blind, placebo-controlled study in outpatients with generalized anxiety disorders found that abecarnil may be clinically efficacious at doses that produce few side effects (Ballenger et al. 1991). It is unclear whether the development of this drug will go forward.

Moclobemide and brofaromine.   Both moclobemide and brofaromine have been shown to be effective in treating social phobia (Fahlen et al. 1995; Versiani et al. 1992). However, the data on moclobemide are somewhat less clear; a large recent study (Noyes et al. 1997) showed no difference from placebo. On the other hand, a recent study found that brofaromine (Lott et al. 1997) produced a significant reduction in anxiety compared with placebo in patients with social phobia.

Brofaromine, in addition to inhibiting the A isoenzyme of monoamine oxidase, also inhibits the reuptake of serotonin. Because SSRIs, particularly fluvoxamine (van Vliet et al. 1994) and sertraline (Katzelnick et al. 1995), have been reported to be effective in treating social phobia, it is unclear which of brofaromine's qualities is most related to its efficacy in treating social phobia.

SUMMARY

In this chapter, we identify several medications that we believe show particular promise. However, there are a multitude of reasons, both medical and economic, that any or all of these medications may never be used as psychopharmacological agents in the United States. Let us add these observations: Expert clinicians tend to be biased toward efficacy over safety. Because they are called on to treat the most difficult cases, and because of their own expert knowledge, they tend to be eager to have new agents available and are less troubled by potential hazards. Regulators are obligated to be biased in the direction of safety. Interestingly, pharmaceutical manufacturers are often in a middle ground, having strong economic incentives to provide new medications but keeping a serious eye toward the potential for hazard.

REFERENCES

Andrews CO, Fischer JH: Gabapentin: a new agent for the management of epilepsy. Ann Pharmacother 28:1188–1196, 1994

Angst J, Stabl M: Efficacy of moclobemide in different patient groups: a meta-analysis of studies. Psychopharmacology 106:S109–S113, 1992

Baldwin DS, Montgomery SA: First clinical experience with olanzapine (LY 170053): results of an open-label safety and dose-ranging study in patients with schizophrenia. Int Clin Psychopharmacol 10:239–244, 1995

Ballenger JC, McDonald S, Noyes R, et al: The first double-blind, placebo-controlled trial of a partial benzodiazepine agonist, abecarnil (ZK 112–119), in generalized anxiety disorder. Psychopharmacol Bull 27:171–179, 1991

Barnas C, Stuppack CH, Miller C, et al: Zotepine in the treatment of schizophrenic patients with prevailingly negative symptoms: a double-blind trial vs. haloperidol. Int Clin Psychopharmacol 7:23–27, 1992

Ben-Menachem E, Henriksen O, Dam M, et al: Double-blind, placebo-controlled trial of topiramate as add-on therapy in patients with refractory partial seizures. Epilepsia 37:539–543, 1996

Bennett J, Goldman WT, Suppes T: Gabapentin for treatment of bipolar and schizoaffective disorder. J Clin Psychopharmacol 17:141–142, 1997

Berzewski H, Van Joffaert M, Cagiano CA: Efficacy and tolerability of reboxetine compared with imipramine in a double-blind study in patients suffering from major depressive episodes. Eur Neuropsychopharmacol 7:S23, 1997

Borison RL: Clinical efficacy of serotonin-dopamine antagonists relative to classic neuroleptics. J Clin Psychopharmacol 15:24S–29S, 1995

Borison RL, Diamond BI, Pathiraja AP, et al: Clinical overview of risperidone, in Novel Antipsychotics. Edited by Meltzer HY. New York, Raven, 1992, pp 233–240

Borison RL, Arvanitis LA, Miller BG, et al: ICI 204,636, an atypical antipsychotic: efficacy and safety in a multicenter, placebo-controlled trial in patients with schizophrenia. J Clin Psychopharmacol 16:158–169, 1996

Bowden CL: Treatment of bipolar disorder, in The American Psychiatric Press Textbook of Psychopharmacology. Edited by Schatzberg AF, Nemeroff CB. Washington, DC, American Psychiatric Press, 1995, pp 603–614

Brodie MJ: Tiagabine pharmacology in profile. Epilepsia 36:57–59, 1995

Brosen K: Are pharmacokinetic drug interactions with the SSRIs an issue? Int Clin Psychopharmacol 11:23–28, 1996

Brown SD, Wolf HH, Swinyard RE, et al: The novel anticonvulsant topiramate enhances GABA-mediated chloride flux (abstract). Epilepsia 34:122–123, 1993

Calabrese JR, Fatemi SH, Woyshville MJ: Antidepressant effects of lamotrigine in rapid cycling bipolar disorder. Am J Psychiatry 153:9, 1996

Casey DE: Seroquel (quetiapine): preclinical and clinical findings of a new atypical antipsychotic. Exp Opin Invest Drugs 5:939–957, 1996

Chouinard G, Saxena BM, Nair NPV, et al: Brofaromine in depression: a Canadian multicenter placebo trial and a review of standard drug comparative studies. Clin Neuropharmacol 16:S52–S54, 1993

Cole JO: Where are those new antidepressants we were promised? Arch Gen Psychiatry 45:193–197, 1988

Coulter DA, Sombati S, DeLorenzo RJ: Selective effects of topiramate on sustained repetitive firing and spontaneous bursting in hippocampal neurons (abstract). Epilepsia 34:123, 1993

Cyr M, Brown C: Nefazodone: its place among the antidepressants. Ann Pharmacother 30:1006–1012, 1996

Dalery J, Dagens-Lafant V, DeBodinat C: Value of tianeptine in treating major recurrent unipolar depression: study versus placebo for 16½ months of treatment. Encephale 23:56–64, 1997

Daniel D, Swann A, Silber C, et al: The long term cardiovascular safety of sertindole. Poster presented at the convention of the American College of Neuropsychopharmacology, San Juan, Puerto Rico, December 1996

Davis R, Wilde M: Mirtazapine: a review of its pharmacology and therapeutic potential in the management of major depression. CNS Drugs 5(5):384–402, 1996

DeBattista C, Solvason HB, Belanoff J, et al: Treatment in psychotic depression. Am J Psychiatry 154:1625–1626, 1997

de Boer T: The effects of mirtazapine on central noradrenergic and serotonergic neurotransmission. Int Clin Psychopharmacol 10:19–23, 1995

Fahlen T, Nilsson H, Borg K, et al: Social phobia: the clinical efficacy and tolerability of the monoamine oxidase A and serotonin uptake inhibitor brofaromine. Acta Psychiatr Scand 92:351–358, 1995

Fleischhacker WW, Barnas C, Stuppack CH: Zotepine vs. haloperidol in paranoid schizophrenia: a double-blind trial. Psychopharmacol Bull 25:97–100, 1989

Gilman JT: Lamotrigine: an antiepileptic agent for the treatment of partial seizures. Ann Pharmacother 29:144–151, 1995

Glick ID, Lecrubier Y, Montgomery SA, et al: Efficacious and safe psychotropics not available in the United States. Psychiatric Annals 26:354–361, 1996

Gram L: Tiagabine: a novel drug with a GABAergic mechanism of action. Epilepsia 35:585–587, 1994

Gram L, Koasterkov P, Dam M: Gamma-vinyl GABA: a double-blind, placebo-controlled trial in partial epilepsy. Ann Neurol 17:262–266, 1985

Grof P, Joffe R, Kennedy S, et al: An open study of oral flesinoxan, a 5-HT1A receptor agonist, in treatment-resistant depression. Int Clin Psychopharmacol 8:167–172, 1993

Hirsch SR, Link CGG, Goldstein JM, et al: ICI 204,636: a new atypical antipsychotic drug. Br J Psychiatry 168:45–56, 1996

Invernizzi G, Aguglia E, Bertolina A, et al: The efficacy and safety of tianaptine in the treatment of depressive disorder: results of a controlled double-blind multicentre study vs. amitriptyline. Neuropsychobiology 30:85–93, 1994

Kasper S: Efficacy of antidepressants in the treatment of severe depression: the place of mirtazapine. J Clin Psychopharmacol 17:19S–28S, 1997

Katzelnick DJ, Kobak KA, Greist MH, et al: Sertraline for social phobia: a double-blind, placebo-controlled crossover study. Am J Psychiatry 152:1368–1371, 1995

Kehne JH, Baron BM, Carr AA, et al: Preclinical characterization of the potential of the putative atypical antipsychotic MDL 100,907 as a potent 5-HT2A antagonist with a favorable CNS safety profile. J Pharmacol Exp Ther 277:968–981, 1996

Kondo T, Otani K, Ishida M, et al: Adverse effects of zotepine and their relationship to serum concentrations of the drug and prolactin. Ther Drug Monit 16:120–124, 1994

Lader M: Citalopram—a new antidepressant. Primary Care Psychiatry 2:49–58, 1996

Lewander T, Westbergh S-E, Morrison D: Clinical profile of remoxipride—a combined analysis of a comparative, double blind multicentre trial programme. Acta Psychiatr Scand 358:92–98, 1990

Lewander T, Uppfeldt G, Kohler C, et al: Remoxipride and raclopride: pharmacological background and clinical outcome, in Novel Antipsychotics. Edited by Meltzer HY. New York, Raven, 1992, pp 67–78

Lippert B, Metcalf BW, Jung MJ, et al: 4-Amino-hex-5-enoic acid, a selective catalytic inhibitor of 4-aminobutyric-acid aminotransferase in mammalian brain. Eur J Biochem 74:441–445, 1977

Loiseau P, Hardenberg JP, Pestre M, et al: Double-blind, placebo-controlled study of vigabatrin (gamma-vinyl GABA) in drug-resistant epilepsy. Epilepsia 27:115–120, 1986

Lott M, Greist JH, Jefferson JW, et al: Brofaromine for social phobia: a multicenter, placebo-controlled, double-blind study. J Clin Psychopharmacol 17:255–260, 1997

Marder SR, Meibach RC: Risperidone in the treatment of schizophrenia. Am J Psychiatry 151:825–835, 1994

Mengel H: Tiagabine. Epilepsia 35:581–584, 1994

Mitchell PB: Novel antidepressants report: novel French antidepressants not available in the United States. Psychopharmacol Bull 31:509–519, 1995

Montgomery SA: Safety of mirtazapine: a review. Int Clin Psychopharmacol 10:37–45, 1995

Montgomery S, Djarv L: The antidepressant efficacy of citalopram. Int Clin Psychopharmacol 11:29–33, 1996

Montgomery S, Kasper S: Comparison of compliance between serotonin reuptake inhibitors and tricyclic antidepressants: a meta-analysis. Int Clin Psychopharmacol 9:33–40, 1995

Muldoon C: The safety and tolerability of citalopram. Int Clin Psychopharmacol 11:35–40, 1996

Noyes R, Moroz G, Davidson JRT, et al: Moclobemide in social phobia: a controlled dose-response trial. J Clin Psychopharmacol 17:247–254, 1997

Otsuka Pharmaceuticals: Investigator's Brochure. Rockville, MD, America Pharma, 1997

Ott C: Zotepin—ein Neuroleptikum mit neuartigem wirkungsmechanismus. Fundamenta Psychiatrica 6:216–224, 1992

Overall JE, Gorham DR: The Brief Psychiatric Rating Scale. Psychol Rep 10:799–812, 1962

Paillere-Martinot M-L, Lecrubier Y, Martinot J-L, et al: Improvement of some schizophrenic deficit symptoms with low doses of amisulpride. Am J Psychiatry 152:130–133, 1995

Patris M, Bouchard J-M, Bougerol T, et al: Citalopram versus fluoxetine: a double-blind, controlled, multicentre, phase III trial in patients with unipolar major depression treated in general practice. Int Clin Psychopharmacol 11:129–136, 1996

Perrault GH, Depoortere R, Morel E: Psychopharmacological profile of amisulpride: an antipsychotic drug with presynaptic D2/D3 dopamine receptor antagonist activity and limbic selectivity. J Pharmacol Exp Ther 280:73–82, 1997

Rahbeeni Z, Ozand PT, Rashed M: 4-Hydroxybutyric aciduria. Brain Dev 16 (suppl):64–71, 1994

Ramsay RE: Clinical efficacy and safety of gabapentin. Neurology 44:S23–S30, 1994

Rangel RJ, Penry JK, Wilder BJ, et al: Topiramate: a new antiepileptic drug for complex partial seizures—first use in epileptic patients (abstract). Neurology 38:234, 1988

Ranjan R, Meltzer H: Acute and long-term effectiveness of clozapine in treatment-resistant psychotic depression. Biol Psychiatry 40:253–258, 1996

Reeves K, Harrigan EP: Efficacy and safety of ziprasidone. Poster presented at the convention of the American College of Neuropsychopharmacology, San Juan, Puerto Rico, December 1996

Rihmer Z, Barsi J, Vad G, et al: Moclobemide (Aurorix) in primary major depression. Neuropsychopharmacol Biol Psychiatry 18:367–372, 1994

Satoh K, Someya T, Shibasaki M: Nemonapride for the treatment of schizophrenia. Am J Psychiatry 154:292, 1997

Schotte A, Janssen PFM, Gommeren W, et al: Risperidone compared with new and reference antipsychotic drugs: in vitro and in vivo receptor binding. Psychopharmacology 124:57–73, 1996

Seeger TF, Seymour PA, Schmidt AW: Ziprasidone (CP-88,059): a new antipsychotic with combined dopamine and serotonin receptor antagonist activity. J Pharmacol Exp Ther 275:101–103, 1995

Singh L, Field M, Oles R: Anxiolytic effects of gabapentin in preclinical tests. Poster presented at the convention of the American College of Neuropsychopharmacology, San Juan, Puerto Rico, December 1996

Sramek JJ, Elkins L, Church L: A bridging study of MDL 100,907 in schizophrenic patients. Poster presented at the convention of the American College of Neuropsychopharmacology, San Juan, Puerto Rico, December 1996

Stimmel GL, Dopheide JA, Stahl SM: Mirtazapine: an antidepressant with noradrenergic and specific serotonergic effects. Pharmacotherapy 17:10–12, 1997

Svartengren J, Celander M: The limbic functional selectivity of amperozide is not mediated by dopamine D2 receptors as assessed by in vitro and in vivo binding. Eur J Pharmacol 254:73–81, 1994

Tartara A, Manni R, Galimberti CA, et al: Vigabatrin in the treatment of epilepsy: a double-blind, placebo-controlled study. Epilepsia 27:717–223, 1986

Tassinari CA, Michelucci R, Ambrosetto G: Double-blind study of vigabatrin in the treatment of drug-resistant epilepsy. Arch Neurol 44:907–910, 1987

Tassinari CA, Michelucci R, Chauvel P: Double-blind, placebo-controlled trial of topiramate (600 mg daily) for the treatment of refractory partial epilepsy. Epilepsia 37:763–768, 1996

Tollefson GD, Sanger TM, Lieberman JA: Olanzapine versus haloperidol in the treatment of first episode psychosis (abstract). Schizophr Res 24:193, 1997a

Tollefson GD, Tran PV, Hamilton S, et al: Olanzapine versus risperidone in the treatment of psychosis: preliminary report. Schizophr Res 24:191–192, 1997b

van Vliet IM, den Boer JA, Westenberg HG: Psychopharmacological treatment of social phobia: a double-blind placebo-controlled study with fluvoxamine. Psychopharmacology 115:128–134, 1994

Versiani M, Nardi AEW, Mundim FD, et al: Pharmacotherapy of social phobia, a controlled study with moclobemide and phenelzine. Br J Psychiatry 161:353–360, 1992

Volz HP, Faltus F, Magyar I, et al: Brofaromine in treatment-resistant depressed patients: a comparative trial versus tranylcypromine. J Affective Disord 30:209–217, 1994

Walden J, Hesslinger B, van Calker D, et al: Addition of lamotrigine to valproate may enhance efficacy in the treatment of bipolar affective disorder. Pharmacopsychiatry 29:193–195, 1996

Wetzel H, Szegedi A, Hain C, et al: Seroquel (ICI 204 636), a putative "atypical" antipsychotic, in schizophrenia with positive symptomatology: results of an open clinical trial and changes of neuroendocrinological and EEG parameters. Psychopharmacology 119:231–238, 1995

Wilde M, Benfield P: Tianeptine: a review of its pharmacodynamic and pharmacokinetic properties, and therapeutic efficacy in depression and coexisting anxiety and depression. Drugs 49:411–439, 1995

Wilder BJ, Penry JK, Rangel RJ, et al: Topiramate: efficacy, toxicity and dose/plasma concentrations (abstract). Epilepsia 29:698, 1988

Yamamoto M, Usuda S, Tachikawa S, et al: Pharmacological studies on a new benzamide derivative, YM-09151–2, with potential neuroleptic properties. Neuropharmacology 21:945–951, 1982

Index

Page numbers printed in **boldface** *type refer to tables or figures.*